U0332236

MD安德森肿瘤学

The MD Anderson Manual of Medical Oncology

THIRD EDITION

HAGOP M. KANTARJIAN
ROBERT A. WOLFF

第3版（双语版）

编译委员会主任委员　詹启敏

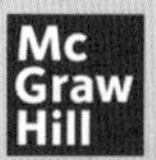

湖南科学技术出版社

《西医经典名著集成》丛书编译委员会

MD安德森肿瘤学

第3版（双语版）

编译委员会

主任委员	詹启敏	北京大学
副主任委员	张小田	北京大学肿瘤医院
	王晰程	北京大学肿瘤医院
	徐崇锐	广东省人民医院
	燕　翔	中国人民解放军总医院
	邱海波	中山大学肿瘤防治中心
	殷文瑾	上海交通大学医学院附属仁济医院
委　　员	（按贡献量和姓氏拼音排序）	
	刘　静	上海交通大学医学院附属瑞金医院
	李　伟	苏州大学附属第一医院
	刘思初	广东省人民医院
	杜跃耀	上海交通大学医学院附属仁济医院
	王耀辉	上海交通大学医学院附属仁济医院
	朱　芳	华中科技大学同济医学院附属协和医院
	曹彦硕	北京大学肿瘤医院
	陈祎霏	北京大学肿瘤医院
	邓　磊	美国罗斯韦尔公园癌症研究中心
	高　山	中国人民解放军总医院
	韩　颖	天津市肿瘤医院
	雷源源	香港中文大学威尔斯亲王医院
	李丹妮	中国医科大学附属第一医院
	李际盛	山东大学齐鲁医院
	梁婷婷	吉林大学第一医院
	刘小军	兰州大学第一医院
	卢瑗瑗	空军军医大学西京消化病医院
	马德宁	中国科学院大学附属肿瘤医院（浙江省肿瘤医院）
	孟　睿	华中科技大学同济医学院附属协和医院
	齐长松	北京大学肿瘤医院
	邱　红	华中科技大学同济医院
	孙　婧	江苏省人民医院
	孙丽斌	青岛大学附属医院

The MD Anderson Manual of Medical Oncology

Third Edition

Editors

Hagop M. Kantarjian, MD

Professor of Medicine
Chair, Department of Leukemia
The University of Texas MD Anderson Cancer Center
Houston, Texas

Robert A. Wolff, MD

Professor of Medicine
Department of Gastrointestinal Medical Oncology
The University of Texas MD Anderson Cancer Center
Houston, Texas

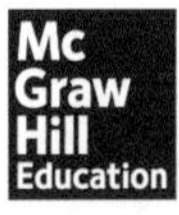

New York Chicago San Francisco Athens London Madrid Mexico City
Milan New Delhi Singapore Sydney Toronto

Dedication

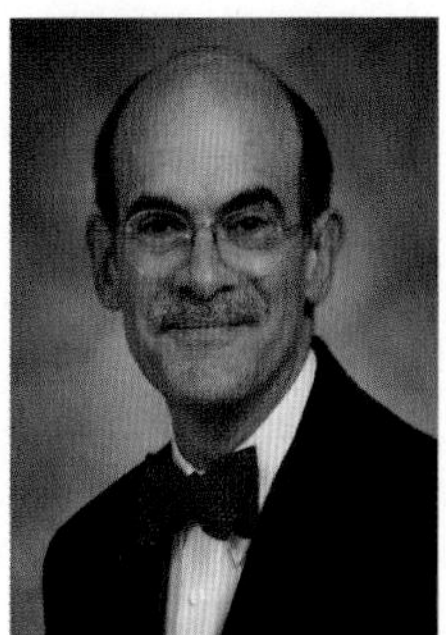

Charles A. Koller, MD
1948-2013

This third edition of *The MD Anderson Manual of Medical Oncology* is dedicated to Charles A. Koller, a valued member of MD Anderson's Leukemia Department for nearly three decades, a committed physician, and an editor of the first and second editions of *The MD Anderson Manual of Medical Oncology*.

Contributors

James P. Allison, PhD
Professor of Immunology
Chair, Department of Immunology
The University of Texas MD Anderson Cancer Center
Houston, Texas

Hesham M. Amin, MD
Professor of Hematopathology Adm.
The University of Texas MD Anderson Cancer Center
Houston, Texas

Borje Andersson, MD, PhD
Professor of Stem Cell Transplantation
The University of Texas MD Anderson Cancer Center
Houston, Texas

Joann Ater, MD
Professor of Pediatrics
Department of Pediatrics
The University of Texas MD Anderson Cancer Center
Houston, Texas

Rony Avritscher, MD
Associate Professor
Interventional Radiology
The University of Texas MD Anderson Cancer Center
Houston, Texas

Muhamed Baljevic, MD
Fellow, Hematology and Medical Oncology
Department of Cancer Medicine
The University of Texas MD Anderson Cancer Center
Houston, Texas

Nishin A. Bhadkamkar, MD
Assistant Professor
General Oncology
The University of Texas MD Anderson Cancer Center
Houston, Texas

Mehmet A. Bilen, MD
Fellow, Cancer Medicine - Fellowship Program
The University of Texas MD Anderson Cancer Center
Houston, Texas

Jonathan E. Brammer, MD
Instructor
Department of Stem Cell Transplantation and Cellular Therapy
The University of Texas MD Anderson Cancer Center
Houston, Texas

Jubilee Brown, MD
Department of Gynecologic Oncology
The University of Texas MD Anderson Cancer Center
Houston, Texas

Eduardo Bruera, MD
Department of Palliative Care and Rehabilitation Medicine
The University of Texas MD Anderson Cancer Center
Houston, Texas

Carlos Bueso-Ramos, MD, PhD
Professor of Hematopathology
The University of Texas MD Anderson Cancer Center
Houston, Texas

Naifa Lamki Busaidy, MD
Associate Professor of Endocrine Neoplasia and HD
The University of Texas MD Anderson Cancer Center
Houston, Texas

Matthew T. Campbell, MD
Assistant Professor of Genitourinary Medical Oncology
The University of Texas MD Anderson Cancer Center
Houston, Texas

Tina Cascone, MD, PhD
Fellow, Hematology and Medical Oncology
Division of Cancer Medicine
The University of Texas MD Anderson Cancer Center
Houston, Texas

Richard E. Champlin, MD
Chairman of Department of Stem Cell Transplantation and Cellular Therapy
The University of Texas MD Anderson Cancer Center
Houston, Texas

Nikolaos Charalampakis, MD, PhD
Former Postdoctoral Fellow
Department of Gastrointestinal Medical Oncology
The University of Texas MD Anderson Cancer Center
Houston, Texas
Oncology Unit, Department of 2nd Internal Medicine Propedeutics
Attikon University Hospital - National Kapodistrian University of Athens
Athens, Greece

Chan Yoon Cheah, MBBS, DMedSc
Fellow, Lymphoma and Myeloma Research
The University of Texas MD Anderson Cancer Center
Houston, Texas

Roy F. Chemaly, MD, MPH, FIDSA, FACP
Professor of Medicine
Chair, Infection Control Committee
Department of Infectious Diseases, Infection Control, and Employee Health
The University of Texas MD Anderson Cancer Center
Houston, Texas

Dai Chihara, MD
Fellow, Leukemia
The University of Texas MD Anderson Cancer Center
Houston, Texas

Stefan O. Ciurea, MD
Associate Professor
Department of Stem Cell Transplantation and Cellular Therapy
The University of Texas MD Anderson Cancer Center
Houston, Texas

Anthony Conley, MD
Assistant Professor
Department of Sarcoma Medical Oncology
The University of Texas MD Anderson Cancer Center
Houston, Texas

Paul G. Corn, MD, PhD
Associate Professor of Genitourinary Medical Oncology
The University of Texas MD Anderson Cancer Center
Houston, Texas

Jorge Cortes, MD
Jane and John Justin Distinguished Chair in Leukemia Research
Chief, CML and AML Sections
Deputy Chair, Department of Leukemia
The University of Texas MD Anderson Cancer Center
Houston, Texas

Christopher H. Crane, MD
Professor
Program Director and Section Chief, Gastrointestinal Section
Department of Radiation Oncology
The University of Texas MD Anderson Cancer Center
Houston, Texas

Bogdan Czerniak, MD, PhD
Professor of Pathology
Department of Pathology
The University of Texas MD Anderson Cancer Center
Houston, Texas

Prajnam Das, MD
Associate Professor, Radiation Oncology Department
The University of Texas MD Anderson Cancer Center
Houston, Texas

Michael A. Davies, MD, PhD
Department of Melanoma Medical Oncology
Department of Systems Biology
The University of Texas MD Anderson Cancer Center
Houston, Texas

Rony Dev, DO
Associate Professor, Palliative Care Medicine
The University of Texas MD Anderson Cancer Center
Houston, Texas

Sunny S. Dhah, DO
Fellow, Department of Palliative Care and Rehabilitation Medicine
The University of Texas MD Anderson Cancer Center
Houston, Texas

Colin P. N. Dinney, MD
Chair Department of Urology
The University of Texas MD Anderson Cancer Center
Houston, Texas

Madeleine Duvic, MD
Professor of Medicine and Dermatology
Blanche Bender Professorship in Cancer Research
Deputy Chair, Department of Dermatology
The University of Texas MD Anderson Cancer Center
Houston, Texas

George A. Eapen, MD
Professor of Pulmonary Medicine
The University of Texas MD Anderson Cancer Center
Houston, Texas

Elena Elimova , MD, MSc, FRCPC
Staff Physician, Division of Medical Oncology Assistant Professor, Department of Medicine University of Toronto Princess Margaret Cancer Centre
Toronto, Ontario

Cathy Eng, MD, FACP
Professor
Associate Medical Director, Colorectal Center
Director, Network Clinical Research, Gastro-intestinal Medical Oncology
Department of Gastrointestinal Medical Oncology
The University of Texas MD Anderson Cancer Center
Houston, Texas

Saadia A. Faiz, MD
Associate Professor of Pulmonary Medicine
The University of Texas MD Anderson Cancer Center
Houston, Texas

Michelle Fanale, MD
Associate Professor of Lymphoma and Myeloma
The University of Texas MD Anderson Cancer Center
Houston, Texas

Luis E. Fayad, MD
Associate Professor of Medicine
Department of Lymphoma and Myeloma
The University of Texas MD Anderson Cancer Center
Houston, Texas

Tamer M. Fouad, MD, PhD
Assistant Professor (Adjunct)
Department of Breast Medical Oncology
The University of Texas MD Anderson Cancer Center
Houston, Texas

Keith Fournier, MD
Assistant Professor of Surgery
Department of Surgical Oncology
The University of Texas MD Anderson Cancer Center
Houston, Texas

Nathan H. Fowler, MD
Associate Professor
Department of Lymphoma and Myeloma
The University of Texas MD Anderson Cancer Center
Houston, Texas

Jack B. Fu, MD
Assistant Professor
Department of Palliative Care and Rehabilitation Medicine
The University of Texas MD Anderson Cancer Center
Houston, Texas

Andy Futreal, PhD
Chair Ad Interim of Genomic Medicine
The University of Texas MD Anderson Cancer Center
Houston, Texas

Sameh Gaballa, MD, MS
Fellow, Department of Stem Cell Transplantation and Cellular Therapy
The University of Texas MD Anderson Cancer Center
Houston, Texas

Guillermo Garcia-Manero, MD
Professor of Leukemia
The University of Texas MD Anderson Cancer Center
Houston, Texas

Jeffrey E. Gershenwald, MD
Department of Surgical Oncology
Department of Cancer Biology
The University of Texas MD Anderson Cancer Center
Houston, Texas

Don L. Gibbons, PhD
Assistant Professor
Department of Thoracic/Head and Neck Medical Oncology, Department of Molecular and Cellular Oncology
The University of Texas MD Anderson Cancer Center
Houston, Texas

Bonnie S. Glisson, MD
Professor of Medicine
Thoracic/Head and Neck Medical Oncology
The University of Texas MD Anderson Cancer Center
Houston, Texas

Kathryn A. Gold, MD
Assistant Professor
Department of Thoracic/Head and Neck Medical Oncology
The University of Texas MD Anderson Cancer Center
Houston, Texas

Jennifer B. Goldstein, MD
Instructor of Gastrointestinal Medical Oncology-Research
The University of Texas MD Anderson Cancer Center
Houston, Texas

Diogo Bugano Diniz Gomes, MD
Medical Oncology
Hospital Israelita Albert Einstein
Brazil

Sangeeta Goswami, MD, PhD
Fellow, Medical Oncology
Department of Cancer Medicine
The University of Texas MD Anderson Cancer Center
Houston, Texas

Bruno P. Granwehr, MD, MS
Associate Professor of Infectious Diseases
The University of Texas MD Anderson Cancer Center
Houston, Texas

John de Groot, MD
Department of Neuro-Oncology
The University of Texas MD Anderson Cancer Center
Houston, Texas

Horiana B. Grosu, MD
Assistant Professor of Pulmonary Medicine
The University of Texas MD Anderson Cancer Center
Houston, Texas

G. Brandon Gunn, MD
Associate Professor
Department of Radiation Oncology
The University of Texas MD Anderson Cancer Center
Houston, Texas

Mouhammed Amir Habra, MD
Associate Professor
Department of Endocrine Neoplasia and Hormonal Disorders
The University of Texas MD Anderson Cancer Center
Houston, Texas

Danielle El-Haddad, MD
Clinical Research Resident
Department of Cardiology
The University of Texas MD Anderson Cancer Center
Houston, Texas

Fredrick B. Hagemeister, MD
Professor of Lymphoma and Myeloma
The University of Texas MD Anderson Cancer Center
Houston, Texas

Daniel M. Halperin, MD
Assistant Professor
Department of Gastrointestinal Medical Oncology
The University of Texas MD Anderson Cancer Center
Houston, Texas

Gabriel N. Hortobagyi, MD, FACP, FASCO
Professor, Department of Breast Medical Oncology
The University of Texas MD Anderson Cancer Center
Houston, Texas

Chitra Hosing, MD
Professor of Medicine
Stem Cell Transplantation and Cellular Therapy
The University of Texas MD Anderson Cancer Center
Houston, Texas

Xuelin Huang, PhD
Professor
Department of Biostatistics
The University of Texas MD Anderson Cancer Center
Houston, Texas

David Hui, MD, MSc
Department of Palliative Care and Rehabilitation Medicine
The University of Texas MD Anderson Cancer Center
Houston, Texas

Maria D. Iniesta
Senior Coordinator of Research Data, Gynecology Oncology and Reproductive Medicine
The University of Texas MD Anderson Cancer Center
Houston, Texas

Elias Jabbour
Department of Leukemia
The University of Texas MD Anderson Cancer Center
Houston, Texas

Nitin Jain, MD
Assistant Professor
Department of Leukemia
The University of Texas MD Anderson Cancer Center
Houston, Texas

Milind M. Javle, MD
Professor
Department of Gastrointestinal Medical Oncology
The University of Texas MD Anderson Cancer Center
Houston, Texas

Amir A. Jazaeri, MD
Department of Gynecologic Oncology
The University of Texas MD Anderson Cancer Center
Houston, Texas

Faye Johnson, MD, PhD
Associate Professor of Thoracic/Head and Neck Medical Oncology
The University of Texas MD Anderson Cancer Center
Houston, Texas

Eric Jonasch, MD
Professor of Genitourinary Medical Oncology
The University of Texas MD Anderson Cancer Center
Houston, Texas

Hagop M. Kantarjian, MD
Professor of Medicine
Chair, Department of Leukemia
The University of Texas MD Anderson Cancer Center
Houston, Texas

Meghan Karuturi, MD
Assistant Professor of Breast Medical Oncology
The University of Texas MD Anderson Cancer Center
Houston, Texas

Ahmed Kaseb, MD
Associate Professor
Department of Gastrointestinal Medical Oncology
The University of Texas MD Anderson Cancer Center
Houston, Texas

Partow Kebriaei, MD
Department of Stem Cell Transplantation and Cellular Therapy
Division of Cancer Medicine
The University of Texas MD Anderson Cancer Center
Houston, Texas

Joseph Khoury, MD
Assistant Professor of Hematopathology Adm.
The University of Texas MD Anderson Cancer Center
Houston, Texas

Merrill S. Kies, MD
Clinical Professor of Thoracic/Head and Neck Medical Oncology
The University of Texas MD Anderson Cancer Center
Houston, Texas

Dae Won Kim, MD
Department of Melanoma Medical Oncology
The University of Texas MD Anderson Cancer Center
Houston, Texas

Peter Kim, MD
Assistant Professor of Medicine
Department of Cardiology
The University of Texas MD Anderson Cancer Center
Houston, Texas

Piyanuch Kongtim, MD
Department of Stem Cell Transplantation and Cellular Therapy
The University of Texas MD Anderson Cancer Center
Houston, Texas

Sergej N. Konoplev, MD, PhD
Associate Professor
Department of Hematopathology
The University of Texas MD Anderson Cancer Center
Houston, Texas

Dimitrios P. Kontoyiannis, MD, ScD
Professor of Infectious Disease
The University of Texas MD Anderson Cancer Center
Houston, Texas

Scott Kopetz, MD, PhD.
Associate Professor of Gastro-Intestinal Medical Oncology
The University of Texas MD Anderson Cancer Center
Houston, Texas

Sunil Krishnan, MD
Professor
Department of Radiation Oncology
The University of Texas MD Anderson Cancer Center
Houston, Texas

Michael H. Kroll
Section of Benign Hematology
The University of Texas MD Anderson Cancer Center
Houston, Texas

Lily Kwatampora, MBChB, MPH
Fellow, Clinical Research
Department of Endocrinology
The University of Texas MD Anderson Cancer Center
Houston, Texas

Hans C. Lee, MD
Department of Lymphoma and Myeloma
The University of Texas MD Anderson Cancer Center
Houston, Texas

Christopher H. Lieu, MD
Assistant Professor of Medicine
University of Colorado Cancer Center
Aurora, Colorado

Pei Lin, MD
Department of Hematopathology
The University of Texas MD Anderson Cancer Center
Houston, Texas

J. Andrew Livingston, MD
Fellow, Medical Oncology
Division of Cancer Medicine
The University of Texas MD Anderson Cancer Center
Houston, Texas

Christopher J. Logothetis, MD
Chair, Genitourinary Medical Oncology
The University of Texas MD Anderson Cancer Center
Houston, Texas

Karen H. Lu, MD
Chair and Professor, Department of Gynecologic Oncology and Reproductive Medicine
The University of Texas MD Anderson Cancer Center
Houston, Texas

Anita Mahajan, MD
Department of Radiation Oncology
The University of Texas MD Anderson Cancer Center
Houston, Texas

Mariana Chavez-MacGregor, MD
Assistant Professor of Health Services Research-Clinical
The University of Texas MD Anderson Cancer Center
Houston, Texas

Elisabet E. Manasanch, MD, MHSc
Department of Lymphoma and Myeloma
The University of Texas MD Anderson Cancer Center
Houston, Texas

Ellen F. Manzullo, MD, FACP
Professor of Medicine
Deputy Division Head (Clinical)
The University of Texas MD Anderson Cancer Center
Houston, Texas

David J. McConkey, PhD
Professor of Urology Research
The University of Texas MD Anderson Cancer Center
Houston, Texas

Jennifer L. McQuade, MD
Fellow, Medical Oncology
Division of Cancer Medicine
The University of Texas MD Anderson Cancer Center
Houston, Texas

L. Jeffrey Medeiros, MD
Chair and Professor, Department of Hematopathology
The University of Texas MD Anderson Cancer Center
Houston, Texas

Rohtesh S. Mehta, MD, MPH, MS
Fellow, Department of Stem Cell Transplantation and Cellular Therapy
The University of Texas MD Anderson Cancer Center
Houston, Texas

Zahi Mitri, MD
Fellow, Hematology and Medical Oncology
Department of Cancer Medicine
The University of Texas MD Anderson Cancer Center
Houston, Texas

Van Morris, MD
Assistant Professor, Department of Gastrointestinal Medical Oncology
The University of Texas MD Anderson Cancer Center
Houston, Texas

Elie Mouhayar, MD, FACC, FSVM
Associate Professor of Medicine
Department of Cardiology
The University of Texas MD Anderson Cancer Center
Houston, Texas

Stacy Moulder-Thompson, MD, MSCI
Associate Professor
Chief, Section of Clinical Research and Drug Development
Department of Breast Medical Oncology
The University of Texas MD Anderson Cancer Center
Houston, Texas

M. Blum Murphy, MD
Assistant Professor of Gastrointestinal Medical Oncology
The University of Texas MD Anderson Cancer Center
Houston, Texas

Loretta J. Nastoupil, MD
Assistant Professor
Department of Lymphoma and Myeloma
The University of Texas MD Anderson Cancer Center
Houston, Texas

Kate J. Newberry
Senior Research Scientist of Leukemia Research
The University of Texas MD Anderson Cancer Center
Houston, Texas

Barbara O'Brien, MD
Department of Neuro-Oncology
The University of Texas MD Anderson Cancer Center
Houston, Texas

Susan O'Brien, MD
Associate Director for Clinical Science
Chao Family Comprehensive Cancer Center
Medical Director
Sue and Ralph Stern Center for Clinical Trials and Research
Professor of Medicine
Division of Hematology/ Oncology
Department of Medicine
University of California
Irvine, California

Yasuhiro Oki, MD
Associate Professor
Department of Lymphoma and Myeloma
The University of Texas MD Anderson Cancer Center
Houston, Texas

Michaela A. Onstad, MD
Fellow, Gynecologic Oncology and Reproductive Medicine
The University of Texas MD Anderson Cancer Center
Houston, Texas

Betul Oran, MD
Assistant Professor
Department of Stem Cell Transplantation and Cellular Therapy
Division of Cancer Medicine
The University of Texas MD Anderson Cancer Center
Houston, Texas

Michael J. Overman, MD
Associate Professor of Medicine
Department of Gastrointestinal Medical Oncology
The University of Texas MD Anderson Cancer Center
Houston, Texas

Levent Ozsari
Istanbul, Turkey

Lance C. Pagliaro, MD
Professor of Oncology
Mayo Clinic College of Medicine
Senior Associate Consultant
Department of Oncology, Division of Medical Oncology
Mayo Clinic
Rochester, Minnesota

Janelle B. Pakish, MD
Fellow, Gynecologic Oncology and Reproductive Medicine
The University of Texas MD Anderson Cancer Center
Houston, Texas

Simrit Parmar, MD
Department of Stem Cell Transplantation and Cellular Therapy
The University of Texas MD Anderson Cancer Center
Houston, Texas

Krina Patel, MD
Department of Stem Cell Transplantation and Cellular Therapy
The University of Texas MD Anderson Cancer Center
Houston, Texas

Sapna P. Patel, MD
Department of Melanoma Medical Oncology
The University of Texas MD Anderson Cancer Center
Houston, Texas

Shreyaskumar Patel, MD
Professor
Department of Sarcoma Medical Oncology
The University of Texas MD Anderson Cancer Center
Houston, Texas

Alexandria T. Phan, MD
Professor, Gastrointestinal Medical Oncology
Hematology-Oncology
Houston Methodist Cancer Center
Houston, Texas

Katherine M. Pisters, MD
Professor of Thoracic/Head and Neck Medical Oncology
The University of Texas MD Anderson Cancer Center
Houston, Texas

Sujit S. Prabhu, MD
Department of Neurosurgery
The University of Texas MD Anderson Cancer Center
Houston, Texas

Muzaffar H. Qazilbash, MD
Department of Stem Cell Transplantation and Cellular Therapy
The University of Texas MD Anderson Cancer Center
Houston, Texas

Kanwal Raghav, MD
Assistant Professor of Medicine
Department of Gastrointestinal Medical Oncology
The University of Texas MD Anderson Cancer Center
Houston, Texas

Pedro T. Ramirez, MD
Professor
Director of Minimally Invasive Surgical Research and Education
Department of Gynecologic Oncology and Reproductive Medicine
The University of Texas MD Anderson Cancer Center
Houston, Texas

Jasleen K. Randhawa, MD
Fellow, Department of Leukemia
The University of Texas MD Anderson Cancer Center
Houston, Texas

Ravin Ratan, MD
Fellow, Cancer Medicine
The University of Texas MD Anderson Cancer Center
Houston, Texas

Farhad Ravandi-Kashani, MD
Professor of Medicine
Chief, Section of Developmental Therapeutics
Department of Leukemia
The University of Texas MD Anderson Cancer Center
Houston, Texas

Vinod Ravi, MD
Associate Professor
Department of Sarcoma Medical Oncology
The University of Texas MD Anderson Cancer Center
Houston, Texas

Suresh K. Reddy, MD
Professor of Palliative Care Medicine
The University of Texas MD Anderson Cancer Center
Houston, Texas

Katayoun Rezvani, MD, PhD
Department of Stem Cell Transplantation and Cellular Therapy
Division of Cancer Medicine
The University of Texas MD Anderson Cancer Center
Houston, Texas

Alyssa G. Rieber, MD
Assistant Professor
Department of Oncology
Lyndon B. Johnson Hospital
The University of Texas MD Anderson Cancer Center
Houston, Texas

Kari L. Ring, MD
Department of Gynecologic Oncology
The University of Texas MD Anderson Cancer Center
Houston, Texas

Adan Rios, MD
Associate Professor of Medicine
Oncologist, Division of Oncology
Department of Internal Medicine
The University of Texas MD Anderson Cancer Center
Houston, Texas

Maria Alma Rodriguez, MD
Vice President, Medical Affairs
Professor
Department of Lymphoma and Myeloma
The University of Texas MD Anderson Cancer Center
Houston, Texas

Aron S. Rosenstock, MD
Fellow, Clinical
Division of Cancer Medicine
The University of Texas MD Anderson Cancer Center
Houston, Texas

Rachel A. Sanford
Section of Benign Hematology
The University of Texas MD Anderson Cancer Center
Houston, Texas

Kathleen M. Schmeler, MD
Associate Professor of Gynecology, Oncology and Reproductive Medicine
The University of Texas MD Anderson Cancer Center
Houston, Texas

Maryam N. Shafaee, MD
Fellow, Cancer Medicine - Fellowship Program
The University of Texas MD Anderson Cancer Center
Houston, Texas

Vickie R. Shannon, MD
Professor of Medicine
Director, Pulmonary Rehabilitation Program
The University of Texas MD Anderson Cancer Center
Houston, Texas

Padmanee Sharma, MD, PhD
Professor of Genitourinary Medical Oncology and Immunology
Department of Genitourinary Medical Oncology
The University of Texas MD Anderson Cancer Center
Houston, Texas

Kaoswi Shih, MD
Hospice and Palliative Medicine Fellow
Department of Palliative Care and Rehabilitation Medicine
The University of Texas MD Anderson Cancer Center
Houston, Texas

Ki Y. Shin, MD
Professor, Rehabilitation Medicine
The University of Texas MD Anderson Cancer Center
Houston, Texas

Elizabeth J. Shpall, MD
Professor
Department of Stem Cell Transplantation and Cellular Therapy
Division of Cancer Medicine
The University of Texas MD Anderson Cancer Center
Houston, Texas

Rachna Shroff, MD
Assistant Professor
Department of Gastro-Intestinal Medical Oncology
The University of Texas MD Anderson Cancer Center
Houston, Texas

Arlene O. Siefker-Radtke, MD
Associate Professor of Genitourinary Medical Oncology
The University of Texas MD Anderson Cancer Center
Houston, Texas

Ishwaria M. Subbiah
Fellow, Palliative Care Medicine
The University of Texas MD Anderson Cancer Center
Houston, Texas

Ryuma Tanaka, MD
Department of Pediatrics-Patient Care
The University of Texas MD Anderson Cancer Center
Houston, Texas

Nizar M. Tannir, MD, FACP
Professor of Medicine
Deputy Chair, Department of Genitourinary Medical Oncology
The University of Texas MD Anderson Cancer Center
Houston, Texas

Sheeba Thomas, MD
Department of Lymphoma and Myeloma
The University of Texas MD Anderson Cancer Center
Houston, Texas

Kara Thompson, MD
Assistant Professor of Medicine
Department of Cardiology
The University of Texas MD Anderson Cancer Center
Houston, Texas

Philip A. Thompson, MD
Department of Leukemia
Division of Cancer Medicine
The University of Texas MD Anderson Cancer Center
Houston, Texas

Apostolia-Maria Tsimberidou, MD, PhD
Department of Investigational Cancer Therapeutics
The University of Texas MD Anderson Cancer Center
Houston, Texas

Marc Uemura, MD, MBA
Fellow, Hematology and Oncology
The University of Texas MD Anderson Cancer Center
Houston, Texas

Naoto T. Ueno, MD, PhD, FACP
Professor of Medicine
Executive Director of Morgan Welch Inflammatory Breast Cancer Research Program and Clinic
Department of Breast Medical Oncology
The University of Texas MD Anderson Cancer Center
Houston, Texas

Vicente Valero, MD
Professor of Breast Medical Oncology
The University of Texas MD Anderson Cancer Center
Houston, Texas

Gauri R. Varadhachary, MD
Professor
Department of Gastrointestinal Medical Oncology
Medical Director
Gastrointestinal Medical Center
The University of Texas MD Anderson Cancer Center
Houston, Texas

Srdan Verstovsek, MD, PhD
Professor of Medicine
Director, Hanns A. Pielenz Clinical Research Center for Myeloproliferative Neoplasms
Department of Leukemia
The University of Texas MD Anderson Cancer Center
Houston, Texas

Roopma Wadhwa, MD, MHA
Oklahoma Health Sciences Center
Oklahoma, Oklahoma

Casey Wang
University of Alabama
Tuscaloosa, Alabama

Shiao-Pei Weathers, MD
Department of Neuro-Oncology
The University of Texas MD Anderson Cancer Center
Houston, Texas

Steven P. Weitzman, MD
Assistant Professor of Medicine
Department of Endocrine Neoplasia and Hormonal Disorders
The University of Texas MD Anderson Cancer Center
Houston, Texas

Jason R. Westin, MD
Assistant Professor of Lymphoma/Myeloma
The University of Texas MD Anderson Cancer Center
Houston, Texas

William G. Wierda, MD, PhD
Professor of Medicine
Center Medical Director
CLL Section Chief
Department of Leukemia
The University of Texas MD Anderson Cancer Center
Houston, Texas

William N. William Jr., MD
Associate Professor
Head and Neck Section Chief
Department of Thoracic and Head and Neck Medical Oncology
The University of Texas MD Anderson Cancer Center
Houston, Texas

Robert A. Wolff, MD
Professor of Medicine
Department of Gastrointestinal Medical Oncology
The University of Texas MD Anderson Cancer Center
Houston, Texas

Christopher G. Wood, MD
Professor of Urology
The University of Texas MD Anderson Cancer Center
Houston, Texas

James C. Yao, MD
Chair and Professor, Department of Gastrointestinal Medical Oncology
The University of Texas MD Anderson Cancer Center
Houston, Texas

Sai-Ching Jim Yeung, MD, PhD
Professor of Emergency Medicine
The University of Texas MD Anderson Cancer Center
Houston, Texas

Zhijing Zhang
Fellow, Post-doctoral
The University of Texas Health Science Center at Houston
Houston, Texas

Patrick A. Zweidler-McKay, MD, PhD
Associate Professor
Section Chief for Pediatric Leukemia and Lymphoma
Division of Pediatrics
The University of Texas MD Anderson Cancer Center
Houston, Texas

A Brief History of MD Anderson Cancer Center

Houston's evolution into the fourth largest city in the United States was propelled by four seminal events. First was the Great Galveston Hurricane of 1900, which destroyed the city port of Galveston and led to the realization that Houston could become a viable and safer deep-water port; this led to the widening of the Ship Channel to offer direct access to Houston. Second was the discovery of oil at Spindletop in Beaumont, Texas in 1901. This prompted the development of the oil industry in Texas and transformed Houston from a small town into a large city. Third was (of course) the commercialization of air conditioning in 1950's, which made Houston (and many Southern cities of the United States) more livable. And lastly, the allocation of land for the Texas Medical Center created the largest medical center in the world with one of the highest densities of clinical facilities for patient care, basic science, and translational research. The Texas Medical Center is a major contributor to Houston's economy and growth.

Several additional factors contributed to the creation of The University of Texas MD Anderson Cancer Center in Houston and its development into one of the most important cancer centers in the world. First was the generous philanthropy of visionary Texans such as Monroe Dunaway Anderson (Fig. 1) (his nephew died of leukemia in 1936) and his partner Will Clayton, who founded the charitable MD Anderson Foundation, which helped create the Texas Medical Center in 1945. The charter of the Anderson Foundation did not specify how the money should be used, but Mr. Anderson's trustees and close friends—Colonel William Bates, John Freeman and Horace Williams—leaned strongly in favor of health care. Soon after taking possession of the estate from its executors, the trustees turned to Dr. Ernest Bertner (Fig. 2) for advice. Dr. Bertner was a prominent Houston surgeon and gynecologist who was well known to the trustees because of his care for cancer patients, despite inadequate facilities and treatment options (he was later called the "father of the Texas Medical Center").

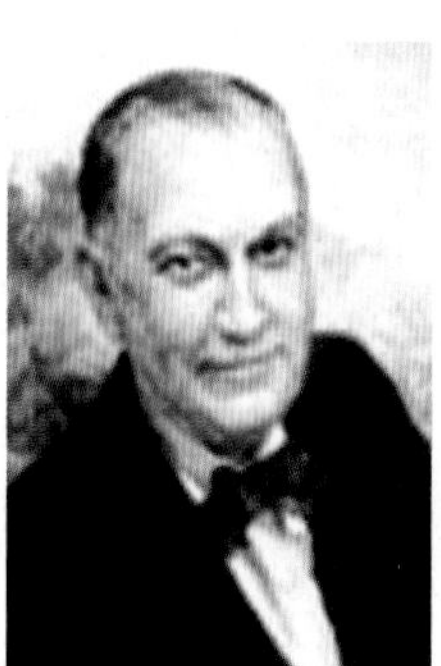

FIGURE 1.

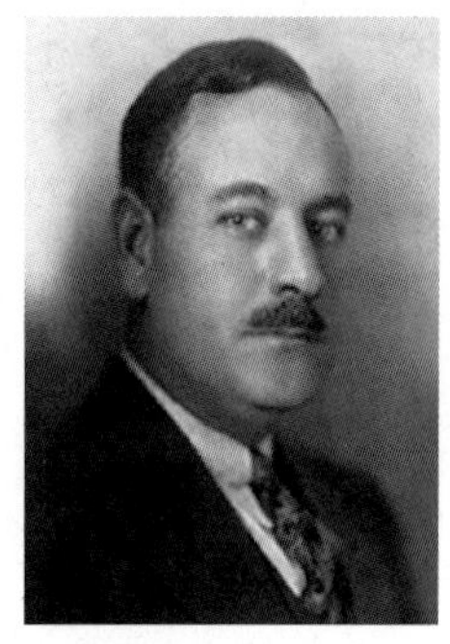

FIGURE 2.

The trustees and Dr. Bertner noted that the 1941 Texas legislature authorized the University of Texas to create a hospital for cancer research and treatment, allocating $500,000 for the purpose. Today, that figure would be approximately $8 million. The Anderson trustees, with Dr. Bertner's guidance, seized the opportunity and offered to match the $500,000 legislative appropriation, if the hospital was to be named for Monroe Dunaway Anderson and located in Houston. The legislature accepted their offer. The trustees then purchased 134 acres of mosquito-infested land to create the Texas Medical Center, stating that the new cancer hospital would be located there. They made it known that the new state hospital should be an academic institution. In fact, MD Anderson was the first comprehensive cancer hospital to be associated with a major university as an independent free-standing unit.

In 1942, The University of Texas Board of Regents appointed Dr. Bertner as the director of the new hospital. A 6-acre property near downtown was purchased from the estate of Captain James A. Baker, grandfather of former Secretary of State James Baker III, and became the first campus of the hospital. An empty carriage house became the office and stables were the research laboratories. Twelve surplus army barracks were procured for patient clinics (Figs. 3A-C). With the addition of 22 leased beds at Hermann Hospital, the dream became reality, and the "MD Anderson Hospital and Tumor Institute" was created. A small

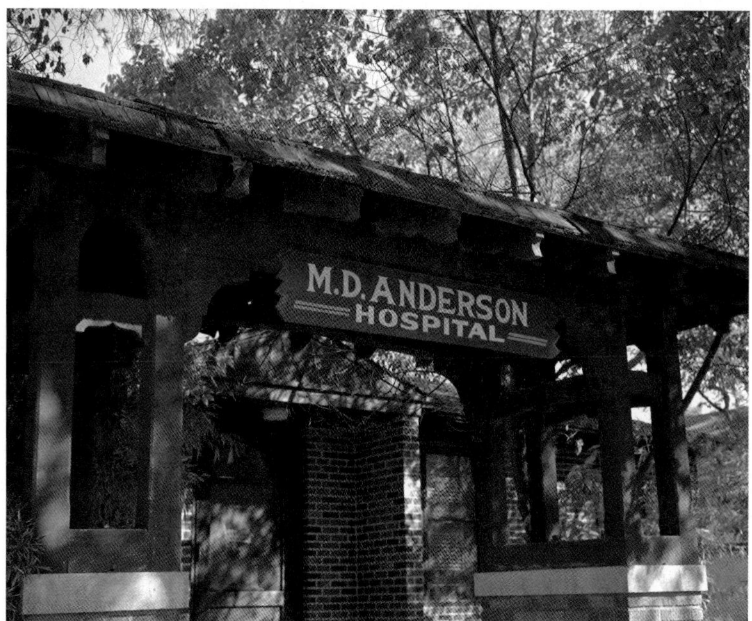

FIGURE 3A.

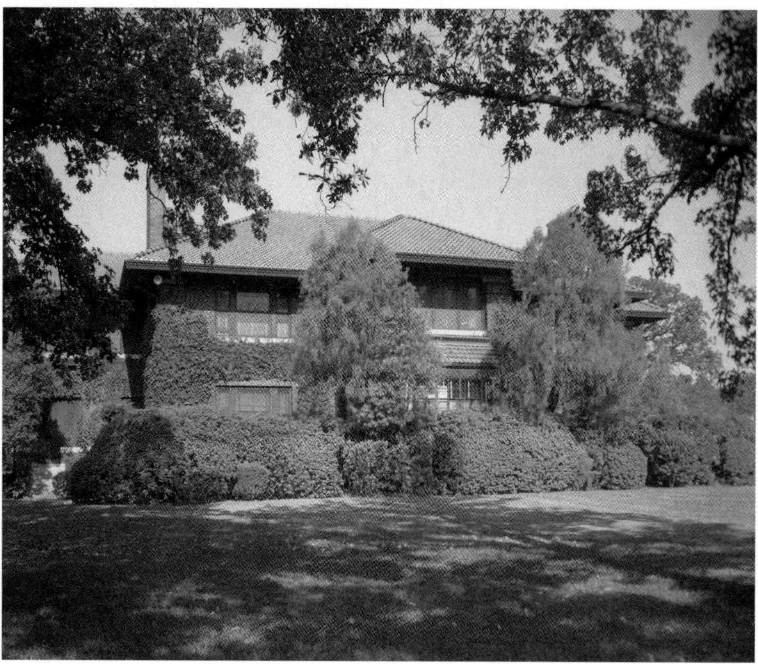

FIGURE 3B.

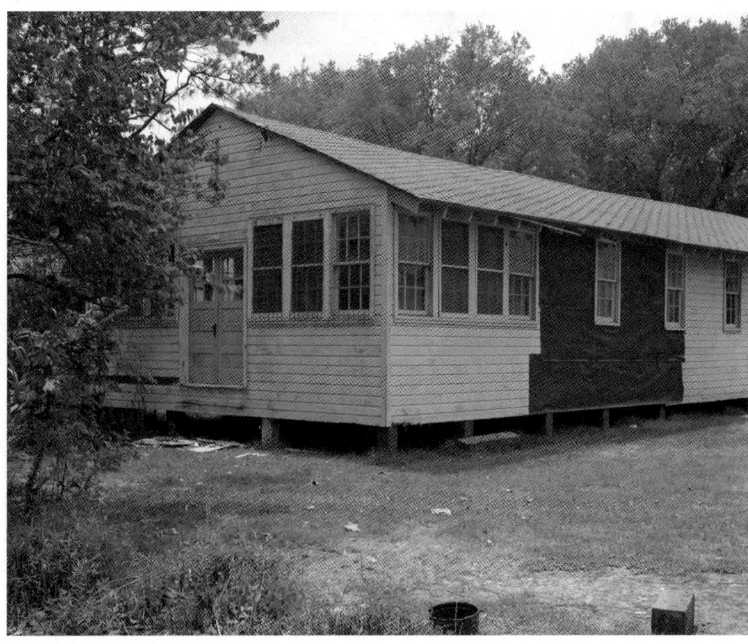

FIGURE 3C.

faculty of physicians and scientists was recruited from the University of Texas Medical Branch in Galveston, and cancer patients finally had a home. It was renamed "MD Anderson Hospital for Cancer Research" in 1942.

In 1946, Dr. Bertner persuaded Dr. Randolph Lee Clark, a native Texan, to become president of what was to become The University of Texas MD Anderson Cancer Center. Dr. Clark, a widely recognized surgeon, concentrated on recruiting an excellent surgical faculty and then set upon acquiring all the basic and clinical scientists and clinicians. From the outset, all efforts, whether administrative, clinical or research, were focused on developing excellence in research-driven cancer care. Forty-six patients were receiving treatment in these early quarters when the hospital moved to its current site in March 1954 (Figs. 4A and B).

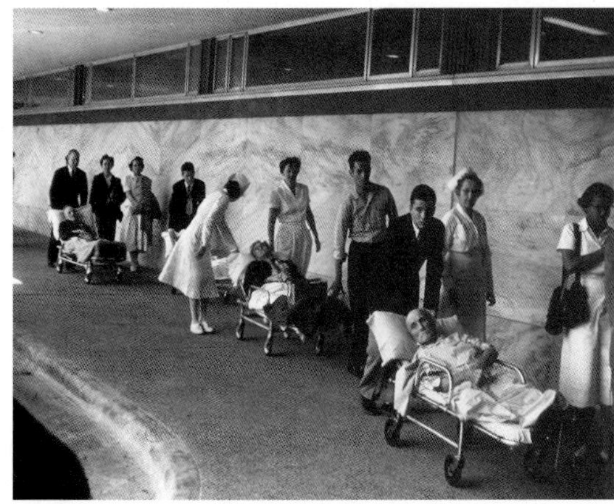

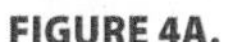

FIGURE 4A.

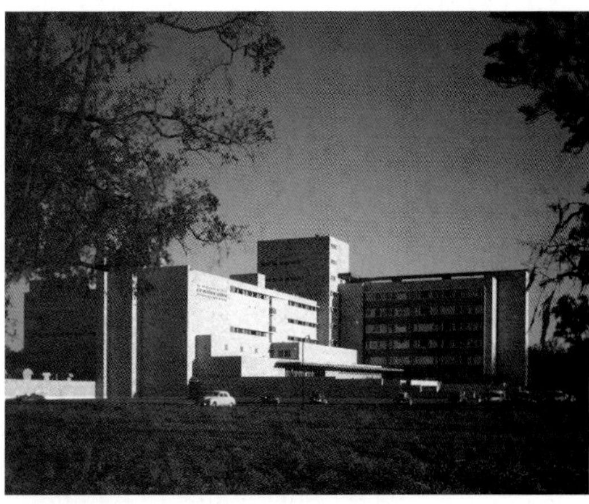

FIGURE 4B.

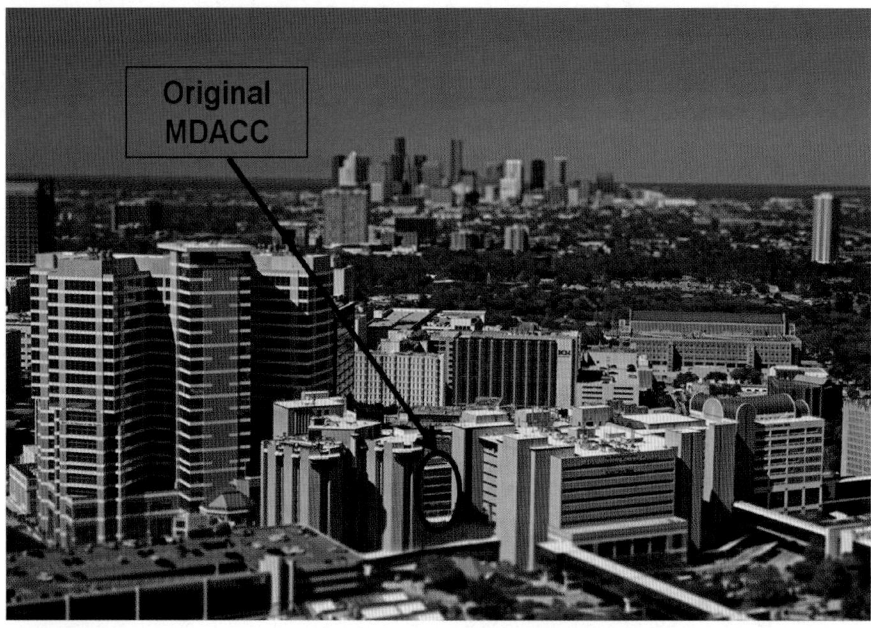

FIGURE 5.

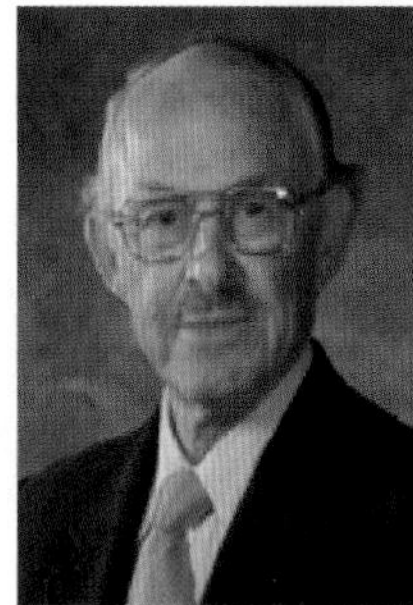

FIGURE 6A.

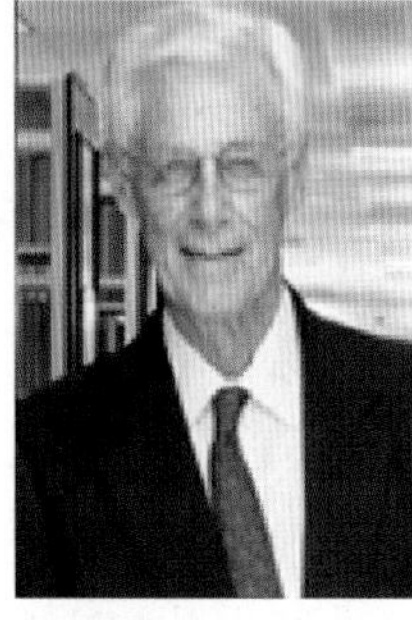

FIGURE 6B.

Additional resources to expand the MD Anderson infrastructure (Fig. 5) and research capacities came from several venues: (1) generous donations from the oil industry; (2) the visionary research and administrative leadership under its four presidents, Drs. Randolph Lee Clark (1946–1978) (Fig. 6A), Charles A. LeMaistre (1978–1996) (Fig. 6B), John Mendelsohn (1996–2011) (Fig. 6C), and Ronald DePinho (2011–present) (Fig. 6D); (3) the recruitment of world-renowned cancer research pioneers (some of the early legends included Drs. Emil J. Freireich, Emil Frei, Gilbert Fletcher, James Butler, Felix Rutledge, Gerald Dodd, and Sidney Wallace); and (4) the relentless research efforts of the cancer experts on the MD Anderson's faculty.

Today, MD Anderson is one of the largest cancer centers in the world, with more than 21,000 employees and 1800 faculty; serving more than 150,000 patients with cancer in Houston every year; operating a 700-bed cancer hospital; and being ranked as the No. 1 hospital for cancer care by the *U.S. News and World Report* in 11 of the past 14 years. The MD Anderson Cancer Center research has resulted in numerous discoveries that became standards of care across many types of cancers, and that have saved the lives and/or improved survivals and outcomes of millions of patients with cancer around the world.

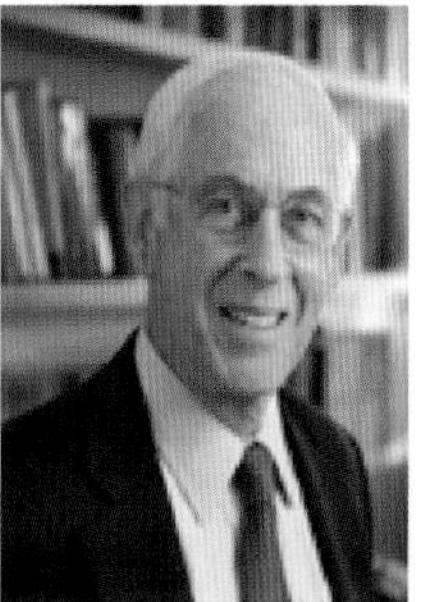

FIGURE 6C.

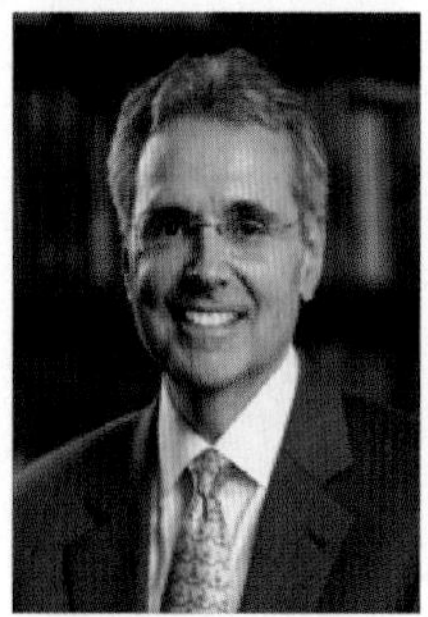

FIGURE 6D.

One component of MD Anderson's mission is to spread its knowledge about cancer research and discoveries across the globe. This educational mission is furthered by the hematology/oncology fellowship that currently trains more than 40 medical hematology-oncology cancer specialists on its premises. *The MD Anderson Manual of Medical Oncology*, created as part of our educational mission, is written by our fellows as first authors and supported in depth by senior tumor specialty faculty as co-authors. We envision this third edition expanding into a continuously updated electronic version that educates and spreads knowledge and discoveries in cancer research and therapy rapidly and widely.

Charles A. LeMaistre, M.D.
John Mendelsohn, M.D.
Ronald A. DePinho, M.D.

Foreword

The MD Anderson Manual of Medical Oncology, third edition, articulates the personalized, multidisciplinary approach to cancer management pioneered by the University of Texas MD Anderson Cancer Center. This approach has contributed to our ranking as number one in cancer care in 11 of the past 14 years in the *US News & World Report's* "America's Best Hospitals" survey. Our unique perspective has evolved from decades of clinical practice and research with more than a million patients treated. The book is designed to bring a pragmatic approach to cancer management that may serve as a guide for oncologists around the world. The text reflects how MD Anderson currently operates, including many patient care practices that would not have been recognized by practitioners just a decade ago. In a single year, 96,500 people with cancer—33,200 of them new patients—seek care at MD Anderson. Since the first edition, we have improved our ability to identify biomarkers that are predictive for survival, a major triumph in medical oncology that is demonstrated throughout the text.

The current edition emphasizes and discusses recent developments in precision medicine and immunotherapies.

Reflecting new advances in our approach to cancer management, the third edition of *The MD Anderson Manual of Medical Oncology* features several new chapters. For example, there are new chapters on important aspects of stem cell transplantation: cord blood transplant, haploidentical stem cell transplantation, and cellular therapy in allogeneic hematopoietic cell transplantation. In addition, new chapters on pediatric cancers, molecular biomarkers and cancer, immuno-oncology, targeted therapies in cancer, applied biostatistics, oncocardiology, pulmonary complications of cancer therapy, and cancer-associated thrombosis have been added.

To help clinicians quickly assess cancer management options, every chapter includes abundant tables, diagrams, and imaging photos. These include, for example, treatment algorithms and decision trees developed at MD Anderson for specific cancers or disease subtypes; promising novel therapy targets and the latest clinical trial phase of drugs targeting them; and new molecular therapies recommended to overcome resistance to previously effective therapies.

The new era of novel personalized, targeted therapeutics has also sparked the recent evolution of another crucial advancement in management of metastatic disease: the transition from sequential care culminating in the sole delivery of palliative care, to integration of ongoing active disease treatment with simultaneous interdisciplinary symptom control, palliative care, and rehabilitation to improve quality of life. Clinicians at MD Anderson no longer approach advanced metastatic disease management with palliative care goals alone; now, these patients are often offered frontline cancer treatment and the opportunity to participate in clinical trials for investigational drugs.

In recognition of the growing pool of patients who are surviving their cancer, MD Anderson has greatly expanded programs for cancer survivors since the publication of the first edition.

Waun Ki Hong, MD
American Cancer Society Professor
Samsung Distinguished University Chair Emeritus in Cancer Medicine
Former Division Head, Cancer Medicine
Professor, Thoracic/Head and Neck Medical Oncology
The University of Texas MD Anderson Cancer Center
Houston, Texas
May 2016

Preface

When we first envisioned *The MD Anderson Manual of Medical Oncology*, we hoped that it would fill an important void in oncology reference material by serving as a hands-on resource for the practicing oncologist. The first edition, published in 2006, was written exclusively by our faculty and fellows with the idea of giving a bird's-eye view of how multidisciplinary care was practiced at our institution. We were proud of that initial effort and pleased that the book received positive reviews from several high-impact journals, including *JAMA*, *The Lancet*, and *The New England Journal of Medicine*.

The second edition, published in 2011, moved closer to the aims of providing more illustrations, figures, tables, and algorithms. In addition, the second edition included new chapters on myelodysplastic syndromes, Philadelphia chromosome-negative myeloproliferative neoplasms, T-cell lymphomas, small bowel cancer and appendiceal tumors, inflammatory breast cancer, and penile cancer.

In the third edition, we have continued the tradition of including evidence-based management algorithms in the form of flowcharts and diagrams, shaped by the clinical experience of our world-class faculty at MD Anderson. Readers are also provided with a practical guide to the diagnostic and therapeutic strategies used at MD Anderson.

The new edition of *The MD Anderson Manual of Medical Oncology* contains new chapters on cord blood transplant, haploidentical stem cell transplantation, cellular therapy in allogeneic hematopoietic cell transplantation, pediatric cancers, molecular biomarkers and cancer, immuno-oncology, targeted therapies in cancer, applied biostatistics, oncocardiology, pulmonary complications of cancer therapy, and cancer-associated thrombosis. In addition, there is expanded coverage of the rapidly growing areas of biological and immune therapies of cancer.

The new edition of *The MD Anderson Manual of Medical Oncology* will also be a continually updated version of the book, online, with the latest science and clinical recommendations from the world-renowned clinical investigators at MD Anderson.

We hope that this edition serves to help oncologists everywhere provide high-quality, state-of-the-art cancer care to their patients.

Hagop M. Kantarjian, MD
Robert A. Wolff, MD

Contents 目　录

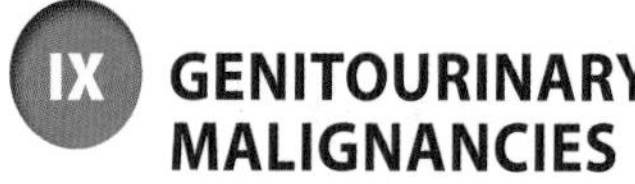

IX GENITOURINARY MALIGNANCIES

Section Editor: Nizar M. Tannir

第九篇 泌尿生殖系统恶性肿瘤

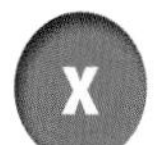

X NEUROLOGIC TUMORS

Section Editors: John de Groot and Michael Fisch

第十篇 神经系统肿瘤

XI MELANOMA AND SARCOMAS

Section Editors: Michael A. Davies and Sapna P. Patel

第十一篇 黑色素瘤和肉瘤

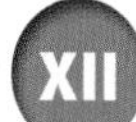

XII OTHER TUMORS

Section Editors: Michael Fisch and John de Groot

第十二篇 其他肿瘤

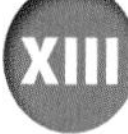

XIII NOVEL AND OTHER CANCER TOPICS OF INTEREST

Section Editors: Apostolia-Maria Tsimberidou and Nizar M. Tannir

第十三篇 前沿和其他有趣的肿瘤话题

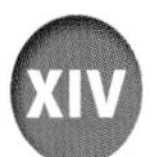

XIV SUPPORTIVE CARE

Section Editor: Karen H. Lu

第十四篇 支持治疗

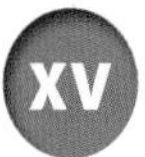

XV PALLIATIVE CARE AND SYMPTOM MANAGEMENT

Section Editors: Eduardo Bruera and Michael Fisch

第十五篇 姑息治疗和症状管理

Section I

Leukemia

Section Editor: William G. Wierda

第一篇 白血病

1

Acute Lymphoblastic Leukemia

第一章　急性淋巴细胞白血病

Muhamed Baljevic
Elias Jabbour
Susan O'Brien
Hagop M. Kantarjian

中文导读

急性淋巴细胞白血病的特征是在血液、骨髓和其他组织中淋巴样祖细胞的异常增殖。本章介绍了该病的流行病学、病因学、临床症状、诊断标准和治疗策略。诊断方面，本病的确诊与分型高度依赖于流式细胞仪免疫表型检测技术，细胞和分子遗传学检测在急性淋巴细胞白血病的诊断及治疗过程中也有重要的作用，通常可用于疾病风险和预后的预测，本章对这两部分内容进行了详细的介绍。对于急性淋巴细胞白血病的治疗分为两个阶段：初次确诊后的初始治疗和复发后的解救治疗，具体的治疗方案选择需要结合本病的分型和预后风险综合考虑。初始治疗主要包括以下几个阶段：诱导缓解、强化治疗、维持治疗和预防中枢神经系统浸润，在强化治疗阶段可以考虑进行异基因造血干细胞移植。复发后的患者预后普遍欠佳，解救治疗的目的是重新诱导疾病完全缓解，然后再进行异基因造血干细胞移植，以达到控制疾病的目的。此外，本章也简述了急性淋巴细胞白血病免疫治疗的新策略以及目前正在进行的临床试验项目，从而为本病的治疗提供更为全面的诊疗参考。

EPIDEMIOLOGY AND ETIOLOGY

Acute lymphoblastic leukemia (ALL) is characterized by the proliferation and accumulation of lymphoid progenitor cells in the blood, bone marrow, and other tissues. It has a bimodal distribution. The overall age-adjusted incidence is 1.7 per 100,000 persons, but ALL affects 4 to 5 per 100,000 persons during age 4 to 5 years and half that number around the fifth decade of life. Approximately 60% of cases are diagnosed in patients ≤20 years old, with a median age at diagnosis of 14 years. In 2014, the American Cancer Society estimated that approximately 6,000 individuals would be diagnosed with ALL that year ([1,2]). Acute lymphoblastic leukemia represents 20% of adult leukemias but is the most common childhood acute leukemia, representing approximately 80% of cases ([1,2]).

The etiology of ALL is unknown in most cases ([3-7]). Chromosomal translocations occurring in utero during fetal hematopoiesis have suggested genetic factors as the primary cause for pediatric ALL and postnatal genetic events as secondary contributors. Monozygotic and dizygotic twins of patients with ALL and individuals with genetic disorders, such as Klinefelter (XXY and variants) and Down (trisomy 21) syndromes, or inherited diseases with excessive chromosomal fragility, such as Bloom syndrome, Fanconi anemia, and ataxia telangiectasia, have all been found to have higher incidence of ALL, implicating a possible genetic predisposition. Additional studies have postulated infectious etiologies ([4]). Human T-cell lymphotropic virus type-1 is known to cause adult T-cell leukemia/lymphoma ([5]); Epstein-Barr virus has been associated with lymphoproliferative disorders, including Burkitt lymphoma and mature B-cell ALL ([6]); and varicella has been linked to childhood ALL ([7]).

CLINICAL PRESENTATION AND LABORATORY ABNORMALITIES

Presenting symptoms can be nonspecific, particularly in children. They largely reflect bone marrow failure and include malaise, fatigue, bleeding or bruising, and secondary infections. The B symptoms, such as fever, night sweats, and weight loss, are frequent. White blood cell (WBC) count at presentation varies widely, and circulating blasts are generally noted. Symptoms related to hyperleukocytosis are rare in ALL, given the lymphoblast morphology, even when WBC counts are high.

Leukemic involvement of the central nervous system (CNS) ranging from cranial neuropathies to meningeal infiltration occurs in <10% of patients at presentation. It is more common in mature B-cell ALL (Burkitt leukemia) ([8]). A history or findings of abdominal masses, significant spontaneous tumor lysis syndrome, and chin numbness (mental nerve) indicating cranial nerve involvement are also more common in this subtype of ALL ([9]). Lymphadenopathy and hepatosplenomegaly, although rarely symptomatic, are noted in approximately 20% of patients ([9]).

DIAGNOSIS

Immunophenotyping

The diagnosis of ALL is largely based on flow cytometric immunophenotyping, although identification of cytogenetic-molecular abnormalities plays a significant role (Fig. 1-1). The World Health Organization (WHO) proposed new guidelines for the diagnosis of neoplastic diseases of hematopoietic and lymphoid tissues ([10]). The French-American-British (FAB) Cooperative Group diagnostic approach, which recognizes L1 to L3 morphologic subtypes, has been essentially abandoned. A blast count of ≥20% was established as sufficient for diagnosis.

Flow cytometric analysis successfully assigns lineage in more than 95% of cases. True mixed phenotype acute leukemia is rare ([11]). Concomitant expression of markers from more than one lineage is seen in 15% to 50% of adult and 5% to 35% of pediatric ALL ([12-14]), but this is not prognostically relevant. Targeted genomic profiling may further define ALL subtypes with different response profiles to therapy and prognoses, which are only partially discriminated by current diagnostic tools.

Immunophenotypically, ALL blasts are negative for myeloperoxidase (MPO), although low-level MPO positivity (3%-5%) may occur in rare cases that otherwise lack expression of myeloid markers by flow cytometry ([15]). Terminal deoxynucleotidyl transferase (TdT), although not a specific marker of ALL, helps separate malignant lymphocytosis from reactive processes and distinguish L3 ALL (TdT negative) from other ALL subtypes ([16]).

Both the prior FAB and current WHO classification systems rely heavily on morphologic assessment ([17]), which accounts for cell size, cytoplasm, nucleoli, basophilia, and vacuolation. The former FAB L3 morphology, characterized by a high rate of cell turnover, is associated with mature B-cell ALL (Burkitt leukemia) and gives rise to the "starry sky" pattern on marrow biopsies.

Three broad immunophenotypic ALL groups can be distinguished: precursor B-cell, mature B-cell, and T-cell ALL (Table 1-1). Precursor B-cell ALL (B-ALL) stains positive for TdT, HLA-DR, CD19, and CD79a. According to the stages of maturation, further B-cell

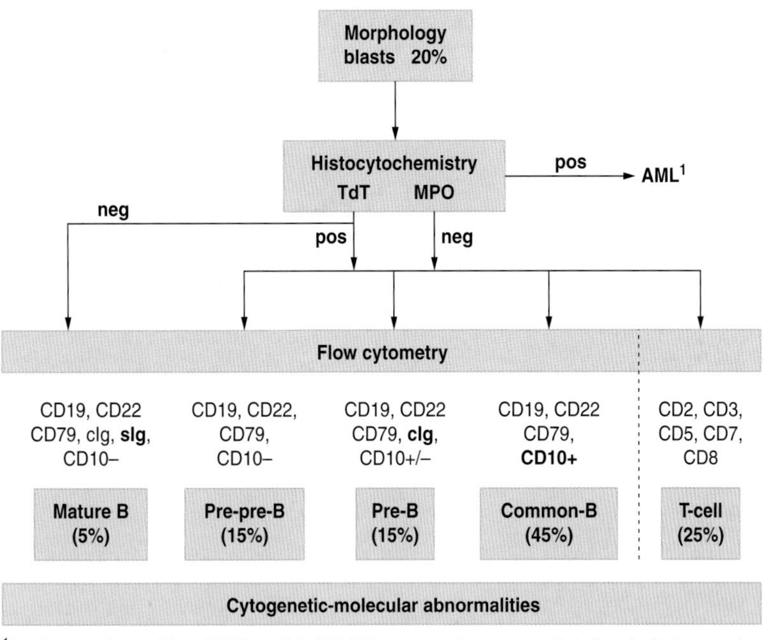

FIGURE 1-1 Diagnosis of acute lymphoblastic leukemia. AML, acute myeloid leukemia.

subgroups have been defined as pre-pre-B-ALL (pro–B-ALL), common ALL, and pre–B-ALL. Although they all stain positive for CD19, CD79a, or CD22, expression of CD10 (common ALL antigen [CALLA]) distinguishes common ALL (early pre–B-ALL), and cytoplasmic immunoglobulins with or without CD10 identify pre–B-ALL. Mature B-ALL (Burkitt leukemia) is TdT negative but expresses surface immunoglobulins (usually immunoglobulin M), as well as κ or λ light chains in a clonal fashion. It has almost ubiquitous expression of CD20, which has therapeutic implications ([18]).

T-cell ALL (T-ALL) further stratifies into subtypes based on different stages of thymic differentiation ([19]). As the most lineage-specific marker for T-cell differentiation, surface CD3 (sCD3) is typically positive in mature T-ALL, which is also positive for either CD4 or CD8, but not both. However, pre–T-ALL is negative for CD4, CD8, and sCD3 but may still express cytoplasmic CD3. A more simplified classification divides T-ALL into early T-ALL ($sCD3^-$, $CD1a^-$), thymic T-ALL ($sCD3^{+/-}$, $CD1a^+$), and mature T-ALL ($sCD3^+$, $CD1a^+$). Only thymic T-ALL has excellent outcome with chemotherapy alone.

Cytogenetic-Molecular Profiling

Frequent cytogenetic and molecular abnormalities associated with adult ALL offer insight into the events leading to leukemic progression (Table 1-2) ([20]). They are of both prognostic and predictive significance and have varying frequencies in children and adults, which explains some of the differences in outcomes in these two groups. This is particularly true in the case of ALL

Table 1-1 Immunophenotypic Classification of ALL

B Lineage		T Lineage	
CD19/CD79a/CD22		CD3 (Surface/Cytoplasmic)	
Pre-pre-B-ALL (pro–B-ALL)	—	Precursor T-ALL	CD1a, CD2, CD5, CD7, CD8, cCD3
Common ALL	CD10 (CALLA)	Mature T-ALL	Surface CD3 (plus any other T-cell markers)
Pre–B-ALL	Cytoplasmic IgM		
Mature B-ALL	Cytoplasmic or surface Ig κ or λ		

Table 1-2 Cytogenetic and Molecular Abnormalities in ALL

Category	Cytogenetics	Involved Genes	Adults Frequency (%)	Children Frequency (%)
Hyperdiploid			2-15	10-26
Hypodiploid			5-10	5-10
Pseudodiploid	t(9;22)(q34;q11)	*BCR-ABL1*	15-25	2-6
	del(9)(q21-22)	*p15, p16*	6-30	20
	t(4;11);t(9;11); t(11;19); t(3;11)	*MLL*	5-10	<5
	del(11)(q22-23)	*ATM*	25-30[a]	15[a]
	t(12;21)(p12;q22)	*TEL-AML1*	<1[b]	20-25[b]
	t(1;19)	*E2A-PBX1*	<5	<5
	t(17;19)	*E2A-HLF*	<5	<5
	t(1;14)(p32;q11)	*TAL1*	10-15	5-10
	t(7;9)(q34;q32)	*TAL2*	<1	<1
	t(10;14)(q24;q11)	*HOX11*	5-10	<5
	t(5;14)(q35;q32)	*HOX11L2*	1	2-3
	t(1;14)(p32;q11)	*TCR*	20-25[c]	20-25[c]
	del(13)(q14)	*miR15/miR16*	<5	<5
	t(8;14); t(8;22); t(2;8)	*C-MYC*	5	2-5
	+8	?	10-12	2
	del(7p)	?	5-10	<5
	del(5q)	?	<2	<2
	del(6q); t(6;12)	?	5	<5

[a]As determined by loss of heterozygosity.
[b]As determined by polymerase chain reaction.
[c]In T-cell ALL, overall incidence <10%.

harboring Philadelphia chromosome [t(9;22)] (Ph) or other chromosomal changes with prognostic relevance such as Burkitt karyotypes [t(8;14), t(2;8), t(8;22)] or t(4;11). Next-generation sequencing, expression proteomics, and oligonucleotide microarrays have transformed our understanding of the genomic landscape of ALL and are yielding new molecular subgroups with actionable defects ([21-23]).

Recently, a Ph-like signature in 10% of children with standard-risk ALL and as many as 25% to 30% of young adults with ALL has been defined using genome-wide gene expression arrays. This subgroup lacks the expression of BCR-ABL1 fusion protein but does have a gene expression profile similar to BCR-ABL1 ALL ([24-26]). The vast majority of these patients have deletions in key transcription factors involved in B-cell signaling, such as IKZF1, TCF3, EBF1, PAX5, and VPREB1, as well as kinase-activating alterations involving ABL1, ABL2, CRLF2, CSF1R, EPOR, JAK2, NTRK3, PDGFRB, PTK2B, TSLP, or TYK2 and sequence mutations involving *FLT3*, *IL7R*, or *SH2B3*. The most common alterations (~50%) are rearrangements of CRLF2, which activate downstream signaling through JAK kinases, and approximately half of these cases have activating mutations in *JAK1* or *JAK2* (Fig. 1-2). Importantly, patients with ABL1, ABL2, CSF1R, and PDGFRB expression fusions were sensitive in in vitro and in vivo human xenograft models to ABL class tyrosine kinase inhibitors (TKIs; eg, dasatinib); rearrangements in *EPOR*, *IL-7R*, and *JAK2* mutations and fusions were sensitive to JAK kinase inhibitors (eg, ruxolitinib); and patients with ETV6-NTRK3 fusion were sensitive to ALK kinase inhibitors (eg, crizotinib) ([25]), further expanding therapeutic options in this subgroup with poor outcome.

Observations of epigenetic alterations regulating distinct molecular pathways that occur frequently at presentation and relapse have identified a "hypermethylator" phenotype of ALL ([27]). These patients may respond favorably to treatment with hypomethylating agents (azacitidine or decitabine). Identification of these and other molecular and cytogenetic changes in adult ALL drives the development of risk-adapted and targeted therapies, particularly in high-risk groups (Table 1-3) ([28]).

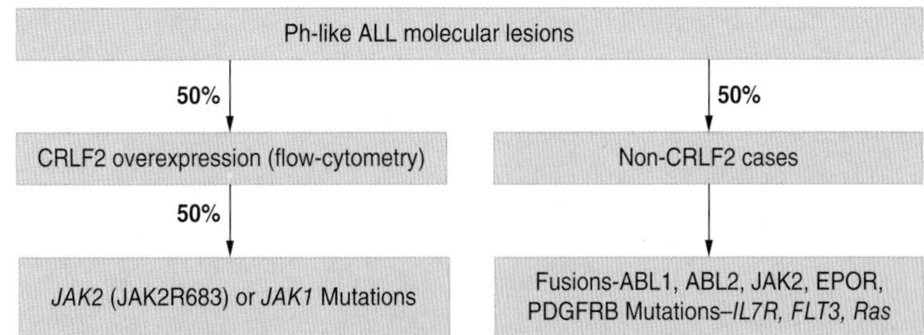

FIGURE 1-2 Ph-like acute lymphoblastic leukemia (ALL) molecular lesions and associated molecular fusions or mutations.

FRONTLINE THERAPY

Therapy for ALL consists of complex and comprehensive regimens consisting of several phases: induction, intensified consolidation, maintenance, and CNS prophylaxis ([9,29]). Each involves the use of a core group of agents considered the backbone of therapy in a time- and dose-dependent manner, with a goal of restoring normal hematopoiesis, eradicating resistant subclones, providing adequate prophylaxis of sanctuary sites (eg, CNS, testicles), and eliminating minimal residual disease (MRD) during the consolidation and maintenance phases ([9,30]). Combining anthracyclines (eg, daunorubicin or doxorubicin), vincristine, and dexamethasone (for better CNS penetration), often coupled with cyclophosphamide or asparaginase with growth factor support, represents the cornerstone of ALL induction regimens. This results in complete remission (CR) rates of 70% to 90% and median remission durations of 18 months ([30,31]). Patients who achieve CR subsequently transition to the consolidation phase, which, depending on the risk-oriented subtype, may consist of consolidation chemotherapy (cytarabine, methotrexate, cyclophosphamide, and 6-mercaptopurine) or allogeneic hematopoietic stem-cell transplantation (AHSCT). Consolidation is followed by prolonged maintenance therapy with daily 6-mercaptopurine, weekly methotrexate, and monthly pulses of vincristine and prednisone or dexamethasone, given over 2 to 3 years (POMP or DOMP, depending on corticosteroid

Table 1-3 Recent Genetic Determinants in ALL by Lineage

ALL Lineage	Cytogenetic Aberration	Involved Genes	Protein	Comments
B cell	BCR/ABL+ (Ph+)	*IKZF1*	Ikaros	Poor outcome. 80% of Ph+ cases.
		CRLF2 + the Ig heavy chain locus; or an interstitial *PAR1* deletion	CRLF2	5%-10% of cases with no molecular rearrangement. Poor outcome. 50% of children with Down syndrome.
	BCR/ABL-like	*IKZF1* deletions; rearrangements/mutations in *CRLF2*, *IGH-CRLF2*, and *NUP214-ABL1*; in-frame fusions of *EBF1-PDGFRB*, *BCR-JAK2*, or *STRN3-JAK2*; cryptic *IGH-EPOR* rearrangements		15% of cases. Potential use of TKIs and/or mTOR and JAK2 inhibitors.
	Near hypodiploid	*NRAS*, *KRAS*, *FLT3*, and *NF1*		70% of cases.
	Low hypodiploid	*IKZF2*, and by *TP53* disruptions, *CDKN2A/B* locus deletion		91% of cases.
	Hyperdiploid	*CREBBP*		
		NT5C2 mutations	NT5C2	
		TP53 mutations		6% of cases.
T cell		*PICALM-MLLT10*, *NUP214-ABL1* fusion, *EML-ABL1*, *SET-NUP214* fusion, *MLL*, *NOTCH1*, *FBW7*, *BCL11B*, *JAK1*, *PTPN2*, *IL7R*, *PHF6*, *RAS/PTEN*		*NOTCH1* (>60%) and/or *FBW7* (~20%) mutations associated with a favorable outcome. *RAS/PTEN* and *JAK1* usually poor outcome.

mTOR, mammalian target of rapamycin; TKI, tyrosine kinase inhibitor.

used) ([30-32]). Maintenance, which is omitted in mature B-ALL due to high cure rates, may also involve the use of TKIs for patients with Ph-positive ALL. Primary CNS involvement at diagnosis is rare (<10%) but is as high as 50% to 75% at 1 year without prophylactic administration of intrathecal chemotherapy (IT) ([31]). Although high-dose cytarabine (1-7.5 mg/m^2) and methotrexate (5-8 g/m^2) successfully penetrate the blood-brain barrier, they are too toxic to serve as the sole CNS prophylaxis. The inclusion of IT prophylaxis (methotrexate, cytarabine, liposomal cytarabine, hydrocortisone, or thiotepa) reduces the incidence of CNS relapse to 4% by allowing sustained therapeutic concentration of the agents in the cerebrospinal fluid. The number of ITs varies according to protocol (usually 8 for standard risk, 12 for Ph positive, and 16 for Burkitt), and in rare cases of extramedullary disease spread (eg, masses or chloromas), IT may even be supplemented by radiation therapy.

One extensively studied regimen used in treatment of adult ALL is the hyper-CVAD (HCVAD) regimen, where patients receive hyperfractionated cyclophosphamide, vincristine, doxorubicin, and dexamethasone alternating with high-dose methotrexate and cytarabine for a total of eight alternating cycles approximately every 3 to 4 weeks (Table 1-4) ([30,31]). This is followed by 2 years of POMP maintenance therapy, interspersed with intensification courses during months 6, 7, 18, and 19. The number of IT injections (two per course) depends on the risk of CNS relapse, which has been identified as high for patients with mature B-ALL. Our current approach is giving 8 ITs for nonmature B-ALL and 16 ITs for mature B-ALL, resulting in a 5-year overall survival (OS) between 38% and 50% ([30]). Due the improved cure rates of Ph-positive ALL patients, an increase in the CNS relapse rate was observed, which is the reason the protocol was modified to include 12 ITs for Ph-positive ALL.

Table 1-4 Doses and Schedule of the Hyper-CVAD Regimen

Therapy Segment	Dose and Schedule
Induction and intensified consolidation	Hyper-CVAD (courses 1, 3, 5, and 7)
	• Cyclophosphamide 300 mg/m^2 IV over 3 h every 12 h for 6 doses on days 1-3
	• Mesna 600 mg/m^2 as an IV continuous infusion over 24 h daily on days 1-3 (starting approximately 1 h prior to cyclophosphamide and finishing 12 h after the last dose)
	• Doxorubicin 50 mg/m^2 IV continuous infusion over 24 h on day 4
	• Vincristine 2 mg IV on days 4 and 11
	• Dexamethasone 40 mg daily on days 1-4 and 4-11
	Methotrexate (MTX) and high-dose cytarabine (courses 2, 4, 6, and 8)
	• MTX 200 mg/m^2 IV over 2 h followed by 800 mg/m^2 IV over 22 h on day 1
	• Leucovorin rescue 15 mg every 6 h for eight doses (starting 12 h after completion of MTX)
	• Cytarabine 3 g/m^2 IV over 2 h every 12 h for 4 doses on days 2 and 3
	• Methylprednisolone 50 mg IV twice daily on days 1-3
CNS prophylaxis	IT MTX 12 mg (6 mg if via Omaya reservoir) on day 2 and cytarabine 100 mg on day 7 of each course
	Low risk: 6 IT
	High risk: 8 IT
	Mature B cell: 16 IT
Maintenance therapy	POMP
	• 6-Mercaptopurine 50 mg orally three times per day
	• MTX 20 mg/m^2 orally weekly
	• Prednisone 200 mg orally days 1-5 every month
	• Vincristine 2 mg IV every month
	• Intensification with four additional courses of hyper-CVAD plus MTX/cytarabine
Supportive care	• Antibiotic prophylaxis (levofloxacin, fluconazole, valacyclovir)
	• Hematopoietic growth factor support during induction and consolidation
	• Laminar air flow rooms (for patients ≥60 years old)

CNS, central nervous system; IT, intrathecal; IV, intravenous.

Mature B-Cell and Burkitt Acute Lymphoblastic Leukemia

The addition of rituximab to short intensive chemotherapy has also improved outcome in adult Burkitt and Burkitt-type lymphoma or ALL ([29, 33, 34]). Hoelzer and colleagues have recently reported the benefit of adding rituximab to short intensive chemotherapy in 363 patients with Burkitt lymphoma/leukemia; the addition of rituximab resulted in CR and 5-year survival rates of 88% and 80%, respectively ([33]). Higher rates of survival were reported in adolescents compared to adults and elderly patients (90% vs 84% vs 62%, respectively) ([33]). Low-intensity chemotherapy with infused etoposide, doxorubicin, and cyclophosphamide with vincristine, prednisone, and rituximab (EPOCH-R) was recently tested in 30 adult patients with Burkitt lymphoma ([35]). The progression-free survival (PFS) and OS rates were 90% and 100%, respectively. Of note, marrow involvement was present in only 13% of patients, and CNS involvement was present in only 3% of patients ([35]).

CD20-Positive Pre–B-Cell Acute Lymphoblastic Leukemia

There have been several alterations to traditional protocols with further refining of the disease. Expression of cell surface marker CD20 in adult ALL ranges from 35% to ubiquitous depending on the subtype and has been associated with an inferior prognosis ([18]). The addition of two doses of monoclonal CD20 antibody (rituximab) administered with the first four cycles of chemotherapy and during maintenance intensification at months 6 and 18 resulted in improved OS in younger patients compared with similar chemotherapy historical controls (75% vs 47% at 3 years; $P = .003$) ([36]). Improvement in the 5-year remission duration and survival rates was also reported in patients <55 years old by the German Multicenter Study Group for ALL (GMALL) when rituximab was added to standard induction and consolidation therapy ([37]).

Ofatumumab is a more potent second-generation anti-CD20 monoclonal antibody that binds to a membrane proximal small-loop epitope on the CD20 protein. A phase II study in CD20-positive pre–B-ALL combined ofatumumab with HCVAD during induction, resulting in a 96% rate of both CR and MRD negativity. At a median follow-up of 14 months, the 1-year PFS and OS rates were 94% and 92%, respectively ([38]).

Philadelphia-Positive Acute Lymphoblastic Leukemia

Philadelphia-positive ALL used to have a very poor outcome in general. The incorporation of TKIs into treatment regimens has significantly improved patient outcomes, as supported by several reports ([39-42]). Incorporation of early, daily, and concurrent TKI with chemotherapy has proven more effective than intermittent pulses ([41, 42]).

Second-generation TKIs, such as the dual src and abl inhibitor dasatinib, which is more potent than imatinib and crosses the blood-brain barrier ([43]), have also been investigated in combination with chemotherapy. In an attempt to improve on the outcomes with imatinib, dasatinib was administered at 100 mg daily for 14 days with induction chemotherapy, followed by 70 mg continuous dosing with the consolidation cycles, and at 100 mg daily continuously during the maintenance phase ([44]). Overall, 94% of patients achieved CR, 96% achieved complete cytogenetic response (CCyR), and 65% achieved complete molecular response (CMR). Allogeneic hematopoietic stem-cell transplantation was performed in 22 patients (12 in first CR and 10 in second CR), with 3-year disease-free survival (DFS) and OS rates of 49% and 61%, respectively.

Attempting to reduce exposure to cytotoxic chemotherapy by intensifying chemotherapy with TKIs can be very effective but toxic ([45, 46]). Patients in the GRAAPH-2005 study were randomized to imatinib 800 mg daily for 4 weeks combined with weekly vincristine and dexamethasone versus imatinib 800 mg daily for 2 weeks combined with HCVAD chemotherapy ([45]). The CR rate was higher in the low-intensity group due to induction-related mortality in the HCVAD group (7% vs <1%; $P = .01$). An equal number of patients in each group proceeded to autologous stem cell transplantation and allogeneic stem cell transplantation, and at 3 years, OS was similar between the two arms (53% for low intensity vs 49% for HCVAD; $P = .61$).

Studies have also evaluated the use of dasatinib and nilotinib with low-intensity chemotherapy ([46-48]). In the EWALL-Ph-01 study, dasatinib with low-intensity chemotherapy was administered to 71 patients with newly diagnosed Ph-positive ALL age ≥55 years ([46]). Dasatinib was dosed at 140 mg once daily during induction and at 100 mg daily during consolidation, yielding a CR rate of 94%. The estimated 3-year OS was 45%.

Many Ph-positive ALL patients can relapse with threonine-to-isoleucine mutation at position 315 (T315I), which is refractory to imatinib and second-generation TKIs. A third-generation TKI, ponatinib, which has activity against T315I, was evaluated in phase I and II trials in patients with Ph-positive leukemias and was shown to have significant antileukemic activity ([49, 50]). More recently, 39 patients with newly diagnosed Ph-positive ALL were treated with HCVAD and ponatinib 45 mg daily for 14 days during induction and then continuously thereafter until CCyR and CMR were obtained, when decreases to 30 mg and 15 mg daily could be instituted, respectively. The CR, CCyR, and CMR rates were 100%, 100%, and 74%, respectively. After a median follow-up of 20 months, 1-year PFS and OS were 97% and 87%, respectively ([51]).

Although current standard of care still advocates AHSCT consolidation in first CR ([39]), new information regarding the status of MRD in Ph-positive ALL has raised a question as to who should be referred for it. The predictive value of MRD assessment by quantitative reverse transcriptase polymerase chain reaction (RT-PCR) and multiparameter flow cytometry (FCM) was recently assessed in patients with Ph-positive ALL treated with combination chemotherapy and TKIs who did not undergo AHSCT. Achieving major molecular response at 3, 6, 9, and 12 months (P = .02, .04, .05, and .01, respectively) and having negative FCM at 3 and 12 months were associated with improved survival (P = .04 and .001, respectively) ([52]). This information suggests that patients with early and sustained molecular response may not need consolidation with AHSCT.

T-Cell Acute Lymphoblastic Leukemia

Treatment of adult T-ALL and T-cell lymphoblastic lymphoma (T-LL) results in a long-term survival rate of 40% to 60%, and the outcome is strongly associated with T-cell phenotype ([53, 54]). Adding nelarabine, a selective anti–T-ALL agent may further improve the outcome. In a single-arm, phase II study, 48 patients with newly diagnosed T-ALL or T-LL were treated with HCVAD and neralabine ([55]). The CR rate was 93%; the 5-year survival rate was 66% after a median follow-up of 41 months. These rates were 38% and 70% for patients with early T-cell precursor (ETP) and mature T-ALL, respectively. Indeed, ETP-ALL is a distinct T-cell entity characterized by the absence of CD1a, sCD3, and CD8 expression; weak CD5 expression; and expression of one or more myeloid or stem cell–associated markers ([54]). It confers poor prognosis with the use of standard intensive chemotherapy, which results in high rates of remission failure and relapse compared to patients with typical T-ALL (72% at 10 years vs 10% at 10 years). This phenotype is in part a reflection of the higher degree of genomic instability (number and size of genetic defects) that ETP-ALL harbors, with over 60% of adult patients carrying mutations in *DNMT3A*, *FLT3*, or *NOTCH1*, which may allow for tailored induction regimens with targeted therapies ([56]). Following induction, AHSCT should be considered in first remission for all ETP-ALL patients.

Adolescent and Young Adult Acute Lymphoblastic Leukemia

Retrospective studies have shown that pediatric regimens resulted in better outcomes than adult regimens (which had deviated significantly from the established principles of ALL therapy in pediatric regimens). Pediatric-inspired regimens, such as the Berlin-Frankfurt-Münster (BFM) regimen (Table 1-5), deliver more intensive nonmyelosuppressive agents like vincristine, asparaginase, corticosteroids, and CNS therapy ([54, 55]).

The Group for Research on Adult Acute Lymphoblastic Leukemia (GRAALL) evaluated a pediatric-inspired regimen in patients up to age 60 years and compared the results to a historical control group treated with an adult regimen. In patients treated with the pediatric-inspired regimen, the CR rate was 93%, and at 42 months, event-free survival (EFS) and OS rates were 55% (95% CI, 48%-52%) and 60% (95% CI, 53%-66%), respectively ([57]). Although the pediatric-inspired regimen resulted in improved survival compared with the control (66% vs 44%; $P < .001$), the cumulative incidence of treatment-related death in patients age 40 to 60 years old was 23%, erasing the margin of benefit gained with enhanced activity of pediatric regimens. Thus, the toxicity threshold can be reached and crossed in the adult population in attempts to reach higher cure rates, limiting the usefulness of intensifying chemotherapy to the pediatric-inspired strength.

The UKALL14 study of 91 adults with a median age of 47 years (range, 25-65 years) used PEG-asparaginase at a dose of 1,000 units/m^2 on days 4 and 18 during induction, resulting in a CR rate of 66%, with induction-related mortality rate of 20% and hepatotoxicity rate of 56%, prompting the omission of PEG-asparaginase in patients ≥40 years old ([58]).

A recent US Intergroup study of 318 adolescent and young adult (AYA) patients (median age, 24 years) treated with a pediatric-inspired regimen was reported. With a median follow-up of 28 months, the estimated 5-year EFS and OS rates were 45% and 55%, respectively ([59]). Presence of MRD at day 28 following initiation of induction therapy and presence of a Ph-like gene expression signature were significantly associated with worse EFS and OS. The Ph-like signature, which was detected in 28% of patients, resulted in 2-year EFS of only 52%, compared to 81% for those without Ph-like disease.

Our internal review of 85 AYA patients up to age 40 (median age, 21 years) treated with pediatric-like augmented BFM showed CR and MRD negativity rates of 94% and 69%, respectively ([60]). The 5-year CR rate was 58%, and the 5-year OS rate was 62%. Compared with a historical control group of similar patients who received HCVAD with or without rituximab, 3-year OS rates were 72% and 71%, respectively. However, in patients age 25 years and older, the pediatric-inspired regimen was inferior and caused more liver dysfunction, pancreatitis, osteonecrosis, and thrombosis compared to HCVAD with CD20-targeted therapies.

Hence, HCVAD-based regimens that use the backbone ALL agents but eliminate or reduce the exposure to asparaginase show similar CR and remission rates

Table 1-5 Doses and Schedule of the Augmented Berlin-Frankfurt-Münster (BFM) Regimen

Therapy Segment	Dose and Schedule
Induction (4 weeks)	IT cytarabine 100 mg within 3 days prior to start of induction
	Daunorubicin 25 mg/m^2 IV weekly for 4 doses
	Vincristine 2 mg IV weekly for 4 doses
	Prednisone 60 mg/m^2/d orally in divided doses on days 1-28
	PEG-asparaginase 2,500 international units/m^2 IV during week 1
	IT Methotrexate 12 mg during weeks 2 and 5
Extended induction (2 weeks)	Daunorubicin 25 mg/m^2 IV during week 1
	Vincristine 2 mg IV weekly for 2 doses
	Prednisone 60 mg/m^2/day orally in divided doses for 14 days
	PEG-asparaginase 2500 international units/m^2 IV during week 1
Consolidation 1 (8 weeks)	Cyclophosphamide 1 g/m^2 IV during weeks 1 and 5
	Cytarabine 75 mg/m^2 subcutaneously or IV on days 1-4 and 8-11 of each month
	6-Mercaptopurine 60 mg/m^2/day orally on days 1-14 of each month
	Vincristine 2 mg IV during weeks 3 and 4 of each month
	PEG-asparaginase 2500 international units/m^2 IV during weeks 3 and 6
	IT methotrexate 12 mg weekly for 4 weeks
Consolidation 2 (7 weeks)	Vincristine 2 mg IV every 10 days for 5 doses
	Methotrexate, starting at 100 mg/m^2 and escalating by 50 mg/m^2/dose every 10 days for 5 doses
	PEG-asparaginase 2,500 IU/m^2 IV during weeks 1 and 4
	IT methotrexate 12 mg during weeks 1 and 5
Consolidation 3–part A (4 weeks)	Vincristine 2 mg IV weekly for 3 doses
	Dexamethasone 10 mg/m^2/d orally in divided doses on days 1-7 and days 15-21
	Doxorubicin 25 mg/m^2 IV weekly for 3 doses
	PEG-asparaginase 2,500 IU/m^2 IV during week 1
	IT methotrexate 12 mg during week 1
Consolidation 3–part B (4 weeks)	Cyclophosphamide 1 g/m^2 IV during week 1
	Cytarabine 75 mg/m^2 subcutaneously or IV for 4 consecutive days during weeks 1 and 2
	Thioguanine 60 mg/m^2/d orally for 14 days
	Vincristine 2 mg IV during weeks 3 and 4
	PEG-asparaginase 2,500 IU/m^2 IV during week 3
	IT methotrexate 12 mg during weeks 1 and 2
Maintenance (24 months)	Vincristine 2 mg IV monthly
	Dexamethasone 6 mg/m^2/d orally for 5 days every month
	6-Mercaptopurine 75 mg/m^2/d in divided doses
	Methotrexate 20 mg/m^2 orally weekly
	IT methotrexate 12 mg every 3 months for the first 12 months of maintenance
Supportive care	Antibiotic prophylaxis (levofloxacin, trimethoprim/sulfamethoxazole [start week 2 of induction], fluconazole, valacyclovir)

Slow early responders repeat consolidation 2 and consolidation 3A and 3B prior to maintenance therapy. If central nervous system disease is present at start of therapy, then give methotrexate 12 mg IT weekly until negative for blasts, methotrexate 12 mg IT every other week for 8 doses, and then methotrexate 12 mg IT monthly for 6 months.
IT, intrathecal; IV, intravenous.

CHAPTER 1

and survival outcomes compared with the pediatric-inspired regimens in similar patient populations.

Acute Lymphoblastic Leukemia in Elderly Patients

Conventional ALL chemotherapy is associated with high mortality rates (30%-35%) during consolidation/maintenance in elderly patients (>60 years) ([60]). A low-intensity regimen may improve outcome. In a phase II study with inotuzumab ozogamicin and low-intensity hyper-CVD therapy, 26 patients with a median age of 67 years (range, 60-79 years) were treated for newly diagnosed ALL ([61]). Inotuzumab, which is a CD22-directed monoclonal antibody bound to calicheamicin (chemotoxin), was administered at a dose of 1.3 to 1.8 mg/m^2 once with each of the first four courses; doxorubicin was eliminated in induction; cyclophosphamide and steroids were 50% reduced; methotrexate was reduced to 250 mg/m^2 on day 1 and cytarabine to 0.5 mg/m^2 × 4 on days 2 and 3 of even courses. The overall response rate (ORR) was 96% (CR, 79%; CR with incomplete platelet recovery [CRp], 17%), with all patients with cytogenetic abnormalities achieving CCyR. All responders also achieved MRD-negative status, 75% of which occurred after cycle 1. The 1-year PFS and OS rates were 86% and 81%, respectively. The 1-year survival rate was superior to previous results obtained with HCVAD with or without rituximab in similar patient populations (1-year OS, 81% vs 60%, respectively).

Role of Allogeneic Stem Cell Transplantation

Allogeneic stem cell transplantation has traditionally been reserved for patients with high-risk features including B-lineage with WBC ≥30 × 10^9/L, T-lineage with WBC ≥100 × 10^9/L, hypodiploid, Ph-positive, or mixed-lineage leukemia translocation ALL [eg, t(4;11)]. However, there has been some debate regarding who should be referred for AHSCT in first CR based on recent data that indicate that patients with standard-risk disease, and not high-risk disease, benefit the most ([62]). As an alternative, many centers have incorporated MRD via FCM or RT-PCR after induction or consolidation to stratify patients based on their response to chemotherapy ([63]). In fact, when controlled for other known risk factors, failure to achieve MRD has emerged as a powerful indicator of future relapse ([52]) and therapeutic approach (ie, AHSCT vs more chemotherapy). In one study, MRD status at various time points after CR was used to guide treatment in adult patients with ALL ([64]). Patients who remained MRD positive at the end of consolidation were deemed to be higher risk and underwent AHSCT instead of receiving prolonged maintenance therapy. Patients who achieved MRD-negative status had a significantly improved 5-year OS (75% vs 33%; P = .001). Furthermore, in a recent update of the GRAALL experience in 423 younger adults with Ph-negative ALL in first remission (265 B-cell precursor ALL and 158 T-ALL patients), postinduction MRD level ≥10^{-4} and unfavorable genetic characteristics (ie, *MLL* gene rearrangement or focal *IKZF1* gene deletion in B-cell precursor ALL and no *NOTCH1/FBXW7* mutation and/or *N/K-RAS* mutation and/or *PTEN* gene alteration in T-ALL) were independently associated with worse outcome ([65]). Therefore, for patients with standard-risk ALL, MRD status should guide the postremission therapy, whereby patients who fail to achieve MRD negativity can be transplanted in first CR. In addition to the MRD status, new genomic and immunophenotyping technologies were essential in identifying patients with poor prognosis. Patient with Ph-like ALL and ETP-ALL should be considered for AHSCT in first CR ([24, 54]).

Minimal Residual Disease

Postinduction assessment for persistence or reemergence of MRD in patients with ALL is the most important adverse prognostic factor and identifies chemorefractory disease ([64, 66, 67]). Virtually all adults with ALL and molecular failure exhibit poor prognosis despite continued chemotherapy and are candidates for stem-cell transplantation and targeted therapies ([68]).

The Programa Español de Tratamientos en Hematología (PETHEMA) ALL-AR-03 trial in adolescent and adult patients with high-risk Ph-negative ALL showed poor MRD clearance by FCM after early consolidation and identified the pattern of MRD clearance as the only prognostic factor for DFS and OS ([69]).

Blinatumomab is a bispecific T-cell engaging (BiTE) antibody and is the first agent in its class that engages host T cells to the target cell surface antigen–expressing cancer cells. It contains the variable domains of a CD19 and a CD3 antibody, joined via nonimmunogenic linker ([70]). Cytotoxic T cells are activated upon binding to CD19, inducing cell death through the perforin system. Given the pharmacokinetics of the construct (short half-life and the mechanism of action), continuous infusion over several weeks resulted in significantly improved drug activity in ALL and minimization of side effects. Twenty-one patients in hematologic and morphologic CR with persistent or reappearing MRD during consolidation were first studied with a blinatumomab dose of 15 μg/m^2/d as a continuous infusion for 28 days every 6 weeks for a total of 4 cycles or proceeded to AHSCT if a donor was available ([71]). Minimal residual disease conversion following one cycle of therapy was seen in 80% of patients. After a median follow-up of 33 months,

60% of patients remained in CR, with the same percentage of patients experiencing estimated 3-year refractory-free survival ([72]). Nontransplanted patients had a similar favorable outcome compared to the nine patients who underwent AHSCT.

A recent confirmatory, open-label, multicenter, phase II trial of blinatumomab in 116 patients with MRD-positive B-cell precursor ALL in CR resulted in overall MRD eradication in 80% of patients, almost all (78%) after a single cycle of therapy ([73]). As a result, the MD Anderson Cancer Center (MDACC) will open a trial evaluating the role of blinatumomab in patients with positive MRD in CR.

SALVAGE THERAPY

The prognosis of adult patients with relapsed ALL remains poor, with limited effective therapies available. Relapsed disease carries a median survival of only 24 weeks, and patients who have short duration of first CR or primary refractory disease do particularly poorly, with a median OS of less than 5 months ([74]). The goal of salvage therapy is to reinduce CR and consolidate with an AHSCT. Given that we currently lack agents or regimens that can singularly achieve cure in the relapsed setting, patients should be enrolled on a clinical trial if possible. Choice of salvage is contingent upon the previous treatment history, remission duration, ongoing comorbidities, and the relapse-specific features that may be targetable.

Asparaginase could be incorporated into salvage for patients without previous exposure to it. This can be achieved through the augmented HCVAD protocol designed at MDACC, which intensifies the standard vincristine and corticosteroid backbone and adds the pegylated asparaginase ([75]). In an initial study, 80% of 88 evaluable patients initially received conventional HCVAD and 76% were receiving this regimen in first salvage. The ORR was 64%; 47% of patients achieved CR, whereas the remainder achieved partial response (PR) or CRp. Twenty-eight patients (32%) underwent AHSCT, 19 of whom were in CR at the time of transplantation. Despite the favorable response rate, median OS was 6 months, with some long-term responders. As such, regardless of whether they have received conventional HCVAD previously, this regimen represents a reasonable choice for relapsed patients with good performance status who can tolerate intensive chemotherapy.

Clofarabine is a new-generation purine nucleoside analog modeled after fludarabine and cladribine that is approved as a third-line therapy for pediatric ALL ([76]). Attempts have been made in both pediatric and adult population to build on its modest activity as a single agent by combining it with other chemotherapeutics ([77-79]). In a phase II multicenter study evaluating clofarabine added to cyclophosphamide and etoposide in 25 heavily relapsed refractory pediatric patients, ORR was 44% (7 patients with CR), and 10 patients eventually underwent AHSCT ([77]). Patients with prior AHSCT were excluded due to a high rate of veno-occlusive disease (VOD). In the adult population, a French group evaluated clofarabine in patients with relapsed ALL by combining it with dexamethasone, mitoxantrone, etoposide, and asparaginase (VANDEVOL, n = 37) or with cyclophosphamide (ENDEVOL, n = 18) ([78]). Complete remission was achieved in 41% and 50% of patients, respectively, and less than one-third of patients received subsequent AHSCT. The median OS was 6.5 months. The PETHEMA group reported on 31 heavily pretreated relapsed/refractory adult ALL patients, of whom 84% had received two or more previous treatment regimens ([79]). Complete remission was achieved in 26% of patients, with a median OS of approximately 3 months.

Nelarabine is soluble prodrug of 9-β-D-arabinofuranosylguanine and is approved as a nucleoside analog. It has predominant activity in patients with relapsed T-ALL who have failed two prior regimens. By selectively accumulating in T cells, it lends itself as particularly useful in this subset of patients. The GMALL group analyzed 126 patients with relapsed T-ALL/lymphoma who received two cycles of nelarabine as a single agent, with a goal to consolidate patients in CR with AHSCT (partial responders appeared to have potential to achieve CR with continued therapy) ([80]). After one to three cycles, the CR rate was 36%, with 80% receiving AHSCT. Median OS for the entire cohort was only 6 months, with a 12% probability of survival at 3 years; those who underwent AHSCT after CR had a far better outcome, with a 3-year OS probability of 36%. The major toxicity of nelarabine is neurotoxicity; however, this study noted a low rate of grade 3/4 neurotoxicity, even in patients with prior heavy exposure to vincristine. Nelarabine remains a viable salvage option, and its use continues to be optimized in the frontline combination setting or with alternative dosing schedules ([81]).

Vincristine is a standard component of almost all regimens in both adult and pediatric ALL and is frequently capped at 2 mg due to compromising dose-limiting neurotoxicity manifested as peripheral neuropathy or moderate to severe constipation. In an effort to optimize its pharmacodynamics and delivery, a liposomal formulation was synthesized. A phase II study evaluated 65 patients with relapsed and refractory ALL with vincristine sulfate liposome administered as a weekly intravenous infusion at 2.25 mg/m^2 with no capping parameter ([82]). In this heavily pretreated population, the ORR was 35%, and 12 patients underwent AHSCT. Grade 3 peripheral neuropathy was observed in 15% of patients, and the median OS was 4.6 months (five patients were alive at 12 months).

NOVEL STRATEGIES WITH IMMUNOTHERAPY

Monoclonal Antibodies

Further intensification of conventional regimens has been limited by unfavorable toxicity/antileukemic profile. The development of monoclonal antibodies directed against cell surface antigens that are better tolerated has since led to significant improvement in outcomes for a number of malignancies, including ALL.

Blinatumomab, a bispecific antibody (anti-CD3 and anti-CD19), was studied in patients with relapsed/refractory ALL as a continuous infusion for 28 days every 6 weeks. The ORR (CR or CRp) with two cycles of therapy was 68%, with an estimated median OS of 9 months ([83]). In an open-label, single-arm, multicenter phase II study in 189 patients with relapsed/refractory disease, the ORR was 43%, with 80% of the responses during the first cycle. The median response duration and OS were 9 and 6 months, respectively ([84]). Blinatumomab causes constitutional symptoms (fever, chills) that coincide with a rapid rise in activated T cells, leading to secondary cytokine release syndrome (CRS) that occurs shortly after the start of therapy ([85]). It can be mitigated with the short course of steroids. Blinatumomab is currently being evaluated in a phase II study in patients with relapsed Ph-positive ALL and in a phase III trial in patients with ALL in first or second relapse (blinatumomab vs investigator's choice of therapy). In a priority review designated by the US Food and Drug Administration, blinatumomab was granted accelerated approval in December 2014 for the treatment of patients with Ph–negative, relapsed or refractory B-ALL.

Inotuzumab ozogamicin is a CD22 immunoconjugate linked to calicheamicin, which is a potent cytotoxic inducer of double-strand DNA breaks. A single-institution phase II study of inotuzumab in 49 patients with highly relapsed/refractory ALL (73%

Table 1-6 Ongoing Trials at MD Anderson Cancer Center and Elsewhere Available for Patients With ALL (Frontline and Salvage Setting)

	Trial Characteristics	
ALL Subgroup	**Frontline Setting**	**Salvage Setting**
Pre–B-cell ALL	*Age <40 years* 1. Ofatumumab + augmented BFM *Age 40-59 years* 1. Hyper-CVAD + ofatumumab 2. Hyper-CVAD + liposomal vincristine *Elderly (≥60 years)* 1. Mini-hyper-CVD + inotuzumab	1. Mini-hyper-CVD + inotuzumab 2. Low-dose inotuzumab (0.9 mg/m^2) 3. Chimeric antigen receptor (CAR) T-cell therapies
Pre–B-cell ALL, MRD+ disease	Blinatumomab	
T-cell ALL	Hyper-CVAD + nelarabine	
Burkitt leukemia, de novo or relapsed refractory	1. Dose-adjusted EPOCH + ofatumumab/rituximab 2. Hyper-CVAD + ofatumumab	
Philadelphia-positive ALL	Hyper-CVAD + ponatinib	Inotuzumab + bosutinib
Philadelphia-like ALL		A phase II study assessing the combination of ruxolitinib or dasatinib + chemotherapy for refractory/relapsed disease
Mixed phenotype acute leukemia (MPAL), de novo and relapsed	Clofarabine, idarubicin, cytarabine, vincristine, and corticosteroid +/– rituximab	
Novel treatment strategies	1. Nelarabine (single-agent) continuous infusion 2. BMS-906024 (NOTCH inhibitor) 3. Ibrutinib 4. Intrathecal rituximab in patients with lymphoid malignancies involving the central nervous system	

BFM, Berlin-Frankfurt-Münster; CVAD, cyclophosphamide, vincristine, doxorubicin, dexamethasone; CVD, cyclophosphamide, vincristine, dexamethasone; EPOCH, etoposide, prednisolone, vincristine, cyclophosphamide, doxorubicin; MRD, minimal residual disease.

receiving two or more salvage therapies) treated every 3 to 4 weeks resulted in an ORR of 57%, with a median OS of 5.1 months. Survival was comparable between patients who underwent a subsequent AHSCT and those who did not. Serious toxicity in the transplant group included the development of VOD in five patients (23%), although four of these patients had multiple prior alkylating therapies. A modified weekly dosing schedule developed based on preclinical studies yielded a similar ORR to the single-dose schedule (59% vs 57%), with a median survival of 9.5 months. This mode of delivery was less toxic, and hepatotoxicity was also significantly reduced, including a 7% incidence of VOD after autologous stem cell transplantation. An additional multicenter phase I/II study of 37 patients with relapsed/refractory ALL, in which 54% of patients were receiving two or more salvage therapies, also evaluated weekly inotuzumab. The CR and CRp rates were 79% (19/24) and 46% (6/13) in the dose-expansion and dose-escalation cohorts, respectively. Among the responders, 22 patients achieved MRD negativity. Furthest along in the development process, inotuzumab was investigated and compared in a randomized trial to physician's choice of therapy in patients with ALL in first and second salvage. Early results have shown a significant improvement in the response rate (CR/CR with incomplete hematologic recovery) favoring inotuzumab versus standard-of-care intensive chemotherapy (80.7% vs 33.3%, $P < .0001$) ([86]). Survival data are maturing.

Chimeric Antigen Receptor T Cells

Autologous T cells can be engineered to express a receptor directed at CD19. Response can be durable given the ability of T cells to expand and persist in vivo. As such, chimeric antigen receptor (CAR) T cells have become an effective approach for targeting lymphoid malignancies ([87, 88]). In a pilot study with 25 children and 5 adults who were treated for relapsed/refractory ALL with CTL019, 27 patients (90%) achieved CR, with 6-month EFS and OS rates of 67% and 78%, respectively ([89]). In a recent phase I trial of 21 children and young adults with relapsed/refractory ALL treated with CAR T cells after lymphodepletion, 21 evaluable patients (70%) achieved CR, with 12 (60%) achieving MRD negativity. At a median follow-up of 10 months, the OS rate was 52% ([90]). In another study of relapsed refractory ALL with antecedent detectable disease before T-cell infusion, 14 patients (88%) showed response, 10 (63%) with CR and 4 (25%) with CRp. Overall, 75% of treated patients achieved MRD negativity ([91]). Patients responding to this form of therapy invariably develop some degree of CRS, which is usually very manageable with steroids or tocilizumab. Ongoing research is trying to identify the most optimal use of this innovative therapeutic strategy.

EMERGING THERAPIES: MD ANDERSON APPROACH

A number of innovative therapies for various stages of disease, tailored to risk-adapted strategies, are transforming the treatment of adult ALL and are beginning to result in significant improvements in long-term outcomes. There are several ongoing trials available for patients with ALL at our institution and elsewhere in the frontline and salvage setting (Table 1-6). Our choice of therapy for particular ALL subtypes is outlined in Table 1-7.

CONCLUSION

Therapeutic capabilities in adult ALL have rapidly reached new heights over the past decade with the introduction of highly promising monoclonal antibodies, immune conjugates, CAR T cells, and new-generation TKIs. Rituximab has repeatedly been shown to improve OS, and blinatumomab and inotuzumab have demonstrated significant activity in a highly relapsed/refractory population. Genomic profiling has identified new prognostic markers (eg, *IKZF1*), as well as new therapeutic targets (eg, ABL, JAK, ETV6-NTRK3) that are amenable to targeted therapies that can improve the adverse prognosis of Ph-like

Table 1-7 MD Anderson Cancer Center Choice of Therapy for ALL Subtypes

Subtype of ALL	Therapy
Pre–B-cell ALL CD20+	Hyper-CVAD + ofatumumab
T-cell ALL	Hyper-CVAD + nelarabine
Elderly (≥60 years) B-cell ALL	Mini-hyper-CVD + inotuzumab
Burkitt lymphoma/ leukemia	Hyper-CVAD + ofatumumab/ Dose adjusted EPOCH-ofatumumab/ rituximab
Ph-positive ALL	Hyper-CVAD + ponatinib
Ph-like–positive ALL	Chemotherapy + ruxolitinib/ dasatinib
Mixed phenotype acute leukemia	Clofarabine, idarubicin, cytarabine, vincristine, corticosteroids +/− rituximab
Adolescent and young adult	Hyper-CVAD + ofatumumab Augmented BFM + ofatumumab

CVAD, cyclophosphamide, vincristine, doxorubicin, dexamethasone; CVD, cyclophosphamide, vincristine, dexamethasone; EPOCH, etoposide, prednisolone, vincristine, cyclophosphamide, doxorubicin.

ALL. As many of the newer agents advance through the final stages of development, we will be seeking to determine optimal combination and order of delivery and the role of cytotoxic chemotherapy in the safest achievement of durable cure rates. Although the role of these agents still continues to be defined, frontline introduction of most effective therapies can be expected to increase the rate of MRD negativity, optimizing responses and closing the outcome gap separating pediatric from adult ALL. Harnessing the full potential of the immune system with the durable presence of autologous T-cell constructs may ultimately lead to obviation of stem cell transplantation in search of better cure rates in adult ALL.

REFERENCES

1. American Cancer Society. *American Cancer Society: Cancer Facts and Figures 2014*. Altanta, GA: American Cancer Society; 2014.
2. Siegel R, Naishadham D, Jemal A. Cancer statistics, 2012. *CA Cancer J Clin*. 62(1):10-29. doi:10.3322/caac.20138.
3. Lightfoot TJ, Roman E. Causes of childhood leukaemia and lymphoma. *Toxicol Appl Pharmacol*. 2004;199(2):104-117. doi:10.1016/j.taap.2003.12.032.
4. Richardson RB. Promotional etiology for common childhood acute lymphoblastic leukemia: the infective lymphoid recovery hypothesis. *Leuk Res*. 2011;35(11):1425-1431. doi:10.1016/j.leukres.2011.07.023.
5. Chevalier SA, Durand S, Dasgupta A, et al. The transcription profile of Tax-3 is more similar to Tax-1 than Tax-2: insights into HTLV-3 potential leukemogenic properties. *PLoS One*. 2012;7(7):e41003. doi:10.1371/journal.pone.0041003.
6. Lombardi L, Newcomb EW, Dalla-Favera R. Pathogenesis of Burkitt lymphoma: expression of an activated c-myc oncogene causes the tumorigenic conversion of EBV-infected human B lymphoblasts. *Cell*. 1987;49(2):161-170.
7. Vianna NJ, Polan AK. Childhood lymphatic leukemia: prenatal seasonality and possible association with congenital varicella. *Am J Epidemiol*. 1976;103(3):321-332.
8. Cortes J. Central nervous system involvement in adult acute lymphocytic leukemia. *Hematol Oncol Clin North Am*. 2001;15(1):145-162.
9. Faderl S, O'Brien S, Pui C-H, et al. Adult acute lymphoblastic leukemia: concepts and strategies. *Cancer*. 2010;116(5):1165-1176. doi:10.1002/cncr.24862.
10. Harris NL, Jaffe ES, Diebold J, et al. World Health Organization classification of neoplastic diseases of the hematopoietic and lymphoid tissues: report of the Clinical Advisory Committee meeting-Airlie House, Virginia, November 1997. *J Clin Oncol*. 1999;17(12):3835-3849.
11. Matutes E, Morilla R, Farahat N, et al. Definition of acute biphenotypic leukemia. *Haematologica*. 1997;82(1):64-66.
12. Preti HA, Huh YO, O'Brien SM, et al. Myeloid markers in adult acute lymphocytic leukemia. Correlations with patient and disease characteristics and with prognosis. *Cancer*. 1995;76(9):1564-1570.
13. Putti MC, Rondelli R, Cocito MG, et al. Expression of myeloid markers lacks prognostic impact in children treated for acute lymphoblastic leukemia: Italian experience in AIEOP-ALL 88-91 studies. *Blood*. 1998;92(3):795-801.
14. Pui CH, Rubnitz JE, Hancock ML, et al. Reappraisal of the clinical and biologic significance of myeloid-associated antigen expression in childhood acute lymphoblastic leukemia. *J Clin Oncol*. 1998;16(12):3768-3773.
15. Serrano J, Román J, Sánchez J, Torres A. Myeloperoxidase gene expression in acute lymphoblastic leukaemia. *Br J Haematol*. 1997;97(4):841-843.
16. Faber J, Kantarjian H, Roberts MW, Keating M, Freireich E, Albitar M. Terminal deoxynucleotidyl transferase-negative acute lymphoblastic leukemia. *Arch Pathol Lab Med*. 2000;124(1):92-97. doi:10.1043/0003-9985(2000)124<0092:TDTNAL>2.0.CO;2.
17. Foa R, Vitale A. Towards an integrated classification of adult acute lymphoblastic leukemia. *Rev Clin Exp Hematol*. 2002;6(2):181-202.
18. Thomas DA, O'Brien S, Jorgensen JL, et al. Prognostic significance of CD20 expression in adults with de novo precursor B-lineage acute lymphoblastic leukemia. *Blood*. 2009;113(25):6330-6337. doi:10.1182/blood-2008-04-151860.
19. Onciu M, Lai R, Vega F, Bueso-Ramos C, Medeiros LJ. Precursor T-cell acute lymphoblastic leukemia in adults: age-related immunophenotypic, cytogenetic, and molecular subsets. *Am J Clin Pathol*. 2002;117(2):252-258. doi:10.1309/08DJ-GPBH-H0VR-RC6F.
20. Mancini M, Scappaticci D, Cimino G, et al. A comprehensive genetic classification of adult acute lymphoblastic leukemia (ALL): analysis of the GIMEMA 0496 protocol. *Blood*. 2005;105(9):3434-3441. doi:10.1182/blood-2004-07-2922.
21. Kohlmann A, Schoch C, Schnittger S, et al. Pediatric acute lymphoblastic leukemia (ALL) gene expression signatures classify an independent cohort of adult ALL patients. *Leukemia*. 2004;18(1):63-71. doi:10.1038/sj.leu.2403167.
22. Ferrando AA, Neuberg DS, Staunton J, et al. Gene expression signatures define novel oncogenic pathways in T cell acute lymphoblastic leukemia. *Cancer Cell*. 2002;1(1):75-87.
23. Yeoh E-J, Ross ME, Shurtleff SA, et al. Classification, subtype discovery, and prediction of outcome in pediatric acute lymphoblastic leukemia by gene expression profiling. *Cancer Cell*. 2002;1(2):133-143.
24. Den Boer ML, van Slegtenhorst M, De Menezes RX, et al. A subtype of childhood acute lymphoblastic leukaemia with poor treatment outcome: a genome-wide classification study. *Lancet Oncol*. 2009;10(2):125-134. doi:10.1016/S1470-2045(08)70339-5.
25. Roberts KG, Li Y, Payne-Turner D, et al. Targetable kinase-activating lesions in Ph-like acute lymphoblastic leukemia. *N Engl J Med*. 2014;371(11):1005-1015. doi:10.1056/NEJMoa1403088.
26. Harvey RC, Mullighan CG, Chen I-M, et al. Rearrangement of CRLF2 is associated with mutation of JAK kinases, alteration of IKZF1, Hispanic/Latino ethnicity, and a poor outcome in pediatric B-progenitor acute lymphoblastic leukemia. *Blood*. 2010;115(26):5312-5321. doi:10.1182/blood-2009-09-245944.
27. Garcia-Manero G, Daniel J, Smith TL, et al. DNA methylation of multiple promoter-associated CpG islands in adult acute lymphocytic leukemia. *Clin Cancer Res*. 2002;8(7):2217-2224.
28. Roberts KG, Morin RD, Zhang J, et al. Genetic alterations activating kinase and cytokine receptor signaling in high-risk acute lymphoblastic leukemia. *Cancer Cell*. 2012;22(2):153-166. doi:10.1016/j.ccr.2012.06.005.
29. Thomas DA, Faderl S, O'Brien S, et al. Chemoimmunotherapy with hyper-CVAD plus rituximab for the treatment of adult Burkitt and Burkitt-type lymphoma or acute lymphoblastic leukemia. *Cancer*. 2006;106(7):1569-1580. doi:10.1002/cncr.21776.
30. Kantarjian H, Thomas D, O'Brien S, et al. Long-term follow-up results of hyperfractionated cyclophosphamide, vincristine, doxorubicin, and dexamethasone (hyper-CVAD), a dose-intensive regimen, in adult acute lymphocytic leukemia. *Cancer*. 2004;101(12):2788-2801. doi:10.1002/cncr.20668.
31. Kantarjian HM, O'Brien S, Smith TL, et al. Results of treatment with hyper-CVAD, a dose-intensive regimen, in adult acute lymphocytic leukemia. *J Clin Oncol*. 2000;18(3):547-561.
32. Pui C-H, Evans WE. Treatment of acute lymphoblastic leukemia. *N Engl J Med*. 2006;354(2):166-178. doi:10.1056/NEJMra052603.
33. Hoelzer D, Walewski J, Döhner H, et al. Improved outcome of adult Burkitt lymphoma/leukemia with rituximab and chemotherapy: report of a large prospective multicenter trial. *Blood*.

2014;124(26):3870-3879. doi:10.1182/blood-2014-03-563627.

34. Rizzieri DA, Johnson JL, Byrd JC, et al. Improved efficacy using rituximab and brief duration, high intensity chemotherapy with filgrastim support for Burkitt or aggressive lymphomas: Cancer and Leukemia Group B study 10002. *Br J Haematol.* 2014;165(1):102-111. doi:10.1111/bjh.12736.
35. Dunleavy K, Pittaluga S, Shovlin M, et al. Low-intensity therapy in adults with Burkitt's lymphoma. *N Engl J Med.* 2013;369(20):1915-1925. doi:10.1056/NEJMoa1308392.
36. Thomas DA, O'Brien S, Faderl S, et al. Chemoimmunotherapy with a modified hyper-CVAD and rituximab regimen improves outcome in de novo Philadelphia chromosome-negative precursor B-lineage acute lymphoblastic leukemia. *J Clin Oncol.* 2010;28(24):3880-3889. doi:10.1200/JCO.2009.26.9456.
37. Hoelzer D, Gökbuget N. Chemoimmunotherapy in acute lymphoblastic leukemia. *Blood Rev.* 2012;26(1):25-32. doi:10.1016/j.blre.2011.08.001.
38. Jabbour E, Kantarjian H, Thomas D, et al. Phase II study of the hyper-CVAD regimen in combination with ofatumumab as frontline therapy for adults with CD-20 positive acute lymphoblastic leukemia. *Blood.* 2013;122:2664.
39. Tanguy-Schmidt A, Rousselot P, Chalandon Y, et al. Long-term follow-up of the imatinib GRAAPH-2003 study in newly diagnosed patients with de novo Philadelphia chromosome-positive acute lymphoblastic leukemia: a GRAALL study. *Biol Blood Marrow Transplant.* 2013;19(1):150-155. doi:10.1016/j.bbmt.2012.08.021.
40. Bassan R, Rossi G, Pogliani EM, et al. Chemotherapy-phased imatinib pulses improve long-term outcome of adult patients with Philadelphia chromosome-positive acute lymphoblastic leukemia: Northern Italy Leukemia Group protocol 09/00. *J Clin Oncol.* 2010;28(22):3644-3652. doi:10.1200/JCO.2010.28.1287.
41. Fielding AK, Rowe JM, Buck G, et al. UKALLXII/ECOG2993: addition of imatinib to a standard treatment regimen enhances long-term outcomes in Philadelphia positive acute lymphoblastic leukemia. *Blood.* 2014;123(6):843-850. doi:10.1182/blood-2013-09-529008.
42. Wassmann B, Pfeifer H, Goekbuget N, et al. Alternating versus concurrent schedules of imatinib and chemotherapy as front-line therapy for Philadelphia-positive acute lymphoblastic leukemia (Ph+ ALL). *Blood.* 2006;108(5):1469-1477. doi:10.1182/blood-2005-11-4386.
43. Hu Y, Liu Y, Pelletier S, et al. Requirement of Src kinases Lyn, Hck and Fgr for BCR-ABL1-induced B-lymphoblastic leukemia but not chronic myeloid leukemia. *Nat Genet.* 2004;36(5):453-461. doi:10.1038/ng1343.
44. Ravandi F, O'Brien S, Thomas D, et al. First report of phase 2 study of dasatinib with hyper-CVAD for the frontline treatment of patients with Philadelphia chromosome-positive (Ph+) acute lymphoblastic leukemia. *Blood.* 2010;116(12):2070-2077. doi:10.1182/blood-2009-12-261586.
45. Chalandon Y, Thomas X, Hayette S, et al. Is less chemotherapy detrimental in adults with Philadelphia chromosome-positive acute lymphoblastic leukemia treated with high-dose imatinib? Results of the prospective randomized GRAAPH-2005 study. Paper presented at: 54th Annual Meeting of the American Society of Hematology; December 8-11, 2012; Atlanta, GA.
46. Rousselot P, Coude MM, Huguet F, et al. Dasatinib and low intensity chemotherapy for first-line treatment in patients with de novo Philadelphia positive ALL aged 55 and over: final results of the EWALL-Ph-01 study. Paper presented at: 54th Annual Meeting of the American Society of Hematology; December 8-11, 2012; Atlanta, GA.
47. Ottman OG, Pfeifer H, Cayuela JM, et al. Nilotinib (Tasigna) and chemotherapy for first-line treatment in elderly patients with de novo Philadelphia chromosome/BCR-ABL1 positive acute lymphoblastic leukemia (ALL): a trial of the European Working Group for Adult ALL (EWALL-PH-02). *Blood.* 2014;124:798.
48. Chiaretti S, Vitale A, Elia L, et al. First results of the multicenter total therapy GIMEMA LAL 1509 protocol for de novo adult Philadelphia chromosome positive acute lymphoblastic leukemia (ALL) patients. *Blood.* 2014;124:797.
49. Cortes JE, Kantarjian H, Shah NP, et al. Ponatinib in refractory Philadelphia chromosome-positive leukemias. *N Engl J Med.* 2012;367(22):2075-2088. doi:10.1056/NEJMoa1205127.
50. Cortes JE, Kim D-W, Pinilla-Ibarz J, et al. A phase 2 trial of ponatinib in Philadelphia chromosome-positive leukemias. *N Engl J Med.* 2013;369(19):1783-1796. doi:10.1056/NEJMoa1306494.
51. O'Brien S, Jabbour E, Thomas D, et al. Phase II study of combination of hyperCVAD with ponatinib in frontline therapy of patients with Philadelphia chromosome positive acute lymphoblastic leukemia. *J Clin Oncol.* 2013;31(suppl):7024.
52. Ravandi F, Jorgensen JL, Thomas DA, et al. Detection of MRD may predict the outcome of patients with Philadelphia chromosome-positive ALL treated with tyrosine kinase inhibitors plus chemotherapy. *Blood.* 2013;122(7):1214-1221. doi:10.1182/blood-2012-11-466482.
53. Zhang J, Ding L, Holmfeldt L, et al. The genetic basis of early T-cell precursor acute lymphoblastic leukaemia. *Nature.* 2012;481(7380):157-163. doi:10.1038/nature10725.
54. Coustan-Smith E, Mullighan CG, Onciu M, et al. Early T-cell precursor leukaemia: a subtype of very high-risk acute lymphoblastic leukaemia. *Lancet Oncol.* 2009;10(2):147-156. doi:10.1016/S1470-2045(08)70314-0.
55. Jain P, Kantarjian H, Ravandi F, et al. The combination of hyper-CVAD plus nelarabine as frontline therapy in adult T-cell acute lymphoblastic leukemia and T-lymphoblastic lymphoma: MD Anderson Cancer Center experience. *Leukemia.* 2014;28(4):973-975. doi:10.1038/leu.2013.312.
56. Neumann M, Heesch S, Schlee C, et al. Whole-exome sequencing in adult ETP-ALL reveals a high rate of DNMT3A mutations. *Blood.* 2013;121(23):4749-4752. doi:10.1182/blood-2012-11-465138.
57. Huguet F, Leguay T, Raffoux E, et al. Pediatric-inspired therapy in adults with Philadelphia chromosome-negative acute lymphoblastic leukemia: the GRAALL-2003 study. *J Clin Oncol.* 2009;27(6):911-918. doi:10.1200/JCO.2008.18.6916.
58. Patel B, Kirkwood A, Day A, et al. Feasibility of pegylated-asparaginase (PEG-ASP) during induction in adults with acute lymphoblastic leukaemia (ALL): results from the UK phase 3 multicentre trial UKALL 14. *Blood.* 2013;122:3900.
59. Stock W, Luger SM, Advani AS, et al. Favorable outcomes for older adolescents and young adults (AYA) with acute lymphoblastic leukemia (ALL): early results of U.S. intergroup trial C10403. Paper presented at: 56th Annual Meeting of the American Society of Hematology; December 6-9, 2014; San Francisco, CA.
60. Rytting ME, Thomas DA, O'Brien SM, et al. Augmented Berlin-Frankfurt-Münster therapy in adolescents and young adults (AYAs) with acute lymphoblastic leukemia (ALL). *Cancer.* 2014;120(23):3660-3668. doi:10.1002/cncr.28930.
61. Jabbour E, O'Brien S, Nitin J, et al. Inotuzumab ozogamicin (IO) in combination with low-intensity chemotherapy as front-line therapy for older patients and as salvage therapy for adult with relapse/refractory acute lymphoblastic leukemia. *Clin Lymphoma Myeloma Leuk.* 2015;15(suppl):S171.
62. Goldstone AH, Richards SM, Lazarus HM, et al. In adults with standard-risk acute lymphoblastic leukemia, the greatest benefit is achieved from a matched sibling allogeneic transplantation in first complete remission, and an autologous transplantation is less effective than conventional consolidation. *Blood.* 2008;111(4):1827-1833. doi:10.1182/blood-2007-10-116582.
63. Campana D. Minimal residual disease in acute lymphoblastic leukemia. *Hematology Am Soc Hematol Educ Program.* 2010;2010:7-12. doi:10.1182/asheducation-2010.1.7.
64. Bassan R, Spinelli O, Oldani E, et al. Improved risk classification

for risk-specific therapy based on the molecular study of minimal residual disease (MRD) in adult acute lymphoblastic leukemia (ALL). *Blood.* 2009;113(18):4153-4162. doi:10.1182/blood-2008-11-185132.
65. Beldjord K, Chevret S, Asnafi V, et al. Oncogenetics and minimal residual disease are independent outcome predictors in adult patients with acute lymphoblastic leukemia. *Blood.* 2014;123(24):3739-3749. doi:10.1182/blood-2014-01-547695.
66. Van der Velden VHJ, Corral L, Valsecchi MG, et al. Prognostic significance of minimal residual disease in infants with acute lymphoblastic leukemia treated within the Interfant-99 protocol. *Leukemia.* 2009;23(6):1073-1079. doi:10.1038/leu.2009.17.
67. Conter V, Bartram CR, Valsecchi MG, et al. Molecular response to treatment redefines all prognostic factors in children and adolescents with B-cell precursor acute lymphoblastic leukemia: results in 3184 patients of the AIEOP-BFM ALL 2000 study. *Blood.* 2010;115(16):3206-3214. doi:10.1182/blood-2009-10-248146.
68. Gökbuget N, Kneba M, Raff T, et al. Adult patients with acute lymphoblastic leukemia and molecular failure display a poor prognosis and are candidates for stem cell transplantation and targeted therapies. *Blood.* 2012;120(9):1868-1876. doi:10.1182/blood-2011-09-377713.
69. Ribera J-M, Oriol A, Morgades M, et al. Treatment of high-risk Philadelphia chromosome-negative acute lymphoblastic leukemia in adolescents and adults according to early cytologic response and minimal residual disease after consolidation assessed by flow cytometry: final results of the PETHEMA ALL-AR-03 trial. *J Clin Oncol.* 2014;32(15):1595-1604. doi:10.1200/JCO.2013.52.2425.
70. Nagorsen D, Kufer P, Baeuerle PA, Bargou R. Blinatumomab: a historical perspective. *Pharmacol Ther.* 2012;136(3):334-342. doi:10.1016/j.pharmthera.2012.07.013.
71. Topp MS, Kufer P, Gökbuget N, et al. Targeted therapy with the T-cell-engaging antibody blinatumomab of chemotherapy-refractory minimal residual disease in B-lineage acute lymphoblastic leukemia patients results in high response rate and prolonged leukemia-free survival. *J Clin Oncol.* 2011;29(18):2493-2498. doi:10.1200/JCO.2010.32.7270.
72. Topp MS, Gökbuget N, Zugmaier G, et al. Long-term follow-up of hematologic relapse-free survival in a phase 2 study of blinatumomab in patients with MRD in B-lineage ALL. *Blood.* 2012;120(26):5185-5187. doi:10.1182/blood-2012-07-441030.
73. Goekbuget N, Dombret H, Bonifacio M, et al. BLAST: a confirmatory, single-arm, phase 2 study of blinatumomab, a bispecific T-cell engager (BiTE) antibody construct, in patients with minimal residual disease B-precursor acute lymphoblastic leukemia (ALL). Paper presented at: 56th Annual Meeting of the American Society of Hematology; December 6-9, 2014; San Francisco, CA.
74. Kantarjian HM, Thomas D, Ravandi F, et al. Defining the course and prognosis of adults with acute lymphocytic leukemia in first salvage after induction failure or short first remission duration. *Cancer.* 2010;116(24):5568-5574. doi:10.1002/cncr.25354.
75. Faderl S, Thomas DA, O'Brien S, et al. Augmented hyper-CVAD based on dose-intensified vincristine, dexamethasone, and asparaginase in adult acute lymphoblastic leukemia salvage therapy. *Clin Lymphoma Myeloma Leuk.* 2011;11(1):54-59. doi:10.3816/CLML.2011.n.007.
76. Sanofi. Clolar (clofarabine) Package Insert. Cambridge, MA: Sanofi; 2015.
77. Hijiya N, Thomson B, Isakoff MS, et al. Phase 2 trial of clofarabine in combination with etoposide and cyclophosphamide in pediatric patients with refractory or relapsed acute lymphoblastic leukemia. *Blood.* 2011;118(23):6043-6049. doi:10.1182/blood-2011-08-374710.
78. Pigneaux A, Sauvezie M, Vey N, et al. Clofarabine combinations in adults with refractory/relapsed acute lymphoblastic leukemia (ALL): a GRAAL report. *Blood.* 2011;118:2586.
79. Barba P, Sampol A, Calbacho M, et al. Clofarabine-based chemotherapy for relapsed/refractory adult acute lymphoblastic leukemia and lymphoblastic lymphoma. The Spanish experience. *Am J Hematol.* 2012;87(6):631-634. doi:10.1002/ajh.23167.
80. Gökbuget N, Basara N, Baurmann H, et al. High single-drug activity of nelarabine in relapsed T-lymphoblastic leukemia/lymphoma offers curative option with subsequent stem cell transplantation. *Blood.* 2011;118(13):3504-3511. doi:10.1182/blood-2011-01-329441.
81. Jain P, Kantarjian HM, Thomas DA, et al. Phase II study of nelarabine with Hyper-CVAD in patients with previously untreated T-cell acute lymphoblastic leukemia (T-ALL) and lymphoblastic lymphoma (LL). Paper presented at: 54th Annual Meeting of the American Society of Hematology; December 8-11, 2012; Atlanta, GA.
82. O'Brien S, Schiller G, Lister J, et al. High-dose vincristine sulfate liposome injection for advanced, relapsed, and refractory adult Philadelphia chromosome-negative acute lymphoblastic leukemia. *J Clin Oncol.* 2013;31(6):676-683. doi:10.1200/JCO.2012.46.2309.
83. Topp M, Gokbuget N, Zugmaier G, et al. Effect of anti-CD19 BiTE blinatumomab on complete remission rate and overall survival in adult patients with relapsed/refractory B-precursor ALL. *J Clin Oncol.* 2012;30(suppl):6500.
84. Topp MS, Goekbuget N, Stein AS, et al. Confirmatory open-label, single-arm, multicenter phase 2 study of the BiTE antibody blinatumomab in patients (pts) with relapsed/refractory B-precursor acute lymphoblastic leukemia (r/r ALL). *J Clin Oncol.* 2014;32(suppl):7005.
85. Klinger M, Brandl C, Zugmaier G, et al. Immunopharmacologic response of patients with B-lineage acute lymphoblastic leukemia to continuous infusion of T cell-engaging CD19/CD3-bispecific BiTE antibody blinatumomab. *Blood.* 2012;119(26):6226-6233. doi:10.1182/blood-2012-01-400515.
86. DeAngelo DJ, Stelljes M, Martinelli G, et al. Efficacy and safety of inotuzumab ozogamicin (ino) vs standard of care (soc) in salvage 1 or 2 patients with acute lymphoblastic leukemia (all): an ongoing global phase 3 study. Paper presented at: 20th Congress of the European Hematology Association; June 14, 2015; Vienna, Austria.
87. Porter DL, Levine BL, Kalos M, Bagg A, June CH. Chimeric antigen receptor-modified T cells in chronic lymphoid leukemia. *N Engl J Med.* 2011;365(8):725-733. doi:10.1056/NEJMoa1103849.
88. Grupp SA, Kalos M, Barrett D, et al. Chimeric antigen receptor-modified T cells for acute lymphoid leukemia. *N Engl J Med.* 2013;368(16):1509-1518. doi:10.1056/NEJMoa1215134.
89. Maude SL, Frey N, Shaw PA, et al. Chimeric antigen receptor T cells for sustained remissions in leukemia. *N Engl J Med.* 2014;371(16):1507-1517. doi:10.1056/NEJMoa1407222.
90. Lee DW, Kochenderfer JN, Stetler-Stevenson M, et al. T cells expressing CD19 chimeric antigen receptors for acute lymphoblastic leukaemia in children and young adults: a phase 1 dose-escalation trial. *Lancet.* 2015;385(9967):517-528. doi:10.1016/S0140-6736(14)61403-3.
91. Davila ML, Riviere I, Wang X, et al. Efficacy and toxicity management of 19-28z CAR T cell therapy in B cell acute lymphoblastic leukemia. *Sci Transl Med.* 2014;6(224):224ra25. doi:10.1126/scitranslmed.3008226.

2 Adult Acute Myeloid Leukemia

第二章　成人急性髓细胞白血病

Jasleen K. Randhawa
Joseph Khoury
Farhad Ravandi-Kashani

中文导读

急性髓细胞白血病是由外周血、骨髓和髓外组织中髓系细胞异常克隆性增殖所导致的一组非特异性血液肿瘤。尽管我们对急性髓细胞白血病的分子生物学的理解有一些进展，但其治疗仍存在不足，结果因细胞遗传学和分子特征以及年龄和合并症情况的不同而存在较大差异。本章在简单介绍了急性髓细胞白血病的流行病学特点、病因学机制、危险因素分类、临床表现以及诊断与分型之后，详细总结了该病治疗方面的内容。针对患者的个体差异以及基因学和分子生物学特点，急性髓细胞白血病的治疗包括传统诱导化学药物治疗（简称化疗）、分子靶向治疗和免疫治疗，本章分别进行了详细的阐述。本章还介绍了针对不同人群的治疗，包括青少年人群、老年人群、FMS样酪氨酸激酶3（FLT3）融合人群、再次复发人群，以及适合造血干细胞移植治疗的人群。急性髓细胞白血病可能导致多种并发症，因此，最佳对症支持治疗尤其重要。最后，本章对急性早幼粒细胞白血病和微小残留病灶也进行了简单介绍。

Acute myeloid leukemia (AML) consists of a heterogeneous group of hematologic neoplasms characterized by clonal proliferation of myeloid blasts in the peripheral blood, bone marrow, and extramedullary tissues. Despite advances in our understanding of the molecular biology of AML, its treatment remains challenging and outcomes vary greatly depending on the cytogenetic and molecular features as well as age and comorbidities.

INTRODUCTION

Acute myeloid leukemia is thought to be the culmination of genetic mutations and chromosomal aberrations within myeloid precursors resulting in disrupted differentiation, excessive proliferation, and suppressed apoptosis of neoplastic cells referred to as *blasts*.

Over the last several decades, improvements in chemotherapeutic regimens and supportive care have resulted in significant but modest progress in treating AML. Better understanding of the biology of AML has resulted in the identification of new therapeutic targets. Despite this, currently, the majority of patients with AML die from the complications of their disease. With better definition of molecular abnormalities and elucidation of the pathogenic events in various AML subtypes and with the development of novel targeted agents, a better outcome for patients with AML may be achievable in the future.

EPIDEMIOLOGY, ETIOLOGY, AND RISK FACTORS

Approximately 13,000 individuals are diagnosed annually in the United States with leukemia. The incidence of AML is 4.3 per 100,000 ([1]). The median age at presentation is about 65 years. The incidence of AML, as well as myelodysplastic syndrome (MDS), appears to be rising, particularly in individuals over 60 years of age. The incidence of AML is slightly higher in males and in populations of European descent. Acute promyelocytic leukemia (APL), a distinct subtype of AML, has been reported to be more common among populations of Hispanic background ([2]).

An increased incidence of AML is seen in patients with disorders associated with increased chromatin fragility such as Bloom syndrome, Fanconi anemia, Kostmann syndrome, and Wiskott-Aldrich syndrome or ataxia-telangiectasia. Other syndromes, such as Down (trisomy of chromosome 21), Klinefelter (XXY and variants), and Patau (trisomy of chromosome 13) syndromes, have also been associated with a higher incidence of AML ([3]).

Therapeutic radiation increases AML risk, particularly if given concomitantly with alkylating agents. Two categories of therapy-related AML have been described. Patients exposed to alkylating agents (eg, cyclophosphamide, melphalan, nitrogen mustard) can develop AML after a latency period of 4 to 8 years, which is often associated with abnormalities of chromosomes 5 and/or 7. Exposure to agents that inhibit the DNA repair enzyme topoisomerase II (eg, etoposide) is also associated with secondary AML with a shorter latency period, usually 1 to 3 years ([4]). Benzene, smoking, dyes, herbicides, and pesticides have been implicated as potential risk factors for development of AML ([5]).

Acute myeloid leukemia may also be secondary to transformation of an antecedent myeloid disorder, such as MDS, myeloproliferative neoplasm (MPN), or MDS/MPN, or other bone marrow disorders, such as aplastic anemia.

CLINICAL PRESENTATION

Fatigue, bruising or bleeding, fever, and infection, reflecting a state of bone marrow failure, are common in AML. Only 10% of patients present with white blood cell (WBC) count greater than $100 \times 10^9/L$ ([1]). These patients are at higher risk of tumor lysis syndrome, central nervous system involvement, and leukostasis. Leukostasis may manifest as dyspnea, chest pain, headaches, altered mental status, cranial nerve palsies, or priapism. Leukostasis and tumor lysis syndrome are oncologic emergencies and require prompt recognition and management.

Physical findings other than bleeding and infection may include organomegaly, lymphadenopathy, sternal tenderness, retinal hemorrhages, and infiltration of gingivae, skin, soft tissues, or meninges (more common with monocytic variants, M4 or M5). Disseminated intravascular coagulopathy (DIC) with bleeding diathesis is a common presentation in APL.

DIAGNOSIS AND CLASSIFICATION

The diagnosis of AML is typically based on the presence of 20% myeloid blasts in the bone marrow or peripheral blood in accordance with World Health Organization (WHO) classification criteria (Table 2-1) ([6]). Acute myeloid leukemia subtypes in the WHO classification are defined on the basis of morphology, immunophenotype, and molecular/genetic features. In some patients, AML presents as a mass in extramedullary tissues (myeloid sarcoma). Patients who have the cytogenetic abnormalities t(8;21)(q22;q22),

Table 2-1 Acute Myeloid Leukemia and Related Precursor Neoplasms and Acute Leukemias of Ambiguous Lineage (World Health Organization 2008)

Myeloproliferative neoplasms (MPN)
- Chronic myelogenous leukemia, *BCR-ABL1*–positive
- Chronic neutrophilic leukemia
- Polycythemia vera
- Primary myelofibrosis
- Essential thrombocythemia
- Chronic eosinophilic leukemia, not otherwise specified
- Mastocytosis
- Myeloproliferative neoplasms, unclassifiable

Myeloid and lymphoid neoplasms associated with eosinophilia and abnormalities of *PDGFRA*, *PDGFRB*, or *FGFR1*
- Myeloid and lymphoid neoplasms associated with *PDGFRA* rearrangement
- Myeloid neoplasms associated with *PDGFRB* rearrangement
- Myeloid and lymphoid neoplasms associated with *FGFR1* abnormalities

Myelodysplastic/myeloproliferative neoplasms (MDS/MPN)
- Chronic myelomonocytic leukemia
- Atypical chronic myeloid leukemia, *BCR-ABL1*–negative
- Juvenile myelomonocytic leukemia
- Myelodysplastic/myeloproliferative neoplasm, unclassifiable
  - *Provisional entity: refractory anemia with ring sideroblasts and thrombocytosis*

Myelodysplastic syndrome (MDS)
- Refractory cytopenia with unilineage dysplasia
  - Refractory anemia
  - Refractory neutropenia
  - Refractory thrombocytopenia
- Refractory anemia with ring sideroblasts
- Refractory cytopenia with multilineage dysplasia
- Refractory anemia with excess blasts
- Myelodysplastic syndrome with isolated del(5q)
- Myelodysplastic syndrome, unclassifiable
- Childhood myelodysplastic syndrome
  - *Provisional entity: refractory cytopenia of childhood*

Acute myeloid leukemia and related neoplasms
- Acute myeloid leukemia with recurrent genetic abnormalities
  - AML with t(8;21)(q22;q22); *RUNX1-RUNX1T1*
  - AML with inv(16)(p13.1q22) or t(16;16)(p13.1;q22); *CBFB-MYH11*
  - APL with t(15;17)(q22;q12); *PML-RARA*
  - AML with t(9;11)(p22;q23); *MLLT3-MLL*
  - AML with t(6;9)(p23;q34); *DEK-NUP214*
  - AML with inv(3)(q21q26.2) or t(3;3)(q21;q26.2); *RPN1-EVI1*
  - AML (megakaryoblastic) with t(1;22)(p13;q13); *RBM15-MKL1*
  - *Provisional entity: AML with mutated NPM1*
  - *Provisional entity: AML with mutated CEBPA*
- Acute myeloid leukemia with myelodysplasia-related changes
- Therapy-related myeloid neoplasms
- Acute myeloid leukemia, not otherwise specified
  - AML with minimal differentiation
  - AML without maturation
  - AML with maturation
  - Acute myelomonocytic leukemia
  - Acute monoblastic/monocytic leukemia
  - Acute erythroid leukemia
    - Pure erythroid leukemia
    - Erythroleukemia, erythroid/myeloid
  - Acute megakaryoblastic leukemia
  - Acute basophilic leukemia
  - Acute panmyelosis with myelofibrosis
- Myeloid sarcoma
- Myeloid proliferations related to Down syndrome
  - Transient abnormal myelopoiesis
  - Myeloid leukemia associated with Down syndrome
- Blastic plasmacytoid dendritic cell neoplasm

Acute leukemias of ambiguous lineage
- Acute undifferentiated leukemia
- Mixed phenotype acute leukemia with t(9;22)(q34;q11.2); *BCR-ABL1*
- Mixed phenotype acute leukemia with t(v;11q23); *MLL* rearranged
- Mixed phenotype acute leukemia, B-myeloid, NOS
- Mixed phenotype acute leukemia, T-myeloid, NOS
- *Provisional entity: natural killer* (*NK*) *cell lymphoblastic leukemia/lymphoma*

B lymphoblastic leukemia/lymphoma
- B lymphoblastic leukemia/lymphoma, NOS
- B lymphoblastic leukemia/lymphoma with recurrent genetic abnormalities
  - B lymphoblastic leukemia/lymphoma with t(9;22)(q34;q11.2);*BCR-ABL 1*
  - B lymphoblastic leukemia/lymphoma with t(v;11q23); *MLL* rearranged
  - B lymphoblastic leukemia/lymphoma with t(12;21)(p13;q22) *TEL-AML1* (*ETV6-RUNX1*)
  - B lymphoblastic leukemia/lymphoma with hyperdiploidy
  - B lymphoblastic leukemia/lymphoma with hypodiploidy
  - B lymphoblastic leukemia/lymphoma with t(5;14)(q31;q32) *IL3-IGH*
  - B lymphoblastic leukemia/lymphoma with t(1;19)(q23;p13.3);*TCF3-PBX1*

T lymphoblastic leukemia/lymphoma

inv(16)(p13q22) or t(16;16)(p13;q22), and t(15;17)(q22;q12) are diagnosed with AML regardless of the blast percentage.

Bone marrow sampling is essential for the initial workup of a patient with suspected acute leukemia. Sampling should include a core biopsy as well as aspiration material. The core biopsy should be used to perform touch preparations, which are invaluable in case of a dry tap. The aspiration material is used to prepare a clot and aspirate smears, in addition to having portions submitted for flow cytometry, cytogenetics, and molecular diagnostics.

Confirmation of myeloid lineage is commonly accomplished using flow cytometry. In most AML cases, blasts express one or more markers of immature hematopoietic precursors such as CD34 and HLA-DR, in addition to dim CD45 (common leukocyte antigen). Myeloid lineage is predicated on the expression of antigens associated with granulocytic, monocytic, erythroid, and/or megakaryocytic differentiation by blasts (Table 2-2). Expression of myeloperoxidase (MPO) is considered specific for myeloid differentiation, although AML blasts may lack MPO expression. Although aberrant expression of lymphoid antigens is commonly seen in some cases with a bona fide AML phenotype, such expression is generally limited to one or a few lymphoid antigens. Acute leukemia with ambiguous lineage is beyond the scope of this discussion; briefly, it refers to acute leukemia with overlapping expression of myeloid and lymphoid antigens or lack of both.

Molecular diagnostics play a critical role in the laboratory workup of AML. Whereas the scope of known molecular alterations in AML was limited until a few years ago, the advent of next-generation sequencing (NGS) has dramatically increased our understanding of the molecular landscape of AML. As a result, the limited number of polymerase chain reaction (PCR)–based assays that used to be performed during AML workup have been gradually replaced at most large facilities by NGS-based panels that simultaneously assess the mutation status of tens to hundreds of genes. The current NGS mutation panel for new and relapsed myeloid malignancies used at our institution assesses the coding sequences of the 28 genes listed in Table 2-3.

RISK STRATIFICATION OF ACUTE MYELOID LEUKEMIA

Once a diagnosis of AML has been made, the next step is to risk stratify the patient. Several variables are predictive of outcome, including patient-related variables, such age and performance status, as well as disease-related predictors, such as cytogenetic and molecular characteristics.

The karyotype remains one of the best predictors of outcome in patients with AML. The European LeukemiaNet (ELN) guidelines have proposed a risk stratification system based on cytogenetics and molecular analysis [7]. As listed in Table 2-4, the patients are classified as having favorable-, intermediate-, and unfavorable-risk disease. The drawback of this classification system is that it takes into account few mutations for prognostication. More recent data suggest that the favorable prognosis attributed to mutant *CEBPA* is true in cases of bilallelic *CEBPA* mutation rather than the monoallelic mutation [8]. Of note, in patients with *FLT3*-negative/*NPM1*-positive AML, *DNMT3A* assessment is of importance. Loghavi et al showed that in patients with karyotypically normal AML with *NPM1* mutations, presence of concurrent *DNMT3A* mutation has an adverse effect on outcomes, with the effect being more detrimental than either *FLT3-ITD* or *FLT3-TKD* mutations [9]. This analysis showed that of patients with de novo karyotypically normal AML, particularly those <60 years old, AML$^{DNMT3A/FLT3/NPM1}$ patients seem to have the worst clinical outcomes, followed by those with AML$^{FLT3/DNMT3A}$ and then those with AML$^{NPM1/DNMT3A}$ [9]. Currently, normal karyotype AML patients with *NPM1*-positive/*FLT3*-negative disease are considered favorable risk according to the ELN guidelines.

The presence of *TP53* mutations is associated with a poor outcome. A recent report by German/Austrian investigators indicated that the outcome of patients with *TP53* mutations is worse than that of patients with the monosomal karyotype known to be an adverse prognostic indicator [10]. In this study, the analysis showed that the *TP53* mutation was commonly associated with older patients and a monosomal karyotype and correlated with a low complete remission (CR) rate and shorter relapse-free survival (RFS), event-free survival (EFS), and overall survival (OS). On multivariate analysis, *TP53* mutations were associated with the worst prognosis [10].

Several novel molecular aberrations, including mutations of the *IDH*, *ASXL1*, *DNMT3A*, *TET2*, *MLL*, and *PHF6* genes, have been described, particularly in patients with a normal karyotype [11]. However, their utility in clinical practice remains limited, and they have limited value in determining best treatment strategies for patients.

TREATMENT OF ACUTE MYELOID LEUKEMIA

In the 1960s, Freireich et al demonstrated the significance of achieving a CR to improve survival [12]. Since then, the objective of therapy has been to produce and

Table 2-2 Immunophenotypic Markers of Hematopoietic Lineage Differentiation Commonly Used in Flow Cytometry Analysis

Myeloid				Lymphoid	
Granulocytic	Monocytic	Erythroid	Megakaryocytic	B Cell	T Cell
MPO	CD4	CD41	CD42b	CD19	cCD3
CD13	CD14	CD71	CD61	cCD79a	
CD15	CD64			cIgM	
CD33					
CD117					

Table 2-3 Next-Generation Sequencing–Based Mutation Analysis Panel for Myeloid Neoplasms Currently Used for Frontline Assessment at the MD Anderson Cancer Center

ABL1	*EGFR*	*GATA2*	*IKZF2*	*MDM2*	*NOTCH1*	*RUNX1*
ASXL1	*EZH2*	*HRAS*	*JAK2*	*MLL*	*NPM1*	*TET2*
BRAF	*FLT3*	*IDH1*	*KIT*	*MPL*	*NRAS*	*TP53*
DNMT3A	*GATA1*	*IDH2*	*KRAS*	*MYD88*	*PTPN11*	*WT11*

Table 2-4 Risk Stratification of AML European LeukemiaNet Criteria

Genetic group	Subsets
Favorable	t(8;21)(q22;q22); *RUNX1-RUNX1T1*
	inv(16)(p13.1q22) or t(16;16)(p13.1;q22); *CBFB-MYH11*
	Mutated *NPM1* without *FLT3*-ITD (normal karyotype)
	Mutated *CEBPA* (normal karyotype)
Intermediate-I[a]	Mutated *NPM1* and *FLT3*-ITD (normal karyotype)
	Wild-type *NPM1* and *FLT3*-ITD (normal karyotype)
	Wild-type *NPM1* without *FLT3*-ITD (normal karyotype)
Intermediate-II	t(9;11)(p22;q23); *MLLT3-MLL*
	Cytogenetic abnormalities not classified as favorable or adverse[b]
Adverse	inv(3)(q21q26.2) or t(3;3)(q21;q26.2); *RPN1-EVI1*
	t(6;9)(p23;q34); *DEK-NUP214*
	t(v;11)(v;q23); *MLL* rearranged
	–5 or del(5q); –7; abnl(17p); complex karyotype[c]

Frequencies, response rates, and outcome measures should be reported by genetic group, and, if sufficient numbers are available, by specific subsets indicated; excluding cases of acute promyelocytic leukemia.

[a] Includes all AMLs with normal karyotype except for those included in the favorable subgroup; most of these cases are associated with poor prognosis, but they should be reported separately because of the potential different response to treatment.

[b] For most abnormalities, adequate numbers have not been studied to draw firm conclusions regarding their prognostic significance.

[c] Three or more chromosome abnormalities in the absence of one of the WHO designated recurring translocations or inversions, that is, t(15;17), t(8;21), inv(16) or t(16;16), t(9;11), t(v;11)(v;q23), t(6;9), inv(3) or t(3;3); indicate how many complex karyotype cases have involvement of chromosome arms 5q, 7q, and 17p.

Reproduced with permission from Dohner H, Estey EH, Amadori S, et al. Diagnosis and management of acute myeloid leukemia in adults: recommendations from an international expert panel, on behalf of the European LeukemiaNet, *Blood*. 2010 Jan 21;115(3):453-474.

maintain CR, the only currently accepted approach to AML cure. Criteria for CR have been defined by the International Working Group and are followed in the clinic and in clinical trials for response assessment ([13]). After 3 years in CR, the probability of AML recurrence sharply declines to less than 10% ([14]), and patients in continuous CR for 3 or more years can be considered "potentially cured." However, clearly the definition of CR is an arbitrary one, and with improved technology, the precision for detection of residual disease after the initial therapy has increased. Whether this improved detection and application of novel strategies to eradicate the residual leukemia will translate to improved cure rates will be the subject of future trials.

Once AML is diagnosed, the need for emergency therapy must be assessed. Emergency treatment is required (1) in cases of APL, (2) if the circulating blast count is >50 to 100 × 10^9/L, and (3) in the presence of DIC or organ dysfunction (especially pulmonary) attributed to leukemic infiltration (mostly seen in patients with >10 × 10^9/L circulating blasts and/or M4 or M5 French-American-British [FAB] morphology). In the latter situation, it is important to initiate immediate chemotherapy. Leukapheresis for severe leukocytosis and/or leukostasis should also be considered ([15]). In patients with low presenting WBC count, several studies have demonstrated that initiation of therapy can delayed for several days until all the necessary diagnostic information is available ([16]).

At University of Texas MD Anderson Cancer Center (MDACC), most patients are enrolled on clinical trials, if eligible. The therapy is tailored to the individual patient characteristics including their cytogenetic and molecular profile. We discuss here the therapies for the various patient groups with AML.

INDUCTION THERAPY IN ACUTE MYELOID LEUKEMIA

Conventional treatment for AML, divided into remission induction and postremission therapy, has been with combinations of anthracyclines and cytarabine (ara-C).

Anthracyclines and Cytarabine

At MDACC, young patients with AML (<60 years old) are treated with idarubicin (IDA) plus cytarabine-based regimens. The dose of IDA is 12 mg/m^2 for 3 days, and ara-C is given as a continuous infusion at a dose of 1.5 g/m^2 for 4 days. An alternative used by many cooperative groups is the "3+7 regimen," where the anthracycline (ie, IDA or daunorubicin [DNR]) is usually given daily for 3 days and ara-C is given at 100 to 200 mg/m^2 daily for 7 days by continuous infusion.

In clinical practice, a bone marrow aspirate is usually obtained 2 to 3 weeks after beginning therapy. A biopsy is needed only if the quality of the aspirate does not permit determination of cellularity. If the day 21 marrow is hypoplastic, therapy is usually delayed until it is clear that leukemia has reappeared, at which time the second course begins. A second repeated course of therapy can produce remissions, but these are usually of shorter duration than remissions produced after one course of therapy. The timing of a second course with persistent AML is controversial. Several cooperative groups advocate starting a second course if there is persistent AML on days 10 to 15 of chemotherapy. With high-dose ara-C (HDAC), a delay of a second course with persistent disease on days 21 to 28 may be indicated if the blasts are decreasing because most (90%) CRs are obtained after the first course and response to a second course is poor. It is important to recognize that the initial marrow obtained after a period of hypoplasia may demonstrate up to 30% to 50% blasts as a reflection of the regeneration of normal, not "leukemic," marrow recovery. In this circumstance, follow-up (eg, at 1- to 2-week intervals) marrows may show reduction in blast percentages concomitant with a rise in neutrophils and platelets.

Typically, once in remission after treatment with the induction course, patients receive postremission therapy, with the same drugs administered at approximately monthly intervals for 4 to 12 months.

Choice of Anthracyclines

Randomized trials have attempted to identify which anthracycline (eg, IDA, DNR, mitoxantrone [MTZ], aclarubicin) is better ([17]). In a three-arm randomized study comparing DNR, IDA, and MTZ as part of the induction regimen for older patients, there was no advantage for any one arm ([18]). In contrast, in a three-arm randomized trial conducted by the European Organization for Research and Treatment of Cancer (EORTC) and Italian Group for Hematological Diseases in Adults (GIMEMA) comparing the same three agents, the 5-year disease-free survival (DFS) and OS were significantly better for patients receiving IDA and MTZ (P = .03 and .02, respectively). The recovery time was longer with IDA and MTZ (P < .0001) ([19]). Gardin et al analyzed pooled data from trials conducted in AML patients age ≥50 years ([20]). These trials compared the efficacy of IDA versus DNR in induction and consolidation. They assessed the outcomes of these patients and showed that IDA resulted in a higher CR rate of 69% (vs 61% with DNR, P = .02) but did not lead to superior OS (median OS, 14.2 months; P = .13) ([20]).

Different doses of DNR have been evaluated in several trials, in addition to standard-dose ara-C (100 or 200 mg/m^2 daily for 7 days). Two studies showed that using DNR 90 mg/m^2 had better outcomes than DNR 45 mg/m^2, regardless of age. Both studies showed higher CR rates and OS in patients receiving a higher dose of DNR, without any additional toxicity. The beneficial effect was mostly seen in patients less than 50 years old and with more favorable cytogenetics ([21,22]). More recently, a French group also showed that DNR 60 mg/m^2 had similar relapse rate, RFS, and OS compared to DNR 90 mg/m^2 ([23]).

Even though the studies do not show survival advantage with IDA over DNR, the CR rates are definitely higher with IDA. Hence, at MDACC, IDA is the preferred anthracycline of choice.

CPX-351

CPX-351 is a novel formulation for delivery of ara-C and DNR synergistically to the leukemic cells. In this formulation, ara-C and DNR are encapsulated in a 5:1 fixed molar ratio that was found to be consistently synergistic in vitro. A multicenter, open-label, phase II study was conducted across 18 centers in the United States in the first-line setting. Patients >60 years old with de novo AML were randomized to receive the CPX-351 versus the 7+3 regimen. Higher response rates were noted with CPX-351, with an overall response rate (ORR) of 66.7% (vs 57.6%, $P = .06$). Patients with adverse cytogenetics had an improved response with CPX-351 (77% vs 38%). Improvements in the median OS (14.7 months vs 12.9 months) and EFS (6.5 months vs 2 months) were noted in the CPX-351 cohort ([24]). A phase III trial is currently ongoing.

High-Dose Cytarabine

Several randomized trials have assessed the efficacy of HDAC (1-3 g/m^2) versus standard-dose ara-C (SDAC) (100-200 mg/m^2) for induction therapy. The Cancer and Leukemia Group B (CALGB) and the Eastern Cooperative Oncology Group (ECOG) restricted their analysis to patients in CR, whereas the Southwestern Oncology Group (SWOG) compared HDAC with SDAC during induction and randomized SDAC patients to SDAC or HDAC once the patients were in CR ([25]). Finally, the Australian Leukemia Study Group (ALSG) randomized patients to HDAC or SDAC during induction only (Table 2-5) ([26]). These trials concluded that (1) the toxicity of HDAC (eg, cerebellar) outweighs the anti-AML effect in patients >65 years; (2) patients >60 years benefit from HDAC given during induction (SWOG, ALSG), in CR (CALGB, ECOG), and perhaps both (SWOG); and (3) HDAC potentially increases the cure rates to 70% to 80% in patients with inversion 16 or t(8;21) and to 30% to 40% in patients with normal karyotype, but little, if at all, in patients with adverse karyotypes. In a meta-analysis of three trials in 1,691 patients, induction with HDAC was compared to SDAC. Although there was no difference in CR rates, the 4-year RFS ($P = .03$), 4-year OS ($P = .0005$), and 5-year EFS ($P < .0001$) were better with HDAC ([27]).

Gemtuzumab Ozogamicin

Gemtuzumab ozogamicin (GO) is a CD33-targeted immunoconjugate linking an anti-CD33 antibody to calicheamicin. It received an accelerated approval by the US Food and Drug Administration for use in relapsed/refractory elderly AML patients but was withdrawn voluntarily by the manufacturer from the market in 2010 due to toxicity concerns. However, in a recent trial by the French Leukemia Association, patients age 50 to 70 years with previously untreated de novo AML were randomized to receive standard chemotherapy with 7+3 (DNR, ara-C) with or without GO. Gemtuzumab was administered in fractionated doses. The ORR was 78%, with 73% achieving CR and 5% achieving CR with incomplete platelet recovery (CRp). The OS (34 months vs 19 months, $P = .036$), EFS (15.6 months vs 9.7 months, $P = .0003$), and RFS (28 months vs 11 months, $P = .0003$) were significantly better in the GO group. Another study by the Medical Research Council (MRC) in the United Kingdom showed a benefit for the addition of GO to ara-C and anthracycline-based induction regimens ([28]). A recent meta-analysis examined five randomized trials in untreated patients with AML and demonstrated a benefit of GO in the frontline therapy of some subsets of patients with AML. The available data suggest utility of GO in patients with AML allowing the argument for the reconsideration of its approval in the United States.

Table 2-5 Standard Versus High-Dose Cytarabine (HDAC) in Newly Diagnosed AML

Study	HDAC During:	No. of Patients	Beneficial Effect of HDAC
ALSG	Induction	279	CR duration
SWOG	Induction and/or consolidation	723	Event-free survival
ECOG	Consolidation	170	If age <60 years
CALGB	Consolidation	596	If age <60 years

ALSG, Australian Leukemia Study Group; CALGB, Cancer and Leukemia Group B; CR, complete response; ECOG, Eastern Cooperative Oncology Group; SWOG, Southwest Oncology Group.

TREATMENT OF YOUNGER PATIENTS WITH ACUTE MYELOID LEUKEMIA

Clofarabine, Idarubicin, and Cytarabine

Clofarabine is a second-generation nucleoside analogue that has activity in adult patients with AML. A phase I trial of clofarabine, conducted at MDACC, in combination with IDA alone versus IDA and ara-C (CIA) in patients with relapsed, refractory AML showed a CR rate of 13% versus 48%, respectively. The median duration of remission was also longer with the CIA combination (15 months) as compared to clofarabine and IDA (4.5 months) ([29]). This was followed by a phase II trial that investigated the CIA regimen in patients ≤60 years old with newly diagnosed AML. Patients who achieved a response (CR or CRp) went on to receive up to six cycles of consolidation therapy. The cycles were administered every 4 to 6 weeks. All patients received prophylactic antibiotics, antifungals, and antivirals. The median age of the patients was 48 years (range, 19-60 years), 66% had intermediate-risk cytogenetics, and 36% had diploid and 34% adverse karyotype. The ORR was 79%, with 74% CR and 3% CRp. Eighteen percent of patients received two induction cycles to achieve a CR/CRp, and 42% went on to receive an allogeneic stem cell transplantation (SCT) in first CR. The median OS and RFS were not reached, whereas the median EFS was 13.5 months. A subset analysis showed better OS ($P = .04$) and EFS ($P = .04$) in patients ≤40 years old as compared to >40 years old ([30]).

Purine Analogues

The addition of purine analogues, cladribine and fludarabine, to anthracyclines and ara-C has been associated with improved outcomes in a number of studies.

Cladribine/Fludarabine

Holowiecki et al conducted a randomized phase III trial evaluating the addition of cladribine or fludarabine to DNR/ara-C in younger patients with untreated AML. Six hundred fifty-two patients, with a median age of 47 years (range, 17-60 years), were randomized to receive DNR plus ara-C (DA), DA plus cladribine (DAC), and DA plus fludarabine (DAF). The consolidation regimen was the same for all arms and included two consecutive courses of ara-C (1.5 g/m^2 intravenously [IV] days 1-3) plus MTZ (10 mg/m^2 IV days 3-5) and HDAC (2 g/m^2 IV twice a day on days 1, 3, and5). Overall CR rate was 61%, with 56% achieving a CR after one cycle of induction and 5% after two cycles. The CR rate was higher in the DAC arm compared to the DA arm (62% vs 51%, $P = .02$). The CR rates were similar in the DA and DAF arms. The median OS was significantly higher in the DAC arm (24 months) compared to the DA arm (14 months, $P = .02$). There was no significant difference in the median OS between the DAF and DA arms ([31]).

Vorinostat

Vorinostat is an oral histone deacetylase inhibitor that has been shown to have single-agent activity in AML ([32]). It was studied in combination with the IDA plus ara-C regimen at MDACC in a phase II trial in the frontline setting in patients with AML or intermediate-2/high-risk MDS. Induction was given as vorinostat 500 mg orally three times a day (days 1-3) along with IDA (12 mg/m^2 days 4-6) and ara-C (1.5 mg/m^2 continuous infusion days 4-7). Subsequently, patients achieving a remission could be treated with five cycles of consolidation and up to 12 months of single-agent vorinostat for maintenance. At a median follow-up of 82 weeks, the median OS was 82 weeks (range, 3-134 weeks) and median EFS was 47 weeks (range, 3-134 weeks). There was trend for a longer survival in the *FLT3-ITD*–mutated patients (91 weeks; range 6-134 weeks). The overall remission rate was 85%, with 76% achieving a CR and 9% achieving a CRp; 25% of the patients went on to undergo an allogeneic SCT in first CR.

TREATMENT OF PATIENTS ≥60 YEARS OLD

Acute myeloid leukemia in older adults (≥60 years) is considered a biologically and clinically distinct entity. The outcomes of older AML patients are poor with the standard anti-AML therapies. The analysis of the Swedish Acute Leukemia Registry (1976-2005) showed that the early death rates in all AML patients, regardless of age, were lower with intensive therapy compared to palliative therapy ([33]).

Acute myeloid leukemia in the elderly has adverse biologic features such as higher frequency of stem-cell–like phenotype of leukemic blasts, higher frequency of multilineage involvement with dysplastic features, higher frequency of antecedent hematologic disorders, and higher frequency of *MDR-1* gene expression, which leads to higher potential for cytotoxic drug extrusion by the leukemic blasts, causing resistance to chemotherapeutic agents ([34]). Acute myeloid leukemia in older patients is more frequently associated with poor-risk cytogenetics (up to 50% vs 10%-15% in younger patients) ([35]). Hence, the majority of elderly AML patients should be considered for investigational clinical trials. Other factors contributing to worse outcome in elderly patients include poor performance status, organ dysfunction, and a higher incidence of an antecedent hematologic disorders. In general, patients with three or more of these factors have expected CR rates of less than 20%, 8-week mortality rates greater than 50%, and 1-year survival rates of less than 10% using conventional regimens. These patients constitute 25% to 30% of elderly patients with AML. Approximately 20% of elderly patients have none or one of these adverse factors and have a reasonable outcome with expected CR rates above 60%, 8-week mortality rates of 10%, and 1-year survival rates of ≥50% ([36]).

Low-Dose Cytarabine

Low-dose ara-C (LDAC) was superior to hydroxyurea in a randomized trial enrolling 204 elderly patients with AML considered unfit for chemotherapy ([37]). The CR rates were 15% with LDAC and 1% with hydroxyurea ($P = .0003$); the 1-year survival rates were 27% versus 3% ($P = .0004$).

Clofarabine

A randomized phase II study compared clofarabine (30 mg/m^2 IV × 5 days) versus clofarabine and ara-C (20 mg/m^2 subcutaneously daily × 14 days) in 70 elderly patients with AML ([38]). Combination therapy achieved a better CR (63% vs 31%; $P = .025$) and better EFS (7.1 months vs 1.7 months; $P = .04$) but did not improve OS (11.4 months vs 5.8 months; $P = .1$).

Hypomethylating Agents

Kantarjian et al conducted a randomized phase III trial comparing decitabine 20 mg/m^2 for 10 days with physician's choice in 485 patients ([39]). This study showed that decitabine improved CR/CRp rates compared with physician's choice (18% vs 8%; $P = .001$). Decitabine was well tolerated with a good safety profile. The primary analysis showed a nonsignificant improvement in the OS, but an unplanned analysis 2 years later demonstrated an improvement in the OS in the decitabine arm ($P = .03$) ([39]). Quintas-Cardama et al showed that patients with newly diagnosed AML who are >65 years old have an ORR of 47% (CR rate, 42%) with intensive chemotherapy and an ORR of 29% (CR rate, 28%) with epigenetic therapy (azacitidine, decitabine) ($P \leq .001$) ([40]). The median OS was similar in both the groups (6.5 months; $P = .413$) ([40]). These studies show that hypomethylating agents have similar survival outcomes in elderly AML patients when compared to intensive chemotherapy.

Recently, the results of the AML-AZA001 trial were presented. Four hundred forty-eight patients ≥65 years old with newly diagnosed de novo or secondary AML who were deemed ineligible for transplant and with intermediate- or poor-risk cytogenetics were enrolled. Patients were randomized to receive either azacitidine or a conventional care regimen. Azacitidine was administered at 75 mg/m^2/d for 7 days subcutaneously. A prolongation in the median OS was observed in the azacitidine arm (6.4 months vs 3.2 months; $P = .0185$). The conventional care regimen included best supportive care in 18%, LDAC in 64%, and intensive chemotherapy in 18% ([41]). Several groups have consistently shown a CR rate of 31% to 47% with decitabine 20 mg/m^2 administered daily for 10 days, with a median OS of 9 to 12 months. However, the associated increased myelosuppression leads to increased rates of hospitalization for infections ([42]).

Vosaroxin

Vosaroxin is an anticancer quinolone that was shown to have activity in older patients with poor-risk AML in the REVEAL-1 study ([43]). In this study, patients ≥ 60 years old with unfavorable-risk AML were treated with single-agent vosaroxin. An ORR of 32% was observed including 29% CR and 32% CR/CRp. The median OS was about 7 months, and the 1-year OS rate was 38% ([43]). Overall, vosaroxin resulted in low early mortality and an encouraging response rate. Subsequently, a combination of vosaroxin and decitabine was evaluated in older patients with newly diagnosed AML and high-risk MDS. The ORR was 76% (including 59% CR, 14% CRp, and 3% CR with incomplete blood count recovery [CRi]). Interestingly, the response rate in the patients with adverse cytogenetics was 69%. The median OS was 8.3 months, and the median remission duration had not been reached ([44]).

Volasertib

Polo-like kinases (Plks) are serine/threonine protein kinases that play a role in mitotic checkpoint regulation and cell division. The Plk-1 is expressed in dividing cells, and its expression peaks during the G_2/M phase of cell cycle. It has been shown to be overexpressed in AML cells ([45]). Volasertib is a Plk inhibitor that was evaluated in a phase II trial in older patients with AML considered not to be candidates for intensive induction therapy ([46]). Patients were randomized to LDAC 20 mg subcutaneously twice a day for 10 days with or without volasertib 350 mg IV on days 1 to 15 every 4 weeks. Eighty-seven patients with a median age of 76 years (range, 57-86 years) were enrolled. The ORR (CR+CRi) was 13.3% for the LDAC alone arm versus 31% for the LDAC plus volasertib arm ($P = .052$). The time to response was a median of 63.5 days (range, 30-120 days). Patients received a median of 8 cycles of therapy (range, 2-22 cycles) in the combination arm compared with

7 in the LDAC alone arm (range, 5-11 cycles). At a median follow-up of 28.2 months, the median EFS was 5.6 months in the LDAC plus volasertib arm compared with 2.3 months in the LDAC alone arm (P = .021). The addition of volasertib led to a longer RFS of 18.5 months (vs 10 months) and a longer median OS of 8 months (vs 5.2 months; P = .047). A higher incidence of grade 3 gastrointestinal toxicity, febrile neutropenia, and infections was noted in the combination arm, but there was no difference in early mortality noted between the two arms.

Nonchemotherapy Options

Nonchemotherapy options are also being explored for this subset of patients with AML. Pollyea et al reported the results of upfront combination of azacitidine (75 mg/m^2 × 7 days) and lenalidomide (escalating doses, starting at day 8 of each cycle, every 6 weeks) in patients ≥60 years old ([47]). They reported an ORR of 40%, with a median time to response of 3 months and median duration of response of 7 months. The median OS was 5 months for all patients ([47]). Wetzler et al evaluated octogenarian patients with AML who had been enrolled in cooperative group trials and concluded that intensive induction (7+3 or similar) is effective therapy, with a 30% CR rate ([48]). In these patients, *FLT3-ITD* did not impact median OS (10 months; P = .31) in contrast to *NPM1* mutations, which were associated with a prolonged median OS (91 months; P = .002) ([48]).

Several groups have proposed predictive models for geriatrics assessment prior to determining what therapy to assign older patients ([49, 50]). These models look at several prognostic factors, including functional status, cytogenetics, age, and molecular status, to predict mortality and survival with therapy. This suggests that a careful assessment of the patient and disease characteristics is needed before assigning therapy to older patients.

Investigational treatment and palliative care options are more plausible in poorer-prognosis elderly patients, and the patients and their families should be involved in discussions of treatment decisions.

Consolidation Therapy

There is debate as to the best therapy for consolidation following achievement of CR after initial induction therapy. The number of cycles of therapy is also not agreed upon. However, for patients treated with hypomethylating agents, it is recommended that the treatment is continued indefinitely until disease progression, as is the practice for patients with MDS.

TREATMENT OF *FLT3*-MUTATED ACUTE MYELOID LEUKEMIA

FMS-like tyrosine kinase 3 (*FLT3*) is a member of the class III receptor tyrosine kinase family that plays an important role in the survival, proliferation, and differentiation of hematopoietic progenitor cells. *FLT3* is overexpressed in most patients with AML, and activating mutations of *FLT3* are among the most prevalent molecular abnormalities in AML, with internal tandem duplication (ITD) occurring in 25% to 35% of patients with normal karyotype ([51]). In addition, 5% to 7% of patients may have point mutations within the activation loop of the kinase domain or in the juxtamembrane domain. Patients with *FLT3* activating mutations have an inferior outcome with a shorter RFS and OS. In addition, after exposure to *FLT3* inhibitors, nearly a quarter of patients with *FLT3-ITD* develop mutations in the kinase domain as a mechanism of resistance. The major *FLT3* inhibitors are summarized in Table 2-6. Table 2-7 lists the *FLT3* inhibitors currently under development.

TREATMENT OF CORE-BINDING FACTOR ACUTE MYELOID LEUKEMIA

Core-binding factor (CBF) AML is a distinct entity. It is considered a favorable karyotype. It includes patients with a pericentric inversion of chromosome 16 (inversion 16; associated with FAB subtype M4EO) and

Table 2-6 Major *FLT3* Inhibitors

FLT3 Inhibitor	Patient Characteristics	Regimen	CR	OS
Sorafenib	Relapsed, refractory ([93])	IA + sorafenib	93% in *FLT3*-mutated	74% at 1 year
	Frontline ([94])	7+3 + sorafenib	60%	63% at 3 years
Quizartinib	Relapsed, refractory ([95])	Single agent	13%	14 weeks
	Relapsed, refractory ([96])	Quizartinib + LDAC/AZA	60%	—
Crenolanib	Relapsed, refractory ([97])	Single agent	*FLT3-ITD*: 23% *FLT3-TKD*: 20%	6 months

AZA, azacitidine; CR, complete response; IA, idarubicin plus cytarabine; LDAC, low-dose cytarabine; OS, overall survival.

Table 2-7 *FLT3* Inhibitors Under Development

Preclinical	Phase I	Phase II	Phase III
VX-322	IMC-EB10	Sorafenib	Lestaurtinib
VX-398	KW-2449	MLN-518	Midostaurin
MC-2002	Ponatinib	Crenolanib	Quizartinib
MC-2006	CHIR-258	PLX3397	
	ASP2215		

translocation (16;16) or a translocation between chromosomes 8 and 21 (t[8;21]; associated with FAB subtype M2). Each of these abnormalities disrupts the function of a transcription factor (CBF), regulating the expression of genes important in hematopoietic differentiation. inv(16) and t(16;16) lead to the formation of the *CBF-MYH11* fusion gene. t(8;21) leads to the formation of the *RUNX1-RUNXT1* fusion gene. The *CBF-MYH11*– and *RUNX1-RUNXT1*–related leukemias represent CBF-AML. These leukemias are very sensitive to induction and consolidation and have high response rates. About 10% of unselected patients (typically younger patients) have CBF-AML. At MDACC, all newly diagnosed patients with CBF-AML are treated with fludarabine (30 mg/m^2/d on days 1-5) and HDAC (2 g/m^2/d on days 1-5) regimens with or without the addition of granulocyte colony-stimulating factor (G-CSF). This is followed by up to six courses of an HDAC-containing regimen. A CR rate of 93% and an EFS of 20 months in 114 newly diagnosed CBF-AML patients were previously reported ([52]). A frontline regimen of fludarabine, ara-C, and G-CSF (FLAG)-GO was evaluated at MDACC and showed a remission rate of 95% and a 3-year OS and RFS of 78% and 85%, respectively ([53]). In the UK MRC-AML15 trial, 1,113 patients with AML were randomized to receive or not receive a small dose of GO (3 mg/m^2) with their induction therapy. A benefit for adding GO to the induction regimen was seen in patients with CBF-AML ([28]). In a meta-analysis of five clinical trials wherein addition of GO to induction chemotherapy was evaluated, a significant improvement in OS was noted in patients with favorable- and intermediate-risk cytogenetics (P = .01). The improvement in survival was attributed to reduced relapse (P = .00006) ([54]). All of these studies strongly support the use of FLAG-based regimens for CBF-AML and advocate the addition of GO to the induction to improve survival and RFS in these patients.

Approximately 25% of CBF-AML patients carry a gain-of-function mutation in the *KIT* gene, which results in a constitutively activated tyrosine kinase. Hence, the CALGB 10801 alliance and a group in Germany are evaluating the addition of a *KIT* inhibitor, dasatinib, to the standard induction therapy. The initial results showed a 92% CR rate and 1-year DFS and OS rates of 90% and 87%, respectively. Long-term outcomes of this study are awaited ([55]).

The treatment for newly diagnosed AML is summarized in Figs. 2-1 and 2-2.

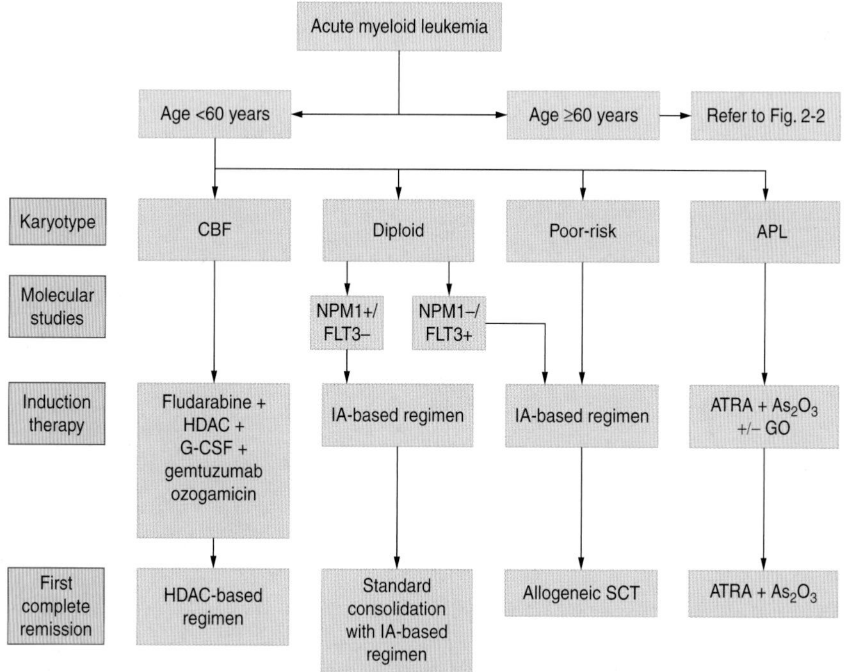

FIGURE 2-1 A proposed approach to the management of newly diagnosed adult acute myeloid leukemia. APL, acute promyelocytic leukemia; As_2O_3, arsenic trioxide; ATRA, all-*trans*-retinoic acid; CBF, core-binding factor leukemias (including inv[16], t[8;21]); FLT3, fms-like tyrosine kinase 3; G-CSF, granulocyte colony-stimulating factor; GO, gemtuzumab ozogamicin; HDAC, high-dose cytarabine; IA, idarubicin and cytarabine; NPM1, nucleophosmin; SCT, stem-cell transplantation.

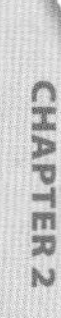

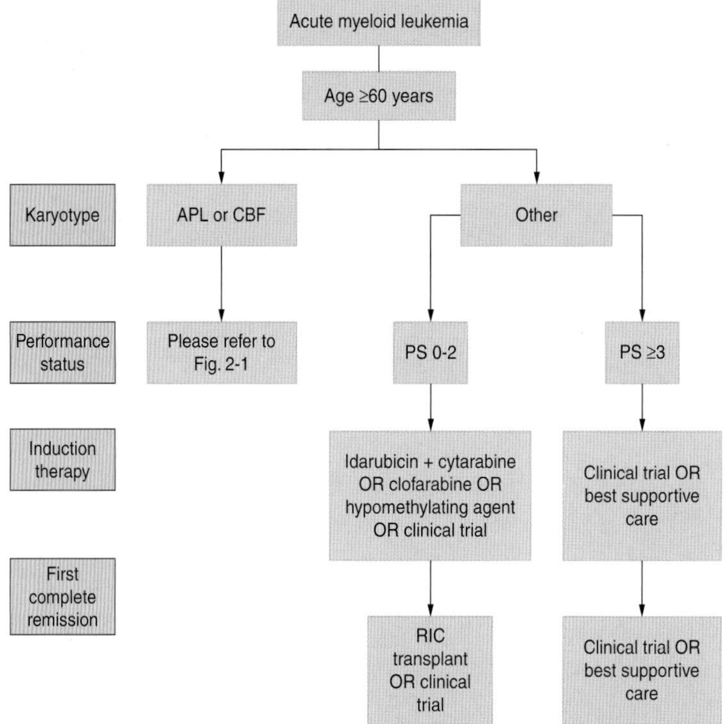

FIGURE 2-2 A proposed approach to the management of newly diagnosed adult acute myeloid leukemia in patients ≥60 years. APL, acute promyelocytic leukemia; CBF, core-binding factor leukemias (including inv[16], t[8;21]); PS, performance status according to the Eastern Cooperative Oncology Group; RIC transplant, reduced-intensity conditioning transplant.

TREATMENT OF RELAPSED/REFRACTORY ACUTE MYELOID LEUKEMIA

Although the outcome of patients with AML has improved, relapse remains frequent and constitutes the leading cause of mortality. Breems et al defined a prognostic score for patients with AML in first relapse based on the following variables: (1) relapse-free interval from first CR; (2) cytogenetics at diagnosis; (3) age at first relapse; and (4) SCT before first relapse ([56]). In an analysis of 594 patients who underwent second salvage therapy for relapsed AML at MDACC, 13% achieved CR (median CR duration, 7 months), and 1-year survival was 8% ([57]) (Fig. 2-3).

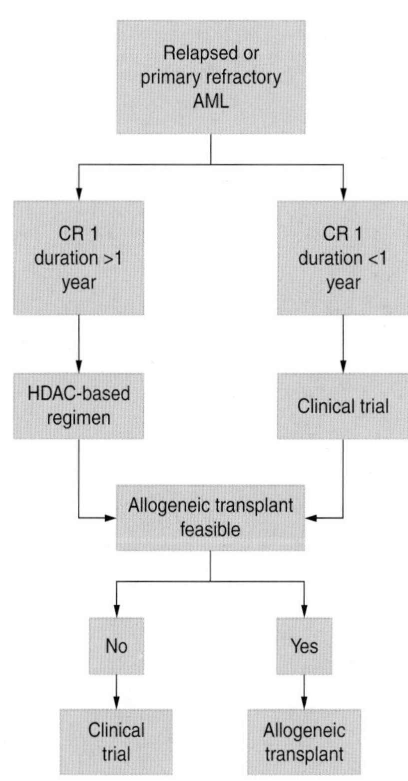

FIGURE 2-3 A proposed algorithm for management of relapsed/refractory acute myeloid leukemia (AML). CR1, first complete remission; HDAC, high-dose cytarabine.

Allogeneic transplant appears superior to HDAC- or intermediate-dose ara-C–containing regimens in patients with duration of first CR less than 1 year; the great majority of these transplants were from a human leukocyte antigen (HLA)–matched sibling donor ([58, 59]). However, because few patients are cured with conventional therapy, all patients with relapsed or refractory AML should be treated in clinical trials. Gemtuzumab, a conjugate composed of a humanized anti-CD33 antibody linked to the antitumor antibiotic calicheamicin, was the only approved treatment for relapsed AML in patients older than 60 years of age with the CR1 duration (CRD1) of 3 months or longer. Complete response rates of 30% were reported with this agent. Veno-occlusive disease was observed in 5% to 10% of patients. Gemtuzumab is no longer commercially available.

For relapsed/refractory AML patients, enrollment in a clinic trial remains the first consideration. Recently, results of VALOR, a phase III trial of vosaroxin or placebo with ara-C in patients with refractory AML or in first relapse, were reported ([60]). The vosaroxin and ara-C arm had a higher complete CR rate of 30% (vs 16%; $P < 0.0001$). The median OS was statistically prolonged in the patients ≥60 years old who received vosaroxin and ara-C (7.1 months vs 5 months; $P = 0.003$). The 30- and 60-day mortality rates were similar in both arms. These results suggest that the combination of vosaroxin and ara-C could become a new standard for treatment of older patients with refractory or relapsed AML.

STEM-CELL TRANSPLANTATION

High-dose chemotherapy with or without radiation followed by SCT is increasingly used as therapy for AML patients in first CR. In prospective, nonrandomized trials in Europe and the United States, patients younger than age 55 years in first CR with an HLA-matched sibling were assigned to allogeneic transplantation or, if no donor, to autologous transplantation or one further course of HDAC (with DNR in the European study) (Table 2-8) ([61-64]).

In a meta-analysis of 24 prospective clinical trials involving more than 6,000 patients with AML in first CR, Koreth et al showed that allogeneic SCT has significant survival benefit in patients with intermediate- and poor-risk AML but not with good-risk AML ([65]). This finding contrasts with the retrospective review of 999 patients by Ferrant et al that observed similar benefit with allogeneic and autologous transplantation for patients with poor-risk karyotype and a benefit with allogeneic SCT only in patients with good- and intermediate-risk cytogenetics ([66]). However, further stratification of risk groups based on molecular markers within individual karyotypes suggests that only specific subsets of patients may benefit from allogeneic SCT. Schlenk et al demonstrated superior OS with allogeneic SCT compared to intensive chemotherapy in only the following groups of normal karyotype de novo AML patients: (1) *FLT3-ITD* positive and (2) *NPM1/CEBPA/FLT3-ITD* negative ([67]). Patients with inversion 16 or t(8;21) do better with chemotherapy ([68]). Patients with AML who are younger than 20 years old have relatively low transplant-related mortality and may do better with allogeneic SCT.

New concepts in both transplantation and chemotherapy have emerged. These include the use of peripheral blood rather than marrow as the source of SCT ([69]), the use of nonmyeloablative regimens to allow engraftment and take advantage of the graft-versus-leukemia effect, and the use of IV busulfan to overcome the erratic pharmacology of the oral form ([70]). In particular, nonmyeloablative regimens (reduced-intensity conditioning or "mini-transplant") have gained particular traction in elderly patients who have traditionally experienced high treatment-related mortality with conventional myeloablative regimens. The principles of this approach include reduction of regimen-related toxicities and shifting the burden of tumor cell kill from high-dose cytotoxic therapy to graft-versus-leukemia effects. A number of recent studies have reported 2- to 5-year survival rates of 25% to 64% after nonmyeloablative allogeneic SCT for older patients with high-risk MDS and AML. Survival was similar for recipients of related and unrelated HLA-matched grafts. The nonrelapse mortality was 16% to 39%, resulting mainly from complications of graft-versus-host disease and comorbidities preceding SCT. Relapse rates ranged from 16% to 53% and were influenced both by disease burden and cytogenetics at the time of SCT ([71]). Further details on this subject are beyond the scope of this chapter.

Table 2-8 Allogeneic Stem-Cell Transplantation (ASCT) Versus Chemotherapy in AML in First Complete Remission (CR)

Study	No. of Patients	% Match	% ASCT in CR	Significant Difference Favoring ASCT
Archimbaud et al ([61])	58	74	34	No
Zittoun et al ([62])	294	63	23	LFS
Cassileth et al ([63])	238	88	23	No
Burnett et al ([64])	656	58	23	No

LFS, leukemia-free survival.

CHAPTER 2

SUPPORTIVE CARE

Adequate and close supportive care is extremely important in the care of acute leukemia. Both G-CSF and granulocyte-macrophage colony-stimulating factor (GM-CSF) have reduced the median time to neutrophil recovery by an average of 5 to 7 days ([72]). Antileukemic therapeutic efficacy is not compromised by these agents. Therapy of acute leukemia often results in rapid reduction of elevated WBC counts. This is often associated with the development of tumor lysis, characterized by hyperuricemia, hyperkalemia, hyperphosphatemia, hypocalcemia, acidosis, and renal failure. Prevention of tumor lysis syndrome requires administration of IV fluids and allopurinol (or rasburicase) if the blast count is above 10×10^9/L. Saline or steroid eye drops daily should be given to patients undergoing HDAC therapy until 24 hours after completion of chemotherapy. In these patients, neurologic assessments for cerebellar neurotoxicity should be performed before each dose of HDAC.

Acute pulmonary failure during induction therapy for AML is a serious complication. Predictive factors identified at diagnosis include male sex, diagnosis of APL, poor ECOG performance status, lung infiltrates at diagnosis, and an increased serum creatinine. Fluid restriction, high-dose steroids, and continuous venovenous hemofiltration have been shown to be effective strategies in treating acute pulmonary failure.

Infectious complications are a major cause of morbidity and death. Prophylactic administration of antibiotics in the absence of fever is usually offered. The development of fever (>101°F), unrelated to administration of chemotherapy, calls for administration of broad-spectrum antibiotics, such as imipenem or a third- (eg, ceftazidime) or fourth-generation cephalosporin (eg, cefepime). Antibiotic selection should be prompt, individualized, and in accordance with the updated antibiotic susceptibility profile of each institution. If infection persists, G-CSF should be started, and if indicated, granulocyte transfusions, using G-CSF to increase the donors' granulocyte counts, should be given. Close fluid balance is critical because fluid retention is common, can radiologically mimic pneumonia, and may increase the risk of diffuse alveolar hemorrhage during induction.

Another controversial area is whether adherence to a neutropenic diet (avoidance of fresh fruits and vegetables) during induction chemotherapy decreases the risk of infection. One hundred fifty-three patients with AML diagnosed at MDACC were admitted to a high-efficiency particulate air-filtered room for induction chemotherapy ([73]). They were randomized to receive a diet containing no raw fruits or vegetables (cooked diet) or to a diet containing fresh fruits and vegetables (raw diet). Twenty-nine percent of patients in the cooked group and 35% of patients in the raw group developed a major infection ($P = .60$). Time to major infection and survival time were similar in the two groups, thereby suggesting that a neutropenic diet did not prevent major infection or death.

INVESTIGATIONAL AGENTS

In the new era of molecular prognostication, targeted therapies and immunotherapies are the new kids on the block. *FLT3* inhibitors have been discussed earlier in the section on *FLT3* AML.

IDH Inhibitors

IDH mutations occur in approximately 20% of AML. The reported frequency is 6% to 16% for *IDH1* and 8% to 18% for *IDH2* mutations. The majority (85%) occur in patients with diploid or trisomy 8 cytogenetics. The prevalence increases with increasing age, and these mutations are strongly associated with *NPM1*-positive and MPN-derived AML (21%-31%) ([74]). AG221 is an oral *IDH2* inhibitor that has been shown to have the ability to trigger differentiation of leukemic blast cells, leading to objective durable responses, including CRs. At the American Society of Hematology 2014 annual meeting, Stein et al reported response rates of 62% (CR, CRp, CRi, and partial response) in AML patients treated with AG221 in a phase I trial ([75]). The median duration of response was 3 months, noted in 90% of the patients.

Venetoclax (ABT199)

ABT199 (venetoclax) is a selective, oral, BCL-2 inhibitor that was evaluated in a phase II trial at MDACC in relapsed/refractory AML patients unfit for intensive chemotherapy. Thirty-two patients were enrolled, of whom 11 had *IDH* mutations. An ORR of 19% (CR and marrow CR) was noted, with a suggestion that patients with *IDH* mutations might benefit more than other patients ([76]).

Immunotherapy with monoclonal antibodies in AML is also an area of interest in the treatment of AML. Newer agents are being developed in this area, and we should have more agents in the arsenal to treat AML in the near future.

ACUTE PROMYELOCYTIC LEUKEMIA

Acute promyelocytic leukemia is a distinct subtype of AML accounting for 5% to 15% of cases, with unique clinical, morphologic, and cytogenetic features. It results from a translocation between the retinoic acid receptor α (RARα) locus on chromosome 17 and the promyelocytic leukemia protein (PML) locus located on chromosome 15 ([77]). This *PML-RARα* fusion is demonstrable in 95% to 100% of cases. Independent risk factors for a diagnosis of APL in a patient with AML are younger age, Hispanic ethnicity, and obesity ([2]). The main clinical presentation is bleeding diathesis resulting both from plasmin-dependent primary fibrinolysis and DIC ([78]). Cytogenetic analysis detects the distinctive t(15;17). In the rare case where such analysis does not show the t(15;17) but the clinical or morphologic picture is suggestive, molecular test for *PML-RARα* can be confirmatory. The POD test, an immunohistochemical test that can be performed in few hours, can detect the characteristic disruption of PML in virtually all cases and is a rapid and reliable quick test for APL. Recognition of APL is crucial because appropriate treatment with all-*trans*-retinoic acid (ATRA) and arsenic trioxide is different than for other types of AML and is curative in most patients ([79]). A stratification system has been developed that distinguishes newly diagnosed patients with APL as low, intermediate, or high risk. Low-risk patients present with WBC count less than 10 × 10^9/L and platelet count above 40 × 10^9/L; a WBC count above 10 × 10^9/L identifies high-risk patients. Others are at intermediate risk. Anticipated cure rates are close to 100%, 90%, and 70% in low-, intermediate-, and high-risk patients, respectively ([80]) (Table 2-9).

Several findings have contributed recently to the increased cure rates in APL. Anthracyclines were historically the first effective treatment, inducing a cure rate of 30% to 40% in APL. The role of ara-C is questionable and probably beneficial only in the setting of suboptimal anthracycline therapy. Addition of ATRA 45 mg/m^2 twice daily to chemotherapy (eg, IDA 12 mg/m^2 on days 2, 4, 6, and 8) increases CR rate and, more dramatically, increases the cure rate from 40% to 70%. The major toxicity of ATRA is a potentially fatal APL differentiation syndrome characterized by fever and leakage of fluid into the extravascular space producing fluid retention, effusions, dyspnea, and hypotension; it is effectively treated with dexamethasone (10 mg IV twice a day for 3-5 days, with a rapid taper) ([81]). A molecular test (*PML-RARAα* fusion transcript by PCR) that detects molecular evidence of the t(15;17) provides a relatively sensitive and highly specific means to document minimal residual disease negativity and detect impending relapse ([82]).

Table 2-9 Risk Stratification of APL

Risk Group	WBC Count (× 10^9/L)	Platelet Count (× 10^9/L)	% RFS
Low	≤10	>40	98
Intermediate	≤10	≤40	89
High	>10		70

RFS, relapse-free survival; WBC, white blood cell.

Once a diagnosis of APL is suspected, it is imperative that the patient be given ATRA, even before the diagnosis is confirmed. All-*trans*-retinoic acid is given at a dose of 45 mg/m^2/d in divided doses. It serves to prevent coagulopathy and start induction therapy ([83]).

Arsenic trioxide (ATO) was shown to be at least noninferior, and possibly superior, to ATRA and chemotherapy in low-/intermediate-risk APL. In the Italian-German APL 0406 trial, Lo-Coco et al showed that the CR rate was 100% in the ATRA+ATO arm versus 95% in the ATRA plus chemotherapy (IDA) arm, with a superior OS of 98.7% versus 91.1% (P = .02) ([84]).

The regimens generally used for treatment of APL, according to risk category, are summarized in Tables 2-10, 2-11, and 2-12.

Ravandi et al evaluated outcomes of newly diagnosed APL patients treated with ATRA and ATO with or without GO without traditional cytotoxic chemotherapy ([85]). The regimen is summarized in Table 2-13. They reported CR rates of 95% and 81%, respectively, for low-risk and high-risk patients. The estimated 3-year survival rate was 85%.

Hence, in the modern era of APL treatment, it is possible to have long-term cure for APL without the use of conventional chemotherapy, which is a tremendous achievement for modern-day oncology.

MINIMAL RESIDUAL DISEASE

Minimal residual disease (MRD) is defined as any measurable disease detectable above a certain level of detection, depending on the methodology applied. Minimal residual disease predicts a failure to maintain CR, and its detection is critical to assess the quality of response after induction therapy and to outline postremission therapy based on the individual risk of relapse. As mentioned in the section on APL, the detection of *PML-RARAα* fusion transcript after achieving CR and its subsequent monitoring to detect early relapse has become the standard of care for patients with APL. Detection of MRD in non-APL AML is an upcoming field where guidelines and standard of care need to be defined. Several methods are being assessed to determine the best method for detection of MRD in patients with AML. There are several issues with the detection of MRD, including lack of a standardized methodology to measure MRD, inconsistency in MRD thresholds, and uncertainty of the ideal time for evaluation of MRD.

Konopleva et al reported that in patients with newly diagnosed AML who have abnormal cytogenetics at presentation, determination of cytogenetics in the

Table 2-10 Treatment of High-Risk APL

Study	Induction	Consolidation	Maintenance
CALGB ([98])	ATRA 45 mg/m² PO every day until CR + Dauno 50 mg/m² D3-6 + cytarabine 200 mg/m² D3-9	ATO 0.15 mg/kg/d × 5 d/wk for 5 wk × 2 (C2 after 2-wk rest), then ATRA 45 mg/m² PO D1-7 + Dauno 50 mg/m² D1-3	ATRA 45 mg/m² × 7 d every other week + MP 60 mg/m²/d PO + MTX 20 mg/m² weekly (1 year)
French ([99])	ATRA 45 mg/m² PO every day + Dauno 60 mg/m² × 3 + cytarabine 200 mg/m² × 7	Dauno 60 mg/m² × 3 d + cytarabine 200 mg/m² × 7 d, then cytarabine 1.5-2 g/m² every 12 h × 5d + Dauno 45 mg/m² × 3 d 5 doses of IT chemotherapy	ATRA 45 mg/m² × 15 d every 3 months + MP 90 mg/m²/d PO + MTX 15 mg/m² weekly PO (2 years)
PETHEMA ([100])	ATRA 45 mg/m²/d until CR + idarubicin 12 mg/m² D2,4,6,8	ATRA 45 mg/m²/d × 15 d + idarubicin 5 mg/m²/d × 4 d + cytarabine 1 g/m²/d × 4 d, then ATRA 45 mg/m²/d × 15 d + mitoxantrone 10 mg/m²/d × 5 d, then ATRA 45 mg/m²/d × 15 d + idarubicin 12 mg/m²/d × 1 dose + cytarabine 150 mg/m²/8 h × 4 d	ATRA 45 mg/m² × 15 d every 3 months + MP 50 mg/m²/d PO + MTX 15 mg/m² IM weekly (2 years)

ATO, arsenic trioxide; ATRA, all-*trans*-retinoic acid; CALGB, Cancer and Leukemia Group B; CR, complete remission; D, day; Dauno, daunorubicin; IM, intramuscular; IT, intrathecal; MP, mercaptopurine; MTX, methotrexate; PO, oral; PETHEMA, Programa Español de Tratamientos en Hematología.

Table 2-11 Treatment of Low-/Intermediate-1–Risk APL

Study	Induction	Consolidation	Maintenance
CALGB ([98])	ATRA 45 mg/m² PO every day until CR + Dauno 50 mg/m² D3-6 + cytarabine 200 mg/m² D3-9	ATO 0.15 mg/kg/d × 5 d/wk for 5 wk × 2 (C2 after 2-wk rest), then ATRA 45 mg/m² PO D1-7 + Dauno 50 mg/m² D1-3	ATRA 45 mg/m² × 7 d every other week + MP 60 mg/m²/d PO + MTX 20 mg/m² weekly (1 year)
French ([99])	ATRA 45 mg/m² PO every day + Dauno 60 mg/m² × 3 + cytarabine 200 mg/m² × 7	Dauno 60 mg/m² × 3 d + cytarabine 200 mg/m² × 7 d, then cytarabine 1 g/m² every 12 h × 4 d + Dauno 45 mg/m² × 3 d	ATRA 45 mg/m² × 15 d every 3 months + MP 90 mg/m²/d PO + MTX 15 mg/m² weekly PO (2 years)
PETHEMA ([100])	ATRA 45 mg/m²/d until CR + idarubicin 12 mg/m² D2,4,6,8	ATRA 45 mg/m²/d × 15 d + idarubicin 5 mg/m² × 4 d, then ATRA 45 mg/m²/d × 15 d + mitoxantrone 10 mg/m²/d × 3 d, then ATRA 45 mg/m²/d × 15 d + idarubicin 12 mg/m²/d × 1 dose	ATRA 45 mg/m² × 15 d every 3 months + MP 50 mg/m²/d PO + MTX 15 mg/m² IM weekly (2 years)
		ATRA 45 mg/m² × 15 d + idarubicin **7** mg/m² × 4 d, then ATRA 45 mg/m² × 15 d + mitoxantrone 10 mg/m² × 3 d, then ATRA 45 mg/m² × 15 d + idarubicin 12 mg/m² × 2 doses	

ATO, arsenic trioxide; ATRA, all-*trans*-retinoic acid; CALGB, Cancer and Leukemia Group B; CR, complete remission; D, day; Dauno, daunorubicin; IM, intramuscular; IT, intrathecal; MP, mercaptopurine; MTX, methotrexate; PO, oral; PETHEMA, Programa Español de Tratamientos en Hematología.

marrow at day 21 of induction chemotherapy predicts RFS independent of the number of blasts ([86]). Chen et al from MDACC demonstrated that persistence of cytogenetic abnormalities at the time of morphologic CR portends a worse outcome ([87]). They looked at patients with abnormal cytogenetics at time of diagnosis who achieved a morphologic CR after induction. Twenty-eight percent of patients in CR had abnormal karyotype (ACCR) and the remaining 72% had normal cytogenetic CR (NCCR). Patients with ACCR had a shorted RFS and OS compared to patients with NCCR (6 months vs 21 months; $P < .001$; and 11 months vs 46 months; $P < .001$, respectively). The RFS and OS for patients with unfavorable cytogenetics at diagnosis who were NCCR were similar to those in patients with favorable/intermediate risk at diagnosis who were ACCR. The ACCR patients who underwent an allogeneic SCT had a significantly longer 3-year RFS

Table 2-12 Treatment of APL with ATRA+ATO+GO

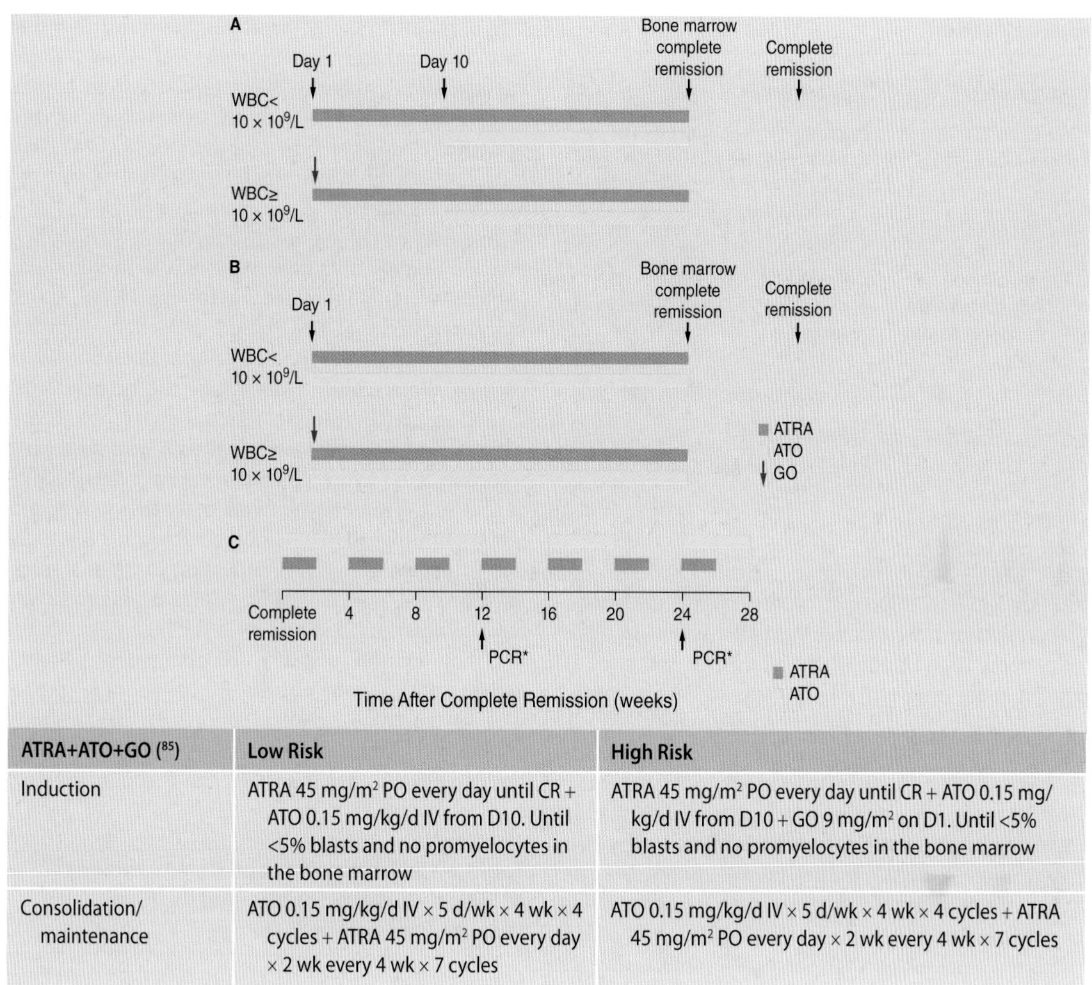

ATRA+ATO+GO ([85])	Low Risk	High Risk
Induction	ATRA 45 mg/m^2 PO every day until CR + ATO 0.15 mg/kg/d IV from D10. Until <5% blasts and no promyelocytes in the bone marrow	ATRA 45 mg/m^2 PO every day until CR + ATO 0.15 mg/kg/d IV from D10 + GO 9 mg/m^2 on D1. Until <5% blasts and no promyelocytes in the bone marrow
Consolidation/ maintenance	ATO 0.15 mg/kg/d IV × 5 d/wk × 4 wk × 4 cycles + ATRA 45 mg/m^2 PO every day × 2 wk every 4 wk × 7 cycles	ATO 0.15 mg/kg/d IV × 5 d/wk × 4 wk × 4 cycles + ATRA 45 mg/m^2 PO every day × 2 wk every 4 wk × 7 cycles

ATO, arsenic trioxide; ATRA, all-*trans*-retinoic acid; CR, complete remission; D, day; GO, gemtuzumab ozogamicin; IV, intravenous; PCR, polymerase chain reaction; PO, oral; WBC, white blood cell.

Table 2-13 Monitoring of APL Therapy

• Document MR at end of consolidation
• Monitor PCR (BM or PB) every 3 mo × 2 y – High risk – Age >60 – Long treatment delays during consolidation
• If PCR becomes positive from negative => confirm!
• If confirmed, intervene
• Try to use the same lab for PCR

BM, bone marrow; MR, molecular response; PB, peripheral blood; PCR, polymerase chain reaction.

(33% vs 9%; *P* = .04) and a 3-year OS (33% vs 8%; *P* = .06) than the patients who did not undergo an SCT. Interestingly, the RFS and OS achieved by patients with ACCR, who underwent an allogeneic SCT, was similar to the NCCR patients who did not undergo an SCT. This suggests a role for individualizing AML therapy based on cytogenetic MRD status.

Another method of quantitative detection of MRD in AML is real-time PCR (RT-PCR) (Table 2-14). Real-time PCR rapidly quantifies PCR products by reverse transcriptase fluorescent signals during exponential amplification. The sensitivity of molecular detection of fusion transcripts ranges from 1 leukemic cell in 1,000 to 100,000 normal cells, that is, 0.1% to 0.001% The fusion transcripts most extensively used to monitor MRD in AML (in addition to *PML-RARα* for APL) are *AML1-ETO*, *CBFβ-MYH11*, and *MLL-AF9*, which are present in approximately one-third of non-APL AML cases ([88]). Various mutations, such as *FLT3*, *NPM1*, and c-*KIT*, can also be assessed by RT-PCR to determine the residual disease status. Polymerase chain reaction analysis of *NPM1* mutations after therapy is prognostic

CHAPTER 2

Table 2-14 Advantages and Disadvantages of Real-Time Reverse Transciptase Polymeras Chain Reaction

Advantages	Disadvantages
Very sensitive reactions	Applicable to a limited number of molecular targets - *PML-RARα* - CBF leukemias - *NPM1*
Mutations and translocations are commonly found in AML	CBF-AML may have persistence of qualitative assay positivity for years
	Can miss therapy-related AML
	Expensive
	Longer turnaround time

CBF, core-binding factor.

and can be used to predict relapse. *NPM1* mutations are present in 30% of all AML patients and in 50% of patients with normal-karyotype AML. Chou et al looked at the role of MRD analysis of *NPM1* mutations by PCR and the impact on outcomes ([89]). One hundred ninety-four samples from 38 patients with de novo AML and *NPM1* mutations were analyzed over 10 years. The samples were taken 1 month after induction and 3 months after consolidation. Any rise in the mutant signals during follow-up was associated with a 3.2 times increased risk of relapse. Of the relapsed patients, the rise in the mutation levels predicted a relapse at a median of 4.9 months (range, 1-12.3 months) prior to a clinical relapse being seen. This analysis also showed that the degree of reduction in mutation levels affects outcomes and that there is a co-relation between MRD after consolidation and OS and RFS (but not after induction). The Wilms tumor 1 gene (*WT1*) is highly expressed in most acute leukemias, and its detection in bone marrow has been associated with the presence, persistence, or relapse of leukemia. Recently, investigators from Turin, Italy, systematically applied their best-performing *WT1* RT-PCR assay on 620 patient samples and demonstrated that application of a standardized *WT1* assay can indeed provide independent prognostic information in AML ([90]). Studies are ongoing to further elucidate the role of the *WT1* gene assay to risk stratify patients who might benefit from intensification of therapy to improve outcomes.

Leukemic cells express abnormal patterns of cellular markers, and these aberrant immunophenotypes can be identified by multiparameter flow cytometry. To yield a sensitivity of 0.01% (10^{-4}), at least 200,000 cells are needed per tube (at least 200,000 events are required to detect 20 aberrant blasts), and three to four tubes are run per patient; 0.1% is the commonly used threshold in most studies in the literature. An advantage of flow cytometry–based studies of MRD is that they can accurately quantify residual leukemic cells and can also distinguish aberrant blasts from normal myeloid precursors. An immunophenotypic fingerprint of the AML can be established for MRD analysis for follow-up. However, there are several advantages and disadvantages with this technique (Table 2-15).

Rubnitz et al reported outcomes with MRD-directed therapy in childhood AML ([91]). In this study, patients were randomized to receive HDAC-based induction versus LDAC-based induction. Minimal residual disease levels, on day 22 after induction, were used to allocate GO to determine the timing of the second induction. Minimal residual disease was determined, and GO was given to patients with poor early response, and high-risk patients were allocated to allogeneic SCT. This study showed that MRD was no different with high-dose chemotherapy versus low-dose chemotherapy at day 22 of induction 1. Minimal residual disease >1% on day 22 was a significant prognostic factor influencing OS and EFS in the high-risk patients but not in the standard-/favorable-risk patients. Patients with low-level MRD (0.1% to <1%) did as well as the MRD-negative cohort. An Italian group analyzed the outcomes of adult AML patients based on MRD levels after induction and consolidation and

Table 2-15 Advantages and Disadvantages of Flow Cytometry for Minimal Residual Disease Assessment

Advantages	Disadvantages
Widely applicable (90%-95% of cases) Relatively rapid turnaround time	Interpretation often challenging, requires experience Can be expensive Lack of standardization Leukemia-associated immunophenotypes (LAIPs) may not cover all leukemic blasts, partial overlap with normal Antigen shift resulting from selection/emergence of subclones - A complete change in LAIPs in about 20% of AML, with 80% having at least one LAIP similar to the original Posttherapy sample is hypocellular; not enough cells/events Use of a comprehensive panel of antibodies to establish baseline

reported that the MRD status at the end of consolidation was the most important predictor of prognosis. In the MRD-positive group, patients who underwent an allogeneic SCT had improved outcomes ([92]).

In general, a lack of standardization among different laboratories, identification of thresholds, and time points during follow-up represent the major subjects of controversy for the routine implementation of MRD detection in non-APL AML at this time.

CONCLUSION

After a period of paucity in discoveries, new strategies are finally evolving that may help patients with AML. The biology of the disease is now better understood. Patients with CBF-AML have a high cure rate with HDAC. Patients with APL have benefited from newer treatment with ATRA and arsenical derivatives. Better definition of the complex process initiating and sustaining the leukemic process will lead to a better definition of targets for therapeutic intervention that may translate into improved cure rates. Specific attention must be given to prognostic factors that identify subsets of AML in which specific tailored therapies will be helpful.

REFERENCES

1. Foon KA, Casciato DA. Acute leukemia. In: Casciato DA, Lowitz BB, eds. Manual of Clinical Oncology. 3rd ed. Boston, MA: Little, Brown and Company; 1995:431-445.
2. Estey E, Thall P, Kantarjian H, Pierce S, Kornblau S, Keating M. Association between increased body mass index and a diagnosis of acute promyelocytic leukemia in patients with acute myeloid leukemia. *Leukemia.* 1997;11:1661-1664.
3. Crane MM, Strom SS, Halabi S, et al. Correlation between selected environmental exposures and karyotype in acute myelocytic leukemia. *Cancer Epidemiol Biomarkers Prev.* 1996;5:639-644.
4. Armstrong SA, Staunton JE, Silverman LB, et al. MLL translocations specify a distinct gene expression profile that distinguishes a unique leukemia. *Nat Genet.* 2002;30:41-47.
5. West RR, Stafford DA, White AD, Bowen DT, Padua RA. Cytogenetic abnormalities in the myelodysplastic syndromes and occupational or environmental exposure. *Blood.* 2000;95:2093-2097.
6. Vardiman JW, Thiele J, Arber DA, et al. The 2008 revision of the World Health Organization (WHO) classification of myeloid neoplasms and acute leukemia: rationale and important changes. *Blood.* 2009;114:937-951.
7. Dohner H, Estey EH, Amadori S, et al. Diagnosis and management of acute myeloid leukemia in adults: recommendations from an international expert panel, on behalf of the European LeukemiaNet. *Blood.* 2010;115:453-474.
8. Taskesen E, Bullinger L, Corbacioglu A, et al. Prognostic impact, concurrent genetic mutations, and gene expression features of AML with CEBPA mutations in a cohort of 1182 cytogenetically normal AML patients: further evidence for CEBPA double mutant AML as a distinctive disease entity. *Blood.* 2011;117:2469-2475.
9. Loghavi S, Zuo Z, Ravandi F, et al. Clinical features of de novo acute myeloid leukemia with concurrent DNMT3A, FLT3 and NPM1 mutations. *J Hematol Oncol.* 2014;7:74.
10. Rucker FG, Schlenk RF, Bullinger L, et al. TP53 alterations in acute myeloid leukemia with complex karyotype correlate with specific copy number alterations, monosomal karyotype, and dismal outcome. *Blood.* 2012;119:2114-2121.
11. Patel JP, Gonen M, Figueroa ME, et al. Prognostic relevance of integrated genetic profiling in acute myeloid leukemia. *N Engl J Med.* 2012;366:1079-1089.
12. Freireich EJ, Gehan EA, Sulman D, Boggs DR, Frei E 3rd. The effect of chemotherapy on acute leukemia in the human. *J Chronic Dis.* 1961;14:593-608.
13. Cheson BD, Bennett JM, Kopecky KJ, et al. Revised recommendations of the International Working Group for Diagnosis, Standardization of Response Criteria, Treatment Outcomes, and Reporting Standards for Therapeutic Trials in Acute Myeloid Leukemia. *J Clin Oncol.* 2003;21:4642-4649.
14. de Lima M, Strom SS, Keating M, et al. Implications of potential cure in acute myelogenous leukemia: development of subsequent cancer and return to work. *Blood.* 1997;90:4719-4724.
15. Giles FJ, Shen Y, Kantarjian HM, et al. Leukapheresis reduces early mortality in patients with acute myeloid leukemia with high white cell counts but does not improve long-term survival. *Leuk Lymphoma.* 2001;42:67-73.
16. Sekeres MA, Elson P, Kalaycio ME, et al. Time from diagnosis to treatment initiation predicts survival in younger, but not older, acute myeloid leukemia patients. *Blood.* 2009;113:28-36.
17. Berman E, Heller G, Santorsa J, et al. Results of a randomized trial comparing idarubicin and cytosine arabinoside with daunorubicin and cytosine arabinoside in adult patients with newly diagnosed acute myelogenous leukemia. *Blood.* 1991;77:1666-1674.
18. Rowe JM, Neuberg D, Friedenberg W. A phase III study of daunorubicin vs idarubicin vs mitoxantrone for older adult patients (>55 yrs) with acute myelogenous leukemia (AML): a study of the Eastern Cooperative Oncology Group (E3993) [abstract]. *Blood.* 1998;92:1284.
19. Vignetti M, de Witte T, Suciu S, et al. Daunorubicin (DNR) vs mitoxantrone (MTZ) vs idarubicin (IDA) administered during induction and consolidation in acute myelogenous leukemia (AML) followed by autologous or allogeneic stem transplantation (SCT): results of the EORTC-GIMEMA [abstract 611]. *Blood.* 2003;102:175a.
20. Gardin C, Chevret S, Pautas C, et al. Superior long-term outcome with idarubicin compared with high-dose daunorubicin in patients with acute myeloid leukemia age 50 years and older. *J Clin Oncol.* 2013;31:321-327.
21. Fernandez HF, Sun Z, Yao X, et al. Anthracycline dose intensification in acute myeloid leukemia. *N Engl J Med.* 2009;361:1249-1259.
22. Lowenberg B, Ossenkoppele GJ, van Putten W, et al. High-dose daunorubicin in older patients with acute myeloid leukemia. *N Engl J Med.* 2009;361:1235-1248.
23. Devillier R, Bertoli S, Prebet T, Recher C, Vey N. Induction therapy for AML patients with daunorubicin dose of 60 mg/m^2 and 90 mg/m^2 results in similar complete response rate, relapse-free and overall survival. *Blood.* 2013;122(21):66.
24. Lancet JE, Cortes JE, Hogge DE, et al. Phase 2 trial of CPX-351, a fixed 5:1 molar ratio of cytarabine/daunorubicin, vs cytarabine/daunorubicin in older adults with untreated AML. *Blood.* 2014;123:3239-3246.
25. Mayer RJ, Davis RB, Schiffer CA, et al. Intensive postremission chemotherapy in adults with acute myeloid leukemia. Cancer and Leukemia Group B. *N Engl J Med.* 1994;331:896-903.
26. Bishop JF, Matthews JP, Young GA, Bradstock K, Lowenthal RM. Intensified induction chemotherapy with high dose cytarabine and etoposide for acute myeloid leukemia: a review and updated results of the Australian Leukemia Study Group. *Leuk*

Lymphoma. 1998;28:315-327.

27. Kern W, Estey EH. High-dose cytosine arabinoside in the treatment of acute myeloid leukemia: review of three randomized trials. *Cancer*. 2006;107:116-124.
28. Burnett AK, Hills RK, Milligan D, et al. Identification of patients with acute myeloblastic leukemia who benefit from the addition of gemtuzumab ozogamicin: results of the MRC AML15 trial. *J Clin Oncol*. 2011;29:369-377.
29. Faderl S, Ferrajoli A, Wierda W, et al. Clofarabine combinations as acute myeloid leukemia salvage therapy. *Cancer*. 2008;113:2090-2096.
30. Nazha A, Kantarjian H, Ravandi F, et al. Clofarabine, idarubicin, and cytarabine (CIA) as frontline therapy for patients </=60 years with newly diagnosed acute myeloid leukemia. *Am J Hematol*. 2013;88:961-966.
31. Holowiecki J, Grosicki S, Giebel S, et al. Cladribine, but not fludarabine, added to daunorubicin and cytarabine during induction prolongs survival of patients with acute myeloid leukemia: a multicenter, randomized phase III study. *J Clin Oncol*. 2012;30:2441-2448.
32. Garcia-Manero G, Yang H, Bueso-Ramos C, et al. Phase 1 study of the histone deacetylase inhibitor vorinostat (suberoylanilide hydroxamic acid [SAHA]) in patients with advanced leukemias and myelodysplastic syndromes. *Blood*. 2008;111:1060-1066.
33. Juliusson G, Antunovic P, Derolf A, et al. Age and acute myeloid leukemia: real world data on decision to treat and outcomes from the Swedish Acute Leukemia Registry. *Blood*. 2009;113:4179-4187.
34. Leith CP, Kopecky KJ, Godwin J, et al. Acute myeloid leukemia in the elderly: assessment of multidrug resistance (MDR1) and cytogenetics distinguishes biologic subgroups with remarkably distinct responses to standard chemotherapy. A Southwest Oncology Group study. *Blood*. 1997;89:3323-3329.
35. Appelbaum FR, Gundacker H, Head DR, et al. Age and acute myeloid leukemia. *Blood*. 2006;107:3481-3485.
36. Kantarjian H, O'Brien S, Cortes J, et al. Results of intensive chemotherapy in 998 patients age 65 years or older with acute myeloid leukemia or high-risk myelodysplastic syndrome: predictive prognostic models for outcome. *Cancer*. 2006;106:1090-1098.
37. Burnett AK, Milligan D, Prentice AG, et al. A comparison of low-dose cytarabine and hydroxyurea with or without all-trans retinoic acid for acute myeloid leukemia and high-risk myelodysplastic syndrome in patients not considered fit for intensive treatment. *Cancer*. 2007;109:1114-1124.
38. Faderl S, Ravandi F, Huang X, et al. A randomized study of clofarabine versus clofarabine plus low-dose cytarabine as frontline therapy for patients aged 60 years and older with acute myeloid leukemia and high-risk myelodysplastic syndrome. *Blood*. 2008;112:1638-1645.
39. Kantarjian HM, Thomas XG, Dmoszynska A, et al. Multicenter, randomized, open-label, phase III trial of decitabine versus patient choice, with physician advice, of either supportive care or low-dose cytarabine for the treatment of older patients with newly diagnosed acute myeloid leukemia. *J Clin Oncol*. 2012;30:2670-2677.
40. Quintas-Cardama A, Ravandi F, Liu-Dumlao T, et al. Epigenetic therapy is associated with similar survival compared with intensive chemotherapy in older patients with newly diagnosed acute myeloid leukemia. *Blood*. 2012;120:4840-4845.
41. Döhner H, Dombret H. Overall survival in older patients with newly diagnosed acute myeloid leukemia (AML) with >30% bone marrow blasts treated with azacitidine by cytogenetic risk status: results of the AZA-AML-001 study. Paper presented at: 56th Annual Meeting of the American Society of Hematology; December 6-9, 2014; San Francisco, CA.
42. Blum W, Garzon R, Klisovic RB, et al. Clinical response and miR-29b predictive significance in older AML patients treated with a 10-day schedule of decitabine. *Proc Natl Acad Sci U S A*. 2010;107:7473-7478.
43. Stuart RK, Cripe LD, Maris MB, et al. REVEAL-1, a phase 2 dose regimen optimization study of vosaroxin in older poor-risk patients with previously untreated acute myeloid leukaemia. *Br J Haematol*. 2015;168(6):796-805.
44. Naval D, Kantarjian HM, Garcia-Manero G, et al. Phase I/II study of vosaroxin and decitabine in newly diagnosed older patients (pts) with acute myeloid leukemia (AML) and high risk myelodysplastic syndrome (MDS). Paper presented at: 56th Annual Meeting of the American Society of Hematology; December 6-9, 2014; San Francisco, CA.
45. Renner AG, Dos Santos C, Recher C, et al. Polo-like kinase 1 is overexpressed in acute myeloid leukemia and its inhibition preferentially targets the proliferation of leukemic cells. *Blood*. 2009;114:659-662.
46. Dohner H, Lubbert M, Fiedler W, et al. Randomized, phase 2 trial of low-dose cytarabine with or without volasertib in AML patients not suitable for induction therapy. *Blood*. 2014;124:1426-1433.
47. Pollyea DA, Zehnder J, Coutre S, et al. Sequential azacitidine plus lenalidomide combination for elderly patients with untreated acute myeloid leukemia. *Haematologica*. 2013;98:591-596.
48. Wetzler M, Mrozek K, Kohlschmidt J, et al. Intensive induction is effective in selected octogenarian acute myeloid leukemia patients: prognostic significance of karyotype and selected molecular markers used in the European LeukemiaNet classification. *Haematologica*. 2014;99:308-313.
49. Krug U, Rollig C, Koschmieder A, et al. Complete remission and early death after intensive chemotherapy in patients aged 60 years or older with acute myeloid leukaemia: a web-based application for prediction of outcomes. *Lancet*. 2010;376:2000-2008.
50. Kantarjian H, Ravandi F, O'Brien S, et al. Intensive chemotherapy does not benefit most older patients (age 70 years or older) with acute myeloid leukemia. *Blood*. 2010;116:4422-4429.
51. Gilliland DG, Griffin JD. The roles of FLT3 in hematopoiesis and leukemia. *Blood*. 2002;100:1532-1542.
52. Borthakur G, Kantarjian H, Wang X, et al. Treatment of core-binding-factor in acute myelogenous leukemia with fludarabine, cytarabine, and granulocyte colony-stimulating factor results in improved event-free survival. *Cancer*. 2008;113:3181-3185.
53. Borthakur G, Cortes JE, Estey EE, et al. Gemtuzumab ozogamicin with fludarabine, cytarabine, and granulocyte colony stimulating factor (FLAG-GO) as front-line regimen in patients with core binding factor acute myelogenous leukemia. *Am J Hematol*. 2014;89:964-968.
54. Hills RK, Castaigne S, Appelbaum FR, et al. Addition of gemtuzumab ozogamicin to induction chemotherapy in adult patients with acute myeloid leukaemia: a meta-analysis of individual patient data from randomised controlled trials. *Lancet Oncol*. 2014;15:986-996.
55. Marcucci G, Geyer S, Blum W, et al. Adding the KIT inhibitor dasatinib (DAS) to standard induction and consolidation therapy for newly diagnosed patients (pts) with core binding factor (CBF) acute myeloid leukemia (AML): initial results of the CALGB 10801 (Alliance) study. *Blood*. 2013;122:21.
56. Breems DA, Van Putten WL, Huijgens PC, et al. Prognostic index for adult patients with acute myeloid leukemia in first relapse. *J Clin Oncol*. 2005;23:1969-1978.
57. Giles F, O'Brien S, Cortes J, et al. Outcome of patients with acute myelogenous leukemia after second salvage therapy. *Cancer*. 2005;104:547-554.
58. Forman SJ, Schmidt GM, Nademanee AP, et al. Allogeneic bone marrow transplantation as therapy for primary induction failure for patients with acute leukemia. *J Clin Oncol*. 1991;9:1570-1574.

59. Estey E, Kornblau S, Pierce S, Kantarjian H, Beran M, Keating M. A stratification system for evaluating and selecting therapies in patients with relapsed or primary refractory acute myelogenous leukemia. *Blood*. 1996;88:756.
60. Ravandi F, Ritchie E, Sayar H, et al. Improved survival in patients with first relapsed or refractory acute myeloid leukemia (AML) treated with vosaroxin plus cytarabine versus placebo plus cytarabine: results of a phase 3 double-blind randomized controlled multinational study (VALOR) [abstract LBA-6]. Paper presented at: 56th Annual Meeting of the American Society of Hematology; December 6-9, 2014; San Francisco, CA.
61. Archimbaud E, Thomas X, Michallet M, et al. Prospective genetically randomized comparison between intensive postinduction chemotherapy and bone marrow transplantation in adults with newly diagnosed acute myeloid leukemia. *J Clin Oncol*. 1994;12:262-267.
62. Burnett AK, Goldstone AH, Stevens RM, et al. Randomised comparison of addition of autologous bone-marrow transplantation to intensive chemotherapy for acute myeloid leukaemia in first remission: results of MRC AML 10 trial. UK Medical Research Council Adult and Children's Leukaemia Working Parties. *Lancet*. 1998;351:700-708.
63. Cassileth PA, Harrington DP, Appelbaum FR, et al. Chemotherapy compared with autologous or allogeneic bone marrow transplantation in the management of acute myeloid leukemia in first remission. *N Engl J Med*. 1998;339:1649-1656.
64. Zittoun RA, Mandelli F, Willemze R, et al. Autologous or allogeneic bone marrow transplantation compared with intensive chemotherapy in acute myelogenous leukemia. European Organization for Research and Treatment of Cancer (EORTC) and the Gruppo Italiano Malattie Ematologiche Maligne dell'Adulto (GIMEMA) Leukemia Cooperative Groups. *N Engl J Med*. 1995;332:217-223.
65. Koreth J, Schlenk R, Kopecky KJ, et al. Allogeneic stem cell transplantation for acute myeloid leukemia in first complete remission: systematic review and meta-analysis of prospective clinical trials. *JAMA*. 2009;301:2349-2361.
66. Ferrant A, Labopin M, Frassoni F, et al. Karyotype in acute myeloblastic leukemia: prognostic significance for bone marrow transplantation in first remission: a European Group for Blood and Marrow Transplantation study. Acute Leukemia Working Party of the European Group for Blood and Marrow Transplantation (EBMT). *Blood*. 1997;90:2931-2938.
67. Schlenk RF, Dohner K, Krauter J, et al. Mutations and treatment outcome in cytogenetically normal acute myeloid leukemia. *N Engl J Med*. 2008;358:1909-1918.
68. Burnett AK. Transplantation in first remission of acute myeloid leukemia. *N Engl J Med*. 1998;339:1698-1700.
69. Anasetti C, Logan BR, Lee SJ, et al. Peripheral-blood stem cells versus bone marrow from unrelated donors. *N Engl J Med*. 2012;367:1487-1496.
70. Chen YB, Coughlin E, Kennedy KF, et al. Busulfan dose intensity and outcomes in reduced-intensity allogeneic peripheral blood stem cell transplantation for myelodysplastic syndrome or acute myeloid leukemia. *Biol Blood Marrow Transplant*. 2013;19:981-987.
71. Luger S, Ringden O, Perez WS, et al. Similar outcomes using myeloablative versus reduced intensity and non-myeloablative allogeneic transplant preparative regimens for AML or MDS: from the Center for International Blood and Marrow Transplant Research [abstract 348]. *Blood*. 2008;112:136.
72. Godwin JE, Kopecky KJ, Head DR, et al. A double-blind placebo-controlled trial of granulocyte colony-stimulating factor in elderly patients with previously untreated acute myeloid leukemia: a Southwest Oncology Group study (9031). *Blood*. 1998;91:3607-3615.
73. Gardner A, Mattiuzzi G, Faderl S, et al. Randomized comparison of cooked and noncooked diets in patients undergoing remission induction therapy for acute myeloid leukemia. *J Clin Oncol*. 2008;26:5684-5688.
74. Chou WC, Lei WC, Ko BS, et al. The prognostic impact and stability of isocitrate dehydrogenase 2 mutation in adult patients with acute myeloid leukemia. *Leukemia*. 2011;25:246-253.
75. Stein E, Altman JK, DeAngeloa DJ, et al. AG-221, an oral, selective, first-in-class, potent inhibitor of the IDH2 mutant metabolic enzyme, induces durable remissions in a phase I study in patients with IDH2 mutation positive advanced hematologic malignancies [abstract]. Paper presented at: 56th Annual Meeting of the American Society of Hematology; December 6-9, 2014; San Francisco, CA.
76. Konopleva M, Blum W, Stone RM, Kantarjian HM, Letai AG. A phase 2 study of ABT-199 (GDC-0199) in patients with acute myelogenous leukemia (AML). Paper presented at: 56th Annual Meeting of the American Society of Hematology; December 6-9, 2014; San Francisco, CA.
77. Lo Coco F, Diverio D, Falini B, Biondi A, Nervi C, Pelicci PG. Genetic diagnosis and molecular monitoring in the management of acute promyelocytic leukemia. *Blood*. 1999;94:12-22.
78. Tallman MS, Kwaan HC. Reassessing the hemostatic disorder associated with acute promyelocytic leukemia. *Blood*. 1992;79:543-553.
79. Dyck JA, Warrell RP Jr, Evans RM, Miller WH Jr. Rapid diagnosis of acute promyelocytic leukemia by immunohistochemical localization of PML/RAR-alpha protein. *Blood*. 1995;86:862-867.
80. Sanz MA, Lo Coco F, Martin G, et al. Definition of relapse risk and role of nonanthracycline drugs for consolidation in patients with acute promyelocytic leukemia: a joint study of the PETHEMA and GIMEMA cooperative groups. *Blood*. 2000;96:1247-1253.
81. Sanz MA, Montesinos P. How we prevent and treat differentiation syndrome in patients with acute promyelocytic leukemia. *Blood*. 2014;123:2777-2782.
82. Grimwade D, Jovanovic JV, Hills RK, et al. Prospective minimal residual disease monitoring to predict relapse of acute promyelocytic leukemia and to direct pre-emptive arsenic trioxide therapy. *J Clin Oncol*. 2009;27:3650-3658.
83. Sanz MA, Martin G, Gonzalez M, et al. Risk-adapted treatment of acute promyelocytic leukemia with all-trans-retinoic acid and anthracycline monochemotherapy: a multicenter study by the PETHEMA group. *Blood*. 2004;103:1237-1243.
84. Lo-Coco F, Avvisati G, Vignetti M, et al. Retinoic acid and arsenic trioxide for acute promyelocytic leukemia. *N Engl J Med*. 2013;369:111-121.
85. Ravandi F, Estey E, Jones D, et al. Effective treatment of acute promyelocytic leukemia with all-trans-retinoic acid, arsenic trioxide, and gemtuzumab ozogamicin. *J Clin Oncol*. 2009;27:504-510.
86. Konopleva M, Cheng SC, Cortes JE, et al. Independent prognostic significance of day 21 cytogenetic findings in newly-diagnosed acute myeloid leukemia or refractory anemia with excess blasts. *Haematologica*. 2003;88:733-736.
87. Chen Y, Cortes J, Estrov Z, et al. Persistence of cytogenetic abnormalities at complete remission after induction in patients with acute myeloid leukemia: prognostic significance and the potential role of allogeneic stem-cell transplantation. *J Clin Oncol*. 2011;29:2507-2513.
88. van der Velden VH, Hochhaus A, Cazzaniga G, Szczepanski T, Gabert J, van Dongen JJ. Detection of minimal residual disease in hematologic malignancies by real-time quantitative PCR: principles, approaches, and laboratory aspects. *Leukemia*. 2003;17:1013-1034.
89. Chou WC, Tang JL, Wu SJ, et al. Clinical implications of minimal residual disease monitoring by quantitative polymerase chain reaction in acute myeloid leukemia patients bearing nucleophosmin (NPM1) mutations. *Leukemia*. 2007;21:998-1004.
90. Cilloni D, Renneville A, Hermitte F, et al. Real-time quantitative

polymerase chain reaction detection of minimal residual disease by standardized WT1 assay to enhance risk stratification in acute myeloid leukemia: a European LeukemiaNet study. *J Clin Oncol*. 2009;27:5195-5201.

91. Rubnitz JE, Inaba H, Dahl G, et al. Minimal residual disease-directed therapy for childhood acute myeloid leukaemia: results of the AML02 multicentre trial. *Lancet Oncol*. 2010;11:543-552.
92. Maurillo L, Buccisano F, Del Principe MI, et al. Toward optimization of postremission therapy for residual disease-positive patients with acute myeloid leukemia. *J Clin Oncol*. 2008;26:4944-4951.
93. Ravandi F, Cortes JE, Jones D, et al. Phase I/II study of combination therapy with sorafenib, idarubicin, and cytarabine in younger patients with acute myeloid leukemia. *J Clin Oncol*. 2010;28:1856-1862.
94. Röllig C, Muller-Tidow C, Huttmann A, et al. Sorafenib versus placebo in addition to standard therapy in younger patients with newly diagnosed acute myeloid leukemia: results from 267 patients treated in the randomized placebo-controlled SAL-Soraml trial. Paper presented at: 56th Annual Meeting of the American Society of Hematology; December 6-9, 2014; San Francisco, CA.
95. Cortes JE, Kantarjian H, Foran JM, et al. Phase I study of quizartinib administered daily to patients with relapsed or refractory acute myeloid leukemia irrespective of FMS-like tyrosine kinase 3-internal tandem duplication status. *J Clin Oncol*. 2013;31:3681-3687.
96. Borthakur G, Cortes JE, Ravandi F, Kantarjian HM. The combination of quizartinib with azacitidine or low dose cytarabine is highly active in patients (pts) with FLT3-ITD mutated myeloid leukemias: interim report of a phase I/II trial. Paper presented at: 56th Annual Meeting of the American Society of Hematology; December 6-9, 2014; San Francisco, CA.
97. Randhawa J, Kantarjian HM, Borthakur G, et al. Results of a phase II study of crenolanib in relapsed/refractory acute myeloid leukemia patients (pts) with activating FLT3 mutations. Paper presented at: 56th Annual Meeting of the American Society of Hematology; December 6-9, 2014; San Francisco, CA.
98. Powell BL, Moser B, Stock W, et al. Arsenic trioxide improves event-free and overall survival for adults with acute promyelocytic leukemia: North American Leukemia Intergroup Study C9710. *Blood*. 2010;116:3751-3757.
99. Ades L, Chevret S, Raffoux E, et al. Is cytarabine useful in the treatment of acute promyelocytic leukemia? Results of a randomized trial from the European Acute Promyelocytic Leukemia Group. *J Clin Oncol*. 2006;24:5703-5710.
100. Sanz MA, Montesinos P, Rayon C, et al. Risk-adapted treatment of acute promyelocytic leukemia based on all-trans retinoic acid and anthracycline with addition of cytarabine in consolidation therapy for high-risk patients: further improvements in treatment outcome. *Blood*. 2010;115:5137-5146.

3

Chronic Lymphocytic Leukemia and Associated Disorders

第三章　慢性淋巴细胞白血病及相关疾病

Nitin Jain
Carlos Bueso-Ramos
Susan O'Brien
William G. Wierda

中文导读

本章首先简要介绍了慢性淋巴细胞白血病的定义、治疗的现状及近期的研究进展，并介绍了慢性淋巴细胞白血病的流行病学信息。然后从多个方面描述了慢性淋巴细胞白血病的生物学特征，包括表面抗原表型、免疫球蛋白重链可变基因的体细胞突变以及基因组的改变。此后介绍了慢性淋巴细胞白血病的临床特征和实验室检查特征，并详述了该病的诊断标准、鉴别诊断、分期和预后。在治疗部分，首先介绍了慢性淋巴细胞白血病治疗的适应证，然后依次介绍了包括嘌呤类似物、烷化剂、单克隆抗体等一线治疗及该疗法的患者分层和微小残留病变情况；包括B细胞信号通路抑制剂、BCL-2抑制剂、来那度胺、嵌合抗原受体T细胞免疫疗法（CAR-T）等在内的新型靶向治疗；干细胞移植在该病中的应用；支持治疗及自身免疫并发症和低丙种球蛋白血症等常见并发症。在慢性淋巴细胞白血病的转化方面，着重介绍了Richter综合征和向幼淋巴细胞白血病的转化。本章最后介绍了几种特殊类型的慢性淋巴细胞白血病：毛细胞白血病、幼淋巴细胞白血病和大颗粒淋巴细胞白血病的特点及治疗方法。

INTRODUCTION

Chronic lymphocytic leukemia (CLL) is a clonal hematopoietic disorder involving expansion of CD5-positive B cells. Chemoimmunotherapy (CIT) has been the standard first-line treatment for patients with CLL ([1]). In the last several years, major strides have been made in understanding the disease biology of CLL, and, fortunately, several of these discoveries are making their way into the clinic.

EPIDEMIOLOGY

Chronic lymphocytic leukemia is the most common leukemia in the Western Hemisphere, accounting for about 25% of all leukemias in the United States. The estimated number of new CLL cases for 2015 was 14,620, with 8,140 occurring in men and 6,480 in women. Chronic lymphocytic leukemia is uncommon in the Asian population and accounts for only 2.5% of all leukemias in Japan. The incidence is age-related, with an increase from 5.2 per 100,000 persons older than 50 years to 30.4 per 100,000 persons older than 80 years. Population studies have not identified specific occupational or environmental risk factors for developing CLL ([2]). The risk of CLL is not increased in Asians settled in Western countries, indicating that genetic factors play a part in CLL risk ([3]). Up to 15% to 20% of patients with CLL have a family member with CLL or a related lymphoproliferative disorder ([4]). Genome-wide association studies identified several single nucleotide polymorphisms associated with increased risk of CLL ([5,6]).

BIOLOGY

Surface Antigen Phenotype

Chronic lymphocytic leukemia is a clonal B-cell lymphoid leukemia. Chronic lymphocytic leukemia cells morphologically resemble small mature lymphocytes arrested in an intermediate stage of the B-cell differentiation pathway. The hallmark of CLL cells is that they are monoclonal and express CD5, an antigen commonly found on T cells. CD5-positive B cells can be found in the mantle zone of lymphoid follicles, but they constitute a minor fraction of the B-cell population. CD19, CD20, and CD23 are B-cell markers expressed on CLL cells. Surface immunoglobulin, FMC7, CD22, CD11c, and CD79b are either weakly expressed or negative in CLL. Based on the antigen expression profile, CLL appears to arise from an "activated" B cell.

Somatic Hypermutation of Immunoglobulin Heavy-Chain Variable Gene

Normal B-cell development involves an antigen-independent phase and an antigen-dependent phase. During the antigen-independent phase, B cells undergo rearrangement of the variable (V), diversity (D), and joining (J) genes in the bone marrow. Somatic mutation of the heavy- and light-chain variable gene occurs after encounter with antigen in the germinal center. Assessment for somatic hypermutation of immunoglobulin heavy-chain variable gene (*IGHV*) defines two subsets of CLL. Approximately 50% of CLL cases have somatic hypermutation (>2% deviation from germline sequence) of the *IGHV* gene and thus appear to arise from post-germinal B cells, whereas the subset of CLL lacking *IGHV* gene hypermutation (≤2% deviation from germline sequence) appears to arise from naive B cells ([7,8]). The mutation status of CLL cells is fixed, and mutational status is not gained or lost through the course of disease. Several studies showed that unmutated *IGHV* is associated with worse clinical outcomes ([9]).

Because sequencing of the *IGHV* gene to identify the mutational status was labor intensive and not universally available, Damle et al first studied the correlation of *IGHV* mutation status with CD38 expression as a surrogate prognostic marker for *IGHV* mutation status ([7]). A significant association between CD38 expression and unmutated *IGHV* status was noted. Patients with ≥30% CD38 expression had a median survival of 10 years, which was significantly shorter than the median survival not reached for patients with CD38 expression <30% (P = .0001) ([7]). Gene expression profiling of mutated versus unmutated *IGHV* CLL cases showed zeta-associated protein 70 (*ZAP-70*) to be the most differentially expressed gene with higher expression in unmutated *IGHV* cases, providing another surrogate for *IGHV* mutation status ([10]). Higher expression of ZAP-70 (≥20%) was associated with worse clinical outcomes ([10,11]).

Genomic Alterations

Using conventional chromosome banding techniques, cytogenetic abnormalities can be detected in up to 50% of CLL cases. These techniques are hampered by the low mitotic activity of CLL cells; B-cell mitogens may be used to enhance this activity. In addition, metaphases obtained for karyotyping may also arise from normal T cells in the sample, as indicated by sequential immunotyping followed by karyotypic analysis. Fluorescent in situ hybridization (FISH) performed on interphase cells using genomic DNA probes greatly enhanced the ability to detect molecular abnormalities in malignant cells. Fluorescent in situ hybridization demonstrated that molecular abnormalities occur in over 80% of CLL cases. 13q deletion is the most common genetic aberration found in CLL by FISH (55%), followed by 11q deletion (18%), 12q trisomy (16%), and 17p deletion (7%) ([12]). Prior to the use of FISH, trisomy 12 was the most frequently detected chromosomal abnormality in CLL by conventional cytogenetic methods ([13]). Structural abnormalities of 13q were often missed by Giemsa banding, presumably because of the small size of the deletion. The prognosis of CLL varies with the chromosomal abnormality. When divided into five prognostic categories—17p deletion, 11q deletion, 12q trisomy, no observed abnormalities, and 13q deletion (as sole abnormality)—the survival times were 32, 79, 114, 111, and 133 months, respectively ([12]). Patients with 11q deletion tend to have more prominent lymphadenopathy. Patients with 17p and 11q deletion tend to have more advanced disease and respond poorly to conventional therapy ([9]). Clonal evolution can occur over time and with treatment; therefore, FISH assessment should be repeated when therapeutic intervention is being considered.

Whole exome sequencing of CLL cases has identified genes that are recurrently mutated and may contribute to the pathogenesis of the disease ([14, 15]). Recurrently mutated genes include *TP53*, *NOTCH1*, *SF3B1*, *MYD88*, *XPO1*, and *ATM*. Some of these mutations were correlated with clinical outcome ([15, 16]). *TP53* mutations are typically associated with del(17p). *ATM* and *SF3B1* mutations are typically associated with del(11q).

CLINICAL FEATURES

At diagnosis, most patients are older than 60 years, with more than 90% being over 50 years. The diagnosis of CLL is often incidental; routine blood count may reveal an elevated absolute lymphocyte count (ALC). In symptomatic patients, fatigue and infections may be presenting features. B symptoms (fever, weight loss, night sweat) can also occur but are uncommon at initial diagnosis. Exaggerated skin reaction to insect bites (Wells syndrome) is frequent in CLL. Leptomeningeal involvement is rare. Some patients may present with autoimmune hemolytic anemia or immune thrombocytopenia. Physical examination may reveal cervical, axillary, and/or inguinal lymphadenopathy. Splenomegaly and hepatomegaly are not uncommon.

LABORATORY FEATURES

Laboratory findings invariably show lymphocytosis. The ALC can range from $5 \times 10^9/L$ to $>500 \times 10^9/L$. Chronic lymphocytic leukemia cells resemble mature lymphocytes; they have dense chromatin as well as scant cytoplasm and lack nucleoli (Fig. 3-1). Preparation of the blood smear may damage these fragile lymphocytes and produce "smudge" cells. The bone marrow is typically hypercellular for age, and infiltration varies in terms of the percentage of marrow involved as well as in the pattern of involvement, which may be nodular, interstitial, or diffuse (Figs. 3-2A and B). Erythroid, myeloid, and megakaryocytic precursors may be normal or decreased. Anemia or thrombocytopenia may result from marrow infiltration or from immune destruction. Findings of microspherocytes in peripheral blood smear (Fig. 3-3), reticulocytosis, and demonstration of immunoglobulin (Ig) G and/or complement on red cells support the diagnosis of immune hemolytic anemia. Pure red cell aplasia has been described in 1% to 6% of cases. Patients often develop hypogammaglobulinemia, which can progress in severity with advancing disease. Monoclonal gammopathy may also develop. Other laboratory abnormalities include elevated serum β_2-microglobulin (β_2-M); LDH is rarely elevated.

Up to 5% of otherwise normal individuals over the age 40 may harbor a population of monoclonal CD5$^+$/CD19$^+$/CD23$^+$ B cells. These individuals are asymptomatic (absence of cytopenia and lymphadenopathy/organomegaly), and when the absolute monoclonal lymphocyte count is less than 5,000/µL and there is no palpable enlarged lymph node, they are characterized as having monoclonal B lymphocytosis (MBL) ([17]). Individuals with MBL should be monitored. It is estimated that the rate of progression from MBL to CLL is 1% to 2% per year.

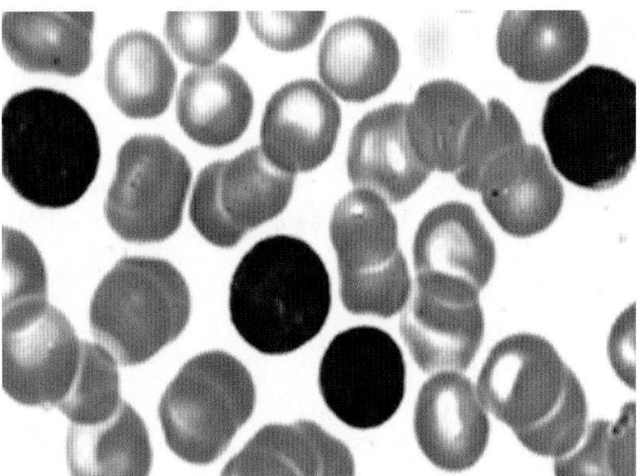

FIGURE 3-1 Chronic lymphocytic leukemia. Peripheral blood smear showing mature-appearing lymphocytes. Note dense chromatin, scant cytoplasm, absence of nucleoli, and smudge cells.

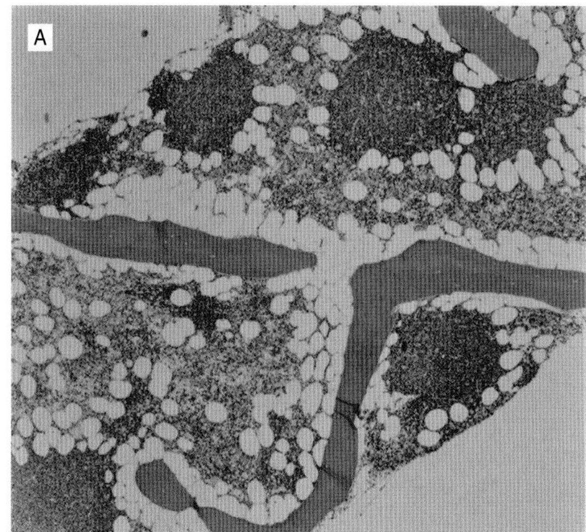

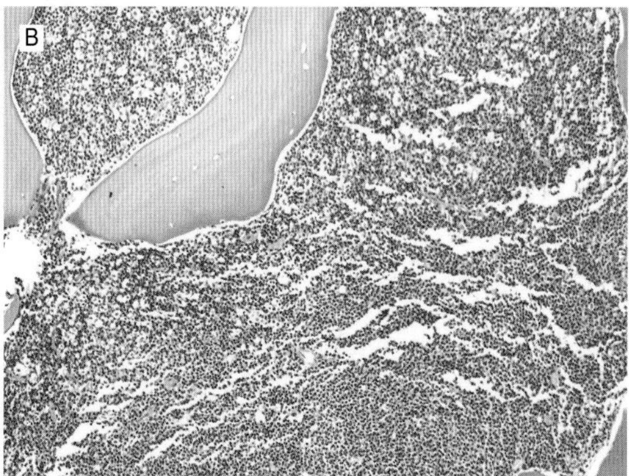

FIGURE 3-2 (A, B) Chronic lymphocytic leukemia. Bone marrow biopsies showing nodular, diffuse, and interstitial patterns of involvement.

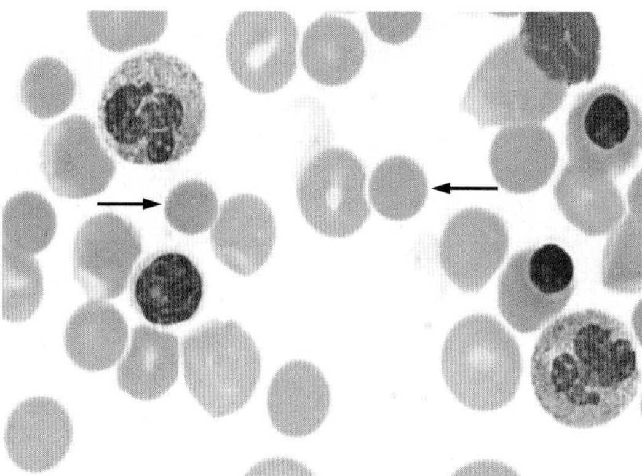

FIGURE 3-3 Immune hemolytic anemia. Presence of microspherocytes (*arrows*) and nucleated red cells indicates immune destruction of red cells. Diagnosis is confirmed by demonstrating the presence of immunoglobulin G (IgG) and/or complement on red cells.

Table 3-1 Diagnostic Criteria for CLL

Parameter	NCI-IWCLL[a]
Diagnosis	
Lymphocytosis	≥5 × 10^9/L B lymphocytes in the peripheral blood
Clonality	Flow cytometry to confirm clonality
Duration of lymphocytosis	Not stated
Bone marrow lymphocytes (%)	Not necessary to make a diagnosis[b]

[a]National Cancer Institute–International Workshop on Chronic Lymphocytic Leukemia ([18]).
[b]Bone marrow aspirate and biopsy can be evaluated for factors contributing to cytopenias that may not be due to leukemia infiltration of the marrow.

DIAGNOSIS

In 2008, the International Workshop on Chronic Lymphocytic Leukemia (IWCLL) updated the recommendations on diagnosis and treatment of CLL (Table 3-1) ([18]). The diagnosis of CLL requires at least 5 × 10^9 clonal B lymphocytes/L in the peripheral blood, with less than 55% of the cells being atypical (prolymphocytes). A monoclonal B-cell count ≥ 5 × 10^9/L was specified to distinguish CLL from small lymphocytic lymphoma in patients with palpable lymph nodes or splenomegaly. B-lymphocyte clonality should be demonstrated by using flow cytometry, which should also confirm expression of B-cell surface antigens (CD19, CD20, CD23), low-density surface immunoglobulin (M or D), and CD5. ZAP-70 (Fig. 3-4) expression in CLL cells has prognostic implication. Distinguishing CLL from mantle cell lymphoma (Figs. 3-5A and B) (see section "Differential Diagnosis") and large granular leukemia (Fig. 3-6) is of utmost importance.

The presence of more than 55% of prolymphocytes would favor a diagnosis of prolymphocytic leukemia (PLL). Prolymphocytes (<55%) can be seen in peripheral blood or bone marrow of patients with CLL (Figs. 3-7A, B, and C).

DIFFERENTIAL DIAGNOSIS

Clinical, morphologic, immunophenotypic, and cytogenetic methods help to distinguish between CLL and other diseases such as mantle cell lymphoma, follicular lymphoma, T-cell PLL (T-PLL), hairy cell leukemia (HCL), marginal zone lymphoma, and Waldenström macroglobulinemia. Table 3-2 summarizes the immunophenotypic features of these disorders. Distinguishing CLL from mantle cell lymphoma is important because both can express CD5 (see Fig. 3-5A). Unlike CLL, mantle cell lymphoma cells are typically CD23 negative,

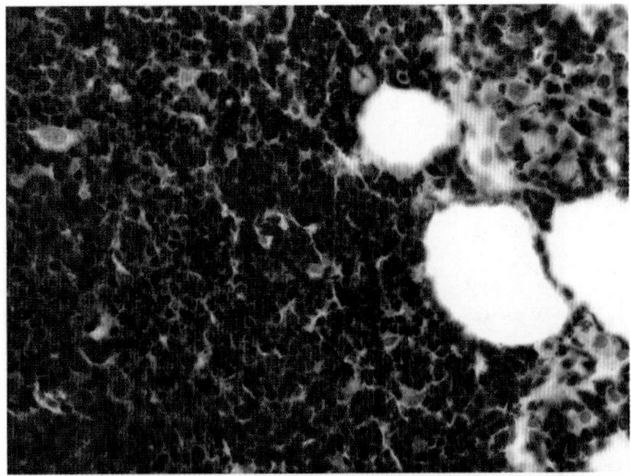

FIGURE 3-4 ZAP-70 expression in chronic lymphocytic leukemia cells indicates poor prognosis. Immunohistochemistry (*above*) or flow cytometry can be used to detect ZAP-70 expression.

FMC-7 positive, and have strong surface immunoglobulin staining. Confirmation of mantle cell lymphoma can be made by detection of the t(11;14) translocation and/or positive nuclear cyclin D1 staining (see Fig. 3-5B).

STAGING

Staging systems for CLL include Rai and Binet staging (Table 3-3). The original Rai classification defined five stages from 0 to IV; this has been modified to three stages by defining Rai stage 0 as low risk, stages I and II as intermediate risk, and stages III and IV as high risk, with median survival times of >12.5, 7, and 1.5 years for each risk group, respectively. Similarly for Binet stages A, B, and C, median survival times are >10, 6, and 2 years, respectively. The diagnostic workup that is undertaken in CLL patients at initial presentation at the University of Texas MD Anderson Cancer Center (MDACC) is listed in Table 3-4.

PROGNOSIS

Both CLL staging systems confer significant prognostic information; however, they are limited by their inability to identify which patient with early-stage disease will develop disease progression. An analysis of the French Cooperative Group trial of Binet stage A patients demonstrated that a subgroup of these stage A patients with a hemoglobin ≥12 g/dL, a lymphocyte count <30 × 10^9/L, and <80% lymphocytes in the bone marrow aspirate was less likely to progress than other stage A patients ([19]). A lymphocyte doubling time of >12 months, Rai stage 0 disease, nondiffuse bone marrow pattern, hemoglobin ≥13 g/dL, and ALC <30 × 10^9/L similarly define a group of CLL with an excellent prognosis ([20]).

Serum factors have been identified as prognostic indicators in early-stage CLL. Patients with early-stage CLL with serum thymidine kinase (TK) levels >7.0

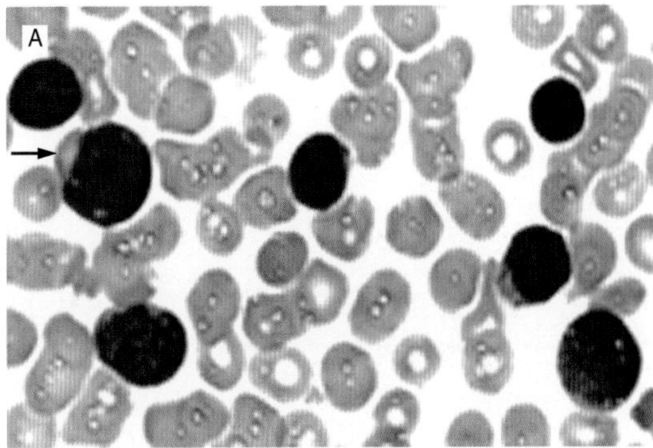

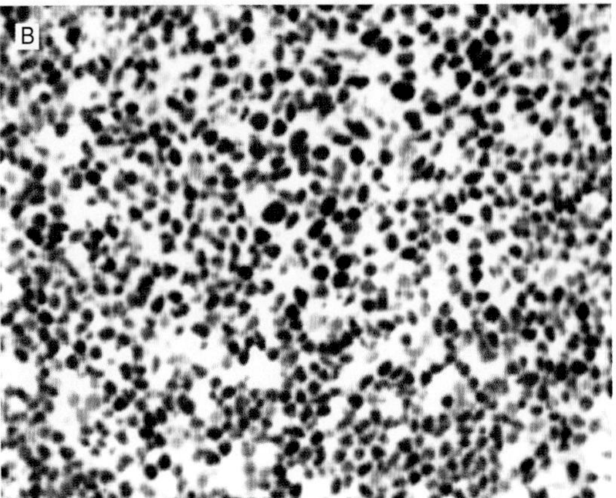

FIGURE 3-5 A. Mantle cell lymphoma (MCL) in leukemic phase. MCL cells (*arrow*) are larger than mature lymphocytes (*center*) with speckled chromatin; some show nuclear cleft. B. Nuclear cyclin D1 staining in mantle cells.

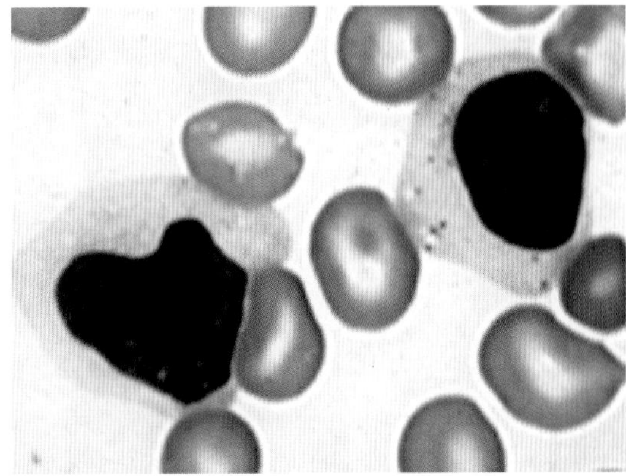

FIGURE 3-6 Large granular lymphocytes with cytoplasmic azurophilic granules.

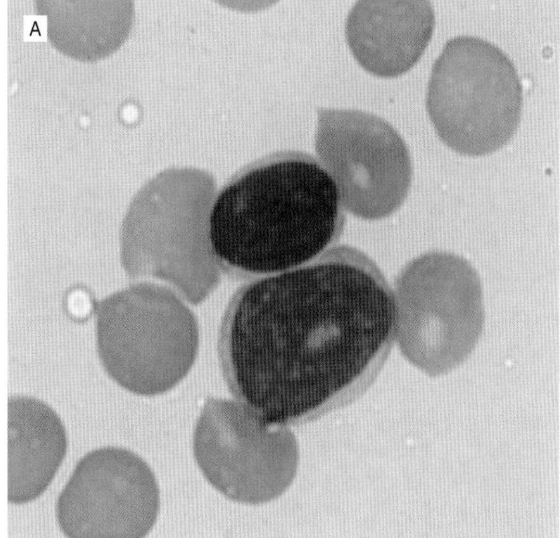

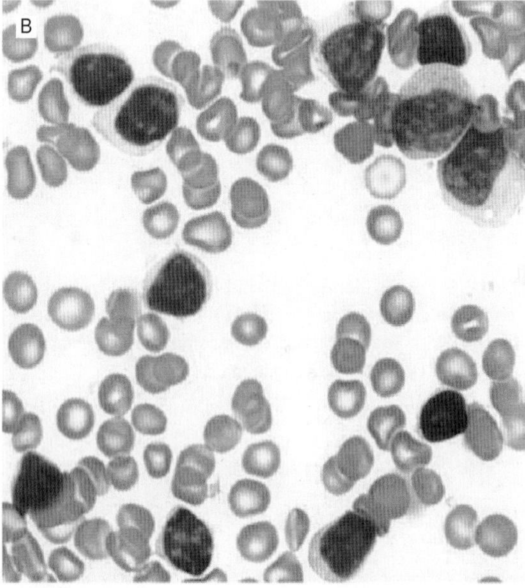

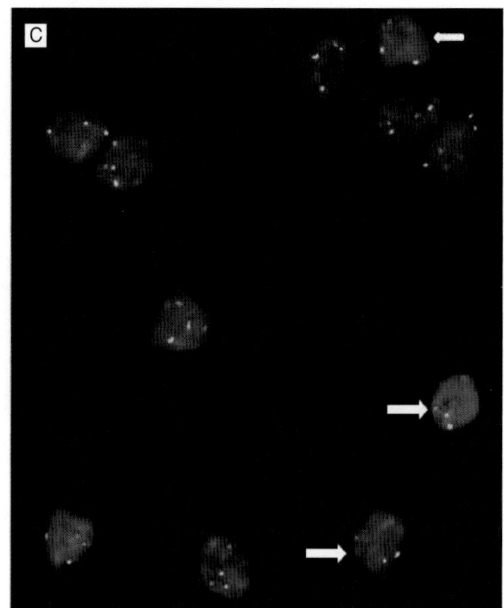

FIGURE 3-7 A. High-power view of a prolymphocyte juxtaposed with a mature-appearing lymphocyte. Note larger size, less condensed chromatin, and prominent nucleolus in prolymphocyte. **B.** Bone marrow smear from a 58-year-old man with a 3-year history of untreated chronic lymphocytic leukemia (CLL). There are small lymphocytes and larger prolymphocytoid lymphocytes with abundant lightly basophilic cytoplasm, fine chromatin, and variably prominent nucleoli. **C.** Interphase FISH. Almost all the lymphocytes show deletion of one locus of D13S319 (*white arrow*) (except two lymphocytes on slide 1, left low), and a large subset of CLL cells also showed trisomy 12 (+12). Interestingly, +12 is almost only seen in prolymphocytoid lymphocytes. The small lymphocytes with clumped chromatin and scant cytoplasm usually do not show +12.

Table 3-2 Immunophenotypic Analysis in Chronic B-Cell Disorders

Disease	sIg	CD5	CD10	CD20	CD22	CD23	CD79B	CD103	FMC7
CLL	Weak	++	–	+	–/+	++	–/+	–	–/+
B-PLL	Strong	–/+	–/+	++	+	–/+	++	–	++
HCL	Strong	–	–	++	++	–	+	+	++
SLVL	Strong	–/+	–	++	++	–/+	++	–	++
FL	Strong	–/+	++	++	++	–/+	++	–	++
MCL	Strong	++	–	++	++	–	++	–	++

B-PLL, prolymphocytic leukemia; CLL, chronic lymphocytic leukemia; FL, follicular lymphoma; HCL, hairy cell leukemia; MCL, mantle cell lymphoma; sIg, surface immunoglobulin; SLVL, splenic lymphoma with villous lymphocytes.

(described in earlier sections). A prognostic model integrating cytogenetic abnormalities identified by FISH with mutated *NOTCH1*, *SF3B1*, *BIRC3*, and *TP53* was proposed ([21]). The established prognostic factors in CLL indicating poorer outcome are listed in Table 3-5.

Table 3-3 Staging of CLL

Rai Stage	Modified Rai Stage	Description	Binet Stage	Description	Median Survival
0	Low risk	Lymphocytosis only	A	Hemoglobin ≥10 g/dL and platelets ≥100 × 10^9/L and <3 enlarged lymphoid-bearing areas	>10 years
1	Intermediate risk	Lymphocytosis and lymphadenopathy	B	Hemoglobin ≥10 g/dL and platelets ≥100 × 10^9/L and ≥3 enlarged lymphoid-bearing areas	5-7 years
2	Intermediate risk	Lymphocytosis and splenomegaly and/or hepatomegaly with/without lymphadenopathy			
3	High risk	Lymphocytosis and anemia (hemoglobin <11 g/dL)	C	Hemoglobin <10 g/dL or platelets <100 × 10^9/L (irrespective of number of lymphoid-bearing areas)	2-3 years
4	High risk	Lymphocytosis and thrombocytopenia (platelets <100 × 10^9/L			

Table 3-4 Initial Evaluation of Patients With CLL at MDACC

History and physical (close attention to lymph node areas, liver/spleen size)
Constitutional symptoms (fever, chills, weight loss, night sweats)
Assessment of performance status
CBC, electrolytes, BUN, creatinine, liver function tests, LDH, quantitative immunoglobulins, β_2-microglobulin
Examination of peripheral blood smear
Bone marrow aspiration and biopsy (in patients with cytopenias or those in need of treatment)
Immunophenotyping of peripheral blood/bone marrow lymphocytes to establish diagnosis
Prognostic marker assessment Flow cytometry for CD38 Immunostaining/flow cytometry for ZAP-70 Interphase FISH (assessment of deletion 17p, deletion 11q, trisomy 12, deletion 13) *IGHV* mutation status
Imaging studies (only if presenting with significant adenopathy or needed treatment); many clinical trials are now incorporating CT scans as per new guidelines, but these are not standard of care outside of a clinical trial. CT scan or PET scan (PET scan preferred if there is a suspicion of Richter transformation)

BUN, blood urea nitrogen; CBC, complete blood count; CLL, chronic lymphocytic leukemia; CT, computed tomography; FISH, fluorescent in situ hybridization; LDH, lactate dehydrogenase; MDACC, MD Anderson Cancer Center; PET, positron emission tomography.

Table 3-5 Established Poor Prognostic Factors in CLL

Male gender
Advanced Rai or Binet staging
Cytogenetic abnormalities [del(17p), del(11q), complex cytogenetics]
Lymphocyte doubling time <12 months
Initial lymphocyte count >50 × 10^9/L
Elevated serum TK
Elevated β_2-microglobulin
Elevated serum-soluble CD23
Higher CD38 expression
Higher ZAP-70 expression
Diffuse pattern of marrow involvement
Unmutated *IGHV* gene
Gene mutations (*TP53*, *BIRC3*, *NOTCH1*, *SF3B1*)

TK, thymidine kinase.

U/L had a significantly shorter progression-free survival (PFS) compared to those with TK levels below that level. Elevated serum β_2-M level is also an adverse prognostic feature that has been shown to correlate with clinical stage and disease progression. High serum LDH levels indicate a poor prognosis.

Fluorescent in situ hybridization, *IGHV* gene mutation status, ZAP-70 expression, and CD38 expression are well-established prognostic factors in CLL

TREATMENT

Indications for Treatment

Unlike most leukemias, an unusual feature of CLL is that making the diagnosis is not necessarily an indication to initiate treatment. Early treatment of asymptomatic CLL with chemotherapy was not shown to prolong survival. In the current era of more effective CIT regimens and targeted therapies, this question will likely be investigated again. The National Cancer Institute (NCI)-IWCLL criteria for treatment of CLL are summarized in Table 3-6. The NCI-IWCLL criteria for response assessment of CLL are summarized in Table 3-7.

First-Line Treatment

Chemoimmunotherapy has been the standard first-line treatment for patients with CLL ([1]).

Table 3-6 Indications for Treatment in CLL (NCI- IWCLL) ([18])

Active disease should be confirmed prior to initiating treatment.
1. Evidence of progressive marrow failure as manifest by the development or worsening of anemia and/or thrombocytopenia
2. Massive (ie, >6 cm below the left costal margin) or progressive or symptomatic splenomegaly
3. Massive nodes or clusters (ie, at least 10 cm in longest diameter) or progressive or symptomatic lymphadenopathy
4. Progressive lymphocytosis with an increase of >50% over a 2-month period or an anticipated doubling time of <6 months[a]
5. Autoimmune anemia and/or thrombocytopenia poorly responsive to corticosteroid therapy or other standard therapy
6. Constitutional symptoms, defined as any one or more of the following disease-related symptoms or signs: a. Unintentional weight loss ≥10% within the previous 6 months b. Significant fatigue (ie, ECOG PS 2 or worse; cannot work or unable to perform usual activities) c. Fevers >100.5°F or 38.0°C for ≥2 weeks without evidence of infection d. Night sweats for >1 month without evidence of infection

ECOG PS, Eastern Cooperative Oncology Group performance status; NCI-IWCLL, National Cancer Institute–International Workshop on Chronic Lymphocytic Leukemia.

[a]In patients with a lymphocyte count of $<30 \times 10^9$/L, lymphocyte doubling time should not be used as a single parameter to define treatment indication. Factors contributing to lymphocytosis or lymphadenopathy other than CLL (ie, infections) should be excluded.

Purine Analogues and Alkylating Agents

Alkylating agents such as chlorambucil or cyclophosphamide, either alone or in combination with corticosteroids, were the cornerstone of treatment of CLL for several decades. In 1988 to 1989, Grever et al and the MDACC group published the first results with fludarabine in patients with CLL ([22, 23]). In the MDACC study, a 5-day schedule of fludarabine in previously treated patients with CLL produced a complete remission (CR) rate of 15% and an overall response rate (ORR) of 44%. Different fludarabine regimens including the addition of prednisone ([24]), a 3-day schedule of fludarabine ([25]), and a once-a-week schedule of fludarabine ([26]) were studied at MDACC. The addition of prednisone to fludarabine did not improve response rates or survival; the incidence of opportunistic infections was increased. The response rate seen with the 3-day schedule of fludarabine was slightly less than that seen with the 5-day schedule but was associated with less immunosuppression and lower morbidity. The once-a-week schedule had an inferior response rate. Fludarabine, when compared to chlorambucil, produced significantly higher response rates in previously untreated patients with CLL (Cancer and Leukemia Group B [CALGB] 9011 trial) ([27]). In this study, 509 patients were randomized to receive fludarabine, chlorambucil, or both in combination. The combination arm was stopped early due to excessive infection-related toxicity. The fludarabine arm had significantly higher CR and ORR compared to patients treated with chlorambucil.

The German CLL Study Group (GCLLSG) CLL5 trial evaluated fludarabine versus chlorambucil as initial treatment for patients older than 65 years ([28]). Although treatment with fludarabine was associated with superior ORR, there was no improvement in PFS or overall survival (OS). The French Cooperative Group on CLL randomized 938 previously untreated patients to one of three treatment regimens: fludarabine, CHOP (cyclophosphamide, doxorubicin, vincristine, prednisone), or CAP (cyclophosphamide, doxorubicin, prednisone) ([29]). Higher ORR and longer time to progression were seen with fludarabine. Fludarabine in combination with cyclophosphamide (FC) was shown to be an effective regimen in CLL. Three large randomized trials (German CLL4 trial [[30]], US Intergroup E2997 trial [[31]], and UK LRF CLL4 trial [[32]]) evaluated the efficacy of FC versus fludarabine monotherapy in treatment-naïve CLL patients and reported superior PFS with the FC combination compared to fludarabine or chlorambucil monotherapy. E2997 was a phase III randomized trial comparing FC versus fludarabine monotherapy in patients with treatment-naïve CLL ([31]). A total of 278 patients were randomly assigned. Fludarabine/cyclophosphamide was

Table 3-7 Definition of Response[a]

Parameter	Complete Remission (CR)	Partial Remission (PR)	Progressive Disease (PD)
Group A			
Lymphadenopathy[b]	None >1.5 cm	Decrease ≥50%	Increase ≥50%
Hepatomegaly or splenomegaly[b]	Normal size	Decrease ≥50%	Increase ≥50%
Blood lymphocytes	$<4 \times 10^9$/L	Decrease ≥50% from baseline	Increase ≥50% from baseline
Bone marrow	Normocellular, <30% lymphocytes, no B-lymphoid nodules Hypocellular marrow defines CRi	50% reduction in marrow infiltrate, or B-lymphoid nodules	
Group B			
Neutrophils	$>1.5 \times 10^9$/L	$>1.5 \times 10^9$/L or 50% improvement from baseline	
Platelet count	$>100 \times 10^9$/L	$>100 \times 10^9$/L or increase ≥50% over baseline	Decrease ≥50% over baseline secondary to CLL
Hemoglobin	>11 g/dL	>11 g/dL or increase ≥50% over baseline	Decrease of >2 g/dL from baseline secondary to CLL

Group A criteria define tumor load, group B criteria define marrow function.
CR: All of the criteria have to be met, and patients have to lack disease-related constitutional symptoms.
CRi: Patients meeting all the criteria of CR except count recovery (unrelated to disease activity). Patients with meeting all CR criteria but with hypocellular marrow are also CRi.
PR: At least two of the group A criteria plus one of the group B criteria have to be met. To define a PR, these parameters need to be documented for at least 2 months.
Nodular PR: Patients meeting all the criteria of CR except with residual marrow nodules. Immunohistochemistry should be performed to define whether these nodules are composed of primarily T cells, lymphocytes other than chronic lymphocytic leukemia (CLL) cells, or CLL cells.
Stable disease (SD): Absence of PD and failure to achieve at least a PR. Stable disease is considered equivalent to nonresponse.
PD: At least one of the above criteria of group A or group B has to be met.
[a]National Cancer Institute—International Workshop Group on CLL ([18]).
[b]As assessed by physical examination (imaging studies for clinical trials).

associated with a higher CR (23.4% *vs* 4.6%; $P < .001$) and higher ORR (74.3% *vs* 59.5%; $P = .013$) compared to fludarabine monotherapy. The PFS was significantly improved for patients treated with FC compared to fludarabine alone (31.6 *vs* 19.2 months; $P < .0001$).

Bendamustine is an alkylating agent that has structural similarities to a purine analog. It consists of both a nitrogen mustard core and purine-like side group. Bendamustine has little cross-resistance with other alkylating agents. A pivotal phase III study comparing bendamustine to chlorambucil in patients with previously untreated CLL led to its approval by the US Food and Drug Administration (FDA) ([33]). A total of 319 patients were randomly assigned. Bendamustine led to a significantly higher ORR (68%) compared to chlorambucil (31%; $P < .0001$). Patients in the bendamustine arm, compared with the chlorambucil arm, had a higher CR rate (31% *vs* 2%) and longer PFS (21.6 *vs* 8.3 months; $P < .0001$).

Cladribine (2-chlorodeoxyadenosine; 2-CDA) and pentostatin have activity in treating CLL. The Polish Adult Leukemia Group (PALG)-CLL2 trial compared cladribine monotherapy, cladribine plus cyclophosphamide, and cladribine, cyclophosphamide, and mitoxantrone as initial therapy for patients with CLL. Although there was a higher CR rate in the mitoxantrone arm, there was no difference in PFS or OS among the three arms ([34]). The PALG-CLL3 phase III trial reported equivalent efficacy of fludarabine/cyclophosphamide versus cladribine/cyclophosphamide in patients with treatment-naïve CLL ([35]).

Monoclonal Antibodies

Rituximab

CD20 is a B-cell–specific surface antigen that is expressed on 95% of B cells. It is tightly bound to the cell surface and is not shed or internalized upon antibody binding. Rituximab is a chimeric antibody that targets the CD20 antigen. Rituximab can mediate cell lysis by various mechanisms, including antibody-dependent cellular cytotoxicity (ADCC), complement-dependent cytotoxicity (CDC), and direct induction of apoptosis. Standard-dose rituximab monotherapy has limited activity in treating patients with CLL. O'Brien et al conducted a dose-escalation study with rituximab; patients received an initial dose of 375 mg/m^2, and the dose was then escalated in cohorts to a maximum of 2,250 mg/m^2 ([36]). The response rate was 36% in patients with CLL, and the response correlated with the dose: 22% for patients treated at 500 to 825 mg/m², 43% for those treated at 1,000 to 1,500 mg/m², and 75% for those treated at the highest dose of 2,250 mg/m². Another dose-intensification strategy with administration of rituximab 375 mg/m² three times a week for 4 weeks yielded an ORR of 45% in patients with CLL ([37]).

Chemoimmunotherapy

A phase II trial (CALGB 9712 study) of sequential versus concurrent administration of fludarabine and rituximab in previously untreated patients with CLL was reported ([38]). Patients were randomized to receive either six monthly courses of fludarabine concurrently with rituximab followed 2 months later by four weekly doses of rituximab as consolidation or fludarabine alone for 6 months followed 2 months later by the same rituximab consolidation therapy. A total of 104 patients were randomized to the concurrent or sequential regimens. The ORR in the sequential arm was 77%, and the CR rate was 28%. The ORR in the concurrent arm was 90%, and the CR rate was 47%.

A CIT protocol developed at MDACC demonstrated the efficacy of combining rituximab with fludarabine and cyclophosphamide ([39, 40]). The regimen was as follows: fludarabine 25 mg/m² per day for 3 days, cyclophosphamide 250 mg/m² per day for 3 days, and rituximab 375 to 500 mg/m² on day 1 (FCR regimen). This was a single-arm study of FCR as initial therapy in 300 patients with progressive or advanced CLL. At a median follow-up of 6 years, the ORR was 95% (CR, 72%; nodular partial remission [PR], 10%; PR, 13%). The 6-year OS and failure-free survival rates were 77% and 51%, respectively. The median time to progression was 80 months. Of note, patients who attained a CR with negative flow cytometry had a superior time to progression (85 *vs* 49 months) and OS (84% *vs* 65% at 6 years).

The GCLLSG group conducted a phase III trial to evaluate the efficacy of FCR versus FC in first-line treatment of patients with advanced CLL (CLL8 trial) ([9]). A total of 817 patients were randomized to receive six courses of either FC (409 patients) or FCR (408 patients). The median age was 61 years (range, 30-81 years). They reported a significantly higher CR rate (44% *vs* 22%; $P < .0001$), ORR (90% *vs* 80%; $P < .0001$), PFS (median PFS, 52 *vs* 33 months; $P < .0001$), and OS (3-year OS, 87% *vs* 83%; $P = .012$) with the addition of rituximab. Treatment with FCR was associated with a higher incidence of grade 3 or 4 neutropenia (33.7% *vs* 21%; $P < .0001$); however, there was no difference in the incidence of grade 3 or 4 infections. This trial established the role of anti-CD20 monoclonal antibody (mAb) in the first-line therapy of CLL.

Bendamustine in combination with rituximab has also been evaluated as first-line treatment for patients with CLL. Fischer et al reported on the outcomes of 117 patients with treatment-naïve CLL who received bendamustine and rituximab (BR) ([41]). Eligibility criteria included creatinine clearance >30 mL/min. The ORR was 88% with a CR rate of 23%. The median PFS was 34 months. Notably, one-third of the patients had a creatinine clearance ≤70 mL/min (these patients are typically excluded from the FCR trials), and these patients did equally as well as patients with a creatinine clearance >70 mL/min.

The GCLLSG recently reported results of the randomized phase III study of FCR versus BR as first-line therapy for patients with CLL (CLL10 trial) ([42]). This trial included patients with CLL [non-del(17p)] and good physical status (Cumulative Illness Rating Scale [CIRS] score ≤6 and creatinine clearance ≥70 mL/min). A total of 282 patients received FCR, and 279 patients received BR. The FCR arm had a significantly higher CR/CR with incomplete count recovery (CRi) rate (39.7 *vs* 30.8; $P = .03$) and significantly improved PFS (median PFS, 55.2 *vs* 41.7 months; $P < .001$). Overall survival was not different between the two groups. Not unexpectedly, patients on the FCR arm experienced more grade 3 or 4 neutropenia (84.2% *vs* 59%; $P < .001$), more thrombocytopenia (21.5% *vs* 14.4%; $P = .03$), and increased risk of grade 3 or 4 infections (39.1% *vs* 26.8%; $P < .001$). However, the treatment-related mortality was similar in the two arms. For patients >65 years of age, there was no improvement in PFS noted with FCR compared to BR; however, there was an increased risk of infections in the older patients. Based on these data, FCR is the standard first-line CIT regimen for patients with CLL who are ≤65 years old. However, for patients who are older than 65 years and deemed fit to receive CIT, BR is the preferred first-line therapy. It is important to note that for patients with moderate renal dysfunction (creatinine clearance, 30-70 mL/min), FCR therapy can lead to significant cytopenias necessitating dose reductions or treatment discontinuations, and therefore, BR may be a better alternative in this group of patients. A list of published CIT trials in the first-line setting in patients with CLL is provided in Table 3-8.

Several studies have been conducted with the intent of modifying the FCR regimen by dose-intensifying rituximab ([43]), adding mitoxantrone ([44]), adding alemtuzumab ([45]), adding granulocyte-macrophage colony-stimulating factor ([46]), or using lower doses of FCR (FCR-Lite) ([47, 48]), but these studies have not shown superior results as compared to those seen with the standard FCR regimen.

Ofatumumab

Ofatumumab is a fully human IgG1 mAb that binds to a different epitope of CD20 than rituximab. Ofatumumab has higher CDC compared with rituximab ([49]).

Table 3-8 First-Line Chemoimmunotherapy Trials for CLL

Regimen	Trial	No. of Patients	Median Age (years)	CR (%)	ORR (%)	PFS (months)
FCR	MDACC ([39, 40])	300	57	72	95	80
	CLL8 trial (FCR arm) ([9])	408	61	44	90	52
	CLL10 trial (FCR arm) ([42])	282	61	40	95	55
	FCR-Lite ([47, 48])	63	58	73	94	70
BR	GCLLSG phase II ([41])	117	64	23	88	34
	CLL10 trial (BR arm) ([42])	279	62	31	96	42
FR	CALGB 9712 ([38])	104	63	47	84	42
PCR	Kay	64	63	41	91	33
FCO	Wierda	61	56	41	75	70% (1 yr)
PCO	Shanafelt	48	65	46	96	NR

BR, bendamustine, rituximab; CALGB, Cancer and Leukemia Group B; CR, complete response; FCO, fludarabine, cyclophosphamide, ofatumumab; FCR, fludarabine, cyclophosphamide, rituximab; FR, fludarabine, rituximab; GCLLSG, German Chronic Lymphocytic Leukemia Study Group; MDACC, MD Anderson Cancer Center; NR, not reported; ORR, overall response rate; PCO, pentostatin, cyclophosphamide, ofatumumab; PCR, pentostatin, cyclophosphamide, rituximab; PFS, progression-free survival.

Wierda et al reported a pivotal trial of ofatumumab monotherapy (weekly for 8 weeks, followed by four monthly infusions) in patients with fludarabine- and alemtuzumab-refractory CLL or fludarabine-refractory CLL with bulky lymph nodes ([50]). In a recent update of this study, the ORR was reported as 49% and 43%, respectively. The median PFS was 4.6 to 5.5 months, and the median OS was 13.9 to 17.4 months. Based on these data, ofatumumab was approved for patients with CLL refractory to fludarabine and alemtuzumab. Ofatumumab has also been combined with chlorambucil as first-line therapy in patients who were deemed ineligible for FCR-based regimens (COMPLEMENT-1 trial) ([51]). A total of 447 patients were randomized to receive chlorambucil +/– ofatumumab. The chlorambucil/ofatumumab combination, compared with chlorambucil alone, significantly improved ORR (82% *vs* 69%; $P < .001$) and PFS (median, 22.4 *vs* 13.1 months; $P < .001$) ([51]). Based on these results, the combination of ofatumumab and chlorambucil was approved for the first-line treatment of patients with CLL for whom fludarabine-based therapy is considered inappropriate.

Obinutuzumab

Obinutuzumab is a humanized type II CD20 mAb with a glycoengineered Fc domain that leads to enhanced ADCC compared with rituximab. This type II CD20 mAb is more effective at direct induction of CLL cell apoptosis, which leads to more effective B-cell depletion than rituximab. In the GCLLSG CLL11 trial, previously untreated patients with CLL with coexisting conditions (CIRS score >6 and/or creatinine clearance 30-69 mL/min) were randomly assigned to receive chlorambucil monotherapy, chlorambucil plus rituximab, or chlorambucil plus obinutuzumab ([52, 53]). A total of 781 patients were enrolled. The median age was 73 years. Treatment with obinutuzumab-chlorambucil, compared to rituximab-chlorambucil, resulted in a higher ORR of 78.4% (CR 20.7% + PR 57.7%) versus 65.1% (CR 7% + PR 58.1%; $P < .001$). Progression-free survival was significantly longer with obinutuzumab-chlorambucil compared to that seen with rituximab-chlorambucil (median PFS, 29.2 *vs* 15.4 months; $P < .001$) ([52, 53]). Infusion-related reactions and neutropenia were more common in the obinutuzumab-chlorambucil arm, but the risk of infection was not increased. Obinutuzumab-chlorambucil was superior to chlorambucil monotherapy for both PFS and OS. This trial established the combination of chlorambucil with a CD20 mAb as a standard of care for first-line therapy in older patients with CLL who have comorbidities. Based on the CLL11 trial, the FDA approved obinutuzumab in combination with chlorambucil for patients with previously untreated CLL.

Alemtuzumab

CD52 is a surface antigen abundantly expressed on CLL cells and normal B and T lymphocytes. Alemtuzumab is a humanized mAb targeting CD52. In the pivotal trial of alemtuzumab, 93 patients, all of whom were refractory to fludarabine, received alemtuzumab ([54]). Alemtuzumab was given intravenously three times weekly for a maximum of 12 weeks. The ORR was 33% (CR, 2%). Response rates were lower among patients with bulky disease. This trial led to FDA approval of this agent for fludarabine-refractory patients with CLL. Subcutaneous administration of alemtuzumab has similar efficacy in CLL as the intravenous administration, unlike in T-PLL ([55]). Hillmen et al conducted a phase III randomized trial (CAM307 trial) to evaluate the efficacy and safety of intravenous alemtuzumab compared with chlorambucil in the first-line treatment of patients with CLL ([56]). In this trial, 297 patients were randomized, 149 to alemtuzumab and 148 to chlorambucil. Alemtuzumab was found to produce a higher ORR (83% *vs* 55%; $P < .0001$) and CR rate (24% *vs* 2%; $P < .0001$) than chlorambucil. It led to superior PFS, with a 42% reduction in risk of progression or death (hazard ratio [HR] = 0.58; $P = .0001$). In addition, the elimination of minimal residual disease (MRD) occurred in 11 of 36 patients treated with alemtuzumab who attained CR compared to none of the patients treated with chlorambucil. Alemtuzumab was well tolerated but did lead to a higher risk of cytomegalovirus (CMV) infection. Because alemtuzumab acts via a p53 independent pathway, it was originally investigated as a promising strategy for patients with del(17p). However, somewhat disappointingly, patients with 17p deletion in the CAM307 trial, although faring better with alemtuzumab than chlorambucil, had a median PFS of only 10.8 months with alemtuzumab. In an attempt to improve upon the efficacy of FCR, a combination of alemtuzumab and FCR (CFAR) has been reported, both in the first-line and in the relapsed setting ([45, 57]). In the first-line CFAR trial, patients <70 years old with serum β_2-M ≥4 mg/L were enrolled. Sixty patients were treated. The ORR was 92%, with a CR rate of 70%. The time-to-event outcomes were comparable to the high-risk FCR-treated patients.

Two recent studies evaluated the combination of alemtuzumab and corticosteroids. In the UK CLL206 trial, the use of alemtuzumab with high-dose pulse methylprednisolone as first-line treatment for patients with del(17p) resulted in a high ORR of 88% with an impressive CR rate of 65%, but the median PFS was only 18.3 months ([58]). The French/German CLL20 trial combined alemtuzumab with dexamethasone followed by consolidation either with alemtuzumab or with an allogeneic stem-cell transplantation (allo-SCT) ([59]). Forty-two patients with del(17p) received first-line therapy with alemtuzumab and dexamethasone in this trial, with an ORR of 97% and a median PFS of 32.8 months. Consolidation with allo-SCT may have contributed to the improved outcomes. However, due to the introduction of novel targeted therapies, potential toxicities with alemtuzumab such as CMV reactivation, and the withdrawal of the drug from the commercial market, alemtuzumab has a limited role in the management of patients with CLL.

Patient Stratification for First-Line Treatment

Based on age, comorbidities, and FISH status, patients can be categorized into several groups:

- Intensive CIT eligible [non-del(17p)]: These are generally patients less than 65 years of age without significant comorbidities. Patients 65 to 70 years of age with good performance status can also be considered in this treatment group. The FCR regimen is the preferred first-line treatment option for these patients. The BR regimen is a reasonable first choice for patients age 65 years or older. For patients with renal impairment (creatinine clearance between 30 and 70 mL/min), BR is preferred over FCR.
- Intensive CIT ineligible [non-del(17p)]: These are generally patients over the age of 65 years or patients with comorbidities. For this group of patients, the combination of chlorambucil and obinutuzumab is the preferred treatment choice. The combination of chlorambucil with ofatumumab is another potential treatment option.
- Patients with del(17p): Patients with del(17p) or *TP53* gene mutation have poor outcomes with conventional CIT regimens such as FCR ([9, 40]). For patients with del(17p), ibrutinib, a Bruton tyrosine kinase (BTK) inhibitor, is the preferred first-line therapy, irrespective of the patient age (see the "Novel Targeted Therapies" section for details).
- Frail patients with significant comorbidities: The median age at the time of first treatment for CLL is around 76 to 77 years. Comorbid conditions and poor performance status can limit the ability of patients in this age group to receive CIT. For such patients, CD20 mAb therapy alone should be considered.

Minimal Residual Disease

Bottcher et al evaluated MRD by four-color flow-cytometry (sensitivity of at least 10^{-4}) in patients enrolled on the CLL8 trial ([60]). Minimal residual disease levels were characterized as low ($<10^{-4}$), intermediate ($\geq 10^{-4}$ to $<10^{-2}$), or high ($\geq 10^{-2}$). After completion of all therapy, there was a significantly higher proportion of patients with low-level MRD (MRD negative per IWCLL) in the FCR arm compared to the FC arm (peripheral blood: 63% *vs* 35%; $P < .0001$; bone marrow: 44% *vs* 28%; $P = .0007$). Achievement of MRD-negative remission was significantly associated with a longer PFS, and in a multivariable model, MRD remained predictive for PFS and OS. The MDACC group reported outcomes for MRD assessment in the bone marrow after first-line FCR therapy ([61]). At the final response assessment, 43% of patients were MRD negative. In a multivariable model, mutated *IGHV* gene and trisomy 12 were independently associated with achievement of MRD-negative remission. Evaluating MRD at the end of treatment is now being incorporated as an endpoint in most clinical trials.

Novel Targeted Therapies

These include B-cell receptor (BCR) inhibitors such as BTK inhibitors, phosphoinositide 3-kinase kinase (PI3K) inhibitors, and spleen tyrosine kinase (Syk) inhibitors.

Targeting Bcl-2, an antiapoptotic protein that is overexpressed in CLL cells, with the small-molecule inhibitor venetoclax represents another important novel strategy. Several studies were done with the immunomodulatory drug lenalidomide in patients with CLL. Immunotherapy with genetically modified T cells (chimeric antigen receptor [CAR]) represents another novel approach to target CLL cells. Preclinical data support the use of checkpoint inhibitors in patients with CLL ([62]), and clinical trials with agents targeting PD-1/PD-L1 are under way.

B-Cell Signaling Pathway Inhibitors

Chronic lymphocytic leukemia cells receive growth and survival signals from the microenvironment of bone marrow, lymph nodes, and spleen. Bruton tyrosine kinase is a central molecule in signal transduction for the BCR as well as CD19, CD38, CD40, CXCR4 chemokine receptor, tumor necrosis factor receptors, and toll-like receptors (TLRs). Other important signal transduction molecules include PI3K and Syk.

BTK Inhibitors

Bruton tyrosine kinase is a nonreceptor tyrosine kinase of the Tec kinase family and plays a crucial role in BCR signaling. Ibrutinib is an oral, selective, and irreversible inhibitor of BTK. It forms a covalent bond with the cysteine-481 of BTK. Byrd et al reported outcomes of 101 patients with relapsed or refractory CLL who received ibrutinib monotherapy ([63]). The median age was 64 years (range, 37-82 years). Thirty-four percent of the patients had del(17p), and 78% had unmutated *IGHV*. Fifty-nine percent of the patients had received four or more prior therapies. The ORR was 90%, with 7% CR, 65% PR, and 9% PR with lymphocytosis (PR-L). The estimated PFS at 30 months was 69%. The median PFS times for patients with del(17p) and del(11q) were 28 and 38.7 months, respectively, and were inferior to the PFS times of patients without del(17p) or del(11q). The most common toxicity was diarrhea, occurring in 55% of patients, the majority of whom had grade 1 or 2 diarrhea. Notable grade ≥3 adverse events were hypertension (20%), pneumonia (25%), neutropenia (18%), thrombocytopenia (10%), bleeding (8%), and atrial fibrillation (6%). In a randomized phase III trial (RESONATE trial), patients with relapsed or refractory CLL were randomized to ibrutinib (n = 195) or ofatumumab (n = 196). The ibrutinib arm had a much higher ORR and superior PFS and OS compared to the ofatumumab arm ([64]). Based on this trial, ibrutinib (420 mg orally once daily) was FDA approved for patients with relapsed/refractory CLL and for patients with del(17p). There are limited data with ibrutinib in the first-line setting. O'Brien et al reported on the outcomes of 31 patients with CLL who received ibrutinib monotherapy in the first-line setting ([65]). The median age was 71 years (range, 65-84 years). After a median follow-up of 35 months, an ORR of 84% was noted, with 23% attaining CR ([66]). The 30-month PFS and OS rates were 96% and 97%, respectively.

It is important to note that most patients will develop lymphocytosis upon initiating ibrutinib. This is expected with ibrutinib and other BCR inhibitors, and it generally resolves over the course of 6 to 9 months with continued treatment. Development of lymphocytosis does not appear to be detrimental to the long-term clinical outcomes.

Mechanisms of ibrutinib resistance remain an area of active research. Several of the patients who progressed on ibrutinib were found to have mutation of *BTK* at cysteine-481 (C481S) and gain-of-function mutations in *PLCγ2*, a signaling molecule downstream of BTK ([67]). Several other BTK inhibitors are in clinical development, including ACP-196 and ONO-4059.

PI3K Inhibitors

PI3K-δ is a critical kinase for activation, proliferation, and survival of B cells and is hyperactive in many B-cell malignancies, including CLL. Idelalisib is a potent, selective, reversible inhibitor of PI3K-δ. A phase I trial of idelalisib was conducted in relapsed and refractory patients with CLL ([68]). A total of 54 patients were enrolled with a median age of 62.5 years (range, 37-82 years). Twenty-four percent of the patients had del(17p) or *TP53* mutation, and 91% had unmutated *IGHV*. The median number of prior therapies was five. Patients were treated at one of six dose levels of oral idelalisib (range, 50-350 mg once or twice daily). The ORR was 72% (39% PR, 33% PR-L). The median PFS was 15.8 months. The most commonly observed grade ≥3 adverse events were pneumonia (20%), neutropenic fever (11%), and diarrhea (6%). Transaminitis of any grade was observed in 15 patients (28%); only one patient experienced a grade ≥3 transaminitis. A phase III clinical trial evaluated the activity of idelalisib/rituximab versus rituximab/placebo in patients with relapsed/refractory CLL in whom rituximab monotherapy would be considered appropriate (not able to receive cytotoxic agents for one or more of the following reasons: severe neutropenia or thrombocytopenia caused by cumulative myelotoxicity from previous therapies, creatinine clearance <60 mL/min, or a CIRS score of >6) ([69]). A total of 220 patients were enrolled. Idelalisib 150 mg was dosed twice daily continuously in 110 patients. Rituximab was administered to all patients at 375 mg/m^2 for the first dose and then at 500 mg/m^2 every 2 weeks for four doses and then every 4 weeks for three doses (eight total doses). This trial demonstrated superior efficacy for combined idelalisib and rituximab over rituximab and placebo, with an HR for PFS of 0.15 ($P < .001$) and HR for OS of 0.28

(P = .02). Pneumonitis was seen in 4% of the patients treated on the idelalisib/rituximab arm. This trial led to the FDA approval of the combination of idelalisib and rituximab for patients with relapsed/refractory CLL in whom rituximab monotherapy would be considered appropriate.

There are limited data in the first-line setting with idelalisib. In a recent report, idelalisib monotherapy (150 mg twice a day) was given as first-line therapy to patients ≥65 years with CLL ([70]). A total of 37 patients were treated. Fourteen percent of the patients had del(17p). In the 27 evaluable patients, an ORR of 81% (all PR/PR-L) was noted. Pneumonitis was seen in two patients. The combination of idelalisib and rituximab has also been reported in the first-line setting for patients ≥65 years old with CLL ([71]). A total of 64 patients were enrolled. The ORR was 97%, with a CR rate of 19%. However, toxicities were common with this regimen; the important grade ≥3 adverse events included diarrhea/colitis (42%), pneumonia (19%), rash (13%), and transaminitis (23%). Colitis is a late event, with a median time to onset of around 9 months. Toxicities observed with idelalisib may be immune-mediated. Besides idelalisib, several other PI3K inhibitors are in clinical development in CLL, including duvelisib (IPI-145) (PI3K-γ and -δ inhibitor) and TGR-1202 (PI3K-δ inhibitor).

BCL-2 Inhibitors

CLL cells express high levels of antiapoptotic proteins of the Bcl-2 family, rendering them long-lived and resistant to senescence and death. Navitoclax (ABT-263) is an orally administered small-molecule inhibitor of Bcl-2, Bcl-w, and Bcl-xL. A phase I/II trial of orally administered navitoclax reported antitumor activity in patients with CLL; however, dose-limiting toxicity was thrombocytopenia ([72]). Thrombocytopenia was secondary to the accelerated platelet senescence from inhibition of Bcl-xL in the platelets. Venetoclax (ABT-199) was designed as a molecule with greater affinity for Bcl-2 and reduced affinity for Bcl-xL ([73]). Preliminary reports suggested monotherapy activity of venetoclax in patients with relapsed/refractory CLL with an ORR of 77% and CR/CRi rate of 23% ([74]). Notably, the CR rate is higher than that seen in BCR inhibitors in relapsed or refractory CLL.

Lenalidomide

Lenalidomide is an immunomodulatory drug with multiple effects on the tumor microenvironment and immune system, including downregulation of immune checkpoint PD-1 on T cells ([75]). Lenalidomide monotherapy was initially studied in relapsed or refractory CLL given either as continuous or interrupted (21 of 28 days) administration of up to 25 mg daily; the reported ORR was 32% to 47%, with 7% to 9% achieving CR, including patients who achieved MRD-negative remission ([76, 77]). Importantly, the responses were independent of the high-risk features including del(17p) and del(11q). Based on these encouraging results, the MDACC group explored lenalidomide monotherapy as first-line therapy for patients with CLL ([78, 79]). Treatment consisted of continuous lenalidomide 5 mg daily. The dose of lenalidomide could be escalated by 5 mg per cycle to the maximum daily dose of 25 mg. A total of 60 patients were enrolled. The ORR was 65%, with 10% CR rate. The median time to best response was 25 months. The estimated 2-year PFS was 60%. Tumor flare, noted in 52% of the patients, was associated with an improved PFS. The MDACC group reported results of the combination of lenalidomide and rituximab, both in the first-line and relapsed setting for patients with CLL ([80]). In the first-line setting, treatment consisted of rituximab 375 mg/m^2 given weekly for 4 weeks then monthly during months 3 to 12 and continuous lenalidomide 10 mg daily from day 9 onward. Forty-eight patients were evaluable. The ORR was 83%, with a CR rate of 15%. Improvement in immunoglobulin levels and T-cell function was noted after lenalidomide treatment, suggesting immune restoration ([75]). Future studies, likely in combination with targeted agents, will further clarify the role of lenalidomide in the treatment of CLL.

Chimeric Antigen Receptor T-Cell Therapy

Chimeric antigen receptors are engineered immune receptors introduced ex vivo into T cells, usually autologous, that redirect these cells to react against CLL cells. The CAR is a recombinant protein composed of an antigen-binding domain derived from single-chain immunoglobulin variable genes and intracellular signaling domains derived from CD3ζ and costimulatory domains derived from CD28 and/or CD137. The transduced T cells are infused into the patient, where they bind to the target antigen and induce T-cell activation and proliferation, cytokine production, and killing of cells expressing the target antigen. CD19 is the most common target of the current CAR T-cell trials, although other targets are being explored as well. Early clinical data are promising, and long-term outcomes are awaited ([81, 82]).

Stem-Cell Transplantation

Because CLL is a disease of older adults, reduced-intensity conditioning (RIC) allo-SCT is the most common type of transplantation offered to patients with CLL. Reduced-intensity conditioning allo-SCT in CLL leads to 5-year event-free survival and OS rates of 35% to 45% and 50% to 60%, respectively ([83]). Khouri et al reviewed outcomes of 86 patients with CLL who underwent RIC allo-SCT at MDACC ([84]). The median age was 58 years. Eighty-three of the 86 patients experienced donor cell engraftment. Overall, the estimated 5-year PFS and OS rates were 36% and 51%, respectively. Notably, immune manipulation by withdrawal of immunosuppression or donor lymphocyte infusions enhanced clinical responses, indicating that CLL is a disease sensitive to immune manipulation. With the introduction of novel targeted therapies, the indications for an allo-SCT in patients with CLL need to be revisited. Allogeneic stem-cell transplantation will likely continue to remain an important strategy for selected group of patients, such as those with high-risk CLL [del(17p) or del(11q) or *TP53* mutation] who have experienced relapse with or are refractory to novel agents.

Supportive Care

Patients with CLL can have a host of complications ranging from immune cytopenias to infectious issues. Supportive care maneuvers are delineated in Table 3-9.

Autoimmune Complications of Chronic Lymphocytic Leukemia

Autoimmune hemolytic anemia (AIHA), autoimmune thrombocytopenia (ITP), and pure red cell aplasia develop in some patients with CLL. The incidence of AIHA is 4% to 11% and that of ITP is 2% to 3% ([85]).

Table 3-9 Supportive Care for Patients With CLL

Situation	Treatment Regimen
Antibiotic prophylaxis	Acyclovir/valacyclovir for herpes virus Trimethoprim/sulfamethoxazole for PCP If getting alemtuzumab: valganciclovir during and 2 months after treatment
Blood transfusions	Blood products should be irradiated (prevents graft-versus-host disease)
Recurrent infections	Antibiotics, antifungals, antiviral agents If IgG <500 mg/dL, and recurrent severe infections, start IVIG every month (0.5 g/kg)

IgG, immunoglobulin G; IVIG, intravenous immunoglobulin; PCP, *Pneumocystis carinii* pneumonia.

Pure red cell aplasia is least common. The autoantibodies in CLL are typically polyclonal and usually IgG, indicating that they are not produced by the leukemic clone. The severity of the autoimmune complications does not necessarily correlate with the severity of CLL, and such events may develop in patients with early stages of the disease. Prednisone is the usual treatment for AIHA and ITP, with a high likelihood of response. However, the majority of patients relapse when treatment is stopped. Intravenous immunoglobulin produces response in 40% of patients, but these responses tend to be transient. CD20 mAb, particularly rituximab, has also been used to treat autoimmune complications of CLL, either as monotherapy or in combination with cyclophosphamide and dexamethasone (RCD regimen) ([86]). Cyclosporine is another option for treatment of immune-mediated cytopenias and can produce responses even in patients with steroid-refractory immune cytopenias ([87]). Splenectomy is reserved for refractory cases.

Hypogammaglobulinemia

Hypogammaglobulinemia is a frequent complication of CLL. The most common cause of morbidity in patients with CLL is infection, in part due to hypogammaglobulinemia. A randomized study evaluated the use of intravenous immunoglobulin (IVIG) versus placebo in patients with CLL and showed significant reduction in bacterial infections, but no difference in the number of life-threatening infections or nonbacterial infections ([88]). Replacement therapy with IVIG is indicated for patients with hypogammaglobulinemia and severe repeated infections.

TRANSFORMATION

Richter Syndrome

The term Richter syndrome (RS) refers to the development of aggressive large-cell lymphoma during the course of CLL. Rarely, disease transformation to Hodgkin lymphoma is seen. Richter syndrome is seen in approximately 5% of patients with CLL. Richter syndrome is usually associated with worsening systemic symptoms, including B symptoms, elevated LDH, rapid tumor growth, and/or extranodal involvement. Diagnosis requires tissue biopsy. Positron emission tomography scans help identify sites to direct tissue biopsy, and every attempt should be made to biopsy the site with the maximum standardized uptake value ([89]). In 80% of patients, the diffuse large B-cell lymphoma (DLBCL) is clonally related to the original CLL, which is a marker of poor prognosis (median survival, approximately 1 year). In the other 20% of patients, the DLBCL is clonally unrelated to the original CLL, possibly representing a new neoplasm, and the prognosis is similar to de novo DLBCL (median survival, approximately 5 years). Risk factors associated with development of RS in a patient with CLL include lymph node size of >3 cm, number of prior therapies, advanced Rai stage (III-IV), del(17p), del(11q), unmutated *IGHV* gene, short telomere length (<5,000 bp), stereotyped B-cell receptors, and expression of CD38, CD49d, or ZAP-70 [90]. Presence of *NOTCH1* mutation is also associated with increased risk of RS. *TP53* mutation is commonly acquired at the time of CLL transformation [90]. Other common genetic abnormalities seen in patients with RS include activation of *C-MYC* and inactivation of *CDKN2A*, indicating possible cell cycle deregulation, and *NOTCH1* mutations (commonly in conjunction with trisomy 12) [91, 92]. The traditional treatment strategy has been intensive CIT such as OFAR (oxaliplatin, fludarabine, cytarabine, and rituximab), Hyper-CVAD (hyperfractionated cyclophosphamide, vincristine, doxorubicin, and dexamethasone), and rituximab plus CHOP [93]. Allogeneic stem-cell transplantation remains the only potentially curative option for patients with RS.

Prolymphocytic Transformation

The NCI-IWCLL criteria allow a diagnosis of CLL to be made in the presence of ≤55% prolymphocytes. The presence of >55% prolymphocytes indicates prolymphocytic transformation. Prolymphocytic leukemia is characterized by a high number of circulating prolymphocytes, splenomegaly, minimal lymphadenopathy, and a median survival of less than 3 years.

HAIRY CELL LEUKEMIA

Hairy cell leukemia is an uncommon B-cell lymphoproliferative disorder affecting adults and represents 2% of all leukemia. There is a marked male preponderance. Most patients have cytopenias; splenomegaly is also frequent at presentation. Hairy cells can be seen in peripheral blood, but their numbers vary. Hairy cells are twice as large as normal lymphocytes, with the nuclei showing a loose chromatin pattern and villus-like cytoplasmic projections (Fig. 3-8) (best viewed under phase-contrast microscopy). Hairy cells typically show positive staining for tartrate-resistant acid phosphatase (TRAP) (Fig. 3-9). Hairy cells infiltrate the bone marrow in an interstitial or focal pattern, with clear zones between cells ("fried-egg" appearance) (Fig. 3-10). Marrow reticulin is increased, and aspirates may result in "dry tap."

Immunophenotypic analysis of hairy cells shows the

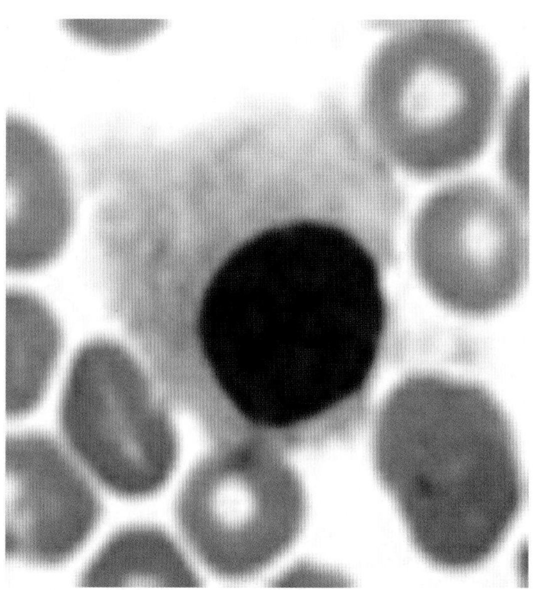

FIGURE 3-8 Hairy cell in peripheral blood with cytoplasmic projections.

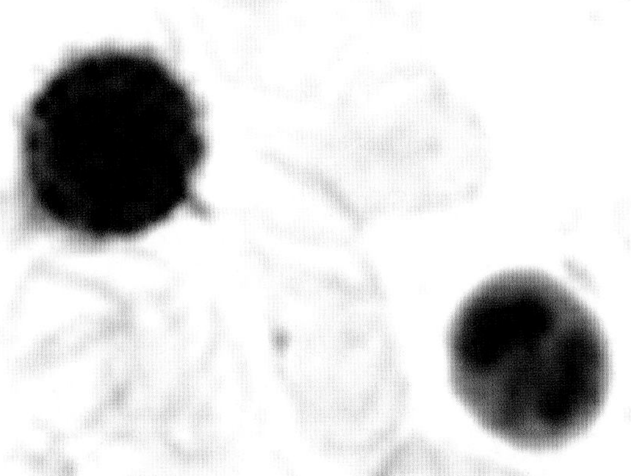

FIGURE 3-9 Hairy cell staining for tartrate-resistant acid phosphatase (*left*). Note the absence of orange-brown staining in a neutrophil.

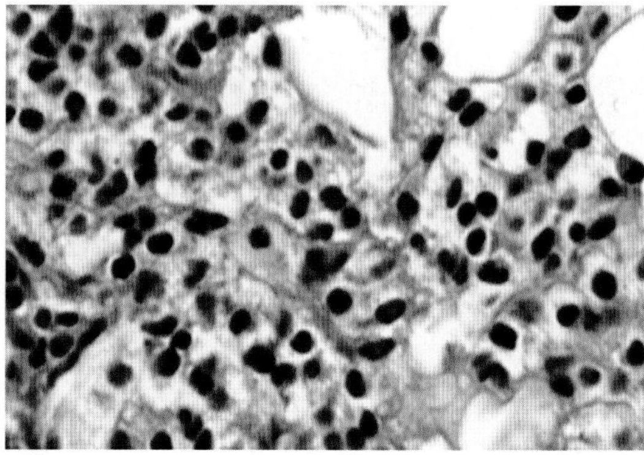

FIGURE 3-10 Bone marrow involvement by hairy cell leukemia showing "fried-egg" appearance (hematoxylin and eosin stain).

presence of CD19, CD20, CD22, CD25, and CD103; in contrast to CLL, hairy cells are negative for CD5 and CD23. Hairy cells also stain strongly for surface immunoglobulin and FMC-7. The *BRAF V600E* mutation was recently found to be present in all patients with HCL ([94]). This may have implications for both diagnosis and treatment of HCL, and vemurafenib, a BRAF inhibitor, is currently in clinical trials as therapy for relapsed or refractory HCL.

Treatment decisions are usually based on the degree of cytopenia and accompanying complications (eg, bleeding, infections, anemia). Pentostatin and cladribine (2-CDA) are the nucleoside analogs that are the mainstay of treatment of HCL. Pentostatin is administered at 4 mg/m^2 every 2 weeks until maximum response, and 2-CDA is given at 0.1 mg/kg/d as a continuous intravenous (IV) infusion for 7 days, or the same total dose can be administered as a 2-hour infusion over 5 days. Because 2-CDA offers a more convenient schedule (single course of therapy) and produces remission rates comparable to those achieved with pentostatin, 2-CDA is more frequently used. Estey et al reported a CR rate of 78% with 2-CDA in patients who had newly diagnosed or previously treated HCL ([95]). One trial evaluated a strategy to improve the initial response to nucleoside analog therapy by adding additional doses of rituximab. Patients received 2-CDA (5.6 mg/m^2 intravenously over 2 hours per day for 5 consecutive days) followed approximately 4 weeks later with rituximab (375 mg/m^2 intravenously weekly for eight doses) ([96]). A CR rate of 100% was reported, and after a median follow-up period of 25 months, the median CR duration, PFS, and OS had not been reached. The majority of relapsed patients achieve second remission when retreated with pentostatin or 2-CDA. The choice of agent may depend on the duration of the first remission: if <3 years, use an alternate agent; if >5 years, use the same agent. Splenectomy, although performed infrequently, can induce hematologic remission. The use of interferon-α is currently limited to patients unresponsive to nucleoside analogs. Rituximab can play a role in patients with relapsed or primary refractory HCL after purine analogs. A percentage of patients may relapse with 2-CDA–resistant disease. In addition, 10% to 20% of patients have a variant form of HCL with high numbers of circulating hairy cells and a poor response to nucleoside analogues. Classic and variant hairy cells strongly express CD22. Recombinant immunotoxin, BL22, has been used in the treatment of chemotherapy-resistant HCL. Moxetumomab pasudotox (HA22 or CAT-8015) is derived from BL22, selected for high-affinity for CD22, and is in clinical trials in patients with HCL.

PROLYMPHOCYTIC LEUKEMIA

Prolymphocytic leukemia is characterized by splenomegaly, a high number of circulating prolymphocytes, minimal lymphadenopathy, and a median survival of less than 3 years. Prolymphocytes are larger and less homogenous than CLL cells; they have abundant clear cytoplasm, clumped chromatin, and a prominent nucleolus (see Figs. 3-7**A**, **B** and **C**). Prolymphocytes can be of either B- or T-cell type. B-cell PLL cells usually do not express CD5 but stain strongly for surface immunoglobulin and FMC-7 (see Table 3-2). T-cell PLL demonstrates postthymic T-cell nature (TdT$^-$, CD1a$^-$, CD5$^+$, CD2$^+$, CD7$^+$). A majority of the cases express CD4$^+$ and are CD8$^-$. Chromosomal abnormalities of chromosome 14 are present in >75% of patients. TCL-1 is commonly overexpressed and detectable by immunohistochemistry.

For T-PLL, alemtuzumab IV is the treatment of choice. Dearden et al reported superior results in the first-line setting with IV alemtuzumab compared to subcutaneous alemtuzumab ([97]). With IV alemtuzumab, an ORR of 91% and CR rate of 81% were reported. Allogeneic stem-cell transplantation is the preferred consolidation regimen. Pentostatin should be considered for patients with poor response to alemtuzumab or relapsed disease. Retreatment with alemtuzumab is a reasonable option if the duration of the first remission was >12 months.

LARGE GRANULAR LYMPHOCYTIC LEUKEMIA

Large granular lymphocytes (LGLs) are larger than normal lymphocytes and contain azurophilic granules in their cytoplasm (see Fig. 3-6). They normally comprise 10% to 15% of peripheral blood mononuclear cells. Clonal expansion of LGLs can arise from either of the normal cellular counterparts and so may have a natural killer (NK)- or T-cell phenotype; the T-cell phenotype composes 80% of LGL leukemias. T-cell LGL cells have a CD3$^+$/CD57$^+$/CD56$^-$ immunophenotype, and NK-cell LGL cells are CD3$^-$/CD56+/CD57$^-$ ([98]). T-cell receptor gene rearrangement studies can help establish the clonality. More recently, around 40% of NK- and T-cell LGL leukemia patients were noted to have mutations in the *STAT3* gene ([99]). Mutations in *STAT5b* were noted in a smaller subset (2%) of patients ([100]). The clinical presentation of LGL leukemia is usually indolent. Cytopenias including neutropenia with accompanying infections, thrombocytopenia, and anemia are common. A small percentage of LGL leukemia patients develop a more aggressive course; these cases tend to have an NK-cell phenotype. Several therapies, including low-dose methotrexate, oral cyclosporine, and oral cyclophosphamide with or without oral prednisone, have all been effective.

REFERENCES

1. Jain N, O'Brien S. Initial treatment of CLL: integrating biology and functional status. *Blood*. 2015;126:463-470.
2. Linet MS, Schubauer-Berigan MK, Weisenburger DD, et al. Chronic lymphocytic leukaemia: an overview of aetiology in light of recent developments in classification and pathogenesis. *Br J Haematol*. 2007;139:672-686.
3. Mak V, Ip D, Mang O, et al. Preservation of lower incidence of chronic lymphocytic leukemia in Chinese residents in British Columbia: a 26-year survey from 1983 to 2008. *Leuk Lymphoma*. 2014;55:824-827.
4. Brown JR. Inherited susceptibility to chronic lymphocytic leukemia: evidence and prospects for the future. *Ther Adv Hematol*. 2013;4:298-308.
5. Berndt SI, Skibola CF, Joseph V, et al. Genome-wide association study identifies multiple risk loci for chronic lymphocytic leukemia. *Nat Genet*. 2013;45:868-876.
6. Speedy HE, Di Bernardo MC, Sava GP, et al. A genome-wide association study identifies multiple susceptibility loci for chronic lymphocytic leukemia. *Nat Genet*. 2014;46:56-60.
7. Damle RN, Wasil T, Fais F, et al. Ig V gene mutation status and CD38 expression as novel prognostic indicators in chronic lymphocytic leukemia. *Blood*. 1999;94:1840-1847.
8. Hamblin TJ, Davis Z, Gardiner A, Oscier DG, Stevenson FK. Unmutated Ig V(H) genes are associated with a more aggressive form of chronic lymphocytic leukemia. *Blood*. 1999;94:1848-1854.
9. Hallek M, Fischer K, Fingerle-Rowson G, et al. Addition of rituximab to fludarabine and cyclophosphamide in patients with chronic lymphocytic leukaemia: a randomised, open-label, phase 3 trial. *Lancet*. 2010;376:1164-1174.
10. Crespo M, Bosch F, Villamor N, et al. ZAP-70 expression as a surrogate for immunoglobulin-variable-region mutations in chronic lymphocytic leukemia. *N Engl J Med*. 2003;348:1764-1775.
11. Rassenti LZ, Huynh L, Toy TL, et al. ZAP-70 compared with immunoglobulin heavy-chain gene mutation status as a predictor of disease progression in chronic lymphocytic leukemia. *N Engl J Med*. 2004;351:893-901.
12. Dohner H, Stilgenbauer S, Benner A, et al. Genomic aberrations and survival in chronic lymphocytic leukemia. *N Engl J Med*. 2000;343:1910-1916.
13. Dohner H, Stilgenbauer S, Dohner K, Bentz M, Lichter P. Chromosome aberrations in B-cell chronic lymphocytic leukemia: reassessment based on molecular cytogenetic analysis. *J Mol Med*. 1999;77:266-281.
14. Puente XS, Pinyol M, Quesada V, et al. Whole-genome sequencing identifies recurrent mutations in chronic lymphocytic leukaemia. *Nature*. 2011;475:101-105.
15. Wang L, Lawrence MS, Wan Y, et al. SF3B1 and other novel cancer genes in chronic lymphocytic leukemia. *N Engl J Med*. 2011;365:2497-2506.
16. Quesada V, Conde L, Villamor N, et al. Exome sequencing identifies recurrent mutations of the splicing factor SF3B1 gene in chronic lymphocytic leukemia. *Nat Genet*. 2012;44:47-52.
17. Strati P, Shanafelt T. Monoclonal B-cell lymphocytosis and early stage CLL: diagnosis, natural history, and risk stratification. *Blood*. 2015;126:454-462.
18. Hallek M, Cheson BD, Catovsky D, et al. Guidelines for the diagnosis and treatment of chronic lymphocytic leukemia: a report from the International Workshop on Chronic Lymphocytic Leukemia updating the National Cancer Institute-Working Group 1996 guidelines. *Blood*. 2008;111:5446-5456.
19. Effects of chlorambucil and therapeutic decision in initial forms of chronic lymphocytic leukemia (stage A): results of a randomized clinical trial on 612 patients. The French Cooperative Group on Chronic Lymphocytic Leukemia. *Blood*. 1990;75:1414-1421.
20. Montserrat E, Vinolas N, Reverter JC, Rozman C. Natural history of chronic lymphocytic leukemia: on the progression and progression and prognosis of early clinical stages. *Nouv Rev Fr Hematol*. 1988;30:359-361.
21. Rossi D, Rasi S, Spina V, et al. Integrated mutational and cytogenetic analysis identifies new prognostic subgroups in chronic lymphocytic leukemia. *Blood*. 2013;121:1403-1412.
22. Grever MR, Kopecky KJ, Coltman CA, et al. Fludarabine monophosphate: a potentially useful agent in chronic lymphocytic leukemia. *Nouv Rev Fr Hematol*. 1988;30:457-459.
23. Keating MJ, Kantarjian H, Talpaz M, et al. Fludarabine: a new agent with major activity against chronic lymphocytic leukemia. *Blood*. 1989;74:19-25.
24. O'Brien S, Kantarjian H, Beran M, et al. Results of fludarabine and prednisone therapy in 264 patients with chronic lymphocytic leukemia with multivariate analysis-derived prognostic model for response to treatment. *Blood*. 1993;82:1695-1700.
25. Robertson LE, O'Brien S, Kantarjian H, et al. A 3-day schedule of fludarabine in previously treated chronic lymphocytic leukemia. *Leukemia*. 1995;9:1444-1449.
26. Kemena A, O'Brien S, Kantarjian H, et al. Phase II clinical trial of fludarabine in chronic lymphocytic leukemia on a weekly low-dose schedule. *Leuk Lymphoma*. 1993;10:187-193.
27. Rai KR, Peterson BL, Appelbaum FR, et al. Fludarabine compared with chlorambucil as primary therapy for chronic lymphocytic leukemia. *N Engl J Med*. 2000;343:1750-1757.
28. Eichhorst BF, Busch R, Stilgenbauer S, et al. First-line therapy with fludarabine compared with chlorambucil does not result in a major benefit for elderly patients with advanced chronic lymphocytic leukemia. *Blood*. 2009;114:3382-3391.
29. Leporrier M, Chevret S, Cazin B, et al. Randomized comparison of fludarabine, CAP, and ChOP in 938 previously untreated stage B and C chronic lymphocytic leukemia patients. *Blood*. 2001;98:2319-2325.
30. Eichhorst BF, Busch R, Hopfinger G, et al. Fludarabine plus cyclophosphamide versus fludarabine alone in first-line therapy of younger patients with chronic lymphocytic leukemia. *Blood*. 2006;107:885-891.
31. Flinn IW, Neuberg DS, Grever MR, et al. Phase III trial of fludarabine plus cyclophosphamide compared with fludarabine for patients with previously untreated chronic lymphocytic leukemia: US Intergroup Trial E2997. *J Clin Oncol*. 2007;25:793-798.
32. Catovsky D, Richards S, Matutes E, et al. Assessment of fludarabine plus cyclophosphamide for patients with chronic lymphocytic leukaemia (the LRF CLL4 Trial): a randomised controlled trial. *Lancet*. 2007;370:230-239.
33. Knauf WU, Lissichkov T, Aldaoud A, et al. Phase III randomized study of bendamustine compared with chlorambucil in previously untreated patients with chronic lymphocytic leukemia. *J Clin Oncol*. 2009;27:4378-4384.
34. Robak T, Blonski JZ, Gora-Tybor J, et al. Cladribine alone and in combination with cyclophosphamide or cyclophosphamide plus mitoxantrone in the treatment of progressive chronic lymphocytic leukemia: report of a prospective, multicenter, randomized trial of the Polish Adult Leukemia Group (PALG CLL2). *Blood*. 2006;108:473-479.
35. Robak T, Jamroziak K, Gora-Tybor J, et al. Comparison of cladribine plus cyclophosphamide with fludarabine plus cyclophosphamide as first-line therapy for chronic lymphocytic leukemia: a phase III randomized study by the Polish Adult Leukemia

Group (PALG-CLL3 Study). *J Clin Oncol.* 2010;28:1863-1869.
36. O'Brien SM, Kantarjian H, Thomas DA, et al. Rituximab dose-escalation trial in chronic lymphocytic leukemia. *J Clin Oncol.* 2001;19:2165-2170.
37. Byrd JC, Murphy T, Howard RS, et al. Rituximab using a thrice weekly dosing schedule in B-cell chronic lymphocytic leukemia and small lymphocytic lymphoma demonstrates clinical activity and acceptable toxicity. *J Clin Oncol.* 2001;19:2153-2164.
38. Woyach JA, Ruppert AS, Heerema NA, et al. Chemoimmunotherapy with fludarabine and rituximab produces extended overall survival and progression-free survival in chronic lymphocytic leukemia: long-term follow-up of CALGB study 9712. *J Clin Oncol.* 2011;29:1349-1355.
39. Keating MJ, O'Brien S, Albitar M, et al. Early results of a chemoimmunotherapy regimen of fludarabine, cyclophosphamide, and rituximab as initial therapy for chronic lymphocytic leukemia. *J Clin Oncol.* 2005;23:4079-4088.
40. Tam CS, O'Brien S, Wierda W, et al. Long-term results of the fludarabine, cyclophosphamide, and rituximab regimen as initial therapy of chronic lymphocytic leukemia. *Blood.* 2008;112:975-980.
41. Fischer K, Cramer P, Busch R, et al. Bendamustine in combination with rituximab for previously untreated patients with chronic lymphocytic leukemia: a multicenter phase II trial of the German Chronic Lymphocytic Leukemia Study Group. *J Clin Oncol.* 2012;30:3209-3216.
42. Eichhorst B, Fink AM, Busch R, et al. Frontline chemoimmunotherapy with fludarabine (F), cyclophosphamide (C), and rituximab (R) (FCR) shows superior efficacy in comparison to bendamustine (B) and rituximab (BR) in previously untreated and physically fit patients (pts) with advanced chronic lymphocytic leukemia (CLL): final analysis of an international, randomized study of the German CLL Study Group (GCLLSG) (CLL10 Study). *Blood.* 2014;124:19a.
43. O'Brien S, Wierda WG, Faderl S, et al. FCR-3 as frontline therapy for patients with chronic lymphocytic leukemia (CLL). *Blood.* 2005;106:2117a.
44. Faderl S, Wierda W, O'Brien S, Ferrajoli A, Lerner S, Keating MJ. Fludarabine, cyclophosphamide, mitoxantrone plus rituximab (FCM-R) in frontline CLL <70 Years. *Leukemia Res.* 2010;34:284-288.
45. Parikh SA, Keating MJ, O'Brien S, et al. Frontline chemoimmunotherapy with fludarabine, cyclophosphamide, alemtuzumab, and rituximab for high-risk chronic lymphocytic leukemia. *Blood.* 2011;118:2062-2068.
46. Strati P, Ferrajoli A, Lerner S, et al. Fludarabine, cyclophosphamide and rituximab plus granulocyte macrophage colony-stimulating factor as frontline treatment for patients with chronic lymphocytic leukemia. *Leuk Lymphoma.* 2014;55:828-833.
47. Foon KA, Mehta D, Lentzsch S, et al. Long-term results of chemoimmunotherapy with low-dose fludarabine, cyclophosphamide and high-dose rituximab as initial treatment for patients with chronic lymphocytic leukemia. *Blood.* 2012;119:3184-3185.
48. Foon KA, Boyiadzis M, Land SR, et al. Chemoimmunotherapy with low-dose fludarabine and cyclophosphamide and high dose rituximab in previously untreated patients with chronic lymphocytic leukemia. *J Clin Oncol.* 2009;27:498-503.
49. Pawluczkowycz AW, Beurskens FJ, Beum PV, et al. Binding of submaximal C1q promotes complement-dependent cytotoxicity (CDC) of B cells opsonized with anti-CD20 mAbs ofatumumab (OFA) or rituximab (RTX): considerably higher levels of CDC are induced by OFA than by RTX. *J Immunol.* 2009;183:749-758.
50. Wierda WG, Kipps TJ, Mayer J, et al. Ofatumumab as single-agent CD20 immunotherapy in fludarabine-refractory chronic lymphocytic leukemia. *J Clin Oncol.* 2010;28:1749-1755.
51. Hillmen P, Robak T, Janssens A, et al. Chlorambucil plus ofatumumab versus chlorambucil alone in previously untreated patients with chronic lymphocytic leukaemia (COMPLEMENT 1): a randomised, multicentre, open-label phase 3 trial. *Lancet.* 2015;385:1873-1883.
52. Goede V, Fischer K, Busch R, et al. Obinutuzumab plus chlorambucil in patients with CLL and coexisting conditions. *N Engl J Med.* 2014;370:1101-1110.
53. Goede V, Fischer K, Engelke A, et al. Obinutuzumab as frontline treatment of chronic lymphocytic leukemia: updated results of the CLL11 study. *Leukemia.* 2015;29:1602-1604.
54. Keating MJ, Flinn I, Jain V, et al. Therapeutic role of alemtuzumab (Campath-1H) in patients who have failed fludarabine: results of a large international study. *Blood.* 2002;99:3554-3561.
55. Stilgenbauer S, Zenz T, Winkler D, et al. Subcutaneous alemtuzumab in fludarabine-refractory chronic lymphocytic leukemia: clinical results and prognostic marker analyses from the CLL2H study of the German Chronic Lymphocytic Leukemia Study Group. *J Clin Oncol.* 2009;27:3994-4001.
56. Hillmen P, Skotnicki AB, Robak T, et al. Alemtuzumab compared with chlorambucil as first-line therapy for chronic lymphocytic leukemia. *J Clin Oncol.* 2007;25:5616-5623.
57. Badoux XC, Keating MJ, Wang X, et al. Cyclophosphamide, fludarabine, alemtuzumab, and rituximab as salvage therapy for heavily pretreated patients with chronic lymphocytic leukemia. *Blood.* 2011;118:2085-2093.
58. Pettitt AR, Jackson R, Carruthers S, et al. Alemtuzumab in combination with methylprednisolone is a highly effective induction regimen for patients with chronic lymphocytic leukemia and deletion of TP53: final results of the national cancer research institute CLL206 trial. *J Clin Oncol.* 2012;30:1647-1655.
59. Stilgenbauer S, Cymbalista F, Leblond V, et al. Alemtuzumab combined with dexamethasone, followed by alemtuzumab maintenance or allo-SCT in "ultra High-risk" CLL: final results from the CLL2O phase II study. *Blood.* 2014;124:1991a.
60. Bottcher S, Ritgen M, Fischer K, et al. Minimal residual disease quantification is an independent predictor of progression-free and overall survival in chronic lymphocytic leukemia: a multivariate analysis from the randomized GCLLSG CLL8 trial. *J Clin Oncol.* 2012;30:980-988.
61. Strati P, Keating MJ, O'Brien SM, et al. Eradication of bone marrow minimal residual disease may prompt early treatment discontinuation in CLL. *Blood.* 2014;123:3727-3732.
62. McClanahan F, Hanna B, Miller S, et al. PD-L1 checkpoint blockade prevents immune dysfunction and leukemia development in a mouse model of chronic lymphocytic leukemia. *Blood.* 2015;126:203-211.
63. Byrd JC, Furman RR, Coutre SE, et al. Targeting BTK with ibrutinib in relapsed chronic lymphocytic leukemia. *N Engl J Med.* 2013;369:32-42.
64. Byrd JC, Brown JR, O'Brien S, et al. Ibrutinib versus ofatumumab in previously treated chronic lymphoid leukemia. *N Engl J Med.* 2014;371:213-223.
65. O'Brien S, Furman RR, Coutre SE, et al. Ibrutinib as initial therapy for elderly patients with chronic lymphocytic leukaemia or small lymphocytic lymphoma: an open-label, multicentre, phase 1b/2 trial. *Lancet Oncol.* 2014;15:48-58.
66. Byrd JC, Furman RR, Coutre SE, et al. Three-year follow-up of treatment-naive and previously treated patients with CLL and SLL receiving single-agent ibrutinib. *Blood.* 2015;125:2497-2506.
67. Woyach JA, Furman RR, Liu TM, et al. Resistance mechanisms for the Bruton's tyrosine kinase inhibitor ibrutinib. *N Engl J Med.* 2014;370:2286-2294.
68. Brown JR, Byrd JC, Coutre SE, et al. Idelalisib, an inhibitor of phosphatidylinositol 3-kinase p110delta, for relapsed/refractory chronic lymphocytic leukemia. *Blood.* 2014;123:3390-3397.
69. Furman RR, Sharman JP, Coutre SE, et al. Idelalisib and

rituximab in relapsed chronic lymphocytic leukemia. *N Engl J Med*. 2014;370:997-1007.

70. Zelenetz AD, Lamanna N, Kipps TJ, et al. A phase 2 study of idelalisib monotherapy in previously untreated patients ≥65 years with chronic lymphocytic leukemia (CLL) or small lymphocytic lymphoma (SLL). *Blood*. 2014;124:1986a.
71. O'Brien S, Lamanna N, Kipps TJ, et al. Update on a phase 2 study of idelalisib in combination with rituximab in treatment-naïve patients ≥65 years with chronic lymphocytic leukemia (CLL) or small lymphocytic lymphoma (SLL). *Blood*. 2014;124:1994a.
72. Roberts AW, Seymour JF, Brown JR, et al. Substantial susceptibility of chronic lymphocytic leukemia to BCL2 inhibition: results of a phase I study of navitoclax in patients with relapsed or refractory disease. *J Clin Oncol*. 2012;30:488-496.
73. Souers AJ, Leverson JD, Boghaert ER, et al. ABT-199, a potent and selective BCL-2 inhibitor, achieves antitumor activity while sparing platelets. *Nat Med*. 2013;19:202-208.
74. Seymour JF, Davids MS, Pagel JM, et al. ABT-199: novel Bcl-2 specific inhibitor updated results confirm substantial activity and durable responses in high-risk CLL. Paper presented at: European Hematology Association Annual Meeting; June 12-15, 2014; Milan, Italy. Abstract S702.
75. Ramsay AG, Johnson AJ, Lee AM, et al. Chronic lymphocytic leukemia T cells show impaired immunological synapse formation that can be reversed with an immunomodulating drug. *J Clin Invest*. 2008;118:2427-2437.
76. Chanan-Khan A, Miller KC, Musial L, et al. Clinical efficacy of lenalidomide in patients with relapsed or refractory chronic lymphocytic leukemia: results of a phase II study. *J Clin Oncol*. 2006;24:5343-5349.
77. Ferrajoli A, Lee BN, Schlette EJ, et al. Lenalidomide induces complete and partial remissions in patients with relapsed and refractory chronic lymphocytic leukemia. *Blood*. 2008;111:5291-5297.
78. Badoux XC, Keating MJ, Wen S, et al. Lenalidomide as initial therapy of elderly patients with chronic lymphocytic leukemia. *Blood*. 2011;118:3489-3498.
79. Strati P, Keating MJ, Wierda WG, et al. Lenalidomide induces long-lasting responses in elderly patients with chronic lymphocytic leukemia. *Blood*. 2013;122:734-737.
80. Thompson PA, Keating MJ, Hinojosa C, et al. Lenalidomide and rituximab in combination as initial treatment of chronic lymphocytic leukemia: initial results of a phase II study. *Blood*. 2014;124:1988a.
81. Brentjens RJ, Riviere I, Park JH, et al. Safety and persistence of adoptively transferred autologous CD19-targeted T cells in patients with relapsed or chemotherapy refractory B-cell leukemias. *Blood*. 2011;118:4817-4828.
82. Porter DL, Levine BL, Kalos M, Bagg A, June CH. Chimeric antigen receptor-modified T cells in chronic lymphoid leukemia. *N Engl J Med*. 2011;365:725-733.
83. Dreger P, Schetelig J, Andersen N, et al. Managing high-risk CLL during transition to a new treatment era: stem cell transplantation or novel agents? *Blood*. 2014;124:3841-3849.
84. Khouri IF, Bassett R, Poindexter N, et al. Nonmyeloablative allogeneic stem cell transplantation in relapsed/refractory chronic lymphocytic leukemia: long-term follow-up, prognostic factors, and effect of human leukocyte histocompatibility antigen subtype on outcome. *Cancer*. 2011;117:4679-4688.
85. Dearden C. Disease-specific complications of chronic lymphocytic leukemia. *Hematology Am Soc Hematol Educ Program*. 2008:450-456.
86. Kaufman M, Limaye SA, Driscoll N, et al. A combination of rituximab, cyclophosphamide and dexamethasone effectively treats immune cytopenias of chronic lymphocytic leukemia. *Leuk Lymphoma*. 2009;50:892-899.
87. Cortes J, O'Brien S, Loscertales J, et al. Cyclosporin A for the treatment of cytopenia associated with chronic lymphocytic leukemia. *Cancer*. 2001;92:2016-2022.
88. Molica S, Musto P, Chiurazzi F, et al. Prophylaxis against infections with low-dose intravenous immunoglobulins (IVIG) in chronic lymphocytic leukemia. Results of a crossover study. *Haematologica*. 1996;81:121-126.
89. Falchi L, Keating MJ, Marom EM, et al. Correlation between FDG/PET, histology, characteristics, and survival in 332 patients with chronic lymphoid leukemia. *Blood*. 2014;123:2783-2790.
90. Rossi D, Cerri M, Capello D, et al. Biological and clinical risk factors of chronic lymphocytic leukaemia transformation to Richter syndrome. *Br J Haematol*. 2008;142:202-215.
91. Chigrinova E, Rinaldi A, Kwee I, et al. Two main genetic pathways lead to the transformation of chronic lymphocytic leukemia to Richter syndrome. *Blood*. 2013;122:2673-2682.
92. Fabbri G, Khiabanian H, Holmes AB, et al. Genetic lesions associated with chronic lymphocytic leukemia transformation to Richter syndrome. *J Exp Med*. 2013;210:2273-2288.
93. Tsimberidou AM, Wierda WG, Wen S, et al. Phase I-II clinical trial of oxaliplatin, fludarabine, cytarabine, and rituximab therapy in aggressive relapsed/refractory chronic lymphocytic leukemia or Richter syndrome. *Clin Lymphoma Myeloma Leuk*. 2013;13:568-574.
94. Tiacci E, Trifonov V, Schiavoni G, et al. BRAF mutations in hairy-cell leukemia. *N Engl J Med*. 2011;364:2305-2315.
95. Estey EH, Kurzrock R, Kantarjian HM, et al. Treatment of hairy cell leukemia with 2-chlorodeoxyadenosine (2-CdA). *Blood*. 1992;79:882-887.
96. Ravandi F, O'Brien S, Jorgensen J, et al. Phase 2 study of cladribine followed by rituximab in patients with hairy cell leukemia. *Blood*. 2011;118:3818-3823.
97. Dearden CE, Khot A, Else M, et al. Alemtuzumab therapy in T-cell prolymphocytic leukemia: comparing efficacy in a series treated intravenously and a study piloting the subcutaneous route. *Blood*. 2011;118:5799-5802.
98. Steinway SN, LeBlanc F, Loughran TP Jr. The pathogenesis and treatment of large granular lymphocyte leukemia. *Blood Rev*. 2014;28:87-94.
99. Koskela HL, Eldfors S, Ellonen P, et al. Somatic STAT3 mutations in large granular lymphocytic leukemia. *N Engl J Med*. 2012;366:1905-1913.
100. Rajala HL, Eldfors S, Kuusanmaki H, et al. Discovery of somatic STAT5b mutations in large granular lymphocytic leukemia. *Blood*. 2013;121:4541-4550.

4

Chronic Myeloid Leukemia

第四章　慢性粒细胞白血病

Muhamed Baljevic
Elias Jabbour
Jorge Cortes
Hagop M. Kantarjian

中文导读

慢性粒细胞白血病是一种起源于多能造血干细胞的恶性克隆性疾病，病程发展较缓慢，白血病细胞中可找到Ph染色体和/或BCR-ABL1融合基因。本章首先介绍了慢性粒细胞白血病的流行病学特征和病因学，由于该病发病率呈逐年上升趋势，对该疾病进行深入了解尤为重要。在介绍了慢性粒细胞白血病的生物学机制后，本章进一步阐述了其临床表现和病程演变。慢性粒细胞白血病患者一般会经历慢性期、加速期和急变期。患者的诊断基于临床检查和实验室检查。临床检查主要评估是否存在器官肿大（如脾大）和髓外造血。实验室检查主要包括血常规、骨髓象、细胞遗传学及分子生物学改变等。慢性粒细胞白血病一旦进入急变期，治疗效果欠佳，因此,应着重于慢性期的治疗。常用的治疗方法有酪氨酸激酶抑制剂、化疗和造血干细胞移植。酪氨酸激酶抑制剂包括用于一线治疗的伊马替尼、达沙替尼和尼洛替尼，以及二、三代药物博舒替尼和帕纳替尼，本章分别简述了相关的临床试验、推荐剂量和副作用，同时为一线和二、三线酪氨酸激酶抑制剂的选择做出指导。化疗部分简述了高三尖杉酯碱的相关研究结果。造血干细胞移植是加速期和急性变期的重要治疗手段，该部分主要阐述了其在慢性粒细胞白血病中的作用和应用时机。治疗反应的评估通过血液学反应标准来判断，对患者的监测包括差异血细胞计数、细胞遗传学和对BCR-ABL1转录水平及激酶域突变的分子检测等。最后，本章对慢性期、加速期、急变期的用药策略和停药原则给出了指导和建议。

INTRODUCTION

Chronic myeloid leukemia (CML) is a myeloproliferative disorder of pluripotent hematopoietic stem cells, characterized by the molecular *BCR-ABL1* rearrangement, which drives a proliferative and survival advantage of the leukemic clone. About 30% to 50% of patients with CML are asymptomatic at diagnosis and are incidentally diagnosed during routine examination. Patients may also present with characteristic clinical findings secondary to large numbers of myeloid circulating progenitors, leading to splenomegaly, leukocytosis, or even isolated thrombocytosis. The landscape of CML has had a dramatic course, with a host of findings that have elucidated the biology and molecular pathology of the disease. The understanding of the molecular events led to the creation of the first targeted therapy—imatinib mesylate. Its impact on therapy and survival propelled CML as a model for modern molecular medicine in the fast-developing era of personalized targeted therapy.

EPIDEMIOLOGY AND ETIOLOGY

The incidence of CML is 1 to 2 cases per 100,000 adults with a slight male predominance and rising incidence with age, accounting for approximately 15% of newly diagnosed cases of leukemia in adults ([1]). Chronic myeloid leukemia is uncommon in children, with a median age at diagnosis of 67 years. There are no known hereditary, geographic, familial, or ethnic associations. No chemical or infectious associations have been established, although an increased risk has been linked with exposure to ionizing radiation ([2]).

In 2014, in the United States, an estimated 6,000 cases of CML were diagnosed. Since 2000, the year of introduction of imatinib, the annual mortality in CML has decreased from 10% to 20% to 1% to 2%. Consequently, the prevalence of CML in the United States, which was estimated at about 25,000 to 30,000 cases in 2000, has increased to an estimated 80,000 to 100,000+ cases in 2015 and will reach a plateau of about 180,000 cases by 2030 ([3]). The overall survival (OS) of patients over the recent decade has greatly improved. The exact mechanism of initiation of the defining molecular event in CML—Philadelphia (Ph) chromosome translocation—remains elusive.

BIOLOGY OF CHRONIC MYELOID LEUKEMIA

Chronic myeloid leukemia is defined by a unique cytogenetic and/or molecular abnormality—the Ph chromosome—originating in a pluripotent stem cell, with a balanced translocation between the long arms of chromosomes 9 and 22, t(9,22)(q34,q11.2) ([4]). Detectable by routine cytogenetics or by fluorescent in situ hybridization (FISH), the Ph chromosome is noted in 90% to 95% of patients with the clinical and laboratory features of CML. In the remaining 5% to 10% of patients, the molecular *BCR-ABL1* rearrangement can be recognized with high-sensitivity reverse transcriptase polymerase chain reaction (RT-PCR). All remaining cases with unknown biology deemed as true Ph-negative CML or atypical CML carry a poor prognosis. The Ph chromosome joins the proto-oncogene *c-abl* from chromosome 9 to the breakpoint cluster region (*BCR*) gene in chromosome 22, generating a novel fusion *BCR-ABL1* oncogene. Depending on the breakpoint region in *BCR*, several variants including those of 190, 210 (most common; 95% of Ph-positive cases), or 230 kDa molecular weight can be formed. The translation product is a chimeric protein with constitutively active tyrosine kinase activity that activates multiple downstream pathways, including PI3 kinase, NF-κB, JAK/STAT, RAS, RAF, ERK, MYC, and JNK.

Following the 2005 discovery of the *JAK2* V617F mutation as the molecular abnormality common to polycythemia vera, essential thrombocytosis, and idiopathic myelofibrosis, CML has been segregated into a separate group of myeloproliferative neoplasms categorized as *BCR-ABL1* positive/*JAK2* V617F negative.

Roughly 10% to 15% of patients, typically at a more advanced stage of disease, experience clonal evolution with additional chromosomal aberrations including trisomy 8, monosomy 7, isochrome 17, a double Ph chromosome, or additional loss of material from 22q. Clonal evolution is considered a criterion of accelerated phase, particularly when it occurs during the course of the disease. Corresponding molecular alterations that follow these changes include deregulation of *p53*, *RB1*, *C-MYC*, and *AML-EVI1*.

CLINICAL FEATURES AND NATURAL HISTORY

There are three separate phases of CML: chronic phase (CP), intermediate or accelerated phase (AP), and terminal or blast phase (BP). Even though all three represent a stepwise progression of disease in terms of aggressiveness from CP to BP, the natural course of the disease may not progress from one to the other, nor will disease always include all three. The vast majority of patients are diagnosed as asymptomatic in the CP. Splenomegaly is the most consistent presenting sign, detected in 50% to 60% of cases. Previously defined criteria indicating progression from CP to AP include 15% or more blasts, 30% or more blasts plus promyelocytes, 20% or more

Table 4-1 Criteria for Accelerated Phase According to MDACC, IBMTR, and WHO

	MDACC	IBMTR	WHO
Blasts	≥15%	≥10%	10-19[a]
Blasts+Pros	≥30%	≥20%	NA
Basophils	≥20%	≥20%[b]	≥20%
Platelets (× 10^9/L)	<100	Unresponsive ↑, persistent ↓	<100 or >1000 unresponsive
Cytogenetics	CE	CE	CE not at diagnosis
WBC	NA	Difficult to control, or doubling <5 days	NA
Anemia	NA	Unresponsive	NA
Splenomegaly	NA	Increasing	NA
Other	NA	Chloromas, myelofibrosis	Megakaryocyte proliferation, fibrosis

CE, clonal evolution; IBMTR, International Bone Marrow Transplant Registry; MDACC, University of Texas MD Anderson Cancer Center; NA, not applicable; Pros, promonocytes; WHO, World Health Organization.
[a]Blast phase ≥20% blasts (≥30% for MDACC and IBMTR).
[b]Basophils + eosinophils.

basophils, platelets <100 × 10^9/L unrelated to therapy, or cytogenetic clonal evolution ([5]). Other criteria have been proposed (Table 4-1). Compared to CP, median survival in AP is significantly shorter, although a significant improvement in survival has been observed with the availability of tyrosine kinase inhibitors (TKIs), particularly among early responders ([6]).

Most patients evolve into AP prior to BP, but 20% progress to BP without AP warning signals. Blast phase is considered an acute leukemia. It is defined by the presence of at least 30% blasts in the peripheral blood or bone marrow or the presence of extramedullary disease (chloroma or granulocytic sarcoma). Half of the patients in BP carry a myeloid phenotype, whereas the other half is split evenly between lymphoid and undifferentiated ([7]). Median survival in BP CML remains poor; a combination of TKI with chemotherapy followed by allogeneic stem-cell transplantation is recommended.

DIAGNOSIS AND CLINICAL WORKUP

Initial evaluation aims to elicit signs and/or symptoms of disease, whereas physical examination evaluates for any presence of organomegaly or extramedullary hematopoiesis. Diagnosing typical CML requires documentation of the Ph chromosome abnormality by routine cytogenetic evaluation (karyotype), FISH, or molecular studies (RT-PCR) ([8]). Bone marrow aspiration and biopsy are required, because they will not only confirm the diagnosis (eg, cytogenetic analysis), but also provide information needed for staging and classification. Although FISH, which relies on co-localization of large genomic probes specific to the *BCR* and *ABL* genes, or RT-PCR from peripheral blood can both confirm the presence of the Ph chromosome or the *BCR-ABL1* rearrangement, only bone marrow cytogenetics can reveal additional chromosomal abnormalities that are important in the initial diagnosis and staging.

True Ph- and *BCR-ABL1*–negative patients are considered to have Ph-negative CML or chronic myelomonocytic leukemia. In a few instances, a patient may be diagnosed with Ph-positive acute myeloid leukemia (AML) or acute lymphoblastic leukemia (ALL). It may be impossible to determine whether these cases represent de novo Ph-positive acute leukemias or a BP of a previously unrecognized CML.

LABORATORY FEATURES

The most common laboratory finding in CP CML is leukocytosis, with myeloid cells in all stages of maturation seen in the peripheral blood. Frequently, there is an increase of basophils and eosinophils. The bone marrow is markedly hypercellular, with the myeloid-to-erythroid ratio significantly increased (Figs. 4-1 to 4-5) ([9]).

A marrow aspiration and chromosomal analysis are needed to identify any variances in marrow blasts or basophils and to identify the Ph chromosome and possible cytogenetic clonal evolution (Fig. 4-6). Fluorescent in situ hybridization and PCR should be done at diagnosis in all patients. FISH may identify the presence of the *BCR-ABL1* rearrangement, even when the Ph chromosome is not found by conventional cytogenetic analysis. Furthermore, FISH can be performed on peripheral blood interphase cells (Fig. 4-7). Reverse transcriptase PCR testing amplifies the region around

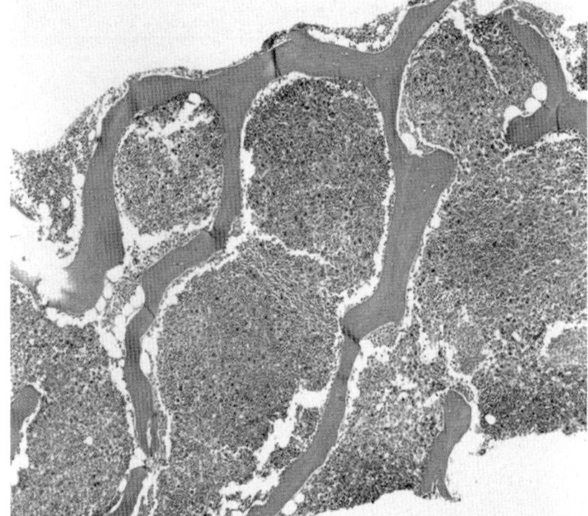

FIGURE 4-1 Chronic myeloid leukemia, chronic phase. The bone marrow biopsy is 100% cellular with granulocytic and megakaryocytic hyperplasia.

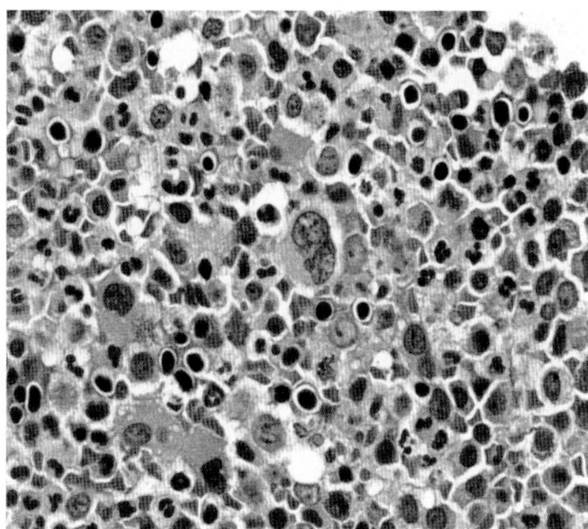

FIGURE 4-2 Chronic myeloid leukemia, chronic phase. Myeloid progenitors with increased immature cells in a hypercellular bone marrow.

the splice junction between *BCR* and *ABL* and is highly sensitive for detecting CML, identifying the initial type of *BCR-ABL1* transcript (important for follow-up), and especially quantifying minimal residual disease (MRD). In general, simultaneous peripheral blood and marrow quantitative PCRs have a high level of concordance, although false-positive and false-negative results can be seen (false-negative results due to poor-quality material or failure of the reaction; false-positive results due to contamination). Quantitative PCR assesses the amount *of BCR-ABL1* transcripts and is universally performed. Table 4-2 presents a summary of the proposed evaluation at diagnosis and during follow-up for patients with CML.

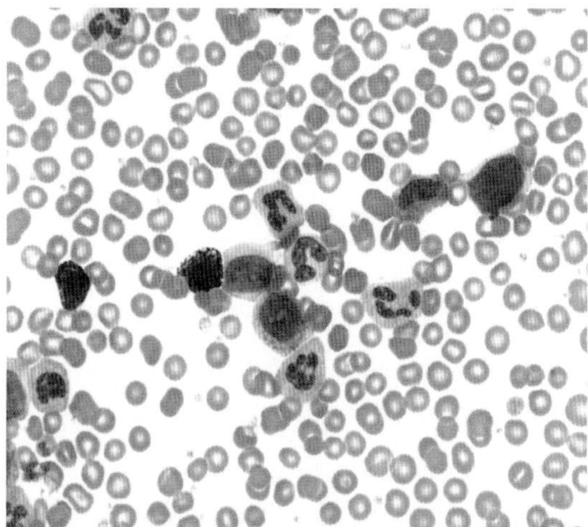

FIGURE 4-3 Chronic myeloid leukemia in accelerated phase. Aspirate smear shows increased blasts and basophils.

PROGNOSIS

As the newer generation agents became available, the prognostic significance of certain clinical characteristics changed. Achieving a complete cytogenetic response (CCyR) is the most important prognostic factor for long-term survival ([10]). It has become evident that achieving a cytogenetic response, particularly during the first 3 to 6 months of therapy, translates into the best probability of long-term outcome.

RESPONSE AND EVALUATION OF MINIMAL RESIDUAL DISEASE

Response to therapy is initially judged by measurement of hematologic response criteria. A complete hematologic response (CHR) is defined as normalization of white blood cell (WBC) counts to <10 × 10^9/L

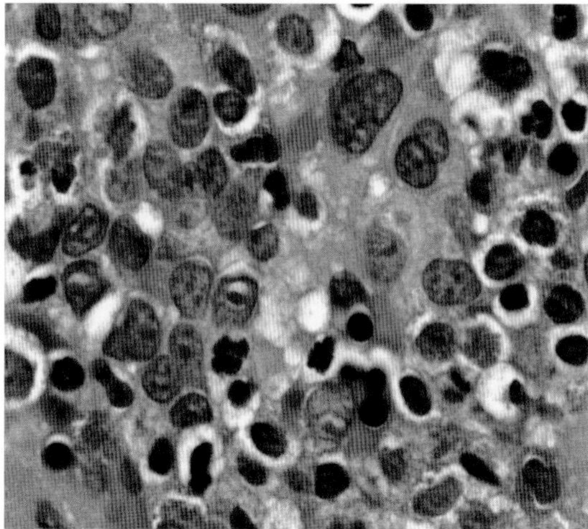

FIGURE 4-4 Chronic myeloid leukemia, accelerated phase. Bone marrow biopsy section demonstrate foci of blasts.

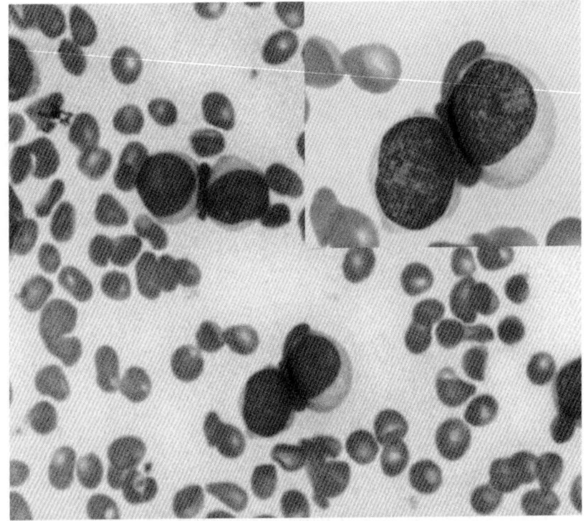

FIGURE 4-5 Chronic myeloid leukemia in blast phase. The majority of evaluable white cells are immature (blasts).

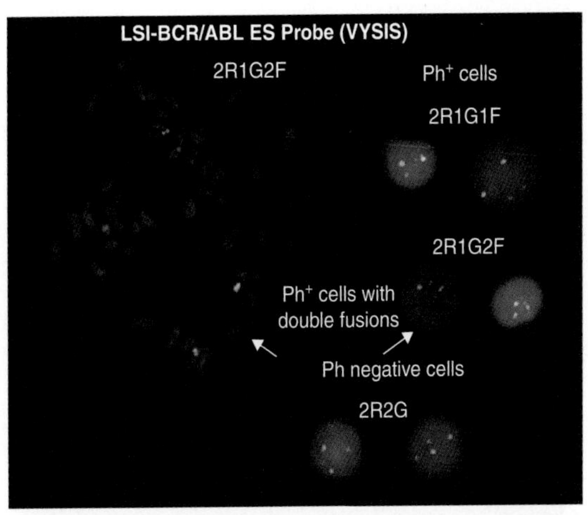

FIGURE 4-7 Fluorescent in situ hybridization (in metaphase in left panel; in interphase in right panel) image showing the *BCR-ABL* rearrangement.

with a normal differential, platelet count <450 × 10^9/L, and disappearance of splenomegaly and other symptoms of CML. Patients who achieve a CHR are further classified according to the type of cytogenetic response attained (Table 4-3).

Cytogenetic responses are divided into complete, partial, and minor. Complete cytogenetic response corresponds to 0% of all metaphases remaining Ph positive; partial cytogenetic response is defined as 1% to 35% of metaphases being Ph positive; and minor cytogenetic response is defined as 35% to 95% Ph-positive metaphases. An analysis involving review of at least 20 metaphases is necessary to evaluate a cytogenetic response. Although FISH results correlate well with the karyotypic evaluation, cytogenetic response criteria have not been validated with FISH.

Molecular response is assessed by quantitative PCR (usually RT-PCR) in the peripheral blood or bone

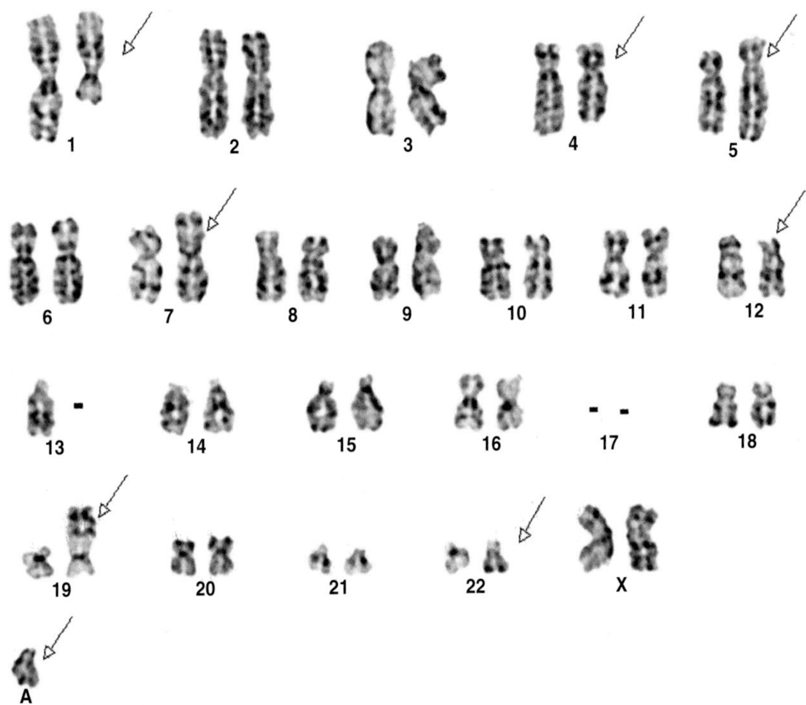

FIGURE 4-6 Karyotype from a patient with blast-phase chronic myeloid leukemia demonstrating clonal evolution. Reciprocal translocation involving chromosomes 9 and 22 has occurred. Additional chromosomal abnormalities are present indicating clonal evolution.

CHAPTER 4

Table 4-2 Monitoring of CML Patients

Status	Diagnostic Testing
At diagnosis	• Bone marrow evaluation with cytogenetics and RT-PCR
During therapy	• Cytogenetics at 3, 6, and 12 months of therapy, then every 6-12 months. Once the patient achieves a stable CCyR, every 12-36 months or closer if the transcript level changes significantly
	• FISH if insufficient metaphases or to monitor cytogenetic response in between bone marrows
	• After achieving durable CCyR, quantitative RT-PCR every 3-6 months for the first year, then every 6 months for patients in MMR
	• ABL kinase domain mutation screening for any of the following patients: failing to achieve CHR at 3 months, PCyR at 6 months and CCyR at 12 months; hematologic or cytogenetic relapse; sustained 1-log increase in *BCR-ABL1* transcript ratio; progression to AP or BP

AP, accelerated phase; BP, blast phase; CCyR, complete cytogenic response; CHR, complete hematologic response; CML, chronic myeloid leukemia; FISH, fluorescent in situ hybridization; MMR, major molecular response; PCyR, partial cytogenic response; RT-PCR, reverse transcriptase polymerase chain reaction.

Table 4-3 Response Criteria in CML

Hematologic remission	
Complete	Normalization of peripheral counts and differential, and disappearance of all signs and symptoms of CML including splenomegaly
Cytogenetic remission[a]	
Complete	0% Ph-positive metaphases
Partial	1%-35% Ph-positive metaphases
Minor	36%-95% Ph-positive metaphases
None	>95% Ph-positive metaphases
(Complete and partial remissions together constitute major cytogenetic remissions, ie, 0%-34% Ph-positive metaphases)	
Molecular remission[b]	
Complete	Undetectable *BCR-ABL* transcripts[c]
Major	*BCR-ABL/ABL* ratio of <0.1% (International Scale)

[a]Cytogenetic response is based on a routine karyotype analyzing at least 20 metaphases.
[b]Molecular responses is based on quantitative polymerase chain reaction (PCR; usually real-time PCR).
[c]PCR with a sensitivity of at least 4.5-log.

marrow ([11]). A major molecular response (MMR) is considered when the *BCR-ABL1/ABL1* ratio is ≤0.1% on the international scale (IS). A complete molecular response (CMR) represents achievement of undetectable transcripts of *BCR-ABL1* in an assay with a sensitivity of at least 4.5 logs. For correlative purposes, *BCR-ABL1* transcript levels (IS) of ≤1% are equivalent to a CCyR; levels of ≤10% are equivalent to a partial cytogenetic response.

THERAPY

Three commercially available TKIs are approved for the frontline treatment of CML: imatinib, dasatinib, and nilotinib. Available guidelines support all three as viable frontline options for the initial management of CP CML.

Imatinib Mesylate

Prior to the development of targeted therapy, CML was treated with busulfan or hydroxyurea for many years, with a poor prognosis and inability to delay disease progression. The introduction of interferon-alfa (IFN-α) improved survival in CML and resulted in CCyRs in 5% to 25% of patients with CP CML.

Imatinib mesylate (STI-571 or Gleevec) is a selective and potent competitive inhibitor of the adenosine triphosphate (ATP)–binding site of the Bcr-Abl oncoprotein, as well as c-kit, PDGFRα and PDGFRβ, and abl-related gene (*ARG*) ([12]). It is taken orally with 98% bioavailability and a half-life of 13 to 16 hours. It was first used in CML patients who developed resistance or intolerance to IFN-α and resulted in a CCyR of 60% and an estimated 5-year OS of 76% ([13]).

Based on these results, the large International Randomized Study of Interferon and STI571 (IRIS) trial evaluated imatinib versus IFN-α and low-dose cytarabine as frontline therapy in patients with newly diagnosed CP CML. Patients were randomized to receive imatinib 400 mg/d or INF-α plus low-dose subcutaneous cytarabine, which was standard of care at the time ([10]). After a median follow-up of 19 months, planned outcome analyses were significantly better in almost all categories for patients receiving imatinib. The rates of CCyR (74% vs 9%; $P < .001$) and freedom from progression to AP or BP at 12 months (99% vs 93%; $P < .001$) were improved. There was a high crossover rate to imatinib. The responses to imatinib were durable, as outlined in an 8-year follow-up of the original study ([14]). Estimated event-free survival was 81%, and OS was 93% when only CML-related deaths were considered. With an annual mortality of 2%, the estimated median survival of a newly diagnosed patient with CML may be in the range of 20 to 30 years.

Imatinib Dose

A phase I imatinib study in patients who had failed prior IFN-α therapy established a clear relationship between dose and response ([15]). No significant responses were observed at doses <300 mg daily. An arbitrary dose of 400 mg daily for CP was selected in phase II studies, despite the lack of dose-limiting toxicity at doses up to 1,000 mg daily (maximum-tolerated dose was not defined). The Rationale and Insight for Gleevec High-Dose Therapy (RIGHT) trial studied imatinib 400 mg twice a day as initial therapy in 115 patients with newly diagnosed CML ([16]). The rate of CCyR was 85% at 12 months and 83% at 18 months, with corresponding rates of MMR of 54% at 12 months and 63% at 18 months.

These results led to a randomized phase III open-label study, the Tyrosine Kinase Inhibitor Optimization and Selectivity Trial (TOPS), comparing 400 and 800 mg of imatinib in 476 patients. The trial showed significant superiority for the 800-mg dose in terms of MMR rate at 3 months (3% vs 12%), 6 months (17% vs 34%), and 9 months (33% vs 45%) but not at 12 months (40% vs 46%) ([17]). A final update of the trial showed no significant difference in MMR rates at 24 months (52% vs 50%) ([18]). Another European study also reported no benefit with imatinib 800 mg compared to 400 mg in high-risk CML (CCyR rates were 64% and 58% and MMR rates were and 40% and 33%, respectively) ([19]).

The French SPIRIT study evaluated the impact of adding IFN or cytarabine in a randomized study where 636 patients with untreated CP CML received one of the following: imatinib 400 mg daily alone, imatinib 400 mg daily with cytarabine (20 mg/m²/d on days 15-28 of each 28-day cycle) or pegylated IFN-α-2a (90 μg weekly), or imatinib 600 mg daily alone ([20]). The rates of cytogenetic response at 12 months were similar among the four groups, whereas the rate of molecular response (a decrease in the ratio of *BCR-ABL1/ABL1* of ≤0.01%) was significantly higher in patients receiving imatinib and pegylated IFN-α-2a compared with imatinib 400 mg alone arm (30% vs 14%, respectively; $P = .001$). This rate was also significantly higher in patients treated for more than 12 months compared to treatment lasting ≤12 months. However, this high rate of early and deep responses did not translate into long-term improvement due to the poor tolerance of pegylated IFN.

Imatinib 400 mg daily is the regimen of choice for newly diagnosed patients with CP CML, with an emphasis on maintaining adequate dose intensity with minimal treatment interruptions or dose reductions for the best outcome.

Management of Toxicity

Imatinib is well tolerated, although adverse events not requiring treatment interruptions or decrease in dosing may occur in 30% to 40% of patients. A list of some of the most frequently encountered side effects and suggestions for management are included in Table 4-4. Any grade 3 or 4 toxicities related to imatinib require treatment interruption and resumption

Table 4-4 Recommended Management of the Most Common Adverse Events Associated With Imatinib

Adverse Events	Management
Nausea/vomiting	Take with food, fluids
	Antiemetics
Diarrhea	Loperamide
	Diphenoxylate atropine
Peripheral edema	Diuretics
Periorbital edema	Steroid-containing cream
Skin rash	Avoid sun exposure
	Topical steroids
	Systemic steroids
	(Early intervention important)
Muscle cramps	Tonic water or quinine
	Electrolyte replacement as needed
	Calcium gluconate
Arthralgia, bone pain	Nonsteroidal anti-inflammatory agents
Elevated transaminases (uncommon)	Hold therapy and monitor closely
	Dose reduction upon resolution
Myelosuppression	
Anemia	Treatment interruption/dose reduction usually not indicated
	Erythropoietin or darbepoetin
Neutropenia	Hold therapy if grade ≥3 (ie, ANC <1 × 10⁹/L)
	Restart at lower dose if recovery takes >2 weeks
	Consider G-CSF if recurrent/persistent, or sepsis
Thrombocytopenia	Hold therapy if grade ≥3 (ie, platelets <50 × 10⁹/L)
	Restart at lower dose if recovery takes >2 weeks
	Consider IL-11 10 μg/kg 3-7 days/week

ANC, absolute neutrophil count; G-CSF, granulocyte colony-stimulating factor; IL-10, interleukin-10.

upon resolution of toxicity or its decrease to grade 1 or less. Subsequent dose should be reduced if recurring or long-lasting adverse effects are encountered, keeping in mind that doses below 300 mg daily are not recommended due to lack of adequate activity. Only 2% to 3% of patients exhibit true intolerance to imatinib and require permanent discontinuation. Early recognition and intervention targeting toxicities greatly reduce the need for unnecessary treatment interruptions and dose reductions.

Myelosuppression is common and frequently seen within the first 2 to 3 months of therapy. It is generally self-limited, and dose interruptions are not recommended unless grade 3 neutropenia or thrombocytopenia (ie, neutrophils <1 × 10^9/L, platelets <50 × 10^9/L) develops. Anemia alone usually does not require interruptions or dose adjustments. Treatment is restarted when counts recover above specified thresholds. Following treatment interruption, WBC should be monitored at least once weekly, and if recovery occurs within 2 weeks, treatment would be resumed with the same dose at which myelosuppression occurred. If recovery takes longer than 2 weeks, the dose could be reduced in increments (eg, from 800 to 600 mg, from 600 to 400 mg, or from 400 to 300 mg). Hematopoietic growth factors may be beneficial with recurrent or prolonged myelosuppression (eg, erythropoietin or darbepoetin and filgrastim).

Dasatinib

Dasatinib (Sprycel) is an oral second-generation TKI that is a piperazinyl derivative. It has an excellent oral bioavailability and is 350 times more potent in vitro than imatinib ([21, 22]) (in vitro sensitivity of different *BCR-ABL1* mutants to different TKIs is presented in Table 4-5) ([23]). Dasatinib exhibits significant activity against most imatinib-resistant *BCR-ABL1* mutations, with the exception of T315I, as well as a few others, including V299L and F317L ([24]). In contrast to imatinib, dasatinib binds to both the active and inactive conformations of *BCR-ABL1* and also inhibits the Src family of kinases, which may be important in suppressing critical cell signaling pathways ([25]).

Following evaluation in the salvage setting after imatinib failure, dasatinib was assessed in the frontline setting. The DASISION trial was a phase III randomized study that compared imatinib 400 mg once daily to dasatinib 100 mg once daily in 519 patients with newly diagnosed CP CML ([26]). The primary end point was confirmed CCyR at 12 months. The dasatinib arm resulted in higher confirmed CCyR at 12 months (77% vs 66%; *P* = .007). The rates of molecular response were significantly higher with dasatinib (MMR, 76% vs 64%, *P* = .002; molecular response with a 4.5-log reduction in *BCR-ABL* transcripts from baseline [$MR^{4.5}$], 42% and 33%, *P* = .025). Dasatinib induced deeper responses at early time points (3, 6, or 12 months) compared to imatinib. The rate of transformation to AP or BP was lower in patients treated with dasatinib (4.6% and 7.3%, respectively). There was no progression-free survival (PFS) or OS difference at 5 years. Relevant toxicities included pleural effusion rate of 29% with dasatinib (mostly grade 1 or 2; 15 patients discontinued dasatinib due to pleural effusion). Arterial ischemic events were slightly higher with dasatinib (5% vs 2%, respectively). Pulmonary hypertension was reported in 14 dasatinib-treated patients, with 6 discontinuing the drug. Comparison of the phase III trials in the frontline treatment of CP CML with imatinib, dasatinib, and nilotinib is outlined in Table 4-6.

A randomized phase II trial compared dasatinib 100 mg daily with imatinib 400 mg daily in 253 patients with newly diagnosed CP CML. Higher rates of CCyR (84% vs 69%) and 12-month MMR (59% vs 44%; *P* = .059) were reported in patients receiving dasatinib. No difference in PFS or OS was reported. Grade 3 and 4 toxicities were most commonly hematologic, including thrombocytopenia, which was more common with dasatinib (18% vs 8%) ([27]).

The results of the SPIRIT-2 trial were recently reported ([28]). More than 800 patients with newly diagnosed CML were treated in a phase III trial and were randomized to either dasatinib 100 mg daily or imatinib 400 mg daily ([28]). The 12-month CCyR and MMR rates were higher with dasatinib (CCyR: 51% vs 40%, *P* = .002; MMR: 58% vs 43%, *P* < .001). Among 40 patients who discontinued therapy due to suboptimal response, only three patients (1%) received dasatinib. The PFS and OS were not significantly different. The rate of grade 3 or 4 thrombocytopenia was higher with dasatinib (13% vs 4%). Pleural effusions were observed in 78 patients (19%) treated with dasatinib (13 required drainage). The rate of cardiovascular events was slightly higher with dasatinib (2% vs 0.5%).

Dasatinib is otherwise well tolerated. Myelosuppression occurs frequently, with grade 3 or 4 neutropenia or thrombocytopenia in 20% of patients. The most common nonhematologic grade 3 or 4 toxicities at the same dose were pleural effusion (9%), dyspnea (6%), bleeding (4%), diarrhea (3%), and fatigue (3%).

Nilotinib

Nilotinib (Tasigna) is a structural analog of imatinib with 50 times more potent affinity for the ATP-binding site in vitro ([29]) and more selective activity against unmutated and most mutated forms of *BCR-ABL1* ([29, 30]). It is approved at a dose of 400 mg twice daily for patients with CP or AP CML who have resistance or intolerance to imatinib.

Table 4-5 In Vitro Sensitivity of Different *BCR-ABL1* Mutants to Different Tyrosine Kinase Inhibitors

BCR-ABL Mutant	Ponatinib	Imatinib	Nilotinib	Dasatinib	Bosutinib
Native	3	201	15	2	71
M244V	3	287	12	2	147
L248R	8	10000	549	6	874
L248V	4	586	26	5	182
G250E	5	1087	41	4	85
Y253H	5	4908	179	3	40
E255K	6	2487	127	9	181
E255V	16	8322	784	11	214
V299L	4	295	24	16	1228
T315A	4	476	50	59	122
T315I	6	9773	8091	10000	4338
F317C	3	324	16	45	165
F317I	7	266	25	40	232
F317L	4	675	21	10	82
F317V	10	1023	26	104	1280
M351T	4	404	15	2	97
E355A	7	441	18	3	74
F359C	6	728	47	2	70
F359I	11	324	64	3	76
F359V	4	346	41	2	59
H396R	4	395	23	2	60
E459K	5	612	38	4	127
Criteria Used to Classify Drug Potency					
	Ponatinib	**Imatinib**	**Nilotinib**	**Dasatinib**	**Bosutinib**
Effective C_{ave} at recommended dose	28[a]	444	131	11	159
IC_{50} <75% of C_{ave}	<21	<333	<98	<8	<119
IC_{50} 75%-150% of C_{ave}	21-32	333-500	98-147	8-12	119-179
IC_{50} 150%-300% of C_{ave}	33-95	501-1499	148-442	13-37	180-537
IC_{50} >300% of C_{ave}	>95	>1499	>442	>37	>537

C_{ave}, average concentration; IC_{50}, half maximal inhibitory concentration.
[a]Ponatinib 45 mg dose. Data shown as mean IC_{50} (nM) from three separate experiments.

After approval for patients who failed imatinib therapy, nilotinib was evaluated in newly diagnosed CML in CP. The ENESTnd study was a randomized phase III trial comparing two different dose schedules of nilotinib (300 and 400 mg twice daily) to imatinib 400 mg once daily as initial therapy for patients with early CP CML ([31]). The primary end point was the rate of MMR at 12 months, which was higher with both doses of nilotinib compared to imatinib (44% and 43% vs 22%; $P < .001$). The rate of transformation to AP or BP by 12 months of therapy was significantly lower with nilotinib (<1%) compared to imatinib (4%). The adverse effect profiles showed a higher rate of cardiovascular events with nilotinib (10% with nilotinib 300 mg twice a day; 16% with nilotinib 400 mg twice a day; and 2% with imatinib). The 6-year follow-up continues to demonstrate higher rates of early and deeper sustained molecular response with nilotinib, a reduced risk of progression to AP and BP, and an acceptable safety profile ([32]). Nilotinib is well tolerated, with grade 3 or 4 myelosuppression as the most common adverse event (neutropenia or thrombocytopenia observed in 10%-20% of patients). Nonhematologic toxicity includes liver function abnormalities in 10% to 15% of patients and asymptomatic elevation of lipase and amylase in 10% to 15% of patients. Vascular adverse events were

CHAPTER 4

Table 4-6 Comparison of the Phase III Trials in the Frontline Treatment of CP CML

Trial	Treatment	CCyR (%)	MMR (%)	*BCR-ABL* <10% at 3 Months (%)	EFS/PFS (%)	OS (%)	Longest Follow-Up (years)
		At 6 years			*At 6 years*		
IRIS	Imatinib (n = 304)	83	86	NR	81	85	8
		At 2 years	*At 5 years*		*At 5 years*		
DASISION	Dasatinib (n = 259)	86	76	84	85	91	5
	Imatinib (n = 260)	82	64	64	86	90	
		At 2 years	*At 5 years*		*At 5 years*	*At 6 years*	
ENESTnd	Nilotinib 300 mg (n = 282)	87	77	91	95	92	6
	Nilotinib 400 mg (n = 281)	85	77	89	97	96	
	Imatinib (n = 283)	77	60	67	93	91	

CCyR, complete cytogenetic response; CP CML, chronic phase chronic myelogenous leukemia; EFS/PFS, event-free survival/progression-free survival; MMR, major molecular response; NR, not reported; OS, overall survival.

reported at an cumulative rate of 10% over 6 years. Rare cases (<1%) of pancreatitis have been reported. Nilotinib has the potential for QTc prolongation, and a baseline electrocardiogram is required prior to the start of therapy. Diabetes may be exacerbated with nilotinib.

Selecting a Frontline Therapy

With multiple TKIs available for newly diagnosed CP CML, there are several considerations when choosing a starting agent, such as efficacy, patient status (eg, age; comorbidities; history of diabetes, hypertension, pancreatitis, chronic lung disease, pulmonary hypertension, cardiac history), and treatment value. The high prices of TKIs are of concern, given that patients can now remain on TKIs and expect to live normal lives ([33]). The prices for the second-generation dasatinib and nilotinib are comparable, both costing more than $100,000 annually. Once imatinib becomes available as a generic drug, the choice of TKIs in relation to value (benefit-to-price) needs to be considered, particularly in patients with low-risk disease.

For patients with baseline cardiopulmonary comorbidities such as chronic obstructive pulmonary disease, congestive heart failure, or uncontrolled hypertension or pulmonary arterial hypertension, a TKI other than dasatinib may be favored, given the risk of pleural effusions. Dasatinib also impairs platelet function, and patients on concomitant anticoagulants may be at an increased risk for hemorrhagic complications ([34]).

Nilotinib has been linked with hyperglycemia and QT interval prolongation, and should be used with caution in uncontrolled diabetics and in patients with baseline QT prolongation (routine monitoring of the QT interval is essential). Potassium and magnesium should be repleted to optimal serum levels prior to starting nilotinib, and the drug should be taken on an empty stomach twice daily. Recently, nilotinib has been associated with a low but significant incidence of peripheral artery disease, cerebrovascular accidents, and cardiovascular syndromes ([35]). Therefore, it is reasonable to choose other TKIs for patients with cardiovascular morbidities. Nilotinib rarely causes pancreatitis and should be avoided in patients with prior history of pancreatic inflammations. Imatinib is associated with the development of peripheral edema as one of its major side effects. Among patients with significant baseline peripheral edema, nilotinib or dasatinib may be favored as first options; close monitoring and intermittent use of loop diuretics might mitigate the effects of fluid retention.

MONITORING PATIENTS

Monitoring involves routine blood counts with differentials, cytogenetics, and molecular testing for *BCR-ABL1* transcript levels and for *BCR-ABL1* kinase domain mutations. Blood counts should be performed every 1 to 2 weeks until CHR and at least every 3 months thereafter or more frequently as clinically indicated ([36]). Cytogenetic analysis is the only test that gives reliable information regarding the presence of additional chromosomal aberrations.

At baseline, all patients undergo a marrow analysis to establish the diagnosis and provide a sample for cytogenetic testing. This also allows for proper staging in terms of the blast and basophil percentage. Presently, it is recommended that patients have a follow-up bone marrow study at 3, 6, and 12 months after starting therapy ([37]). An alternative method to determine cytogenetic response is with the use of FISH on peripheral blood. If a patient is responding optimally, and the FISH study is negative at 6 or 12 months, it may be reasonable to omit further marrow exams, as the patient is likely to be in stable CCyR ([38, 39]). Once a patient achieves a stable CCyR, particularly if associated with MMR, bone marrow aspirations with cytogenetics are recommended only every 1 to 3 years or if there are significant changes in the transcript levels or peripheral blood counts.

For patients in durable CCyR, periodic molecular monitoring every 3 to 6 months using quantitative RT-PCR is acceptable and useful, but may lead to erroneous changes in treatment due to discordance in results between labs or even within the same lab. This is harmful to patients because it leads to potentially discontinuing a useful therapy that the patient may have been tolerating well. One strategy to minimize this is to use interphase FISH as a complementary diagnostic test along with the molecular test to detect possible false-positive or false-negative results generated by either assay ([39]). For patients in CCyR, the achievement and maintenance of an MMR is questionable. Studies evaluating patients receiving imatinib or second-generation TKIs found that patients in CCyR have similar survival whether there is achievement of MMR or not ([40-42]). For patients in MMR, periodic molecular monitoring every 6 months is useful.

The value of early molecular response has been shown in a number of studies to have strong prognostic value. This has been applied to each of the TKIs appropriate for use in the frontline setting. A *BCR-ABL1* transcript level of less than 10% at 3 months has been shown to separate groups into high- and low-risk categories for long-term outcomes (ie, progression, survival) ([40, 43, 44]). An important question is what to do with a patient who does not meet the 3-month benchmark. One option is to switch TKIs early, but there are currently no data showing this would alter long-term outcome. Several experts have suggested that a follow-up measurement at 6 months will help define patients clearly in need of a change in therapy ([37]). This has been retrospectively analyzed with conflicting results ([45-47]). At least two independent studies suggested that patients with *BCR-ABL1* transcript levels greater than 10% at 3 months do not necessarily have an inferior outcome ([46, 47]). Patients who continued on therapy and achieved transcripts levels less than 10% by 6 months had the same long-term favorable outcome as patients with optimal molecular responses at 3 months.

Although achieving undetectable or the lowest possible transcript level is desirable, molecular positivity above the levels of MMR in the context of a CCyR is not an indication of failure of therapy. Some studies have suggested that increasing transcript levels may increase the risk of developing mutations or failure of therapy, but the magnitude of the increase that may predict for such events is variable, partly due to the variability of the testing in different laboratories. This may lead to erroneous changes in treatment, which is harmful, as it leads to potential discontinuation of viable and tolerable therapy. A single elevation in transcript levels should be confirmed in a subsequent determination 1 to 3 months later, and incremental increase in *BCR-ABL1* transcript levels should be determined to be greater than the variability of the laboratory test. In such situations, compliance with therapy should first be revisited. The risk of relapse or emergence of mutations is mostly associated with a sizeable (five- to tenfold) increase in the *BCR-ABL1* transcript levels that is associated with a loss of MMR or occurs in a patient who never achieved an MMR. Changes still below the level of MMR have little if any prognostic significance. Several studies evaluating patients receiving imatinib or second-generation TKIs showed that patients in CCyR have similar survival with or without MMR ([40, 41]). ABL kinase domain mutation screening should be performed in patients who have an inadequate initial response (defined as failure to achieve CHR at 3 months, partial cytogenetic response at 6 months, and CCyR at 12 months), in patients who show hematologic or cytogenetic relapse, or in patients with sustained 1-log increase in *BCR-ABL1* transcript ratio ([36]). All patients who progress to AP or BP CML should have ABL kinase mutations tested (Table 4-7).

Table 4-7 Main Features of the Monitoring Techniques Available for CML

Parameter	Cytogenetics	FISH	PCR
No cells evaluated	20	200	>10,000
Rapidity (days)	14-21	1-3	7-10
Source	BM	BM/PB	BM/PB
Clonal evolution	Yes	No	No
False negativity	NA	Yes	Yes
False positivity	No	≤10%	NA

BM, bone marrow; FISH, fluorescent in situ hybridization; NA, not applicable; PB, peripheral blood; PCR, polymerase chain reaction.

CHAPTER 4

When to Switch Therapy

Achievement of CCyR should be expected by 12 months of therapy, especially for standard-dose imatinib, whereas it may be reasonable to expect CCyR for second-generation TKIs within 3 to 6 months of treatment ([48]). Patients who do not achieve a CHR by 3 months should be considered for a change in therapy. If considering a change in therapy at 3 or 6 months for *BCR-ABL1* transcript level greater than 10% for patients on imatinib or second-generation TKIs, it is worth noting that very early switching has not yet been shown to influence the long-term outcomes ([49]). As such, it can be advocated that if the transcript level at 3 months is greater than 10%, providers should perform serial molecular monitoring between 3 and 6 months for definitive treatment response evaluation ([37]). If patients retain >10% transcript level at 6 months, change in therapy is indicated, because the chance of CCyR would be low. Patients who meet all of the relevant responses by the first 12 months are monitored periodically using FISH and PCR testing, and if there are clear signs of possible relapse or failure, bone marrow examination with conventional cytogenetics and kinase domain sequencing should be performed. Not achieving CCyR by 12 months or any extent of later cytogenetic relapse requires a change in therapy. Fluctuating molecular levels during concurrent CCyR should only prompt closer monitoring and a compliance assessment.

Response definitions recommended by the 2013 European LeukemiaNet guidelines are summarized in Table 4-8. Lack of MMR or CMR should not be interpreted as signal for change in TKI therapy. Achieving CMR allows for possibility of treatment discontinuation, which is only recommended in the setting of a clinical trial.

MANAGEMENT OF RESISTANCE

A subset of patients treated with imatinib may develop resistance. Among patients treated in CP, the rate of resistance is less than 4% per year and decreases after the first 3 years to approximately 0.5% to 1% per year. Following achievement of CCyR, the rate of resistance after year 3 of imatinib therapy is less than 1%, suggesting a durable CCyR on imatinib and the predictability of the CML course once such a response is obtained.

Mechanisms of resistance to imatinib can be *BCR-ABL1* dependent or independent. The first, more common group includes amplification or overexpression of BCR-ABL1 or its protein product ([50]) and point mutations of the *ABL* sequence ([51]). The second group includes multidrug-resistance expression and overexpression of Src kinases ([52]). *BCR-ABL1*–dependent mutations have been identified in approximately 50% of patients who develop clinical resistance to imatinib ([53]). More than 90 different mutations with varied significance and imatinib sensitivity have been described in relevant kinase domains, including the ATP-binding domain (P-loop), the catalytic domain, the activation loop, and amino acids that direct interact with imatinib. The "gatekeeper" mutation of particular importance

Table 4-8 Response Definitions to Imatinib in Chronic Phase CML (2013 European LeukemiaNet Guidelines)

	Response		
Evaluation Time Point	Optimal Response	Warning (close monitoring)	Failure (switch TKI)
Baseline	—	CCA in Ph+ cells High-risk Sokal (>1.2), Euro Score (>1,480) or Eutos-Score (>87)	—
3 months	BCR/ABL1[IS] ≤10% and/or Ph+ ≤35% (PCyR)	BCR/ABL1[IS] >10% and/or Ph+ 36%-95%	No CHR and/or Ph+ >95%
6 months	BCR/ABL1[IS] ≤1% and/or Ph+ 0% (CCyR)	BCR/ABL1[IS] 1%-10% and/or Ph+ 1%-35%	BCR/ABL1[IS] >10% and/or Ph >35%
12 months	BCR/ABL1[IS] ≤0.1% (MMR)	BCR-ABL1[IS] 0.1%-1%	BCR/ABL1[IS] >1% and/or Ph >0%
Any time	MMR or better	CCA in Ph− cells (−7 or 7q−)	Loss of CHR Loss of CCyR Loss of MMR confirmed[a] Mutations CCA in Ph+ cells

CCA, clonal chromosomal abnormalities; CCyR, complete cytogenic response; CHR, complete hematologic response; IS, BCR-ABL1 on International Scale; MMR, major molecular response; PCyR, partial cytogenetic response; TKI, tyrosine kinase inhibitor.
[a]In two consecutive tests, of which one was ≥1%.

is the T315I, which is resistant to all available TKIs except ponatinib. Most of the clinically relevant mutations develop in a few residues in the P-loop (G250E, Y253F/H, and E255K/V), the contact site (T315I), and the catalytic domain (M351T and F359V) ([54]). A list of mutations following imatinib resistance with their half-maximal inhibitory concentration values is shown in Table 4-5 ([23]). The long-term outcome of patients with CML treated with second-generation TKIs after imatinib failure is predicted by the in vitro sensitivity of *BCR-ABL1* kinase domain mutations ([55]). It is unclear if the identification of small mutated clones is clinically relevant ([56, 57]).

Although the sequential use of kinase inhibitor therapy often rescues a response, it can also result in further gain of mutations by the same (compound mutations) or different (polyclonal mutations) Ph clones, which represents a significant hurdle in the treatment of CML ([58]). High molecular dynamics in particular yield compound *BCR-ABL1* kinase domain mutations (polymutants), which represent two or more codon changes in the same *BCR-ABL* mRNA transcript ([59]). Ultra-deep sequencing to resolve qualitative and quantitative complexity of mutated populations surviving TKIs has recently suggested that conventional Sanger sequencing might be inadequate for this evaluation ([60]), although a recent report argues that many *BCR-ABL1* compound mutations may actually be artifacts due to PCR-mediated recombination ([61]).

Before labeling a patient as having TKI resistance and modifying therapy, treatment compliance and drug-drug interactions must be evaluated. Lower adherence rates observed more commonly in younger individuals, patients with adverse effects on treatment, and patients who have required dose escalations correlate with worse outcomes ([62]). Mutation analysis should be carried out only in instances of failure criteria.

Imatinib Dose Escalation

Imatinib escalation was the main option for managing suboptimal responses and treatment failures before the era of second-generation TKIs. In a phase II study that reported a 2-year follow-up after high-dose imatinib (400 mg twice daily; n = 49) for patients with CP CML and resistance to imatinib at doses from 400 to 600 mg, the major cytogenetic response (MCyR), CCyR, and MMR were 33%, 18%, and 12%, respectively, with an estimated PFS of 65% at 2 years ([63]). In another dose-escalation study from the University of Texas MD Anderson Cancer Center, 84 patients with CP CML were dose escalated to imatinib 600 to 800 mg/d after developing hematologic failure (n = 21) or cytogenetic failure (n = 63) to standard-dose imatinib ([55]). Among patients who met the criteria for cytogenetic failure, 75% (47 of 63 patients) responded to imatinib dose escalation. In contrast, in patients in whom imatinib was dose escalated because of hematologic failure, 48% achieved a CHR and only 14% (3 of 21 patients) achieved a cytogenetic response. Patients more likely to respond to imatinib dose increase are those who have previously achieved a cytogenetic response and then lost it and who have not developed any mutations unresponsive to imatinib. With mutations, a switch to a second-generation TKI is preferable.

SECOND- AND THIRD-GENERATION TYROSINE KINASE INHIBITORS

Dasatinib was first approved by the US Food and Drug Administration at a dose of 70 mg orally twice daily based on its efficacy and safety in a series of phase II trials in patients with all stages of CML (and those with Ph-positive ALL) who were resistant to, or intolerant of, imatinib ([64-66]). Over 50% of patients treated with dasatinib in CP after imatinib failure achieved a CCyR. Responses to dasatinib, nilotinib, bosutinib, and ponatinib among patients in CP, AP, and BP after imatinib failure or resistance are summarized in Table 4-9.

A randomized trial of dasatinib versus higher dose imatinib (800 mg daily) among patients who failed prior therapy with imatinib (400-600 mg) showed a significantly higher rate of response and PFS for patients receiving dasatinib, particularly among those who were already receiving imatinib 600 mg, those with *BCR-ABL1* mutations, and those who had never achieved a cytogenetic response with imatinib, establishing second-generation TKIs as the preferred approach after failure to imatinib standard-dose therapy ([63]).

In a long-term, 6-year follow-up of a phase III trial of 670 CP CML patients who were resistant (74%) or intolerant (24%) to imatinib, patients were randomized to receive dasatinib 100 mg once daily, 50 mg twice daily, 140 mg once daily, or 70 mg twice daily ([67]). At 6 years, PFS rates were 49%, 51%, 50%, and 47%, respectively, and OS rates were 71%, 74%, 77%, and 70%, respectively. The 6-year MMR rates were 43% and 40% in patients treated in the 100 mg once daily arm and all other arms combined, respectively. Dasatinib 100 mg once daily retained high activity and was associated with less toxicity, particularly pleural effusions and myelosuppression (grade 3 or 4 neutropenia or thrombocytopenia, 30% each), and the lowest rate of drug discontinuation for toxicity. Based on these results, the standard dasatinib dose for patients in CP became 100 mg daily. Similar results established 140 mg once daily as the preferred dose in advanced-stage disease.

Table 4-9 Important Phase II Trials of Second- and Third-Generation TKIS After Prior TKI Failure

	Percent Response													
	Dasatinib				Nilotinib				Bosutinib			Ponatinib		
	CP	AP	MyBP	LyBP	CP	AP	MyBP	LyBP	CP	AP	BP	CP	AP	BP
	N = 167	N = 174	N = 109	N = 48	N = 321	N = 137	N = 105	N = 31	N = 200	N = 51	N = 38	N = 270	N = 79	N = 94
Median follow-up (mo)	24	14	12	12	48	9	3	3	24	6	3	36	36	36
% resistant to imatinib	74	93	91	88	70	80	82	82	69	NR	NR	75	96	
% hematologic response		79	50	40	94	56	22	19	85	54	36	NR	NR	NR
CHR	92	45	27	29	76	31	11	13	81	54	36	NR	MaHR: 57	MaHR: 34
NEL		19	7	6		12	1	0		0	NR		NR	NR
% cytogenetic response		44	36	52	NR	NR	NR	NR		NR	NR		NR	NR
Complete	50	32	26	46	45	20	29	32	46	27	35	53	55	36
Partial	13	7	7	6	14	12	10	16	12	20	18	30	NR	NR
% survival	*At 6 years*				*At 4 years*				*At 4 years*			*At 3 years*		
	91	82	50	50	87	67	42	42	98	60	50	81	59	9

AP, accelerated phase; BP, blast phase; CHR, complete hematologic response; CP, chronic phase; LyBP, lymphoid blast phase; MyBP, myeloid blast phase; NEL, no evidence of leukemia; MaHR, major hematologic response; NR, not reported; TKI, tyrosine kinase inhibitor.

In a phase II study, 321 CP CML patients who were resistant or intolerant to imatinib were treated with nilotinib 400 mg twice daily ([68]). At the 48-month follow-up, 45% of the patients achieved CCyR; the PFS and OS rates were 57% and 78%, respectively ([69]). Deeper levels of molecular responses at 3 and 6 months correlated with improved long-term outcomes. In the expanded access ENACT trial, 1,422 patients in CML CP or AP after imatinib failure were treated with nilotinib 400 mg twice daily ([70]). After a median follow-up of 18 months, the CCyR rate was 50% and the PFS rate was 80%.

Bosutinib

Bosutinib (SKI606) is an orally available dual Src/Abl inhibitor that is 30 to 50 times more potent than imatinib against unmutated *BCR-ABL1*. It has activity against most imatinib-resistant *BCR-ABL1* mutants with the exception of T315I. In contrast to other available TKIs, bosutinib has minimal inhibitory activity against C-Kit and PDGFR. It was initially studied in patients resistant or intolerant to imatinib ([71]). Among 288 patients treated in a phase I/II trial, more than two-thirds of the patients had imatinib-resistant CML. The primary end point, MCyR at 6 months, was achieved in 31%. Overall, 41% of patients achieved a CCyR, and 64% of them achieved MMR. The 2-year PFS and OS rates were 79% and 92%, respectively. Responses to bosutinib in CP, AP, and BP after imatinib resistance or failure are summarized in Table 4-9.

Bosutinib also was assessed as third- or fourth-line therapy in 118 patients with CP CML who had been previously treated with imatinib followed by nilotinib and/or dasatinib ([72]). Bosutinib resulted in a CCyR rate of 24%. The 24-month PFS and OS rates were 73% and 83%, respectively. Clinical efficacy in the relapse setting led to the evaluation of bosutinib as frontline therapy.

Treatment with bosutinib has been generally well tolerated with no pleural effusions and modest myelosuppression. The most common adverse events were gastrointestinal (nausea, vomiting, diarrhea) and were usually grade 1 or 2, manageable, and transient and diminished in frequency and severity after the first 3 to 4 weeks of treatment ([72]). A multicenter phase III randomized trial is ongoing to compare a lower dose (400 mg daily) of bosutinib and standard-dose imatinib (400 mg) in patients with newly diagnosed CP CML.

Ponatinib

Ponatinib (formerly AP24534) is a rationally designed third-generation TKI that efficiently inhibits Bcr-Abl as well as *FLT3*, *PDGFR*, *VEGF*, and *C-KIT* ([73]). It is more than 500 times more potent than imatinib at inhibiting *BCR-ABL1* and is the first compound in the class to inhibit T315I mutation ([73]). Ponatinib was approved following the phase II PACE trial, in which 449 patients with heavily pretreated CML or Ph-positive ALL, resistant to or intolerant to dasatinib or nilotinib or with the T315I mutation, were enrolled ([74]). The dose of ponatinib was 45 mg once daily. Among the 267 patients who received ponatinib in CP, 56% achieved an MCyR by 12 months (MCyR rate of 70% in patients with a T315I mutation). Patients responded more favorably if they had received fewer TKIs. After a median follow-up of 3.5 years, 59% of patients achieved MCyR; 83% of those remained in MCyR at 3 years. Furthermore, 39% of patients achieved an MMR or better. The 3-year PFS and OS rates were 60% and 81%, respectively ([75]). Arterial occlusive events occurred in 28% of patients (23% serious). The most common all-grade treatment-emergent adverse events were abdominal pain (46%), rash (46%), thrombocytopenia (45%), headache (43%), constipation (41%), and dry skin (41%) ([75]). Grade 3 or 4 toxicities included myelosuppression (48% overall, observed less commonly in CP CML patients), hepatotoxicity (8%), pancreatitis (5%), hemorrhagic events associated mostly with grade 4 thrombocytopenia (5%), treatment-emergent symptomatic hypertension (2%), neuropathy (2%), and cranial neuropathy (<1%).

As of early 2014, ponatinib labeling included a revised warning regarding risk of thrombotic events (13% per year), vascular occlusions, heart failure, and hepatotoxicity; revised dosing information; and indications limited to adults with T315I mutation and those for whom no other TKI is indicated ([76]). Vascular occlusion adverse events were more frequent with increasing age and in patients with prior history of ischemia, hypertension, diabetes, or hyperlipidemia ([77]). Factors associated with increased risk of vascular occlusion events include older age, higher dose, history of myocardial infarction or prior vascular events, and longer duration of CML ([78]).

Choosing a Second- or Third-Line Option

When faced with treatment failure, a bone marrow with cytogenetic assessment should be completed to determine disease phase and possible clonal evolution. Mutational testing for *BCR-ABL1* kinase domain mutations should also be performed, because it helps guide the decision on TKI selection. Dasatinib, nilotinib, and bosutinib are effective against most mutations known to elicit resistance to imatinib ([71, 79]). For dasatinib, bosutinib, and nilotinib, in vitro and in vivo data have identified mutations that have differential responses to different agents: dasatinib and bosutinib perform better with Y253H, E255K/V, or F359C/V mutations, whereas nilotinib has activity with V299L and F317L mutations, which confer resistance to dasatinib and bosutinib ([80, 81]). If mutational information is not available, one can resort to considerations regarding toxicity. Bosutinib is a valid choice for patients who fail imatinib and who have pulmonary and vascular risk factors. Ponatinib should be considered the agent of choice for any patient with T315I mutation or compound mutations, in patients who have failed prior second-generation TKIs, and in patients with advanced-phase disease. Vascular thrombotic events represent a serious risk but are likely outweighed by the risks of T315I-mutated disease, for which effective treatment options are scarce.

NON–TYROSINE KINASE INHIBITORS

Omacetaxine mepesuccinate is a cephalotaxine ester and a derivative of homoharringtonine that has a mechanism of action independent of tyrosine kinase inhibition. It is a multitarget protein synthesis inhibitor with an excellent bioavailability through the subcutaneous route. Unaffected by the presence of mutations, it has been in clinical development for several years with activity against CML ([82]). It has recently also been found to affect the leukemic stem cell compartment, making it an attractive option for the potential total elimination of the leukemic burden and potential cure.

Omacetaxine was approved in the United States for the treatment of patients with CP or AP CML with resistance and/or an intolerance to two or more TKIs on the basis of pooled data from two phase II, open-label, international, multicenter studies (CML-202 and CML-203), in which patients were treated with omacetaxine 1.25 mg/m^2 twice daily for 14 days every 28 days until response, followed by maintenance for 7 days every 28 days ([83, 84]). Initial results showed that 20% of patients with CP CML achieved a durable MCyR with a median response duration of 17.7 months ([83]) and 27% of patients with AP CML achieved a major hematologic response (MHR) that was maintained for a median of 9 months ([84]). After a minimum follow-up of 24 months, 18% of patients in CP CML achieved a MCyR with a median duration of 12.5 months and 14% of patients in AP CML achieved or maintained an MHR for a median of 4.7 months (MCyR was not achieved); median OS times for CP CML (n = 50) and AP CML (n = 14) patients who received more than three cycles of treatment were 49 and 25 months, respectively ([85]). Grade 3 or higher hematologic toxicities (including thrombocytopenia, anemia, or neutropenia) were the major side effects (79% and 73% for CP CML and AP CML, respectively), with discontinuation due to toxicity in 10% of CP and 5% of AP patients. Further analyses of CP and AP CML patients with the T315I mutation (n = 16 and n = 2, respectively), showed that three CP patients achieved MCyR, whereas one AP patient achieved no evidence of leukemia ([85]).

ALLOGENEIC STEM CELL TRANSPLANTATION

After the successful introduction of TKIs, there has been a paradigm shift in the approach to CML therapy. An allogeneic stem cell transplant (ASCT) is no longer recommended as a first-line therapy and is instead reserved as a third-line or later strategy. It still has an important role in patients who evolve to AP or BP. Transplantation carries significant risks of acute and chronic graft-versus-host disease (GVHD), veno-occlusive disease, life-threatening infections, secondary malignancy, and poorer overall quality of life, although recent advances in the field have significantly improved some of these risks. Current recommendations for an ASCT are restricted to patients who are in AP or BP CML, those in CP who have failed at least two TKIs and acquired compound mutations, and patients harboring the T315I mutation after a trial of ponatinib therapy ([86]). Prior exposure to TKIs does not have a negative impact on the transplant outcome; in fact, patients referred to transplant may have a better outcome if undergoing transplant with less CML burden ([87]). Recommendations for the role and timing of ASCT CML are outlined in the Table 4-10 ([76]).

TREATMENT DISCONTINUATION

Few studies have addressed the issue of discontinuing TKI therapy. The Stop Imatinib (STIM) trial evaluated the risk of relapse in patients who stopped treatment with imatinib after being in CMR (MR$^{4.5}$) for longer than 2 years. At the most recent follow-up of 50 months, among 100 patients monitored, 61% developed molecular relapse, with most of these events occurring within 7 months of imatinib discontinuation. Nearly all patients regained CMR on retreatment with imatinib (one patient lost CCyR and was treated with dasatinib) ([88, 89]). This study suggested that approximately 40% of patients with durable CMR might be cured with TKI alone. Overall, low-risk Sokal score and duration of imatinib therapy greater than 60 months predicted for preservation of CMR following discontinuation of therapy.

The TWISTER study followed 40 patients who stopped imatinib after greater than 2 years of undetectable MRD (MR$^{4.5}$) ([90]). During the median follow-up of 43 months (minimum, 15 months), 22 patients (55%) became molecularly positive, and nearly 70% of molecular relapses occurred within the first 6 months

Table 4-10 Recommendations for Role and Timing of Allogeneic HSCT in CML

Status	TKIs	Allogeneic HSCT
AP, BP	Interim treatment to MRD	If in remission
Imatinib or first-line second-generation TKI treatment failure in CP, with T315I mutation	Ponatinib	If not responding well to ponatinib
Imatinib or first-line second-generation TKI treatment failure in CP, no clonal evolution, no mutations, good initial response to imatinib	Long-term treatment with TKI in second-line setting	Third-line, after second TKI treatment failure
Imatinib or first-line second-generation TKI treatment failure in CP, with clonal evolution, with mutations resistant to second-generation TKIs, no CyR to imatinib	Interim treatment with ponatinib eventually to MRD	As soon as possible if no response to ponatinib
Elderly patients, age >70 years, after imatinib treatment failure	Long-term treatment with TKI in second-line setting	Forego allogeneic HSCT for many years (maximize quality of life)

AP, accelerated phase; BP, blast phase; CML, chronic myeloid leukemia; CP, chronic phase; CyR, cytogenetic response; HSCT, hematopoietic stem cell transplantation; MRD, minimal residual disease; TKI, tyrosine kinase inhibitor.

of treatment cessation. Following the resumption of TKIs, patients regained molecular responses. None of the relapsing patients developed kinase domain mutation, AP, or BP.

A pan-European Stop Tyrosine Kinase Inhibitor trial (EURO-SKI study) aimed to define factors associated with durable deep MR after stopping TKI. An interim analysis of 200 patients with 6-month follow-up of molecular events was reported ([91]). Adults in CP CML on TKI treatment in confirmed deep molecular response (molecular response with a 4-log reduction in *BCR-ABL* transcripts from baseline [MR^4]; *BCR-ABL* <0.01%) for at least 1 year (>4 log reduction on TKI therapy for >12 months confirmed by three consecutive PCR tests) and on TKI treatment for at least 3 years were eligible. Median duration of TKI treatment was 8 years (range, 3-12.6 years), and median duration of MR^4 before TKI cessation was 5.4 years (range, 1-11.7 years). Overall, 123 of the 200 patients remained without relapse in the first 6 months. Recurrence of CML, defined as loss of MMR, was observed in 47 (47%) of 114 patients treated for <8 years, as compared to 27 (27%) of 86 patients treated for >8 years (P = .003). The duration of MR^4 >5 years versus <5 years was predictive for a lower relapse rate (P = .03).

The feasibility of second-generation TKI discontinuation has also been tested in the French STOP 2G-TKI study for patients treated with nilotinib or dasatinib as frontline therapy or after imatinib failure or intolerance ([92]). Twenty-four months of persistent MR$^{4.5}$ was a requirement for discontinuation of TKI. Interim outcome of 52 patients with a median follow-up of 32 months (range, 12-56 months) reported treatment-free survival of 54% (majority of relapses occurred early, with a median duration of 4 months).

At present, given the uncertainty in selecting the best candidate patients for discontinuation of TKI therapy and the lack of long-term follow up, TKI discontinuation should not be recommended outside the context of a clinical trial.

ADVANCED-STAGE (ACCELERATED PHASE/BLAST PHASE) CHRONIC MYELOID LEUKEMIA

Patients in AP or BP CML may receive initial therapy with newer generation TKIs (preferred over imatinib) to reduce the disease burden and may be considered for early ASCT ([93-95]). Nonlymphoid BP response rate is 40% with a combination of TKIs and chemotherapy, with a median OS of 6 to 12 months. With TKI and antilymphoid therapy, the response rate in lymphoid BP is 70% to 80%, and the median OS is 12 to 24 months ([96, 97]). Tyrosine kinase inhibitors provide hematologic responses in 80% of patients, with an estimated 4-year OS of 40% to 55% in AP, but only a 40% response rate with a median OS of 9 to 12 months in BP. De novo AP responds better to frontline TKI therapy compared to AP transformed from antecedent CP, with a 6- to 8-year OS on TKI therapy of 60% to 80% ([98]). These patients may continue on TKI therapy indefinitely, provided they attain CCyR. Currently, the only curative therapy for AP or BP CML is ASCT, with a cure rate of 15% to 40% for AP and 5% to 20% for BP ([37]). Patients in both phases should be encouraged to participate in clinical trials.

CHAPTER 4

RECOMMENDATIONS FOR TREATMENT

Chronic Phase

Standard-of-care, category 1 recommendation for the treatment of patients with newly diagnosed CP CML includes any of the three TKIs: imatinib, dasatinib, or nilotinib. Comorbidities, disease risk factors, side effect profiles, and cost may help in choosing one over another. Second-generation TKIs have demonstrated higher rates of early optimal responses; however, their impact on long-term OS remains to be evaluated. Achievement of CCyR is the primary goal of TKI therapy, and it may be desired by 3 to 6 months of therapy with dasatinib or nilotinib. Patients should be carefully monitored with an emphasis on compliance as well as treatment of side effects to minimize unnecessary treatment interruptions and dose reductions. Allogeneic stem cell transplantation or other chemotherapy agents are no longer recommended as frontline treatments given the excellent responses and long-term OS achieved with TKIs. Kinase domain mutation profile is of relevance in the CML cytogenetic or hematologic relapse setting only and should be considered for patients who are failing imatinib or second-generation TKIs or who progress to AP or BP.

Accelerated and Blast Phase

Newer generation TKIs are preferred over imatinib as the frontline therapy. Allogeneic stem-cell transplantation, ideally in second CP, should be considered early for all AP patients based on response to TKI therapy. De novo AP may be treated long-term with TKI therapy alone provided CCyR is achieved. Tyrosine kinase inhibitor monotherapy or combination with chemotherapy (hyperfractionated cyclophosphamide, vincristine, doxorubicin, and dexamethasone [hyper-CVAD] for lymphoid, AML-type for myeloid phenotype) may be considered for patients who are poor transplant candidates or as a bridge to ASCT.

FUTURE DIRECTIONS

In 2016, multiple TKIs are available for the treatment of CML, including imatinib, dasatinib, nilotinib, bosutinib, and ponatinib, in addition to omacetaxine and other older therapeutic agents. Following the dramatic refinement of therapeutic options for CML over the last 15 years, the majority of patients with CML are expected to have a normal life expectancy, provided that compliance with therapy is maintained and optimal monitoring is closely implemented, modifying therapy for early signs of resistance or treatment failure. The prevalence of CML will continue to increase over the next two decades. This will offer an opportunity to celebrate this success, but also will be a burden in terms of potential long-term side effects and costs of care. Future efforts will address improving complete molecular eradication of CML and achieving durable CMRs, even after therapy discontinuation (molecular cure). New-generation TKIs in novel combinations with available agents (eg, omacetaxine, decitabine, pegylated IFN) or with new investigational therapies (eg, JAK2 inhibitors, hedgehog inhibitors, stem cell toxins or vaccines, bcl2 inhibitors, other immune approaches) are likely to play a key role in the ultimate cure of CML.

REFERENCES

1. Jemal A, Siegel R, Xu J, Ward E. Cancer statistics, 2010. *CA Cancer J Clin*. 2011;60(5):277-300.
2. Corso A, Lazzarino M, Morra E, et al. Chronic myelogenous leukemia and exposure to ionizing radiation—a retrospective study of 443 patients. *Ann Hematol*. 1995;70(2):79-82.
3. Huang X, Cortes J, Kantarjian H. Estimations of the increasing prevalence and plateau prevalence of chronic myeloid leukemia in the era of tyrosine kinase inhibitor therapy. *Cancer*. 2012;118(12):3123-3127.
4. Kurzrock R, Gutterman JU, Talpaz M. The molecular genetics of Philadelphia chromosome-positive leukemias. *N Engl J Med*. 1988;319(15):990-998.
5. Kantarjian HM, Dixon D, Keating MJ, et al. Characteristics of accelerated disease in chronic myelogenous leukemia. *Cancer*. 1988;61(7):1441-1446.
6. Cortes J, Kantarjian H. Advanced-phase chronic myeloid leukemia. *Semin Hematol*. 2003;40(1):79-86.
7. Cortes JE, Talpaz M, Kantarjian H. Chronic myelogenous leukemia: a review. *Am J Med*. 1996;100(5):555-570.
8. Jabbour E, Cortes JE, Kantarjian HM. Molecular monitoring in chronic myeloid leukemia: response to tyrosine kinase inhibitors and prognostic implications. *Cancer*. 2008;112(10):2112-2118.
9. Knox WF, Bhavnani M, Davson J, Geary CG. Histological classification of chronic granulocytic leukaemia. *Clin Lab Haematol*. 1984;6(2):171-175.
10. O'Brien SG, Guilhot F, Larson RA, et al. Imatinib compared with interferon and low-dose cytarabine for newly diagnosed chronic-phase chronic myeloid leukemia. *N Engl J Med*. 2003;348(11):994-1004.
11. Guo JQ, Lin H, Kantarjian H, et al. Comparison of competitive-nested PCR and real-time PCR in detecting BCR-ABL fusion transcripts in chronic myeloid leukemia patients. *Leukemia*. 2002;16(12):2447-2453.
12. Druker BJ, Tamura S, Buchdunger E, et al. Effects of a selective inhibitor of the Abl tyrosine kinase on the growth of Bcr-Abl positive cells. *Nat Med*. 1996;2(5):561-566.
13. Kantarjian H, Sawyers C, Hochhaus A, et al. Hematologic and cytogenetic responses to imatinib mesylate in chronic myelogenous leukemia. *N Engl J Med*. 2002;346(9):645-652.
14. Deininger M, O'Brien SG, Guilhot F, et al. International randomized study of interferon *v* STI571 (IRIS) 8-year follow up: sustained survival and low risk for progression of events in patients with newly diagnosed chronic myeloid leukemia in chronic phase (CML-CP) treated with imatinib. *Blood*. 2009;114:1126.
15. Druker BJ, Talpaz M, Resta DJ, et al. Efficacy and safety of a specific inhibitor of the BCR-ABL tyrosine kinase in chronic

myeloid leukemia. *N Engl J Med.* 2001;344(14):1031-1037.
16. Cortes JE, Kantarjian HM, Goldberg SL, et al. High-dose imatinib in newly diagnosed chronic-phase chronic myeloid leukemia: high rates of rapid cytogenetic and molecular responses. *J Clin Oncol.* 2009;27(28):4754-4759.
17. Cortes JE, Baccarani M, Guilhot F, et al. Phase III, randomized, open-label study of daily imatinib mesylate 400 mg versus 800 mg in patients with newly diagnosed, previously untreated chronic myeloid leukemia in chronic phase using molecular end points: tyrosine kinase inhibitor optimization and selectivity study. *J Clin Oncol.* 2010;28(3):424-430.
18. Baccarani M, Druker BJ, Branford S, et al. Long-term response to imatinib is not affected by the initial dose in patients with Philadelphia chromosome-positive chronic myeloid leukemia in chronic phase: final update from the Tyrosine Kinase Inhibitor Optimization and Selectivity (TOPS) study. *Int J Hematol.* 2014;99(5):616-624.
19. Baccarani M, Rosti G, Castagnetti F, et al. Comparison of imatinib 400 mg and 800 mg daily in the front-line treatment of high-risk, Philadelphia-positive chronic myeloid leukemia: a European LeukemiaNet Study. *Blood.* 2009;113(19):4497-4504.
20. Preudhomme C, Guilhot J, Nicolini FE, et al. Imatinib plus peginterferon alfa-2a in chronic myeloid leukemia. *N Engl J Med.* 2010;363(26):2511-2521.
21. O'Hare T, Walters DK, Stoffregen EP, et al. In vitro activity of Bcr-Abl inhibitors AMN107 and BMS-354825 against clinically relevant imatinib-resistant Abl kinase domain mutants. *Cancer Res.* 2005;65(11):4500-4505.
22. Tokarski JS, Newitt JA, Chang CYJ, et al. The structure of dasatinib (BMS-354825) bound to activated ABL kinase domain elucidates its inhibitory activity against imatinib-resistant ABL mutants. *Cancer Res.* 2006;66(11):5790-5797.
23. Gozgit JM, Schrock A, Chen TH, et al. Comprehensive analysis of the in vitro potency of ponatinib, and all other approved BCR-ABL tyrosine kinase inhibitors (TKIs), against a panel of single and compound BCR-ABL mutants. *Blood.* 2013;122:3992.
24. Lombardo LJ, Lee FY, Chen P, et al. Discovery of N-(2-chloro-6-methyl-phenyl)-2-(6-(4-(2-hydroxyethyl)-piperazin-1-yl)-2-methylpyrimidin-4-ylamino)thiazole-5-carboxamide (BMS-354825), a dual Src/Abl kinase inhibitor with potent antitumor activity in preclinical assays. *J Med Chem.* 2004;47(27):6658-6661.
25. Shah NP, Tran C, Lee FY, Chen P, Norris D, Sawyers CL. Overriding imatinib resistance with a novel ABL kinase inhibitor. *Science.* 2004;305(5682):399-401.
26. Kantarjian H, Shah NP, Hochhaus A, et al. Dasatinib versus imatinib in newly diagnosed chronic-phase chronic myeloid leukemia. *N Engl J Med.* 2010;362(24):2260-2270.
27. Radich JP, Kopecky KJ, Appelbaum FR, et al. A randomized trial of dasatinib 100 mg versus imatinib 400 mg in newly diagnosed chronic-phase chronic myeloid leukemia. *Blood.* 2012;120(19):3898-3905.
28. O'Brien SG, Hedgley C, Adams S, et al. Spirit 2: an NCRI randomised study comparing dasatinib with imatinib in patients with newly diagnosed CML. *Blood.* 2014;632:517 (ASH Annual Meeting Abstracts).
29. Weisberg E, Manley PW, Breitenstein W, et al. Characterization of AMN107, a selective inhibitor of native and mutant Bcr-Abl. *Cancer Cell.* 2005;7(2):129-141.
30. Golemovic M, Verstovsek S, Giles F, et al. AMN107, a novel aminopyrimidine inhibitor of Bcr-Abl, has in vitro activity against imatinib-resistant chronic myeloid leukemia. *Clin Cancer Res.* 2005;11(13):4941-4947.
31. Saglio G, Kim D-W, Issaragrisil S, et al. Nilotinib versus imatinib for newly diagnosed chronic myeloid leukemia. *N Engl J Med.* 2010;362(24):2251-2259.
32. Larson, RA, Kim D-W, Issaragrisil S, et al. Efficacy and safety of nilotinib (NIL) vs imatinib (IM) in patients (pts) with newly diagnosed chronic myeloid leukemia in chronic phase (CML-CP): long-term follow-up (f/u) of ENESTnd [abstract]. *Blood.* 2014;632:4541.
33. Jabbour E, Kantarjian H. Chronic myeloid leukemia: 2014 update on diagnosis, monitoring, and management. *Am J Hematol.* 2014;89(5):547-556.
34. Quintás-Cardama A, Han X, Kantarjian H, Cortes J. Tyrosine kinase inhibitor-induced platelet dysfunction in patients with chronic myeloid leukemia. *Blood.* 2009;114(2):261-263.
35. Quintás-Cardama A, Kantarjian H, Cortes J. Nilotinib-associated vascular events. *Clin Lymphoma Myeloma Leuk.* 2012;12(5):337-340.
36. Baccarani M, Cortes J, Pane F, et al. Chronic myeloid leukemia: an update of concepts and management recommendations of European LeukemiaNet. *J Clin Oncol.* 2009;27(35):6041-6051.
37. Baccarani M, Deininger MW, Rosti G, et al. European LeukemiaNet recommendations for the management of chronic myeloid leukemia: 2013. *Blood.* 2013;122(6):872-884.
38. Testoni N, Marzocchi G, Luatti S, et al. Chronic myeloid leukemia: a prospective comparison of interphase fluorescence in situ hybridization and chromosome banding analysis for the definition of complete cytogenetic response: a study of the GIMEMA CML WP. *Blood.* 2009;114(24):4939-4943.
39. Kantarjian H, Cortes J. Considerations in the management of patients with Philadelphia chromosome-positive chronic myeloid leukemia receiving tyrosine kinase inhibitor therapy. *J Clin Oncol.* 2011;29(12):1512-1516.
40. Jabbour E, Kantarjian HM, Saglio G, et al. Early response with dasatinib or imatinib in chronic myeloid leukemia: 3-year follow-up from a randomized phase 3 trial (DASISION). *Blood.* 2014;123(4):494-500.
41. Hehlmann R, Lauseker M, Jung-Munkwitz S, et al. Tolerability-adapted imatinib 800 mg/d versus 400 mg/d versus 400 mg/d plus interferon-α in newly diagnosed chronic myeloid leukemia. *J Clin Oncol.* 2011;29(12):1634-1642.
42. Kantarjian HM, Shan J, Jones D, et al. Significance of increasing levels of minimal residual disease in patients with Philadelphia chromosome-positive chronic myelogenous leukemia in complete cytogenetic response. *J Clin Oncol.* 2009;27(22):3659-3663.
43. Marin D, Ibrahim AR, Lucas C, et al. Assessment of BCR-ABL1 transcript levels at 3 months is the only requirement for predicting outcome for patients with chronic myeloid leukemia treated with tyrosine kinase inhibitors. *J Clin Oncol.* 2012;30(3):232-238.
44. Jain P, Kantarjian H, Nazha A, et al. Early responses predict better outcomes in patients with newly diagnosed chronic myeloid leukemia: results with four tyrosine kinase inhibitor modalities. *Blood.* 2013;121(24):4867-4874.
45. Neelakantan P, Gerrard G, Lucas C, et al. Combining BCR-ABL1 transcript levels at 3 and 6 months in chronic myeloid leukemia: implications for early intervention strategies. *Blood.* 2013;121(14):2739-2742.
46. Nazha A, Kantarjian H, Jain P, et al. Assessment at 6 months may be warranted for patients with chronic myeloid leukemia with no major cytogenetic response at 3 months. *Haematologica.* 2013;98(11):1686-1688.
47. Branford S, Roberts N, Yeung DT, et al. Any BRC-ABL reduction below 10% at 6 months of therapy significantly improves outcome for CML patients with a poor response at 3 months [abstract]. *Blood.* 2013;122:254.
48. Jabbour E, Kantarjian HM, O'Brien S, et al. Front-line therapy with second-generation tyrosine kinase inhibitors in patients with early chronic phase chronic myeloid leukemia: what is the optimal response? *J Clin Oncol.* 2011;29(32):4260-4265.
49. Cortes JE, De Souza CA, Lopez JL, et al. Switching to nilotinib in patients with chronic myeloid leukemia in chronic phase with

suboptimal cytogenetic response on imatinib: first results of the LASOR trial [abstract]. *Blood.* 2013;122:95.

50. Le Coutre P, Tassi E, Varella-Garcia M, et al. Induction of resistance to the Abelson inhibitor STI571 in human leukemic cells through gene amplification. *Blood.* 2000;95(5):1758-1766.
51. Gorre ME, Mohammed M, Ellwood K, et al. Clinical resistance to STI-571 cancer therapy caused by BCR-ABL gene mutation or amplification. *Science.* 2001;293(5531):876-880.
52. Weisberg E, Griffin JD. Mechanism of resistance to the ABL tyrosine kinase inhibitor STI571 in BCR/ABL-transformed hematopoietic cell lines. *Blood.* 2000;95(11):3498-3505.
53. Branford S, Rudzki Z, Walsh S, et al. Detection of BCR-ABL mutations in patients with CML treated with imatinib is virtually always accompanied by clinical resistance, and mutations in the ATP phosphate-binding loop (P-loop) are associated with a poor prognosis. *Blood.* 2003;102(1):276-283.
54. Soverini S, Colarossi S, Gnani A, et al. Contribution of ABL kinase domain mutations to imatinib resistance in different subsets of Philadelphia-positive patients: by the GIMEMA Working Party on Chronic Myeloid Leukemia. *Clin Cancer Res.* 2006;12(24):7374-7379.
55. Jabbour E, Jones D, Kantarjian HM, et al. Long-term outcome of patients with chronic myeloid leukemia treated with second-generation tyrosine kinase inhibitors after imatinib failure is predicted by the in vitro sensitivity of BCR-ABL kinase domain mutations. *Blood.* 2009;114(10):2037-2043.
56. Quintás-Cardama A, Cortes J. Molecular biology of Bcr-Abl1-positive chronic myeloid leukemia. *Blood.* 2009;113(8):1619-1630.
57. Willis SG, Lange T, Demehri S, et al. High-sensitivity detection of BCR-ABL kinase domain mutations in imatinib-naive patients: correlation with clonal cytogenetic evolution but not response to therapy. *Blood.* 2005;106(6):2128-2137.
58. Shah NP, Skaggs BJ, Branford S, et al. Sequential ABL kinase inhibitor therapy selects for compound drug-resistant BCR-ABL mutations with altered oncogenic potency. *J Clin Invest.* 2007;117(9):2562-2569.
59. Gibbons DL, Pricl S, Posocco P, et al. Molecular dynamics reveal BCR-ABL1 polymutants as a unique mechanism of resistance to PAN-BCR-ABL1 kinase inhibitor therapy. *Proc Natl Acad Sci USA.* 2014;111(9):3550-3555.
60. Soverini S, De Benedittis C, Machova Polakova K, et al. Unraveling the complexity of tyrosine kinase inhibitor-resistant populations by ultra-deep sequencing of the BCR-ABL kinase domain. *Blood.* 2013;122(9):1634-1648.
61. Parker WT, Phillis SR, Yeung DTO, Hughes TP, Scott HS, Branford S. Many BCR-ABL1 compound mutations reported in chronic myeloid leukemia patients may actually be artifacts due to PCR-mediated recombination. *Blood.* 2014;124(1):153-155.
62. Marin D, Bazeos A, Mahon F-X, et al. Adherence is the critical factor for achieving molecular responses in patients with chronic myeloid leukemia who achieve complete cytogenetic responses on imatinib. *J Clin Oncol.* 2010;28(14):2381-2388.
63. Kantarjian H, Pasquini R, Lévy V, et al. Dasatinib or high-dose imatinib for chronic-phase chronic myeloid leukemia resistant to imatinib at a dose of 400 to 600 milligrams daily: two-year follow-up of a randomized phase 2 study (START-R). *Cancer.* 2009;115(18):4136-4147.
64. Cortes J, Rousselot P, Kim D-W, et al. Dasatinib induces complete hematologic and cytogenetic responses in patients with imatinib-resistant or -intolerant chronic myeloid leukemia in blast crisis. *Blood.* 2007;109(8):3207-3213.
65. Guilhot F, Apperley J, Kim DW, et al. Dasatinib induces significant hematologic and cytogenetic responses in patients with imatinib-resistant or -intolerant chronic myeloid leukemia in accelerated phase. *Blood.* 2007;109(10):4143-4150.
66. Hochhaus A, Baccarani M, Deininger M, et al. Dasatinib induces durable cytogenetic responses in patients with chronic myelogenous leukemia in chronic phase with resistance or intolerance to imatinib. *Leukemia.* 2008;22(6):1200-1206.
67. Shah NP, Guilhot F, Cortes JE, et al. Long-term outcome with dasatinib after imatinib failure in chronic-phase chronic myeloid leukemia: follow-up of a phase 3 study. *Blood.* 2014;123(15):2317-2324.
68. Kantarjian HM, Giles FJ, Bhalla KN, et al. Nilotinib is effective in patients with chronic myeloid leukemia in chronic phase after imatinib resistance or intolerance: 24-month follow-up results. *Blood.* 2011;117(4):1141-1145.
69. Giles FJ, le Coutre PD, Pinilla-Ibarz J, et al. Nilotinib in imatinib-resistant or imatinib-intolerant patients with chronic myeloid leukemia in chronic phase: 48-month follow-up results of a phase II study. *Leukemia.* 2012;27(1):107-112.
70. Nicolini FE, Turkina A, Shen Z-X, et al. Expanding Nilotinib Access in Clinical Trials (ENACT): an open-label, multicenter study of oral nilotinib in adult patients with imatinib-resistant or imatinib-intolerant Philadelphia chromosome-positive chronic myeloid leukemia in the chronic phase. *Cancer.* 2012;118(1):118-126.
71. Cortes JE, Kantarjian HM, Brümmendorf TH, et al. Safety and efficacy of bosutinib (SKI-606) in chronic phase Philadelphia chromosome-positive chronic myeloid leukemia patients with resistance or intolerance to imatinib. *Blood.* 2011;118(17):4567-4576.
72. Khoury HJ, Cortes JE, Kantarjian HM, et al. Bosutinib is active in chronic phase chronic myeloid leukemia after imatinib and dasatinib and/or nilotinib therapy failure. *Blood.* 2012;119(15):3403-3412.
73. O'Hare T, Shakespeare WC, Zhu X, et al. AP24534, a pan-BCR-ABL inhibitor for chronic myeloid leukemia, potently inhibits the T315I mutant and overcomes mutation-based resistance. *Cancer Cell.* 2009;16(5):401-412.
74. Cortes JE, Kim D-W, Pinilla-Ibarz J, et al. A phase 2 trial of ponatinib in Philadelphia chromosome-positive leukemias. *N Engl J Med.* 2013;369(19):1783-1796.
75. BusinessWire: ARIAD announces long-term safety and efficacy data of ponatinib from phase 2 pace clinical trial median follow-up now approximately 3.5 years for chronic phase CML patients. http://www.businesswire.com/news/home/20150612005041/en/ARIAD-Announces-Long-Term-Safety-Efficacy-Data-Ponatinib#.VYnbHRNVhBc. Accessed June 30, 2015.
76. Jabbour E, Kantarjian H, Cortes J. Use of second- and third-generation tyrosine kinase inhibitors in the treatment of chronic myeloid leukemia: an evolving treatment paradigm. *Clin Lymphoma Myeloma Leuk.* 2015;15(6):323-334.
77. Iclusig (ponatinib) [prescribing information]. Cambridge, MA: ARIAD Pharmaceuticals, Inc; 2014.
78. Kantarjian HM, Kim DW, Pinilla-Ibarz J, et al. Ponatinib (PON) in patients (pts) with philadelphia chromosome-positive (Ph+) leukemias resistant or intolerant to dasatinib or nilotinib, or with the T315I mutation: longer-term follow up of the PACE trial [abstract]. *J Clin Oncol.* 2014;325:7081.
79. Jabbour E, Branford S, Saglio G, Jones D, Cortes JE, Kantarjian HM. Practical advice for determining the role of BCR-ABL mutations in guiding tyrosine kinase inhibitor therapy in patients with chronic myeloid leukemia. *Cancer.* 2011;117(9):1800-1811.
80. Müller MC, Cortes JE, Kim D-W, et al. Dasatinib treatment of chronic-phase chronic myeloid leukemia: analysis of responses according to preexisting BCR-ABL mutations. *Blood.* 2009;114(24):4944-4953.
81. Hughes T, Saglio G, Branford S, et al. Impact of baseline BCR-ABL mutations on response to nilotinib in patients with chronic myeloid leukemia in chronic phase. *J Clin Oncol.* 2009;27(25):4204-4210.
82. Kantarjian HM, Talpaz M, Santini V, Murgo A, Cheson B, O'Brien SM. Homoharringtonine: history, current research, and future direction. *Cancer.* 2001;92(6):1591-1605.

83. Cortes JE, Nicolini FE, Wetzler M, et al. Subcutaneous omacetaxine mepesuccinate in patients with chronic-phase chronic myeloid leukemia previously treated with 2 or more tyrosine kinase inhibitors including imatinib. *Clin Lymphoma Myeloma Leuk.* 2013;13(5):584-591.
84. Nicolini FE, Khoury HJ, Akard L, et al. Omacetaxine mepesuccinate for patients with accelerated phase chronic myeloid leukemia with resistance or intolerance to two or more tyrosine kinase inhibitors. *Haematologica.* 2013;98(7):e78-e79.
85. Cortes JE, Kantarjian HM, Rea D, et al. Final analysis of the efficacy and safety of omacetaxine mepesuccinate in patients with chronic- or accelerated-phase chronic myeloid leukemia: results with 24 months of follow-up. *Cancer.* 2015;121(10):1637-1644.
86. Jabbour E, Cortes J, Santos FPS, et al. Results of allogeneic hematopoietic stem cell transplantation for chronic myelogenous leukemia patients who failed tyrosine kinase inhibitors after developing BCR-ABL1 kinase domain mutations. *Blood.* 2011;117(13):3641-3647.
87. Lee SJ, Kukreja M, Wang T, et al. Impact of prior imatinib mesylate on the outcome of hematopoietic cell transplantation for chronic myeloid leukemia. *Blood.* 2008;112(8):3500-3507.
88. Mahon F-X, Réa D, Guilhot J, et al. Discontinuation of imatinib in patients with chronic myeloid leukaemia who have maintained complete molecular remission for at least 2 years: the prospective, multicentre Stop Imatinib (STIM) trial. *Lancet Oncol.* 2010;11(11):1029-1035.
89. Mahon FX, Rea D, Guilhot J, et al. Long term follow-up after imatinib cessation for patients in deep molecular response: the updated results of the STIM1 study [abstract]. *Blood.* 2013;122:255.
90. Ross DM, Branford S, Seymour JF, et al. Safety and efficacy of imatinib cessation for CML patients with stable undetectable minimal residual disease: results from the TWISTER study. *Blood.* 2013;122(4):515-522.
91. Mahon F-X, Richter J, Guilhot J, et al. Interim analysis of a pan European stop tyrosine kinase inhibitor trial in chronicmyeloid leukemia: The EURO-SKI study [abstract]. *Blood.* 2014;632:151.
92. Rea D, Nicolini FE, Tulliez M, et al. Dasatinib or nilotinib discontinuation in chronic phase (CP)-chronic myeloid leukemia (CML) patients (pts) with durably undetectable BCR-ABL Transcripts: interim analysis of the STOP 2G-TKI study with a minimum follow-up of 12 months—on behalf of the French CML group [abstract]. *Blood.* 2014;632:811.
93. Apperley JF, Cortes JE, Kim D-W, et al. Dasatinib in the treatment of chronic myeloid leukemia in accelerated phase after imatinib failure: the START a trial. *J Clin Oncol.* 2009;27:3472-3479.
94. Oehler VG, Gooley T, Snyder DS, et al. The effects of imatinib mesylate treatment before allogeneic transplantation for chronic myeloid leukemia. *Blood.* 2007;109(4):1782-1789.
95. Le Coutre PD, Giles FJ, Hochhaus A, et al. Nilotinib in patients with Ph+ chronic myeloid leukemia in accelerated phase following imatinib resistance or intolerance: 24-month follow-up results. *Leukemia.* 2012;26(6):1189-1194.
96. Ravandi F, O'Brien S, Thomas D, et al. First report of phase 2 study of dasatinib with hyper-CVAD for the frontline treatment of patients with Philadelphia chromosome-positive (Ph+) acute lymphoblastic leukemia. *Blood.* 2010;116(12):2070-2077.
97. Quintás-Cardama A, Kantarjian H, Garcia-Manero G, et al. A pilot study of imatinib, low-dose cytarabine and idarubicin for patients with chronic myeloid leukemia in myeloid blast phase. *Leuk Lymphoma.* 2007;48(2):283-289.
98. Ohanian M, Kantarjian HM, Quintas-Cardama A, et al. Tyrosine kinase inhibitors as initial therapy for patients with chronic myeloid leukemia in accelerated phase. *Clin Lymphoma Myeloma Leuk.* 2014;14(2):155-162.e1.

5

Myelodysplastic Syndromes: The MD Anderson Cancer Center Approach

第五章　骨髓增生异常综合征：MD安德森癌症中心策略

Carlos Bueso-Ramos
Guillermo Garcia-Manero

中文导读

本章总结了MD安德森癌症中心的专家对骨髓增生异常综合征的认识和了解以及常用的治疗策略。骨髓增生异常综合征是一组造血系统疾病，以造血功能障碍为主要特征，并伴有向急性髓细胞白血病转化的风险。本章首先介绍了MD 安德森癌症中心诊治的该病患者情况；在骨髓增生异常综合征的流行病学和病因学中，最常见的危险因素是癌症治疗而导致的化疗和放射治疗（简称放疗）暴露史；进而分析了骨髓增生异常综合征患者的临床和实验室特征及全血细胞的形态学特征，从细胞和分子遗传学的角度探讨了与治疗和预后有关的基因突变；并描述了世界卫生组织（WHO）的分类标准，主要依据该疾病的所有生物学特征，包括形态学、细胞遗传学、免疫表型和临床表现等。随后，基于WHO的分类标准，本章进一步探讨了该病的诊断及由生物学指标衍生的预后评分系统，并详细剖析了骨髓增生异常综合征患者的生存预后。在治疗部分，基于患者年龄、合并症和疾病风险的考虑，强调了治疗目的的差异性；并对该病主要的治疗手段，包括支持治疗、造血生长因子、来那度胺、低甲基化试剂、细胞毒性化疗、免疫治疗和造血干细胞移植等进行了详细的解读。最后，本章对一些特殊临床状况患者的治疗进行了简明扼要的解释和指引。

Myelodysplastic syndromes (MDS) refer to a group of hematopoietic disorders characterized by ineffective hematopoiesis and increased risk of transformation to acute myelogenous leukemia (AML). Most patients with MDS succumb to causes related to the disease. The median age of patients with MDS is 70 to 75 years. It is likely that environmental factors play an important role in the pathogenesis of this disease. Myelodysplastic syndromes are classified according to the World Health Organization (WHO) criteria, and a number of prognostic scores can be used to calculate survival and risk of transformation. Cytogenetic, genomic, and epigenetic alterations are common in MDS and help in the prediction of prognosis and potentially in the selection of therapy. Over the last decade, we have witnessed significant improvements in supportive care and therapeutic modalities for patients with MDS. These include growth factors, immune modulatory agents (lenalidomide), and hypomethylating agents (5-azacitidine and decitabine). We also better understand patient subgroups, such as those with hypomethylating failure disease. In this chapter, we summarize our knowledge of MDS and the treatment approach we use at MD Anderson Cancer Center.

THE MD ANDERSON APPROACH TO THE PATIENT WITH MDS

Every year, approximately 350 to 400 patients are referred to our center with a diagnosis of MDS. Nearly 20% of patients referred with a diagnosis of MDS receive a different diagnosis in our center. In most instances, the final diagnosis is that of AML or a form of higher-risk MDS. Other benign and malignant conditions can also be observed. In a study of 915 patients referred between 2005 and 2009 and using very strict criteria, 12% were reclassified when initially evaluated here ([1]). This justifies our practice to repeat a confirmatory bone marrow aspiration and biopsy at the time of initial MDS evaluation at MD Anderson.

Once the diagnosis is confirmed, the next important step is to calculate the "risk" of the patient. Most clinicians and investigators still use the International Prognostic Scoring System (IPSS) ([2]) score to perform such analysis, but newer potentially more precise models, such as the Revised International Prognostic Scoring System (IPSS-R), have been developed ([3-5]). In general, patients with low or intermediate-1 risk by the IPSS or those with less than 10% blasts in the bone marrow are considered as having "lower" risk disease, whereas those with excess blasts or intermediate-2 or high-risk disease are considered as having "higher" risk disease.

Patients with lower risk disease can be candidates for a wide range of interventions, depending on their specific characteristics and transfusion needs. Patients with minimal cytopenias, who are transfusion independent, who have a low percentage of blasts in the bone marrow, and have diploid cytogenetics are more frequently observed, as their 4-year survival is close to 80% ([4]). At the end of the spectrum, older patients with significant cytopenias and transfusion needs can have very poor prognosis, particularly if their cytogenetics are abnormal ([4]). The median survival of these patients is less than 12 months; around 60% to 70% of patients with MDS are in this category, but there are few interventions known to alter the natural history of these patients. Transfusion and growth factor support are usually started. Interventions such as lenalidomide have significant activity in improving red cell counts in patients with deletion of chromosome 5 ([6]) but are significantly less active in patients without this alteration ([7]). The role of the hypomethylating agents 5-azacitidine or decitabine is less clear in this situation, although they are frequently used. Allogeneic stem cell transplantation (alloSCT) is not frequently used up front in patients with lower risk disease ([8]). It is currently accepted that delaying transplantation until the time of progression is associated with longer survival even if transplant outcomes are poorer when performed at that time. A new subset of patients has emerged that is constituted by patients with lower risk disease but with hypomethylating failure. We recently described their natural history ([9]). New investigational strategies are needed for this subset of patients.

Treatment decisions are relatively simpler for patients with higher risk MDS. The data with the hypomethylating agents indicate that treatment with these agents improves survival significantly when compared to supportive care or low-dose chemotherapy approaches. The optimal approach for younger (those less than 60 to 65 years) patients with MDS is unclear. These patients can be treated with hypomethylating agents or an AML-like induction therapy or can be considered for up-front alloSCT. No study has compared these treatments in younger patients. An approach followed by our group is to stratify patients based on cytogenetics. Younger patients with normal karyotype are usually offered induction therapy with an AML-like approach followed when possible by alloSCT. In contrast, younger patients with abnormal karyotypes are offered hypomethylating agent-based therapy followed by alloSCT. It is not our routine to proceed with transplant up front in patients with excess blasts. Older patients benefit significantly from the use of hypomethylating agents, and there is basically no upper age limit that may contraindicate their use ([10]). Finally, the group of patients with higher risk disease and hypomethylating failure constitute a major medical need ([11]).

A comprehensive review of current knowledge in MDS is provided next. Current areas of intense research are the development of newer forms of therapy for patients with newly diagnosed disease and strategies for patients who have relapsed or not responded to hypomethylating agent-based therapy.

EPIDEMIOLOGY AND ETIOLOGY

The incidence of MDS increases with age. Most patients diagnosed with this condition are more than 60 years old; the median age at diagnosis is 75 years ([12]). The incidence is higher in males than females, with a 2:1 ratio ([12]). The incidence in the United States is 30 to 35 individuals per million per year with a relative yearly increase in the reported incidence, probably related to increase awareness of the disease and reporting efforts ([13]).

The risk of developing MDS is related to the individual's racial background. In the United States, the incidence is highest in the white population ([12]). Patients with MDS from Asia present at a younger age ([14]). The underlying cause of this phenomenon is not known but may reflect genetic differences between different racial groups. Asian patients have a similar frequency of karyotype abnormality as European and American cohorts, although they may have less frequent alterations of chromosomes 5 and 7 ([14-16]). The combination of younger age at diagnosis and lack of chromosome 7 alterations can explain the longer survival observed in patients from Asia.

There is no known cause of MDS. Genetic or environmental risk factors may contribute to MDS. Genetic syndromes, such as Down syndrome, Bloom syndrome, and Fanconi anemia, are associated with an increased risk of MDS, which often presents earlier in life ([17, 18]). Genetic polymorphisms that influence the activity of enzymes responsible for metabolizing toxic chemicals or chemotherapy drugs may influence an individual's predisposition to MDS. Polymorphisms have been described in the cytochrome p450 3A, glutathione-*S*-transferase, and NAD(P)H quinine oxidoreductase enzyme systems that increase the risk of developing myeloid malignancy ([19-21]).

Environmental agents may contribute to the development of MDS by causing toxic damage to hematopoietic stem cells. A causal relationship between occupational exposures to benzene and radiation and the development of myeloid malignancy has been demonstrated ([22]). Exposure to organic solvents and pesticides has also been implicated in the development of MDS ([23-25]). There is no correlation between MDS and socioeconomic status ([24]).

The most significant risk factor for the development of MDS is previous exposure to chemotherapy or radiotherapy used to treat other cancers. Treatment-related MDS (t-MDS) constitutes a minority of MDS diagnoses but may be increasing in prevalence with improved survival rates after successful cancer therapies for tumors. Usually, t-MDS presents 5 to 6 years after initial cancer treatment and generally has a poor prognosis ([26]). Patients treated for lymphoma are at risk of this long-term complication ([27]). Patients who undergo autologous hematopoietic stem cell transplantation have a higher risk (10%-15%) of developing treatment-related MDS or AML, with incidence rates in some centers of up to 10% ([28]). In our experience with t-MDS at MD Anderson in 281 patients, most of the risk was associated with complex cytogenetics or presence and alteration of chromosome 7 ([29]).

CLINICAL AND LABORATORY FEATURES

Most patients with MDS are diagnosed incidentally during routine complete blood cell count (CBC) analysis or because of nonspecific symptoms. Anemia is the most common cytopenia in MDS and is associated with fatigue. A lower percentage of patients presents with bleeding or bruising secondary to thrombocytopenia or with infections related to neutropenia. Physical examination is often normal. Hepatosplenomegaly may be present in patients with chronic myelomonocytic leukemia (CMML) or overlap myeloproliferative neoplasms. A change in the severity of cytopenia or rapid worsening of symptoms may indicate disease transformation. Patients suspected to have MDS transformation require prompt investigation because 20% to 30% of patients will develop acute leukemia throughout their disease course ([2]).

Initial assessment should include a CBC, reticulocyte count, and serum chemistry, including evaluation of B_{12} and folate, iron studies (ferritin), and erythropoietin level examination. Other causes of cytopenias or MDS-mimicking syndromes (eg, HIV [human immunodeficiency virus], other infections, autoimmune disorders, or copper deficiency) should be ruled out through appropriate tests. A bone marrow aspirate and biopsy with samples taken for an iron stain and cytogenetic studies are required. Morphological assessment of the disease is still required for MDS. Cytogenetic studies may confirm the presence of clonal hematopoiesis and provide additional important prognostic information. Analysis of specific gene mutations, such as *TET2*, *DNMT3A*, *ASXL1*, *TP53*, splicing factors, *NRAS*, *FLT-3*, *IDH1*, *IDH2*, and *JAK2* may improve our prognostic and predictive evaluation and may in time allow for the use of targeted interventions using selective inhibitors (eg, *FLT3*, *JAK2*, or *IDH1/2* inhibitors) or allow earlier consideration of alloSCT. However, it should also be noted that these molecular abnormalities ([30]) may be present in older individuals with or without cytopenias and may not necessarily point to an MDS diagnosis ([31, 32]). In general, no patient should be diagnosed as having MDS without knowledge of the clinical and drug history or while on growth factor therapy, including erythropoietin.

MORPHOLOGICAL FEATURES

Morphological classification of MDS is based on a 500-cell differential count on the bone marrow aspirate and leukocyte differential performed on the blood smear ([33]). Table 5-1 shows the different subsets of MDS under the newly revised WHO MDS classification. This analysis determines the percentage of blasts present in the blood and bone marrow and provides an assessment of the number of myeloid lineages involved in the dysplastic process, and the iron stain determines the presence and number of ring sideroblasts (Fig. 5-1) ([33]).

Blood cell abnormalities on the peripheral blood smear are variable ([33]) (see Fig. 5-1). Red cells may be macrocytic and frequently display anisopoikilocytosis. Polychromasia or basophilic stippling may be present. Dysplastic granulocytes may show abnormal folding of the nucleus, and cytoplasmic granules are often reduced or absent. Platelets are of variable size and may also be hypogranular. The presence of circulating blast cells or an excess of monocytes is important for the classification of high-risk MDS and CMML, respectively.

Definitive diagnosis requires a bone marrow aspirate and biopsy. The bone marrow is usually normocellular or hypercellular, reflecting that hematopoiesis is ineffective. Abnormal maturation of hematopoietic cells results in a variable proportion of myeloblasts that are significantly increased in the more aggressive MDS. Morphological abnormalities found in the nucleus of erythroblasts include nuclear budding, internuclear bridging, karyorrhexis, multinuclearity, and megaloblastoid changes (see Fig. 5-1). Cytoplasmic features include the presence of ring sideroblasts and abnormal vacuolization. Abnormal or absent granulation is a common feature of dysplastic granulocyte series. Aberrant nuclear folding of the neutrophil precursor can produce a dysplastic bilobed nucleus, the pseudo–Pelger-Huet anomaly. Megakaryocytes may have a very variable morphology, and a small dysplastic form called the micromegakaryocyte is a typical finding. A normal megakaryocyte has a polyploid nucleus that can be altered with dysplasia to produce hypolobulation or nuclei that are dispersed throughout the cell. The bone marrow biopsy provides the best assessment of the overall cellularity and allows examination of the architecture of the marrow and surrounding bone (Fig. 5-2). The presence of fibrosis can be assessed on biopsy with specific stains for reticulin and collagen. In normal bone marrow, the immature blast cells are frequently located near the endosteal surface. In MDS, these cells may be distant to this site and form aberrant clusters referred to as abnormal localization of immature precursors (ALIP). Immunohistochemical staining of biopsies can aid diagnosis, with CD34 staining to identify blast and progenitor cells and CD42 or CD62 for quantitation and assessment of megakaryocytes ([34]) (see Fig. 5-2).

Nonclonal diseases may cause dysplastic morphological changes in blood cells. Secondary causes of dysplasia should be excluded in the initial assessment and can potentially complicate the diagnosis. Blood cell dysplasia is seen with exposure to heavy metals or antituberculous therapies, B_{12} and folate deficiency, HIV infection, excessive alcohol consumption ([33]), and occasionally normal aging ([35]). Dysplastic features are commonly observed after chemotherapy or with the therapeutic use of granulocyte colony-stimulating factor (G-CSF). These diagnoses should be assessed in the history and may require exclusion with further laboratory testing. Diagnostic difficulties may occur in patients with marked hypocellularity of the bone marrow and in patients with prominent fibrosis as there are often very few cells in the aspirate sample to allow morphological assessment of dysplasia. For patients with prominent hypocellularity of the marrow, it may be difficult to distinguish from aplastic anemia, for which morphological dysplasia of the erythroid lineage may also be observed. In cases of marked fibrosis, bone marrow aspiration is often unsuccessful. Some patients with mild dysplastic changes in the bone marrow and a diploid karyotype may be difficult to definitively diagnose at initial presentation and may require a period of observation to confirm the underlying diagnosis. These patients require review with repeat investigations performed in 3 to 6 months.

Table 5-1 Classification of MDS According to World Health Organization Criteria

• Refractory cytopenia with unilineage dysplasia (RCUD)
• Refractory anemia (RA)
• Refractory neutropenia (RN)
• Refractory thrombocytopenia (RT)
• Refractory anemia with ring sideroblasts (RARS)
• Refractory cytopenia with multilineage dysplasia (RCMD)
• Refractory anemia with excess blasts (RAEB-1, -2)
• Myelodysplastic syndrome with isolated del(5q)
• Myelodysplastic syndrome, unclassifiable (MDS,U)
• Childhood myelodysplastic syndrome
• Refractory cytopenia of childhood (RCC)

Data from Vardiman JW, Thiele J, Arber DA, et al. The 2008 revision of the World Health Organization (WHO) classification of myeloid neoplasms and acute leukemia: rationale and important changes. *Blood*. 2009;114(5):937-951.

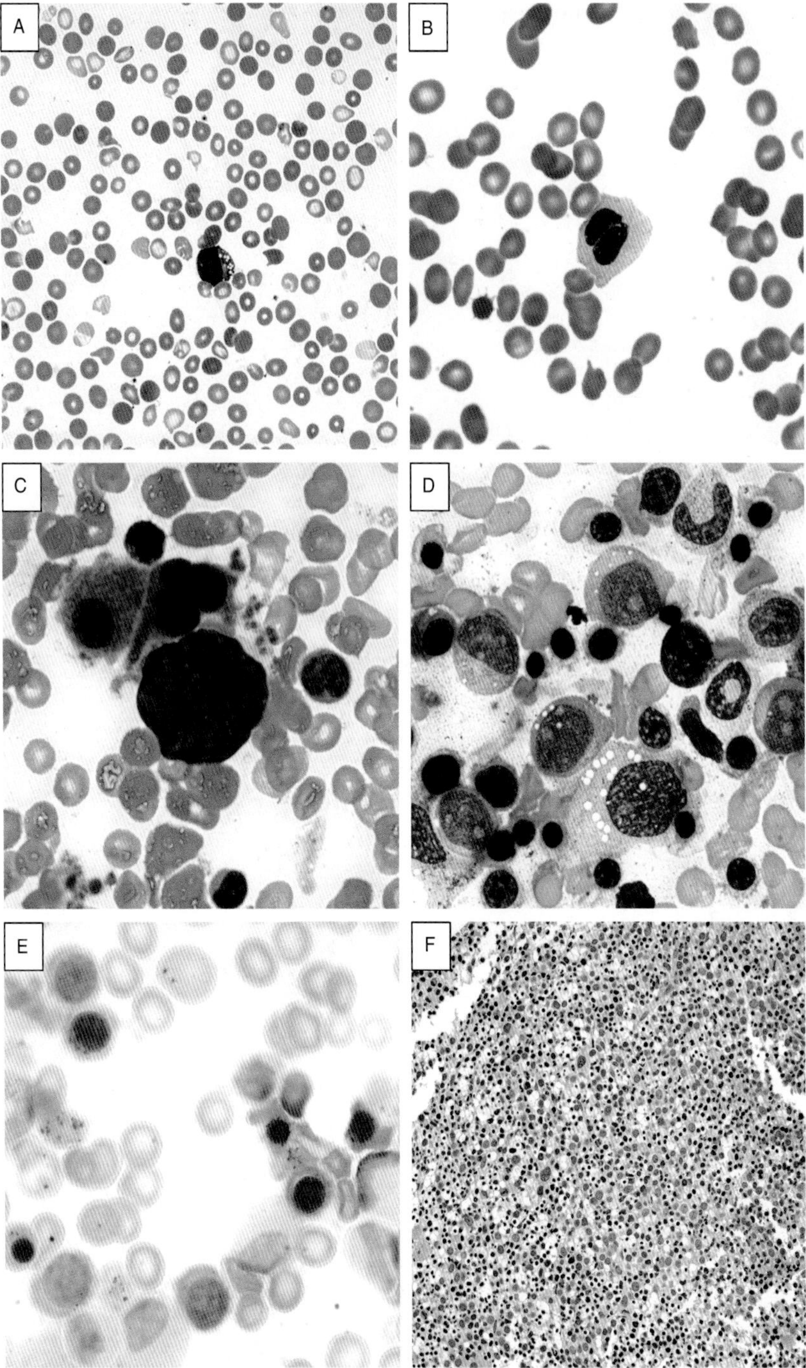

FIGURE 5-1 Morphological features of peripheral blood and bone marrow in the myelodysplastic syndromes. **A.** Peripheral blood film from a patient with refractory anemia with excess blasts-1. The erythrocytes show hypochromasia, anisocytosis, and macroovalocytes. There is also an occasional blast (*center*). **B.** Peripheral blood film from a patient with refractory cytopenia with multilineage dysplasia demonstrating pseudo–Pelger-Huet cell (*center*) with hypercondensed chromatin and bilobed nuclei and hypogranular cytoplasm. **C.** Dysplastic small megakaryocytes, some with monolobated or with separated nuclei and mature granular cytoplasm in the bone marrow aspirate from a patient with refractory anemia with excess blasts. **D.** Increased blasts, dysgranulopoiesis, and dyserythropoiesis in the bone marrow aspirate from a patient with refractory anemia with excess blasts. **E.** Ring sideroblasts and Pappenheimer bodies from a patient with refractory anemia with ring sideroblasts. **F.** Hypercellular (100%) bone marrow biopsy with increased immature cells and dysplastic megakaryocytes in a 70-year-old male with refractory anemia with excess blasts.

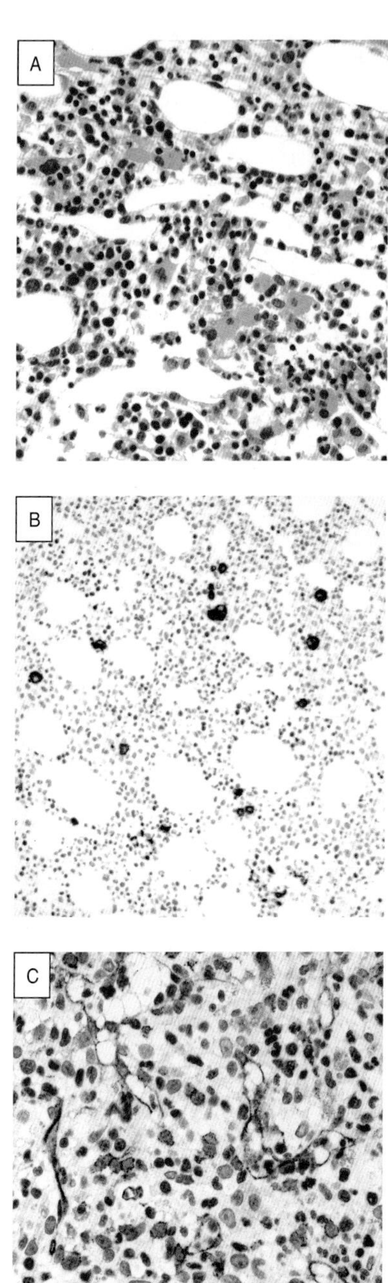

FIGURE 5-2 Morphological and immunohistochemical feature of bone marrow biopsy in the myelodysplastic syndromes. **A.** Trephine bone marrow biopsy with numerous dysplastic monolobated megakaryocytes in a 60-year-old female patient with refractory anemia with excess blasts type 1. **B.** CD61 immunohistochemical stain highlighting many dysplastic micromegakaryocytes. CD61 may be helpful in detecting dysplastic micromegakaryocytes to aid in confirming dysmegakaropoiesis and abnormal translocation of megakaryocytes to endosteal surfaces. **C.** CD34 immunohistochemical staining highlighting the presence of an increased number of blasts and increased blood vessels.

CYTOGENETIC AND MOLECULAR ANALYSIS

A cytogenetic abnormality is found in 40% to 50% of patients with primary MDS and lower risk disease; it is higher in patients with more advanced MDS. Cytogenetic analysis of hematopoietic cells derived from the bone marrow aspirate provides important prognostic and predictive information and may direct therapy (eg, lenalidomide therapy with deletion 5q or earlier alloSCT with complex or adverse karyotypes). A karyotypic abnormality provides evidence for the presence of a clonal blood disorder, which may be particularly important if the morphological changes are not clear. Typically, cytogenetic analysis will assess 20 bone marrow metaphases ([34]). Multiple different cytogenetic abnormalities have been described ([36]). These are summarized in Table 5-2. No specific cytogenetic abnormalities characterize MDS. Unlike AML and chronic myeloid leukemia, genetic translocations are rare in MDS, but deletions are common.

The presence or absence of a cytogenetic abnormality has a marked influence on prognosis ([36]). Median survival of patients with normal karyotypes is approximately 53 months, compared to less than 12 months for patients with three or more cytogenetic abnormalities (complex). Del(5q) and del(20q) are associated with a favorable prognosis. However, when these abnormalities are present in association with other cytogenetic abnormalities, especially as a component of a complex karyotype, the prognosis is poor. Abnormalities of chromosome 7, usually deletions, are associated with poor prognosis regardless of the presence or absence of other abnormalities. Complex cytogenetic abnormalities are more frequently observed in patients with increased marrow blasts. A progressively worse prognosis is observed with increasing complexity. Patients with six or more abnormalities have a very poor median survival of 5 months ([36]). In 2012, a new comprehensive scoring cytogenetic system was developed using data from 2,902 patients ([37]). This analysis resulted in 19 new cytogenetic categories and 5 prognostic subgroups (Fig. 5-3). This scoring system serves as the basis for the IPSS-R ([5]).

Treatment-related MDS has a particularly high incidence of cytogenetic abnormalities, with karyotypic changes observed in 70% to 90% of cases ([26, 29, 36]). A high incidence of abnormalities is associated with an unfavorable prognosis for this group of patients. Abnormalities of chromosomes 5 and 7 are frequently observed after exposure to alkylating agents ([38, 39]). Translocations involving 11q23 are seen after treatment with topoisomerase II inhibitors ([38]).

Table 5-2 Frequency of Common Karyotypic Abnormalities Among World Health Organization (WHO) and French-American-British (FAB) Subgroups ([35])

		Karyotype, No. (%)					
Classification	No.	Normal	del(5q)	-7/del(7q)	+8	-20/del(20q)	Complex
All FAB	1949	942 (48.3)	295 (15.1)	209 (10.7)	162 (8.3)	86 (4.4)	282 (14.5)
RA	573	267 (46.6)	139 (24.3)	30 (5.2)	37 (6.5)	31 (5.4)	47 (8.2)
RARS	252	147 (58.3)	23 (9.1)	24 (9.5)	14 (5.6)	9 (3.6)	20 (7.9)
RAEB	415	179 (43.1)	71 (17.1)	60 (23.8)	39 (9.4)	21 (5.1)	98 (23.6)
RAEB-t	305	132 (43.3)	38 (12.5)	50 (16.4)	30 (9.8)	16 (5.2)	68 (22.3)
CMML	272	170 (62.5)	4 (1.5)	23 (8.5)	18 (6.6)	2 (<1)	12 (4.4)
MDS-AL	132	47 (30.9)	20 (15.2)	22 (16.7)	25 (18.9)	7 (5.3)	37 (28.0)
All WHO	595	285 (47.8)	110 (18.5)	53 (8.9)	40 (6.7)	22 (3.7)	71 (11.9)
5q- syndrome	61	0 (0.0)	61 (100.0)	0 (0.0)	0 (0.0)	0 (0.0)	0 (0.0)
RA	56	38 (67.9)	3 (6.5)	5 (10.9)	1 (2.2)	1 (2.2)	6 (13.0)
RARS	26	23 (88.5)	0 (0.0)	0 (0.0)	1 (3.8)	0 (0.0)	0 (0.0)
RCMD	164	88 (53.7)	11 (6.7)	20 (12.2)	12 (7.3)	8 (4.8)	18 (11.0)
RSCMD	77	34 (44.2)	8 (10.4)	8 (10.4)	8 (10.4)	3 (3.9)	12 (15.6)
RAEB-I	90	42 (45.7)	16 (17.8)	10 (11.1)	5 (5.6)	4 (4.4)	15 (16.7)
RAEB-II	121	60 (49.6)	11 (9.1)	8 (6.6)	13 (10.7)	5 (4.1)	19 (15.7)

Data from Bain BJ. The bone marrow aspirate of healthy subjects. *Br J Haematol.* 1996;94(1):206-209.

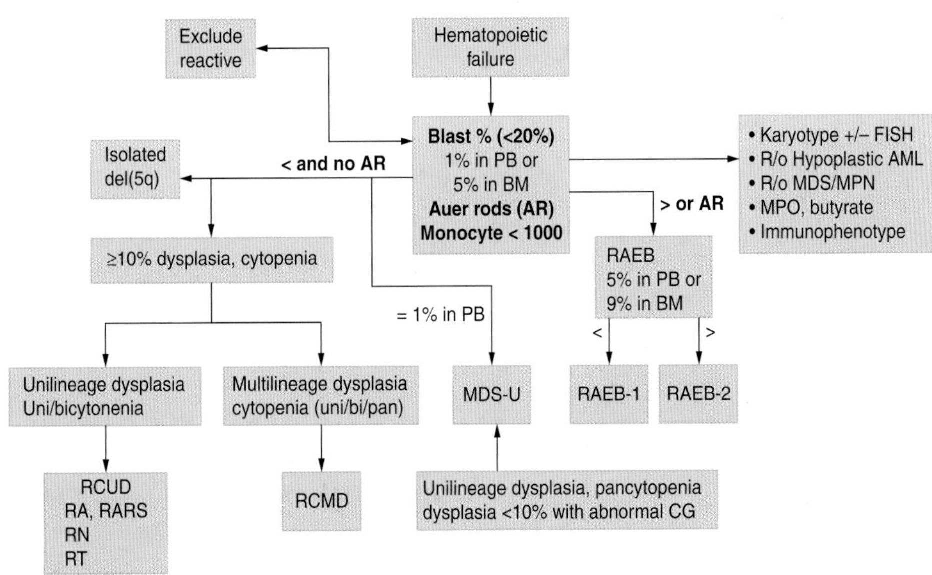

FIGURE 5-3 Algorithm for the classification of adult-onset primary myelodysplastic syndromes (MDS). This classification system is based on the 2008 criteria of the World Health Organization. AML, acute myeloid leukemia; FISH, fluorescence in situ hybridization; RAEB, refractory anemia with excess blasts; RARS, refractory anemia with ring sideroblasts that are equal to or greater than 15% of bone marrow erythroid precursors; RCMD, refractory cytopenia with multilineage dysplasia; RCUD, refractory cytopenia with unilineage dysplasia.

The high frequency of chromosomal deletions has prompted interest in the identification of epigenetic repressive alterations, such as aberrant DNA methylation in MDS. Aberrant DNA methylation of multiple promoter CpG islands has been associated with poor prognosis in MDS ([40]). At this point, we do not have evidence of specific molecular pathways that are epigenetically inactivated in MDS.

An association between a genetic abnormality and disease phenotype was reported in a few specific subsets of MDS. An example is the 5q- syndrome. A minority of patients with an interstitial deletion of chromosome 5q display an indolent anemia with relative preservation of the platelet count associated with hypolobated megakaryocytes in the bone marrow. This array of findings is called the 5q- syndrome ([41]) and is recognized as a separate diagnostic entity in the current WHO classification. The genetic defect within the deleted region that is responsible for the disease is not known. Research has focused on one candidate gene, *SPARC*, that may potentially contribute to the malignant phenotype ([42]). *CTNNA1* is another gene on chromosome 5q identified to be important in MDS and AML but without specific features of the 5q- syndrome ([43]). Ebert et al. reported the identification of *RPS14* as haploinsufficient in 5q- MDS. *RPS14* is involved in ribosomal biogenesis, and its deficiency has a role in anemia in this syndrome ([44]). It is likely that a complex network of genes cooperate in the pathogenesis of this syndrome. Indeed, microRNA 145 and 146a have been found to be involved in the biology of 5q- syndrome ([45]).

A small number of patients have been described with a deletion of 17p associated with abnormalities in the *p53* gene. This specific disorder has a poor prognosis and may be suspected when morphological characteristics of prominent dysgranulopoiesis, including neutrophils exhibiting the Pelger-Huet anomaly and abnormal vacuolization, are present ([46]). Acquired hemoglobin H disease produces red cell changes on the blood smear reminiscent of α-thalassemia. This red cell phenotype is secondary to decreased expression of α-globin within the bone marrow MDS clone and is associated with a mutation in the *ATRX* gene in most cases ([47]). These rare syndromes represent a small minority of patients with MDS, and specific gene defects are not identified in most patients.

Several groups have used large-scale single-nucleotide polymorphism (SNP) arrays in MDS ([48]). This has allowed the identification of areas of microdeletions and uniparenteral disomy in MDS ([49]). It is likely that these genomic regions harbor genes important in MDS, such as *c-CBL* ([50]). Over the last 5 years, we have accumulated significant information regarding genomic alterations in MDS ([30, 51]). The data are summarized in Fig. 5-4 from a study reported by a consortium of European investigators ([51]). Common mutations affect genes involved in gene splicing, epigenetic regulators (eg, *TET2*, *DNMT3A*, *ASXL1*, and *EZH2*), and other pathways, such as *TP53*. The presence of mutations in *TP53* and *EZH2* is associated with poor prognosis ([30]). A recent analysis correlated specific genomic alterations with gene expression patterns that may explain some of the phenotypic features of the disease ([52]).

OTHER LABORATORY STUDIES

Flow cytometry is not required for the routine diagnosis of MDS, but it may sometimes provide valuable supplementary information. Flow cytometry can confirm the presence of specific myeloid lineages within the marrow and may also identify aberrant expression of cell surface markers indicative of a clonal cell population. This may have diagnostic significance in confirming abnormal hematopoiesis, particularly in the setting of inconclusive morphological changes and a normal karyotype. Quantitation of the number of CD34-positive cells in the bone marrow may assist in the differentiation of hypoplastic MDS from aplastic anemia. In MDS, the number of CD34 cells is usually normal or increased, compared to aplastic anemia, for which it is frequently reduced ([53]).

Fluorescent in situ hybridization (FISH) techniques using probes specific for specific chromosomes (ie, covering chromosomes 5, 7, 8, 20) have not been fully standardized in MDS. Their use should not be consider standard of care in MDS and cannot yet replace conventional cytogenetics.

DIAGNOSIS

The classification systems used to group different MDS have evolved over time with increased understanding

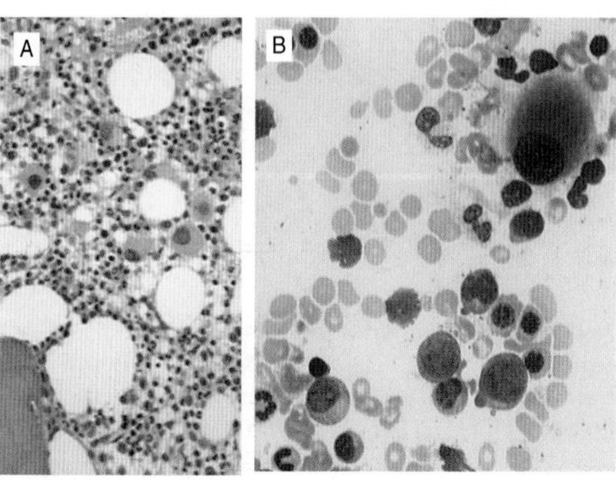

FIGURE 5-4 Bone marrow morphology of MDS with deletion of chromosome 5.

of the biology and genetics of the disease. The first widely accepted classification was that proposed by the French-American-British (FAB) study group ([54]). The FAB categorized MDS primarily on the percentage of blasts in the peripheral blood and bone marrow, with disease entities defined by increased numbers of blasts associated with a more aggressive clinical course. Patients with a bone marrow blast percentage greater than 30% were considered to have acute myeloid leukemia. This classification used only morphological criteria to define disease groups and provided a framework that allowed the study of the natural history of MDS and its response to therapy.

The WHO classification of MDS was developed with the objective of using all features of disease biology, including morphology, cytogenetics, immunophenotype, and clinical behavior ([55]). This classification was updated in 2008 ([56]) (see Table 5-1). Figure 5-5 shows an algorithm for the morphological diagnosis of MDS. In the original WHO classification, the importance of morphological assessment of blast percentage within the bone marrow and peripheral blood was retained, although the threshold level for the diagnosis of acute leukemia was altered. Patients with more than 20% bone marrow blasts were considered to have AML. Patients with 20% to 29% blasts had a similar prognosis as patients with greater than 30% blasts. Within the WHO MDS categories with an increased blast percentage, the magnitude of the blast elevation was quantified between refractory anemia with excess blasts (RAEB) types 1 and 2, reflecting the worse prognosis of patients with an elevated blast count ([2]). In patients with a normal proportion of blast cells within the bone marrow, the relatively indolent refractory anemia (RA) and RA with ring sideroblasts (RARS) introduced in the FAB system were further delineated by assessment for the presence of multilineage dysplasia. Patients with dysplastic maturation limited to the erythroid lineage have a more favorable prognosis than patients with cytopenia and dysplasia present in multiple myeloid lineages. Also, WHO introduced the 5q- syndrome as a separate diagnostic entity primarily on the basis of a genetic abnormality rather than morphological features alone. Deletions involving chromosome 5q are relatively common in MDS, and the WHO classification tightly defined the syndrome as an isolated del(5q) associated with anemia, a preserved or increased platelet count, and hypolobated megakaryocytes on the bone marrow biopsy (Fig. 5-6). The WHO classification has been validated by a number of independent groups ([57, 58]). The most recent WHO classification ([56]) included the following changes: (1) specific guidelines for the requirement of specimen collection and blast and blast lineage assessment, as well as for the analysis of genetic alterations; (2) an effort to report new changes in the diagnosis and classification of MDS/MPN; (3) inclusion of patients with cytopenias but not clear morphological evidence of MDS in the bone marrow as presumptive MDS; (4) inclusion of refractory cytopenia with unilineage dysplasia; and (5) disappearance of the category of refractory cytopenia with multilineage dysplasia and ring sideroblasts (RCMD-RS) ([56]).

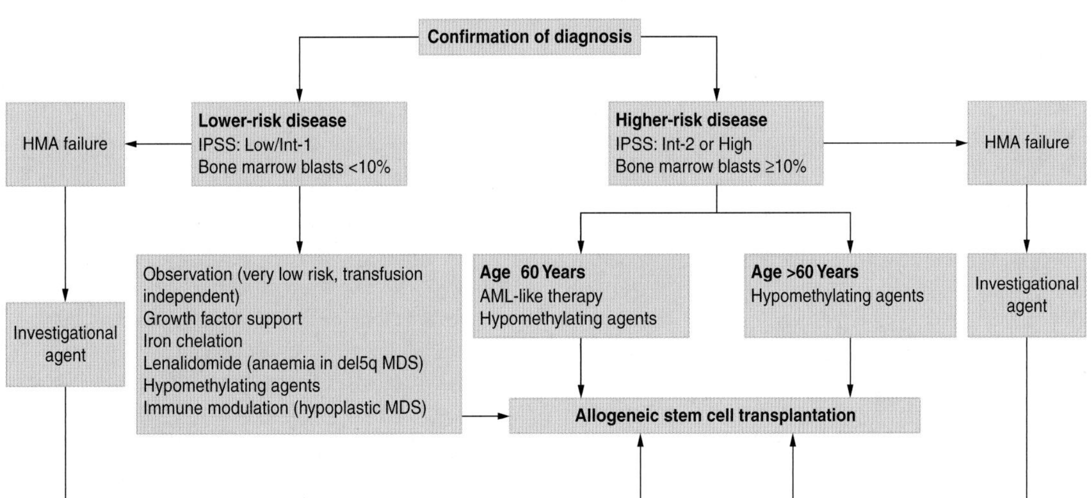

FIGURE 5-5 An approach to the management of MDS.

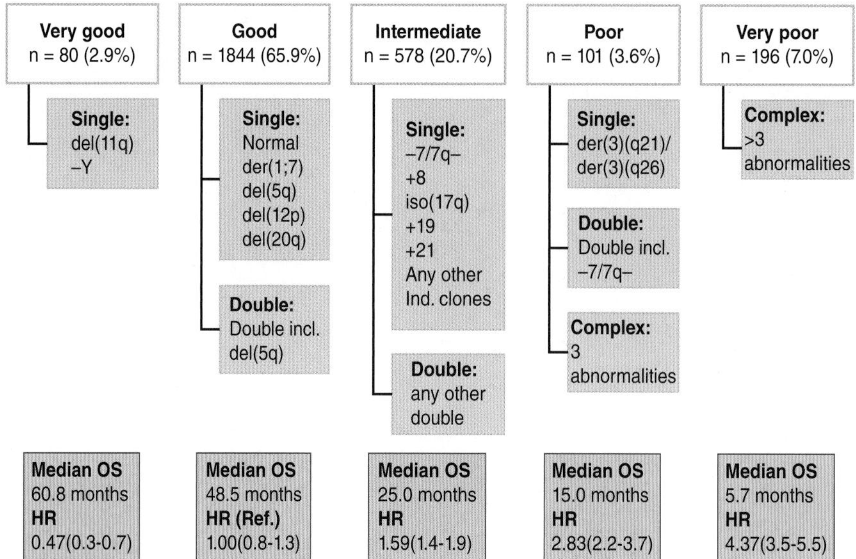

FIGURE 5-6 Cytogenetic score.

PROGNOSIS

The prognosis of patients with MDS is heterogeneous. The development of clinical systems that allow accurate prognostication of individual patients into low- and high-risk categories has proven essential to guide rational management decisions and allow the introduction of investigational drug protocols. The IPSS ([2]) is the most widely used system for assessment of prognosis and treatment planning. It provides an assessment of the prognosis of patients with primary MDS at the time of initial diagnosis. It was designed by the retrospective analysis of a large pool of 816 patients with MDS and followed the natural history of the disease to determine important factors related to patient outcome. Overall survival and the risk of transformation to acute leukemia were related to the number of blood cytopenias, the percentage of myeloblasts in the bone marrow, and the presence of specific cytogenetic abnormalities. The risk associated with cytogenetic abnormalities was determined to be good if a normal diploid karyotype, isolated del(5q), isolated del(20q), or isolated -Y were present. Poor risk abnormalities were defined as abnormalities involving chromosome 7 or complex karyotypes with the presence of three or more karyotypic abnormalities. All other cytogenetic abnormalities were considered intermediate risk. The IPSS weighed these variables to produce a score that stratifies patients into four separate risk groups: low, intermediate-1, intermediate-2, and high risk (Table 5-3). Survival and risk of transformation to acute leukemia are then predicted from cohorts of different ages as illustrated in Table 5-3B. Patients classified as IPSS low and intermediate-1 risks are generally considered to have low-risk MDS, and patients classified as having IPSS intermediate-2 and high are grouped into those with high-risk MDS.

Low-risk MDS are typically treated more conservatively than higher risk MDS. Prognostication in this low-risk group may be particularly important as it is unclear at this time whether some low-risk patients may benefit from early therapeutic intervention. To determine which low-risk patients should be considered for treatment protocols investigating early intervention, patients with low-risk MDS at MD Anderson were analyzed to further stratify prognosis in low and intermediate-1 IPSS groupings ([4]). Factors associated with worse prognosis in this low-risk group included thrombocytopenia (platelets <50 × 10^9/L), anemia (hemoglobin concentration <10 g/dL), age (>60 years), blast count >4%, and a karyotype that was not diploid or del(5q). This model stratified low-risk patients into three subgroups with a median survival of 80, 27, and 14 months, respectively. Increased ferritin and β_2-microglobulin were also associated with worse survival, but these factors were not included in the prognostic model. As patient survival was significantly different between these low-risk categories, investigation of early intervention protocols in low-risk patients with relatively poor survival may be warranted (Table 5-4). We described the cause of death of patients with lower risk MDS ([59]). Approximately 80% of patients died from a complication intrinsic to MDS and not due to disease progression, which only occurred in 10% to 20% of patients. The most frequent cause of death was infection, followed by bleeding. Patients with increased percentage of blasts and a monosomy 7 had an increased risk of transformation to AML ([59]).

The IPSS determines risk at the time of initial

Table 5-3 International Prognostic Scoring System ([1])

A: IPSS Score Is the Sum of the Three Listed Prognostic Factors					
Score	0	0.5	1	1.5	2
BM blasts (%)	<5	5-10	–	11-20	21-30
Karyotype[a]	Good	Intermediate	Poor		
Cytopenias	0/1	2/3			
B: Prognosis Determined by IPSS Score					
		Median Survival (Years)			
Risk Group	IPSS Score	≤60 years	>60 years	≤70 years	>70 years
Low	0	11.8	4.8	9	3.9
Intermediate-1	0.5-1.0	5.2	2.7	4.4	2.4
Intermediate-2	1.5-2.0	1.8	1.1	1.3	1.2
High	≤2.5	0.3	0.5	0.4	0.4

Cytopenias defined as hemoglobin concentration <10 g/dL, neutrophils $<1.5 \times 10^9$/L, and platelets $<100 \times 10^9$/L.
[a]Good: normal, -Y, del(5q), del(20q); poor: complex (≤3 abnormalities) or chromosome 7 anomalies; intermediate: other abnormalities.

diagnosis, but it does not provide information regarding changes in risk as patients progress through the course of their disease. A dynamic prognostication system has been developed to address this deficiency and provides a score that is predictive of survival and leukemic transformation over time. The WHO classification-based Prognostic Scoring System (WPSS) weights three variables: WHO diagnostic classification, karyotype abnormalities categorized according to the IPSS criteria, and transfusion requirement ([3]). This stratifies patients into five disease groups that demonstrate different survival and risk of evolution to acute leukemia over time. Very low-risk patients in this classification have an overall mortality rate that was not different from the general population. This model incorporates changes in the disease risk profile over time, allowing further refinement in prediction of survival and leukemic progression as the disease progresses. A model has been developed by the MD Anderson group that accounts for both de novo and secondary disease and includes CMML. It also allows prognostication at diagnosis or any time during the course of MDS ([60]). The characteristics of this model are shown in Tables 5-5, 5-6, and 5-7.

Table 5-4 A Low-Risk MDS-Specific Model

A			
Adverse Factor	Coefficient	*P* Value	Assigned Score
Unfavorable cytogenetics	0.203	<.0001	1
Age ≤60 years	0.348	<.0001	2
Hemoglobin <10 (g/dL)	0.216	<.0001	1
Plt $<50 \times 10^9$/L	0.498	<.0001	2
$(50\text{-}200) \times 10^9$/L	0.277	.0001	1
BM blasts ≤4%	0.195	.0001	1
B			
Score	No. of Patients	Median Survival (Months)	4-Year Survival (%)
0	11	NR	78
1	58	83	82
2	113	51	51
3	185	36	40
4	223	22	27
5	166	14	9
6	86	16	7
7	13	9	NA

The score is calculated in patients with MDS and an IPSS score of low or intermediate-1. **A.** Significant characteristics by multivariate analysis. Each one has an assigned score. The calculated total score can then be used in **B** to predict median and 4-year survivals ([3]).

The presence of fibrosis on the bone marrow biopsy occurs in a minority of patients with MDS, but this pathological feature is not incorporated into routine diagnostic classifications or prognostic systems. Fibrosis is more frequently observed in patients with multilineage dysplasia or with karyotype abnormalities and, when present, is associated with a more rapid progression to severe bone marrow failure and shortened survival ([61]). In younger patients, it may warrant early consideration of alloSCT.

Recently, an international consortium developed a new MDS classification known as IPSS-R, or Revised IPSS ([5]). The basis for this effort was to improve on known limitations of the initial IPSS. IPSS-R includes a refined cytogenetic annotation and newer thresholds

CHAPTER 5

Table 5-5 MDACC Model—Simplified Myelodysplastic Syndrome Risk Score

Prognostic Factor	Coefficient	Points
Performance status		
≤2	0.267	2
Age (years)		
60-64	0.179	1
≤65	0.336	2
Platelets (×10⁹/L)		
<30	0.418	3
30-49	0.270	2
50-199	0.184	1
Hemoglobin <12 g/dL	0.274	2
Bone marrow blasts (%)		
5-10	0.222	1
11-29	0.260	2
White blood cells >20 × 10⁹/L	0.258	2
Karyotype: Chromosome 7 abnormality or complex ≤3 abnormalities	0.479	3
Prior transfusion, yes	0.107	1

MDACC, MD Anderson Cancer Center. Score points were obtained by dividing the coefficients by 0.15 and rounding to the nearest integer.

of cytopenias and blast percentages. Tables 5-8 and 5-9 show the characteristics of this new classification. The IPSS-R divides patients into five categories (very low, low, intermediate, high, and very high). Algorithms have been developed to calculate expected survival and time to progression based age and IPSS-R score.

Although IPSS-R is the classification that the MDS expert community wishes it used when reporting on patients with MDS, practically and clinically it has not been adopted by MD Anderson. The main issues are the complexity of the score and the fact that it is unclear how to approach patients with intermediate risk disease. Furthermore, all drugs currently used in MDS were approved under IPSS or FAB criteria. Finally, it is likely that all these classifications will soon be modified to incorporate newer molecular data.

Patients with MDS are older and may suffer from other comorbidities. We have calculated the impact of comorbidities using the ACE-27 (Adult Comorbidity Evaluation-27) comorbidity score on the outcome of patients with MDS ([62]). This analysis indicated synergism between the presence of comorbidity and disease score. The same was observed when ACE-27 was calculated with IPSS-R ([63]).

THERAPY

The number of effective drug treatments available to treat MDS has expanded in recent years, providing a range of management alternatives. Some treatments improve hematopoietic function and alleviate symptoms related to blood cytopenia; other therapies alter the natural history of the disease and improve survival. Both approaches may be appropriate in different clinical contexts, and many patients receive different combinations of treatments throughout their disease course.

The goals of therapy in MDS vary in different patient populations. A management plan should consider the patient's age, comorbidities, and disease risk. Patients with low-risk MDS most commonly

Table 5-6 MDS MDACC Model—Estimated Overall Survival by Prognostic Score

		Survival		
Score	No. of Patients (%)	Median (Months)	% At 3 Years	% At 6 Years
Low				
0-4	157 (16)	54	63	38
Int-1				
5	111 (12)	30	40	14
6	116 (12)	23	29	14
Int-2				
7	127 (13)	14	19	8
8	106 (11)	13	13	4
High				
9	97 (10)	10	10	2
≤10	244 (25)	5	2	0

Int, intermediate.

Table 5-7 MDS MDACC Model—Estimated Overall Survival by Four Levels of Prognostic Score Points

		Survival		
Score	No. of Patients (%)	Median (Months)	Score	No. of Patients (%)
0-4	157 (16)	54	63	38
5-6	227 (24)	25	34	13
7-8	233 (24)	14	16	6
≤9	341 (36)	6	4	0.4

Adapted with permission from Kantarjian H, O'Brien S, Ravandi F, et al. Proposal for a new risk model in myelodysplastic syndrome that accounts for events not considered in the original International Prognostic Scoring System, Cancer 2008 Sep 15;113(6):1351-1361.

Table 5-8 IPSS-R Prognostic Score Values

Prognostic Variable	0	0.5	1	1.5	2	3	4
Cytogenetics	Very good	–	Good	–	Intermediate	Poor	Very poor
BM blast (%)	≤2	–	>2% to < 5%	–	5%-10%	>10%	–
Hemoglobin	≥10	–	8 to <10	<8	–	–	–
Platelets	≥100	50 to <100	<50	–	–	–	–
ANC	≥0.8	<0.8	–	–	–	–	–

–, not applicable.
Data from Schanz J, Tuchler H, Sole F, et al. New comprehensive cytogenetic scoring system for primary myelodysplastic syndromes (MDS) and oligoblastic acute myeloid leukemia after MDS derived from an international database merge. *J Clin Oncol*. 2012;30(8):820-829.

Table 5-9 IPSS-R Prognostic Risk Categories/Scores

Risk Category	Risk Score					
Very low	≤1.5					
Low	>1.5-3					
Intermediate	>3-4.5					
High	>4.5-6					
Very High	>6					
	No. of Patients	Very Low	Low	Intermediate	High	Very high
Patients (%)	7,012	19	38	20	13	10
Survival, all[a]		8.8	5.3	3.0	1.6	0.8
		(7.8-9.9)	(5.1-5.7)	(2.7-3.3)	(1.5-1.7)	(0.7-0.8)
Hazard ratio		0.5	1.0	2.0	3.2	8.0
(95% CI)		(0.46-0.59)	(0.93-1.1)	(1.8-2.1)	(2.9-3.5)	(7.2-8.8)
Patients (%)	6,485	19	37	20	13	11
AML/25%[a,b]		NR	10.8	3.2	1.4	0.73
		(14.5-NR)	(9.2-NR)	(2.8-4.4)	(1.1-1.7)	(0.7-0.9)
Hazard ratio		0.5	1.0	3.0	6.2	12.7
(95% CI)		(0.4-0.6)	(0.9-1.2)	(2.7-3.5)	(5.4-7.2)	(10.6-15.2)

NR, indicates not reached. [a]Medians, years (95% CI), $P < .001$. [b]Median time to 25% AML evolution (95% CIs), $P < .001$.

experience problems related to chronic anemia, and the disease may remain stable for prolonged periods. If these patients are elderly, they may best be managed with relatively nontoxic therapies that aim to maintain quality of life. Treatment options include transfusions of blood products, growth factor therapies (erythropoietin with or without colony-stimulating factors), and non–growth factor therapies with immune modulators (lenalidomide) and epigenetic drug treatment (azacitidine and decitabine). High-risk MDS has a poor prognosis and forms a continuum with acute myeloid leukemia. Aggressive therapies may be warranted in these high-risk patients to eradicate the malignant clone and improve survival. Intensive therapies may include high-dose chemotherapy and consideration of alloSCT in younger patients. Intensive treatment protocols are not suitable for all patients because they expose the patient to significant risks of treatment-related morbidity and mortality. An algorithm for treatment approaches at MD Anderson Cancer Center is shown in Fig. 5-7.

Assessing response to treatment in MDS can be complex as treatment goals in low- and high-risk disease may be different. Clinical response criteria in low-risk disease usually measure improvements in peripheral blood cell counts and quality-of-life factors. Response in high-risk disease is typically more stringent, with measures of resolution of bone marrow changes by morphological and cytogenetic criteria. Standardized criteria are available to assess response to treatment in MDS and are particularly useful to allow comparisons between drug trials [64].

Supportive Care

Chronic blood cytopenia is a principal characteristic of MDS. Therapies aimed at alleviating problems related to anemia, neutropenia, and thrombocytopenia are an essential component of management. Bacterial infections require aggressive treatment with antibiotics. Platelet transfusions are administered for episodes of bleeding or for prophylaxis in patients with severe thrombocytopenia. Transfusion thresholds at MD Anderson include a hemoglobin level of 8 g/dL (unless the patient is otherwise symptomatic) and a platelet count of less than 10 K/UL (unless there is evidence of bleeding). Additional hemostatic support with the use of antifibrinolytic agents may be considered for problematic mucosal bleeding or for surgical procedures. The role of prophylactic antibiotics is less established in neutropenic patients. It is our practice at MD Anderson to use triple therapy (antibacterial with a quinolone, antiviral, and antifungal) in all patients with severe neutropenia who are receiving therapy.

Symptomatic anemia is often the major clinical problem in patients with low-risk MDS. In this group, red cell transfusion is effective symptomatic therapy, but a prolonged transfusion program may cause problems with transfusion-related hemosiderosis, alloantibody formation, and volume overload in patients

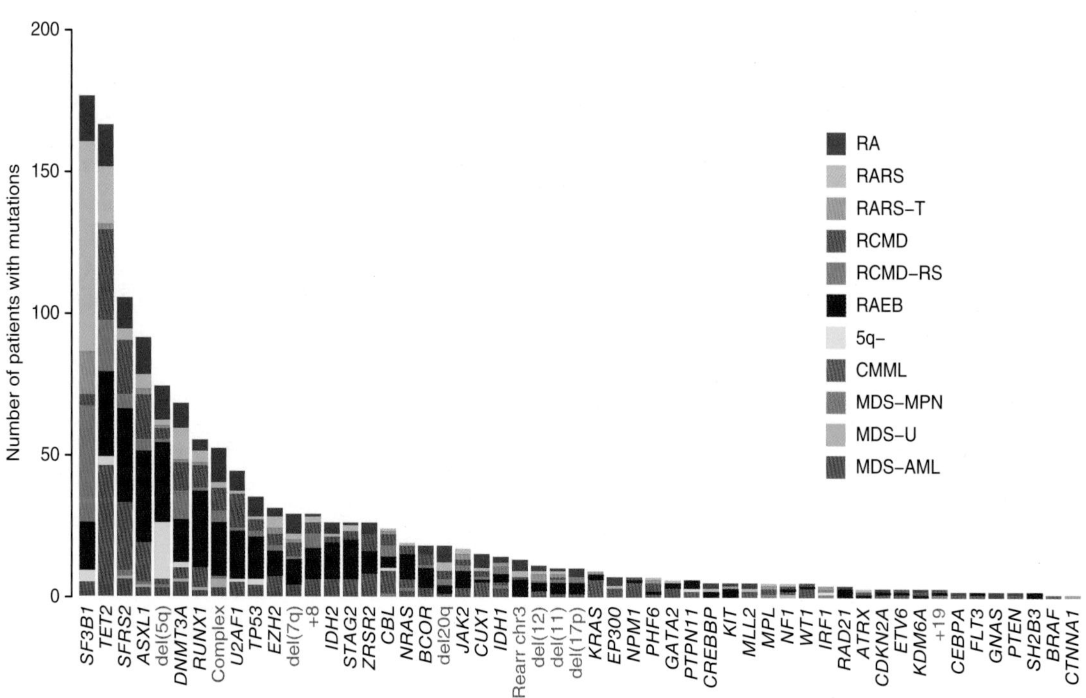

FIGURE 5-7 Molecular data.

with impaired cardiac function. Deposition of iron in body tissues is treated with iron chelation. The efficacy of iron chelation therapy is best demonstrated in thalassemia major, where regular deferoxamine therapy reduces iron deposition in organs and improves survival [65]. In MDS, it is hypothesized to have similar advantages [66], but this needs to be confirmed in ongoing randomized clinical trials. The parenteral administration of deferoxamine is inconvenient. The development of effective oral iron-chelating drugs, such as deferasirox, has allowed iron chelation to be performed more easily [67]. Iron chelation should start with parenteral deferoxamine or oral deferasirox after 20 to 40 units of red cells have been administered, particularly if there is an expectation of prolonged survival and continued transfusion therapy. Serum ferritin may be used as a guide to chelation therapy, with a ferritin concentration greater than 1,000 μg/L typically attained after transfusion of 20 red cell units [58]. Iron chelation therapy should also be considered in a younger patient who may be a candidate for allogeneic transplantation. An elevated pretransplant ferritin has been associated with a lower overall survival after allogeneic transplantation and an increase in the hepatic transplant complication of veno-occlusive disease [68].

Hematopoietic Growth Factors

Hematopoietic growth factors are the primary regulators of blood progenitor cell proliferation and are used therapeutically to promote effective hematopoiesis. Erythropoietin therapy has been explored as an alternative to red cell transfusion in patients with low-risk MDS. Recombinant erythropoietin (rEPO) in various forms, including epoetin α, epoetin β, and the long-acting darbepoetin, has been studied in different cohorts of patients. Overall, erythroid responses in unselected patients were modest, in the range of 10% to 20% [69]. The best responses were identified in patients with low-risk MDS, a low serum EPO level (<200 IU/L), and no red cell transfusion requirement [70]. In this favorable subgroup of patients with MDS, an erythroid response to rEPO therapy was observed in 40% to 60% of patients [70]. The median duration of response was 2 years, and therapy was associated with improved quality of life [71]. Data suggest that patients who respond to growth factor therapy have better survival than historical control cohorts who received supportive care alone [70].

Erythropoietin in combination with G-CSF is also effective, with response rates of 40% to 50% in selected cohorts [71, 72]. The combination of these two hematopoietic cytokines appears to offer a synergistic clinical benefit and allows improvements in hemoglobin levels in some patients who fail to respond to EPO monotherapy. The benefit of this combination may be most marked in RARS and RCMD, but this has not been confirmed [70]. Disease transformation is a theoretical risk in patients receiving chronic hematopoietic growth factors, but long-term observations of these patients suggested that these cytokines do not promote leukemic transformation [70, 72]. Hematopoietic growth factor therapy should be considered to treat anemia in patients with low-risk MDS associated with a low serum EPO. Erythropoietin can be initiated as monotherapy with the addition of G-CSF if there is no objective response in 2 to 3 months.

Thrombopoietin has been used to promote platelet production and minimize the bleeding complications related to severe thrombocytopenia. Initial trials with recombinant thrombopoietin were disappointing. New second-generation thrombomimetic agents are now being tested [73]. These drugs should not be used outside the context of clinical trials due to potential concerns of increased blasts and fibrosis.

Lenalidomide

Lenalidomide is a chemical analogue of thalidomide with diverse biological actions that encompass immune modulation and antiangiogenic effects. Selective activity of lenalidomide against MDS associated with an interstitial deletion on the long arm of chromosome 5 was first suggested in a study examining the effects of this drug on anemia in patients with low-risk MDS [74]. Erythroid responses were noted in 56% of the cohort, with the most significant response found in the subgroup with a del(5q) abnormality. This observation was confirmed in a larger multicenter phase II study of lenalidomide [6]. This second trial demonstrated an overall erythroid response in 76% of patients with the del(5q) abnormality. Responses were prolonged and occurred rapidly, with a median time to a hematologic response of 4 to 5 weeks. A cytogenetic response was documented in 73% of patients, with 44% developing complete cytogenetic remission. Cytogenetic responses were observed in patients with the del(5q) abnormality alone and in patients with the del(5q) abnormality associated with additional cytogenetic defects. This clearly demonstrated that the activity of lenalidomide was not limited to patients with the 5q- syndrome but was also observed in patients with low-risk MDS, with a variety of WHO classifications associated with a del(5q) abnormality on cytogenetic studies. A randomized trial comparing different doses of lenalidomide versus observation further confirmed the activity of the drug at a dose of 10 mg daily [75]. Although none of these studies was powered to document improvement in survival, a recent analysis indicated that achieving a cytogenetic response with lenalidomide was associated with prolonged survival [76].

Lenalidomide therapy in MDS is usually started at 10 mg daily. A favorable response is typically characterized by normalization of anemia and cytogenetic response ([6]). The most important side effect of therapy with lenalidomide is myelosuppression, which may necessitate dose reduction in patients with persistent thrombocytopenia and neutropenia. Interestingly, the degree of myelosuppression has been associated with response. Thrombocytopenia at diagnosis (platelet count <100 × 10^9/L) has been associated with a worse response to lenalidomide treatment. This may reflect repeated or prolonged treatment interruptions secondary to myelosuppression.

Lenalidomide and thalidomide also demonstrated activity in low-risk MDS without the del(5q) abnormality. Lenalidomide has been studied in 214 patients with low-risk MDS (IPSS low and intermediate-1) and predominantly a normal karyotype ([7]). In this cohort, 26% of patients achieved transfusion independence, and 17% developed a reduction in transfusion requirement. The median duration of transfusion independence was 41 weeks, and cytogenetic responses were documented in 19% of patients with karyotypic abnormalities. These results were confirmed in a randomized trial ([77]).

Hypomethylating Agents

5-Azacitidine and 5-aza-2′-deoxycytidine (decitabine) are chemically related drugs with a spectrum of activity that includes both low- and high-risk MDS. The mechanism of action of these drugs is uncertain, although both agents reverse abnormal promoter DNA methylation that surrounds the promoter of some tumor-suppressor genes in cancer cells. Aberrant promoter methylation is associated with transcriptional repression, or silencing, and may contribute to the loss of tumor-suppressor gene function in MDS. Decitabine and 5-azacitidine are both cytidine analogues that incorporate into DNA and form covalent bonds with DNA methyltransferase enzymes. Depletion of methyltransferase activity within the cell then causes newly synthesized DNA to be hypomethylated compared to the parent strand. After at least two cycles of cell division, DNA becomes globally hypomethylated with alteration in gene expression within the leukemic cell. Both agents display cytotoxicity at high doses, while hypomethylating activity remains prominent at lower doses. These biochemical changes are an attractive target for drug therapy as normal tissues have little gene promoter methylation, so hypomethylating therapy may have some degree of specificity for the malignant clone.

5-Azacitidine first demonstrated broad-spectrum activity in MDS. Comparison of azacitidine (75 mg/m^2 subcutaneously for 7 days every 28 days) to best supportive care in a randomized control trial demonstrated an overall response rate of 48% with azacitidine compared to 5% with supportive care ([78, 79]). Azacitidine therapy was associated with a prolongation in the time to leukemic transformation and better quality of life. The median time to response was three cycles, and response rates were independent of MDS classification. Complete responses were observed in relatively few patients (10%), with most patients experiencing hematologic improvement. A report of a multicenter phase III study of azacitidine in patients with high-risk MDS demonstrated an increase in overall survival of approximately 9 months for patients receiving azacitidine compared to other standard therapies ([80]). This was the first drug trial that demonstrated a survival advantage in MDS. A subset analysis of the trial data suggested that azacitidine may have significant activity in MDS associated with abnormalities in chromosome 7, a cytogenetic abnormality associated with a poor outcome.

Decitabine has similar clinical activity to azacitidine and has been studied in various dose regimes in predominantly high-risk MDS and AML. Comparison of decitabine (45 mg/m^2 in three divided doses administered for 3 consecutive days every 6 weeks) to best supportive care in a randomized trial demonstrated an overall response rate of 17%, with complete remissions in 9% of patients with predominantly high-risk MDS ([81]). Subgroup analysis revealed that patients who received decitabine had a longer median time to transformation to AML or death if they were treatment naïve or had high-risk MDS. Myelosuppression was the major drug toxicity. Data from this trial may underestimate the efficacy of the drug as a significant proportion of patients on decitabine received a small number of treatment cycles, which may have been insufficient to demonstrate a response. This is supported by previous phase II trial data that suggested decitabine had an overall response rate similar to azacitidine ([82]). Subsequent clinical trial development with decitabine has focused on improving response rates by lowering the daily dose and lengthening administration schedules. One such schedule of intravenous administration of decitabine for 5 days every 4 weeks demonstrated a complete response rate of 39% in a high-risk MDS cohort ([83, 84]). Improvements in hematopoietic function are often delayed after the initiation of azacitidine or decitabine therapy, and drug treatment should continue for four to six cycles before cessation because of poor response.

Chemical modification of histone proteins by acetylation contributes to the regulation of gene expression and probably interacts with abnormal DNA methylation to cause transcriptional suppression of tumor-suppressor genes. Histone deacetylase inhibitors alter chromatin structure to promote gene transcription, and their combination with hypomethylating agents demonstrates significant in vitro synergy ([85]). Initial clinical drug trials in MDS and AML at MD Anderson indicated increased clinical activity with this type of combination ([86, 87]) azacitidine. None of the randomized trials (hypomethylating agent with or without HDAC inhibitor) showed a survival improvement ([88]).

Cytotoxic Chemotherapy

The relatively poor prognosis associated with high-risk MDS has initiated intensive treatment strategies incorporating high-dose chemotherapy in the same protocols used to treat acute myeloid leukemia. In high-risk MDS, AML-type treatments produce a complete response rate of about 40% to 60%, but remissions are brief ([89, 90]). This poor response to high-dose chemotherapy is due, at least in part, to the relatively greater proportion of patients diagnosed with RAEB having poor prognosis cytogenetics involving complex changes of chromosomes 5 and 7. Elderly patients with significant comorbidities tolerate high-dose chemotherapy poorly.

Patients with high-risk MDS have been treated with a variety of intensive chemotherapy regimens at MD Anderson Cancer Center ([91, 92]). Studies have examined using intermediate- to high-dose cytosine arabinoside (ara-C) (A) in various combinations with idarubicin (I), cyclophosphamide (C), fludarabine (F), and topotecan (T), as regimens: IA, FA, FAI, TA, and CAT. The overall complete response rate for these regimens was 55% to 58%. A short antecedent history of hematological disorder, a normal karyotype, performance status, age, and treatment in a laminar airflow environment were all predictive of attaining a complete response. This intensive approach was beneficial in some patients as those who developed a complete response within 6 weeks of chemotherapy obtained a survival advantage. However, these regimens were toxic, with significant treatment-related mortality in the first 6 weeks, ranging from 5% with TA to 21% with FAI. Consolidation chemotherapy was used in most cases where a remission was achieved with a regimen containing the drugs used in induction but at a reduced intensity of 50% to 66% of the initial dose. Survival of patients treated with IA and TA therapies were comparable and superior to those patients treated with FA, FAI, and CAT regimens, but prognosis remained poor. Nevertheless, this approach does benefit some younger individuals (<65 years) with a normal karyotype, achieving an encouraging 5-year survival rate of 27% with intensive treatment. For older patients, the TA combination can be considered as it has a relatively low treatment-related mortality and it does not contain anthracycline drugs (relatively contraindicated in the presence of heart disease).

Immunosuppressive Therapy

Immune dysfunction contributes to blood cytopenia in some patients with MDS, producing a clinical overlap with aplastic anemia. Immunosuppressive therapy with antithymocyte globulin (ATG) with or without the addition of cyclosporine has been explored in small numbers of patients with MDS. Response rates of 30% to 50% have been observed in selected cohorts of patients with low-risk MDS administered a course of ATG, with a minority of patients experiencing prolonged remission ([93-95]). Features that may predict a good response to immunosuppressive therapy include younger age, HLA-DR status, shorter duration of red cell transfusion, low-risk IPSS, and bone marrow hypocellularity ([95-97]). Selection of appropriate patients for immunosuppression is important as ATG therapy is poorly tolerated in an older population with low-risk MDS ([98]). The PD-1 axis is expressed in patients with MDS. This may allow the development of new forms of therapy and combinations using inhibitors of this pathway ([99]).

Hematopoietic Stem Cell Transplantation

In MDS, alloSCT is potentially, but the therapy carries significant risk associated with treatment toxicity, prolonged cytopenia, infection, and graft-versus-host disease. In young patients with suitable donors, the transplant procedure offers the best chance of cure, with a long-term disease-free survival of 30% to 50% ([100-104]). Given the risks associated with this procedure, patient suitability and timing of the transplant are important issues.

Allogeneic transplantation with myeloablative conditioning has been examined exclusively in younger patients (median age in the mid-30s) in most studies. Patients with low-risk disease (RA/RARS) have experienced the best survival rate. However, this is also the subgroup of patients predicted to experience prolonged survival without aggressive therapies. This procedure is associated with a significant treatment-related mortality of up to 30% to 50% in some studies ([102, 103]). Relapse after transplantation occurs in approximately 20%, and the relapsed disease has a relatively poor response to donor lymph ocyte infusion ([102, 103, 105]). Increased risk of allogeneic transplantation mortality in MDS is associated with older age, poor risk cytogenetics (particularly abnormalities of chromosome 7 or a complex karyotype), the presence of excess blasts in the bone marrow, and longer duration of disease ([106, 107]). Patients with treatment-related MDS also have a poor transplant outcome, but this is related to the frequency of high-risk cytogenetic changes ([107, 108]).

The development of nonmyeloablative allogeneic

transplantation with reduced-intensity conditioning has allowed allogeneic transplantation to be considered in older patients with MDS and in patients whose comorbidities or organ dysfunction would exclude them from myeloablative treatment ([109]). This procedure has reduced the transplant-related mortality, the major problem limiting the availability of this potentially curative therapy to older patients. This therapy aims to minimize organ toxicity related to initial chemo- or radiotherapy and allow stable engraftment of donor cells that provide the curative potential associated with the graft-versus-leukemia effect. Comparison of reduced-intensity conditioning transplantation with standard myeloablative conditioning showed reduced transplant-related mortality but increased relapse rate, resulting in comparable rates of overall survival between the two transplantation strategies ([106, 110, 111]).

Statistical modeling based on historical allogeneic transplantation outcomes for matched sibling transplantation suggested that the maximal overall survival is achieved by different transplant strategies in different MDS risk groups ([112]). Patients with low-risk disease (IPSS low and intermediate-1 groups) maximize overall survival by delaying transplantation after diagnosis until evidence of disease progression but before the development of overt acute leukemia. This delayed transplant approach provided the greatest survival benefit to younger patients (<40 years).

Specific features of disease progression have not been defined, but evidence of new cytogenetic abnormalities, progressive cytopenia, and increasing blast percentage in the bone marrow are suggested as potential triggers for transplantation. Patients with high-risk disease (IPSS intermediate-2 and high) should ideally receive the transplant as soon as possible after diagnosis. The presence of bone marrow fibrosis delays engraftment in allogeneic transplantation and its presence is an additional risk factor in transplant outcome in high-risk MDS. In this group, fibrosis considerably increases transplantation risk.

Early consideration of transplantation is suggested in a younger patient with significant MDS-associated fibrosis ([108]). The IBMTR studied the outcomes of patients older than 60 years of age with MDS treated with either reduced-intensity transplantation or hypomethylating agents ([8]). The results of this analysis indicated that transplant should not be considered as first-line therapy in lower risk MDS. Of interest, in higher risk MDS it appears that there is a benefit toward transplant compared to hypomethylating-based therapy, but survival curves cross significantly later than after 24 months of therapy. This indicated that there is probably a specific group of patients, not yet defined, that derive the maximal benefit from transplantation.

SPECIFIC CLINICAL SITUATIONS

Despite the clinical activity of several agents described earlier, most patients with MDS will eventually succumb to their disease. This emphasizes the need to develop better strategies both up-front and in patients who have failed prior therapies.

Treating Patients With Lower-Risk Disease and Poor Prognosis

It is now demonstrated that the prognosis of patients with lower-risk MDS is very heterogeneous, with a significant subset of patients having poor prognosis ([4]). Because most of these patients die as a consequence of MDS, introducing therapy early in this selected group of patients may help. This has significant implications not only for the role of alloSCT in MDS but also for the incorporation of disease-modifying strategies. We have studied the role of very low-dose or oral schedules of hypomethylating agents in this setting ([113, 114]). Randomized phase III trials are being conducted to investigate the impact of these interventions on survival.

Hypermethylator Failure MDS

One of the major problems is the treatment of patients who have failed therapy with a hypomethylating agent. Data from MD Anderson indicated that prognosis is very poor for patients with higher risk disease and hypomethylating failure with a median survival of less than 5 months ([11]). The survival of patients with lower risk disease and hypomethylating failure is less than 17 months ([11]). In general, this group of patients is refractory to most conventional antileukemia agents available, such as cytarabine. These patients should be treated with investigational new agents or be considered for alloSCT as soon as possible. Agents currently being studied include nucleoside analogues (clofarabine and sapacitabine) and the multikinase inhibitor ON1910. Following encouraging pilot data, a phase II randomized trial of ON01910 versus best standard of care (2:1) in patients with MDS and failure of hypomethylation therapy showed a trend for survival benefit with ON01910 (median survival 8.5 vs 5.5 months; $P = .08$), which was significant in the subsets of patients with primary resistance to hypomethylating agent therapy or with higher risk MDS ([115]). Additional studies of ON01910 in MDS are under consideration. Other investigational agents of interest include vosaroxin (topoisomerase inhibitor), volasertib (polo-like kinase inhibitor), omacetaxine, checkpoint inhibitors (eg, PD-1 and PDL1 inhibitors), ACE11, and others.

REFERENCES

1. Naqvi K, Jabbour E, Bueso-Ramos C, et al. Implications of discrepancy in morphologic diagnosis of myelodysplastic syndrome between referral and tertiary care centers. *Blood.* 2011;118(17):4690-4693. PMID: 21868570. PMCID: 4081364.
2. Greenberg P, Cox C, LeBeau MM, et al. International scoring system for evaluating prognosis in myelodysplastic syndromes. *Blood.* 1997;89(6):2079-2088. PMID: 9058730.
3. Malcovati L, Germing U, Kuendgen A, et al. Time-dependent prognostic scoring system for predicting survival and leukemic evolution in myelodysplastic syndromes. *J Clin Oncol.* 2007;25(23):3503-3510. PMID: 17687155.
4. Garcia-Manero G, Shan J, Faderl S, et al. A prognostic score for patients with lower risk myelodysplastic syndrome. *Leukemia.* 2008;22(3):538-543. PMID: 18079733.
5. Greenberg PL, Tuechler H, Schanz J, et al. Revised International Prognostic Scoring System for myelodysplastic syndromes. *Blood.* 2012;120(12):2454-2465. PMID: 22740453.
6. List A, Dewald G, Bennett J, et al. Lenalidomide in the myelodysplastic syndrome with chromosome 5q deletion. *N Engl J Med.* 2006;355(14):1456-1465. PMID: 17021321.
7. Raza A, Reeves JA, Feldman EJ, et al. Phase 2 study of lenalidomide in transfusion-dependent, low-risk, and intermediate-1 risk myelodysplastic syndromes with karyotypes other than deletion 5q. *Blood.* 2008;111(1):86-93. PMID: 17893227.
8. Koreth J, Pidala J, Perez WS, et al. Role of reduced-intensity conditioning allogeneic hematopoietic stem-cell transplantation in older patients with de novo myelodysplastic syndromes: an international collaborative decision analysis. *J Clin Oncol.* 2013;31(21):2662-2670. PMID: 23797000. PMCID: 3825320.
9. Jabbour EJ, Garcia-Manero G, Strati P, et al. Outcome of patients with low-risk and intermediate-1-risk myelodysplastic syndrome after hypomethylating agent failure: A report on behalf of the MDS Clinical Research Consortium. *Cancer.* 2014. PMID: 25410759.
10. Fenaux P, Mufti GJ, Hellstrom-Lindberg E, et al. Azacitidine prolongs overall survival compared with conventional care regimens in elderly patients with low bone marrow blast count acute myeloid leukemia. *J Clin Oncol.* 2010;28(4):562-569. PMID: 20026804.
11. Jabbour E, Garcia-Manero G, Batty N, et al. Outcome of patients with myelodysplastic syndrome after failure of decitabine therapy. *Cancer.* 2010;116(16):3830-3834. PMID: 20564137. PMCID: 4295788.
12. Ma X, Does M, Raza A, Mayne ST. Myelodysplastic syndromes: incidence and survival in the United States. *Cancer.* 2007;109(8):1536-1542. PMID: 17345612.
13. Rollison DE, Howlader N, Smith MT, et al. Epidemiology of myelodysplastic syndromes and chronic myeloproliferative disorders in the United States, 2001-2004, using data from the NAACCR and SEER programs. *Blood.* 2008;112(1):45-52. PMID: 18443215.
14. Matsuda A, Germing U, Jinnai I, et al. Difference in clinical features between Japanese and German patients with refractory anemia in myelodysplastic syndromes. *Blood.* 2005;106(8): 2633-2640. PMID: 15972453.
15. Morel P, Hebbar M, Lai JL, et al. Cytogenetic analysis has strong independent prognostic value in de novo myelodysplastic syndromes and can be incorporated in a new scoring system: a report on 408 cases. *Leukemia.* 1993;7(9):1315-1323. PMID: 8371581.
16. Chen B, Zhao WL, Jin J, et al. Clinical and cytogenetic features of 508 Chinese patients with myelodysplastic syndrome and comparison with those in Western countries. *Leukemia.* 2005;19(5):767-775. PMID: 15759035.
17. Poppe B, Van Limbergen H, Van Roy N, et al. Chromosomal aberrations in Bloom syndrome patients with myeloid malignancies. *Cancer Genet Cytogenet.* 2001;128(1):39-42. PMID: 11454428.
18. Luna-Fineman S, Shannon KM, Atwater SK, et al. Myelodysplastic and myeloproliferative disorders of childhood: a study of 167 patients. *Blood.* 1999;93(2):459-466. PMID: 9885207.
19. Allan JM, Wild CP, Rollinson S, et al. Polymorphism in glutathione S-transferase P1 is associated with susceptibility to chemotherapy-induced leukemia. *Proc Natl Acad Sci USA.* 2001;98(20):11592-11597. PMID: 11553769. PMCID: 58774.
20. Felix CA, Walker AH, Lange BJ, et al. Association of CYP3A4 genotype with treatment-related leukemia. *Proc Natl Acad Sci USA.* 1998;95(22):13176-13181. PMID: 9789061. PMCID: 23750.
21. Larson RA, Wang Y, Banerjee M, et al. Prevalence of the inactivating 609C-->T polymorphism in the NAD(P)H:quinone oxidoreductase (NQO1) gene in patients with primary and therapy-related myeloid leukemia. *Blood.* 1999;94(2):803-807. PMID: 10397748.
22. Descatha A, Jenabian A, Conso F, Ameille J. Occupational exposures and haematological malignancies: overview on human recent data. *Cancer Causes Control.* 2005;16(8):939-953. PMID: 16132803.
23. West RR, Stafford DA, Farrow A, Jacobs A. Occupational and environmental exposures and myelodysplasia: a case-control study. *Leuk Res.* 1995;19(2):127-139. PMID: 7869741.
24. Rigolin GM, Cuneo A, Roberti MG, et al. Exposure to myelotoxic agents and myelodysplasia: case-control study and correlation with clinicobiological findings. *Br J Haematol.* 1998;103(1):189-197. PMID: 9792307.
25. Nagata C, Shimizu H, Hirashima K, et al. Hair dye use and occupational exposure to organic solvents as risk factors for myelodysplastic syndrome. *Leuk Res.* 1999;23(1):57-62. PMID: 9933136.
26. Kantarjian HM, Keating MJ, Walters RS, et al. Therapy-related leukemia and myelodysplastic syndrome: clinical, cytogenetic, and prognostic features. *J Clin Oncol.* 1986;4(12):1748-1757. PMID: 3783201.
27. Josting A, Wiedenmann S, Franklin J, et al. Secondary myeloid leukemia and myelodysplastic syndromes in patients treated for Hodgkin's disease: a report from the German Hodgkin's Lymphoma Study Group. *J Clin Oncol.* 2003;21(18):3440-3446. PMID: 12668650.
28. Traweek ST, Slovak ML, Nademanee AP, Brynes RK, Niland JC, Forman SJ. Clonal karyotypic hematopoietic cell abnormalities occurring after autologous bone marrow transplantation for Hodgkin's disease and non-Hodgkin's lymphoma. *Blood.* 1994;84(3):957-963. PMID: 8043877.
29. Quintas-Cardama A, Daver N, Kim H, et al. A prognostic model of therapy-related myelodysplastic syndrome for predicting survival and transformation to acute myeloid leukemia. *Clin Lymphoma Myeloma Leuk.* 2014;14(5):401-410. PMID: 24875590. PMCID: 4167474.
30. Bejar R, Stevenson K, Abdel-Wahab O, et al. Clinical effect of point mutations in myelodysplastic syndromes. *N Engl J Med.* 2011;364(26):2496-2506. PMID: 21714648. PMCID: 3159042.
31. Jaiswal S, Fontanillas P, Flannick J, et al. Age-related clonal hematopoiesis associated with adverse outcomes. *N Engl J Med.* 2014;371(26):2488-2498. PMID: 25426837. PMCID: 4306669.
32. Kwok B, Reddy P, Lin K, et al. Next-generation sequencing-based profiling of idiopathic cytopenia of undetermined significance identifies a subset of patients with genomic similarities to lower-risk myelodysplastic syndrome. *Blood.* 2014;124(21):166.
33. Jaffe ES, Harris NL, Stein H, Vardiman JW. *World Health Organization Classification of Tumours: Pathology and Genetics of Tumours*

of Haematopoietic and Lymphoid Tissues. Lyon, France: IARC Press; 2001.
34. Valent P, Horny HP, Bennett JM, et al. Definitions and standards in the diagnosis and treatment of the myelodysplastic syndromes: Consensus statements and report from a working conference. *Leuk Res*. 2007;31(6):727-736. PMID: 17257673.
35. Bain BJ. The bone marrow aspirate of healthy subjects. *Br J Haematol*. 1996;94(1):206-209. PMID: 8757536.
36. Haase D, Germing U, Schanz J, et al. New insights into the prognostic impact of the karyotype in MDS and correlation with subtypes: evidence from a core dataset of 2124 patients. *Blood*. 2007;110(13):4385-495. PMID: 17726160.
37. Schanz J, Tuchler H, Sole F, et al. New comprehensive cytogenetic scoring system for primary myelodysplastic syndromes (MDS) and oligoblastic acute myeloid leukemia after MDS derived from an international database merge. *J Clin Oncol*. 2012;30(8):820-829. PMID: 22331955.
38. Pedersen-Bjergaard J, Pedersen M, Roulston D, Philip P. Different genetic pathways in leukemogenesis for patients presenting with therapy-related myelodysplasia and therapy-related acute myeloid leukemia. *Blood*. 1995;86(9):3542-3552. PMID: 7579462.
39. Rowley JD, Golomb HM, Vardiman JW. Nonrandom chromosome abnormalities in acute leukemia and dysmyelopoietic syndromes in patients with previously treated malignant disease. *Blood*. 1981;58(4):759-767. PMID: 7272506.
40. Shen L, Kantarjian H, Guo Y, et al. DNA methylation predicts survival and response to therapy in patients with myelodysplastic syndromes. *J Clin Oncol*. 2010;28(4):605-613. PMID: 20038729. PMCID: 2815995.
41. Sokal G, Michaux JL, Van Den Berghe H, et al. A new hematologic syndrome with a distinct karyotype: the 5 q-chromosome. *Blood*. 1975;46(4):519-533. PMID: 1174689.
42. Pellagatti A, Jadersten M, Forsblom AM, et al. Lenalidomide inhibits the malignant clone and up-regulates the SPARC gene mapping to the commonly deleted region in 5q- syndrome patients. *Proc Natl Acad Sci USA*. 2007;104(27):11406-11411. PMID: 17576924. PMCID: 1892786.
43. Liu TX, Becker MW, Jelinek J, et al. Chromosome 5q deletion and epigenetic suppression of the gene encoding alpha-catenin (CTNNA1) in myeloid cell transformation. *Nat Med*. 2007;13(1):78-83. PMID: 17159988.
44. Ebert BL, Pretz J, Bosco J, et al. Identification of RPS14 as a 5q- syndrome gene by RNA interference screen. *Nature*. 2008;451(7176):335-339. PMID: 18202658. PMCID: 3771855.
45. Starczynowski DT, Kuchenbauer F, Argiropoulos B, et al. Identification of miR-145 and miR-146a as mediators of the 5q- syndrome phenotype. *Nat Med*. 2010;16(1):49-58. PMID: 19898489.
46. Lai JL, Preudhomme C, Zandecki M, et al. Myelodysplastic syndromes and acute myeloid leukemia with 17p deletion. An entity characterized by specific dysgranulopoiesis and a high incidence of P53 mutations. *Leukemia*. 1995;9(3):370-381. PMID: 7885035.
47. Gibbons RJ, Pellagatti A, Garrick D, et al. Identification of acquired somatic mutations in the gene encoding chromatin-remodeling factor ATRX in the alpha-thalassemia myelodysplasia syndrome (ATMDS). *Nat Genet*. 2003;34(4):446-449. PMID: 12858175.
48. Maciejewski JP, Mufti GJ. Whole genome scanning as a cytogenetic tool in hematologic malignancies. *Blood*. 2008;112(4): 965-974. PMID: 18505780. PMCID: 2515145.
49. Heinrichs S, Kulkarni RV, Bueso-Ramos CE, et al. Accurate detection of uniparental disomy and microdeletions by SNP array analysis in myelodysplastic syndromes with normal cytogenetics. *Leukemia*. 2009;23(9):1605-1613. PMID: 19387468. PMCID: 2950785.
50. Dunbar AJ, Gondek LP, O'Keefe CL, et al. 250K single nucleotide polymorphism array karyotyping identifies acquired uniparental disomy and homozygous mutations, including novel missense substitutions of c-Cbl, in myeloid malignancies. *Cancer Res*. 2008;68(24):10349-10357. PMID: 19074904. PMCID: 2668538.
51. Papaemmanuil E, Gerstung M, Malcovati L, et al. Clinical and biological implications of driver mutations in myelodysplastic syndromes. *Blood*. 2013;122(22):3616-3627; quiz 99. PMID: 24030381. PMCID: 3837510.
52. Gerstung M, Pellagatti A, Malcovati L, et al. Combining gene mutation with gene expression data improves outcome prediction in myelodysplastic syndromes. *Nat Commun*. 2015;6:5901. PMID: 25574665.
53. Matsui WH, Brodsky RA, Smith BD, Borowitz MJ, Jones RJ. Quantitative analysis of bone marrow CD34 cells in aplastic anemia and hypoplastic myelodysplastic syndromes. *Leukemia*. 2006;20(3):458-462. PMID: 16437138.
54. Bennett JM, Catovsky D, Daniel MT, et al. Proposals for the classification of the myelodysplastic syndromes. *Br J Haematol*. 1982;51(2):189-199. PMID: 6952920.
55. Vardiman JW, Harris NL, Brunning RD. The World Health Organization (WHO) classification of the myeloid neoplasms. *Blood*. 2002;100(7):2292-2302. PMID: 12239137.
56. Vardiman JW, Thiele J, Arber DA, et al. The 2008 revision of the World Health Organization (WHO) classification of myeloid neoplasms and acute leukemia: rationale and important changes. *Blood*. 2009;114(5):937-951. PMID: 19357394.
57. Howe RB, Porwit-MacDonald A, Wanat R, Tehranchi R, Hellstrom-Lindberg E. The WHO classification of MDS does make a difference. *Blood*. 2004;103(9):3265-3270. PMID: 14684416.
58. Malcovati L, Porta MG, Pascutto C, et al. Prognostic factors and life expectancy in myelodysplastic syndromes classified according to WHO criteria: a basis for clinical decision making. *J Clin Oncol*. 2005;23(30):7594-7603. PMID: 16186598.
59. Dayyani F, Conley AP, Strom SS, et al. Cause of death in patients with lower-risk myelodysplastic syndrome. *Cancer*. 2010;116(9):2174-2179. PMID: 20162709. PMCID: 3753205.
60. Kantarjian H, O'Brien S, Ravandi F, et al. Proposal for a new risk model in myelodysplastic syndrome that accounts for events not considered in the original International Prognostic Scoring System. *Cancer*. 2008;113(6):1351-1361. PMID: 18618511. PMCID: 4188533.
61. Buesche G, Teoman H, Wilczak W, et al. Marrow fibrosis predicts early fatal marrow failure in patients with myelodysplastic syndromes. *Leukemia*. 2008;22(2):313-322. PMID: 18033321.
62. Naqvi K, Garcia-Manero G, Sardesai S, et al. Association of comorbidities with overall survival in myelodysplastic syndrome: development of a prognostic model. *J Clin Oncol*. 2011;29(16):2240-2246. PMID: 21537048. PMCID: 3107743.
63. Daver N, Naqvi K, Jabbour E, et al. Impact of comorbidities by ACE-27 in the revised-IPSS for patients with myelodysplastic syndromes. *Am J Hematol*. 2014;89(5):509-516. PMID: 24458781. PMCID: 4221257.
64. Cheson BD, Greenberg PL, Bennett JM, et al. Clinical application and proposal for modification of the International Working Group (IWG) response criteria in myelodysplasia. *Blood*. 2006;108(2):419-425. PMID: 16609072.
65. Brittenham GM, Griffith PM, Nienhuis AW, et al. Efficacy of deferoxamine in preventing complications of iron overload in patients with thalassemia major. *N Engl J Med*. 1994;331(9):567-573. PMID: 8047080.
66. Jensen PD, Heickendorff L, Pedersen B, et al. The effect of iron chelation on haemopoiesis in MDS patients with transfusional iron overload. *Br J Haematol*. 1996;94(2):288-299. PMID: 8759889.

67. Neufeld EJ. Oral chelators deferasirox and deferiprone for transfusional iron overload in thalassemia major: new data, new questions. *Blood*. 2006;107(9):3436-3441. PMID: 16627763. PMCID: 1895765.
68. Armand P, Kim HT, Cutler CS, Ho VT, Koreth J, Alyea EP, et al. Prognostic impact of elevated pretransplantation serum ferritin in patients undergoing myeloablative stem cell transplantation. *Blood*. 2007;109(10):4586-4588. PMID: 17234738. PMCID: 1885508.
69. Hellstrom-Lindberg E. Efficacy of erythropoietin in the myelodysplastic syndromes: a meta-analysis of 205 patients from 17 studies. *Br J Haematol*. 1995;89(1):67-71. PMID: 7833279.
70. Park S, Grabar S, Kelaidi C, et al. Predictive factors of response and survival in myelodysplastic syndrome treated with erythropoietin and G-CSF: the GFM experience. *Blood*. 2008;111(2):574-582. PMID: 17940203.
71. Hellstrom-Lindberg E, Gulbrandsen N, Lindberg G, et al. A validated decision model for treating the anaemia of myelodysplastic syndromes with erythropoietin + granulocyte colony-stimulating factor: significant effects on quality of life. *Br J Haematol*. 2003;120(6):1037-1046. PMID: 12648074.
72. Jadersten M, Montgomery SM, Dybedal I, Porwit-MacDonald A, Hellstrom-Lindberg E. Long-term outcome of treatment of anemia in MDS with erythropoietin and G-CSF. *Blood*. 2005;106(3):803-811. PMID: 15840690.
73. Kantarjian H, Fenaux P, Sekeres MA, et al. Safety and efficacy of romiplostim in patients with lower-risk myelodysplastic syndrome and thrombocytopenia. *J Clin Oncol*. 2010;28(3):437-444. PMID: 20008626.
74. List A, Kurtin S, Roe DJ, et al. Efficacy of lenalidomide in myelodysplastic syndromes. *N Engl J Med*. 2005;352(6):549-557. PMID: 15703420.
75. Fenaux P, Giagounidis A, Selleslag D, et al. A randomized phase 3 study of lenalidomide versus placebo in RBC transfusion-dependent patients with Low-/Intermediate-1-risk myelodysplastic syndromes with del5q. *Blood*. 2011;118(14):3765-3776. PMID: 21753188.
76. List AF, Bennett JM, Sekeres MA, et al. Extended survival and reduced risk of AML progression in erythroid-responsive lenalidomide-treated patients with lower-risk del(5q) MDS. *Leukemia*. 2014;28(5):1033-1040. PMID: 24150217. PMCID: 4017258.
77. Santini V, Almeida A, Giagounidis A, et al. Efficacy and safety of lenalidomide (LEN) versus placebo (PBO) in RBC-transfusion dependent (TD) patients (Pts) with IPSS low/intermediate (Int-1)-risk myelodysplastic syndromes (MDS) without Del(5q) and unresponsive or refractory to erythropoiesis-stimulating agents (ESAs): results from a randomized phase 3 study (CC-5013-MDS-005). *Blood*. 2014;124(21):409.
78. Silverman LR, Demakos EP, Peterson BL, et al. Randomized controlled trial of azacitidine in patients with the myelodysplastic syndrome: a study of the cancer and leukemia group B. *J Clin Oncol*. 2002;20(10):2429-2440. PMID: 12011120.
79. Silverman LR, McKenzie DR, Peterson BL, et al. Further analysis of trials with azacitidine in patients with myelodysplastic syndrome: studies 8421, 8921, and 9221 by the Cancer and Leukemia Group B. *J Clin Oncol*. 2006;24(24):3895-3903. PMID: 16921040.
80. Fenaux P, Mufti GJ, Hellstrom-Lindberg E, Santini V, Finelli C, Giagounidis A, et al. Efficacy of azacitidine compared with that of conventional care regimens in the treatment of higher-risk myelodysplastic syndromes: a randomised, open-label, phase III study. *Lancet Oncol*. 2009;10(3):223-232. PMID: 19230772. PMCID: 4086808.
81. Kantarjian H, Issa JP, Rosenfeld CS, et al. Decitabine improves patient outcomes in myelodysplastic syndromes: results of a phase III randomized study. *Cancer*. 2006;106(8):1794-1803. PMID: 16532500.
82. Wijermans P, Lubbert M, Verhoef G, et al. Low-dose 5-aza-2'-deoxycytidine, a DNA hypomethylating agent, for the treatment of high-risk myelodysplastic syndrome: a multicenter phase II study in elderly patients. *J Clin Oncol*. 2000;18(5):956-962. PMID: 10694544.
83. Issa JP, Garcia-Manero G, Giles FJ, et al. Phase 1 study of low-dose prolonged exposure schedules of the hypomethylating agent 5-aza-2'-deoxycytidine (decitabine) in hematopoietic malignancies. *Blood*. 2004;103(5):1635-1640. PMID: 14604977.
84. Kantarjian H, Oki Y, Garcia-Manero G, et al. Results of a randomized study of 3 schedules of low-dose decitabine in higher-risk myelodysplastic syndrome and chronic myelomonocytic leukemia. *Blood*. 2007;109(1):52-57. PMID: 16882708.
85. Cameron EE, Bachman KE, Myohanen S, Herman JG, Baylin SB. Synergy of demethylation and histone deacetylase inhibition in the re-expression of genes silenced in cancer. *Nat Genet*. 1999;21(1):103-107. PMID: 9916800.
86. Garcia-Manero G, Kantarjian HM, Sanchez-Gonzalez B, et al. Phase 1/2 study of the combination of 5-aza-2'-deoxycytidine with valproic acid in patients with leukemia. *Blood*. 2006;108(10):3271-3279. PMID: 16882711. PMCID: 1895437.
87. Soriano AO, Yang H, Faderl S, et al. Safety and clinical activity of the combination of 5-azacytidine, valproic acid, and all-trans retinoic acid in acute myeloid leukemia and myelodysplastic syndrome. *Blood*. 2007;110(7):2302-2308. PMID: 17596541.
88. Prebet T, Sun Z, Figueroa ME, et al. Prolonged administration of azacitidine with or without entinostat for myelodysplastic syndrome and acute myeloid leukemia with myelodysplasia-related changes: results of the US Leukemia Intergroup trial E1905. *J Clin Oncol*. 2014;32(12):1242-1248. PMID: 24663049. PMCID: 3986386.
89. Wattel E, De Botton S, Luc Lai J, et al. Long-term follow-up of de novo myelodysplastic syndromes treated with intensive chemotherapy: incidence of long-term survivors and outcome of partial responders. *Br J Haematol*. 1997;98(4):983-891. PMID: 9326199.
90. Bernasconi C, Alessandrino EP, Bernasconi P, et al. Randomized clinical study comparing aggressive chemotherapy with or without G-CSF support for high-risk myelodysplastic syndromes or secondary acute myeloid leukaemia evolving from MDS. *Br J Haematol*. 1998;102(3):678-683. PMID: 9722293.
91. Kantarjian H, Beran M, Cortes J, et al. Long-term follow-up results of the combination of topotecan and cytarabine and other intensive chemotherapy regimens in myelodysplastic syndrome. *Cancer*. 2006;106(5):1099-1109. PMID: 16435387.
92. Beran M, Shen Y, Kantarjian H, et al. High-dose chemotherapy in high-risk myelodysplastic syndrome: covariate-adjusted comparison of five regimens. *Cancer*. 2001;92(8):1999-2015. PMID: 11596013.
93. Molldrem JJ, Caples M, Mavroudis D, Plante M, Young NS, Barrett AJ. Antithymocyte globulin for patients with myelodysplastic syndrome. *Br J Haematol*. 1997;99(3):699-705. PMID: 9401087.
94. Killick SB, Mufti G, Cavenagh JD, et al. A pilot study of antithymocyte globulin (ATG) in the treatment of patients with "low-risk" myelodysplasia. *Br J Haematol*. 2003;120(4):679-684. PMID: 12588356.
95. Lim ZY, Killick S, Germing U, et al. Low IPSS score and bone marrow hypocellularity in MDS patients predict hematological responses to antithymocyte globulin. *Leukemia*. 2007;21(7):1436-1441. PMID: 17507999.
96. Saunthararajah Y, Nakamura R, Nam JM, et al. HLA-DR15 (DR2) is overrepresented in myelodysplastic syndrome and aplastic anemia and predicts a response to immunosuppression in myelodysplastic syndrome. *Blood*. 2002;100(5):1570-1574. PMID: 12176872.
97. Saunthararajah Y, Nakamura R, Wesley R, Wang QJ, Barrett AJ. A simple method to predict response to immunosuppressive

therapy in patients with myelodysplastic syndrome. *Blood.* 2003;102(8):3025-3027. PMID: 12829603.

98. Steensma DP, Dispenzieri A, Moore SB, Schroeder G, Tefferi A. Antithymocyte globulin has limited efficacy and substantial toxicity in unselected anemic patients with myelodysplastic syndrome. *Blood.* 2003;101(6):2156-2158. PMID: 12411290.
99. Yang H, Bueso-Ramos C, DiNardo C, et al. Expression of PD-L1, PD-L2, PD-1 and CTLA4 in myelodysplastic syndromes is enhanced by treatment with hypomethylating agents. *Leukemia.* 2014;28(6):1280-1288. PMID: 24270737. PMCID: 4032802.
100. Arnold R, de Witte T, van Biezen A, et al. Unrelated bone marrow transplantation in patients with myelodysplastic syndromes and secondary acute myeloid leukemia: an EBMT survey. European Blood and Marrow Transplantation Group. *Bone Marrow Transplant.* 1998;21(12):1213-1216. PMID: 9674854.
101. Runde V, de Witte T, Arnold R, et al. Bone marrow transplantation from HLA-identical siblings as first-line treatment in patients with myelodysplastic syndromes: early transplantation is associated with improved outcome. Chronic Leukemia Working Party of the European Group for Blood and Marrow Transplantation. *Bone Marrow Transplant.* 1998;21(3):255-261. PMID: 9489648.
102. Sierra J, Perez WS, Rozman C, et al. Bone marrow transplantation from HLA-identical siblings as treatment for myelodysplasia. *Blood.* 2002;100(6):1997-2004. PMID: 12200358.
103. Castro-Malaspina H, Harris RE, Gajewski J, et al. Unrelated donor marrow transplantation for myelodysplastic syndromes: outcome analysis in 510 transplants facilitated by the National Marrow Donor Program. *Blood.* 2002;99(6):1943-1951. PMID: 11877264.
104. Deeg HJ, Storer B, Slattery JT, et al. Conditioning with targeted busulfan and cyclophosphamide for hemopoietic stem cell transplantation from related and unrelated donors in patients with myelodysplastic syndrome. *Blood.* 2002;100(4):1201-1207. PMID: 12149198.
105. Campregher PV, Gooley T, Scott BL, et al. Results of donor lymphocyte infusions for relapsed myelodysplastic syndrome after hematopoietic cell transplantation. *Bone Marrow Transplant.* 2007;40(10):965-971. PMID: 17846603.
106. Martino R, Iacobelli S, Brand R, et al. Retrospective comparison of reduced-intensity conditioning and conventional high-dose conditioning for allogeneic hematopoietic stem cell transplantation using HLA-identical sibling donors in myelodysplastic syndromes. *Blood.* 2006;108(3):836-846. PMID: 16597592.
107. Armand P, Kim HT, DeAngelo DJ, et al. Impact of cytogenetics on outcome of de novo and therapy-related AML and MDS after allogeneic transplantation. *Biol Blood Marrow Transplant.* 2007;13(6):655-664. PMID: 17531775. PMCID: 2743535.
108. Chang C, Storer BE, Scott BL, et al. Hematopoietic cell transplantation in patients with myelodysplastic syndrome or acute myeloid leukemia arising from myelodysplastic syndrome: similar outcomes in patients with de novo disease and disease following prior therapy or antecedent hematologic disorders. *Blood.* 2007;110(4):1379-1387. PMID: 17488876. PMCID: 1939908.
109. Giralt S, Thall PF, Khouri I, et al. Melphalan and purine analog-containing preparative regimens: reduced-intensity conditioning for patients with hematologic malignancies undergoing allogeneic progenitor cell transplantation. *Blood.* 2001;97(3):631-637. PMID: 11157478.
110. Scott BL, Sandmaier BM, Storer B, et al. Myeloablative vs nonmyeloablative allogeneic transplantation for patients with myelodysplastic syndrome or acute myelogenous leukemia with multilineage dysplasia: a retrospective analysis. *Leukemia.* 2006;20(1):128-135. PMID: 16270037.
111. Sorror ML, Sandmaier BM, Storer BE, et al. Comorbidity and disease status based risk stratification of outcomes among patients with acute myeloid leukemia or myelodysplasia receiving allogeneic hematopoietic cell transplantation. *J Clin Oncol.* 2007;25(27):4246-4254. PMID: 17724349.
112. Cutler CS, Lee SJ, Greenberg P, et al. A decision analysis of allogeneic bone marrow transplantation for the myelodysplastic syndromes: delayed transplantation for low-risk myelodysplasia is associated with improved outcome. *Blood.* 2004;104(2): 579-585. PMID: 15039286.
113. Garcia-Manero G, Gore SD, Cogle C, et al. Phase I study of oral azacitidine in myelodysplastic syndromes, chronic myelomonocytic leukemia, and acute myeloid leukemia. *J Clin Oncol.* 2011;29(18):2521-2527. PMID: 21576646. PMCID: 3675699.
114. Garcia-Manero G, Jabbour E, Borthakur G, et al. Randomized open-label phase II study of decitabine in patients with low- or intermediate-risk myelodysplastic syndromes. *J Clin Oncol.* 2013;31(20):2548-2553. PMID: 23733767.
115. Garcia-Manero G, Fenaux P, Aref A-K, et al. Overall survival and subgroup analysis from a randomized phase III study of intravenous rigosertib versus best supportive care in patients with higher-risk myelodysplastic syndrom after failing hypomethylating agents. *Blood.* 2014;124(21):163.

6

Philadelphia Chromosome-Negative Myeloproliferative Neoplasms

第六章　费城染色体阴性骨髓增殖性肿瘤

Srdan Verstovsek
Kate J. Newberry
Hesham M. Amin

中文导读

本章首先阐述了骨髓增殖性疾病的共有的疾病特征，并介绍了WHO对于骨髓增殖性疾病的系统分类更新及骨髓增殖性肿瘤定义的由来。随后，本章主要解析了经典骨髓增殖性肿瘤的病理生理学机制、临床特征、诊断标准、预后评分体系以及目前的治疗手段和进展。这类疾病具体包括：真性红细胞增多症、原发性血小板增多症、原发性骨髓纤维化、慢性嗜酸性粒细胞白血病/高嗜酸性粒细胞综合征、慢性中性粒细胞白血病和肥大细胞疾病。通过本章的系统讲解，旨在于更加全面地让我们了解不同骨髓增殖性肿瘤的特征与临床相关进展，从而进一步提升对于此类疾病的临床管理能力。

INTRODUCTION

The field of myeloproliferative disorders (MPDs) has evolved considerably since the sentinel observations made by William Dameshek in 1951. He had commented in an editorial in the journal *Blood:* "To put together such apparently dissimilar diseases as chronic granulocytic leukemia, polycythemia, myeloid metaplasia and di Guglielmo's syndrome may conceivably be without foundation, but for the moment at least, this may prove useful and even productive. What more can one ask of a theory¿" ([1]).

The central feature among the MPDs is effective clonal myeloproliferation without dysplasia. Other features shared by most MPDs include involvement of a multipotent hematopoietic progenitor cell, marrow hypercellularity, predisposition to thrombosis, hemorrhage, and marrow fibrosis, and more recently, mutations in different tyrosine kinases (TKs), for example, JAK2 (Janus kinase 2), platelet-derived growth factor receptor (PDGFR), and KIT ([2-5]). When the concept of MPDs was first proposed, it consisted of five disorders: chronic myelogenous leukemia (CML), polycythemia vera (PV), essential thrombocythemia (ET), chronic idiopathic myelofibrosis (CIMF), and erythroleukemia. Over the years, erythroleukemia was reclassified under acute myeloid leukemia (AML). The remaining four (CML, PV, ET, CIMF) are recognized as classic MPDs.

The World Health Organization (WHO) 2001 classification assigned the classic MPDs to a broader category of chronic MPDs that also included atypical MPDs, namely, chronic neutrophilic leukemia (CNL), chronic eosinophilic leukemia/hypereosinophilic syndrome (CEL/HES), and chronic MPD, unclassifiable (MPD-U). The MPDs were, in turn, classified among one of the five categories of myeloid neoplasms, the others being: (1) AML, (2) myelodysplastic syndromes (MDS), (3) MDS/MPD, and (4) mast cell disease (MCD).

In the revised 2008 WHO classification system for chronic myeloid neoplasms, the phrase *disease* in both MPD and MDS/MPD has been replaced by *neoplasm,* reflecting the neoplastic nature of these conditions, so that MPD is now referred to as myeloproliferative neoplasm (MPN) ([6]). In addition, MCD is now included within the MPN category (Table 6-1). Also, CIMF has recently been renamed as primary myelofibrosis (PMF). Chronic myelogenous leukemia, characterized by the reciprocal translocation of chromosomes 9 and 22, is discussed elsewhere. Here, we discuss classic MPNs, as well as CEL/HES, CNL, and MCD, for which important advances have been made, both in the understanding the disease pathology and in clinical management.

POLYCYTHEMIA VERA

Polycythemia vera is a clonal disorder characterized by an accumulation of phenotypically normal red cells, granulocytes, and platelets. The word *polycythemia* is composed of the Greek words *poly* ("many"), *cyt* ("cells"), and *hemia* ("blood"), indicating too many blood cells (red, white, and platelets). The term *vera* is from the Latin word meaning true, making a distinction between PV and a host of other conditions that can result in an increase in the number of red blood cells. The main feature of the disease is elevated red cell mass (RCM) associated with predisposition to thrombosis. Polycythemia vera occurs mainly in older adults. In a large observational study of 1,638 patients with PV, median age at diagnosis was 62.1 years, and only 4% of patients were younger than 40 years ([7]). The median survival is long, approximately 20 years (although inferior to the general population).

Table 6-1 2008 World Health Organization Classification Scheme for Myeloid Neoplasms

1.	Acute myeloid leukemia
2.	Myelodysplastic syndromes (MDS)
3.	Myeloproliferative neoplasms (MPNs)
	3.1 Chronic myelogenous leukemia
	3.2 Polycythemia vera
	3.3 Essential thrombocythemia
	3.4 Primary myelofibrosis
	3.5 Chronic neutrophilic leukemia
	3.6 Chronic eosinophilic leukemia, not otherwise categorized
	3.7 Hypereosinophilic syndrome
	3.8 Mast cell disease
	3.9 MPNs, unclassifiable
4.	MDS/MPN
	4.1 Chronic myelomonocytic leukemia
	4.2 Juvenile myelomonocytic leukemia
	4.3 Atypical chronic myeloid leukemia
	4.4 MDS/MPN, unclassifiable
5.	Myeloid neoplasms associated with eosinophilia and abnormalities of PDGFRA, PDGFRB, or FGFR1
	5.1 Myeloid neoplasms associated with PDGFRA rearrangement
	5.2 Myeloid neoplasms associated with PDGFRB rearrangement
	5.3 Myeloid neoplasms associated with FGFR1 rearrangement (8p11 myeloproliferative syndrome)

The JAK2–signal transducers and activators of transcription (JAK2-STAT) pathway has been known to play an important role in hematopoiesis, which is mediated in part by erythropoietin (Epo) and thrombopoietin (Tpo) via their cognate receptors. In 2005, four different groups identified an activating mutation in the *JAK2* gene in up to 97% of patients with PV ([2-5]). The JAK proteins are bound to the cytoplasmic domains of type I cytokine receptors (eg, the Epo and Tpo receptors), and the binding of cytokines or growth factors (eg, Epo and Tpo) to the receptors induces dimerization and phosphorylation of the JAKs. The activated JAK then phosphorylates the cytoplasmic domains of the cytokine receptors. STATs bind to these phosphorylated receptor sites and in turn are phosphorylated by the JAKs. These phosphorylated and activated STAT molecules regulate the transcription of the target genes in the nucleus. JAK2 has two domains: JH1 (the active kinase domain) and JH2 (pseudokinase domain: inhibits kinase activity of JAK2). The most common mutation in PV is a guanine-to-thymine substitution in exon 14, resulting in a valine-to-phenylalanine substitution at position 617 (JAK2V617F). This gain of function mutation, which renders JAK2 constitutively active, results in Epo-independent proliferation of erythroid precursors. The pathologic nature of this mutation has been illustrated by many studies. Mice that receive bone marrow (BM) cells expressing the JAK2 mutation develop erythrocytosis ([3]). In contrast to wild-type JAK2, mutated JAK2 allows for the Epo-independent growth of cell lines in culture ([3-5]). The JAK2V617F mutation is present in approximately 95% to 97% of patients with PV and is not present in secondary polycythemia. Mutations in exon 12 of *JAK2* have been identified in the remaining patients with PV who are negative for JAK2V617F mutation ([8]). Therefore, with current sensitive testing, almost all patients with PV should have mutations in either exon 14 or exon 12 of *JAK2*.

Clinical Features

Presenting constitutional symptoms (seen in 30%-50% of patients) include headache, weakness, pruritus, fatigue, dizziness, and sweating. Thrombosis and hemorrhage due to increased blood viscosity and reduced blood flow are the most common serious complications. Mild splenomegaly is seen in up to 70% of patients. Mild leukocytosis can occur with PV, as can thrombocytosis. Thrombocytosis can lead to ocular migraine and erythromelalgia (burning pain in feet or hands associated with warmth and erythema). Some patients are asymptomatic and are diagnosed after abnormal findings on a routine blood examination. The BM is typically hypercellular with megakaryocyte pleomorphism. In the polycythemia vera study group (PVSG01) study, cellularity of the pretreatment BMs (n = 281) ranged from 36% to 100% (mean 82%), with absence of stainable iron in 94% of the patients ([9]). Cytogenetic abnormalities are infrequent. In two large retrospective studies of patients with PV (n = 137 and n = 133), cytogenetic studies were abnormal in 11% to 14% (trisomy 8 being the most common) and had no impact on either thrombosis risk or survival ([10, 11]).

Thrombosis and Bleeding

Thrombosis is the most serious complication of PV (Table 6-2) and is a presenting manifestation in 15% to 20% of patients ([9, 12]). In a large study of 1,213 patients with PV, thrombosis (both arterial and venous) occurred in 41% of patients overall (64% of thrombotic events were at presentation or before diagnosis and 36% during follow-up) ([12]). In a more recent study of 1,545 patients diagnosed using 2008 WHO diagnostic criteria, thrombosis occurred in 23% of patients before diagnosis and in 21% during follow-up ([13, 14]). Arterial thrombosis is more common overall than venous thrombosis. Ischemic stroke and transient ischemic attacks account for a majority of arterial thromboses at diagnosis ([12, 13]). The overall rate of thrombotic events was estimated to occur in 2.6% to 4.4% of patients per year ([12, 13, 15]). The rate of thrombotic events increases with age (1.8/100 patients per year for those in the <40 year age group to 5.1/100 patients per year for those >70 years) ([12]). Older age and a previous history of thrombosis have been established as risk factors for thrombosis ([12, 13]). In the PVSG studies, one-third of the individuals who survived the initial thrombotic event had recurrent thrombosis ([16]). Budd-Chiari syndrome (BCS) can be a presenting manifestation of PV. PV is the underlying cause in 50% of patients with BCS ([17]), and JAK2 mutation has been found in 40% to 58% of patients with BCS ([18]).

The development of myelofibrosis (MF; called post-PV MF) and AML are the two major late complications of PV. Post-PV MF develops in 10% to 20% of patients with PV and is characterized by clinical features similar to PMF (anemia, cytopenias, leukoerythroblastosis, and progressive splenomegaly). Trisomy 1q is the most common chromosomal abnormality in post-PV MF. A longer disease duration (>10 years) is associated with a 15-fold higher risk of transformation to MF ($P < .0001$) ([15]). Passamonti et al reported outcomes on a series of 647 patients with PV; 68 patients developed MF after a median of 13 years ([18]). The median survival for post-PV MF was 5.7 years ([19]). In the Efficacy and Safety of Low-Dose Aspirin and Polycythemia Vera (ECLAP) study, 22 of the 1,638 patients (1.3%) developed AML after a median of 8.4 years from the diagnosis of PV. Older age and exposure to chemotherapy (^{32}P,

Table 6-2 Thrombosis and Bleeding in Polycythemia Vera (at Diagnosis and at Follow-Up)

	At Diagnosis				At Follow-Up				
Study	**No. of Patients**	**Asymptomatic**	**Major Thrombosis (%) (Arterial %, Venous %)**	**Bleeding (%)**	**Major Thrombosis (%) (Arterial %, Venous %)**	**Bleeding (%)**	**Major Thrombosis Rate**	**Deaths From Thrombosis (%)**	**Deaths From Bleeding (%)**
PVSG01	431	NR	13.9 (61, 39)	14.9	27.6 (NR, NR)	2.7		31	5
Groupo Italiano Studio Policitemia (GISP)	1,213	NR	34 (67, 33)	NR	19 (63, 37)	NR	3.4%/y	29.7	2.6
ECLAP	1,638	NR	36 (75, 25)	8.1	10.3 (70, 30)	7.1	4.4%/y	26	3.7
Passamonti (2000[a])	163	37	34 (64, 36)	3	18 (80, 20)	NR		19	6
CYTO-PV	365	NR	25 (60, 40)	4.9	7.4 (56, 44)	1.9	2.7%/y	44	NR
IWG-MRT	1,545	NR	23 (68, 32)	4.2	21 (57, 43)	4.2	2.6%/y	21	1.4

[a]Data from Passamonti F, Brusamolino E, Lazzarino M, et al. Efficacy of pipobroman in the treatment of polycythemia vera: long-term results in 163 patients, *Haematologica* 2000;85(10):1011-1018.

busulfan, and pipobroman; $P = .002$), but not hydroxyurea (HU) alone, was associated with an increased risk of AML ([7]). In a prospective study of 338 patients, 8 developed MF and 10 developed AML after a median of 3.2 years. JAK2V617F allele burden was significantly related to the risk of developing MF but not AML ([20]).

The most common fatal complication in PV is thrombosis, accounting for 19% to 31% of deaths during follow-up (see Table 6-2). In a study of 1,213 patients, the most frequent fatal complications were thrombosis (30%) and cancer (15% AML, 15% other cancers) ([12]). In the ECLAP study (n = 1,638), the most common causes of death were cardiovascular diseases, AML, and solid tumors in 45%, 13%, and 19.5%, respectively ([15]). In the International Working Group for Myelofibrosis Research and Treatment (IWG-MRT) IWG-MRT study (n = 1,545), the most common causes of death were cancer (22% AML, 22% other cancers) and thrombotic complications (19.5%). As is the case with thrombotic risk, older age and history of thrombosis were associated with increased mortality ([15]). Leukocytosis (white blood cell [WBC] count >15 × 10^9/L) at diagnosis of PV has been correlated with an increased risk of thrombosis (especially myocardial infarction) ([21]), leukemic transformation ([22]), development of post-PV MF ([19]), and worse survival ([22]). In a prospective study of 338 patients with PV, only age greater than 60 had a significant effect on thrombosis risk or survival; neither leukocytosis (WBC count >11 × 10^9/L) nor the JAK2V617F allele burden correlated with the risk of thrombosis ([20]), but JAK2V617F allele burden was associated with transformation to MF. A study from the IWG-MRT suggested a new prognostic model using data from 1,545 patients with PV ([14]). The final model included age (57-66 or ≥67), leukocytosis (≥15 × 10^9/L), or venous thrombosis as independent predictors of worse survival. Independent risk factors for shorter leukemia-free survival included age greater than 61 years, abnormal karyotype, and leukocyte count ≥15 × 10^9/L. Previous arterial thrombosis and hypertension were associated with an increased risk of arterial thrombosis, while previous venous thrombosis and age of 65 or older were risk factors for venous thrombosis ([13]).

Diagnosis

As our understanding of PV has improved with development of newer molecular markers such as JAK2 mutation, so have the diagnostic criteria for PV (Table 6-3). As JAK2V617F or similar activating mutations, such as exon 12 mutations, are present in almost 100% of patients with PV, the 2008 WHO classification appropriately incorporated JAK2 mutation as a major criterion for the diagnosis of PV. Compared to the PVSG criteria, for which RCM measurement was mandatory, the WHO criteria have placed less reliance on direct RCM measurement

Table 6-3 2008 World Health Organization Diagnostic Criteria for Polycythemia Vera

Major criteria
• Hb >18.5 g/dL in men or Hb >16.5 g/dL in women or other evidence of increased red cell volume
• Presence of JAK2V617F or other functionally similar mutations, such as JAK2 exon 12 mutation
Minor criteria
• Bone marrow biopsy showing hypercellularity for age with panmyelosis with prominent erythroid, granulocytic, and megakaryocytic proliferation
• Serum erythropoietin level below the reference range for normal
• Endogenous erythroid colony formation in vitro
Diagnosis: Both major criteria with one minor or first major with any two minor criteria

Reproduced with permission from Tefferi A, Thiele J, Orazi A, et al. Proposals and rationale for revision of the World Health Organization diagnostic criteria for polycythemia vera, essential thrombocythemia, and primary myelofibrosis: recommendations from an ad hoc international expert panel. *Blood.* 2007;110(4):1092-1097.

and established hemoglobin (Hb) cutoffs (Hb >18.5 g/dL in men or Hb >16.5 g/dL in women; Hb >17 g/dL in men and >15 g/dL in women if associated with a documented and sustained increase of at least 2 g/dL from an individual's baseline value that cannot be attributed to correction of iron deficiency) for diagnostic purposes. This view is not universally held, and some experts still advocate use of direct RCM measurement ([23]). For patients suspected to have PV (based on elevated Hb/hematocrit [Hct], presence of symptoms or thrombotic/hemorrhagic complications), initial evaluation should include an analysis of peripheral blood for the JAK2 mutation and measurement of serum EPO (Fig. 6-1). As red cell proliferation is autonomous in PV, serum Epo is generally low, and erythroid colonies can grow in vitro without the addition of exogenous Epo. For patients who have not received prior chemotherapy, the endogenous (Epo-independent) erythroid colony formation test has sensitivity and specificity approaching 100%; however, the test is not commercially available. Classical morphologic features seen in BM biopsies in PV and post-PV MF are shown in Figs. 6-2 to 6-4.

TREATMENT

The main goal of therapy is to prevent thrombotic events. The cornerstone of therapy is phlebotomy. This was established by the PVSG01 trial, in which patients were randomized to phlebotomy alone, phlebotomy plus chlorambucil, or phlebotomy plus ^{32}P. The incidence of thrombosis during the first 2 years of the trial

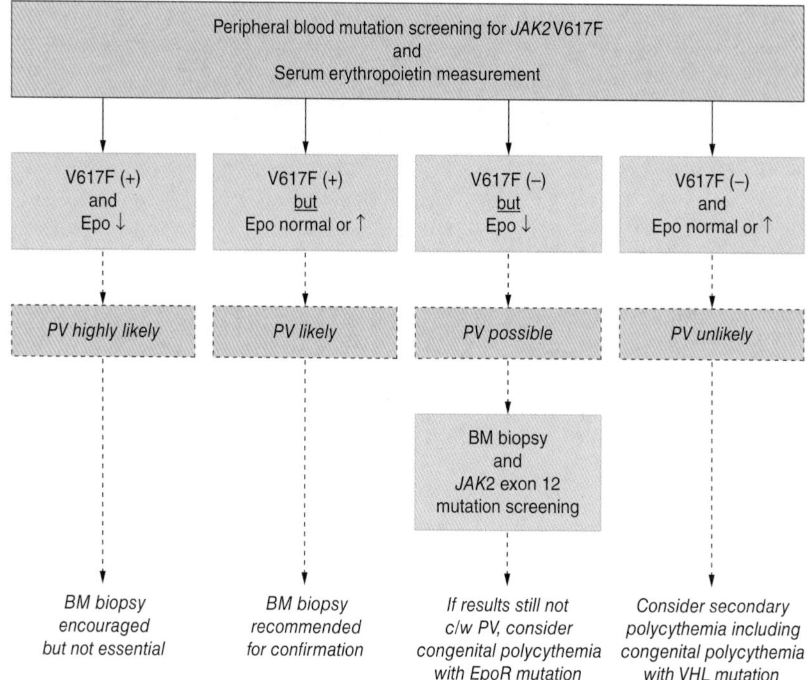

FIGURE 6-1 Diagnostic algorithm for suspected polycythemia vera. (Reproduced with permission from Tefferi A, Vardiman JW. Classification and diagnosis of myeloproliferative neoplasms: the 2008 World Health Organization criteria and point-of-care diagnostic algorithms. *Leukemia.* 2008;22:14-22.)

was significantly higher in the phlebotomy arm (23%) than in the ^{32}P arm (16%). However, median survival was significantly higher in the phlebotomy only arm (12.6 years vs 10.9 years in the ^{32}P arm and 9.1 in the chlorambucil arm). In addition, the AML risk was 1.5%, 9.6%, and 13.2% in the phlebotomy only, ^{32}P, and chlorambucil arms, respectively. The incidence of MF was similar in all three arms. Given the increased risk of AML and reduced survival in the chlorambucil arm, further use of chlorambucil in PV was abandoned. The desired goal of phlebotomy is to reduce the Hct to 45% or less for males and 42% or less for females. Regular phlebotomy also induces iron deficiency, which has not been shown to be detrimental in the absence

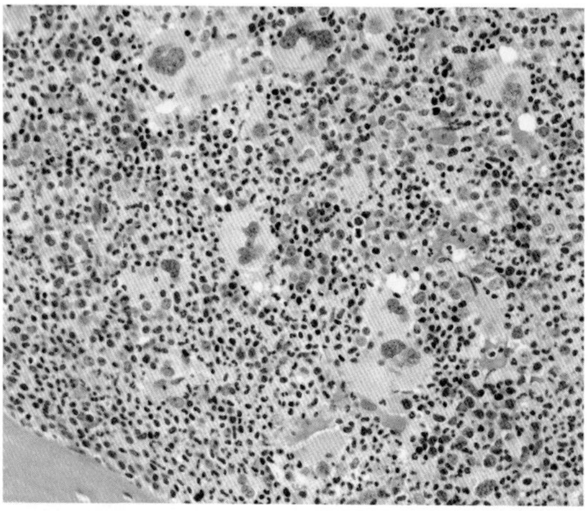

FIGURE 6-2 Bone marrow biopsy from a patient with PV shows remarkable hypercellularity because of myeloid hyperplasia and markedly increased megakaryocytes. Although morphologically some of the megakaryocytes demonstrate slight size variations, most of the megakaryocytes are unremarkble (×200).

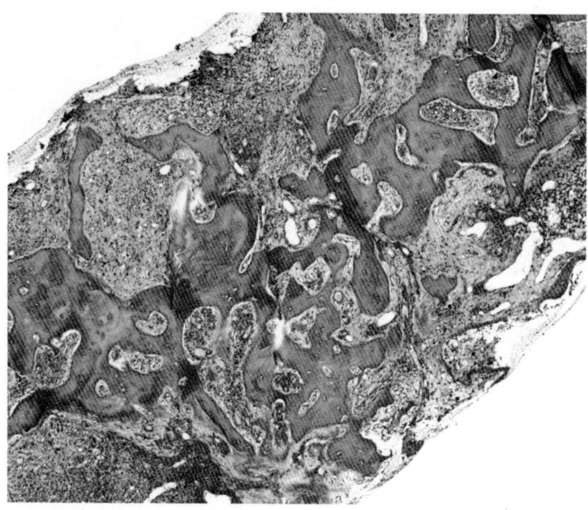

FIGURE 6-3 Extensive bone remodeling and osteosclerosis are occasionally encountered features in bone marrow biopsies during the postpolycythemic myelofibrosis phase of PV (×40).

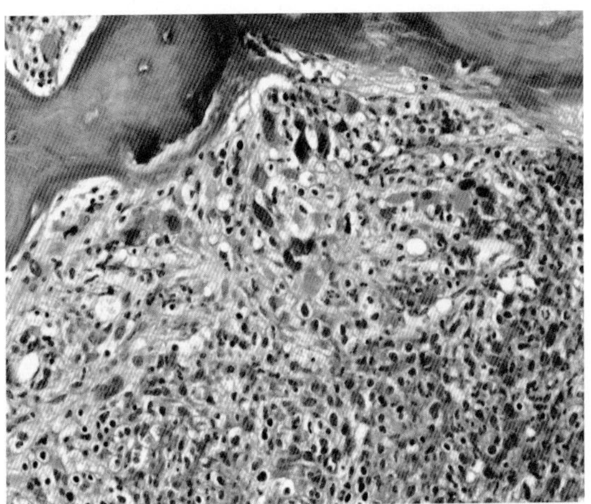

FIGURE 6-4 In contrast to the relatively normal megakaryocytes seen during early stages of PV, megakaryocytes become markedly atypical during postpolycythemic myelofibrosis phase. The atypical morphologic features include pronounced size variations, usually because of the presence of numerous small forms. Classically, megakaryocytes nuclei become hyperchromatic during this advanced stage of PV (×200).

of anemia. Patients with PV who become iron deficient due to phlebotomy use should not receive iron supplementation.

The use of high-dose aspirin (acetylsalicylic acid, ASA) (900 mg daily), initially studied by PVSG, was found to increase the risk of gastrointestinal bleeding and was not pursued further ([24]). Low-dose ASA was proposed as an alternative after it was discovered that thrombosis in PV is mediated in part by increased thromboxane synthesis ([25]), and that low-dose ASA can effectively suppress its production. In the ECLAP study, Landolfi et al randomized 518 patients with PV to low-dose ASA (100 mg daily) or placebo ([26]). All patients had been previously treated with phlebotomy, cytoreductive therapy, or both. The use of ASA resulted in a 60% reduction in the risk of nonfatal myocardial infarction, nonfatal stroke, pulmonary embolism, major venous thrombosis, and death from cardiovascular causes (P = .03). Overall mortality, cardiovascular mortality, major venous thrombosis, and pulmonary embolism were not statistically different between the two groups. Major cerebrovascular events were less frequent in the low-dose ASA group, but the difference was not significant (3.8 vs 1.2%; P = .08). The incidence of major bleeding episodes was not significantly increased in the low-dose ASA group. A subgroup analysis indicated that ASA was more effective in patients with a disease duration of 5 years or less, platelet count less than 334 × 10^9/L, and Hct of 48% or greater and those who had not been treated with cytoreductive therapy. The median Hct achieved during the study was 46%, higher than the recommended targets for PV, leading to the argument that effective Hct control may lessen the beneficial effects of ASA. A recent meta-analysis from the Cochrane Hematological Malignancies Group in 630 patients with PV randomized to low-dose ASA versus placebo found nonsignificant lowering of fatal thrombotic events (odds ratio [OR] 0.20, 95% confidence interval [CI], 0.03-1.14), without excess major bleeding ([27]). They predicted that 19 fatal thrombotic events will be prevented for every 1,000 people treated with ASA. Therefore, all patients with PV should receive low-dose ASA unless contraindicated.

Target Hct values (<45% for men, <42% for women) for patients treated with phlebotomy or cytoreductive therapy were based on a retrospective study showing that thrombotic events increased at Hct levels greater than 44% ([28]). The CYTO-PV trial then evaluated the benefit of maintaining stringent control of Hct (target Hct <45%). The study randomized 365 patients with PV treated with phlebotomy or HU into two arms: one with a target Hct less than 45% and another with a target Hct between 45% and 50% ([29]). Patients with tight control of Hct (<45%) had a significantly lower rate of major thrombosis and death from cardiovascular causes. Hydroxyurea is the preferred cytoreductive therapy for PV patients; however, resistance or intolerance can develop in up to 13% of patients ([30]). Aggressive chemotherapy is not recommended. In a large study with 1,213 patients, the risk of death due to cancer was four times higher in patients who had received ^{32}P or myelosuppressive (alkylating or nonalkylating) agents compared with those receiving phlebotomy or other pharmacological treatments (6.7% vs 1.6%; P = .06), supporting PVSG01 data ([12]). Similarly, in a study of 1,545 patients, exposure to pipobroman or P^{32}/chlorambucil was associated with leukemic transformation, while exposure to HU or busulfan was not ([14]). In a population-based study from Sweden, exposure to two or more cytoreductive treatments (commonly HU followed by alkylating agents) was associated with a 2.9-fold increased risk of transformation to AML. However, exposure to HU alone, even at the highest dose levels, was not significantly associated with an increased risk of AML ([31]).

Interferon alfa (IFN-α), has been reported to be effective at suppressing erythrocytosis in 82% of patients, with a similar number reporting reduction in spleen size and alleviation of pruritus ([32]). Interferon alfa is not teratogenic, making it the cytoreductive therapy of choice in pregnancy. It is also nonleukemogenic ([7]). However, up to one-third of patients discontinue treatment due to side effects (fever, malaise, and depression).

Longer-acting pegylated forms of IFN-α (PEG-IFN-α-2a) have also been studied. Kiladjian et al reported the results of a phase II multicenter French study of PEG-IFN-α-2a in 40 patients ([33]). At 12 months, all 37 evaluable patients had a hematologic response, including 94.6% complete hematologic responses (CHRs), the study end point. Sequential samples tested for JAK2V617F allele burden in 29 patients showed a decrease in 26 (90%). Complete molecular response (CMR; undetectable JAK2V617F) was achieved in seven (24%) patients. Similar results were reported from another phase II study of 40 patients treated with PEG-IFN-α-2a ([34]). The overall hematologic response was 80%; the CHR was 70%. Of 35 patients evaluable for JAK2V617F allele burden, 54% showed a reduction and 14% achieved a CMR. After a median time on treatment of 42 months, 76% of patients had achieved a CHR and 18% a CMR ([35]). A newer, longer-acting form of pegylated IFN-α (PEG-proline-IFN-α-2b), which allows for subcutaneous dosing every 2 weeks, is being tested in Europe in a randomized phase III trial against HU.

The oral JAK1/2 inhibitor ruxolitinib was approved by the Food and Drug Administration (FDA) for the treatment of myelofibrosis in 2011 and for PV in December 2014, based on the results of a randomized phase III clinical trial. In the phase II trial, 34 patients refractory to HU were treated with ruxolitinib; 97% had rapid and durable normalization of Hct (<45%) by week 24. After a median follow-up of 35 months, 59% had achieved a CR ([36]). Responses were defined by European Leukemia Network criteria established in 2009: A CR was defined as normalization of Hct (<45% males, <42% females), leukocyte counts, platelets, and spleen size in the absence of phlebotomies and thrombotic events. There was rapid and sustained normalization of WBC and platelet counts, reduction in spleen size, and improvement in systemic symptoms (pruritus, bone pain, night sweats). Five patients experienced grade 3 or higher anemia or thrombocytopenia. The pivotal phase III RESPONSE trial randomized patients refractory to, or intolerant of, HU requiring therapy to receive either ruxolitinib 10 mg twice daily (n = 110) or best-available therapy (BAT; n = 112) ([37]). Twenty-one percent of patients in the ruxolitinib arm achieved the primary end point (Hct control without phlebotomy and a ≥35% reduction in spleen volume from baseline by magnetic resonance imaging at week 32) versus 1% in the HU arm. Overall, 77% of patients in the ruxolitinib group achieved one or more of the criteria for the primary end point, and 49% (vs 1% of BAT patients) had a 50% or greater improvement in the MPN-Symptom Assessment Form total symptom score, a validated measure of patient-reported symptoms ([38]). Ninety-six patients crossed over to the ruxolitinib arm after week 32. Grade 3/4 anemia or thrombocytopenia occurred in 1.8% and 5.5% of patients, respectively, compared with 0% and 3.6% of BAT patients, respectively. Ruxolitinib has been approved as therapy for PV after resistance to or intolerance of HU.

Treatment Conclusions

All patients with PV should undergo phlebotomy and receive low-dose ASA unless contradicted. Patients who are at high risk for thrombosis (age >60 years or history of thrombosis) should receive cytoreductive therapy (HU preferred; IFN-α can be considered, especially PEG-IFN-α-2a, in younger patients). The goal Hct is 45% or less for males and 42% or less for females. With the approval of ruxolitinib for PV, patients resistant or intolerant to HU should be offered ruxolitinib, a JAK2 inhibitor.

ESSENTIAL THROMBOCYTHEMIA

Essential thrombocythemia is characterized by persistent thrombocytosis with a predisposition to thrombosis and bleeding. Essential thrombocythemia is not a cytogenetically or a morphologically defined disease entity and remains a diagnosis of exclusion. It is a disease of the elderly; the median age of diagnosis is 55 to 60 years. The female-to-male ratio is 2:1.

Reactive causes of thrombocytosis should be excluded. Most often, the underlying cause is apparent (postsplenectomy, acute infection, blood loss). Other MPNs, such as PV or CML, can also present with thrombocytosis and should be ruled out. In a population-based study (ages 18 to 65 years), 99 of the 9,998 persons studied (1%) had a platelet count greater than 400 × 10^9/L at baseline, of whom only 8 (0.1% of the population studied) had persistent thrombocytosis at greater than 6 months ([39]). Three of the eight patients were confirmed to have ET at baseline, with one additional case of ET diagnosed after 5 years of follow-up. In another study of 732 patients with thrombocytosis (>500 × 10^9/L), ET was present in 5.5% and reactive thrombocytosis in 87% patients ([40]). The magnitude of elevation in the platelet count does not distinguish between reactive and clonal thrombocytosis. In 280 consecutive patients with extreme thrombocytosis (platelet count >1 million), reactive thrombocytosis was noted in 82%, and 14% had MPNs, including ET in 4% ([41]). Reactive thrombocytosis, irrespective of the degree of elevation of platelet counts, does not increase the risk of thromboembolic or bleeding complications. Such complications, if seen, are the results of underlying disease conditions (malignancy, iron deficiency from gastrointestinal bleeding) rather than of elevated platelets.

Pathophysiology

Thrombopoietin regulates the differentiation and proliferation of megakaryocytes. It is produced primarily by the liver parenchymal cells. The gene for Tpo is located on chromosome 3q27-28. It binds to the c-Mpl receptors on platelets and megakaryocytes. When the platelet count is low, more free Tpo is available to bind to megakaryocytes to stimulate proliferation, leading to a rise in the platelet count and vice versa. In most cases of reactive thrombocytosis, Tpo is increased via acute phase reactants, such as interleukin 6. Unlike PV, for which Epo levels are generally low, Tpo levels are high normal or abnormally increased in ET ([42]). This may be due to the increased BM stromal production of Tpo or decreased clearance, as expression of platelet c-Mpl is markedly reduced in ET ([42]). Approximately 50% of patients with ET harbor the JAK2V617F mutation, and 3% to 5% have a mutation in the thrombopoietin receptor (MPL) (W515L/K; tryptophan to leucine or lysine substitution at residue 515) ([43]), both of which lead to dysregulated JAK-STAT signaling. Most patients with ET have JAK2V617F allele burdens less than 50%, suggesting that lower JAK2V617F gene dosage may lead to the development of ET versus PV, for which the allele burden is generally higher ([44]).

Recently, mutations in the gene encoding calreticulin (CALR) have been found in nearly 70% of patients with ET negative for JAK2 or MPL mutations (~25% of all patients with ET) ([45, 46]). The CALR mutation may define a distinct subset of ET. In a series of 717 patients with ET, those with CALR mutations were younger and predominantly male and had a lower incidence of thrombosis, lower hemoglobin levels, lower leukocyte counts, and higher platelet counts than those with the JAK2V617F mutation ([47]). Additional studies are needed to fully elucidate the implications of molecular studies in clinical practice.

Clinical Features

With the increasing use of automated blood counters and routine blood count screenings, more patients with ET are being diagnosed while asymptomatic. Constitutional symptoms are uncommon in ET. Vasomotor manifestations such as dizziness, lightheadedness, acral paresthesia, livedo reticularis, and erythromelalgia were noted in 34% of patients in one study of 147 patients with ET ([48]). Mild splenomegaly (<5 cm) was noted in up to 40% of patients, leukocytosis in 30% to 40%, and mild anemia in 10% to 20%. Thromboembolic and bleeding complications are the major cause of morbidity and mortality in ET. A series of 322 patients with ET from one institution reported a 26% incidence of major thrombosis and 11% incidence of major bleeding at diagnosis ([49]). Hemorrhagic complications increase with extreme thrombocytosis (platelet count >1.5 million/μL) and with the use of antiplatelet therapy such as ASA.

Most serious late complications of ET include transformation to AML and MF (post-ET MF). In a study of 605 patients with ET, the incidence of AML transformation was 3.3%, with a median time to transformation of 11.5 years ([50]). Risk factors for transformation included anemia, platelet count greater than 1,000 × 10^9/L, and increasing age. JAK2 mutational status or the type of therapy (including HU) did not influence the risk of leukemic transformation. In another series of 195 patients with ET, the median time to transformation to MF was 8 years, with an actuarial probability of 2.7% at 5 years, 8.3% at 10 years, and 15.3% at 15 years ([51]). In a large series from seven centers in Europe, patients were reclassified using 2008 WHO criteria ([52]). The diagnosis of ET was confirmed in 891 patients and revised to early/prefibrotic MF in 180 patients. Among patients with ET, the incidence of transformation to AML and MF was 1% and 4%, respectively. The 15-year cumulative incidence of transformation to AML or MF was 2.1% and 9.3%, respectively. In another series of 576 patients with ET, the cumulative incidence of AML was 3.8% and of transformation to MF was 9.5% ([53]).

Diagnosis

Essential thrombocythemia remains a diagnosis of exclusion. Reactive thrombocytosis must be excluded. An important change in the 2008 WHO classification was lowering the platelet count for ET diagnosis from 600 × 10^9/L to 450 × 10^9/L (Table 6-4). Bone marrow biopsy is mandatory for diagnosis to rule out PMF

Table 6-4 2008 WHO Criteria for Diagnosis of Essential Thrombocythemia

1. Sustained platelet count ≥450 × 10^9/L
2. Bone marrow biopsy specimen showing proliferation mainly of the megakaryocytic lineage with increased numbers of enlarged, mature megakaryocytes; no significant increase or left shift of neutrophil granulopoiesis or erythropoiesis
3. Not meeting WHO criteria for PV, PMF, CML, MDS, or other myeloid neoplasm
4. Demonstration of JAK2V617F or other clonal marker, or in the absence of a clonal marker, no evidence for reactive thrombocytosis
Diagnosis of ET requires meeting all four criteria

Reproduced with permission from Tefferi A, Thiele J, Orazi A, et al. Proposals and rationale for revision of the World Health Organization diagnostic criteria for polycythemia vera, essential thrombocythemia, and primary myelofibrosis: recommendations from an ad hoc international expert panel. *Blood.* 2007;110(4):1092-1097.

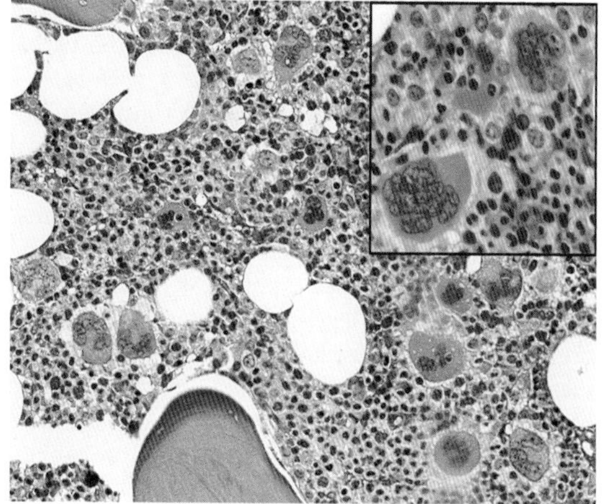

FIGURE 6-5 Essential thrombocytosis is characterized by increased bone marrow cellularity, myeloid hyperplasia, and notably increased megakaryocytes (×200). The megakaryocytes in ET tend to display larger than normal size, and they also contain large hyperlobulated nuclei (inset; ×400).

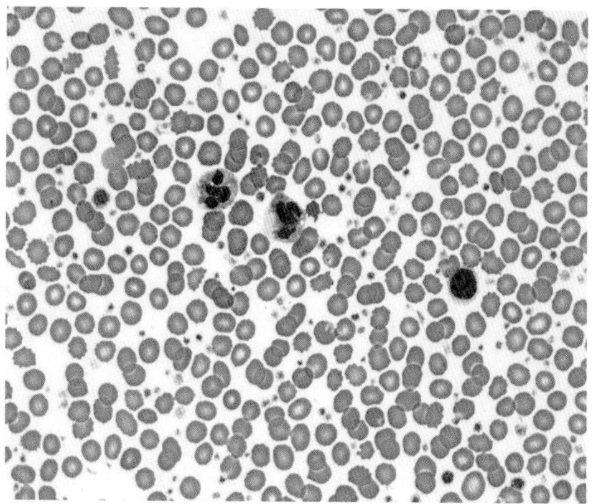

FIGURE 6-6 Peripheral blood smear from a patient with ET shows markedly increased platelets with scattered large forms (×400).

and MDS/MPN. A BM biopsy typically shows large but mature-appearing megakaryocytes with deeply lobulated or hyperlobulated nuclei (Fig. 6-5). The peripheral smear is significant for markedly increased platelets (Fig. 6-6). Reticulin staining should be done to rule out any underlying fibrosis. The presence of megakaryocytic dysplasia in the BM biopsy suggests "prefibrotic" MF, which implies a higher risk of transformation to overt MF or AML ([52]). Chronic neutrophilic leukemia should be ruled out by testing for the *Bcr-Abl* fusion gene. Testing for the JAK2, MPL, or CALR mutations is recommended to establish the clonal nature of the disease, ruling out reactive thrombocytosis (Fig. 6-7).

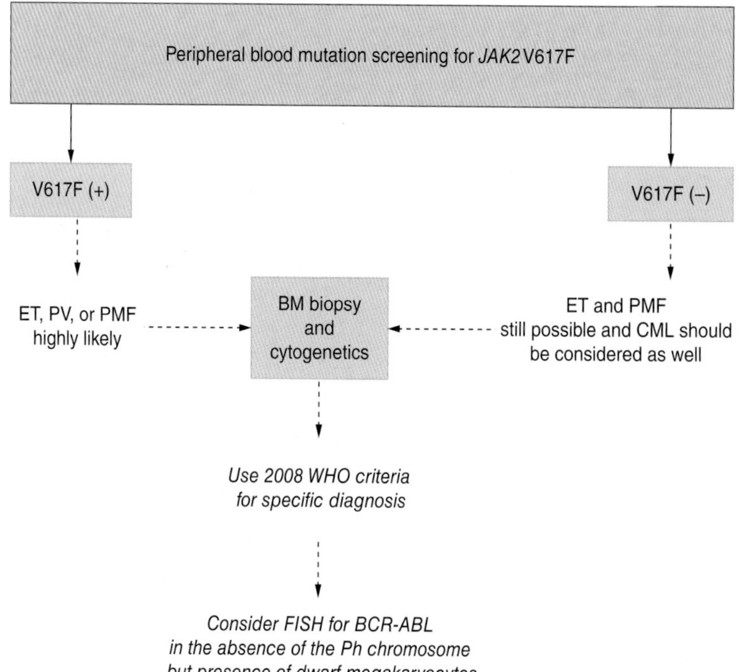

FIGURE 6-7 Diagnostic algorithm for suspected essential thrombocytosis. FISH, fluorescence in situ hybridization. (Reproduced with permission from Tefferi A, Vardiman JW. Classification and diagnosis of myeloproliferative neoplasms: the 2008 World Health Organization criteria and point-of-care diagnostic algorithms. *Leukemia.* 2008;22:14-22.)

Prognosis

Like in PV, thrombosis and hemorrhage are the main complications of ET. Older age and history of prior thrombosis have been shown to predict for future thrombotic events in most studies, whereas cardiovascular risk factors have been predictive in only some. Platelet count does not correlate with risk of thrombosis in ET (Table 6-5). Some studies have found an inverse relationship between the platelet count and the thrombotic risk. This is thought to be due to acquired von Willebrand factor (vWF) disease with elevated platelet counts (eg, >1.5 million/μL), predisposing to more bleeding and protection from thrombosis.

Recent studies from the IWG-MRT of a series of 891 patients, from seven centers in Europe diagnosed with ET using 2008 WHO criteria, reported a 6% incidence of major bleeding at a rate of 0.79 patients/year ([54]). The incidence of thrombosis (fatal and nonfatal events) was 25% at a rate of 1.9% of patients/year ([52, 55]). The rate of nonfatal arterial events (1.2% of patients/year) was higher than that of venous events (0.6% patient/year) ([55]). Factors independently associated with bleeding included previous hemorrhage and ASA therapy ([54]). Factors independently associated with major thrombosis included age greater than 60 years; cardiovascular risk factors (diabetes, hypertension, or smoking); previous thrombosis; and JAK2V617F mutation ([55]). Leukocytosis (>11 × 10^9/L) was an additional independent risk factor for arterial thrombosis; male gender increased the risk of venous thrombosis. Extreme thrombocytosis (platelet count > 1,000 × 10^9/L) was independently associated with a reduced risk of arterial thrombosis ([55]). This is thought to be due to acquired vWF disease with elevated platelet counts, predisposing to more bleeding and protection from thrombosis, which is consistent with previous reports showing an inverse relationship between platelet count and thrombotic risk ([56]).

Using these risk factors, a new prognostic model was proposed to predict risk of thrombosis in patients with ET (International Prognostic Score of Thrombosis in Essential Thrombocythemia [IPSET-Thrombosis]) ([57]). The prognostic score assigned weights to the four risk factors, and the patients could be stratified in three risk categories, with an annual risk of thrombosis ranging from 1.03% of patients/year for the low-risk group to 3.56% of patients/year for the high-risk group (Table 6-6).

Data from the same cohort of patients were used to develop a new possible score to predict overall survival at diagnosis (IPSET) ([58]). The final prognostic score included age 60 years or greater, leukocyte count 11 × 10^9/L or greater, and prior thrombosis as independent risk factors for survival (see Table 6-6). The model stratified patients into three risk categories with median survival ranging from more than 25 years in the low-risk group to 14.7 years for the high-risk group. While the JAK2V617F mutation was associated with increased thrombosis risk ([52]), it was not predictive of survival, which was consistent with findings from other studies ([53]). In another study, JAK2V617F was identified as an independent predictor of pregnancy complications ([59]). Cytogenetic abnormalities are uncommon in ET (<10% at diagnosis) and have not been correlated with survival or transformation risk ([60]).

Treatment

The goal of therapy in ET is to prevent the major cause of morbidity and mortality: thromboembolic events. As the majority of patients have a normal life expectancy, excess treatment that could cause potentially dangerous side effects should be avoided. Cardiovascular risk factors should be aggressively managed in all patients. Smoking was an important risk factor for thrombosis in many studies; all patients should be advised about smoking cessation. The two major classes of drugs used in ET are antiplatelet therapy and cytoreductive therapy (Table 6-7).

Antiplatelet Therapy

Antiplatelet therapy with ASA is useful in treating the microvascular symptoms of ET, especially erythromelalgia. The role of antiplatelet therapy in reducing thrombotic episodes in ET is less clear as no placebo-controlled, randomized trial is available. In a retrospective study, Van Genderen et al showed decreased thrombosis risk and improvements in microvascular symptoms with ASA monotherapy ([61]). Extrapolating from the ECLAP study results in PV ([26]), the general consensus is to use low-dose ASA (75-100 mg daily) in patients with ET unless contraindicated by bleeding history. ASA also provides control of underlying ET-related systemic symptoms. Caution should be exercised in using ASA in patients with a very high platelet count (>1500 × 10^9/L) due to the increased risk of bleeding from acquired von Willebrand disease ([62]). In the UK Medical Research Council Primary Thrombocythemia 1 (MRC PT-1) trial comparing HU and anagrelide in ET, all patients received antiplatelet therapy unless contraindicated ([63]). Possibly because of the synergistic effect of ASA with anagrelide, an increased risk of bleeding was noted in the anagrelide arm compared to HU. It has been suggested that low-dose ASA given twice a day may be effective in patients whose symptoms are not controlled with once-a-day dosing. A study with once-daily ASA found that most patients had incomplete inhibition of thromboxane A_2, and that twice-daily dosing improved the response ([64]).

Table 6-5 Risk Factors for Thrombosis in ET Patients

		Risk Factors Studied					
Study	No. of Patients	Age >60 Years, Odds Ratio/Hazard Ratio/ Significance Level	History of Thrombosis	Risk Factors for CV Events (Smoking, Diabetes, Hypertension, Hyperlipidemia)	Platelet Count >1,000 × 10^9/L	Leukocytosis	JAK-2 Status
Colombi (1991) ([60a])	103	NS	$P < .001$	–	NS	–	–
Cortelazzo (1990) ([60b])	100	10.3	13	NS	NS	–	–
Besses (1999) ([60c])	148	3.3	3.0	4.7	NS	–	–
Bazzan (1999) ([60d])	187	NS	–	NS	NS	–	–
Jantunen (2001) ([60e])	132	NS	–	$P = .01$	NS	–	–
Chim (2005) ([60f])	231	$P = .01$	NS	–	NS	–	–
Wolanskyj ([49])	322	1.51	2.3 (arterial only)	NS	–	1.74 (WBC > 15,000)	NS
Carobbio (2007) ([60g])	439	2.3 (age and previous thrombosis evaluated together)	2.3	–	NS	2.3 (WBC > 8,700)	NS
Alvarez- Larran (2007) ([60h])	126 (<40 y)	NA	NS	Smoking	NS	–	NS
Radaelli (2007) ([60i])	306	NS	7.6	$P < .05$	NS	–	–
Tefferi (2007) ([60j])	605	NS	$P < .001$	NS	–	WBC (≥15,000) $P < .01$ for thrombosis at baseline (NS for thrombosis on follow-up)	NS
Passamonti (2008) ([60k])	605	$P < .001$	$P = .03$	NS	NS	NS	–
Carobbio ([56])	1,063	1.7 (age and previous thrombosis evaluated together)	1.7	–	Patients with WBC <11,000 and platelet <1,000: most likely to have JAK-2 mutation and highest risk of thrombosis		
Carobbio ([55])	891	1.5	1.93	1.56	0.50	1.14	2.04

NS, nonsignificant; (–), not studied.

Table 6-6 International Prognostic Score for Essential Thrombocythemia (IPSET) and IPSET-Thrombosis

Risk Factor	IPSET	IPSET-Thrombosis
Age >60 years	2	1
Previous thrombosis	1	2
WBC count ≥11 × 10^9/L	1	
Cardiovascular risk factors		1
JAK2V617F positive		2
Prognostic score (median survival or rate of thrombosis)		
Low	0 points (not reached)	<2 points (1.03% patients/y)
Intermediate	1-2 points (24.5 y)	2 points (2.35% patients/y)
High	3-4 points (14.7 y)	>2 points (3.56% patients/y)

Cytoreductive Therapy

Hydroxyurea and anagrelide are the two main cytoreductive agents currently used in patients with ET. Hydroxyurea is a nonspecific, cytotoxic, and myelosuppressive drug. Anagrelide has a selective effect on megakaryocyte lineage. Two randomized studies in ET have established the role of HU. In the Italian study by Cortelazzo et al, 114 patients with high-risk ET (age >60 years, history of thrombosis, or both) were randomized to receive either placebo or HU, with a goal platelet count to less than 600 × 10^9/L ([65]). After a median follow-up of 27 months, 3.6% in the HU group had thrombotic episodes compared with 24% in the placebo group (P = .003). This study established the antithrombotic effect of HU in ET. Harrison et al reported concerning the UK MRC PT-1 study with 809 high-risk patients randomized to receive HU plus ASA or anagrelide plus ASA ([63]). The goal platelet count was less than 400 × 10^9/L. Anagrelide therapy was associated with higher rates of arterial thrombosis, serious hemorrhage, or death from these complications but a lower rate of venous thrombosis compared with the HU arm. Serious hemorrhage with anagrelide was likely due to a synergistic effect with ASA. The risk of MF was significantly higher in the anagrelide arm (5-year risk 7% vs 2% in the HU arm), and significantly more patients in the anagrelide arm withdrew from the study because of side effects (22% vs 11%, P = .001). The risk of developing MDS/AML was similar in the two arms.

Table 6-7 Treatment of Essential Thrombocythemia

Risk Category	Intervention
High risk (age <60 years or history of thrombosis)	Cytoreduction[a] and low-dose ASA
Intermediate risk (age <60 years and no history of thrombosis) with cardiovascular risk factors, especially smoking and/or platelet count >1,000 × 10^9/L	Low-dose ASA (caution ASA use with extreme thrombocytosis; rule out von Willebrand disease first)
	Cytoreduction[a] if bleeding present; role of cytoreduction in absence of bleeding unclear
Low risk (age <60 years and no history of thrombosis)	Observation or low-dose ASA

[a]Cytoreduction: HU first choice; low-dose aspirin (ASA) indicated for microvascular symptoms for any risk group.

Based on this trial, HU is now considered the standard first-line treatment in ET. However, the debate over the long-term safety of HU (especially potential leukemogenic risk) coupled with the recently reported ANAHYDRET study showing noninferiority of anagrelide monotherapy compared with HU monotherapy have reignited the debate about the optimal first-line therapy in ET ([66]).

Interferon alfa has been used to treat patients with ET, with a greater than 75% hematological response rate in various series. The average starting dose is 3 to 5 million units given subcutaneously daily or three times a week. Side effects (depression, flu-like symptoms) limit frontline use in ET. Because of its nonteratogenic nature, IFN-α is mainly used in pregnant women and women of childbearing age with high-risk ET.

Once-weekly PEG-IFN-α-2a has been evaluated in 39 patients ([34]). A CHR (defined as normalization of platelet count in the absence of thromboembolic events) was noted in 76% of patients. Among 16 patients with serial samples available for testing JAK2V617F allele burden, 38% had some decease in JAK2 allele burden; 6% achieved CMR. These results suggested PEG-IFN-α-2a may be useful in ET. An ongoing randomized trial is comparing PEG-INF-α-2a versus ASA plus HU in patients with PV or ET (NCT01259856).

Special Issues

Management of Extreme Thrombocytosis (Platelet Count >1.5 Million/μL)

Aspirin should be avoided due to risk of bleeding secondary to acquired von Willebrand disease. The use of cytoreductive agents is suggested, especially when bleeding is present, to lower platelets counts and decrease the risk of bleeding. Many experts regard extreme thrombocytosis as a high-risk category and treat all such patients with cytoreduction; others reserve it for those with bleeding complications.

Management of Young Patients With Extreme Thrombocytosis

Ruggeri et al prospectively studied 65 asymptomatic patients who were younger than 60 years of age and with a platelet count less than 1,500 × 10^9/L ([67]). No prophylactic cytoreduction was given, and ASA was used only for erythromelalgia symptoms. The risk of thromboembolic complications was found to be similar to the control population. The occurrence of pregnancy or minor surgical intervention was not associated with an increased risk of thrombosis. Cytoreductive therapy was needed in 27% of patients at a median of 34 months. Tefferi et al studied 74 young women (<50 years of age) with ET ([68]). The risk of thrombosis and major hemorrhage was lower (7% at diagnosis and 18% at follow-up for thrombosis; 4% major hemorrhage at diagnosis and follow-up) than in the general ET population. Patients with a history of thrombosis had a 45% rate of subsequent thrombosis compared with 13% in those without prior thrombosis, indicating the need for cytoreduction with a history of thrombosis, even in younger patients. None of the 34 pregnancies in this study group was associated with a major thrombotic complication.

PRIMARY MYELOFIBROSIS

Primary myelofibrosis is a clonal disorder of a multipotent hematopoietic progenitor cell of unknown etiology; it is characterized by myeloid cell proliferation, megakaryocytic atypia, BM fibrosis, a leukoerythroblastic peripheral blood picture, extramedullary hematopoiesis (EMH), and splenomegaly. Primary myelofibrosis was previously called CIMF, MF with myeloid metaplasia (MMM), or agnogenic myeloid metaplasia (AMM). The disease can occur either de novo or as a late complication of PV or ET. In either case, it manifests as progenitor cell–derived clonal myeloproliferation accompanied by intense marrow stromal reaction, including collagen fibrosis, osteosclerosis, and angiogenesis.

Pathophysiology

Fibrogenesis and angiogenesis are thought to develop consequent to the release of growth-promoting factors (such as vascular endothelial growth factor [VEGF], PDGF, basic fibroblast growth factor [bFGF] and transforming growth factor β [TGF-β]) from proliferating atypical megakaryocytes in the BM. The JAK2V617F mutation is found in 50% to 60% of patients with PMF. Persistent JAK-STAT signaling, resulting in the overproduction of proinflammatory cytokines, has been observed in all patients with PMF ([69, 70]). Proinflammatory cytokines have been associated with many of the symptoms of MF, including splenomegaly, transfusion dependence, thrombocytopenia, and shortened survival ([71]). Mutations in the thrombopoietin receptor (MPL) are found in 5% to 10% of patients, and CALR mutations in an additional 25% ([45, 46]). Rare inactivating mutations in negative regulators of JAK-STAT signaling (eg, LNK, SOCS, and CBL) also contribute to the dysregulated JAK-STAT signaling in PMF ([72]).

The exact contributions of mutations in JAK2, MPL, and CALR to disease pathogenesis remain unclear. Recent studies suggested that the heterogeneity of mutations in PMF may underlie the heterogeneity of its clinical phenotype; that is, these mutations may be associated with distinct clinical features. In a study of 617 patients with PMF, those with CALR mutations had a lower risk of anemia, thrombocytopenia, and leukocytosis ([73]). In another series of 428 patients with PMF, CALR mutations were associated with younger age, lower leukocyte count, and higher platelet count, while MPL W515K/L mutations were associated with younger age and lower leukocyte count when compared with JAK2V617F mutations ([53]). A number of other mutations have also been found in PMF, albeit at much lower frequencies than JAK2 and CALR mutations (eg, mutations in ASXL1, EZH2, SRSF2, CBL, IDH1/IDH2, TP53, TET2, and DNMT3) ([72]). Unlike the JAK2/CALR/MPL mutations, which are mutually exclusive, the other less-frequent mutations may coexist with each other or with the three driver mutations.

Clinical Features

PMF is a heterogeneous disorder with variable age of onset, presenting features, phenotypic manifestations, and prognosis. The incidence of PMF increases with age. In a series of 1,054 patients, the median age at diagnosis was 64 years; 17% of patients were younger than 50 years and 5% younger than 40 years ([74]). Clinical presentation can range from no or minimal symptoms, where disease is discovered during a workup for leukocytosis or splenomegaly, to severe symptoms. Severe fatigue is the most common presenting symptom. Constitutional symptoms (fatigue, weight loss, pruritus, low-grade fever, night sweats) are a prominent feature of PMF and can be debilitating. Myeloproliferation is one of the major features of the disease and can lead to sequestration of immature cells and production of blood cells in sites other than the BM, a phenomenon known as EMH. This commonly manifests as marked hepatosplenomegaly, with associated pain, early satiety, portal hypertension, and anemia and thrombocytopenia. Splenomegaly is present in 80% of patients and may extend into the pelvis. Hepatomegaly is seen in 40% to 70% of patients. EMH might cause symptoms in various other organs, leading to respiratory distress, pulmonary hypertension, ascites, pericardial tamponade, cord compression, and paralysis. Peripheral smear generally provides the first clue toward a diagnosis of PMF, with the presence of characteristic teardrop red cells and a leukoerythroblastic picture (presence of immature myeloid cells including blasts in the peripheral blood). Progressive anemia generally develops, requiring transfusions. Some patients may present with leukocytosis and thrombocytosis; however, most develop leukopenia and thrombocytopenia in later stages of the disease. Among the most feared complications of PMF is transformation to AML, occurring in 10% to 20% of patients in the first 10 years from diagnosis. The outcome after transformation is poor, with a median survival of 5 months. Transformation to AML is the most common cause of death in MF, followed by MF progression without acute transformation, thrombosis, and cardiovascular complications, infection, bleeding, and portal hypertension.

Table 6-8 2008 WHO Criteria for Diagnosis of Primary Myelofibrosis (PMF)

Major criteria
1. Presence of megakaryocyte proliferation and atypia, usually accompanied by either reticulin and/or collagen fibrosis, or, in the absence of significant reticulin fibrosis, the megakaryocyte changes must be accompanied by an increased bone marrow cellularity characterized by granulocytic proliferation and often decreased erythropoiesis (ie, prefibrotic cellular-phase disease)
2. Not meeting WHO criteria for PV, CML, MDS, or other myeloid neoplasm
3. Demonstration of JAK2617VF or other clonal marker (eg, MPL515WL/K) or, in the absence of a clonal marker, no evidence of bone marrow fibrosis due to underlying inflammatory or other neoplastic diseases
Minor criteria
1. Leukoerythroblastosis
2. Increase in serum lactate dehydrogenase level
3. Anemia
4. Palpable splenomegaly
Diagnosis of PMF requires meeting all three major criteria and at least two minor criteria

Reproduced with permission from Tefferi A, Thiele J, Orazi A, et al. Proposals and rationale for revision of the World Health Organization diagnostic criteria for polycythemia vera, essential thrombocythemia, and primary myelofibrosis: recommendations from an ad hoc international expert panel. *Blood.* 2007;110(4):1092-1097.

Diagnosis

A diagnosis of PMF is made using the 2008 WHO criteria (see Table 6-8) ([6]). Symptoms such as splenomegaly, leukoerythroblastosis, anemia, poor quality of life, and BM megakaryocyte hyperplasia are suggestive of PMF. Marrow fibrosis by itself is not specific for a diagnosis of PMF. Various degrees of fibrosis are observed in other MPNs, and MDS with fibrosis must be excluded. Morphologic features of the BM during the prefibrotic (cellular) phase of PMF are shown in Fig. 6-8, and those during the fibrotic phase are depicted in Figs. 6-9 to 6-11. Classical morphological features consistent with PMF and seen in the peripheral blood smear are demonstrated in Fig. 6-12. Bone marrow histology, especially megakaryocyte morphology, is a critical diagnostic criterion for PMF (Fig. 6-13). All patients suspected of having PMF should undergo bone marrow biopsy with reticulin and collagen staining and testing for JAK2V617F, CALR, and MPL mutations. Chronic myelogenous leukemia should be ruled out by testing for Bcr-Abl.

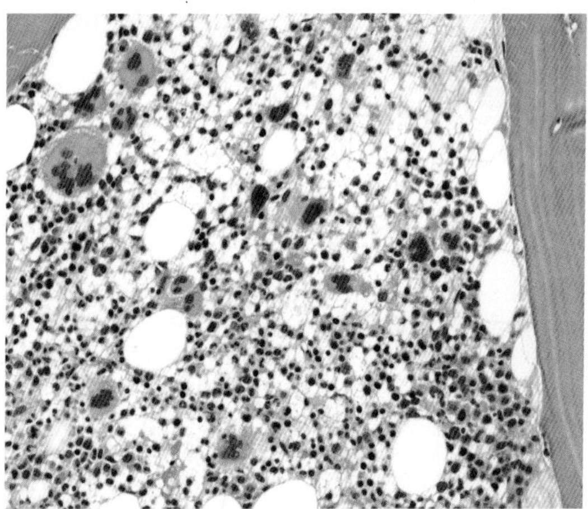

FIGURE 6-8 It is difficult to distinguish the prefibrotic (cellular) phase of PMF from other types of chronic myeloproliferative neoplasms based on morphological criteria alone. However, careful microscopic examination of the bone marrow biopsy usually reveals scattered atypical megakaryocytes with morphological criteria classical for PMF in the fibrotic phase. As shown, some of the megakaryocytes in this bone marrow biopsy are remarkably variable in size and shape and characteristically contain markedly hyperchromatic nuclei (×200).

Prognosis

The median survival is 5 years. In a review of 1,054 patients with PMF, the median survival was

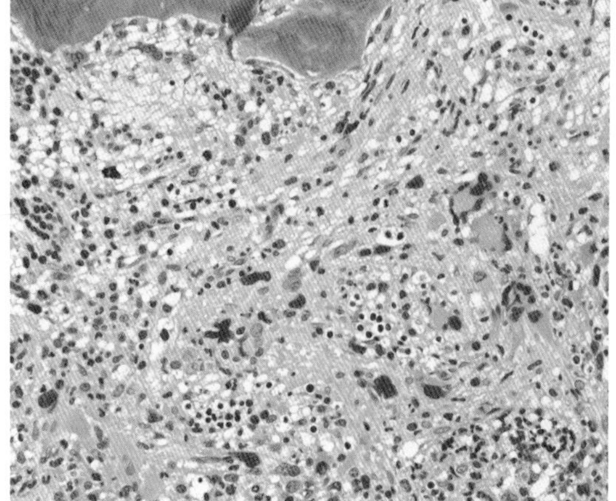

FIGURE 6-9 During the fibrotic phase of PMF, bone marrow hematopoietic cellular elements tend to decrease in number with interstitial infiltration of the bone marrow by fibroblasts that leads to a streaming effect. Characteristically, the megakaryocytes demonstrate variability in size and shape, and megakaryocytes containing hyperchromatic and hyperlobulated nuclei are frequently encountered during the fibrotic phase of PMF (×200).

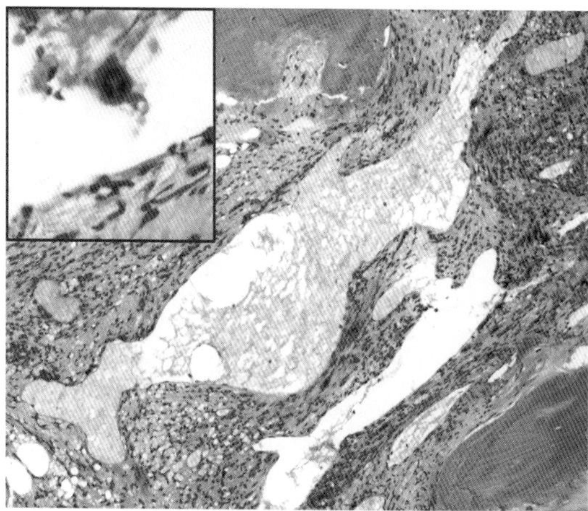

FIGURE 6-10 Another common feature of the bone marrow during the fibrotic phase is marked expansion of bone marrow sinusoids, which are usually rudimentary under normal conditions (×100). Hematopoietic cellular elements can be detected within the bone marrow sinuses; a megakaryocyte is shown, comprising what is known as intrasinusoidal hematopoiesis (inset; ×400).

69 months ([74]). Younger patients with good prognostic features may have a life expectancy exceeding 10 years. The most commonly used prognostic scoring systems are the International Prognostic Scoring System (IPSS), designed to be used at diagnosis, and the Dynamic IPSS (D-IPSS), which can be used at any point in the patient's disease course ([74, 75]) (Table 6-9). Both prognostic scoring systems are based on clinical and laboratory characteristics: age (>65 years), constitutional symptoms (yes/no), hemoglobin (<10 g/dL), leukocyte counts (>25 × 10^9/L), and circulating blasts (≥1%). In the IPSS system, all factors are given a score of 1, while in the D-IPSS, hemoglobin below 10 g/dL is given 2 points. On the basis of these risk factors, patients are separated into four risk groups: low risk (0 points); intermediate-1 risk (1 point IPSS; 1-2 points D-IPSS); intermediate-2 risk (2 points IPSS; 3-4 points D-IPSS); and high risk (≥3 points IPSS; 5-6 points D-IPSS). Cytogenetic abnormalities are found in about half of the patients with PMF. Common abnormalities include del(13q), del(20q), trisomy 8 or 9, and abnormalities of chromosome 1 [partial trisomy and der(6)t(1;6)] ([76]). Tam et al analyzed 256 patients with PMF; 36% had chromosomal abnormalities ([77]). They categorized patients into those with favorable cytogenetics (sole deletion of 13q or 20q, trisomy 9 +/– one other abnormality); diploid cytogenetics; unfavorable cytogenetics (abnormalities of chromosomes 5 or 7, or complex [≥3]

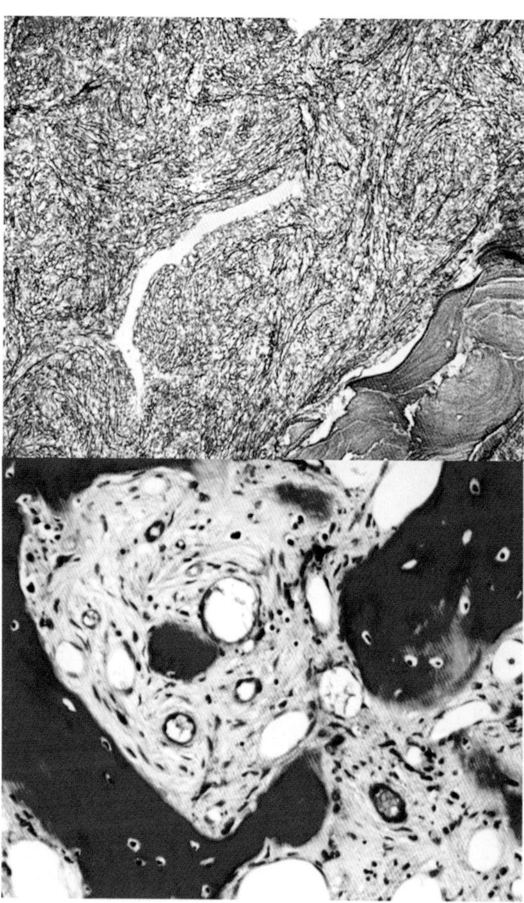

FIGURE 6-11 During the fibrotic phase of PMF, the bone marrow is characterized by increased interstitial reticulin fibrosis (upper panel; ×100), which might be associated with the abnormal presence of collagen fibers that are detected by trichrome staining (lower panel; ×200).

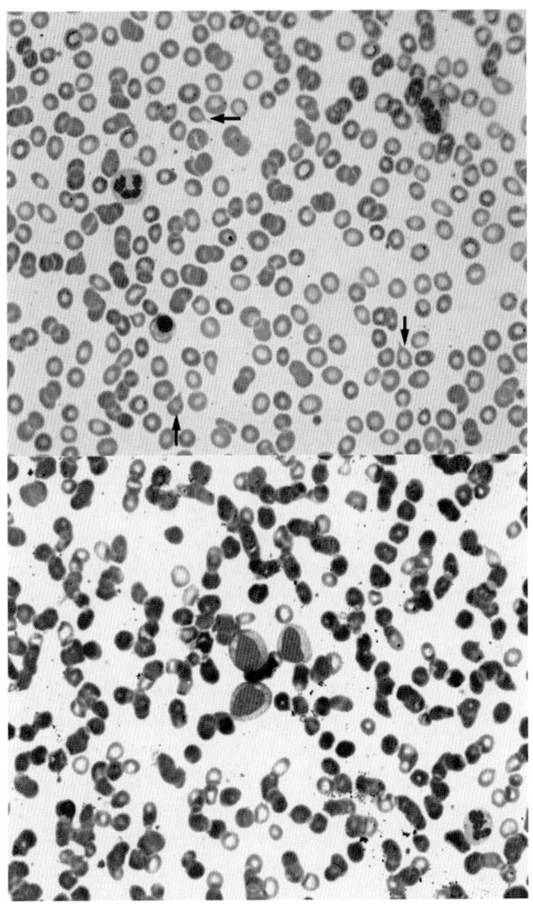

FIGURE 6-12 Careful examination of peripheral blood smears from patients with PMF usually reveals teardrop red blood cells (*arrows*, upper panel; ×400). In addition, nucleated red blood cells (upper panel) and left-shifted granulopoiesis (lower panel; ×400) are seen, two morphologic criteria collectively described as leukoerythroblastosis.

Table 6-9 Prognostic Scoring Systems for Myelofibrosis

Factors	IPSS	D-IPSS	D-IPSS-plus
Age >65 years	1	1	1
Constitutional symptoms	1	1	1
Hemoglobin <10 g/dL	1	2	1
Leukocytes >25 × 10^9/L	1	1	1
Blood blasts ≥1%	1	1	1
Platelet count < 100 × 10^9/L			1
Transfusion dependence			1
Unfavorable karyotype			1
Risk stratification *(median survival)*			
Low	0 points (11.2 y)	0 points (not reached)	0 points (15.4 y)
Intermediate-1	1 point (7.9 y)	1-2 points (14.2 y)	1 point (6.5 y)
Intermediate-2	2 points (4 y)	3-4 points (4 y)	2-3 points (2.9 y)
High	≥3 points (2.3 y)	5-6 points (1.5 y)	≥4 points (1.3 y)

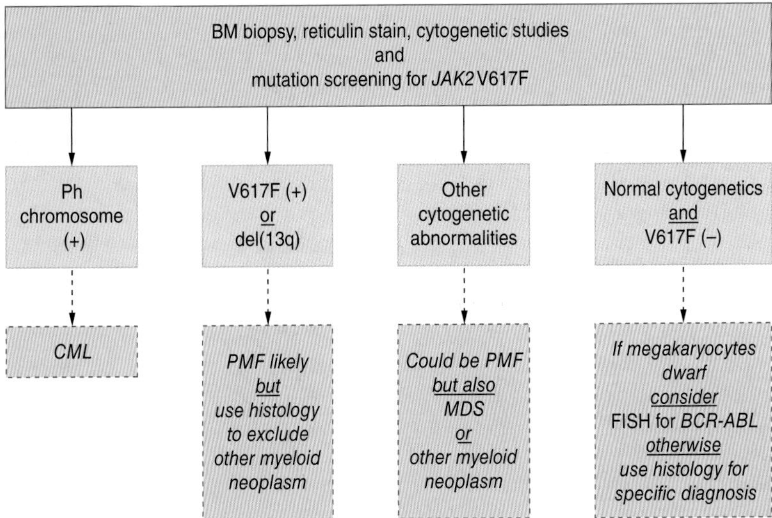

FIGURE 6-13 Diagnostic algorithm for suspected primary myelofibrosis. (Reproduced with permission from Tefferi A, Vardiman JW. Classification and diagnosis of myeloproliferative neoplasms: the 2008 World Health Organization criteria and point-of-care diagnostic algorithms. *Leukemia.* 2008;22:14-22.)

cytogenetics); and very unfavorable cytogenetics (any abnormality of chromosome 17). The median survival times (for patients with assessment at diagnosis) were 63, 46, 15, and 5 months, respectively. Gangat et al added unfavorable karyotype, platelet count below 100×10^9/L, and transfusion dependence as independent risk factors for inferior survival in another prognostic model (DIPSS-plus) ([78]).

Recent studies have explored the prognostic relevance of various mutations. In a study of 617 patients with PMF, CALR mutations were associated with longer survival (median 17.7 years) ([73]). Patients without any mutation in JAK2, MPL, or CALR ("triple negative") had a higher incidence of transformation to AML and a shorter survival (median 3.2 years). When the CALR, JAK2, and MPL mutations were added to the IPSS, patients could be further subdivided into five risk groups, with significantly different median survivals ([73]). Another study of 428 patients with PMF reported similar findings ([53]). Patients with CALR mutations had the longest survival (median 15.9 years), while patients without any of these mutations (triple negative) had the shortest survival (median 2.3 years) ([53]). Mutations in epigenetic modulators (ASXL1, SRSF2, and EZH2) were associated with worse survival and increased risk of transformation to AML ([72]). The negative prognostic impact of ASXL1 was shown in another series of 570 patients ([79]). Patients who had ASXL1 mutations in the absence of CALR mutations had the worst survival (median 2.3 years). Future studies will explore further how to best implement the molecular information in everyday practice.

Treatment

Before the approval by the FDA of the JAK1/2 inhibitor ruxolitinib in 2011, treatment of MF was unsatisfactory. Cytoreductive drugs such as HU or cladribine were used to control hyperproliferation, although their effects are transient and rarely result in complete spleen regression. Oral alkylating agents have also been used, but often induce severe myelosuppression and are associated with an increased risk of transformation to AML. Corticosteroids, erythroid-stimulating agents, and androgens have proven helpful in treatment of anemia. Patients with low serum Epo (<125 U/L) can be given subcutaneous injections of Epo (40,000 U/week). Corticosteroids (prednisone 0.5 to 1.0 mg/kg/day) or androgens (testosterone enanthate injections 400-600 mg/week; oral danazol 200 mg two or three times/day) have also been useful. Immunomodulatory agents (low-dose thalidomide and lenalidomide) have anticytokine and antiangiogenic effects and have been shown to reduce splenomegaly and improve anemia. They are usually used with tapering doses of prednisone for 3 months. Interferon alfa has been used with some success, but significant toxicity prevents its use in many patients. It may slow disease progression in patients with early MF, as well as reverse BM fibrosis in some patients ([80]). A recent retrospective study of Peg-IFN-α-2a in 62 patients with MF reported improvements in anemia and constitutional symptoms, normalization of platelet and leukocyte counts, and reduction in splenomegaly ([81]). In selected patients, splenectomy or splenic radiation may help with symptom control or may improve blood cell count but these procedures carry significant side effects.

JAK Inhibitors

Two pivotal phase III randomized trials provided evidence for the regulatory approval of the oral JAK1/2 inhibitor ruxolitinib. COMFORT-I randomized patients to ruxolitinib (n = 155) or placebo (n = 154) ([82]), while COMFORT-II compared ruxolitinib (n = 146) to BAT (n = 73) ([83]). Significantly more patients in the ruxolitinib arms had 35% or more reduction in spleen volume (approximately 50% reduction by palpation) from baseline at week 24 (COMFORT-I) or week 48 (COMFORT-II). Both studies showed significantly better improvements in MF-related symptoms and quality of life in patients treated with ruxolitinib. Thrombocytopenia and anemia were the most common toxicities associated with ruxolitinib therapy. These effects mostly appeared within the first 3 to 6 months of treatment and were managed with dose reductions or transfusions.

Long-term follow-up analyses have demonstrated that the effects of ruxolitinib are durable. After a median follow-up of 2 years, more than 80% of patients treated with ruxolitinib in COMFORT-I who had achieved a 35% or greater reduction in spleen volume had maintained at least a 10% reduction ([84]). In COMFORT-II, at 144 weeks, the Kaplan-Meier estimated probability of maintaining a spleen response was 50% ([85]). Ruxolitinib also improved survival ([85, 86]). Long-term treatment with ruxolitinib may delay progression of or reverse BM fibrosis in some patients ([87]). Two case reports showed nearly complete resolution of marrow fibrosis and a reduction in JAK2V617F allele burden after long-term treatment with ruxolitinib ([88, 89]).

In our experience, most patients with symptomatic splenomegaly or systemic MF-related symptoms, even those with transfusion-dependent anemia, can be successfully treated with ruxolitinib for long periods of time if the patient is carefully monitored (particularly during the first 3-6 months) and the dose adjusted to avoid therapy interruptions. Recommended starting doses are 20 mg twice per day in patients with platelets above 200×10^9/L, 15 mg twice a day in patients with platelets between 100 and 200×10^9/L, and 5 mg twice a day in patients with platelet counts below 100×10^9/L. The dose can be increased to a maximum of 25 mg twice a day if tolerated. Avoidance of treatment interruption is important for treatment success, as symptoms return to baseline within 7 to 10 days. Ruxolitinib doses of 10 mg twice a day or higher are effective maintenance doses. Other JAK inhibitors, which appear to be less myelosuppressive (pacritinib) and may possibly reduce the need for red blood cell transfusions (momelotinib), are in late-phase clinical development for MF.

Allogeneic Stem Cell Transplantation

Allogeneic stem cell transplant (alloSCT) is curative in MF; however, fewer than 10% of patients undergo alloSCT due to older age or severe comorbidities. Reduced-intensity conditioning regimens are an option in older patients and those with comorbidities [90]. Spleen size influences the rate of engraftment after transplant, but splenectomy before alloSCT is not recommended. The use of ruxolitinib pretransplant to reduce splenomegaly is being evaluated. A study of 14 patients treated with ruxolitinib (median duration 6.5 months) before alloSCT showed that, at the time of transplantation, 7 of 11 patients with splenomegaly had a 41% median reduction in palpable spleen size as well as improvement in disease-related symptoms [91]. Thirteen (93%) patients had engraftment, and 11 were alive after a median follow-up of 9 months. Treatment-related mortality was 7%. In a prospective study of 22 patients pretreated with ruxolitinib, 69% had reductions in spleen size, 86% had improvement in symptoms, engraftment was seen in all cases, and the estimated 1-year survival was 81% [92]. Although the numbers were small, survival was longer in patients who responded to ruxolitinib (n = 10) than in those who did not (n = 10) (100% vs 60% estimated 1-year survival; $P = .02$).

Combination and Novel Therapies

Other targeted agents, such as epigenetic modifying agents (azacitidine, decitabine, panobinostat, and pracinostat); hedgehog inhibitors (LDE-225, IPI-926); PI3 kinase inhibitors (BKM120); antifibrotic agents (PRM-151); or telomenase inhibitor (imetelstat) have been tested. Most have not shown significant efficacy as single agents. Preclinical studies have shown synergistic effects when some of these agents were combined with ruxolitinib, suggesting a useful strategy to improve outcomes. Clinical trials testing ruxolitinib in combination with pracinostat, panobinostat, lenalidomide, decitabine, azacytidine, BEZ235, and LDE-225 are ongoing results of these trials are eagerly awaited.

Treatment Conclusions

Patients with MF should first be assigned to a risk category using one of the standard prognostic tools (IPSS, D-IPSS). For patients with low-risk disease, a watch-and-wait approach is acceptable. Patients in the intermediate or high-risk groups should be treated based on their symptoms. In most cases, with careful titration and monitoring, ruxolitinib can be safely used. For younger patients in the intermediate-2 and high-risk categories, alloSCT can be offered. For patients who are not eligible for alloSCT or are intolerant or lose their response to other therapies, enrollment in clinical trials is recommended. Ruxolitinib and other JAK inhibitors have been effective in reducing splenomegaly, in improving symptoms and quality of life, and in prolonging survival in patients with MF. JAK inhibitors have not been shown to eradicate the mutant clone, and patients lose their response to therapy over time. Results from ongoing trials of new targeted agents and their combinations are eagerly awaited.

CHRONIC EOSINOPHILIC LEUKEMIA/HYPEREOSINOPHILIC SYNDROME

Hypereosinophilic syndrome is characterized by chronic eosinophil overproduction in the absence of obvious reactive or clonal causes of eosinophilia. Eosinophilic tissue infiltration may involve the heart, skin, central and peripheral nervous systems, lungs, spleen, liver, and gastrointestinal tract. A diagnosis of HES requires the presence of an absolute eosinophil count of more than 1.5×10^9/L for at least 6 months and evidence of end-organ damage. Patients with hypereosinophilia who are found to have clonal disease (ie, a cytogenetic or molecular abnormality proving the existence of a malignant clone), peripheral blood blasts greater than 2%, or bone marrow blasts greater than 5% have CEL [93]. Hypereosinophilic syndrome and CEL have similar clinical presentations, and distinguishing between the two can be difficult unless proper testing for a molecular/cytogenetic marker is done. As most common causes of eosinophilia are reactive, conditions such as infections (especially parasitic), atopy, drug reactions, connective tissue disorders, or vasculitis must be ruled out.

In 2003, Cools et al described a karyotypically occult but fluorescent in situ hybridization (FISH)–apparent molecular aberrancy in a subset of patients with HES/CEL [94]. This abnormality consisted of an interstitial deletion of chromosome 4q12, leading to the fusion of the FIP1-like 1 (FIP1L1) gene to the PDGFRα gene. The resultant product, FIP1L1-PDGFRα, is a constitutively active TK highly amenable to inhibition by imatinib. Other molecularly defined HES/CEL subtypes include mutations involving the genes that encode for PDGFRβ (located on chromosome 5q31-q33) and fibroblast growth factor receptor 1 (FGFR1; located on chromosome 8p11) [95]. All such patients have been reclassified using the new 2008 WHO classification into separate groups, as the resulting rearranged genes have become markers of disease clonality (see Table 6-1): myeloid neoplasms associated with eosinophilia and abnormalities of PDGFRα, PDGFRβ, or FGFR1.

Hypereosinophilic syndrome is more common in men than women, and patients are usually younger (20-50 years old). The continuous presence of a large number of eosinophils in the blood can eventually cause multiple organ tissue damage due to tissue infiltration by eosinophils. The disease can range from presenting with minimal symptoms and a long survival to being rapidly fatal due to sudden, severe heart failure or acute leukemia. Clinical manifestations include pruritus, urticaria, angioedema, erythematous papules, valvular heart disease, mural thrombi, cardiomyopathy, polyneuropathies, optic neuritis, pulmonary infiltrates, and pleural effusion.

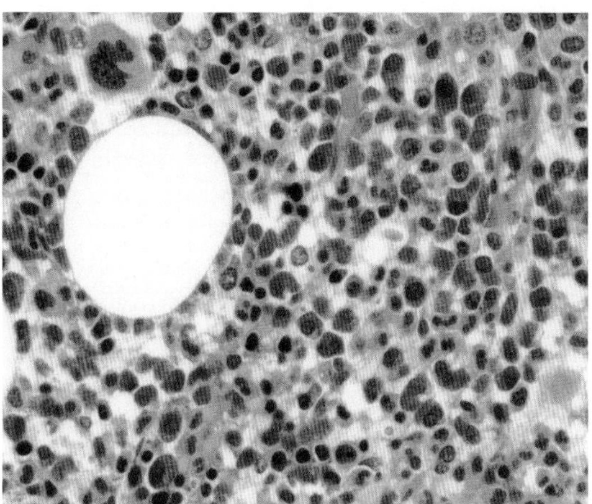

FIGURE 6-14 In CEL/HES, bone marrow typically shows increased cellularity with striking interstitial infiltration by eosinophils (×400).

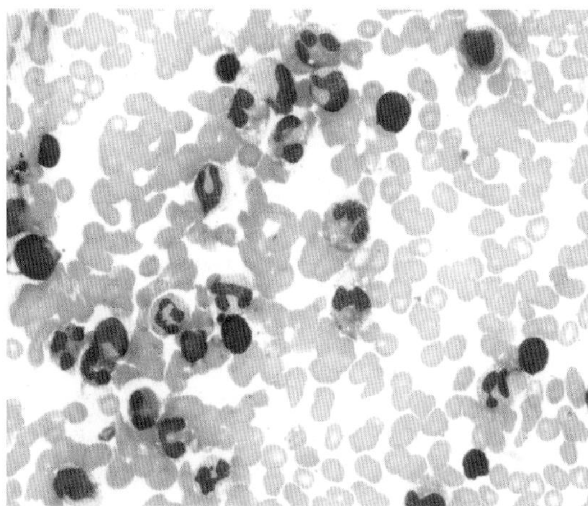

FIGURE 6-15 Markedly increased, morphologically unremarkable eosinophils are typically detected in the bone marrow aspirate smears from patients with CEL/HES (×400).

Diagnosis

Patients suspected to have HES must undergo bone marrow evaluation, cytogenetic analysis, and testing for FIP1L1-PDGFRα, as treatment modalities for patients with this mutation are different. Figures 6-14 and 6-15 illustrate the morphological findings in HES/CEL. The incidence of the FIP1L1—PDGFRα rearrangement is low in patients with hypereosinophilia. In the initial study by Cools et al, FIP1L1-PDGFRα was found in 56% of the patients [94]. Other studies have reported a frequency ranging from 3% to 88%, likely reflecting the intrinsic heterogeneity among patients with hypereosinophilia and the impact of referral bias [94,96]. In the largest study to date, FISH analysis aimed at detecting a deletion/excision of the CHIC2 locus at chromosome 4q12 (indirect test for FIP1L1-PDGFRα abnormality) was performed in 741 unselected patients with eosinophilia; only 21 (3%) were positive [96]. In another study of 376 patients with persistent unexplained eosinophilia, 40 patients (11%) were FIP1L1-PDGFRα positive [97]. T-cell immunophenotyping and T-cell receptor gene rearrangement analysis should be performed in all patients, and if either clonal or immunophenotypically aberrant T cells are identified, a diagnosis of lymphoproliferative variant of HES is preferred. Chest x-ray, pulmonary function tests, echocardiogram, and measurement of serum troponin levels should be performed at diagnosis. An increased level of serum cardiac troponin correlates with the presence of cardiomyopathy in HES. A diagnostic algorithm for primary eosinophilia is presented in Fig. 6-16.

Treatment

For asymptomatic patients with no organ damage and normal troponin levels, no active HES therapy is recommended. These patients should be followed closely. For patients with symptomatic disease or evidence of end-organ damage, therapy for HES generally entails the use of corticosteroids, IFN-α, or cytoreductive agents such as HU, vincristine, or cyclosporine. The first-line treatment of HES is usually prednisone (starting dose of 1 mg/kg/day), with a response rate of 70%. Relapses often occur with cessation of therapy, requiring alternative options, such as IFN-α or HU. Vincristine is useful for acute reductions when total eosinophil count is very high (≥50 × 10^9/L).

For patients refractory to conventional therapies, the use of monoclonal antibody therapy should be considered. Two drugs are currently available: mepolizumab, which targets interleukin 5, and alemtuzumab, which targets the CD52 antigen expressed by

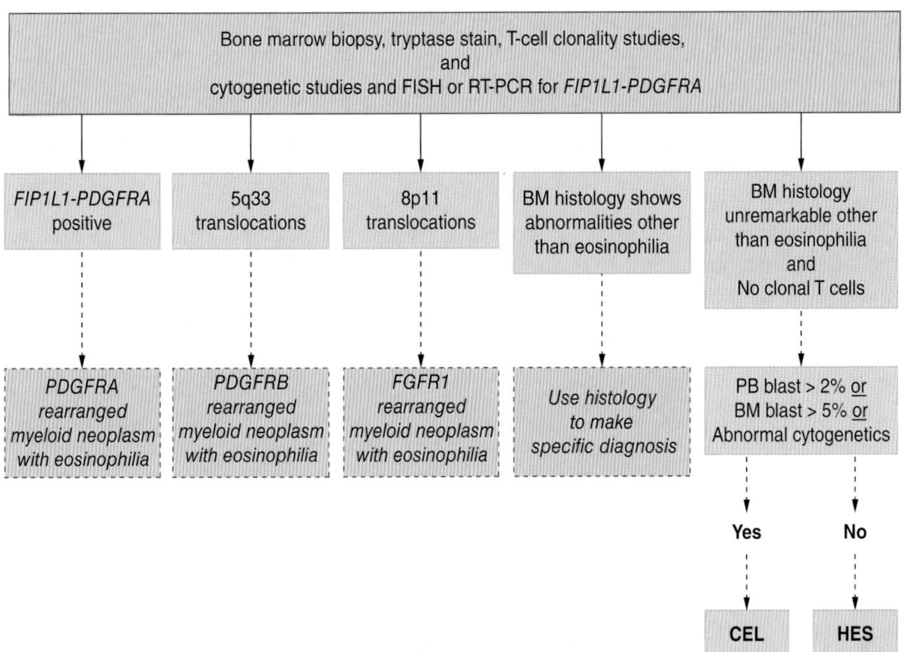

FIGURE 6-16 Diagnostic algorithm for suspected primary eosinophilia. BM, bone marrow; PB, peripheral blood; PDGFRA, platelet-derived growth factor receptor alpha; PDGFRB, platelet-derived growth factor beta. RT-PCR, reverse transcriptase polymerase chain reaction. (Reproduced with permission from Tefferi A, Vardiman JW. Classification and diagnosis of myeloproliferative neoplasms: the 2008 World Health Organization criteria and point-of-care diagnostic algorithms. *Leukemia.* 2008;22:14-22.)

eosinophils but not neutrophils. Rothenberg et al conducted a randomized, placebo-controlled trial evaluating the safety and efficacy of mepolizumab in patients with stable HES on steroids without life-threatening complications as a steroid-sparing agent ([98]). The primary end point (reduction of the prednisone dose to ≤10 mg/day for ≥8 consecutive weeks) was achieved in 84% of patients receiving mepolizumab compared with 43% of patients in the placebo group ($P < .001$). In a long-term extension study, 78 patients received mepolizumab for a median 251 weeks (range, 4-302 weeks), and 69% were still receiving mepolizumab at the end of the study. Sixty-two percent of patients were free of prednisone or other HES treatments for 12 weeks or more ([99]).

Mepolizumab is currently available on a compassionate use basis. Among 11 patients with HES/CEL (9 previously treated) treated with alemtuzumab ([100]), 10 (91%) achieved CHR (defined as the reduction of the absolute eosinophil count and the percentage of eosinophils in peripheral blood to normal values) after a median of 2 weeks, and symptoms completely resolved in 9 patients. Bone marrow eosinophilia resolved in four of the seven evaluable patients. The median duration of CHR was short lived (3 months), and 7 of the 10 CHRs relapsed. Although effective in eliminating the disease, therapy with alemtuzumab requires a maintenance phase, with alemtuzumab given periodically every few weeks or months on the first evidence of recurrent symptoms and signs of the disease. A long-term follow-up of nine of the original patients and three additional patients was recently published ([101]). Ten of twelve patients treated with alemtuzumab achieved CHR and elimination of disease symptoms after a median of 1 week; this was sustained for a median duration of 66 weeks. Five patients with CHR receiving maintenance alemtuzumab for a median duration of 20 weeks (range, 1-266 weeks) had a significantly longer time to disease progression than those who were not given maintenance therapy ($P = .01$). Eleven patients eventually relapsed (only one who was on maintenance therapy). Five of six patients achieved a second CHR after rechallenge with alemtuzumab, with three of five receiving maintenance therapy.

Imatinib mesylate is a potent adenosine triphosphate (ATP)–competitive tyrosine kinase inhibitor (TKI) that is highly active against ABL, PDGFR, and KIT protein kinases. Imatinib therapy for patients with eosinophilia carrying the FIP1L1-PDGFRα has been established as effective in multiple studies ([94, 102]). Baccarani et al reported a CHR of 99% in patients carrying FIP1L1-PDGFRα compared with 19% in patients without this mutation ([102]). Imatinib is standard of care for this subset of patients with hypereosinophilia, and therapy with imatinib is recommended even in the absence of symptoms to prevent the risk of end-organ damage.

In the United States, imatinib is approved for the treatment of adults with HES/CEL associated with the

FIP1L1-PDGFRα kinase (starting dose of 100 mg daily with a dose increase to 400 mg daily if suboptimal response and lack of side effects) and for patients with HES/CEL whose FIP1L1-PDGFRα status is negative or unknown (recommended dose is 400 mg daily). As the response to imatinib in FIP1L1-PDGFRα–negative patients is limited, frontline therapy with imatinib for patients with HES should not be indiscriminate and should be reserved for patients who fail conventional therapy. Imatinib is also approved therapy for patients with eosinophilia and PDGFRβ involvement, which is usually discovered on cytogenetic testing, as it involves chromosomal translocations involving 5q31-q33. In some academic centers, a assay based on polymerase chain reaction (PCR) for PDGFRβ gene expression is available and should be used as part of the workup of eosinophilia.

Treatment Conclusions

All patients suspected of having primary eosinophilia should undergo testing for a PDGFRα fusion gene. This is usually done using PCR to test for PDGFRα expression. Alternatively, FISH analysis can be performed to test for the absence of the *CHIC2* gene. Patients with this rearranged gene should be treated with imatinib 100 mg daily. PDGFRβ gene overexpression can be documented by specific PCR or suspected by the presence of chromosome translocation involving 5q31-q33. For PDGFRα/β-negative patients, prednisone is the first line of treatment. For patients refractory to steroids or relapsing on steroids, IFN-α or HU can be used as second-line agents. Mepolizumab or alemtuzumab can be considered for refractory patients. Combination chemotherapy using cladribine and cytarabine has also been used.

CHRONIC NEUTROPHILIC LEUKEMIA

Chronic neutrophilic leukemia is extremely rare and was first included as a distinct entity in the 2001 WHO classification system ([103]). The disease is characterized by the chronic overproduction of mature neutrophils and an increased number of granulocytes in the bone marrow. Diagnostic criteria were not revised in 2008 (Table 6-10). The recent identification of mutations in the colony-stimulating factor 3 receptor (CSF3R) in most patients with WHO-defined CNL is likely to result in a revision in the next edition. Deep sequencing of coding regions of 1,862 genes in patients with CNL (n = 9) and atypical CML (aCML) (n = 20) identified mutations in the CSF3R gene in eight of nine patients with CNL ([104]). Most mutations were found in the membrane proximal region (T618I or T615A). Some cases also had nonsense mutations leading to a truncated cytoplasmic tail. Under normal conditions, CSF3R, which is activated by binding its ligand granulocyte colony-stimulating factor, promotes the differentiation of granulocyte progenitor cells into neutrophils. Mutations in the membrane proximal region lead to constitutive activation of the JAK-STAT pathway, while truncation mutations result in ligand hypersensitivity and activation of the downstream SRC kinase pathway.

Studies in mice support the role of CSF3R mutations in CNL: Deletion of CSFR3 in mice leads to neutropenia, and mice transplanted with CSF3RT618I-positive hematopoietic cells develop a CNL-like phenotype, with mature granulocytosis, marrow hypercellularity, and infiltration of the spleen and liver with mature granulocytes ([105]). In another study, the coding region of CSF3R was sequenced in patients with clinically suspected CNL (n = 35) or aCML (n = 19), as well as 170 cases of CMML and PMF ([106]). The diagnoses were reevaluated using WHO criteria. Twelve cases of CNL were confirmed, 5 were associated with a monoclonal gammopathy-associated CNL, and 9 were confirmed as aCML. Of the 13 patients found to have the CSF3R mutation, 12 had WHO-defined CNL, and 1 had unconfirmed CNL. All mutations were found in the membrane proximal region, with CSF3RT618I being the most common (10 patients). None of the cases of monoclonal gammopathy-associated CNL had CSF3R mutations, suggesting that patients with evidence of a plasma cell dyscrasia should not be classified as having CNL.

Clinical Features

As with other MPNs, the clinical presentation of CNL is heterogeneous. In a long-term study of 12 cases of WHO-defined CNL and 28 cases from a critical

Table 6-10 World Health Organization Diagnostic Criteria for Chronic Neutrophilic Leukemia

1. Peripheral blood leukocytosis ≥25 × 10^9/L, with >80% neutrophils, <10% immature granulocytes, and <1% myeloblasts
2. Hypercellular bone marrow with granulocytic hyperplasia, without dysplasia and <5% myeloblasts
3. Hepatosplenomegaly
4. No identifiable cause of physiologic neutrophilia or demonstration of clonality of myeloid cells
5. Negative for the BCR-ABL1 fusion gene and rearrangements of PDGFRA, PDGFRB, or FGFR1
6. No evidence of PV, ET, or PMF
7. No evidence of MDS or MDS/MPN; no granulocytic dysplasia or myelodysplastic changes in other myeloid lineages; monocytes <1 × 10^9/L

literature review, the median age at diagnosis was 66 years (range, 15-86). Clinical manifestations included fatigue, palpable splenomegaly, weight loss, easy bruising, bone pain, and night sweats. Most patients have mild anemia, and platelet counts are usually normal or slightly low. The median survival in CNL is less than 2 years [106, 107]. Intracranial hemorrhage is the most common cause of death, followed by leukemic transformation [107]. Transformation was seen in 20% of patients after a median of 21 months from diagnosis. Genome sequencing studies suggested that SET binding protein 1 (SETBP1) may be associated with accelerated or blast phase disease [106].

Diagnosis

Most patients are asymptomatic at presentation and are diagnosed after a finding of leukocytosis on routine blood testing. The diagnosis is generally one of exclusion. The absence of Bcr-Abl1 and rearrangement of PDGFRα, PDGFRβ, and FGFR1 are key diagnostic criteria.

Other diagnostic criteria include sustained peripheral blood leukocytosis with more than 80% neutrophils, less than 10% mature granulocytes, and less than 1% myeloblasts and a hypercellular bone marrow (>90% cellularity) due to granulocytic hyperplasia, with no dysplastic features (see Table 6-10). Unlike other MPNs, megakaryocytic hyperplasia or clusters of large atypical megakaryocytes is not seen. Most patients have normal cytogenetics.

Treatment

There is no standard treatment for CNL. Hydroxyurea is commonly used to control leukocytosis and splenomegaly. Interferon alfa has also been used. These agents can reduce leukocytosis but do not modify the natural disease course. Splenic radiation and splenectomy have been used, but splenectomy has been associated with further increases in neutrophil counts [107]. Induction chemotherapy has been used to treat patients in the blastic phase; however, outcomes are poor. Stem cell transplantation was used with some success in selected cases [107, 108]. Ruxolitinib has been reported as a therapy in two cases [104, 109].

MAST CELL DISEASE

Mast cell disease is a heterogeneous group of disorders characterized by clonal expansion of mast cells (MCs) and their excessive accumulation in various organs such as skin, bone marrow, gastrointestinal tract, lymph nodes, liver, and spleen. Its clinical course can vary from no/minimal symptoms to diffuse systemic involvement. Mastocytosis has been classified into seven subtypes by the 2001 WHO guidelines: cutaneous mastocytosis, indolent systemic mastocytosis (ISM), systemic mastocytosis (SM) with an associated clonal hematological non-MC-lineage disease (SM-AHNMD), aggressive SM (ASM), MC leukemia, MC sarcoma, and extracutaneous mastocytoma [110]. Systemic mastocytosis is defined by the presence of one major and one minor or three minor diagnostic criteria (Table 6-11). Patients with SM are further characterized with regard to the presence of so-called B and C findings (assessing disease burden and disease aggressiveness, respectively) (Table 6-12). Patients with SM with no findings are identified as having ISM, those with B findings as smoldering SM (SSM, a subtype of ISM with possibly more aggressive clinical course), and those with C findings as ASM. The 2008 WHO guidelines redefined mastocytosis as "mast cell disease," reclassifying it as an MPN, with SM a subtype with bone marrow involvement.

Clinical Features

Symptoms of mastocytosis can be divided into those caused by the release of MC mediators or those caused by MC organ infiltration. Vasoactive mediators (histamine, leukotrienes, prostaglandins) released from MCs can lead to itching, flushing, light-headedness, syncope, palpitations, diarrhea, heartburn, fatigue, and headache and can be exacerbated by infections, alcohol, exercise, and medications. Common sites of organ infiltration include skin and gastrointestinal tract.

Table 6-11 World Health Organization Diagnostic Criteria for Systemic Mastocytosis

Major Criteria
1. Multifocal, dense infiltrates of mast cells (≥15 mast cells in aggregates) in bone marrow biopsy sections and/or in other extracutaneous organ(s)
Minor Criteria
1. Greater than 25% mast cells in bone marrow or other extracutaneous organ(s) show an atypical morphology (typically spindle shaped)
2. *c-kit* mutation at codon 816 is present in extracutaneous tissues
3. Mast cells in bone marrow coexpress CD117 and either CD2, CD25, or both (by flow cytometry)
4. Serum tryptase persistently is ≥20 ng/mL (not accounted for in patients with an associated, clonal, hematologic, nonmast cell disorder)
Diagnosis requires meeting either one major criteria and one minor criteria or three minor criteria

Data from Valent P, Horny HP, Escribano L, et al. Diagnostic criteria and classification of mastocytosis: a consensus proposal, *Leukemia Res* 2001 Jul;25(7):603-625.

CHAPTER 6

Table 6-12 B and C Findings in Systemic Mastocytosis

B Findings: Indication of High MC Burden and Expansion of the Genetic Defect Into Various Myeloid Lineages
1. Infiltration grade of mast cells in bone marrow >30% on histology and serum total tryptase levels >200 ng/mL
2. Hypercellular bone marrow with loss of fat cells, discrete signs of dysmyelopoiesis without substantial cytopenias, or World Health Organization criteria for myelodysplastic syndrome or myeloproliferative disorder
3. Organomegaly: Palpable hepatomegaly, splenomegaly, or lymphadenopathy (>2 cm on computed tomography or ultrasound) without impaired organ function
C Findings: Indication of Impaired Organ Function Because of MC Infiltration (Confirmed by Biopsy in Most Patients)
1. Cytopenia(s): Absolute neutrophil count <1,000/μL, or hemoglobin <10 g/dL, or platelets <100,000/μL
2. Hepatomegaly with ascites and impaired liver function
3. Palpable splenomegaly with hypersplenism
4. Malabsorption with hypoalbuminemia and weight loss
5. Skeletal lesions: Large osteolyses and/or severe osteoporosis causing pathologic fractures
6. Life-threatening organomegaly in other organ systems that definitively is caused by an infiltration of the tissue by neoplastic mast cells

Urticaria pigmentosa is the most common skin manifestation, characterized by reddish-brown macules and papules. Scratching of affected skin characteristically leads to development of urticaria and erythema (Darier sign). Gastrointestinal involvement can present as chronic diarrhea, steatorrhea, malabsorption, and ascites. Anemia is the most common hematological abnormality due to bone marrow infiltration, and peripheral eosinophilia is seen in around 20% of patients. Bone pain and fractures can also occur.

Diagnosis

Diagnosis relies primarily on the identification of neoplastic MCs in various organs (see Table 6-11). Bone marrow examination is imperative for diagnosis of SM, as most adults with mastocytosis have underlying bone marrow involvement. Figures 6-17 and 6-18 illustrate a case of SM detected in the bone marrow. Neoplastic MCs are characteristically spindle shaped and present in multifocal aggregates, and unlike normal MCs, neoplastic MCs express surface markers CD2 or CD25. Serum tryptase and urinary histamine levels are generally increased. Screening for the KIT D816V mutation should be considered for all patients. KIT is a TK receptor encoded by the *c-kit* gene located on chromosome 4q12 in humans. Binding of stem cell factor (SCF) to KIT leads to receptor dimerization and phosphorylation of the downstream signaling molecules ([111]). KIT plays an important role in normal hematopoiesis, and its expression declines in hematopoietic cell lines with maturation, except in MCs. Furitsu et al first showed that KIT was constitutively activated and expressed in the absence of SCF in a MC line derived from a patient with MC leukemia ([112]). Using a sensitive PCR-based assay, a point mutation, resulting in the substitution of valine for aspartate at codon 816 (D816V) in the TK

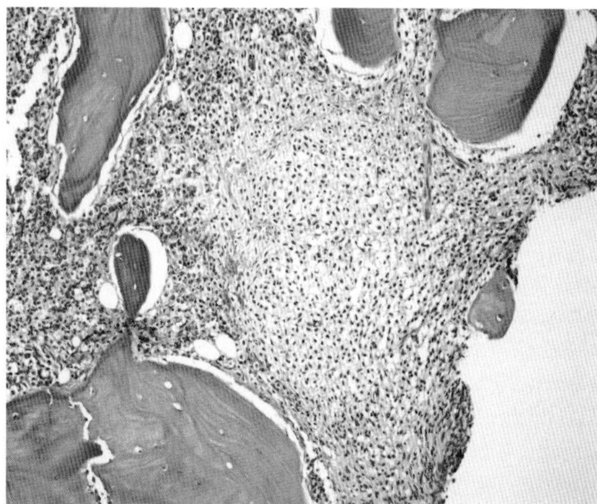

FIGURE 6-17 Bone marrow biopsy from a patient with SM demonstrates total focal replacement of the normal cellular elements by mast cells (×100). Immunohistochemical staining performed on this specimen demonstrated that the neoplastic mast cells aberrantly expressed CD2 and CD25.

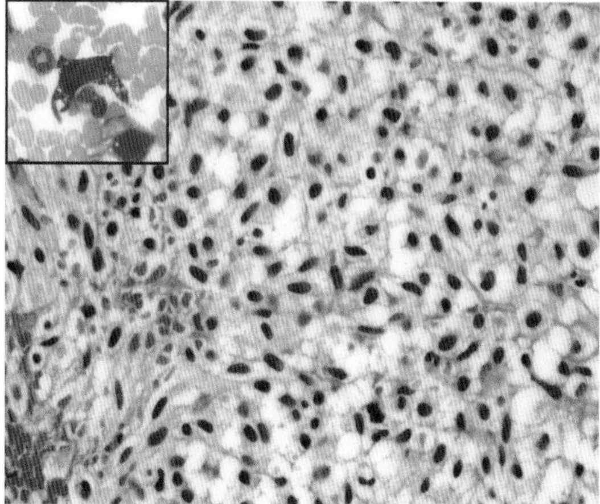

FIGURE 6-18 In SM, mast cells tend to have abundant, colorless cytoplasm and contain elongated-to-oval nuclei (×400). In the bone marrow aspirate smears, the mast cells are increased in number and size and attain a spindle shape (inset; ×400).

domain of the KIT receptor, is noted in more than 90% of patients with SM ([113]). Recently, TET2 mutation (a candidate tumor suppressor gene on chromosome 4q24) was reported in 29% of patients with SM and correlated with the presence of the KITD816V mutation, monocytosis, and female gender ([114]).

Treatment

There is a lack of effective treatment for SM. Symptomatic treatments include the use of oral antihistamines and MC stabilizers such as cromolyn sodium ([115]). Patients should avoid factors that can trigger MC degranulation, such as emotional stress, cold exposure, alcohol use, strenuous exercise, and the use of nonsteroidal anti-inflammatory drugs. Both sedating and nonsedating H1 antihistamines can be used to alleviate pruritus and itching. Randomized controlled trials evaluating the efficacy of antihistamines in SM are lacking. Cetirizine has been shown to be equivalent to hydroxyzine in relieving pruritus in patients with chronic urticaria, with the advantage that it does not cause sedation ([116]). Therefore, most patients initially are treated with nonsedating H1 antihistamines. Higher doses of sedating antihistamines could be used for those with severe symptoms.

As both H1 and H2 receptors are present in skin (85% cutaneous histamine receptors are H1 and 15% are H2), the addition of an H2 blocker should be considered for those not responding to H1 antihistamines alone ([116]). Cromolyn sodium is beneficial in patients with gastrointestinal symptoms (diarrhea, vomiting, abdominal pain). Short courses of prednisone can be considered for patients with severe symptoms, especially malabsorption and ascites. Aspirin can cause MC degranulation but may help with flushing. Therefore, patients should be on H1 and H2 antihistamine therapy before starting ASA therapy ([115]). Patients with a history of anaphylaxis or cardiovascular collapse should carry an epinephrine pen. Omalizumab (a humanized murine monoclonal antibody that inhibits immunoglobulin E binding to MCs and basophils) is effective in patients with SM and syncopal episodes and skin manifestations. For patients with osteoporosis, bisphosphonate therapy may help. Cytoreductive therapies (IFN-α and cladribine) are used for severe disease symptoms. In a multicenter trial in 20 patients with SM, IFN-α-2b led to a partial or minor response in 13 ([117]). The combination of IFN-α-2b plus prednisone has also been studied. The use of cladribine in 33 patients with mastocytosis produced major response in 24 ([118]). Cladribine may be the best therapy for patients with ASM.

Various TKIs targeting KIT are now being studied in clinical trials. Imatinib is a potent inhibitor of various TKs, including wild-type KIT, but is not effective against the most common KIT mutation in SM, D816V. Imatinib binds KIT only in its inactive configuration, and the D816V mutation leads to stabilization of the active open configuration. Clinical experience with imatinib corresponded to the in vitro data, with no significant responses in patients with the KITD816V mutation ([119]). An important subgroup of patients with SM and imatinib responsiveness is the subset with the FIP1L1-PDGFRα mutation. Peripheral blood eosinophilia is seen in approximately 20% of patients (SM-eos) and bone marrow eosinophilia in 25%. In a study by Pardanani et al, 56% of patients with SM and eosinophilia had the FIP1L1-PDGFRα fusion oncogene ([120]). In that study, all treated SM-eos patients with the FIP1L1-PDGFRα mutation responded to imatinib 100 mg daily, while those without the FIP1L1-PDGFRα mutation did not respond (irrespective of the KITD816V mutation status). All patients with SM and eosinophilia should undergo testing for the FIP1L1-PDGFRα mutation. Imatinib is approved by the FDA for patients with ASM without the KITD816V mutation or unknown KIT mutation status (at 400 mg daily) and for ASM associated with eosinophilia (starting dose 100 mg daily with dose escalation to 400 mg daily if insufficient response and absence of side effects). Other TKIs under investigation in patients with the KITD816V mutation are dasatinib, nilotinib, and midostaurin. The clinical results have been modest.

REFERENCES

1. Dameshek W. Some speculations on the myeloproliferative syndromes. *Blood.* 1951;6(4):372-375.
2. Baxter EJ, Scott LM, Campbell PJ, et al. Acquired mutation of the tyrosine kinase JAK2 in human myeloproliferative disorders. *Lancet.* 2005;365(9464):1054-1061.
3. James C, Ugo V, Le Couedic JP, et al. A unique clonal JAK2 mutation leading to constitutive signalling causes polycythaemia vera. *Nature.* 2005;434(7037):1144-1148.
4. Kralovics R, Passamonti F, Buser AS, et al. A gain-of-function mutation of JAK2 in myeloproliferative disorders. *N Engl J Med.* 2005;352(17):1779-1790.
5. Levine RL, Wadleigh M, Cools J, et al. Activating mutation in the tyrosine kinase JAK2 in polycythemia vera, essential thrombocythemia, and myeloid metaplasia with myelofibrosis. *Cancer Cell.* 2005;7(4):387-397.
6. Tefferi A, Vardiman JW. Classification and diagnosis of myeloproliferative neoplasms: the 2008 World Health Organization criteria and point-of-care diagnostic algorithms. *Leukemia.* 2007;22(1):14-22.
7. Finazzi G, Caruso V, Marchioli R, et al. Acute leukemia in polycythemia vera: an analysis of 1,638 patients enrolled in a prospective observational study. *Blood.* 2005;105(7):2664-2670.
8. Scott LM, Tong W, Levine RL, et al. JAK2 exon 12 mutations in polycythemia vera and idiopathic erythrocytosis. *N Engl J Med.* 2007;356(5):459-468.
9. Wasserman LR. The treatment of polycythemia vera. *Semin Hematol.* 1976;13(1):57-78.
10. Gangat N, Strand J, Lasho TL, et al. Cytogenetic studies at diagnosis in polycythemia vera: clinical and JAK2V617F allele burden correlates. *Eur J Haematol.* 2008;80(3):197-200.

11. Sever M, Quintas-Cardama A, Pierce S, Zhou L, Kantarjian H, Verstovsek S. Significance of cytogenetic abnormalities in patients with polycythemia vera. *Leuk Lymphoma*. 2013:1-4.
12. Polycythemia vera: the natural history of 1,213 patients followed for 20 years. Gruppo Italiano Studio Policitemia. *Ann Intern Med*. 1995;123(9):656-664.
13. Barbui T, Carobbio A, Rumi E, et al. In contemporary patients with polycythemia vera, rates of thrombosis and risk factors delineate a new clinical epidemiology. *Blood*. 2014;124(19):3021-3023.
14. Tefferi A, Rumi E, Finazzi G, et al. Survival and prognosis among 1,545 patients with contemporary polycythemia vera: an international study. *Leukemia*. 2013;27(9):1874-1881.
15. Marchioli R, Finazzi G, Landolfi R, et al. Vascular and neoplastic risk in a large cohort of patients with polycythemia vera. *J Clin Oncol*. 2005;23(10):2224-2232.
16. Berk PD, Goldberg JD, Donovan PB, Fruchtman SM, Berlin NI, Wasserman LR. Therapeutic recommendations in polycythemia vera based on Polycythemia Vera Study Group protocols. *Semin Hematol*. 1986;23(2):132-143.
17. De Stefano V, Teofili L, Leone G, Michiels JJ. Spontaneous erythroid colony formation as the clue to an underlying myeloproliferative disorder in patients with Budd-Chiari syndrome or portal vein thrombosis. *Semin Thromb Hemost*. 1997;23(5):411-418.
18. Kiladjian JJ, Cervantes F, Leebeek FW, et al. The impact of JAK2 and MPL mutations on diagnosis and prognosis of splanchnic vein thrombosis: a report on 241 cases. *Blood*. 2008;111(10):4922-4929.
19. Passamonti F, Rumi E, Caramella M, et al. A dynamic prognostic model to predict survival in post-polycythemia vera myelofibrosis. *Blood*. 2008;111(7):3383-3387.
20. Passamonti F, Rumi E, Pietra D, et al. A prospective study of 338 patients with polycythemia vera: the impact of JAK2 (V617F) allele burden and leukocytosis on fibrotic or leukemic disease transformation and vascular complications. *Leukemia*. 2010;24(9):1574-1579.
21. Landolfi R, Di Gennaro L, Barbui T, et al. Leukocytosis as a major thrombotic risk factor in patients with polycythemia vera. *Blood*. 2007;109(6):2446-2452.
22. Gangat N, Strand J, Li CY, Wu W, Pardanani A, Tefferi A. Leucocytosis in polycythaemia vera predicts both inferior survival and leukaemic transformation. *Br J Haematol*. 2007;138(3):354-358.
23. Spivak JL, Silver RT. The revised World Health Organization diagnostic criteria for polycythemia vera, essential thrombocytosis, and primary myelofibrosis: an alternative proposal. *Blood*. 2008;112(2):231-239.
24. Tartaglia AP, Goldberg JD, Berk PD, Wasserman LR. Adverse effects of antiaggregating platelet therapy in the treatment of polycythemia vera. *Semin Hematol*. 1986;23(3):172-176.
25. Landolfi R, Ciabattoni G, Patrignani P, et al. Increased thromboxane biosynthesis in patients with polycythemia vera: evidence for aspirin-suppressible platelet activation in vivo. *Blood*. 1992;80(8):1965-1971.
26. Landolfi R, Marchioli R, Kutti J, et al. Efficacy and safety of low-dose aspirin in polycythemia vera. *N Engl J Med*. 2004; 350(2):114-124.
27. Squizzato A, Romualdi E, Passamonti F, Middeldorp S. Antiplatelet drugs for polycythaemia vera and essential thrombocythaemia. *Cochrane Database Syst Rev*. 2013;4:CD006503.
28. Pearson TC, Wetherley-Mein G. Vascular occlusive episodes and venous haematocrit in primary proliferative polycythaemia. *Lancet*. 1978;2(8102):1219-1222.
29. Marchioli R, Finazzi G, Specchia G, et al. Cardiovascular events and intensity of treatment in polycythemia vera. *N Engl J Med*. 2013;368(1):22-33.
30. Alvarez-Larrán A, Pereira A, Cervantes F, et al. Assessment and prognostic value of the European LeukemiaNet criteria for clinicohematologic response, resistance, and intolerance to hydroxyurea in polycythemia vera. *Blood*. 2012;119(6):1363-1369.
31. Bjorkholm M, Derolf AR, Hultcrantz M, et al. Treatment-related risk factors for transformation to acute myeloid leukemia and myelodysplastic syndromes in myeloproliferative neoplasms. *J Clin Oncol*. 2011;29(17):2410-2415.
32. Silver RT. Recombinant interferon-alpha for treatment of polycythaemia vera. *Lancet*. 1988;2(8607):403.
33. Kiladjian JJ, Cassinat B, Chevret S, et al. Pegylated interferon-alfa-2a induces complete hematologic and molecular responses with low toxicity in polycythemia vera. *Blood*. 2008;112(8):3065-3072.
34. Quintas-Cardama A, Kantarjian H, Manshouri T, et al. Pegylated interferon alfa-2a yields high rates of hematologic and molecular response in patients with advanced essential thrombocythemia and polycythemia vera. *J Clin Oncol*. 2009;27(32):5418-5424.
35. Quintás-Cardama A, Abdel-Wahab O, Manshouri T, et al. Molecular analysis of patients with polycythemia vera or essential thrombocythemia receiving pegylated interferon alpha-2a. *Blood*. 2013;122(6):893-901.
36. Verstovsek S, Passamonti F, Rambaldi A, et al. A phase 2 study of ruxolitinib, an oral JAK1 and JAK2 inhibitor, in patients with advanced polycythemia vera who are refractory or intolerant to hydroxyurea. *Cancer*. 2014;120(4):513-520.
37. Vannucchi AM, Kiladjian JJ, Griesshammer M et al. Ruxolitinib versus standard therapy for the treatment of polycythemia vera. *N Engl J Med*. 2015;372(5):426-435.
38. Scherber R, Dueck AC, Johansson P, et al. The Myeloproliferative Neoplasm Symptom Assessment Form (MPN-SAF): international prospective validation and reliability trial in 402 patients. *Blood*. 2011;118(2):401-408.
39. Ruggeri M, Tosetto A, Frezzato M, Rodeghiero F. The rate of progression to polycythemia vera or essential thrombocythemia in patients with erythrocytosis or thrombocytosis. *Ann Intern Med*. 2003;139(6):470-475.
40. Griesshammer M, Bangerter M, Sauer T, Wennauer R, Bergmann L, Heimpel H. Aetiology and clinical significance of thrombocytosis: analysis of 732 patients with an elevated platelet count. *J Intern Med*. 1999;245(3):295-300.
41. Buss DH, Cashell AW, O'Connor ML, Richards F, 2nd, Case LD. Occurrence, etiology, and clinical significance of extreme thrombocytosis: a study of 280 cases. *Am J Med*. 1994;96(3):247-253.
42. Horikawa Y, Matsumura I, Hashimoto K, et al. Markedly reduced expression of platelet c-mpl receptor in essential thrombocythemia. *Blood*. 1997;90(10):4031-4038.
43. Beer PA, Campbell PJ, Scott LM, et al. MPL mutations in myeloproliferative disorders: analysis of the PT-1 cohort. *Blood*. 2008;112(1):141-149.
44. Kittur J, Knudson RA, Lasho TL, et al. Clinical correlates of JAK2V617F allele burden in essential thrombocythemia. *Cancer*. 2007;109(11):2279-2284.
45. Klampfl T, Gisslinger H, Harutyunyan AS, et al. Somatic mutations of calreticulin in myeloproliferative neoplasms. *N Engl J Med*. 2013;369(25):2379-2390.
46. Nangalia J, Massie CE, Baxter EJ, et al. Somatic CALR mutations in myeloproliferative neoplasms with nonmutated JAK2. *N Engl J Med*. 2013;369(25):2391-2405.
47. Rumi E, Pietra D, Ferretti V, et al. JAK2 or CALR mutation status defines subtypes of essential thrombocythemia with substantially different clinical course and outcomes. *Blood*. 2014;123(10):1544-1551.
48. Fenaux P, Simon M, Caulier MT, Lai JL, Goudemand J, Bauters F. Clinical course of essential thrombocythemia in 147 cases. *Cancer*. 1990;66(3):549-556.

49. Wolanskyj AP, Schwager SM, McClure RF, Larson DR, Tefferi A. Essential thrombocythemia beyond the first decade: life expectancy, long-term complication rates, and prognostic factors. *Mayo Clin Proc.* 2006;81(2):159-166.
50. Gangat N, Wolanskyj AP, McClure RF, et al. Risk stratification for survival and leukemic transformation in essential thrombocythemia: a single institutional study of 605 patients. *Leukemia.* 2007;21(2):270-276.
51. Cervantes F, Alvarez-Larran A, Talarn C, Gomez M, Montserrat E. Myelofibrosis with myeloid metaplasia following essential thrombocythaemia: actuarial probability, presenting characteristics and evolution in a series of 195 patients. *Br J Haematol.* 2002;118(3):786-790.
52. Barbui T, Thiele J, Passamonti F, et al. Survival and disease progression in essential thrombocythemia are significantly influenced by accurate morphologic diagnosis: an international study. *J Clin Oncol.* 2011;29(23):3179-3184.
53. Tefferi A, Guglielmelli P, Larson DR, et al. Long-term survival and blast transformation in molecularly-annotated essential thrombocythemia, polycythemia vera and myelofibrosis. *Blood.* 2014.
54. Finazzi G, Carobbio A, Thiele J, et al. Incidence and risk factors for bleeding in 1104 patients with essential thrombocythemia or prefibrotic myelofibrosis diagnosed according to the 2008 WHO criteria. *Leukemia.* 2012;26(4):716-719.
55. Carobbio A, Thiele J, Passamonti F, et al. Risk factors for arterial and venous thrombosis in WHO-defined essential thrombocythemia: an international study of 891 patients. *Blood.* 2011;117(22):5857-5859.
56. Carobbio A, Finazzi G, Antonioli E, et al. Thrombocytosis and leukocytosis interaction in vascular complications of essential thrombocythemia. *Blood.* 2008;112(8):3135-3137.
57. Barbui T, Finazzi G, Carobbio A, et al. Development and validation of an International Prognostic Score of thrombosis in World Health Organization-essential thrombocythemia (IPSET-thrombosis). *Blood.* 2012;120(26):5128-5133; quiz 5252.
58. Passamonti F, Thiele J, Girodon F, et al. A prognostic model to predict survival in 867 World Health Organization-defined essential thrombocythemia at diagnosis: a study by the International Working Group on Myelofibrosis Research and Treatment. *Blood.* 2012;120(6):1197-1201.
59. Passamonti F, Randi ML, Rumi E, et al. Increased risk of pregnancy complications in patients with essential thrombocythemia carrying the JAK2 (617V>F) mutation. *Blood.* 2007;110(2):485-489.
60. Gangat N, Tefferi A, Thanarajasingam G, et al. Cytogenetic abnormalities in essential thrombocythemia: prevalence and prognostic significance. *Eur J Haematol.* 2009;83(1):17-21.
    a. Colombi M, Radaelli F, Zocchi L et al. Thrombotic and hemorrhagic complications in essential thrombocythemia. A retrospective study of 103 patients. *Cancer.* 1991;67(11)2926-2930.
    b. Cortelazzo S, Viero P, Finazzi G et al. Incidence and risk factors for thrombotic complications in a historical cohort of 100 patients with essential thrombocythemia. *J Clin Oncol.* 1990;8(3):556-562.
    c. Besses C, Cervantes F, Pereira A et al. Major vascular complications in essential thrombocythemia: a study of the predictive factors in a series of 148 patients. *Leukemia.* 1999;13(2):150-154.
    d. Bazzan M, Tamponi G, Schinco P et al. Thrombosis-free survival and life expectancy in 187 consecutive patients with essential thrombocythemia. *Ann Hematol.* 1999;78(12):539-543.
    e. Jantunen R, Juvonen E, Ikkala E et al. The predictive value of vascular risk factors and gender for the development of thrombotic complications in essential thrombocythemia. *Ann Hematol.* 2001;80(2):74-78.
    f. Chim CS, Kwong YL, Lie AK et al. Long-term outcome of 231 patients with essential thrombocythemia: prognostic factors for thrombosis, bleeding, myelofibrosis, and leukemia. *Arch Intern Med.* 2005;165(22):2651-2658.
    g. Carobbio A, Finazzi G, Guerini V et al. Leukocytosis is a risk factor for thrombosis in essential thrombocythemia: interaction with treatment, standard risk factors, and Jak2 mutation status. *Blood.* 2007;109(6):2310-2313.
    h. Alvarez-Larran A, Cervantes F, Bellosillo B et al. Essential thrombocythemia in young individuals: frequency and risk factors for vascular events and evolution to myelofibrosis in 126 patients. *Leukemia.* 2007;21(6):1218-1223.
    i. Radaelli F, Colombi M, Calori R et al. Analysis of risk factors predicting thrombotic and/or haemorrhagic complications in 306 patients with essential thrombocythemia. *Hematol Oncol.* 2007;25(3):115-120.
    j. Tefferi A, Gangat N, Wolanskyj A. The interaction between leukocytosis and other risk factors for thrombosis in essential thrombocythemia. *Blood.* 2007;109(9):4105.
    k. Passamonti F, Rumi E, Arcaini L et al. Prognostic factors for thrombosis, myelofibrosis, and leukemia in essential thrombocythemia: a study of 605 patients. *Haematologica.* 2008;93(11):1645-1651.
61. van Genderen PJ, Mulder PG, Waleboer M, van de Moesdijk D, Michiels JJ. Prevention and treatment of thrombotic complications in essential thrombocythaemia: efficacy and safety of aspirin. *Br J Haematol.* 1997;97(1):179-184.
62. Budde U, Scharf RE, Franke P, Hartmann-Budde K, Dent J, Ruggeri ZM. Elevated platelet count as a cause of abnormal von Willebrand factor multimer distribution in plasma. *Blood.* 1993;82(6):1749-1757.
63. Harrison CN, Campbell PJ, Buck G, et al. Hydroxyurea compared with anagrelide in high-risk essential thrombocythemia. *N Engl J Med.* 2005;353(1):33-45.
64. Pascale S, Petrucci G, Dragani A, et al. Aspirin-insensitive thromboxane biosynthesis in essential thrombocythemia is explained by accelerated renewal of the drug target. *Blood.* 2012;119(15):3595-3603.
65. Cortelazzo S, Finazzi G, Ruggeri M, et al. Hydroxyurea for patients with essential thrombocythemia and a high risk of thrombosis. *N Engl J Med.* 1995;332(17):1132-1136.
66. Gisslinger H, Gotic M, Holowiecki J, et al. Anagrelide compared with hydroxyurea in WHO-classified essential thrombocythemia: the ANAHYDRET Study, a randomized controlled trial. *Blood.* 2013;121(10):1720-1728.
67. Ruggeri M, Finazzi G, Tosetto A, Riva S, Rodeghiero F, Barbui T. No treatment for low-risk thrombocythaemia: results from a prospective study. *Br J Haematol.* 1998;103(3):772-777.
68. Tefferi A, Fonseca R, Pereira DL, Hoagland HC. A long-term retrospective study of young women with essential thrombocythemia. *Mayo Clin Proc.* 2001;76(1):22-28.
69. Anand S, Stedham F, Gudgin E, et al. Increased basal intracellular signaling patterns do not correlate with JAK2 genotype in human myeloproliferative neoplasms. *Blood.* 2011;118(6):1610-1621.
70. Rampal R, Al-Shahrour F, Abdel-Wahab O, et al. Integrated genomic analysis illustrates the central role of JAK-STAT pathway activation in myeloproliferative neoplasm pathogenesis. *Blood.* 2014;123(22):e123-e133.
71. Tefferi A, Vaidya R, Caramazza D, Finke C, Lasho T, Pardanani A. Circulating interleukin (IL)-8, IL-2R, IL-12, and IL-15 levels are independently prognostic in primary myelofibrosis: a comprehensive cytokine profiling study. *J Clin Oncol.* 2011;29(10):1356-1363.
72. Vannucchi AM, Lasho TL, Guglielmelli P, et al. Mutations and prognosis in primary myelofibrosis. *Leukemia.* 2013; 27(9):1861-1869.
73. Rumi E, Pietra D, Pascutto C, et al. Clinical effect of driver mutations of JAK2, CALR, or MPL in primary myelofibrosis. *Blood.* 2014;124(7):1062-1069.
74. Cervantes F, Dupriez B, Pereira A, et al. New prognostic scoring

CHAPTER 6

system for primary myelofibrosis based on a study of the International Working Group for Myelofibrosis Research and Treatment. *Blood*. 2009;113(13):2895-2901.

75. Passamonti F, Cervantes F, Vannucchi AM, et al. A dynamic prognostic model to predict survival in primary myelofibrosis: a study by the IWG-MRT (International Working Group for Myeloproliferative Neoplasms Research and Treatment). *Blood*. 2010;115(9):1703-1708.
76. Hussein K, Van Dyke DL, Tefferi A. Conventional cytogenetics in myelofibrosis: literature review and discussion. *Eur J Haematol*. 2009;82(5):329-338.
77. Tam CS, Abruzzo LV, Lin KI, et al. The role of cytogenetic abnormalities as a prognostic marker in primary myelofibrosis: applicability at the time of diagnosis and later during disease course. *Blood*. 2009;113(18):4171-4178.
78. Gangat N, Caramazza D, Vaidya R, et al. DIPSS plus: a refined Dynamic International Prognostic Scoring System for primary myelofibrosis that incorporates prognostic information from karyotype, platelet count, and transfusion status. *J Clin Oncol*. 2011;29(4):392-397.
79. Tefferi A, Guglielmelli P, Lasho TL, et al. CALR and ASXL1 mutations-based molecular prognostication in primary myelofibrosis: an international study of 570 patients. *Leukemia*. 2014;28(7):1494-1500.
80. Silver RT, Vandris K, Goldman JJ. Recombinant interferon-alpha may retard progression of early primary myelofibrosis: a preliminary report. *Blood*. 2011;117(24):6669-6672.
81. Ianotto JC, Kiladjian JJ, Demory JL, et al. PEG-IFN-alpha-2a therapy in patients with myelofibrosis: a study of the French Groupe d'Etudes des Myelofibroses (GEM) and France Intergroupe des syndromes Myeloproliferatifs (FIM). *Br J Haematol*. 2009;146(2):223-225.
82. Verstovsek S, Mesa RA, Gotlib J, et al. A double-blind, placebo-controlled trial of ruxolitinib for myelofibrosis. *N Engl J Med*. 2012;366(9):799-807.
83. Harrison C, Kiladjian JJ, Al-Ali HK, et al. JAK inhibition with ruxolitinib versus best available therapy for myelofibrosis. *N Engl J Med*. 2012;366(9):787-798.
84. Verstovsek S, Mesa RA, Gotlib J, et al. Efficacy, safety and survival with ruxolitinib in patients with myelofibrosis: results of a median 2-year follow-up of COMFORT-I. *Haematologica*. 2013;98(12):1865-1871.
85. Cervantes F, Vannucchi AM, Kiladjian JJ, et al. Three-year efficacy, safety, and survival findings from COMFORT-II, a phase 3 study comparing ruxolitinib with best available therapy for myelofibrosis. *Blood*. 2013;122(25):4047-4053.
86. Vannucchi AM, Hagop K, Kiladjian J-J, et al. A pooled overall survival analysis of the COMFORT studies: 2 randomized phase 3 trials of ruxolitinib for the treatment of myelofibrosis. *Blood*. 2013;122(21):2820.
87. Kvasnicka HM, Thiele J, Bueso-Ramos CE, et al. Effects of five-years of ruxolitinib therapy on bone marrow morphology in patients with myelofibrosis and comparison with best available therapy. *Blood*. 2013;122(21):4055-4055.
88. Molica M, Serrao A, Saracino R, et al. Disappearance of fibrosis in secondary myelofibrosis after ruxolitinib treatment: new endpoint to achieve? *Ann Hematol*. 2014;93(11):1951-1952.
89. Wilkins BS, Radia D, Woodley C, Farhi SE, Keohane C, Harrison CN. Resolution of bone marrow fibrosis in a patient receiving JAK1/JAK2 inhibitor treatment with ruxolitinib. *Haematologica*. 2013;98(12):1872-1876.
90. Kroger N, Holler E, Kobbe G, et al. Allogeneic stem cell transplantation after reduced-intensity conditioning in patients with myelofibrosis: a prospective, multicenter study of the Chronic Leukemia Working Party of the European Group for Blood and Marrow Transplantation. *Blood*. 2009;114(26):5264-5270.
91. Jaekel N, Behre G, Behning A, et al. Allogeneic hematopoietic cell transplantation for myelofibrosis in patients pretreated with the JAK1 and JAK2 inhibitor ruxolitinib. *Bone Marrow Transplant*. 2014;49(2):179-184.
92. Stubig T, Alchalby H, Ditschkowski M, et al. JAK inhibition with ruxolitinib as pretreatment for allogeneic stem cell transplantation in primary or post-ET/PV myelofibrosis. *Leukemia*. 2014;28(8):1736-1738.
93. Bain B, Pierre P, Imbert M, Vardiman JW, Brunning RD, Flandrin G. Chronic eosinophillic leukaemia and the hypereosinophillic syndrome. In: Jaffe ES, Harris NL, Stein H, et al., eds., *Pathology and Genetics of Tumours of Haematopoeitic and Lymphoid Tissues*. Lyon, France: IARC Press; 2001:29-31.
94. Cools J, DeAngelo DJ, Gotlib J, et al. A tyrosine kinase created by fusion of the PDGFRA and FIP1L1 genes as a therapeutic target of imatinib in idiopathic hypereosinophilic syndrome. *N Engl J Med*. 2003;348(13):1201-1214.
95. Pardanani A, Verstovsek S. Hypereosinophilic syndrome, chronic eosinophilic leukemia, and mast cell disease. *Cancer J*. 2007;13(6):384-391.
96. Pardanani A, Ketterling RP, Li CY, et al. FIP1L1-PDGFRA in eosinophilic disorders: prevalence in routine clinical practice, long-term experience with imatinib therapy, and a critical review of the literature. *Leuk Res*. 2006;30(8):965-970.
97. Jovanovic JV, Score J, Waghorn K, et al. Low-dose imatinib mesylate leads to rapid induction of major molecular responses and achievement of complete molecular remission in FIP1L1-PDGFRA-positive chronic eosinophilic leukemia. *Blood*. 2007; 109(11):4635-4640.
98. Rothenberg ME, Klion AD, Roufosse FE, et al. Treatment of patients with the hypereosinophilic syndrome with mepolizumab. *N Engl J Med*. 2008;358(12):1215-1228.
99. Roufosse FE, Kahn J-E, Gleich GJ, et al. Long-term safety of mepolizumab for the treatment of hypereosinophilic syndromes. *J Allergy Clin Immunol*. 2013;131(2):461-467.e465.
100. Verstovsek S, Tefferi A, Kantarjian H, et al. Alemtuzumab therapy for hypereosinophilic syndrome and chronic eosinophilic leukemia. *Clin Cancer Res*. 2009;15(1):368-373.
101. Strati P, Cortes J, Faderl S, Kantarjian H, Verstovsek S. Long-term follow-up of patients with hypereosinophilic syndrome treated with Alemtuzumab, an anti-CD52 antibody. *Clin Lymphoma Myeloma Leuk*. 2013;13(3):287-291.
102. Baccarani M, Cilloni D, Rondoni M, et al. The efficacy of imatinib mesylate in patients with FIP1L1-PDGFRalpha-positive hypereosinophilic syndrome. Results of a multicenter prospective study. *Haematologica*. 2007;92(9):1173-1179.
103. Jaffe ES, World Health Organization. *Pathology and Genetics of Tumours of Haematopoietic and Lymphoid Tissues*. Lyon, France, and Oxford, UK: IARC Press; Oxford University Press (distributor); 2001.
104. Maxson JE, Gotlib J, Pollyea DA, et al. Oncogenic CSF3R mutations in chronic neutrophilic leukemia and atypical CML. *N Engl J Med*. 2013;368(19):1781-1790.
105. Fleischman AG, Maxson JE, Luty SB, et al. The CSF3R T618I mutation causes a lethal neutrophilic neoplasia in mice that is responsive to therapeutic JAK inhibition. *Blood*. 2013;122(22):3628-3631.
106. Pardanani A, Lasho TL, Laborde RR, et al. CSF3R T618I is a highly prevalent and specific mutation in chronic neutrophilic leukemia. *Leukemia*. 2013;27(9):1870-1873.
107. Elliott MA, Hanson CA, Dewald GW, Smoley SA, Lasho TL, Tefferi A. WHO-defined chronic neutrophilic leukemia: a long-term analysis of 12 cases and a critical review of the literature. *Leukemia*. 2005;19(2):313-317.
108. Piliotis E, Kutas G, Lipton JH. Allogeneic bone marrow transplantation in the management of chronic neutrophilic leukemia. *Leuk Lymphoma*. 2002;43(10):2051-2054.
109. Lasho TL, Mims A, Elliott MA, Finke C, Pardanani A, Tefferi A. Chronic neutrophilic leukemia with concurrent CSF3R and

SETBP1 mutations: single colony clonality studies, in vitro sensitivity to JAK inhibitors and lack of treatment response to ruxolitinib. *Leukemia*. 2014;28(6):1363-1365.

110. Valent P, Horny HP, Escribano L, et al. Diagnostic criteria and classification of mastocytosis: a consensus proposal. *Leuk Res*. 2001;25(7):603-625.
111. Lemmon MA, Pinchasi D, Zhou M, Lax I, Schlessinger J. Kit receptor dimerization is driven by bivalent binding of stem cell factor. *J Biol Chem*. 1997;272(10):6311-6317.
112. Furitsu T, Tsujimura T, Tono T, et al. Identification of mutations in the coding sequence of the proto-oncogene c-kit in a human mast cell leukemia cell line causing ligand-independent activation of c-kit product. *J Clin Invest*. 1993;92(4):1736-1744.
113. Garcia-Montero AC, Jara-Acevedo M, Teodosio C, et al. KIT mutation in mast cells and other bone marrow hematopoietic cell lineages in systemic mast cell disorders: a prospective study of the Spanish Network on Mastocytosis (REMA) in a series of 113 patients. *Blood*. 2006;108(7):2366-2372.
114. Tefferi A, Levine RL, Lim KH, et al. Frequent TET2 mutations in systemic mastocytosis: clinical, KITD816V and FIP1L1-PDGFRA correlates. *Leukemia*. 2009;23(5):900-904.
115. Worobec AS. Treatment of systemic mast cell disorders. *Hematol Oncol Clin North Am*. 2000;14(3):659-687, vii.
116. Kaplan AP. Clinical practice. Chronic urticaria and angioedema. *N Engl J Med*. 2002;346(3):175-179.
117. Casassus P, Caillat-Vigneron N, Martin A, et al. Treatment of adult systemic mastocytosis with interferon-alpha: results of a multicentre phase II trial on 20 patients. *Br J Haematol*. 2002;119(4):1090-1097.
118. Lortholary O, Vargaftig J, Feger F, et al. Efficacy and safety of cladribine in adult systemic mastocytosis: a French multicenter study of 33 patients. *ASH Annu Meeting Abstr*. 2004;104(11):661.
119. Pardanani A, Elliott M, Reeder T, et al. Imatinib for systemic mast-cell disease. *Lancet*. 2003;362(9383):535-536.
120. Pardanani A, Brockman SR, Paternoster SF, et al. FIP1L1-PDGFRA fusion: prevalence and clinicopathologic correlates in 89 consecutive patients with moderate to severe eosinophilia. *Blood*. 2004;104(10):3038-3045.

Section II

Lymphoma and Myeloma

Section Editor: Nathan H. Fowler

第二篇 淋巴瘤和骨髓瘤

7 Indolent Lymphomas

第七章　惰性淋巴瘤

Loretta J. Nastoupil
Chan Yoon Cheah
L. Jeffrey Medeiros
Nathan H. Fowler

中文导读

本章首先简介了惰性非霍奇金淋巴瘤的分类情况及疾病特点，然后针对滤泡性淋巴瘤、慢性淋巴细胞白血病/小淋巴细胞淋巴瘤、边缘区淋巴瘤、淋巴浆细胞淋巴瘤/巨球蛋白血症4种主要的病理类型逐一进行了介绍。在滤泡性淋巴瘤部分，介绍了其流行病学、临床特点、组织学、免疫表型特征和分子特征，阐明了其诊断和分期策略、预后判断指标、治疗后监测策略，介绍了局限期滤泡性淋巴瘤的治疗策略，并详细阐述了进展期滤泡性淋巴瘤的药物治疗策略及其维持治疗、巩固治疗和解救治疗策略。在慢性淋巴细胞白血病/小淋巴细胞淋巴瘤部分，介绍了其临床特点和治疗策略，阐明了其组织学特征、免疫表型特征和分子特征。在边缘区B细胞淋巴瘤部分，详细介绍了MALT淋巴瘤的临床特点、组织学特点、免疫表型特征、细胞遗传学特征、分子特征以及其诊断和治疗策略，并简要介绍了淋巴结边缘区淋巴瘤和脾边缘区淋巴瘤的临床特点、治疗策略、组织学、免疫表型特征和分子特征。在淋巴浆细胞淋巴瘤/巨球蛋白血症部分，介绍了其临床特点、组织学、免疫表型特征、分子特征和治疗策略。目前大多数进展期惰性淋巴瘤仍不可治愈，本章最后对惰性淋巴瘤的新型治疗策略进行了展望。

The indolent non-Hodgkin lymphomas (NHLs) represent approximately one-third of all malignant lymphomas [1, 2]; most are of B-cell lineage. Follicular lymphoma (FL) is the most common indolent lymphoma. Other indolent B-cell lymphomas include small lymphocytic lymphoma/chronic lymphocytic leukemia (SLL/CLL), the marginal zone B-cell lymphomas (MZLs; extranodal, nodal, and splenic), and lymphoplasmacytic lymphoma (LPL), most cases of which are more specifically classified as Waldenström macroglobulinemia (WM) (Table 7-1) [2]. Mantle cell lymphoma can morphologically resemble indolent B-cell lymphomas, but it is often clinically more aggressive and therefore is not covered in this chapter. Indolent T-cell NHLs, such as mycosis fungoides, are also not covered in this chapter.

FOLLICULAR LYMPHOMAS

Epidemiology

Follicular lymphomas, the second most commonly occurring lymphoma in the United States, represents 22% of all NHLs [1] and 80% of indolent B-cell lymphomas. Follicular lymphoma occurs almost exclusively in adults, with an equal frequency in men and women. The incidence rates are highest among Caucasians, and median age at diagnosis is approximately 58 years [3]. Risk of FL has been shown to be increased in persons with a first-degree relative with NHL or who worked as spray painters and among women with Sjögren syndrome [3]. Of FL cases, 2% to 3% transform annually to diffuse large B-cell lymphoma (DLBCL) [4]. Survival for patients with FL is improving, with a median survival of 8 to 10 years in the prerituximab era [2, 5, 6]; in more modern eras, median survival has been reported to be greater than 18 years [7].

Clinical Features

Patients with FL most often present with asymptomatic lymphadenopathy. Constitutional symptoms such as fever, drenching night sweats, and significant weight loss occur in approximately 15% of patients. Patients may have symptoms related to lymph node enlargement, especially when there are bulky masses in the retroperitoneum. Other symptoms can include fatigue and, occasionally, end-organ consequences such as obstructive uropathy or bone marrow compromise. Central nervous system (CNS) disease is rare. Urgent situations, such as superior vena cava syndrome or spinal cord compression, are rare, in part related to the usual slow pace of growth of lymphadenopathy in FL. Spontaneous regression of lymphadenopathy can occur in FL. Such regressions, however, are usually partial and are typically short-lived. The potential of FL to wax and wane provides one of several clues that suggest that the host immune system can play an important role in the disease course in FL. Consequently, FL has been a prime focus for immunotherapy approaches.

Approximately 80% to 90% of patients with FL present with advanced-stage disease (stage III or IV) with generalized lymphadenopathy. The bone marrow is involved in approximately 50% of patients. Clinical features suspicious for transformation to DLBCL include rapidly progressive lymphadenopathy, systemic (B) symptoms, localized pain, and a rise in serum lactate dehydrogenase (LDH) level.

Histologic, Immunophenotypic, and Molecular Features

In FL, the normal lymph node architecture is partially or completely replaced by lymphoma, which typically forms follicles but rarely can be diffuse, composed of centrocytes (small, cleaved cells) and centroblasts (large, noncleaved cells). The method currently recommended in the World Health Organization (WHO)

Table 7-1 Indolent Lymphomas

Entities included	Follicular lymphoma Small lymphocytic lymphoma/chronic lymphocytic leukemia Extranodal marginal zone B-cell lymphoma (MALT lymphoma) Splenic B-cell marginal zone lymphoma Nodal marginal zone lymphoma Lymphoplasmacytic lymphoma (including Waldenström macroglobulinemia)
Age	Mostly a disease of older adults (usually over the age of 40 years)
Extent of disease	Often disseminated (except MALT lymphoma), with >80% having stage III-IV disease. Bone marrow involvement common
Natural history	Low proliferation fraction. Slow-growing; may have a waxing and waning course. Patients typically survive for many years. Transformation to large cell lymphoma can occur.
Curability	Although current therapy such as radiotherapy or chemotherapy can often control the disease, it usually fails to eradicate the tumor except for early-stage disease (including MALT lymphoma). This is reflected in a continuous downward slope of relapse-free survival curves for patients with these lymphomas.

classification to grade FL is based on a count of the centroblasts ([2, 8]). In grade 1 FL, centroblasts are rare, less than 5 per ×400 microscopic field. Grade 2 FL contains 5 or more but less than 15 centroblasts per ×400 microscopic field. The current WHO classification states that there is no prognostic benefit derived from distinguishing grade 1 from grade 2 cases and designates these tumors as FL grade 1 or 2. At least two types of grade 3 FL are described. In grade 3a, more than 15 centroblasts per ×400 microscopic field are present. In grade 3b, sheets of centroblasts are present with rare or absent centrocytes ([2]). Recent data suggested that FL grade 3b has more features in common with DLBCL than with the indolent FL ([9]).

Some patients with B-cell lymphoma of germinal center cell origin may have histologic discordance (ie, low-grade FL in the bone marrow and DLBCL in a lymph node) ([10]). In addition, different lymph nodes biopsied in a given patient or a single lymph node can comprise different grades of FL.

Follicular lymphoma is a neoplasm of mature B-cell lineage. Most grade 1 and 2 tumors express immunoglobulin (Ig), but a subset of FLs, mostly grade 3, may be Ig negative. All FLs express pan B-cell markers and typically express Ig and B-cell antigens at high density ("bright" immunofluorescence by flow cytometry). These neoplasms also express the germinal center-associated markers CD10, Bcl-6, and LMO2 and are negative for T-cell antigens. *Bcl-2* is expressed in 80% to 90% of FLs but can be negative, most often in grade 3 neoplasms ([2]). Because *Bcl-2* is negative in reactive germinal centers, this marker is helpful in differential diagnosis (Fig. 7-1).

Using conventional cytogenetic analysis, approximately 75% of FL cases grow in culture and can be successfully karyotyped. The cytogenetic hallmark of FL is t(14;18)(q32;q21), which is identified in 80% to 90% of cases. A small subset of FLs lack the t(14;18), suggesting that a minor pathway of follicular lymphomagenesis may exist that is independent of t(14;18). This appears to apply particularly to grade 3b nodal FL, FLs arising in extranodal sites such as skin, and rare FLs that occur in children, which commonly lack the t(14;18).

As a result of the t(14;18), the Bcl-2 oncogene on chromosome 18q21 is translocated adjacent to the joining region of the immunoglobulin heavy chain (IgH) gene on chromosome 14q32. The *Bcl-2* gene is deregulated by being placed under the influence of IgH gene regulatory elements (enhancer region). Insights about the role of the *Bcl-2* gene in FL were a gateway to the identification of a large family of proapoptotic and antiapoptotic genes, which play a role in a wide variety of hematopoietic and solid neoplasms ([11-13]).

The breakpoints on chromosome 18 are primarily clustered at two sites, the major (MBR) and minor (mcr) breakpoint cluster regions, involved in 50% to 60% and 10% to 20% of cases, respectively ([14]). Other breakpoint clusters have also been described, for example, the intermediate cluster region (ICR). The ICR is involved in approximately 5% of cases; there may be geographic variations in the frequencies of t(14;18) breakpoints ([15]).

The Bcl-2 protein is a 25-kDa molecule that is overexpressed in FL and protects cells from programmed cell death (apoptosis) ([11, 12, 16]). Inhibition of apoptosis prolongs cell life, resulting in an expanded compartment of B cells, thereby providing more opportunity for additional molecular defects, which presumably are involved in histologic transformation. The presence of the t(14;18) alone appears not to be sufficient for neoplastic transformation. The t(14;18) has been identified in rare cells in the tonsils and lymph nodes of normal individuals without clinical evidence of lymphoma ([17]).

Other cytogenetic abnormalities have been reported in FL. Of these, trisomy 7 and 18, abnormalities of 3q27-28 and 6q23-26, and 17p deletions are most frequent. Abnormalities of 3q27-28 involve the *Bcl-6* gene

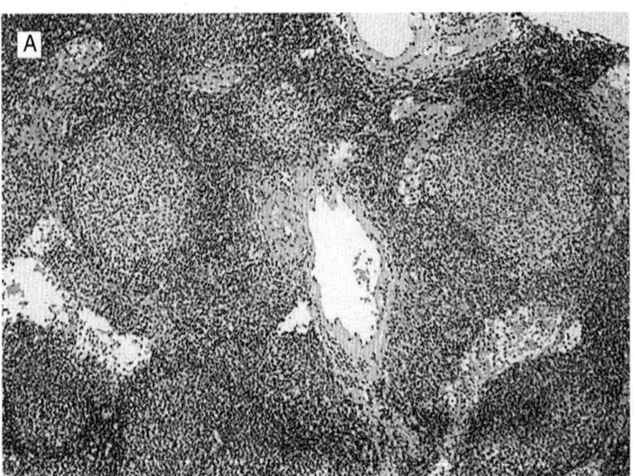

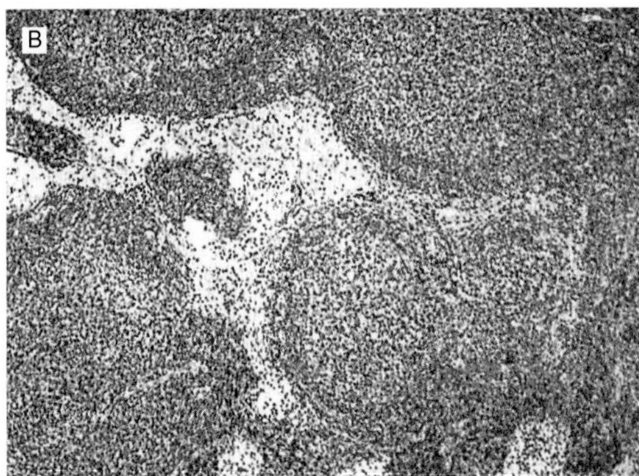

FIGURE 7-1 Follicular lymphoma, grade 1. A. In this needle biopsy specimen, neoplastic follicles partially replace architecture. B. The neoplastic cells are Bcl-2 positive, supporting lymphoma (A, hematoxylin and eosin, ×100; B, Bcl-2 immunostain ×100).

and most often occur in the form of translocations. Secondary cytogenetic and molecular genetic abnormalities have also been extensively studied, including in the context of transformation of FL to DLBCL ([18-20]).

The importance of the immunologic microenvironment in the clinical behavior of FL has been an area of intensive study. Gene expression profiling methods have shown molecular signatures attributable to subsets of T cells and macrophages in FLs that influence the risk of disease progression and prognosis ([21-24]).

Follicular Lymphoma In Situ

Follicular lymphoma in situ (FLIS) is thought to be a preneoplastic or possibly very early stage of FL ([25]). Most often, FLIS is an incidental finding that occurs in lymph nodes excised for a variety of reasons (eg, axillary lymph nodes in a patient with breast carcinoma). The overall frequency of FLIS is low, approximately 2%.

Morphologically, FLIS is difficult to recognize in routine, tissue sections stained with hematoxylin-eosin. The lymph node architecture is normal, with widely scattered follicles that are of normal size and inconspicuous. The germinal centers have a sharp peripheral margin and are monotonous, composed almost exclusively of centrocytes, a morphologic clue to the diagnosis of FLIS ([26]). Immunohistochemical analysis is essential for the recognition of FLIS. The germinal center cells are strongly positive for BCL2 and CD10 ([26, 27]). Typically, BCL2 expression by the FLIS cells is brighter than the expression level by mantle zone cells surrounding the germinal center. The cells of FLIS also express pan B-cell antigens and other germinal center B-cell markers, such as BCL-6 and LMO2. Cytogenetic and molecular studies have shown that the cells of FLIS carry t(14;18)(q32;q21) and monoclonal Ig gene rearrangements. Array comparative genomic hybridization and other methods performed on FLIS lesions have shown that the cells of FLIS carry the t(14;18) but have relatively few secondary genetic abnormalities, in contrast with fully developed FL ([28]). *EZH2* mutations have been detected in FLIS, suggesting this is another early lesion in FL pathogenesis.

Evidence of overt lymphoma at another anatomic site also is present in a small subset of patients with FLIS ([26]). In addition, some patients with FLIS subsequently develop a histologically discordant type of lymphoma. These cases suggest that FLIS could be a marker of genetic instability or a marker of genetic predisposition to lymphoma. Lymphomas most often reported in association with FLIS include classical Hodgkin lymphoma, splenic marginal zone lymphoma, and SLL/CLL ([27]).

In aggregate, the data suggest that FLIS is a neoplastic process representing an early step in FL pathogenesis that is unlikely to affect patient survival if it is an isolated finding. However, because a subset of some patients with FLIS also has or may develop overt lymphoma at other anatomic sites, staging studies are indicated. If FLIS is the only disease discovered, overtreatment is to be avoided.

Diagnostic Workup and Staging

Clinical evaluation requires a comprehensive history, including age; sex; presence of B symptoms (fevers, chills, drenching night sweats, unexplained weight loss of more than 10% of body mass over 6 months, pruritus); fatigue; and a history of malignancy. Physical examination should include identification and measurement of all accessible lymph node sites, including epitrochlear and occipital lymph nodes, and assessment of the abdomen for splenomegaly or hepatomegaly.

The diagnosis is best established by an excisional lymph node biopsy to provide adequate tissue for assessment of the lymph node architecture. The most easily accessible lymph node may not be the most informative or representative one. For example, if a small peripheral lymph node shows grade 1 FL but the patient has a large abdominal mass, a high serum LDH level, and other features suggestive of transformation, then an additional biopsy to exclude higher-grade disease should be considered because this would influence the selection of appropriate therapy. Core needle biopsies guided by radiographic or imaging techniques may be performed on masses that are not easily accessible. Fine-needle aspiration (FNA) can be misleading for initial diagnosis; complete classification may not be possible because the limited tissue sample prevents the assessment of architecture, and there is the possibility of sampling error. In the initial staging evaluation, FNA may play a role in documenting and defining sites of involvement.

Once the diagnosis of FL has been established, patients should undergo testing to determine stage, assess prognostic risk factors, and evaluate their general health. A complete blood cell count may show anemia or thrombocytopenia, which can result from bone marrow involvement or occasionally from hypersplenism or autoimmune problems. Leukemic involvement can occur in 10% of patients. Serum LDH and β_2-microglobulin (B2M) levels may be elevated and are of prognostic significance. Bilateral bone marrow biopsies with unilateral aspiration are recommended for the staging workup because of the patchy nature of involvement. In FL, the bone marrow characteristically shows a paratrabecular pattern of involvement (Fig. 7-2). Because the lymphoma cells are associated with stroma and are not easily aspirated, bone marrow aspirate smears assessed by routine light microscopy may not be informative. Flow cytometry and molecular assessment (eg, polymerase chain reaction, PCR) of

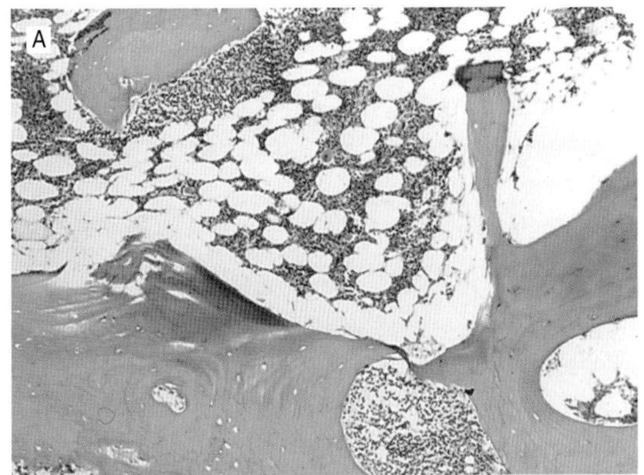

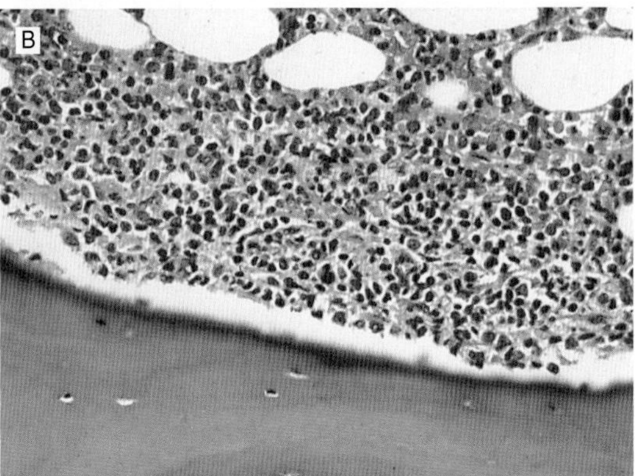

FIGURE 7-2 Follicular lymphoma involving bone marrow. A. The neoplasm is infiltrating the bone marrow with a paratrabecular pattern. B. Neoplastic small-cleaved cells adjacent to bone are seen in this field (A, B, hematoxylin and eosin; A, ×100; B, ×400).

aspirate material can increase the sensitivity of bone marrow assessment, but in the absence of morphologic abnormalities, positive PCR or flow findings are traditionally not taken as evidence to warrant assignment of stage IV ([29]). For example, it is well established that patients at Ann Arbor stage I or II can have cells with the t(14;18) detected in the peripheral blood or bone marrow by PCR.

Imaging studies should include neck and chest computed tomography (CT) for delineation of lymphadenopathy. Abdominal and pelvic CT scans are essential for assessing lymphadenopathy as well as organomegaly. Positron emission tomography (PET) using fluorine-18 fluorodeoxyglucose (FDG) is a useful tool for assessing patients with FDG-avid lymphomas and Hodgkin lymphoma. The field is evolving, and PET combined with CT (PET-CT) is replacing PET alone. Compared with CT scans, PET-CT can improve the accuracy of staging for nodal and extranodal sites and leads to a change in stage in 10% to 30% of patients, more often upstaging these patients ([30]). Improving staging accuracy is important to ensure patients are appropriately treated. Although most lymphomas are FDG avid, there is great variability in FDG uptake ([31-33]). Imaging by PET can be less reliable in indolent lymphoma. Therefore, adoption of PET scanning for staging patients with indolent lymphoma has not been embraced to the same extent that it has for DLBCL and Hodgkin lymphoma. Recent consensus guidelines recommend the use of PET-CT for staging in clinical practice and clinical trials for patients with FL and may be used to select the best site to biopsy.

Prognostic Factors

The prognostic importance of histologically distinguishing grade 1 or 2 FL from the more aggressive grade 3 FL is well accepted. However, most investigators have not found a clear difference in long-term survival between patients with grades 1 and 2 FL, although older literature suggested that FL grade 2 (nodular mixed-cell lymphoma, in older nomenclature) was more prone to early progression than grade 1 if therapy was deferred ([34]). Higher degrees of nodularity have been associated in some reports with improved outcome. An increased proliferation rate is associated with a poorer prognosis ([35, 36]).

Variables that have been shown to correlate with survival in patients with FL include tumor burden, host factors, and response to therapy. Tumor burden can be estimated by assessing stage of disease, size of nodal disease, bone marrow involvement, serum B2M, LDH levels, and number of nodal sites. Adverse host factors include advanced age, B symptoms, low hemoglobin level, male gender, and poor performance status. The background cells in the diagnostic lymph node biopsy may also provide prognostic information, as shown in gene expression profiling studies ([22, 24]).

The International Prognostic Index (IPI) was devised for aggressive lymphomas and consists of five variables: age, performance status, Ann Arbor stage, extranodal involvement, and serum LDH level ([37]). The IPI is also a useful predictor of survival in patients with indolent B-cell lymphomas. One important limitation of this system is that only 11% of the patients fell into the high-risk group, and most of these patients had poor performance status and would be poor candidates for aggressive therapy.

Partly for that reason, a Follicular Lymphoma International Prognostic Index (FLIPI) was developed. Initially, an eight-parameter model (age ≥60 years, male gender, Ann Arbor stages III and IV, nodal sites ≥5, bone marrow involvement, serum LDH level greater than normal, hemoglobin level <12 g/dL, and lymphocytes ≥1000/mL) was proposed ([38]). However, a simplified version of this model was found to be comparably predictive, using the five parameters of age, Ann Arbor

CHAPTER 7

stage, serum LDH, hemoglobin level, and number of nodal sites ([39]). This prognostic model separates patients into three prognostic groups: good risk with 0 to 1 factors, intermediate risk with 2 factors, and poor risk with 3 or more factors. The overall 5-year survival was 90% for the good-risk group, 78% for the intermediate-risk group, and 53% for the poor-risk group ([39]). The validity of the FLIPI model has been demonstrated in rituximab-treated patients ([40]). A FLIPI-2 model was developed through the prospective collection of prognostic data, producing a five-factor model that incorporates age (>60 years adverse); hemoglobin level (<12 g/dL adverse); serum B2M level (adverse if above normal range); bone marrow (adverse if involved); and size of lymphadenopathy (>6 cm adverse), which has not been validated ([41]).

There are more similarities than differences in these models. For instance, the importance of serum B2M was shown in the univariate analyses of both the IPI and FLIPI data sets, but the B2M data were collected prospectively only in the FLIPI-2 report. The importance of sampling the bone marrow, as shown in the FLIPI-2 report, deserves particular emphasis, because practice patterns indicate that the important data offered are often not collected. Easily applied models such as the IPI, FLIPI, or FLIPI-2 can provide a framework for selecting the timing or intensity of therapy, and can facilitate the interpretation of clinical trials, by providing a tool to assess for disparities in patient selection when results of various trials are compared (Table 7-2).

At the time of relapse, favorable predictors for survival in patients with FL include having achieved a complete response with initial therapy, having had a durable remission of more than 1 year following initial therapy, and being less than 60 years of age.

Table 7–2 Prognostic Models for Lymphoma

	Model		
Prognostic Factor	*IPI*	*FLIPI*	*FLIPI-2*
Age	√	√	√
PS	√		
Stage	√	√	
No. of E sites	√		
Bone marrow			√
No. of nodal sites		√	
Size of nodes			√
LDH	√	√	
Hgb		√	√
B2M			√

PS, performance status; B2M, serum β-2-microglobulin.

Posttreatment Monitoring

An international working group has recommended end-of-treatment assessment and defined response criteria for NHL. These criteria have recently been updated, with important modifications, including incorporation of PET-CT ([30]). In FDG-avid FL, PET-CT should be used for response assessment, using the 5-point scale (1, no uptake above background; 2, uptake ≤ mediastinum; 3, uptake > mediastinum but ≤ liver; 4, uptake moderately > liver; 5, uptake markedly higher than liver and/or new lesions). The criteria based on PET-CT eliminate complete response unconfirmed (CRu) evaluation and improve the prognostic value of a partial response (PR). A complete metabolic response (PET-CT), even with a persistent mass, is considered a complete remission (CR). With CT-based assessment, a complete radiologic response is determined by nodal masses regressing to 1.5 cm or less in the longest diameter and no extralymphatic sites of disease. Bone marrow reevaluation is performed to confirm clinical remission if the bone marrow was initially positive.

Although the monitoring of patients with molecular studies is not currently considered standard practice, detection of the t(14;18)/*IGH-BCL2* by PCR techniques has been useful in the monitoring of subclinical disease. "Molecular remission," the disappearance of cells with the t(14;18) detected by PCR, used to be considered a rarity in patients with FL treated with standard therapy. Gribben et al reported that only 1 of 212 (0.5%) patients achieved molecular remission following conventional chemotherapy ([42]). With high-dose therapy and stem cell transplantation (SCT), however, molecular remissions could be attained, and those with molecular remission experienced more durable remissions. Improvements in therapy have changed this picture. Even before the advent of anti-CD20 monoclonal antibody (MAb) therapy, more potent chemotherapy regimens were capable of inducing molecular remission in over half of patients. With the availability of rituximab, which can largely eradicate B cells from the blood and bone marrow, it is now common to see molecular remission. Some recent studies continued to show that molecular remission correlates with more durable clinical remission([43, 44]), but other studies did not ([45]).

Surveillance Imaging

There are limited data supporting patient benefit from surveillance imaging in FL. As a consequence, there is considerable variation in practice. Zinzani et al performed one of the only prospective studies of surveillance imaging, which included 78 patients with FLs in first CR following induction therapy ([46]). Patients received PET-CT scans every 6 months for 2 years, with annual scans thereafter. The relapse rate was 8% to 10% as shown by scans performed until 36 months and decreased after that time. As the purpose of the study was to describe specificity of scans, the impact on management and subsequent outcome was not reported. Gerlinger et al performed surveillance with annual CT scans and bone marrow biopsies in 71 patients with FL in second or subsequent remission following SCT ([47]). Although approximately half of relapses were CT detected, few such patients required immediate treatment; there was no difference in overall survival between patients in whom disease relapse was detected by imaging compared with clinical presentation. Their conclusion was surveillance imaging was futile in this setting. Surveillance CT scans result in radiation exposure, patient anxiety, and significant health-care costs, which should be carefully weighed against any potential benefit. The National Comprehensive Cancer Network (NCCN) guidelines suggest "surveillance CT scan up to every 6 months for the first 2 years following completion of therapy, and not more than annually thereafter." In contrast, the European Society for Medical Oncology (ESMO) guidelines are more conservative, suggesting minimal adequate radiological or ultrasound investigations every 6 months for 2 years and annually thereafter. Regular CT scans are not mandatory outside clinical trials, and PET-CT should not be used for surveillance ([48]).

Treatment of Limited-Stage Follicular Lymphomas

At diagnosis, approximately 15% to 20% of patients with FL have limited-stage disease (stages I and II). This stage of disease is associated with a favorable outcome, and up to half of these patients may be cured. Consequently, seizing the opportunity for cure should be strongly considered, even though some advocate deferral of therapy ([49]). Several series have reported long-term disease-free survival of approximately 35% to 50% for stage I to II patients treated with involved-field radiotherapy (RT), so it appears that many of these patients are cured ([49-53]). Studies with extended-field or total lymphoid RT, in an attempt to increase cure rates, have not shown convincing additional benefit.

The integration of chemotherapy with involved-field RT has shown promising results in some trials. Investigators at MD Anderson Cancer Center (MDACC) prospectively treated 85 patients with stage I or II FL with 10 cycles of COP-Bleo (cyclophosphamide, vincristine, prednisone, and bleomycin) or CHOP-Bleo (COP-Bleo plus doxorubicin) and involved-field RT "sandwiched" after the third cycle. The disease-free survival at 5 and 10 years was 80% and 72%, respectively—an apparent improvement over results with RT alone ([54]). Analysis of the National LymphoCare Study also demonstrated improvement in progression free survival (PFS) in patients who received systemic therapy in combination with RT ([55]). The role of rituximab in stage I or II disease is not clearly defined; efficacy has been extrapolated from the advanced-stage literature. A prospective, randomized study is being conducted here at MDACC to investigate the addition of rituximab to RT in limited stage, previously untreated patients with FL; results are yet to come.

In summary, patients with limited-stage FL appear to be potentially curable. The role of RT in these patients is well established, so involved-field RT remains the standard treatment (see Table 7-2). Despite the established role of involved-field RT and its endorsement by experts, RT appears to be underutilized in practice ([55,56]). Total lymphoid RT and combined-modality therapy approaches remain controversial and are seldom used.

Management of Advanced-Stage Follicular Lymphomas

For decades, the treatment of patients with advanced stage FL has been built on two pillars that lean in opposite directions. First, there are numerous effective therapeutic options that can induce remission (Table 7-3); second, relapse appears to be inevitable. If and when therapeutic advances lead to more comprehensive control of FL, then there may be consensus about early intervention because a smaller tumor burden would presumably be more easily treatable, analogous to the stage I or II situation. Until then, it is still the case that deferral of therapy is a common consideration for many asymptomatic patients with low tumor burden.

Table 7–3 Management Strategies for Follicular Lymphoma and Other Indolent Lymphomas

Stages I-II	IF RT RT and CT[a]
Stages III-IV	Deferral of therapy (if no threatening disease) Single-agent alkylators Single-agent MoAb COP and variants, with MoAb CHOP and variants,[a] with MoAb FND and variants,[a] with MoAb RT (stage III) CT and RT[a] (stage III) Consolidation (see text) Maintenance (see text)

COP, cyclophosphamide, vincristine, and prednisone; CHOP, COP and doxorubicin; CT, chemotherapy; FND, fludarabine, mitoxantrone, and dexamethasone; IF, involved field; MoAb, monoclonal antibody; RT, radiation therapy.

[a]MDACC protocol approaches over the years (see text).

CHAPTER 7

When treatment is deemed appropriate, there are a number of considerations in choosing an initial management strategy. With advances in supportive care, we have seen improvement in the tolerability of chemotherapy and SCT. With a better understanding of B-cell lymphomagenesis and the role of the microenvironment, noncytotoxic therapeutic strategies are being incorporated into front-line clinical trials. The range of therapeutic options for patients with advanced-stage FL remains broad (see Table 7-3). The therapeutic goals continue to focus on minimizing toxicity, providing palliation, and attaining durable CR. Consideration of a clinical trial when available is advisable.

Rituximab Monotherapy

For patients with asymptomatic FL with a low tumor burden, deferment of therapy until the development of symptoms or high tumor burden has been accepted based on three randomized trials demonstrating survival equivalent to that with immediate therapy in the prerituximab era ([57-59]). With the long-term safety and efficacy of rituximab established, observation has been challenged in the modern era with rituximab monotherapy in patients with low tumor burden. The goal is to delay the first cytotoxic chemotherapy and to have an impact on health-related quality of life.

The findings of a randomized trial of rituximab versus a watch-and-wait approach in asymptomatic, nonbulky patients with FL suggested patients who received rituximab monotherapy had a delay in progression in comparison to those with an initial watch-and-wait approach ([60]). Those who received rituximab maintenance following rituximab induction also reported improved quality of life. No significant difference in overall survival was reported.

The RESORT study was a randomized cooperative group trial evaluating two dosing strategies of rituximab monotherapy in patients with untreated, grade I or II FL of low tumor burden ([61]). There were 289 patients randomized to either rituximab maintenance or retreatment after responding to rituximab induction (4 weekly doses). The median time to treatment failure (FFS) was similar (3.9 vs 4.3 years), quality of life was similar, and significant toxicity was infrequent among both strategies. For patients with FL with a low tumor burden, rituximab monotherapy followed by a retreatment strategy was associated with less rituximab use while providing comparable disease control to that achieved with a maintenance strategy.

For patients with untreated FL of low tumor burden not eligible for a clinical trial or deemed appropriate for more intensive therapy, an initial management strategy of rituximab monotherapy was associated with a delay in the need for cytotoxic therapy, was well tolerated, and was perceived by some to enhance their health-related well-being. Hence, the decision between observation and rituximab monotherapy should be made following a detailed discussion about the goals of treatment.

Rituximab Plus Chemotherapy

Several trials have shown convincingly that the addition of rituximab to chemotherapy leads to improved outcomes (Table 7-4). Incorporation of rituximab (R) has become standard. Suitable partners for rituximab in induction regimens include cyclophosphamide, vincristine, and prednisone (CVP); cyclophosphamide, doxorubicin, vincristine, and prednisone (CHOP); bendamustine (B); and fludarabine-based regimens (such as FND [fludarabine, mitoxantrone, and dexamethasone]) ([57, 60-66]). Few randomized studies have been conducted to inform selection of frontline chemoimmunotherapy. Bendamustine-rituximab (BR) has been compared with R-CHOP in a randomized trial; BR appeared to be better tolerated and modestly more effective than R-CHOP ([66]). A randomized study comparing R-CVP versus R-CHOP versus R-FM (fludarabine and mitoxantrone) reported R-CHOP and R-FM were superior to R-CVP in regard to time to treatment failure and PFS; however, both, particularly R-FM, were associated with a higher rate of adverse events ([67]). A global phase III study randomized patients with indolent or mantle

Table 7–4 Front-Line Rituximab-Plus-Chemotherapy Trials in Indolent Lymphoma

Regimen	Trial Design	% CR	% PR	% FFS (@ Time)	% Survival @ Time)
R-CVP[a]	Phase III	41[a]	40	52 (3 years)[a]	89 (30 months)
R-CHOP[a]	Phase III	20	77	75 (3 years)[a]	96 (2 years)
R-MCP[a]	Phase III	50[a]	42	71 (4 years)[a]	87 (4 years)[a]
R-Bendamustine[a,b]	Phase III	40[a]	53	58 (4 years)[a]	–
R-FND[c]	Phase III	88	12	76 (3 years)	96 (3 years)
R-FCM	Phase II	83	11	58 (5 years)	89 (5 years)

[a]Significantly better than comparator arm. For R-CVP, survival benefit noted in 2008 update.
[b]Comparator arm R-CHOP.
[c]Comparator arm FND, followed by rituximab (maintenance).

cell lymphoma to either BR or the standard therapy of R-CHOP or R-CVP, finding BR was noninferior and associated with an acceptable safety profile ([68]).

The most common initial management strategy in the United States is currently chemoimmunotherapy ([56]). A phase II study conducted here at MDACC reported on the efficacy and safety of a novel, nonchemotherapeutic strategy of rituximab and lenalidomide in untreated FL with high response rates (overall response rate [ORR] 98%, CR 87%) and manageable toxicity ([69]). This study provided the rationale for conducting a large, global phase III, randomized study investigating rituximab chemotherapy (R-CVP, R-CHOP, or BR) versus rituximab-lenalidomide in patients with untreated FL. Enrollment has completed; results are yet to come. The findings of this study may lead to a change in the treatment paradigm of previously untreated FL.

Maintenance Therapy

Rituximab maintenance (Table 7-5) has been widely utilized after frontline chemoimmunotherapy with the goal of extending the disease-free interval after induction. A randomized study investigated the efficacy of 2 years of rituximab maintenance following rituximab chemotherapy in patients with previously untreated FL ([70]). Rituximab maintenance after chemoimmunotherapy significantly improved PFS (HR [hazard ratio] = 0.55, 95% CI [confidence interval] 0.44-0.68) and was generally well tolerated but had no significant impact on overall survival. Factors influencing the decision to pursue a maintenance strategy should include consideration of the patient's risk of early relapse, the response to induction therapy, and the financial burden of extended dosing.

Consolidation Therapy

A large multicenter randomized trial of radioimmunotherapy (RIT) consolidation therapy has shown a significant failure-free survival benefit when used after a variety of induction therapy regimens ([71]). Notably, the induction therapy included rituximab in only a minority of the patients. Still, the feasibility and impact of such a strategy is noteworthy. Prolongation of disease control was significant in subset analyses of both complete and partial responders to the induction therapy. Patients who attained only partial remission after chemotherapy commonly attained CR after RIT (77%).

Other trials have also studied RIT consolidation. A Southwest Oncology Group trial compared CHOP followed by RIT versus R-CHOP in patients with advanced-stage FL ([72]). With a follow-up of 4.9 years, there was no significant difference in the 2-year PFS (80% vs 76%) or OS (overall survival) (93% vs. 97%) rates. With the benefits and safety profile of rituximab as part of induction or as maintenance established, the role of RIT in the modern era is unclear.

Salvage Therapy

There are many effective therapeutic options for patients with relapsed disease. The efficacy of single-agent rituximab has been demonstrated reproducibly, although most responses to salvage rituximab are PR rather than CR. Attempts at improving the rate of CRs and enhancing the duration of response are evolving (Table 7-6).

Newer anti-CD20 MAbs are being investigated, with modifications that theoretically represent enhancements over rituximab, such as fully humanized MAbs as opposed to a chimeric mouse–human construct; MAbs with enhanced capacity for mediation of complement-dependent cytotoxicity; MAbs with enhanced mediation of antibody-dependent cellular cytotoxicity; and other modifications. Monoclonal antibodies that target antigens other than CD20 have been developed. CD19 and CD22 are B-cell-specific antigens that internalize following antibody binding. The development of therapeutic antibodies

CHAPTER 7

Table 7–5 Maintenance Rituximab

		Induction Response		↑ FFS With
	Induction	% CR	% PR	Maintenance[a]
A. Front-line trials	Rituximab	9	58	Yes
	CVP	13	60	Yes
	Various + R	–	–	Yes
B. Salvage	Rituximab	0	28	Yes[b]
	R-CHOP	30	55	Yes
	R-FCM	41	54	Yes

[a]Maintenance schedules and duration variable (see text).
[b]Benefit of maintenance was matched by re-treatment at time of progression.

Table 7–6 Consolidation Therapy Approaches

Induction	Consolidation	% CR After Induction	% CR After Consolidation	% CR + PR	% FFS (@ Times)
CHOP	Rituximab[a]	57	[a]	94	44 (3 years)
FN	Rituximab[a]	68	[a]	96	63 (3 years)
CHOP	Tositumomab	39	69	98	67 (5 years)
Various	Ibritumomab/Y-90	51[b]	87[b]	100[b]	53 (3 years[a])
R-FND	Ibritumomab/Y-90	69	89	89	73 (3 years)
Fludarabine	Tositumomab/I-131	9	86	100	60 (5 years)

[a]In these trials, rituximab crossover only for subset who did not attain molecular response: conversion to molecular remission occurred in 74% and 61% in the two trials.

[b]Trial design accepted only CR and PR patients for RIT. FFS measured from study entry, before RIT but after induction chemotherapy.

against these targets has included their use both alone and as immunotoxins, that is, as delivery systems for toxins, analogous to the delivery of isotopes with RIT.

Many therapeutic options under study in the past decade have been developed against specific cell growth regulatory pathways. These include targets of the B-cell receptor pathway: Bruton tyrosine kinase (BTK) inhibitors (eg, ibrutinib) ([73]), phosphatidylinositol-3-kinase delta (PI3Kδ) inhibitors (eg, idelalisib) ([74]), and inhibitors of the proteasome or nuclear factor kappa B (NF-κB) pathway (eg, bortezomib) ([75]). As previously discussed, immune modulation is an attractive approach particularly in indolent lymphoma. Rituximab in combination with lenalidomide in the relapsed setting has been reported to be an effective salvage and bridge to SCT ([76]). Enhancement of the endogenous antitumor response by targeting the microenvironment may be achieved with immune checkpoint inhibitors such as anti-PD1 MAbs. A recent study investigated the activity of pidilizumab with rituximab in 32 patients with relapsed FL and reported an ORR of 66% and CR rate of 52% with no autoimmune or treatment-related grade 3 or 4 adverse events ([77]). With some of these agents, their categorization as "biological" or "targeted" therapy, rather than conventional cytotoxic therapy, may be arguable. Some of these targeted therapies are associated with myelosuppressive toxicity, as is seen with conventional chemotherapy.

Numerous non–cross-resistant chemotherapeutic agents can be effective in indolent lymphomas (Table 7-7). Typically, those not chosen for a patient's frontline treatment are candidates for salvage use. It is notable that retreatment of previously responsive patients is a legitimate option. Long-term follow-up studies have shown that second and later responses can be attained, even with the same agents, but the ensuing clinical remissions become progressively more brief. Because some physicians advocate the avoidance of the toxicities of certain agents (eg, doxorubicin or the nucleoside analogs) in the frontline setting, their role in the salvage setting is an important consideration. Selected salvage chemotherapy regimens are listed in Table 7-7.

Novel agents such as idelalisib (PI3Kδi) have demonstrated efficacy (ORR 57%, CR 6%) with a manageable safety profile (grade ≥3 neutropenia, 27%; transaminitis, 13%; pneumonia, 7%) in relapsed/refractory FL, leading to Food and Drug Administration approval for use in patients who have had at least two prior lines of systemic therapy ([74]). As a result, a number of B-cell receptor pathway inhibitors and immune modulators are currently under investigation either as monotherapy or in combination with chemotherapy and MAbs. With minimal additive toxicity, combination approaches are under way in an attempt to obtain higher complete response rates and extend disease-free intervals. Consideration of a clinical trial in the setting of relapsed or refractory FL is strongly recommended given the vast trial options available and evolving management strategies.

Table 7–7 Selected Salvage Chemotherapy Regimens

Ara C – Cisplatin backbone ESHAP (etoposide; methylprednisone, ara C; cisplatin) ASHAP[a] (doxorubicin; methylprednisone; ara C; cisplatin)
Fludarabine-based FND (fludarabine; mitoxantrone; dexamethasone) R-FCM (rituximab; fludarabine; cyclophosphamide; mitoxantrone)
Others MINE (mesna; ifosfamide; mitoxantrone; etoposide) R-GemOx[a] (rituximab; gemcitabine; oxaliplatin) ICE[a] (ifosfamide; carboplatin; etoposide) B-R (bendamustine; rituximab)

[a]Most extensive literature in aggressive lymphoma, and/or as lead-in to stem cell transplant.

Stem cell transplantation approaches can be arduous, but deserve strong consideration in patients with recurrent high-risk-FL. Autologous SCT strategies result in substantially more durable remissions than conventional-dose salvage therapy ([78]). Allogeneic SCT is a strategy that is contingent on availability of a donor, and it is a complex undertaking that includes real risks of treatment-related mortality. Nonetheless, allogeneic SCT not only can result in long-term remission but also can potentially lead to cure, presumably through its graft-versus-lymphoma effect. Data suggest that non–myeloablative allogeneic SCT is associated with less toxicity than conventional myeloablative allogeneic SCT, and augmentation of the conditioning regimen, including incorporation of bendamustine, has resulted in reduced myelosuppression and graft-versus-host disease ([79]). With improved tolerance of SCT and the potential for cure, this remains a management strategy for eligible patients.

Palliative treatment for FL can include involved-field RT to sites of problematic disease (eg, for obstructive uropathy). Among chemotherapy options, one historically mild option is chlorambucil. Observation without therapy is of course also an option, even at the time of initial diagnosis, in patients with active disease but no threatening or symptomatic disease. The approach of deferral of therapy is common, but it should be done thoughtfully and with monitoring. Because elderly patients are often selected for the "watch-and-wait" strategy, that option should be weighed against the observation that elderly patients with FL have a 10-fold increased risk of dying within 1 year compared with age-matched controls ([41]).

SMALL LYMPHOCYTIC LYMPHOMA/ CHRONIC LYMPHOCYTIC LEUKEMIA

Small lymphocytic lymphoma represents approximately 7% of all NHLs ([1, 2]). The WHO classification restricts SLL to tumors involving lymph nodes with the same B-cell immunophenotype as CLL without leukemic involvement and considers SLL to be the nodal or tissue counterpart of CLL ([2]). Cases of SLL and CLL, combined, represent about 12% of all B-cell NHLs.

Clinical Features and Management

Patients with SLL often present with asymptomatic lymphadenopathy. The B symptoms are uncommon and are observed in less than 10% of patients. Splenomegaly is common. Bone marrow is often involved, affecting approximately 70% of patients ([1, 2]). Although the traditional staging systems for SLL and CLL differ, these systems share common features, and the prognosis of patients with SLL is similar to that of patients with CLL.

Management strategies for patients with FL and CLL are often applicable to patients with SLL, but there are some caveats. For instance, as CD20 is usually dimly expressed by SLL/CLL, anti-CD20 antibody therapy for SLL may be better modeled on the results in the CLL literature rather than the results of patients with FL. Conversely, the response to anti-CD52 antibody therapy (alemtuzumab) seems to depend greatly on tissue penetration, and response is often inadequate at sites of bulky disease in patients with SLL/CLL ([80]).

Histologic, Immunophenotypic, and Molecular Features

The lymph node architecture is diffusely and usually totally effaced by SLL/CLL ([2]). The neoplastic cells are predominantly small, round lymphocytes. Vague pale areas composed of lymphocytes, prolymphocytes, and paraimmunoblasts, known as proliferation centers (or pseudofollicles), are usually present and are diagnostic of this neoplasm. In 5% to 10% of SLL/CLL cases, residual reactive lymphoid follicles are present, surrounded by neoplasm; this represents the so-called interfollicular pattern of SLL/CLL. In this morphologic variant, proliferation centers can surround benign follicles, mimicking nodal MZL.

The SLL/CLL cells express monotypic immunoglobulin light chain, IgM, usually IgD, pan–B-cell antigens, and Bcl-2. CD23 is usually positive in 90% to 95% of cases, and CD22, CD79B, and FMC7 are negative in most cases. The density of Ig and CD20 antigen expression on the surface of SLL/CLL cells is characteristically low ("dim" immunofluorescence by flow cytometry). These neoplasms almost invariably express the CD5 antigen, a pan–T-cell antigen that is not expressed on normal B cells. Other T-cell antigens are negative. CD38 and ZAP70 are expressed by a subset of cases, and expression correlates with unmutated Ig genes and poorer prognosis ([81]). The neoplastic cells are negative for CD10 and Bcl-6 ([2]).

Conventional cytogenetic analysis has shown chromosomal abnormalities in 50% to 60% of SLL/CLL cases. This low frequency is partly attributable to poor cell growth in culture. Translocations involving the Ig genes are rare in SLL/CLL. The t(14;19)(q32;q13) involving the *bcl*-3 gene at 19q13 is most common but is present in less than 5% of SLL/CLL cases. The t(14;19) is associated with atypical morphologic or immunophenotypic features and a poorer prognosis.

Fluorescence in situ hybridization (FISH) analysis has shown a higher frequency of abnormalities in SLL/CLL because this technique can assess interphase as well as metaphase nuclei and does not require cell growth in culture. At our center, SLL/CLL cases are routinely assessed by FISH with a panel of probes, including those specific for 6q, 11q (ATM), trisomy 12,

13q14, and 17p (*p53*). Deletion of the 13q14 locus is the most common abnormality in SLL/CLL. Trisomy 12 is detected in approximately 15% to 20% of cases and appears to be a secondary event, as it is usually found in only a subset of the neoplastic cells ([82]). Both del (11q) and trisomy 12 have been correlated with poorer prognosis. Abnormalities of the *p53* or *MYC* genes correlate with increased risk of histologic transformation (Richter syndrome) and poorer prognosis.

Monoclonal B-Cell Lymphocytosis

Monoclonal B-cell lymphocytosis (MBL) is defined as a monotypic B-cell expansion in peripheral blood that is less than 5×10^9/L in a patient with no evidence of other signs or symptoms of a lymphoproliferative disorder (eg, lymphadenopathy or related autoimmune disease) ([83]). An older name used for MBL was *monoclonal B-cell lymphocytosis of uncertain significance*. This term is analogous to monoclonal gammopathy of undetermined significance, an early precursor of plasma cell myeloma that is detected in the bone marrow.

Cases of MBL have been further subclassified into three categories: CLL-like immunophenotype (CD5$^+$, CD20 dim positive), atypical CLL immunophenotype (CD5$^+$, CD20 bright positive), and non-CLL (CD5$^-$, CD20 bright positive) immunophenotype. The CLL-like category is most common, representing at least 75% of all cases of MBL, and the overall frequency of CLL-like MBL in the general population has ranged in various studies from 3.5% to 12%. The frequency of CLL-like MBL increases with age, and over half of all patients over 90 years of age have CLL-like MBL.

Monoclonal B-cell lymphocytosis is covered elsewhere in this volume. The concept of CLL-like MBL, however, is relevant to lymph node diagnosis because a small percentage of patients who undergo surgery for carcinoma (or other nonlymphoid tumors) can have an incidentally detected CD5$^+$ B-cell lymphoproliferative disorder in a lymph node, usually removed for staging purposes. Typically, the lesions only partially replace the architecture of the lymph node biopsy specimen, and there is no evidence of other sites of lymphadenopathy, hepatosplenomegaly, or absolute lymphocytosis. In one study, approximately 10% of patients with these findings progressed to overt CLL/SLL. Gibson and colleagues ([84]) proposed that the concept of clinical CLL-like MBL can be extended to lymph node biopsy specimens. The authors suggested that a lymph node biopsy specimen involved (usually partially) by a B-cell infiltrate with a CLL immunophenotype, but without proliferation centers, is the tissue equivalent of clinical CLL-like MBL if the patient had a peripheral blood monoclonal B-cell count of less than 5×10^9/L and lymph nodes were less than 1.5 cm as shown by imaging studies ([84]).

MARGINAL ZONE B-CELL LYMPHOMAS

Although their names are similar, the MZLs are not closely related to MBLs at the genetic level and have different pathogeneses. The MZLs include extranodal MZL of mucosa-associated lymphoid tissue (MALT lymphoma), nodal marginal zone lymphoma, and splenic B-cell marginal zone lymphoma (SMZL). Prior to the advent of immunophenotypic and molecular methods, MALT lymphomas were often classified as *pseudolymphomas*. Immunophenotypic and gene rearrangement studies showed that most pseudolymphomas express monotypic immunoglobulin light chain or carry monoclonal Ig gene rearrangements.

The MALT lymphomas represent 7% to 8% of all NHLs ([1, 2]). Nodal marginal zone lymphomas represent approximately 2% of all NHLs. Splenic MZL is rare, representing less than 1% of all NHLs ([1]). Splenic MZL can be associated with circulating lymphocytes with villous cytoplasmic projections. The entity previously described as splenic lymphoma with villous lymphocytes is, in most cases, SMZL.

Extranodal Marginal Zone B-Cell Lymphoma

Clinical Features

Patients with MALT lymphoma present with extranodal disease that is often localized (stage I-E or II-E). There may be a history of infection or autoimmune disease, and the disease is usually indolent. Peripheral lymph node involvement is uncommon in patients with MALT lymphoma. The most common site of involvement is the stomach, but numerous other extranodal locations can be involved, including lung, skin, orbit, salivary glands, other parts of the gastrointestinal tract, thyroid gland, and other rare sites. Dissemination occurs in up to 30% of cases, most often in patients with nongastric MALT lymphoma, often to other extranodal sites. In patients with nongastric MALT lymphomas, subclinical gastric involvement is not uncommon. The bone marrow is involved in only 10% to 20% of patients

The stomach is the best-studied site of involvement. Patients often present with signs and symptoms suggestive of peptic ulcer disease, such as epigastric pain and dyspepsia. Anemia, weight loss, and gastrointestinal bleeding can be seen in patients with more advanced disease. *Helicobacter pylori* is present in the gastric mucosa of many patients with MALT lymphoma. Antibiotic eradication of *H. pylori* has resulted in regression of MALT lymphoma in over half of treated patients ([85, 86]). Thus, *H. pylori* is thought to be essential to lymphomagenesis in gastric MALT lymphoma.

In nongastric MALT lymphomas, symptoms are related to the anatomic site involved. Disseminated disease is generally more common in these patients than in patients with gastric MALT lymphoma. Despite the higher frequency of stage IV disease, the 5-year survival is 90% with a variety of therapies.

Histologic Features

Four findings are present in most MALT lymphomas: a population of neoplastic small lymphoid (centrocyte-like) cells that may have monocytoid features, occasional large lymphoid cells (blasts), lymphoepithelial lesions, and reactive lymphoid follicles (Figs. 7-3 to 7-5).

The neoplastic small lymphoid cells exhibit a range of cytologic appearances. In some cases, the cells resemble small lymphocytes with or without plasmacytoid differentiation. In other cases, the neoplasm appears biphasic: One component is a population of small lymphoid cells, and the other is a population of cells with extensive plasmacytoid differentiation, resembling mature plasma cells (see Fig. 7-5). In other cases, the cells have markedly irregular nuclear contours and resemble small-cleaved cells. All of these cell types may have abundant pale cytoplasm, imparting a monocytoid appearance. In most MALT lymphomas, occasional large lymphoid cells (blasts) are also present. However, when large cells are numerous and form confluent sheets, the neoplasm has evolved to DLBCL.

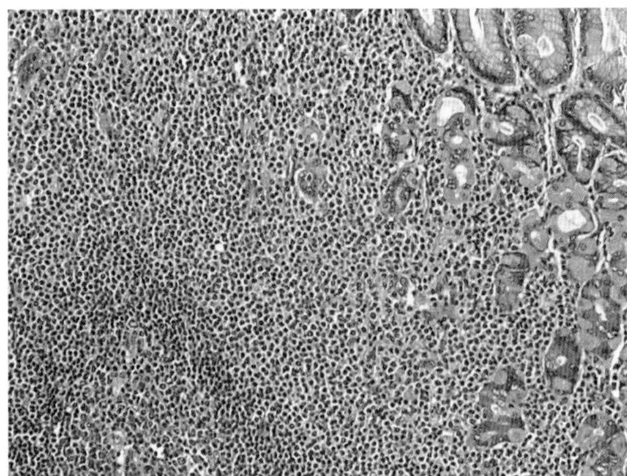

FIGURE 7-3 Extranodal marginal zone B-cell lymphoma of MALT (MALT lymphoma) involving the stomach. The neoplasm partially replaces gastric mucosa and infiltrates epithelium. A reactive follicle is present at the bottom left of the field.

The small neoplastic cells have a marked tendency to infiltrate epithelium, forming so-called lymphoepithelial lesions (see Fig. 7-4). In well-formed lesions, aggregates of neoplastic cells are found within the epithelium. Reactive lymphoid follicles are also usually present in MALT lymphomas, generally surrounded by neoplastic small lymphoid cells. Neoplastic cells can also accumulate in these follicles (termed *colonization*), imparting a vaguely nodular appearance at low-power magnification.

Anatomic site-specific histologic findings are also observed in MALT lymphomas, involving chronic antigenic stimulation as a result of either an infectious organism or autoimmune disease. For example, normal lymphoid tissue is not usually present in the stomach. However, more benign forms of MALT are likely acquired, probably in response to *H. pylori* infection. *Chlamydia psittaci*, *Borrelia burgdorferi*, and *Campylobacter jejuni* are other infectious agents that have been associated with orbital, skin, and small intestinal MALT lymphomas, respectively, although the data linking *B. burgdorferi* to skin lymphomas does not appear to be strong. Like the stomach, normal lymphoid tissue is also poorly developed in the lung. However, two inflammatory diseases are frequently associated with lung MALT lymphoma: Sjögren syndrome and

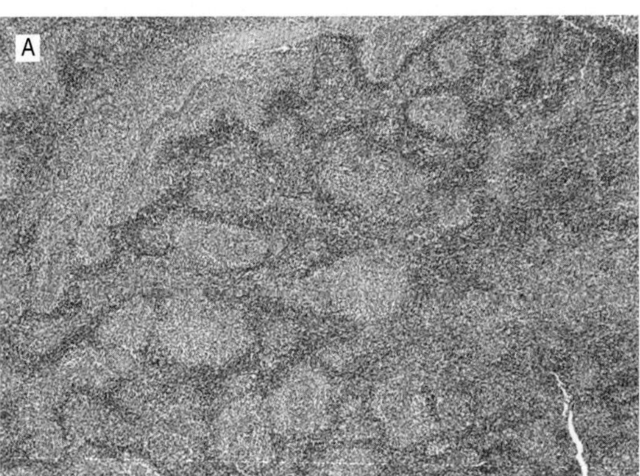

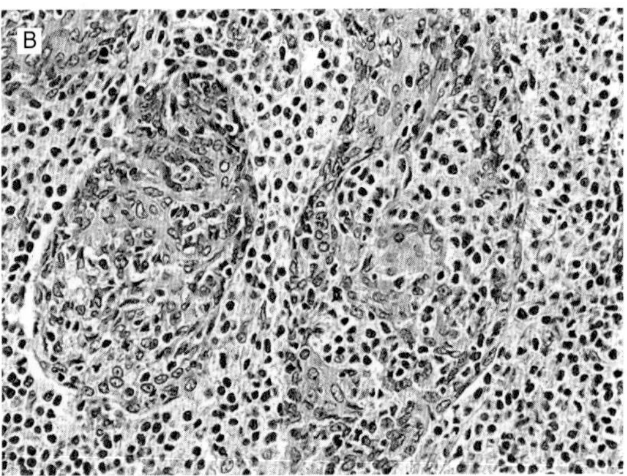

FIGURE 7-4 A MALT lymphoma of a salivary gland. A. The neoplastic cells have a pale (monocytoid) low-power appearance and surround ducts. B. Lymphoepithelial lesions are prominent in this case (A, B, hematoxylin and eosin; A, ×20; B, ×400).

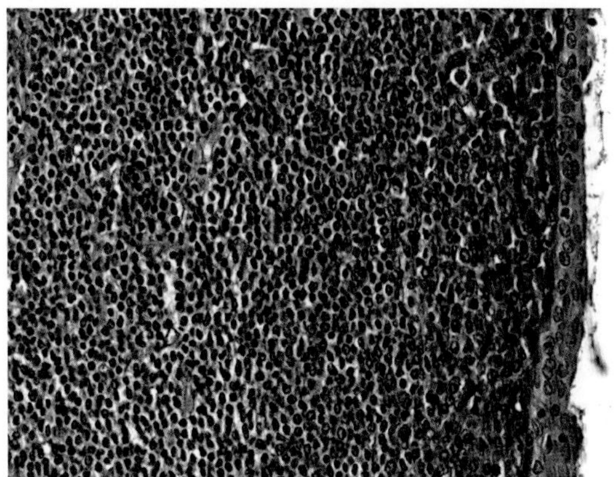

FIGURE 7-5 A MALT lymphoma of the conjunctiva. In this field, the neoplasm has a biphasic pattern, with the subepithelial portion exhibiting extensive plasmacytoid differentiation (periodic acid–Schiff, ×400).

lymphoid interstitial pneumonia. Similarly, MALT lymphomas of the salivary gland are usually associated with Sjögren syndrome, and Hashimoto's thyroiditis usually precedes MALT lymphoma of the thyroid gland.

Immunophenotypic, Cytogenetic, and Molecular Features

The MALT lymphomas express monotypic Ig light chain, pan B-cell antigens, and Bcl-2. These tumors typically do not express IgD, CD10, CD21, CD23, Bcl-6, cyclin D1, or T-cell antigens, including CD5. Four chromosomal translocations are well characterized in MALT lymphomas: t(11;18), t(14;18), t(1;14), and t(3;14).

Finally, t(11;18)(q21;q21) has been identified in approximately 20% to 30% of MALT lymphomas. In this translocation, the *birc*3 (formerly known as *api*2) gene on 11q21 and the *malt*1 gene on chromosome 18q21 are disrupted and recombine to form a novel *birc*3-*malt*1 fusion gene. The *birc*3 gene belongs to the inhibitor of apoptosis protein (IAP) gene family that is evolutionarily conserved and plays a role in regulating apoptosis. *Malt*1 is a novel gene that is critical to the function of BIRC3-MALT1. The t(11;18) is most common in MALT lymphomas of the lung and stomach.

The t(14;18)(q32;q21) has been identified in approximately 10% to 20% of MALT lymphomas. In this translocation, the *Malt*1 gene is juxtaposed next to the IgH gene on the derivative chromosome 14. As a result, MALT1 is overexpressed. The t(14;18) appears to be most common in MALT lymphomas, arising in the ocular adnexal region and liver.

The t(1;14)(p22;q32) is an uncommon translocation in MALT lymphomas, occurring in less than 5% of cases; it juxtaposes the *bcl*-10 gene at 1p22 adjacent to the IgH gene. This translocation truncates *bcl*-10, and thus Bcl-10 protein loses its proapoptotic function. Mutations of the *bcl*-10 gene also occur outside the context of the t(1;14) in 7% to 10% of MALT lymphomas. These mutations consist predominantly of deletions or insertions and are predicted to result in truncated proteins.

The t(3;14)(p14;q32) has also been described in MALT lymphomas. This translocation juxtaposes the *foxp*1 gene at 3p14.1 with the IgH gene. The t(3;14) appears to be most common in MALT lymphomas arising in the thyroid gland, ocular adnexal region, and skin. Vinatzer et al identified additional chromosomal translocations or partner genes in MALT lymphomas, including t(1;14)/IgH-CNN3, t(5;14)/IgH-ODZ2, t(3;14)/IgH-Bcl6, t(9;14)/IgH-JMJD2C, and t(6;7)(q25;q11) ([87]).

Activation of NF-κB may be a final common pathway in MALT lymphomas. API2-MALT1 is known to activate NF-κB. Similarly, overexpression of MALT1 or Bcl-10, by binding with each other, can form a complex in the cell and act to activate NF-κB ([88]).

Workup and Management

The diagnosis of gastric MALT lymphoma is established by endoscopy, with multiple biopsies obtained from abnormal and normal mucosa ([85]). Endoscopic ultrasound may also be helpful in determining the depth of the lesion and for staging. Early-stage disease can be successfully treated initially with antibiotic therapy, with complete regression in 35% to 100% of patients and a low rate of recurrence ([88]). Therefore, the recommended therapy for stage I or II disease is a standard regimen of antibiotic therapy for *H. pylori* with follow-up endoscopy 2 to 3 months later to document *H. pylori* eradication. If patients remain *H. pylori* positive, a second-line anti-*Helicobacter* regimen is administered until they are *H. pylori* negative. The time between *H. pylori* eradication and CR of gastric MALT lymphoma varies and can take longer than 1 year. More extensive disease, as documented by endoscopic ultrasound demonstrating lymphoma involvement beyond the mucosa and in regional nodes, is less likely to respond to antibiotic therapy ([85]). Lack of response has been correlated with the presence of the t(11;18).

Surgery, RT, chemotherapy, and anti-CD20 MAb therapy have been used for both MALT lymphomas and other MZLs. The treatment of choice is dependent on the site of disease, the stage, and the patient's clinical presentation. Surgery and RT are prime therapeutic approaches for localized MALT lymphoma, including gastric MALT lymphoma that does not respond adequately to antibiotic therapy. Chemotherapy and MAb therapy are also options, especially for widespread disease. Conconi et al studied rituximab in patients with MALT lymphoma and found significant activity in both untreated and relapsed patients ([89]). By extrapolation from SLL/CLL data, combinations that include nucleoside analogues have been explored [90]. The best systemic treatment option is not clear.

Nodal Marginal Zone Lymphoma

Clinical Features and Management

Patients with nodal MZL typically present with peripheral or para-aortic lymphadenopathy and bone marrow involvement. The 5-year overall and failure-free survival rates are lower for patients with nodal MZL compared to patients with MALT lymphoma (56% vs 81% and 28% vs 65%, respectively). The majority of effective treatment regimens and outcomes of patients with nodal MZL are similar to that of patients with advanced FL.

Histologic, Immunophenotypic, and Molecular Features

Nodal MZLs have a propensity to involve the marginal zones of a lymph node. In most cases, however, the neoplasm also expands into the perifollicular compartments with sparing of germinal centers, or it completely replaces lymph node architecture. The cytologic features of nodal MZL are the most distinctive aspect of this neoplasm. The tumor cell cytoplasm is relatively abundant and pale, with well-delineated cell borders (Fig. 7-6). The tumor cell nuclei are small, chromatin is relatively clumped, and mitotic figures are infrequent. Rare large cells are also present.

Nodal MZLs are mature B-cell neoplasms that express monotypic Ig, pan B-cell antigens, and Bcl-2. These tumors do not express CD10, CD21, CD23, Bcl-6, cyclin D1, or T-cell antigens, including CD5. Conventional cytogenetics and FISH studies have identified a variety of abnormalities, most often trisomy 3. However, there are no unique recurrent chromosomal abnormalities in nodal MZL. The t(11;18), t(14;18), and t(1;14) have not been identified.

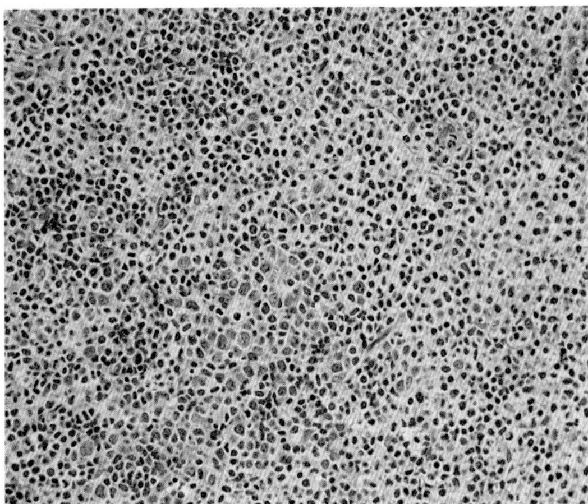

FIGURE 7-6 Nodal marginal zone lymphoma. In this field, the neoplastic cells have abundant pale cytoplasm and surround a reactive germinal center composed of large cells (center of field) (hematoxylin and eosin, ×400).

Splenic Marginal Zone Lymphoma

Clinical Features and Management

Patients with SMZL usually present with splenomegaly, cytopenias, and circulating malignant lymphocytes. They commonly have modest abdominal lymphadenopathy and bone marrow involvement. Monoclonal gammopathy, usually of IgM type, can be observed in 10% to 20% of patients. Peripheral lymphadenopathy and B-type symptoms are uncommon. The clinical course is indolent, with the 5-year overall survival rate ranging from 65% to 78%.

Approximately one-third of patients with SMZL will never require therapy. Splenectomy is indicated in patients with symptomatic splenomegaly or cytopenias secondary to hypersplenism. If splenectomy is contraindicated, splenic irradiation may be an alternative. Alkylating agents have been used, but responses are usually partial and not durable. Patients treated with fludarabine demonstrate a higher response rate and longer-lasting remission than those treated with alkylating agents. Rituximab has significant activity in SMZL.

Histologic, Immunophenotypic, and Molecular Features

In SMZL, the white pulp is expanded by a neoplasm that initially replaces the marginal and mantle zones and then eventually replaces the white pulp (Fig. 7-7). Lesser red pulp involvement is also usually present. At high-power magnification, the neoplastic cells are small lymphocytes with abundant pale (monocytoid) cytoplasm. The neoplastic cells may exhibit plasmacytoid differentiation. Occasional large lymphoid cells are present. In a peripheral blood smear, the neoplastic cells can have villous cytoplasmic projections.

Splenic MZL is a mature B-cell neoplasm that expresses monotypic immunoglobulin, pan B-cell antigens, and Bcl-2. A subset of cases is positive for IgD or CD5 (dim intensity by flow cytometry). These neoplasms are negative for CD10, Bcl-6, cyclin D1, and T-cell antigens (other than CD5).

Conventional cytogenetics and FISH analysis have identified a variety of abnormalities, most often trisomy of chromosomes 3 and 7. Deletion of 7q is present in approximately 50% of cases. A recent study using array-based comparative genomic hybridization has shown del(7q36.2) involving the sonic hedgehog (SHH) gene and del(7q31.32) involving the protection of telomere 1 (POT1) genes in SMZL [91]. MYD88 L265P mutations have been identified in 10% to 20% of cases of SMZL and correlate with IgM gammopathy [92].

LYMPHOPLASMACYTIC LYMPHOMA AND WALDENSTRÖM MACROGLOBULINEMIA

In the current version of the WHO classification, LPL is defined as a neoplasm composed of small lymphocytes, plasmacytoid lymphocytes, and plasma cells and most often involves the bone marrow but can also involve lymph nodes and spleen. Often, LPL is associated with a serum IgM paraprotein, but this feature is *not* required for the diagnosis of LPL ([2]). Patients with LPL also can have a serum paraprotein composed of IgA or IgG, and the relationship of these cases to WM is not clear. In contrast, patients with WM have LPL involving the bone marrow associated with a serum IgM paraprotein of any level ([93, 94]). Using these definitions, all patients with WM have LPL, but not all patients with LPL have WM.

Patients with LPL not meeting the criteria for WM are rare, and there is poor characterization. Furthermore, a serum IgM paraprotein can be observed in patients with other types of indolent B-cell lymphoma ([95]), and there is morphologic and immunophenotypic overlap with MZLs. For these reasons, our focus here is on WM.

Clinical Features

Some patients with WM can be asymptomatic, but many have symptoms of anemia, which is a common presenting feature. Only about 15% of patients have splenomegaly, hepatomegaly, or lymphadenopathy ([2, 94]). The hyperviscosity syndrome—characterized by mucosal hemorrhage, visual disturbances, neurologic changes, and cardiac failure—is dramatic and classic but occurs in only a minority of patients with WM. Other even less-common manifestations include cryoglobulinemia, cold-agglutinin hemolysis, autoimmune thrombocytopenia, amyloidosis, and light-chain nephropathy ([93, 94]).

Histologic, Immunophenotypic, and Molecular Features

The bone marrow is always involved in WM ([93]). Bone marrow aspirate smears show increased small lymphocytes, plasmacytoid small lymphocytes, and mature plasma cells, in varying proportions. Mast cells are commonly increased (Fig. 7-8). In the so-called polymorphous type of WM, large lymphoid cells are increased, 5% to 10%. Although the large cells do not form sheets and thus the criteria for large B-cell lymphoma are not met, patients with the polymorphous type have a poorer prognosis, suggesting that this is may be an early stage of large-cell transformation ([96]).

The cells of WM are composed of essentially two immunophenotypically distinct cell populations corresponding to lymphocytes and plasma cells. The lymphocytes cells express monotypic surface Ig light chain, IgM, and pan B-cell antigens such as CD19 and CD20 and are negative for CD3 and Bcl-6. In most cases, the lymphocytes are negative for CD5, CD10, and CD23 by immunohistochemical staining; however, dim expression of CD5 and CD23 is not uncommon when assessed by flow cytometry. The plasma cells express CD19, CD38, and CD138 and are negative for CD20.

Conventional cytogenetics has shown no characteristic chromosomal abnormalities in WM. The most common cytogenetic abnormality is deletion (6q). The t(9;14)(p13;q32) is a rare abnormality reported in a subset of nodal small B-cell lymphomas with plasmacytoid differentiation, previously presumed to be LPL/WM.

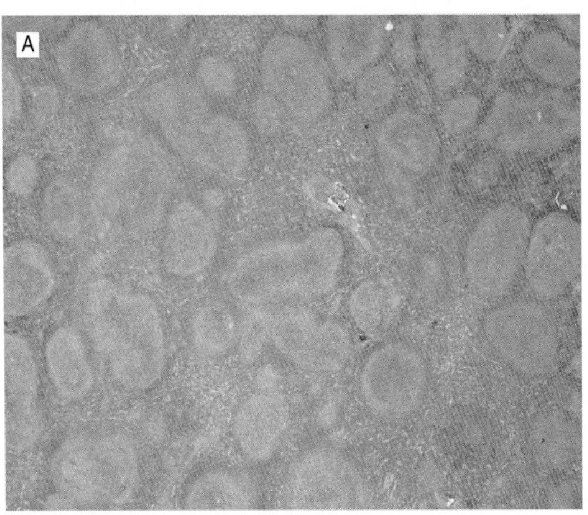

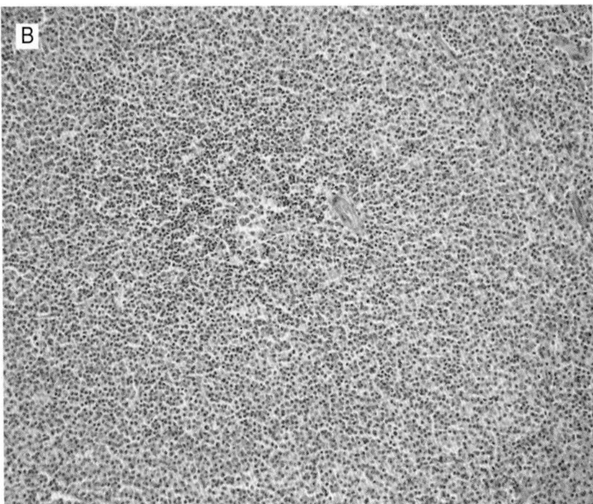

FIGURE 7-7 Splenic marginal zone lymphoma. A. At low power, the while pulp of the spleen is markedly expanded by lymphoma, which has a biphasic pattern. B. One white pulp nodule at higher magnification (A, B, hematoxylin and eosin; A, ×20; B, ×200).

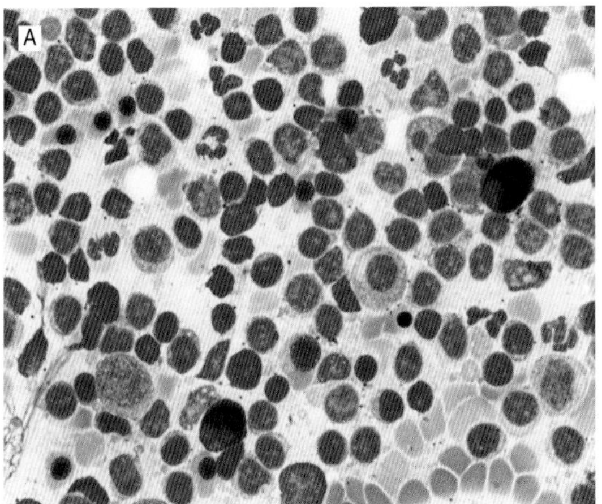

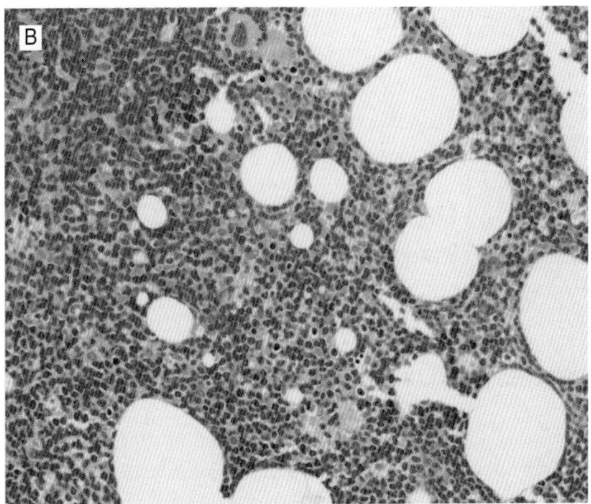

FIGURE 7-8 Waldenström macroglobulinemia involving bone marrow. A. The bone marrow aspirate smear shows numerous small neoplastic lymphocytes with occasional benign mast cells. B. The bone marrow biopsy specimen shows an interstitial and diffuse pattern of involvement by the neoplasm. (A, Wright-Giemsa, ×1,000; B, hematoxylin and eosin, ×400).

However, studies using conventional cytogenetics or FISH have not detected the t(9;14) in any case of WM.

The MYD88 L265P mutation is commonly present in cases of WM, ranging from about 80% to up to 95% of cases ([92, 97]). This finding is now considered a part of the definition of WM by many observers and may be included as part of the disease definition in future versions of the WHO classification. Other gene mutations have been reported in WM. Of these, CXCR4 mutations are most common and correlate with tumor burden ([98]). The MYD88 L265P mutations also occur, at low frequency, in other indolent B-cell lymphomas, including SLL/CLL and MZLs. The MYD88 L265P mutation also seems to correlate with the presence of IgM gammopathy in other indolent B-cell lymphomas.

Management

A prognostic scoring system for patients with WM based on age, albumin, and number of cytopenias has been developed that stratifies patients into low-, intermediate-, and high-risk groups. Other prognostic variables include performance status and serum B2M level. Patients in the low-risk group can be observed.

Alkylating agents such as chlorambucil or bendamustine, nucleoside analogues such as cladribine or fludarabine, and the anti-CD20 antibody rituximab, either as single agents or in various combinations, have been used as initial therapy for the treatment of patients with WM. Important novel options include incorporation of the proteasome inhibitor bortezomib or monotherapy with ibrutinib. Individual patient characteristics need to be weighed in choosing therapy, including the age of the patient, the need for rapid disease control, and consideration of the patient's later candidacy for an autologous transplant approach. For patients with relapsed or refractory disease whose initial remission lasted more than 1 year, retreatment with the same therapy can be considered. Transplantation, both autologous and allogeneic, can be considered for patients with relapsed or primary refractory disease who have good performance status.

Plasmapheresis is indicated for the management of hyperviscosity syndrome and may be helpful for other IgM-related disorders, such as cryoglobulinemia, neuropathy, amyloidosis, and light-chain nephropathy. Plasmapheresis is typically used on a short-term basis until chemotherapy takes effect. In patients with autoimmune conditions or clinical symptoms from cryoglobulinemia, corticosteroids may be helpful.

CONCLUSIONS

To date, most advanced-stage indolent B-cell lymphomas remain incurable. Novel approaches to therapy are continuing to be explored, including next-generation MAbs, pathway inhibitors, and immune modulators. These approaches to therapy and novel combinations will likely play an increasingly important role in the management of patients with indolent B-cell lymphomas. Allogeneic transplantation in indolent B-cell lymphomas continues to be an area of heightened interest, especially with the development of the better tolerated miniallogeneic transplant strategies. The importance of the graft-versus-lymphoma effect reflects our growing knowledge that the host's immune response is a potentially powerful tool that we have not yet fully exploited. As emerging therapies become integrated with the best of conventional therapies, it is optimistic that a curative approach for more patients with indolent B-cell lymphomas is achievable. Equally promising is widespread use of well-tolerated therapy that is associated with durable disease control resulting in chronic management. Also worthwhile of clinical exploration is identifying the most effective sequencing of therapy over an individual's disease course. With so many unanswered questions and emerging novel strategies, consideration of clinical trials for indolent lymphoma is strongly recommended to facilitate the translation of important scientific breakthroughs.

REFERENCES

1. A clinical evaluation of the International Lymphoma Study Group classification of non-Hodgkin's lymphoma. The Non-Hodgkin's Lymphoma Classification Project. *Blood.* 1997;89(11):3909-3918. PMID: 9166827.
2. Swerdlow SH, Campo E, Harris N, et al. *WHO Classification of Tumors of the Hematopoietic and Lymphoid Tissues.* Lyon, France: IARC; 2008.
3. Linet MS, Vajdic CM, Morton LM, et al. Medical history, lifestyle, family history, and occupational risk factors for follicular lymphoma: the InterLymph Non-Hodgkin Lymphoma Subtypes Project. *J Natl Cancer Inst Monogr.* 2014;2014(48):26-40. PMID: 25174024. PMCID: 4155461.
4. Link BK, Maurer MJ, Nowakowski GS, et al. Rates and outcomes of follicular lymphoma transformation in the immunochemotherapy era: a report from the University of Iowa/MayoClinic Specialized Program of Research Excellence Molecular Epidemiology Resource. *J Clin Oncol.* 2013;31(26):3272-3278.
5. Armitage JO, Weisenburger DD. New approach to classifying non-Hodgkin's lymphomas: clinical features of the major histologic subtypes. Non-Hodgkin's Lymphoma Classification Project. *J Clin Oncol.* 1998;16(8):2780-2795. PMID: 9704731.
6. National Cancer Institute sponsored study of classifications of non-Hodgkin's lymphomas: summary and description of a working formulation for clinical usage. The Non-Hodgkin's Lymphoma Pathologic Classification Project. *Cancer.* 1982; 49(10):2112-2135. PMID: 6896167.
7. Tan D, Horning SJ, Hoppe RT, et al. Improvements in observed and relative survival in follicular grade 1-2 lymphoma during 4 decades: the Stanford University experience. *Blood.* 2013 8;122(6):981-987. PMID: 23777769. PMCID: 3739040.
8. Mann RB, Berard CW. Criteria for the cytologic subclassification of follicular lymphomas: a proposed alternative method. *Hematol Oncol.* 1983;1(2):187-192. PMID: 6376315.
9. Bosga-Bouwer AG, van den Berg A, Haralambieva E, et al. Molecular, cytogenetic, and immunophenotypic characterization of follicular lymphoma grade 3B; a separate entity or part of the spectrum of diffuse large B-cell lymphoma or follicular lymphoma? *Hum Pathol.* 2006;37(5):528-533. PMID: 16647949.
10. Conlan MG, Bast M, Armitage JO, Weisenburger DD. Bone marrow involvement by non-Hodgkin's lymphoma: the clinical significance of morphologic discordance between the lymph node and bone marrow. Nebraska Lymphoma Study Group. *J Clin Oncol.* 1990;8(7):1163-1172.
11. Reed JC. Bcl-2-family proteins and hematologic malignancies: history and future prospects. *Blood.* 2008;111(7):3322-3330. PMID: 18362212. PMCID: 2275002.
12. Baliga BC, Kumar S. Role of Bcl-2 family of proteins in malignancy. *Hematol Oncol.* 2002;20(2):63-74.
13. Danial NN, Korsmeyer SJ. Cell death: critical control points. *Cell.* 2004;116(2):205-219.
14. Cleary ML, Galili N, Sklar J. Detection of a second t(14;18) breakpoint cluster region in human follicular lymphomas. *J Exp Med.* 1986;164(1):315-320.
15. Albinger-Hegyi A, Hochreutener B, Abdou M-T, et al. High frequency of t(14;18)-translocation breakpoints outside of major breakpoint and minor cluster regions in follicular lymphomas: improved polymerase chain reaction protocols for their detection. *Am J Pathol.* 2002;160(3):823-832.
16. Tsujimoto Y, Finger LR, Yunis J, Nowell PC, Croce CM. Cloning of the chromosome breakpoint of neoplastic B cells with the t(14;18) chromosome translocation. *Science.* 1984;226(4678): 1097-1099.
17. Ladetto M, Drandi D, Compagno M, et al. PCR-detectable nonneoplastic Bcl-2/IgH rearrangements are common in normal subjects and cancer patients at diagnosis but rare in subjects treated with chemotherapy. *J Clin Oncol.* 2003;21(7):1398-1403.
18. Cheung KJJ, Shah SP, Steidl C, et al. Genome-wide profiling of follicular lymphoma by array comparative genomic hybridization reveals prognostically significant DNA copy number imbalances. *Blood.* 2009;113(1):137-148.
19. Berglund M, Enblad G, Thunberg U, et al. Genomic imbalances during transformation from follicular lymphoma to diffuse large B-cell lymphoma. *Mod Pathol.* 2007;20(1):63-75.
20. Glas AM, Knoops L, Delahaye L, et al. Gene-expression and immunohistochemical study of specific T-cell subsets and accessory cell types in the transformation and prognosis of follicular lymphoma. *J Clin Oncol.* 2007;25(4):390-398.
21. Bende RJ, Smit LA, van Noesel CJM. Molecular pathways in follicular lymphoma. *Leukemia.* 2007;21(1):18-29.
22. de Jong D. Molecular pathogenesis of follicular lymphoma: a cross talk of genetic and immunologic factors. *J Clin Oncol.* 2005;23(26):6358-6363. PMID: 16155020.
23. Farinha P, Al-Tourah A, Gill K, Klasa R, Connors JM, Gascoyne RD. The architectural pattern of FOXP3-positive T cells in follicular lymphoma is an independent predictor of survival and histologic transformation. *Blood.* 2010;115(2):289-295.
24. Dave SS, Wright G, Tan B, et al. Prediction of survival in follicular lymphoma based on molecular features of tumor-infiltrating immune cells. *N Engl J Med.* 2004;351(21):2159-2169.
25. Mamessier E, Song JY, Eberle FC, et al. Early lesions of follicular lymphoma: a genetic perspective. *Haematologica.* 2014;99(3): 481-488. PMID: 24162788. PMCID: 3943311.
26. Jegalian AG, Eberle FC, Pack SD, et al. Follicular lymphoma in situ: clinical implications and comparisons with partial involvement by follicular lymphoma. *Blood.* 2011;118(11):2976-2984. PMID: 21768298. PMCID: 3175777.
27. Carbone A, Gloghini A. Emerging issues after the recognition of in situ follicular lymphoma. *Leuk Lymphoma.* 2014;55(3):482-490. PMID: 23713483.
28. Schmidt J, Salaverria I, Haake A, et al. Increasing genomic and epigenomic complexity in the clonal evolution from in situ to manifest t(14;18)-positive follicular lymphoma. *Leukemia.* 2014; 28(5):1103-1112. PMID: 24153014.
29. Cheson BD, Horning SJ, Coiffier B, et al. Report of an international workshop to standardize response criteria for non-Hodgkin's lymphomas. NCI Sponsored International Working Group. *J Clin Oncol.* 1999;17(4):1244. PMID: 10561185. Epub 1999/11/24.
30. Cheson BD, Fisher RI, Barrington SF, et al. Recommendations for initial evaluation, staging, and response assessment of Hodgkin and non-Hodgkin lymphoma: The Lugano Classification. *J Clin Oncol.* 2014;32(27):3059-3068. PMID: 25113753.
31. Weiler-Sagie M, Bushelev O, Epelbaum R, et al. (18)F-FDG avidity in lymphoma readdressed: a study of 766 patients. *J Nucl Med.* 2010;51(1):25-30.
32. Noy A, Schoder H, Gonen M, et al. The majority of transformed lymphomas have high standardized uptake values (SUVs) on positron emission tomography (PET) scanning similar to diffuse large B-cell lymphoma (DLBCL). *Ann Oncol.* 2009;20(3):508-512.
33. Schoder H, Noy A, Gonen M, et al. Intensity of 18-fluorodeoxyglucose

CHAPTER 7

uptake in positron emission tomography distinguishes between indolent and aggressive non-Hodgkin's lymphoma. *J Clin Oncol.* 2005;23(21):4643-4651.
34. Portlock CS, Rosenberg SA. No initial therapy for stage III and IV non-Hodgkin's lymphomas of favorable histologic types. *Ann Intern Med.* 1979;90(1):10-13.
35. Koster A, Tromp HA, Raemaekers JMM, et al. The prognostic significance of the intra-follicular tumor cell proliferative rate in follicular lymphoma. *Haematologica.* 2007;92(2):184-190.
36. Martin AR, Weisenburger DD, Chan WC, et al. Prognostic value of cellular proliferation and histologic grade in follicular lymphoma. *Blood.* 1995;85(12):3671-3678.
37. A predictive model for aggressive non-Hodgkin's lymphoma. The International Non-Hodgkin's Lymphoma Prognostic Factors Project. *N Engl J Med.* 1993;329(14):987-994. PMID: 8141877. Epub 1993/09/30.
38. Solal-Celigny P. Internation Prognostic Index for follicular lymphoma. *Proc Am Soc Clin Oncol.* 2002;21:281.
39. Solal-Celigny P, Roy P, Colombat P, et al. Follicular lymphoma international prognostic index. *Blood.* 2004;104(5):1258-1265.
40. Buske C, Hoster E, Dreyling M, Hasford J, Unterhalt M, Hiddemann W. The Follicular Lymphoma International Prognostic Index (FLIPI) separates high-risk from intermediate- or low-risk patients with advanced-stage follicular lymphoma treated front-line with rituximab and the combination of cyclophosphamide, doxorubicin, vincristine, and prednisone (R-CHOP) with respect to treatment outcome. *Blood.* 2006;108(5):1504-1508.
41. Federico M, Bellei M, Marcheselli L, et al. Follicular Lymphoma International Prognostic Index 2: a new prognostic index for follicular lymphoma developed by the International Follicular Lymphoma Prognostic Factor Project. *J Clin Oncol.* 2009;27(27): 4555-4562.
42. Gribben JG, Neuberg D, Barber M, et al. Detection of residual lymphoma cells by polymerase chain reaction in peripheral blood is significantly less predictive for relapse than detection in bone marrow. *Blood.* 1994;83(12):3800-3807.
43. Johnson PW, Swinbank K, MacLennan S, et al. Variability of polymerase chain reaction detection of the bcl-2-IgH translocation in an international multicentre study. *Ann Oncol.* 1999; 10(11):1349-1354.
44. van Oers MHJ, Tonnissen E, Van Glabbeke M, et al. BCL-2/IgH polymerase chain reaction status at the end of induction treatment is not predictive for progression-free survival in relapsed/resistant follicular lymphoma: results of a prospective randomized EORTC 20981 phase III intergroup study. *J Clin Oncol.* 2010;28(13):2246-2252.
45. Darby AJ, Lanham S, Soubeyran P, Johnson PWM. Variability of quantitative polymerase chain reaction detection of the bcl-2-IgH translocation in an international multicenter study. *Haematologica.* 2005;90(12):1706-1707.
46. Zinzani PL, Stefoni V, Tani M, et al. Role of [18F]fluorodeoxyglucose positron emission tomography scan in the follow-up of lymphoma. *J Clin Oncol.* 2009;27(11):1781-1787. PMID: 19273712.
47. Gerlinger M, Rohatiner AZ, Matthews J, Davies A, Lister TA, Montoto S. Surveillance investigations after high-dose therapy with stem cell rescue for recurrent follicular lymphoma have no impact on management. *Haematologica.* 2010;95(7):1130-1135. PMID: 20107155. PMCID: Pmc2895037. Epub 2010/01/29.
48. Dreyling M, Ghielmini M, Marcus R, Salles G, Vitolo U, Ladetto M. Newly diagnosed and relapsed follicular lymphoma: ESMO clinical practice guidelines for diagnosis, treatment and follow-up. *Ann Oncol.* 2014;25(suppl 3):iii76-iii82.
49. Soubeyran P, Eghbali H, Trojani M, Bonichon F, Richaud P, Hoerni B. Is there any place for a wait-and-see policy in stage I0 follicular lymphoma? A study of 43 consecutive patients in a single center. *Ann Oncol.* 1996;7(7):713-718.
50. Gospodarowicz MK, Bush RS, Brown TC, Chua T. Prognostic factors in nodular lymphomas: a multivariate analysis based on the Princess Margaret Hospital experience. *Int J Radiat Oncol Biol Phys.* 1984;10(4):489-497.
51. Mac Manus MP, Hoppe RT. Is radiotherapy curative for stage I and II low-grade follicular lymphoma? Results of a long-term follow-up study of patients treated at Stanford University. *J Clin Oncol.* 1996;14(4):1282-1290.
52. Wilder RB, Jones D, Tucker SL, et al. Long-term results with radiotherapy for stage I-II follicular lymphomas. *Int J Radiat Oncol Biol Phys.* 2001;51(5):1219-1227.
53. Peterson PM, Gospodarowicz M, Tsang R. Long-term outcome in stage I and II follicular lymphoma following treatment with involved field radiation therapy alone. *ASCO Meeting Abstracts.* 2004:563.
54. Seymour JF, Pro B, Fuller LM, et al. Long-term follow-up of a prospective study of combined modality therapy for stage I-II indolent non-Hodgkin's lymphoma. *J Clin Oncol.* 2003;21(11): 2115-2122.
55. Friedberg JW, Byrtek M, Link BK, et al. Effectiveness of first-line management strategies for stage I follicular lymphoma: analysis of the National LymphoCare Study. *J Clin Oncol.* 2012;30(27): 3368-3375.
56. Friedberg JW, Taylor MD, Cerhan JR, et al. Follicular lymphoma in the United States: first report of the National LymphoCare Study. *J Clin Oncol.* 2009;27(8):1202-1208. PMID: PMC2738614.
57. Ardeshna KM, Smith P, Norton A, et al. Long-term effect of a watch and wait policy versus immediate systemic treatment for asymptomatic advanced-stage non-Hodgkin lymphoma: a randomised controlled trial. *Lancet.* 2003;362(9383):516-522. PMID: 12932382.
58. Young RC, Longo DL, Glatstein E, Ihde DC, Jaffe ES, DeVita VT Jr. The treatment of indolent lymphomas: watchful waiting v aggressive combined modality treatment. *Semin Hematol.* 1988;25(2 suppl 2):11-16. PMID: 2456618.
59. Brice P, Bastion Y, Lepage E, et al. Comparison in low-tumor-burden follicular lymphomas between an initial no-treatment policy, prednimustine, or interferon alfa: a randomized study from the Groupe d'Etude des Lymphomes Folliculaires. Groupe d'Etude des Lymphomes de l'Adulte. *J Clin Oncol.* 1997;15(3): 1110-1117. PMID: 9060552.
60. Ardeshna KM, Qian W, Smith P, et al. Rituximab versus a watch-and-wait approach in patients with advanced-stage, asymptomatic, non-bulky follicular lymphoma: an open-label randomised phase 3 trial. *Lancet Oncol.* 2014;15(4):424-435.
61. Kahl BS, Hong F, Williams ME, et al. Rituximab extended schedule or re-treatment trial for low-tumor burden follicular lymphoma: eastern cooperative oncology group protocol e4402. *J Clin Oncol.* 2014;32(28):3096-3102.
62. Herold M, Haas A, Srock S, et al. Rituximab added to first-line mitoxantrone, chlorambucil, and prednisolone chemotherapy followed by interferon maintenance prolongs survival in patients with advanced follicular lymphoma: an East German Study Group Hematology and Oncology Study. *J Clin Oncol.* 2007;25(15):1986-1992.
63. Hiddemann W, Kneba M, Dreyling M, et al. Frontline therapy with rituximab added to the combination of cyclophosphamide, doxorubicin, vincristine, and prednisone (CHOP) significantly improves the outcome for patients with advanced-stage follicular lymphoma compared with therapy with CHOP alone: results of a prospective randomized study of the German Low-Grade Lymphoma Study Group. *Blood.* 2005;106(12):3725-3732.
64. Marcus R, Imrie K, Solal-Celigny P, et al. Phase III study of R-CVP compared with cyclophosphamide, vincristine, and prednisone alone in patients with previously untreated advanced follicular lymphoma. *J Clin Oncol.* 2008;26(28):4579-4586. PMID: 18662969.

65. McLaughlin P, Hagemeister F, Rodriguez M. Safety of fludarabine, mitoxantrone, and dexamethasone combined with rituximab in the treatment of stage IV indolent lymphoma. *Semin Oncol.* 2000;27(6, S12):37-41.
66. Rummel MJ, Niederle N, Maschmeyer G, et al. Bendamustine plus rituximab versus CHOP plus rituximab as first-line treatment for patients with indolent and mantle-cell lymphomas: an open-label, multicentre, randomised, phase 3 non-inferiority trial. *Lancet.* 2013;381(9873):1203-1210.
67. Federico M, Luminari S, Dondi A, et al. R-CVP versus R-CHOP versus R-FM for the initial treatment of patients with advanced-stage follicular lymphoma: results of the FOLL05 trial conducted by the Fondazione Italiana Linfomi. *J Clin Oncol.* 2013;31(12): 1506-1513.
68. Flinn IW, van der Jagt R, Kahl BS, et al. Randomized trial of bendamustine-rituximab or R-CHOP/R-CVP in first-line treatment of indolent NHL or MCL: the BRIGHT study. *Blood.* 2014;123(19):2944-2952. PMID: 24591201. PMCID: 4260975.
69. Fowler NH, Davis RE, Rawal S, et al. Safety and activity of lenalidomide and rituximab in untreated indolent lymphoma: an open-label, phase 2 trial. *Lancet Oncol.* 2014;15(12):1311-1318.
70. Salles G, Seymour JF, Offner F, et al. Rituximab maintenance for 2 years in patients with high tumour burden follicular lymphoma responding to rituximab plus chemotherapy (PRIMA): a phase 3, randomised controlled trial. *Lancet.* 2011;377(9759): 42-51. PMID: 21176949.
71. Morschhauser F, Radford J, Van Hoof A, et al. Phase III trial of consolidation therapy with yttrium-90-ibritumomab tiuxetan compared with no additional therapy after first remission in advanced follicular lymphoma. *J Clin Oncol.* 2008;26(32):5156-5164.
72. Press OW, Unger JM, Rimsza LM, et al. Phase III randomized Intergroup trial of CHOP plus rituximab compared with CHOP chemotherapy plus 131iodine-tositumomab for previously untreated follicular non-Hodgkin lymphoma: SWOG S0016. *J Clin Oncol.* 2013;31(3):314-320.
73. Advani RH, Buggy JJ, Sharman JP, et al. Bruton tyrosine kinase inhibitor ibrutinib (PCI-32765) has significant activity in patients with relapsed/refractory B-cell malignancies. *J Clin Oncol.* 2013;31(1):88-94. PMID: 23045577.
74. Gopal AK, Kahl BS, de Vos S, et al. PI3Kδ inhibition by idelalisib in patients with relapsed indolent lymphoma. *N Engl J Med.* 2014;370(11):1008-1018.
75. de Vos S, Goy A, Dakhil SR, et al. Multicenter randomized phase II study of weekly or twice-weekly bortezomib plus rituximab in patients with relapsed or refractory follicular or marginal-zone B-cell lymphoma. *J Clin Oncol.* 2009;27(30):5023-5030.
76. Wang ML, Rule S, Martin P, et al. Targeting BTK with ibrutinib in relapsed or refractory mantle-cell lymphoma. *N Engl J Med.* 2013;369(6):507-516. PMID: 23782157.
77. Westin JR, Chu F, Zhang M, et al. Safety and activity of PD1 blockade by pidilizumab in combination with rituximab in patients with relapsed follicular lymphoma: a single group, open-label, phase 2 trial. *Lancet Oncol.* 2014;15(1):69-77. PMID: 24332512. PMCID: 3922714.
78. Rohatiner AZS, Nadler L, Davies AJ, et al. Myeloablative therapy with autologous bonerow transplantation for follicular lymphoma at the time of second or subsequent remission: long-term follow-up. *J Clin Oncol.* 2007;25(18):2554-2559.
79. Khouri IF, Wei W, Korbling M, et al. BFR (bendamustine, fludarabine, and rituximab) allogeneic conditioning for chronic lymphocytic leukemia/lymphoma: reduced myelosuppression and GVHD. *Blood.* 2014;124(14):2306-2312.
80. Ferrajoli A, O'Brien S, Keating MJ. Alemtuzumab: a novel monoclonal antibody. *Expert Opin Biol Ther.* 2001;1(6):1059-1065. PMID: 11728236.
81. Admirand JH, Rassidakis GZ, Abruzzo LV, Valbuena JR, Jones D, Medeiros LJ. Immunohistochemical detection of ZAP-70 in 341 cases of non-Hodgkin and Hodgkin lymphoma. *Mod Pathol.* 2004;17(8):954-961.
82. Aoun P, Blair HE, Smith LM, et al. Fluorescence in situ hybridization detection of cytogenetic abnormalities in B-cell chronic lymphocytic leukemia/small lymphocytic lymphoma. *Leuk Lymphoma.* 2004;45(8):1595-1603.
83. Rawstron AC, Bennett FL, O'Connor SJ, et al. Monoclonal B-cell lymphocytosis and chronic lymphocytic leukemia. *N Engl J Med.* 2008;359(6):575-583. PMID: 18687638.
84. Gibson SE, Swerdlow SH, Ferry JA, et al. Reassessment of small lymphocytic lymphoma in the era of monoclonal B-cell lymphocytosis. *Haematologica.* 2011;96(8):1144-1152. PMID: 21546505. PMCID: 3148908.
85. Steinbach G, Ford R, Glober G, et al. Antibiotic treatment of gastric lymphoma of mucosa-associated lymphoid tissue. An uncontrolled trial. *Ann Intern Med.* 1999;131(2):88-95.
86. Wotherspoon AC, Doglioni C, Diss TC, et al. Regression of primary low-grade B-cell gastric lymphoma of mucosa-associated lymphoid tissue type after eradication of *Helicobacter pylori. Lancet.* 1993;342(8871):575-577.
87. Vinatzer U, Gollinger M, Mullauer L, Raderer M, Chott A, Streubel B. Mucosa-associated lymphoid tissue lymphoma: novel translocations including rearrangements of ODZ2, JMJD2C, and CNN3. *Clin Cancer Res.* 2008;14(20):6426-6431.
88. Isaacson PG, Du MQ. MALT lymphoma: from morphology to molecules. *Nat Rev Cancer.* 2004;4(8):644-653. PMID: 15286744.
89. Conconi A, Martinelli G, Thieblemont C, et al. Clinical activity of rituximab in extranodal marginal zone B-cell lymphoma of MALT type. *Blood.* 2003;102(8):2741-2745.
90. Samaniego F, Fanale M, Pro B, et al. Pentostatin, cyclophosphamide, and rituximab (PCR) achieve high response rates in indolent B-cell lyphoma without prolonged myelosuppression. ASH Annual Meeting Abstracts. 2008;112(11):835.
91. Vega F, Cho-Vega JH, Lennon PA, et al. Splenicginal zone lymphomas are characterized by loss of interstitial regions of chromosome 7q, 7q31.32 and 7q36.2 that include the protection of telomere 1 (POT1) and sonic hedgehog (SHH) genes. *Br J Haematol.* 2008;142(2):216-226.
92. Martinez-Lopez A, Curiel-Olmo S, Mollejo M, et al. MYD88 (L265P) Somatic mutation in marginal zone B-cell lymphoma. *Am J Surg Pathol.* 2015;39(5):644-651. PMID: 25723115.
93. Owen RG, Treon SP, Al-Katib A, et al. Clinicopathological definition of Waldenstrom's macroglobulinemia: consensus panel recommendations from the Second International Workshop on Waldenstrom's Macroglobulinemia. *Semin Oncol.* 2003;30(2): 110-115.
94. Dimopoulos MA, Gertz MA, Kastritis E, et al. Update on treatment recommendations from the Fourth International Workshop on Waldenstrom's Macroglobulinemia. *J Clin Oncol.* 2009; 27(1):120-126. PMID: 19047284.
95. Lin P, Hao S, Handy BC, Bueso-Ramos CE, Medeiros LJ. Lymphoid neoplasms associated with IgM paraprotein: a study of 382 patients. *Am J Clin Pathol.* 2005;123(2):200-205.
96. Lin P, Mansoor A, Bueso-Ramos C, Hao S, Lai R, Medeiros LJ. Diffuse large B-cell lymphoma occurring in patients with lymphoplasmacytic lymphoma/Waldenstrom macroglobulinemia. Clinicopathologic features of 12 cases. *Am J Clin Pathol.* 2003; 120(2):246-253.
97. Treon SP, Xu L, Yang G, et al. MYD88 L265P somatic mutation in Waldenstrom's macroglobulinemia. *N Engl J Med.* 2012;367(9): 826-833. PMID: 22931316.
98. Treon SP, Cao Y, Xu L, Yang G, Liu X, Hunter ZR. Somatic mutations in MYD88 and CXCR4 are determinants of clinical presentation and overall survival in Waldenstrom macroglobulinemia. *Blood.* 2014;123(18):2791-2796. PMID: 24553177.

8 Aggressive B-Cell Lymphomas

第八章　侵袭性B细胞淋巴瘤

Jason R. Westin
Sergej N. Konoplev
Luis E. Fayad
L. Jeffrey Medeiros

中文导读

作为淋巴瘤中最常见的发病类型，随着医学探索及经验积累，对侵袭性B细胞淋巴瘤的研究有了进一步的深入和发展。本章主要介绍了侵袭性B细胞淋巴瘤的流行病学、病因学、临床表现、病理诊断、临床特征等内容，同时针对侵袭性B细胞淋巴瘤的主要亚型，如弥漫大B细胞淋巴瘤、套细胞淋巴瘤、伯基特淋巴瘤，从发病率、诊断、组织病理学、生存率等方面进行了详细描述。本章随后重点阐述了影像学检查及骨髓活检在侵袭性B细胞淋巴瘤初诊和临床分期中的应用、预后因素以及不同分期和特殊类型侵袭性B细胞淋巴瘤的治疗方案选择。围绕复发/难治性淋巴瘤、高级别B细胞淋巴瘤、老年侵袭性B细胞淋巴瘤这些热点问题，本章也对其诊疗现状进行了概述和治疗推荐。此外本章对疗效评估、生存期随访、复发/难治淋巴瘤的判定都进行了详细的描述，并强调关注侵袭性B细胞淋巴瘤患者诊疗的全程管理。本章最后探讨了新药和临床试验，揭示了侵袭性B细胞淋巴瘤分子生物学、转化医学方面的研究将迎来新的发展机遇。

It is clinically useful to divide non-Hodgkin lymphomas (NHL) into indolent and aggressive based on their clinical behavior ([1]). Patients with indolent NHL typically have a survival of many years, even if untreated, but paradoxically are usually incurable. Patients with aggressive NHL have a survival time measured in weeks to months if untreated yet are usually chemosensitive and frequently curable. In this chapter, we focus on the clinical characteristics, pathology, and treatment of aggressive NHL.

EPIDEMIOLOGY

The incidence of NHL has increased over the last five decades, as reported by US and international registries ([2-4]). During the years 1993 to 1995, the age-adjusted incidence increased 3% per year according to data from the Surveillance, Epidemiology, and End Results (SEER) program of the National Cancer Institute ([2]). Some of this increased incidence can be attributed to the acquired immunodeficiency syndrome (AIDS), but this epidemic does not explain the increase of NHL before 1980. In the elderly population, there has also been a marked increase of NHL, largely the indolent NHLs, which are discussed in Chapter 7.

An estimated 71,850 new cases of NHL will be diagnosed in the United States in 2015, and 19,790 NHL-related deaths will occur. In 2014, NHL was the ninth largest cause of death among men and the eighth largest cause in women (3% of all cancer-related deaths). Diffuse large B-cell lymphoma (DLBCL), the most common NHL subtype, has an aggressive behavior and is more common in whites than African Americans in the United States; however, 5-year survival outcomes are worse in African Americans ([5]).

ETIOLOGY

Most cases of aggressive NHL do not have a well-defined cause. Recent work has shown that the lifetime risk for many cancers correlates with the total number of divisions of normal self-renewing cells ([6]). The implications of these findings suggest that many cancers may not be due to hereditable genetic aberrancies, environmental exposures, infectious etiologies, or other known causes, but instead are attributable to a combination of factors that may include chance. For the NHLs that appear to have currently identifiable drivers, there are four groups of drivers: immune suppression (both acquired and primary), infectious agents, toxic exposure, and familial (Table 8-1).

The strongest association is with immune suppression, both primary and acquired ([7]). Examples of primary immunodeficiency include inherited immune disorders, such as Wiskott-Aldrich syndrome, severe combined immune deficiency, common variable immune deficiency, and ataxia-telangiectasia ([8]). These and other inherited disorders are associated with an increased lifetime risk of developing NHL, with aggressive B-cell NHL being most common.

Table 8-1 Risk Factors Associated With Aggressive Non-Hodgkin Lymphomas

Inherited and acquired immune deficiency
Wiskott-Aldrich syndrome
Ataxia-telangiectasia
Chédiak-Higashi syndrome
X-linked immunoproliferative disorder
Severe combined immunodeficiency
Common variable immune deficiency
Iatrogenic immune suppression
Solid organ or bone marrow transplant
Toxic exposures
Prior chemotherapy
Phenoxyherbicides
Dioxin
Radiation or radiation therapy
Infectious exposures
Epstein-Barr virus
Human T-cell leukemia/lymphoma virus
Human herpesvirus type 8 (HHV-8)
Human immunodeficiency virus (HIV)
Autoimmune disorders
Sjögren syndrome
Celiac sprue
Systemic lupus erythematosus
Rheumatoid arthritis

Patients who are immunosuppressed for therapeutic reasons—for example, after transplantation—are also at increased risk of NHL, especially if treated with cyclosporine, azathioprine, prednisone, or monoclonal antibodies for the removal of T cells ([9]). A loose association can be drawn between the level of immune suppression and lymphoma risk. Transplant patients treated with the highest doses of immunosuppressive agents, such as heart transplant recipients, are at greater risk of developing lymphomas. These lesions are also more likely to be aggressive, extranodal forms. Individuals treated with pharmacologic immune suppression for autoimmune disorders—such as systemic lupus erythematosus, Sjögren syndrome, or rheumatoid arthritis—are also at increased risk for NHL, including the tumor necrosis factor antagonists ([10]). A subset of these NHLs is histologically aggressive and associated with Epstein-Barr virus (EBV). These lesions may regress following withdrawal of the immunosuppressive agent, speaking to the complex interaction between the immune system and an immune clonal population ([11]).

CHAPTER 8

Infectious agents associated with development of aggressive NHL include human immunodeficiency virus (HIV), EBV, human herpesvirus type 8, and human T-cell lymphotropic virus type 1 ([12]). The greatest factor involved in the worldwide increase in NHL, although lessened with the advent of highly active antiretroviral therapy (HAART), is HIV infection ([13]). The risk of NHL is increased by up to 300% in untreated HIV-infected patients, rising in proportion to the duration of the HIV infection. Although the risk of NHL in HIV-infected patients appears to be decreased by HAART, the relative risk of NHL remains much higher than that for those not infected with HIV. Aggressive NHL can occur in HIV-infected patients at any stage of infection, but the risk increases as CD4 counts drop to $<100 \times 10^3/\mu L$, and NHL is considered an AIDS-defining illness.

EBV also plays a role in lymphomagenesis, due in part to chronic antigenic stimulation ([14]). EBV is virtually always associated with certain types of NHL, such as endemic (African) Burkitt lymphoma (BL) and extranodal T-cell/natural killer (NK)-cell lymphoma of nasal type, with many other NHL subtypes occasionally involved. Many patients with HIV-related lymphomas are co-infected by EBV, including HIV-associated primary central nervous system (CNS) lymphoma, which is infected in essentially 100% of cases ([15]). Human herpesvirus type 8 is associated with primary effusion lymphoma (PEL), which tends to occur in HIV-infected patients. Human T-cell lymphotropic virus type 1 is associated with adult T-cell lymphoma/leukemia.

Environmental and occupational exposures to toxins are associated with an increased risk of NHL ([16]). Herbicides, especially phenoxyacetic acid derivatives, are associated with NHL, especially in the farming belts of the United States. Occupations held by individuals reported to be at increased risk for NHL include farming, metalworking, forestry, aircraft maintenance, woodworking, and dry cleaning. One of the common exposures in these industries is the use of organic solvents.

Family history of NHL is also a potential risk factor for some lymphomas. Individuals who have relatives with NHL may have a slightly higher risk of developing NHL, but data are inconclusive and mechanisms are unclear ([17]).

CLINICAL PRESENTATION

The clinical presentation of patients with aggressive NHL varies substantially based on histologic type and anatomic site of disease. The likelihood of B symptoms, including fever greater than 38°C, night sweats, or weight loss greater than 10% of body weight in the preceding 6 months, increases with NHL aggressiveness. Approximately 50% of patients present with these B symptoms, often with fatigue, malaise, and pruritus, although these are less common initially.

Most patients present with painless lymphadenopathy, which is often first treated with antibiotics for presumed infection and eventually biopsied when lymph nodes fail to regress. The most common scenario involves a diagnosis based on examination of peripheral lymph nodes, which may be detectable prior to internal lymph nodes becoming enlarged and causing symptoms. Peripheral lymph nodes are not usually painful, unless they are rapidly enlarging or are massive. Symptoms vary with the anatomic site of internal lymphadenopathy. Patients with mediastinal lymphadenopathy frequently experience cough, chest pain, and less commonly superior vena cava syndrome. Patients with large nodal masses in the abdomen or retroperitoneum frequently experience pain, abdominal fullness, or early satiety. Retroperitoneal lymphadenopathy can cause back pain and discomfort.

Extranodal disease is common in patients with aggressive NHL. The most common extranodal sites are the intestines, tonsils, and skin, although the frequency of involvement of these sites varies across reports. Disease in the gastrointestinal (GI) tract can present with nonspecific symptoms, including obstruction, blood loss with subsequent anemia, or diarrhea. Other extranodal sites include liver, lung, testis, bones, CNS, and spleen; however, aggressive extranodal NHL may involve nearly any organ system.

CLINICOPATHOLOGIC CHARACTERISTICS

Diffuse Large B-Cell Lymphoma, Not Otherwise Specified

Diffuse large B-cell lymphoma is the most common type of NHL ([1, 18]). It occurs mainly in adults, with a median age in the sixth decade. Men are affected slightly more often than women. B-type symptoms or bulky disease occurs in one-third of patients. Nodal presentation is most common, but extranodal sites are involved in approximately 40% of patients (Figs. 8-1 and 8-2), and more than one-third of patients have more than one extranodal site of disease. Slightly more than half of patients have stage III or IV disease ([19]). Bone marrow involvement occurs in approximately 10% to 20% of patients. Diffuse large B-cell lymphoma uncommonly involves privileged sites, such as the testis and CNS, of which the latter portends a poor prognosis.

If untreated, DLBCL is invariably fatal, but DLBCL is generally sensitive to chemotherapy, at least initially.

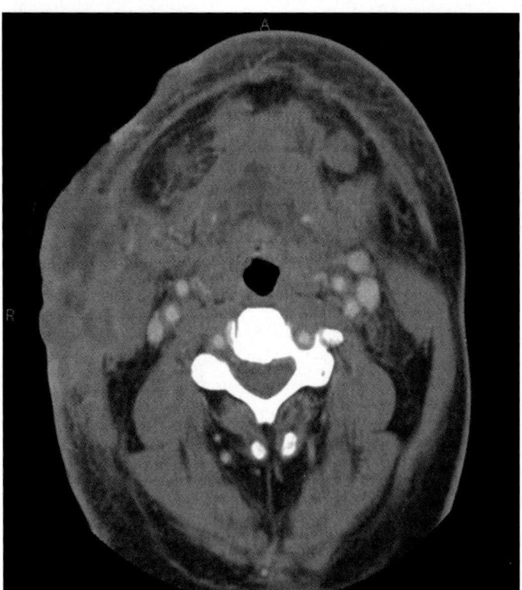

FIGURE 8-1 Computed tomography scan showing diffuse large B-cell lymphoma with extensive lymph node involvement in the neck.

With current immune-chemotherapy approaches, a slight majority of patients will be cured of their disease, with 2-year event-free survival of approximately 70% ([20]). The International Prognostic Index (IPI) score remains a widely used prognostic model, despite not accounting for any tumor-specific biologic features. With rituximab plus chemotherapy–based disease management, the 4-year progression-free and overall survival rates for DLBCL patients with a Revised IPI (R-IPI) of 0, 1 to 2, and 3 to 5 are as shown in Table 8-2 ([21]).

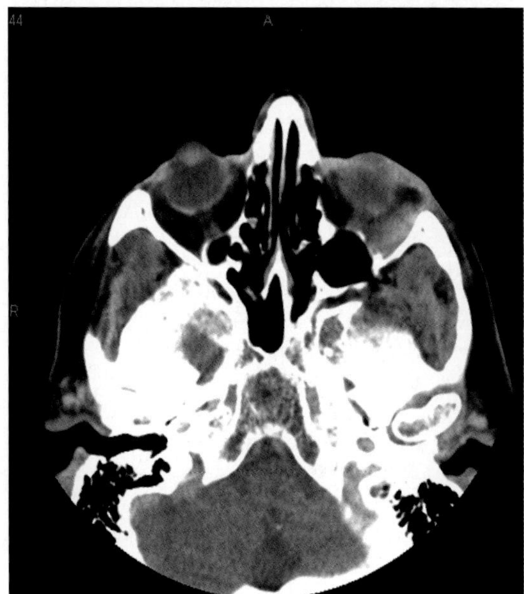

FIGURE 8-2 Computed tomography scan showing diffuse large B-cell lymphoma as a periorbital mass.

These data are generally useful but unfortunately are not predictive of outcomes for an individual patient. Nearly half of patients will have a poor-risk R-IPI, and of these patients, approximately half will be cured and half will die of disease. Few patients with relapsed disease are cured.

The diagnosis of DLBCL is based on its diffuse growth pattern and large neoplastic cells, with frequent mitotic figures ([1]). Cytologically, the neoplastic cells can be subdivided as large centrocytes, centroblasts, or immunoblasts. Large centrocytes range from 13 to 30 mm in size and have irregular or cleaved nuclear contours, relatively small, indistinct nucleoli, and a thin rim of eosinophilic cytoplasm. Centroblasts are 20 to 30 mm in size and have round or oval vesicular nuclei with two or three nucleoli and more abundant amphophilic cytoplasm (Figs. 8-3 and 8-4). Immunoblasts are larger than centroblasts, with an eccentrically located vesicular round or oval nucleus containing a prominent target-like central nucleolus and relatively abundant amphophilic, often plasmacytoid cytoplasm (Fig. 8-5). Elevated proliferation (Ki-67) rates and immunoblastic features appear to correlate with *MYC* rearrangements ([22]).

Immunophenotypic studies have shown that DLBCLs are of mature B-cell lineage. Approximately two-thirds of cases express monotypic immunoglobulin (Ig). These tumors express pan-B-cell antigens, 60% to 70% express BCL2, and a subset is positive for CD10 and BCL6.

Diffuse large B-cell lymphomas are heterogeneous at the molecular level. A subset of cases carries the t(14;18) involving *BCL2*, as shown by conventional cytogenetic or molecular studies ([23,24]). Another subset of DLBCLs has translocations or other abnormalities involving *BCL6* at chromosome 3q27. *BCL6* is rearranged in approximately 20% to 40% of DLBCLs, more often in tumors arising at extranodal sites ([25]). Recently, DLBCLs with translocations involving both

Table 8-2 Survival Rates for Diffuse Large B-Cell Lymphoma Patients

Revised IPI	No. of Factors Present	% of Patients	4-Year PFS	4-Year OS
Very good	0	10	94	94
Good	1-2	45	80	79
Poor	3-5	45	53	55

IPI, International Prognostic Index; OS, overall survival; PFS, progression-free survival.

MYC and *BCL2* or *BCL6*, representing approximately 5% to 10% of DLBCL, have been shown to have an extremely aggressive behavior and are commonly referred to as "double-hit" DLBCL ([26]). Diffuse large B-cell lymphomas with overexpression of MYC and BCL2 or BCL6 protein levels are more common and are designated double-positive DLBCLs. These tumors are still adverse compared to DLBCLs without protein overexpression but less so than translocation-defined double-hit DLBCLs ([27-29]).

Gene expression profiling (GEP) can molecularly divide DLBCL into three groups: germinal center B-cell like (GCB), activated B-cell like (ABC), and a third noncharacteristic group. Patients with the GCB type of DLBCL have a better prognosis independent of the IPI ([30, 31]). Despite the initial GEP studies of DLBCL occurring approximately 15 years ago, this technology is not routinely used in clinical practice due to logistical issues and need for significant bioinformatic analysis. Fortunately, new technologies may allow these issues to finally be overcome by limiting the number of genes analyzed, such as in the Lymph-2Cx Nanostring assay (Nanostring, Seattle, WA) ([32]). In lieu of GEP, a limited number of immunohistochemical markers, including CD10, MUM-1, BCL6, GCET1, and FOXP1, can subclassify DLBCL into GCB and non-GCB with relatively good concordance with GEP ([33, 34]).

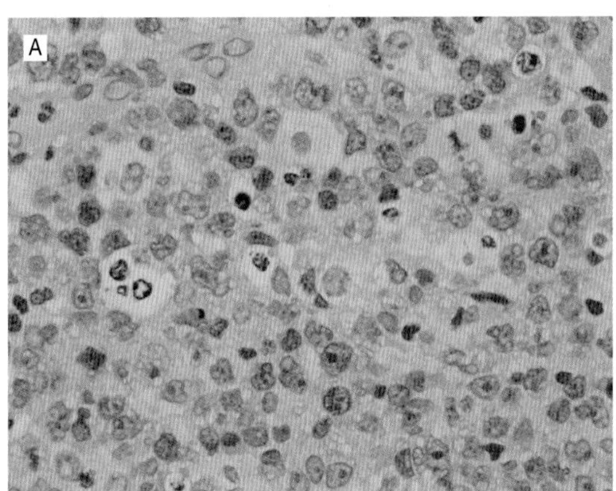

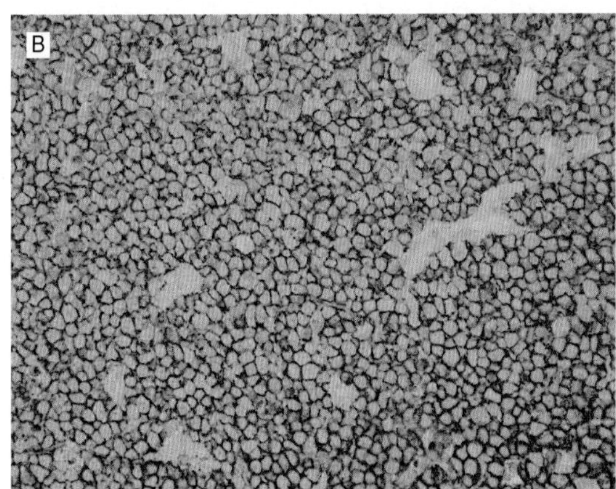

FIGURE 8-3 Diffuse large B-cell lymphoma. A. The neoplastic cells are large with vesicular chromatin and are arranged in a diffuse pattern. B. The neoplastic cells are positive for CD20. (A, hematoxylin-eosin, 1,000×; B, immunohistochemistry, 400×.)

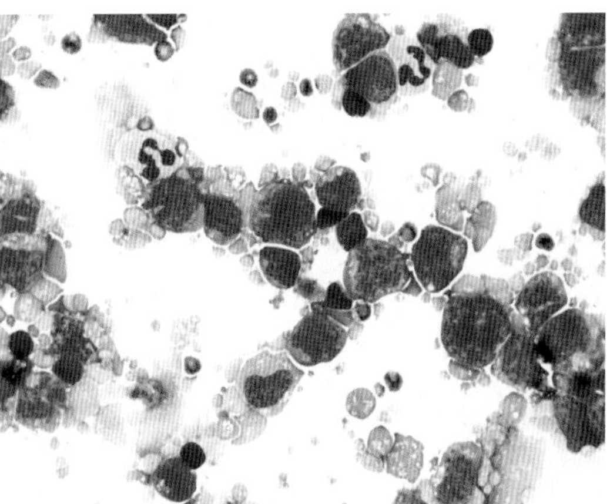

FIGURE 8-4 Diffuse large B-cell lymphoma. Fine-needle aspiration of cervical lymph node. The neoplastic cells are large (compared with neutrophils in field) with abundant basophilic cytoplasm (Wright-Giemsa, 1,000×).

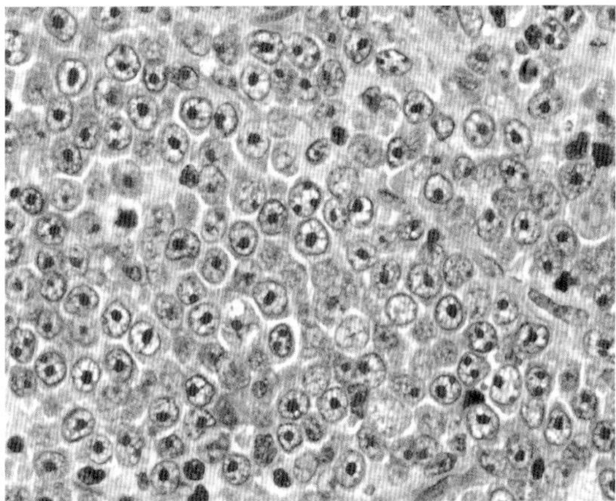

FIGURE 8-5 Diffuse large B-cell lymphoma, immunoblastic variant. The neoplastic cells are large with prominent central nucleoli imparting a "target-like" appearance (hematoxylin-eosin, 1,000×).

Diffuse Large B-Cell Lymphoma Clinicopathologic Subtypes

T-Cell/Histiocyte-Rich B-Cell Lymphoma

T-cell/histiocyte-rich (TCHR) DLBCL is a diffuse neoplasm in which most of the cells are reactive T cells and histiocytes and the large, neoplastic B cells represent <10% of all cells in the infiltrate (Fig. 8-6). Patients with TCHR-DLBCL commonly have a history of nodular lymphocyte-predominant Hodgkin lymphoma, and TCHR-DLBCL may represent a transformation event in some patients.

Primary Diffuse Large B-Cell Lymphoma of the Central Nervous System

This entity includes all primary intracerebral or intraocular lymphomas. Although these lymphomas are remarkable for their unique clinical presentation, histologically and at the immunophenotypic level, these neoplasms closely resemble other cases of systemic DLBCL. In HIV-positive patients, the neoplastic cells commonly have immunoblastic features and are positive for EBV. Approximately, one-third of the cases demonstrate translocations involving the *BCL6* gene.

Primary Cutaneous Diffuse Large B-Cell Lymphoma, Leg Type

As the name suggests, DLBCL, leg type, presents as cutaneous lesions originally described in the lower extremities, although all skin sites may be affected. Lesions often are initially confused with an insect bite, but eventually become diffuse and ulcerated, and the clinical course is aggressive. Histologic sections show diffuse sheets of monotonous neoplastic cells with centroblastic or immunoblastic morphology with frequent mitotic figures ([36]). The neoplastic cells have a non–germinal center B-cell immunophenotype, and fluorescence in situ hybridization studies often detect rearrangements of *BCL6*, *IGH*, and/or *MYC* ([37]).

Epstein-Barr Virus–Positive Diffuse Large B-Cell Lymphoma of the Elderly

This DLBCL is most common in the elderly, defined arbitrarily as >50 years of age but can occur in younger patients and often presents at an advanced stage. Epstein-Barr virus is a defining feature. Histologically, these neoplasms have a diffuse pattern and show a spectrum of features, and two morphologic variants are recognized: polymorphous, with a broad range of B-cell maturation in the reactive background, and monomorphous, which contains mostly large cells ([1]). Geographic necrosis is common, and the neoplastic cells usually have a non–germinal center B-cell immunophenotype.

Intravascular Large B-Cell Lymphomas

These are rare neoplasms in which the lymphoma cells are confined to intravascular spaces ([1]). The histologic diagnosis can be subtle, and therefore, diagnosis can be delayed. The neoplastic cells are large, express B-cell antigens, and usually have a non–germinal center B-cell immunophenotype. The molecular basis of intravascular large B-cell lymphoma is unknown (Fig. 8-7).

Primary Effusion Lymphoma

Primary effusion lymphoma, also known as body cavity–based lymphoma, is a very rare neoplasm of large B cells that involves a body cavity and is almost always associated with AIDS ([38]). The prognosis for patients with PEL is poor. Human herpesvirus type 8 (also known as Kaposi sarcoma–associated herpesvirus) is present in virtually all cases of PEL, and its presence selects for a distinct cellular gene expression profile ([1]). EBV is also present in most cases of PEL. An extracavitary (solid) variant of PEL also can occur, involving lymph nodes or extranodal sites ([39]).

Primary Mediastinal (Thymic) B-Cell Lymphoma

These neoplasms are thought to arise in the thymus, are usually localized to the thoracic cavity, and occur more frequently in young women, with a female-to-male ratio of 2:1 ([1]). Patients with primary mediastinal B-cell

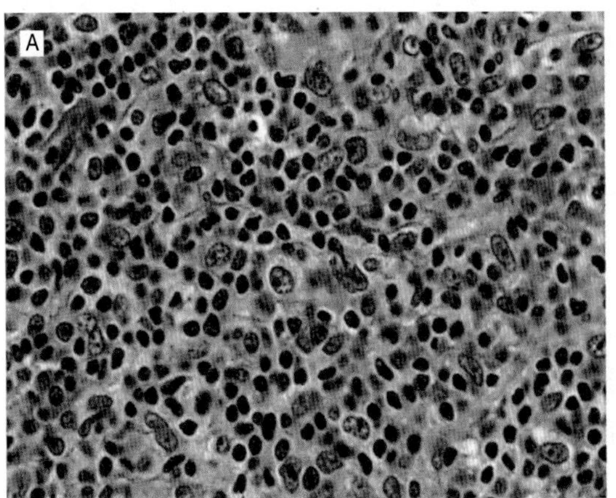

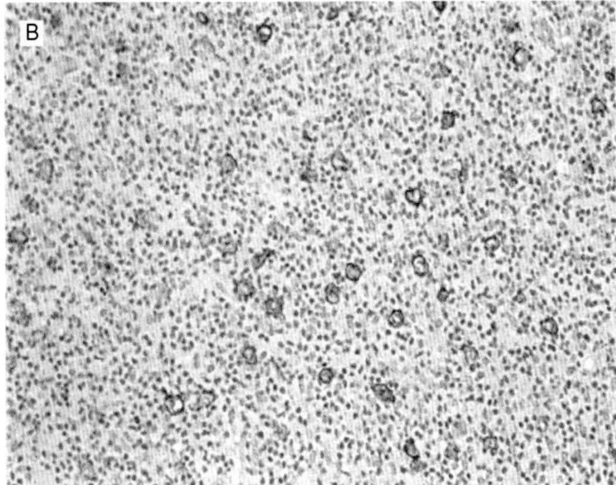

FIGURE 8-6 T-cell/histiocyte-rich large B-cell lymphoma. **A.** Scattered large neoplastic lymphoid cells in a background of numerous small lymphocytes. **B.** The large neoplastic cells are positive for CD20, and the small lymphocytes are T cells (immunostain not shown [**A**, hematoxylin-eosin, 630×]; **B**, immunohistochemistry, 200×).

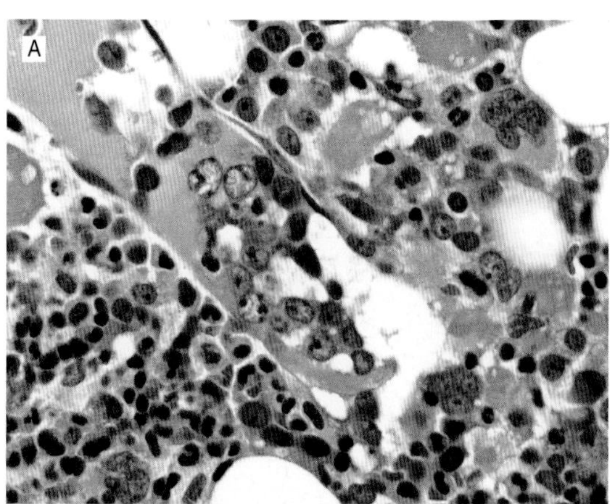

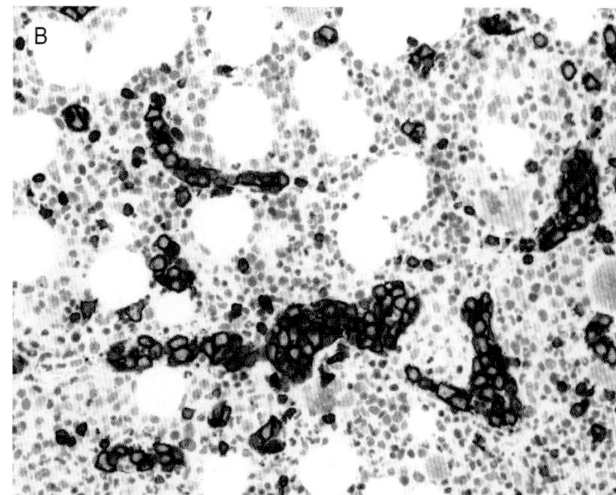

FIGURE 8-7 Intravascular large B-cell lymphoma involving bone marrow. A. Large neoplastic cells are present with a small blood vessel. B. The anti-CD20 antibody highlights numerous large neoplastic cells within many blood vessels. (A, hematoxylin-eosin, 1,000×; B, immunohistochemistry, 400×.)

lymphoma (PMBL) present frequently with cough and dyspnea mimicking a respiratory infection or, rarely, superior vena cava syndrome. Histologically, PMBL has a diffuse pattern and is composed of large lymphoid cells that exhibit a spectrum of cytologic appearances: centroblastic, immunoblastic, or a mixture. Sclerosis is common, mitotic figures are usually numerous, and the tumor cells can have clear or pale cytoplasm. Immunophenotypic studies have shown that PMBLs are frequently Ig negative and commonly lack major histocompatibility complex class II antigens. Gene expression profiling analysis of PMBL has shown significant overlap with classical Hodgkin lymphoma ([40]). Rearrangements of *CIITA* occur in about 40% of PMBLs, and amplification of the chromosome 9p24.1 locus (site of programmed death ligands) and mutations of *PTPN1* have been reported in about 25% of cases ([41]). These molecular abnormalities highlight the interaction between the immune system and PMBL in pathogenesis and suggest potential therapeutic targets.

Mantle Cell Lymphoma

Mantle cell lymphoma (MCL) represents approximately 6% of all NHLs ([19]). Patients with MCL have a median age in the seventh decade, and MCL has a male-to-female ratio of approximately 3:1 ([42]). Most patients present with advanced-stage disease, with bone marrow involvement in approximately 60% of patients, and most patients have low-level involvement of the peripheral blood. Overt leukemia may be associated with a poorer prognosis. Although GI symptoms are uncommon, 85% to 90% of MCL patients have GI involvement ([43]). Blastoid MCLs have a more aggressive clinical course and often have occult CNS involvement. In the peripheral blood, MCL can sometimes resemble B-cell prolymphocytic leukemia.

Histologically, in classical MCL, the lymph node architecture is replaced by a diffuse or vaguely nodular neoplasm (Fig. 8-8) ([1]). In a subset of cases, a mantle zone pattern results when the neoplasm selectively involves the follicular mantle zones surrounding normal or reactive germinal centers (Fig. 8-9). Cytologically, MCL is composed of a monotonous population of small lymphoid cells with slightly or clearly irregular nuclear contours (Fig. 8-10). In about 15% of cases, MCL may show blastoid (lymphoblastic-like) or pleomorphic (large cell–like) features. These neoplasms are associated with a poorer prognosis and have a high frequency of *TP53* or *TP16* mutations.

Mantle cell lymphomas express monotypic Ig light chain IgM, IgD, pan-B-cell antigens, BCL2, SOX11, alkaline phosphatase, and CD5 ([21]). A high proliferation rate, most often assessed by Ki-67 immunohistochemical analysis, predicts a poorer prognosis. t(11;14)

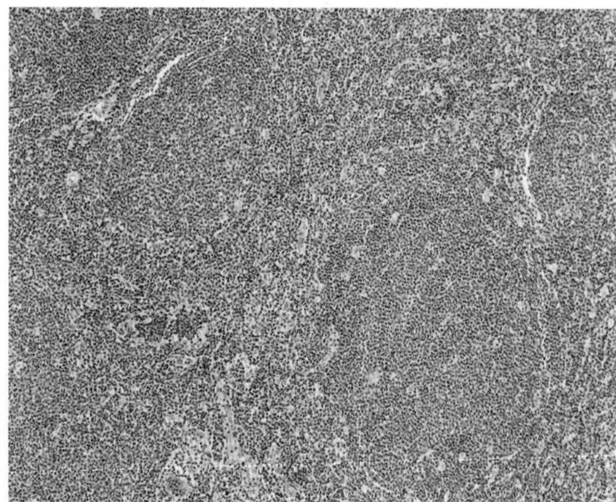

FIGURE 8-8 Mantle cell lymphoma, nodular pattern (hematoxylin-eosin, 50×).

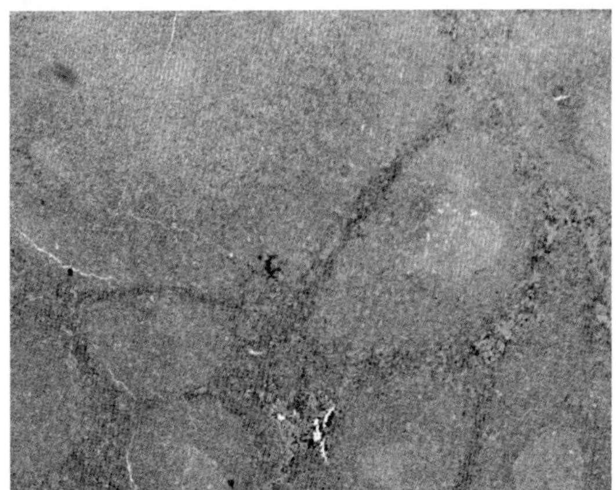

FIGURE 8-9 Mantle cell lymphoma, mantle zone pattern (hematoxylin-eosin, 50×).

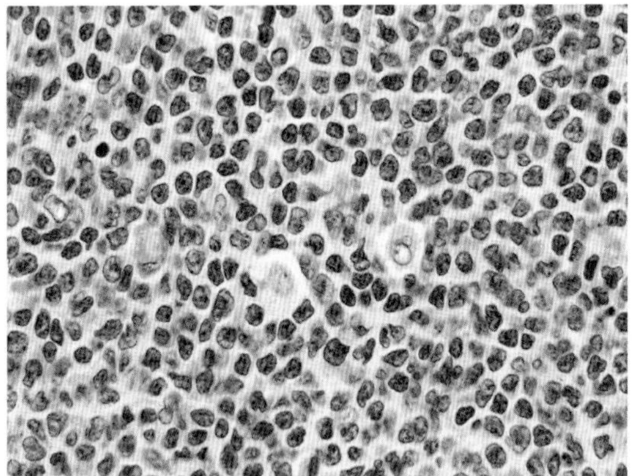

FIGURE 8-10 Mantle cell lymphoma. In this field, a uniform population of small, irregular lymphoid cells can be seen (hematoxylin-eosin, 400×).

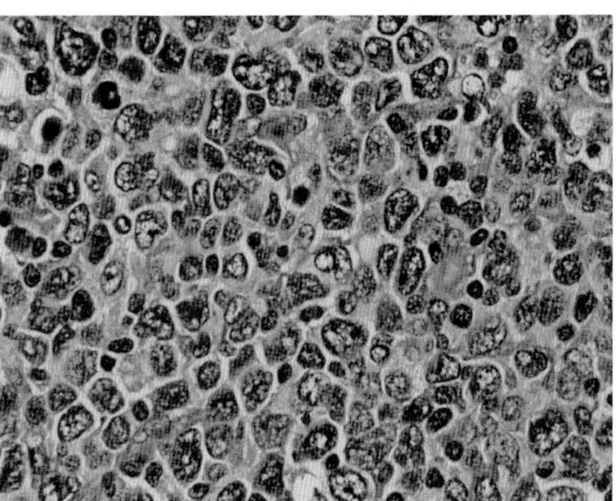

FIGURE 8-11 Mantle cell lymphoma, blastoid variant. The neoplastic cells are large and pleomorphic and were cyclin D1 positive (immunostain not shown) (hematoxylin-eosin, 1,000×).

(q13;q32) is present in virtually all cases of MCL ([44]). In this translocation, *CCND1* on 11q13 is juxtaposed with *IGH* on 14q32, resulting in overexpression of cyclin D1 (Fig. 8-11). Cyclin D1 facilitates cell cycle transition from G_1 to S phase ([45]). Although t(11;14) is central to the pathogenesis of MCL, t(11;14) is insufficient to cause lymphomagenesis. Conventional cytogenetic studies have shown a number of additional abnormalities ([46,47]), and a number of gene mutations have been reported.

Burkitt Lymphoma

There are three variants of BL: endemic (African), sporadic (nonendemic), and AIDS-associated ([21,48]). Endemic BL was first described in equatorial Africa and is associated with EBV infection in 95% of patients ([48]). The median age of patients is approximately 7 years, with a 3:1 male-to-female ratio ([49]). Abdominal and retroperitoneal lymph nodes, the GI tract, and the gonads can be involved.

Sporadic BL occurs in industrialized nations and is associated with EBV infection in approximately 25% of patients. Patients are usually in the second or third decade of life, with a male-to-female ratio of 3:1. Involvement of the jaw is uncommon, and patients may present with large masses in the abdomen, peripheral lymph nodes, pleura, or pharynx ([19]). In endemic or sporadic BL, bone marrow and CNS involvement are uncommon at presentation, but they are frequent sites of subsequent dissemination.

Burkitt lymphoma can also occur in the clinical setting of immunosuppression, including HIV infection, posttransplant, or congenital immune deficiency setting ([19]). Epstein-Barr virus infection occurs in 30% to 40% of cases.

Morphologically, all variants are similar. The relatively clear histiocytes in a background of blue lymphoma cells imparts a "starry sky" appearance (Fig. 8-12**A**). This pattern results from rapid cell turnover with individual cell necrosis and scavenging of debris by macrophages. The neoplastic cells are round to ovoid, uniform in shape, and approximately the size of benign histiocyte nuclei. The chromatin is coarse, with two to five prominent basophilic nucleoli. Mitotic figures are numerous.

Burkitt lymphomas of endemic, sporadic, and AIDS-associated types are of mature B-cell lineage and express Ig, pan-B-cell antigens, CD10, and BCL6 ([23]). Burkitt lymphomas have a very high proliferation rate (>99%) using an antibody specific for Ki-67 (Fig. 8-12**B** and **C**) and are negative for BCL2. *MYC* translocations are characteristic of BL. Approximately, 80% of

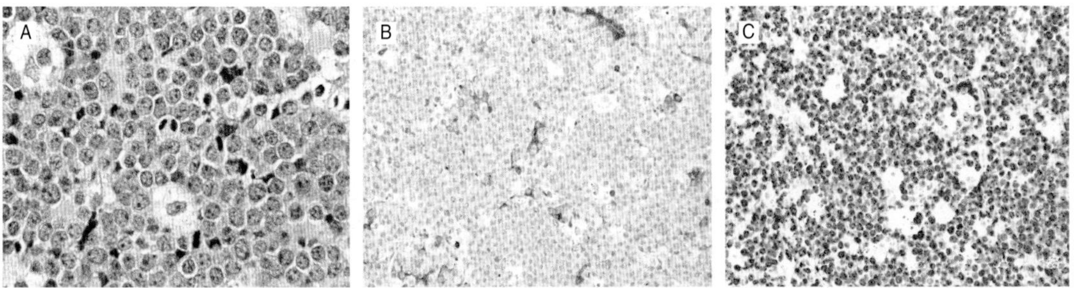

FIGURE 8-12 Burkitt lymphoma. **A.** The neoplastic cells are intermediate in size, similar to that of benign histiocyte nuclei, with multiple small nucleoli. A starry sky pattern is also seen in this field. **B and C.** The neoplastic cells are negative for BCL-2 (**B**) and are >99% positive for Ki-67 (**C**). (**A**, hematoxylin-eosin, 1,000×; **B**, **C**, immunohistochemistry, 400×.)

cases carry the t(8;14)(q24;q32), with the remaining cases having one of two variant translocations, t(2;8)(p11;q24) or t(8;22) (q24;q11) ([50-52]). Common to each of these translocations is involvement of chromosome region 8q24, the site of the *MYC*, which is deregulated. Via these translocations, *MYC* is juxtaposed with the IgH or the Ig light chain genes.

B-Cell Lymphoma With Features Intermediate Between Diffuse Large B-Cell Lymphoma and Burkitt Lymphoma

This entity in the 2008 edition of the World Health Organization (WHO) classification of hematopoietic neoplasms is designed for cases that do not fit either DLBCL or BL ([1]). In the past, these cases were designated as atypical Burkitt/Burkitt-like lymphoma or as high-grade B-cell lymphoma or B-cell lymphoma with high-grade features. This group often exhibits morphologic and immunophenotypic deviation from typical cases of BL and DLBCL. These neoplasms have a diffuse pattern, often with a starry sky appearance, and a high proliferation rate (Fig. 8-13) ([53, 54]). A significant number of cases demonstrate *MYC* rearrangement, although in some of the cases, *MYC* rearrangement involves one of the non-Ig partners ([55]). Many cases of so-called double-hit lymphoma fit within this category. These cases commonly demonstrate strong BCL2 expression and a complex karyotype ([56]). The algorithm for diagnosis of high-grade B-cell lymphoma is illustrated in Fig. 8-14.

STAGING AND INITIAL EVALUATION

The Ann Arbor Staging system, developed in 1971 for Hodgkin lymphoma, is used to stage NHL (Table 8-3) ([19]). NHLs are often disseminated at diagnosis, unlike Hodgkin lymphoma. Of interest, there does not appear to be any meaningful difference in the outcomes of patients with stage III or IV disease, and thus the purpose of staging is to identify the patients with localized NHL who may benefit from additional local therapy.

A careful history and physical examination, including the presence of systemic symptoms, is essential. Performance status and comorbid conditions should be assessed. Physical examination should include a complete survey of all external lymph node groups

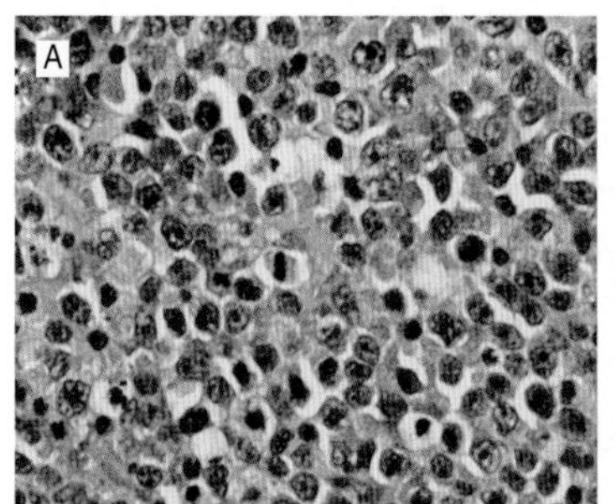

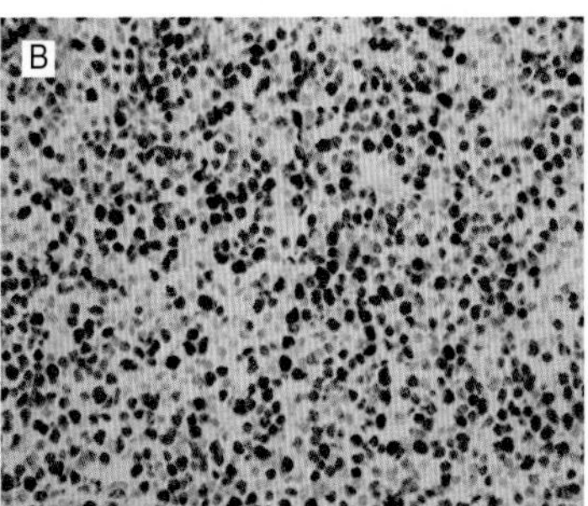

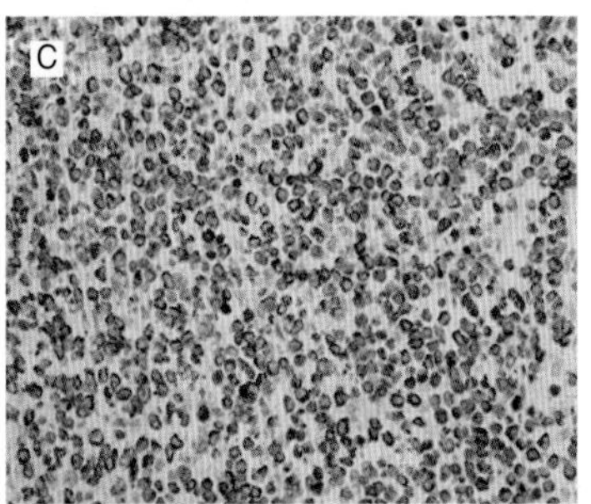

FIGURE 8-13 B-cell lymphomas with features intermediate between diffuse large B-cell lymphoma and Burkitt lymphoma. Similar to Burkitt lymphoma, the neoplastic cells are intermediate-sized and demonstrate brisk mitotic activity, but unlike Burkitt lymphoma, cells have prominent single nucleoli (**A**). While the proliferative rate is similar to Burkitt lymphoma (**B**), the neoplastic cells strongly express Bcl-2 (**C**). In this case, fluorescence in situ hybridization detected both translocations t(8;14) and t(14;18), so-called double-hit lymphoma (Lymph node, **A**, hematoxylin-eosin, 1,000×; **B**, Ki-67 (Mib-1), 400×; **C**, Bcl-2, 400×).

The Diagnostic Approach to High-Grade B-cell Lymphoma
Sheets of CD20-positive cells with many mitotic figures and high Ki-67. Tingible body macrophages ("starry-sky appearance" and areas of necrosis are commonly seen)
History of CLL/SLL
Yes
Richter Syndrome
No
TdT Expression
Yes
B Lymphoblastic Leukemia/Lymphoma
No
Cyclin D1 Expression or CCND1/IgH Rearrangement
Yes
Blastiod Mantle Cell Lymphoma
Cell Size
Large
Intermediate/Medium
MYC and BCL2 or BCL6 Rearrangement!
Homogeneous Cell Size, BCL-2-Negative, BCL-6–Strongly Positive
No
Yes
No
Yes
High-grade DLBCL, NOS
DLBCL, double-hit[1]
B-cell lymphoma,[1] unclassifiable, with features intermediate between DLBCL and Burkitt lymphoma
Burkitt lymphoma
[1]In the current WHO classification, B-cell lymphoma, unclassifiable, with features intermediate between DLBCL and Burkitt lymphoma, also includes DLBCL, double-hit.

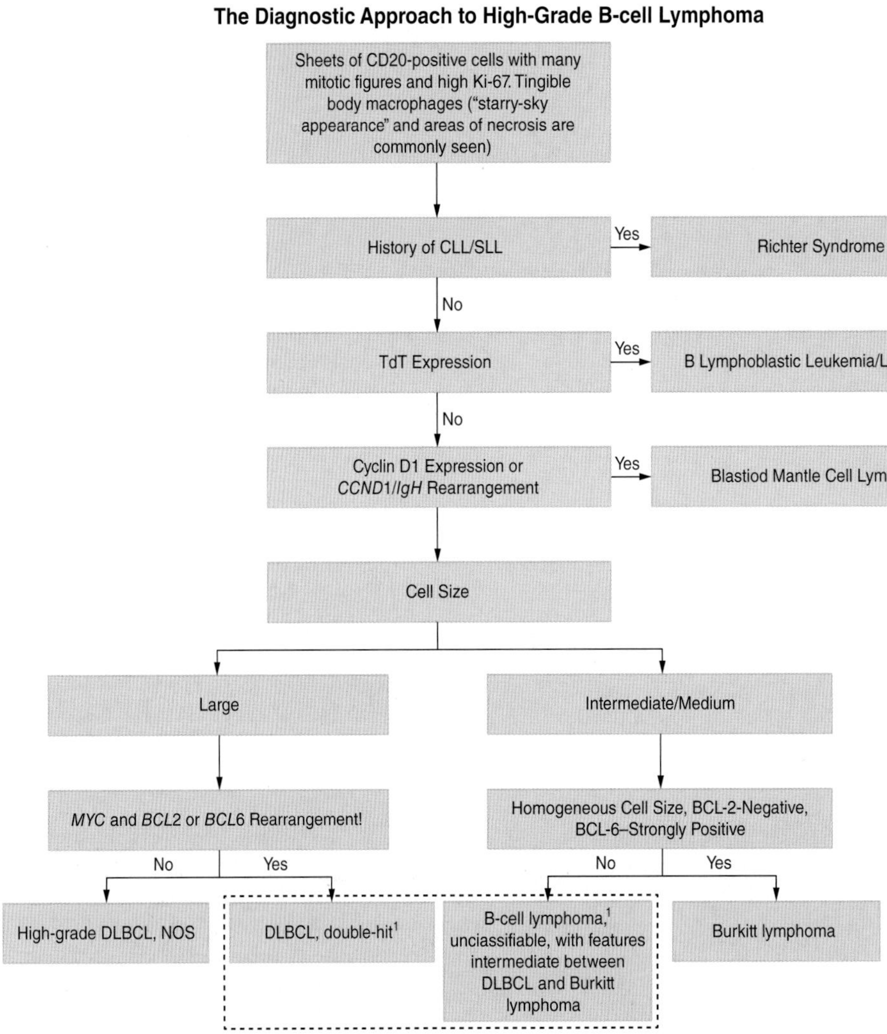

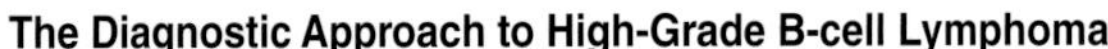

FIGURE 8-14 Algorithm for diagnosis of high-grade B-cell lymphoma. CLL, chronic lymphocytic leukemia; DLBCL, diffuse large B-cell lymphoma; NOS, not otherwise specified; SLL, small lymphocytic lymphoma; WHO, World Health Organization.

including cervical, supraclavicular, axillary, epitrochlear, inguinal, and popliteal areas. Examination of abdomen for organomegaly is necessary, and in men, the testes should be examined. A complete neurologic examination must also be performed. Laboratory evaluation includes a complete blood count with differential, lactate dehydrogenase (LDH), β_2-microglobulin, kidney and liver function tests, albumin, calcium, and uric acid. Testing for hepatitis B is indicated prior to rituximab therapy, as the virus may reactivate during or after treatment. Testing for HIV should always be performed, as should bone marrow aspiration and biopsy (bilateral biopsies for certain NHL types; also see comments on fluorodeoxyglucose [FDG] positron emission tomography [PET] and bone marrow findings below). Examination of the cerebrospinal fluid (CSF) should be strongly considered for patients with highly aggressive NHL; DLBCL associated with spinal or paraspinal masses; renal or adrenal, ovarian, breast, or skull lesions; bone marrow involvement; testicular lymphoma; or nasal or sinus lymphomas; or any patient with clinical symptoms leading to suspicion of CNS involvement ([57]).

Additional clinical evaluation is guided by the histologic type of NHL, symptoms, and anatomic sites involved by NHL. Lymphomas of the GI tract, especially in the stomach, require endoscopy for diagnosis unless other disease sites can be found to biopsy. It is especially important that multiple biopsies of different areas of the stomach be obtained because sampling error is frequent. There is no utility to gastrectomy or other surgical management for extranodal

Table 8-3 ANN ARBOR Staging System for Non-Hodgkin Lymphomas[a]

Stage I	Involvement of a single nodal group or extranodal site (I_E)
Stage II	Involvement of two or more nodal groups on the same side of the diaphragm or localized involvement of an extranodal site or organ (II_E) and one or more nodal groups on the same side of the diaphragm
Stage III	Involvement of nodal groups on both sides of the diaphragm, which may be accompanied by localized involvement of an extranodal region or site (III_E) of spleen (III_S) or both (III_{SE})
Stage IV	Diffuse or disseminated involvement of one or more distant extranodal sites

[a]Temperature >38°C, weight loss >10% of body weight in the last 6 months, night sweats preceding diagnosis are defined as "B" symptoms and designated by the suffix B. Others are designated by the suffix A.

disease. Other types of aggressive NHL can involve the GI tract, especially MCL [43]. Evaluation of primary CNS lymphoma requires biopsy of the lesion, but a vigorous search for additional disease sites should be undertaken concurrently, because therapy for CNS and systemic disease will need to account directly for both.

Imaging Studies for Initial Staging

The use of imaging studies for evaluating lymphoma patients has evolved greatly. In 2014, FDG-PET–computed tomography (CT) scans were named the preferred imaging technique for FDG-avid lymphomas (essentially all aggressive NHLs) [58]. Based on these new guidelines, referred to as the Lugano criteria, a routine chest x-ray is no longer required. These guidelines also recommend that bone marrow biopsy could be omitted if the bone or marrow is FDG-avid on initial PET/CT scans. There still is significant controversy regarding the opposite situation: If the PET/CT scan does not show bone or marrow involvement, what is the utility of a bone marrow biopsy? Scant infiltration of DLBCL in the bone marrow (10%) may be missed with lack of FDG avidity, and thus, routine bone marrow biopsy may still be required for staging DLBCL patients (Figs. 8-15 and 8-16).

Limitations of PET/CT scan for staging of aggressive lymphoma include the fact that uptake of FDG is not specific to tumors and that infection and inflammatory processes are common false-positive findings on PET. As a result, an unexpected FDG-avid lesion that will result in a significant change in management should be confirmed by biopsy. The presence of high normal background activity in an organ, for example, in the kidneys or testes, may also make it difficult to identify abnormal FDG sites in that region. Although there is usually high normal metabolic activity within the brain, CNS lymphomas are often positive on FDG-PET scans, showing greater metabolic activity than the adjacent brain. However, additional imaging with magnetic resonance imaging (MRI) may be indicated for confirmation.

Bone Marrow Evaluation

Bone marrow aspiration and biopsy should be performed as part of the initial staging evaluation because involvement suggests widespread disease (stage IV) that affects treatment and prognosis, with the caveat mentioned above (see previous section). Bilateral iliac crest assessment is preferred because sensitivity of detection is higher than unilateral biopsy [59]. Although several studies found high accuracy of FDG-PET for predicting bone marrow involvement, a recent analysis concluded that the positive predictive value is high, but a negative FDG-PET is not completely concordant with the results of bone marrow biopsy [60]. Of note, the pattern of uptake within the bone marrow spaces on FDG-PET is important, because a diffuse pattern is

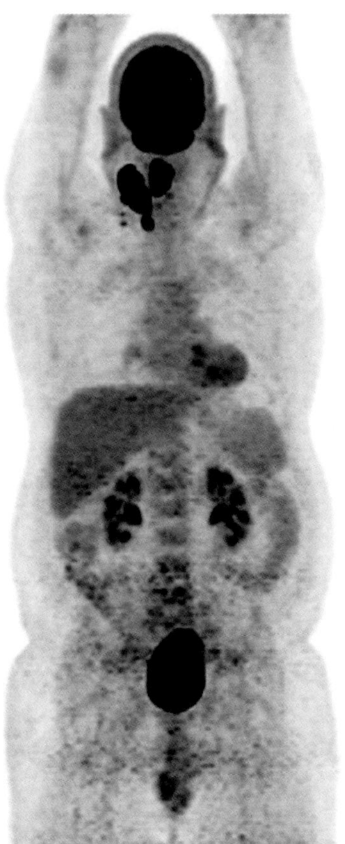

FIGURE 8-15 Positron emission tomography (PET) scan showing right cervical lymph nodes involved by diffuse large B-cell lymphoma.

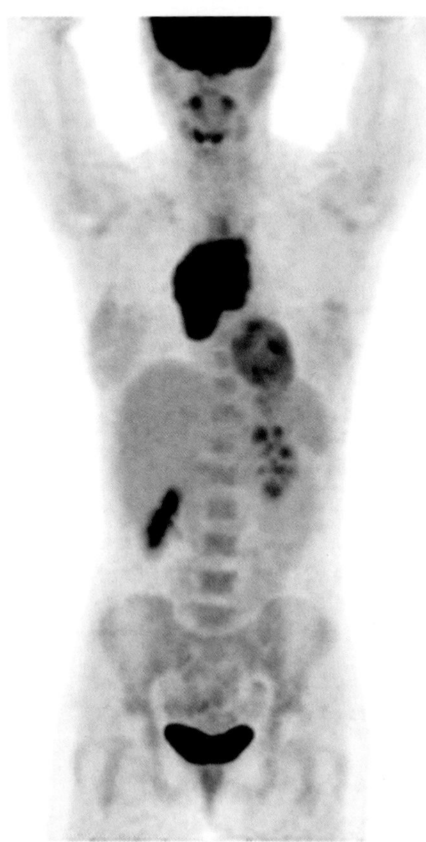

FIGURE 8-16 Extranodal lymphoma on fluorodeoxyglucose positron emission tomography (FDG-PET)/computed tomography (CT). The patient presented with mediastinal lymphoma; this is easily seen on a maximum intensity projection (MIP) image from FDG-PET/CT. However, an additional focus is present in the right kidney; although not confirmed by biopsy, the renal lesion disappeared after chemotherapy, and the stage was changed from stage I to stage IV.

commonly seen with activation (eg, with underlying anemia or infection, or after chemotherapy or growth factor treatment), and caution should be taken in interpreting this as diffuse bone marrow involvement by tumor. In contrast, focal or nodular uptake within osseous structures is suspicious (Fig. 8-17).

PROGNOSTIC FACTORS

Pretreatment

Prognostic factors in patients with aggressive NHL can be broadly grouped into pretreatment (tumor-related) and treatment-related characteristics. Tumor-related genetic characteristics of importance, as noted earlier, include germinal (GCB) or non-GCB origin genetic profile and presence of *MYC* and *BCL2* translocations ("double-hit"). Other tumor-related characteristics reported to be of prognostic value include a complex karyotype shown by conventional cytogenetics, high proliferation rate (high Ki-67 expression), and BCL2 and/or MYC expression shown by immunohistochemical staining ([1]).

High serum LDH level is a measure of anaerobic metabolism and/or cell turnover and tumor bulk and is associated with a lower probability of complete remission and poorer long-term survival in patients with aggressive NHL. Other pretreatment prognostic factors include serum β_2-microglobulin level, stage, number of disease sites, bulky disease, presence of bone marrow involvement, poor performance status, and age ([61]). Of these pretreatment factors, age appears to be the most important, with patients over the age of 60 having lower response rates and a higher rate of relapse ([62]).

The most commonly used system to provide pretreatment prognostic information in patients with aggressive NHL is the IPI, first developed in 1993 (Table 8-4) ([63]). These initial data resulted from a cohort of 2,031 patients treated with doxorubicin-containing regimens analyzed for the presence of factors that independently predicted survival. The most commonly used doxorubicin-based regimen at that time was CHOP (cyclophosphamide, doxorubicin, vincristine, and prednisone) (Table 8-5). Significant prognostic factors were serum LDH (abnormal vs normal), age (<60 vs >60), number of extranodal sites (<2 vs >2), performance status (Eastern Cooperative Oncology Group [ECOG] 0-1 vs 2-4), and stage (I and II vs III and IV). Each of the five factors had an equal impact on survival. Risk groups identified were low (zero to one factor), low/intermediate (two factors), high/intermediate (three factors), and high (four to five factors), with 5-year survival rates of 73%, 51%, 43%, and 26%, respectively. Stage, serum LDH level, and performance status were independent predictive prognostic factors in a simplified subanalysis of 1,274 subjects ≤60 years of age in the same study. In this subgroup, the 5-year survival rate was 83% for zero risk factors, 69% for one risk factor, 46% for two risk factors, and 32% for three risk factors. In patients over 60 years of age, the 5-year survival rates were 56%, 44%, 37%, and 21%, respectively. These data highlight the prognostic significance of age on the survival of patients with aggressive NHL.

The IPI has been broadly applied as the standard for prognosis in patients with aggressive NHL, although corrections or changes to the IPI have been proposed including the National Comprehensive Cancer Network IPI ([64]), the IPI24 ([65]), and the R-IPI, which accounts for the addition of rituximab to the frontline treatment of DLBCL ([21]). In the R-IPI, there are only three groups—low risk with zero risk factors, intermediate risk with one or two risk factors, and high risk with three or more factors—with 4-year progression-

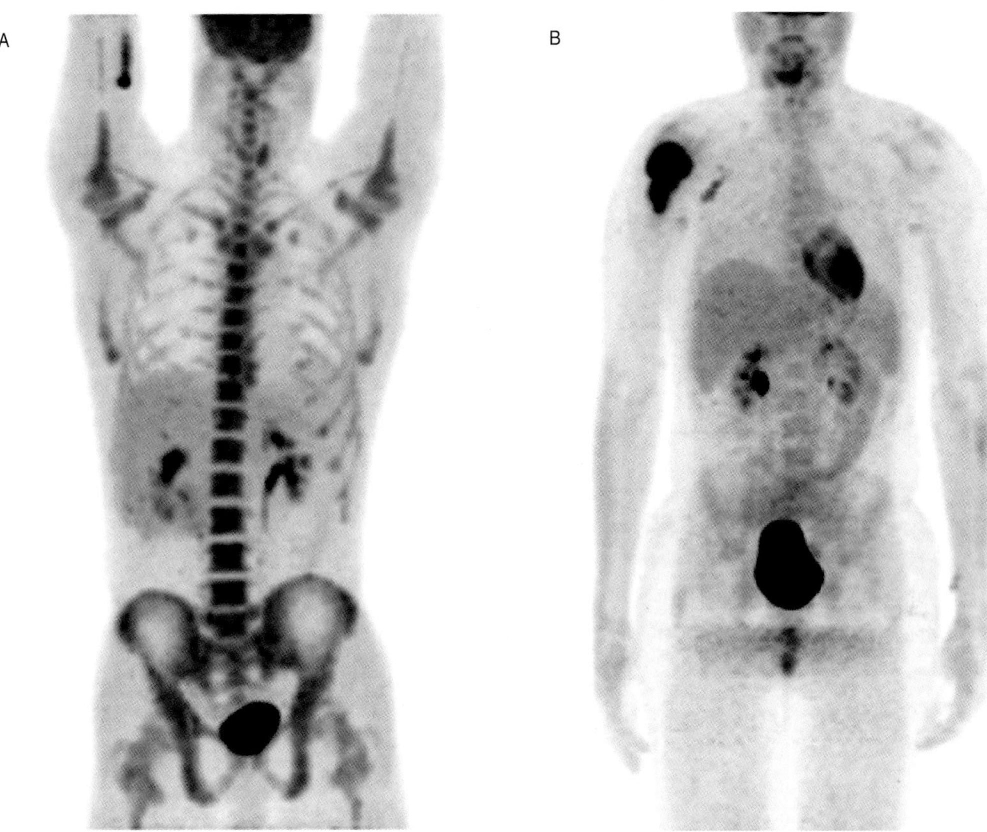

FIGURE 8-17 Bone and bone marrow uptake on fluorodeoxyglucose positron emission tomography (FDG-PET)/computed tomography (CT). **A.** Typical pattern of marrow activation, commonly seen after chemotherapy or with growth factor treatment. This is diffuse but homogenous. In contrast (**B**), another patient had negative bilateral iliac crest biopsies but had focal activity in a destructive lesion involving the right humerus. Directed biopsy of this site was positive for bone involvement.

Table 8-4 International Prognostic Index With Age-Adjusted Index

FACTORS					
Age	≤60 versus >60				
Serum LDH	Normal versus high				
Performance status	0 or 1 versus 2-4				
Extranodal disease	≤1 or less versus >1				
Stage	I or II versus III or IV				
INTERNATIONAL INDEX					
GROUP	RISK FACTORS	RELAPSE-FREE SURVIVAL		SURVIVAL	
		2 Years (%)	*5 Years (%)*	*2 Years (%)*	*5 Years (%)*
All ages	0-1	79	70	84	73
	2	66	50	66	51
	3	59	49	54	43
	4-5	52	40	34	26
Age adjusted ≤60	0	88	86	90	83
	1	74	66	79	69
	2	62	53	59	46
	3	61	58	37	32
Age adjusted >60	0	75	46	80	56
	1	64	45	68	44
	2	60	41	48	37
	3	47	37	31	21

Table 8-5 Most Commonly Used Chemotherapeutic Regimens in Diffuse Large B-Cell Lymphomas

Regimen	Dose/Route	Days	Interval
FRONTLINE			
R-CHOP			
Cyclophosphamide	750 mg/m² IV	1	21 days
Doxorubicin	50 mg/m² IV	1	
Prednisone	100 mg PO	1-5	
Vincristine	1.4 mg/m² IV	1	
Rituximab	375 mg/m² IV	1	
SALVAGE (first salvage, preautologous SCT)			
RICE			
Rituximab	375 mg/m² IV	1	14-21 days
Ifosfamide	5 g/m² IV CI	2	
Mesna concurrent with Ifosfamide	5 g/m² IVCI 2 over 24 h, then 2 g/m² over 12 h	2-3	
Carboplatin[a]	Maximum 800 mg	2	
Etoposide	100 mg/m² IV	2-4	
GCSF	5 mcg/kg/day SC	7-14	

[a]Calculate Carboplatin dose using Calvert equation: AUC = 5 g/mL/min; dose = 5 × [25+Cl_{cr}] capped at 800 mg.

free survival (PFS) rates of 94%, 80%, and 53%, respectively.

Prognostic Factors in Mantle Cell Lymphoma

The same prognostic factors in the IPI for aggressive lymphomas are of utility in patients with MCL. Other adverse prognostic factors include *p53* mutations or deletion, elevated Ki-67, and blastoid histology. A prognostic model for MCL patients treated with chemotherapy followed by high-dose chemotherapy followed by autologous stem cell transplantation (Mantle Cell International Prognostic Index) was proposed using age, performance status, LDH, and leukocyte count ([66]). Patients were divided in low-, intermediate-, and high-risk groups, with overall survival (OS) times of not reached, 51 months, and 29 months, respectively. In patients receiving rituximab plus hyperfractionated cyclophosphamide, vincristine, doxorubicin, and dexamethasone (R-hyper-CVAD), alternating with rituximab-methotrexate and cytarabine, this model could not be reproduced ([67]). However, it was reproducible in patients treated with CHOP-rituximab–like regimens consolidated with high-dose chemotherapy with stem cell transplantation ([68]).

Prognostic Factors in Primary Central Nervous System Lymphoma

Age and LDH are important prognostic factors in patients with HIV-negative primary CNS lymphoma; however, the most important factor is performance status at the time of treatment. Elevated LDH, CSF protein, and tumor mass location(s) are also contributors to prognosis ([69]). Many patients can improve their condition by use of corticosteroids and thus be candidates for intensive chemotherapy-based regimens that are potentially curative.

Therapy-Associated Prognostic Factors

An important posttreatment prognostic indicator is tumor response to induction chemotherapy. In patients with aggressive NHL, dramatic response to induction with early complete remission (by the third cycle of therapy) is associated with a superior outcome ([70]). Fluorodeoxyglucose PET has been found to be highly sensitive for the detection of aggressive NHL in posttreatment residual masses, but its ability to detect interim therapy response is controversial. Moskowitz et al found that DLBCL patients with persistent FDG avidity after four cycles of rituximab plus CHOP (R-CHOP) had an 86% false-positive rate (PET/CT positive, biopsy negative for persistent disease) ([71]). Similar data have been shown by many others, highlighting the need for biopsy confirmation of a positive PET/CT scan prior to therapeutic decisions.

Patients who fail to achieve at least a good partial response to induction chemotherapy have primary refractory disease and short survival despite all efforts. Another important indicator of prognosis is duration of remission obtained after induction chemotherapy, because patients with relapses occurring at <1 year have a worse outcome ([72]).

APPROACH TO THERAPY

Early-Stage Aggressive Non-Hodgkin Lymphoma

Early-stage (localized) aggressive NHLs (stages I and contiguous II) were historically treated with radiation therapy (RT) alone, and the results were highly variable ([73]). The 5-year survival with involved-field RT for stage I/II disease was approximately 50%. Patients with bulky disease (>5 cm) suffered a higher relapse rate. Although many studies were undertaken to improve results by adjusting dosages and field coverage, it was the addition of combination chemotherapy to RT regimens that improved outcome most dramatically. Four randomized trials were conducted in patients with early-stage aggressive NHL before rituximab therapy was incorporated into the CHOP regimen. The first study was by the Southwest Oncology Group (SWOG); eight cycles of CHOP were compared to three cycles of CHOP followed by involved-field RT (40-55 Gy) in limited-stage DLBCL ([74]). The combined-modality arm achieved an OS of 82%, versus 72% for the CHOP alone arm. The ECOG randomized patients with bulky stage I or II disease to eight cycles of CHOP with or without involved-field RT. Patients achieving a complete remission were randomized to involved-field RT (30 Gy) or no further therapy. Patients achieving partial remission received involved-field RT at a higher dose (40 Gy). Disease-free survival at 5 years was higher in patients who received radiation (73% vs 58%) after achieving complete remission ([75]). The Groupe d'Etude des Lymphomes de l'Adulte (GELA) conducted a similar study comparing aggressive chemotherapy (dose-intensified doxorubicin, cyclophosphamide, vindesine, bleomycin, and prednisone [ACVBP]) alone versus abbreviated chemotherapy (three cycles of CHOP) followed by involved-field RT for stage I or II mostly low-risk aggressive lymphoma. All patients in this study were younger than age 60 years. Both the 5-year event-free survival (82%) and OS (90%) rates were significantly better in the chemotherapy group than in the combined-modality group (74% and 81%, respectively); however, the chemotherapy group had significant toxicity and ACVBP is not available in the United States. Although the addition of RT reduced relapses at the initial disease sites, this was not enough to overcome the excessive number of relapses in the abbreviated chemotherapy group ([76]). Despite these results indicating the inability of abbreviated chemotherapy plus RT to prevent out-of-field relapses, the GELA group conducted another trial, GELA LNH 93-4, comparing CHOP with CHOP plus involved-field RT to 40 Gy, this time for patients older than 60 years ([77]). The use of ACVBP had been dropped by the time this trial was undertaken because of excessive toxicity. At a median follow-up time of 7 years, no significant differences were evident in 5-year event-free survival rates (61% for chemotherapy alone vs 64% for chemoradiation) or OS rates (72% vs 68%, respectively). The results in the chemotherapy-only group were similar to the results from the group that received eight cycles of CHOP in the SWOG trial discussed earlier. However, because relapses could appear beyond 5 years, another 5 to 10 years should be allowed to elapse before any approach is widely adopted. A SWOG trial evaluated the addition of rituximab to three cycles of CHOP, followed by involved field RT, for localized DLBCL and found favorable comparisons to nonrituximab historical controls ([78]). The MD Anderson Cancer Center (MDACC) approach to the treatment of DLBCL is shown in Fig. 8-18.

Localized MCL in general has been treated in the same way as extensive disease, but the use of RT with or without chemotherapy has been reported by investigators in British Columbia to be effective as well ([79]).

CHAPTER 8

Advanced-Stage Aggressive Non-Hodgkin Lymphoma

Initial cures using chemotherapy for patients with large-cell lymphoma were reported in the 1970s ([80, 81]). The SWOG initially reported that CHOP induced complete response in 50% of patients, with long-term disease-free survival in 35%, and CHOP has since represented the standard of care in the treatment of patients with aggressive NHL despite intensive research into newer regimens. Subsequent trials of combination chemotherapy over the last 25 years can be thought of as "generations" ([82]). The initial generation included CHOP, M-BACOD (methotrexate, bleomycin, doxorubicin, cyclophosphamide, etoposide, and leucovorin), BACOD, ProMACE-MOPP (addition of etoposide), ProMACE-CytaBOM (addition of cytarabine), and MACOP-B (methotrexate with leucovorin rescue, doxorubicin, cyclophosphamide, vincristine, prednisone, and bleomycin). These regimens showed an increased rate of complete remission of nearly 80% in early studies with greater than 60% long-term disease-free survival. The SWOG undertook a landmark phase III trial comparing CHOP, MACOP-B, M-BACOD, and ProMACE-CytaBOM, which showed that, despite early reports of improved response, OS at 3 years varied from 50% to 54%, with disease-free survival ranging from 41% to 46%. In this trial, there was no apparent advantage to increased intensity of therapy. Another finding noted in the 1980s was that inclusion of an anthracycline in the chemotherapy regimen was important to long-term disease-free survival.

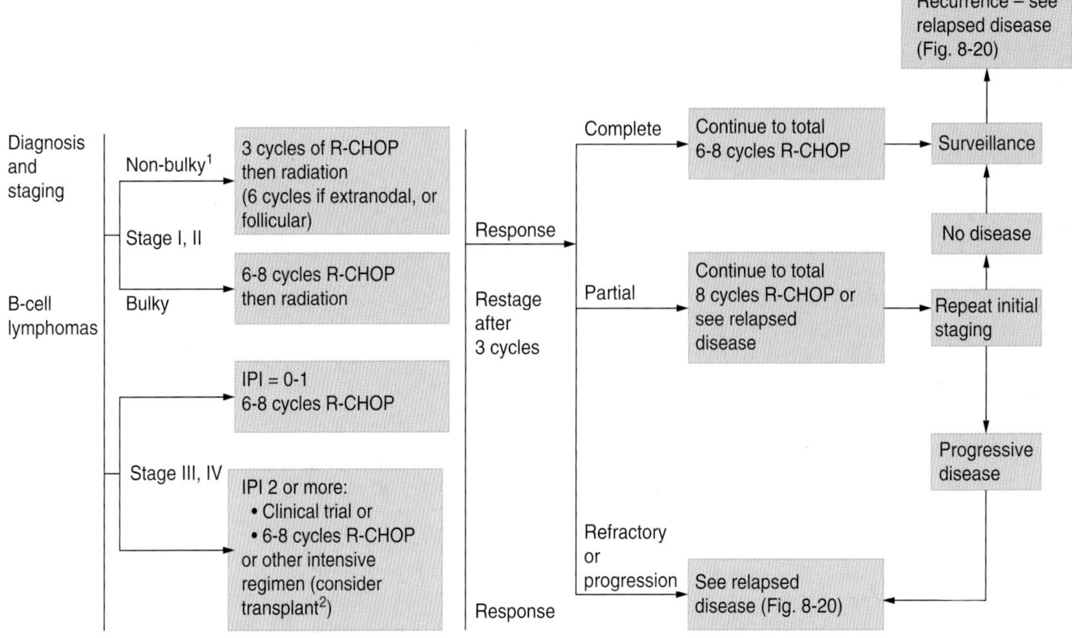

[1]Bulky disease is >5 cm by definition at MD Anderson Cancer Center. [2]Especially if bone marrow disease is present.

FIGURE 8-18 Algorithm for treatment of diffuse large B-cell lymphoma.

Other approaches have included alternating regimens, higher dose therapy, and dose-dense therapy. The first two have not been shown to have a survival benefit, whereas the third is still under scrutiny.

Dose-dense therapy was reported to be feasible in 2003 by the German High-Grade NHL Study Group (DSHNHL) ([83]). Three variants of CHOP-like therapy were evaluated, including CHOP-14, CHOEP-14 (addition of etoposide 100 mg/m^2 on days 1-3), and CHOP-21, each with hematopoietic growth factor support. An interim analysis of 959 patients showed that adherence to the dose-dense regimens was excellent, although dose reductions were more frequently required for the addition of etoposide. To evaluate younger patients, 710 patients with good-prognosis aggressive NHL age 18 to 60 years were randomized to receive six cycles of CHOP-21, CHOP-14, CHOEP-21, or CHOEP-14 ([84]). Patients in the 2-week regimens received granulocyte colony-stimulating factor (G-CSF) from day 4. Initial sites of bulky or extranodal disease were treated with 36 Gy of RT. Patients receiving CHOEP achieved a higher complete response rate (87.6% vs 79.4%) and 5-year event-free survival (69.2% vs 57.6%) than patients treated with CHOP. Dose density (the 2-week regimens) improved OS in a multivariate analysis. Patients receiving CHOEP had a higher rate of myelosuppression, but generally, the regimen was well tolerated.

While the German group was exploring dose density, GELA reported their results of trial LNH98-5 in which 399 patients with DLBCL were randomized to receive either R-CHOP every 21 days or standard CHOP alone for a total of eight cycles. Patients with stage II to IV DLBCL who were between 60 and 80 years old were eligible for this trial. No RT or intrathecal chemotherapy was administered. The complete response rate (76% vs 63%) and the 5-year PFS, disease-free survival, and OS rates were better in the rituximab arm ([85]).

Based on the GELA LNH98-5 results and their own data, the DSHNHL designed a four-arm randomized study in patients older than 60 years (RICOVER-60) that compared CHOP-14 with or without rituximab for six cycles versus CHOP-14 for eight cycles with or without rituximab (in the six-cycle R-CHOP arm, the patients received a total of eight doses of rituximab) ([86]). The CHOP alone group was inferior, and six cycles of R-CHOP plus two cycles of rituximab were as effective as eight cycles of R-CHOP. Of note, this trial also found that patients who achieved a partial response after four cycles received no additional benefit from receiving a total of eight cycles, as compared to the standard six cycles. Subsequent to this study, two other studies addressing the question of R-CHOP every 21 days versus every 14 days in DLBCL, one from the United Kingdom and the other from GELA, have not shown any benefit in the dose-dense group compared to standard R-CHOP every 21 days ([87, 88]).

An ongoing trial is directly comparing rituximab plus etoposide, prednisone, vincristine, cyclophosphamide, doxorubicin (R-EPOCH) versus R-CHOP in patients with DLBCL, with highly anticipated results expected in 2016. In addition, there are numerous phase II and III trials evaluating the effect of novel agents, including lenalidomide and ibrutinib, when added to standard-of-care therapies. At MDACC, our preference is that all patients with DLBCL be evaluated for a clinical trial at each treatment stage.

Special Types and Situations in Diffuse Large B-Cell Lymphoma

Primary Central Nervous System and Ocular Lymphoma

The treatment of patients with primary CNS lymphoma is limited to drugs that can cross the blood-brain barrier. Standard chemotherapies such as R-CHOP do not cross to the brain, and they have limited activity in this condition. The initial evaluation must include slit-lamp evaluation of the eyes, MRI of the brain and spine, lumbar puncture, and the standard studies for any other lymphoma to exclude systemic disease. The most common histology in primary CNS lymphoma is DLBCL, and the most important drug is high-dose methotrexate, in general at doses higher than 3.0 g/m^2. The combination of chemoimmunotherapy using rituximab, high-dose methotrexate, procarbazine, and vincristine is generally considered the standard of care ([89]). In this approach, patients have historically received consolidation with low-dose RT if in complete remission, although there is controversy regarding the role of RT. Lower doses of radiation have decreased the long-term neurotoxicity seen in prior studies ([90]). In the most widely used approach, patients receive consolidation with high-dose cytarabine after completion of RT. Recent studies have shown promising results without the use of RT, although larger studies are required to evaluate whether omitting RT due to concerns about neurotoxicity is viable ([91]). The use of intrathecal chemotherapy is controversial in patients with no evidence of leptomeningeal involvement, but it is used in patients with CSF disease. Radiation fields should include the eyes if those are thought to be involved.

Testicular Lymphomas

Most patients with testicular lymphoma have DLBCL, but other lymphoma types can be seen. Patients with testicular lymphoma often have a worse prognosis compared to other DLBCL patients without testicular involvement. The treatment in this group of patients should include prophylaxis of CNS relapses with intrathecal chemotherapy and RT to the contralateral testicle to decrease the risk for localized relapses ([19]).

Intravascular Lymphomas

These lymphomas are traditionally considered to have poor prognosis. They have better outcomes with the addition of rituximab to the standard chemotherapy regimen. They have a high incidence of CNS relapse, but there are no standard CNS prophylaxis recommendations in this group of patients ([19]).

Primary Mediastinal B-Cell Lymphoma

Historically, PMBL had been an NHL subtype with a poor prognosis, despite intensive therapy and young fit patients ([92]). These tumors are usually CD20$^+$, and thus rituximab is now incorporated with standard-of-care chemotherapy. Consolidation with RT after chemotherapy has been a standard practice, but investigators from the National Institutes of Health have shown that dose-adjusted R-EPOCH without radiotherapy can achieve excellent results ([93]). These data have not yet been confirmed in a multicenter trial, and thus controversy exists regarding whether RT can be omitted in all patients or may still play a role in patients with a residual large non–FDG-avid mass. At MDACC, our current practice is treat PMBL patients with dose-adjusted R-EPOCH and omit RT for all patients who achieve a complete response.

Treatment of Advanced Mantle Cell Lymphoma

Mantle cell lymphoma is considered a special case because of its recognized aggressiveness and frequent refractory behavior (Fig. 8-19). In many studies of patients with MCL, the disease has been shown to be the NHL type with the poorest prognosis overall, with complete and partial response rates of 29% and 45%, respectively, when treated with a CHOP-like regimen. Investigators at MDACC have investigated hyper-CVAD, a regimen of fractionated cyclophosphamide and continuous infusion doxorubicin, vincristine, and dexamethasone alternating with methotrexate and cytarabine, which had previously been used for patients with acute lymphoblastic leukemia (Table 8-6) ([94]). In long-term follow-up of R-hyper-CVAD alternating with rituximab plus methotrexate and cytarabine in untreated MCL, Romaguera and colleagues reported a 97% response rate, 87% complete response rate, and median time to treatment failure of 4.6 years ([94]). The median OS had not been reached at a median follow-up of 8 years. Because the most toxic portion of this treatment is the high-dose methotrexate-cytarabine cycle, Kahl et al used a modified R-hyper-CVAD with maintenance rituximab for 2 years, obtaining a 77% overall response rate, a complete response rate of 64%, and a median PFS of 37 months ([95]). Many other groups have incorporated a

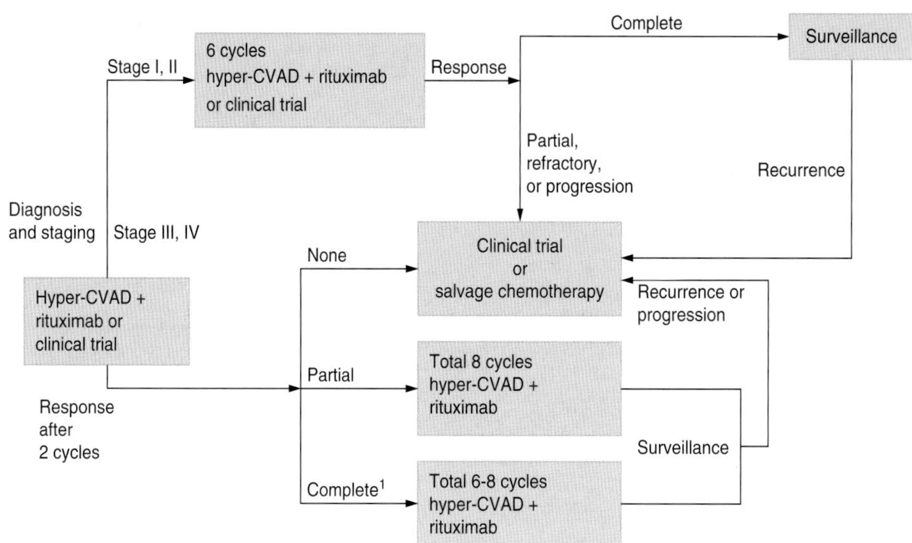

FIGURE 8-19 Algorithm for treatment of mantle cell lymphoma.

Table 8-6 R-Hyper-CVAD Regimen Used in Mantle Cell Lymphoma and Highly Aggressive Lymphomas[a]

Regimen	Dose/Route	Days	Interval
Hyper-CVAD/Methotrexate/ Ara-C			21-28 days
Cycles 1,3,5,7			
Rituxan	375 mg/m^2 IV by slow infusion	1	
Cyclophosphamide	300 mg/m^2/dose over 3 h q 12 h × 6 doses	1-3	
Mesna	600 mg/m^2/day CIV over 24 h daily (Start 1 h prior to cyclophosphamide and complete by 12 h after last dose of cyclophosphamide)	1-3	
Doxorubicin	25 mg/m^2/day CIV over 24 h daily (Begin at 12 h after last dose of cyclophosphamide)	4-5	
Vincristine	1.4 mg/m^2 IV (max 2 mg) (Give 12 h after last dose of cyclophosphamide and on day 11)	4 and 11	
Dexamethasone	40 mg PO daily	1-4 and 11-14	
Cycles 2, 4, 6, 8			
Methotrexate	200 mg/m^2 IV over 2 h then 800 mg/m^2 IV over 22 h	1	
Solumedrol	50 mg IV q 12 h × 6 doses	1-3	
Ara-C	3 g/m^2 IV over 2 h every 12 h × 4 doses	2-3	
Leucovorin	50 mg IV followed by 15 mg IV q 6 h × 8 doses (Start 12 h after completion of methotrexate)		
Intrathecal therapy[b]			
Ara-C	100 mg	2	
Methotrexate	12 mg (6 mg if Ommaya reservoir)	7	

[a]Dose reductions for renal insufficiency, age, and previous toxicity are required. Intrathecal chemotherapy is more frequent for proven CNS disease.
[b]Mantle cell lymphoma is not typically treated with intrathecal therapy.

consolidation phase with autologous stem cell transplantation after induction chemotherapy with various regimens with remarkable results ([96]). Bendamustine with rituximab, in comparison to R-CHOP, achieved a statistically significant prolongation in PFS and thus has become a new standard-of-care option for patients unfit to undergo more intensive approaches ([97]).

Special Considerations

Patients with double-hit lymphomas, defined as the presence of *MYC* translocation with *BCL2* or *BCL6* or another oncogene, have a very poor outcome even with aggressive treatments ([29]). Consolidation with transplant in first response should be considered, even though transplant outcome data have not shown clear benefit due to small sample sizes in the largest retrospective series ([98, 99]). At MDACC, our approach to double-hit DLBCL currently includes dose-adjusted R-EPOCH and consideration of autologous stem cell transplantation consolidation if the patient is fit, but clinical trials are always preferred. The best treatment approach for patients with DLBCL with double protein expression is unclear ([100]), and additional clinical trials are needed.

Central nervous system prophylaxis remains controversial. However, it is recommended in patients with high-grade lymphomas or BL, bone marrow involvement with DLBCL, renal or adrenal involvement, two or more extranodal sites, testicular involvement, and disease involvement in areas close to the CNS ([19, 57]).

With the widespread use of effective antiretroviral therapy, patients with HIV-associated lymphomas have an improved prognosis and should be treated with curative intent ([101]). Standard treatments with rituximab-containing regimens, such as R-CHOP, dose-adjusted R-EPOCH, or continuous infusion cyclophosphamide, doxorubicin, and etoposide, reported acceptable results, especially in the era of the HAART. In HIV-associated BL, investigators from the National Cancer Institute (NCI) have shown that a short course of R-EPOCH can be highly effective ([102]). It is important to note, however, that when EPOCH-based treatments are used, it is often recommended that HAART be stopped while on treatment.

REFRACTORY OR RELAPSED AGGRESSIVE NON-HODGKIN LYMPHOMA

Treatment of Recurrent/Refractory Diffuse Large B-Cell Lymphoma

Approximately 10% of patients treated for aggressive NHL fail to achieve a complete remission after induction therapy; their disease is termed *primary refractory* (Fig. 8-20). A larger portion of patients with aggressive NHL, up to a third of all patients, will relapse after initially responding to chemotherapy. Although these patients may be sensitive to a second chemotherapy regimen, most patients with refractory and relapsed aggressive NHL have a poor prognosis. Conventional salvage therapy includes rituximab combined with

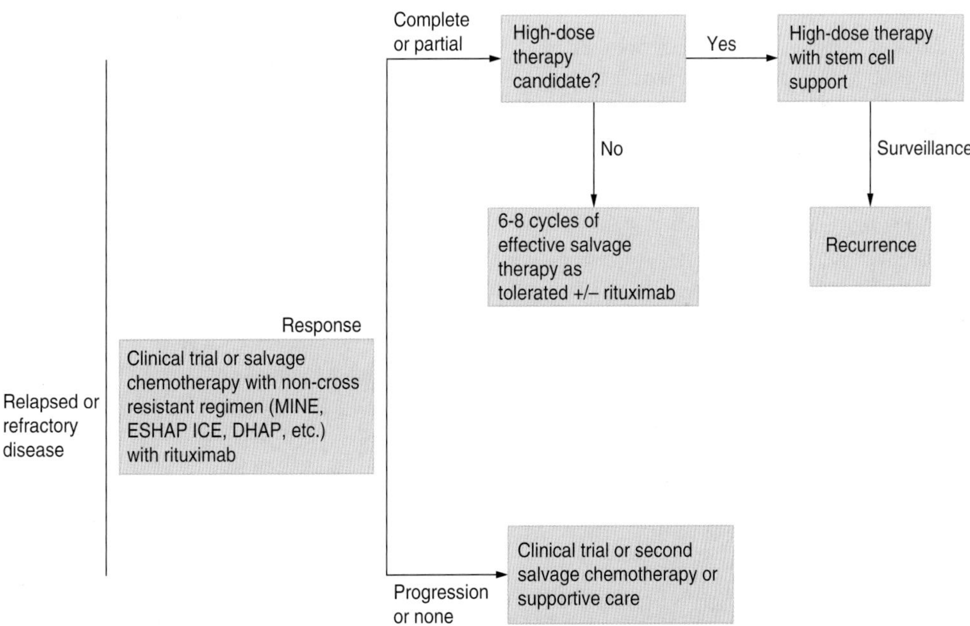

FIGURE 8-20 Algorithm for treatment of relapsed aggressive lymphomas (except high-grade or mantle cell lymphoma). MINE, mesna, ifosfamide, mitoxantrone, etoposide.

standard chemotherapeutics such as ifosfamide, etoposide, taxanes, and platinum compounds. Among the most commonly used are DHAP (dexamethasone, cytarabine, and cisplatin), ICE (carboplatin replacing cisplatin), GDP (gemcitabine, dexamethasone, and cisplatin), TTR (paclitaxel, topotecan, and rituximab) and ESHAP (etoposide, methylprednisolone, cytarabine, and cisplatin) ([103-105]). The salvage regimens tend to have higher toxicity and require greater support for administration, often including hospitalization.

Because of the poor prognosis in patients with relapsed disease, the purpose of many of the chemotherapy regimens offered in this clinical setting is to attain remission followed by high-dose chemotherapy with stem cell support. The Parma trial examined autologous bone marrow transplantation versus salvage chemotherapy in patients with relapsed, chemotherapy-sensitive NHL ([106]). Patients were randomized to four more cycles of DHAP versus high-dose therapy with stem cell support, showing an event-free survival rate of 46% in the high-dose arm but only 12% in the DHAP alone arm. This is considered strong evidence that high-dose therapy with stem cell support is the treatment of choice for patients with chemosensitive relapsed or primary refractory aggressive NHL.

Gisselbrecht et al reported a GELA study known as the CORAL trial for second-line treatment for 400 recurrent/refractory CD20$^+$ DLBCL patients randomized to receive rituximab plus DHAP (R-DHAP) versus rituximab plus ICE (R-ICE); responding patients received autologous stem cell transplantation. No difference in the response rates (~50% in prior rituximab-exposed patients), PFS, and OS were noted between the R-ICE and R-DHAP groups ([103]).

Patients who do not respond to a second-line treatment or are unfit for an aggressive approach should be evaluated for a clinical trial. If not eligible for a trial, they should then be considered for a palliative treatment that may provide meaningful transient benefit or palliative care. Patients who are responding to second-line treatment, but who are unable to mobilize stem cell treatment, should be considered for alternative donor transplant. Treatment response failure beyond second relapse indicates an incurable disease. A small portion of patients, however, may be rescued with salvage chemotherapy and a second stem cell transplantation, often of allogeneic donor origin; however, this is unlikely, and investigational agents should be prioritized over further chemotherapy. At MDACC, our priority for patients who are either unfit for aggressive therapy or resistant to second-line chemotherapy is to aggressively pursue a clinical trial.

Patients with a history of follicular lymphoma with subsequent transformation to DLBCL, who had prior doxorubicin-based treatment, should be treated with salvage therapy for recurrent DLBCL.

Treatment of Recurrent Mantle Cell Lymphoma

Decisions regarding salvage therapy for patients with recurrent MCL should be individualized, depending on their candidacy for stem cell transplantation. Aside from aggressive combination chemotherapy, targeted therapy agents are active against MCL, and bortezomib, lenalidomide, and ibrutinib have each been approved by the US Food and Drug Administration (FDA) for relapsed MCL.

Recurrent Primary Central Nervous System and Ocular Lymphoma

The treatment of recurrent primary CNS lymphoma is limited because of the inability of many drugs to penetrate into the CNS. Retreatment with high-dose methotrexate can be attempted if there was a long duration of the first remission. Patients with recent prior whole-brain RT may be at high risk for methotrexate-induced encephalopathy. Reports using temozolomide in combination with rituximab have been encouraging. Responding patients may benefit with consolidation with high-dose chemotherapy (especially with preparative regimens including thiotepa), followed by autologous stem cell transplantation.

HIGHLY AGGRESSIVE (HIGH-GRADE) NON-HODGKIN LYMPHOMA

Patients with highly aggressive NHL have largely benefited from the successful application of pediatric therapy regimens to the adult population, with long-term remissions approaching 80% to 90% in some series (Fig. 8-21). The most important principle for treating patients with highly aggressive NHL is prompt systemic therapy, as these are medical emergencies. Attempts should be made to maintain dose intensity and density using supportive therapies, such as growth factor support, prophylaxis for tumor lysis syndrome, and CNS prophylaxis.

Patients with BL should not be treated with CHOP or CHOP-like regimens due to poor long-term disease-free survival ([19]). Combined-modality therapy appears to add toxicity without any proven benefit. Patients at MDACC have been treated with the hyper-CVAD/methotrexate/cytarabine regimen, with intrathecal methotrexate/cytarabine CNS prophylaxis with some success ([107]) (see Table 8-6). The NCI has developed an alternating regimen of cyclophosphamide, doxorubicin, vincristine, methotrexate, leucovorin, and ifosfamide, etoposide, and cytarabine with intrathecal cytarabine and methotrexate called CODOX-M/

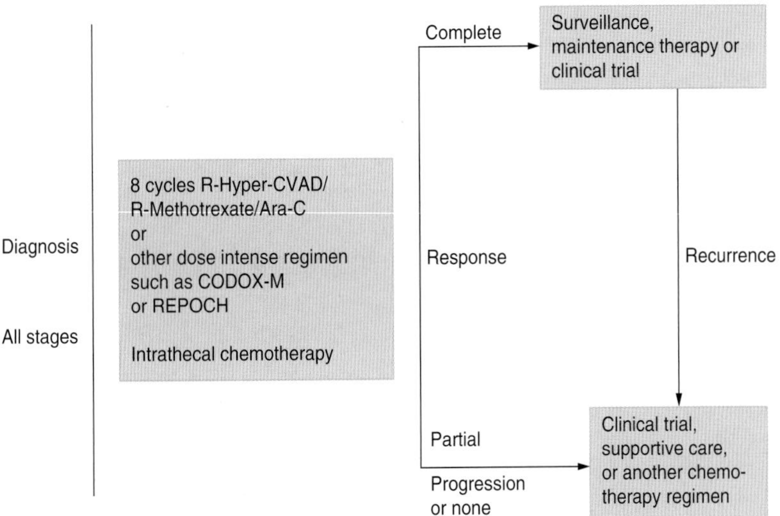

FIGURE 8-21 Algorithm for treatment of Burkitt and Burkitt-like lymphoma. Ara-C, cytarabine.

IVAC ([108]). This is administered for four cycles, with CODOX-M as cycles 1 and 3 and IVAC as cycles 2 and 4. A complete remission rate of 92% was reported, with a 3-year event-free survival rate of 85%. At MDACC, rituximab was added to standard hyper-CVAD alternating with methotrexate-cytarabine (see Table 8-6), resulting in impressive long term outcomes. Adverse risk factors for these patients include elevated LDH, age, and leukemic presentation ([109]). Finally, the EPOCH chemotherapy regimen developed at the NCI has recently shown great promise in a small phase II trial, in both HIV-positive and HIV-negative BL, with freedom from progression rates in excess of 90% with 5 years of follow-up ([102]).

THERAPY IN ELDERLY PATIENTS

As has been repeatedly shown, patients with aggressive NHL over the age of 60 years have a worse prognosis ([21, 110]). Unfortunately, more than 50% of patients with aggressive NHL are over 60 years old, and most of these patients do not experience extended long-term survival. Treatment of older patients is complicated by higher overall toxicity rates and lower tolerance of aggressive therapies. At MDACC, our practice is to screen older patients with DLBCL for clinical trials with novel therapies.

Although it is sometimes necessary to reduce the doses of chemotherapeutic regimens to treat elderly patients with comorbid conditions, CHOP is generally well tolerated by patients without contraindications to doxorubicin. Growth factor support should be used. Unfortunately, patients with a contraindication to doxorubicin also frequently have contraindications to other therapies, such as platinum-containing regimens. The substitution of etoposide for doxorubicin in patients who have contraindications to anthracyclines appears to be highly effective in a population-based retrospective review ([111]). A multicenter trial found that R-mini-CHOP, a significantly reduced dosing of conventional R-CHOP, resulted in an acceptable compromise between efficacy and toxicity in patients age 80 years and older ([112]).

NEW DRUGS

The field of new cancer drugs has evolved rapidly and is difficult to adequately capture in a book chapter. Since 2000, there has been an incredible number of new drugs evaluated in clinical trials for patients with aggressive lymphomas. The typical pattern of drug development includes an evaluation of toxicity and dosing in the relapsed/refractory setting. If tolerable and an early signal of efficacy is found, drugs are then evaluated in larger phase II trials, often in a population enriched for likely responders. The authors of this chapter believe that the evaluation of efficacy in heavily pretreated, refractory aggressive NHL may actually underestimate the true response rate of targeted therapies ([113]).

The drugs listed here are not yet FDA approved for DLBCL, BL, or MCL, but appear promising thus far in clinical trials ([61]). The goal of this section is not to recommend use of these nonapproved drugs off of a clinical trial but to serve as an indication of the large progress on the horizon. The Bruton tyrosine kinase inhibitor ibrutinib has now been approved for several B-cell malignancies, including MCL. Early trials confirmed a pathway-based prediction of increased efficacy in the non-GCB subtype of DLBCL ([114]). Based on promising efficacy and acceptable toxicity, ibrutinib is now being evaluated in a randomized clinical trial with R-CHOP (vs R-CHOP + placebo) ([115]).

Other inhibitors of the B-cell receptor pathway, including Syk, are ongoing but to date have demonstrated modest results in heavily pretreated patients. Inhibitors of the PI3K/Akt/mTOR pathway have shown significant promise across lymphoma subtypes, although as single agents, they have proven more effective in indolent lymphomas ([116]). Inhibitors of the various isoforms of PI3K are in numerous clinical trials in various B-cell malignancies, with idelalisib already being approved for some NHL subtypes. Inhibitors of TORC1 have shown response rates in the 30% response range across NHL subtypes, and temsirolimus has received an orphan drug approval for MCL in Europe. Newer inhibitors that block both TORC1 and TORC2 may prove more effective, but further trials are needed. Lenalidomide is a drug with a diverse impact on numerous targets and cell types but is often described as a potent immunomodulatory drug and recently was approved for relapsed MCL. In the ABC subtype of DLBCL, lenalidomide blocks expression of interferon regulatory factor 4 (IRF4 or MUM1) and leads to a synthetic lethal response ([117]). Based on these and other findings, two randomized phase III trials are planned to evaluate R-CHOP with lenalidomide or placebo ([118]). Other agents appear to have great promise but are at a very early stage of clinical trial development, including selinexor, BCL2 inhibitors including venetoclax, and immune checkpoint inhibitor therapies.

RESPONSE AND FOLLOW-UP

Definitions of Response

Response to therapy is assessed according to criteria based on the anatomic and metabolic changes that occur in disease-involved nodal and extranodal sites ([119]). A recent consensus statement was issued by leading clinical investigators to attempt standardization of response criteria to be used in clinical trials. There remains controversy about what constitutes an abnormal PET, and it is generally recommended that uptake be compared to the mediastinal blood pool and liver as internal controls and that the results be scored based on these results ([120]) (Table 8-7).

Table 8-7 Response Definitions for Clinical Trials

Response	Definition	Nodal Masses	Spleen, Liver	Bone Marrow
CR	Disappearance of all evidence of disease	(a) FDG-avid or PET positive prior to therapy; mass of any size permitted if PET is negative (b) Variably FDG-avid or PET negative; regression to normal size on CT	Not palpable, nodules disappeared	Infiltrate cleared on repeat biopsy; if indeterminate by morphology, immunohistochemistry should be negative
PR	Regression of measurable disease and no new sites	≥50% decrease in SPD of up to six largest dominant masses; no increase in size of other nodes (a) FDG-avid or PET positive prior to therapy; one or more PET positive at previously involved site (b) Variably FDG-avid or PET negative; regression on CT	≥50% decrease in SPD of nodules (for single nodule in greatest transverse diameter); no increase in size of liver or spleen	Irrelevant if positive prior to therapy; cell type should be specified
SD	Failure to attain CR/PR or PD	(a) FDG-avid or PET positive prior to therapy; PET positive at prior sites of disease and no new sites on CT or PET (b) Variably FDG-avid or PET negative; no change in size of previous lesions on CT		
Relapsed disease or PD	Any new lesion or increase by ≥50% of previously involved sites from nadir	Appearance of a new lesion(s) >1.5 cm in any axis, ≥50% increase in longest diameter of a previously identified node >1 cm in short axis Lesions PET positive if FDG-avid lymphoma or PET positive prior to therapy	>50% increase from nadir in the SPD of any previous lesions	New or recurrent involvement

CR, complete remission; CT, computed tomography; FDG, [^{18}F] fluorodeoxyglucose; PD, progressive disease; PET, positron emission tomography; PR, partial remission; SD, stable disease; SPD, sum of the product of the diameters.
Reproduced with permission from Cheson BD, Pfistner B, Juweid ME, et al: Revised response criteria for malignant lymphoma, *J Clin Oncol.* 2007 Feb 10;25(5):579-586.

Restaging

Fluorodeoxyglucose PET has proven very useful in assessing responses to therapy and is now considered standard of care for initial posttherapy restaging in FDG-avid lymphomas. Despite this recommendation, FDG-PET/CT should not be used for long-term follow-up imaging after initial response is confirmed ([121]) (Figure 8-22).

Surveillance

Follow-up of patients with aggressive NHL after complete remission and cessation of therapy is typically done every 3 to 6 months for 2 years, then annually until year 5, although there is significant controversy about optimal use of surveillance imaging ([19]). A large retrospective evaluation of the utility of surveillance imaging to detect recurrence, as compared to patient-reported complaints, found that most DLBCL recurrences were identified based on symptoms and not imaging alone and that outcomes were not different between imaging and symptom-identified recurrences ([122]). The emergence of blood-based minimal residual disease detection techniques may ultimately make the debate about the utility of imaging moot.

Relapse or Recurrence

The presence of a new lesion, either by anatomic criteria or on FDG-PET scan, is considered relapsed or progressive disease, but at MDACC, we view a biopsy to confirm imaging findings to be essential. Fluorodeoxyglucose PET is nonspecific, and uptake may occur in both benign and malignant tumors, in inflammatory or infectious lesions, and with normal physiologic processes. Sarcoidosis and fungal infections may mimic lymphoma, and biopsy is often necessary to exclude recurrence (Fig. 8-23). A single persistent or new focus of activity, with paradoxical response at other sites of disease, requires further evaluation with a biopsy, because findings may represent a premalignant lesion, such as a thyroid or colonic adenoma, or an incidental second malignant tumor (Fig. 8-24).

NEW DIRECTIONS

Over the last 20 years, remarkable advances have been made in the diagnosis, characterization, and treatment of patients with aggressive NHL. The molecular characterization of disease is finally gaining clinical traction, due in large part to efficacy in clinical trials being preferential for a particular disease subtype. The future is bright for basic science, translational, and clinical research for aggressive lymphomas with a multitude of new therapeutic agents. It is our strong recommendation that all patients be considered for clinical trials to move the field forward.

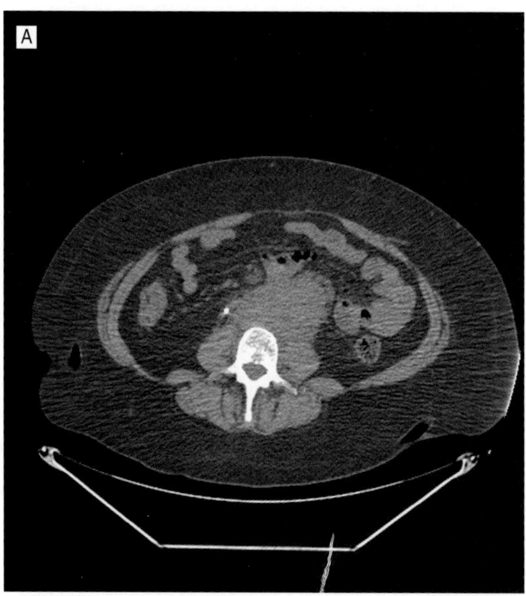

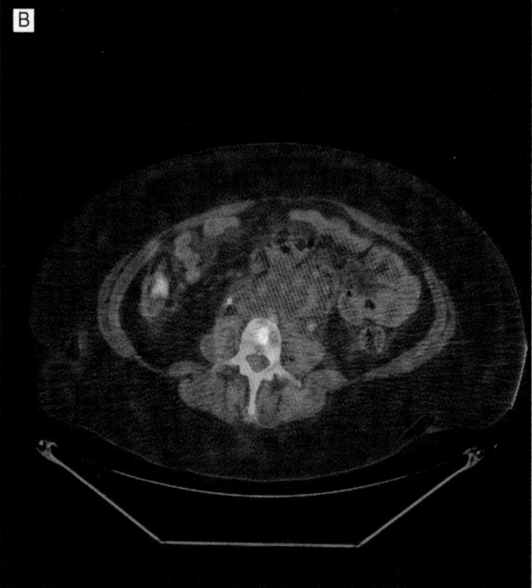

FIGURE 8-22 Residual mass, not residual lymphoma. After completing chemotherapy, this patient had a residual soft tissue abnormality in the retroperitoneum. **A.** This was previously positive on fluorodeoxyglucose positron emission tomography (FDG-PET) but now does not have activity above background levels and is considered negative. **B.** Biopsy of this mass was negative, and it was stable on follow-up studies. Previously, this would be considered a partial response (PR) or unconfirmed complete response (CRu). Under the revised criteria, taking into account the FDG-PET findings, this is considered a complete response (CR).

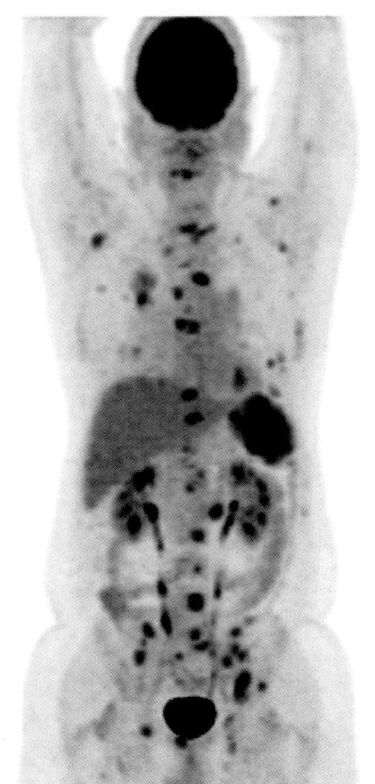

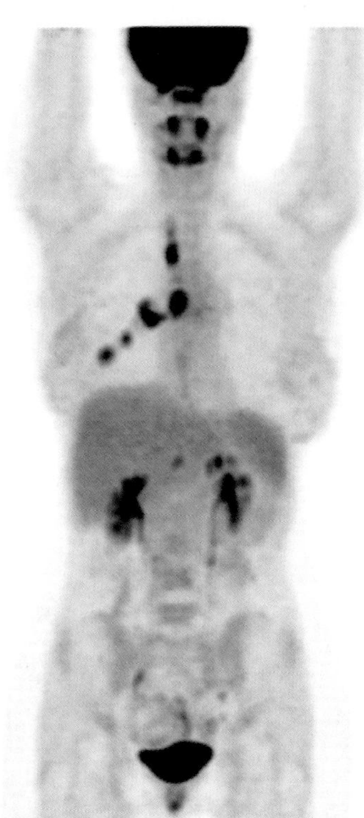

FIGURE 8-23 Examples of false-positive fluorodeoxyglucose positron emission tomography (FDG-PET). Restaging study is suspicious for recurrent lymphoma. **A.** With predominantly osseous involvement; however, biopsy revealed nonnecrotizing granulomas thought to be due to sarcoidosis. Two months later, nearly all of the FDG-avid sites resolved without any therapy. **B.** A second patient presented over 10 years after successful treatment for lymphoma, with new lymphadenopathy and lung opacities that were positive on FDG-PET. Biopsy revealed fungal lymphadenitis.

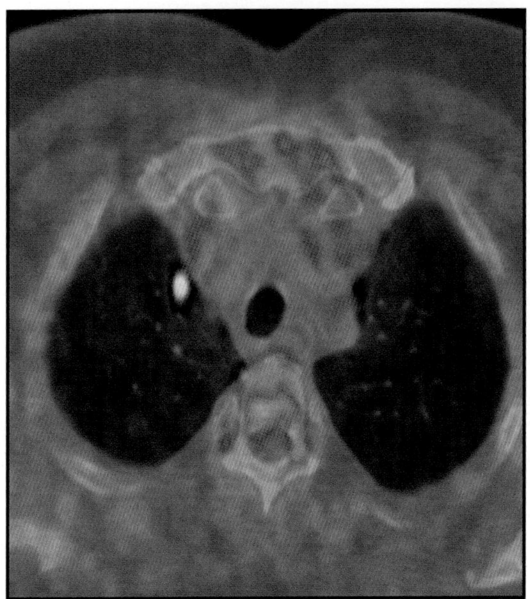

FIGURE 8-24 Incidental significant finding on fluorodeoxyglucose positron emission tomography (FDG-PET)/computed tomography (CT). An enlarging metabolically active lung nodule is seen. Biopsy revealed non–small-cell lung cancer, and the patient went on to have lobectomy for stage I lung cancer.

REFERENCES

1. Swerdlow SH, Campo E, Harris NL, et al. *WHO Classification of Tumours of Haematopoietic and Lymphoid Tissues*. 4th ed. Geneva, Switzerland: World Health Organization; 2008.
2. Groves FD, Linet MS, Travis LB, Devesa SS. Cancer surveillance series: non-Hodgkin's lymphoma incidence by histologic subtype in the United States from 1978 through 1995. *J Natl Cancer Inst*. 2000;92(15):1240-1251.
3. Clarke CA, Glaser SL. Changing incidence of non-Hodgkin lymphomas in the United States. *Cancer*. 2002;94(7):2015-2023.
4. Siegel RL, Miller KD, Jemal A. Cancer statistics, 2015. *CA Cancer J Clin*. 2015;65(1):5-29.
5. Li Y, Wang Y, Wang Z, Yi D, Ma S. Racial differences in three major NHL subtypes: descriptive epidemiology. *Cancer Epidemiol*. 2015;39(1):8-13.
6. Tomasetti C, Vogelstein B. Variation in cancer risk among tissues can be explained by the number of stem cell divisions. *Science*. 2015;347(6217):78-81.
7. Filipovich AH, Mathur A, Kamat D, Shapiro RS. Primary immunodeficiencies: genetic risk factors for lymphoma. *Cancer Res*. 1992;52(19 Suppl):5465s-5467s.
8. Mueller N. Overview of the epidemiology of malignancy in immune deficiency. *J Acquir Immune Defic Syndr*. 1999;21(Suppl 1):S5-10.
9. Opelz G, Dohler B. Lymphomas after solid organ transplantation: a collaborative transplant study report. *Am J Transplant*. 2004;4(2):222-230.
10. Brown SL, Greene MH, Gershon SK, Edwards ET, Braun MM.

Tumor necrosis factor antagonist therapy and lymphoma development: twenty-six cases reported to the Food and Drug Administration. *Arthritis Rheum*. 2002;46(12):3151-3158.
11. Salloum E, Cooper DL, Howe G, et al. Spontaneous regression of lymphoproliferative disorders in patients treated with methotrexate for rheumatoid arthritis and other rheumatic diseases. *J Clin Oncol*. 1996;14(6):1943-1949.
12. Lyons SF, Liebowitz DN. The roles of human viruses in the pathogenesis of lymphoma. *Semin Oncol*. 1998;25(4):461-475.
13. Cote TR, Biggar RJ, Rosenberg PS, et al. Non-Hodgkin's lymphoma among people with AIDS: incidence, presentation and public health burden. AIDS/Cancer Study Group. *Int J Cancer*. 1997;73(5):645-650.
14. Young LS, Murray PG. Epstein-Barr virus and oncogenesis: from latent genes to tumours. *Oncogene*. 2003;22(33):5108-5121.
15. Goedert JJ. The epidemiology of acquired immunodeficiency syndrome malignancies. *Semin Oncol*. 2000;27(4):390-401.
16. McDuffie HH, Pahwa P, McLaughlin JR, et al. Non-Hodgkin's lymphoma and specific pesticide exposures in men: cross-Canada study of pesticides and health. *Cancer Epidemiol Biomarkers Prev*. 2001;10(11):1155-1163.
17. Chatterjee N, Hartge P, Cerhan JR, et al. Risk of non-Hodgkin's lymphoma and family history of lymphatic, hematologic, and other cancers. *Cancer Epidemiol Biomarkers Prev*. 2004;13(9):1415-1421.
18. Westin JR, Fayad LE. Beyond R-CHOP and the IPI in large-cell lymphoma: molecular markers as an opportunity for stratification. *Curr Hematol Malig Rep*. 2009;4(4):218-224.
19. National Comprehensive Cancer Network. *Non-Hodgkin Lymphoma: NCCN Clinical Practice Guidelines in Oncology*. Version 2. 2015. Fort Washington, PA: National Comprehensive Cancer Network; 2015.
20. Maurer MJ, Ghesquieres H, Jais JP, et al. Event-free survival at 24 months is a robust end point for disease-related outcome in diffuse large B-cell lymphoma treated with immunochemotherapy. *J Clin Oncol*. 2014;32(10):1066-1073.
21. Sehn LH, Berry B, Chhanabhai M, et al. The revised International Prognostic Index (R-IPI) is a better predictor of outcome than the standard IPI for patients with diffuse large B-cell lymphoma treated with R-CHOP. *Blood*. 2007;109(5):1857-1861.
22. Horn H, Staiger AM, Vohringer M, et al. Diffuse large B-cell lymphomas of immunoblastic type are a major reservoir for MYC-IGH translocations. *Am J Surg Pathol*. 2015;39(1):61-66.
23. Thieblemont C, Brière J. MYC, BCL2, BCL6 in DLBCL: impact for clinics in the future? *Blood*. 2013;121(12):2165-2166.
24. Horn H, Ziepert M, Becher C, et al. MYC status in concert with BCL2 and BCL6 expression predicts outcome in diffuse large B-cell lymphoma. *Blood*. 2013;121(12):2253-2263.
25. Lenz G, Staudt LM. Aggressive lymphomas. *N Engl J Med*. 2010;362(15):1417-1429.
26. Oki Y, Noorani M, Lin P, et al. Double hit lymphoma: the MD Anderson Cancer Center clinical experience. *Br J Haematol*. 2014;166(6):891-901.
27. Johnson NA, Slack GW, Savage KJ, et al. Concurrent expression of MYC and BCL2 in diffuse large B-Cell lymphoma treated with rituximab plus cyclophosphamide, doxorubicin, vincristine, and prednisone. *J Clin Oncol*. 2012;30(28):3452-3459.
28. Green TM, Young KH, Visco C, et al. Immunohistochemical double-hit score is a strong predictor of outcome in patients with diffuse large B-cell lymphoma treated with rituximab plus cyclophosphamide, doxorubicin, vincristine, and prednisone. *J Clin Oncol*. 2012;30(28):3460-3467.
29. Cheah CY, Oki Y, Westin JR, Turturro F. A clinician's guide to double hit lymphomas. *Br J Haematol*. 2015;168(6):784-795.
30. Alizadeh AA, Eisen MB, Davis RE, et al. Distinct types of diffuse large B-cell lymphoma identified by gene expression profiling. *Nature*. 2000;403(6769):503-511.
31. Rosenwald A, Wright G, Chan WC, et al. The use of molecular profiling to predict survival after chemotherapy for diffuse large-B-cell lymphoma. *N Engl J Med*. 2002;346(25):1937-1947.
32. Scott DW, Wright GW, Williams PM, et al. Determining cell-of-origin subtypes of diffuse large B-cell lymphoma using gene expression in formalin-fixed paraffin-embedded tissue. *Blood*. 2014;123(8):1214-1217.
33. Hans CP, Weisenburger DD, Greiner TC, et al. Confirmation of the molecular classification of diffuse large B-cell lymphoma by immunohistochemistry using a tissue microarray. *Blood*. 2004;103(1):275-282.
34. Visco C, Li Y, Xu-Monette ZY, et al. Comprehensive gene expression profiling and immunohistochemical studies support application of immunophenotypic algorithm for molecular subtype classification in diffuse large B-cell lymphoma: a report from the International DLBCL Rituximab-CHOP Consortium Program Study. *Leukemia*. 2012;26(9):2103-2113.
35. Lin CH, Kuo KT, Chuang SS, et al. Comparison of the expression and prognostic significance of differentiation markers between diffuse large B-cell lymphoma of central nervous system origin and peripheral nodal origin. *Clin Cancer Res*. 2006;12(4):1152-1156.
36. Grange F, Bekkenk MW, Wechsler J, et al. Prognostic factors in primary cutaneous large B-cell lymphomas: a European multicenter study. *J Clin Oncol*. 2001;19(16):3602-3610.
37. Dijkman R, Tensen CP, Jordanova ES, et al. Array-based comparative genomic hybridization analysis reveals recurrent chromosomal alterations and prognostic parameters in primary cutaneous large B-cell lymphoma. *J Clin Oncol*. 2006;24(2):296-305.
38. Chen Y-B, Rahemtullah A, Hochberg E. Primary effusion lymphoma. *Oncologist*. 2007;12(5):569-576.
39. Pan ZG, Zhang QY, Lu ZB, et al. Extracavitary KSHV-associated large B-Cell lymphoma: a distinct entity or a subtype of primary effusion lymphoma? Study of 9 cases and review of an additional 43 cases. *Am J Surg Pathol*. 2012;36(8):1129-1140.
40. Steidl C, Gascoyne RD. The molecular pathogenesis of primary mediastinal large B-cell lymphoma. *Blood*. 2011;118(10):2659-2669.
41. Steidl C, Shah SP, Woolcock BW, et al. MHC class II transactivator CIITA is a recurrent gene fusion partner in lymphoid cancers. *Nature*. 2011;471(7338):377-381.
42. Campo E, Rule S. Mantle cell lymphoma: evolving management strategies. *Blood*. 2015;125(1):48-55.
43. Romaguera JE, Medeiros LJ, Hagemeister FB, et al. Frequency of gastrointestinal involvement and its clinical significance in mantle cell lymphoma. *Cancer*. 2003;97(3):586-591.
44. Vaandrager JW, Schuuring E, Zwikstra E, et al. Direct visualization of dispersed 11q23 chromosomal translocations in mantle cell lymphoma by multicolor DNA fiber fluorescence in situ hybridization. *Blood*. 1996;88:1177-1182.
45. Bertoni F, Zucca E, Cotter FE. Molecular basis of mantle cell lymphoma. *Br J Haematol*. 2004;124:130-140.
46. Wlodorska I, Pittaluga S, Hagemeijer A, et al. Secondary chromosome changes in mantle cell lymphoma. *Haematologica*. 1999;84:594-599.
47. Onciu M, Schlette E, Medeiros LJ, et al. Cytogenetic findings in mantle cell lymphoma cases with a high level of peripheral blood involvement have a distinct pattern of abnormalities. *Am J Clin Pathol*. 2001;116:886-892.
48. Magrath IT. African Burkitt's lymphoma: history, biology, clinical features, and treatment. *Am J Pediatr Hematol Oncol*. 1991;13:222-246.
49. Burkitt D. A sarcoma involving the jaws in African children. *Br J Surg*. 1958;46(197):218-223.
50. Ioachim HL, Dorsett B, Cronin W, et al. Acquired

immunodeficiency syndrome-associated lymphomas: clinical pathologic, immunologic, and viral characteristics of 111 cases. *Hum Pathol.* 1991;22:659-673.
51. Berard CW, O'Conor GT, Thomas LB, et al. Histopathological definition of Burkitt's tumour. *Bull WHO.* 1969;40:601-607.
52. Hecht JL, Aster JC. Molecular biology of Burkitt's lymphoma. *J Clin Oncol.* 2000;18:3707-3721.
53. Braziel RM, Arber DA, Slovak ML, et al. The Burkitt-like lymphomas: a Southwest Oncology Group study delineating phenotypic, genotypic, and clinical features. *Blood.* 2001;97(12):3713-3720.
54. Haralambieva E, Boerma EJ, van Imhoff GW, et al. Clinical, immunophenotypic, and genetic analysis of adult lymphomas with morphologic features of Burkitt lymphoma. *Am J Surg Pathol.* 2005;29(8):1086-1094.
55. Le Gouill S, Talmant P, Touzeau C, et al. The clinical presentation and prognosis of diffuse large B-cell lymphoma with t(14;18) and 8q24/c-MYC rearrangement. *Haematologica.* 2007; 92(10):1335-1342.
56. Kanungo A, Medeiros LJ, Abruzzo LV, Lin P. Lymphoid neoplasms associated with concurrent t(14;18) and 8q24/c-MYC translocation generally have a poor prognosis. *Mod Pathol.* 2006;19(1):25-33.
57. Savage KJ, Zeynalova S, Kansara RR, et al. Validation of a prognostic model to assess the risk of CNS disease in patients with aggressive B-cell lymphoma [abstract]. *Blood.* 2014;394.
58. Cheson BD, Fisher RI, Barrington SF, et al. Recommendations for initial evaluation, staging, and response assessment of Hodgkin and non-Hodgkin lymphoma: the Lugano Classification. *J Clin Oncol.* 2014;32(27):3059-3068.
59. Coller BS, Chabner BA, Gralnick HR. Frequencies and patterns of bone marrow involvement in non-Hodgkin lymphomas: observations on the value of bilateral biopsies. *Am J Hematol.* 1977;3:105-119.
60. Khan AB, Barrington SF, Mikhaeel NG, et al. PET-CT staging of DLBCL accurately identifies and provides new insight into the clinical significance of bone marrow involvement. *Blood.* 2013;122(1):61-67.
61. Cai Q, Westin J, Fu K, et al. Accelerated therapeutic progress in diffuse large B cell lymphoma. *Ann Hematol.* 2014;93(4):541-556.
62. Vose JM, Armitage JO, Weisenburger DD, et al. The importance of age in survival of patients treated with chemotherapy for aggressive non-Hodgkin's lymphoma. *J Clin Oncol.* 1988;6(12):1838-1844.
63. The International Non-Hodgkin's Lymphoma Prognostic Factors Project. A predictive model for aggressive non-Hodgkin's lymphoma. *N Engl J Med.* 1993;329(14):987-994.
64. Zhou Z, Sehn LH, Rademaker AW, et al. An enhanced International Prognostic Index (NCCN-IPI) for patients with diffuse large B-cell lymphoma treated in the rituximab era. *Blood.* 2014;123(6):837-842
65. Maurer MJ, Ghesquieres H, Jais J-P, et al. IPI24: An international study to create an IPI for the event-free survival at 24 months (EFS24) endpoint for DLBCL in the immunochemotherapy era [abstract]. *Blood.* 2013;362.
66. Hoster E, Dreyling M, Klapper W, et al. A new prognostic index (MIPI) for patients with advanced-stage mantle cell lymphoma. *Blood.* 2008;111(2):558-565.
67. Shah JJ, Fayad L, Romaguera J. Mantle Cell International Prognostic Index (MIPI) not prognostic after R-hyper-CVAD. *Blood.* 2008;112(6):2583.
68. Geisler CH, Kolstad A, Laurell A, et al. The Mantle Cell Lymphoma International Prognostic Index (MIPI) is superior to the International Prognostic Index (IPI) in predicting survival following intensive first-line immunochemotherapy and autologous stem cell transplantation (ASCT). *Blood.* 2010;115(8):1530-1533.
69. Ferreri AJM. How I treat primary CNS lymphoma. *Blood.* 2011;118(3):510-522.
70. Armitage JO, Weisenburger DD, Hutchins M, et al. Chemotherapy for diffuse large-cell lymphoma—rapidly responding patients have more durable remissions. *J Clin Oncol.* 1986;4(2):160-164.
71. Moskowitz CH, Schoder H, Teruya-Feldstein J, et al. Risk-adapted dose-dense immunochemotherapy determined by interim FDG-PET in Advanced-stage diffuse large B-Cell lymphoma. *J Clin Oncol.* 2010;28(11):1896-1903.
72. Gisselbrecht C, Schmitz N, Mounier N, et al. Diffuse large B-cell lymphoma (DLBCL) Patients failing second-line R-DHAP Or R-ICE chemotherapy included in the Coral study. *Blood.* 2013;122(21):764.
73. Chen MG, Prosnitz LR, Gonzalez-Serva A, Fischer DB. Results of radiotherapy in control of stage I and II non-Hodgkin's lymphoma. *Cancer.* 1979;43(4):1245-1254.
74. Miller TP, Dahlberg S, Cassady JR, et al. Chemotherapy alone compared with chemotherapy plus radiotherapy for localized intermediate- and high-grade non-Hodgkin's lymphoma. *N Engl J Med.* 1998;339(1):21-26.
75. Horning SJ, Weller E, Kim K, et al. Chemotherapy with or without radiotherapy in limited-stage diffuse aggressive non-Hodgkin's lymphoma: Eastern Cooperative Oncology Group study 1484. *J Clin Oncol.* 2004;22(15):3032-3038.
76. Reyes F, Lepage E, Ganem G, et al. ACVBP versus CHOP plus radiotherapy for localized aggressive lymphoma. *N Engl J Med.* 2005;352(12):1197-1205.
77. Bonnet C, Fillet G, Mounier N, et al. CHOP alone compared with CHOP plus radiotherapy for localized aggressive lymphoma in elderly patients: a study by the Groupe d'Etude des Lymphomes de l'Adulte. *J Clin Oncol.* 2007;25(7):787-792.
78. Persky DO, Unger JM, Spier CM, et al. Phase II study of rituximab plus three cycles of CHOP and involved-field radiotherapy for patients with limited-stage aggressive B-cell lymphoma: Southwest Oncology Group study 0014. *J Clin Oncol.* 2008;26(14):2258-2263.
79. Leitch HA, Gascoyne RD, Chhanabhai M, Voss NJ, Klasa R, Connors JM. Limited-stage mantle-cell lymphoma. *Ann Oncol.* 2003;14(10):1555-1561.
80. DeVita VT Jr, Canellos GP, Chabner B, Schein P, Hubbard SP, Young RC. Advanced diffuse histiocytic lymphoma, a potentially curable disease. *Lancet.* 1975;1(7901):248-250.
81. McKelvey EM, Gottlieb JA, Wilson HE, et al. Hydroxyldaunomycin (Adriamycin) combination chemotherapy in malignant lymphoma. *Cancer.* 1976;38(4):1484-1493.
82. Fisher RI, Gaynor ER, Dahlberg S, et al. Comparison of a standard regimen (CHOP) with three intensive chemotherapy regimens for advanced non-Hodgkin's lymphoma. *N Engl J Med.* 1993;328(14):1002-1006.
83. Wunderlich A, Kloess M, Reiser M, et al. Practicability and acute haematological toxicity of 2- and 3-weekly CHOP and CHOEP chemotherapy for aggressive non-Hodgkin's lymphoma: results from the NHL-B trial of the German High-Grade Non-Hodgkin's Lymphoma Study Group (DSHNHL). *Ann Oncol.* 2003;14(6):881-893.
84. Pfreundschuh M, Trumper L, Kloess M, et al. Two-weekly or 3-weekly CHOP chemotherapy with or without etoposide for the treatment of young patients with good-prognosis (normal LDH) aggressive lymphomas: results of the NHL-B1 trial of the DSHNHL. *Blood.* 2004;104(3):626-633.
85. Feugier P, Van Hoof A, Sebban C, et al. Long-term results of the R-CHOP study in the treatment of elderly patients with diffuse large B-cell lymphoma: a study by the Groupe d'Etude des Lymphomes de l'Adulte. *J Clin Oncol.* 2005;23(18):4117-4126.
86. Pfreundschuh M, Schubert J, Ziepert M, et al. Six versus eight cycles of bi-weekly CHOP-14 with or without rituximab in elderly patients with aggressive CD20+ B-cell lymphomas:

a randomised controlled trial (RICOVER-60). *Lancet Oncol.* 2008;9(2):105-116.

87. Cunningham D, Hawkes EA, Jack A, et al. Rituximab plus cyclophosphamide, doxorubicin, vincristine, and prednisolone in patients with newly diagnosed diffuse large B-cell non-Hodgkin lymphoma: a phase 3 comparison of dose intensification with 14-day versus 21-day cycles. *Lancet.* 2013;381(9880):1817-1826.
88. Delarue R, Tilly H, Mounier N, et al. Dose-dense rituximab-CHOP compared with standard rituximab-CHOP in elderly patients with diffuse large B-cell lymphoma (the LNH03-6B study): a randomised phase 3 trial. *Lancet Oncol.* 2013; 14(6):525-533.
89. Shah GD, Yahalom J, Correa DD, et al. Combined immunochemotherapy with reduced whole-brain radiotherapy for newly diagnosed primary CNS lymphoma. *J Clin Oncol.* 2007; 25(30):4730-4735.
90. Correa DD, Rocco-Donovan M, DeAngelis LM, et al. Prospective cognitive follow-up in primary CNS lymphoma patients treated with chemotherapy and reduced-dose radiotherapy. *J Neurooncol.* 2009;91(3):315-321.
91. Rubenstein JL, Hsi ED, Johnson JL, et al. Intensive chemotherapy and immunotherapy in patients with newly diagnosed primary CNS lymphoma: CALGB 50202 (Alliance 50202). *J Clin Oncol.* 2013;31(25):3061-3068.
92. Johnson PW, Davies AJ. Primary mediastinal B-cell lymphoma. *Hematology Am Soc Hematol Educ Program.* 2008:349-358.
93. Dunleavy K, Pittaluga S, Maeda LS, et al. Dose-adjusted EPOCH-rituximab therapy in primary mediastinal B-cell lymphoma. *N Engl J Med.* 2013;368(15):1408-1416.
94. Romaguera JE, Fayad LE, Feng L, et al. Ten-year follow-up after intense chemoimmunotherapy with rituximab-hyperCVAD alternating with rituximab-high dose methotrexate/cytarabine (R-MA) and without stem cell transplantation in patients with untreated aggressive mantle cell lymphoma. *Br J Haematol.* 2010;150(2):200-208.
95. Kahl BS, Longo WL, Eickhoff JC, et al. Maintenance rituximab following induction chemoimmunotherapy may prolong progression-free survival in mantle cell lymphoma: a pilot study from the Wisconsin Oncology Network. *Ann Oncol.* 2006; 17(9):1418-1423.
96. Geisler CH, Kolstad A, Laurell A, et al. Long-term progression-free survival of mantle cell lymphoma after intensive front-line immunochemotherapy with in vivo-purged stem cell rescue: a nonrandomized phase 2 multicenter study by the Nordic Lymphoma Group. *Blood.* 2008;112(7):2687-2693.
97. Rummel MJ, Niederle N, Maschmeyer G, et al. Bendamustine plus rituximab versus CHOP plus rituximab as first-line treatment for patients with indolent and mantle-cell lymphomas: an open-label, multicentre, randomised, phase 3 non-inferiority trial. *Lancet.* 2013;381(9873):1203-1210.
98. Oki Y, Noorani M, Lin P, et al. Double hit lymphoma: the MD Anderson Cancer Center clinical experience. *Br J Haematol.* 2014;166(6):891-901.
99. Petrich AM, Gandhi M, Jovanovic B, et al. Impact of induction regimen and stem cell transplantation on outcomes in double-hit lymphoma: a multicenter retrospective analysis. *Blood.* 2014;124(15):2354-2361.
100. Green TM, Young KH, Visco C, et al. Immunohistochemical double-hit score is a strong predictor of outcome in patients with diffuse large B-cell lymphoma treated with rituximab plus cyclophosphamide, doxorubicin, vincristine, and prednisone. *J Clin Oncol.* 2012;30(28):3460-3467.
101. Dunleavy K, Wilson WH. How I treat HIV-associated lymphoma. *Blood.* 2012;119(14):3245-3255.
102. Dunleavy K, Pittaluga S, Shovlin M, et al. Low-intensity therapy in adults with Burkitt's lymphoma. *N Engl J Med.* 2013;369(20):1915-1925.
103. Gisselbrecht C, Glass B, Mounier N, et al. Salvage regimens with autologous transplantation for relapsed large B-cell lymphoma in the rituximab era. *J Clin Oncol.* 2010;28(27):4184-4190.
104. Crump M, Kuruvilla J, Couban S, et al. Randomized comparison of gemcitabine, dexamethasone, and cisplatin versus dexamethasone, cytarabine, and cisplatin chemotherapy before autologous stem-cell transplantation for relapsed and refractory aggressive lymphomas: NCIC-CTG LY.12. *J Clin Oncol.* 2014;32(31):3490-3496.
105. Westin JR, McLaughlin P, Romaguera J, et al. Paclitaxel, topotecan and rituximab: long term outcomes of an effective salvage programme for relapsed or refractory aggressive B-cell non-Hodgkin lymphoma. *Br J Haematol.* 2014;167(2):177-184.
106. Philip T, Guglielmi C, Hagenbeek A, et al. Autologous bone marrow transplantation as compared with salvage chemotherapy in relapses of chemotherapy-sensitive non-Hodgkin's lymphoma. *N Engl J Med.* 1995;333(23):1540-1545.
107. Oki Y, Westin JR, Vega F, et al. Prospective phase II study of rituximab with alternating cycles of hyper-CVAD and high-dose methotrexate with cytarabine for young patients with high-risk diffuse large B-cell lymphoma. *Br J Haematol.* 2013;163(5):611-620.
108. Mead GM, Sydes MR, Walewski J, et al. An international evaluation of CODOX-M and CODOX-M alternating with IVAC in adult Burkitt's lymphoma: results of United Kingdom Lymphoma Group LY06 study. *Ann Oncol.* 2002;13(8):1264-1274.
109. Thomas DA, Faderl S, O'Brien S, et al. Chemoimmunotherapy with hyper-CVAD plus rituximab for the treatment of adult Burkitt and Burkitt-type lymphoma or acute lymphoblastic leukemia. *Cancer.* 2006;106(7):1569-1580.
110. Ziepert M, Hasenclever D, Kuhnt E, et al. Standard International Prognostic Index remains a valid predictor of outcome for patients with aggressive CD20+ B-cell lymphoma in the rituximab era. *J Clin Oncol.* 2010;28(14):2373-2380.
111. Moccia AA, Schaff K, Hoskins P, et al. R-CHOP with etoposide substituted for doxorubicin (R-CEOP): excellent outcome in diffuse large B cell lymphoma for patients with a contraindication to anthracyclines. *Blood.* 2009;114(22):408.
112. Peyrade F, Jardin F, Thieblemont C, et al. Attenuated immunochemotherapy regimen (R-miniCHOP) in elderly patients older than 80 years with diffuse large B-cell lymphoma: a multicentre, single-arm, phase 2 trial. *Lancet Oncol.* 2011;12(5):460-468.
113. Westin JR, Kurzrock R. It's about time: lessons for solid tumors from chronic myelogenous leukemia therapy. *Mol Cancer Ther.* 2012;11(12):2549-2555.
114. Wilson WH. Treatment strategies for aggressive lymphomas: what works? *Hematology Am Soc Hematol Educ Program.* 2013;2013:584-590.
115. Younes A, Thieblemont C, Morschhauser F, et al. Combination of ibrutinib with rituximab, cyclophosphamide, doxorubicin, vincristine, and prednisone (R-CHOP) for treatment-naive patients with CD20-positive B-cell non-Hodgkin lymphoma: a non-randomised, phase 1b study. *Lancet Oncol.* 2014;15(9):1019-1026.
116. Westin JR. Status of PI3K/Akt/mTOR pathway inhibitors in lymphoma. *Clin Lymphoma Myeloma Leuk.* 2014;14(5):335-342.
117. Yang Y, Shaffer AL 3rd, Emre NC, et al. Exploiting synthetic lethality for the therapy of ABC diffuse large B cell lymphoma. *Cancer Cell.* 2012;21(6):723-737.
118. Nowakowski GS, LaPlant B, Macon WR, et al. Lenalidomide combined with R-CHOP overcomes negative prognostic impact of non-germinal center B-cell phenotype in newly diagnosed diffuse large B-Cell lymphoma: a phase II study. *J Clin Oncol.* 2015;33(3):251-257.
119. Cheson BD, Fisher RI, Barrington SF, et al. Recommendations for initial evaluation, staging, and response assessment of

Hodgkin and non-Hodgkin lymphoma: the Lugano classification. *J Clin Oncol*. 2014;32(27):3059-3068.
120. Moskowitz CH. Interim PET-CT in the management of diffuse large B-cell lymphoma. *Hematology Am Soc Hematol Educ Program*. 2012;2012(1):397-401.
121. Schnipper LE, Lyman GH, Blayney DW, et al. American Society of Clinical Oncology 2013 top five list in oncology. *J Clin Oncol*. 2013;31(34):4362-4370.
122. Thompson CA, Ghesquieres H, Maurer MJ, et al. Utility of routine post-therapy surveillance imaging in diffuse large B-cell lymphoma. *J Clin Oncol*. 2014;32(31):3506-3512.

9

T-Cell Lymphomas

第九章　T细胞淋巴瘤

Dai Chihara
Casey Wang
Madeleine Duvic
L. Jeffrey Medeiros
Yasuhiro Oki

中文导读

T细胞淋巴瘤是一类异质性较高的恶性肿瘤，包括多种类型，且侵袭性强，外周T细胞淋巴瘤是T细胞淋巴瘤中常见的发病类型。本章节阐述了几种外周T细胞淋巴瘤亚型的流行病学、临床表现、组织病理学特征、发病机制，其中包括：外周T细胞淋巴瘤（非特指型）、间变性大细胞淋巴瘤、血管免疫母T细胞淋巴瘤以及其他罕见类型T细胞淋巴瘤。对外周T细胞淋巴瘤的分子细胞学和预后因素都进行了详细分析。在外周T细胞淋巴瘤治疗方面，尤其关注一线化疗方案、挽救化疗方案、自体/异基因造血干细胞移植方案的选择，也简述了针对复发/难治性外周T细胞淋巴瘤的新型靶向药物的作用机制和选择原则。另外，皮肤T细胞淋巴瘤是一类罕见的T细胞淋巴，随着近年该病的发病率增长，也引起了越来越多的关注。本章节在皮肤T细胞淋巴瘤部分，围绕分类、临床表现、诊断、预后等进行了全面解析，讲述了早/中期、难治或发生转化的蕈样肉芽肿以及Sézary综合征的治疗推荐，以及不同类型靶向药物的选择。除了ALK阳性间变性大细胞淋巴瘤，其余的外周T细胞淋巴瘤亚型和皮肤T细胞淋巴瘤的预后均较差，未来期盼有更多临床试验和新型靶向药物能为患者带来新的治疗选择。

PERIPHERAL (MATURE) T-CELL LYMPHOMAS

Peripheral T-cell lymphoma (PTCL) is a heterogeneous group of lymphomas derived from a mature T cell (Fig. 9-1). Currently, the World Health Organization (WHO) classification combines mature T- and natural killer (NK)-cell neoplasms under the umbrella term PTCL, and the category is composed of 23 different entities (Table 9-1), based on the different morphologic, phenotypic, molecular, and clinical features, including disease site ([1]). Most PTCLs lack distinct genetic or biologic alterations that are seen in B-cell lymphomas, such as t(14;18) in follicular lymphoma and t(11;14) in mantle cell lymphoma. Compared with B-cell lymphomas, many types of PTCL develop not in lymph nodes, but in specific extranodal sites such as extranodal NK/T-cell lymphoma, nasal type (ENKL) in the nasal cavity, enteropathy-associated T-cell lymphoma (EATL) in the small intestine, and hepatosplenic T-cell lymphoma (HSTL) in the liver and spleen.

EPIDEMIOLOGY

Peripheral T-cell lymphoma represents 5% to 10% of all lymphomas in the United States ([2]). The most common histologic subtype is PTCL, not otherwise specified (PTCL-NOS), followed by angioimmunoblastic T-cell lymphoma (AITL) or anaplastic large-cell lymphoma (ALCL), either ALK positive or ALK negative. The three types account for about 60% of all cases of PTCLs ([3]). The age-adjusted incidence in the United States for PTCL-NOS, AITL, and ALCL is 0.30, 0.05, and 0.25 per 100,000 person-years, respectively ([2]). Previous studies have indicated that some Asian countries have a higher incidence of PTCL ([3]). However, age-adjusted incidence estimated by population-based cancer registry data showed a similar incidence of PTCL in the United States and Japan except for NK/T-cell lymphoma (NKTCL) and adult T-cell leukemia/lymphoma (ATLL) ([4]). The incidence of cutaneous T-cell lymphoma (CTCL) is higher in the United States, particularly in African Americans.

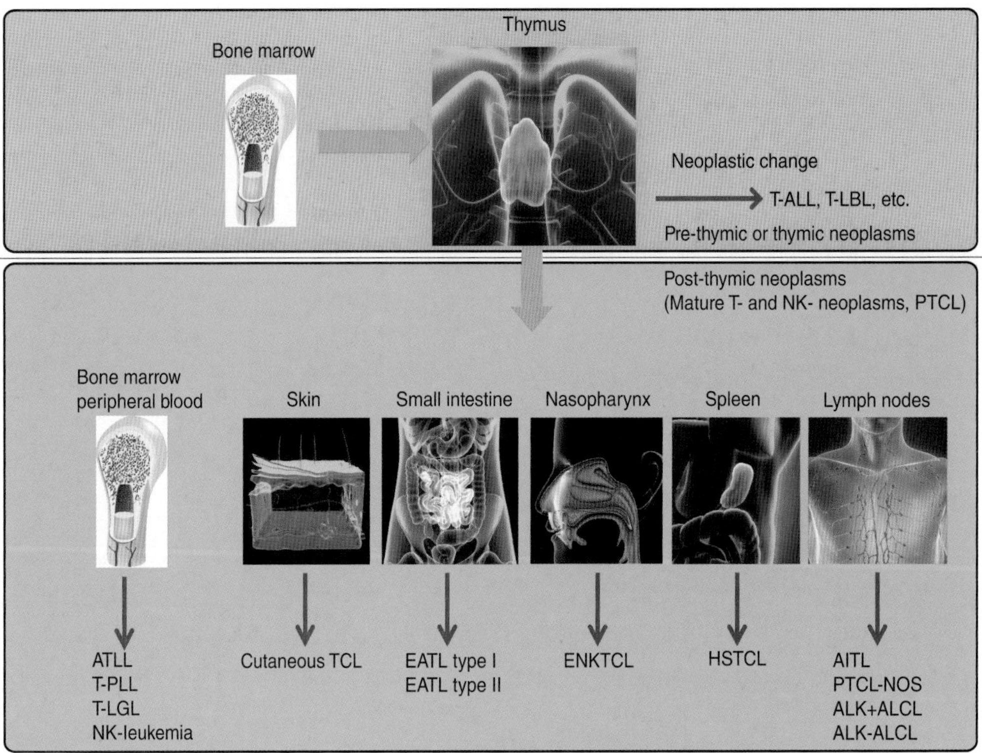

FIGURE 9-1 Peripheral T-cell lymphoma: T-cell maturation and organ of involvement. AITL, angioimmunoblastic T-cell lymphoma; ALCL, anaplastic large T-cell lymphoma; ATLL, adult T-cell lymphoma/leukemia; EATL, enteropathy associated T-cell lymphoma; ENKTCL, extranodal NK/T-cell lymphoma; HSTCL, hepatosplenic T-cell lymphoma; NK, natural killer; PTCL, peripheral T-cell lymphoma; PTCL-NOS, PTCL, not otherwise specified; T-ALL, T-cell acute lymphoblastic leukemia; TCL, T-cell lymphoma; T-LBL, T-cell lymphoblastic lymphoma; T-LGL, T-cell large granular lymphocytic leukemia; T-PLL, T-cell prolymphocytic leukemia.

Table 9-1 Peripheral T-Cell Lymphomas in World Health Organization Classification, 4th Edition

Mature T-cell and NK-cell neoplasms
T-cell prolymphocytic leukemia
T-cell large granular lymphocytic leukemia
Chronic lymphoproliferative disorder of NK cells
Aggressive NK-cell lymphoma
Extranodal NK/T-cell lymphoma, nasal type
Systemic EBV-positive T-cell lymphoproliferative disease of childfood
Hydroa vacciniforme-like lymphoma
Adult T-cell leukemia/lymphoma
Enteropathy-associated T-cell lymphoma
Hepatosplenic T-cell lymphoma
Subcutaneous panniculitis-like T-cell lymphoma
Mycosis fungoides
Sézary syndrome
Primary cutaneous CD30-positive T-cell lymphoproliferative disorders
Lymphomatoid papulosis
Primary cutaneous anaplastic large-cell lymphoma
Primary cutaneous gamma-delta T-cell lymphoma
Primary cutaneous CD8-positive aggressive epidermotropic cytotoxic T-cell lymphoma
Primary cutaneous CD4-positive small/medium T-cell lymphoma
Peripheral T-cell lymphoma, unspecified
Angioimmunoblastic T-cell lymphoma
Anaplastic large-cell lymphoma, ALK positive
Anaplastic large-cell lymphoma, ALK negative

EBV, Epstein-Barr virus; NK, natural killer.

PRESENTATION AND HISTOPATHOLOGIC FINDINGS

The presentation of patients with T-cell lymphoma largely depends on the subtype. Peripheral T-cell lymphoma, not otherwise specified, AITL, and ALCL often present with generalized lymphadenopathy, and there is also frequent involvement of the skin, gastrointestinal tract, liver, spleen, and bone marrow. In contrast, a number of rare specific subtypes, such as NKTCL, HSTL, and EATL, present primarily with extranodal disease, and other subtypes, such as NKTCL and ATLL, may have a leukemic presentation. Advanced-stage disease (stages III and IV) is common: PTCL-NOS, 69%; AITL, 89%; ALK-positive ALCL, 65%; ALK-negative ALCL, 58%; EATL, 69%; and HSTL, 90%.

The histopathologic and immunophenotypic findings may vary within a given subtype. Therefore, the diagnosis should be made based on a combination of clinical presentation and histopathologic findings. T-cell receptor rearrangements are found in most cases of PTCL, but a negative result does not necessarily exclude the disease.

Peripheral T-Cell Lymphoma, Not Otherwise Specified

Peripheral T-cell lymphoma, not otherwise specified, represents the largest subtype and accounts for 25% to 30% of all PTCLs ([1, 3]). Its definition in the current WHO classification is a "mature T-cell lymphoma which does not correspond to any of the specifically defined entities." The diagnosis of PTCL-NOS should be made only when other specific entities have been excluded, and, therefore, it is a heterogeneous category at the genetic level.

There is male predominance (male-to-female ratio of approximately 2:1). Patients most often present with lymph node enlargement and with advanced-stage disease (60%-70%) with B symptoms. Extranodal presentation is also common (30%-40%), with the bone marrow, skin, and gastrointestinal tract being the most commonly affected sites ([5, 6]).

Histologically, the lymph node architecture is diffusely effaced ([1]). The cytologic spectrum is extremely broad ranging from highly polymorphous to monomorphous presentations. Most cases exhibit a spectrum of cell sizes from medium to large and can have abundant clear cytoplasm with irregular, pleomorphic, and hyperchromatic nuclei and high mitotic figures (Figs. 9-2 and 9-3). Reed-Sternberg–like cells may also be found.

Immunophenotypic studies show aberrant T-cell phenotype, typically marked by downregulation of CD5 and CD7. Nodal cases most often show $CD4^+$/$CD8^-$ phenotype. T-cell receptor (TCR) β-chain (βF1) is usually expressed, allowing the distinction from γδ T-cell lymphomas and NK-cell lymphomas. Cytotoxic molecules, such as TIA-1 and granzyme B, are expressed in 40% of nodal PTCL-NOS, and expression is associated with younger age at presentation, aggressive features, treatment resistance, and inferior survival ([7]). CD30 expression is observed in 3% to 50% of cases ([5, 8, 9]). Lymphoma cells may occasionally express CD15, but the phenotypic profile and morphology allow the distinction from ALCL and Hodgkin lymphoma ([9]). Cytogenetic abnormalities in PTCLs are common, and karyotypes are often complex. Recurrent chromosomal gains have been observed in chromosomes 7q, 8q, 17q, and 22q, and recurrent losses in chromosomes 4q, 5q, 6q, 9p, 10q, 12q, and 13q, with del 5q, 10q, and 12q being associated with better outcome ([10, 11]).

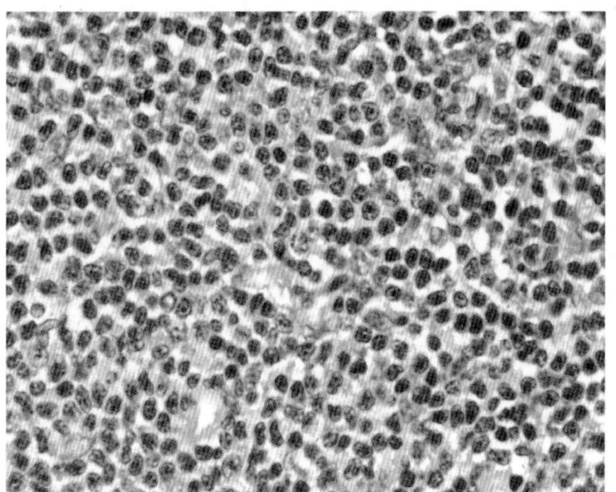

FIGURE 9-2 Peripheral T-cell lymphoma, not otherwise specified. The neoplastic cells in this case are predominantly small (hematoxylin-eosin, 1,000×).

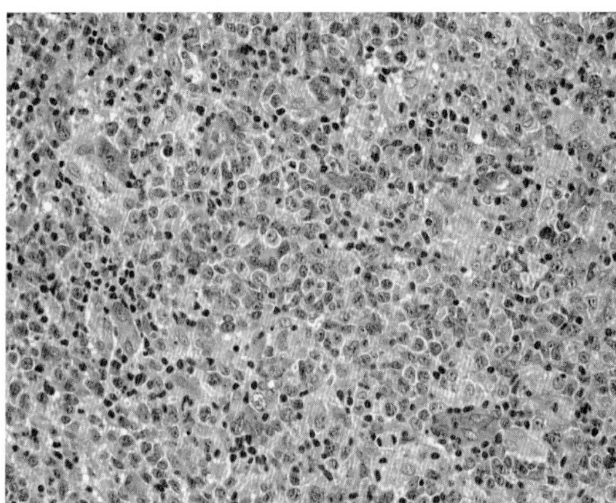

FIGURE 9-3 Peripheral T-cell lymphoma, not otherwise specified. The neoplastic cells in this case are small and large (hematoxylin-eosin, 1,000×).

Gene expression profiling analysis has confirmed the molecular heterogeneity of the PTCL-NOS category. Using expression signatures, about one-third of PTCL-NOS cases can be classified as other known T-cell entities, such as AITL. In addition, cases of PTCL-NOS that remain can be divided into two groups characterized by high expression of GATA3 or TBX21, with the GATA3 group having poor survival ([12]).

Follicular T-Helper Cell Lymphoma

These tumors are currently considered a variant of PTCL-NOS, but they have a distinctive follicular pattern and are thought to be derived for follicular T-helper cells, a small T-cell population that is $CD10^+$, $BCL6^+$, and $PD\text{-}1/CD279^+$ in normal follicles. A recurrent t(5;9)(q33;q22), resulting in the *ITK-SYK* fusion gene, has been described in a subset of patients with follicular histology ([13]).

Anaplastic Large-Cell Lymphoma

In the current WHO classification, two types of systemic ALCL are recognized. One type associated with translocations involving the *ALK* gene and leading to ALK overexpression is well established. The other category, morphologically similar to ALK-positive ALCL but lacking ALK abnormalities of overexpression, is considered a provisional category and designated as ALK-negative ALCL. However, there are recent data that show that the ALK-negative ALCL category is highly heterogeneous at the genetic level and that genetic abnormalities correlate with prognosis, calling into question the validity of the ALK-negative ALCL category.

ALK-Positive Anaplastic Large-Cell Lymphoma

Patients with ALK-positive ALCL are younger, with a median age in the low 30s, and children are commonly affected ([14,15]). Anaplastic large-cell lymphoma accounts for 3% to 5% of all non-Hodgkin lymphomas (NHLs) and for 10% to 20% of childhood lymphomas ([1]). Patients with ALK-positive ALCL generally present with lymph node enlargement and frequent extranodal involvement of skin, bone, soft tissue, lung, and liver. More than half present with B symptoms at diagnosis, particularly fever.

Histologically, ALK-positive ALCL exhibits a wide histologic spectrum (Fig. 9-4). A number of morphologic patterns have been recognized: common type, lymphohistiocytic, small cell, Hodgkin-like, sarcoma-like, and others, as well as mixed or composite patterns. About 80% of cases exhibit the common pattern, characterized by large lymphoma cells infiltrating sinuses and/or showing cohesive features. The lymphohistiocytic and small-cell patterns each represent 5% to 10% of cases of ALK-positive ALCL. In all variants, the lymphoma cells have eccentric, horseshoe- or kidney-shaped nuclei, often with an eosinophilic region near the nucleus (so-called hallmark cells). The cytoplasm is abundant and usually basophilic (see Fig. 9-4).

ALK-positive ALCL is a lymphoma of T/null-cell lineage that is characterized by strong and diffuse CD30 and ALK expression. Most of cases are $CD2^+$, $CD4^+$, $CD43^+$, $CD3^-$, $CD8^-$, and $BCL2^-$. CD15 and PAX5 are negative (unlike classical Hodgkin lymphoma). The pattern of ALK expression, in part, can predict molecular abnormalities involving ALK. Cytoplasmic and nuclear expression correlates with the t(2;5)(p23;q35)/NPM1/ALK ([16]). Other cases with ALK abnormalities show a cytoplasmic restricted or, rarely, a membranous pattern of expression [17].

ALK-Negative Anaplastic Large-Cell Lymphoma

Patients with ALK-negative ALCL are older, with a median age in the late 50s. Clinically patients present with aggressive disease, with lymph node enlargement, frequent extranodal involvement, and B symptoms. The morphologic spectrum of ALK-negative ALCL is similar to ALK-positive ALCL, except that the neoplastic cells may be more pleomorphic. The neoplastic cells have a T/null-cell immunophenotype and strongly and uniformly express CD30 but are negative for ALK.

A recent study has shown that ALK-negative ALCL is molecularly heterogeneous. Rearrangement of *DUSP22*, marked by t(6;7), was found in 30% of cases and is associated with excellent prognosis with 90% long-term survival, whereas *TP63* rearrangement, marked by inv(3), was seen in 8% of cases and is associated with poor prognosis with only 17% long-term survival. The remaining cases are still poorly characterized.

Angioimmunoblastic T-Cell Lymphoma

Angioimmunoblastic T-cell lymphoma was first described as angioimmunoblastic lymphadenopathy with dysproteinemia in 1974 and was thought to be a preneoplastic process. Evidence now indicates that AITL is a de novo PTCL. Angioimmunoblastic T-cell lymphoma represents the second most common subtype, accounting for 15% to 20% of PTCLs [3].

The median age of patients with AITL is 65 years [18, 19]. Most patients present with advanced disease. Generalized lymphadenopathy and extranodal presentations, including hepatosplenomegaly, bone marrow involvement, rash with pruritus, ascites, and pleural effusion are frequent. B symptoms (fever, night sweats, weight loss) are common. Laboratory abnormalities include polyclonal hypergammaglobulinemia (sometimes with a positive direct Coombs

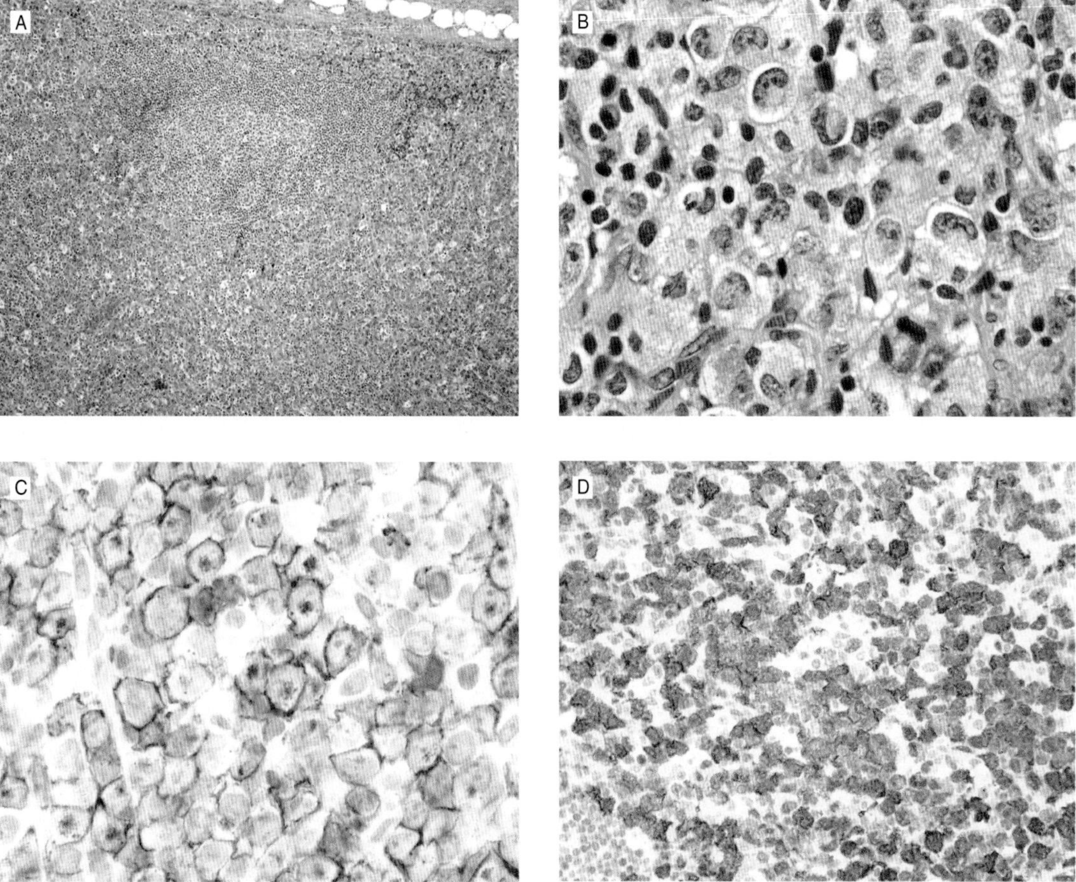

FIGURE 9-4 ALK-positive anaplastic large-cell lymphoma. **A.** In this field, the neoplasm is paracortical and spares a central lymphoid follicle. **B.** The neoplastic cells are large with horseshoe-shaped nuclei. **C, D.** The neoplastic cells express CD30 (**C**) and ALK (**D**). (**A, B,** hematoxylin-eosin; **A,** 100×; **B,** 1,000×; **C, D,** immunohistochemistry; **C,** 1,000×; **D,** 400×).

test), anemia, hypereosinophilia, thrombocytopenia, and positive autoantibodies for cold agglutinin, rheumatoid factor, antinuclear factor, and anti–smooth muscle antibody are also common ([18, 19]).

Histologically, the lymph node architecture is replaced by a diffuse, polymorphous population of cells associated with a proliferation of branching high endothelial venules. The neoplastic cells are small to medium in size, often with abundant clear cytoplasm, and can form small clusters surrounding the follicles and high endothelial venules (Fig. 9-5). Reactive cells are numerous in AITL, such as lymphocytes, eosinophils, plasma cells, histiocytes, and $CD21^+$ follicular dendritic cell networks. Most cases also show expansion of B cells positive for Epstein-Barr virus (EBV), which is thought to be related to immune dysfunction.

In AITL, lymphoma cells usually express T-cell antigens such as CD3, CD2, and CD5, and have a T-helper cell immunophenotype characterized by expression of CD4, CD10, BCL6, CXCL13, and PD-1. Follicular dendritic cells ($CD21^+$, $CD23^+$) are expanded, usually surrounding high endothelial venules.

Chromosomal abnormalities have been identified in AITL, with trisomy 3 and trisomy 5 being most common ([20]). Recent studies have shown mutations in *TET2*, *IDH2*, *DNMT3A*, and *RHOA* ([21]). Among 243 patients in the International T-Cell Lymphoma Project, 5-year failure-free survival and overall survival (OS) rates were 18% and 32%, respectively, which was very similar to the outcome of patients with PTCL-NOS ([18]).

Rare Types of T-Cell Lymphoma

Adult T-Cell Lymphoma/Leukemia

Adult T-cell lymphoma/leukemia is a distinct clinicopathologic entity associated with infection by the human T-cell lymphotropic virus type-1 (HTLV-1) ([1]). The HTLV-1 is a single-stranded RNA retrovirus that is lymphotropic for T lymphocytes. Infection with HTLV-1 is endemic in Africa, Iran, the Caribbean islands, Central and South America, and the southern part of Japan ([22]). Approximately 10 to 20 million

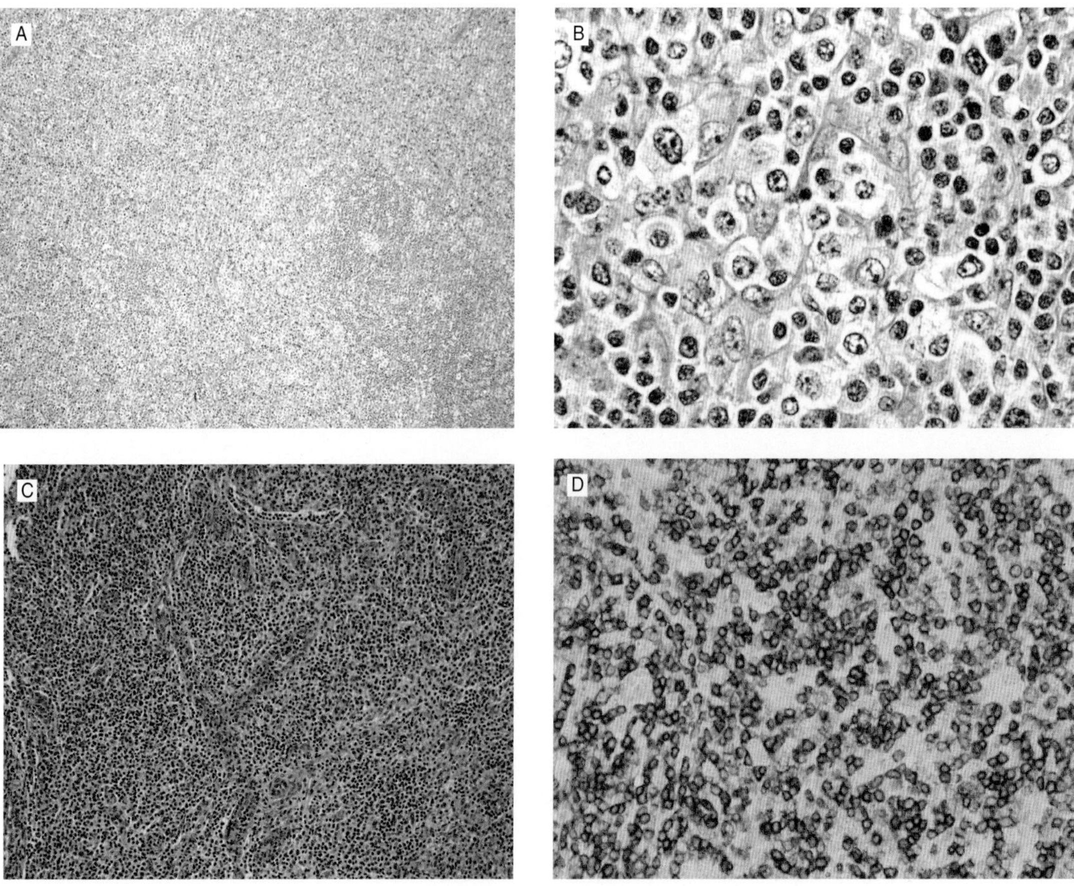

FIGURE 9-5 Angioimmunoblastic T-cell lymphoma. **A.** The neoplasm has a paracortical distribution. **B.** The neoplasm is composed of numerous cells with clear cytoplasm. **C.** In this field, arborizing blood vessels are shown. **D.** The neoplastic cells are positive for CD3. (**A-C**, hematoxylin-eosin; **A**, 100×; **B**, 1,000×; **C**, 200×; **D**, immunohistochemistry, 400×).

people are infected by HTLV-1 worldwide. Three major routes of HTLV-1 infection have been established: vertical transmission by breastfeeding, parental transmission, and sexual transmission. The lifetime cumulative incidence of ATLL in an HTLV-1 carrier is 2% to 3% for women and 6% to 7% for men ([23]). The median age at the time ATLL develops is the seventh decade of life. Risk factors for developing ATLL include high proviral load, advanced age, family history of ATLL, and types of human leukocyte antigen alleles ([24]). Individuals infected in adulthood rarely, if ever, develop ATLL, suggesting that the latency of infection is very long and age at the time of HTLV-1 infection is important ([25]). Adult T-cell lymphoma/leukemia accounts for less than 1% of NHL in the United States but accounts for around 35% to 40% of NHL in the endemic area in Japan ([4]). However, there seems to be an increasing trend in the incidence of ATLL in the United States, possibly due to the emigration of people from endemic areas ([26]). The prognosis is extremely poor with conventional chemotherapy ([27]). Median OS is less than 1 year without allogeneic stem cell transplantation.

Adult T-cell lymphoma/leukemia is classified into four subtypes based on clinicopathologic features and prognosis: acute, lymphoma, chronic, and smoldering ([28]). Patients with acute ATLL, the most common form of the disease, have generalized lymphadenopathy, hepatosplenomegaly, skin lesions, peripheral blood involvement, lytic bone lesions, and hypercalcemia. Hypercalcemia may also develop in the absence of bone lesions, secondary to secretion of parathyroid hormone–related peptide by the neoplastic cells (Fig. 9-6).

In the peripheral blood, the neoplastic cells are medium-sized, with basophilic cytoplasm and markedly irregular, multilobulated nuclei, including cloverleaf shapes (also known as flower cells) ([1]). The neoplastic cells in lymph nodes and viscera exhibit a spectrum of cell sizes, including small, medium, and large, with relatively round or markedly irregular nuclear contours. Histopathologic findings are not specific for ATLL, and testing for HTLV-1 antibody is needed for suspicious cases even in non-endemic areas.

Immunophenotypic studies show a mature T-cell immunophenotype. The neoplastic cells intensely express CD25 antigen. They also frequently express the chemokine receptor CCR4 and FOXP3, suggesting that regulatory T cells are the closest normal counterpart ([29]).

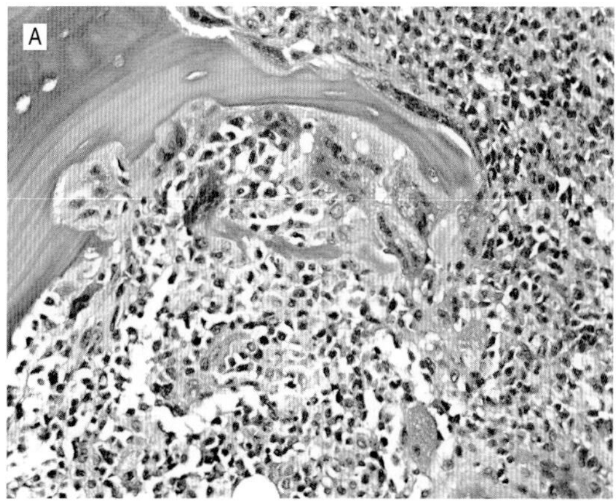

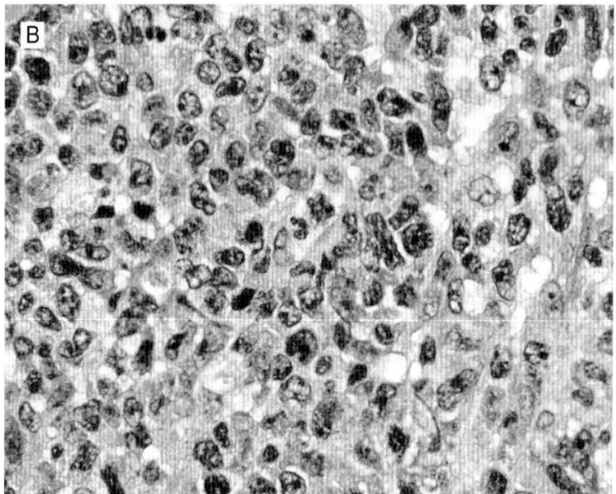

FIGURE 9-6 Adult T-cell leukemia/lymphoma involving bone. A. In this field, numerous osteoclasts are surrounding and resorbing bone. B. The neoplastic cells are large. (A, B, hematoxylin-eosin; A, 400×; B, 1,000×).

Extranodal NK/T-Cell Lymphoma, Nasal Type

Extranodal NK/T-cell lymphoma is an aggressive lymphoma that can have an NK-cell or cytotoxic T-cell immunophenotype and may arise from a precursor cell of NK/T cells. It occurs predominantly in the nasal/paranasal area and much less often at nonnasal sites, such as skin/soft tissue and the gastrointestinal tract ([1]). Extranodal NK/T-cell lymphoma is more prevalent in Asians and Native Americans in Central and South America ([4]). Its pathogenesis is unknown; however, the lymphoma cells in essentially all cases are positive for EBV-encoded RNA (EBER), suggesting a very strong association between EBV infection and oncogenesis. Patients with nasal involvement present with symptoms of nasal congestion or epistaxis. With locally advanced disease, the tumor erodes the palate and bone, causing pain, fistula, and infection. Some cases may be complicated by hemophagocytic syndrome ([30]).

Histologically, ENKL shows a diffuse proliferation of lymphoma cells, often with an angiocentric or angiodestructive growth pattern, associated with a mixture of reactive lymphocytes and histiocytes. Fibrinoid change can be seen in the blood vessels.

Granulocytes are rare unless associated with necrotic changes (Fig. 9-7).

Typically, the lymphoma cells express the NK-cell marker CD56, CD2, and cytoplasmic CD3 and are negative for surface CD3, CD5, and TCR. Cytotoxic molecules such as TIA-1, granzyme B, and perforin are also positive. Deletion of chromosome 6 is the most frequent cytogenetic aberration ([31]). Chromosome 6 includes two genes named *PRDM1* and *FOXO3*, which may play a role in lymphomagenesis ([32]). Outcome with conventional chemotherapy is poor, with a median OS of 1 to 2 years ([33]). High EBV DNA load in plasma is associated with lower response rate to chemotherapy and worse outcome ([34]).

Enteropathy-Associated T-Cell Lymphoma

Enteropathy-associated T-cell lymphoma is a rare primary intestinal lymphoma often localized (but diffusely infiltrating) in the small intestine ([1]). Two types of EATL are recognized. Type I accounts for 80% to 90% of EATL, shows large lymphoid cells with an inflammatory background, and is strongly associated with celiac disease. Type II EATL accounts for 10% to 20% of EATL, shows monomorphic medium-sized lymphoma cells, and occurs sporadically, often without a history of celiac disease. Type I is predominant in Europe whereas type II is more common in Asia ([35]). Patients present frequently with abdominal pain, weight loss, and sometimes intestinal perforation ([36]).

Grossly, the involved intestine demonstrates multiple ulcers (Fig. 9-8), which may extend deeply into the bowel wall, often resulting in perforation; a distinct mass may not be found. The jejunum is the most common site of involvement. Histologically, the neoplasms are diffuse, and the neoplastic cells are a mixture of small, medium, and large lymphoid cells (see Fig. 9-8).

The intestine not involved by neoplasm may exhibit blunting of villi, as is seen in celiac disease.

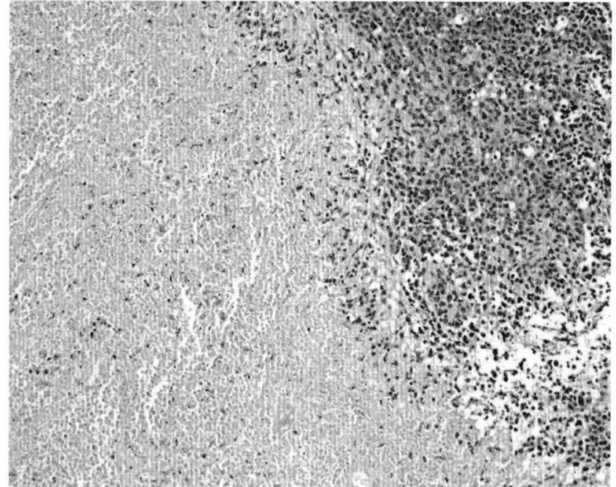

FIGURE 9-7 Extranodal NK/T-cell lymphoma, nasal type, involving nasopharynx. Extensive necrosis (left of field) is common in these neoplasms (hematoxylin-eosin, 200×).

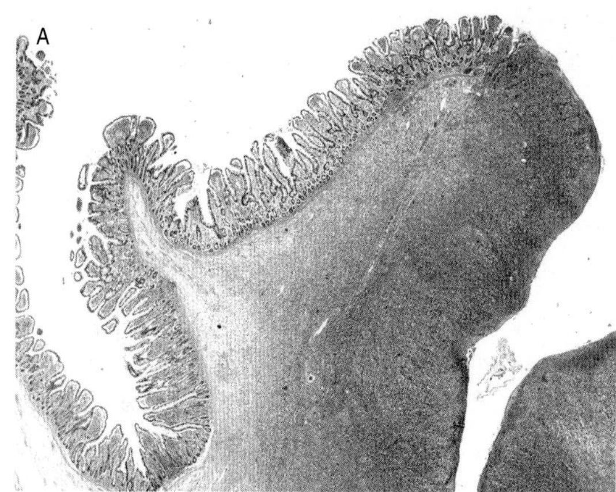

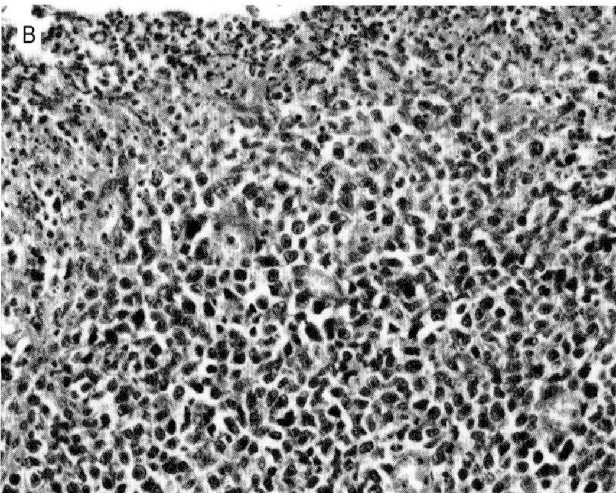

FIGURE 9-8 Enteropathy-associated T-cell lymphoma. A. This field shows the transition from benign mucosa (left of field) to lymphoma and ulcer. B. The neoplastic cells are large. (A, B, hematoxylin-eosin; A, 20×; B, 400×).

Enteropathy-associated T-cell lymphoma expresses pan-T-cell antigens and usually has a cytotoxic profile positive for TIA-1, granzyme B, and perforin. Type II EATL expresses CD56 more often than type I EATL ([35]). Comparative genomic hybridization analysis often shows amplification of chromosome 9p31.3-qter and deletions of chromosome 16q12.1. The prognosis is poor, with a median OS of 10 months ([35]).

Hepatosplenic T-Cell Lymphoma

Hepatosplenic T-cell lymphoma accounts for less than 1% of all NHL and is derived from cytotoxic T cells. Most cases express the gamma-delta (γδ) TCR, but a minority of cases express the alpha-beta (αβ) TCR ([1]). Lymphoma cells predominantly involve the spleen, liver, and bone marrow. Peak incidence is in adolescents and young adults with a median age of 35 years. There is strong male predominance ([1, 37]).

Patients typically present with hepatosplenomegaly

(abdominal pain) and B symptoms. Because of the hepatosplenomegaly and bone marrow involvement, patients often manifest marked cytopenia, most prominently thrombocytopenia. Chronic immune suppression seems to be associated with the risk of HSTL; up to 20% of patients develop the disease after solid organ transplantation or chronic antigenic stimulation.

Histologically, these neoplasms are composed of medium-sized lymphoid cells with slightly irregular nuclear contours, condensed chromatin, and small nucleoli ([1]). In the liver, HSTL infiltrates sinusoids and spares portal tracts. In the spleen, the red pulp is involved and the white pulp spared (Fig. 9-9). In the bone marrow, the neoplastic cells can resemble blasts in aspirate smears and are commonly intrasinusoidal in core biopsy specimens.

Hepatosplenic T-cell lymphomas have a mature but aberrant T-cell immunophenotype. Most cases are positive for CD3 but negative for CD4 and CD8. CD56 is often positive, and most HSTLs are positive for TIA-1 but negative for granzyme B and perforin. Isochromosome (7q) and trisomy of chromosome 8 are common in HSTL ([38]). Hepatosplenic T-cell lymphoma is extremely aggressive and chemoresistant. The median OS duration is less than 2 years ([37]).

Subcutaneous Panniculitis-Like T-Cell Lymphoma

Subcutaneous panniculitis-like T-cell lymphoma (SPTCL) is a rare cytotoxic T-cell lymphoma that arises in subcutaneous tissue. The previous WHO classification included both αβ and γδ type as SPTCL, but the recent WHO classification separated these diseases, and γδ type is now classified as cutaneous γδ T-cell lymphoma ([1]). Cutaneous γδ T-cell lymphoma is much more aggressive than SPTCL, which occurs in younger patients (median age of 35 years) ([39]). Patients present with multiple subcutaneous nodules, most commonly in the extremities and trunk. Patients can develop a hemophagocytic syndrome, causing systemic symptoms with pancytopenia, fever, and hepatosplenomegaly ([39]).

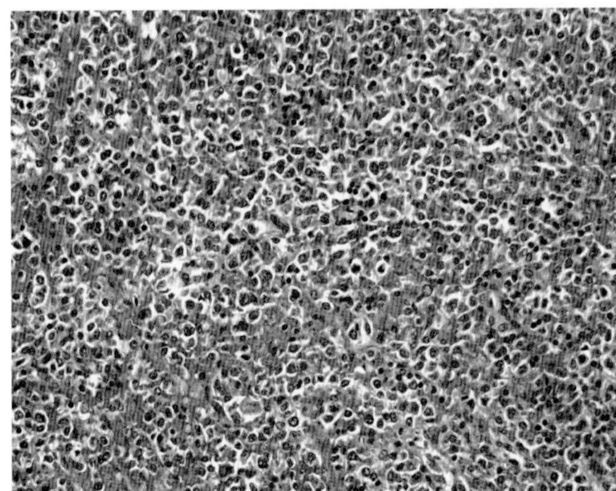

FIGURE 9-9 Hepatosplenic T-cell lymphoma involving spleen (hematoxylin-eosin, 400×).

Histologically, SPTCLs involve subcutaneous tissue, without involvement of the overlying dermis. The neoplastic cells infiltrate fat lobules, usually sparing septa. Marked coagulative necrosis and fat necrosis are common, resembling panniculitis (Fig. 9-10). Lymphoma cells have irregular and hyperchromatic nuclei with pale-staining cytoplasm and can be surrounded by fat cells, often with some admixed histiocytes.

Subcutaneous panniculitis-like T-cell lymphoma has an αβ T-cell phenotype, usually $CD3^+$, $CD8^+$, and $CD4^-$ with expression of cytotoxic molecules, including TIA-1, granzyme B, and perforin ([1]). Survival of patient is highly dependent on whether the patient has a hemophagocytic syndrome or not. The 5-year OS rates with and without a hemophagocytic syndrome were 46% and 91%, respectively ([39]).

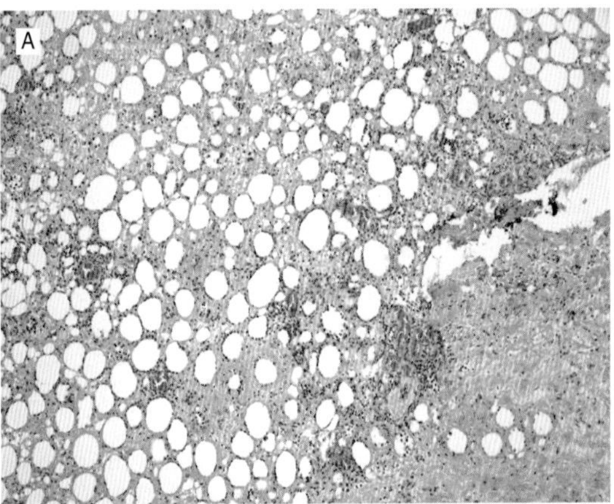

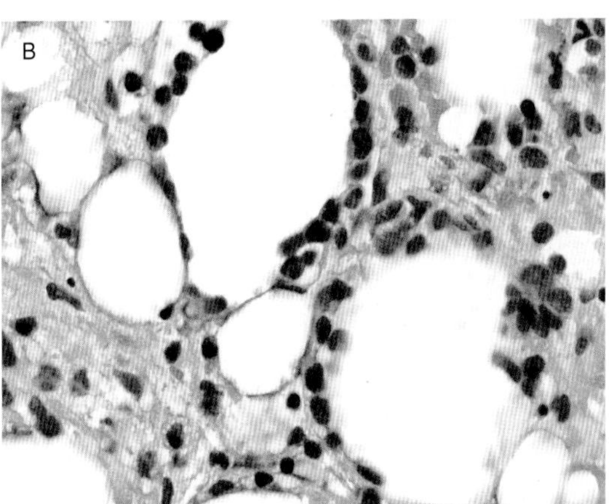

FIGURE 9-10 Subcutaneous panniculitis-like T-cell lymphoma. **A.** The neoplasm involves adipose tissue and is associated with extensive fat necrosis in this field. **B.** The neoplastic lymphocytes surround fat spaces. (Hematoxylin-eosin; **A,** 100×; **B,** 1,000×).

MOLECULAR ANALYSIS OF PERIPHERAL T-CELL LYMPHOMA

Gene expression profiling of PTCL has revealed that certain molecular signatures can discriminate histopathologic subtypes and, in addition, may divide cases into several subgroups based on genes that are found in clusters, including the follicular helper T-cell type of PTCL-NOS that has similarities to AITL ([40]). In addition, next-generation sequencing and a comprehensive search for recurrent somatic mutations in PTCL have identified genes that are frequently mutated in PTCL, and the most highly mutated genes are responsible for epigenetic regulation, such as *TET2, IDH2,* and *DNMT3A* ([12]). Interestingly *IDH2* mutation seems particularly detected in cases of AITL. Such molecular analysis may help to determine molecular targets of therapy in patients with PTCL.

PROGNOSTIC FACTORS

Prognosis varies according to the PTCL subtype. With the exception of patients with AL-positive ALCL, long-term survival is approximately 30% to 35% ([3]). The International Prognostic Index (IPI) provides a prognostic score based on clinical and laboratory factors but was developed for aggressive lymphomas and does not incorporate immunophenotypic results ([41]). Prognostic factors for T-cell lymphomas have been analyzed in a retrospective review of a large cohort of patients with PTCL-NOS, AITL, and ALCL. The prognostic index for PTCL-NOS (PIT) includes age >60 years, Eastern Cooperative Oncology Group performance status ≥2, elevated lactate dehydrogenase (LDH), and bone marrow involvement, with each factor given a score of 1 ([6]). Five-year OS ranged from 62% (PIT = 0) to 18% (PIT = 3-4). The AITL prognostic index is calculated using aging >60 years, white blood cell (WBC) count $>10^4/\mu L$, anemia, platelet count $<15 \times 10^4/\mu L$, immunoglobulin (Ig) A level >400 mg/dL, and extranodal involvement >1 ([19]). Three-year OS rates of low-risk patients (score 0-1) and high-risk patients (score 4-6) were 85% and 12%, respectively. ALK-positive ALCL is associated with generally good prognosis ([3]). However, the prognosis of patients with ALK-negative ALCL is worse than that of patients with ALK-positive ALCL, but seems better than those with other subtypes of PTCL ([3]). The Group d'Etude des Lymphomes de l'Adulte (GELA) group reported that age (<40 or ≥40) and β_2-microglobulin were good prognostic indicators of ALK-negative ALCL ([14]). The 8-year OS rates of patients in group 1 (age <40 years and β_2-microglobulin <3 mg/L) and group 4 (age ≥40 years and β_2-microglobulin ≥3 mg/L) were 84% and 22%, respectively. These prognostic models are clinically convenient and useful in estimating the prognosis of patients with PTCLs. However, there has not been an effective strategy to determine treatment approaches based on such prognostic indicators.

THERAPY

First-Line Therapy

CHOP (cyclophosphamide, doxorubicin, vincristine, and prednisone) has been the most commonly used chemotherapy. The overall response rate (ORR) after CHOP is 70% to 80%, with complete response (CR) rates of 50%. Long-term progression-free survival (PFS) rate for PTCL-NOS, AITL, and ALK-negative ALCL after CHOP is only 30% ([3, 42, 43]). ALK-positive ALCL is an exception in PTCL and has a relatively favorable outcome, with 5-year PFS exceeding 60%. The benefit of anthracycline in the treatment of PTCLs has been questioned ([3]).

Given the poor outcome with conventional chemotherapy, more intensive approaches and/or upfront autologous stem cell transplantation (ASCT) were investigated. Retrospective study at the MD Anderson Cancer Center (MDACC) showed that patients treated with dose-intensified regimens (hyper-CHOP, hyper-CVAD [hyperfractionated cyclophosphamide, vincristine, doxorubicin, and dexamethasone]) had similar survival as those treated with CHOP ([44]). Other studies showed a benefit from adding etoposide to CHOP ([45, 46]). The German High-Grade Non-Hodgkin Lymphoma Study Group (DSHNHL) evaluated the outcome of 320 patients with T-cell lymphoma enrolled in clinical trials ([46]). The addition of etoposide to CHOP improved response rates and was associated with longer event-free survival (EFS) in younger patients with normal LDH (18-60 years). The 3-year EFS rates with or without etoposide in the regimen were 75% and 51%, respectively. Ellin et al evaluated 755 patients with PTCL in the Swedish Lymphoma Registry and confirmed that the addition of etoposide to CHOP was associated with superior PFS in patients age ≤60 years ([45]). Based on these studies, CHOEP (etoposide 100 mg/m^2 intravenously [IV] on days 1-3 in addition to standard CHOP) is now increasingly used as first-line treatment of PTCLs. The role of upfront ASCT is described later.

Salvage Chemotherapy

Commonly used traditional salvage chemotherapy regimens for relapsed/refractory PTCLs are platinum-containing regimens such as ICE (ifosfamide, carboplatin, and etoposide), GDP (gemcitabine, dexamethasone, and cisplatin), or GemOx (gemcitabine and oxaliplatin). The ORR with ICE ranges from 20% to 70%, with a median PFS of 6 months ([47]). The ORR was 40% with GDP ([48]) and 38% with GemOx with a median PFS of 10 months ([49]). It should be noted that the outcome of patients with relapsed/refractory PTCLs is dismal if stem cell transplantation is not an option. In a study by the British Columbia Cancer Agency, the median durations of PFS and OS were 3.1 and 5.5 months, respectively, in patients with PTCLs who relapsed or progressed after first-line treatment and did not undergo stem cell transplantation ([50]). Thus, previously mentioned combination salvage chemotherapy regimens are primarily offered for patients who are to undergo stem cell transplantation after such salvage therapy. For those who are not transplantation candidates, single-agent chemotherapy or other novel therapeutic options are to be considered over combination chemotherapy, as detailed later in this chapter.

Hematopoietic Stem Cell Transplantation

Frontline Autologous Stem Cell Transplantation

The role of frontline ASCT in patients with PTCL who achieve CR after induction therapy has only been evaluated either in single-arm nonrandomized studies or in randomized studies including a minority of patients with PTCL ([51]). The German group evaluated CHOP followed by upfront ASCT in patients with newly diagnosed PTCLs (excluding ALK-positive ALCL) ([43]). Among 83 patients treated, the ORR after high-dose chemotherapy was 66% with a CR rate of 56%. The 3-year OS and PFS rates were 48% and 36%, respectively. For patients who actually underwent transplant (66% of patients), the 3-year OS rate was 71% ([43]). The Nordic group evaluated six cycles of CHOEP (etoposide was omitted for patients >60 years old) followed by upfront ASCT in patients with PTCLs (excluding ALK-positive ALCL) ([52]). Among 160 patients treated, the ORR after CHOEP was 82%, with a CR rate of 51%. The 5-year OS and PFS rates were 51% and 44%, respectively. By the subtype-stratified analysis, 5-year OS rates of PTCL-NOS, AITL, ALK-negative ALCL, and EATL were 47%, 52%, 70%, and 48%, respectively. These outcomes seem better than those of historical patients treated by conventional chemotherapy like CHOP ([53]). Based on these studies, upfront ASCT in PTCLs other than ALK-positive ALCL is considered a reasonable option in clinical practice. For other subtypes of PTCL such as ATLL and HSTL, upfront ASCT is not associated with prolonged remission ([54]).

Frontline Allogeneic Stem Cell Transplantation

A recent study demonstrated the potential benefit of upfront allogeneic stem cell transplantation (alloSCT) for PTCLs in first remission ([55]). Among 49 patients (PTCL-NOS, n = 33; AITL, n = 4; ALK-negative ALCL, n = 7) who underwent upfront alloSCT, the 2-year OS was 72.5% and 1-year nonrelapse mortality (NRM) was 8.2%. Previous studies of alloSCT had generally shown NRM as high as 30%. Given this, the treatment is still considered investigational. In some subtypes of PTCL, such as ATLL, upfront alloSCT has been tested extensively, showing relatively good outcome ([56]).

Autologous Stem Cell Transplantation for Relapsed or Refractory Disease

The benefit of ASCT is rather disappointing, with 5-year PFS <20% ([57]). Patients who experience excellent response to salvage chemotherapy may be considered for ASCT consolidation ([58]), particularly if there is no alloSCT option. Although the most commonly used regimen is BEAM (carmustine, etoposide, cytarabine, and melphalan), alternative conditioning regimens may improve outcome.

Allogeneic Stem Cell Transplantation for Relapsed or Refractory Disease

Likely due to the graft-versus-lymphoma effect, alloSCT may provide effective disease control in relapsed/refractory PTCLs ([59-61]). The French group has reported the outcome of 77 patients who received alloSCT. The 5-year NRM rate was 33%, and 5-year OS and EFS rates were 57% and 53%, respectively ([61]). In a Japanese study, 354 patients (PTCL-NOS, n = 200; AITL, n = 77; ALCL, n = 77) who received alloSCT were analyzed ([62]). The 3-year NRM rates and the 3-year OS rates in younger patients (16-49 years old) who received myeloablative regimen versus a reduced-intensity conditioning regimen were 22% versus 14% and 43% versus 56%, respectively ([62]). We generally consider alloSCT for young patients achieving second remission.

NK/T-Cell Lymphoma

Historically, NKTCL is refractory to conventional treatment like CHOP. Combined-modality approach for early-stage disease (concurrent chemoradiation therapy) and different multiagent chemotherapy for advanced-stage disease have shown some success.

For limited-stage ENKL, platinum-containing chemotherapy given concurrently with high-dose radiation is promising. In a phase II Japanese study of concurrent DeVIC (dexamethasone, etoposide, ifosfamide, and carboplatin) therapy with 50 Gy of radiation, the 5-year OS rate was 70% ([63]). In a phase II study from Korea, patients first received concurrent radiation with weekly cisplatin and then received three cycles of VIPD (etoposide, ifosfamide, cisplatin, and dexamethasone). The ORR after concurrent therapy was 100%, with a CR rate of 73%, and the 3-year PFS and OS rates were 85% and 86%, respectively ([64]). Based on these studies, concurrent platinum-based chemotherapy and radiation therapy is an accepted standard approach for localized-stage ENKL.

For advanced-stage disease, there are no effective combination chemotherapies. Because ENKL highly expresses P-glycoprotein (multidrug-resistant protein), combination regimens using agents independent of P-glycoprotein were investigated. The most promising combination therapy is SMILE (methotrexate, ifosfamide, dexamethasone, etoposide, and L-asparaginase) ([65]), yielding an ORR of 79%, CR rate of 45%, and a 2-year OS rate of 50%. The French group treated 19 patients with L-asparaginase, methotrexate, and dexamethasone (AspaMetDex). The ORR was 78%, with a CR rate of 61%, and the median survival was 12.2 months ([66]).

Novel Treatments

Table 9-2 shows the new agents used to treat peripheral T-cell lymphoma.

Brentuximab Vedotin

Brentuximab vedotin (BV) is an intravenously administered antibody-drug conjugate that consists of the CD30-specific monoclonal antibody conjugated with monomethyl auristatin E by linker peptide. Binding of the antibody-drug conjugate to CD30 on the cell surface causes internalization of the drug by endocytosis. The drug subsequently travels to the lysosome, causing cell cycle arrest and apoptotic death. Brentuximab vedotin was studied for the treatment of relapsed/refractory systemic ALCL, which uniformly expresses CD30. In a pivotal phase II study in patients with relapsed/refractory systemic ALCL, the ORR was 86%, and the CR rate was 57%. The median PFS was 26.3 months in patients who achieved CR ([67]). Grade ≥3 adverse events included neutropenia (21%), thrombocytopenia (14%), peripheral sensory neuropathy (12%), and anemia (7%). The US Food and Drug Administration (FDA) approved BV for the treatment of patients with ALCL in whom at least one prior multidrug chemotherapy regimen had failed.

Brentuximab vedotin was also investigated in rather small number of patients with other PTCLs expressing CD30 ([68]). In PTCL-NOS, ORR was 33%, with a CR rate of 14%, and median PFS was 7.6 months. The ORR in patients with AITL was 54%, with a CR rate of 38%, and median PFS was 5.5 months.

Interestingly, there was no correlation between immunohistochemical CD30 expression and clinical response. A multicenter double-blind phase III study of CHP (CHOP without vincristine) plus BV (A+CHP) versus standard CHOP for CD30^{+} PTCLs (10% or higher) is ongoing (ClinicalTrials.gov identifier: NCT01777152).

Table 9-2 New Agents in Peripheral T-Cell Lymphoma

Agent	Dose/Schedule	No.	ORR (%)	CR (%)	Median DOR (months)	Median PFS (months)	Reference
Brentuximab vedotin	1.8 mg/kg, IV, day 1, every 21 d						
ALCL		58	86	57	12.6	13.3	67
PTCL-NOS		21	33	14	7.6	1.6	68
AITL		13	54	38	5.5	6.7	68
Pralatrexate	30 mg/m^2, IV, weekly x 6, every 49 d	111	29	11	10.1	3.5	69
Romidepsin	14 mg/m^2, IV, weekly x 3, every 28 d	131	25	15	17.0	4.0	70
Belinostat	1,000 mg/m^2, IV, d 1-5, every 21 d	129	26	10	8.3		71
Bendamustine	120 mg/m^2, IV, d 1-2, every 21 d	60	50	28	3.5	3.6	72
Mogamulizumab	1.0 mg/kg, IV, weekly x 8	37	35	14		3.0	74
Alisertib	50 mg, PO BID, 7 d, every 21 d	8	57	43			75

AITL, angioimmunoblastic T-cell lymphoma; ALCL, anaplastic large-cell lymphoma; BID, twice a day; CR, complete response rate; d, day; DOR, duration of response; IV, intravenous; ORR, overall response rate; PFS, progression-free survival; PO, oral; PTCL-NOS, peripheral T-cell lymphoma, not otherwise specified.

Pralatrexate

Pralatrexate, an inhibitor of dihydrofolate reductase, is more than 10-fold more cytotoxic than methotrexate. A pivotal phase II study (PROPEL trial) enrolled 115 patients with relapsed or refractory PTCL. The ORR was 29%, with a CR rate of 11% ([69]). When response rates are analyzed based on histology, the ORRs of patients with PTCL-NOS (n = 59), AITL (n = 13), and ALCL (n = 17) were 31%, 8%, and 29%, respectively. The median PFS was 3.5 months in all patients and 10.1 months in responding patients. Severe mucositis (grade 3-4 in 22%) often leads to dose delays or interruption.

Histone Deacetylase Inhibitors

Histone deacetylase (HDAC) inhibitors are considered epigenetic modulating agents that induce accumulation of acetylated nucleosomal histones and induce differentiation and/or apoptosis in transformed cells. Two FDA-approved HDAC inhibitors for relapsed PTCLs are romidepsin and belinostat.

Romidepsin was approved for the treatment of CTCL in 2009 and for the treatment of recurrent PTCLs in 2011. A phase II study (n = 130) in relapsed/refractory PTCLs showed ORR of 25%, with a CR rate of 15% ([70]). The median PFS was 4 months overall. It should be noted, however, that responses were frequently durable, with a median duration of response of 28 months. The most common grade 3 or 4 adverse events were thrombocytopenia, neutropenia, and infections. A multicenter phase III study of CHOP with or without romidepsin in patients with previously untreated PTCLs is ongoing (NCT01796002).

Belinostat was approved in 2014 by the FDA for the treatment of recurrent or refractory PTCL, based on the result of a phase II study (BELIEF trial) ([71]). This study enrolled patients with PTCLs after a failure of one or more prior systemic therapies. Among 129 patients enrolled, the ORR was 26%, with a CR rate of 10%. The median response duration was 8.3 months. Grade 3 or 4 toxicity included thrombocytopenia (13%), neutropenia (13%), and anemia (10%). This drug is also being tested in combination with standard CHOP therapy in the frontline settings (NCT01839097).

Other Agents

Bendamustine is nitrogen mustard, consisting of chloroethylamine, an alkylating group, attached to a benzimidazole ring, a purine analog. In a phase II study (BENTLY trial) of 60 patients with relapsed PTCL or CTCL, the ORR was 50%, with a CR rate of 28% ([72]). Median PFS was 3.6 months. The dose used in the trial for PTCLs was 120 mg/m^2 every 21 days, which is more intensive than the dose used in low-grade B-cell lymphoma (90 mg/m^2 every 28 days in combination with rituximab).

Mogamulizumab is a defucosylated anti-cc chemokine receptor 4 (CCR4) antibody that was initially developed for the treatment of ATLL. In a phase II study (n = 28) of patients with relapsed CCR4-positive ATLL, single-agent mogamulizumab showed an ORR of 50%, with a CR rate of 31%. Median PFS was 5.2 months ([73]). Because CCR4 is also expressed in various proportions of PTCLs, mogamulizumab was evaluated in patients with CCR4-positive relapsed PTCL or CTCL. Of the 38 patient treated, ORR was 35%, with a CR rate of 14%. Median PFS of responders was 5.5 months ([74]).

Alisertib is an aurora A kinase inhibitor. In a phase II study of 48 patients with relapsed/refractory NHL treated with alisertib, 8 had PTCL. The ORR was 57%, with a CR rate of 14% ([75]). A phase III study comparing alisertib to investigator's choice single-agent drug (pralatrexate, gemcitabine, or romidepsin) in relapsed/refractory PTCL is ongoing (NCT01482962).

CUTANEOUS T-CELL LYMPHOMAS

Cutaneous T-cell lymphomas are a clinically heterogeneous group of mature T-cell lymphomas, accounting for most lymphomas arising in skin. Mycosis fungoides (MF) and Sézary syndrome (SS) are defined by their cutaneous lesions that result from the accumulation of a T-helper memory/effector subset with a CD4$^+$, CD8$^-$, CD45RO$^+$CLA$^+$ phenotype in skin and blood ([1]). Most commonly, MF starts as an indolent and chronic dermatitis in the sun-shielded areas. A diagnostic biopsy specimen is difficult to obtain in early MF because of similarities with eczema and contact dermatitis.

CLASSIFICATION

Mycosis fungoides is staged using the tumor-node-metastasis (TNM) classification schema for the purpose of predicting disease prognosis (Fig. 9–11). Mycosis fungoides and SS, the most common variants, are still rare with an annual incidence of 3 to 4 new cases per million individuals, or 1,200 new cases per year in the United States ([76]). The next most common entities are the CD30$^+$ lymphoproliferative disorders: lymphomatoid papulosis (LyP) and primary cutaneous anaplastic large-cell lymphoma (pcALCL). Subcutaneous panniculitic T-cell lymphoma, cutaneous γ/δ T-cell lymphoma, and NK/T-cell lymphomas are rare and more aggressive (see Table 9-1).

PRESENTATION AND DIAGNOSIS

The International Society for Cutaneous Lymphomas (ISCL) has developed an algorithm to diagnose

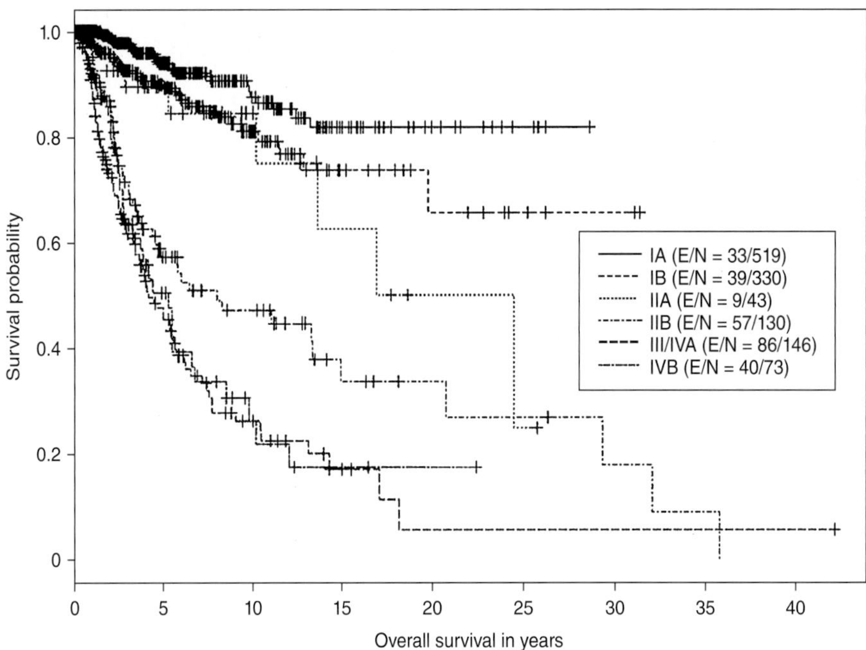

FIGURE 9–11 Mycosis fungoides (MF) and Sézary syndrome: disease-specific survival by clinical stage. Disease-specific survival of 1263 patients with MF and Sézary syndrome was measured according to clinical stage at diagnosis. (Reproduced, with permission, from Talpur R, Singh L, Daulat S, et al. Long-term outcomes of 1263 patients with mycosis fungoides and Sézary syndrome from 1982 to 2009. *Clin Cancer Res*. 2012;18(18):5051-5060.)

early-stage MF. The clinical diagnosis is based on a scoring system consisting of clinical, histopathologic, molecular, and immunopathologic criteria. A score of 4 is needed to make the diagnosis (77).

Clinically, patients have persistent or progressive patches and thin plaques on sun-shielded areas. Lesion morphology is variable, and patients can also exhibit poikiloderma. Histologically, MF is characterized by an atypical lymphocytic infiltrate in the superficial dermis and epidermis (epidermotropism). Epidermotropism is not always seen, especially in folliculotropic mycosis fungoides and SS. There is a predominance of $CD4^{+}CD8^{-}$ cells evidenced by an increased CD4:8 ratio and reduced CD7 expression. The finding of clonality with *TCR* gene rearrangement is not diagnostic but helps to support the diagnosis of lymphoma over a reactive process and is given 1 point under the ISCL algorithm. Mycosis fungoides may progress to a leukemic and erythrodermic condition called SS. Sézary syndrome is defined by erythroderma involving >80% of the body and the presence of >1,000/mL of atypical cells in the peripheral blood. By flow cytometry, most patients have increased numbers of $CD4^{+}CD26^{-}$ "Sézary cells." In the skin, the atypical cells have lost epidermotropism and are found around the dermal vessels rather than in the epidermis. Sézary cells secrete Th2 cytokines, interleukin (IL)-4, and IL-10, causing loss of cellular immunity due to decreased production of Th1 cytokines, interferon-γ, and IL-2 (78). This results in atopy characterized by erythroderma, peripheral eosinophilia, increased IgE production, and intractable pruritus. *Staphylococcus aureus* colonization can worsen erythroderma and pruritus. Molecular studies in MF show emergence of one or more clones of skin-homing $CD4^{+}$ T cells with progression to SS; these appear in the blood and can be detected by flow cytometry (79).

PROGNOSIS

The predictive factors for survival are the T classification, presence of extracutaneous manifestations, and patient age (80). Independent adverse prognostic factors are large-cell transformation, follicular mucinosis, thickness of the tumor infiltrate, and elevated LDH and β_2-microglobulin (81). Patients with SS have worse prognosis. A high Sézary cell count, loss of T-cell subset markers such as CD5 and CD7, and chromosomal abnormalities in T cells are also associated with poor outcome (82).

THERAPY

Figure 9-12 summarizes the primary treatment map for CTCL.

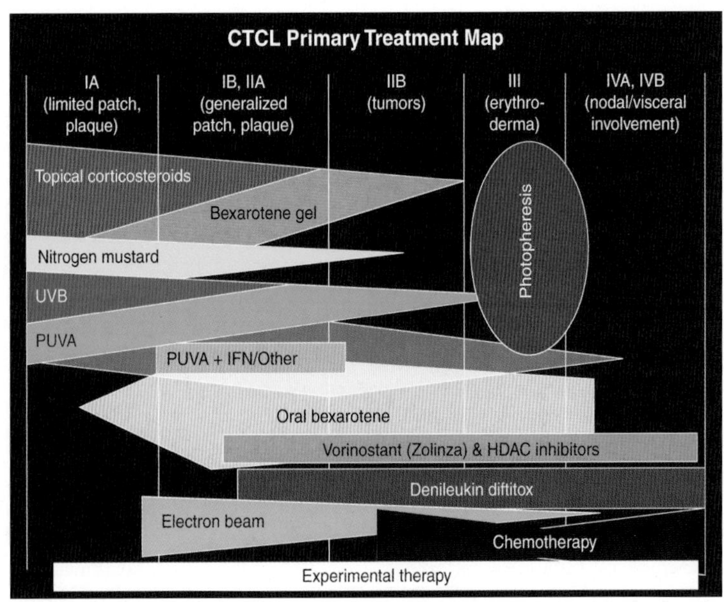

FIGURE 9-12 Cutaneous T-cell lymphoma (CTCL) primary treatment map. HDAC, histone deacetylase; IFN, interferon; PUVA, psoralen plus ultraviolet A; UVB, ultraviolet B.

Treatment of Early Mycosis Fungoides

A number of FDA-approved therapies are available to treat MF/SS. Therapies are divided into skin-directed and systemic categories. Many of these agents are also used for eczema, psoriasis, and other forms of lymphoma.

Early MF (stages IA, IB, and IIA) is characterized by eczematous or psoriasiform dermatitis covering <80% body surface area without evidence of blood or visceral involvement. Early MF is treated with combination skin-directed therapy. The first therapy is topical steroids. For hypertrophic plaque lesions, the topical retinoid gels or creams may help restore normal epidermal differentiation and reduce the time of clearing when used in combination with phototherapy. The response rate for 1% bexarotene (Targretin) gel was 76% in patients not previously treated; this agent is the only topical therapy approved for MF ([83]). We have also found this gel to be useful for MF on the hands or feet ([84]) and for aborting LyP lesions ([85]) or MF tumors. Mechlorethamine (Valchlor) is a topical nitrogen mustard compound widely used for early-stage MF. Mechlorethamine gel and ointment have response rates of 46.9% and 46.2%, respectively, in stage IA to IIA MF. Faster responses are seen with the gel formulation ([86]).

Treatment of Intermediate-Stage, Refractory, or Transformed Mycosis Fungoides and Sézary Syndrome

Patients with MF who do not respond to first-line single-agent topical treatment need more potent therapy such as combinations of skin-directed and systemic therapy. These can include topical steroids, topical and systemic retinoids, topical nitrogen mustard, interferon-α, and chemotherapies (Table 9-3). For patch disease, narrowband ultraviolet B is effective and can be combined with topical steroids, retinoids, or interferon-α or -γ. Thick plaque lesions or folliculotropic MF lesions are more difficult to clear and are treated with psoralen–ultraviolet A (PUVA) plus interferon or an oral retinoid (bexarotene, acitretin, or isotretinoin) but often require radiation. Total skin electron beam radiation (TSEB) is effective against plaque and tumor lesions but is reserved for patients with extensive skin involvement who have failed to respond to skin-directed therapies or are planning to undergo stem cell transplantation ([87]). Low-dose TSEB of 10 to 20 Gy has good efficacy compared to the standard dose of 30 to 36 Gy ([88]). After TSEB, patients use a form of maintenance therapy such as Mustargen, PUVA, or oral bexarotene.

Intravenous denileukin diftitox (Ontak) and oral bexarotene have received FDA approval in 1998 and 1999, respectively, for the treatment of MF. Both are used in the setting of more advanced skin disease. Denileukin diftitox received FDA approval for treatment of all states of CTCL based on a randomized two-dose arm trial showing a response rate of 30%. Complete responses were seen in 10% of patients ([89]). Capillary leak syndrome is a side effect seen in 20% to 30% of patients treated with denileukin diftitox and may be prevented with hydration. Acute infusion reactions are blocked by steroid premedication. High expression of $CD25^+$ in >20% of tumor cells is associated with a higher response rate of 60%

compared to 20% with low expression. However, denileukin diftitox is currently unavailable; it was taken off the market recently by the FDA for inconsistent batches. E7777, a new fusion protein of human interleukin-2 and diphtheria toxin fragments, is undergoing clinical trials. Bexarotene and steroids may increase T-cell CD25 expression and could suggest synergism ([90]). Bexarotene monotherapy has a response rate of 54% at a dose of 300 mg/m^2 in early-stage disease and a response rate of 45% in more advanced stages. Its dose-limiting toxicity is hypertriglyceridemia, which can be controlled with the addition of an 3-hydroxy-3-methylglutaryl-coenzyme A reductase and/or a statin ([91]).

Patients with transformed MF, tumors, or nodal disease respond to local radiation, denileukin diftitox, nucleoside analogues (gemcitabine, pentostatin), doxorubicin, HDAC inhibitors, or combination chemotherapy. Often, the duration of response is limited. Multiagent chemotherapy combinations, although effective for a limited time, can also induce immunosuppression, leading to line-induced sepsis or opportunistic infections.

Table 9-3 Overview of Current Therapeutic Options for MF/SS

Skin-Directed Therapy
• Topical corticosteroids • Topical chemotherapy (eg, nitrogen mustard, carmustine) • Topical retinoids (bexarotene, tazarotene) • Topical imiquimod • Phototherapy (UVB, NbUVB, PUVA) • Electron beam therapy
Biological Therapy
RXR retinoid (bexarotene) • RAR retinoid (isotretinoin) • Interferons • Granulocyte-macrophage colony-stimulating factor • Extracorporeal photopheresis • Fusion protein/toxin (denileukin difitox)
Other Systemic Therapies
Cytotoxic chemotherapy (methotrexate, Doxil, gemcitabine, etoposide, pentostatin) • Bone marrow/stem cell transplantation
Experimental Therapies
HDAC inhibitors (vorinostat, depsipeptide) • Transimmunization extracorporeal photopheresis • Targeted monoclonal antibodies (CD52, CCR4, CD4) • Cytokines (IL-12, IL-2) • TLR agonists (CpG oligodeoxynucleotides) • Tumor vaccines

UVB, ultraviolet B light; NbUVB, narrow-band ultraviolet B light; PUVA, psoralen plus ultraviolet A light; RXR, retinoid X receptor; RAR, retinoic acid receptor; TLR, toll-like receptor 9; IL, interleukin.
Data from Kim EJ, Hess S, Richardson SK, et al. Immunopathogenesis and therapy of cutaneous T cell lymphoma. *J Clin Invest.* 2005;115:798-812.

Generalized exfoliative erythroderma (EE) is found in patients with blood involvement (SS). Extracorporeal photopheresis was approved in 1987 for the treatment of CTCL, and significant responses were seen in erythrodermic patients ([92]). Extracorporeal photopheresis is usually combined with biologic response modifiers, especially interferon-α or -γ, and retinoids. Responses approach 60% to 70% in SS ([93]). Extracorporeal photopheresis is also effective in early MF when used alone or in combination with biologic response modifiers (interferon-α or oral bexarotene) ([94]).

NOVEL TREATMENTS

The recently FDA-approved HDAC inhibitors, vorinostat (Zolinza) in 2006, depsipeptide (Romidepsin) in 2009, and belinostat (Beleodaq) in 2014, represent a new strategy for targeted therapy of CTCL and are effective in patients highly refractory to chemotherapy and other agents. Their mechanism of action, like retinoids, involves inducing transcription of genes that control differentiation and apoptosis selectively in malignant cells. Oral vorinostat is well tolerated at a dose of 400 mg daily and has a rapid onset of action. Vorinostat yields a response rate of 30%. The response rate is higher (36%) in patients with SS compared to other stages. The drug improves skin, nodal, and blood involvement and reduces pruritus ([95]). Romidepsin (previously known as depsipeptide or FK228) is approved for the treatment of CTCL after at least one prior systemic therapy. The response rate is 34% (CR, 6%) in MF ([96]). The recommended dose and schedule of romidepsin is 14 mg/m^2 intravenously over 4 hours on days 1, 8, and 15 of a 28-day cycle. Most patients (63%) with moderate or severe pruritus experienced significant relief, which significantly impacted quality of life in SS and MF patients ([97, 98]).

Gemcitabine therapy yields a response rate of 70%, and doxorubicin has a response rate of 80% ([99, 100]). A phase II study of gemcitabine and bexarotene showed a lower response rate than gemcitabine alone ([101]).

Pralatrexate was used at a lower dose of 15 mg/m^2 in MF and produced a response rate of 57% ([102]). Pralatrexate in combination with bexarotene achieved similar efficacy ([103]).

Targeted therapy with monoclonal antibodies against T-cell molecules is under investigation. Zanolimumab (HuMax-CD4) induced responses in 24% of patients and had an acceptable safety profile at a dose of 980 mg weekly ([104]). Alemtuzumab (Campath-H), targeting CD52, is useful in SS, especially in the elderly. It can be given subcutaneously but is extremely immunosuppressive, because it depletes T cells, B cells, and NK cells for years. Diphtheria fusion protein coupled to CD3 is under investigation. Forodesine is a nucleoside analogue that inhibits purine nucleoside phosphorylase and deoxyguanosine triphosphate buildup, causing T-cell apoptosis. A randomized phase II trial showed oral forodesine to achieve partial response in 11% of 144 patients at a daily dose of 200 mg ([105]). Intravenous forodesine also showed activity in relapsed-refractory NKTCL ([106]).

Other agents in trials for MF include CpG (activate Toll-like receptors), lenalidomide, sapacitabine (oral nucleoside inhibitor), and enzastaurin (PKC/AKT inhibitor). Lenalidomide 25 mg daily for 21 daily every month produces a response rate of 28% ([107]).

FUTURE DIRECTIONS

T-cell lymphomas are rare and represent a heterogenous group of diseases with poor prognosis. It is strongly recommended that patients with non–ALK-positive ALCL PTCLs and CTCLs receive treatment on clinical trials so that progress can be made in the management of these rare neoplasms. Targeted therapies may offer more selective activity with reduced immunosuppression.

REFERENCES

1. Swerdlow S, Campo E, Harris N, et al. *WHO Classification of Tumours of Haematopoietic and Lymphoid Tissues*. Lyon, France: International Agency for Research on Cancer (IARC); 2008.
2. Morton LM, Wang SS, Devesa SS, Hartge P, Weisenburger DD, Linet MS. Lymphoma incidence patterns by WHO subtype in the United States, 1992-2001. *Blood*. 2006;107(1):265-276.
3. Vose J, Armitage J, Weisenburger D. International peripheral T-cell and natural killer/T-cell lymphoma study: pathology findings and clinical outcomes. *J Clin Oncol*. 2008;26(25):4124-4130.
4. Chihara D, Ito H, Matsuda T, et al. Differences in incidence and trends of haematological malignancies in Japan and the United States. *Br J Haematol*. 2014;164(4):536-545.
5. Weisenburger DD, Savage KJ, Harris NL, et al. Peripheral T-cell lymphoma, not otherwise specified: a report of 340 cases from the International Peripheral T-cell Lymphoma Project. *Blood*. 2011;117(12):3402-3408.
6. Gallamini A, Stelitano C, Calvi R, et al. Peripheral T-cell lymphoma unspecified (PTCL-U): a new prognostic model from a retrospective multicentric clinical study. *Blood*. 2004;103(7):2474-2479.
7. Asano N, Suzuki R, Kagami Y, et al. Clinicopathologic and prognostic significance of cytotoxic molecule expression in nodal peripheral T-cell lymphoma, unspecified. *Am J Surg Pathol*. 2005;29(10):1284-1293.
8. Sabattini E, Pizzi M, Tabanelli V, et al. CD30 expression in peripheral T-cell lymphomas. *Haematologica*. 2013;98(8):e81-e82.
9. Went P, Agostinelli C, Gallamini A, et al. Marker expression in peripheral T-cell lymphoma: a proposed clinical-pathologic prognostic score. *J Clin Oncol*. 2006;24(16):2472-2479.
10. Thorns C, Bastian B, Pinkel D, et al. Chromosomal aberrations in angioimmunoblastic T-cell lymphoma and peripheral T-cell lymphoma unspecified: a matrix-based CGH approach. *Genes Chromosomes Cancer*. 2007;46(1):37-44.
11. Zettl A, Rudiger T, Konrad MA, et al. Genomic profiling of peripheral T-cell lymphoma, unspecified, and anaplastic large T-cell lymphoma delineates novel recurrent chromosomal alterations. *Am J Pathol*. 2004;164(5):1837-1848.
12. Iqbal J, Wright G, Wang C, et al. Gene expression signatures delineate biological and prognostic subgroups in peripheral T-cell lymphoma. *Blood*. 2014;123(19):2915-2923.
13. Streubel B, Vinatzer U, Willheim M, Raderer M, Chott A. Novel t(5;9)(q33;q22) fuses ITK to SYK in unspecified peripheral T-cell lymphoma. *Leukemia*. 2006;20(2):313-318.
14. Sibon D, Fournier M, Briere J, et al. Long-term outcome of adults with systemic anaplastic large-cell lymphoma treated within the Groupe d'Etude des Lymphomes de l'Adulte trials. *J Clin Oncol*. 2012;30(32):3939-3946.
15. Savage KJ, Harris NL, Vose JM, et al. ALK- anaplastic large-cell lymphoma is clinically and immunophenotypically different from both ALK+ ALCL and peripheral T-cell lymphoma, not otherwise specified: report from the International Peripheral T-Cell Lymphoma Project. *Blood*. 2008;111(12):5496-5504.
16. Duyster J, Bai RY, Morris SW. Translocations involving anaplastic lymphoma kinase (ALK). *Oncogene*. 2001;20(40):5623-5637.
17. Falini B, Pulford K, Pucciarini A, et al. Lymphomas expressing ALK fusion protein(s) other than NPM-ALK. *Blood*. 1999;94(10):3509-3515.
18. Federico M, Rudiger T, Bellei M, et al. Clinicopathologic characteristics of angioimmunoblastic T-cell lymphoma: analysis of the international peripheral T-cell lymphoma project. *J Clin Oncol*. 2013;31(2):240-246.
19. Tokunaga T, Shimada K, Yamamoto K, et al. Retrospective analysis of prognostic factors for angioimmunoblastic T-cell lymphoma: a multicenter cooperative study in Japan. *Blood*. 2012;119(12):2837-2843.
20. Dogan A, Attygalle AD, Kyriakou C. Angioimmunoblastic T-cell lymphoma. *Br J Haematol*. 2003;121(5):681-691.
21. Sakata-Yanagimoto M, Enami T, Yoshida K, et al. Somatic RHOA mutation in angioimmunoblastic T cell lymphoma. *Nat Genet*. 2014;46(2):171-175.
22. Proietti FA, Carneiro-Proietti AB, Catalan-Soares BC, Murphy EL. Global epidemiology of HTLV-I infection and associated diseases. *Oncogene*. 2005;24(39):6058-6068.
23. Tokudome S, Tokunaga O, Shimamoto Y, et al. Incidence of adult T-cell leukemia/lymphoma among human T-lymphotropic virus type I carriers in Saga, Japan. *Cancer Res*. 1989;49(1):226-228.
24. Iwanaga M, Watanabe T, Utsunomiya A, et al. Human T-cell leukemia virus type I (HTLV-1) proviral load and disease progression in asymptomatic HTLV-1 carriers: a nationwide prospective study in Japan. *Blood*. 2010;116(8):1211-1219.
25. Iwanaga M, Watanabe T, Yamaguchi K. Adult T-cell leukemia: a review of epidemiological evidence. *Front Microbiol*. 2012;3:322.
26. Chihara D, Ito H, Katanoda K, et al. Increase in incidence of adult T-cell leukemia/lymphoma in non-endemic areas of Japan and the United States. *Cancer Sci*. 2012;103(10):1857-1860.
27. Tsukasaki K, Utsunomiya A, Fukuda H, et al. VCAP-AMP-VECP compared with biweekly CHOP for adult T-cell leukemia-lymphoma: Japan Clinical Oncology Group Study JCOG9801. *J Clin Oncol*. 2007;25(34):5458-5464.
28. Shimoyama M. Diagnostic criteria and classification of clinical subtypes of adult T-cell leukaemia-lymphoma. A report from the Lymphoma Study Group (1984-87). *Br J Haematol*. 1991;79(3):428-437.
29. Karube K, Ohshima K, Tsuchiya T, et al. Expression of FoxP3, a key molecule in CD4CD25 regulatory T cells, in adult T-cell leukaemia/lymphoma cells. *Br J Haematol*. 2004;126(1):81-84.
30. Medeiros LJ, Jaffe ES, Chen YY, Weiss LM. Localization of Epstein-Barr viral genomes in angiocentric immunoproliferative

CHAPTER 9

lesions. *Am J Surg Pathol.* 1992;16(5):439-447.
31. Wong KF, Chan JK, Kwong YL. Identification of del(6)(q21q25) as a recurring chromosomal abnormality in putative NK cell lymphoma/leukaemia. *Br J Haematol.* 1997;98(4):922-926.
32. Karube K, Nakagawa M, Tsuzuki S, et al. Identification of FOXO3 and PRDM1 as tumor-suppressor gene candidates in NK-cell neoplasms by genomic and functional analyses. *Blood.* 2011;118(12):3195-3204.
33. Au WY, Weisenburger DD, Intragumtornchai T, et al. Clinical differences between nasal and extranasal natural killer/T-cell lymphoma: a study of 136 cases from the International Peripheral T-Cell Lymphoma Project. *Blood.* 2009;113(17):3931-3937.
34. Suzuki R, Yamaguchi M, Izutsu K, et al. Prospective measurement of Epstein-Barr virus-DNA in plasma and peripheral blood mononuclear cells of extranodal NK/T-cell lymphoma, nasal type. *Blood.* 2011;118(23):6018-6022.
35. Delabie J, Holte H, Vose JM, et al. Enteropathy-associated T-cell lymphoma: clinical and histological findings from the international peripheral T-cell lymphoma project. *Blood.* 2011;118(1):148-155.
36. Gale J, Simmonds PD, Mead GM, Sweetenham JW, Wright DH. Enteropathy-type intestinal T-cell lymphoma: clinical features and treatment of 31 patients in a single center. *J Clin Oncol.* 2000;18(4):795-803.
37. Belhadj K, Reyes F, Farcet JP, et al. Hepatosplenic gammadelta T-cell lymphoma is a rare clinicopathologic entity with poor outcome: report on a series of 21 patients. *Blood.* 2003;102(13):4261-4269.
38. Alonsozana EL, Stamberg J, Kumar D, et al. Isochromosome 7q: the primary cytogenetic abnormality in hepatosplenic gammadelta T cell lymphoma. *Leukemia.* 1997;11(8):1367-1372.
39. Willemze R, Jansen PM, Cerroni L, et al. Subcutaneous panniculitis-like T-cell lymphoma: definition, classification, and prognostic factors: an EORTC Cutaneous Lymphoma Group Study of 83 cases. *Blood.* 2008;111(2):838-845.
40. Piccaluga PP, Agostinelli C, Tripodo C, et al. Peripheral T-cell lymphoma classification: the matter of cellular derivation. *Exp Rev Hematol.* 2011;4(4):415-425.
41. A predictive model for aggressive non-Hodgkin's lymphoma. The International Non-Hodgkin's Lymphoma Prognostic Factors Project. *N Engl J Med.* 1993;329(14):987-994.
42. Simon A, Peoch M, Casassus P, et al. Upfront VIP-reinforced-ABVD (VIP-rABVD) is not superior to CHOP/21 in newly diagnosed peripheral T cell lymphoma. Results of the randomized phase III trial GOELAMS-LTP95. *Br J Haematol.* 2010;151(2):159-166.
43. Reimer P, Rudiger T, Geissinger E, et al. Autologous stem-cell transplantation as first-line therapy in peripheral T-cell lymphomas: results of a prospective multicenter study. *J Clin Oncol.* 2009;27(1):106-113.
44. Escalon MP, Liu NS, Yang Y, et al. Prognostic factors and treatment of patients with T-cell non-Hodgkin lymphoma: the M. D. Anderson Cancer Center experience. *Cancer.* 2005; 103(10):2091-2098.
45. Ellin F, Landstrom J, Jerkeman M, Relander T. Real-world data on prognostic factors and treatment in peripheral T-cell lymphomas: a study from the Swedish Lymphoma Registry. *Blood.* 2014;124(10):1570-1577.
46. Schmitz N, Trumper L, Ziepert M, et al. Treatment and prognosis of mature T-cell and NK-cell lymphoma: an analysis of patients with T-cell lymphoma treated in studies of the German High-Grade Non-Hodgkin Lymphoma Study Group. *Blood.* 2010;116(18):3418-3425.
47. Mikesch JH, Kuhlmann M, Demant A, et al. DexaBEAM versus ICE salvage regimen prior to autologous transplantation for relapsed or refractory aggressive peripheral T cell lymphoma: a retrospective evaluation of parallel patient cohorts of one center. *Ann Hematol.* 2013;92(8):1041-1048.
48. Emmanouilides C, Colovos C, Pinter-Brown L, et al. Pilot study of fixed-infusion rate gemcitabine with cisplatin and dexamethasone in patients with relapsed or refractory lymphoma. *Clin Lymphoma.* 2004;5(1):45-49.
49. Yao YY, Tang Y, Zhu Q, et al. Gemcitabine, oxaliplatin and dexamethasone as salvage treatment for elderly patients with refractory and relapsed peripheral T-cell lymphoma. *Leuk Lymphoma.* 2013;54(6):1194-1200.
50. Mak V, Hamm J, Chhanabhai M, et al. Survival of patients with peripheral T-cell lymphoma after first relapse or progression: spectrum of disease and rare long-term survivors. *J Clin Oncol.* 2013;31(16):1970-1976.
51. Stiff PJ, Unger JM, Cook JR, et al. Autologous transplantation as consolidation for aggressive non-Hodgkin's lymphoma. *N Engl J Med.* 2013;369(18):1681-1690.
52. d'Amore F, Relander T, Lauritzsen GF, et al. Up-front autologous stem-cell transplantation in peripheral T-cell lymphoma: NLG-T-01. *J Clin Oncol.* 2012;30(25):3093-3099.
53. Abouyabis AN, Shenoy PJ, Sinha R, Flowers CR, Lechowicz MJ. A systematic review and meta-analysis of front-line anthracycline-based chemotherapy regimens for peripheral T-cell lymphoma. *ISRN Hematol.* 2011;2011:623924.
54. Tanase A, Schmitz N, Stein H, et al. Allogeneic and autologous stem cell transplantation for hepatosplenic T-cell lymphoma: a retrospective study of the EBMT Lymphoma Working Party. *Leukemia.* 2015;29(3):686-688.
55. Loirat M, Chevallier P, Leux C, et al. Upfront allogeneic stem-cell transplantation for patients with nonlocalized untreated peripheral T-cell lymphoma: an intention-to-treat analysis from a single center. *Ann Oncol.* 2015;26(2):386-392.
56. Hishizawa M, Kanda J, Utsunomiya A, et al. Transplantation of allogeneic hematopoietic stem cells for adult T-cell leukemia: a nationwide retrospective study. *Blood.* 2010;116(8):1369-1376.
57. Smith SD, Bolwell BJ, Rybicki LA, et al. Autologous hematopoietic stem cell transplantation in peripheral T-cell lymphoma using a uniform high-dose regimen. *Bone Marrow Transplant.* 2007;40(3):239-243.
58. Kim MK, Kim S, Lee SS, et al. High-dose chemotherapy and autologous stem cell transplantation for peripheral T-cell lymphoma: complete response at transplant predicts survival. *Ann Hematol.* 2007;86(6):435-442.
59. Kim SW, Yoon SS, Suzuki R, et al. Comparison of outcomes between autologous and allogeneic hematopoietic stem cell transplantation for peripheral T-cell lymphomas with central review of pathology. *Leukemia.* 2013;27(6):1394-1397.
60. Jacobsen ED, Kim HT, Ho VT, et al. A large single-center experience with allogeneic stem-cell transplantation for peripheral T-cell non-Hodgkin lymphoma and advanced mycosis fungoides/Sezary syndrome. *Ann Oncol.* 2011;22(7):1608-1613.
61. Le Gouill S, Milpied N, Buzyn A, et al. Graft-versus-lymphoma effect for aggressive T-cell lymphomas in adults: a study by the Societe Francaise de Greffe de Moelle et de Therapie Cellulaire. *J Clin Oncol.* 2008;26(14):2264-2271.
62. Aoki K, Suzuki R, Chihara D, et al. Reduced-intensity conditioning of allogeneic transplantation for nodal peripheral T-cell lymphomas [abstract]. *Blood.* 2015:2585.
63. Yamaguchi M, Tobinai K, Oguchi M, et al. Concurrent chemoradiotherapy for localized nasal natural killer/T-cell lymphoma: an updated analysis of the Japan clinical oncology group study JCOG0211. *J Clin Oncol.* 2012;30(32):4044-4046.
64. Kim SJ, Kim K, Kim BS, et al. Phase II trial of concurrent radiation and weekly cisplatin followed by VIPD chemotherapy in newly diagnosed, stage IE to IIE, nasal, extranodal NK/T-cell lymphoma: Consortium for Improving Survival of Lymphoma study. *J Clin Oncol.* 2009;27(35):6027-6032.
65. Yamaguchi M, Kwong YL, Kim WS, et al. Phase II study of

SMILE chemotherapy for newly diagnosed stage IV, relapsed, or refractory extranodal natural killer (NK)/T-cell lymphoma, nasal type: the NK-Cell Tumor Study Group study. *J Clin Oncol.* 2011;29(33):4410-4416.

66. Jaccard A, Gachard N, Marin B, et al. Efficacy of L-asparaginase with methotrexate and dexamethasone (AspaMetDex regimen) in patients with refractory or relapsing extranodal NK/T-cell lymphoma, a phase 2 study. *Blood.* 2011;117(6):1834-1839.
67. Pro B, Advani R, Brice P, et al. Brentuximab vedotin (SGN-35) in patients with relapsed or refractory systemic anaplastic large-cell lymphoma: results of a phase II study. *J Clin Oncol.* 2012;30(18):2190-2196.
68. Horwitz SM, Advani RH, Bartlett NL, et al. Objective responses in relapsed T-cell lymphomas with single agent brentuximab vedotin. *Blood.* 2014;123(20):3095-3100.
69. O'Connor OA, Pro B, Pinter-Brown L, et al. Pralatrexate in patients with relapsed or refractory peripheral T-cell lymphoma: results from the pivotal PROPEL study. *J Clin Oncol.* 2011;29(9):1182-1189.
70. Coiffier B, Pro B, Prince HM, et al. Results from a pivotal, open-label, phase II study of romidepsin in relapsed or refractory peripheral T-cell lymphoma after prior systemic therapy. *J Clin Oncol.* 2012;30(6):631-636.
71. O'Connor OA, Masszi T, Savage KJ, et al. Belinostat, a novel pan-histone deacetylase inhibitor (HDACi), in relapsed or refractory peripheral T-cell lymphoma (R/R PTCL): results from the BELIEF trial [asbtract]. *Blood.* 2013:8507.
72. Damaj G, Gressin R, Bouabdallah K, et al. Results from a prospective, open-label, phase II trial of bendamustine in refractory or relapsed T-cell lymphomas: the BENTLY trial. *J Clin Oncol.* 2013;31(1):104-110.
73. Ishida T, Joh T, Uike N, et al. Defucosylated anti-CCR4 monoclonal antibody (KW-0761) for relapsed adult T-cell leukemia-lymphoma: a multicenter phase II study. *J Clin Oncol.* 2012;30(8):837-842.
74. Ogura M, Ishida T, Hatake K, et al. Multicenter phase II study of mogamulizumab (KW-0761), a defucosylated anti-cc chemokine receptor 4 antibody, in patients with relapsed peripheral T-cell lymphoma and cutaneous T-cell lymphoma. *J Clin Oncol.* 2014;32(11):1157-1163.
75. Friedberg JW, Mahadevan D, Cebula E, et al. Phase II study of alisertib, a selective aurora A kinase inhibitor, in relapsed and refractory aggressive B- and T-cell non-Hodgkin lymphomas. *J Clin Oncol.* 2014;32(1):44-50.
76. Girardi M, Heald PW, Wilson LD. The pathogenesis of mycosis fungoides. *N Engl J Med.* 2004;350(19):1978-1988.
77. Pimpinelli N, Olsen EA, Santucci M, et al. Defining early mycosis fungoides. *J Am Acad Dermatol.* 2005;53(6):1053-1063.
78. Kim EJ, Hess S, Richardson SK, et al. Immunopathogenesis and therapy of cutaneous T cell lymphoma. *J Clin Invest.* 2005;115(4):798-812.
79. Vega F, Luthra R, Medeiros LJ, et al. Clonal heterogeneity in mycosis fungoides and its relationship to clinical course. *Blood.* 2002;100(9):3369-3373.
80. Kim YH, Liu HL, Mraz-Gernhard S, Varghese A, Hoppe RT. Long-term outcome of 525 patients with mycosis fungoides and Sezary syndrome: clinical prognostic factors and risk for disease progression. *Arch Dermatol.* 2003;139(7):857-866.
81. Diamandidou E, Colome M, Fayad L, Duvic M, Kurzrock R. Prognostic factor analysis in mycosis fungoides/Sezary syndrome. *J Am Acad Dermatol.* 1999;40(6 Pt 1):914-924.
82. Scarisbrick JJ, Whittaker S, Evans AV, et al. Prognostic significance of tumor burden in the blood of patients with erythrodermic primary cutaneous T-cell lymphoma. *Blood.* 2001;97(3):624-630.
83. Breneman D, Duvic M, Kuzel T, Yocum R, Truglia J, Stevens VJ. Phase 1 and 2 trial of bexarotene gel for skin-directed treatment of patients with cutaneous T-cell lymphoma. *Arch Dermatol.* 2002;138(3):325-332.
84. Lain T, Talpur R, Duvic M. Long-term control of mycosis fungoides of the hands with topical bexarotene. *Int J Dermatol.* 2003;42(3):238-241.
85. Krathen RA, Ward S, Duvic M. Bexarotene is a new treatment option for lymphomatoid papulosis. *Dermatology.* 2003;206(2):142-147.
86. Lessin SR, Duvic M, Guitart J, et al. Topical chemotherapy in cutaneous T-cell lymphoma: positive results of a randomized, controlled, multicenter trial testing the efficacy and safety of a novel mechlorethamine, 0.02%, gel in mycosis fungoides. *JAMA Dermatol.* 2013;149(1):25-32.
87. Duvic M, Donato M, Dabaja B, et al. Total skin electron beam and non-myeloablative allogeneic hematopoietic stem-cell transplantation in advanced mycosis fungoides and Sezary syndrome. *J Clin Oncol.* 2010;28(14):2365-2372.
88. Harrison C, Young J, Navi D, et al. Revisiting low-dose total skin electron beam therapy in mycosis fungoides. *Int J Radiat Oncol Biol Phys.* 2011;81(4):e651-e657.
89. Olsen E, Duvic M, Frankel A, et al. Pivotal phase III trial of two dose levels of denileukin diftitox for the treatment of cutaneous T-cell lymphoma. *J Clin Oncol.* 2001;19(2):376-388.
90. Foss F, Demierre MF, DiVenuti G. A phase-1 trial of bexarotene and denileukin diftitox in patients with relapsed or refractory cutaneous T-cell lymphoma. *Blood.* 2005;106(2):454-457.
91. Assaf C, Bagot M, Dummer R, et al. Minimizing adverse side-effects of oral bexarotene in cutaneous T-cell lymphoma: an expert opinion. *Br J Dermatol.* 2006;155(2):261-266.
92. Lim HW, Edelson RL. Photopheresis for the treatment of cutaneous T-cell lymphoma. *Hematol Oncol Clin North Am.* 1995;9(5):1117-1126.
93. McGinnis KS, Ubriani R, Newton S, et al. The addition of interferon gamma to oral bexarotene therapy with photopheresis for Sezary syndrome. *Arch Dermatol.* 2005;141(9):1176-1178.
94. Talpur R, Demierre MF, Geskin L, et al. Multicenter photopheresis intervention trial in early-stage mycosis fungoides. *Clin Lymphoma Myeloma Leuk.* 2011;11(2):219-227.
95. Duvic M, Vu J. Vorinostat: a new oral histone deacetylase inhibitor approved for cutaneous T-cell lymphoma. *Expert Opin Investig Drugs.* 2007;16(7):1111-1120.
96. Whittaker SJ, Demierre MF, Kim EJ, et al. Final results from a multicenter, international, pivotal study of romidepsin in refractory cutaneous T-cell lymphoma. *J Clin Oncol.* 2010;28(29):4485-4491.
97. Kim YH, Demierre MF, Kim EJ, et al. Clinically meaningful reduction in pruritus in patients with cutaneous T-cell lymphoma treated with romidepsin. *Leuk Lymphoma.* 2013;54(2):284-289.
98. Piekarz RL, Frye R, Turner M, et al. Phase II multi-institutional trial of the histone deacetylase inhibitor romidepsin as monotherapy for patients with cutaneous T-cell lymphoma. *J Clin Oncol.* 2009;27(32):5410-5417.
99. Marchi E, Alinari L, Tani M, et al. Gemcitabine as frontline treatment for cutaneous T-cell lymphoma: phase II study of 32 patients. *Cancer.* 2005;104(11):2437-2441.
100. Wollina U, Dummer R, Brockmeyer NH, et al. Multicenter study of pegylated liposomal doxorubicin in patients with cutaneous T-cell lymphoma. *Cancer.* 2003;98(5):993-1001.
101. Illidge T, Chan C, Counsell N, et al. Phase II study of gemcitabine and bexarotene (GEMBEX) in the treatment of cutaneous T-cell lymphoma. *Br J Cancer.* 2013;109(10):2566-2573.
102. Horwitz S, Duvic M, Kim Y. Pralatrexate is active in cutaneous T-cell lymphoma (CTCL): results of a multicenter, dose-finding trial [abstract]. *Blood.* 2009;114:919.
103. Talpur R, Thompson A, Gangar P, Duvic M. Pralatrexate alone or in combination with bexarotene: long-term tolerability in

relapsed/refractory mycosis fungoides. *Clin Lymphoma Myeloma Leuk*. 2014;14(4):297-304.

104. d'Amore F, Radford J, Relander T, et al. Phase II trial of zanolimumab (HuMax-CD4) in relapsed or refractory non-cutaneous peripheral T cell lymphoma. *Br J Haematol*. 2010;150(5):565-573.
105. Dummer R, Duvic M, Scarisbrick J, et al. Final results of a multicenter phase II study of the purine nucleoside phosphorylase (PNP) inhibitor forodesine in patients with advanced cutaneous T-cell lymphomas (CTCL) (mycosis fungoides and Sezary syndrome). *Ann Oncol*. 2014;25(9):1807-1812.
106. Ogura M, Tsukasaki K, Nagai H, et al. Phase I study of BCX1777 (forodesine) in patients with relapsed or refractory peripheral T/natural killer-cell malignancies. *Cancer Sci*. 2012;103(7):1290-1295.
107. Querfeld C, Rosen ST, Guitart J, et al. Results of an open-label multicenter phase 2 trial of lenalidomide monotherapy in refractory mycosis fungoides and Sezary syndrome. *Blood*. 2014;123(8):1159-1166.

10

Hodgkin Lymphoma

第十章　霍奇金淋巴瘤

Dai Chihara
Fredrick B. Hagemeister
L. Jeffrey Medeiros
Michelle A. Fanale

中文导读

本章首先概述了霍奇金淋巴瘤的流行病学、病理分类、霍奇金淋巴瘤的放疗剂量和放射野大小的更新等治疗进展；其次，详细介绍了不同病理类型霍奇金淋巴瘤的临床表现、组织学特征和免疫表型；进而系统地介绍了MD安德森癌症中心对霍奇金淋巴瘤的诊断、分期、治疗、预后判断、疗效评价和随访流程；最后，重点阐述了近年来霍奇金淋巴瘤的治疗进展，包括结节性淋巴细胞为主型霍奇金淋巴瘤和经典型霍奇金淋巴瘤的治疗方案选择。在经典型霍奇金淋巴瘤部分，主要分别介绍了早期预后良好患者、早期预后不良患者、晚期患者和复发/难治性霍奇金淋巴瘤患者的方案选择，并介绍了大剂量化疗联合自体干细胞移植对复发/难治性霍奇金淋巴瘤患者的疗效，以及自体干细胞移植治疗失败后复发患者的药物选择。本章最后介绍了新型靶向药物在霍奇金淋巴瘤中的应用前景。

INTRODUCTION

Hodgkin lymphoma (HL) was recognized in the first half of the nineteenth century by Thomas Hodgkin and Samuel Wilks ([1]). HL usually arises in lymph nodes, preferentially in the cervical area, and the majority of HLs manifest clinically in young adults in their third and fourth decades of life. The incidence of HL is 3.0 per 100,000 person-year in the United States; it is higher in the Western countries than Asian countries ([2, 3]). Biological and clinical studies have shown that HLs are comprised of two disease entities: nodular lymphocyte-predominant HL (NLPHL) and classical HL (cHL) ([1]). The two entities differ in their clinical features and behavior. Within cHL, four subtypes have been described: nodular sclerosis, mixed cellularity, lymphocyte-rich, and lymphocyte-depleted. These four subtypes differ in their clinical features, growth pattern, presence of fibrosis, and frequency of Epstein-Barr virus infection but share the immunophenotype of tumor cells.

The management of HL continues to evolve. Before the widespread use of modern polychemotherapy, large-field radiation therapy was able to cure cHL patients. However, reliance on radiation alone required extensive radiation portals to treat nearly the entire lymphatic system with radiation doses up to 44 Gy. With long-term follow-up, many patients developed heart toxicity and second malignancies. Therefore, efforts have been made to reduce the long-term toxicities of treatment for HL while maintaining excellent cure rates. With modern chemotherapy, multiple randomized studies have shown that radiation portals can be safely reduced from extended-field radiation to involved-field radiation and, now, even smaller fields of radiation, including involved-node radiation.

Currently, the treatment of cHL is stratified by risk groups—early-stage favorable, early-stage unfavorable, and advanced-stage disease—according to the clinical stage and the presence or absence of adverse clinical features. In this chapter, we will review advances in the management of HL, including recent publications about strategies of management of the rarer diagnosis of NLPHL.

TYPES OF HODGKIN LYMPHOMA

Over the past decade, investigators have made significant progress in the diagnosis, classification, staging, prognosis, and treatment of HL. In past years, the true lineage of the neoplastic cells in HL was unknown; hence, the term *Hodgkin disease* was used. It is now recognized that almost all cases of HL are of B-cell lineage; hence, the name changed to Hodgkin lymphoma.

The classification of HL has remained relatively stable over the past 40 years, and the World Health Organization (WHO) classification of lymphoid neoplasms was updated in 2008 ([1]) (Table 10-1). The current WHO classification recognizes that NLPHL is distinct from the other types that can be grouped together under the rubric of cHL ([1]).

In 2015, it was estimated that 9,050 Americans would be diagnosed with HL, with a median age at diagnosis of 39 years ([4]). Hodgkin lymphoma has been traditionally defined as a hematopoietic neoplasm composed of diagnostic Hodgkin and Reed-Sternberg (HRS) cells within a reactive cell background. An HRS cell is large, 30 to 60 μm, containing a bilobed vesicular nucleus, with each lobe containing a prominent round eosinophilic nucleolus surrounded by a clear zone or halo; it also has abundant cytoplasm. However, HRS cells often comprise less than 1% of the involved tumor tissue and are absent in NLPHL. Hodgkin and Reed-Sternberg cells are believed to be derived from germinal center (GC) B cells that have unfavorable immunoglobulin V gene mutations, whereas lymphocyte-predominant (LP) cells, which were previously termed lymphocytic and histiocytic (LH) cells, are thought to originate from antigen-selected GC B cells ([5]).

Nodular Lymphocyte-Predominant Hodgkin Lymphoma

Clinical Features

Approximately 5% of patients with HL have NLPHL. This disease is usually localized and most often involves cervical or axillary lymph nodes ([1, 6]). The disease affects patients of all ages, males more often than females, and is clinically indolent (Table 10-2). Systemic symptoms—such as fever, weight loss, and nights sweats (also known as B symptoms)—are infrequent. Patients with NLPHL are characterized as having a more indolent course with delayed relapse compared with cHL, analogous to low-grade non-HL ([6]). Patients with NLPHL are at 5% to 6% risk for developing diffuse large B-cell lymphoma (DLBCL) or T-cell/histiocyte-rich large B-cell lymphoma ([1]).

Table 10-1 World Health Organization Classification of Hodgkin Lymphoma

Nodular lymphocyte predominant
Classical Hodgkin lymphoma Nodular sclerosis Lymphocyte rich Mixed cellularity Lymphocyte depleted

Table 10-2 Comparison of Clinical Features of Nodular Lymphocyte-Predominant (NLPHL) and Classical Hodgkin Lymphoma (HL)

Clinical Feature	NLPHL	Classical HL
Frequency	5%	95%
Age distribution	Unimodal: equal in children and adults	Bimodal: peak in second and third decades
Male	70%	50%
Sites involved	Lymph nodes with sparing mediastinum	Mediastinum, cervical lymph nodes
Stage at diagnosis[a]	I	II or III
B symptoms	<20%	40%
Clinical course	Indolent, late relapses	Aggressive, curable

[a]Most common stage at time of diagnosis.

The German Hodgkin Lymphoma Study Group (GHSG) has reported a large retrospective study of 394 patients with NLPHL. Patients were predominantly men (75%), only 9% had B symptoms, and 79% had early-stage disease ([7]). With a median follow-up of 50 months, tumor control (freedom from treatment failure) and overall survival were 88% and 96%, respectively, slightly better than in cHL (82% and 92%, respectively).

Histologic Features

Nodular lymphocyte-predominant Hodgkin lymphoma is characterized by effacement of nodal architecture by variably sized, vague nodules composed of numerous small lymphocytes, histiocytes, and characteristic neoplastic LP cells (Fig. 10-1**A**) ([1, 8]). These cells are typically large, with pale cytoplasm and polyploid vesicular nuclei containing inconspicuous nucleoli resembling kernels of popped corn, hence the nickname popcorn cells (Fig. 10-1**B**). However, LP cells can exhibit a range of cytologic appearances. These cells can be round and/or have relatively prominent nucleoli. Eosinophils, neutrophils, and plasma cells are usually absent in NLPHL, and there is no associated necrosis or fibrosis.

Cases of NLPHL can also have diffuse areas. When diffuse areas are large, their presence often correlates with more aggressive disease. To reflect this change in clinical behavior, many pathologists diagnose such cases as NLPHL with progression to T-cell/histiocyte-rich large B-cell lymphoma, also described as T-cell–rich B-cell lymphoma (TCRBCL). Other pathologists use the term *NLPHL with large diffuse areas* and suggest that the diffuse areas may represent the beginning stages of progression to DLBCL. The boundary between NLPHL with diffuse areas and TCRBCL remains blurred. Most cases previously designated as diffuse LPHL, as defined previously ([9]), are now classified differently. With appropriate workup, these cases are usually classified as NLPHL with large diffuse areas, lymphocyte-rich cHL, or TCRBCL.

Gene expression profiling of NLPHL to determine the origin and pathogenesis of LP cells found significant similarities between NLPHL, TCRBCL, and cHL ([10]). Overall, LP cells are thought to derive from antigen-selected GC B cells ([5]). LP cells also demonstrate deregulation of numerous apoptosis regulators and putative oncogenes and a partial loss of their B-cell phenotype. In addition, there is constitutive activation of nuclear factor-κB (NF-κB), Janus kinases/signal transducers and activator of transcription (JAK/STAT) pathway, and aberrant extracellular-regulated kinase signaling.

Immunophenotypic Findings

Nodular lymphocyte-predominant Hodgkin lymphoma is immunophenotypically distinct from other types of HL. The LP cells usually express leukocyte common antigen (LCA; CD45), immunoglobulin J chain, B-cell antigens (CD19, CD20, CD22, CD79A, and BCL-6), and epithelial membrane antigen (EMA) and are negative for CD15 and CD30 (Figs. 10-1**C** and **D**). These results suggest that the LP cells are B cells that arise from the GC. The LP cells are negative for T-cell antigens but are often surrounded by a rosette of small, reactive T cells that may be positive for pan-T-cell antigens and CD57 (Fig. 10-1**E**). Epstein-Barr virus is almost always absent in the LP cells of NLPHL.

Lymphocyte-Rich Classical Hodgkin Lymphoma

Lymphocyte-rich cHLs (LRHLs) have been recognized that resemble NLPHL histologically but are cHL immunophenotypically ([1, 6, 8]). The frequency of this type of HL is not well known but is most likely low (<5%). Clinically, patients with LRHL are similar to patients with other subtypes of cHL or have clinical findings intermediate between NLPHL and cHL. Unlike patients with NLPHL, late relapse is uncommon in patients with LRHL.

Histologically, these tumors are rich in small lymphocytes and histiocytes. Granulocytes and plasma cells are usually infrequent. Necrosis is usually not present. Lymphocyte-rich cHL may be either nodular or diffuse. The nodular type closely resembles NLPHL. Vague nodules of numerous small lymphocytes are present, and the nodules may have a small

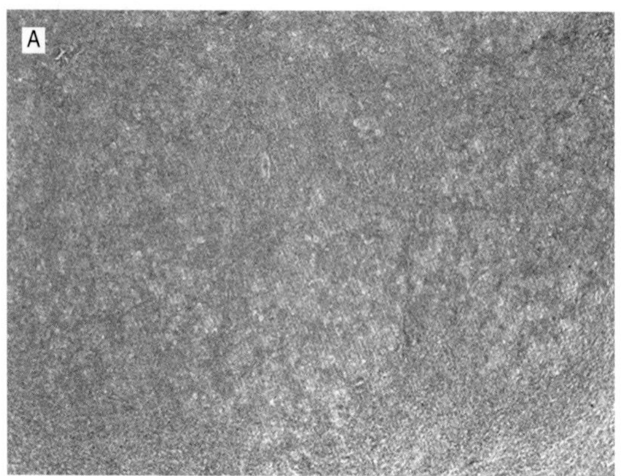

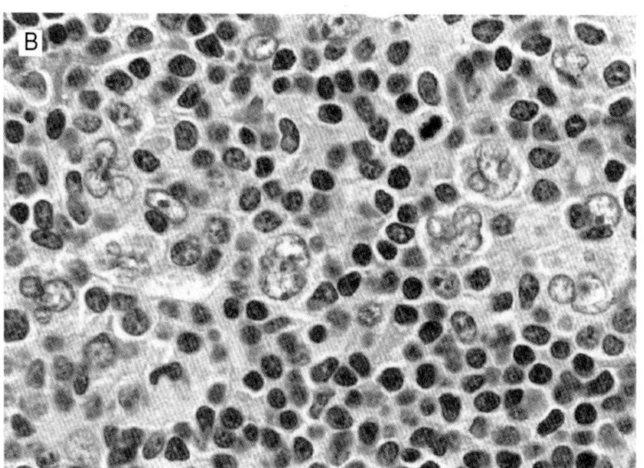

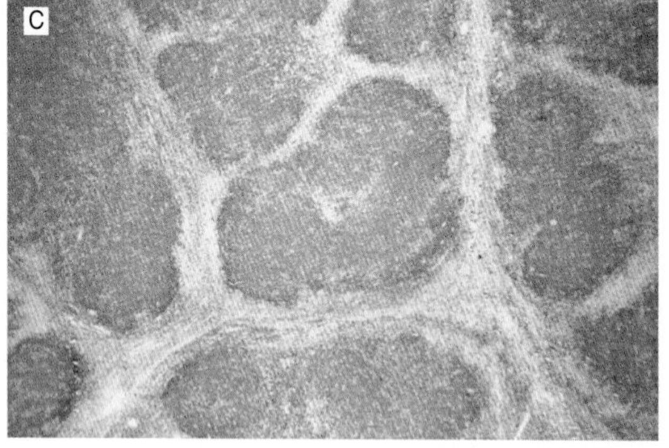

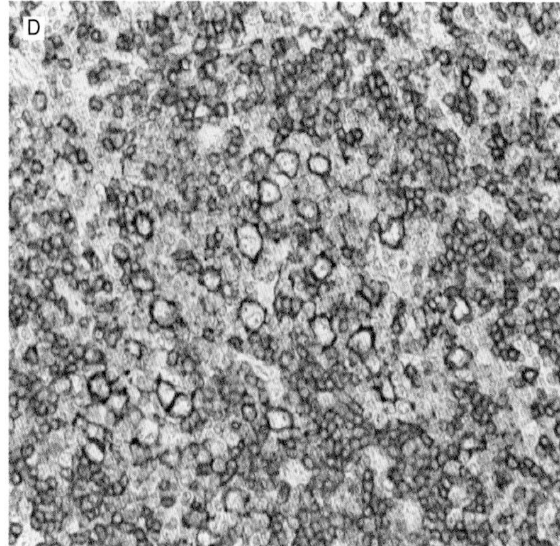

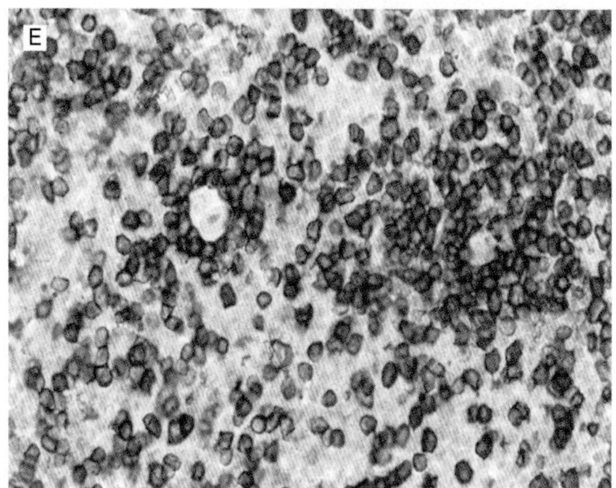

FIGURE 10-1 Nodular lymphocyte-predominant Hodgkin lymphoma. **A.** At low-power magnification, the neoplasm is vaguely nodular. **B.** At high-power magnification, large lymphocytic and histiocytic (LH) cells, resembling popped kernels of corn, are identified in a background of reactive lymphocytes and histiocytes. **C** and **D.** Immunohistochemical stain for CD20. **C.** At low-power magnification, this immunostain highlights the nodular pattern and shows numerous B cells in the nodules. **D.** At high-power magnification, large LH cells and small reactive B cells are positive for CD20. **E.** Immunohistochemical stain for CD3. Scattered small reactive T cells are present and focally surround the LH cells (so-called rosetting).

compressed GC (Figs. 10-2A and B). The neoplastic cells are present in the mantle zones of the nodules. These neoplastic cells usually resemble Reed-Sternberg and typical mononuclear variant cells (so-called Hodgkin cells) rather than LP cells. The cell composition is similar in diffuse cases of LRHL, but nodularity is minimal or absent. Immunohistochemical studies of LRHL show that the large neoplastic cells have an immunophenotype similar to that of all cHL cases, positive for CD15 and CD30 and negative for LCA (CD45) (Figs. 10-2C to E).

In a study of NLPHL by the European Task Force on Lymphoma ([8]), a large number of tumors that had been classified as NLPHL were reviewed; the diagnosis was confirmed in only half of these cases. Most of those excluded were reclassified as LRHL.

Nodular Sclerosis Hodgkin Lymphoma

Clinical Features

Nodular sclerosis (NS) is the most common form of cHL, representing 60% to 70% of all cases in Western countries; it is also the most common type of cHL in patients younger than age 50 years. Whites are affected more often than others, and nodular sclerosis HL (NSHL) is much less frequent in Asian countries ([2, 3]). The age-adjusted incidence rate of NSHL has been stable since 1993 to 2008 in the United States according to the National Cancer Institute (NCI) Surveillance, Epidemiology, and End Results (SEER) data ([2]). The male-to-female ratio is approximately equal. Nodular sclerosis HL has a marked predilection for involving mediastinal, supraclavicular, and cervical lymph nodes. A mediastinal mass is very common, and the thymus may be involved.

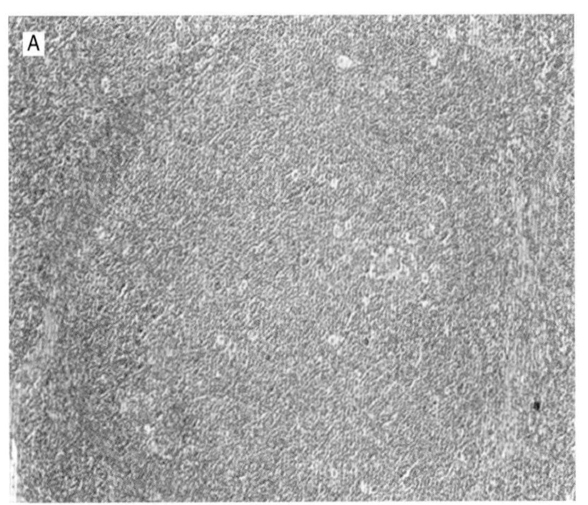

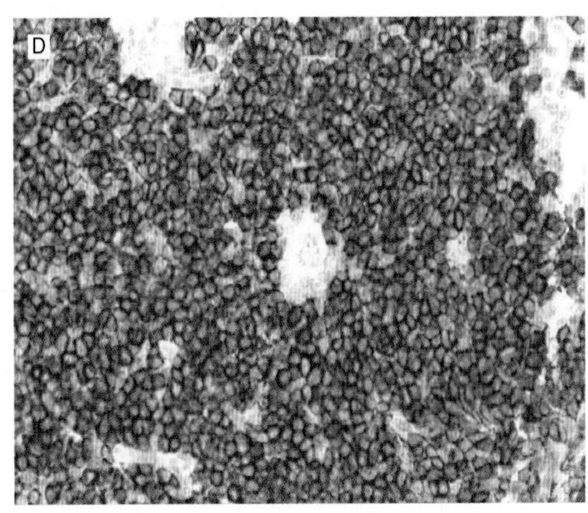

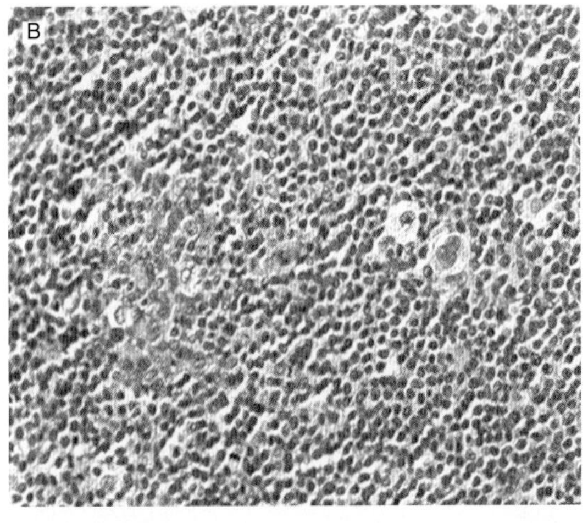

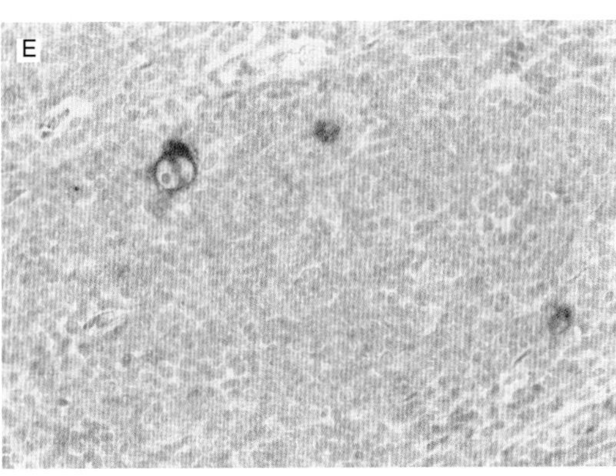

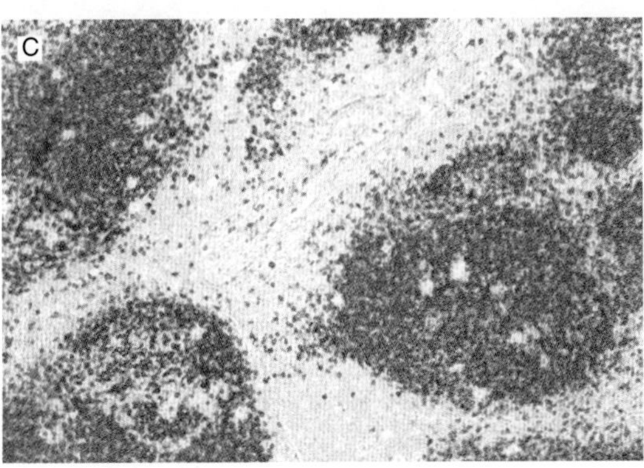

FIGURE 10-2 Lymphocyte-rich classical Hodgkin lymphoma, nodular variant. **A.** At low-power magnification, the neoplasm has a nodular pattern and is rich in reactive small lymphocytes (resembling nodular lymphocyte-predominant Hodgkin lymphoma). **B.** At high-power magnification, large neoplastic cells (so-called Hodgkin cells) are identified in the mantle zone of the follicle (note reactive germinal center to left of field). **C** and **D.** Immunohistochemical stain for CD20. **C.** The nodules contain numerous small reactive B cells. **D.** The Hodgkin cells are negative for CD20. **E.** Immunohistochemical stain for CD30. The Hodgkin cells are positive.

Histologic Features

Nodular sclerosis HL is characterized by a triad of findings: (1) a nodular pattern, (2) broad bands of fibrosis that outline the nodules, and (3) characteristic mononuclear cell variants known as lacunar cells (Fig. 10-3). A lacunar cell has abundant clear cytoplasm with a sharply demarcated cell membrane. In formalin-fixed tissue, a characteristic artifact occurs. The cell cytoplasm retracts, leaving a clear space or lacuna surrounding the cell, hence the origin of the name. The typical lacunar cell has a polylobulated nucleus with one or multiple small nucleoli. However, lacunar cells can show great morphologic variability and can be round with prominent nucleoli, or they may resemble large noncleaved cells. A heterogeneous mixture of reactive cells may be seen in HL, including small lymphocytes, histiocytes, eosinophils, neutrophils, and plasma cells in variable numbers.

Nodular sclerosis HL has been graded (as 1 or 2) by the British National Lymphoma Investigation (BNLI) group ([11]) according to the numbers of neoplastic cells and reactive cells present, and this grading system has been adopted by the WHO classification ([1]). Grade 2 cases of NSHL show numerous neoplastic (lacunar) cells and depletion of reactive lymphocytes. Lymphocyte-depleted and syncytial variants (Fig. 10-4) of NSHL have been described; these cases are the outermost examples of grade 2 NSHL. The syncytial variant of NSHL is composed of sheets of neoplastic cells and necrosis.

Mixed Cellularity Hodgkin Lymphoma

Clinical Features

The mixed cellularity variant of HL (MCHL), the second most common type, affects 15% to 25% of all patients with the disease and is the most common form in patients older than age 50 years ([1, 12]). Males are affected more often than females. According to NCI SEER data, MCHL is relatively more common in African Americans and Hispanic Americans than in whites in the United States. A substantial percentage of patients with MCHL have clinical stage III or stage IV disease and B symptoms.

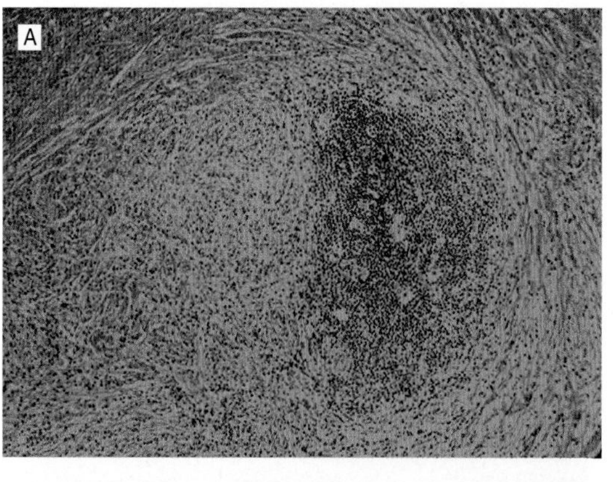

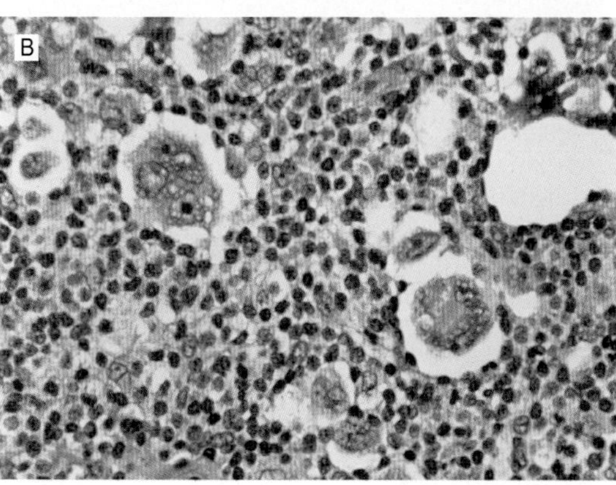

FIGURE 10-3 Nodular sclerosis Hodgkin lymphoma. **A.** The neoplasm is nodular, and the nodules are surrounded by dense fibrous bands. **B.** The large neoplastic cells (lacunar cells) lie within lacunar spaces, and many are multinucleated in this field. Reactive cells are present in the background.

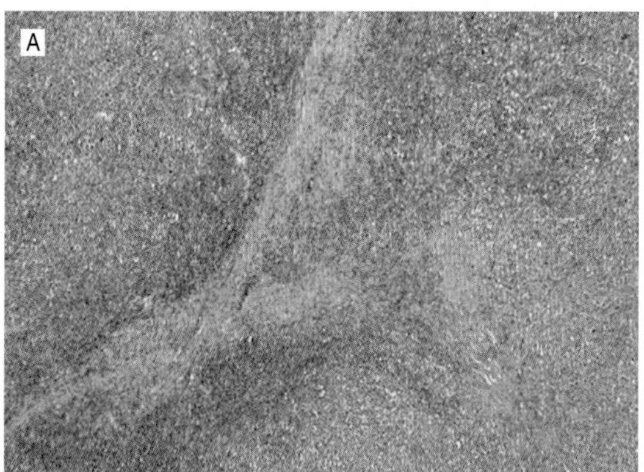

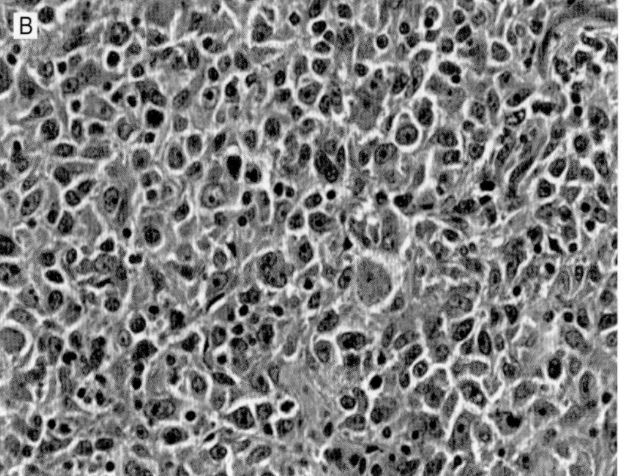

FIGURE 10-4 Syncytial variant of nodular sclerosis Hodgkin lymphoma. **A.** Nodularity and a fibrous bond can be appreciated in this field. **B.** The nodules are composed of many neoplastic cells with depletion of small lymphocytes.

Histologic Features

Mixed cellularity HL is characterized by a large number of Reed-Sternberg cells and Hodgkin cells in a background of numerous eosinophils, plasma cells, histiocytes, and granulocytes in varying proportions ([1]) (Fig. 10-5). The lymph node architecture is usually diffusely replaced. Partially involved lymph nodes show selective paracortical infiltration. Disorderly fibrosis may be seen, but the broad fibrous bands and capsular fibrosis characteristic of NSHL are absent.

Two variants of MCHL can be relatively more difficult to diagnose. In the interfollicular variant, which most likely represents partial involvement of lymph nodes by HL, the tumor is located in the interfollicular region and is often associated with reactive follicular hyperplasia and marked plasmacytosis. In the epithelioid histiocyte-rich variant, numerous epithelioid histiocytes and granulomas are present; these can be so numerous as to obscure the neoplastic cells. The importance of these variants of MCHL lies in their unusual histologic findings.

Lymphocyte-Depleted Hodgkin Lymphoma

Clinical Features

Lymphocyte-depleted HL (LDHL) is the least common type, representing 1% of all cases ([12]). In the NCI SEER study, it was shown that the age-adjusted incidence rate for LDHL has decreased. This decrease is most likely explained by the recognition by pathologists that many tumors previously classified as LDHL are, in fact, non-HLs (such as anaplastic large-cell lymphoma). Improved classification is the result of application of immunohistochemical and molecular methods to the study of these tumors.

Patients with LDHL are usually elderly, and LDHL is rare in individuals younger than 40 years old. There is a slight male predominance. Whites and African Americans are equally affected. Most patients have advanced clinical stage and B symptoms. Patients commonly have a large contiguous mass of matted lymph nodes or diffuse visceral involvement. The diffuse fibrosis type of LDHL commonly has a subdiaphragmatic distribution. Lymphocyte-depleted HL has the poorest prognosis of all types of HL ([12]).

Histologic Features

The LDHL category includes two variants originally recognized by Lukes and Butler: diffuse fibrosis and reticular (Fig. 10-6). The diffuse fibrosis variant of LDHL is characterized by an extensive proliferation of disordered, hypocellular fibrosis. Diagnostic HRS cells can be difficult to find and may be spindled within

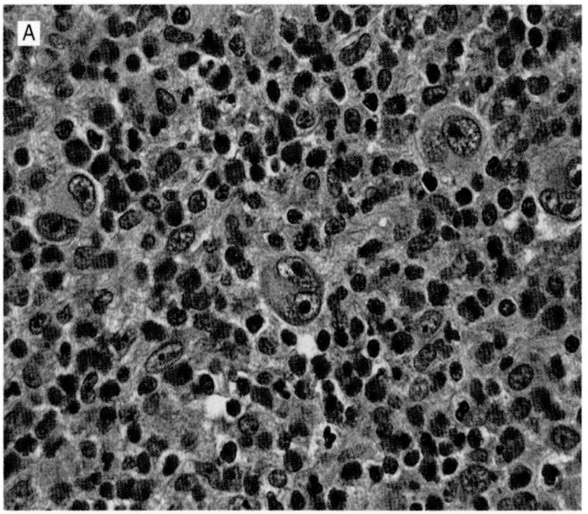

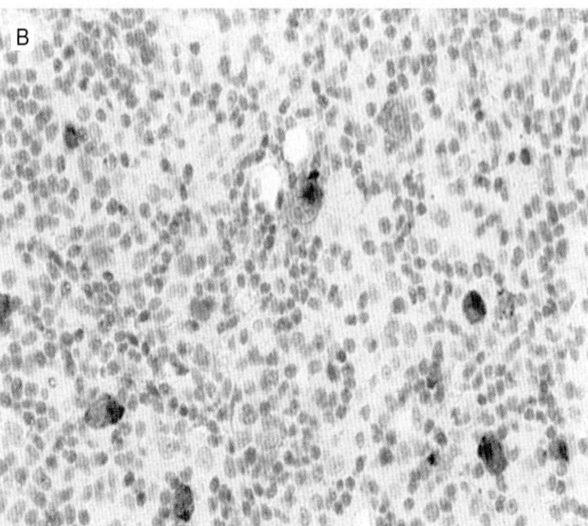

FIGURE 10-5 Mixed cellularity Hodgkin lymphoma. A. Classic Reed-Sternberg cell (center of field) and mononuclear Hodgkin cells can be appreciated in a background of reactive lymphocytes, histiocytes, and eosinophils. B. Immunostain for Epstein-Barr virus latent membrane protein type 1. The neoplastic cells are positive.

dense collagen. Reactive inflammatory cells are relatively few. The reticular variant of LDHL has numerous HRS cells and bizarre variants that have been termed pleomorphic variants. These cells may exhibit marked variations in nuclear number and shape, often with giant nucleoli. Normal small lymphocytes are infrequent compared with the other subtypes of HL. Necrosis is common and may be extensive. The HRS cells and pleomorphic variants may be found in sheets. Mitotic figures are usually numerous.

Immunophenotypic Findings in Classical Hodgkin Lymphoma

Overall the mature B-cell origin of the HRS cells is not readily apparent because HRS cells have a very unusual

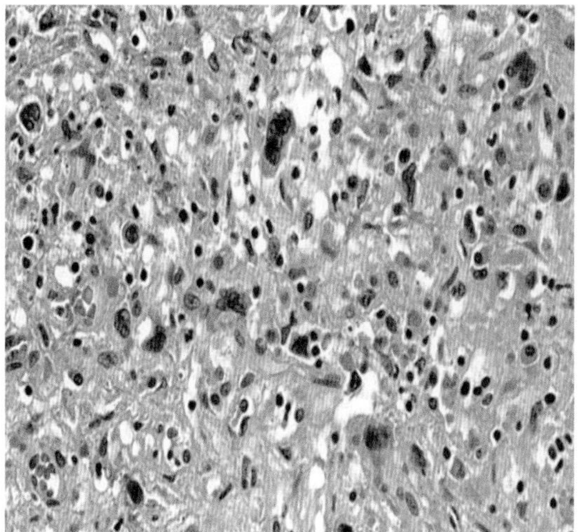

FIGURE 10-6 Lymphocyte-depleted Hodgkin lymphoma. Large neoplastic cells in the background of loose, nonpolarized fibrosis and lymphocyte depletion.

phenotype and have expression of genes that are seen on many hematopoietic cell types. The neoplastic cells are positive for CD15 and CD30 and negative for LCA (CD45) (Fig. 10-7) and EMA ([1]). B-cell antigens, such as CD20, CD79A, PAX-5/BSAP, and MUM1/IRF4, are expressed in a subset of cases. CD20 expression is often weak. T-cell antigens are usually not expressed by the neoplastic cells. BCL-2 is positive in up to half the cases and has been correlated with poorer prognosis ([13]). Epstein-Barr virus is relatively common in cHL, but its frequency varies greatly among different types.

HODGKIN LYMPHOMA: STAGING AND THERAPY

The University of Texas MD Anderson Cancer Center (MDACC) diagnostic and treatment algorithms for HL are shown in Fig. 10-8.

Staging of the Patients

The Ann Arbor system for staging patients with HL at the time of initial presentation forms the basis for the treatment of disease and has allowed comparison of results achieved by different investigators for more than two decades. Important modifications of the Ann Arbor system were developed at the Cotswold Conference in 1989 (Table 10-3) ([14]). Since then, the staging evaluation has been changing. A recent recommendation for the staging procedure in lymphoma described the importance of positron emission tomography (PET)–computed tomography (CT) scan for fluorodeoxyglucose (FDG)-avid lymphomas, of which HL is one example ([15]). For HL and other FDG-avid lymphomas, PET-CT improves the accuracy of staging compared to CT scans for nodal and extranodal sites ([16]).

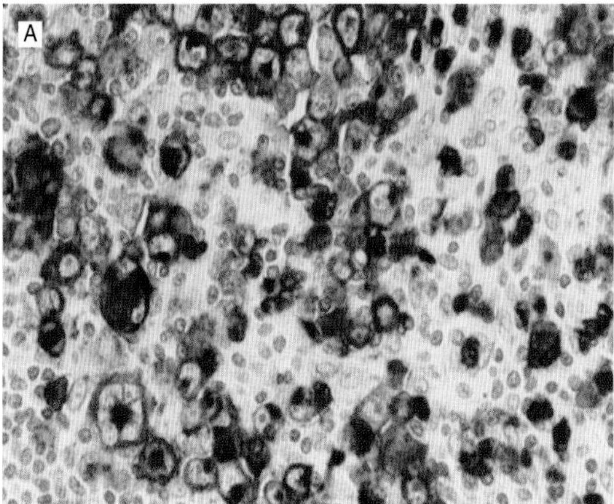

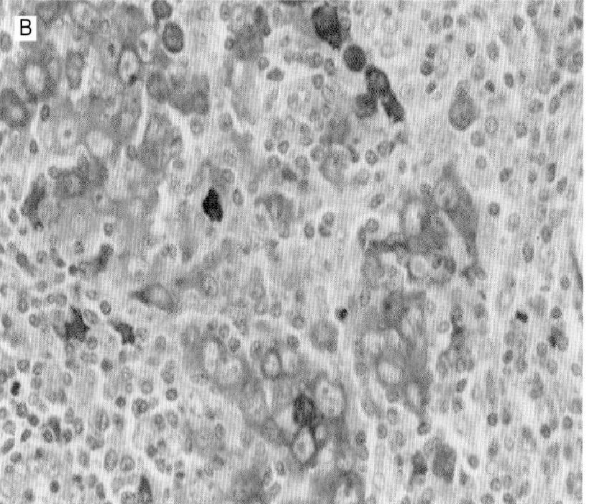

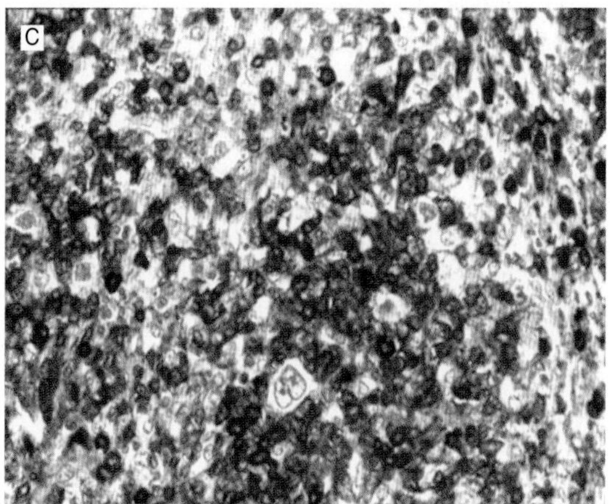

FIGURE 10-7 Typical immunohistochemical findings in classic Hodgkin lymphoma. The Hodgkin cells are positive for CD15 (A) and CD30 (B). The Hodgkin cells in (C) are negative for LCA (CD45RB).

Positron emission tomography–CT leads to change in stage in 10% to 30% of patients, more often upstaging, although alteration in treatment occurs in fewer patients with no demonstrated impact on overall outcome. However, PET-CT is critical as a baseline measurement before therapy to increase the accuracy of subsequent response assessment ([17]). In addition, contrast-enhanced CT scan should be included for a more accurate measurement of nodal size if required for clinical trials.

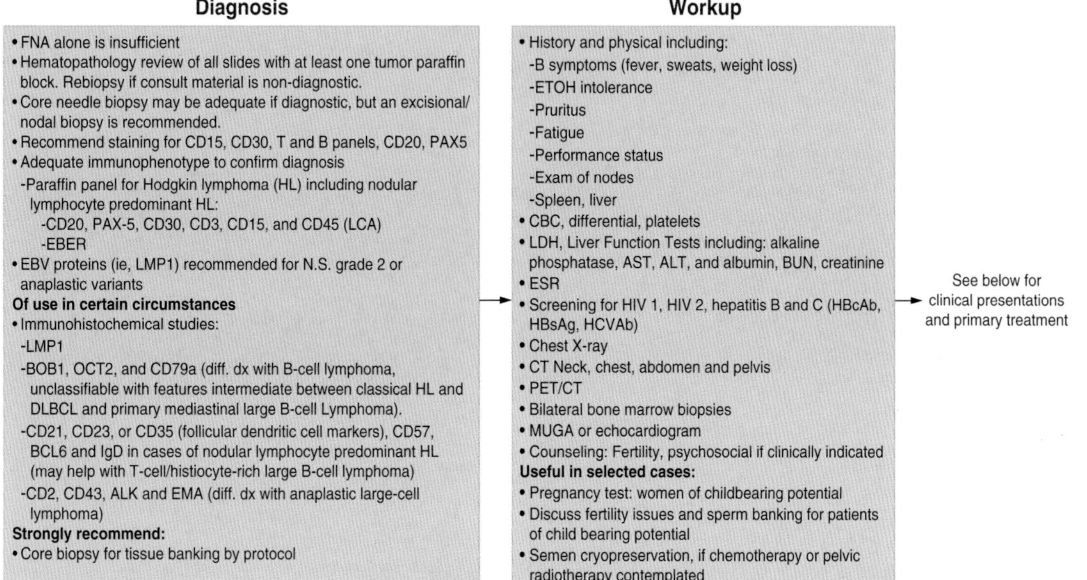

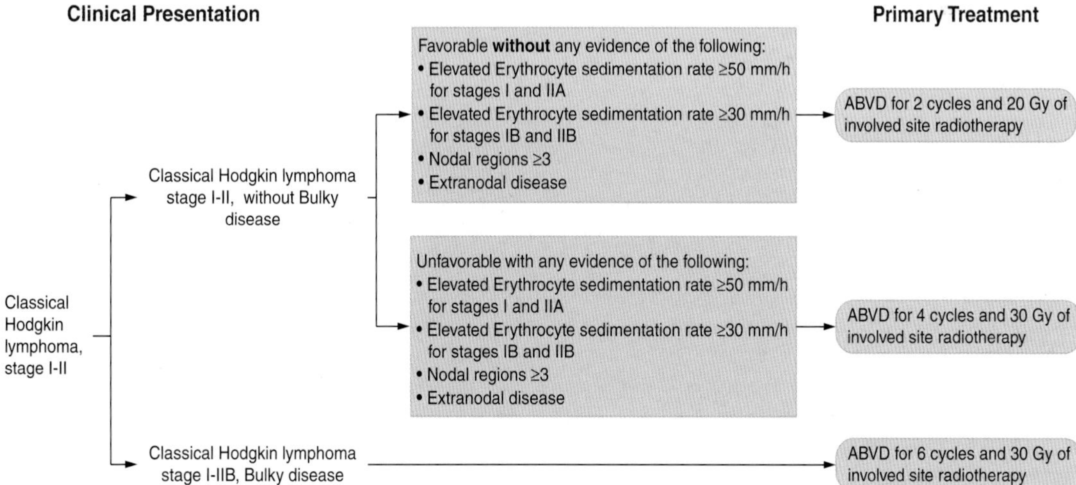

FIGURE 10-8 A-I. MD Anderson Cancer Center algorithms for Hodgkin lymphoma. ABVD: Doxorubicin, bleomycin, vinblastine, dacarbazine; R-CHOP: Rituximab, cyclophosphamide, doxorubicin, vincristine, prednisone; R-ABVD: Rituximab, Doxorubicin, bleomycin, vinblastine, dacarbazine; ICE: Ifosfamide, Carboplatin, and Etoposide; DHAP: High dose cytarabine, cisplatin and dexamethasone; IGEV: Ifosfamide, gemcitabine, vinorelbine and prednisone; GND: Gemcitabine, Navelbine and Doxil. © 2014 The University of Texas MD Anderson Cancer Center.

Clinical Presentation	Primary Treatment	
Classic Hodgkin disease advance stages, IIB, III, IV[1]	ABVD for 6 cycles with or without 30 Gy of involved site radiotherapy	See below for response assessment
Lymphocyte predominate Hodgkin disease stages, I, II	Involved site radiotherapy	See below for response assessment
Lymphocyte predominate Hodgkin disease stages, III, IV	• R-CHOP for 6 cycles Or • R-ABVD for 6 cycles	See below for response assessment

[1]Advanced stage is consistent with an International Prognostic Score (IPS); Consider BEACOPP Chemotherapy regimens for advanced-stage clinical Hodgkin

End-of-Therapy Response Assessment and Treatment of Classical Hodgkin and Lymphocyte-Predominate Hodgkin

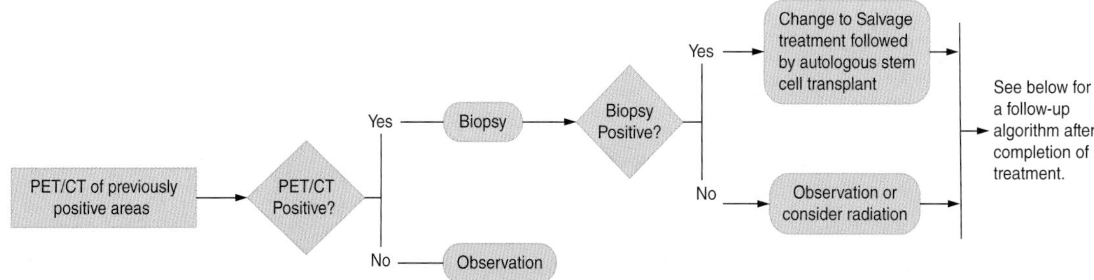

Follow-Up After Completion of Treatment

- Follow-up with an oncologist is recommended
- Interim H&P: every 4 months for years 1 and 2 then every 6 months for years 3-5, then annually
- Pneumococcal and meningococcal revaccination every 6 years, if patient treated with splenic radiotherapy
- Annual influenza vaccine (especially if patient treated with bleomycin or chest radiotherapy)
- Laboratory studies:
  -CBC, platelets, Chemistry profile (LDH, Liver Function Tests including: alkaline phosphatase, AST, ALT, albumin, BUN, and creatinine) every 4 months for years 1 and 2, then every 6 months for years 3-5, then annually
  -TSH every 6 months if radiotherapy to neck and optional for all other cases
- Imaging study one during the first 12 months, then as clinically indicated.
- Annual breast screening: initiate alternating mammography and MRI 8 years post therapy or at age 35, whichever is sooner, if radiotherapy above diaphragm
- Counseling: reproduction, health habits, psychosocial, cardiovascular, breast self-exam, skin cancer risk, end-of-treatment discussion
- Recommend written follow-up instructions for the patient

FIGURE 10-8 (Continued)

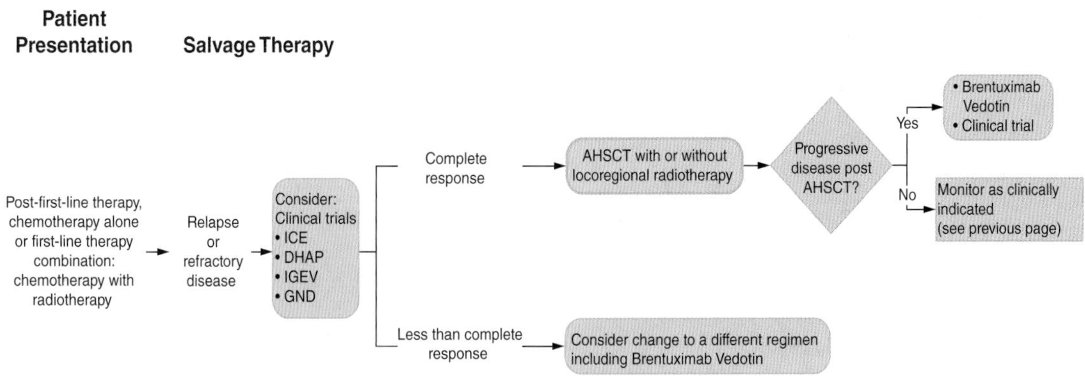

FIGURE 10-8 (Continued)

Table 10-3 Ann Arbor Staging System With Cotswold Modifications for Hodgkin Lymphoma

Stage I	Involvement of a single lymph node region or lymphoid structure (eg, spleen, thymus, Waldeyer ring) or a single extralymphatic site.
Stage II	Involvement of two or more lymph node regions on the same side of the diaphragm; localized contiguous involvement of only one extralymphatic organ or site and lymph node region on the same side of the diaphragm (IIE). The number of anatomic regions involved should be indicated by a subscript (eg, II_3).
Stage III	Involvement of lymph node regions on both sides of the diaphragm (III), which may also be accompanied by spleen involvement (IIIS) or by localized contiguous involvement of only one extralymphatic organ or site (IIIE) or both (IIISE).
Stage IV	Diffuse or disseminated involvement of one or more extranodal organs or tissues, with or without associated lymph node involvement.
Modifying Features	
A	No symptoms
B	Fever (>38°C), drenching night sweats, unexplained weight loss of >10% body weight within the preceding 6 months
X	Bulky disease: greater than one-third widening of the mediastinum, >10 cm maximum diameter of a nodal mass
E	Involvement of a single extranodal site that is contiguous or proximal to the known nodal site
CS	Clinical stage
PS	Pathologic stage (as determined by laparotomy)

Patient Evaluation

The initial evaluation of patients with HL has both prognostic and therapeutic significance (see Fig. 10-8). Routine studies that should be performed include a complete blood cell count with differential, electrolytes, blood urea nitrogen (BUN), creatinine, liver function tests, lactate dehydrogenase (LDH), albumin, pregnancy test in women of childbearing age, erythrocyte sedimentation rate (ESR), pulmonary function test (PFT) with carbon monoxide diffusing capacity (DLCO), evaluation of cardiac ejection fraction, chest x-ray, CT of neck, chest, abdomen, and pelvis, and PET-CT (Table 10-4).

Bone marrow biopsy has been standard in lymphoma staging. However, the high sensitivity of PET-CT for bone marrow involvement has recently led to questioning the use of bone marrow biopsy as a staging procedure in several common histologies, including HL ([15]). In one study in HL, 18% of patients had focal skeletal lesion on PET-CT, but only 6% had positive

Table 10-4 Recommended Procedures for Staging of Hodgkin Lymphoma

History and examination	Identification of B symptoms
Radiologic and other assessments	Chest radiograph
	Computed tomographic (CT) scans including neck, chest, abdomen, and pelvis whole-body positron emission tomography (PET) scan
	Echocardiogram or multigated acquisition (MUGA) scan
	Pulmonary function tests
	Human immunodeficiency virus serology
	Pregnancy test in women of childbearing age
Hematologic procedures	Complete blood count with differential
	Erythrocyte sedimentation rate (ESR)
	Bilateral bone marrow aspiration and biopsy
Biochemical procedures	Liver function tests
	Serum albumin
	Lactate dehydrogenase
Procedures for use under special circumstances	Ultrasound scanning
	Magnetic resonance imaging

bone marrow biopsy, all with advanced-stage disease on PET-CT ([18]). Patients with early-stage disease rarely have marrow involvement in the absence of a suggestive PET finding, and those with advanced-stage disease rarely have marrow involvement in the absence of disease-related symptoms. Although the issue is controversial and some institutions still perform bone marrow biopsy for the initial staging evaluation, almost all patients would not have been allocated to another treatment based on bone marrow biopsy results. Thus, the recommendation states that bone marrow biopsy is no longer indicated for the routine staging of HL.

Magnetic resonance imaging (MRI) has not superseded CT scanning of the chest and abdomen in the evaluation of HL. It is largely restricted to the assessment of specific situations such as bony involvement and spinal cord compression as well as in lieu of CT scans in pregnant patients.

Prognostic Factors

In HL patients at a low clinical stage (CS)—that is, CS I or CS II—several prognostic factors, based largely on patients treated only with radiotherapy, have been identified through retrospective studies. Adverse factors are: (1) advanced age, which correlates with the presence of occult abdominal disease and with poor results of salvage therapy; (2) male sex; (3) MC histologic type, which is associated with the presence of occult abdominal disease; (4) B symptoms, also associated with the presence of occult abdominal disease; (5) large mediastinal mass, defined as a mass measuring greater than one-third the chest diameter on a standard chest radiograph; (6) a larger number of involved nodal regions; (7) an elevated ESR; (8) anemia; and (9) a low serum albumin level ([19, 20]).

International organizations have defined various systems that calculate the risk of recurrence of disease or, in some cases, death, after treatment for HL. The European Organization for the Research and Treatment of Cancer (EORTC) has defined CS I and CS II patients as having an unfavorable risk of development of recurrence if any of the following factors apply: (1) age >50 years, (2) no symptoms present with ESR >50 mm/h or B symptoms with ESR >30 mm/h, (3) large mediastinal mass, (4) stage II, or (5) at least four nodal regions involved ([21]). The GHSG has assigned CS I and CS II patients to the category of unfavorable disease with any of the following adverse factors: (1) large mediastinal mass, (2) at least three nodal regions involved, (3) no symptoms present with ESR >50 mm/h or B symptoms with ESR >30 mm/h, or (4) localized extranodal infiltration (so-called E lesions) (Table 10-5) ([22]). In advanced disease, the International Prognostic Score (IPS) was developed on the basis of an analysis of 5,141 patients most of whom were initially treated with an anthracycline-containing chemotherapy regimen. Seven factors were identified, as shown in Table 10-6 ([23]).

Response Assessment

Prior to 1999, the criteria used to assess response to therapy were not routinely standardized. The International Working Group (IWG) formulated guidelines for the assessment of response to therapy in 1999 ([24]). The criteria were based on CT scan and have been used internationally. With the introduction of the PET scan, the guideline has been updated twice, in 2007 and in 2014 ([15, 25]). Based on the high negative predictive value (95%-100%) and positive predictive value (>90%) of PET scan in the response evaluation for HL ([26]), current recommendations for response evaluation clearly state that PET-CT is more accurate than CT for end-of-treatment assessment. Previous guidelines for reviewing PET scan were based on imprecise visual

Table 10-5 Prognostic Classification of the EORTC and GHSG Groups for Clinical Stage I/II Hodgkin Lymphoma

EORTC Unfavorable (presence of *any* of the following): Age ≤50 years ESR >50 mm/h without B symptoms, ESR >30 mm/h with B symptoms ≤4 nodal sites of involvement Bulky mediastinal mass
GHSG Unfavorable (presence of *any* of the following): ESR >50 mm/h without B symptoms, ESR >30 mm/h with B symptoms ≤3 nodal sites of involvement Bulky mediastinal mass Extranodal involvement

EORTC, European Organization for the Research and Treatment of Cancer; ESR, erythrocyte sedimentation rate; GHSG, German Hodgkin Lymphoma Study Group.

Table 10-6 International Prognostic Score (IPS) for Hodgkin Lymphoma

Hemoglobin <10.5 g/dL
Age ≤45 years
Male sex
Lymphocyte count <600/μL or <8% of white blood cell count
Serum albumin <4 g/dL
White blood cell count ≤15,000/μL
Stage IV disease (Ann Arbor system)

Data from Moccia AA, Donaldson J, Chhanabhai M, et al: International Prognostic Score in advanced-stage Hodgkin's lymphoma: altered utility in the modern era, *J Clin Oncol*. 2012 Sep 20;30(27):3383-3388.

interpretation, whether the scan is positive or negative, and whether it is intended for end-of-treatment evaluation using mediastinal blood pool as the comparator ([27]). More recent guidelines recommend using a 5-point scale assessment (Deauville criteria, Table 10-7) for clinical trials including interim analysis and end-of-treatment assessment. A score of 1 or 2 is considered to represent complete metabolic response. A score of 4 or 5 is considered to be treatment failure at the end-of-treatment evaluation. There are difficulties in the interpretation of a score of 3, in which the uptake is higher than mediastinum but less than or equivalent to liver. Recent data suggest that most patients with a score of 3 have good prognosis at the end of treatment ([28]). However, in response-adapted trials exploring treatment de-escalation, a more cautious approach may be preferred.

Treatment of Hodgkin Lymphoma

Nodular Lymphocyte-Predominant Hodgkin Lymphoma

Because of the rarity of this disease, it is difficult to derive the information by randomized prospective clinical trials. Recently, several well-designed single-arm phase II trials and large retrospective analyses have been reported.

Early-Stage Disease

Although radiation as a single modality for treatment would be considered inferior treatment for patients with early-stage cHL, multiple studies have observed excellent outcomes using radiation therapy (RT) alone for early-stage NLPHL.

In the retrospective review by the GHSG on the HD-4 and HD-7 trials, the 2-year freedom from treatment failure (FFTF) and overall survival (OS) rates were 92% and 100% respectively, with involved-field RT (IFRT), compared with 100% and 94% respectively, for extended-field RT (EFRT) ([29]). Also, our center (MDACC) reported excellent outcomes with RT alone for stage IA and IIA patients ([30]). With a median follow-up of 8.8 years, only 1 of 20 patients who received limited-field RT experienced relapse. The best outcome was noted in stage IA patients, who had a 5-year relapse-free survival rate of 95%. The Harvard study group reported a retrospective analysis of long-term outcomes of 113 patients with early-stage NLPHL ([31]). Ten-year progression-free survival (PFS) and OS rates were 64% and 100%, respectively, with limited-field RT, and 81% and 95%, respectively, with EFRT. Of note, 86% of patients who received chemotherapy alone had relapse of disease.

These observations indicate that: (1) chemotherapy alone is not indicated for NLPHL, (2) RT alone would be accepted as the standard of management for early-stage NLPHL without bulky disease or B symptoms, and (3) limited-field RT is appropriate to reduce the

Table 10-7 Five-Point Deauville Criteria

Score 1: no uptake
Score 2: uptake ≤ mediastinum
Score 3: uptake > mediastinum but ≤ liver
Score 4: moderately increased uptake > liver
Score 5: markedly increased uptake > liver and/or new lesions related to lymphoma
Score X: New areas of uptake unlikely to be related to lymphoma

toxicity and mortality. With these retrospective studies, no improvement was seen with combined-modality treatment (chemotherapy and RT) compared with RT alone. However, the data from the British Columbia Cancer Agency (BCCA) have suggested a potential improvement in the outcomes for adding a brief course of ABVD (doxorubicin, bleomycin, vinblastine, and dacarbazine) before RT in patients with early-stage NLPHL ([32]). Ten-year PFS and OS rates were 65% and 84%, respectively, for RT alone, and 91% and 93%, respectively, for combined-modality treatment. As with retrospective studies, cautious interpretation is needed because of possible selection bias, variable staging procedures, availability of supportive care, and differences in duration of follow-up for the different treatments.

Because of high CD20 expression in NLPHL, rituximab monotherapy was evaluated for the treatment of early-stage NLPHL. Two prospective studies have been reported by the GHSG and the Stanford group ([33, 34]). Overall response rates (ORRs) were high (100% in both studies). However, the responses were not durable. Currently, the National Comprehensive Cancer Network (NCCN) guidelines recommend IFRT alone for early-stage NLPHL without B symptom. B symptom and bulky disease are uncommon presentations for NLPHL and would be treated with combined-modality treatment as for cHL.

CHAPTER 10

Advanced-Stage Disease

Because at least 70% to 80% of patients with NLPHL are diagnosed with early-stage disease, defining the optimal treatment regimen for advanced-stage disease is challenging. Chemotherapy is the mainstay of treatment for advanced-stage disease.

The GHSG compared the outcome of patients with NLPHL and cHL enrolled in prospective trials ([7]). There were no significant differences in FFTF between NLPHL and cHL, with 50-month FFTF rates of 77% and 75%, respectively. Of note, the chemotherapy regimens used in the GHSG trials were COPP (cyclophosphamide, vincristine, procarbazine, and prednisone), COPP/ABVD, and BEACOPP (bleomycin, etoposide, doxorubicin, cyclophosphamide, vincristine, procarbazine, and prednisone), which contain higher dose of alkylating agents than ABVD. The BCCA reported a matched-control analysis of patients with NLPHL and cHL treated with ABVD or ABVD-like chemotherapy ([35]). Although not statistically significant, there was a trend toward an inferior PFS for patients with NLPHL versus cHL (44% vs 77% at 15 years; $P = 0.096$). These studies have suggested that alkylating agents may provide some therapeutic advantage. We have reported the results of R-CHOP (rituximab plus cyclophosphamide, doxorubicin, vincristine, and prednisone) in patients with advanced-stage NLPHL ([36]). The ORR with R-CHOP was 100%, with a complete response (CR) rate of 90%, and no relapses or transformations have been observed at a median follow-up of 42 months.

Currently, NCCN guidelines list therapeutic options such as CVP (cyclophosphamide, vincristine, and prednisone), CHOP, and ABVD with or without rituximab. The standard approach to patients with advanced-stage NLPHL at MDACC is R-CHOP based on our data.

Relapsed and Transformed Disease

Patients with NLPHL may have late relapse or transform to B-cell lymphoma, for which standard treatment is not well defined. Rituximab has been evaluated for treatment of relapsed NLPHL. In a study by the GHSG that enrolled 14 patients, rituximab therapy resulted in an ORR of 100%, a CR rate of 57%, and a median time to progression of 33 months ([37]). The Stanford group examined the benefit of limited versus extended rituximab therapy in the frontline and relapsed settings ([33]). Eighteen patients with relapsed NLPHL were enrolled in the study. The ORR with rituximab monotherapy was 100%, and the 5-year PFS was 71.4% with rituximab maintenance therapy of 4 weekly infusions every 6 months for 2 years. These results indicate that rituximab monotherapy is effective in relapsed NLPHL.

Transformation at time of relapse can also occur. In a retrospective study by the BCCA, 95 patients were identified as diagnosed with NLPHL over a 40-year time period ([38]). Median time of follow-up was 6.5 years, and 14% of patients experienced transformation. Median time to transformation was 8.1 years, with 4:1 ratio of DLBCL to TCRBCL. In the 10 patients with transformed lymphoma, the 10-year PFS and OS rates were 52% and 62%, respectively.

The rarity of the disease makes it difficult to prospectively evaluate the role of autologous stem cell transplantation (ASCT) for patients with relapsed or refractory NLPHL. However, patients who relapse with transformation should be managed according to algorithms for DLBCL. An MDACC retrospective study reviewed the outcomes for 26 patients who underwent ASCT. At time of transplantation, many had transformation to TCRBCL. At time of ASCT, 85% were in remission, with 35% in CR. At a median follow-up of 50 months, the event-free survival (EFS) rate was 69% ([39]).

MD Anderson Approach

We treat stage IA and IIA LPHL patients with IFRT. It is rare for a stage I or II patient to present with B symptoms, but if a patient does, we treat the patient with (particularly for stage IIB) combined-modality therapy with an anthracycline-containing chemotherapy regimen followed by IFRT. Our preferred regimen is R-CHOP. For advanced-stage patients, we treat with R-CHOP for six cycles. Patients who relapse can be considered for extended rituximab therapy. For patients with evidence of transformation to DLBCL or TCRBCL, if anthracycline-containing chemotherapy had already been given, we use salvage chemotherapy with regimens such as rituximab plus ICE (ifosfamide, carboplatin, and etoposide) followed by ASCT.

Classical Hodgkin Lymphoma

The common practice for treatment and participation in clinical trials is to divide cHL patients into three treatment groups: early stage favorable, early stage unfavorable, and advanced stage.

Early-Stage Favorable Hodgkin Lymphoma

Treatment of early-stage favorable HL is evolving. Historically, wide-field RT or EFRT without chemotherapy was the standard of care ([40]). Extended-field RT produced superior disease-free survival (DFS) compared with IFRT ([41]). More than 90% of patients achieved CR with this approach; however, the relapse rate was unacceptably high (≥30%). In addition, EFRT had considerable long-term side effects. In a large prospective analysis of over 15,000 HL patients, the actuarial risk of developing a solid tumor was 21.9% at 25 years after HL diagnosis, with the absolute risk being nearly 50%. Common secondary solid tumors were female breast and lung cancers ([42]). The key studies comparing RT alone with combined-modality strategies were conducted by the GHSG and EORTC. In the GHSG HD-7 trial, patients were randomly assigned to receive either 30 Gy of EFRT alone or two cycles of ABVD followed by the same RT ([43]). Although, response rates did not differ between the two treatment arms, the 7-year FFTF rate was significantly better in the combined-modality arm (88% vs 67%). The results of the randomized EORTC H8F trial were similar. Treatment arms consisted of three cycles of MOPP (mechlorethamine, vincristine, procarbazine, prednisone)/ABV (doxorubicin, bleomycin, vinblastine) followed by IFRT or subtotal nodal irradiation (STNI) alone ([44]). Patients receiving combined-modality treatment had a significantly superior 5-year EFS (98% vs 74%) and better 10-year OS estimates (97% vs 92%). As a result of these two large randomized controlled trials and the recognition of notable long-term side effects and high relapse rates, EFRT monotherapy has now been abandoned in favor of combined-modality therapy, which is now the standard treatment for early-stage HL.

Combined-modality therapy has evolved based on the premise that this approach results in high freedom from recurrence in early-stage HL and that efficacy can be maintained using less toxic chemotherapy and RT regimens. At MDACC, investigators performed a retrospective analysis of 286 patients with early-stage HL treated with chemotherapy followed by IFRT or EFRT with a median dose of 40 Gy ([45]). Five-year relapse-free survival (RFS) and OS rates were 88% and 93%, respectively. The type and number of chemotherapy cycles used did not significantly affect RFS and OS. However, the 5-, 10-, and 15-year cumulative risks of developing solid tumors in patients treated with chemotherapy and IFRT were 0%, 6.9%, and 11.4%, respectively. These results were strikingly more favorable than those of chemotherapy plus EFRT (2.7%, 11.1%, and 28.7%, respectively).

There are many completed and ongoing trials addressing issues of the best modality, best RT field, optimal dose of RT, optimal combination of drugs, number of cycles, and optimal timing of chemotherapy, with the goals being to maintain efficacy and minimize toxicities ([22, 46-50]) (Table 10-8).

The key study in combined-modality therapy for the current standard treatment is the HD-10 trial by the GHSG ([22]). The GHSG HD-10 trial had four arms testing two versus four cycles of ABVD followed by 20 versus 30 Gy of IFRT in patients with favorable early-stage HL. This trial addressed both the optimal dose of RT and the optimal number of cycles of chemotherapy. The ABVD two- and four-cycle arms both had CR rates of 97%. The 20- and 30-Gy IFRT groups had CR rates of 97% and 98%, respectively. With a median follow-up of 7.5 years, there were no differences among the four groups in PFS, FFTF, and OS. The four-cycle ABVD and 30-Gy IFRT treatment groups had more toxicity than the less intensive treatment groups. Based on these data, the least toxic regimen, two cycles of ABVD and 20 Gy of IFRT, is the current standard approach for favorable early-stage HL.

In the next trial by the GHSG, the HD-13 trial, the aim was to determine whether bleomycin or dacarbazine can be omitted from chemotherapy ([47]). This four-arm trial investigated ABVD, AVD (doxorubicin, vinblastine, dacarbazine), ABV, and AV (doxorubicin, vinblastine) plus 30 Gy of IFRT. In this trial, the ABV and AV plus IFRT arms were closed because of concern for higher relapses. Five-year FFTF rates were 93%, 81%, 89%, and 77% with ABVD, ABV, AVD, and AV, respectively. Based on this trial, both dacarbazine and bleomycin cannot be omitted from ABVD without a substantial loss of efficacy. The standard treatment for patients with early-stage favorable HL should remain ABVD followed by IFRT.

Recently, several studies have evaluated the use of interim PET scan for treatment stratification. The EORTC/Lymphoma Study Association (LYSA)/Fondazione Italiana Linfomi (FIL) H10 trial was conducted to assess whether involved-node radiotherapy (INRT) could be omitted without compromising PFS in patients attaining a negative early PET scan after two

Table 10-8 Key Trials for Patients With Favorable Early-Stage Hodgkin Lymphoma

Trial	Trial Design
Milan 1990 to 1997	ABVD × 4 → STLI
	ABVD × 4 → IFRT
Stanford	Stanford V × 8 weeks → IFRT
EORTC/GELA H9F	EBVP × 6 → IFRT 20 Gy
	EBVP × 6 → IFRT 30 Gy
	EBVP × 6 alone
GHSG HD-10	ABVD × 2 → IFRT 2 Gy
	ABVD × 4 → IFRT 20 Gy
	ABVD × 2 → IFRT 30 Gy
	ABVD × 4 → IFRT 30 Gy
GHSG HD-13	ABVD × 2 → IFRT 30 Gy
	ABV × 2 → IFRT 30 Gy
	AVD × 2 → IFRT 30 Gy
	AV × 2 → IFRT 30 Gy
EORTC/LYSA/FIL H10F	ABVD × 3 → INRT 30 Gy (+ 6 Gy)
	ABVD × 2 → then PET scan
	• If PET negative → ABVD × 2
	• If PET positive → BEACOPP escalated × 2 → INRT 30 Gy (+ 6 Gy)
GHSG HD-16	ABVD × 2 → IFRT 20 Gy
	ABVD × 2 → then PET scan
	• If PET negative → stop treatment
	• If PET positive → IFRT 20 Gy

ABV, doxorubicin, bleomycin, vinblastine; ABVD, doxorubicin, bleomycin, vinblastine, dacarbazine; AV, doxorubicin, vinblastine; AVD, doxorubicin, vinblastine, dacarbazine; BEACOPP, bleomycin, etoposide, doxorubicin, cyclophosphamide, vincristine, procarbazine, prednisone; EBVP, epirubicin, bleomycin, vinblastine, prednisone; EORTC, European Organization for Research and Treatment of Cancer; FIL, Fondazione Italiana Linfomi; GELA, Groupe d'Etude des Lymphomes de l'Adulte; GHSG, German Hodgkin Lymphoma Study Group; IFRT, involved-field radiotherapy; INRT, involved-node radiotherapy; LYSA, Lymphoma Study Association; PET, positron emission tomography; Stanford V, mechlorethamine, doxorubicin, vinblastine, vincristine, bleomycin, etoposide, prednisone; STLI, subtotal lymphoid irradiation.

cycles of ABVD as compared with standard combined-modality treatment ([46]). The patients were randomized to a standard treatment giving RT irrespective of PET status after two cycles of ABVD or to an experimental arm that omitted RT if the PET was negative after two cycles of ABVD. Patients with a positive interim PET continued treatment with two cycles of escalated BEACOPP. The chemotherapy-only arm (four cycles of ABVD) was closed due to an increased number of events, and all patients with a negative PET received additional RT. Although the median follow-up time was very short (1.1 years), 1-year PFS was significantly lower in the experimental arm than the standard arm (94.9% vs 100.0%). In contrast, the UK RAPID trial showed noninferior outcome for patients who omitted RT after negative PET scan ([51]). In this trial, patients were randomized to IFRT or to the no further treatment arm if they had a negative PET scan after three cycles of ABVD. The 3-year PFS rates were 93.8% versus 90.7%, and the 3-year OS rates in an intent-to-treat analysis were 97.0% and 99.5% in patients who received IFRT and no further treatment, respectively. Thus, there was a trend toward improved PFS for patients who received IFRT. Another trial is ongoing by the GHSG. The randomized GHSG HD-16 trial resembles the H10 trial. Patients are randomized to a standard treatment arm or an experimental arm that omits RT if the PET scan is negative after two cycles of ABVD. The question of whether treatment can be further reduced based on the results of the PET scan is the subject of ongoing clinical trials.

The MD Anderson Approach

The treatment for favorable early-stage HL is still evolving. Patients are typically screened for clinical protocol options if available. As standard therapy, we use two cycles of ABVD plus 20 Gy of IFRT for this group of patients.

Early-Stage Unfavorable Hodgkin Lymphoma

Combined-modality approaches consisting of four cycles of chemotherapy followed by IFRT represent the standard of care for patients with early-stage unfavorable HL. Multiple trials have shown that reduction of radiation field does not lead to inferior clinical outcomes. In a retrospective analysis conducted at MDACC, 286 patients (1980-1995) with early-stage HL were treated with chemotherapy followed by IFRT or EFRT. The type and number of chemotherapy regimens used did not significantly affect RFS and OS. There was a trend toward higher risks of secondary tumors in the EFRT group ([45]). In the EORTC H8U trial, three different regimens were randomly compared ([44]). Patients were assigned to receive either six cycles of MOPP/ABV plus IFRT, four cycles of MOPP/ABV plus IFRT, or four cycles of MOPP/ABV plus subtotal nodal plus spleen irradiation. The MOPP/ABV regimen followed by IFRT resulted in 88% EFS at 5 years and 85% OS at 10 years with no difference noted compared to the other treatment arms. Thus, four cycles of chemotherapy is the standard for patients with early-stage unfavorable HL. Similar to early-stage favorable HL, ABVD alone was more effective than MOPP and equally as effective as, but less toxic than, the alternating regimen MOPP/ABVD ([52]). Given the relapse rates with ABVD, there is interest in evaluating alternative more intensive regimens ([46, 53-56]) (Table 10-9).

To address whether ABVD or the Stanford V regimen (mechlorethamine, doxorubicin, vinblastine,

Table 10-9 Key Trials for Patients With Unfavorable Early-Stage Hodgkin Lymphoma

Trial	Trial Design
SWOG/ECOG 2496	ABVD × 6 → IFRT 36 Gy to >5 cm disease
	Stanford V × 12 weeks → IFRT 36 Gy to >5 cm disease
EORTC/GELA H9U	ABVD × 6 → IFRT (36–40 Gy)
	ABVD × 4 → IFRT (36–40 Gy)
	BEACOPP × 4 → IFRT (36–40 Gy)
GHSG HD11	ABVD × 4 → IFRT 30 Gy
	ABVD × 4 → IFRT 20 Gy
	BEACOPP baseline × 4 → IFRT 30 Gy
	BEACOPP baseline × 4 → IFRT 20 Gy
GHSG HD-14	ABVD × 4 → IFRT 30 Gy
	BEACOPP escalated + ABVD × 2 → IFRT 30 Gy
EORTC/LYSA/ FIL H10U	ABVD × 4 → INRT 30Gy (+ 6 Gy)
	ABVD × 2 → then PET scan
	• If PET negative → ABVD × 4
	• If PET positive → BEACOPP escalated × 2 → INRT 30 Gy (+ 6 Gy)
GHSG HD-17	BEACOPP escalated + ABVD × 2 → IFRT 30 Gy
	BEACOPP escalated + ABVD × 2 → then PET scan
	• If PET negative → stop treatment
	• If PET positive → INRT 30 Gy

ABVD, doxorubicin, bleomycin, vinblastine, dacarbazine; BEACOPP, bleomycin, etoposide, doxorubicin, cyclophosphamide, vincristine, procarbazine, prednisone; ECOG, Eastern Cooperative Oncology Group; EORTC, European Organization for Research and Treatment of Cancer; FIL, Fondazione Italiana Linfomi; GELA, Groupe d'Etude des Lymphomes de l'Adulte; GHSG, German Hodgkin Lymphoma Study Group; IFRT, involved-field radiotherapy; INRT, involved-node radiotherapy; LYSA, Lymphoma Study Association; PET, positron emission tomography; Stanford V, mechlorethamine, doxorubicin, vinblastine, vincristine, bleomycin, etoposide, prednisone; SWOG, Southwest Oncology Group.

vincristine, bleomycin, etoposide, prednisone) would be the best approach for patients with early-stage bulky unfavorable HL, the intergroup Southwest Oncology Group (SWOG)/Eastern Cooperative Oncology Group (ECOG) 2496 trial was conducted ([53]). In this trial, patients with early-stage bulky unfavorable disease (they also included advanced-stage disease in the trial) were randomized to six cycles of ABVD followed by IFRT at 36 Gy to bulk greater than 5 cm versus 12 weeks of Stanford V followed by the same IFRT plan of care. In this patients group, there were no difference in ORR and FFS between ABVD and Stanford V.

To improve the tumor control in this patient group, the BEACOPP regimen was compared to ABVD in trials by both the GHSG and the EORTC. In the EORTC H9U trial, patients were randomized to receive either six cycles of ABVD followed by IFRT, four cycles of ABVD followed by IFRT, or four cycles of BEACOPP baseline followed by IFRT. All patients received 30 Gy of IFRT. At a median follow-up of 4 years, EFS and OS remain statistically equivalent in all arms, with EFS ranging from 87% to 91% and OS ranging from 93% to 95% ([56]). Although the final results of this trial are pending, BEACOPP could not show a benefit over ABVD at the time of analysis. The GHSG HD-11 trial randomized patients to four arms of therapy and evaluated four cycles of ABVD followed by 30 versus 20 Gy of IFRT and compared outcomes to four cycles of BEACOPP baseline followed by 30 versus 20 Gy of IFRT. The FFTF with BEACOPP was superior in patients who received 20 Gy of IFRT, whereas there were no differences between BEACOPP and ABVD in patients who received 30 Gy of IFRT. Overall survival did not differ significantly between the four treatment arms. Thus, BEACOPP was not adopted as a standard chemotherapy regimen for patients with early-stage unfavorable HL due to increased toxicity observed in comparison with ABVD ([55]).

The GHSG HD-14 trial introduced escalated BEACOPP to evaluate a more intensive regimen ([54]). Patients received four cycles of ABVD followed by 30 Gy of IFRT or two cycles of BEACOPP escalated followed by two cycles of ABVD (2 + 2) and then 30 Gy of IFRT. At a median follow-up of 43 months, there was better tumor control (5-year FFTF estimate of 94.8%) with the 2 + 2 protocol, compared with the ABVD arm (5-year FFTF of 87.7%). There was no significant difference in OS between the two arms. Based on these trials, ABVD remains the standard chemotherapy for patients with early-stage unfavorable HL.

Similar to early-stage favorable HL, current trials for patients with early-stage unfavorable HL, such as the EORTC/Groupe d'Etude des Lymphomes de l'Adulte H10U and GHSG HD-17, are evaluating the treatment stratification according to the result of an interim PET scan. The standard arm in the EORTC/LYSA/FIL H10U trial consisted of four cycles of ABVD followed by 30 Gy of INRT irrespective of the result of an interim PET scan performed after the second cycle of ABVD. In the experimental arm, patients with a negative PET received a total of six cycles of ABVD without consolidation RT, whereas patients with a positive PET continued treatment with two cycles of escalated BEACOPP before receiving INRT. However, as for patients with early-stage favorable HL, the chemotherapy-only arm (six cycles of ABVD) was closed due to an increased number of events, so that all patients with a negative PET received additional RT. There was no difference in the 1-year PFS between the standard and experimental arms (97.3% vs 94.7%). In the GHSG HD-17 trial, all patients received chemotherapy according to the 2 + 2 regimen before a PET scan was performed. In the standard arm, patients received an additional 30 Gy of IFRT irrespective of the results of the PET scan. In the experimental arm, patients with a negative PET scan stopped treatment, whereas patients with a positive PET scan received 30 Gy of INRT. This ongoing trial plans to evaluate whether it is possible to spare RT in patients with a negative PET scan after intensive escalated BEACOPP.

A trial conducted by the National Cancer Institute of Canada (NCIC) and the ECOG indicated that chemotherapy-only approaches appear possible in patients with early unfavorable HL, at least in patients with nonbulky disease ([57]). The trial randomized patients with early-stage unfavorable clinical features to receive either four to six cycles of ABVD or two cycles of ABVD followed by STNI. At a median follow-up of 11.3 years, freedom from disease progression was better in patients who receiving combined-modality treatment; however, OS was better for patients treated with chemotherapy alone. This was mainly caused by the increased number of deaths from secondary neoplasia among patients who had received combined-modality treatment. Nevertheless, we should keep in mind that STNI is outdated and no longer used. Chemotherapy alone might be a treatment option in patients with nonbulky early-stage unfavorable HL, but combined-modality therapy should remain standard until further data support that the chemotherapy-only approach is feasible.

The MD Anderson Approach

In summary, treatment with four cycles of ABVD plus 30 Gy of IFRT is presently a standard-of-care option for early-stage unfavorable HL. We screen patients for any available clinical protocols. If a patient has a bulky mediastinal mass of 10 cm or greater, we typically treat with six cycles of ABVD followed by IFRT.

Advanced-Stage Hodgkin Lymphoma

Treatment of advanced-stage HL usually consists of six to eight cycles of chemotherapy. The ABVD regimen was shown to be effective and less toxic than MOPP and MOPP/ABVD in a randomized clinical trial by the Cancer and Leukemia Group B (CALGB) ([52]). With ABVD, MOPP, and MOPP/ABVD, 5-year failure-free survival rates were 61%, 50%, and 65%, and 5-year OS rates were 73%, 66%, and 75%, respectively. Based on the trial, the chemotherapy regimen most often used in the United States is ABVD. However, the GHSG has established escalated BEACOPP as a standard treatment for advanced-stage HL. Many trials are addressing whether one regimen may be more suitable for the treatment of advanced HL than another, and the issue has been the subject of ongoing debate for more than decade. Various chemotherapy regimens have been developed in an attempt to improve outcomes ([26, 52, 58-61]) (Table 10-10).

The GHSG HD-9 trial, a three-arm randomized trial, evaluated four cycles of COPP/ABVD versus eight cycles of BEACOPP baseline versus eight cycles of BEACOPP escalated ([61, 62]). The BEACOPP escalated regimen showed significantly better survival than the other two arms. With BEACOPP escalated, COPP/ABVD, and BEACOPP baseline, 5-year FFTF rates were 87%, 69%, and 76%, respectively. The 5-year OS rates were 91%, 83%, and 88%, respectively.

The GHSG HD-12 trial investigated whether the number of cycles of BEACOPP escalated could be de-escalated by evaluating eight cycles of BEACOPP escalated versus four cycles of BEACOPP escalated plus four cycles of BEACOPP baseline (4 + 4) and what the potential added benefit of consolidation RT would be in treating sites of initial bulk or residual disease ([60]). Severe toxicity and therapy-related death rates were similar in both arms, and the survival outcome was slightly inferior in the 4 + 4 regimen. Thus, the trial could not address how to decrease the toxicity while maintaining the efficacy of eight cycles of BEACOPP escalated.

The next GHSG trial also aimed to reduce treatment toxicity without compromising efficacy ([26]). The trial evaluated the role of response evaluation based on PET scan in assessing the need for IFRT. Chemotherapy consisted of eight cycles of BEACOPP escalated, six cycles of BEACOPP escalated, or eight cycles of BEACOPP-14, a time-dense variant of the BEACOPP baseline protocol. Additional localized RT was only applied to patients who had PET-positive residual lymphoma larger than 2.5 cm at the end of chemotherapy. With eight cycles of BEACOPP escalated, six cycles of BEACOPP escalated, and eight cycles of BEACOPP-14, the 5-year FFTF rates were 85%, 89%, and 85%, respectively, and the 5-year OS rates were 92%, 95%, and 95%, respectively. The negative predictive value for the postchemotherapy PET scan so that IFRT to PET-negative lesions would be omitted was very high (94.1% at 12 months). This superiority for six cycles of BEACOPP escalated was mainly attributed to the lower rate of treatment-related adverse events and fewer deaths due to secondary neoplasia. Based on this trial, treatment with six cycles of BEACOPP escalated was adopted as a standard chemotherapy for advanced-stage HL by the GHSG.

The interim analysis of the most recent trial by the GHSG, HD-18, was presented ([63]). In this trial, patients initially receive two cycles of BEACOPP escalated. Then, interim PET scan is performed, and patients are randomized. The standard arm consists of a total of six cycles of BEACOPP escalated irrespective of the

Table 10-10 Key Trials for Advanced-Stage Hodgkin Lymphoma

Trials	Design
CALGB	ABVD × 6 to 8
	ABVD/MOPP × 12
	MOPP × 6 to 8
GHSG HD-9	COPP/ABVD × 8
	BEACOPP baseline × 8
	BEACOPP escalated × 8
GHSG HD-12	BEACOPP escalated × 8 → IFRT to bulk/residual mass
	BEACOPP escalated × 8
	BEACOPP escalated × 4 + BEACOPP baseline × 4 → IFRT to bulk/residual mass
	BEACOPP escalated × 4 + BEACOPP baseline × 4
GHSG HD-15	BEACOPP escalated × 8 → IFRT to PET-positive residual masses ≤2.5 cm
	BEACOPP escalated × 6 → IFRT to PET-positive residual masses ≤2.5 cm
	BEACOPP-14 × 8 → IFRT to PET-positive residual masses ≤2.5 cm
LYSA H34	ABVD × 8
	BEACOPP escalated × 4 + BEACOPP baseline × 4
GITIL	ABVD × 6 to 8 depends on the response after four cycles
	BEACOPP escalated × 4 + BEACOPP baseline × 4
	• High-dose chemotherapy is planned by protocol at the time of progression or relapse
GHSG HD-18	BEACOPP escalated × 2 → then PET scan
	• If PET negative
	• Additional BEACOPP escalated × 4
	• Additional BEACOPP escalated × 2
	• If PET positive
	• Additional BEACOPP escalated × 4
	• Additional BEACOPP escalated × 4 + rituximab

ABVD, doxorubicin, bleomycin, vinblastine, dacarbazine; BEACOPP, bleomycin, etoposide, doxorubicin, cyclophosphamide, vincristine, procarbazine, prednisone; CALGB, Cancer and Leukemia Group B; COPP, cyclophosphamide, vincristine, procarbazine, prednisone; GHSG, German Hodgkin Lymphoma Study Group; GITIL, Gruppo Italiano Terapie Innovative nei Linfomie; IFRT, involved-field radiotherapy; LYSA, Lymphoma Study Association; MOPP, mechlorethamine, vincristine, procarbazine, prednisone; PET, positron emission tomography.

result of the interim PET. In the experimental treatment arm, patients with a CR by interim PET scan are randomized to receive either four or two cycles of BEACOPP escalated. Patients with PET-positive residual disease after two cycles of chemotherapy are randomized to receive either a total of four additional cycles of BEACOPP escalated or rituximab plus BEACOPP escalated. There were no significant differences in the survival between the rituximab plus BEACOPP escalated and the BEACOPP escalated arms. The PFS in PET-positive patients receiving standard treatment with BEACOPP escalated was higher than expected, with a 3-year PFS of over 90%. In this trial, PET result after cycle 2 of therapy was not able to determine a high-risk patient group.

In the SWOG S0816 trial, patients with stage III or IV disease underwent a baseline PET scan ([64]). They then received two cycles of ABVD, and the PET scan (PET-2) was repeated. If the PET-2 scan was negative, four further cycles of ABVD were given. If the PET-2 scan was positive, treatment was changed and intensified to BEACOPP escalated for six cycles for patients who were human immunodeficiency virus (HIV) negative and to BEACOPP standard for six cycles for patients who were HIV positive. This trial was also the first American study to use centralized real-time intergroup review (SWOG, ECOG, CALGB) of the PET scan results for treatment decisions. Response-adapted therapy with centralized interim PET review was highly feasible, even in an intergroup setting. However, the 2-year PFS of PET-2–positive patients was still lower than that of PET-2–negative patients of (61% vs 79%), even though they received six more cycles of BEACOPP escalated after PET-2.

The Gruppo Italiano Terapie Innovative nei Linfomie (GITIL) conducted a similar trial ([65]). In

GITIL HD0607, patients started with two cycles of ABVD chemotherapy, and then the PET-2 scan was performed. If the patients were PET negative, they received another four cycles of ABVD with or without RT. If the patients were PET positive, they received four cycles of BEACOPP escalated and two cycles of BEACOPP baseline. The 1-year PFS rates of patients with PET-2–positive and PET-2–negative scans were 81% and 95%, respectively.

At this point, response-adapted therapy based on interim PET scan should be performed in well-designed clinical trials, and longer follow-up data of the completed trials are essential.

Even with the results of the GHSG HD-9 trial, first-line chemotherapy for advanced-stage HL is still a matter of debate. The standard arm used in the HD-9 trial was COPP/ABVD, not ABVD alone. Three randomized trials have been conducted to address this issue. One Italian group conducted the HD2000 trial and LYSA conducted the H34 trial to compare the outcome between BEACOPP and ABVD ([58, 66]). In the HD2000 trial, patients were randomly assigned to receive six cycles of ABVD, four cycles of BEACOPP escalated plus two cycles of BEACOPP baseline, or six courses of CEC (cyclophosphamide, lomustine, vindesine, melphalan, prednisone, epidoxorubicin, vincristine, procarbazine, vinblastine, and bleomycin). Patients who received BEACOPP had higher PFS and OS rates than patients who received ABVD (5-year PFS, 81% vs 68%; 5-year OS, 92% vs 84%). In the H34 trial, patients were randomly assigned to receive eight cycles of ABVD or four cycles of BEACOPP escalated plus four cycles of BEACOPP baseline. Both PFS and OS were higher in the BEACOPP arm than the ABVD arm (5-year PFS, 93% vs 75%; 5-year OS, 99% vs 92%). These two trials showed a higher efficacy with BEACOPP than ABVD.

However, GITIL reported that ABVD has a similar efficacy to BEACOPP if high-dose chemotherapy (HDCT) is planned at the time of relapse of refractory disease ([59]). In the GITIL trial, patients were randomly assigned to either four cycles of BEACOPP escalated plus four cycles of BEACOPP baseline or to six to eight cycles of ABVD, each followed by local RT when indicated. Patients with residual or progressive disease after the initial therapy were to be treated with high-dose salvage therapy with ASCT. The 7-year FFTF was significantly better with BEACOPP than ABVD (85% vs 73%); however, there was no significant difference in the 7-year OS between arms after completion of the overall planned treatment (89% vs 84%). Although two out of three randomized trials showed some benefit in survival with BEACOPP, longer follow-up is essential to confirm the conclusion because the toxicities such as secondary malignancy would be an issue for the long-term survival in young patients. Most of the institutes in the United States are still using ABVD as first-line chemotherapy, mostly because of its high efficacy, high tolerability, and lower toxicities compared with BEACOPP escalated ([66a]).

The MD Anderson Approach

We screen patients for available protocols for initial treatment of advanced-stage disease. As a standard approach off clinical protocol, we treat these patients with six to eight cycles of ABVD. Although the data supporting IFRT for advanced-stage disease is controversial, we sometimes consider IFRT for patients who have presented with an initial bulky mass and who continue to have a residual mass at the end of therapy with PET-negative status.

The Value of Positron Emission Tomography Scan in Hodgkin Lymphoma

A PET scan is useful not only for staging but also for response evaluation and evaluation of expected outcome in patients with HL. An interim PET scan obtained after two cycles of therapy (PET-2) was a stronger prediction of outcome than the IPS, with 2-year PFS for patients with a positive PET-2 of 13% compared with 95% for those with a negative PET-2 ([67]). The PET-2 also strongly predicts treatment failure ([68]). In a meta-analysis, a positive PET-2 in low-intermediate–risk advanced HL patients was a reliable predictor of poor response ([69]). The value of the interim PET scan is now being evaluated in prospective clinical trials. The SWOG S0816 phase II intergroup trial is evaluating interim PET in stage III or IV cHL patients treated with two cycles of ABVD. Patients who have a negative PET receive four additional cycles of ABVD; PET-positive patients receive BEACOPP baseline if HIV positive and BEACOPP escalated if HIV negative.

The HD-15 trial showed a negative predictive value of 94% for PET after BEACOPP-based therapy in advanced-stage HL ([70]). The PFS at 12 months was 96% for PET-negative patients and 86% for PET-positive patients. At the time of posttreatment examination, PET has higher diagnostic and prognostic value than conventional CT ([71-73]). The role of PET prior to transplantation was also evaluated: a negative PET prior to ASCT is significantly associated with higher EFS. In a study by the Memorial Sloan-Kettering Cancer Center, the 5-year EFS was 80% in patients with PET-negative status and 40% in patients with PET-positive status before transplantation ([74]).

Refractory or Relapsed Hodgkin Lymphoma

Although many patients with HL are cured with frontline therapy, 10% to 15% of patients with early-stage disease with unfavorable risk factors and 40% of patients with advanced-stage disease with high-risk factors can develop relapse or refractory disease.

Relapsed HL can be divided into three subgroups: early relapse within 12 months of CR after first-line chemotherapy; late relapse after CR >12 months after first-line chemotherapy; and primary refractory HL (ie, patients who never achieve a CR). Moskowitz et al identified the following three prognostic factors associated with EFS in patients receiving ICE, followed by HDCT and ASCT: CR less than 1 year, extranodal disease, and presence of B symptoms. The 5-year EFS was 83% in patients with zero to one factor compared with 10% if all three factors were present ([75]).

For patients with relapsed or refractory disease after standard frontline management, additional salvage chemotherapy followed by HDCT plus ASCT is the standard approach. One of the key goals of salvage chemotherapy is to achieve CR prior to ASCT. The response rates of multiple salvage regimens are listed in Table 10-11. It is difficult to directly compare these regimens because they have not been evaluated in randomized clinical trials.

Although we screen all patients for available protocols at relapse, the most common salvage chemotherapies outside clinical trials are the platinum-containing regimens such as ICE or DHAP (cisplatin, cytarabine, dexamethasone). With ICE, the ORR was 84% and the CR rate was 26%. The DHAP regimen showed similar results, with ORR of 89% and CR rate of 21%. Gemcitabine-containing regimens are also effective. With GND (gemcitabine, vinorelbine, pegylated liposomal doxorubicin), the ORR was 70%, with a CR rate of 19%. With GDP (gemcitabine, dexamethasone, platinum), the ORR was 62%, with a CR rate of 10%.

Table 10-11 Salvage Chemotherapy Regimens for Hodgkin Lymphoma

Regimen	ORR (%)	CR (%)
DHAP	88	21
ASHAP	70	34
ESHAP	73	41
MINE	73	34
ICE	85	26
IGEV	81	54
GND	70	19
GDP	62	10

ASHAP, doxorubicin, methylprednisolone, cytarabine, cisplatin; CR, complete response; DHAP, dexamethasone, cytarabine, cisplatin; ESHAP, etoposide, methylprednisolone, cytarabine, cisplatin; GDP, gemcitabine, dexamethasone, cisplatin; GND, gemcitabine, vinorelbine, pegylated liposomal doxorubicin; ICE, ifosfamide, carboplatin, etoposide; IGEV, ifosfamide, gemcitabine, vinorelbine; MINE, mitoguazone, ifosfamide, vinorelbine, etoposide; ORR, overall response rate.

High-Dose Chemotherapy With Autologous Stem Cell Transplantation for Relapsed Hodgkin Lymphoma

For patients with chemotherapy-sensitive disease, the treatment of choice after relapse is HDCT followed by ASCT. This recommendation is based on reports from two randomized clinical trials ([76, 77]). In the BNLI study, patients with relapsed or refractory HL received BEAM (carmustine, etoposide, cytarabine, and melphalan) at high doses followed by an ASCT or at lower doses (mini-BEAM) without an ASCT. The 3-year freedom from second treatment failure was significantly better for patients who received HDCT (53% vs 10%). The GHSG/European Group for Blood and Marrow Transplantation (EBMT) randomized trial compared four cycles of Dexa-BEAM (dexamethasone plus BEAM) versus two cycles of Dexa-BEAM followed by ASCT. At 3 years, the FFTF in the high-dose therapy group was 55% versus 34% with four cycles of chemotherapy.

Multiple investigators have shown that response to salvage chemotherapy is a strong predictor of long-term outcome after ASCT. The 5-year OS for patients who were in CR at the time of ASCT was 79% compared with 59% for those in PR and 17% for those with resistant disease at the time of ASCT ([78]). Studies have shown the impact of pre-ASCT PET scan results on EFS. Patients with negative pre-ASCT PET scans have significantly higher EFS and failure-free survival rates compared to patients with positive pre-ASCT PET scans ([79, 80]). A European intergroup evaluated a dose-intensified regimen before ASCT ([81]). Patients were randomly assigned after two cycles of DHAP to ASCT or sequential cyclophosphamide, methotrexate, and etoposide before ASCT. There were no significant differences between the two treatment arms in terms of mortality, FFTF, and OS. Thus, the less toxic approach consisting of two cycles of DHAP (or other salvage regimen such as ICE) followed by HDCT and ASCT remains the standard of care for patients with relapsed HL.

Treatment of Relapse After Autologous Stem Cell Transplantation

Patients with disease progression after ASCT uniformly have a poor outcome. In a study of HL patients who failed ASCT, the median time to progression after the next therapy was only 3.8 months, and the median survival after ASCT failure was 26 months ([82]). An international multicenter retrospective study showed that the survival of patients who relapsed after an ASCT did not improve from 1981 to 2007 ([83]). However, there has been a major advance in the treatment of relapsed or refractory HL in the last 5 years.

Brentuximab Vedotin

CD30 was considered an ideal target for monoclonal antibody therapy for HL, because its expression is highly restricted to the HRS cells. Brentuximab vedotin (BV), or SGN-35, is an intravenously administered antibody-drug conjugate that consists of the CD30-specific monoclonal antibody conjugated with monomethyl auristatin E (MMAE) by linker peptide. Binding of the antibody-drug conjugate to CD30 on the cell surface causes internalization of the drug by endocytosis, and the drug subsequently travels to the lysosome, where proteases cleave the linker and release MMAE to the cytosol ([84]). Released MMAE binds to tubulin and disrupts the microtubule polymerization, resulting in cell cycle arrest and apoptotic death of CD30-expressing cells. After efficacy was shown in a phase I trial including 45 patients with relapsed or refractory CD30-positive hematologic malignancies, a pivotal phase II study with 102 patients with HL who had relapsed after HDCT and ASCT was conducted ([85, 86]). Patients received BV 1.8 mg/kg every 3 weeks up to a maximum of 16 cycles. The ORR was 75%, with a CR rate of 34%. These data led to the first drug approval by the US Food and Drug Administration (FDA) for the treatment of HL in more than 30 years. Durable remission was reported with longer follow-up ([87]), and the median OS and PFS were 40.5 months and 9.3 months, respectively. The 3-year PFS rate of patients who achieved CR with BV was 58%. This survival outcome is notable considering that the patients enrolled in this trial had disease progression after ASCT.

Achieving CR before ASCT is the key to better outcomes in patients with relapsed or refractory HL. Therefore, BV is often used as a third-line therapy in patients who have not achieved CR after second-line salvage chemotherapy such as ICE. The Seattle group retrospectively evaluated the efficacy of BV in patients who were refractory to platinum-based salvage chemotherapy ([88]). Fifteen patients who had PET-positive disease after platinum-based salvage therapy were treated with a median of four cycles of BV. Normalization of PET scan occurred in 8 (53%) of 15 patients but was only observed in patients who had achieved partial remission or stable disease after salvage therapy. This suggests that BV can achieve PET-CR in a considerable subset of patients with platinum-refractory HL prior to ASCT.

BV is also effective in patients who relapse after allogeneic stem cell transplantation (allo-SCT). Twenty-five patients who relapsed after allo-SCT received BV. The ORR and CR rates were 50% and 38%, respectively. The median PFS was 7.8 months, and the median OS was not reached.

Many clinical trials are ongoing to evaluate BV in various settings; these include as salvage combinations with chemotherapy prior to ASCT, as initial therapy in combinations with chemotherapy and as maintenance therapy after ASCT for high-risk patients.

A phase II study evaluating single-agent BV and augmented ICE salvage therapy prior to ASCT was conducted. Patients received BV for two cycles, followed by PET. Patients who achieved PET-CR proceeded to ASCT. Patients who failed to achieve PET-CR received two cycles of augmented ICE prior to consideration for ASCT. Preliminary results showed that among 28 patients who underwent ASCT, 9 patients (32%) achieved PET-CR with two cycles of BV ([89]). Maintenance therapy with BV after ASCT was evaluated in a placebo-controlled randomized phase III study (AETHERA) ([90]). Patients were enrolled in this study if they were (1) refractory to frontline therapy, (2) had relapse <12 months after frontline therapy, or (3) had relapse ≥12 months after frontline therapy with extranodal disease. The median PFS was 43 months with BV and 24 months with placebo. This represents a significant 43% reduction in the risk of disease progression with BV. Once finalized, these results will potentially change the standard treatment of high-risk patients who relapse after first-line chemotherapy.

A phase III trial comparing BV plus AVD (ABVD without bleomycin) versus standard ABVD in patients with newly diagnosed advanced-stage HL is ongoing (NCT01712490). A phase I study comparing BV in combination with ABVD or AVD treatment showed a high CR rate of 96%. However, BV combined with bleomycin resulted in a high rate of pulmonary toxicity (44%) ([91]). Based on this phase I trial, BV is combined with AVD. This BV+AVD combination, if superior to ABVD, may change the standard of care in patients with newly diagnosed advanced-stage HL.

Gemcitabine

Gemcitabine-containing regimens are effective. A phase II study of single-agent gemcitabine, 200 mg/m^2 given on days 1, 8, and 15 of a 28-day schedule, showed an ORR of 43% with a CR rate of 14% ([92]). The GVD regimen (gemcitabine, vinorelbine, and pegylated liposomal doxorubicin) was evaluated by the CALGB in 91 patients with relapsed or refractory HL. The ORR was 70%, with a CR rate of 19% ([93]). The 4-year PFS and OS rates in transplant-naive patients treated with GVD followed by ASCT were 52% and 70%, respectively. In patients in whom prior transplant failed, the 4-year DFS and OS rates were 10% and 34%, respectively. The GDP regimen produced similar results, with an ORR of 62% and a CR rate of 10%. A combination regimen named IGEV (ifosfamide, gemcitabine, vinorelbine) was evaluated in 91 patients and produced an ORR of 81% with a high CR rate of 54%; 60% of primary refractory patients responded to IGEV ([94]).

Bendamustine

Bendamustine is a bifunctional alkylating agent derived from 2-chloroethylamine that had been a standard chemotherapy for indolent lymphoma (follicular lymphoma and mantle cell lymphoma) ([95, 96]). The Memorial Sloan-Kettering Cancer Center conducted a phase II trial of bendamustine in patients with HL who relapsed after ASCT or who were not eligible for ASCT ([97]). Patients received bendamustine of 120 mg/m^2 on days 1 and 2 of a 28-day cycle, for six planned cycles. The ORR was 53%, including a 33% CR rate; the median PFS was 5.2 months. Preliminary data of a phase I/II study for the combination of bendamustine and BV for relapsed/refractory transplant-naïve patients showed an ORR of 94% with CR rate of 82% ([98]). At the time of report, 20 of 34 patients who had a response to this combination had undergone ASCT.

Allogeneic Stem Cell Transplantation

The main advantage of an allo-SCT is its graft-versus-HL effect. Retrospective studies have shown this benefit by documenting lower relapse rates in allo-SCT patients who have chronic graft-versus-host disease (GVHD) and by showing that donor lymphocyte infusion (DLI) can induce relatively long-lasting remissions ([99]). Initial studies of allo-SCT in HL patients described high rates of nonrelapse mortality (NRM), up to 61%. More recent studies evaluated reduced-intensity conditioning (RIC) and have shown decreases in treatment-related mortality (TRM). Overall, RIC allo-SCT induces modest long-term remissions with a PFS rate of 30% ([100, 101]).

The EBMT reviewed 168 patients who had undergone allo-SCT ([101]). Seventy-nine patients received myeloablative conditioning, and 89 patients received RIC. Fifty-two percent of patients had undergone a prior ASCT and 45% had chemosensitive disease. The NRM was significantly lower and OS was significantly better with RIC versus myeloablative conditioning. One-year NRM was 23%, and 5-year PFS and OS were 18% and 28%, respectively, in patients who received RIC.

At MDACC, we reviewed the outcomes of 58 patients who received RIC with fludarabine-melphalan in preparation for allo-SCT ([102]). Overall, 83% of patients had undergone a prior ASCT and 52% had chemotherapy-sensitive disease at the time of allo-SCT. The TRM at 2 years was 15%, with nearly half of the TRM occurring within the first 100 days after allo-SCT. The incidence of chronic GVHD was 73%. The 2-year PFS and OS rates were 32% and 64%, respectively. There was a trend toward improvement in PFS for those with chemotherapy-sensitive disease but not for OS. Allogeneic stem cell transplantation is still an important option for eligible patients who relapse after ASCT.

Novel Agents

Advances in our understanding of HL pathology and biology have led to the development of promising targeted agents.

Programmed Death-1 Inhibitors

Nivolumab is a programmed death (PD)-1 immune checkpoint inhibitor antibody that selectively blocks the interaction between PD-1 and its ligands PD-L1 and PD-L2. This PD-1 pathway has a mechanism that normally leads to downregulation of cellular immune response. By inhibiting this interaction, nivolumab can enhance T-cell function, which may result in antitumor activity. Nivolumab has been evaluated in a phase II trial for patients with relapsed or refractory HL ([103]). Twenty-three patients were treated; 78% had received ASCT and 78% had received BV before nivolumab. Nivolumab was given at a dose of 3 mg/kg every 2 weeks. The ORR was 87%, with a CR rate of 17%. The 6-month PFS rate was 86%. Nivolumab thus showed substantial therapeutic activity and an acceptable safety profile in patients with previously heavily treated relapsed or refractory HL. Nivolumab has been granted "Breakthrough Therapy Designation" by the FDA, and a pivotal trial is ongoing (NCT02181738).

Another PD-1 inhibitor, pembrolizumab, was evaluated in a phase IB trial in patients who had disease progression or relapse with BV ([104]). Similar to nivolumab, a promising level of efficacy was seen, with an ORR of 53% and a CR rate of 20% at 12 weeks in 15 patients who were evaluable for response at the time of the preliminary report.

Histone Deacetylase Inhibitor

Histone deacetylases (HDACs) act on lysine amino acid groups on multiple proteins including many transcription factors. The HDACs are grouped into four classes, with classes I, II, and IV being zinc dependent. Several HDAC inhibitors are being investigated as therapies for relapsed or refractory HL. Panobinostat is an HDAC class I and II or pan-HDAC inhibitor and has been evaluated in a phase II trial in patients with relapsed or refractory HL after ASCT ([105]). Patients received panobinostat 40 mg orally three times a week for 21-day cycles. For the 129 patients enrolled in the trial, the ORR was 21%, with a CR rate of 4%. Treatment was well tolerated; the most common grade 3 to 4 adverse event was thrombocytopenia. The median PFS was 6.1 months, and 1-year OS was 78%.

We have conducted a phase I/II randomized trial of ICE with or without panobinostat in patients with relapsed or refractory HL (NCT01169636). Preliminary results of the trial showed an ORR of 86% with a CR rate of 71%. All patients who achieved response were able to proceed to ASCT.

Mocetinostat, another HDAC inhibitor, was evaluated in a phase II trial in patients with relapsed or refractory HL. The initial dose of 110 mg orally three times a week for 28-day cycles was reduced to 85 mg because 70% of patients required dose reduction for toxicity. Among 51 patients treated, 60% had a reduction in tumor measurements, with 24% achieving partial response. Toxicities included thrombocytopenia, fatigue, pneumonia, anemia, and pericardial effusion.

Mammalian Target of Rapamycin Inhibitors

Everolimus is an oral agent that targets the mammalian target of rapamycin (mTOR) complex 1 (mTORC1). Hodgkin lymphoma cells have an activated PI3K pathway (upstream of mTOR) and may be susceptible to inhibition of this pathway. Everolimus was evaluated in a phase II trial in patients with relapsed HL ([106]). Nineteen patients were enrolled, and 87% had received ASCT before everolimus. The ORR was 47%, with eight partial responses and one CR. The median time to progression was 7.2 months, with four responders remaining progression free at 12 months. Synergistic activity between everolimus and panobinostat was suggested by in vitro studies. We conducted a phase I trial of everolimus plus panobinostat in patients with relapsed or refractory lymphoma ([107]). Among the 30 patients treated, 14 patients had HL. The ORR was 43%, with a CR rate of 15%. However, grade 3 to 4 thrombocytopenia was reported in 64% of patients, limiting the future development of this combination.

Several clinical trials evaluating the combination of mTOR inhibitors and other drugs are ongoing. Sirolimus was evaluated in combination with an HDAC inhibitor, vorinostat, in a phase I trial at MDACC ([108]). The ORR was 57%, with a CR rate of 32% in heavily pretreated patients. Brentuximab vedotin will be evaluated in combination with mTOR inhibitors such as sirolimus, temsirolimus, and everolimus (NCT01902160, NCT02254239).

The MD Anderson Approach

Patients with relapsed or refractory HL are planned for second-line or salvage chemotherapy followed by an ASCT. We screen patients who have relapsed or refractory HL for current clinical trial options including our current randomized phase II clinical trial of panobinostat plus ICE (P-ICE) versus ICE. Patients who respond to salvage chemotherapy are planned to undergo ASCT. The role of BV for maintenance in patients with high risk of relapse after ASCT is an evolving topic. Based on the positive data recently presented for the AETHERA trial, this could become a standard of care. We screen patients with relapsed HL after an ASCT for novel agent clinical trial options. The preference is to treat with either BV if not previously given before ASCT or with a BV combination treatment on protocol including our planned BV plus dual mTORC1 inhibitor MLN0128 phase I trial. For patients who have early disease relapse or refractory disease after BV treatment, we consider novel agent protocols such as the PD-1 inhibitor trials. For patients not eligible or who do not wish to enroll in clinical trials, we consider chemotherapy regimens such as GND, bendamustine, or others. Given the benefits versus risks of allo-SCT, a subset of patients can be potentially considered for this approach, particularly otherwise healthy patients who achieve complete remission with addition therapies.

CONCLUSION

Although standard frontline chemotherapy with or without radiation therapy offers a high cure rate for cHL, approximately 20% of patients will develop refractory or relapsed disease. Thus, the challenge that remains is how to best develop strategies of therapy that increase the cure rates for the refractory/relapsed group of patients, while decreasing both short- and long-term toxicities, including secondary malignancies, for patients who are cured of their disease with current standard approaches. Huge recent achievements have occurred on both fronts, including a decrease of both the number of cycles of chemotherapy and the doses of RT for patients with early-stage disease, and introduction of novel therapeutics such as BV into frontline regimens paired with chemotherapy. Despite the fact that BV is a clear therapeutic advance, there remains a continued need to develop new therapies. Recently completed trials have shown significant promise for several new molecularly targeted therapeutic agents, with the PD-1 inhibitors demonstrating the ability to have significant efficacy even in patients with BV-resistant disease. Future directions are anticipated to increase the focus on evaluating the efficacy of combinations of targeted agents, with likely future trials exploring the potential activity of chemotherapy-free targeted treatment combinations in the frontline setting. Better understanding of the molecular biology of both cHL and NLPHL will also lead to more rationally designed novel agent trials and allow us to best select treatment strategies. The future of HL treatment has evolved significantly over the past decade, and these successes will only be significantly multiplied over the next decade to follow.

REFERENCES

1. Swerdlow S, Campo E, Harris N, et al. *WHO Classification of Tumours of Haematopoietic and Lymphoid Tissues*. Lyon, France:

International Agency for Research on Cancer (IARC); 2008.
2. Chihara D, Ito H, Matsuda T, et al. Differences in incidence and trends of haematological malignancies in Japan and the United States. *Br J Haematol*. 2014;164(4):536-545.
3. Morton LM, Wang SS, Devesa SS, Hartge P, Weisenburger DD, Linet MS. Lymphoma incidence patterns by WHO subtype in the United States, 1992-2001. *Blood*. 2006;107(1):265-276.
4. National Cancer Institute: Surveillance, Epidemiology, and End Results (SEER) Program. National Cancer Institute, DCCPS. Released April 2014 [Cancer Statistics Branch]. www.seer.cancer.gov. Accessed September 14, 2015.
5. Schmitz R, Stanelle J, Hansmann ML, Kuppers R. Pathogenesis of classical and lymphocyte-predominant Hodgkin lymphoma. *Annu Rev Pathol*. 2009;4:151-174.
6. Diehl V, Sextro M, Franklin J, et al. Clinical presentation, course, and prognostic factors in lymphocyte-predominant Hodgkin's disease and lymphocyte-rich classical Hodgkin's disease: report from the European Task Force on Lymphoma Project on Lymphocyte-Predominant Hodgkin's Disease. *J Clin Oncol*. 1999;17(3):776-783.
7. Nogova L, Reineke T, Brillant C, et al. Lymphocyte-predominant and classical Hodgkin's lymphoma: a comprehensive analysis from the German Hodgkin Study Group. *J Clin Oncol*. 2008;26(3):434-439.
8. Anagnostopoulos I, Hansmann ML, Franssila K, et al. European Task Force on Lymphoma project on lymphocyte predominance Hodgkin disease: histologic and immunohistologic analysis of submitted cases reveals 2 types of Hodgkin disease with a nodular growth pattern and abundant lymphocytes. *Blood*. 2000;96(5):1889-1899.
9. Lukes RJ, Butler JJ. The pathology and nomenclature of Hodgkin's disease. *Cancer Res*. 1966;26(6):1063-1083.
10. Brune V, Tiacci E, Pfeil I, et al. Origin and pathogenesis of nodular lymphocyte-predominant Hodgkin lymphoma as revealed by global gene expression analysis. *J Exp Med*. 2008;205(10):2251-2268.
11. MacLennan KA, Bennett MH, Tu A, et al. Relationship of histopathologic features to survival and relapse in nodular sclerosing Hodgkin's disease. A study of 1659 patients. *Cancer*. 1989;64(8):1686-1693.
12. Medeiros LJ, Greiner TC. Hodgkin's disease. *Cancer*. 1995;75(1 Suppl):357-369.
13. Kuppers R. Molecular biology of Hodgkin's lymphoma. *Adv Cancer Res*. 2002;84:277-312.
14. Lister TA, Crowther D, Sutcliffe SB, et al. Report of a committee convened to discuss the evaluation and staging of patients with Hodgkin's disease: Cotswolds meeting. *J Clin Oncol*. 1989;7(11):1630-1636.
15. Cheson BD, Fisher RI, Barrington SF, et al. Recommendations for initial evaluation, staging, and response assessment of Hodgkin and non-Hodgkin lymphoma: the Lugano Classification. *J Clin Oncol*. 2014;32(27):3059-3068.
16. Cheson BD. Role of functional imaging in the management of lymphoma. *J Clin Oncol*. 2011;29(14):1844-1854.
17. Barrington SF, Mackewn JE, Schleyer P, et al. Establishment of a UK-wide network to facilitate the acquisition of quality assured FDG-PET data for clinical trials in lymphoma. *Ann Oncol*. 2011;22(3):739-745.
18. El-Galaly TC, d'Amore F, Mylam KJ, et al. Routine bone marrow biopsy has little or no therapeutic consequence for positron emission tomography/computed tomography-staged treatment-naive patients with Hodgkin lymphoma. *J Clin Oncol*. 2012;30(36):4508-4514.
19. Mauch P, Tarbell N, Weinstein H, et al. Stage IA and IIA supradiaphragmatic Hodgkin's disease: prognostic factors in surgically staged patients treated with mantle and paraaortic irradiation. *J Clin Oncol*. 1988;6(10):1576-1583.
20. Tubiana M, Henry-Amar M, van der Werf-Messing B, et al. A multivariate analysis of prognostic factors in early stage Hodgkin's disease. *Int J Radiat Oncol Biol Phys*. 1985;11(1):23-30.
21. Cosset JM, Henry-Amar M, Meerwaldt JH, et al. The EORTC trials for limited stage Hodgkin's disease. The EORTC Lymphoma Cooperative Group. *Eur J Cancer*. 1992;28A(11):1847-1850.
22. Engert A, Plutschow A, Eich HT, et al. Reduced treatment intensity in patients with early-stage Hodgkin's lymphoma. *N Engl J Med*. 2010;363(7):640-652.
23. Hasenclever D, Diehl V. A prognostic score for advanced Hodgkin's disease. International Prognostic Factors Project on Advanced Hodgkin's Disease. *N Engl J Med*. 1998;339(21):1506-1514.
24. Cheson BD, Horning SJ, Coiffier B, et al. Report of an international workshop to standardize response criteria for non-Hodgkin's lymphomas. NCI Sponsored International Working Group. *J Clin Oncol*. 1999;17(4):1244.
25. Cheson BD, Pfistner B, Juweid ME, et al. Revised response criteria for malignant lymphoma. *J Clin Oncol*. 2007;25(5):579-586.
26. Engert A, Haverkamp H, Kobe C, et al. Reduced-intensity chemotherapy and PET-guided radiotherapy in patients with advanced stage Hodgkin's lymphoma (HD15 trial): a randomised, open-label, phase 3 non-inferiority trial. *Lancet*. 2012;379(9828):1791-1799.
27. Juweid ME, Stroobants S, Hoekstra OS, et al. Use of positron emission tomography for response assessment of lymphoma: consensus of the Imaging Subcommittee of International Harmonization Project in Lymphoma. *J Clin Oncol*. 2007;25(5): 571-578.
28. Biggi A, Gallamini A, Chauvie S, et al. International validation study for interim PET in ABVD-treated, advanced-stage Hodgkin lymphoma: interpretation criteria and concordance rate among reviewers. *J Nucl Med*. 2013;54(5):683-690.
29. Nogova L, Reineke T, Eich HT, et al. Extended field radiotherapy, combined modality treatment or involved field radiotherapy for patients with stage IA lymphocyte-predominant Hodgkin's lymphoma: a retrospective analysis from the German Hodgkin Study Group (GHSG). *Ann Oncol*. 2005;16(10):1683-1687.
30. Schlembach PJ, Wilder RB, Jones D, et al. Radiotherapy alone for lymphocyte-predominant Hodgkin's disease. *Cancer J*. 2002;8(5):377-383.
31. Chen RC, Chin MS, Ng AK, et al. Early-stage, lymphocyte-predominant Hodgkin's lymphoma: patient outcomes from a large, single-institution series with long follow-up. *J Clin Oncol*. 2010;28(1):136-141.
32. Savage KJ, Skinnider B, Al-Mansour M, Sehn LH, Gascoyne RD, Connors JM. Treating limited-stage nodular lymphocyte predominant Hodgkin lymphoma similarly to classical Hodgkin lymphoma with ABVD may improve outcome. *Blood*. 2011;118(17):4585-4590.
33. Advani RH, Horning SJ, Hoppe RT, et al. Mature results of a phase II study of rituximab therapy for nodular lymphocyte-predominant Hodgkin lymphoma. *J Clin Oncol*. 2014;32(9): 912-918.
34. Eichenauer DA, Fuchs M, Pluetschow A, et al. Phase 2 study of rituximab in newly diagnosed stage IA nodular lymphocyte-predominant Hodgkin lymphoma: a report from the German Hodgkin Study Group. *Blood*. 2011;118(16):4363-4365.
35. Xing KH, Connors JM, Al-Mansour M, Gascoyne RD, Skinnider B, Savage KJ. The outcome of advanced stage nodular lymphocyte predominant Hodgkin's lymphoma (NLPHL) compared to classical Hodgkin's lymphoma (CHL): a matched pair analysis [abstract]. *Blood*. 2012;120:1531.
36. Fanale M, Lai CM, MacLaughlin P, et al. Outcomes of nodular lymphocyte predominant Hodgkin's lymphoma (NLPHL) patients treated with R-CHOP [abstract]. *Blood*. 2010;116:2812.
37. Schulz H, Rehwald U, Morschhauser F, et al. Rituximab in relapsed lymphocyte-predominant Hodgkin lymphoma:

long-term results of a phase 2 trial by the German Hodgkin Lymphoma Study Group (GHSG). *Blood*. 2008;111(1):109-111.
38. Al-Mansour M, Connors JM, Gascoyne RD, Skinnider B, Savage KJ. Transformation to aggressive lymphoma in nodular lymphocyte-predominant Hodgkin's lymphoma. *J Clin Oncol*. 2010;28(5):793-799.
39. Karuturi M, Hosing C, Fanale M, et al. High-dose chemotherapy and autologous stem cell transplantation for nodular lymphocyte-predominant Hodgkin lymphoma. *Biol Blood Marrow Transplant*. 2013;19(6):991-994.
40. Rosenberg SA, Kaplan HS. The evolution and summary results of the Stanford randomized clinical trials of the management of Hodgkin's disease: 1962-1984. *Int J Radiat Oncol Biol Phys*. 1985;11(1):5-22.
41. Specht L, Gray RG, Clarke MJ, Peto R. Influence of more extensive radiotherapy and adjuvant chemotherapy on long-term outcome of early-stage Hodgkin's disease: a meta-analysis of 23 randomized trials involving 3,888 patients. International Hodgkin's Disease Collaborative Group. *J Clin Oncol*. 1998;16(3):830-843.
42. Dores GM, Metayer C, Curtis RE, et al. Second malignant neoplasms among long-term survivors of Hodgkin's disease: a population-based evaluation over 25 years. *J Clin Oncol*. 2002;20(16):3484-3494.
43. Engert A, Franklin J, Eich HT, et al. Two cycles of doxorubicin, bleomycin, vinblastine, and dacarbazine plus extended-field radiotherapy is superior to radiotherapy alone in early favorable Hodgkin's lymphoma: final results of the GHSG HD7 trial. *J Clin Oncol*. 2007;25(23):3495-3502.
44. Ferme C, Eghbali H, Meerwaldt JH, et al. Chemotherapy plus involved-field radiation in early-stage Hodgkin's disease. *N Engl J Med*. 2007;357(19):1916-1927.
45. Chronowski GM, Wilder RB, Tucker SL, et al. Analysis of in-field control and late toxicity for adults with early-stage Hodgkin's disease treated with chemotherapy followed by radiotherapy. *Int J Radiat Oncol Biol Phys*. 2003;55(1):36-43.
46. Raemaekers JM, Andre MP, Federico M, et al. Omitting radiotherapy in early positron emission tomography-negative stage I/II Hodgkin lymphoma is associated with an increased risk of early relapse: clinical results of the preplanned interim analysis of the randomized EORTC/LYSA/FIL H10 trial. *J Clin Oncol*. 2014;32(12):1188-1194.
47. Behringer K, Goergen H, Hitz F, et al. Omission of dacarbazine or bleomycin, or both, from the ABVD regimen in treatment of early-stage favourable Hodgkin's lymphoma (GHSG HD13): an open-label, randomised, non-inferiority trial. *Lancet*. 2015;385(9976):1418-1427.
48. Advani RH, Hoppe RT, Baer D, et al. Efficacy of abbreviated Stanford V chemotherapy and involved-field radiotherapy in early-stage Hodgkin lymphoma: mature results of the G4 trial. *Ann Oncol*. 2013;24(4):1044-1048.
49. Noordijk EM, Thomas J, Ferme C. First results of the EORTC-GELA H9 randomized trials: the H9-F trial (comparing 3 radiation dose levels) and H9-U trial (comparing 3 chemotherapy schemes) in patients with favorable or unfavorable early stage Hodgkin's lymphoma (HL) [abstract]. *J Clin Oncol*. 2005;561:6505.
50. Bonadonna G, Bonfante V, Viviani S, Di Russo A, Villani F, Valagussa P. ABVD plus subtotal nodal versus involved-field radiotherapy in early-stage Hodgkin's disease: long-term results. *J Clin Oncol*. 2004;22(14):2835-2841.
51. Radford J, Barrington SF, Counsell N, et al. Involved field radiotherapy versus no further treatment in patients with clinical stages IA and IIA Hodgkin lymphoma and a 'negative' PET scan after 3 cycles ABVD. Results of the UK NCRI RAPID trial [abstract]. *Blood*. 2012:547.
52. Canellos GP, Anderson JR, Propert KJ, et al. Chemotherapy of advanced Hodgkin's disease with MOPP, ABVD, or MOPP alternating with ABVD. *N Engl J Med*. 1992;327(21):1478-1484.
53. Gordon LI, Hong F, Fisher RI, et al. Randomized phase III trial of ABVD versus Stanford V with or without radiation therapy in locally extensive and advanced-stage Hodgkin lymphoma: an intergroup study coordinated by the Eastern Cooperative Oncology Group (E2496). *J Clin Oncol*. 2013;31(6):684-691.
54. von Tresckow B, Plutschow A, Fuchs M, et al. Dose-intensification in early unfavorable Hodgkin's lymphoma: final analysis of the German Hodgkin Study Group HD14 trial. *J Clin Oncol*. 2012;30(9):907-913.
55. Eich HT, Diehl V, Gorgen H, et al. Intensified chemotherapy and dose-reduced involved-field radiotherapy in patients with early unfavorable Hodgkin's lymphoma: final analysis of the German Hodgkin Study Group HD11 trial. *J Clin Oncol*. 2010;28(27):4199-4206.
56. Ferme C, Divine M, Vranovsky A, Morschhauser F, Bouabdallah R, Gabarre J. Four ABVD and involved-field radiotherapy in unfavorable supradiaphragmatic clinical stages (CS) I-II Hodgkin's lymphoma (HL): preliminary results of the EORTC-GELA H9-U trial [abstract]. *Blood*. 2005;106:813.
57. Meyer RM, Gospodarowicz MK, Connors JM, et al. ABVD alone versus radiation-based therapy in limited-stage Hodgkin's lymphoma. *N Engl J Med*. 2012;366(5):399-408.
58. Mounier N, Brice P, Bologna S, et al. ABVD (8 cycles) versus BEACOPP (4 escalated cycles >/= 4 baseline): final results in stage III-IV low-risk Hodgkin lymphoma (IPS 0-2) of the LYSA H34 randomized trial. *Ann Oncol*. 2014;25(8):1622-1628.
59. Viviani S, Zinzani PL, Rambaldi A, et al. ABVD versus BEACOPP for Hodgkin's lymphoma when high-dose salvage is planned. *N Engl J Med*. 2011;365(3):203-212.
60. Borchmann P, Haverkamp H, Diehl V, et al. Eight cycles of escalated-dose BEACOPP compared with four cycles of escalated-dose BEACOPP followed by four cycles of baseline-dose BEACOPP with or without radiotherapy in patients with advanced-stage Hodgkin's lymphoma: final analysis of the HD12 trial of the German Hodgkin Study Group. *J Clin Oncol*. 2011;29(32):4234-4242.
61. Engert A, Diehl V, Franklin J, et al. Escalated-dose BEACOPP in the treatment of patients with advanced-stage Hodgkin's lymphoma: 10 years of follow-up of the GHSG HD9 study. *J Clin Oncol*. 2009;27(27):4548-4554.
62. Diehl V, Franklin J, Pfreundschuh M, et al. Standard and increased-dose BEACOPP chemotherapy compared with COPP-ABVD for advanced Hodgkin's disease. *N Engl J Med*. 2003;348(24):2386-2395.
63. Borchmann P, Haverkamp H, Lohri A, Kreissl S, Greil R, Markova J. Addition of rituximab to BEACOPP escalated to improve the outcome of early interim PET positive advanced stage Hodgkin lymphoma patients: second planned interim analysis of the HD18 study [abstract]. *Blood*. 2014:500.
64. Press OW, LeBlanc M, Rimsza L, Schoder H, Friedberg JW, Evens AM. A phase II trial of response-adapted therapy of stages III–IV Hodgkin lymphoma using early interim FDG-PET imaging: US Intergroup S0816 [abstract]. *Hematol Oncol*. 2013;31:124.
65. Gallamini A, Rossi A, Patti C, Picardi M, Di Raimondo F, Cantonetti M. Early treatment intensification in advanced-stage high-risk Hodgkin lymphoma (HL) patients, with a positive FDG-PET scan after two ABVD courses: first interim analysis of the GITIL/FIL HD0607 clinical trial [abstract]. *Blood*. 2012;120:550.
66. Federico M, Luminari S, Iannitto E, et al. ABVD compared with BEACOPP compared with CEC for the initial treatment of patients with advanced Hodgkin's lymphoma: results from the HD2000 Gruppo Italiano per lo Studio dei Linfomi Trial. *J Clin Oncol*. 2009;27(5):805-811.
66a. Merli F, Luminari S, Gobbi PG, et al. Long-Term Results of the HD2000 Trial Comparing ABVD Versus BEACOPP Versus

CHAPTER 10

COPP-EBV-CAD in Untreated Patients With Advanced Hodgkin Lymphoma: A Study by Fondazione Italiana Linfomi. J Clin Oncol. 2015; e-pub

67. Gallamini A, Hutchings M, Rigacci L, et al. Early interim 2-[18F]fluoro-2-deoxy-D-glucose positron emission tomography is prognostically superior to international prognostic score in advanced-stage Hodgkin's lymphoma: a report from a joint Italian-Danish study. *J Clin Oncol*. 2007;25(24):3746-3752.
68. Hutchings M, Loft A, Hansen M, et al. FDG-PET after two cycles of chemotherapy predicts treatment failure and progression-free survival in Hodgkin lymphoma. *Blood*. 2006;107(1):52-59.
69. Terasawa T, Lau J, Bardet S, et al. Fluorine-18-fluorodeoxyglucose positron emission tomography for interim response assessment of advanced-stage Hodgkin's lymphoma and diffuse large B-cell lymphoma: a systematic review. *J Clin Oncol*. 2009;27(11):1906-1914.
70. Kobe C, Dietlein M, Franklin J, et al. Positron emission tomography has a high negative predictive value for progression or early relapse for patients with residual disease after first-line chemotherapy in advanced-stage Hodgkin lymphoma. *Blood*. 2008;112(10):3989-3994.
71. de Wit M, Bohuslavizki KH, Buchert R, Bumann D, Clausen M, Hossfeld DK. 18FDG-PET following treatment as valid predictor for disease-free survival in Hodgkin's lymphoma. *Ann Oncol*. 2001;12(1):29-37.
72. Jerusalem G, Beguin Y, Fassotte MF, et al. Whole-body positron emission tomography using 18F-fluorodeoxyglucose for posttreatment evaluation in Hodgkin's disease and non-Hodgkin's lymphoma has higher diagnostic and prognostic value than classical computed tomography scan imaging. *Blood*. 1999;94(2):429-433.
73. Devizzi L, Maffioli L, Bonfante V, et al. Comparison of gallium scan, computed tomography, and magnetic resonance in patients with mediastinal Hodgkin's disease. *Ann Oncol*. 1997;8(Suppl 1):53-56.
74. Moskowitz AJ, Yahalom J, Kewalramani T, et al. Pretransplantation functional imaging predicts outcome following autologous stem cell transplantation for relapsed and refractory Hodgkin lymphoma. *Blood*. 2010;116(23):4934-4937.
75. Moskowitz CH, Nimer SD, Zelenetz AD, et al. A 2-step comprehensive high-dose chemoradiotherapy second-line program for relapsed and refractory Hodgkin disease: analysis by intent to treat and development of a prognostic model. *Blood*. 2001;97(3):616-623.
76. Schmitz N, Pfistner B, Sextro M, et al. Aggressive conventional chemotherapy compared with high-dose chemotherapy with autologous haemopoietic stem-cell transplantation for relapsed chemosensitive Hodgkin's disease: a randomised trial. *Lancet*. 2002;359(9323):2065-2071.
77. Linch DC, Winfield D, Goldstone AH, et al. Dose intensification with autologous bone-marrow transplantation in relapsed and resistant Hodgkin's disease: results of a BNLI randomised trial. *Lancet*. 1993;341(8852):1051-1054.
78. Sirohi B, Cunningham D, Powles R, et al. Long-term outcome of autologous stem-cell transplantation in relapsed or refractory Hodgkin's lymphoma. *Ann Oncol*. 2008;19(7):1312-1319.
79. Filmont JE, Gisselbrecht C, Cuenca X, et al. The impact of pre- and post-transplantation positron emission tomography using 18-fluorodeoxyglucose on poor-prognosis lymphoma patients undergoing autologous stem cell transplantation. *Cancer*. 2007;110(6):1361-1369.
80. Svoboda J, Andreadis C, Elstrom R, et al. Prognostic value of FDG-PET scan imaging in lymphoma patients undergoing autologous stem cell transplantation. *Bone Marrow Transplant*. 2006;38(3):211-216.
81. Josting A, Muller H, Borchmann P, et al. Dose intensity of chemotherapy in patients with relapsed Hodgkin's lymphoma. *J Clin Oncol*. 2010;28(34):5074-5080.
82. Kewalramani T, Nimer SD, Zelenetz AD, et al. Progressive disease following autologous transplantation in patients with chemosensitive relapsed or primary refractory Hodgkin's disease or aggressive non-Hodgkin's lymphoma. *Bone Marrow Transplant*. 2003;32(7):673-679.
83. Arai S, Fanale M, DeVos S, et al. Defining a Hodgkin lymphoma population for novel therapeutics after relapse from autologous hematopoietic cell transplant. *Leuk Lymphoma*. 2013;54(11):2531-2533.
84. Sutherland MS, Sanderson RJ, Gordon KA, et al. Lysosomal trafficking and cysteine protease metabolism confer target-specific cytotoxicity by peptide-linked anti-CD30-auristatin conjugates. *J Biol Chem*. 2006;281(15):10540-10547.
85. Younes A, Gopal AK, Smith SE, et al. Results of a pivotal phase II study of brentuximab vedotin for patients with relapsed or refractory Hodgkin's lymphoma. *J Clin Oncol*. 2012;30(18):2183-2189.
86. Younes A, Bartlett NL, Leonard JP, et al. Brentuximab vedotin (SGN-35) for relapsed CD30-positive lymphomas. *N Engl J Med*. 2010;363(19):1812-1821.
87. Gopal AK, Chen R, Smith SE, et al. Durable remissions in a pivotal phase 2 study of brentuximab vedotin in relapsed or refractory Hodgkin lymphoma. *Blood*. 2015;125(8):1236-1243.
88. Onishi M, Graf SA, Holmberg L, et al. Brentuximab vedotin administered to platinum-refractory, transplant-naive Hodgkin lymphoma patients can increase the proportion achieving FDG PET negative status. *Hematol Oncol*. 2014: doi: 10.1002/hon.2166.
89. Moskowitz A, Schoder H, Gerecitano JF, et al. FDG-PET adapted sequential therapy with brentuximab vedotin and augmented ICE followed by autologous stem cell transplant for relapsed and refractory Hodgkin lymphoma. *Clin Adv Hematol Oncol*. 2014;12(2 Suppl 6):7.
90. Moskowitz CH, Nadamanee A, Masszi T, et al. The Aethera trial: results of a randomized, double-blind, placebo-controlled phase 3 study of brentuximab vedotin in the treatment of patients at risk of progression following autologous stem cell transplant for Hodgkin lymphoma [abstract]. *Blood*. 2014:673.
91. Younes A, Connors JM, Park SI, et al. Brentuximab vedotin combined with ABVD or AVD for patients with newly diagnosed Hodgkin's lymphoma: a phase 1, open-label, dose-escalation study. *Lancet Oncol*. 2013;14(13):1348-1356.
92. Zinzani PL, Bendandi M, Stefoni V, et al. Value of gemcitabine treatment in heavily pretreated Hodgkin's disease patients. *Haematologica*. 2000;85(9):926-929.
93. Bartlett NL, Niedzwiecki D, Johnson JL, et al. Gemcitabine, vinorelbine, and pegylated liposomal doxorubicin (GVD), a salvage regimen in relapsed Hodgkin's lymphoma: CALGB 59804. *Ann Oncol*. 2007;18(6):1071-1079.
94. Santoro A, Magagnoli M, Spina M, et al. Ifosfamide, gemcitabine, and vinorelbine: a new induction regimen for refractory and relapsed Hodgkin's lymphoma. *Haematologica*. 2007;92(1):35-41.
95. Flinn IW, van der Jagt R, Kahl BS, et al. Randomized trial of bendamustine-rituximab or R-CHOP/R-CVP in first-line treatment of indolent NHL or MCL: the BRIGHT study. *Blood*. 2014;123(19):2944-2952.
96. Rummel MJ, Niederle N, Maschmeyer G, et al. Bendamustine plus rituximab versus CHOP plus rituximab as first-line treatment for patients with indolent and mantle-cell lymphomas: an open-label, multicentre, randomised, phase 3 non-inferiority trial. *Lancet*. 2013;381(9873):1203-1210.
97. Moskowitz AJ, Hamlin PA Jr, Perales MA, et al. Phase II study of bendamustine in relapsed and refractory Hodgkin lymphoma. *J Clin Oncol*. 2013;31(4):456-460.
98. LaCasce A, Bociek RG, Matous J, et al. Brentuximab vedotin

in combination with bendamustine for patients with Hodgkin lymphoma who are relapsed or refractory after frontline therapy. *Blood*. 2014;124(21):293.

99. Peggs KS, Hunter A, Chopra R, et al. Clinical evidence of a graft-versus-Hodgkin's-lymphoma effect after reduced-intensity allogeneic transplantation. *Lancet*. 2005;365(9475):1934-1941.
100. Devetten MP, Hari PN, Carreras J, et al. Unrelated donor reduced-intensity allogeneic hematopoietic stem cell transplantation for relapsed and refractory Hodgkin lymphoma. *Biol Blood Marrow Transplant*. 2009;15(1):109-117.
101. Sureda A, Robinson S, Canals C, et al. Reduced-intensity conditioning compared with conventional allogeneic stem-cell transplantation in relapsed or refractory Hodgkin's lymphoma: an analysis from the Lymphoma Working Party of the European Group for Blood and Marrow Transplantation. *J Clin Oncol*. 2008;26(3):455-462.
102. Anderlini P, Saliba R, Acholonu S, et al. Fludarabine-melphalan as a preparative regimen for reduced-intensity conditioning allogeneic stem cell transplantation in relapsed and refractory Hodgkin's lymphoma: the updated M.D. Anderson Cancer Center experience. *Haematologica*. 2008;93(2):257-264.
103. Ansell SM, Lesokhin AM, Borrello I, et al. PD-1 blockade with nivolumab in relapsed or refractory Hodgkin's lymphoma. *N Engl J Med*. 2015;372(4):311-319.
104. Moskowitz CH, Ribrag V, Michot J-M, et al. PD-1 blockade with the monoclonal antibody pembrolizumab (MK-3475) in patients with classical Hodgkin lymphoma after brentuximab vedotin failure: preliminary results from a phase 1b study (KEYNOTE-013) [abstract]. *Blood*. 2014:290.
105. Younes A, Sureda A, Ben-Yehuda D, et al. Panobinostat in patients with relapsed/refractory Hodgkin's lymphoma after autologous stem-cell transplantation: results of a phase II study. *J Clin Oncol*. 2012;30(18):2197-2203.
106. Johnston PB, Inwards DJ, Colgan JP, et al. A phase II trial of the oral mTOR inhibitor everolimus in relapsed Hodgkin lymphoma. *Am J Hematol*. 2010;85(5):320-324.
107. Oki Y, Buglio D, Fanale M, et al. Phase I study of panobinostat plus everolimus in patients with relapsed or refractory lymphoma. *Clin Cancer Res*. 2013;19(24):6882-6890.
108. Janku F, Oki Y, Falchook GS, et al. Activity of the mTOR inhibitor sirolimus and HDAC inhibitor vorinostat in heavily pretreated refractory Hodgkin lymphoma patients [abstract]. *J Clin Oncol*. 2014;32:8508.

11

Multiple Myeloma and Other Plasma Cell Dyscrasias

第十一章　多发性骨髓瘤和其他浆细胞疾病

Hans C. Lee
Krina Patel
Piyanuch Kongtim
Simrit Parmar
Pei Lin
Muzaffar H. Qazilbash
Sheeba Thomas
Elisabet E. Manasanch

中文导读

本章重点介绍了多发性骨髓瘤和其他浆细胞疾病的病因学、遗传学、生物学、诊断、临床特征和治疗进展。在多发性骨髓瘤部分，首先概述了多发性骨髓瘤的分类、流行病学、危险因素、病理生理学和遗传/分子分型；进而详细介绍了多发性骨髓瘤的临床表现、实验室检查、影像学检查、诊断标准、分期、危险分层、疗效评价标准；最后重点介绍了多发性骨髓瘤治疗方案的选择，主要包括：可移植患者和不可移植患者的一线治疗方案选择、自体干细胞移植和异体干细胞移植在多发性骨髓瘤患者中的应用、维持治疗的方案选择以及复发/难治性多发性骨髓瘤患者的治疗方案选择；并对意义未明单克隆丙种球蛋白病，冒烟型骨髓瘤及孤立性骨浆细胞瘤的流行病学、诊断标准及治疗方案做了简明介绍。在其他浆细胞疾病方面，主要介绍了华氏巨球蛋白血症、轻链淀粉样变、POEMS综合征、TEMPI综合征、免疫球蛋白重链疾病等浆细胞疾病的临床特征、诊断标准和治疗方案选择。最后，本章对新型靶向药物在多发性骨髓瘤及其他浆细胞疾病中的应用前景做了简要介绍。

INTRODUCTION

Plasma cell dyscrasias are heterogeneous disorders arising from the proliferation of a monoclonal population of plasma cells. Some of these disorders can present serendipitously as benign processes that can be observed; others are highly aggressive and require immediate intervention. The most common plasma cell dyscrasia is monoclonal gammopathy of undetermined significance (MGUS), a benign condition that can be observed. Related disorders include smoldering multiple myeloma (SMM), multiple myeloma (MM), solitary plasmacytoma of the bone, extramedullary plasmacytoma, Waldenström macroglobulinemia (WM), primary amyloid light-chain (AL) amyloidosis, heavy-chain disease, POEMS (polyneuropathy, organomegaly, endocrinopathy, monoclonal gammopathy, and skin changes) syndrome, and the recently recognized TEMPI (telangiectasias, elevated erythropoietin and erythrocytosis, monoclonal gammopathy, perinephric fluid collection, and intrapulmonary shunting) syndrome. The spectrum of MGUS, SMM, and MM represents a natural progression of the same disease. This chapter focuses on the etiology, genetics, biology, diagnosis, clinical features, and current therapy of MM and other plasma cell disorders.

Major recent discoveries have changed the way we understand, diagnose, and treat plasma cell dyscrasias. The initial sequencing of the myeloma genome and single-cell genetic analysis paved the way for the concept of intraclonal heterogeneity and Darwinian selection of clones. Increasingly sensitive diagnostic and monitoring techniques allow for more accurate diagnosis, minimal residual disease monitoring, and detection of early relapse. New diagnostic criteria for MM have been implemented, and the introduction of novel classes of agents such as immunomodulatory drugs and proteasome inhibitors has led to improved overall survival. Additionally, immunotherapy using monoclonal antibodies against different myeloma targets has shown promising activity in clinical trials. Major advances have also occurred in WM as a highly recurrent single point mutation of the *MYD88* gene has been identified, and new treatments that abrogate this highly active pathway are already in use. Finally, a new paraneoplastic syndrome, the TEMPI syndrome, has been identified and described.

MULTIPLE MYELOMA

Multiple myeloma is a malignant proliferation of plasma cells. In virtually all cases, myeloma cells (as well as their precursors MGUS and SMM) secrete immunoglobulins. Usually, myeloma cells secrete immunoglobulin (Ig) G (60%); other types are less common (IgA 20%, IgD 2%, IgE <0.1%, biclonal <1%). Light chain–only secretion is noted in 18%; <5% of patients do not secrete a heavy- or light-chain immunoglobulin (nonsecretory MM).

Epidemiology and Risk Factors

In 2014, approximately 24,000 people were diagnosed with MM in the United States, and 11,090 died from the disease. The median age at diagnosis is 69 years. The incidence is highest in the age range of 65 to 74 years (27.7%), followed by the 75- to 84 year-old range (24.7%). The annual age-adjusted incidence of the disease per 100,000 population is 7.2 among white men and 4.3 among white women. Among African Americans, the frequency doubles to 14.8 in men and 10.5 in women. There is also a difference in mortality by racial group. The annual age-adjusted mortality rate per 100,000 is 4.0 and 2.5 in white men and women, respectively, and 7.7 and 5.3 in African American men and women, respectively. The incidence and mortality rates are lowest among Asians and Pacific Islanders.

Risk factors that predispose to MGUS and MM point toward common shared etiologic environmental and genetic factors. Age is a risk factor for MGUS, because its prevalence is four times higher among individuals ≥80 years old than among those 50 to 59 years old. Increased risk of MGUS has also been reported in first-degree family members of patients with MGUS and MM (risk ratio between 2 and 3). In a study of black and white women of similar socioeconomic status, obesity, black race, and increasing age conferred an increased risk of MGUS. Personal and family history of autoimmune or inflammatory disorders as well as infections have been linked to an increased risk of MGUS and MM. Exposure to infections has been hypothesized to be involved in the malignant transformation of MM, or it could represent impaired immunity associated with MGUS and SMM, which often precedes a diagnosis of MM. Radiation exposure, pesticides, and cleaners are also associated with an increased risk of MGUS and MM.

Although MM is not an inherited disease, more than a hundred familial cases have been reported in the literature. The largest series described 39 unique families with 79 MM cases. Both dominant and recessive inherited traits may play a role in familial MM. Large genomic studies have identified low penetrant genetic variants that confer a modest increase in the risk of developing MM ([1, 2]). Based on epidemiologic and familial aggregation studies, most of the inherited risk of developing MM may result from different genetic polymorphisms, each of which has only a small effect on the predisposition to develop disease ([3]).

Pathophysiology and Genetics/Molecular Classification

Multiple myeloma arises from terminally differentiated B cells or even early committed B cells (germinal center B cells) that manifest clinically as more differentiated plasma cells. The major role of normal differentiated plasma cells is to produce immunoglobulins (antibodies) to fight infections. To become an effective part of the adaptive immune system, B cells must undergo immunoglobulin gene rearrangement and affinity maturation in response to antigens presented by antigen-presenting cells within the lymph node germinal center. For this to occur, hypervariable regions in the immunoglobulin heavy chain locus (IGH in chromosome 14q32) undergo programmed mutations (somatic hypermutation) through which, among others, double DNA strand breaks and chromosomal translocations are generated. The primary etiology of MM has been linked to *IGH* translocations and increased copies of odd-numbered chromosomes (hyperdiploidy), which result in cyclin D dysregulation. These events can be observed early in the course of monoclonal gammopathies (such as in MGUS or SMM) as well as in MM, suggesting that they are primary genetic events. Initial whole-genome and exome sequencing in 38 MM patients confirmed the complexity of genetic alterations seen in MM and uncovered secondary mechanisms of transformation to MM ([4]). Secondary events included mutations in the oncogene *MYC* (most commonly observed in plasma cell leukemia or aggressive forms of MM), mutations in the nuclear factor-κβ (NF-κβ) pathway, including *BRAF* and *RAS*, and chromosome copy number abnormalities such as deletions, amplifications, or additions. Changes in DNA methylation patterns are also important secondary events leading to increased tumor diversity and more aggressive forms of plasma cell dyscrasias (Table 11-1).

Different tests for gene expression profiling (GEP) are available for molecular classification of MM. Currently, molecular profiling of MM is mostly used for research purposes (eg, identification of high-risk MM for inclusion in clinical trials). These tests may become increasingly important as we develop more personalized treatment for MM.

Serial genomic analysis during the disease course of myeloma patients has identified different MM subclones within the same tumor. This has been termed intraclonal heterogeneity. In this model, different myeloma subclones compete for selection as they are exposed to the microenvironment and therapeutic pressures ([5]). Single-cell genetic analysis at diagnosis confirmed that MM is highly heterogeneous and characterized by the accumulation of a diverse range of mutations at the subclonal level ([6]). In this scenario, the acquisition of new mutations leads to new subclones with different clinical phenotypes and sensitivities to therapy. Intraclonal heterogeneity in myeloma has many potential implications for therapy, suggesting that subclonal targeting in combination therapies may be needed to eradicate the multiple subclones. Increasing genetic complexity is seen with progression from MGUS to MM and plasma cell leukemia, which may suggest that earlier treatment may result in improved clinical outcomes.

The bone marrow microenvironment also plays a role in the etiology of MM and its related disorders. Plasma cells communicate effectively with the microenvironment in a process called cell trafficking. Upregulation of cytokines that increase vascular permeability, proliferation, or cell homing (interleukin [IL]-6, vascular endothelial growth factor, and insulin-like growth factor) have been involved in the progression to MM. Gene expression profiling has revealed that modulation of certain genes can lead to a permissive microenvironment that promotes growth of myeloma subclones leading to active disease ([7]). Thus, targeting the microenvironment is an area of extensive research that, combined with therapeutic targeting of myeloma subclones, may lead to improved outcomes. New and effective antimyeloma combination therapies and well-designed clinical trials are needed to test these hypotheses.

Clinical Presentation

The clinical presentation of MM and its precursors is variable. Patients with MGUS or SMM usually do not present with specific myeloma-related symptoms. Their diagnosis is often incidental based on workup for

Table 11-1 Genetic Alterations Found in Monoclonal Gammopathies, From Monoclonal Gammopathy of Undetermined Significance to Plasma Cell Leukemia

Primary genetic events
IGH translocations [t(4:14), t(6:14), t(14:20), t(14;16), t(11,14)]
Hyperdiploidy (trisomies of chromosomes 3, 5, 7, 9, 11, 15, 21)
Secondary genetic events
Additions (1q, 17q, 12p)
Deletions (1p, 13, 11q, 14q, 17p, 6q, 8p)
Translocations [t(8;14)]
Methylation changes (global hypomethylation and gene-specific hypermethylation)
Mutations in NF-κβ pathway (*TRAF3*, I-κβ)
Proliferation (*NRAS, KRAS, BRAF, MYC, MAPK, PI3K, MET*)

CHAPTER 11

a low albumin-to-globulin ratio, high serum protein, or other conditions such as autoimmune diseases, peripheral neuropathy, skin rashes, or hemolytic anemias.

In contrast, patients initially presenting with MM usually have at least one of the CRAB criteria (hyper**C**alcemia, **R**enal disease, **A**nemia, and **B**one disease) classically used to define symptomatic MM. Anemia is the most common finding, occurring in 73% of patients, and is typically a normocytic, normochromic anemia. Anemia can be due to a variety of factors, including marrow replacement or cytokine production by plasma cells, which lead to decreased erythropoiesis, or decreased erythropoietin levels due to renal disease ([8]).

Bone pain is common, occurring in 60% of patients, and related to increased resorption of bone, leading to lytic bone lesions. Painful vertebral compression fractures can occur and may represent a medical emergency when associated with symptoms of cord compression. Increased bone resorption has been attributed to factors such as RANK ligand (RANKL), osteoprotegerin (OPG), macrophage inflammatory protein (MIP)-1α, IL-6, and IL-3, which stimulate osteoclast activity in areas infiltrated by plasma cells as a result of interactions between plasma cells and the microenvironment (Fig. 11-1).

An elevated creatinine is a presenting sign in 50% of patients. Renal disease is often attributed to light-chain cast nephropathy resulting from precipitation of light chains that bind to Tamm-Horsfall mucoproteins secreted by cells in the ascending loop of Henle. These precipitated complexes obstruct the distal convoluted tubules and collecting ducts, leading to tubular atrophy and interstitial fibrosis. Other causes of renal failure include hypercalcemia, leading to nephrocalcinosis, as well as amyloidosis, heavy-chain disease, and light-chain disease.

Hypercalcemia >11 mg/dL is present in 10% of patients and represents a medical emergency requiring hydration with isotonic saline and bisphosphonate therapy with zoledronic acid or pamidronate in moderate or severe cases. Calcitonin can also be used to rapidly reduce serum calcium levels.

Other common presenting symptoms include fatigue (32%) and weight loss (20%). Due to immune dysfunction, patients are at risk for infections. About 7% to 18% of patients may present with extramedullary plasmacytomas. Less common symptoms include fever, splenomegaly, hepatomegaly, and lymphadenopathy.

Diagnostic Workup

Once a plasma cell dyscrasia is suspected, a comprehensive diagnostic workup should be initiated to demonstrate the presence or absence of a clonal plasma cell disorder, to determine if end-organ damage is present, and to evaluate laboratory markers related to prognosis. These should include the following components.

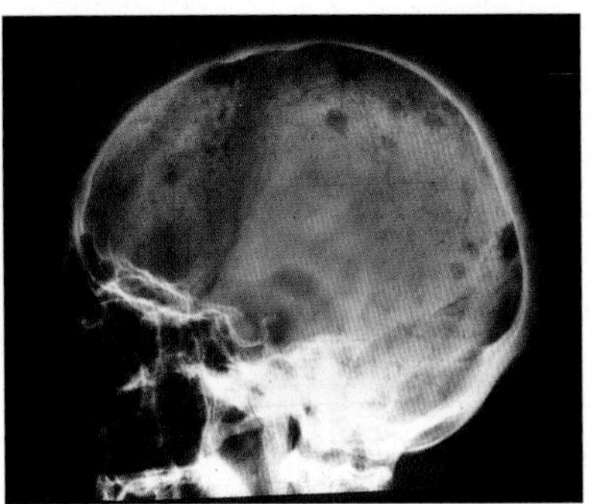

FIGURE 11-1 **Radiographic image of the skull showing "punched out" osteolytic lesions characteristic of multiple myeloma.**

Laboratory Studies

- Complete blood count (CBC)
- Serum chemistries including creatinine, calcium, albumin, lactate dehydrogenase (LDH), β_2-microglobulin, and immunoglobulin levels (IgG, IgA, IgM)
- Serum protein electrophoresis with immunofixation to quantify monoclonal protein (M-protein) and determine immunoglobulin isotype
- Serum free light-chain assay to evaluate the ratio of serum kappa to lambda light chains
- Urinalysis with 24-hour urine collection with protein electrophoresis and immunofixation (Fig. 11-2)

Imaging Studies

- Skeletal survey with plain films of the axial and appendicular skeleton is the minimum standard of care to evaluate lytic bone lesions.
- Advanced imaging with either whole-body low-dose computed tomography (CT), positron emission

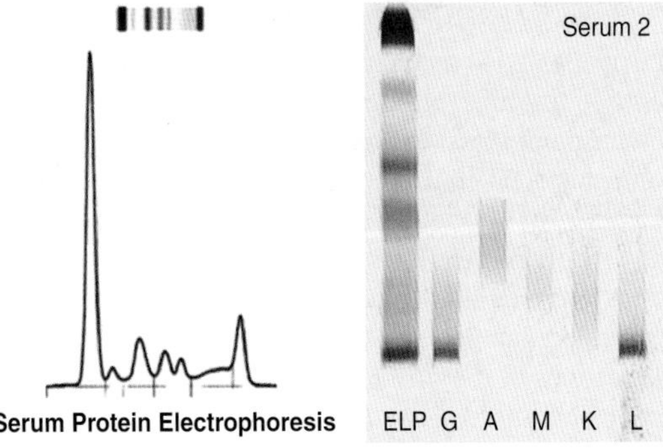

FIGURE 11-2 **Serum protein electrophoresis demonstrates an M-protein peak (*left*). Immunofixation confirms it to be monoclonal IgG lambda type.**

tomography–computed tomography (PET-CT), or magnetic resonance imaging (MRI) can detect up to 80% more lesions compared with plain film x-rays.
  - An advanced imaging modality is particularly recommended in the diagnosis of SMM to detect subtle bone lesions that would warrant the initiation of treatment. It is also helpful in assessing baseline disease burden as an adjunct to serum and urine markers prior to initiation of treatment in MM.
  - A CT scan can be helpful in the characterization of soft tissue masses in the case of extramedullary plasmacytomas and can direct to an area to be biopsied.
  - An MRI scan is useful for evaluating the axial skeleton in the presence of symptoms and assessing for spinal cord compression. It can also identify abnormal marrow uptake as T1-weighted images will show a diffuse decrease in marrow signal intensity but will enhance with the administration of contrast.
  - Positron emission tomography–computed tomography can be prone to false-positive findings but has more specificity due to increased metabolic uptake at the site of lytic lesions and is the preferred initial baseline advanced imaging modality at the University of Texas MD Anderson Cancer Center (MDACC) in combination with skeletal surveys.
- There is no role for nuclear bone imaging because bone scan isotopes are not taken up by lytic lesions.

Bone Marrow Aspiration and Biopsy

- Morphologic review and immunohistochemistry (Fig. 11-3)
- Flow cytometry for immunophenotyping of plasma cells:
  - Plasma cells are positive for CD38 and CD138.
  - Normal plasma cells have higher expression of CD19 and CD45; malignant plasma cells typically lack these surface antigens.
  - Malignant plasma cells have increased expression of CD56 and CD117; normal plasma cells have weak expression of these markers.
- Conventional cytogenetic karyotyping
- Fluorescent in situ hybridization (FISH) for recurrent chromosomal deletions, amplifications, and translocations that have prognostic significance; these include:
  - Deletion 13q14, deletion 17p13 (*TP53*), and deletion of 1p32
  - Amplification of 1q21
  - Translocations involving the immunoglobulin heavy-chain locus on chromosome 14q32 and its common partners, including 11q13 (*CCND1*), 4p16 (*FGFR3* and *MMSET*), 16q23 (*c-MAF*), 6p21 (*CCND3*), and 20q12 (*MAFB*)
- Gene expression profiling of the CD138$^+$ bone marrow aspirate plasma cells to identify high-risk MM and to facilitate inclusion in clinical trials

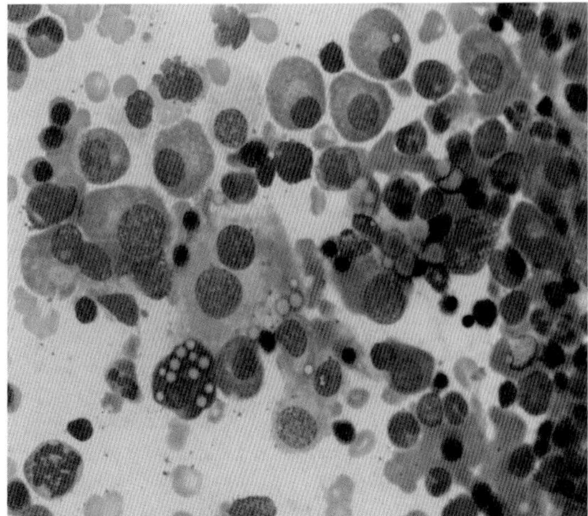

FIGURE 11-3 Multiple myeloma bone marrow aspirate. Some plasma cells have cytoplasmic immunoglobulin inclusions (Wright-Giemsa, 500×).

Other Tests

- Abdominal wall fat pad biopsy (warranted if there are signs and symptoms suggestive of amyloidosis; see separate discussion), which should be stained with Congo red stain. Amyloid fibrils show green birefringence under polarized light.
- Serum viscosity (if there are concerns for hyperviscosity usually due to elevated IgM levels in WM; see separate discussion). Hyperviscosity should be a clinical diagnosis, and therapeutic plasma exchange should not be delayed while waiting for the results of serum viscosity level.

Myeloma Diagnostic Criteria

Based on the above workup, a diagnosis of a plasma cell dyscrasia may be made, which can span the spectrum of the premalignant MGUS stage to SMM to full malignant transformation to MM. Definitions of these clinical stages according to the International Myeloma Working Group (IMWG) criteria are summarized in Table 11-2 ([9]). Historically, SMM and MM have been distinguished by the presence of end-organ damage as defined by CRAB criteria. The 2014 updated IMWG criteria were revised to reclassify some SMM patients as having MM (even in the absence of symptoms) if certain biomarkers were present that might indicate impending development of CRAB features. These include clonal bone marrow plasmacytosis ≥60%, an involved-to-uninvolved serum free light chain ratio

Table 11-2 Definitions of MGUS, SMM, and MM by 2014 IMWG Criteria

		Definition	Progression Rate
Premalignant	Monoclonal gammopathy of undetermined significance (MGUS)	• Monoclonal protein <3 g/dL • Clonal bone marrow plasma cells <10% • Absence of CRAB[a] criteria related to plasma cell clonal disorder • In light-chain MGUS[b], urinary monoclonal protein must be <500 mg/24 h	• 1% per year for MGUS • 0.3% per year for light-chain MGUS
	Smoldering multiple myeloma (SMM)	• Serum monoclonal protein ≥3 g/dL or urinary monoclonal protein ≥500 mg/24 h and/or bone marrow plasmacytosis 10%-60% • Absence of CRAB criteria[a] or amyloidosis	10% per year (see Table 11-9 for risk stratification in SMM)
	Multiple myeloma (MM)	• Clonal bone marrow plasma cells ≥10% or biopsy-proven bony or extramedullary plasmacytoma AND • Evidence of end-organ damage attributed to a plasma cell disorder as defined by CRAB[a] criteria OR ≥1 biomarker of malignancy, which includes bone marrow clonal plasmacytosis ≥60%, involved-to-uninvolved serum free light chains ≥100, or >1 focal lesion on magnetic resonance imaging studies that is at least 5 mm in size	Not applicable

[a]CRAB criteria:
1. HyperCalcemia: Serum calcium >1 mg/dL above the upper limit of normal or >11 mg/dL.
2. Renal insufficiency: creatinine clearance <40 mL/min or serum creatinine >2 mg/dL.
3. Anemia: hemoglobin <2 g/dL below the lower limit of normal or <10 g/dL.
4. Bone lesions: one or more osteolytic lesions on skeletal survey, computed tomography (CT) scan, or positron emission tomography–CT.

[b]Defined as abnormal free light-chain ratio (<0.26 or >1.65) in the absence of immunoglobulin heavy-chain expression on immunofixation.

Adapted with permission from Rajkumar SV, Dimopoulos MA, Palumbo A, et al. International Myeloma Working Group updated criteria for the diagnosis of multiple myeloma, *Lancet Oncol* 2014 Nov;15(12):e538-e548.

≥100, or more than one focal lesion on MRI studies of at least 5 mm in size. Patients with SMM and at least one of these biomarkers have a 70% to 80% chance of progression to MM at 2 years compared to 20% (10% per year) in the absence of these high-risk features. Initiating therapy in these patients may delay the onset of MM-defining end-organ damage events and associated morbidity and adverse effects on quality of life.

Staging and Risk Stratification

The course of MM is heterogeneous. Risk stratification using staging and prognostic tools may yield insights into the underlying disease biology and expected course. Prognostic studies can help stratify patients in clinical trials and may help guide therapy [eg, bortezomib in t(4;14) and del 13q].

International Staging System

The International Staging System (ISS) was established in 2005 by the IMWG after a retrospective analysis of the outcomes of >10,000 patients across 17 different centers. In this study, β_2-microglobulin and albumin were powerful correlates of median survival, and patients could be categorized into three stages based on serum levels at diagnosis (Table 11-3). Because β_2-microglobulin is renally excreted, high levels may be found in the presence of renal failure, which makes the interpretation of the ISS in this setting challenging. The ISS is the current preferred staging method and has supplanted the previously used Durie-Salmon staging system, which was confounded by observer-dependent variables, such as degree of lytic bone lesions, that

Table 11-3 International Staging System

• Stage I **Parameters:** Albumin >3.5 g/dL and β_2-microglobulin <3.5 mg/L **Median Overall Survival:** 62 months
• Stage II **Parameters:** Neither stage I nor stage III **Median Overall Survival:** 44 months
• Stage III **Parameters:** β_2-microglobulin >5.5 mg/L **Median Overall Survival:** 29 months

added subjectivity in its assessment. It is important to note that the ISS has only been validated at the time of diagnosis in patients with MM and should not be extrapolated to patients with MGUS or SMM.

Risk Stratification

In addition to the ISS, patients can be stratified into standard-, intermediate-, and high-risk categories based on cytogenetic findings by both conventional karyotyping and FISH. Other high-risk features include elevated serum LDH, extramedullary disease, circulating plasma cells, and a high-risk GEP pattern as defined by a 70-gene panel. Risk stratification based on these criteria is summarized in Table 11-4.

Table 11-4 Risk Stratification of Newly Diagnosed Multiple Myeloma

Standard Risk	Intermediate Risk	High Risk
t(11;14) t(6;14) Hyperdiploid karyotype	t(4;14) Del 13q Hypodiploid karyotype	Del 17p13 Amplification of 1q21 t(14;20) t(14;16) Lactate dehydrogenase ≥2× institutional upper limit of normal Plasma cell leukemia High-risk gene expression profiling signature

Response Criteria

International Myeloma Working Group Uniform Response Criteria

The IMWG proposed new guidelines in 2006 to standardize response criteria in MM and to define disease progression to facilitate comparisons of outcomes between treatment centers and for reporting results in clinical trials. These International Uniform Response Criteria guidelines are summarized in Table 11-5. Assessment of response with M-protein measurements using serum protein electrophoresis, urine protein electrophoresis, and serum free light-chain assay is recommended prior to each cycle of therapy. Bone marrow biopsy is necessary to monitor disease in the

Table 11-5 IMWG International Uniform Response Criteria

Response Category	Criteria
sCR	Meets criteria for CR PLUS Normal FLC ratio AND No clonal cells in bone marrow by immunohistochemistry or immunofluorescence
CR	Negative serum and urine immunofixation AND Disappearance of any soft tissue plasmacytomas AND ≤5% plasma cells in bone marrow
VGPR	Serum and urine M-protein detectable by immunofixation but negative M-protein OR ≥90% reduction in serum M-protein plus urine M-protein level <100 mg per 24 h
PR	≥50% reduction of serum M-protein and reduction in 24-h urinary M-protein by ≥90% or to <200 mg per 24 h If unmeasurable serum and urine M-protein, ≥50% decrease in the difference between involved and uninvolved FLC levels If unmeasurable serum and urine M-protein serum FLC assay, ≥50% reduction in plasma cells is required in place of M-protein, as long as baseline bone marrow plasma cell percentage was ≥30% In addition to above criteria, a ≥50% reduction in the size of any baseline soft tissue plasmacytoma is required
SD	Not meeting criteria for CR, VGPR, PR, or progressive disease
PD	Increase of ≥25% from baseline in at least one of the following: Serum M-component (the absolute increase must be ≥0.5 g/dL) Urine M-component (the absolute increase must be ≥200 mg/24 h Difference between involved and uninvolved FLC levels if serum and urine M-protein are unmeasurable (the absolute increase must be >10 mg/dL) Bone marrow plasma cell percentage (the absolute % must be ≥10%) Development of new bone lesions or soft tissue plasmacytomas or definite increase in size of existing bone lesions or soft tissue plasmacytomas Development of hypercalcemia >11.5 mg/dL related to plasma cell dyscrasia

CR, complete response; FLC, free light chain; IMWG, International Myeloma Working Group; M-protein, monoclonal protein; PD, progressive disease; PR, partial response; sCR, stringent complete response; SD, stable disease; VGPR, very good partial response.

Adapted with permission from Durie BG, Harousseau JL, Miguel JS, et al. International uniform response criteria for multiple myeloma, *Leukemia* 2006 Sep;20(9):1467-1473.

absence of a measurable M-protein in the serum or urine or to document a complete or stringent complete response. Serial imaging assessments may be required if soft tissue plasmacytomas are present at baseline.

Minimal Residual Disease

In recent years, the fraction of patients achieving deep responses, including complete remission, after initial MM therapy has increased significantly. This correlates with improved progression-free survival (PFS) and overall survival (OS) in several studies ([10]). With a deepened level of remission, more sensitive methods to assess and monitor minimal residual disease (MRD) have been investigated. These include flow cytometry, allele-specific polymerase chain reaction (ASO-PCR), and next-generation sequencing (NGS)–based assays ([11]). MRD may soon be used as a valid surrogate end point to compare treatment strategies and advise on consolidation and maintenance therapies. At present, MRD assessment by multiparameter flow cytometry is the most reproducible method in MM. It has a sensitivity of 10^{-5} if at least 2×10^6 cells from bone marrow aspirates are analyzed. An international effort to adopt standardized or harmonized MRD detection assay and analysis by multiparameter flow cytometry in clinical practice and in clinical trials is ongoing.

Treatment of Newly Diagnosed Multiple Myeloma

After the diagnostic workup and risk stratification are complete, patients who meet the criteria for MM as defined by IMWG criteria should initiate therapy. The most important initial assessment is whether a patient is a candidate for high-dose chemotherapy and autologous stem cell transplantation (SCT), largely based on existing comorbidities and age. In the transplant-eligible population, current MM standard of care involves frontline chemotherapy, followed by consolidative high-dose melphalan and autologous SCT, followed by maintenance therapy. Some chemotherapy agents (eg, melphalan) may adversely affect stem cell collection and should be avoided in the initial therapy of transplant-eligible patients. Melphalan may be included in the frontline therapy of transplant-ineligible patients.

Frontline Therapy for Transplant-Eligible Patients

A number of different regimens can be used in the frontline setting for transplant-eligible patients. These usually consist of two- or three-drug combinations, and the choice of therapy is individualized based on factors such as patient comorbidities (neuropathy, diabetes), preferred route of administration (oral, intravenous, or subcutaneous), and underlying disease biology [eg, bortezomib in t(4;14) and del 13q]. Patients are usually given two to four cycles of therapy prior to stem cell collection to reduce disease burden before proceeding to high-dose chemotherapy and autologous stem cell rescue. Given the evidence that the depth and duration of response may translate into improved long-term outcomes, we generally prefer the three-drug regimens over the two-drug regimens as initial therapy in newly diagnosed patients.

Lenalidomide and Dexamethasone

The efficacy of the second-generation immunomodulatory drug (IMiD) lenalidomide combined with dexamethasone (Len/Dex) was initially demonstrated in the relapsed and refractory setting. Subsequently, a randomized phase III study in newly diagnosed MM compared lenalidomide plus high-dose dexamethasone versus placebo plus high-dose dexamethasone ([12]). Overall response rates (ORR), defined as a partial response or greater, and very good partial response (VGPR) rates were significantly higher in the Len/Dex arm (78% and 63%, respectively) versus the placebo/Dex arm (48% and 16%, respectively). The 1-year PFS rate was also higher in the Len/Dex arm (78% vs 52%), although there was no significant difference in OS between the two groups (94% vs 88%). Grade 3 or 4 neutropenia was higher with Len/Dex (21% vs 5%), as was the rate of venous thromboembolism (VTEs) (23.5% vs 5%) despite aspirin prophylaxis.

To possibly decrease the dexamethasone dose while retaining efficacy, a randomized study was conducted with lenalidomide in combination with high-dose dexamethasone (40 mg on days 1-4, 8-11, and 17-20 every 4 weeks) versus low-dose dexamethasone (40 mg on days 1, 8, 15, and 22 every 4 weeks) ([13]). Patients receiving high-dose dexamethasone achieved a higher ORR (79% vs 68%) after four cycles of therapy. However, a second interim analysis at 1 year demonstrated a statistically significant superior OS in the low-dose dexamethasone arm compared to the high-dose arm (96% vs 87%). This was attributed to increased toxicities of high-dose dexamethasone therapy including VTEs and infections. Based on this study, lenalidomide is recommended to be given in combination with low-dose dexamethasone.

Bortezomib and Dexamethasone

The proteasome inhibitor bortezomib in combination with dexamethasone was studied as frontline therapy in a large phase III trial comparing bortezomib and dexamethasone versus vincristine, doxorubicin, and dexamethasone (VAD) therapy prior to autologous SCT ([14]). Postinduction ORR (78.5% vs 62.8%), ≥VGPR rates (37.7% vs 15.1%), and complete response (CR) or near complete response (nCR) rates (14.8% vs 6.4%) all favored the bortezomib and dexamethasone arm over the VAD arm. There was also a trend toward improved median PFS in the bortezomib and dexamethasone arm (36.0 vs 29.7 months) but no difference in OS. In a separate analysis, initial treatment with bortezomib and dexamethasone prior to autologous SCT was shown to overcome the adverse prognostic features of t(4;14) in relation to event-free survival (EFS) and OS compared to VAD, although del 17p remained a poor prognostic factor regardless of the treatment regimen. Herpes simplex prophylaxis with acyclovir or valacyclovir should be given with bortezomib-containing regimens. Subcutaneous administration of bortezomib is preferred because it has similar efficacy as the intravenous route with decreased peripheral neuropathy ([15]).

Cyclophosphamide, Bortezomib, and Dexamethasone

The addition of oral cyclophosphamide to bortezomib and dexamethasone (CyBorD) was studied in phase II trials. In the EVOLUTION phase II trial, patients were randomized to receive bortezomib, lenalidomide, and dexamethasone (VRD); bortezomib, lenalidomide, cyclophosphamide, and dexamethasone (VDCR); or CyBorD, all followed by maintenance bortezomib for four 6-week cycles ([16]). The study was later amended to add an additional day 15 dose of cyclophosphamide, in addition to days 1 and 8, in patients receiving CyBorD. Patients receiving the modified CyBorD regimen achieved an ORR of 82%, with a VGPR or better rate of 53% and a CR rate of 47%. The 1-year PFS rate was 100%.

In another phase II study, standard twice-weekly (days 1, 4, 8, and 11) bortezomib was compared to weekly bortezomib (days 1, 8, 15, and 22) in combination with weekly cyclophosphamide and dexamethasone ([17]). ORR (88% vs 93%) and VGPR rates (60% vs 61%) were similar in both the twice-weekly and weekly bortezomib groups. In addition to demonstrating the efficacy of the three-drug combination of CyBorD, this study also suggested that weekly (instead of twice-weekly) bortezomib could be used to reduce treatment-related toxicity because it resulted in fewer grade 3 and 4 adverse events compared to the twice-weekly schedule (37% and 3% vs 48% and 12%, respectively).

Bortezomib, Lenalidomide, and Dexamethasone

The efficacy of VRD has also been demonstrated in several phase II trials. A phase I/II study evaluating the safety and efficacy of VRD resulted in an impressive 100% ORR in the phase II part, with 74% of patients achieving VGPR or better ([18]). As mentioned, VRD was also included as one of the arms in the phase II EVOLUTION trial, which resulted in an 85% ORR, with a VGPR or better rate of 51% and a CR rate of 24% ([16]). Phase III studies are ongoing comparing VRD with bortezomib and dexamethasone (NCT00522392) or lenalidomide and dexamethasone (NCT00644228) in the frontline setting. In addition, the role and timing of autologous SCT are being reexamined in the era of novel agents in a large international phase III trial of frontline VRD followed by lenalidomide maintenance therapy (with the option of SCT at the time of relapse) versus VRD followed by autologous SCT as per the current standard of care (NCT01208662). Phase II studies are also evaluating the efficacy of the second-generation proteasome inhibitor carfilzomib in combination with lenalidomide and dexamethasone (CRD) in the frontline setting with delayed autologous SCT; early results show rapid and deep responses with less peripheral neuropathy ([19, 20]). These studies will clarify the role of novel triplet combinations in the frontline setting and provide insight as to whether deeper responses, including molecular responses, with the multiple novel agents in combination, ultimately translate into improved long-term outcomes (Table 11-6).

Frontline Therapy for Transplant-Ineligible Patients

Initial treatment regimens for transplant-eligible patients can also be used in transplant-ineligible patients. Without the need to collect autologous stem cells, the alkylating agent melphalan can be incorporated into frontline therapy in nontransplant candidates. For 40 years, melphalan and prednisone (MP) represented the standard of care for transplant-ineligible patients. However, the addition of novel agents to the MP backbone and non–melphalan-containing combinations now form the new standard of preferred regimens.

Thalidomide/Lenalidomide, Melphalan, and Prednisone

The Gruppo Italiano Malattie Ematologiche dell'Adult (GIMEMA) compared melphalan, prednisone, and thalidomide (MPT) with MP ([21]). The ORR (76% vs 47.6%) and nCR/CR rates (27.9% vs 7.2%) favored the MPT arm. The median PFS was better in the MPT arm (21.8 vs 14.5 months), although the median OS was similar (45.0 vs 47.6 months). Subsequent phase III studies also demonstrated improved ORR and PFS with MPT compared to MP, with both the Intergroupe Francophone du Myélome (IFM) 99-06 and IFM 01-01 studies also showing a higher OS rate with MPT compared to MP.

Melphalan, prednisone, and lenalidomide (MPL) was also compared with MP alone in a phase III trial comparing MPL with lenalidomide maintenance (MPL-L) versus MPL versus MP ([22]). The ORR was significantly higher in patients receiving MPL-L or MPL (77% and 68%, respectively) compared to those receiving MP (50%). Although MPT and MPL are superior to MP

Table 11-6 Phase II and III Clinical Trials for Selected Frontline Regimens in Transplant-Eligible Multiple Myeloma Patients

Author	Phase	Treatment (No.)	% ORR (CR)	PFS	OS
Zonder et al ([12])	III	Len + HD Dex (97) HD Dex (95)	78 (26)[a] 48 (4)	1-year: 78%[a] 1-year: 52%	3-year: 79% 3-year: 73%
Rajkumar et al ([13])	III	Len + HD Dex (223) Len + LD Dex (222)	81 (5)[a] 70 (4)	19.1 mo 25.3 mo[a]	1-year: 87% 1-year: 97%[a]
Harousseau et al ([14])	III	VAD (242) VD (240)	63 (3) 79 (13)[a]	29.7 mo 36.0 mo	3-year: 77% 3-year: 81%
Kumar et al ([16])	II	CyBorD (33) VRD (42) VRDC (48) CyBorD-mod (17)	75 (22) 85 (24) 88 (25) 100 (47)	1-year: 93% 1-year: 83% 1-year: 86% 1-year: 100%	1-year: 100% 1-year: 100% 1-year: 92% 1-year: 100%
Richardson et al ([18])	II	VRD (35)	100 (37)	18-month: 75%[b]	18-month: 97%[b]

CR, complete response; CyBorD, cyclophosphamide, bortezomib, dexamethasone; CyBorD-mod, modified CyBorD with additional day 15 cyclophosphamide dose; HD Dex, high-dose dexamethasone; LD Dex, low-dose dexamethasone; Len, lenalidomide; ORR, overall response rate; OS, overall survival; PFS, progression-free survival; VAD, vincristine, doxorubicin, dexamethasone; VD, bortezomib, dexamethasone; VRD, bortezomib, lenalidomide, dexamethasone; VRDC, bortezomib, lenalidomide, dexamethasone, cyclophosphamide.

[a]Statistically significant.

[b]Includes patients in phase I portion of study.

CHAPTER 11

alone in terms of ORR and PFS, increased toxicity with the addition of a third drug must be carefully balanced with enhanced efficacy, because grade 3 and 4 adverse events were more pronounced in the MPT and MPL arms compared to MP. Although not compared head-to-head, nonhematologic grade 3 and 4 adverse events were less frequent with MPL compared to MPT ([22, 23]).

Bortezomib, Melphalan, and Prednisone

Bortezomib plus MP (VMP) was also compared with MP alone in a large randomized phase III trial. The ORR and CR rates were 71% and 30%, respectively, in patients receiving VMP versus 35% and 4%, respectively, in the MP arm. Median PFS was better with VMP (24.0 vs 16.6 months). An OS benefit for VMP versus MP (median, 56.4 vs 43.1 months) was also reported in the final analysis ([24]). Again, the benefits of efficacy must be weighed carefully against toxicity, as grade 3 and 4 adverse events, particularly peripheral neuropathy, were greater in the VMP arm (13%).

Non–Melphalan-Based Regimens

The role of melphalan-containing regimens in transplant-ineligible patients has been challenged. Lenalidomide and low-dose dexamethasone (Rd) in four-week cycles until disease progression versus the same regimen for a fixed duration of 72 weeks versus MPT in 6-week cycles for 72 weeks were compared in a randomized phase III study in over 1,500 transplant-ineligible patients ([25]). Although the ORRs were similar between the three arms, median PFS favored continuous Rd (25.5 months) versus 18 cycles of Rd (20.7 months) and MPT (21.2 months). There was a trend toward improved 3-year OS with continuous Rd (59%) versus fixed-duration Rd (56%) and MPT (51%). There was also a trend toward fewer grade 3 and 4 adverse events in the continuous Rd arm (70%) compared to the MPT arm (78%), in particular grade 3 and 4 neutropenia and neuropathy. However, there was a higher incidence of grade 3 and 4 infections with continuous Rd (29%), likely related to the longer duration of glucocorticoid use.

A community-based phase IIIB trial compared bortezomib and dexamethasone (BD) versus bortezomib, thalidomide, and dexamethasone (BTD) versus melphalan, prednisone, and bortezomib (MPB) followed by maintenance bortezomib ([26]). The ORR, PFS, and OS were similar across all three arms. Discontinuation due to adverse events was highest in the BTD arm (35%) compared to BD (24%) and MPB (30%). This demonstrates the safety and efficacy of the use of BD in the elderly population. In general, the incorporation of novel agents to combination therapy has improved ORR and long-term outcomes in elderly, transplant-ineligible patients. However, treatment must be individualized based on comorbidities and disease characteristics as well as the patient's own goals of care (Table 11-7).

Stem Cell Transplantation

Autologous Stem Cell Transplantation

High-dose melphalan without autologous SCT was first reported in 1983 by McElwain and colleagues from the Royal Marsden Hospital. Compared with chemotherapy alone, intensified chemotherapy followed by autologous SCT appears to prolong OS in previously untreated patients with MM. One comparative study and two randomized trials showed that autologous SCT provided survival benefits of approximately 12 months.

In the French IFM 90 trial, high-dose chemotherapy supported by autologous SCT was compared with conventional chemotherapy in 200 previously untreated patients with MM <65 years of age ([27]). The results showed a higher CR rate (22% vs 5%) and higher rates of 5-year EFS (28% vs 10%) and OS (52% vs 12%) in the autologous SCT group. The median OS in patients assigned to the SCT arm was 13 months longer (57 vs 44 months).

The Medical Research Council Myeloma VII trial compared conventional-dose chemotherapy with high-dose therapy and autologous SCT in 401 previously untreated patients with MM <65 years old ([28]). The rates of CR were significantly higher in the autologous SCT group (44% vs 8%). Intent-to-treat analysis showed a significant higher rate of OS and PFS with SCT. Compared with standard therapy, autologous SCT increased median OS by almost 12 months (54.1 vs 42.3 months). There was a trend toward a greater survival benefit in patients with poor prognosis (defined by β_2-microglobulin level >8 mg/L).

In three other randomized studies, however, there has been no survival benefit with autologous SCT ([29-31]). Comparison among these trials is difficult due to the variability in patient eligibility including age, induction chemotherapy, conditioning regimen for SCT, and definitions of response. Subsequent trials have confirmed that autologous SCT deepens the response obtained with primary therapy. Thus, autologous SCT has become standard of care for eligible patients based on performance status and organ function. Most recently, a retrospective analysis of 1,038 patients with MM treated at the Mayo Clinic (2001-2010) reported a superior OS after autologous SCT. The median OS was 4.9 years without autologous SCT and not reached with autologous SCT ([32]).

Many different preparative regimens have been assessed over the last 20 years, but only one prospective randomized trial by the IFM has directly compared two different preparative regimens ([33]). In 282 newly diagnosed patients <65 years old, high-dose melphalan at 200 mg/m^2 was shown to be superior to a combination of melphalan 140 mg/m^2 plus 8 Gy of total-body irradiation (TBI), mainly due to reduced toxicity including

Table 11-7 Phase III Trials for Selected Frontline Regimens in Transplant-Ineligible Multiple Myeloma Patients

Author	Treatment (No.)	% ORR (CR)	Median PFS (months)	Median OS (months)
Facon et al ([103])	MPT (125) MP (196)	76 (13)[a] 35 (2)	27.5[a] 17.8	51.6[a] 33.2
Palumbo et al ([21, 104])	MPT (129) MP (126)	76 (16)[a] 48 (2)	21.8[a] 14.5	45 47.6
Hulin et al ([23])	MPT (115) MP (117)	62 (7)[a] 31 (1)	24.1[a] 18.5	44[a] 29.1
Waage et al ([105])	MPT (184) MP (179)	57 (13)[a] 40 (4)	15 14	29 32
Wijermans et al ([106])	MPT (165) MP (168)	66 (NR)[a] 45 (NR)	15[a] 11	40[a] 31
Palumbo et al ([22])	MPR-R (152) MPR (153) MP (154)	77 (10)[a] 68 (3)[a] 50 (3)	31[a] 14 13	3-year: 70% 3-year: 62% 3-year: 66%
San Miguel et al ([24, 107])	VMP (344) MP (338)	71 (30)[a] 35 (4)	24[a] 16.6	56.4[a] 43.1
Benboubker et al ([25])	RD to PD (535) RD × 72 weeks (541) MPT × 72 weeks (547)	75 (15)[a] 73 (14)[a] 62 (9)	25.5[a] 20.7 21.2	4 year: 59% 4 year: 56% 4-year: 51%
Niesvizky et al ([26])	BD (146) BTD (133) VMP (144)	73 (30) 80 (40) 69 (33)	13.8 14.7 17.3	1-year: 87% 1-year: 86% 1-year: 89%

BD, bortezomib, dexamethasone; BTD, bortezomib, thalidomide, dexamethasone; CR, complete response; MP, melphalan, prednisone; MPR, melphalan, prednisone, lenalidomide; MPR-R, MPR with lenalidomide maintenance; MPT, melphalan, prednisone, thalidomide; NR, not reported; ORR, overall response rate; OS, overall survival; PD, pomalidomide plus low-dose dexamethasone; PFS, progression-free survival; RD, lenalidomide, dexamethasone; VMP, bortezomib plus MP.
[a]Statistically significant.

CHAPTER 11

mucositis and transplant-related mortality. Melphalan remains the standard of care, but the addition of novel agents to conditioning is being investigated.

Transplantation can be performed either early after induction therapy or later at disease progression. Fermand et al compared early and late autologous SCT and reported a similar OS ([31]). However, the average time without symptoms, treatment, and treatment toxicity were significantly better with early autologous SCT. A retrospective study of 167 patients who received induction therapy containing at least one of three novel agents (lenalidomide, thalidomide, or bortezomib) followed by autologous SCT either within 12 months of diagnosis or later found a higher CR rate in the early autologous SCT arm but no difference in PFS or OS. The potential benefit of early versus late autologous SCT was assessed in a trial randomizing patients between 55 and 65 years of age to either conventional chemotherapy alone or chemotherapy followed by autologous SCT. With a median follow-up of 120 months, a trend toward better EFS, but no OS benefit, was observed in patients undergoing early transplantation ([31]). Finally, the US Intergroup Trial S9321 found no PFS or OS benefit with early SCT ([29]). A recent cost analysis study by Pandya et al suggests that early autologous SCT is cost-effective compared to delayed autologous SCT ([34]).

At MDACC, we offer autologous SCT to all eligible patients after induction therapy regardless of age. We use a preparative regimen of melphalan 200 mg/m^2 (unless the patient is treated on a clinical trial with a novel preparative regimen). In selected patients (>70 years old or dialysis dependent), we lower the melphalan dose to 140 mg/m^2. We offer tandem autologous SCT only in the setting of a clinical trial or if there is significant residual disease after first autologous SCT. A second salvage transplant is an option for patients with relapsed disease; we offer this mainly to patients whose benefit from transplant was >1 year and whose disease burden can be significantly reduced by salvage chemotherapy. We offer maintenance therapy after transplantation (discussed later).

Allogeneic Stem Cell Transplantation

The curative potential of allogeneic SCT results from a graft-versus-tumor effect and dose-intense therapy rescued with a tumor-free graft. The existence of a graft-versus-myeloma effect was first documented by Tricot and colleagues and later confirmed in large single- and multi-institutional series of donor lymphocyte infusions. High-dose therapy is toxic but potentially curative. To overcome toxicity from high-dose regimens and to extend applicability to older patients with significant comorbidities, allogeneic SCT with reduced-intensity conditioning regimens has been attempted.

Two prospective trials investigated a tandem autologous plus reduced-intensity allogeneic SCT approach as part of the initial therapy for MM, with conflicting results. The IFM group reported on the outcomes of patients with high-risk disease (defined at the time as high levels of β_2-microglobulin and deletion of chromosome 13 by FISH) who received initial autologous SCT with melphalan 200 mg/m^2 ([35]). Sixty-five patients had an human leukocyte antigen (HLA)-identical sibling donor, of whom 46 received a reduced-intensity conditioning regimen consisting of fludarabine, busulfan, and antithymocyte globulin (ATG). Patients without an HLA sibling donor received a second autologous SCT prepared with melphalan 220 mg/m^2. On an intent-to-treat basis, the OS and the EFS did not differ significantly between the two groups (median OS and EFS, 35 and 25 months with allogeneic SCT vs 41 and 30 months with autologous SCT, respectively). There was a trend toward better OS with tandem autologous SCT (median, 47.2 vs 35 months) for patients who actually received a reduced-intensity allogeneic SCT.

The Italian Cooperative Group performed a similar study ([36]). After a median follow-up of 3 years, nonrelapse mortality was 11% for the autologous-plus-allogeneic group versus 4% for the tandem autologous group (P = 0.09). The CR rates were significantly higher in the autologous-plus-allogeneic group than the tandem autologous group (46% vs 16%), as was OS (84% vs 62%) and EFS (75% vs 41%). A follow-up analysis at 7 years further suggests a long-term survival and disease-free survival advantage with allogeneic SCT over standard autologous SCT (median OS, not reached vs 5.3 years; median EFS, 39 vs 33 months) ([37]). The Bone Marrow Transplant Clinical Trials Network (BMT CTN) enrolled 710 patients, of whom 625 had standard-risk disease; 156 patients received autologous SCT followed by allogeneic SCT, whereas 366 patients underwent tandem autologous SCT. The 3-year PFS was 43% with autologous-allogeneic SCT and 46% with autologous-autologous SCT. No OS difference was seen ([38]). A long-term follow-up analysis of the NMAM2000 study by the European Society for Blood and Marrow Transplantation demonstrated that PFS and OS with autologous SCT followed by reduced-intensity allogeneic SCT were improved at 96 months compared to autologous SCT alone (PFS and OS: 22% and 49% vs 12% and 36%, respectively) ([39]). Specifically, autologous SCT followed by reduced-intensity conditioning allogeneic SCT seemed to overcome the poor prognostic impact of del 13q.

At MDACC, we only perform reduced-intensity allogeneic SCT. We use the tandem autologous plus allogeneic SCT approach only in the setting of a clinical trial. Allogeneic SCTs are offered to patients with relapsed, chemotherapy-sensitive disease who are <70 years old, have an HLA-identical sibling or unrelated donor, and are in good general physical condition. Our preparative regimen is a combination of fludarabine and melphalan (100 or 140 mg/m^2), with ATG added for unrelated donor SCT.

To improve outcomes of autologous transplantation by adding a graft-versus-myeloma component, current laboratory research and clinical trials at MDACC are focused on eradicating MRD after autologous SCT using cellular therapy and vaccines.

Maintenance Therapy

The curability of MM has long been a matter of discussion. A small proportion of patient may achieve long-term survival and possibly a cure, but most patients relapse even after initial complete remission is achieved ([40]). To delay the time to disease recurrence, maintenance therapy following autologous SCT has been explored to limit growth of residual malignant plasma cells. Initial maintenance strategies included interferon-α, although treatment-related toxicities such as flu-like symptoms and malaise made it challenging to administer. The approval of thalidomide in the late 1990s renewed interest in maintenance therapy. Multiple trials showed improvements in PFS and sometimes OS with thalidomide maintenance after autologous SCT. Toxicities related to long-term therapy, notably peripheral neuropathy, made it difficult to tolerate.

Given its more favorable side effect profile, lenalidomide maintenance therapy after autologous SCT was next explored. The Cancer and Leukemia Group B (CALGB) study randomized patients to lenalidomide or placebo maintenance starting 100 days following autologous SCT ([41]). PFS was significantly greater in the lenalidomide arm (46 vs 27 months); OS was also significantly better. The IFM reported a similar trial in which patients received two 4-week cycles of consolidation with lenalidomide 25 mg after autologous SCT before being randomized to lenalidomide maintenance versus placebo ([42]). PFS also favored lenalidomide maintenance (median PFS, 41 vs 23 months), but there was no difference in OS. Both studies reported an increase in second primary malignancies with lenalidomide maintenance (8% in the CALGB and IFM studies) versus placebo (3% in CALGB and 4% in IFM). However, when all competing factors for death are considered (including death from relapsed MM), patients have a much higher risk of mortality from other causes rather than secondary malignancies ([43, 44]). Potential risks and benefits of lenalidomide maintenance should be discussed with patients to make informed decisions. Lenalidomide maintenance can also be considered in nontransplant patients after initial therapy based on the phase III MPL-L versus MPL versus MP study described earlier ([22]).

Bortezomib maintenance therapy was investigated in the phase III Hemato-Oncologie voor Volwassenen Nederland (HOVON)-65/German Multicenter Myeloma Group (GMMG)-HD4 trial, where patients were randomized to receive either VAD or bortezomib, doxorubicin, and dexamethasone (PAD) induction, followed by high-dose melphalan and autologous SCT ([45]). Patients were then randomized again to receive either thalidomide or bortezomib maintenance therapy for 2 years. The CR rates, PFS, and OS all favored bortezomib-containing induction and maintenance regimens, and benefit was also noted in high-risk patients with del 17p. In general, we offer patients lenalidomide maintenance therapy following autologous SCT at MDACC. In the setting of high-risk cytogenetic features, bortezomib consolidation/maintenance should be considered based on the HOVON data.

Treatment of Relapsed/Refractory Multiple Myeloma

We recommend enrollment in clinical trials when possible for all patients with relapsed/refractory MM. Alternatively, there are a number of therapeutic options that have gained regulatory approval that may be considered in this setting.

Immunomodulatory Drugs

Many patients may already be on maintenance lenalidomide at the time of disease recurrence. Increasing to standard-dose lenalidomide (25 mg daily for 21 out of 28 days) with or without dexamethasone is an option. Two large phase III trials demonstrated the efficacy of lenalidomide and dexamethasone compared to dexamethasone alone, with ORR, PFS, and OS favoring the combination. Although high-dose dexamethasone was used in these trials, low-dose dexamethasone is typically given in combination with lenalidomide in this setting, extrapolating from data comparing these approaches in frontline therapy.

Pomalidomide is a third-generation IMiD with greater in vivo potency than thalidomide and lenalidomide. In a phase III study in relapsed/refractory MM, patients were randomized to receive either pomalidomide plus low-dose dexamethasone (Pd) versus only high-dose dexamethasone ([46]). Around 75% patients were double refractory to both lenalidomide and bortezomib. The ORR was 35% with Pd versus 10% with high-dose dexamethasone. The median PFS was 4.0 months with Pd versus 1.9 months with high-dose dexamethasone. Based on these results, pomalidomide gained US Food and Drug Administration (FDA) approval in 2013 for MM refractory to last therapy and prior bortezomib and lenalidomide exposure.

Proteasome Inhibitors

Bortezomib has shown efficacy in relapsed MM in two large randomized phase III trials. The APEX phase III trial compared intravenous bortezomib to high-dose dexamethasone; ORR, PFS, and OS were all superior in the bortezomib arm. As mentioned, subcutaneous bortezomib is favored over the intravenous route due to similar efficacy and less peripheral neuropathy ([15]).

Bortezomib has also been studied in combination with other agents. The addition of pegylated liposomal doxorubicin in combination with bortezomib gained regulatory approval after demonstrating superior PFS compared to bortezomib monotherapy in relapsed/refractory bortezomib-naïve MM patients, although the ORRs were not statistically different between the two groups ([47]). Phase II data of VRD in relapsed/refractory MM resulted in an ORR of 64%. Median PFS was 8.5 months, and median OS was 30 months ([48]). The CyBorD regimen may also be considered in relapsed MM based on phase II data.

The second-generation proteasome inhibitor carfilzomib recently gained regulatory approval for patients exposed to bortezomib and an IMiD and whose disease was refractory to last therapy. Like bortezomib, carfilzomib inhibits the chymotrypsin-like activity of the 20S proteasome, but its unique structural properties allow for greater specificity and irreversible binding to its target. The efficacy of carfilzomib in relapsed/refractory MM was established in a single-arm phase II trial of 266 patients, all of whom received prior IMiD therapy, and all but one patient received prior bortezomib ([49]). The ORR was 24%. Among 169 patients refractory to both bortezomib and lenalidomide, the ORR was 15%. Only 12% of patients reported any grade of treatment-emergent peripheral neuropathy.

The role of carfilzomib in relapsed and/or refractory MM continues to evolve, as it is being tested in combination with other novel agents. Interim results of a phase III study comparing carfilzomib, lenalidomide, and dexamethasone (CRd) with lenalidomide and dexamethasone (Rd) were recently reported ([50]). In this study, 66% of patients received prior bortezomib and 20% received prior lenalidomide. The median PFS was significantly longer with CRd compared with Rd (26.3 vs 17.6 months). The combination of carfilzomib, pomalidomide, and dexamethasone has also shown promising results ([51]). However, the impact of carfilzomib on OS is uncertain. An interim analysis of a phase III study that randomized relapsed/refractory patients to carfilzomib versus glucocorticoid therapy did not meet its primary end point of OS benefit ([52]). Finally, although earlier studies established the maximum-tolerated dose of carfilzomib at 20 mg/m^2 for cycle 1 and 27 mg/m^2 for subsequent cycles, phase I and II data have emerged demonstrating the safety and efficacy of higher doses of carfilzomib up to 56 mg/m^2 administered over 30 minutes compared to a 2- to 10-minute intravenous bolus given in earlier studies ([53]). An ongoing Southwest Oncology Group randomized phase II study is comparing high-dose versus low-dose carfilzomib (with dexamethasone in both arms).

Investigational Agents

Although IMiDs and proteasome inhibitors now form the backbone of most MM regimens, both in the upfront and relapsed settings, several promising new classes of investigational agents have shown both safety and promising efficacy in phase I and II clinical trials. These include novel immunotherapeutic approaches with the anti-CD38 antibody daratumumab ([54]) and the anti-SLAMF7 antibody elotuzumab in combination with lenalidomide and low-dose dexamethasone ([55]), both of which have garnered "breakthrough therapy" designations from the FDA based on early efficacy data. Phase III studies are comparing lenalidomide and low-dose dexamethasone with or without elotuzumab in both relapsed/refractory (NCT01239797) and newly diagnosed MM (NCT01891643). These same combinations with lenalidomide and low-dose dexamethasone are also being tested in phase III trials with daratumumab in both relapsed/refractory (NCT02076009) and frontline MM (NCT02252172).

Histone deacetylase (HDAC) inhibitors have also shown promising activity. Although they only have modest activity as single agents, the potential of HDAC inhibitors has been most pronounced in combination with other anti-MM drugs, namely bortezomib. Disruption of aggresome formation by HDAC inhibition may provide potent synergy with proteasome inhibition by interfering with protein turnover and inducing the unfolded protein response. Based on this rationale, the pan-deacetylase inhibitor panobinostat was studied in combination with bortezomib and dexamethasone and compared to placebo, bortezomib, and dexamethasone in a large phase III trial ([56]). At interim analysis, PFS was significantly higher with panobinostat compared to placebo (11.99 vs 8.08 months); OS was similar. The ORR did not differ between the arms, although the depth of response (CR or nCR) was significantly higher in the panobinostat arm. Concerns have been raised about drug efficacy (measured only by PFS) in the setting of significant toxicities, particularly grade 3 and 4 thrombocytopenia, diarrhea, and fatigue. In the future, more selective HDAC inhibitors with fewer off-target effects may need to be developed and tested for the full potential of this therapeutic approach to be realized.

ARRY-520, a novel antimitotic, inhibits the kinesin-spindle protein (KSP). In a phase II study, ARRY-520 was given with or without low-dose dexamethasone in relapsed/refractory MM ([57]). Patients in the cohort with low-dose dexamethasone were all refractory to lenalidomide and bortezomib; the ORR was 22%. A phase II trial with ARRY-520 in combination with carfilzomib or bortezomib is ongoing (Table 11-8).

Monoclonal Gammopathy of Undetermined Significance

The 2014 IMWG guidelines define MGUS as a serum M-protein <3 g/dL, <10% clonal marrow plasma cells, and absence of end-organ damage (CRAB criteria and myeloma-defining events; see Table 11-2) attributed to an underlying plasma cell proliferative disorder. The 2014 standard of care for MGUS is surveillance every 6 to 12 months with a physical exam and typical MM serum and urine studies. Patients with MGUS can also be risk stratified for progression to MM according to established models (Table 11-9).

Smoldering Multiple Myeloma

Smoldering MM is defined as having a serum M-protein of ≥3.0 g/dL and/or ≥10% more marrow plasma cells without evidence of end-organ damage as defined by CRAB criteria and MM-defining events (see Table 11-2). Compared with MGUS, this premalignant clonal plasma cell proliferation carries a higher risk of progression to overt MM. In a large retrospective study of 276 patients with SMM followed over 26 years, the risk of progression to MM was 10% per year for the first 5 years, 3% per year for the next 5 years, and 1% per year for the last 10 years.

There is great heterogeneity in the SMM disease course. Some patients may remain asymptomatic for the rest of their lives, whereas others may rapidly develop disease that meets MM criteria. Efforts have been made to risk stratify SMM to help predict the clinical course, guide surveillance strategies, and design trials for early intervention. One prognostic model found that patients with both clonal bone marrow plasmacytosis ≥10% and serum M-protein ≥3 g/dL had an 87% chance of MM progression at 15 years compared to 70% with only ≥10% marrow plasma cells (but monoclonal protein of <3 g/dL) and 39% with only monoclonal protein ≥3 g/dL (but <10% bone marrow plasma cells) ([58]). Later, a serum free light-chain ratio of <0.125 or >8 was suggested as an independent prognostic factor for disease progression and incorporated into the prognostic score for SMM. A number of other factors have been shown to increase the risk of progression such as high-risk cytogenetics [del 17p, t(4;14), amplification of 1q], ≥95% aberrant marrow plasma cells by flow cytometry, IgA M-protein, immunoparesis of uninvolved immunoglobulins, circulating

Table 11-8 Phase II and III Clinical Trials Leading to Regulatory Approval of Novel Agents for Relapsed and/or Refractory Multiple Myeloma Patients

Author	Phase	Treatment (No.)	% ORR (CR)	Median PFS	OS
Richardson et al ([108])	III	Bortezomib (333) HD-Dex (336)	38 (6)[a] 18 (1)	6.2[a] 3.5	80% at 1 year[a] 66% at 1 year
Orlowski et al ([47])	III	Bortezomib + PLD (324) Bortezomib (322)	44 (4) 41 (2)	9.3[a] 6.5	76% at 15 months[a] 65% at 15 months
Weber et al ([109])	III	Lenalidomide + HD-Dex (177) HD-Dex (176)	61 (14)[a] 20 (1)	11.1[a] 4.1	29.6[a] 20.2
Dimopoulos et al ([110])	III	Lenalidomide + HD-Dex (176) HD-Dex (175)	60 (16)[a] 24 (3)	11.3[a] 4.7	NYR[a] 20.6
San Miguel et al ([46])	III	Pomalidomide + LD-Dex (302) HD-Dex (153)	31 (1)[a] 10 (0)	4.0[a] 1.9	12.7[a] 8.1
Siegel et al ([49])	II	Carfilzomib (257)	24 (0)	3.7	15.6

CR, complete response; HD-Dex, high-dose dexamethasone; LD-Dex, low-dose dexamethasone; NYR, not yet reached; ORR, overall response rate; OS, overall survival; PFS, progression-free survival; PLD, pegylated liposomal doxorubicin.
[a]Statistically significant.

CHAPTER 11

Table 11-9 Risk Stratification Models for MGUS and SMM

MGUS			
Mayo Clinic ([111])	**No. of Risk Factors**	**No. of Patients**	**20-Year Progression (%)**
Risk factors:	0	449	5%
1) M-protein >1.5 g/dL	1	420	21%
2) Non-IgG MGUS	2	226	37%
3) FLC ratio <0.26 or >1.65	3	53	58%
	Total	1148	20%
PETHEMA ([112])			5-year progression (%)
Risk factors	0	127	2%
1) ≥95% abnormal PCs by bone marrow flow cytometry	1	133	10%
	2	16	46%
2) DNA aneuploidy	Total	276	8.5%
SMM			
Mayo Clinic ([113])	No. of Risk Factors	No. of Patients	5-Year Progression (%)
Risk factors:	1	76	25%
1) Bone marrow plasma cells ≥ 10%	2	115	51%
2) M-protein ≥ 3g/dL	3	82	76%
3) FLC ratio <0.125 or > 8	Total	273	51%
PETHEMA ([112])			
Risk factors:	0	28	4%
1) ≥95% abnormal PC	1	22	46%
2) Immunoparesis	2	39	72%
	Total	89	46%
SWOG ([114])			2-Year Progression (%)
Risk factors:	0	33	3%
1) GEP70 score >–0.26 ([115])	1	29	29.1%
2) M-protein >3 g/dL	≥2	17	70.6%
3) Involved serum FLC >25 mg/dL	Total	79	34.2%

FLC, free light chain; GEP70, gene expression profiling 70; IgG, immunoglobulin G; immunoparesis, decreased in uninvolved immunoglobulins below the lower limit of normal; MGUS, monoclonal gammopathy of undetermined significance; PC, plasma cells; PETHEMA, Program para el Tratamiento de Hemopatias Malignas; SMM, smoldering multiple myeloma; SWOG, Southwest Oncology Group.

plasma cells by slide-based immunofluorescence, and proteinuria ([59]).

Through these studies, a very-high-risk group was identified, with a 2-year progression risk of 70% to 80%, when there is at least one of the following risk factors: ≥60% bone marrow plasmacytosis, an involved-to-uninvolved serum free light-chain ratio ≥100, or more than one focal lesion on MRI that is at least 5 mm in size. This prompted revisiting the classical definition of SMM and led the IMWG in 2014 to recategorize asymptomatic patients with SMM who meet these criteria as having active MM requiring therapy ([9]).

The benefits of preemptive treatment of high-risk SMM are still unclear. Until this is further clarified, treatment of high-risk SMM should be undertaken preferentially through clinical trials. A phase III trial comparing lenalidomide and dexamethasone versus observation in high-risk patients found an improvement in median PFS in the treatment arm (median PFS, not reached vs 26 months) and a significant 3-year OS benefit (94% vs 80%, $P = 0.03$) ([60]). However, results have not yet been replicated in other studies, and an excessive mortality rate in the observation arm for SMM patients has raised concerns about the interpretation of these results.

At MDACC, we recommend that patients with high-risk SMM be enrolled in a clinical trial. In the absence of clear data, we would otherwise recommend observation and close surveillance in these patients, although this practice may change soon as we gather data from relevant trials focused on high-risk SMM.

Solitary Plasmacytoma of Bone

A solitary plasmacytoma of bone is defined by the presence of a plasmacytoma without bone marrow evidence of monoclonal plasma cells, lytic bony lesions, or other clinically significant sequelae of MM. About 24% to 72% of patients with a solitary plasmacytoma have a monoclonal protein in the serum or urine. Initial workup should include all of the aforementioned serum and urine laboratory studies used in evaluation of MM, as well as advanced imaging with PET-CT or MRI to rule out multifocal disease that would upstage the disease to MM. Biopsy of the solitary plasmacytoma to demonstrate clonal plasma cells and a unilateral bone marrow biopsy to rule out systemic disease are necessary. Treatment should include radiation therapy of at least 40 Gy, although one may consider a dose of up to 50 Gy for lesions greater than 5 cm. After radiation therapy, surveillance should be performed with serial measurements of serum and urine M-protein levels and imaging studies, initially every 3 months and then less frequently. Patients who progress to overt MM during surveillance should follow the treatment guidelines for MM.

Patients with solitary plasmacytoma of bone often progress to MM within 2 to 4 years, with a median OS of 7.5 to 12 years. In one study, persistence of a serum M-protein 1 year after radiation therapy was an adverse prognostic factor predicting a 10-year myeloma-free survival of 29% compared to 91% with undetectable M-protein. Another study found that an abnormal free light-chain ratio and a serum M-protein >0.5 g/dL were significant adverse factors for disease progression at 5 years.

OTHER PLASMA CELL DYSCRASIAS

Waldenström Macroglobulinemia

Background

Waldenström macroglobulinemia is an uncommon, low-grade malignancy characterized by the presence of lymphoplasmacytic cells together with the presence of a monoclonal IgM paraprotein. The median age at diagnosis is between 63 and 68 years. Men are more commonly affected, and the disease is more common among whites than other populations. Recent data show that 67% to 100% of WM cases are associated with a mutation of the myeloid differentiation primary response 88 (*MYD88*) gene located on chromosome 3p22 ([61]).

Clinical Presentation and Diagnostic Workup

Many patients are asymptomatic at diagnosis. When symptoms develop, they are caused by tumor infiltration (cytopenias, hepatomegaly, splenomegaly), circulating IgM (hyperviscosity, cryoglobulinemia, and/or cold agglutinin anemia), and/or tissue deposition of IgM (neuropathy, glomerular disease, and/or amyloidosis). Symptomatic hyperviscosity syndrome may be associated with visual disturbances, dizziness, cardiopulmonary symptoms, decreased consciousness, and a bleeding diathesis. Polyneuropathies are common. Some are associated with antigenic targets of the monoclonal serum IgM, including myelin-associated glycoprotein (MAG) and sulphatide. Others are caused by direct tumor infiltration, tissue deposition of IgM, the amount and properties of the circulating monoclonal IgM, or binding of unidentified antigens. Patients may also present with cold or warm autoimmune hemolytic anemia, iron deficiency anemia, or dilutional anemia.

Initial evaluation (Table 11-10) in suspected WM should include a CBC, serum chemistries, liver function tests, viral hepatitis serologies, serum protein electrophoresis (SPEP) and immunofixation, quantitative immunoglobulin levels, and a β_2-microglobulin. In patients suspected of having a cryoglobulinemia, a cryocrit should be drawn and, together with SPEP and quantitative immunoglobulin specimens, should immediately be placed in a 37°C water bath to facilitate accurate assessment. A serum viscosity level and cold agglutinin titer/Coombs test should be drawn if hyperviscosity or a hemolytic anemia, respectively, is suspected. Iron studies should be considered for patients having a microcytic anemia. Bone marrow biopsy should be performed to demonstrate infiltration by lymphoplasmacytic cells and can help determine the cause of an existing anemia. Flow cytometry

Table 11-10 Initial Workup for Waldenström Macroglobulinemia

Essential Testing	Useful Under Certain Circumstances
History and physical CBC with differential, BUN, creatinine, electrolytes, liver function tests Quantitative immunoglobulins Serum protein electrophoresis (SPEP) and immunofixation Urine protein electrophoresis (UPEP) and immunofixation Serum viscosity[a] Hepatitis B and C serology Cryocrit[b] Cold agglutinin titer Unilateral bone marrow aspirate and biopsy	*MYD88* L265P AS-PCR testing of bone marrow biopsy Funduscopic examination[c] Coombs test Anti-myelin associated glycoprotein (anti-MAG) antibody/anti-GM1 antibody electromyogram Congo red staining of abdominal fat pad biopsy and/or bone marrow biopsy

AS-PCR, allele-specific polymerase chain reaction; BUN, blood urea nitrogen; CBC, complete blood count.
[a]Most patients with serum viscosity of less than 4 cP will not have symptoms of hyperviscosity.
[b]If cryocrit positive, then initial and follow-up cryocrit and SPEP samples should be measured under warm conditions.
[c]When hyperviscosity is suspected.

will typically show a pattern of sIgM⁺, CD19⁺, CD20⁺, CD22⁺, and CD79⁺. Testing for the *MYD88* L265 gene mutation in the marrow or peripheral blood can help distinguish WM from marginal zone lymphoma and MM, where the incidence of this mutation is low ([61]). Patients should have baseline CT scans (chest, abdomen, and pelvis) to evaluate for extramedullary disease. An ophthalmologic examination should be performed to look for retinal changes (hemorrhages or "sausage vessels") in patients with suspected hyperviscosity syndrome.

Asymptomatic patients can be followed every 3 months during the first year, with longer follow-up intervals thereafter, in the setting of disease stability ([62]). In such patients, the risk of developing symptomatic disease is about 6% in the first year, 39% at 3 years, and 55% at 5 years, so lifelong follow-up is necessary ([62]). Higher M-protein and marrow infiltration have been associated with increased risk of progression to symptomatic disease ([62]).

At MDACC, therapy is initiated for symptomatic hyperviscosity, hemoglobin <10 g/dL, platelet count ≤100,000/μL, bulky adenopathy, symptomatic organomegaly, symptomatic cryoglobulinemia, or significant peripheral neuropathy (Table 11-11) ([63]). Therapy for hyperviscosity consists of prompt initiation of plasma exchange followed by chemotherapy. Because of the risk of precipitating symptomatic hyperviscosity in patients with high levels of circulating IgM, packed red cell transfusions should be used conservatively and should preferably be administered after plasma exchange in high-risk patients.

Frontline Therapy

When autologous SCT may be considered at relapse, nucleoside analogs should be avoided prior to stem cell harvest, and primary therapy with a proteasome inhibitor or alkylator, together with rituximab with or without dexamethasone, should be considered ([64, 65]). Combinations of bortezomib-rituximab with or without dexamethasone result in an ORR of 57% to 83%.

Table 11-11 Treatment Indications for Waldenström Macroglobulinemia

• Symptomatic hyperviscosity (eye grounds, neurologic changes)
• Hemoglobin <10 g/dL
• Platelet count ≤100,000/μL
• Bulky adenopathy
• Symptomatic organomegaly
• Symptomatic cryoglobulinemia
• Amyloidosis
• Neuropathy

Carfilzomib-rituximab-dexamethasone showed an ORR of 68% ([65, 66]). Comparable ORRs (77%-96%) have been seen with alkylating agent–based regimens (rituximab plus rituximab, cyclophosphamide, doxorubicin, vincristine, and prednisone [CHOP]; rituximab-cyclophosphamide-vincristine-prednisone; rituximab-cyclophosphamide-dexamethasone; and rituximab-bendamustine) ([67]). The use of single-agent rituximab should be reserved for patients unable to tolerate combination chemotherapy, because ORRs are low (20%-50%).

When future autologous SCT is not a consideration, nucleoside analog–based combinations may be considered. In a trial by the Waldenström Macroglobulinemia Clinical Trials Group, fludarabine-rituximab demonstrated an ORR of 96% and median PFS of 51.2 months ([68]). In a phase II trial of 18 patients, two cycles of cladribine, cyclophosphamide, and rituximab yielded an ORR of 94%, and at a median follow-up of 8 years, median OS was not reached ([69]).

Rituximab is integral to the treatment of WM but must be used with caution in patients with highly elevated IgM levels due to the potential for an associated IgM flare. In these cases, it is prudent to delay administration of rituximab until after the patient has received some cytoreductive therapy. Because this phenomenon can confound interpretation of results, disease response should be assessed after two cycles of induction therapy unless there is clear progression of extramedullary disease.

Treatment at Disease Relapse

At relapse, patients may be re-treated with a previously successful regimen if their initial remission lasted at least 1 year. When the initial disease-free-interval is shorter, use of one of the other frontline regimens (detailed above) should be considered.

Another effective option is the Bruton tyrosine kinase (BTK) inhibitor ibrutinib. In a phase II trial of 63 patients, ibrutinib showed an ORR of 57% and was well tolerated ([70]). Immunomodulatory agents with or without rituximab have shown efficacy. Thalidomide-rituximab and lenalidomide-rituximab resulted in a major response rate of 64% and 25%, respectively. Pomalidomide monotherapy is associated with a ≥ minor response rate of 33%.

For patients intolerant to rituximab, the fully humanized monoclonal anti-CD20 antibody ofatumumab may be useful. In patients who have previously received rituximab, two cycles of ofatumumab were associated with an ORR of 52% ([71]).

Alemtuzumab can also be considered because WM cells express CD52. In a phase II study of 28 previously treated patients with either lymphoplasmacytic lymphoma or WM, alemtuzumab-rituximab yielded an

ORR of 76% ([72]). However, this regimen is rarely used due to the associated high risk of CMV reactivation.

The role of SCT in WM is still being defined. In a retrospective review of 158 patients (32% had at least three prior lines of therapy), the 5-year PFS and OS rates with autologous SCT were 39.7% and 68.5%, respectively ([73]). Several groups have also studied allogeneic SCT in WM. The 5-year PFS was between 49% and 56% but with notable treatment-related mortality ([74]).

Future Directions

Next-generation proteasome inhibitors (eg, ixazomib, oprozomib), new anti-CD20 monoclonal antibodies (eg, GA-101), the HDAC inhibitor panobinostat, the toll-like receptor antagonist IMO-8400, and second-generation BTK inhibitors are under study in WM. Emerging knowledge about the *MYD88* gene and *CXCR4* mutations may allow more rational disease-targeted therapies.

Systemic Light-Chain Amyloidosis

Background

Systemic light-chain (AL) amyloidosis is a rare plasma cell proliferative disorder. It results from organ deposition of amyloid fibrils that consist of the NH_2-terminal amino acid residues of the variable portion of the light-chain immunoglobulin molecule. The estimated age-adjusted incidence is 5.1 to 12.8 cases per million person-years. About 75% of cases are derived from lambda light chain. AL amyloidosis may result primarily from a small plasma cell clone in the bone marrow or may be associated with an underlying plasma cell dyscrasia or other B-cell malignancies. Coexisting AL amyloid deposits are identified in 10% to 15% of patients with MM.

The commonly affected organs include the heart, kidneys, liver, gastrointestinal tract, and peripheral nervous system. This leads to clinical symptomatology of nephrotic syndrome, cardiomyopathy, hepatomegaly, neuropathy, macroglossia, anemia, carpal tunnel syndrome, and periorbital purpura. The exact pathophysiology of organ or tissue damage in AL amyloidosis is not completely understood, but the reduction of serum free light-chain concentration after chemotherapy treatment results in improved cardiac function and suggests that free light chain plays an important role in organ dysfunction.

Clinical Presentation and Diagnostic Workup

The clinical presentation of AL amyloidosis depends on the spectrum and severity of organ involvement. The common clinical features at diagnosis include nephrotic syndrome with or without renal insufficiency, cardiomyopathy, autonomic neuropathy, and hepatosplenomegaly. Many patients have multisystem involvement at diagnosis (Table 11-12). The diagnosis requires histologic evidence of amyloid deposition in tissues either by aspiration of abdominal subcutaneous fat and/or biopsy of the organs involved, with the demonstration of clonal plasma cell disorder and abnormal free light chain in serum or urine. The pathognomic diagnostic feature of AL amyloidosis a positive tissue stain with Congo red to demonstrate apple-green birefringence under polarized light. Mass spectrometry–based proteomic analysis of amyloid tissue should be pursued when available. This helps confirm the type of amyloid protein, because more than 10 forms of systemic amyloidosis are currently known, and correct typing is imperative for appropriate treatment (Table 11-13).

Prognosis and Staging

Even though patients commonly have a low burden of clonal plasma cells, long-term survival outcome is dismal due to organ impairment from amyloid deposition. The presence of cardiac involvement is a detrimental factor for survival. The median survival time is 4 months in patients presenting with congestive heart failure versus 16 months in those without it ([75]).

Table 11-12 Clinical Presentations of Al Amyloidosis

Organ Involvement	Clinical Presentation
Kidney	Nephrotic syndrome Renal failure
Heart	Abnormal electrocardiogram: low voltages in the standard leads Nondilated cardiomyopathy Arrhythmia
Peripheral and autonomic nervous system	Numbness Muscle weakness Carpal tunnel syndrome Postural hypotension Erectile dysfunction Altered bowel habit Anhidrosis
Gastrointestinal tract	Macroglossia Early satiety Diarrhea Malabsorption Gastrointestinal bleeding Hepatomegaly
Coagulation system	Periorbital purpura (raccoon eyes) Abnormal clotting tests Life-threatening bleeding

Table 11-13 Laboratory and Pathologic Evaluation of AL Amyloidosis

Laboratory evaluation
Complete blood count with differential
Serum creatinine
Liver enzyme and bilirubin
Coagulation tests: prothrombin time, partial thromboplastin time, factor X
Serum protein electrophoresis (SPEP) and immunofixation
Urine protein electrophoresis (UPEP) and immunofixation
Serum free light chains
24-Hour urine protein
Cardiac troponin, brain natriuretic peptide (BNP), or N-terminal pro-BNP
Cardiac testing: electrocardiogram, echocardiogram, cardiac magnetic resonance imaging, chest x-ray
Peripheral nervous system: electromyography, nerve conduction test
Pulmonary function test
Pathologic evaluation
Bone marrow aspiration and biopsy with immunohistochemistry staining for kappa and lambda light chain
Abdominal fat pad aspiration or organ biopsy with Congo red staining for amyloid
Mass spectrometry for amyloid protein identification

Cardiac dysfunction is best assessed by the elevation of cardiac biomarkers: brain natriuretic peptide (BNP), N-terminal pro-brain natriuretic peptide (NT-proBNP), and cardiac troponin T (cTnT) and troponin I (cTnI). Many studies have confirmed the prognostic significance of markers of cardiac injury and dysfunction in AL amyloidosis, and they been incorporated in the staging system for AL amyloidosis ([76]). According to the Revised Prognostic Scoring System from the Mayo Clinic group, patients are assigned a score of 1 for each of the following: difference between involved and uninvolved light chain ≥18 mg/dL, cTnT ≥0.025 ng/mL, and NT-proBNP ≥1,800 pg/mL. The median OS times of patients with Mayo stage I, II, III, and IV (score of 0, 1, 2, and 3, respectively) are 94, 40, 14, and 5.8 months, respectively ([76]).

Treatment

Treatment for AL amyloidosis is similar to that for MM, comprising mainly of various chemotherapy combinations or high-dose therapy with autologous SCT (HDT-ASCT), aimed at eliminating clonal plasma cells. The choice of treatment should be based on risk stratification. Patients with good performance status and normal cardiac markers should be considered for HDT-ASCT.

High-Dose Therapy With Autologous Stem Cell Transplantation

High-dose therapy with autologous SCT has been used since the early 1990s, and it is the only effective treatment modality associated with hematologic and organ responses as well as long-term survival ([77, 78]). It is associated with high treatment-related mortality, ranging from 13% to 43%, especially in patients with cardiac involvement. Careful patient selection based on comorbidity index and cardiac staging is the key to successful outcome of high-dose therapy in AL amyloidosis. A randomized trial comparing HDT-ASCT with standard-dose melphalan plus high-dose dexamethasone showed no differences in hematologic or organ response. Landmark analysis examining only patients surviving more than 6 months after transplantation also showed no survival benefit for HDT-ASCT ([79]). However, almost 25% of the patients in this study received reduced-dose melphalan conditioning, which has been associated with poor transplantation outcomes. A meta-analysis of 12 studies of HDT-ASCT showed no superiority of HDT-ASCT over conventional chemotherapy ([80]). However, in the MDACC experience, improved 10-year survival outcomes were reported in patients undergoing HDT-ASCT compared to conventional chemotherapy ([78]). At centers with extensive experience in treating AL amyloidosis, HDT-ASCT provides promising outcomes with careful patient selection ([79, 81]). Involvement of two or fewer organs and AL amyloidosis with renal involvement show best overall outcome with HDT-ASCT ([78]).

Induction Therapy Before High-Dose Therapy With Autologous Stem Cell Transplantation

With the inclusion of novel agents in induction therapy, improvement in performance status can lead to transplantation eligibility for newly diagnosed patients ([82]). A randomized trial evaluating the role of induction therapy containing bortezomib and dexamethasone followed by HDT-ASCT versus HDT-ASCT in newly diagnosed AL amyloidosis showed better responses and survival outcomes with induction therapy ([83]). In our experience, incorporation of novel-agent induction therapy prior to transplantation is associated with improved survival ([78]). There are no data to support maintenance treatment in AL amyloidosis.

Conventional Chemotherapy

The combination of melphalan and high-dose dexamethasone remains the gold standard for first-line treatment of transplant-ineligible patients and is associated with a good hematologic response (67%) and low toxicity (4%) ([84]). Today, several novel therapeutic combination choices are available for transplant-ineligible patients. Immunomodulatory drugs such as thalidomide and lenalidomide have been investigated in the upfront and relapsed settings with hematologic response rates of 40% to 74% and organ response rates of 20% to 40% ([85, 86]). However, they have also been associated with serious adverse events including bradycardia, fatigue, sedation, and cytopenia ([85, 87]). Bortezomib in combination with conventional chemotherapy such as cyclophosphamide and/or dexamethasone is also effective ([82, 88-90]). Bortezomib has successfully been used as consolidation in patients who did not achieve a CR after HDT-ASCT to improve the quality of response ([91]).

POEMS Syndrome

POEMS syndrome, also known as osteosclerotic myeloma, is a paraneoplastic syndrome related to an underlying clonal plasma cell disorder. The major diagnostic criteria are polyneuropathy, monoclonal gammopathy, sclerotic bone lesions, elevated vascular endothelial growth factor (VEGF), and Castleman disease. Minor features include organomegaly, endocrinopathy, characteristic skin changes, papilledema, extravascular volume overload, and thrombocytosis. The diagnosis of POEMS syndrome is made with three of the major criteria, two of which must include polyneuropathy and a clonal plasma cell neoplasm, and at least one of the minor criteria (Table 11-14) ([92]). Patients may have delays in diagnosis because it is rare and resembles other neurologic diseases, most commonly chronic inflammatory demyelinating polyradiculoneuropathy. The natural history of POEMS syndrome is defined by progressive polyneuropathy and sclerotic bone disease, which leads to significant morbidity, along with mortality if respiratory compromise occurs. POEMS syndrome should be distinguished from the Castleman disease variant of POEMS syndrome, which has no clonal plasma cell association and usually no peripheral neuropathy.

The pathogenesis of this syndrome is not known. Risk stratification is solely based on the clinical phenotype. The extent of plasma cell clonal disease correlates with prognosis in POEMS, but the number of clinical criteria does not. Treatment is aimed at eradicating the underlying plasma cell clone and control of symptoms. With one to three sclerotic plasmacytomas (usually <1 cm in diameter each) without marrow infiltration, localized radiation therapy may suffice. For patients with a dominant sclerotic bone lesion, frontline radiation therapy may be appropriate. Patients with diffuse sclerotic lesions, disseminated marrow involvement, or relapsed disease within 6 months of completing radiation therapy should receive systemic therapy adapted largely from therapy for MM. Alkylators such as melphalan are the mainstay of treatment; lenalidomide has shown promise with manageable toxicity ([93]).

Table 11-14 Diagnostic Criteria for Poems Syndrome

Major criteria	**Polyneuropathy** **Monoclonal plasma cell disorder** Sclerotic bone lesion Castleman disease VEGF elevation
Minor Criteria	Organomegaly Extravascular volume overload Endocrinopathy Skin changes Papilledema Thrombocytosis/polycythemia
Other	Pulmonary hypertension Clubbing Weight loss Hyperhidrosis Thrombosis Low vitamin B_{12} level

Diagnosis of POEMS syndrome is made with three of the major criteria, two of which must include polyneuropathy and a clonal plasma cell neoplasm, and at least one of the minor criteria.
VEGF, vascular endothelial growth factor.

Therapies based on CHOP also show responses. Thalidomide and bortezomib have activity but could exacerbate disease-related peripheral neuropathy. Benefit from anti-VEGF antibodies is unproven ([94]).

High-dose melphalan and autologous SCT can lead to prolonged remissions and significant improvement in clinical symptoms. Seven patients with POEMS syndrome underwent autologous SCT at MDACC ([95]); all had significant or complete resolution of clinical symptoms, and PFS and OS at 5 years were 86% and 100%, respectively. Prompt recognition and institution of supportive care measures and therapy directed against the plasma cell clone result in the best outcomes.

TEMPI Syndrome

In 2011, six patients from the literature were recognized as having common clinical features defining a new multisystem disease characterized by telangiectasias, erythrocytosis with elevated erythropoietin levels, monoclonal gammopathy, perinephric fluid collections, and intrapulmonary shunting. This was termed the TEMPI syndrome ([96]). Bortezomib therapy improved disease-related clinical features, suggesting a pathogenic role of the monoclonal gammopathy ([97, 98]). Bone marrow examination of three patients showed marked erythroid hyperplasia ([99]). Elevated erythropoietin level and a normal VEGF level distinguish TEMPI from POEMS. Due to the disease rarity, patients suspected of having TEMPI syndrome should be referred to academic centers for management.

Immunoglobulin Heavy-Chain Disease

Heavy-chain diseases are plasma cell dyscrasias characterized by the production of heavy-chain immunoglobulin molecules (gamma, alpha, mu) that lack light chains. Alpha-chain disease is the most common variant and can be thought of as an extranodal marginal zone lymphoma of mucosa-associated lymph node tissue. The disease results from lymphocyte and plasma cell infiltration of the mesenteric nodes and small bowel and has features of malabsorption, such as diarrhea, weight loss, abdominal pain, edema, and clubbing. The heavy-chain molecule may be detected in serum, jejunal secretions, and urine ([100]). These patients may be treated with antibiotics or occasionally with surgery. If symptoms persist or if a lymphoma is suspected, chemotherapy may be used.

Gamma heavy-chain disease is similar to lymphoplasmacytoid non-Hodgkin lymphoma ([101]). Patients may present with fever, weakness, lymphadenopathy, hepatosplenomegaly, and Waldeyer ring involvement. Eosinophilia, leukopenia, and thrombocytopenia are common. Treatment with regimens similar to those used for non-Hodgkin lymphoma may be effective ([100]).

Mu heavy-chain disease is extremely rare and often seen in patients with chronic lymphocytic leukemia, although it has been described with underlying WM or MM ([102]). Vacuolated plasma cells are common in the marrow, and many patients have lambda light chains in urine. Therapy choice should follow existing recommendations for the underlying primary disease.

FUTURE DIRECTIONS

The last decade has seen unprecedented advances in the treatment of plasma cell dyscrasias. The advent of novel agents, notably proteasome inhibitors and IMiDs, has resulted in a doubling of the life expectancy in MM. These treatments have been incorporated in standard regimens for primary AL amyloidosis with improved outcomes. Proteasome inhibitors, anti-CD20 monoclonal antibodies, and drugs targeting the B-cell receptor pathway (eg, ibrutinib) have also represented important advances in WM therapy.

Many challenges remain. For example, MM is still considered mostly an incurable disease, and a subgroup of patients with high-risk MM have not benefited substantially from recent therapeutic advances. Promising investigational agents including immunotherapeutic approaches with monoclonal antibodies and rational combinations to overcome resistance are being tested.

Future work involves identifying predictive biomarkers to help individualize therapy in MM and related plasma cell dyscrasias to help maximize efficacy while balancing treatment toxicity. In high-risk SMM, the role of early preemptive therapy needs to be clarified. Improving our understanding of the molecular pathogenesis of MM and its genetic drivers through molecular profiling and refining current risk stratification models remain are key priorities. Another important question is the role and timing of autologous SCT in the era of novel agents. Finally, as new drug combinations induce deeper responses in the frontline setting, significance of achieving molecular remissions is an area of intense research focus. Bridging these knowledge gaps will improve on the advances achieved over the last decade and offer greater individualized treatment approaches, leading to possible cure of MM and its related disorders.

REFERENCES

1. Broderick P, Chubb D, Johnson DC, et al. Common variation at 3p22.1 and 7p15.3 influences multiple myeloma risk. *Nat Genet.* 2012;44(1):58-61.
2. Chubb D, Weinhold N, Broderick P, et al. Common variation at 3q26.2, 6p21.33, 17p11.2 and 22q13.1 influences multiple myeloma risk. *Nat Genet.* 2013;45(10):1221-1225.
3. Morgan GJ, Johnson DC, Weinhold N, et al. Inherited genetic susceptibility to multiple myeloma. *Leukemia.* 2014;28(3):518-524.
4. Chapman MA, Lawrence MS, Keats JJ, et al. Initial genome sequencing and analysis of multiple myeloma. *Nature.* 2011;471(7339):467-472.
5. Keats JJ, Chesi M, Egan JB, et al. Clonal competition with alternating dominance in multiple myeloma. *Blood.* 2012; 120(5):1067-1076.
6. Melchor L, Brioli A, Wardell CP, et al. Single-cell genetic analysis reveals the composition of initiating clones and phylogenetic patterns of branching and parallel evolution in myeloma. *Leukemia.* 2014;28(8):1705-1715.
7. Kaiser MF, Johnson DC, Wu P, et al. Global methylation analysis identifies prognostically important epigenetically inactivated tumor suppressor genes in multiple myeloma. *Blood.* 2013;122(2):219-226.
8. Kyle RA, Gertz MA, Witzig TE, et al. Review of 1027 patients with newly diagnosed multiple myeloma. *Mayo Clinic Proc.* 2003;78(1):21-33.
9. Rajkumar SV, Dimopoulos MA, Palumbo A, et al. International Myeloma Working Group updated criteria for the diagnosis of multiple myeloma. *Lancet Oncol.* 2014;15(12):e538-e548.
10. Paiva B, Gutierrez NC, Rosinol L, et al. High-risk cytogenetics and persistent minimal residual disease by multiparameter flow cytometry predict unsustained complete response after autologous stem cell transplantation in multiple myeloma. *Blood.* 2012;119(3):687-691.
11. Martinez-Lopez J, Lahuerta JJ, Pepin F, et al. Prognostic value of deep sequencing method for minimal residual disease detection in multiple myeloma. *Blood.* 2014;123(20):3073-3079.
12. Zonder JA, Crowley J, Hussein MA, et al. Lenalidomide and high-dose dexamethasone compared with dexamethasone as initial therapy for multiple myeloma: a randomized Southwest Oncology Group trial (S0232). *Blood.* 2010;116(26):5838-5841.
13. Rajkumar SV, Jacobus S, Callander NS, et al. Lenalidomide plus high-dose dexamethasone versus lenalidomide plus low-dose dexamethasone as initial therapy for newly diagnosed multiple

myeloma: an open-label randomised controlled trial. *Lancet Oncol.* 2010;11(1):29-37.

14. Harousseau JL, Attal M, Avet-Loiseau H, et al. Bortezomib plus dexamethasone is superior to vincristine plus doxorubicin plus dexamethasone as induction treatment prior to autologous stem-cell transplantation in newly diagnosed multiple myeloma: results of the IFM 2005-01 phase III trial. *J Clin Oncol.* 2010;28(30):4621-4629.
15. Moreau P, Pylypenko H, Grosicki S, et al. Subcutaneous versus intravenous administration of bortezomib in patients with relapsed multiple myeloma: a randomised, phase 3, non-inferiority study. *Lancet Oncol.* 2011;12(5):431-440.
16. Kumar S, Flinn I, Richardson PG, et al. Randomized, multicenter, phase 2 study (EVOLUTION) of combinations of bortezomib, dexamethasone, cyclophosphamide, and lenalidomide in previously untreated multiple myeloma. *Blood.* 2012;119(19):4375-4382.
17. Reeder CB, Reece DE, Kukreti V, et al. Once- versus twice-weekly bortezomib induction therapy with CyBorD in newly diagnosed multiple myeloma. *Blood.* 2010;115(16):3416-3417.
18. Richardson PG, Weller E, Lonial S, et al. Lenalidomide, bortezomib, and dexamethasone combination therapy in patients with newly diagnosed multiple myeloma. *Blood.* 2010;116(5):679-686.
19. Jakubowiak AJ, Dytfeld D, Griffith KA, et al. A phase 1/2 study of carfilzomib in combination with lenalidomide and low-dose dexamethasone as a frontline treatment for multiple myeloma. *Blood.* 2012;120(9):1801-1809.
20. Korde N, Zingone A, Kwok M, et al. Phase II clinical and correlative study of carfilzomib, lenalidomide, and dexamethasone (CRd) in newly diagnosed multiple myeloma (MM) patients [abstract]. *Blood.* 2012;120(21):732.
21. Palumbo A, Bringhen S, Caravita T, et al. Oral melphalan and prednisone chemotherapy plus thalidomide compared with melphalan and prednisone alone in elderly patients with multiple myeloma: randomised controlled trial. *Lancet.* 2006;367(9513):825-831.
22. Palumbo A, Hajek R, Delforge M, et al. Continuous lenalidomide treatment for newly diagnosed multiple myeloma. *N Engl J Med.* 2012;366(19):1759-1769.
23. Hulin C, Facon T, Rodon P, et al. Efficacy of melphalan and prednisone plus thalidomide in patients older than 75 years with newly diagnosed multiple myeloma: IFM 01/01 trial. *J Clin Oncol.* 2009;27(22):3664-3670.
24. San Miguel JF, Schlag R, Khuageva NK, et al. Persistent overall survival benefit and no increased risk of second malignancies with bortezomib-melphalan-prednisone versus melphalan-prednisone in patients with previously untreated multiple myeloma. *J Clin Oncol.* 2013;31(4):448-455.
25. Benboubker L, Dimopoulos MA, Dispenzieri A, et al. Lenalidomide and dexamethasone in transplant-ineligible patients with myeloma. *N Engl J Med.* 2014;371(10):906-917.
26. Niesvizky R, Flinn IW, Rifkin R, et al. Efficacy and safety of three bortezomib-based combinations in elderly, newly diagnosed multiple myeloma patients: results from all randomized patients in the community-based, phase 3b UPFRONT study [abstract]. *Blood.* 2011;118(21):478.
27. Attal M, Harousseau JL, Stoppa AM, et al. A prospective, randomized trial of autologous bone marrow transplantation and chemotherapy in multiple myeloma. Intergroupe Francais du Myelome. *N Engl J Med.* 1996;335(2):91-97.
28. Child JA, Morgan GJ, Davies FE, et al. High-dose chemotherapy with hematopoietic stem-cell rescue for multiple myeloma. *N Engl J Med.* 2003;348(19):1875-1883.
29. Barlogie B, Kyle RA, Anderson KC, et al. Standard chemotherapy compared with high-dose chemoradiotherapy for multiple myeloma: final results of phase III US Intergroup Trial S9321. *J Clin Oncol.* 2006;24(6):929-936.
30. Blade J, Rosinol L, Sureda A, et al. High-dose therapy intensification compared with continued standard chemotherapy in multiple myeloma patients responding to the initial chemotherapy: long-term results from a prospective randomized trial from the Spanish cooperative group PETHEMA. *Blood.* 2005;106(12):3755-3759.
31. Fermand JP, Katsahian S, Divine M, et al. High-dose therapy and autologous blood stem-cell transplantation compared with conventional treatment in myeloma patients aged 55 to 65 years: long-term results of a randomized control trial from the Group Myelome-Autogreffe. *J Clin Oncol.* 2005;23(36):9227-9233.
32. Kumar SK, Dispenzieri A, Lacy MQ, et al. Continued improvement in survival in multiple myeloma: changes in early mortality and outcomes in older patients. *Leukemia.* 2014;28(5):1122-1128.
33. Moreau P, Facon T, Attal M, et al. Comparison of 200 mg/m(2) melphalan and 8 Gy total body irradiation plus 140 mg/m(2) melphalan as conditioning regimens for peripheral blood stem cell transplantation in patients with newly diagnosed multiple myeloma: final analysis of the Intergroupe Francophone du Myelome 9502 randomized trial. *Blood.* 2002;99(3):731-735.
34. Pandya C, Hashmi S, Khera N, et al. Cost-effectiveness analysis of early vs. late autologous stem cell transplantation in multiple myeloma. *Clin Transplant.* 2014;28(10):1084-1091.
35. Garban F, Attal M, Michallet M, et al. Prospective comparison of autologous stem cell transplantation followed by dose-reduced allograft (IFM99-03 trial) with tandem autologous stem cell transplantation (IFM99-04 trial) in high-risk de novo multiple myeloma. *Blood.* 2006;107(9):3474-3480.
36. Bruno B, Rotta M, Patriarca F, et al. A comparison of allografting with autografting for newly diagnosed myeloma. *N Engl J Med.* 2007;356(11):1110-1120.
37. Giaccone L, Storer B, Patriarca F, et al. Long-term follow-up of a comparison of nonmyeloablative allografting with autografting for newly diagnosed myeloma. *Blood.* 2011;117(24):6721-6727.
38. Krishnan A, Pasquini MC, Logan B, et al. Autologous haemopoietic stem-cell transplantation followed by allogeneic or autologous haemopoietic stem-cell transplantation in patients with multiple myeloma (BMT CTN 0102): a phase 3 biological assignment trial. *Lancet Oncol.* 2011;12(13):1195-1203.
39. Gahrton G, Iacobelli S, Bjorkstrand B, et al. Autologous/reduced-intensity allogeneic stem cell transplantation vs autologous transplantation in multiple myeloma: long-term results of the EBMT-NMAM2000 study. *Blood.* 2013;121(25):5055-5063.
40. Alexanian R, Delasalle K, Wang M, Thomas S, Weber D. Curability of multiple myeloma. *Bone Marrow Res.* 2012;2012:916479.
41. McCarthy PL, Owzar K, Hofmeister CC, et al. Lenalidomide after stem-cell transplantation for multiple myeloma. *N Engl J Med.* 2012;366(19):1770-1781.
42. Attal M, Lauwers-Cances V, Marit G, et al. Lenalidomide maintenance after stem-cell transplantation for multiple myeloma. *N Engl J Med.* 2012;366(19):1782-1791.
43. Thomas A, Mailankody S, Korde N, Kristinsson SY, Turesson I, Landgren O. Second malignancies after multiple myeloma: from 1960s to 2010s. *Blood.* 2012;119(12):2731-2737.
44. Palumbo A, Bringhen S, Kumar SK, et al. Second primary malignancies with lenalidomide therapy for newly diagnosed myeloma: a meta-analysis of individual patient data. *Lancet Oncol.* 2014;15(3):333-342.
45. Sonneveld P, Schmidt-Wolf IG, van der Holt B, et al. Bortezomib induction and maintenance treatment in patients with newly diagnosed multiple myeloma: results of the randomized phase III HOVON-65/ GMMG-HD4 trial. *J Clin Oncol.* 2012;30(24):2946-2955.
46. San Miguel J, Weisel K, Moreau P, et al. Pomalidomide plus low-dose dexamethasone versus high-dose dexamethasone

alone for patients with relapsed and refractory multiple myeloma (MM-003): a randomised, open-label, phase 3 trial. *Lancet Oncol.* 2013;14(11):1055-1066.
47. Orlowski RZ, Nagler A, Sonneveld P, et al. Randomized phase III study of pegylated liposomal doxorubicin plus bortezomib compared with bortezomib alone in relapsed or refractory multiple myeloma: combination therapy improves time to progression. *J Clin Oncol.* 2007;25(25):3892-3901.
48. Richardson PG, Xie W, Jagannath S, et al. A phase 2 trial of lenalidomide, bortezomib, and dexamethasone in patients with relapsed and relapsed/refractory myeloma. *Blood.* 2014;123(10):1461-1469.
49. Siegel DS, Martin T, Wang M, et al. A phase 2 study of single-agent carfilzomib (PX-171-003-A1) in patients with relapsed and refractory multiple myeloma. *Blood.* 2012;120(14):2817-2825.
50. Stewart AK, Rajkumar SV, Dimopoulos MA, et al. Carfilzomib, lenalidomide, and dexamethasone for relapsed multiple myeloma. *N Engl J Med.* 2015;372(2):142-152.
51. Shah JJ, Stadtmauer EA, Abonour R, et al. A multi-center phase I/II trial of carfilzomib and pomalidomide with dexamethasone (Car-Pom-d) in patients with relapsed/refractory multiple myeloma [abstract]. *Blood.* 2012;120(21):74.
52. Hajek R, Bryce R, Ro S, Klencke B, Ludwig H. Design and rationale of FOCUS (PX-171-011): a randomized, open-label, phase 3 study of carfilzomib versus best supportive care regimen in patients with relapsed and refractory multiple myeloma (R/R MM). *BMC Cancer.* 2012;12:415.
53. Lendvai N, Hilden P, Devlin S, et al. A phase 2 single-center study of carfilzomib 56 mg/m2 with or without low-dose dexamethasone in relapsed multiple myeloma. *Blood.* 2014;124(6):899-906.
54. Plesner T, Lokhorst H, Gimsing P, Nahi H, Lisby S, Richardson PG. Daratumumab, a CD38 monoclonal antibody in patients with multiple myeloma: data from a dose-escalation phase I/II study [asbstract]. *Blood.* 2012;120(21):73.
55. Lonial S, Jagannath S, Moreau P, et al. Phase (Ph) I/II study of elotuzumab (Elo) plus lenalidomide/dexamethasone (Len/dex) in relapsed/refractory multiple myeloma (RR MM): updated Ph II results and Ph I/II long-term safety [abstract]. *J Clin Oncol.* 2013;31:8542.
56. San-Miguel JF, Hungria VT, Yoon SS, et al. Panobinostat plus bortezomib and dexamethasone versus placebo plus bortezomib and dexamethasone in patients with relapsed or relapsed and refractory multiple myeloma: a multicentre, randomised, double-blind phase 3 trial. *Lancet Oncol.* 2014;15(11):1195-1206.
57. Shah JJ, Zonder JA, Cohen A, et al. The novel KSP inhibitor ARRY-520 is active both with and without low-dose dexamethasone in patients with multiple myeloma refractory to bortezomib and lenalidomide: results from a phase 2 study [abstract]. *Blood.* 2012;120(21):449.
58. Kyle RA, Remstein ED, Therneau TM, et al. Clinical course and prognosis of smoldering (asymptomatic) multiple myeloma. *N Engl J Med.* 2007;356(25):2582-2590.
59. Dispenzieri A, Stewart AK, Chanan-Khan A, et al. Smoldering multiple myeloma requiring treatment: time for a new definition? *Blood.* 2013;122(26):4172-4181.
60. Mateos MV, Hernandez MT, Giraldo P, et al. Lenalidomide plus dexamethasone for high-risk smoldering multiple myeloma. *N Engl J Med.* 2013;369(5):438-447.
61. Treon SP, Xu L, Yang G, et al. MYD88 L265P somatic mutation in Waldenstrom's macroglobulinemia. *N Engl J Med.* 2012;367(9):826-833.
62. Kyle RA, Therneau TM, Dispenzieri A, et al. Immunoglobulin m monoclonal gammopathy of undetermined significance and smoldering Waldenstrom macroglobulinemia. *Clin Lymphoma Myeloma Leuk.* 2013;13(2):184-186.
63. Kyle RA, Treon SP, Alexanian R, et al. Prognostic markers and criteria to initiate therapy in Waldenstrom's macroglobulinemia: consensus panel recommendations from the Second International Workshop on Waldenstrom's Macroglobulinemia. *Semin Oncol.* 2003;30(2):116-120.
64. Thomas SK, Haygood, TM, Qazilbash MH, et al. A phase II trial of bortezomib-rituximab followed by autologous stem cell harvest (SCH) and cladribine-cyclophosphamide-rituximab (2CdA-Cy-Rit) consolidation as primary therapy of Waldenström's macroglobulinemia (WM). *Blood.* 2013;21:122.
65. Treon SP, Ioakimidis L, Soumerai JD, et al. Primary therapy of Waldenstrom macroglobulinemia with bortezomib, dexamethasone, and rituximab: WMCTG clinical trial 05-180. *J Clin Oncol.* 2009;27(23):3830-3835.
66. Treon SP, Tripsas CK, Meid K, et al. Carfilzomib, rituximab, and dexamethasone (CaRD) treatment offers a neuropathy-sparing approach for treating Waldenstrom's macroglobulinemia. *Blood.* 2014;124(4):503-510.
67. Rummel MJ, Niederle N, Maschmeyer G, et al. Bendamustine plus rituximab versus CHOP plus rituximab as first-line treatment for patients with indolent and mantle-cell lymphomas: an open-label, multicentre, randomised, phase 3 non-inferiority trial. *Lancet.* 2013;381(9873):1203-1210.
68. Treon SP, Branagan AR, Ioakimidis L, et al. Long-term outcomes to fludarabine and rituximab in Waldenstrom macroglobulinemia. *Blood.* 2009;113(16):3673-3678.
69. Thomas SK, Delasalle KB, Shah JJ, Wang L, Orlowski RZ, Weber DM. Impact of rituximab on the treatment of Waldenstrom's macroglobulinemia (WM) [abstract]. *Blood.* 2012;120(21):2734.
70. Treon SP, Tripsas CK, Yang G, et al. A prospective multicenter study of the Bruton's tyrosine kinase inhibitor ibrutinib in patients with relapsed or refractory Waldenstrom's macroglobulinemia [abstract]. *Blood.* 2013;122(21):251.
71. Furman RR, DiRienzo CG, Hayman SR, et al. A phase II trial of ofatumumab in subjects with Waldenstrom's macroglobulinemia [abstract]. *Blood.* 2011;118(21):3701.
72. Treon SP, Soumerai JD, Hunter ZR, et al. Long-term follow-up of symptomatic patients with lymphoplasmacytic lymphoma/Waldenstrom macroglobulinemia treated with the anti-CD52 monoclonal antibody alemtuzumab. *Blood.* 2011;118(2):276-281.
73. Kyriakou C, Canals C, Sibon D, et al. High-dose therapy and autologous stem-cell transplantation in Waldenstrom macroglobulinemia: the Lymphoma Working Party of the European Group for Blood and Marrow Transplantation. *J Clin Oncol.* 2010;28(13):2227-2232.
74. Kyriakou C, Canals C, Cornelissen JJ, et al. Allogeneic stem-cell transplantation in patients with Waldenström macroglobulinemia: report from the Lymphoma Working Party of the European Group for Blood and Marrow Transplantation. *J Clin Oncol.* 2010;28(33):4926-4934.
75. Kyle RA, Gertz MA. Primary systemic amyloidosis: clinical and laboratory features in 474 cases. *Semin Hematol.* 1995;32(1):45-59.
76. Kumar S, Dispenzieri A, Lacy MQ, et al. Revised prognostic staging system for light chain amyloidosis incorporating cardiac biomarkers and serum free light chain measurements. *J Clin Oncol.* 2012;30(9):989-995.
77. Jaccard A, Moreau P, Leblond V, et al. High-dose melphalan versus melphalan plus dexamethasone for AL amyloidosis. *N Engl J Med.* 2007;357(11):1083-1093.
78. Parmar S, Kongtim P, Champlin R, et al. Auto-SCT improves survival in systemic light chain amyloidosis: a retrospective analysis with 14-year follow-up. *Bone Marrow Transplant.* 2014;49(8):1036-1041.
79. Madan S, Kumar SK, Dispenzieri A, et al. High-dose melphalan and peripheral blood stem cell transplantation for light-chain amyloidosis with cardiac involvement. *Blood.*

CHAPTER 11

2012;119(5):1117-1122.

80. Mhaskar R, Kumar A, Behera M, Kharfan-Dabaja MA, Djulbegovic B. Role of high-dose chemotherapy and autologous hematopoietic cell transplantation in primary systemic amyloidosis: a systematic review. *Biol Blood Marrow Transplant.* 2009;15(8):893-902.
81. Dispenzieri A, Kyle RA, Lacy MQ, et al. Superior survival in primary systemic amyloidosis patients undergoing peripheral blood stem cell transplantation: a case-control study. *Blood.* 2004;103(10):3960-3963.
82. Mikhael JR, Schuster SR, Jimenez-Zepeda VH, et al. Cyclophosphamide-bortezomib-dexamethasone (CyBorD) produces rapid and complete hematologic response in patients with AL amyloidosis. *Blood.* 2012;119(19):4391-4394.
83. Huang X, Wang Q, Chen W, et al. Induction therapy with bortezomib and dexamethasone followed by autologous stem cell transplantation versus autologous stem cell transplantation alone in the treatment of renal AL amyloidosis: a randomized controlled trial. *BMC Med.* 2014;12(1):1-10.
84. Palladini G, Russo P, Nuvolone M, et al. Treatment with oral melphalan plus dexamethasone produces long-term remissions in AL amyloidosis. *Blood.* 2007;110(2):787-788.
85. Kumar SK, Hayman SR, Buadi FK, et al. Lenalidomide, cyclophosphamide, and dexamethasone (CRd) for light-chain amyloidosis: long-term results from a phase 2 trial. *Blood.* 2012;119(21):4860-4867.
86. Lichtman EI, Seldin DC, Shelton A, Sanchorawala V. Single agent lenalidomide three times a week induces hematologic responses in AL amyloidosis patients on dialysis. *Am J Hematol.* 2014;89(7):706-708.
87. Palladini G, Perfetti V, Perlini S, et al. The combination of thalidomide and intermediate-dose dexamethasone is an effective but toxic treatment for patients with primary amyloidosis (AL). *Blood.* 2005;105(7):2949-2951.
88. Venner CP, Lane T, Foard D, et al. Cyclophosphamide, bortezomib, and dexamethasone therapy in AL amyloidosis is associated with high clonal response rates and prolonged progression-free survival. *Blood.* 2012;119(19):4387-4390.
89. Reece DE, Hegenbart U, Sanchorawala V, et al. Efficacy and safety of once-weekly and twice-weekly bortezomib in patients with relapsed systemic AL amyloidosis: results of a phase 1/2 study. *Blood.* 2011;118(4):865-873.
90. Kastritis E, Wechalekar AD, Dimopoulos MA, et al. Bortezomib with or without dexamethasone in primary systemic (light chain) amyloidosis. *J Clin Oncol.* 2010;28(6):1031-1037.
91. Landau H, Hassoun H, Rosenzweig MA, et al. Bortezomib and dexamethasone consolidation following risk-adapted melphalan and stem cell transplantation for patients with newly diagnosed light-chain amyloidosis. *Leukemia.* 2013;27(4):823-828.
92. Dispenzieri A. POEMS syndrome: 2014 update on diagnosis, risk-stratification, and management. *Am J Hematol.* 2014;89(2):214-223.
93. Zagouri F, Kastritis E, Symeonidis AS, et al. Immunoglobulin D myeloma: clinical features and outcome in the era of novel agents. *Eur J Haematol.* 2014;92(4):308-312.
94. Sekiguchi Y, Misawa S, Shibuya K, et al. Ambiguous effects of anti-VEGF monoclonal antibody (bevacizumab) for POEMS syndrome. *J Neurol Neurosurg Psychiatry.* 2013;84(12):1346-1348.
95. Patel K, Nusrat M, Shah N, et al. Durable responses with autologous hematopoietic SCT in patients with POEMS syndrome. *Bone Marrow Transplant.* 2014;49(3):465-466.
96. Sykes DB, Schroyens W, O'Connell C. The TEMPI syndrome–a novel multisystem disease. *N Engl J Med.* 2011;365(5):475-477.
97. Kwok M, Korde N, Landgren O. Bortezomib to treat the TEMPI syndrome. *N Engl J Med.* 2012;366(19):1843-1845.
98. Schroyens W, O'Connell C, Sykes DB. Complete and partial responses of the TEMPI syndrome to bortezomib. *N Engl J Med.* 2012;367(8):778-780.
99. Rosado FG, Oliveira JL, Sohani AR, et al. Bone marrow findings of the newly described TEMPI syndrome: when erythrocytosis and plasma cell dyscrasia coexist. *Mod Pathol.* 2015;28(3):367-372.
100. Witzig TE, Wahner-Roedler DL. Heavy chain disease. *Curr Treat Options Oncol.* 2002;3(3):247-254.
101. Wahner-Roedler DL, Kyle RA. Heavy chain diseases. *Best Pract Res Clin Haematol.* 2005;18(4):729-746.
102. Wahner-Roedler DL, Kyle RA. Mu-heavy chain disease: presentation as a benign monoclonal gammopathy. *Am J Hematol.* 1992;40(1):56-60.
103. Facon T, Mary JY, Hulin C, et al. Melphalan and prednisone plus thalidomide versus melphalan and prednisone alone or reduced-intensity autologous stem cell transplantation in elderly patients with multiple myeloma (IFM 99-06): a randomised trial. *Lancet.* 2007;370(9594):1209-1218.
104. Palumbo A, Bringhen S, Liberati AM, et al. Oral melphalan, prednisone, and thalidomide in elderly patients with multiple myeloma: updated results of a randomized controlled trial. *Blood.* 2008;112(8):3107-3114.
105. Waage A, Gimsing P, Fayers P, et al. Melphalan and prednisone plus thalidomide or placebo in elderly patients with multiple myeloma. *Blood.* 2010;116(9):1405-1412.
106. Wijermans P, Schaafsma M, Termorshuizen F, et al. Phase III study of the value of thalidomide added to melphalan plus prednisone in elderly patients with newly diagnosed multiple myeloma: the HOVON 49 Study. *J Clin Oncol.* 2010;28(19):3160-3166.
107. San Miguel JF, Schlag R, Khuageva NK, et al. Bortezomib plus melphalan and prednisone for initial treatment of multiple myeloma. *N Engl J Med.* 2008;359(9):906-917.
108. Richardson PG, Sonneveld P, Schuster MW, et al. Bortezomib or high-dose dexamethasone for relapsed multiple myeloma. *N Engl J Med.* 2005;352(24):2487-2498.
109. Weber DM, Chen C, Niesvizky R, et al. Lenalidomide plus dexamethasone for relapsed multiple myeloma in North America. *N Engl J Med.* 2007;357(21):2133-2142.
110. Dimopoulos M, Spencer A, Attal M, et al. Lenalidomide plus dexamethasone for relapsed or refractory multiple myeloma. *N Engl J Med.* 2007;357(21):2123-2132.
111. Rajkumar SV, Kyle RA, Therneau TM, et al. Serum free light chain ratio is an independent risk factor for progression in monoclonal gammopathy of undetermined significance. *Blood.* 2005;106(3):812-817.
112. Perez-Persona E, Vidriales MB, Mateo G, et al. New criteria to identify risk of progression in monoclonal gammopathy of uncertain significance and smoldering multiple myeloma based on multiparameter flow cytometry analysis of bone marrow plasma cells. *Blood.* 2007;110(7):2586-2592.
113. Dispenzieri A, Kyle RA, Katzmann JA, et al. Immunoglobulin free light chain ratio is an independent risk factor for progression of smoldering (asymptomatic) multiple myeloma. *Blood.* 2008;111(2):785-789.
114. Dhodapkar MV, Sexton R, Waheed S, et al. Clinical, genomic, and imaging predictors of myeloma progression from asymptomatic monoclonal gammopathies (SWOG S0120). *Blood.* 2014;123(1):78-85.
115. Zhan F, Huang Y, Colla S, et al. The molecular classification of multiple myeloma. *Blood.* 2006;108(6):2020-2028.

Section III

Stem Cell Transplantation

Section Editor: Elizabeth J. Shpall

第三篇 干细胞移植

12 Autologous Hematopoietic Progenitor Cell Transplantation

第十二章　自体造血干细胞移植

Riad El Fakih
Nina Shah
Yago Nieto

中文导读

自体造血干细胞移植是恶性血液系统肿瘤及部分实体瘤的有效治疗手段。本章主要系统介绍了自体造血干细胞移植，分类阐述其在不同肿瘤中的应用价值，并对其应用进行展望。在对自体造血干细胞移植的系统介绍部分，从诱导/挽救化疗、干细胞采集、大剂量预处理化疗、干细胞回输、回输后支持治疗等方面详述了自体移植的每一阶段，并提出在部分血液系统肿瘤中自体移植及异基因移植存在的争议。在治疗相关并发症部分，列举了自体移植的常见不良反应，包括感染、黏膜炎、间质性肺炎、出血性膀胱炎，以及心脏系统、神经系统等系统功能损伤等内容。其后，从非霍奇金淋巴瘤、霍奇金淋巴瘤、多发性骨髓瘤、实体瘤等多个病理类型出发，分别论述了自体移植的应用价值。本章的最后展望了自体移植与CART细胞治疗未来发展前景。

BASIC CONCEPTS

High-dose chemotherapy (HDC) with autologous hematopoietic progenitor cell (HPC) transplant is an effective treatment modality for several hematologic malignancies and selected solid tumors. This chapter reviews its current role in the treatment of cancer and outlines promising future directions of progress.

High-dose radiation and chemotherapy are limited by toxicity to normal tissues, particularly the bone marrow. The doses of certain chemotherapeutic agents and radiation can be substantially escalated, with the goal of exploiting their dose-response effect, when followed by autologous or allogeneic transplantation of HPCs to restore hematopoiesis. Pluripotent HPC progenitors present in the graft proliferate and differentiate into the mature blood and immune cells. Autologous transplantation involves collection, cryopreservation, and infusion of the patient's own HPCs.

GENERAL PROCEDURES FOR AUTOLOGOUS TRANSPLANTATION

Preceding Conventional Dose Chemotherapy

Standard chemotherapy is usually given to reduce the tumor burden prior to proceeding with HPC transplantation (Fig. 12-1). In general, the best outcomes are noted in patients with chemosensitive disease, in complete remission (CR), or with minimal tumor burden at time of transplantation.

Stem Cell Collection

Bone marrow is collected via multiple aspirations from the posterior-superior iliac crest in a sterile environment (usually a surgical operating room) while the patient is under anesthesia. Ideally, HPCs should be collected while the patient's marrow is normocellular and uninvolved by the malignancy. Currently, bone marrow HPC collection is rarely, if ever, done for the purpose of autologous transplantation because HPCs can be collected from peripheral blood and engraft more rapidly when collected this way. Hematopoietic progenitor cells are normally infrequent in the blood but are mobilized into the blood during the recovery after chemotherapy and following treatment with granulocyte colony-stimulating factor (G-CSF). Peripheral blood progenitor cells (PBPCs) are collected using apheresis with continuous-flow cell separation. One to four daily apheresis sessions are usually required to achieve the minimal target $CD34^+$ cell dose (at least 2×10^6/kg). The collected PBPCs are subsequently cryopreserved and stored.

Multiple factors have been shown to predict poor success in mobilization and collection, including advanced age; amount of preceding chemotherapy; presence of marrow-infiltrating disease; history of pelvic radiation; prior exposure to certain drugs (melphalan,

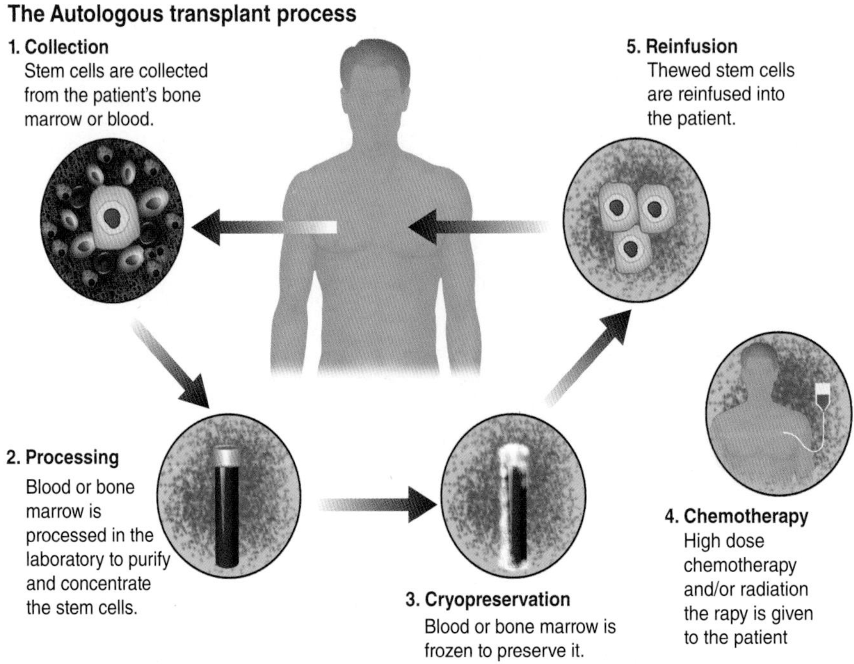

FIGURE 12-1 Autologous hematopoietic progenitor cell transplantation process.

CHAPTER 12

carmustine, bendamustine); low premobilization platelet counts; short intervals from last chemotherapy cycle to mobilization; inadequate chemotherapy-mobilizing regimens or low-dose G-CSF ([1]); and previous treatment with four or more cycles of lenalidomide ([2]). Peripheral blood CD34+ cells more than 10/μL are usually necessary for an adequate collection. Plerixafor has become available as a second PBPC-mobilizing agent, effective for "poor mobilizers," acting synergistically with G-CSF ([3]).

High-Dose Therapy

Autologous transplants are most effective in diseases where up to a three- to fivefold dose escalation of myelosuppressive drugs or radiation leads to a markedly increased cytotoxic effect against the malignancy. The most commonly used drugs are alkylating agents.

The most common cause of failure after autologous HPC transplantation is relapse of the underlying malignancy. This usually occurs because of inadequate systemic cytoreduction, although it may also be caused by reinfusion of malignant cells contaminating the transplant infusion. The optimal HDC regimen is disease specific. Various approaches are being studied to improve the final outcomes, including novel chemotherapy agents ([4, 5]), monoclonal antibodies ([6]), chemoradiotherapy ([7, 8]), and targeted radiation treatments. "Tandem" autologous HPC transplants have been studied in myeloma and germ-cell tumors ([9]). In chemosensitive malignancies, increasing the total dose of therapy may markedly improve the tumor response, but this increases the severity of side effects. Thus, novel HDC regimens must be developed in carefully designed clinical trials to provide the optimal therapeutic index.

Reinfusion of Collected Stem Cells

Stem cells are infused intravenously after HDC is eliminated from the patient's bloodstream, usually 1 to 3 days after completion of the treatment. The cells circulate transiently and home to the bone marrow. Hematopoiesis is restored within a few weeks. Hematopoietic recovery is most rapid with infusion of high doses of CD34+ cells. Most centers require a minimum 2×10^6/kg CD34+ cells per kilogram from peripheral blood ([10]). Neutrophils recover typically in 7 to 10 days and platelets recover in 10 to 14 days after infusion.

Supportive Care

Patients usually receive G-CSF or other hematopoietic growth factors to accelerate neutrophil recovery. Patients are routinely prescribed prophylactic antibiotics and antiviral and antifungal therapy for prevention of infection during the initial phase of marrow engraftment and hematologic recovery.

CONTROVERSIES

Autologous Versus Allogeneic Hematopoietic Progenitor Cell Transplants

The relative role of allogeneic versus autologous transplants has been long debated for specific hematologic malignancies. Autologous HPC transplantation is a process that carries less overall morbidity and mortality because the reinfused cells are not subject to immunologic rejection and do not produce graft-versus-host disease (GVHD). On the other hand, there is a risk of tumor contamination of the autologous HPCs. Some clinical studies have shown that autograft contamination is correlated with shortened disease-free survival (DFS) ([11]) and that the presence of tumor cells or their inadequate purging in autologous samples may correlate with the extent of the disease. Gene-marking studies in neuroblastoma showed that persistent cancer cells in the autograft can contribute to systemic relapse. The risk of contamination of the graft is higher in patients with uncontrolled tumors and known marrow involvement. Perhaps more important, there is no evidence that immune-mediated graft-versus-tumor effect associated with allogeneic HPC transplantation occurs with autologous transplants.

COMPLICATIONS OF HIGH-DOSE CHEMOTHERAPY

High-dose chemotherapy produces profound pancytopenia that usually lasts from 7 to 10 days. Infectious complications can occur in the neutropenic period (ranging from febrile neutropenia to life-threatening septic episodes) and up to 6 months or more posttransplant in the case of *Pneumocystis jirovecii*, fungal infections, or zoster reactivation. Antibacterial prophylaxis with a fluoroquinolone, antiviral prophylaxis with acyclovir/valacyclovir, and antifungal prophylaxis with fluconazole are generally started at the time of stem cell infusion and continued until recovery from neutropenia. *Pneumocystis* prophylaxis (eg, trimethoprim/sulfamethoxazole) is usually started day 30 posttransplant for at least 6 months. Antiviral prophylaxis (acyclovir, valacyclovir) are given for 6 to 12 months ([12]).

High doses of chemotherapy may produce major toxicities in nonhematopoietic tissues. The oral mucosa and the gastrointestinal tract are generally the most sensitive tissues. The lungs, heart, liver, brain, and kidneys are less commonly affected and are generally affected in heavily pretreated patients or those with comorbid conditions. Overall, up to 4% of patients die from regimen-related toxicities or infections. This rate of treatment-related mortality makes autologous transplantation substantially safer than allogeneic transplantation.

Toxic interstitial pneumonitis occurs in up to 40% of patients undergoing high-dose therapy. It has been described with several different chemotherapy agents, such as carmustine ([13, 14]) and total-body irradiation (TBI) ([15]). It is particularly common in patients previously treated with mediastinal radiotherapy ([16, 17]). Steroids constitute the mainstay of treatment of interstitial pneumonitis.

Cardiac toxicity is uncommon. It can be seen after high doses of cyclophosphamide or melphalan. Prior radiation therapy to the mediastinum or left chest wall and advanced age are also predictors of an increased risk of cardiac complications ([18]).

Central nervous system complications are rare, but dementia and leukoencephalopathy have been described as complications of HDC. Hypothyroidism frequently occurs 6 months to 2 years after therapy.

Hemorrhagic cystitis, after high-dose cyclophosphamide or ifosfamide, is uncommon and can be effectively prevented with MESNA (2-mercaptoethanesulfonate) ([19, 20]).

Sinusoidal obstruction syndrome (SOS) (formerly known as veno-occlusive disease or VOD) of the liver is one of the most feared complications associated with HDC. Its clinical syndrome is characterized by fluid retention, hyperbilirubinemia, and hepatomegaly, which can be painful ([21]). Its severity depends on the presence of multiorgan failure and the rapidity of bilirubin rise. Mild cases are often self-limited; severe cases are fatal in more than 80% of patients. Several factors predispose to the development of SOS, including prior liver impairment, older age, and iron overload. The use of oral busulfan and TBI have been most commonly associated with SOS, particularly if used along with cyclophosphamide ([22]). Andersson et al pioneered the use of intravenous busulfan, which decreases the risk of SOS compared with the oral drug formulation ([23]). Pharmacokinetic-guided dosing of busulfan has further decreased the incidence of SOS. Systemic anticoagulant and thrombolytic therapies to treat SOB are ineffective and are associated with major bleeding complications. Defibrotide has emerged as a promising therapy for severe cases of SOS but has not received approval by the Food and Drug Administration yet. Supportive care plays a crucial role, using diuretics and sodium restriction, avoidance of hepatotoxins, oxygen support, and renal replacement therapy if needed.

RESULTS OF AUTOLOGOUS TRANSPLANTATION

Non-Hodgkin Lymphoma

Autologous transplantation has been extensively studied in refractory-relapsed non-Hodgkin lymphoma (NHL).

Aggressive Lymphoma

High-dose chemotherapy and autologous stem cell transplant comprise a standard of care for patients with chemosensitive, relapsed, diffuse large B-cell lymphoma (DLBCL) ([24]) (Fig. 12-2). Resistance to salvage chemotherapy, increased lactic dehydrogenase at the time of relapse or progression, prior complete remission (CR) of less than 12 months, and secondary International Prognostic Index (IPI) (ie, at the time of relapse or progression) greater than 1 have been described as adverse predictors of survival ([25]). In the modern era of exposure to rituximab as part of first-line therapy (R-CHOP), the CORAL study has shown 3-year EFS rates of 25% in chemosensitive relapsed patients undergoing autologous stem cell transplantation ([26]).

High-dose chemotherapy in the first CR has also been evaluated for patients with DLBCL and a high IPI ([27-30]). While some randomized studies have demonstrated an improvement in EFS, none has shown a benefit in overall survival (OS). Thus, autologous transplantation is not routinely used as consolidation in a first remission for DLCL.

Follicular Lymphoma

The role of autologous HPC transplantation remains unclear in the management of patients with chemosensitive, relapsed low-grade lymphoma (eg, follicular lymphoma, FL). The use of high-dose cyclophosphamide ([31]) and TBI ([32]) has resulted in a 5-year EFS of 60% but has been largely abandoned due to the risk of secondary malignancies.

Historically, a major challenge has been the contamination of the autologous graft by malignant cells ([33]). Recently, systemic treatment with rituximab has reduced the numbers of circulating lymphoma cells, thus yielding effective in vivo purging with high likelihood polymerase chain reaction–negative tumor-free PBPC grafts ([34, 35]).

Several randomized trials have shown improved outcomes after HDC for chemosensitive relapsed FL ([36, 37]). However, these studies were largely conducted in the prerituxumab era. The role of HDC in this setting in the current era remains unsettled.

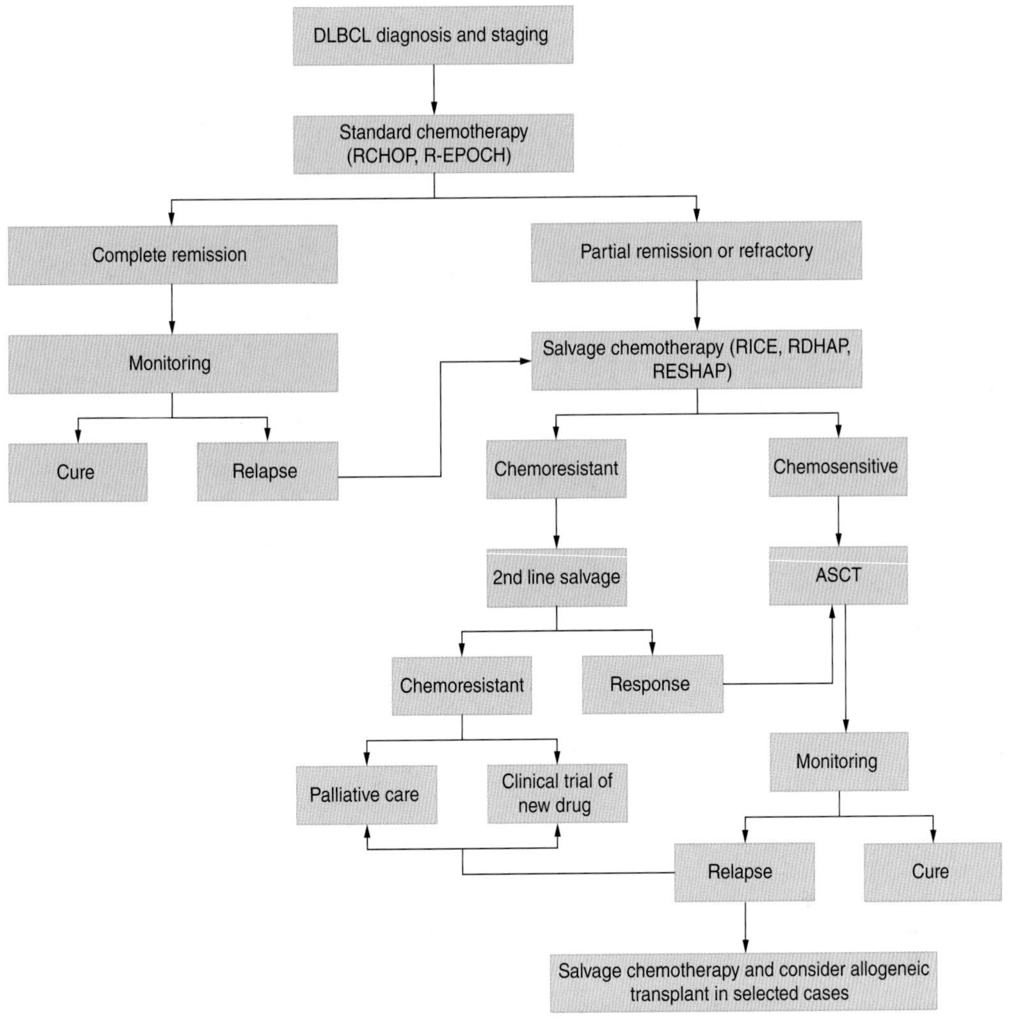

FIGURE 12-2 Algorithm for treatment of DLBCL: stepwise description of DLBCL treatment approach and the role of autologous and allogeneic progenitor cell transplantation after relapse. ASCT, allogeneic stem cell transplant.

Hodgkin Lymphoma

The majority of patients with Hodgkin lymphoma (HL) are curable with first-line therapy (Fig. 12-3). However, up to 20% of patients will not respond to first-line chemotherapy, and 30% will relapse after an initial response ([38, 39]). The use of HDC has been proven to be beneficial in the two settings, with expected long-term EFS of 30% to 40% for patients with primary refractory tumors sensitive to subsequent salvage therapy and of 30% to 65% for patients with chemosensitive relapsed HL ([40, 41]).

Unfavorable prognostic features for autologous transplant include a first CR shorter than 1 year, extranodal relapse, B symptoms at the time of relapse or progression, bulky (>5-cm) lesions at relapse, and relapse within a prior radiation field. Patients without unfavorable prognostic features have 4-year EFS rates of 70%, compared with less than 20% in patients with adverse features ([42]). Positron emission tomographic scan uptake at the time of HD has recently emerged as the main prognostic factor ([43, 44]).

Multiple Myeloma

High-dose therapy with autologous HPC transplantation is an established treatment for multiple myeloma, where the use of high-dose melphalan provides OS benefit as consolidation of a response to first-line therapy ([45-48]) (Fig. 12-4). To date, no other preparative regimen has been shown to be superior to single-agent melphalan (200 mg/m^2) ([49]). The use of a second course of high-dose melphalan ("tandem" autologous transplants) has been shown to be superior to a single transplant in some ([49-51]), but not all, studies ([52]), particularly in patients who do not achieve at least a very good partial remission after the first procedure. The timing of transplant has been prospectively investigated

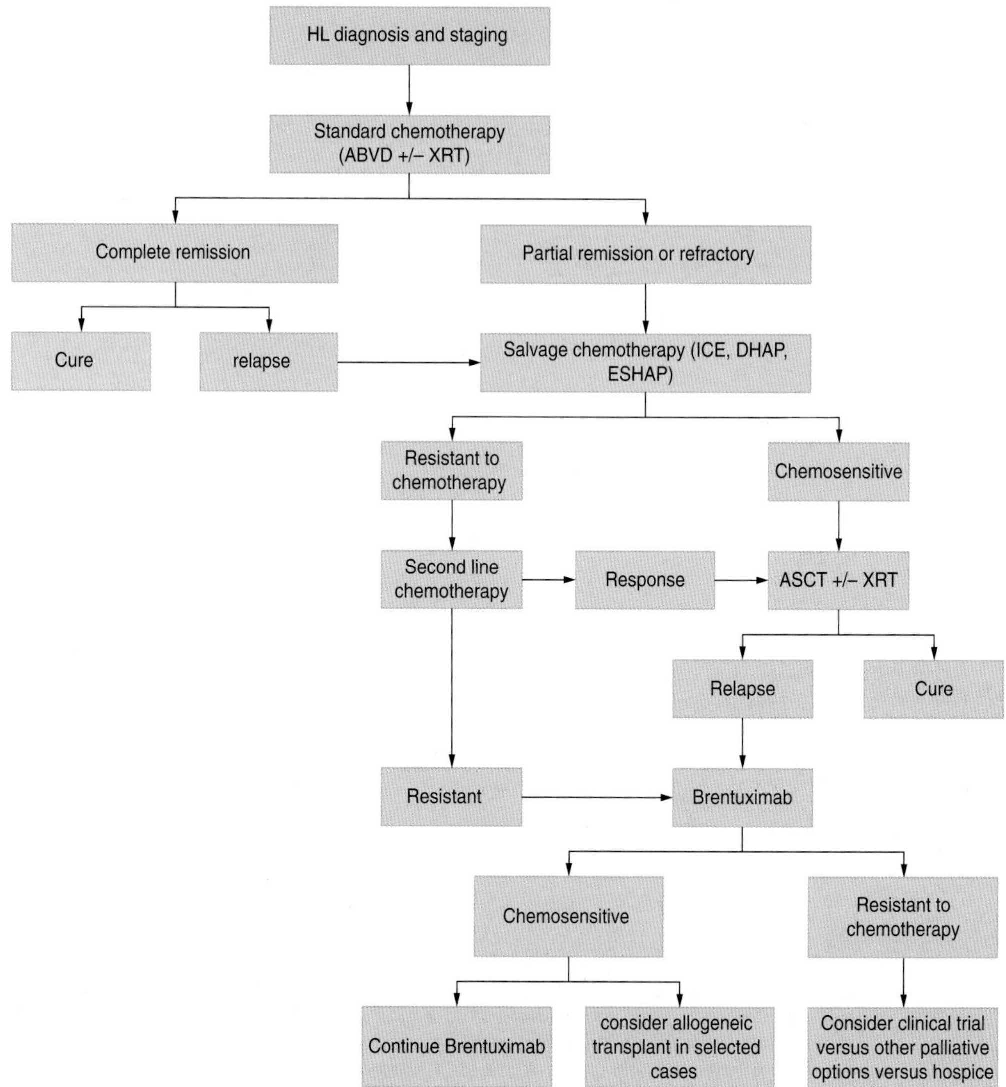

FIGURE 12-3 Algorithm for treatment of HL: stepwise description of HL treatment approach and the role of autologous and allogeneic progenitor cell transplantation after relapse.

in randomized studies. Early (after a brief course of first-line therapy) and late autotransplant (at a time of relapse after prolonged first-line therapy) trials ([53]) resulted in similar OS, with early autotransplantation offering improved quality of life, shorter duration of chemotherapy, and a longer median EFS. Induction therapy, including novel agents such as bortezomib or lenalidomide, appears to be the most effective induction treatment before HDC. Ongoing randomized trials in the United States and Europe are addressing the question of optimal timing of autologous transplant in the present era of novel agents.

Several retrospective analyses have demonstrated durable responses of a second salvage course of HDC with autologous SCT for patients with relapsed disease ([54]). In general, the outcomes appear more favorable for patients who relapse more than 12 months after a first autologous transplant and who respond to subsequent salvage treatment ([55]). More recently, the first randomized controlled trial has been completed comparing salvage HDC and autologous transplant to salvage conventional chemotherapy ([56]). In this study, there was a benefit for the transplant arm, with a significant improvement in time to progression.

Maintenance therapy posttransplant with lenalidomide prolongs EFS and perhaps OS, as shown in several randomized studies ([57, 58]). There is uncertainty about the optimal duration of lenalidomide treatment.

Its use after allogeneic stem cell transplantation has been associated with a small risk of secondary malignancies in the French, but not in the US, study.

Solid Tumors

The use of HDC for breast cancer or ovarian cancer has been abandoned. In contrast, tandem courses of carboplatin-containing HDC have been successful in curing patients with relapsed or refractory germ-cell tumors. Long-term EFS rates range from 10% for patients with cisplatin refractoriness and other poor-prognostic features to 70% for those with good-risk chemosensitive tumors in first relapse ([59]).

FUTURE DIRECTIONS

Patients with rapid recovery of lymphocyte counts have had the best progression-free survival after autologous stem cell transplantation ([60]). Following myeloablative therapy and autologous transplantation, there is homeostatic expansion of lymphocytes. This provides an opportunity for active vaccination or infusion of antigen-specific, tumor-reactive lymphocytes or to infuse genetically modified lymphocytes to enhance antitumor effects. One recent approach utilizes redirecting the specificity of T cells using a chimeric antigen receptor T cell (CAR-T) toward tumor-related antigens such as CD19 or CD20 in lymphomas ([61]).

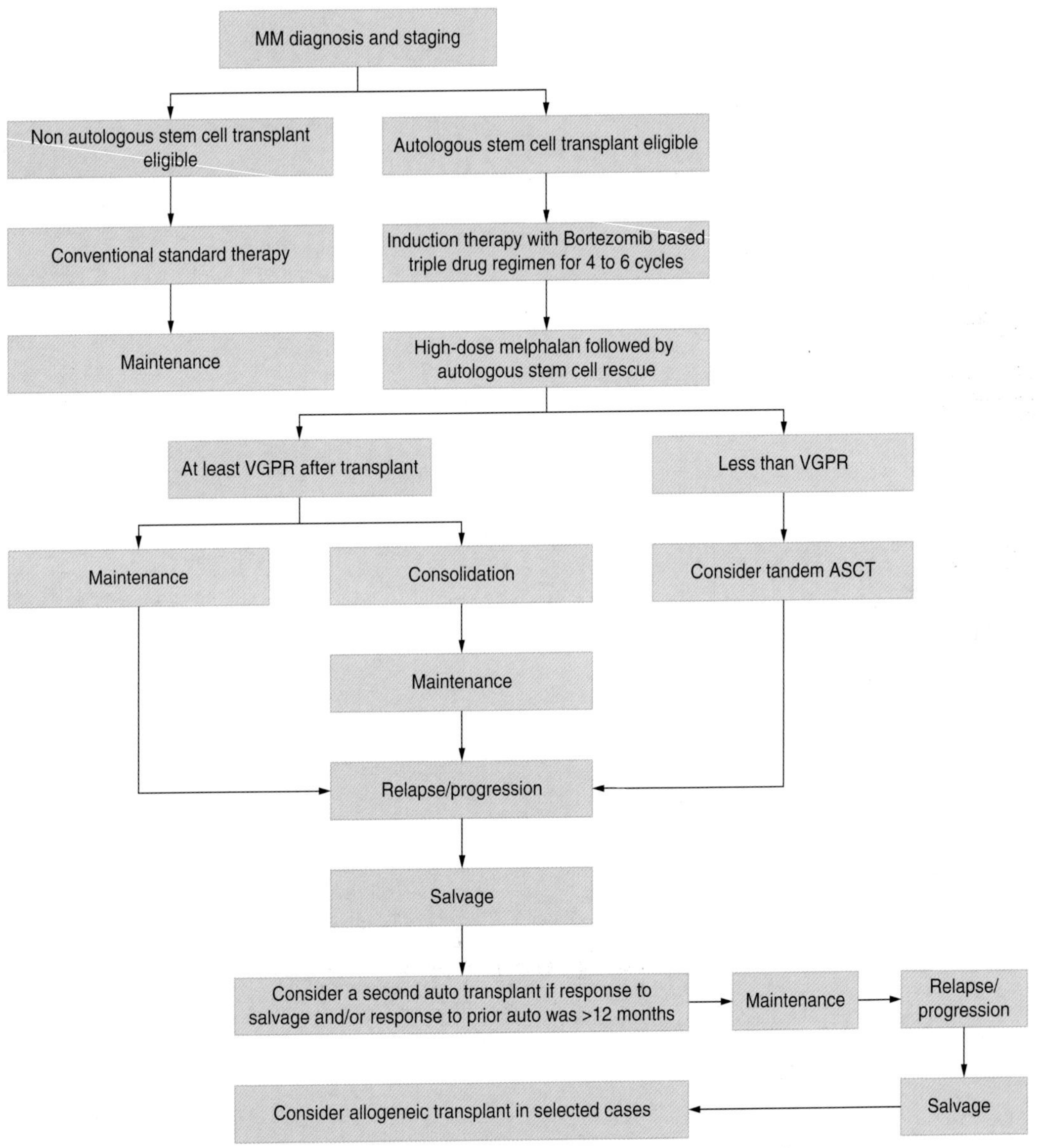

FIGURE 12-4 Algorithm for treatment of multiple myeloma (MM): stepwise description of multiple myeloma treatment approach and the role of autologous and allogeneic progenitor cell transplantation after relapse.

SUMMARY AND CONCLUSIONS

High-dose chemotherapy with autologous HPC transplantation is an effective modality to achieve major antitumor cytoreduction. Autologous transplants need to be integrated into the multimodality management of hematologic malignancies and GCTs. Many current studies focus on posttransplant strategies to prevent regrowth of minimal residual disease, including molecularly targeted approaches and angiogenesis inhibition. Further clinical trials are needed to optimize the use of autologous HPC transplantation in the overall treatment of cancer.

REFERENCES

1. Ikeda K, Kozuka T, Harada M. Factors for PBPC collection efficiency and collection predictors. *Transfus Apher Sci.* 2004;31(3):245-259.
2. Popat U, Saliba R, Thandi R, et al. Impairment of filgrastim-induced stem cell mobilization after prior lenalidomide in patients with multiple myeloma. *Biol Blood Marrow Transplant.* 2009;15(6):718-723.
3. Devine SM, Flomenberg N, Vesole DH, et al. Rapid mobilization of CD34+ cells following administration of the CXCR4 antagonist AMD3100 to patients with multiple myeloma and non-Hodgkin's lymphoma. *J Clin Oncol.* 2004;22:1095–1102.
4. Roussel M, Moreau P, Huynh A, et al. Bortezomib and high dose melphalan as conditioning regimen before autologous stem cell transplantation in patients with de novo multiple myeloma: A phase II study of the Intergroupe Francophone du Myelome (IFM). *Blood.* 2010;115(1):32-37.
5. Barlogie B. Thalidomide and CC-5013 in multiple myeloma: the University of Arkansas experience. *Semin Hematol.* 2003;40 (4 Suppl 4):33-38.
6. Montillo M, Tedeschi A, Miqueleiz S, et al. Alemtuzumab as consolidation after a response to fludarabine is effective in purging residual disease in patients with chronic lymphocytic leukemia. *J Clin Oncol.* 2006;24(15):2337-2342.
7. Vose JM, Bierman PJ, Enke C, et al. Phase I trial of iodine-131 tositumomab with high-dose chemotherapy and autologous stem-cell transplantation for relapsed non-Hodgkin's lymphoma. *J Clin Oncol.* 2005;23(3):461-467.
8. Krishnan A, Nademanee A, Fung HC, et al. Phase II trial of a transplantation regimen of yttrium-90 ibritumomab tiuxetan and high-dose chemotherapy in patients with non-Hodgkin's lymphoma. *J Clin Oncol.* 2008;26(1):90-95.
9. Mehta J. Re: tandem vs single autologous hematopoietic cell transplantation for the treatment of multiple myeloma: a systematic review and meta-analysis. *J Natl Cancer Inst.* 2009;101(20):1430-1431; author reply 1431-1433.
10. Ketterer N, Salles G, Raba M, et al. High CD34 (+) cell counts decrease hematologic toxicity of autologous peripheral blood progenitor cell transplantation. *Blood.* 1998;91(9):3148-3155.
11. Kopp HG, Yildirim S, Weisel KC, et al. Contamination of autologous peripheral blood progenitor cell grafts predicts overall survival after high-dose chemotherapy in multiple myeloma. *J Cancer Res Clin Oncol.* 2009;135(4): 637-642.
12. Tomblyn M, Chiller T, Einsele H, et al. Guidelines for preventing infectious complications among hematopoietic cell transplantation recipients: A global perspective. *Biol Blood Marrow Transplant.* 2009;15(10):1143-1238.
13. Fassas A, Gojo I, Rapoport A, et al. Pulmonary toxicity syndrome following CDEP (cyclophosphamide, dexamethasone, etoposide, cisplatin) chemotherapy. *Bone Marrow Transplant.* 2001;28(4):399-403.
14. Williams L, Beveridge RA, Rifkin RM, et al. Increased pulmonary toxicity results from a 1-day versus 2-day schedule of administration of high-dose melphalan. *Biol Blood Marrow Transplant.* 2002;8(6):334-335.
15. Chen CI, Abraham R, Tsang R, et al. Radiation-associated pneumonitis following autologous stem cell transplantation: predictive factors, disease characteristics and treatment outcomes. *Bone Marrow Transplant.* 2001;27(2):177-182.
16. Alessandrino EP, Bernasconi P, Colombo A, et al. Pulmonary toxicity following carmustine-based preparative regimens and autologous peripheral blood progenitor cell transplantation in hematological malignancies. *Bone Marrow Transplant.* 2000;25(3):309-313.
17. Cao TM, Negrin RS, Stockerl-Goldstein KE, et al. Pulmonary toxicity syndrome in breast cancer patients undergoing BCNU-containing high-dose chemotherapy and autologous hematopoietic cell transplantation. *Biol Blood Marrow Transplant.* 2000;6(4):387-394.
18. Nieto Y, Cagnoni PJ, Bearman SI, et al. Cardiac toxicity following high-dose cyclophosphamide, cisplatin, and BCNU (STAMP-I) for breast cancer. *Biol Blood Marrow Transplant.* 2000;6(2A):198-203.
19. Frustaci S, Foladore S, De Pascale A, et al. Feasibility and efficacy of arginine 2-mercaptoethanesulfonate (ARGIMESNA) in the prevention of hemorragic cystitis from ifosfamide (IFO). *Ann Oncol.* 1992;3(Suppl 2):S115-S118.
20. Khojasteh NH, Zakerinia M, Ramzi M, et al. A new regimen of MESNA (2-mercaptoethanesulfonate) effectively prevents cyclophosphamide-induced hemorrhagic cystitis in bone marrow transplant recipients. *Transplant Proc.* 2000;32(3):596.
21. Bearman SI. The syndrome of hepatic veno-occlusive disease after marrow transplantation. *Blood.* 1995;85:3005-3020.
22. Strasser SI, McDonald GB. Gastrointestinal and hepatic complications. In: Appelbaum FR, Forman SJ, Negrin RS, Blume KG, eds. *Thomas' Hematopoietic Cell Transplantation: Stem Cell Transplantation.* 4th ed. Oxford, UK: Wiley-Blackwell. doi:10.1002/9781444303537.ch95
23. Andersson BS, Madden T, Tran HT, et al. Acute safety and pharmacokinetics of intravenous busulfan when used with oral busulfan and cyclophosphamide as pretransplant conditioning therapy: a phase I study. *Biol Blood Marrow Transplant.* 2000;6:548–554.
24. Philip T, Guglielmi C, Hagenbeek A, et al. Autologous bone marrow transplantation as compared with salvage chemotherapy in relapses of chemotherapy-sensitive non-Hodgkin's lymphoma. *N Engl J Med.* 1995;333(23):1540-1545.
25. Vose JM, Rizzo DJ, Tao-Wu J, et al. Autologous transplantation for diffuse aggressive non-Hodgkin lymphoma in first relapse or second remission. *Biol Blood Marrow Transplant.* 2004;10(2):116-127.
26. Gisselbrecht C, Glass B, Mounier M, et al. Salvage regimens with autologous transplantation for relapsed large B-cell lymphoma in the rituximab era. *J Clin Oncol.* 2010;28(27):4184-4190.
27. Sweetenham JW, Proctor SJ, Blaise D, et al. High-dose therapy and autologous bone marrow transplantation in first complete remission for adult patients with high-grade non-Hodgkin's lymphoma: the EBMT experience. Lymphoma Working Party of the European Group for Bone Marrow Transplantation. *Ann Oncol.* 1994;5(Suppl 2):155-159.
28. Jackson GH, Lennard AL, Taylor PR, et al. Autologous bone marrow transplantation in poor-risk high-grade non-Hodgkin's lymphoma in first complete remission. Newcastle and Northern Lymphoma Group. *Br J Cancer.* 1994;70(3):501-505.
29. Vranovsky A, Ladicka M, Lakota J. Autologous stem cell transplantation in first-line treatment of high-risk aggressive

non-Hodgkin's lymphoma. *Neoplasma*. 2008;55(2):107-112.
30. Tarella C, Gianni AM. Bone marrow transplantation for lymphoma CR1. *Curr Opin Oncol*. 2005;17(2):99-105.
31. Horning SJ, Negrin RS, Hoppe RT, et al. High-dose therapy and autologous bone marrow transplantation for follicular lymphoma in first complete or partial remission: results of a phase II clinical trial. *Blood*. 2001;97(2):404-409.
32. Freedman AS, Ritz J, Neuberg D, et al. Autologous bone marrow transplantation in 69 patients with a history of low-grade B-cell non-Hodgkin's lymphoma. *Blood*. 1991;77(11): 2524-2529.
33. Gribben JG. Autologous hematopoietic transplantation for low-grade lymphomas. *Cytotherapy*. 2002;4:205-215.
34. Kato H, Taji H, Ogura M, et al. Favorable consolidative effect of high-dose melphalan and total-body irradiation followed by autologous peripheral blood stem cell transplantation after rituximab-containing induction chemotherapy with in vivo purging in relapsed or refractory follicular lymphoma. *Clin Lymphoma Myeloma*. 2009;9(6):443-448.
35. Cerny J, Trneny M, Slavickova A, et al. Rituximab based therapy followed by autologous stem cell transplantation leads to superior outcome and high rates of PCR negativity in patients with indolent B-cell lymphoproliferative disorders. *Hematology*. 2009;14(4):187-197.
36. Ladetto M, De Marco F, Benedetti F, et al. Prospective, multicenter randomized GITMO/IIL trial comparing intensive (R-HDS) versus conventional (CHOP-R) chemoimmunotherapy in high-risk follicular lymphoma at diagnosis: the superior disease control of R-HDS does not translate into an overall survival advantag. *Blood*. 2008;111(8):4004-4013.
37. Harry C. Schouten, Wendi Qian, et al. High-dose therapy improves progression-free survival and survival in relapsed follicular non-Hodgkin's lymphoma: results from the randomized European CUP Trial. *J Clin Oncol*. 21:3918-3927.
38. Viviani S, Bonadonna G, Santoro A, et al. alternating versus hybrid MOPP and ABVD combinations in advanced Hodgkin's disease: ten-year results. *J Clin Oncol*. 1996;14(5):1421-1430.
39. Champlin R. Bone marrow transplantation for Hodgkin's disease–recent advances and current issues. *Leuk Lymphoma*. 1993;10(Suppl):103-108.
40. Linch DC1, Winfield D, Goldstone AH, et al. Dose intensification with autologous bone-marrow transplantation in relapsed and resistant Hodgkin's disease: results of a BNLI randomised trial. *Lancet*. 1993;341(8852):1051-1054.
41. Schmitz N, Pfistner B, Sextro M, et al. Aggressive conventional chemotherapy compared with high-dose chemotherapy with autologous haemopoietic stem-cell transplantation for relapsed chemosensitive Hodgkin's disease: a randomised trial of the German Hodgkin's Lymphoma Study Group (GHSG) and the Lymphoma Working Party of the European Group for Blood and Marrow Transplantation (EBMT). *Lancet*. 2002;359(9323):2065-2071.
42. Jagannath S, Armitage JO, Dicke KA, et al. Prognostic factors for response and survival after high-dose cyclophosphamide, carmustine, and etoposide with autologous bone marrow transplantation for relapsed Hodgkin's disease. *J Clin Oncol*. 1989;7(2):179-185.
43. Castagna L, Bramanti S, Balzarotti M, et al. Predictive value of early 18F-fluorodeoxyglucose positron emission tomography (FDG-PET) during salvage chemotherapy in relapsing/refractory Hodgkin lymphoma (HL) treated with high-dose chemotherapy. *Br J Haematol*. 2009;145(3):369-372.
44. Jabbour E, Hosing C, Ayers G, et al. Pretransplant positive positron emission tomography/gallium scans predict poor outcome in patients with recurrent/refractory Hodgkin lymphoma. *Cancer*. 2007;109(12):2481-2489.
45. Attal M, Harousseau JL, Stoppa AM, et al. A prospective, randomized trial of autologous bone marrow transplantation and chemotherapy in multiple myeloma. Intergroupe Francais du Myelome. *N Engl J Med*. 1996;335(2):91-97.
46. Child JA, Morgan GJ, Davies FE, et al. High-dose chemotherapy with hematopoietic stem-cell rescue for multiple myeloma. *N Engl J Med*. 2003;348(19):1875-1883.
47. Lenhoff S, Hjorth M, Holmberg E, et al. Impact on survival of high-dose therapy with autologous stem cell support in patients younger than 60 years with newly diagnosed multiple myeloma: a population-based study. Nordic Myeloma Study Group. *Blood*. 2000;95(1):7-11.
48. Palumbo A, Triolo S, Argentino C, et al. Dose-intensive melphalan with stem cell support (MEL100) is superior to standard treatment in elderly myeloma patients. *Blood*. 1999;94(4):1248-1253.
49. Barlogie B, Shaughnessy J, Tricot G, et al. Treatment of multiple myeloma. *Blood*. 2004;103(1):20-32.
50. Barlogie B, Jagannath S, Desikan KR, et al. Total therapy with tandem transplants for newly diagnosed multiple myeloma. *Blood*. 1999;93(1):55-65.
51. Attal M, Harousseau JL, Facon T, et al. Single versus double autologous stem-cell transplantation for multiple myeloma. *N Engl J Med*. 2003;349(26):2495-2502.
52. Giralt S, Vesole DH, Somlo G, et al. Re: tandem vs single autologous hematopoietic cell transplantation for the treatment of multiple myeloma: a systematic review and meta-analysis. *J Natl Cancer Inst*. 2009;101(13):964; author reply 966-967.
53. Fermand JP1, Ravaud P, Chevret S, et al. High-dose therapy and autologous peripheral blood stem cell transplantation in multiple myeloma: up-front or rescue treatment? Results of a multicenter sequential randomized clinical trial. *Blood*. 1998;92(9):3131-3136.
54. Shah N, Ahmed F, Bashir Q, et al. Durable remission with salvage second autotransplants in patients with multiple myeloma. *Cancer*. 2012;118(14):3549-3555.
55. WI Gonsalves, MA Gertz, MQ Lacy, et al. Second auto-SCT for treatment of relapsed multiple myeloma. *Bone Marrow Transplant*. 2013;48:568–573.
56. Cook G, Williams C, Brown JM, et al. High-dose chemotherapy plus autologous stem-cell transplantation as consolidation therapy in patients with relapsed multiple myeloma after previous autologous stem-cell transplantation (NCRI Myeloma X Relapse [Intensive trial]): a randomised, open-label, phase 3 trial. *Lancet Oncol*. 2014;15(8):874-885.
57. Attal M, Lauwers-Cances V, Marit G, et al. Lenalidomide maintenance after stem-cell transplantation for multiple myeloma. *N Engl J Med*. 2012;366:1782-1791.
58. McCarthy P, Owzar K, Hofmeister C, et al. Lenalidomide after stem-cell transplantation for multiple myeloma. *N Engl J Med*. 2012;366:1770-1781.
59. Nieto, Y. Transplantation for refractory germ cell tumors: does it really make a difference? *Curr Oncol Rep*. 2013;15(3):232-238.
60. Joao C, Porrata LF, Inwards DJ, et al. Early lymphocyte recovery after autologous stem cell transplantation predicts superior survival in mantle-cell lymphoma. *Bone Marrow Transplant*. 2006;37(9):865-871.
61. Singh H, Serrano LM, Pfeiffer T, et al. Combining adoptive cellular and immunocytokine therapies to improve treatment of B-lineage malignancy. *Cancer Res*. 2007;67(6):2872-2880.

13

Allogeneic Transplantation

第十三章　同种异体移植

Jonathan E. Brammer
Borje S. Andersson
Chitra Hosing

中文导读

对于血液系统恶性肿瘤患者，异体干细胞移植对比标准化疗为无法根治的患者提供了一种潜在治愈的手段。过去十余年中，异体干细胞移植技术的发展给很多既往移植高风险的患者带来了根治治疗的机会。本章对异体干细胞移植技术在临床中的运用进行了详细阐述。首先简要回顾了异体干细胞移植的历史发展和相关背景，接着详细介绍了异体干细胞移植的步骤，涵盖了受体的选择、受体的准备、异体干细胞的来源以及移植物抗宿主病的预防等临床应用中的重要环节。随后介绍了移植后的处理流程和常见并发症的处理，包括预防感染、骨髓抑制的治疗、移植失败和肺部感染等并发症处理。急性和慢性移植物抗宿主病是临床工作中移植后常见的并发症，本章对此着重进行了阐述。最后介绍了移植晚期的并发症和移植后复发的处理。

INTRODUCTION

For patients with hematologic malignancies, allogeneic stem cell transplantation (alloSCT) provides potentially curative therapy over standard therapeutic approaches in patients whose disease is incurable with standard chemotherapy. With the development of novel techniques of transplantation, including reduced-intensity conditioning (RIC) and management of transplant-associated toxicities, increasing numbers of patients with advanced age or comorbidities can undergo this potentially lifesaving procedure. According to the most recent statistics from the Center for International Blood and Marrow Transplant Research (CIBMTR), a consortium that collects data from over 400 transplant centers worldwide, over 9,000 patients received alloSCT in 2011, up from 7,500 in 2001 ([1]). Given the increasing frequency of stem cell transplants worldwide, practitioners need to be familiar with the key concepts regarding the indications, procedures, and management of this technique. This chapter reviews the current state of alloSCT, with particular attention to strategies utilized at the MD Anderson Cancer Center (MDACC). The specific indications for alloSCT are briefly discussed, but a more in-depth discussion of indications is found in chapters covering specific disease states.

Background and Rationale

Allogeneic stem cell transplantation was first explored in humans in the late 1950s and early 1960s based on observations in animal models that lethal myelosuppression induced by total-body irradiation (TBI) could be overcome by the infusion of healthy, untreated bone marrow ([2]). The initial experience was limited to patients with terminal leukemia or severe marrow failure states resulting from radiation exposure or disease. Almost all of these early patients died from complications of graft failure, graft-versus-host disease (GVHD), infections, or primary disease ([3]). The first successful allogeneic bone marrow transplant was reported in 1968 in a patient with severe combined immunodeficiency ([4]). Since these initial experiences, alloSCT has been used to treat thousands of patients with historically incurable diseases.

In the early days of the field, it was thought that the curative effect of alloSCT was provided primarily by the high doses of chemotherapy and radiation administered, and that the donor bone marrow simply allowed for hematopoietic recovery in an adequate period of time. However, it was later determined that the stem cell graft, and associated donor immunity, was responsible for the curative potential of alloSCT. This graft-versus-tumor (GVT) effect was first demonstrated in a landmark study published in 1990 ([5]). This study showed decreased rates of relapse in patients who experienced GVHD, an auto-immune syndrome associated with human leukocyte antigen (HLA) mismatch between the donor and recipient. Patients who experienced GVHD had lower rates of relapse compared to patients who either did not experience GVHD or received T-cell-depleted/syngeneic grafts. Patients with GVHD had a strong GVT effect, suggesting that similar mechanisms underlie the immunologic biology of both processes. However, it does not appear that GVHD is necessary for the GVT effect. Separating the adverse effects of GVHD from the therapeutic effect of the GVT effect remains the goal of current efforts to maximize the benefit of alloSCT.

The primary components of all allogeneic hematopoietic transplants are schematically represented in Fig. 13-1 and include recipient, donor, preparative regimen, stem cell source, prophylaxis against GVHD (including posttransplant immune suppression), and posttransplant supportive care. Successful allografting depends on careful consideration of all these components in an effort to minimize the risks of potentially fatal posttransplant complications.

COMPONENTS OF ALLOGENEIC STEM CELL TRANSPLANTATION

Recipient

Allogeneic stem cell transplantation is indicated for a variety of hematologic disorders, although the indication for alloSCT is dependent on the disease, remission status, stage, cytogenetics, and molecular markers in an individual patient. According to the CIBMTR database, the most common indications for alloSCT worldwide

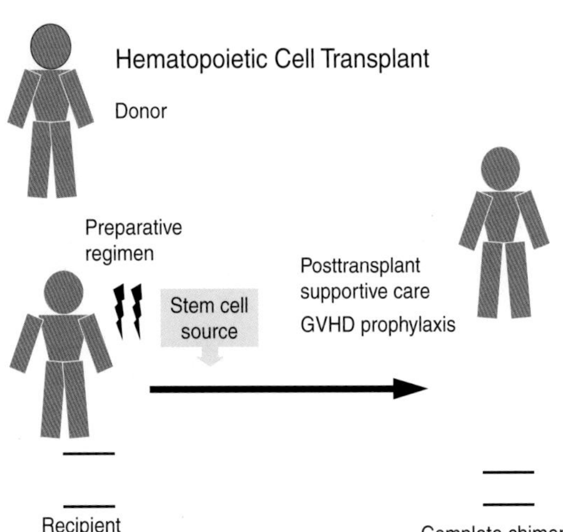

FIGURE 13-1 Components of allogeneic hematopoietic transplantation.

CHAPTER 13

are, in decreasing order: acute myelogenous leukemia (AML), acute lymphoblastic leukemia (ALL), myelodysplasia/myeloproliferative disease, nonmalignant disease, non-Hodgkin lymphoma (NHL), other malignant disease, chronic lymphocytic leukemia (CLL), aplastic anemia, chronic myelogenous leukemia (CML), Hodgkin lymphoma (HL), and multiple myeloma (MM).

The most important recipient-related factors are disease status at transplant and comorbidity status. Over the past 5 years, two risk scores have been developed that enable clinicians to determine who the best transplant recipient is and when transplant should occur. The first is the Armand Disease Risk Index (DRI) ([6]). This analysis identified four risk groups (low, intermediate, high, very high) based on disease type (AML, ALL, cytogenetic classification, etc.) and disease stage (remission status, complete remission [CR], partial remission, induction failure, etc.). Patients in the low, intermediate, high, and very high risk groups had 4-year overall survival (OS) rates of 64%, 46%, 26%, and 6%, respectively, with higher rates of relapse in the higher-risk groups. This scoring system was validated in multivariate analysis as an independent predictor of OS, progression-free survival (PFS), relapse, and nonrelapse mortality (NRM). Subsequent investigators have confirmed the outcomes associations with DRI as well ([7]). The second important tool utilized in selecting patients for alloSCT is the comorbidity index (Hematopoietic Cell Transplantation-Comorbidity Index, HCT-CI), developed by Sorror et al ([8]). Patients' comorbidities were analyzed to determine significant indicators of NRM. Patients with a HCT-CI score of 0, 1 or 2, and 3+ had 2-year NRM of 14%, 21%, and 41%, respectively. Increased pretransplant HCT-CI score has also been shown to predict the severity and mortality of acute GVHD (aGVHD) ([9]). A recent publication from the same group demonstrated that age greater than 40 years combined with the HCT-CI into a "composite comorbidity/age index" correlated with increased NRM for patients with a combined score of 3 or 4 (1 point was added to the HCT-CI for age greater than 40 years) ([10]). The results of this study need to be validated, but the data suggest that the HCT-CI/age index should be considered as part of the evaluation of any patient undergoing transplant. The HCT-CI score can be easily calculated using a validated web-based application (http://www.hctci.org).

At MDACC, all patients undergo an extensive evaluation prior to alloSCT. This includes a complete history and physical, pulmonary function tests (PFTs), echocardiogram, electrocardiogram (ECG), complete blood cell count, and chemistries. The performance status and HCT-CI are documented for each patient. Patients with a HCT-CI score of 0 to 2 are typically considered candidates for myeloablative transplant regimens, whereas patients with HCT-CI scores of 3 or greater are considered for reduced-intensity regimens. Regimen intensity is discussed further in the chapter. There is no specific cutoff for age in evaluating a patient for transplant; rather, a patient's HCT-CI, DRI, age, disease status, family and social support, and personal wishes are all taken into consideration when deciding on proceeding with transplant. A personalized multidisciplinary approach, with a thorough discussion of the risks and benefits of alloSCT, should be undertaken for each patient.

Donor

Most allografts are performed using hematopoietic progenitor cells obtained from an HLA-identical sibling. Transplants using cells procured from volunteer donors, mismatched family members, and cord blood are rapidly becoming more common. The most important factor in selecting an allogeneic donor is HLA compatibility, which is determined by HLA typing. The HLA compatibility is the single most important determinant for the occurrence of severe GVHD after alloSCT.

The HLA system is encoded by a series of genes on chromosome 6. For SCT HLA-A, HLA-B, HLA-C, and HLA-DR are routinely evaluated ([11]). In its strictest sense, *HLA identity* means that the donor and recipient are matched for the amino acid sequence encoded by all HLA loci. Identity is assumed in the setting of related transplant when segregation analysis demonstrates that the donor and recipient have inherited the same maternal and paternal haplotypes (genotypic HLA identity). Otherwise, HLA identity can be verified only by sequencing all HLA loci (phenotypic HLA identity), which is impractical and rarely done.

It is important to note that conventional typing techniques detect a limited number of HLA polymorphic sequences. Therefore, "HLA matched" may not actually be "HLA identical." Conventional serologic typing is based on the complement-dependent microlymphocytotoxicity test and uses selected HLA-specific alloantisera or monoclonal antibodies to identify HLA antigens. A mismatch between cross-reactive antigens is considered minor, whereas a mismatch between non-cross-reactive antigens is considered major. For related patient–donor pairs, a single minor mismatch may be of little biological significance. Molecular typing relies on polymerase chain reaction (PCR) amplification of specific gene segments and can be performed (a) at a level corresponding to the specificities identified by serology (low resolution), (b) at a level where a limited number of alleles are possible (intermediate resolution), or (c) at a level where the specific allele is identified (high resolution). Sequence-based HLA typing is the most precise technique available.

At MDACC, we perform high-resolution typing at HLA-A, HLA-B, HLA-C, DR, DQ, and DP for all related and unrelated donor transplants. Only matching at HLA-A, -B, -C, and DR has been associated with improved survival ([12]). However, patients with DP mismatch have decreased relapse rates, although this is negated by increased GVHD rates. Patients are considered "10/10" if they have identical tissue types for both alleles HLA-A, -B, -C, DR, and DQ, resulting in 10 alleles total. In general, the order of preference at MDACC is matched-related-donor (MRD) sibling, 10/10 matched-unrelated donor (MUD), followed by either cord blood or haploidentical transplantation. The best alternative donor source has not been determined and is the subject of a randomized clinical trial (Bone and Marrow Transplant Clinical Trials Network [BMT CTN] 1101). Discussion of alternative stem cell sources is covered in detail in their respective chapters.

Once identified, the donor must undergo a thorough medical evaluation to determine that (a) he or she may donate safely, (b) the cells will be adequate for the recipient, and (c) the donor understands the risks and benefits of the procedure and provides cells voluntarily.

Preparative Regimen

Preparative regimens are high doses of chemotherapy or TBI administered prior to stem cell infusion with the dual purpose of eradicating the underlying malignancy and inducing a state of immune tolerance that allows for donor cells to engraft and expand. This second effect ultimately gives rise to the GVT effect mediated by donor T cells, which was initially discovered when using donor leukocyte infusions ([13, 14]). Preparative regimens can be categorized into myeloablative conditioning (MAC) versus RIC. RIC can be defined using the CIBMTR criteria: reversible myelosuppression without stem cell support, typically resulting in mixed chimerism in a significant proportion of patients, accompanied by a somewhat decreased rate of nonhematologic toxicity ([15]). The choice between MAC and RIC regimens is based on the underlying disease, the patient's age and comorbid condition(s), and the physician's preference.

CHAPTER 13

Myeloablative Conditioning

Myeloablative conditioning regimens can generally be divided into chemotherapy-based protocols and TBI-based protocols. Total-body irradiation is both immunosuppressive and myeloablative. Single-dose TBI is associated with greater normal-organ toxicity, particularly pulmonary, compared with fractionated regimens ([16]). Therefore, most modern regimens deliver a total dose of 10 to 15 Gy using a variety of fractionation schedules. There is some evidence that higher total doses of TBI may be more effective at preventing relapse, but these benefits are offset by increased NRM. High-dose cyclophosphamide (Cy), a potent immunosuppressive agent, is often given as 60 mg/kg IV on two consecutive days prior to fractionated TBI as part of a Cy-TBI regimen. Although efficacious, TBI is associated with a number of short- and long-term complications, including secondary malignancies, retarded growth and intellectual development, cataracts, and endocrine dysfunction.

The toxicities of TBI-based strategies led to the development of radiation-free conditioning regimens. The most commonly used chemotherapy is the combination of busulfan and cyclophosphamide (BuCy). Busulfan was traditionally administered orally as 4 mg/kg/d divided into four daily doses and given on each of four successive days (total dose, 16 mg/kg), followed by Cy as depicted previously over 2 to 4 days. This was often complicated by excessive toxicity, including veno-occlusive disease (VOD)/sinusoidal obstruction syndrome (SOS), due to the unpredictable bioavailability of oral Bu combined with an adverse interaction with Cy. An intravenous formulation of Bu subsequently has allowed for once- or twice-daily dosing with more predictable systemic drug exposure, especially when coupled with pharmacokinetic targeted dose monitoring (TDM, or "targeted Bu") ([17]). The combination of intravenous Bu and Cy was better tolerated and improved relapse and survival rates ([18]). Further large-scale comparisons of TBI-based versus intravenous Bu-based conditioning in North America and Europe conclusively demonstrated that intravenous Bu-based conditioning is safer and more efficacious than both TBI- and oral Bu-based conditioning for myeloid disorders ([19-21]). These and recently completed studies at MDACC led to targeted Bu becoming the new standard of care when Bu is used as part of an MAC regimen ([22]).

Cyclophosphamide and its metabolites contribute to the development of hemorrhagic cystitis post-transplant and to serious, life-threatening or lethal liver toxicity of the preparative regimen. We sought to substitute Cy with an immunosuppressive agent that would not utilize the GSH/GST and the hepatic cytochrome P450 (CYP450) pathways in its metabolism. The choice came to rely on nucleoside analogues, initially fludarabine (Flu), which replaced Cy in many conditioning regimens. Initial studies with the combination of Flu and Bu (BuFlu) produced high engraftment rates with low levels of toxicity, and this is now considered a standard of care MAC regimen at both MDACC ([23, 24]) and other major transplant centers in North America. In these variant regimens, Flu is typically administered at a dose of 40 to 50 mg/m^2 on days (-7) -6 to -3, and each Flu dose is followed by intravenous Bu at a dose of 130 mg/m^2 over 3 hours on days -6 to -3, adjusted to an average daily systemic exposure (represented by an AUC of 4,000 to 6,000 μmol-min, or total course AUC of 16,000 to 24,000 μmol-min). Alternative regimens under investigation at MDACC include Bu, Flu, and clofarabine, which may result in increased antileukemic activity ([25]). While both Cy-TBI and the variant BuCy regimens provide additive cytotoxic activity from the agents included in the regimen, the beneficial synergistic interaction between the nucleoside analogue Flu and the alkylating agent Bu is highly dependent on optimized sequencing. It is critical that Flu precedes intravenous Bu, both of which are administered once daily ([26]). A summary of conditioning regimens, with disease-specific information and outcomes, can be found in Tables 13-1 and 13-2.

Reduced-Intensity Conditioning

According to the CIBMTR, in 2011 approximately 3,200 RIC transplants were performed, two-thirds of which were in patients over the age of 50. The underlying principle of RIC preparative regimens lies in the immunosuppressive properties of the conditioning regimen to facilitate engraftment, which utilizes immunocompetent donor cells to establish a GVT effect rather than conditioning chemotherapy to attain disease control ([27]). The intensity of the conditioning therapy is generally not enough to control the malignant disease but is sufficient to suppress recipient immunity, promote engraftment, and trigger a subsequent GVT effect. Patients with a history of extensive pretransplantation chemotherapy, prior radiotherapy to the chest or abdomen, prior malignancy, or underlying dysfunction of heart, lung, liver, or kidneys are at increased risk for NRM. This was reflected in the Sorror HCT-CI, in which patients were found to have higher NRM when the HCT-CI was greater than 3. A recent analysis by Sorror et al suggested that a composite HCT-CI/age comorbidity index may be employed, where patients with a score less than 3 had improved 2-year survival and could tolerate MAC or RIC regimens, and patients with HCT-CI of 3 or greater may benefit from a lower-intensity, nonmyeloablative (NMA) regimen, although this hypothesis needs to be prospectively validated. At MDACC, patients with an HCT-CI of 3 or greater generally do not receive standard MAC and are offered an RIC program.

Multiple RIC regimens exist, and they vary in intensity from nearly myeloablative to completely NMA regimens. Like MAC regimens, RIC regimens can be with chemotherapy only or be combined with TBI. Preclinical work in a canine model established that doses as low as 2 Gy were sufficient to allow engraftment of donor stem cells when used in conjunction with postgrafting immunosuppression ([28]). A similar regimen piloted in patients with hematologic malignancies who were more than 50 years old or had significant medical contraindications to standard transplantation demonstrated a lower degree of treatment-related toxicity and a high rate of mixed chimerism by day 28 ([29]).

Table 13-1 Outcomes of Standard MAC/RIC Regimens in Lymphoid Malignancies at MDACC[a]

Disease Type	RIC MAC	Conditioning Regimen	OS	PFS	GVHD Rates
Relapsed/ refractory Hodgkin lymphoma	RIC	Fludarabine/melphalan	64%	32%	aGVHD grade II-IV: 28%
	RIC	Gemcitabine, fludarabine/ melphalan	87% (18 months)	49% (18 months)	NR
Relapsed CLL/NHL	RIC	Fludarabine, bendamustine, rituximab	90% (2 years)	75% (2 years)	aGVHD grade II-IV: 11% Extensive cGVHD: 26%
Relapsed follicular lymphoma	RIC	Fludarabine, cyclophosphamide, rituximab	85%	83%	aGVHD II-IV: 11% Extensive cGVHD: 36%
Acute lymphocytic leukemia	MAC or RIC	Busulfan (AUC 4,000 μM/ min RIC, AUC 5,500 μM/ min MAC), clofarabine	67%	54%	aGVHD II-IV: 38% Extensive cGVHD: 7%
Philadephia chromosome–positive ALL	MAC or RIC	BuMel, Flu/Mel, or TBI based (multiple regimens)	33%	31%	aGVHD II-IV: 30%

Abbreviation: NR, not reported.
[a]Results reported utilized MRD/MUD donors, with standard MDACC GVHD prophylaxis utilizing tacrolimus/minimethotrexate and ATG on days -3, -2, -1 for MUDs.

Table 13-2 Outcomes of Standard MAC/RIC Regimens in Myeloid Malignancies at MDACC[a]

Disease Type	RIC MAC	Conditioning Regimen	OS	PFS	GVHD Rates
Chronic myelogenous leukemia (TKI resistant)[b]	MAC/RIC	MAC:BuFlu, BuFluClo RIC:FluMel, BuFlu based (±TKI, rituxan), others	Mutated: 44% Unmutated: 76%	Mutated: 36% Unmutated: 58%	aGVHD II-IV: 25% Extensive cGVHD: 20%
Acute myelogenous leukemia/MDS/ CML	MAC	Busulfan, fludarabine	68% (CR1) 42% (CR2) 30% (PD)	68% 42% 30%	aGVHD II-IV: 40% cGVHD: 43%
	MAC	Clofarabine, fludarabine, once-daily busulfan[c]	50%	50%	aGVHD II-IV: 39%
Acute myelogenous leukemia/MDS	RIC	Fludarabine, melphalan	71%	68%	aGVHD II-IV: 25% Extensive cGVHD: 29%
Myelofibrosis[d]		Busulfan (dose dense), fludarabine	75%	61%	aGVHD II-IV: 22% cGVHD: 39%

Abbreviation: NR, not reported.
[a]Results reported utilized MRD/MUD donors, with standard MDACC GVHD prophylaxis utilizing tacrolimus/minimethotrexate, and ATG on days -3, -2, -1 for MUDs. NR, not reported.
[b]Patients were stratified based on unmutated or mutated BCR-ABL status.
[c]Preliminary results: current phase II trial ongoing.
[d]This regimen is now a phase II trial open for all MPDs and myeloid malignancies.

A substantial proportion (20%) of patients experienced graft rejection. A later modification to the conditioning regimen included Flu, which improved donor chimerism and decreased graft rejection ([30]). Subsequently, Bu 3.2 mg/kg IV was added to decrease the risk of disease relapse ([31]). Other chemotherapy-based regimens include Bu/Flu, Flu/carmustine/melphalan (Mel), Flu/cytoxan/TBI, and Flu/Mel ([7, 32-35]). The RIC regimen typically used at MDACC, and implemented at many transplant centers, is the Flu/Mel regimen, utilizing Flu 25 mg/m^2 over 5 days and Mel 140 mg/m^2 ([33]). A less-ablative regimen utilizes only 100 mg/m^2 of Mel. A summary of conditioning regimens, with disease-specific information and outcomes, is shown in Tables 13-1 and 13-2.

Sources of Stem Cells

Historically, stem cells used for transplantation were obtained through the harvest of bone marrow cells from the posterior iliac crests of normal donors. Approximately 150 aspirations are necessary to yield 10 to 15 mL/kg of bone marrow, and the procedure is performed under general anesthesia, is associated with a low incidence of complications, and generally is done on an outpatient basis ([36]). Common sequelae of bone marrow harvest include pain and transient postoperative fever. Life-threatening complications occur in less than 1% of patients. In general, total nucleated cell (TNC) doses of 1 to 4 × 10^8 cells per kilogram of recipient weight are required to induce stable engraftment in patients treated with chemotherapy or TBI. Marrow cell dose is an important prognostic factor for survival in both sibling and unrelated donor transplantation ([37]).

Since the early 1990s, the use of peripheral blood-derived stem cells (PBSCs) has become increasingly common. The PBSCs are collected by utilizing recombinant growth factor granulocyte colony-stimulating factor (G-CSF), given for 4 to 6 days at doses of 6 to 16 μg/kg/d, to mobilize hematopoietic stem cells into the peripheral blood, where they may be collected by one or more leukapheresis procedures. A higher dose of CD34$^+$ cells is required when utilizing PBSCs as a stem cell source, with CD34$^+$ cells infused at an average of 2 to 10 × 10^6/kg, 4 × 10^6/kg being the standard of care at MDACC, with a minimum dose of 2 × 10^6/kg.

The rationale for using PBSCs was derived from studies in the autologous setting demonstrating accelerated recovery of hematopoiesis as compared with traditional bone marrow transplantation (BMT) ([38, 39]). Numerous studies, including randomized trials comparing peripheral blood and bone marrow, have now confirmed the efficacy and safety of this approach ([40]). For donors, this has eliminated the risks and morbidities associated with general anesthesia and bone marrow harvest. The PBSC transplantation offers a number of advantages to the recipient. The G-CSF–mobilized PBSCs are enriched for pluripotent CD34$^+$ hematopoietic progenitors when compared with marrow grafts ([41]). This has shortened the duration of neutropenia and thrombocytopenia in recipients by approximately 5 days, with median time to engraftment of 14 days ([40]).

Despite the benefits of more rapid engraftment with PBSCs, a major concern in many studies was an increased rate of GVHD in patients receiving PBSCs. In a major recent study, the incidence of chronic GVHD (cGVHD), but not aGVHD, was higher in recipients of MUD transplants from peripheral blood as opposed to marrow grafts (53% vs 41%, P = .01), although there was no difference in OS (51% vs 46%, P = .29) ([42]). The incidence of graft failure was higher in the bone marrow group versus the PBSC group (9% vs 3%, P = .002). At MDACC, the standard of care for MRDs is PBSC harvest. For MUDs, the standard of care is bone marrow harvest given the increased rates of cGVHD with PBSC harvest. However, for patients who have marrow failure syndromes, particularly myelofibrosis, or for whom rapid engraftment is necessary, PBSC is sometimes utilized.

Umbilical cord blood (UCB) is increasingly utilized as a stem cell source, and its use is discussed in the chapter on alternative donors.

Graft-Versus-Host Disease Prophylaxis

Graft-versus-host disease is a multisystem immunologic disorder that greatly impacts long-term outcomes, including NRM, and quality of life after alloSCT. It continues to represent one of the major obstacles for allogeneic transplantation. The disease is mechanistically linked to the desired outcome of the GVT effect—a concept now universally accepted as a major reason for the success of allogeneic transplantation in reducing disease relapse. Diagnosis and treatment of GVHD are discussed in the section on posttransplant complications. Here, we will discuss the methods of prophylaxis against GVHD.

Two forms of GVHD, acute and chronic, are commonly distinguished based on the timing of occurrence and the clinical manifestations. Chronic GVHD typically presents more insidiously later in the posttransplant period and is associated with sclerosis of the skin, oral ulcerations, xerostomia/xeropthalmia, or bronchiolitis obliterans (BO). However, an "overlap" syndrome, with features of both acute and chronic GVHD, has increasingly been described.

Given the underlying morbidity and mortality associated with GVHD, multiple approaches to reduce the risk of both aGVHD and cGVHD have been implemented. These include posttransplant immune-suppressive chemotherapy (methotrexate, MTX), posttransplant Cy [post-Cy]), immune suppression through T-cell inhibition via calcineurin inhibitors (CNIs) (tacrolimus, cyclosporine), and T-cell depletion (ex vivo and in vivo with antithymocyte globulin [ATG]).

The two CNI inhibitors, tacrolimus and cyclosporine A (CsA), are closely related and are used in combination with MTX for MUDs and MRDs. Cyclosporine prevents T-cell activation by inhibiting the production of interleukin 2 (IL-2) and the expression of IL-2 receptors. It was discovered in the 1980s, initially in the context of aplastic anemia therapy, then in leukemia, that the combination of CsA and MTX was superior in reducing GVHD rates compared with CsA alone ([43]). The combination of CsA with MTX is initiated intravenously 1 to 2 days prior to stem cell infusion and converted to oral twice-daily dosing when possible. The risk of aGVHD increases when cyclosporine blood concentrations drop below a target level, typically 200 to 400 ng/mL. Cyclosporine has myriad drug interactions, which may result in fluctuating levels. Tacrolimus (FK506) is a macrolide lactone closely resembling cyclosporine in mechanism of action, spectrum of toxicities, and pharmacologic interactions. It was found to be effective in the prevention of GVHD from MRDs and MUDs in the 1990s ([44]). In a phase III trial, the combination of tacrolimus and MTX prophylaxis was superior to cyclosporine and MTX in reducing grade II to IV aGVHD and thus is the standard of care at MDACC ([45]). Tacrolimus is initiated at day -2, with goal levels of 6 to 10 ng/mL. A third agent, sirolimus, inhibits the mammalian target of rapamycin (mTOR) pathway and has been utilized as an alternative to CNI. A combination of sirolimus with tacrolimus was equivalent to tacrolimus/mini-MTX for the prevention of GVHD ([46, 47]). At MDACC, sirolimus is typically used for patients unable to tolerate tacrolimus.

Chemotherapy approaches to GVHD prophylaxis include MTX combined with a CNI, or post-transplant cyclophosphamide (post-Cy). Chemotherapy, administered shortly after stem cell infusion but prior to engraftment, is thought to eradicate rapidly proliferating allo-reactive T cells, thus decreasing GVHD. Methotrexate at high doses has the potential for increased severity of regimen-related mucositis and delays in engraftment. These toxicities preclude full dosing of the drug. At MDACC, a modification of the cyclosporine and MTX regimen using mini-MTX was as effective as the full dose, with less toxicity ([48]). Methotrexate was administered on days +1, +3, +6, +11 at a dose of 5 mg/m^2 in combination with methylprednisolone. Subsequently, it was determined that outcomes were identical without methylprednisolone. Thus, mini-MTX, in combination with a CNI, is the standard of care at MDACC for MRDs and MUDs.

In recent years, a calcineurin-free regimen, utilizing post-CY, based on initial success in the haploidentical setting, has become an attractive potential alternative to standard CNI/MTX prophylaxis. Initial studies in the myeloablative setting with BuCy and BuFlu demonstrated comparable rates of GVHD when administering Cytoxan at 50 mg/kg on days +3 and +4 ([49, 50]). However, in a phase II study at MDACC, post-Cy utilized in the RIC setting resulted in increased mortality (unpublished data). Therefore, this regimen should still be considered experimental, and it is the subject of a randomized CTN trial (BMT CTN 1203).

In addition to prophylaxis with CNIs and chemotherapy, T-cell-depleting approaches have demonstrated some success in decreasing the rates of GVHD, both in vivo with ATG and ex vivo with T-cell depletion. The hypothesis is that by depleting allo-reactive T cells (thought to cause GVHD), rates of GVHD will be lower. The use of ATG resulted in decreased rates of severe aGVHD and extensive cGVHD in unrelated donors ([51, 52]). However, the use of ATG remains controversial. A meta-analysis published in 2012 from the Cochrane database showed that ATG did not improve OS, NRM, or relapse, but resulted in decreased incidence of grade II to IV aGVHD ([53]). At MDACC, rabbit ATG is administered on days -3 through -1 (total dose of 4 mg/kg) for MUDs, in combination with mini-MTX/tacrolimus. The MRDs receive mini-MTX/tacrolimus prophylaxis without ATG. An alternate method is ex vivo T-cell depletion prior to marrow infusion; this effectively reduces the incidence and severity of GVHD. However, T-cell depletion also results in increased graft rejection, infectious complications, and relapse rates in a disease-specific manner. Selective depletion of T-cell subsets may be more effective in reducing the risk of acute GVHD while preserving the GVT effect but is not practiced at MDACC ([54, 55]). A summary of the approach to GVHD prophylaxis at MDACC is shown in Fig. 13-2.

POSTTRANSPLANT SUPPORTIVE CARE

The basic principle underlying supportive care is prevention. Most transplant complications have a temporal relationship to the conditioning regimen and the transplant. Appropriate supportive care measures are therefore dependent on anticipated complications. The temporal relationship of common infectious complications is depicted in Fig. 13-3. A summary of posttransplant complications, diagnosis, and management is shown in Table 13-4 and is discussed next.

Infectious Disease Prophylaxis

Infection prophylaxis is provided to guard against bacterial, fungal, and viral pathogens. Based on the high risk of infectious complications and associated significant morbidities, a number of prophylactic and surveillance strategies have been developed. Patients are divided into "high-risk" and "low-risk" categories prior to stem cell transplantation. Standard prophylaxis for low-risk patients (MRD, low-risk MUD with lymphoma, aplastic anemia, myelofibrosis, CML, first and second remission [CR1/CR2] leukemia) is with fluconazole, levofloxacin, and valacyclovir, with trimethoprim/sulfamethoxazole for *Pneumocystis* pneumonia (PCP) prophylaxis. Higher-risk patients, particularly those with known fungal infections, may be treated with posaconazole/voriconazole. A summary of infectious prophylaxis strategies, including for patients being treated for GVHD, is shown in Table 13-3 ([56-62]).

Myelosuppression

Shortly after infusion, hematopoietic stem cells migrate to sites in the lungs, liver, spleen, and marrow. For most patients, a variably cellular marrow can be demonstrated within 14 days. During the time period until growth of stem cells (engraftment), the patient is exposed to significant myelosuppression and pancytopenia as a result of conditioning chemotherapy.

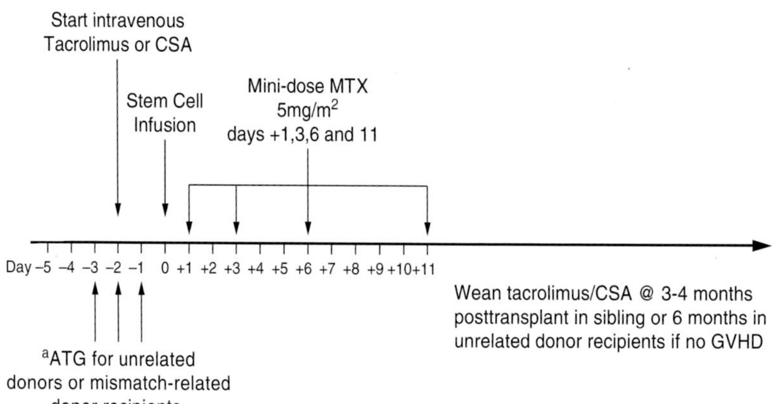

FIGURE 13-2 Standard GVHD prophylaxis at MDACC using tacrolimus, "minidose" methotrexate (MTX), and antithymocyte globulin (ATG). ([a]ATG for mismatched-related and matched-unrelated donor recipients only.)

Engraftment is defined as the first of three consecutive days when the absolute neutrophil count is greater than $0.5 \times 10^3/\mu L$ and the platelet count is greater than $20 \times 10^3/\mu L$. This generally occurs 14 to 24 days after stem cell infusion. Prior to engraftment, patients require aggressive hematologic support with platelet and red blood cell transfusions. All blood products are routinely irradiated to minimize the possibility of graft-versus-host reactions mediated by donor T cells ([63]). For patients experiencing prolonged cytopenias, growth factors may be used to shorten the duration of aplasia without increasing the risk of GVHD or relapse ([64]).

Graft Failure

The failure to recover hematologic function or the loss of marrow function after initial hematopoietic reconstitution constitutes graft failure (rejection). Graft failure can be primary or secondary. Primary graft failure is the failure to reconstitute hematopoiesis after infusion of stem cells. Secondary graft failure is the loss of hematopoiesis after initial engraftment. Rates of graft failure can be as high as 5% to 10% in patients with HLA-mismatched grafts and as low as 0.1% in matched siblings ([65]). Graft failure generally occurs within 60 days of transplantation, although late graft failure may occur. Engraftment is followed by checking "chimerisms" to determine whether a patient's circulating cells are 100% donor or mixed—a "mixed chimera." Chimerism labs include checking for the presence of CD33 (granulocytes) and CD3 (T cells) as a measure of reconstitution of the bone marrow. Typically, patients are considered to be "full donor chimeras" if CD33 and CD3 are more than 95% donor, given an approximately 5% margin of error. Rapid development of full donor chimerism has been associated with decreased relapse and improved OS ([66]). At MDACC, chimerisms typically are checked at days +30, +100, +180, and 1 year.

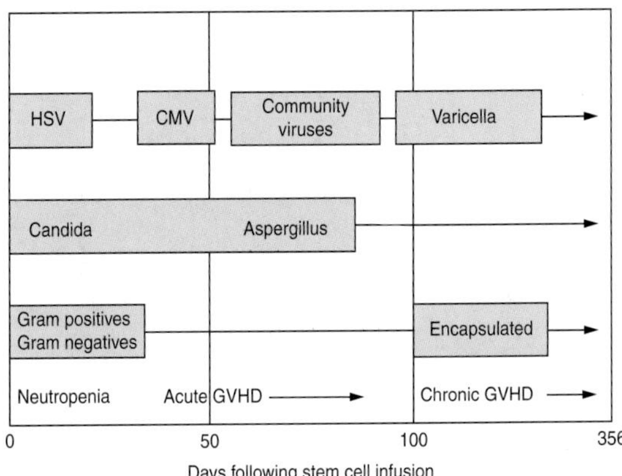

FIGURE 13-3 Timeline of common infectious and noninfectious complications of allogeneic transplantation. CMV, cytomegalovirus; HSV, herpes simplex virus.

Graft failure is due to immunologic graft rejection by the host immune system, infections, drugs, or an inadequate stem cell dose. A number of factors increase the risk of graft failure: a low nucleated cell count infused, T-cell depletion, bone marrow as stem cell source, increasing HLA disparity between donor and host (especially in cord and haploidentical transplantation), and inadequate immunosuppression of the host. Evidence now exists implicating host T cells as the mediators of an active host immune response against the minor alloantigens expressed by the donor cells ([67]).

Veno-Occlusive Disease/Sinusoidal Obstruction Syndrome

One of the most serious complications of high-dose chemotherapy used in preparative regimens is VOD or SOS. This comprises a constellation of findings, including fluid retention with weight gain, painful hepatomegaly, and hyperbilirubinemia. It is caused by endothelial damage to the hepatic sinusoids ([68]). This leads to obstruction of blood flow through hepatic capillaries and venules, which may cause extensive centrilobular necrosis. The incidence of VOD has varied widely. In a systematic review of 135 studies, the incidence was 13.7% ([69]). The spectrum of disease is variable, ranging from mild and transient symptoms to multisystem organ failure (MOF) and death. In severe cases, portal hypertension may result in gastrointestinal (GI) bleeding; similarly, a low-perfusion state may result in prerenal azotemia or overt renal failure. The mortality rate for severe VOD (VOD with MOF) was 84.3%, with multisystem organ failure as the most frequent cause of death.

The diagnosis of VOD is based on clinical findings, requiring two of the following three features within 20 days posttransplant: (a) hyperbilirubinemia >2 mg/dL, (b) painful hepatomegaly, and (c) weight gain >2% of baseline body weight due to fluid retention ([70]). A number of factors contribute to an individual patient's risk for VOD. Preexisting liver disease, elevated transaminases, and Bu/Cy/TBI increase the risk of VOD.

The treatment of VOD is primarily supportive, with management of fluid status, minimizing exposure to hepatotoxic agents, and pain/volume control with narcotics and paracentesis. In severe disease, defibrotide can be considered in addition to supportive care until normalization of bilirubin, although this is still considered investigational ([71]). Urodeoxycholic acid (UDCA or ursadiol) has been demonstrated to prevent VOD and is given 300 mg two or three times daily to all alloSCT recipients at MDACC and continued for 3 months after transplantation. The use of UDCA

Table 13-3 Infectious Disease Prophylaxis in the Allogeneic Transplant Patient

Risk Category	Antibacterial	Antifungal	Antiviral (HSV/VZV)	PCP
Low risk	Levofloxacin 500 mg IV or by mouth daily starting day -1 (or when ANC <1 × 10³/μL) until ANC >1 × 10³/μL	Fluconazole 400 mg IV or by mouth daily until off IST	Valacyclovir 500 mg by mouth daily[a] starting day -1 for 1 year or until off IST OR Acyclovir 250 mg/m² or 5 mg/kg IV piggyback every 12 hours	Bactrim DS 1 tablet by mouth daily Monday, Wednesday, Friday or Bactrim SS daily starting by day +30 for 1 year and until off IST
High risk	Levofloxacin 500 mg IV or by mouth daily starting day -1 (or when ANC <1 × 10³/μL) until ANC >1 × 10³/μL	Voriconazole 200 mg IV or by mouth starting day -1 OR Posaconazole 200 mg by mouth three times daily with food starting day -2 For azole intolerant: Caspofungin 50 mg IV daily starting day -1 OR Micafungin 100-150 mg IV daily starting day -1 OR Liposomal amphotericin 3-5 mg/kg/d Continue until off IST	Valacyclovir 500 mg by mouth daily* starting day -1 for 1 year or off IST OR Acyclovir 250 mg/m² or 5 mg/kg IV piggyback every 12 hours Continue for 1 year or until off IST	Bactrim DS 1 tablet by mouth daily Monday, Wednesday, Friday or Bactrim SS daily starting by day +30 for 1 year and until off IST[c] If sulfa intolerant: Pentamidine 4 mg/kg IV piggyback every 21 days OR Atovaquone 1,500 mg/d by mouth with fatty meal OR Dapsone 100 mg by mouth daily or 50 mg twice daily by mouth (check G6PD status)
aGVHD treatment on steroids	Continue quinolone until prednisone dose ≤0.25 mg/kg/d OR Azithromycin 250 mg by mouth daily (if need continued protection from pneumococcus) OR Penicillin V 500-750 mg by mouth twice daily	Continue antifungal until off IST	Continue antiviral until off IST	Continue PCP prophylaxis until off IST
cGVHD	Continue quinolone until prednisone dose ≤0.25 mg/kg/d OR Azithromycin 250 mg by mouth daily (if need continued protection from pneumococcus) OR Penicillin V 500-750 mg by mouth twice daily	Continue antifungal until off IST	Continue antiviral until off IST	Continue PCP prophylaxis until off IST

Abbreviation: ALT, alanine aminotransferase.

Low risk: MRD, MUD in CR1/CR2 AML, lymphoma, myelofibrosis, no active infections. High risk: hapoloidentical, cord blood transplant, active infection, history of invasive fungal infection.

[a]Consider monitoring posaconazole levels after the first week to ensure adequate absorption. After day +90 if no evidence of infection, consider switching to fluconazole until off IST,

[b]ALT ≥5x ULN, liver GVHD, intolerant to azoles.

[c]In patients who receive alemtuzumab, cord transplants, or haploidentical transplant, duration of PCP prophylaxis should be guided by CD4 counts (continue until absolute CD4 counts are greater than 200 cells/mm³).

Table 13-4 Overview of Management of Major Noninfectious Complications After Allogeneic Stem Cell Transplantation at MDACC

Posttransplant Complication	Diagnosis	Management
Graft failure *Primary*: Failure to recover hematopoiesis after stem cell infusion *Secondary*: Loss of hematopoiesis after initial recovery	Bone marrow biopsy, chimerism studies Rule out infectious causes Review medications; stop stem cell toxic medications like ganciclovir	• Infusion of autologous backup cells if available • Second allogeneic transplant from same or another donor (Cy/ATG, Flu/ATG, alemtuzumab conditioning)
Cytopenias	Complete blood cell count	• Transfuse platelets if <10 × 10^9/L without bleeding and/or without possibility of engraftment • <20 × 10^3/μL for high risk of bleeding, moderate-severe mucositis, invasive procedures • Transfuse 1 unit PRBC if Hg B <8 g/dL • Transfuse 2 units if Hg B <7.5 g/dL
Veno-occlusive disease (VOD)/sinusoidal obstruction syndrome (SOS)	Two of the following: • Bilirubin >2 mg/dL • Painful hepatomegaly • Weight gain/fluid retention	• Ursodeoxycholic acid 300 mg two or three times daily for prophylaxis • Supportive (maintain euvolemia, pain control) • Defibrotide for severe disease with MOF (investigational)
Acute GVHD (aGVHD)	See Table 13-6	• Topical steroids for grade 1 skin involvement only • 2 mg/kg IV or oral prednisone for grades II-IV aGVHD • Continue/resume CNI • Taper steroids first (initially to 1 mg/kg after 1 week, then slow taper thereafter) • Refractory aGVHD options: pentostatin, sirolimus, etanercept, clinical trial
Chronic GVHD	NIH 2005 criteria: 1. Exclude aGVHD 2. Presence of at least 1 diagnostic sign of cGVHD[a] or biopsy of typical organ involvement confirming GVHD 3. Exclusion of other diagnoses	• Prednisone 1 mg/kg daily; begin taper around 2 weeks if resolution of GVHD • If unable to taper steroids by ~2 months, consider adding CNI (sirolimus, CsA, tacrolimus) and taper steroids. Consider ECP, MMF
Bronchiolitis obliterans (BO)	• FEV_1 <75% of predicted • FEV_1/FVC <0.a7 • RV >120% predicted CT: air trapping or bronchiectasis	FAM therapy: • Fluticasone inhaler 440 μg twice a day • Azithromycin 250 mg by mouth twice a day on Monday, Wednesday, Friday • Montelukast 10 mg by mouth daily • Treatment for GVHD with immunosuppression as indicated • Pulmonary consult
Relapse	• Bone marrow biopsy • Chimerisms • Flow cytometry (bone marrow/ blood)	• Consider immune withdrawal • Chemotherapy or disease-directed therapy (ie, TKIs, etc) • Hypomethylating agent +/– donor lymphocyte infusion (DLI) DLI alone (CML)

Cy/ATG, cyclophosphamide + antithymocyte globulin; FEV_1, forced expiratory volume in the first second of expiration; Flu/ATG, fludarabine + antithymocyte globulin; FVC, forced vital capacity; Hg, hemoglobin; PRBC, packed red blood cells.

[a]Diagnostic clinical manifestations specific to cGVHD over aGVHD include lichenification of the skin, mouth, or genitourinary tract and BO.

decreased the rate of VOD significantly (40% vs 15%) in one randomized study and in a meta-analysis ([72, 73]).

Pulmonary Complications

Following alloSCT, patients are at risk for a wide range of pulmonary complications, including pulmonary edema, diffuse alveolar hemorrhage (DAH), and BO. Bronchiolitis obliterans, which may be thought of as "pulmonary cGVHD'," affects 6% to 14% of patients undergoing alloSCT, with an OS of only 13% at 5 years ([74]). It typically presents as increasing shortness of breath and can be detected as moderate-to-severe airflow obstruction on PFTs. Although many cases are

CHAPTER 13

deemed idiopathic or related to an aberrant systemic inflammatory response, the majority are likely related to viral infections. In recent years, the importance of respiratory syncytial virus (RSV), influenza virus, and parainfluenza in the pathogenesis of BO has become more apparent.

Once the diagnosis of BO is made, therapy with inhaled fluticasone, azithromycin, and montelukast (FAM) therapy has been shown to reverse and improve airflow obstruction ([75]). Rapid intervention with FAM therapy or steroids in the setting of respiratory viruses in the posttransplant period may decrease the rate of BO, although this has not been demonstrated in any clinical study. Respiratory infections are covered in the section on infections and are typically managed with antibiotics and supportive care.

INFECTIOUS COMPLICATIONS

Infectious complications result from profound humoral and cellular immune deficiencies that occur shortly after conditioning and may persist for years beyond transplant. Immune deficiencies can be exacerbated by the routine use of immunosuppressive agents for the treatment of GVHD. Immune deficiencies are broadly described in three phases ([76]). Figure 13-3 demonstrates the three phases of posttransplant immune deficiency with associated infectious complications. Table 13-5 discusses posttransplant infectious complications, their diagnosis, and treatment.

ACUTE GRAFT-VERSUS-HOST DISEASE

Acute GVHD typically presents within the first 3 months (100 days) after transplantation and is manifested as a maculopapular skin rash, elevation in liver function tests (LFTs), or GI distress (nausea/vomiting/diarrhea). It occurs in 20% to 70% of patients depending on the conditioning regimen ([77]). Organs may be involved in isolation or simultaneously. A clinical grading system, the Glucksberg Scale, which allows for quantitative estimates of disease severity and response to therapy, is presented in Table 13-6. Severity is described as grade I (mild) to grade IV (severe). Rates of grades II-IV aGVHD vary in different studies. With mini-MTX/tacrolimus prophylaxis with ATG for unrelated/mismatched donors at MDACC, they approach 20% to 30% (see Tables 13-1 and 13-2). Risk factors for aGVHD include MUD transplants, mismatched donors, acute leukemia, TBI, higher HCT-CI score, and female-into-male donor (especially if multiparous) ([78, 79]). An increasingly recognized entity, delayed aGVHD, occurs after the 100-day period, yet still has features of aGVHD. In addition, an overlap syndrome with features of cGVHD and aGVHD occurs.

Acute GVHD can often be diagnosed based on clinical findings. Histologic confirmation can be valuable in excluding other possibilities, such as infection. Mild GVHD of the skin may demonstrate vacuolar degeneration and infiltration of the basal layer by lymphocytes. With more advanced disease, histologic findings of necrotic dyskeratotic cells with acantholysis may progress to frank epidermolysis. In the liver, early GVHD may be difficult to distinguish from hepatitis or other causes.

Mild aGVHD can be treated with topical steroids and slowing of immunosuppressive therapy (IST) taper. Moderate-to-severe aGVHD (grades II-IV) requires systemic treatment. The mainstay of therapy has long been corticosteroid therapy. Methylprednisolone or prednisone, 2 mg/kg/d, achieves responses in 40% to 60% of patients ([80]). Steroid-refractory GVHD responds poorly to second-line therapies and is associated with increased mortality. Novel treatments showing efficacy in preliminary studies include extracorporeal phototherapy, pentostatin, and sirolimus ([81-83]). Acute GVHD of the skin is most responsive to treatment, whereas GVHD of the liver is least responsive. The fatality rate for aGVHD may be as high as 50%. A discussion of MDACC protocols for the treatment of aGVHD is included in Table 13-4.

CHRONIC GRAFT-VERSUS-HOST DISEASE

Chronic GVHD is the single most important factor affecting long-term outcome and quality of life after alloSCT. The incidence of cGVHD is difficult to quantify due to variability in cGVHD definitions and variability in transplant types and procedures. In general, most studies cited rates of 30% to 80%. Figures 13-1 and 13-2 describe the rates of cGVHD in commonly used regimens at MDACC. Chronic GVHD is an alloimmune process (donor graft vs recipient) that results in alloantibody formation as well as antihost T-cell responses and may have single-organ or multisystem involvement. The pathophysiology of cGVHD is incompletely understood, but impaired T-regulatory cell suppression of autoimmunity and loss of B-cell tolerance and B-cell hyperactivity have been implicated ([84, 85]).

The classic definition of cGVHD was a syndrome that developed after day +100, with typical signs including skin, mucosal, or genital lichenification; BO; ocular complications; and significant sclerosis of skin and joints. Disease stage was originally defined as limited versus extensive ([86]). Limited disease was characterized as localized involvement, hepatic dysfunction, or both and was found to have a more favorable

Table 13-5 Overview of Diagnosis and Management of Infectious Complications After Allogeneic Stem Cell Transplantation at MDACC

Infection	Diagnosis	Management
Neutropenic fever	Temperature of 38°C on greater than 2 incidences 1 hour apart or ≥38.2°C AND ANC <0.5 × 10^3/μL or <1 × 10^3/μL expected to fall below 0.5 × 10^3/μL in the next 24 hours	• Blood cultures × 2, urine analysis, chest x-ray Empiric Abs: • Cefepime 2 g IV every 8 hours • Vancomycin 1 g IV every 12 hours • Meropenem 1 g every 8 hours or zosyn 4.5 g IV every 6 hours may be substituted for cefepime • Aztreonam 2 g IV every 8 hours + amikacin for true PCN allergy • Site-specific management, testing
Cytomegalovirus (CMV)	• CMV PCR (two subsequent positive tests) • CMV antigenemia • Follow weekly CMV PCR	Induction phase (until 1 week and CMV antigenemia negative × 2): • Ganciclovir 5 mg/kg IV every 12 hours • Valganciclovir 900 mg by mouth twice daily • Foscarnet 60 mg/kg IV every 8 hours (second line, if significant myelosuppression) • Consider 0.5 mg/kg IVIG for severe infection Maintenance phase (2-3 weeks, longer if end-organ damage): • Ganciclovir 5 m/kg IV every 24 hours • Valganciclovir 900 mg by mouth daily • Foscarnet 60 mg/kg IV every 24 hours • Infectious disease consultation
Human herpesvirus 6 (HHV-6)	• Suspected if viral syndrome/pancytopenia of unclear etiology • Serum PCR for HHV-6	• Cidofovir may have some activity against HHV-6; use with caution due to renal dysfunction • Supportive care
BK virus	• Cystitis, hematuria • Serum BK PCR nonspecific • Urine PCR more specific (with symptoms)	• Supportive care • Ciprofloxacin • Leflunomide • Cidofovir • BK-specific cytotoxic T lymphocytes (investigational) • Taper IST if feasible
Adenovirus	• Typically in severely immunocompromised patients • Symptoms may include FUO, diarrhea/nausea/vomiting, cytopenias, fulminant hepatic failure • Check stool and serum adenovirus PCR.	• Supportive care • Cidofovir • Adenovirus-specific CTLs (investigational) • Taper IST if feasible
Respiratory syncytial virus (RSV)	• Respiratory virus antigen screening • Testing for patients with symptoms of URI (rhinorrhea, fever, cough, SOB)	• Supportive care if URI only • RSV pneumonia: ribavirin 2 g inhaled over 3 hours every 8 hours AND • IVIG 500 mg/kg IV every 48 hours for 3-5 doses
Influenza	• Influenza respiratory antigens	• Oseltamivir 75 mg by mouth twice daily
Clostridium difficile colitis	• Stool sample PCR/ELISA in setting of diarrhea	• Metronidazole 500 mg IV or by mouth every 8 hours × 10-14 days • Vancomycin 125 mg by mouth every 6 hours for severe colitis, instability • Fidaxomicin 200 mg by mouth every 12 hours

(*Continued*)

Table 13-5 Overview of Diagnosis and Management of Infectious Complications After Allogeneic Stem Cell Transplantation at MDACC (Continued)

Infection	Diagnosis	Management
Epstein-Bar virus (EBV)/ posttransplant lymphoproliferative disorder (PTLD)	• EBV PCR monitoring in patients with high titer pretransplant or undergoing haploidentical/cord alloSCT • Any patient with new-onset fever, cytopenias, adenopathy • >3,000 copies/mL on 2 tests required for diagnosis • PET-CT scan	• Rituximab 375 mg/m^2 IV weekly ×4 doses • EBV-specific CTLs (investigational) • Cidofovir • Taper IST if feasible
Invasive *Aspergillus*	• Bronchoscopy if pulmonary; otherwise, CT scan of affected area • FNA/biopsy of affected site	• Infectious disease consult • Switch to voriconazole if on fluconazole
Mucormycosis	• Suspect with sinus infection • Obtain biopsy	• Urgent ear, nose, and throat/infectious disease consult • Switch to posaconazole and/or initiate liposomal amphotericin 5 mg/kg IV daily
Other invasive fungal infection	• Blood cultures • Biopsy of affected site	• Consultation with infectious disease personnel • Amphotericin 5 mg/kg IV daily • Echinocandin therapy for systemic yeast infection (caspofungin, anidulofungin)

ELISA, enzyme-linked immunosorbent assay; FNA, fine-needle aspiration; FUO, fever of unknown origin; IVIG, intravenous immunoglobulin; PCN, penicillin; SOB, shortness of breath; URI, upper respiratory infection.

prognosis. Extensive disease was characterized by generalized skin involvement or localized skin involvement and hepatic dysfunction and ocular or salivary gland involvement or involvement of any other target organ. Patients with extensive cGVHD had a worse prognosis.

In 2005, a National Institutes of Health (NIH) consensus project developed a new definition of cGVHD, for use in future trials, given the inconsistent and incomplete staging using the limited/extensive system ([87]). The criteria eliminated the 100-day requirement. In addition, aGVHD was defined as the existence of classic clinical features (maculopapular rash, GI symptoms, elevated LFTs) within 100 days, or greater

Table 13-6 Clinical Grading of Acute Graft-Versus-Host Disease (Days 1-100)

Extent of Organ Involvement			
Stage	**Skin**	**Liver**	**Gut**
1	Rash on <25% of skin[a]	Bilirubin 2-3 mg/dL[b]	Diarrhea >500 mL/d[c] or persistent nausea[d]
2	Rash on 25%-50% of skin	Bilirubin 3-6 mg/dL	Diarrhea >1,000 mL/d
3	Rash on >50% of skin	Bilirubin 6-15 mg/dL	Diarrhea >1,500 mL/d
4	Generalized erythroderma with bullae	Bilirubin >15 mg/dL	Severe abdominal pain +/– ileus
Grade[e]			
I	Stage I or II	None	None
II	Stage 3 or	Stage 1 or	Stage 1
III	–	Stage 2 or 3 or	Stage 2, 3, or 4
IV[f]	Stage 4 or	Stage 4	–

[a]Use the "rule of nines" or burn chart to determine extent of rash.
[b]Range given as total bilirubin. Downgrade one stage if additional causes of hyperbilirubinemia are documented.
[c]Volume of diarrhea applies to adults. Downgrade one stage if additional causes of diarrhea are documented.
[d]Persistent nausea with histologic evidence of GVHD in the stomach or duodenum.
[e]Criteria for grading given as the minimum degree of organ involvement required to confer that grade.
[f]Grade IV may also include lesser organ involvement but with decrease in performance status.

than 100 days, with the absence of cGVHD symptoms.

The definition of cGVHD must fulfill the following criteria:

1. Exclusion of acute GVHD
2. Presence of at least one diagnostic clinical sign of cGVHD or presence of at least one distinctive manifestation confirmed by biopsy or other testing
3. Exclusion of other diagnoses

Clinical manifestations of cGVHD, which differentiate it from aGVHD, include lichenification of the skin, mouth, or genitourinary tract and BO.

The management of cGVHD is similar to aGVHD, with immune-suppressant agents as the standard therapies. Treatments include systemic and topical steroids, CNIs, mTOR inhibitors, extracorporeal phototherapy, mycophenolate mofetil, and anti–tumor necrosis factor agents. The goal of cGVHD therapy is to relieve symptoms and prolong life long enough for immune tolerance to develop. Once treatment of cGVHD is initiated, the median duration of treatment is typically 2 years ([88]).

The treatment of cGVHD has been outlined by a cGVHD working group series of publications ([89]). Mild cutaneous involvement of cGVHD can be managed with topical steroids alone. Mild manifestations of cGVHD, such as transaminitis, should be managed with systemic corticosteroids, using the lowest effective dose possible. Typically, patients should remain on systemic steroids for 4 to 8 weeks, with tapering doses based on clinical symptoms.

Moderate and severe cGVHD require systemic immunosuppression. The standard first-line therapy is corticosteroids, with a dose of 1 mg/kg/d of prednisone, or equivalent, as the standard of care. Management of corticosteroids and tapering regimens vary widely and are often done on a "trial-and-error" basis. Steroid taper is started 2 weeks after clinical improvement. A dose of 1 mg/kg every other day is continued until resolution of GVHD symptoms. Thereafter, steroids can be tapered by 10% to 20% per week. If symptoms recur, an increase in steroids may yield a response, and a slower taper thereafter is required. If no response is achieved by 3 months, alternative treatments should be considered.

The most frequent clinical problem encountered in the treatment of cGVHD is steroid-dependent or refractory cGVHD, as 50% of patients undergoing therapy for cGVHD will be refractory or dependent on steroids. These patients not only have a worse overall prognosis but also are subject to the long-term effects of high doses of corticosteroids. Second-line treatment of cGVHD is largely focused on reducing steroid requirements and improving quality of life and symptoms ([90]). Steroid-refractory cGVHD was defined by the working group as progression on prednisone 1 mg/kg/d for 2 weeks, stable disease on more than 0.5 mg/kg/d of prednisone for 4 to 8 weeks, or the inability to taper prednisone below 0.5 mg/kg/d. Individual treatments should be tried for at least 4 weeks before being deemed a failure; cutaneous/sclerotic manifestations may require up to 6 months to achieve improvement. Once disease achievement has been improved with the addition of immunosuppressant agents, steroid weaning should be attempted due to the increased toxicities associated with prolonged use.

Multiple agents have been considered in the setting of high-risk or steroid-dependent cGVHD, but as in primary cGVHD, there are limited randomized trial data to justify their use. The most common agents used include CNIs (tacrolimus, cyclosporine), mycophenolate mofetil, mTOR inhibitors (sirolimus), and extracorporeal phototherapy ([83, 91, 92]). These are typically used in combination with prednisone, or with each other, and achieve responses ranging from 35% to 80%. The heterogeneity, combination of drugs, retrospective nature, and lack of randomization in the trials make it difficult to interpret the data; however, there is a clear benefit. Other agents, such as thalidomide, hydroxychloroquine, rituximab, etanercept, azathioprine, and imatinib, have demonstrated a beneficial effect in cGVHD. The optimal treatment regimen in this disease remains to be elucidated. Table 13-4 describes the MDACC approach to cGVHD.

LATE COMPLICATIONS

Patients at MDACC are evaluated annually for several delayed toxicities resulting from alloSCT. These include endocrine toxicities such as hypothyroidism, hypogonadism, or growth hormone deficiency in younger patients. Pulmonary effects may include obstructive lung disease or pulmonary fibrosis. Late infectious complications can occur, including viral reactivation and late fungal infections. These complications are more common in patients who have received alterative donor sources, long-term steroids for GVHD, or both. Patients undergoing alloSCT experience an increased risk for secondary malignancies, about 10% to 13% at 15 years posttransplant ([93, 94]). The spectrum of second malignancies includes NHL, myelodysplastic syndrome (MDS), skin cancer, head and neck cancers, and other solid tumors. Older patient age and IST for chronic GVHD were significantly correlated with the risk of developing a secondary malignancy. The intensive treatment and prolonged recovery from alloSCT can have profound psychosocial implications for patients and their families, and patients often are managed with antidepressants (selective serotonin reuptake inhibitors) to control anxiety and depressive symptoms.

RELAPSE

The major benefit of alloSCT is the reduction in the relapse rate compared with conventional chemotherapy. However, despite aggressive chemotherapy, conditioning, and alloSCT, some patients still relapse. This remains the primary cause of treatment failure after alloSCT and improvement in improving relapse rates remains a priority of the American Society for Bone Marrow Transplantation ([95]).

The management of relapsed disease is complicated and disease and patient specific. Typically, relapse is approached as follows: withdrawal of immune suppression, immune therapy (donor lymphocyte infusions [DLIs] or other immunotherapy), and systemic therapy. In the absence of severe GVHD, immune suppression can be more rapidly weaned in an effort to potentiate the GVT effect ([96]). This may be helpful when there are small amounts (ie, minimal residual disease) or in CML, but is unlikely to result in remission in cases of florid relapse or other more immune-resistant disease types. Systemic therapy options, including chemotherapy, tyrosine kinase inhibitors (TKIs), and other small molecules, are disease specific and often can result in remissions, but without regaining immunologic control are unlikely to result in long-term curative therapy. These approaches are covered in the disease-specific chapters.

Immunotherapy utilizing chimeric antigen receptor T cells is discussed in the novel immune therapies chapter and has demonstrated success in treating relapsed/refractory disease. Immunotherapy in the form of DLIs is frequently used and can result in durable remissions. Donor lymphocyte infusion is an infusion of donor-derived T cells (typically 3×10^7 to 4.5×10^8 $CD3^+$ T cells/kg) aimed to create a GVT effect and regain disease control. This infusion was initially utilized in CML ([13]). It is most effective in CML, but also is effective in other disease types. In the European Bone Marrow Transplant-95 survey, achieving CR with DLI was noted in 80% of patients with CML and cytogenetic relapse, 77% with hematologic relapse, and 36% with transformed CML. In AML/MDS, 26% achieved CR with DLI, whereas only 15% of ALL patients achieved CR ([97]). Donor lymphocyte infusion has been used in combination with chemotherapy, typically lower doses of chemotherapy or hypomethylating agents such as azacitidine, with OS of 29% at 2 years in a recent study ([98]). The most frequent complication of DLI is GVHD, with rates of approximately 50%. At MDACC, DLI is utilized in CML in cases of molecular relapse with detectable BCR-ABL by PCR. It is sometimes utilized in the setting of relapsed leukemia in combination with a hypomethylating agent such as azacitidine. These approaches are not standardized, and there is scant literature to guide our management. Second alloSCT can be considered, particularly in AML/MDS, with potential cure rates around 25% in patients with good performance status ([99]).

Aside from treating active relapse, novel approaches are being investigated to prevent relapse. One of the most promising approaches is a maintenance approach; after transplant, a low dose of an anticancer agent is administered to prevent relapse. This has demonstrated remarkable efficacy in the postautologous transplant setting in MM ([100]). At MDACC, low-dose azacitidine given as maintenance has demonstrated preliminary efficacy in decreasing relapse rates in AML and MDS ([101]). In the setting of molecular or florid relapse of CML, DLI-refractory CML, or Philadelphia chromosome–positive ALL, selective Bcr-Abl TKIs (dasatinib, nilotinib, imatinib) are effective at a lower dose than pretransplant to regain remission ([102, 103]). Table 13-7 describes the management of specific diseases at relapse, as well as maintenance therapy in certain disease types.

DISEASE-SPECIFIC CONSIDERATIONS

The primary benefit of alloSCT is reduction in the risk of disease relapse, and subsequent cure, mediated by the GVT effect in patients for whom cure is unlikely or impossible with standard chemotherapy alone. Given the risk of NRM associated with alloSCT, it is important to distinguish the patients who will most benefit from alloSCT. As discussed, initial considerations include the patient's overall performance status, age, and comorbidity status. Equally important is a consideration of the disease type and status. Table 13-7 provides an overview of disease-specific indications for transplant, disease-specific conditioning regimens, and disease-specific considerations.

In considering an alloSCT, the risk of relapse is weighed against the potential benefits from the GVT effect and potentially curative therapy. Each disease type has a risk classification, typically divided into low-, intermediate-, and high-risk disease. These schemes are outlined in Table 13-7. In general, patients with intermediate- or high-risk disease have an indication for alloSCT, whereas low-risk patients benefit from a watch-and-wait approach. Any relapsed disease, particularly leukemia, is incurable with standard therapies and therefore is high risk. The effectiveness of alloSCT is greatest when the burden of disease is low, given that it takes 3 to 6 months for the full GVT effect to occur given the presence of GVHD prophylaxis/immunosuppression.

Therefore, patients should receive therapy prior to alloSCT to reduce the disease burden. For leukemias, a

Table 13-7 Indications and Current Results of Allografting for Hematologic Malignancies at MD Anderson Cancer Center (MDACC)

Disease/ Stage	Risk Category[a]	Allograft Recommended	Current Results DFS at 5 Years	Standard Conditioning Regimen Agents[a]	Comments
AML CR1	Good	No	N/A		
	Intermediate	Yes	50%-60%	Bu/Flu or Flu/Bu/Clo Flu/Mel (RIC alternative) for high HCT-CI or advanced age Haploidentical/cord blood transplant if no MRD/MUD	Consider maintenance therapy with azacitidine
	Poor (Including FLT3 ITD positive)	Yes	30%-40%	Bu/Flu Flu/Bu/Clo Flu/Mel (RIC alternative) for high HCT-CI or advanced age Haploidentical/cord blood transplant if no MRD/MUD	Consider FLT3 inhibitor as maintenance therapy, ie, sorafenib for FLT3+ AML
AML >CR1		Yes	30%-50% if in remission 10%-20% if active disease	Bu/Flu or Flu/Bu/Clo Flu/Mel (RIC alternative) for high HCT-CI or advanced age Haploidentical/cord blood transplant if no MRD/MUD	Consider maintenance therapy with azacitidine
MDS good risk	IPSS risk: low, intermediate-1	No	N/A		
MDS poor risk	IPSS risk: intermediate-2, high	Yes	35% if in remission 10%-30% if active disease	Bu/Flu or Flu/Bu/Clo Flu/Mel (RIC) for high HCT-CI or advanced age Haploidentical/cord blood transplant if no MRD/MUD	
ALL CR1	Ph+, T-ALL, MRD+ after induction	Yes	40%-50%	Bu/Clo Etoposide-TBI	Consider maintenance TKI (dasatiib, imatinib) if BCR-ABL positivity post-transplant
ALL >CR1		Yes	30% if in remission, 10%-20% if active disease	Bu/Clo Etoposide-TBI RIC regimens for older patients	
CML CP1		No			
CML >CP1	T315I mutation failure/ intolerance of 2 TKI	Yes	60%-80% if chronic phase 30%-40% accelerated phase 10%-20% blast crisis	Bu/Flu or Bu/Flu/Clo Flu/Mel (RIC alternative) for high HCT-CI or advanced age Haploidentical/cord blood transplant if no MRD/MUD	Consider maintenance TKI (dasatinib/imatinib) if BCR-ABL+ posttreatment. Usually lower doses are effective to eliminate MRD t
NHL/CLL CR1		No	N/A		

(*Continued*)

Table 13-7 Indications and Current Results of Allografting for Hematologic Malignancies at MD Anderson Cancer Center (MDACC) (*Continued*)

Disease/ Stage	Risk Category[a]	Allograft Recommended	Current Results DFS at 5 Years	Standard Conditioning Regimen Agents[a]	Comments
NHL first relapse		Autograft not feasible or Less than partial remission to salvage therapy	N/A	RIC regimens (FC, FB) Add rituximab for B-cell malignancies Alternative regimen Flu/Mel Appropriate for alternative stem cell donor transplants (unrelated, mismatched, and cord blood)	
NHL/CLL > first relapse		Yes	10%-50% depending on disease status and chemosensitivity	RIC regimens (FC, FB). Add rituximab for B-cell malignancies Alternative regimen Flu/Mel Appropriate for alternative stem cell donor transplants (unrelated, mismatched, and cord blood)	
Hodgkin disease		Autograft failures	20%-30%	RIC regimens for older patients Flu/004Del/gemcitabine Appropriate for alternative stem cell donor transplants (unrelated, mismatched, and cord blood)	
Myeloma	17p deletion, failure of autotransplant, multiple lines of therapy	Yes only on clinical trial	10%-15%	Bu/Flu Flu/Mel RIC Alternative stem cell donor transplants (unrelated, mismatched, and cord blood) only for patients with high-risk disease	

ALL, acute lymphocytic leukemia; AML, chronic myelogenous leukemia; CLL, chronic lymphocytic leukemia; CR1, first complete remission; DFS, disease-free survival; IV, intravenous; MDS, myelodysplastic syndromes; NHL, non-Hodgkin lymphoma. Bu, busulfan; FBR, fludarabine/bendamustine/rituximab, FCR, fludarabine/cyclophosphamide/rituximab; Flu, fludarabine; IPSS, International Prognostic Scoring System; Mel, melphalan; TKI: tyrosine kinase inhibitor.
[a]Bu/Flu can be administered as a myeloablative regimen (AUC 6,000) or an RIC regime (4,000-5,000); selection of intensity of conditioning regimen is determined based on disease status, patient age, HCT-CI, and risk of relapse.

5% blast value has historically been the threshold for transplant, although in recent years, given improved detection methods, the current optimal patient has a bone marrow free of aberrant blasts and, increasingly, free of low-level minimal residual disease, with no detectable cytogenetic abnormalities ([104, 105]). For lymphomas, the goal is negative positron emission tomographic/computed tomographic (PET/CT) scanning or evidence of decreasing size of lymph nodes (<3 cm) and marrow free of disease (<10% involvement in the case of CLL/indolent lymphoma) in response to chemotherapy. For patients with higher levels of disease prior to alloSCT, the rates of relapse and OS are high. It is increasingly recognized that patients with no detectable residual disease or evidence of leukemia have superior outcomes.

In general, patients who receive MAC have decreased relapse rates and improved survival. Patients with more active or higher-risk disease often receive MAC for this reason. However, there are exceptions to this rule. Patients with indolent lymphoma (follicular lymphoma, CLL) or NHL generally benefit more from a RIC regimen given the disease is slow growing, and there is more time to allow for the GVT effect to develop. In addition, patients with higher HCT-CI of 3+ typically receive RIC regardless of disease status, given that MAC comes at a risk of higher NRM. Figure 13-4 provides a graphical representation of disease type and conditioning intensity. Tables 13-1 and 13-2 provide a breakdown of disease-specific indications by myeloid and lymphoid disease, with survival rates, GVHD rates, and standard-of-care conditioning regimens utilized at MDACC ([25, 35, 106-114]). Table 13-7 provides a more broad consideration of each disease type and outcomes.

CONCLUSIONS

Allogeneic stem cell transplantation provides an important therapeutic approach for the management of hematologic malignancies. Over the past decade, advances in alternative donor transplantation, GVHD prophylaxis, conditioning therapy, supportive care, risk stratification, and management and prevention of disease relapse have advanced the field of transplantation at a time when candidate patients have increasingly

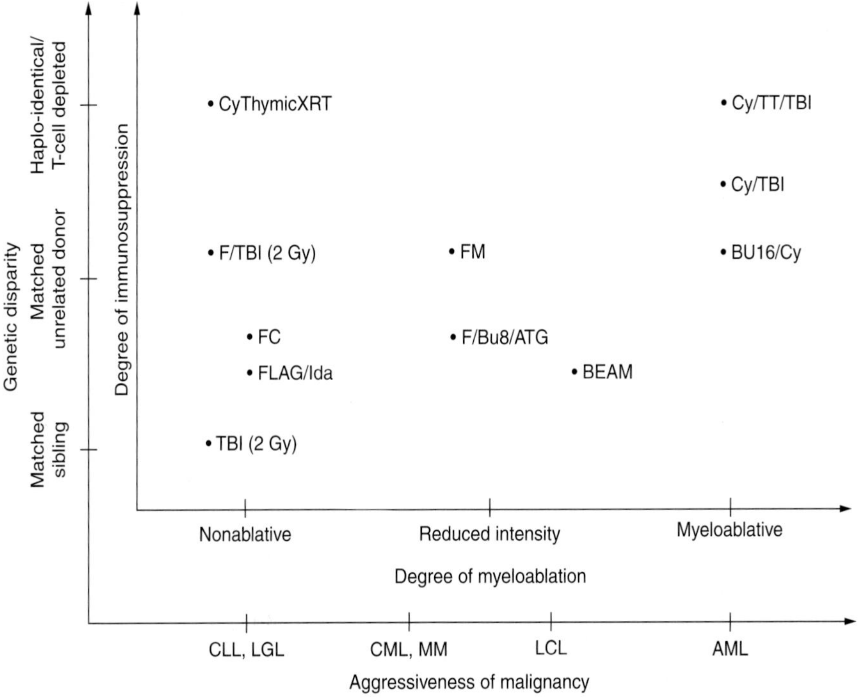

FIGURE 13-4 Relative intensity and use of most commonly reported ablative, reduced intensity, and nonablative conditioning regimens. AML, acute myelogenous leukemia; BEAM, carmustine + etoposide + cytarabine + melphalan; Bu16/Cy, busulfan, 16 mg/kg + cyclophosphamide; CLL, chronic lymphocytic leukemia; CML, chronic myelogenous leukemia; Cy/thymic XRT, cyclophosphamide + thymic irradiation; Cy/TBI, cyclophosphamide + total body irradiation; Cy/TT/TBI, cyclophosphamide + thiotepa + total body irradiation; F/Bu8/ATG, fludarabine + busulfan, 8 mg/kg + antithymocyte globulin; FC, fludarabine + cyclophosphamide; FLAG/Ida, fludarabine + cytarabine + granulocyte colony-stimulating factor + idarubicin; FM, fludarabine + melphalan; F/TBI, fludarabine + total body irradiation; LCL, large-cell lymphoma; LGL, low-grade lymphoma; MM, multiple myeloma; TBI, total body irradiation.

high-risk disease, older age, and more comorbidities. The goal of future investigations will be to decrease NRM and relapse to fully harness the GVT effect and provide optimal therapy for patients with otherwise-incurable disease.

REFERENCES

1. Pasquini MC, WZ. Current use and outcome of hematopoietic stem cell transplantation: CIBMTR summary slides. 2013. http://www.cibmtr.org.
2. Thomas ED, Storb R, Clift RA, et al. Bone-marrow transplantation (second of two parts). *N Engl J Med*. 1975;292(17):895-902. doi:10.1056/NEJM197504242921706.
3. Bortin MM. A compendium of reported human bone marrow transplants. *Transplantation*. 1970;9(6):571-587.
4. Gatti RA, Meuwissen HJ, Allen HD, Hong R, Good RA. Immunological reconstitution of sex-linked lymphopenic immunological deficiency. *Lancet*. 1968;2(7583):1366-1369.
5. Horowitz MM, Gale RP, Sondel PM, et al. Graft-versus-leukemia reactions after bone marrow transplantation. *Blood*. 1990;75(3):555-562.
6. Armand P, Gibson CJ, Cutler C, et al. A disease risk index for patients undergoing allogeneic stem cell transplantation. *Blood*. 2012;120(4):905-913. doi:10.1182/blood-2012-03-418202.
7. Slack JL, Dueck AC, Fauble VD, et al. Reduced toxicity conditioning and allogeneic stem cell transplantation in adults using fludarabine, carmustine, melphalan, and antithymocyte globulin: outcomes depend on disease risk index but not age, comorbidity score, donor type, or human leukocyte antigen mismatch. *Biol Blood Marrow Transplant*. 2013;19(8):1167-1174. doi:10.1016/j.bbmt.2013.05.001.
8. Sorror ML, Maris MB, Storb R, et al. Hematopoietic cell transplantation (HCT)-specific comorbidity index: a new tool for risk assessment before allogeneic HCT. *Blood*. 2005;106(8):2912-2919. doi:10.1182/blood-2005-05-2004.
9. Sorror ML, Martin PJ, Storb RF, et al. Pretransplant comorbidities predict severity of acute graft-versus-host disease and subsequent mortality. *Blood*. 2014;124(2):287-295. doi:10.1182/blood-2014-01-550566.
10. Sorror ML, Storb RF, Sandmaier BM, et al. Comorbidity-age index: a clinical measure of biologic age before allogeneic hematopoietic cell transplantation. *J Clin Oncol*. 2014;32(29):3249-3256. doi:10.1200/JCO.2013.53.8157.
11. Spellman SR, Eapen M, Logan BR, et al. A perspective on the selection of unrelated donors and cord blood units for transplantation. *Blood*. 2012;120(2):259-265. doi:10.1182/blood-2012-03-379032.
12. Lee SJ, Klein J, Haagenson M, et al. High-resolution donor-recipient HLA matching contributes to the success of unrelated donor marrow transplantation. *Blood*. 2007;110(13):4576-4583. doi:10.1182/blood-2007-06-097386.
13. Porter DL, Roth MS, McGarigle C, Ferrara JL, Antin JH. Induction of graft-versus-host disease as immunotherapy for relapsed chronic myeloid leukemia. *N Engl J Med*. 1994;330(2):100-106. doi:10.1056/NEJM199401133300204.
14. Kolb HJ. Graft-versus-leukemia effects of transplantation and donor lymphocytes. *Blood*. 2008;112(12):4371-4383. doi:10.1182/blood-2008-03-077974.
15. Giralt S, Ballen K, Rizzo D, et al. Reduced-intensity conditioning regimen workshop: defining the dose spectrum. Report of a workshop convened by the Center for International Blood and Marrow Transplant Research. *Biol Blood Marrow Transplant*. 2009;15(3):367-369. doi:10.1016/j.bbmt.2008.12.497.
16. Gopal R, Ha CS, Tucker SL, et al. Comparison of two total body irradiation fractionation regimens with respect to acute and late pulmonary toxicity. *Cancer*. 2001;92(7):1949-1958.
17. Andersson BS, Madden T, Tran HT, et al. Acute safety and pharmacokinetics of intravenous busulfan when used with oral busulfan and cyclophosphamide as pretransplantation conditioning therapy: a phase I study. *Biol Blood Marrow Transplant*. 2000;6(5A):548-554.
18. Andersson BS, Kashyap A, Gian V, et al. Conditioning therapy with intravenous busulfan and cyclophosphamide (IV BuCy2) for hematologic malignancies prior to allogeneic stem cell transplantation: a phase II study. *Biol Blood Marrow Transplant*. 2002;8(3):145-154.
19. Bredeson C, LeRademacher J, Kato K, et al. Prospective cohort study comparing intravenous busulfan to total body irradiation in hematopoietic cell transplantation. *Blood*. 2013;122(24):3871-3878. doi:10.1182/blood-2013-08-519009.
20. Copelan EA, Hamilton BK, Avalos B, et al. Better leukemia-free and overall survival in AML in first remission following cyclophosphamide in combination with busulfan compared with TBI. *Blood*. 2013;122(24):3863-3870. doi:10.1182/blood-2013-07-514448.
21. Nagler A, Rocha V, Labopin M, et al. Allogeneic hematopoietic stem-cell transplantation for acute myeloid leukemia in remission: comparison of intravenous busulfan plus cyclophosphamide (Cy) versus total-body irradiation plus Cy as conditioning regimen—a report from the Acute Leukemia Working Party of the European Group for Blood and Marrow Transplantation. *J Clin Oncol*. 2013;31(28):3549-3556. doi:10.1200/JCO.2013.48.8114.
22. Andersson B, de Lima M, Saliba R, et al. Pharmacokinetic dose guidance of IV BUsulfan with fludarabine with allogeneic stem cell transplantation improves progression free survival in patients with AML and MDS; results of a randomized phase III study. *Blood*. 2011;2011:abstract 292.
23. Bornhauser M, Storer B, Slattery JT, et al. Conditioning with fludarabine and targeted busulfan for transplantation of allogeneic hematopoietic stem cells. *Blood*. 2003;102(3):820-826. doi:10.1182/blood-2002-11-3567.
24. Russell JA, Tran HT, Quinlan D, et al. Once-daily intravenous busulfan given with fludarabine as conditioning for allogeneic stem cell transplantation: study of pharmacokinetics and early clinical outcomes. *Biol Blood Marrow Transplant*. 2002;8(9):468-476.
25. Andersson BS, Valdez BC, de Lima M, et al. Clofarabine +/- fludarabine with once daily i.v. busulfan as pretransplant conditioning therapy for advanced myeloid leukemia and MDS. *Biol Blood Marrow Transplant*. 2011;17(6):893-900. doi:10.1016/j.bbmt.2010.09.022.
26. Valdez BC, Li Y, Murray D, Champlin RE, Andersson BS. The synergistic cytotoxicity of clofarabine, fludarabine and busulfan in AML cells involves ATM pathway activation and chromatin remodeling. *Biochem Pharmacol*. 2011;81(2):222-232. doi:10.1016/j.bcp.2010.09.027.
27. Sandmaier BM, Mackinnon S, Childs RW. Reduced intensity conditioning for allogeneic hematopoietic cell transplantation: current perspectives. *Biol Blood Marrow Transplant*. 2007;13(1 Suppl 1):87-97. doi:10.1016/j.bbmt.2006.10.015.
28. Storb R, Yu C, Wagner JL, et al. Stable mixed hematopoietic chimerism in DLA-identical littermate dogs given sublethal total body irradiation before and pharmacological immunosuppression after marrow transplantation. *Blood*. 1997;89(8):3048-3054.
29. McSweeney PA, Niederwieser D, Shizuru JA, et al. Hematopoietic cell transplantation in older patients with hematologic malignancies: replacing high-dose cytotoxic therapy with graft-versus-tumor effects. *Blood*. 2001;97(11):3390-3400.
30. Niederwieser D, Maris M, Shizuru JA, et al. Low-dose total

body irradiation (TBI) and fludarabine followed by hematopoietic cell transplantation (HCT) from HLA-matched or mismatched unrelated donors and postgrafting immunosuppression with cyclosporine and mycophenolate mofetil (MMF) can induce durable complete chimerism and sustained remissions in patients with hematological diseases. *Blood.* 2003;101(4):1620-1629. doi:10.1182/blood-2002-05-1340.

31. Brammer JE, Stentz A, Gajewski J, et al. Nonmyeloablative allogeneic hematopoietic stem cell transplant for the treatment of patients with hematologic malignancies using busulfan, fludarabine, and total body irradiation conditioning is effective in an elderly and infirm population. *Biol Blood Marrow Transplant.* 2015;21(1):89-96. doi:10.1016/j.bbmt.2014.09.024.
32. de Lima M, Couriel D, Thall PF, et al. Once-daily intravenous busulfan and fludarabine: clinical and pharmacokinetic results of a myeloablative, reduced-toxicity conditioning regimen for allogeneic stem cell transplantation in AML and MDS. *Blood.* 2004;104(3):857-864. doi:10.1182/blood-2004-02-0414.
33. Giralt S, Thall PF, Khouri I, et al. Melphalan and purine analog-containing preparative regimens: reduced-intensity conditioning for patients with hematologic malignancies undergoing allogeneic progenitor cell transplantation. *Blood.* 2001;97(3):631-637.
34. Chewning JH, Castro-Malaspina H, Jakubowski A, et al. Fludarabine-based conditioning secures engraftment of second hematopoietic stem cell allografts (HSCT) in the treatment of initial graft failure. *Biol Blood Marrow Transplant.* 2007;13(11):1313-1323. doi:10.1016/j.bbmt.2007.07.006.
35. Alatrash G, de Lima M, Hamerschlak N, et al. Myeloablative reduced-toxicity i.v. busulfan-fludarabine and allogeneic hematopoietic stem cell transplant for patients with acute myeloid leukemia or myelodysplastic syndrome in the sixth through eighth decades of life. *Biol Blood Marrow Transplant.* 2011;17(10):1490-1496. doi:10.1016/j.bbmt.2011.02.007.
36. Buckner CD, Clift RA, Sanders JE, et al. Marrow harvesting from normal donors. *Blood.* 1984;64(3):630-634.
37. Dominietto A, Lamparelli T, Raiola AM, et al. Transplant-related mortality and long-term graft function are significantly influenced by cell dose in patients undergoing allogeneic marrow transplantation. *Blood.* 2002;100(12):3930-3934. doi:10.1182/blood-2002-01-0339
38. To LB, Roberts MM, Haylock DN, et al. Comparison of haematological recovery times and supportive care requirements of autologous recovery phase peripheral blood stem cell transplants, autologous bone marrow transplants and allogeneic bone marrow transplants. *Bone Marrow Transplant.* 1992;9(4):277-284.
39. Sheridan WP, Begley CG, Juttner CA, et al. Effect of peripheral-blood progenitor cells mobilised by filgrastim (G-CSF) on platelet recovery after high-dose chemotherapy. *Lancet.* 1992;339(8794):640-644.
40. Bensinger WI, Martin PJ, Storer B, et al. Transplantation of bone marrow as compared with peripheral-blood cells from HLA-identical relatives in patients with hematologic cancers. *N Engl J Med.* 2001;344(3):175-181. doi:10.1056/NEJM200101183440303.
41. Korbling M, Przepiorka D, Huh YO, et al. Allogeneic blood stem cell transplantation for refractory leukemia and lymphoma: potential advantage of blood over marrow allografts. *Blood.* 1995;85(6):1659-1665.
42. Anasetti C, Logan BR, Lee SJ, et al. Peripheral-blood stem cells versus bone marrow from unrelated donors. *N Engl J Med.* 2012;367(16):1487-1496. doi:10.1056/NEJMoa1203517.
43. Storb R, Deeg HJ, Whitehead J, et al. Methotrexate and cyclosporine compared with cyclosporine alone for prophylaxis of acute graft versus host disease after marrow transplantation for leukemia. *N Engl J Med.* 1986;314(12):729-735. doi:10.1056/NEJM198603203141201.
44. Nash RA, Pineiro LA, Storb R, et al. FK506 in combination with methotrexate for the prevention of graft-versus-host disease after marrow transplantation from matched unrelated donors. *Blood.* 1996;88(9):3634-3641.
45. Ratanatharathorn V, Nash RA, Przepiorka D, et al. Phase III study comparing methotrexate and tacrolimus (prograf, FK506) with methotrexate and cyclosporine for graft-versus-host disease prophylaxis after HLA-identical sibling bone marrow transplantation. *Blood.* 1998;92(7):2303-2314.
46. Cutler C, Logan B, Nakamura R, et al. Tacrolimus/sirolimus vs tacrolimus/methotrexate as GVHD prophylaxis after matched, related donor allogeneic HCT. *Blood.* 2014;124(8):1372-1377. doi:10.1182/blood-2014-04-567164.
47. Ho VT, Aldridge J, Kim HT, et al. Comparison of tacrolimus and sirolimus (Tac/Sir) versus tacrolimus, sirolimus, and mini-methotrexate (Tac/Sir/MTX) as acute graft-versus-host disease prophylaxis after reduced-intensity conditioning allogeneic peripheral blood stem cell transplantation. *Biol Blood Marrow Transplant.* 2009;15(7):844-850. doi:10.1016/j.bbmt.2009.03.017.
48. Yau JC, Dimopoulos MA, Huan SD, et al. An effective acute graft-vs.-host disease prophylaxis with minidose methotrexate, cyclosporine, and single-dose methylprednisolone. *Am J Hematol.* 1991;38(4):288-292.
49. Luznik L, Bolanos-Meade J, Zahurak M, et al. High-dose cyclophosphamide as single-agent, short-course prophylaxis of graft-versus-host disease. *Blood.* 2010;115(16):3224-3230. doi:10.1182/blood-2009-11-251595.
50. Kanakry CG, O'Donnell PV, Furlong T, et al. Multi-institutional study of post-transplantation cyclophosphamide as single-agent graft-versus-host disease prophylaxis after allogeneic bone marrow transplantation using myeloablative busulfan and fludarabine conditioning. *J Clin Oncol.* 2014;32(31):3497-3505. doi:10.1200/JCO.2013.54.0625.
51. Socie G, Schmoor C, Bethge WA, et al. Chronic graft-versus-host disease: long-term results from a randomized trial on graft-versus-host disease prophylaxis with or without anti-T-cell globulin ATG-Fresenius. *Blood.* 2011;117(23):6375-6382. doi:10.1182/blood-2011-01-329821.
52. Finke J, Bethge WA, Schmoor C, et al. Standard graft-versus-host disease prophylaxis with or without anti-T-cell globulin in haematopoietic cell transplantation from matched unrelated donors: a randomised, open-label, multicentre phase 3 trial. *Lancet Oncol.* 2009;10(9):855-864. doi:10.1016/S1470-2045(09)70225-6.
53. Theurich S, Fischmann H, Shimabukuro-Vornhagen A, et al. Polyclonal anti-thymocyte globulins for the prophylaxis of graft-versus-host disease after allogeneic stem cell or bone marrow transplantation in adults. *Cochrane Database Syst Rev.* 2012;9: CD009159. doi:10.1002/14651858.CD009159.pub2.
54. Marmont AM, Horowitz MM, Gale RP, et al. T-cell depletion of HLA-identical transplants in leukemia. *Blood.* 1991;78(8):2120-2130.
55. Champlin R, Giralt S, Przepiorka D, et al. Selective depletion of CD8-positive T-lymphocytes for allogeneic bone marrow transplantation: engraftment, graft-versus-host disease and graft-versus leukemia. *Prog Clin Biol Res.* 1992;377:385-394; discussion 395-388.
56. Tomblyn M, Chiller T, Einsele H, et al. Guidelines for preventing infectious complications among hematopoietic cell transplantation recipients: a global perspective. *Biol Blood Marrow Transplant.* 2009;15(10):1143-1238. doi:10.1016/j.bbmt.2009.06.019.
57. Bucaneve G, Micozzi A, Menichetti F, et al. Levofloxacin to prevent bacterial infection in patients with cancer and neutropenia. *N Engl J Med.* 2005;353(10):977-987. doi:10.1056/NEJMoa044097.

58. Goodman JL, Winston DJ, Greenfield RA, et al. A controlled trial of fluconazole to prevent fungal infections in patients undergoing bone marrow transplantation. *N Engl J Med.* 1992;326(13):845-851. doi:10.1056/NEJM199203263261301.
59. Wingard JR, Carter SL, Walsh TJ, et al. Randomized, double-blind trial of fluconazole versus voriconazole for prevention of invasive fungal infection after allogeneic hematopoietic cell transplantation. *Blood.* 2010;116(24):5111-5118. doi:10.1182/blood-2010-02-268151.
60. Erard V, Guthrie KA, Varley C, et al. One-year acyclovir prophylaxis for preventing varicella-zoster virus disease after hematopoietic cell transplantation: no evidence of rebound varicella-zoster virus disease after drug discontinuation. *Blood.* 2007;110(8):3071-3077. doi:10.1182/blood-2007-03-077644.
61. Stern A, Green H, Paul M, Vidal L, Leibovici L. Prophylaxis for *Pneumocystis* pneumonia (PCP) in non-HIV immunocompromised patients. *Cochrane Database Syst Rev.* 2014;10: CD005590. doi:10.1002/14651858.CD005590.pub3.
62. Link H, Vohringer HF, Wingen F, Bragas B, Schwardt A, Ehninger G. Pentamidine aerosol for prophylaxis of *Pneumocystis carinii* pneumonia after BMT. *Bone Marrow Transplant.* 1993;11(5):403-406.
63. Anderson KC, Weinstein HJ. Transfusion-associated graft-versus-host disease. *N Engl J Med.* 1990;323(5):315-321. doi:10.1056/NEJM199008023230506.
64. Barge AJ. A review of the efficacy and tolerability of recombinant haematopoietic growth factors in bone marrow transplantation. *Bone Marrow Transplant.* 1993;11(Suppl 2):1-11.
65. Mattsson J, Ringden O, Storb R. Graft failure after allogeneic hematopoietic cell transplantation. *Biol Blood Marrow Transplant.* 2008;14(1 Suppl 1):165-170. doi:10.1016/j.bbmt.2007.10.025.
66. Huisman C, de Weger RA, de Vries L, Tilanus MG, Verdonck LF. Chimerism analysis within 6 months of allogeneic stem cell transplantation predicts relapse in acute myeloid leukemia. *Bone Marrow Transplant.* 2007;39(5):285-291. doi:10.1038/sj.bmt.1705582.
67. Voogt PJ, Fibbe WE, Marijt WA, et al. Rejection of bone-marrow graft by recipient-derived cytotoxic T lymphocytes against minor histocompatibility antigens. *Lancet.* 1990;335(8682):131-134.
68. Bearman SI. The syndrome of hepatic veno-occlusive disease after marrow transplantation. *Blood.* 1995;85(11):3005-3020.
69. Coppell JA, Richardson PG, Soiffer R, et al. Hepatic veno-occlusive disease following stem cell transplantation: incidence, clinical course, and outcome. *Biol Blood Marrow Transplant.* 2010;16(2):157-168. doi:10.1016/j.bbmt.2009.08.024.
70. McDonald GB, Sharma P, Matthews DE, Shulman HM, Thomas ED. Venocclusive disease of the liver after bone marrow transplantation: diagnosis, incidence, and predisposing factors. *Hepatology.* 1984;4(1):116-122.
71. Richardson PG, Soiffer RJ, Antin JH, et al. Defibrotide for the treatment of severe hepatic veno-occlusive disease and multiorgan failure after stem cell transplantation: a multicenter, randomized, dose-finding trial. *Biol Blood Marrow Transplant.* 2010;16(7):1005-1017. doi:10.1016/j.bbmt.2010.02.009.
72. Zirakzadeh A MV, Imran H, Litzow M, Kumar S. Ursodiol prophylaxis against hepatic veno-occlusive disease in hematopoietic stem cell transplant recipients: a systematic review and meta-analysis. *Biol Blood Marrow Transplant.* 2006;12(2, Suppl 1): 137-138.
73. Essell JH, Schroeder MT, Harman GS, et al. Ursodiol prophylaxis against hepatic complications of allogeneic bone marrow transplantation. A randomized, double-blind, placebo-controlled trial. *Ann Intern Med.* 1998;128(12 Pt 1):975-981.
74. Williams KM, Chien JW, Gladwin MT, Pavletic SZ. Bronchiolitis obliterans after allogeneic hematopoietic stem cell transplantation. *JAMA.* 2009;302(3):306-314. doi:10.1001/jama.2009.1018.
75. Norman BC, Jacobsohn DA, Williams KM, et al. Fluticasone, azithromycin and montelukast therapy in reducing corticosteroid exposure in bronchiolitis obliterans syndrome after allogeneic hematopoietic SCT: a case series of eight patients. *Bone Marrow Transplant.* 2011;46(10):1369-1373. doi:10.1038/bmt.2010.311.
76. Armitage J, Antman KH. *High Dose Cancer Therapy: Pharmacology, Hematopoietic Stem Cells.* 3rd ed. Philadelphia, PA: Lippincott, Williams & Wilkins; 2000.
77. Glucksberg H, Storb R, Fefer A, et al. Clinical manifestations of graft-versus-host disease in human recipients of marrow from HL-A-matched sibling donors. *Transplantation.* 1974;18(4):295-304.
78. Lee SE, Cho BS, Kim JH, et al. Risk and prognostic factors for acute GVHD based on NIH consensus criteria. *Bone Marrow Transplant.* 2013;48(4):587-592. doi:10.1038/bmt.2012.187.
79. Flowers ME, Inamoto Y, Carpenter PA, et al. Comparative analysis of risk factors for acute graft-versus-host disease and for chronic graft-versus-host disease according to National Institutes of Health consensus criteria. *Blood.* 2011;117(11):3214-3219. doi:10.1182/blood-2010-08-302109.
80. Martin PJ, Rizzo JD, Wingard JR, et al. First- and second-line systemic treatment of acute graft-versus-host disease: recommendations of the American Society of Blood and Marrow Transplantation. *Biol Blood Marrow Transplant.* 2012;18(8):1150-1163. doi:10.1016/j.bbmt.2012.04.005.
81. Alousi AM, Weisdorf DJ, Logan BR, et al. Etanercept, mycophenolate, denileukin, or pentostatin plus corticosteroids for acute graft-versus-host disease: a randomized phase 2 trial from the Blood and Marrow Transplant Clinical Trials Network. *Blood.* 2009;114(3):511-517. doi:10.1182/blood-2009-03-212290.
82. Hoda D, Pidala J, Salgado-Vila N, et al. Sirolimus for treatment of steroid-refractory acute graft-versus-host disease. *Bone Marrow Transplant.* 2010;45(8):1347-1351. doi:10.1038/bmt.2009.343.
83. Greinix HT, Volc-Platzer B, Rabitsch W, et al. Successful use of extracorporeal photochemotherapy in the treatment of severe acute and chronic graft-versus-host disease. *Blood.* 1998;92(9):3098-3104.
84. Teshima T, Maeda Y, Ozaki K. Regulatory T cells and IL-17-producing cells in graft-versus-host disease. *Immunotherapy.* 2011;3(7):833-852. doi:10.2217/imt.11.51.
85. Sarantopoulos S, Blazar BR, Cutler C, Ritz J. B cells in chronic graft-versus-host disease. *Biol Blood Marrow Transplant.* 2015;21(1):16-23. doi:10.1016/j.bbmt.2014.10.029.
86. Shulman HM, Sullivan KM, Weiden PL, et al. Chronic graft-versus-host syndrome in man. A long-term clinicopathologic study of 20 Seattle patients. *Am J Med.* 1980;69(2):204-217.
87. Filipovich AH, Weisdorf D, Pavletic S, et al. National Institutes of Health consensus development project on criteria for clinical trials in chronic graft-versus-host disease: I. Diagnosis and staging working group report. *Biol Blood Marrow Transplant.* 2005;11(12):945-956. doi:10.1016/j.bbmt.2005.09.004.
88. Stewart BL, Storer B, Storek J, et al. Duration of immunosuppressive treatment for chronic graft-versus-host disease. *Blood.* 2004;104(12):3501-3506. doi:10.1182/blood-2004-01-0200.
89. Wolff D, Gerbitz A, Ayuk F, et al. Consensus conference on clinical practice in chronic graft-versus-host disease (GVHD):first-line and topical treatment of chronic GVHD. *Biol Blood Marrow Transplant.* 2010;16(12):1611-1628. doi:10.1016/j.bbmt.2010.06.015.
90. Wolff D, Schleuning M, von Harsdorf S, et al. Consensus Conference on Clinical Practice in Chronic GVHD: second-line treatment of chronic graft-versus-host disease. *Biol Blood Marrow Transplant.* 2011;17(1):1-17. doi:10.1016/j.bbmt.2010.05.011.
91. Koc S, Leisenring W, Flowers ME, et al. Therapy for chronic

graft-versus-host disease: a randomized trial comparing cyclosporine plus prednisone versus prednisone alone. *Blood.* 2002;100(1):48-51.

92. Couriel DR, Saliba R, Escalon MP, et al. Sirolimus in combination with tacrolimus and corticosteroids for the treatment of resistant chronic graft-versus-host disease. *Br J Haematol.* 2005;130(3):409-417. doi:10.1111/j.1365-2141.2005.05616.x.
93. Mohty B, Mohty M. Long-term complications and side effects after allogeneic hematopoietic stem cell transplantation: an update. *Blood Cancer J.* 2011;1(4):e16. doi:10.1038/bcj.2011.14.
94. Kolb HJ, Socie G, Duell T, et al. Malignant neoplasms in long-term survivors of bone marrow transplantation. Late Effects Working Party of the European Cooperative Group for Blood and Marrow Transplantation and the European Late Effect Project Group. *Ann Intern Med.* 1999;131(10):738-744.
95. Bishop MR, Alyea EP 3rd, Cairo MS, et al. National Cancer Institute's First International Workshop on the Biology, Prevention, and Treatment of Relapse After Allogeneic Hematopoietic Stem Cell Transplantation: summary and recommendations from the organizing committee. *Biol Blood Marrow Transplant.* 2011;17(4):443-454. doi:10.1016/j.bbmt.2010.12.713.
96. Elmaagacli AH, Beelen DW, Trenn G, Schmidt O, Nahler M, Schaefer UW. Induction of a graft-versus-leukemia reaction by cyclosporin A withdrawal as immunotherapy for leukemia relapsing after allogeneic bone marrow transplantation. *Bone Marrow Transplant.* 1999;23(8):771-777. doi:10.1038/sj.bmt.1701672.
97. Kolb HJ, Schmid C, Barrett AJ, Schendel DJ. Graft-versus-leukemia reactions in allogeneic chimeras. *Blood.* 2004;103(3):767-776. doi:10.1182/blood-2003-02-0342.
98. Schroeder T, Rachlis E, Bug G, et al. Treatment of acute myeloid leukemia or myelodysplastic syndrome relapse after allogeneic stem cell transplantation with azacitidine and donor lymphocyte infusions—a retrospective multicenter analysis from the German Cooperative Transplant Study Group. *Biol Blood Marrow Transplant.* 2014. doi:10.1016/j.bbmt.2014.12.016.
99. Duncan CN, Majhail NS, Brazauskas R, et al. Long-term survival and late effects among one-year survivors of second allogeneic hematopoietic cell transplantation for relapsed acute leukemia and myelodysplastic syndromes. *Biol Blood Marrow Transplant.* 2015;21(1):151-158. doi:10.1016/j.bbmt.2014.10.006.
100. Attal M, Lauwers-Cances V, Marit G, et al. Lenalidomide maintenance after stem-cell transplantation for multiple myeloma. *N Engl J Med.* 2012;366(19):1782-1791. doi:10.1056/NEJMoa1114138.
101. de Lima M, Giralt S, Thall PF, et al. Maintenance therapy with low-dose azacitidine after allogeneic hematopoietic stem cell transplantation for recurrent acute myelogenous leukemia or myelodysplastic syndrome: a dose and schedule finding study. *Cancer.* 2010;116(23):5420-5431. doi:10.1002/cncr.25500.
102. Hess G, Bunjes D, Siegert W, et al. Sustained complete molecular remissions after treatment with imatinib-mesylate in patients with failure after allogeneic stem cell transplantation for chronic myelogenous leukemia: results of a prospective phase II open-label multicenter study. *J Clin Oncol.* 2005;23(30):7583-7593. doi:10.1200/JCO.2005.01.3110.
103. Pfeifer H, Wassmann B, Bethge W, et al. Randomized comparison of prophylactic and minimal residual disease-triggered imatinib after allogeneic stem cell transplantation for BCR-ABL1-positive acute lymphoblastic leukemia. *Leukemia.* 2013;27(6):1254-1262. doi:10.1038/leu.2012.352.
104. Walter RB, Buckley SA, Pagel JM, et al. Significance of minimal residual disease before myeloablative allogeneic hematopoietic cell transplantation for AML in first and second complete remission. *Blood.* 2013;122(10):1813-1821. doi:10.1182/blood-2013-06-506725.
105. Kroger N, Miyamura K, Bishop MR. Minimal residual disease following allogeneic hematopoietic stem cell transplantation. *Biol Blood Marrow Transplant.* 2011;17(1 Suppl):S94-S100. doi:10.1016/j.bbmt.2010.10.031.
106. Anderlini P, Saliba R, Acholonu S, et al. Fludarabine-melphalan as a preparative regimen for reduced-intensity conditioning allogeneic stem cell transplantation in relapsed and refractory Hodgkin's lymphoma: the updated M.D. Anderson Cancer Center experience. *Haematologica.* 2008;93(2):257-264. doi:10.3324/haematol.11828.
107. Anderlini P, Saliba RM, Ledesma C, et al. Gemcitabine, fludarabine and melphalan as a reduced-intensity conditioning regimen for allogeneic stem cell transplant in relapsed and refractory Hodgkin lymphoma: preliminary results. *Leukemia Lymphoma.* 2012;53(3):499-502. doi:10.3109/10428194.2011.615427.
108. Kebriaei P, Basset R, Ledesma C, et al. Clofarabine combined with busulfan provides excellent disease control in adult patients with acute lymphoblastic leukemia undergoing allogeneic hematopoietic stem cell transplantation. *Biol Blood Marrow Transplant.* 2012;18(12):1819-1826. doi:10.1016/j.bbmt.2012.06.010.
109. Khouri IF, McLaughlin P, Saliba RM, et al. Eight-year experience with allogeneic stem cell transplantation for relapsed follicular lymphoma after nonmyeloablative conditioning with fludarabine, cyclophosphamide, and rituximab. *Blood.* 2008;111(12):5530-5536. doi:10.1182/blood-2008-01-136242.
110. Khouri IF, Wei W, Korbling M, et al. BFR (bendamustine, fludarabine, and rituximab) allogeneic conditioning for chronic lymphocytic leukemia/lymphoma: reduced myelosuppression and GVHD. *Blood.* 2014;124(14):2306-2312. doi:10.1182/blood-2014-07-587519.
111. Popat U, de Lima MJ, Saliba RM, et al. Long-term outcome of reduced-intensity allogeneic hematopoietic SCT in patients with AML in CR. *Bone Marrow Transplant.* 2012;47(2):212-216. doi:10.1038/bmt.2011.61.
112. Popat UR BR, Chen J, Alousi AM, et al. Allogeneic transplantation for myelofibrosis: benefit of dose intensity. *J Clin Oncol.* 2013;31(suppl):abstract 7011.
113. Kebriaei P, Saliba R, Rondon G, et al. Long-term follow-up of allogeneic hematopoietic stem cell transplantation for patients with Philadelphia chromosome-positive acute lymphoblastic leukemia: impact of tyrosine kinase inhibitors on treatment outcomes. *Biol Blood Marrow Transplant.* 2012;18(4):584-592. doi:10.1016/j.bbmt.2011.08.011.
114. Jabbour E, Cortes J, Santos FP, et al. Results of allogeneic hematopoietic stem cell transplantation for chronic myelogenous leukemia patients who failed tyrosine kinase inhibitors after developing BCR-ABL1 kinase domain mutations. *Blood.* 2011;117(13):3641-3647. doi:10.1182/blood-2010-08-302679.

14 Alternative Donor Transplants: Cord Blood Transplant

第十四章　替代供体移植：脐带血移植

Rohtesh S. Mehta
Betul Oran
Elizabeth J. Shpall

中文导读

对于缺少合适骨髓移植供体的患者来说，脐带血移植是非常有意义的方法。本章首先介绍了脐带血移植的背景，以及移植中细胞数量与人白细胞抗原配型的相关内容。脐带血里面的造血干细胞数量不足的情况下，应用两个供体脐带血进行移植也是常用的方案，本章对单脐带与双脐带血移植分别进行了介绍。接下来对于移植前的预处理方案进行了详细的介绍，包括骨髓的预处理方案以及剂量调整的预处理方案。对于移植后并发的移植物抗宿主病和感染也进行了详细的介绍。最后本章分享了MD 安德森癌症中心脐带血移植的完整流程，内容涵盖了患者的选择、预处理、移植物抗宿主病的预防措施以及提高脐带血移植效果的最新进展。

BACKGROUND

The numbers of allogeneic stem cell transplants (SCTs) performed in the United States have increased steadily, from about 7,500 in 1994-1995 to over 13,500 in 2010-2011, in patients above the age of 20 years [1]. Donor identification has been a constant challenge, and only 30% of patients who need allogeneic SCT have a matched sibling donor. The National Marrow Donor Program (NMDP) and its cooperative international registries have about 16 million volunteer donors. It is estimated that 75% of white patients, but only 16% of African Americans and other minority patients, will be able to find a suitably matched unrelated donor (MUD) and proceed to transplantation [2]. Mismatched related (often haploidentical), cord blood (CB) or mismatched unrelated donors (MMUDs) with either peripheral blood (PB) or bone marrow (BM) graft sources are potential options for patients in need of a SCT but lacking a matched related donor (MRD) or unrelated donor.

Using CB as the graft source provides many advantages; CB units are easy to collect with little or no risk to the mother or newborn. Cord blood units can be rapidly obtained for 80% to 95% of the patients 20 years and older across all races and in almost 100% of younger patients [2]. This is particularly advantageous in cases where urgent transplant is mandated. Owing to rapid procurement of CB units, patients can receive CB transplantation (CBT) 4 or 5 weeks earlier than those receiving SCT with a MUD [3]. Further, CBT is associated with low risk of infection transmission, requires less-stringent human leukocyte antigen (HLA)–matching criteria, and has relatively lower risk of graft-versus-host disease (GVHD) with preserved graft-versus-malignancy effects. However, it is associated with a greater risk of graft rejection, delayed engraftment, and delayed immune reconstitution, leading to heightened risk of infection or nonrelapse mortality (NRM) [4-7]. Many of the adverse outcomes noted after CBT are attributed to the naïveté of CB T lymphocytes and the low numbers of total nucleated cells (TNCs) and $CD34^+$ cells in the graft.

CELL DOSE AND HUMAN LEUKOCYTE ANTIGEN MATCHING

The outcomes of CBT depend on the impact of cell dose and the degree of HLA match [8]. The TNC dose available for CBT is a fraction of what is typically used in the PB or BM setting. The median TNC dose obtained from a BM harvest is about 3×10^8 TNCs/kg; the granulocyte colony-stimulating factor (G-CSF)–mobilized PB can yield a median of 7×10^8 TNCs/kg [9]. In contrast, about one-fourth of the CB units contain less than 0.25×10^8 TNCs/kg, and two-thirds of the units have between 0.25×10^8 to 1×10^8 TNCs/kg [8]. The recommended minimum cell dose is typically 2×10^7 TNCs/kg for successful engraftment after a CBT.

The HLA matching criteria between the CB units and the recipient are less stringent compared with other donor sources. Therefore, while unrelated adult donors are selected to be closely matched to recipients at HLA-A, -B, -C, and -DRB1 by high-resolution testing [10, 11], CB units are selected using lower-resolution HLA typing (antigen level) for HLA-A and -B and at the allele level for HLA-DRB1 [12]. In a study of single CBT, Barker et al showed that recipients of 6/6 matched CB units had the lowest transplant-related mortality (TRM) regardless of the dose, followed by 5/6 matched CB units with TNC dose greater than 2.5×10^7/kg or 4/6 matched units with TNC dose greater than 5.0×10^7/kg, and 5/6 matched units with lower TNC dose (<2.5×10^7/kg) [8, 13]. These findings support the notion that both TNC dose and HLA-matching level should be taken into account for CB unit selection.

Although the standard HLA-matching criteria do not require high-resolution typing at class I antigen in CBT, a recent study by the Center for International Blood and Marrow Transplant Research (CIBMTR) and the Eurocord reported better outcomes in single CBT after myeloablative conditioning (MAC) with improved allele-level matching for 4 HLA loci (-A, -B, -C, and -DRB1) [14]. The investigators showed that the frequency of neutrophil recovery was lower for recipients of mismatches at three to five but not at one or two alleles compared with those of HLA-matched units. Nonrelapse mortality was higher with units mismatched at one to five alleles compared with matched units. This retrospective study confirmed the clinical importance of selecting better HLA allele-matched units for single CBT, an observation already well described for BM and PB progenitor cell transplantation. The effect of HLA matching by high-resolution testing is unclear after double CBT (dCBT) and should be investigated.

SINGLE VERSUS DOUBLE CORD BLOOD TRANSPLANTATION

The relatively low number of progenitor cells in a single CB unit resulting in delayed hematopoietic recovery, and engraftment failure limited the use of CBT in adults. Most adults do not have access to a single CB unit containing the recommended nucleated cell dose of 2.5×10^7 TNCs/kg [15]. To overcome the cell-dose limitation, investigators pioneered an approach by which two partially HLA-matched CB units were used to augment the progenitor cell dose when a single unit was considered inadequate and confirmed its feasibility ([15]). A recent CIBMTR analysis investigated the relative risks and benefits of transplanting double CB units compared with an adequately dosed single CB unit. The investigators observed no differences in clinical outcomes after dCBT or adequately dosed single CBT. Both transplant approaches had comparable outcomes with 78% (95% CI, 72-83) versus 81% (95% CI, 74-88, *P* = .83) probabilities of neutrophil engraftment by day 42, and 68% (95% CI, 62-74) versus 63% (95% CI, 53-72; *P* = .34) probabilities of platelet recoveries at 6 months, respectively. There were no differences for grades III or IV acute GVHD (18% [95% CI, 11%-26%] versus 14% [95% CI, 10%-19%], *P* = .64), 2-year probabilities of chronic GVHD (31% [95% CI, 26-37] versus 24% [95% CI, 15-34], *P* = .27), treatment-related mortality (hazard ratio [HR] 0.91; *P* = .63), risk of relapse (HR 0.90, *P* = .64), and overall mortality (HR 0.93, *P* = .62) ([16]).

A unique feature after a dCBT is evidence of mixed chimerism from both the CB units observed during the initial posttransplant period.([17]) In the early post-dCBT period (day +21), both CB units contribute to hematopoiesis in 40% to 50% of patients, but by day +100 one unit predominates in a vast majority ([18, 19]). The factors leading to unit dominance are not well defined. It is however recognized that there is no association with the TNC or CD34$^+$ cell doses, HLA match, gender match, ABO typing, or the order in which CB units are infused ([15, 18-21]). This current lack of evidence is a major limitation to dCBT, and identifying predictive factors for unit dominance would optimize CB unit selection algorithms by allowing for the selection of two CB units with a high probability of long-term engraftment.

CONDITIONING REGIMENS

Myeloablative Conditioning Regimens

High-intensity MAC regimens are reserved for young and otherwise-fit patients who can tolerate the associated regimen morbidity. Such regimens lead to a low risk of relapse at the expense of a high TRM compared with reduced-intensity conditioning (RIC) regimens.

One of the largest registry studies comparing single-unit CB (n = 165) to PB (n = 888) or BM (n = 472) transplants in adults with acute leukemia using MAC regimens from 2002 through 2006 showed promising outcomes with CBT. Total body irradiation (TBI) constituted part of the preparative regimen in about half of patients in the CB group and about two-thirds in the comparative groups. Despite a significantly higher number of patients with fully HLA-matched PB or BM grafts (70%) compared to CB grafts (6%), the rates of disease-free survival (DFS) and relapse were similar among the groups, while the risks of acute or chronic GVHD were significantly lower with CBT. Also, TRM was similar with CBT compared with mismatched PB or BM grafts, but higher in contrast to fully matched PB (HR 1.62; 95% CI, 1.18-2.23; *P* = .003) or BM transplants (HR 1.69; 95% CI, 1.19-2.39; *P* = .003). This was offset by a significantly lower incidence of chronic GVHD compared with fully matched PB (HR 0.38; 95% CI, 0.27-0.53; *P* = .001) or BM transplants (HR 0.63; 95% CI, 0.44-0.90; *P* = .01) ([4]). Therefore, in the absence of matched PB or BM donors, CBT potentially offers better outcomes compared with mismatched alternative donor transplants.

Similar encouraging results were noted in a study that compared 4-6/6 matched dCBT exclusively (using the MAC regimen including fludarabine 75 mg/m^2, cyclophosphamide 120 mg/kg, and TBI 1,200 to 1,320 cGy [Flu/Cy/TBI]) to 8/8 MRD or MUD, or 1 allele–MMUD donors ([7]). This study also noted lower risk of relapse, higher TRM, lower GVHD, and comparable DFS after CBT compared to other groups. The risk of relapse was significantly lower after dCBT (15%, 95% CI, 9%-22%), compared with MRD (43%, 95% CI, 35%-52%) or MUD (37%, 95% CI, 29%-46%) transplants. Higher NRM was noted after dCBT (34%, 95% CI, 25%-42%) compared to MRD (24%, 95% CI, 17%-39%) or MUD (14%, 95% CI, 9%-20%) transplants, which resulted in comparable 5-year DFS between CB (51%, 95% CI, 41%-59%), MRD 33% (95% CI, 26%-41%), and MUD (48%, 95% CI, 40%-56%) transplants. The cumulative incidence of grades II to IV GVHD at day 100 after DCBT, MRD, and MUD was 60% (95% CI, 50%-70%), 65% (95% CI, 57%-73%), and 80% (95% CI, 70%-90%), respectively. The rate of chronic GVHD at 2 years was 26% (95% CI, 15%-35%), 47% (95% CI, 39%-55%), and 43% (95% CI, 34%-52%) respectively ([7]).

In adults with high-risk acute lymphoblastic leukemia (ALL), CBT leads to similar overall survival (OS), TRM, and relapse risk, with significantly lower risk of acute or chronic GVHD, compared with PB or BM transplants. This was demonstrated in a recent registry study that compared outcomes after single or double 4-6/6 matched CB (n = 116) and 7-8/8 matched PB (n = 546) or BM (n =140) transplants after MAC regimens ([22]). More than half of the patients in the CBT group received Flu/Cy/TBI as the conditioning regimen, while about 75% of the patients in the PB or BM groups received TBI/Cy-based regimens. There were no differences in the 3-year OS rates (44%, 44%, and 43%, respectively); relapse risk (22%, 25%, and 28%, respectively); or TRM (42%, 31%, and 39%, respectively) among the groups. However, the risk of acute grades II to IV GVHD (27%, 47%, and 41%, respectively) or grades III and IV acute GVHD (9%, 16%, 24%, respectively) was appreciably lower after CBT compared with 8/8-matched and 7/8-matched PB or BM transplants, respectively ([22]).

Reduced-Intensity Conditioning Regimens

The advent of RIC regimens extended the utility of CBT to older patients and those with comorbid conditions that otherwise restrict the use of the MAC regimens. It is noteworthy that a majority of trials in MRD or MUD transplants used an arbitrary age definition of greater than 55 to 60 years (to define "older patients") as a threshold of using an RIC regimen. However, age greater than 40 to 45 years is generally chosen as a threshold for RIC in the CBT setting.

Barker et al reported that the RIC with fludarabine 200 mg/m^2, cyclophosphamide 50 mg/kg, and 2-Gy TBI (Flu/Cy/2Gy TBI) was well tolerated, with rapid neutrophil recovery, a sustained donor engraftment rate of 94%, and a low incidence of TRM ([23]). This regimen was associated with significantly better DFS compared with other RIC regimens (51% vs 28%, P = .0002, HR 0.53) ([24]). Multiple studies supporting the use of RIC CBT in patients who would not be able to tolerate more intensive preparative regimens have subsequently been reported ([6, 18, 19, 25-27]).

A retrospective single-center study compared the outcomes in patients older than 55 years who underwent CB and MRD SCT with RIC (primarily of Flu/Cy/2Gy TBI). There were no differences in TRM at 180 days (28%, 95% CI, 14%-41% vs 23%, 95% CI, 11%-36%); 3-year DFS (34%, 95% CI, 19%-48% vs 30%, 95% CI, 16%-44%); or 3-year OS (34%, 95% CI, 17%-50% vs 43%, 95% CI, 29%-58%) between the groups ([6]). These findings were confirmed by a registry analysis of patients with acute leukemia comparing the outcomes after CB (n = 161), 8/8-matched (313) and 7/8-matched PB (111) transplants with RIC regimens. Patients with CBT following a Flu/Cy/2 Gy TBI regimen had comparable results with 8/8 HLA-matched PB donors. However, higher TRM and lower OS and LFS were observed in recipients of CBT if they were treated with alternative RIC regimens, including busulfan plus melphalan, or cyclophosphamide with fludarabine and in vivo T-cell depletion with antithymocyte globulin (ATG) ([27]). Similar findings were reported by Eurocord and the European Group for Blood and Marrow Transplantation (EBMT) in patients with lymphoid malignancies. When patients with CB units (n = 104) were compared with 8/8-matched PB MUD (n = 541) transplants, no difference was noted in NRM (29% vs 28%), PFS (28% vs 35%), or OS (56% vs 49%) at 3 years (Fig. 14-1). Further, the risk of chronic GVHD was significantly lower in the CBT group (26% vs 52% at 3 years; P = .0005) ([26]). These studies supported the use of CBT with RIC as a suitable alternative for patients who may benefit from RIC SCT and who do not have a suitable related or unrelated volunteer donor in the time period transplantation is needed.

POSTTRANSPLANT COMPLICATIONS

Disease relapse is the most common cause of mortality after allogeneic SCT, while GVHD and infections are the two leading causes of NRM. Treatment options after SCT relapse include withdrawal of immunosuppression, chemotherapy, or donor lymphocyte

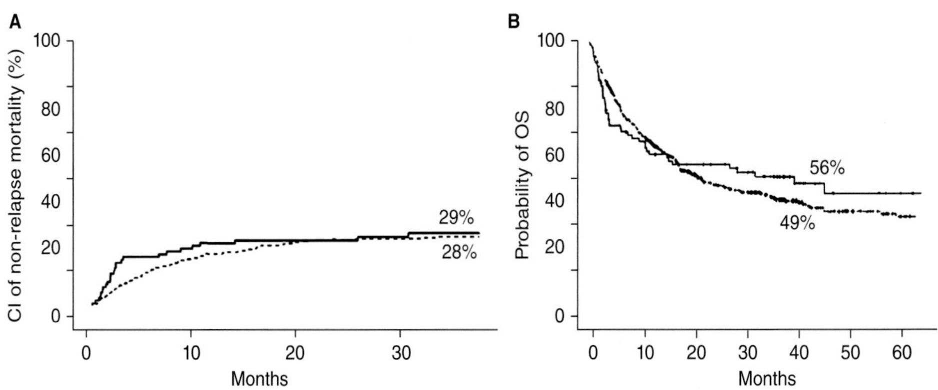

FIGURE 14-1 Comparison of cord blood (*solid line*) and matched unrelated donor transplants (*dotted line*) for lymphoid malignancies. A. Nonrelapse mortality (NRM). B. Overall survival (OS). There were no differences in NRM or OS at 3 -years between the two groups. [Reproduced with permission from Rodrigues CA, Rocha V, Dreger P, et al. Alternative donor hematopoietic stem cell transplantation for mature lymphoid malignancies after reduced-intensity conditioning regimen: similar outcomes with umbilical cord blood and unrelated donor peripheral blood. *Haematologica.* 2014;99(2):370-377.]

infusion (DLI). Although DLI is currently unavailable for CBT patients outside clinical trials, a study showed that in adults who have acute myelogenous leukemia relapse following CB or MRD transplants, DLI in the latter group did not have an impact on OS (19% CB vs 28% MRD at 1 year; $P = .36$), and relapsed patients had poor prognosis independent of the donor source ([28]).

In the CBT setting, infections are the leading cause of early 100-day NRM (27%), while GVHD contributes to most (20%) of the delayed NRM (beyond 100 days) ([4]). The reported probabilities of acute grades III and IV GVHD at day 100 (10%-25%) and chronic GVHD (25%-35%), TRM (20%-50%), risk of relapse (20%-50%), DFS (30%-35%), and OS (30%-45%) at 2 to 3 years varied depending on the conditioning regimens and the study population ([7, 16, 19, 22, 24, 27]). The rates of posttransplant complications are comparable after the use of dCBT and single CBT ([29]).

Early infections (within 100 days) are primarily due to neutropenia and mucosal damage caused by conditioning regimens. Delayed infections are related to the speed of cell-mediated immune reconstitution and use of immunosuppressants. Most early infections are bacterial; more than half of the invasive fungal infections and 45% of cytomegalovirus (CMV) infection occur beyond day +100 ([30]).

The heightened risk of infections in CBT is partly explained by the naïveté of CB T cells and delayed T-lymphocyte immune reconstitution and neutrophil engraftment in contrast to other donor sources ([4,7,27,31,32]). Although significant B-cell recovery starts within 3 to 4 months and may approach normal numbers by 6 months after transplant, T-cell reconstitution is substantially prolonged ([32]). The CD4+ and CD8+ T-cell counts are strikingly reduced after CBT, remain low for up to 6 months, and approach normal values by 1 year. The PB T cells after CBT are more dysfunctional as compared with other types of allogeneic SCTs. Patients also fail to recover thymic function after CBT, in contrast to other allogeneic SCT recipients ([33]) (Fig. 14-2).

A retrospective registry analysis from the CIBMTR comparing CB (n = 150) with matched (n = 367) or antigen-mismatched (n = 83) BM transplants reported higher risk of early (within 100 days) infection-related deaths after CBT compared to other groups (45%, 21%, and 24%, respectively; $P = .01$) ([29]). In another study, the risk of severe infection, especially bacterial infections in the first 100 days, was significantly higher after CBT in contrast to BM or PB graft (85% vs 69%, $P < .01$). The risk of infection-related mortality did not differ at day 100 or at 3 years. In multivariate analysis for CBT, CMV-seropositive recipient, prolonged neutropenia beyond day 30, and low cell dose ($<2 \times 10^7$/kg) were the predictors for infection-related mortality ([30]).

MD ANDERSON APPROACH TO CORD BLOOD TRANSPLANTATION

At the MD Anderson Cancer Center, patients with various hematological malignancies who do not have an MRD or MUD but require SCT are considered for CBT and a search for a CB unit is initiated (Fig. 14-3).

Unit Selection

Within the first days to weeks of the initial donor search, coordinators determine the likelihood of

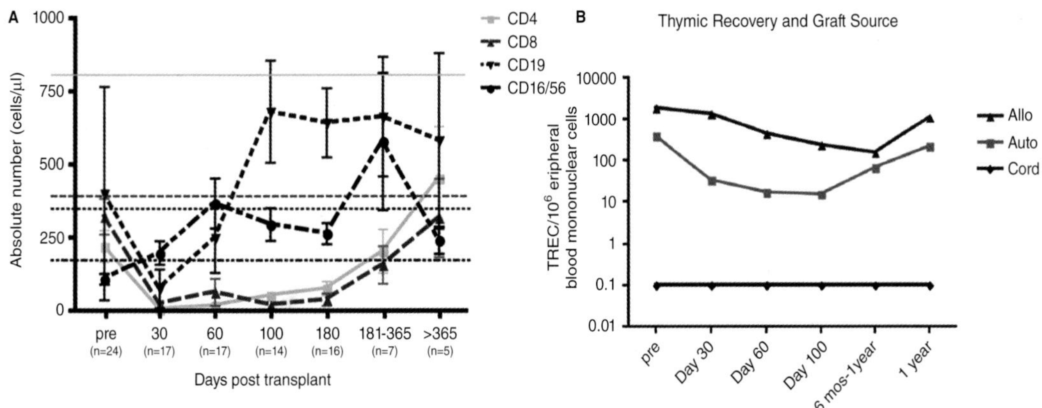

FIGURE 14-2 A. Delayed immune reconstitution after cord blood transplant (CBT). After CBT, NK cells (CD16/CD56) and B cells (CD19) recover early; there is significant decline in CD4 and CD8 T cells, which gradually recovers over several months. Horizontal lines depict normal values. B. Thymic regeneration failure after CBT compared to autologous and allogeneic SCT recipients as determined by the measurement of peripheral recent thymic emigrants by determining the number of T-cell receptor excision circles (TRECs). After CBT, most patients have an undetectable thymopoiesis. [Reproduced with permission from Komanduri KV, St John LS, de Lima M, et al. Delayed immune reconstitution after cord blood transplantation is characterized by impaired thymopoiesis and late memory T-cell skewing. *Blood.* 2007;110(13):4543-4551.]

CHAPTER 14

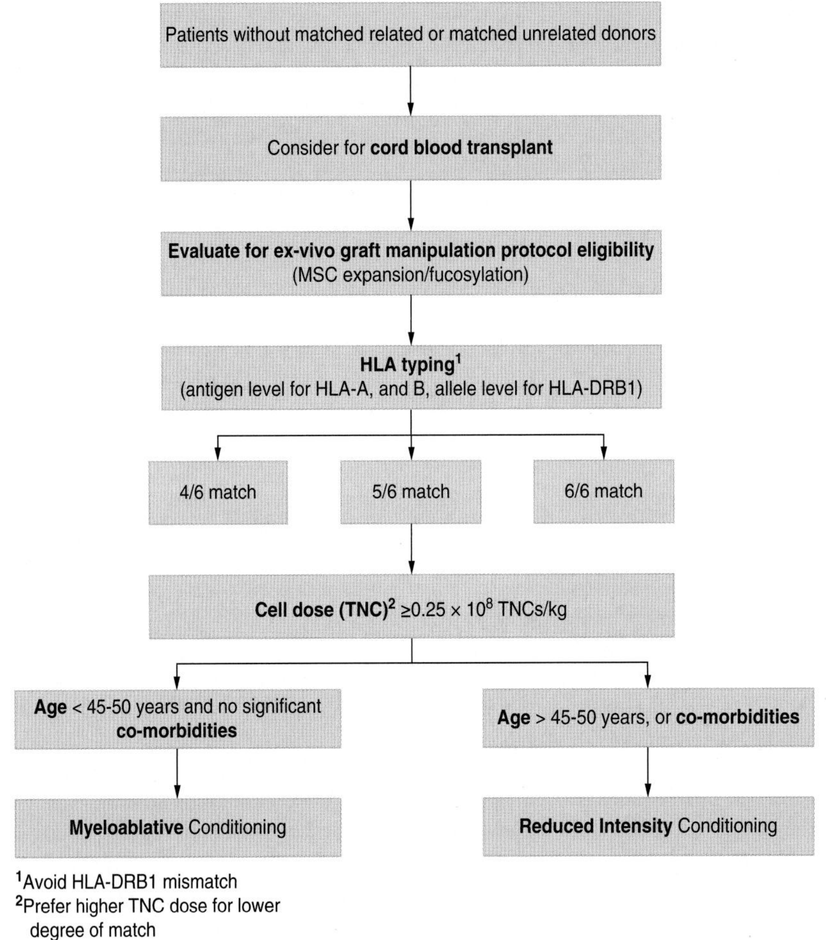

FIGURE 14-3 Approach to a patient for cord blood transplant.

obtaining a suitably matched donor based on the patient's ancestry, the preliminary search results, and review of the HLA typing. If the likelihood of finding a matched donor is deemed to be low, we proceed with confirmatory HLA typing of CB units. Alternatively, we may delay typing of CB units if multiple 10/10 HLA-A, -B, -C, -DRB1, -DQ allele-MUDs are probable or if the transplantation is not urgent. If an unrelated donor collection is delayed because of problems with donor health or availability, a prompt decision is made whether to abandon the unrelated donor search in favor of CB.

To maximize the chance of identifying optimal CB unit(s), we conduct a global search while being aware that there is no global regulatory oversight of CB-banking standards. It is important to know which banks are included in the NMDP consortium of banks, in the Netcord, and in the NMDP Cooperative Registries. We give equal consideration to domestic and international units as the primary units of the graft, whereas we prefer domestic units for backup.

Our current institutional policy is to use a double-unit graft in an effort to augment engraftment and reduce TRM. Given that either unit may engraft after a double-unit CBT, each unit of a double-unit graft is equally important. We give a strong priority to HLA match over precryopreservation TNC threshold of about 2.0×10^7/kg for each unit of a double-unit graft. This approach gives strong priority to HLA match but augments the chance of engraftment by infusing two units with at least an adequate dose in each.

We use novel ex vivo graft manipulation techniques pioneered at the MD Anderson Cancer Center, such as ex vivo CB expansion with mesenchymal stromal cells (MSCs) ([34]) and ex vivo CB fucosylation ([35]). With these, remarkable improvement in engraftment is noted compared with historical controls. The median time to neutrophil engraftment is 15 (range, 9 to 42) days with MSC expansion ([34]) and 14 (range 12-28) days with fucosylation, which is significantly faster than the 24 (range 12-52) days noted in the CIBMTR controls ($P < .001$) ([35]). Similarly, platelet engraftment is 42 (range 15-62) days with MSC expansion and 33 (range 18-100) days with fucosylation, compared with 49 (range 18-264) days in the CIBMTR controls (P = .03) ([34, 35]). We are investigating the impact of CB unit KIR (killer immunoglobulin-like receptor) genotype on transplant outcomes with an aim to integrate KIR information into the CB unit selection algorithm.

Conditioning Regimens

We have investigated various MAC regimens for CBT, which include combinations of (a) melphalan, fludarabine, and thiotepa; (b) busulfan and fludarabine; (c) busulfan, clofarabine, fludarabine, and low-dose TBI given 9 days after chemotherapy; and (d) busulfan, clofarabine, fludarabine, and low-dose TBI given immediately after the chemotherapy ([36]). The most favorable outcomes appear to be associated with the latest regimen, which is well tolerated and associated with prompt engraftment and effective disease control. This regimen consists of fludarabine 10 mg/m^2/d (days -7 through -4), clofarabine 30 mg/m^2/d (days -7 through -4), busulfan at a dose calculated to deliver a daily area under the curve (AUC) of 4,000 μmol/min for 4 days (days -7 through -4) based on an outpatient test dose of 32 mg/m^2, and 2-Gy TBI on day -3. Our preferred RIC regimen consists of fludarabine 40 mg/m^2/d (days -5 through -2) and melphalan 140 mg/m^2 (day -2) in addition to the Flu/Cy/2Gy TBI for patients older than 50 years or not medically fit to tolerate an MAC regimen.

Prophylaxis

Prophylaxis against GVHD is provided with mycophenolate mofetil (MMF) and tacrolimus. We start MMF from day -3 at a dose of 15 mg/kg (maximum of 1 g orally twice daily) and continue it through day +100. Tacrolimus is started from day -2 and taper started at day 180 in the absence of GVHD. We use rabbit ATG 3 mg/kg infused over 2 days on days -4 and -3 in all patients. Patients on azole antifungals require appropriate dose adjustments for tacrolimus. Other drug interactions and creatinine clearance need be considered while calculating the dosing.

Filgrastrim is administered from day 0 until neutrophil engraftment and blood products are transfused as indicated. Standard infectious disease prophylaxis with antibacterial (levofloxacin), antiviral (valacyclovir), and antifungal (voriconazole, posaconazole, or caspofungin—the choice depending on risk factors) and against *Pneumocystis jiroveci* pneumonia are also provided for all CBT patients. The surveillance for CMV using quantitative polymerase chain reaction (qPCR) (or antigenemia assay if absolute neutrophil count is >1 × 10^9/L) is performed routinely twice weekly for the first 100 days after CBT or longer if any complications are present. We routinely perform Epstein-Barr viremia testing using qPCR every 2 weeks from day +30 until day +100. Other viruses, including adenovirus, BK virus, respiratory syncytial virus, influenza, human herpes virus 6, and parainfluenza, are tested as clinically indicated.

Novel Strategies to Improve Cord Blood Transplantation Outcomes

To increase CB cell dose, a variety of ex vivo expansion techniques have been developed that yield significantly higher final numbers of TNCs. These include coculturing the CB cells with cytokine support or MSCs to simulate the BM "hematopoietic niche" ex vivo ([34]) or using nicotinamide analogs ([37]) or copper chelators (such as tetraethylenepentamine) ([38]) and targeting the *Notch* signaling pathway ([39]), all of which block the differentiation of early progenitor cells, leading to expansion of hematopoietic stem cells. Apart from augmenting the cell dose, ex vivo graft manipulation techniques are being explored to improve the inherent homing capacity of CB cells, with an aim to accelerate engraftment. Different methods are being tested in clinical trials, such as fucosylation of the CB progenitor cells ([40]) or the use of prostaglandin E_2 derivatives ([41]) or dipeptidyl peptidase-4 inhibitors. Many of these techniques have demonstrated significantly improved time to neutrophil engraftment (13-17 days) comparable to other donor types (Fig. 14-4).

Ex vivo graft manipulation permitted the generation and clinical use of antivirus and antitumor adoptive immunotherapies as well as cellular therapies for GVHD prevention. A variety of "designer" CB lymphocytes can now be engineered and expanded ex vivo. For instance, these include T cells with specific cytotoxicity against tumors or viruses ([42-44]), chimeric antigen receptor (CAR) T cells ([45]), natural killer (NK) cells ([46]), and regulatory T cells (T_{Regs}) ([47]), which are being tested in clinical trials.

CONCLUSION

Cord blood transplantation is an attractive option for patients who lack a matched PB or BM donor. To overcome the limitation of low cell doses in single-CB units, dCBT has been adopted for many patients and is associated with outcomes comparable to those with other donor sources. There are promising strategies to improve engraftment with ex vivo expansion or homing and to enhance immune reconstitution with the infusion of CB-derived NK cells and cytotoxic T lymphocytes with antiviral and antileukemic specificities.

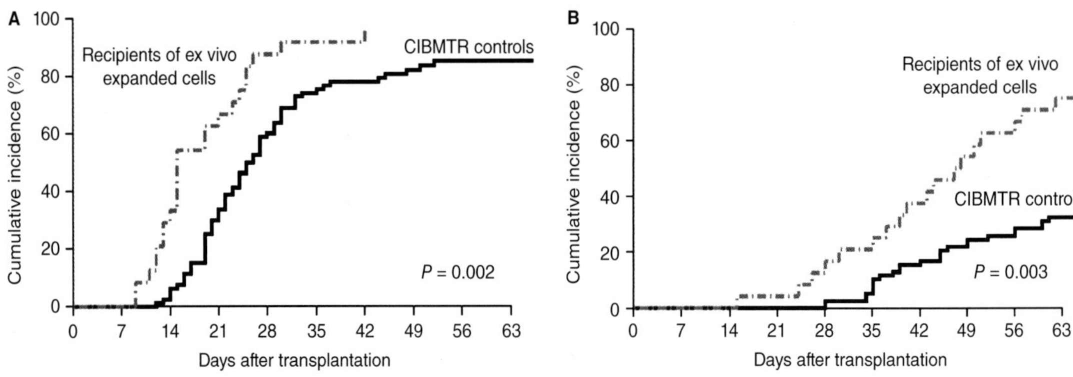

FIGURE 14-4 Cumulative incidences of (A) neutrophil and (B) platelet engraftments after ex vivo CB expansion with mesenchymal stromal cells (MSCs) compared with CIBMTR historical controls. Both neutrophil and platelet engraftments are significantly faster, and a higher proportion of patients engrafts after MSC expansion. [Reproduced with permission from de Lima M, McNiece I, Robinson SN, et al: Cord-blood engraftment with ex vivo mesenchymal-cell coculture, *N Engl J Med* 2012 Dec 13;367(24):2305-2315.]

Prospective multicenter clinical trials are needed to determine the efficacy of these promising technologies.

REFERENCES

1. Pasquini M, Wang Z. *Current use and outcome of hematopoietic stem cell transplantation: CIBMTR Summary Slides, 2013*. http://www.cibmtr.org.
2. Gragert L, Eapen M, Williams E, et al. HLA match likelihoods for hematopoietic stem-cell grafts in the U.S. registry. *N Engl J Med*. 2014;371(4):339-348.
3. Barker JN, Krepski TP, DeFor TE, Davies SM, Wagner JE, Weisdorf DJ. Searching for unrelated donor hematopoietic stem cells: availability and speed of umbilical cord blood versus bone marrow. *Biol Blood Marrow Transplant*. 2002;8(5):257-260.
4. Eapen M, Rocha V, Sanz G, et al. Effect of graft source on unrelated donor haemopoietic stem-cell transplantation in adults with acute leukaemia: a retrospective analysis. *Lancet Oncol*. 2010;11(7):653-660.
5. Jacobson CA, Turki AT, McDonough SM, et al. Immune reconstitution after double umbilical cord blood stem cell transplantation: comparison with unrelated peripheral blood stem cell transplantation. *Biol Blood Marrow Transplant*. 2012;18(4):565-574.
6. Majhail NS, Brunstein CG, Tomblyn M, et al. Reduced-intensity allogeneic transplant in patients older than 55 years: unrelated umbilical cord blood is safe and effective for patients without a matched related donor. *Biol Blood Marrow Transplant*. 2008;14(3):282-289.
7. Brunstein CG, Gutman JA, Weisdorf DJ, et al. Allogeneic hematopoietic cell transplantation for hematologic malignancy: relative risks and benefits of double umbilical cord blood. *Blood*. 2010;116(22):4693-4699.
8. Barker JN, Scaradavou A, Stevens CE. Combined effect of total nucleated cell dose and HLA match on transplantation outcome in 1061 cord blood recipients with hematologic malignancies. *Blood*. 2010;115(9):1843-1849.
9. Singhal S, Powles R, Kulkarni S, et al. Comparison of marrow and blood cell yields from the same donors in a double-blind, randomized study of allogeneic marrow vs blood stem cell transplantation. *Bone Marrow Transplant*. 2000;25(5):501-505.
10. Lee SJ, Klein J, Haagenson M, et al. High-resolution donor-recipient HLA matching contributes to the success of unrelated donor marrow transplantation. *Blood*. 2007;110(13):4576-4583.
11. Petersdorf EW. Optimal HLA matching in hematopoietic cell transplantation. *Curr Opin Immunol*. 2008;20(5):588-593.
12. Gluckman E, Rocha V, Arcese W, et al. Factors associated with outcomes of unrelated cord blood transplant: guidelines for donor choice. *Exp Hematol*. 2004;32(4):397-407.
13. Tucunduva L, Ruggeri A, Sanz G, et al. Impact of myeloablative and reduced intensity conditioning on outcomes after unrelated cord blood transplantation for adults with acute lymphoblastic leukemia. *Biol Blood Marrow Transplant*. 2013;19(2):S127.
14. Eapen M, Klein JP, Ruggeri A, et al. Impact of allele-level HLA matching on outcomes after myeloablative single unit umbilical cord blood transplantation for hematologic malignancy. *Blood*. 2014;123(1):133-140.
15. Barker JN, Weisdorf DJ, DeFor TE, et al. Transplantation of 2 partially HLA-matched umbilical cord blood units to enhance engraftment in adults with hematologic malignancy. *Blood*. 2005;105(3):1343-1347.
16. Scaradavou A, Brunstein CG, Eapen M, et al. Double unit grafts successfully extend the application of umbilical cord blood transplantation in adults with acute leukemia. *Blood*. 2013;121(5):752-758.
17. Hashem H, Lazarus H. Double umbilical cord blood transplantation: relevance of persistent mixed-unit chimerism. *Biol Blood Marrow Transplant*. 2014.
18. Ballen KK, Spitzer TR, Yeap BY, et al. Double unrelated reduced-intensity umbilical cord blood transplantation in adults. *Biol Blood Marrow Transplant*. 2007;13(1):82-89.
19. Brunstein CG, Barker JN, Weisdorf DJ, et al. Umbilical cord blood transplantation after nonmyeloablative conditioning: impact on transplantation outcomes in 110 adults with hematologic disease. *Blood*. 2007;110(8):3064-3070.
20. Arachchillage DR, Dalley CD, Reilly JT, Wilson G, Collins N, Snowden JA. Long-term dual donor derived haematopoietic reconstitution following double unrelated cord blood transplantation—single unit dominance is not always the case. *Br J Haematol*. 2010;149(2):298-299.
21. Gluckman E. Ten years of cord blood transplantation: from bench to bedside. *Br J Haematol*. 2009;147(2):192-199.
22. Marks DI, Woo KA, Zhong X, et al. Unrelated umbilical cord blood transplant for adult acute lymphoblastic leukemia in first and second complete remission: a comparison with allografts from adult unrelated donors. *Haematologica*.

2014;99(2):322-328.
23. Barker JN, Weisdorf DJ, DeFor TE, Blazar BR, Miller JS, Wagner JE. Rapid and complete donor chimerism in adult recipients of unrelated donor umbilical cord blood transplantation after reduced-intensity conditioning. *Blood.* 2003;102(5):1915-1919.
24. Arcese W. Myeloablative versus reduced intensity conditioning regimen cord blood transplants. Paper presented at the 37th Annual Meeting of the European Group for Blood and Marrow Transplantation; April 4, 2011; Paris, France.
25. Miyakoshi S, Yuji K, Kami M, et al. Successful engraftment after reduced-intensity umbilical cord blood transplantation for adult patients with advanced hematological diseases. *Clin Cancer Res.* 2004;10(11):3586-3592.
26. Rodrigues CA, Rocha V, Dreger P, et al. Alternative donor hematopoietic stem cell transplantation for mature lymphoid malignancies after reduced-intensity conditioning regimen: similar outcomes with umbilical cord blood and unrelated donor peripheral blood. *Haematologica.* 2014;99(2):370-377.
27. Brunstein CG, Eapen M, Ahn KW, et al. Reduced-intensity conditioning transplantation in acute leukemia: the effect of source of unrelated donor stem cells on outcomes. *Blood.* 2012;119(23):5591-5598.
28. Bejanyan N, Oran B, Shanley R, et al. Clinical outcomes of AML patients relapsing after matched-related donor and umbilical cord blood transplantation. *Bone Marrow transplant.* 2014;49(8):1029-1035.
29. Laughlin MJ, Eapen M, Rubinstein P, et al. Outcomes after transplantation of cord blood or bone marrow from unrelated donors in adults with leukemia. *N Engl J Med.* 2004;351(22):2265-2275.
30. Parody R, Martino R, Rovira M, et al. Severe infections after unrelated donor allogeneic hematopoietic stem cell transplantation in adults: comparison of cord blood transplantation with peripheral blood and bone marrow transplantation. *Biol Blood Marrow Transplant.* 2006;12(7):734-748.
31. Weisdorf D, Eapen M, Ruggeri A, et al. Alternative donor transplantation for older patients with acute myeloid leukemia in first complete remission: a center for international blood and marrow transplant research-eurocord analysis. *Biol Blood Marrow Transplant.* 2014;20(6):816-822.
32. Szabolcs P, Cairo MS. Unrelated umbilical cord blood transplantation and immune reconstitution. *Semin Hematol.* 2010;47(1):22-36.
33. Komanduri KV, St John LS, de Lima M, et al. Delayed immune reconstitution after cord blood transplantation is characterized by impaired thymopoiesis and late memory T-cell skewing. *Blood.* 2007;110(13):4543-4551.
34. de Lima M, McNiece I, Robinson SN, et al. Cord-blood engraftment with ex vivo mesenchymal-cell coculture. *N Engl J Med.* 2012;367(24):2305-2315.
35. Popat UR, Oran B, Hosing CM, et al. Ex vivo fucosylation of cord blood accelerates neutrophil and platelet engraftment [ASH Abstract 691]. 55th ASH Annual Meeting and Exposition; December 7-10, 2013; New Orleans, LA.
36. Mehta RS, Di Stasi A, Andersson BS, et al. The development of a myeloablative, reduced-toxicity, conditioning regimen for cord blood transplantation. *Clin Lymphoma Myeloma Leuk.* 2014;14(1):e1-e5.
37. Saber W, Cutler CS, Nakamura R, et al. Impact of donor source on hematopoietic cell transplantation outcomes for patients with myelodysplastic syndromes (MDS). *Blood.* 2013;122(11):1974-1982.
38. Ringden O, Pavletic SZ, Anasetti C, et al. The graft-versus-leukemia effect using matched unrelated donors is not superior to HLA-identical siblings for hematopoietic stem cell transplantation. *Blood.* 2009;113(13):3110-3118.
39. Delaney C, Heimfeld S, Brashem-Stein C, Voorhies H, Manger RL, Bernstein ID. Notch-mediated expansion of human cord blood progenitor cells capable of rapid myeloid reconstitution. *Nat Med.* 2010;16(2):232-236.
40. Robinson SN, Thomas MW, Simmons PJ, et al. Fucosylation with fucosyltransferase VI or fucosyltransferase VII improves cord blood engraftment. *Cytotherapy.* 2014;16(1):84-89.
41. Cutler C, Multani P, Robbins D, et al. Prostaglandin-modulated umbilical cord blood hematopoietic stem cell transplantation. *Blood.* 2013;122(17):3074-3081.
42. Hanley P, Leen A, Gee AP, et al. Multi-virus-specific T-cell therapy for patients after hematopoietic stem cell and cord blood transplantation. *Blood.* 2013;122(21):140.
43. Weber G, Gerdemann U, Caruana I, et al. Generation of multi-leukemia antigen-specific T cells to enhance the graft-versus-leukemia effect after allogeneic stem cell transplant. *Leukemia.* 2013;27(7):1538-1547.
44. Micklethwaite KP, Savoldo B, Hanley PJ, et al. Derivation of human T lymphocytes from cord blood and peripheral blood with antiviral and antileukemic specificity from a single culture as protection against infection and relapse after stem cell transplantation. *Blood.* 2010;115(13):2695-2703.
45. Kebriaei P, Huls H, Singh H, et al. First clinical trials employing Sleeping Beauty Gene Transfer System and artificial antigen presenting cells to generate and infuse T cells expressing CD19-specific chimeric antigen receptor. *Blood.* 2013;122(21):166.
46. Shah N, Martin-Antonio B, Yang H, et al. Antigen presenting cell-mediated expansion of human umbilical cord blood yields log-scale expansion of natural killer cells with anti-myeloma activity. *PloS One.* 2013;8(10):e76781.
47. Brunstein CG, Miller JS, Cao Q, et al. Infusion of ex vivo expanded T regulatory cells in adults transplanted with umbilical cord blood: safety profile and detection kinetics. *Blood.* 2011;117(3):1061-1070.

15

Alternative Donor Transplants: Haploidentical Hematopoietic Stem Cell Transplantation

第十五章　替代供体移植：单倍体相合造血干细胞移植

Sameh Gaballa
Richard E. Champlin
Stefan O. Ciurea

中文导读

近10年来，随着大剂量环磷酰胺和新的部分T细胞耗竭技术的出现，单倍体相合造血干细胞移植发展迅速。新技术可以控制强烈的异体反应及促进免疫恢复，减少感染与复发的风险。本章首先介绍了单倍体相合造血干细胞移植技术的背景，接着详细探讨了通过T细胞耗竭技术控制移植物抗宿主病进而降低治疗相关的死亡率，通过移植后使用环磷酰胺平衡移植物抗宿主病与免疫恢复。接着本章介绍了移植后预防再复发的细胞治疗方法，包括有未经修饰的供体淋巴细胞输注、经修饰的供体淋巴细胞输注、嵌合抗原受体T细胞(CART)以及自然杀伤细胞和杀伤免疫球蛋白样受体错配。本章还对供体选择和供体特异性抗体的风险进行了阐述。本章最后展望了这一领域的未来研究方向。

INTRODUCTION

Haploidentical stem cell transplantation (haploSCT) from a first-degree-related haplotype-mismatched donor (siblings, children, parents) could expand allogeneic stem cell transplantation (SCT) to a large proportion of patients with hematologic malignancies without an HLA-matched donor ([1]). As the average family size continues to shrink, the likelihood of finding an HLA-matched related sibling donor continues to decrease ([2]). Moreover, as the population continues to age, finding a young, healthy sibling donor becomes increasingly less likely. The use of matched unrelated donors (MUDs) is limited by the long time to SCT (median 3-4 months), which makes it difficult to treat patients with more advanced disease in rapid need of SCT. The ethnicity/race of the recipient can also limit MUD transplantation as approximately 30% of Caucasians, 70% of Hispanics, and 90% of African Americans do not have a MUD in the worldwide registries ([3]).

In contrast to unrelated donor stem cells, haploidentical (or "half-matched") donors can be available immediately, and there are no costs associated with an unrelated donor search, maintaining a registry, or coordinating logistics with distant donor centers. This is an especially valuable option for the non-Caucasian and mixed-race individuals ([3]). This approach might also be particularly useful in developing countries that may not have the resources to procure unrelated donor transplants or maintain complex unrelated donor registries. Moreover, haploidentical donors offer the possibility to easily collect donor cells for cellular therapy posttransplant. Over the recent decade, significant breakthrough advances in controlling alloreactivity have been made and important steps taken toward graft engineering and posttransplant cellular therapy, approaches that changed dramatically the landscape of haploSCT. Improved haploidentical transplant outcomes represent a major advance in SCT that has practically eliminated the limitation of donor availability for allogeneic SCT.

CHAPTER 15

COMPLETE T-CELL DEPLETION: CONTROL OF GRAFT-VERSUS-HOST DISEASE WITH A HIGH TREATMENT-RELATED MORTALITY

Historically, unmanipulated T-cell-replete haploSCT grafts with conventional graft-versus-host-disease (GVHD) prophylaxis used in the late 1970s were associated with intense bidirectional alloreactivity and unacceptably high morbidity and mortality rates due to hyperacute GVHD and graft rejection ([4-6]). This led in the 1980s to the development of complete ex vivo depletion of T cells using CD34-selected grafts. Complete T-cell depletion has been associated with a lower incidence of acute GVHD (aGVHD); however, this caused delayed immune recovery and was associated with a high nonrelapse mortality (NRM) from infections and higher disease relapse rates given the decreased graft-versus-leukemia effect, as well as a higher rate of graft rejection ([7-9]). While graft rejection was partially overcome with "megadoses" of CD34 cells (typically >10^7 $CD34^+$ cells/kg) and a myeloablative conditioning regimen (including total-body irradiation [TBI], cyclophosphamide, thiotepa) with severe T-cell depletion of the graft, immune recovery remained delayed, leading to high NRM rates in excess of 40% ([10]). Improved results with this approach have been reported in some centers with selective depletion of alpha-beta T cells. T-cell depletion strategies have been most successful in children ([11]). We have used this approach with a different conditioning regimen (fludarabine, melphalan, and thiotepa) and showed that most patients died of NRM related to infectious complications ([12]).

During the last decade, several advances enabled investigators to selectively deplete alloreactive T cells and successfully control GVHD rates while maintaining memory T cells in the graft to accelerate immune recovery and prevent significant infectious complications posttransplant. Table 15-1 summarizes the major contemporaneous approaches to haploSCT. These advances have improved significantly outcomes of patients treated with haploidentical donors, with outcomes now similar to matched transplants (Fig. 15-1) ([12a]). Here, we summarize the recent developments with this type of transplant, focusing on advances made at the MD Anderson Cancer Center (MDACC).

BALANCING GRAFT-VERSUS-HOST DISEASE, IMMUNE RECOVERY, AND THE CONCEPT OF SELECTIVE ALLODEPLETION:POSTTRANSPLANT CYCLOPHOSPHAMIDE

The introduction of high-dose posttransplant cyclophosphamide (HDPTCy) for GVHD prevention represented a major turning point for haploSCT. The concept of inducing immune tolerance with posttransplant cyclophosphamide was introduced by Berenbaum and Brown in 1963, showing that the life of a skin allograft can be prolonged with the use of HDPTCy administered 1 to 3 days after the graft ([13]). Mayumi et al demonstrated that microchimerism and robust tolerance to minor histocompatibility antigens can be achieved in mice receiving allogeneic splenic cells by intraperitoneal high-dose cyclophosphamide

Table 15-1 Current Approaches to HaploSCT

Approach	Rationale	Stage of the Clinical Development
High-dose posttransplantation cyclophosphamide	• Eliminating only the alloreactive T cells • Rapid immune recovery with low infectious complications • Acceptable rates of GVHD • Lower cost	Phase II/III
Selective αβ T-cell depletion	• Removing αβ T cells that are most responsive for aGVHD • Remaining γδ T cells thought to have an innate immune-like response capability without inducing GVHD	Phase I/II
Photodepletion	• Ex vivo depletion of alloreactive T cells with TH9402 that accumulates in activated T cells	Phase I/II
Selective CD45RA+ T-cell depletion	• Elimination of CD45RA+ naïve T cells thought to play a major role in GVHD • Preserves memory T cells that are active against infections	Phase I

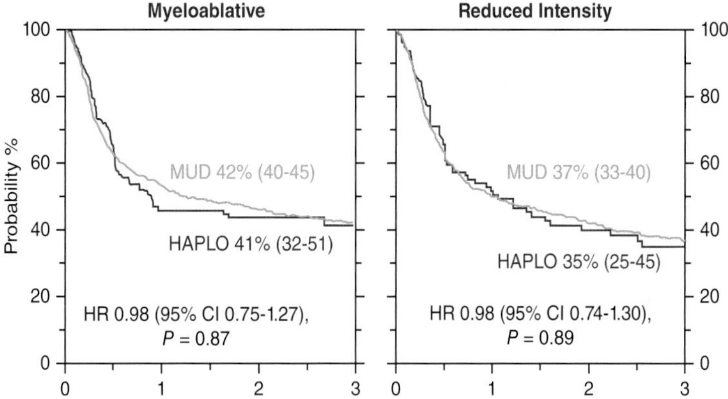

FIGURE 15-1 Progression-free survival at 3 years for patients with haploidentical (n = 192) and 8/8 matched unrelated donor (n = 1,982) with myeloablative conditioning (left) and reduced-intensity conditioning (right) transplantation.

administered on day 2 or 3 posttransplant ([14]). This concept found its best applicability in allogeneic transplantation, particularly in haploidentical transplantation, where HDPTCy induces bidirectional immune tolerance by selectively eliminating the highly dividing alloreactive donor and recipient T cells generated early posttransplant in the setting of a human leukocyte antigen (HLA) mismatched transplant, with decreased rates of GVHD and graft rejection ([15]). HDPTCy spares stem cells (due to high levels of aldehyde dehydrogenase present in the cells), which reconstitute the recipient's hematopoiesis ([16]), and nondividing T cells, including memory T cells. This results in a more rapid immune recovery compared to T-cell-depleted approaches, leading to lower NRM (lower rates of infections) compared with T-cell-depleted haploSCT, as shown by our group ([17]).

We have used HDPTCy since 2009, soon after the first human trials showed the safety of this approach ([18]). Initial studies used a nonmyeloablative conditioning regimen with fludarabine, cyclophosphamide, and 2-Gy TBI, which was associated with a low incidence of grades 2 to 4 aGVHD (35%) and NRM (15%) at 1 year. However, a higher relapse rate was observed ([18]). We then hypothesized that more intense conditioning is needed and can be tolerated, especially for patients with leukemia, and used our melphalan-based conditioning regimen (with fludarabine 120 mg/m^2, melphalan 100 to 140 mg/m^2 with thiotepa 5 to 10 mg/kg [subsequently changed to 2-Gy TBI]) previously used in T-cell-depleted haploSCT, which had been effective in inducing remission in most patients with leukemia even with advanced disease ([12,17]). Updated results for the first 100 patients treated with this regimen showed 3-year PFS rates of 56% to 62% for patients with myeloid malignancies (acute myelocytic leukemia [AML] in complete remission 1/2, myelodysplastic syndrome and chronic myelocytic leukemia in chronic phase) and lymphoma, and 1-year NRM rates of 12% and 22%, respectively ([19]).

With haploSCT, outcomes improved significantly; we and others have subsequently compared transplant outcomes of patients treated with a haploidentical versus a matched related donor or a MUD ([20-22]). These single-institution studies uniformly showed similar outcomes with haploidentical transplant with HDPTCy and HLA-matched donor SCT ([20-22]). To confirm these findings, we compared outcomes of haploidentical with MUD transplants using the Center for International Blood and Marrow Transplant Research (CIBMTR) database. This retrospective analysis of 2,174 patients with AML showed similar 3-year PFS with haploidentical transplants performed with HDPTCy and MUD transplants (41% vs 42% for myeloablative, $P = .87$; 35% vs 37% for reduced-intensity conditioning [RIC], $P = .89$, respectively) (see Fig. 15-1). The incidence of grades 2 to 4 aGVHD was lower for haploidentical compared with MUD transplants (21% vs 42% for myeloablative, 25% vs 35% for RIC) ([23]). Our group has proposed a large prospective multicenter study comparing transplant outcomes using haploidentical and MUDs to the Bone and Marrow Transplant Clinical Trials Network group.

GRAFT ENGINEERING

Several research strategies are being investigated to optimize the haploidentical graft, maximize immune recovery, and minimize GVHD posttransplant. One promising approach is changing complete T-cell depletion to selective depletion of alpha/beta T cells capable of eliciting GVHD while preserving in the graft memory T cells and gamma-delta T cells ([11]). It is currently thought that the gamma-delta T cells possess innate and adaptive immune responses and can function without requiring antigen processing or HLA presentation, making them unlikely to generate GVHD ([24]). Methods to deplete alpha-beta T cells and leaving the gamma-delta subsets intact are being investigated, with encouraging results ([25]). Other novel approaches involve depletion of naïve T cells (CD45RA$^+$) thought to play a major role in the development of GVHD in mouse models ([26-28]) or administration of T-regulatory cells along with the T-cell-depleted graft. These may further reduce the risk of aGVHD and reduce the rate of relapse ([29]). Future trials will explore these approaches at MDACC, as they may control GVHD and facilitate rapid immune recovery without posttransplant immunosuppression.

POSTTRANSPLANT CELLULAR THERAPY TO PREVENT DISEASE RELAPSE

With significant improvements in NRM, disease relapse remains the major cause of death in patients undergoing haploSCT. Several approaches are under investigation at our institution to prevent and treat disease relapse posttransplant (Table 15-2).

Unmodified Donor Lymphocyte Infusion

The readily available haploidentical donors can be sources of posttransplant donor lymphocyte infusion (DLI) administered to prevent or treat early relapse. There is a theoretical higher risk of inducing severe aGVHD with haploidentical DLI; however, the incidence of GVHD was not higher than in matched transplants, possibly due to the tolerizing effect of HDPTCy ([30]). Among 40 patients with hematological malignancies relapsed after a haploSCT who received unmodified

CHAPTER 15

Table 15-2 Posttransplant Cellular Therapies Aimed at Decreasing Disease Relapse in HaploSCT

Approach	Rationale	Pitfalls
Unmodified donor lymphocyte infusion (DLI)	• To fight disease relapse via harnessing graft-versus-malignancy effect	• Limited experience in haploSCT • Potential for GVHD precipitation • Not targeted to specific antigen(s)
Engineered donor lymphocytes with a safety suicide switch	• To fight disease relapse via harnessing graft-versus-malignancy effect • Safety switch allows T-cell suicide in case of GVHD development	• Not targeted to specific antigen(s) • Clinical efficacy not yet demonstrated
Gamma-delta DLI	• Infusion of selected gamma-delta T cells • No GVHD potential	• Graft-versus-malignancy effect not yet demonstrated
T cells with chimeric antigen receptors (CAR-T)	• T cells engineered to recognize specific antigens (eg, CD19) provide graft-versus-malignancy effect without GVHD	• Clinical efficacy after haploSCT not yet demonstrated
Infusion of ex vivo expanded NK cells	• Potential graft-versus-malignancy effect without GVHD	• Clinical efficacy has not yet been demonstrated

haploidentical DLI (1×10^6/kg CD3$^+$ T cells), aGVHD was noted in 25% (grades III-IV aGVHD in 15%). A third of patients achieved a complete response with a median duration of response of 12 months. Most patients received cytoreductive therapy prior to the DLI infusion. Thus, cellular therapy with haploidentical DLI can be effective posttransplant, and future approaches should improve the safety and efficacy of DLI.

Modified Donor Lymphocyte Infusion Using T Cells With a Safety Switch (Suicide Gene)

One approach to control aGVHD post-DLI would be to insert a suicide gene in the haploidentical donor T cells. If significant aGVHD occurs, a "safety off switch" can "turn off" these T cells and avoid excessive aGVHD. This approach has so far been investigated to boost posttransplant immune recovery after T-cell-depleted haploidentical grafts. Ciceri et al infused DLI engineered T cells to express herpes simplex virus–thymidine kinase suicide gene (can be triggered by ganciclovir to induce apoptosis) ([31]). The aim was to boost posttransplant immune reconstitution by adding back T cells after a complete or partial T-cell-depleted haploSCT. Grades 1 to 4 aGVHD developed in 20% of patients and was successfully terminated by inducing the suicide gene with ganciclovir. However, ganciclovir may not be the ideal drug in this setting given that it is commonly used posttransplantation to control cytomegalovirus reactivation. Another approach is to use DLI engineered to express an inducible caspase-9 transgene ([32]). This gene can be induced by a synthetic dimerizing drug, leading to rapid cell death. In a preliminary experience in ten patients, aGVHD developed in five patients and was rapidly reversed with the use of the dimerizing drug.

Chimeric Antigen Receptor T Cells

While the DLI offers nonspecific antitumor activity, the effect is nontargeted. A potential game changer has been the introduction of T cells engineered to express a chimeric receptor, with an extracellular domain that can recognize a specific antigen and an intracellular domain that can activate the cytotoxic T cell. This approach has demonstrated significant activity in tumors expressing CD19, such as acute lymphoblastic leukemia (ALL) or B-cell lymphomas. Maude et al used autologous chimeric antigen receptor (CAR) T cells against CD19 (CTL019) in 30 patients with relapsed-refractory ALL, and complete remission occurred in 90% of patients. They demonstrated that CTL019 cells proliferated in vivo and were detectable in the blood, bone marrow, and cerebrospinal fluid of patients who responded ([33]). We are exploring the use of CAR T cells early after haploidentical transplantation to prevent disease relapse, part of a multiarm clinical trial ([34]). Our center is the only center so far using CAR T cells after haploidentical transplantation. Four patients (three with ALL and one with diffuse large B-cell lymphoma) received CAR T cells generated using the Sleeping Beauty system. The lymphoma patient achieved remission for the first time after transplant and infusion of CAR T cells. Three of these four patients remained in remission at last follow-up. These results are promising and showed that allogeneic CAR T-cell therapy can be safely given without significant GVHD.

Natural Killer Cells and Killer Immunoglobulin-Like Receptor Mismatch

Natural killer (NK) cells are part of the innate immune system and normally are involved in identifying and killing tumor cells or virally infected cells. The NK cells recognize and target "foreign" cells that lack one or more HLA class I alleles specific to the inhibitory receptors (killer immunoglobulin-like receptors, KIRs) ([35]). The NK cells do not contribute to GVHD as they target hematopoietic cells sparing other body organs, making them ideal in the transplant setting. This was first observed in the T-cell-depleted setting, where patients with a KIR "mismatch" had a lower incidence of relapse ([36]). There is great interest in this field to identify haploSCT donors with a KIR mismatch to possibly maximize the graft-versus-tumor effects. Several studies suggested a lower risk of relapse with donors who possess specific activating KIR genes, such as KIR2DS1, KIR2DS2, or the KIR "B" haplotype ([37-39]). We are exploring infusion of ex vivo expanded NK cells using the mb-IL21 method developed at MDACC in haploidentical transplants (protocol 2012-0708) to prevent disease relapse posttransplant in patients with myeloid malignancies ([40]).

DONOR SELECTION FOR HaploSCT AND RISKS FROM DONOR-SPECIFIC ANTIBODIES

Multiple donors may be available to choose from in haploSCT. Several factors are considered when choosing the best donor ([41]). One of the most important factors to evaluate in these patients is the presence of anti-HLA donor-specific antibodies (DSAs) ([42, 43]). Patients may develop antibodies against foreign HLA antigens, particularly parous women or multiply transfused patients. We have shown for the first time that patients with high levels of complement fixing anti-HLA antibodies against donor HLA antigens are at high risk of graft failure ([43]).

Routine evaluation of all donors with HLA mismatches has now been incorporated into standard practice worldwide. Research is currently ongoing to optimize donor selection to improve outcomes ([44]). In general, younger donors are preferred. There is controversy whether the parent gender is important if a parental donor is needed. Some studies suggested using donors selected for maximal NK cell alloreactivity to maximize the graft-versus-malignancy effects. This includes selecting donors with KIR:KIR ligand mismatch or using KIR B haplotype donors (enriched for activating KIR) to exploit the NK cell alloreactivity and decrease relapse rate posttransplant ([37]).

CONCLUSIONS AND FUTURE DIRECTIONS

The field of haploidentical stem cell transplantation has advanced significantly over the past decade with the introduction of HDPTCy and novel methods of partial T-cell depletion. These newer techniques effectively control strong alloreactive reactions in haploSCT and are associated with robust immune recovery, translating into fewer infections and lower NRM. Data from multiple retrospective studies suggested that outcomes are now comparable to MUD SCT, and this type of transplant is expanding worldwide ([23]). Controlled clinical trials are needed to address whether haploidentical transplants are preferred over unrelated donors, at least in some clinical settings. Cellular therapy posttransplant represents a great opportunity to further modulate GVHD and graft-versus-malignancy effects. Future studies will prospectively compare haploSCT to other alternative donor sources and the incorporation of cellular therapy in the treatment of these patients.

CHAPTER 15

REFERENCES

1. Ciurea SO, Bayraktar UD. "No donor"? Consider a haploidentical transplant. *Blood Rev*. 2015;29(2):63-70.
2. Allan DS, Takach S, Smith S, Goldman M. Impact of declining fertility rates in Canada on donor options in blood and marrow transplantation. *Biol Blood Marrow Transplant*. 2009;15(12):1634-1637.
3. Gragert L, Eapen M, Williams E, et al. HLA match likelihoods for hematopoietic stem-cell grafts in the U.S. registry. *N Engl J Med*. 2014;371(4):339-348.
4. Beatty PG, Clift RA, Mickelson EM, et al. Marrow transplantation from related donors other than HLA-identical siblings. *N Engl J Med*. 1985;313(13):765-771.
5. Clift RA, Hansen JA, Thomas ED, et al. Marrow transplantation from donors other than HLA-identical siblings. *Transplantation*. 1979;28(3):235-242.
6. Powles RL, Morgenstern GR, Kay HE, et al. Mismatched family donors for bone-marrow transplantation as treatment for acute leukaemia. *Lancet*. 1983;1(8325):612-615.
7. Ball LM, Lankester AC, Bredius RG, Fibbe WE, van Tol MJ, Egeler RM. Graft dysfunction and delayed immune reconstitution following haploidentical peripheral blood hematopoietic stem cell transplantation. *Bone Marrow Transplant*. 2005;35(Suppl 1):S35-S38.
8. Rizzieri DA, Koh LP, Long GD, et al. Partially matched, nonmyeloablative allogeneic transplantation: clinical outcomes and immune reconstitution. *J Clin Oncol*. 2007;25(6):690-697.
9. Mehta J, Singhal S, Gee AP, et al. Bone marrow transplantation from partially HLA-mismatched family donors for acute leukemia: single-center experience of 201 patients. *Bone Marrow Transplant*. 2004;33(4):389-396.
10. Aversa F, Tabilio A, Velardi A, et al. Treatment of high-risk acute leukemia with T-cell-depleted stem cells from related donors with one fully mismatched HLA haplotype. *N Engl J Med*. 1998;339(17):1186-1193.
11. Bertaina A, Merli P, Rutella S, et al. HLA-haploidentical stem cell transplantation after removal of alphabeta+ T and B cells in children with nonmalignant disorders. *Blood*. 2014;124(5):822-826.
12. Ciurea SO, Saliba R, Rondon G, et al. Reduced-intensity conditioning using fludarabine, melphalan and thiotepa for adult patients undergoing haploidentical SCT. *Bone Marrow Transplant*. 2010;45(3):429-436.
    a. Ciurea SO, Zhang MJ, Bacigalupo AA, et al: Haploidentical transplant with posttransplant cyclophosphamide vs matched unrelated donor transplant for acute myeloid leukemia. *Blood*. 126:1033-40, 2015.
13. Berenbaum MC, Brown IN. Prolongation of homograft survival in mice with single doses of cyclophosphamide. *Nature*. 1963;200:84.
14. Mayumi H, Himeno K, Shin T, Nomoto K. Drug-induced tolerance to allografts in mice. VI. Tolerance induction in H-2-haplotype-identical strain combinations in mice. *Transplantation*. 1985; 40(2):188-194.
15. Luznik L, Jalla S, Engstrom LW, Iannone R, Fuchs EJ. Durable engraftment of major histocompatibility complex-incompatible cells after nonmyeloablative conditioning with fludarabine, low-dose total body irradiation, and posttransplantation cyclophosphamide. *Blood*. 2001;98(12):3456-3464.
16. Jones RJ, Barber JP, Vala MS, et al. Assessment of aldehyde dehydrogenase in viable cells. *Blood*. 1995;85(10):2742-2746.
17. Ciurea SO, Mulanovich V, Saliba RM, et al. Improved early outcomes using a T cell replete graft compared with T cell depleted haploidentical hematopoietic stem cell transplantation. *Biol Blood Marrow Transplant*. 2012;18(12):1835-1844.
18. Luznik L, O'Donnell PV, Symons HJ, et al. HLA-haploidentical bone marrow transplantation for hematologic malignancies using nonmyeloablative conditioning and high-dose, posttransplantation cyclophosphamide. *Biol Blood Marrow Transplant*. 2008;14(6):641-650.
19. Pingali SR, Milton D, di Stasi A, et al. Haploidentical transplantation for advanced hematologic malignancies using melphalan-based conditioning—mature results from a single center. *Biol Blood Marrow Transplant*. 2014;20(2):S40-S41.
20. Di Stasi A, Milton DR, Poon LM, et al. Similar transplantation outcomes for acute myeloid leukemia and myelodysplastic syndrome patients with haploidentical versus 10/10 human leukocyte antigen-matched unrelated and related donors. *Biol Blood Marrow Transplant*. 2014;20(12):1975–1981.
21. Bashey A, Zhang X, Sizemore CA, et al. T-cell-replete HLA-haploidentical hematopoietic transplantation for hematologic malignancies using post-transplantation cyclophosphamide results in outcomes equivalent to those of contemporaneous HLA-matched related and unrelated donor transplantation. *J Clin Oncol*. 2013;31(10):1310-1316.

22. Raiola AM, Dominietto A, di Grazia C, et al. Unmanipulated haploidentical transplants compared with other alternative donors and matched sibling grafts. *Biol Blood Marrow Transplant.* 2014;20(10):1573-1579.
23. Ciurea SO, Zhang MJ, Bacigalupo AA, et al: Haploidentical transplant with posttransplant cyclophosphamide vs matched unrelated donor transplant for acute myeloid leukemia. Blood 126:1033-40, 2015.
24. Bonneville M, O'Brien RL, Born WK. Gammadelta T cell effector functions: a blend of innate programming and acquired plasticity. *Nat Rev Immunol.* 2010;10(7):467-478.
25. Locatelli F, Bauquet A, Palumbo G, Moretta F, Bertaina A. Negative depletion of alpha/beta+ T cells and of CD19+ B lymphocytes: a novel frontier to optimize the effect of innate immunity in HLA-mismatched hematopoietic stem cell transplantation. *Immunol Lett.* 2013;155(1-2):21-23.
26. Anderson BE, McNiff J, Yan J, et al. Memory CD4+ T cells do not induce graft-versus-host disease. *J Clin Invest.* 2003; 112(1):101-108.
27. Chen BJ, Cui X, Sempowski GD, Liu C, Chao NJ. Transfer of allogeneic CD62L- memory T cells without graft-versus-host disease. *Blood.* 2004;103(4):1534-1541.
28. Zheng H, Matte-Martone C, Li H, et al. Effector memory CD4+ T cells mediate graft-versus-leukemia without inducing graft-versus-host disease. *Blood.* 2008;111(4):2476-2484.
29. Martelli MF, Di Ianni M, Ruggeri L, et al. HLA-haploidentical transplantation with regulatory and conventional T-cell adoptive immunotherapy prevents acute leukemia relapse. *Blood.* 2014;124(4):638-644.
30. Zeidan AM, Forde PM, Symons H, et al. HLA-haploidentical donor lymphocyte infusions for patients with relapsed hematologic malignancies after related HLA-haploidentical bone marrow transplantation. *Biol Blood Marrow Transplant.* 2014;20(3): 314-318.
31. Ciceri F, Bonini C, Stanghellini MT, et al. Infusion of suicide-gene-engineered donor lymphocytes after family haploidentical haemopoietic stem-cell transplantation for leukaemia (the TK007 trial): a non-randomised phase I-II study. *Lancet Oncol.* 2009;10(5):489-500.
32. Di Stasi A, Tey SK, Dotti G, et al. Inducible apoptosis as a safety switch for adoptive cell therapy. *N Engl J Med.* 2011; 365(18):1673-1683.
33. Maude SL, Frey N, Shaw PA, et al. Chimeric antigen receptor T cells for sustained remissions in leukemia. *N Engl J Med.* 2014;371(16):1507-1517.
34. Kebriaei P, Huls H, Singh H, et al. Adoptive therapy using Sleeping Beauty Gene Transfer System and artificial antigen presenting cells to manufacture T cells expressing CD19-specific chimeric antigen receptor. Presented at the 56th Annual Meeting and Exposition, American Society of Hematology, December 6-9, 2014, San Francisco, CA.
35. Ruggeri L, Capanni M, Casucci M, et al. Role of natural killer cell alloreactivity in HLA-mismatched hematopoietic stem cell transplantation. *Blood.* 1999;94(1):333-339.
36. Ruggeri L, Capanni M, Urbani E, et al. Effectiveness of donor natural killer cell alloreactivity in mismatched hematopoietic transplants. *Science.* 2002;295(5562):2097-2100.
37. Cooley S, Trachtenberg E, Bergemann TL, et al. Donors with group B KIR haplotypes improve relapse-free survival after unrelated hematopoietic cell transplantation for acute myelogenous leukemia. *Blood.* 2009;113(3):726-732.
38. Sivori S, Carlomagno S, Falco M, Romeo E, Moretta L, Moretta A. Natural killer cells expressing the KIR2DS1-activating receptor efficiently kill T-cell blasts and dendritic cells: implications in haploidentical HSCT. *Blood.* 2011;117(16):4284-4292.
39. Chen DF, Prasad VK, Broadwater G, et al. Differential impact of inhibitory and activating Killer Ig-Like Receptors (KIR) on high-risk patients with myeloid and lymphoid malignancies undergoing reduced intensity transplantation from haploidentical related donors. *Bone Marrow Transplant.* 2012;47(6):817-823.
40. Denman CJ, Senyukov VV, Somanchi SS, et al. Membrane-bound IL-21 promotes sustained ex vivo proliferation of human natural killer cells. *PloS One.* 2012;7(1):e30264.
41. Ciurea SO, Champlin RE. Donor selection in T cell-replete haploidentical hematopoietic stem cell transplantation: knowns, unknowns, and controversies. *Biol Blood Marrow Transplant.* 2013;19(2):180-184.
42. Yoshihara S, Maruya E, Taniguchi K, et al. Risk and prevention of graft failure in patients with preexisting donor-specific HLA antibodies undergoing unmanipulated haploidentical SCT. *Bone Marrow Transplant.* 2012;47(4):508-515.
43. Ciurea SO, de Lima M, Cano P, et al. High risk of graft failure in patients with anti-HLA antibodies undergoing haploidentical stem-cell transplantation. *Transplantation.* 2009;88(8):1019-1024.
44. Wang Y, Chang YJ, Xu LP, et al. Who is the best donor for a related HLA haplotype-mismatched transplant? *Blood.* 2014;124(6):843-850.

16

Cellular Therapy in Allogeneic Hematopoietic Cell Transplantation

第十六章　同种异体造血细胞移植的细胞疗法

Philip A. Thompson
Katayoun Rezvani
Partow Kebriaei

中文导读

自从20世纪50年代末，E.Donnall Thomas博士在一名双胞胎白血病患者身上进行异体干细胞移植以来，随着我们对免疫系统了解的深入，与移植有关的细胞治疗手段为患者带来了更好的疗效。本章对异体造血干细胞移植的细胞疗法进行了背景介绍，并详细探讨了增强移植物抗肿瘤效应以及克服肿瘤逃逸的有关问题，内容包括移植物抗肿瘤效应的病理生理学基础、免疫系统被破坏后的肿瘤逃逸、通过细胞治疗诱导移植物抗肿瘤效应、供体淋巴细胞输注存在的问题与挑战、高风险患者的预防性供体淋巴细胞输注、双特异性T细胞活化抗体、CART、过继转移自然杀伤(NK)细胞以增强抗肿瘤效果、优化NK细胞效率以及PD1/PD-L1抗体。接着本章介绍了通过细胞治疗和过继性转移调节性T细胞以减少移植物抗宿主反应。最后本章介绍了预防和治疗感染的常见措施与方案。

INTRODUCTION

The efficacy of allogeneic hematopoietic cell transplantation (HCT) in hematologic malignancies can in large part be attributed to a graft-versus-tumor (GVT) effect, by which the donor immune system achieves immunologic control of the tumor. As such, it is the prototype of cellular therapy. The human leukocyte antigen (HLA) system is fundamental to transplant biology. The HLAs are highly polymorphic proteins that have a key role in antigen presentation and immunoregulation. Class I HLAs are expressed on the surfaces of all nucleated cells; class II are expressed on specialized antigen-presenting cells (APCs), such as macrophages, dendritic cells, and B cells.

Peptides derived from microbes are presented on class I HLAs to $CD8^+$ T cells and result in immunologic destruction of infected cells; class II HLAs are recognized by $CD4^+$ T cells. T-cell activation requires costimulatory signals from the APC, specifically CD80/86 binding to CD28 or LFA-3 binding to CD2 ([1]). Absence of a costimulatory signal results in T-cell anergy, which is a key mechanism of peripheral immune tolerance to self-antigen in normal immunoregulation. Early posttransplantation, there is a "cytokine storm"; release of proinflammatory cytokines, such as tumor necrosis factor alpha (TNF-α) and interleukin 6 (IL-6), is induced by tissue damage from the conditioning regimen, activating the host innate immune system (Fig. 16-1). Donor T cells interact with host APCs and

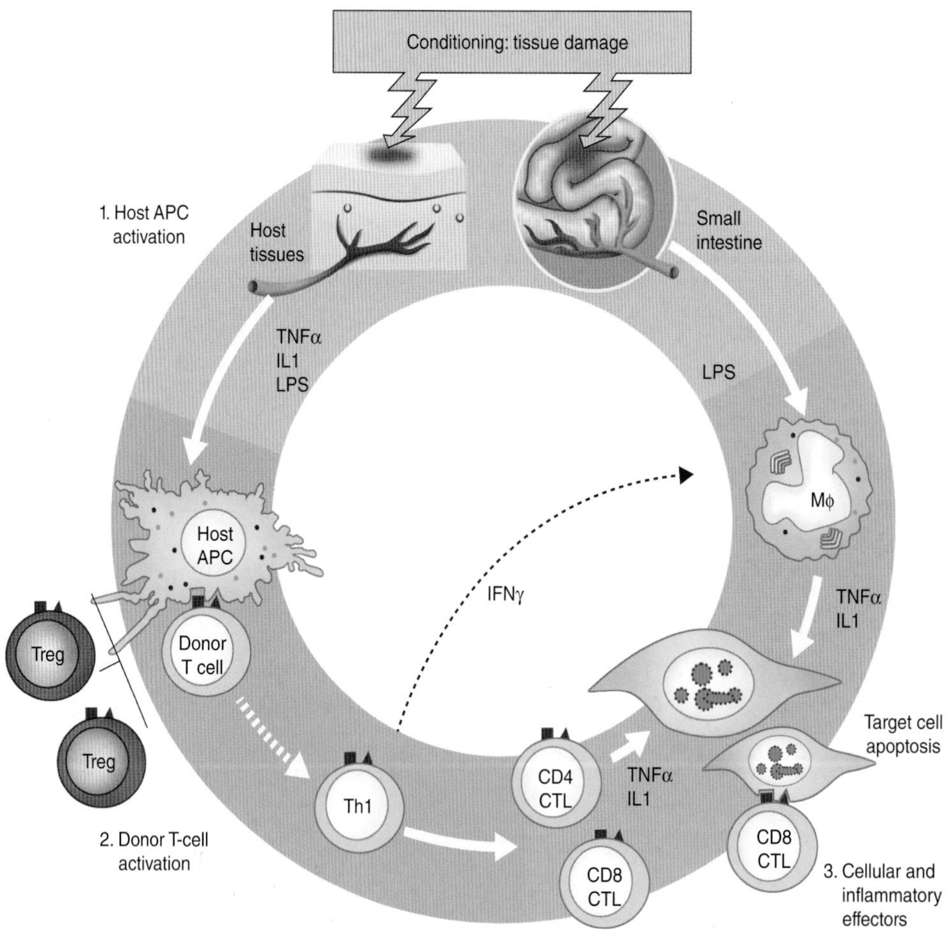

FIGURE 16-1 Pathogenesis of GVHD. In phase I, chemotherapy or radiotherapy as part of transplant conditioning causes host tissue damage and release of inflammatory cytokines such as TNF-α, IL-1, and IL-6, with resulting priming of host antigen-presenting cells (APCs). In phase II, host APCs activate mature donor cells, which subsequently proliferate and differentiate; release of additional effector molecules, such as TNF-α and IL-1, mediates further tissue damage. Lipopolysaccharide (LPS) that has leaked through damaged intestinal mucosa triggers additional TNF-α production. The TNF-α can damage tissue directly by inducing necrosis and apoptosis in the skin and gastrointestinal tract through either TNF receptors or the Fas pathway. Tumor necrosis factor alpha plays a direct role in intestinal GVHD damage, which further amplifies damage in the skin, liver, and lung in a "cytokine storm." The process culminates in death of host cells through CD8-positive cytotoxic T-cell-mediated apoptosis. [Reproduced with permission from Ferrara JL, Levine JE, Reddy P, Holler E. Graft-versus-host disease. *Lancet*. 2009;373(9674):1550-1561].

recognize foreign peptides; helper T cells produce further cytokines, especially IL-2, and prime host APCs via CD40:CD40L interaction. Differentiation of naïve donor T cells into effector cells subsequently occurs, resulting in immunologic attack on host tissues and the potential development of graft-versus-host disease (GVHD) ([2]). Increasing numbers of HLA mismatches are associated with higher incidence of GVHD and transplant-related mortality (TRM) ([3]). However, even in a fully HLA matched HCT, GVHD still occurs due to donor T cells directed against minor histocompatibility antigens (MiHAs), polymorphic peptides displayed on host HLA molecules.

There are three key barriers to successful HCT: GVHD, infectious complications, and relapse due to failure of immunologic control of the underlying disease. Herein, we review these issues in greater detail with an emphasis on recent cellular therapeutic approaches to address these complications.

ENHANCING GRAFT-VERSUS-TUMOR EFFECT TO OVERCOME TUMOR ESCAPE

Pathophysiology of the Graft-Versus-Tumor Effect

The GVT effect occurs due to a predominantly T-cell-mediated immunologic attack on tumor cells. In HLA-identical transplants, GVT effect is mediated by naïve T cells; for development of effector function, these must first be primed by host APCs. This requires the following: presentation of MiHAs or tumor-specific antigens on HLA; appropriate costimulatory molecules, including CD28, OX40, CD40L, and 41BB; and an appropriate "third signal," provided by IL-12, interferon gamma (IFN-γ) or adjuvant ([4]). Restraining influences limiting the degree of immune activation are present to protect the host from an excessive immune response and include expression of CTLA4 (which competes with CD28 for binding to CD80/86) and programmed cell death protein 1 (PD1) and its interactions with its lig and PDL1, which limit T-cell activation and expansion during normal, pathogen-directed immune responses.

Soon after transplant, there is activation and expansion of MiHA-reactive T cells, followed by a decline, similar to that seen in pathogen-directed immune reactions. This may in part relate to the development of peripheral tolerance/anergy and also to replacement of host hematopoiesis, with resulting loss of host APCs. For tumor-associated antigen presentation to continue, there must be cross presentation on donor APCs. In addition, the initial alloresponse to MiHAs results in recruitment of T cells targeting either tumor-associated antigens or nonpolymorphic genes, which are either overexpressed or aberrantly expressed by the tumor ([4]).

Some tumor-associated antigens of importance include pathogenesis related protein (PR1), an epitope shared by proteinase-3 and elastase proteins, which is expressed in normal neutrophils and overexpressed in myeloid leukemias; and PR1-specific CD8+ T-cell responses, which can be detected in a range of myeloid and nonmyeloid malignancies post-HCT and correlate with outcome in chronic myelogenous leukemia (CML) ([5]). CD8+ T-cell responses to WT1, which is frequently overexpressed in acute myelogenous leukemia (AML), can be induced with vaccination strategies in both the autologous and allogeneic settings ([6-8]). Clinical responses from tumor vaccines have thus far been suboptimal.

Natural killer (NK) cells can also mediate antitumor effects; this is discussed in further detail in this chapter.

Tumor Escape From Immunologic Destruction

Tumors utilize numerous mechanisms to escape immunological destruction, including the following:

- Induction of regulatory T cells
- Production of inhibitory cytokines
- Downregulation of costimulatory molecules ([9]) and HLA I ([10])
- Induction of coinhibitory molecules
- Induction of myeloid-derived suppressor cells in the microenvironment that inhibit immune responses through multiple mechanisms.
- Invasion of immunologically privileged sites ([11]).

Cellular therapeutic approaches are designed with the intent to abrogate these escape mechanisms.

Cellular Therapy to Induce Graft-Versus-Tumor Effect

Donor Lymphocyte Infusions

Donor lymphocyte infusion (DLI) may induce remissions in patients with molecular or overt relapse of their malignancy and can reverse CD8+ T-cell exhaustion. ([12]). However, the likelihood of success varies significantly according to the underlying disease. Chronic myelogenous leukemia is most sensitive; follicular lymphoma (FL) and Hodgkin lymphoma (HL) are also highly responsive ([13, 14]). Responses to DLI in AML or myelodysplastic syndrome (MDS) are less frequent, and durability is often poor. Acute lymphoblastic leukemia (ALL) is the least responsive to DLI. Reported response rates are 60% to 73% in CML, 15% to 29% in AML, and 0% to 18% in ALL ([15, 16]).

CHAPTER 16

Problems and Challenges Associated With Donor Lymphocyte Infusion

Development of Graft-Versus-Host Disease

Graft-versus-host disease occurs in 40% to 60% of patients with HCT ([15, 16]) and is more likely to occur in unrelated donor recipients ([13]). Lympho-depleting chemotherapy given prior to DLI enhances alloreactive T-cell proliferation, potentiating the GVT effect but increasing GVHD ([17]). Approaches to reduce the GVHD incidence include the following:

1. Reducing T-cell dose. A dose-response relationship exists for both GVT and GVHD effects. In CML, no increased response is seen with cell doses greater than 4.5×10^8 $CD3^+$ cells/kg. In AML, response rates plateau beyond 1.5×10^8/kg; higher doses increase GVHD. Gradual dose escalation schedules have been successfully utilized in relapses of indolent diseases. Follicular lymphoma appears highly sensitive to DLI after T-cell-depleted HCT, responding to low-dose DLI at doses from 1 to 10×10^6/kg with less than 20% incidence of clinically significant acute GVHD (aGVHD) and chronic GVHD (cGVHD) ([14]). A similar strategy has shown success in HL, mainly in the setting of low-volume disease detected on surveillance positron emission tomographic (PET) imaging ([18]). More sensitive surveillance techniques, such as deep sequencing, to detect low-volume disease may allow earlier institution of DLI and maximize efficacy; utilization of these techniques remains experimental.
2. Transduction of donor lymphocytes with a suicide gene ([19]).
3. Selection of T cells to target tumor-associated antigens/antigens with restricted or differential expression (analogous to the use of viral-specific T cells [VSTs]). Infusion of MiHA-specific T cells was effective at eradicating tumor in mouse models ([20]). In addition, tumor-infiltrating lymphocytes (TILs) recognizing tumor-associated antigens have been successfully used for selected metastatic solid tumors ([21]). However, the technology to isolate TILs remains restricted to a few specialized centers and is yet to be applied in large-scale clinical studies.

Marrow Hypoplasia

If there is insufficient residual donor hematopoiesis prior to DLI, eradication of host hematopoiesis by the infused lymphocytes can result in marrow aplasia; chimerism studies should therefore be performed prior to DLI to ensure adequate donor hematopoiesis ([22]).

Delayed Onset of Action

Responses to DLI may not be seen for up to 2 months ([11]). In indolent diseases (eg, FL), this may not be problematic, but in overt relapse of aggressive diseases (eg, AML), chemotherapy may be required first to achieve disease control ([23]).

Prophylactic Donor Lymphocyte Infusion in High-Risk Patients

The delayed onset of action of DLI has led to the use of preemptive DLI to prevent relapse in high-risk patients. Mixed donor/recipient chimerism within the T-cell lineage is frequently seen in T-cell-depleted transplants and is associated with higher rates of relapse in CML ([24]), FL ([14]), and HL ([18]), likely due to development of bidirectional tolerance with resulting tumor escape from immunologic control. Donor lymphocyte infusion can induce full donor chimerism in both FL and HL, and subsequent relapse rates are low; no formal comparison to similar groups not receiving DLI has been performed.

Bi-Specific T-Cell-Engaging Antibodies

The topic of bi-specific T-cell-engaging antibodies has been discussed in detail elsewhere. Bi-specific T-cell-engaging antibodies are single-chain antibodies that engage T cells via CD3 and direct them to an antigenic target present on tumor cells, typically CD19, resulting in T-cell redistribution, activation, expansion, and perforin-mediated killing of target cells ([25]). Blinatumomab is highly efficacious in ALL in the setting of persistent MRD ([25]), overt relapse, or refractory disease ([26]).

Chimeric Antigen Receptor-Modified T Cells

The ideal cellular therapy for a malignant disease should expand and persist in vivo and selectively target cancer cells. This can be achieved by modifying autologous T cells with a chimeric antigen receptor (CAR). The CAR consists of a single-chain monoclonal antibody (scFv) targeted to a tumor-associated antigen, which is thus recognized in a major histocompatibility complex (MHC)–independent fashion (unlike unmodified T-cell-mediated GVT effect); the scFv is coupled via an extracellular hinge domain and transmembrane domain to an intracellular signaling domain, typically the CD3ζ chain (Fig. 16-2) ([27]). Autologous T cells are collected from peripheral blood (PB) via a steady-state blood draw or apheresis procedure and transduced with the CAR construct via a lentiviral or retroviral vector or using electroporation and a transposon/transposase system ([28]). Cells are cultured and expanded ex

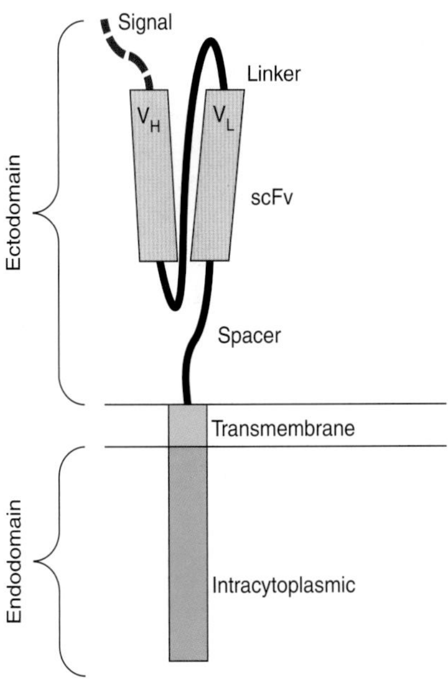

FIGURE 16-2 Schematic of basic chimeric antigen receptor (CAR) construct. The CAR consists of a single-chain monoclonal antibody (scFv) targeted to a tumor-associated antigen, and the scFv is then coupled via an extracellular hinge domain and transmembrane domain to an intracytoplasmic signaling domain, typically the CD3ζ chain.

vivo using either CD3/28 beads [29] or artificial APCs [30] and specific cytokines prior to infusion. The persistence and clinical activity of CAR T cells (CAR-T) in vivo can be enhanced by the addition of a costimulatory molecule to the CAR construct [31], usually CD28 [31, 32]. An initial report in a patient with highly refractory CLL treated with an anti-CD19 CAR-T utilizing CD137 (4-1BB) as the costimulatory domain generated great excitement [33]: Infused T cells expanded more than 3 log, the patient developed a cytokine-release syndrome (CRS) and tumor lysis syndrome (TLS), and achieved complete remission (CR); long-term persistence of CAR-T and persistent normal B-cell aplasia (a predictable, on-target effect when targeting CD19) were demonstrated.

Subsequent results in CLL have been heterogeneous; updated results from the University of Pennsylvania showed that 5 of 24 patients treated achieved durable CRs, 7 had partial responses (PRs), and 12 had no response [34]. The variables underlying response to treatment are not well understood, but in vivo CAR-T expansion is a prerequisite and appears to be more important than the dose of infused cells [30]. In ALL, results have been particularly impressive, with a CR rate of 86% in children treated for relapsed/refractory disease; patients were MRD negative even when tested with highly sensitive deep-sequencing techniques [34]. Long-term survival rates are not yet known, particularly as in many cases the treatment has been used as a "bridge to transplant." At least two patients with ALL have relapsed with CD19-negative disease [34]. Similarly impressive CR rates have been reported by the groups at the National Institutes of Health [35] and Memorial Sloane Kettering Cancer Center [36]. All three groups reported a similar toxicity profile (see Table 16-1). It is unclear whether this treatment can replace HCT in a proportion of patients; long-term survival outcomes in patients ineligible for HCT will be important in answering this question. The CAR-T targeting CD19 have now been used in a range of B-cell malignancies, with responses seen in both aggressive and indolent lymphomas, CLL, and ALL (Table 16-1).

While this therapy shows great promise, many aspects require optimization. Due to the heterogeneity in technique for CAR-T production, it is difficult to compare across trials to determine optimal manufacturing methods. The controversies are numerous: First, while it has been shown that addition of a costimulatory domain to the CAR enhances expansion and persistence [31], it is unclear whether CD28 or 4-1BB, or both, is superior. Second, lympho-depleting chemotherapy may enhance CAR-T expansion and persistence [32], but the optimal drugs and schedule are unknown. Third, the epitope targeted by the antibody fragment is likely important, in terms of both the spatial location of epitope binding and binding affinity. Fourth, the hinge and transmembrane domains are important in determining interaction with antigen and formation of the immunologic synapse, but little is known about optimizing this aspect of the CAR design. Fifth, the method of T-cell transduction (viral vs transposon) may be important in determining efficacy. Sixth, the ex vivo culture technique and duration (eg, CD3/28 beads vs artificial APCs and which supplemental cytokines to provide) may be important; for example, culture after transduction using the Sleeping Beauty system is relatively prolonged, which is problematic in kinetically active diseases such as ALL [37]. The dose and composition (unselected vs specific ratios of CD4/8 cells) of T-cell product infused are also variables requiring consideration. Finally, the bulk of tumor present at the time of CAR-T infusion may potentially affect the in vivo proliferation of the infused CAR-T, and the ideal time of infusion (eg, in an MRD state vs overt relapse) has not been elucidated.

Adverse Events and Optimizing Safety

All responding patients have had some degree of CRS and have developed B-cell aplasia [38]. Cytokine-release syndrome is characterized by fever with variable systemic symptoms, including hypotension, and high levels of inflammatory cytokines, of which IL-6 appears particularly important [37]. Macrophage activation

Table 16-1 Summary of Reported Studies Using Chimeric Antigen Receptor (CAR) T Cells Directed Against CD19 in Hematologic Malignancies

Reference	Cancer	CAR Endodomains	Number of Patients	Clinical Outcome	Toxicities
Kochenderfer et al, 2014 (91)	CLL, DLBCL, NHL, PMBCL, SMZL	CD28 & CD3ζ	15	8 CR, 4 PR, 1 SD, 2 NE	Fever, hypotension, renal failure, confusion, aphasia
Maude et al, 2014 (35)	ALL	CD28 & CD3ζ	30	90% CR (15 prior HCT); 67% EFS, 78% OS at 6 mo.	SIRS 27%, B-cell aplasia 73%
Lee et al, 2014 (36)	ALL	CD28 & CD3ζ	21	70% CR	33% severe SIRS
Davila et al, 2014 (35)	ALL	CD28 & CD3ζ	16	88% CR	43% severe SIRS
Kochenderfer et al, 2013 (92)	CLL, Lymphoma	CD28 & CD3ζ	10	1 CR, 1 PR, 2 PD, 6 SD	Fever, SIRS, TLS
Brentjens et al, 2013 (93)	ALL	CD28 & CD3ζ	5	5 CR	SIRS
Grupp et al, 2013 (94)	ALL	4-1BB & CD3ζ	2	2 CR	SIRS, central nervous system toxicity
Kochenderfer et al, 2012 (38)	CLL, Lymphoma	CD28 & CD3ζ	8	1 CR, 5 PR, 1 SD, 1 died (influenza)	Mild SIRS
Brentjens et al, 2011 (32)	CLL, ALL	CD28 & CD3ζ	8	1 PR, 2 SD, 3 NR, 1 PD, 1 died (sepsis-like disease)	Fever, death
Savoldo et al, 2011 (31)	NHL	CD28 & CD3ζ versus CD3ζ	6	2 SD, 4 NR	None
Porter et al, 2011 (33)	CLL	4-1BB & CD3ζ	1	CR	TLS, SIRS
Kalos et al, 2011 (95)	CLL	4-1BB & CD3ζ	3	2 CR, 1 PR	Fever, rigors, dyspnea, cardiac dysfunction, febrile syndrome, hypotension
Kochenderfer et al, 2010 (96)	Lymphoma	CD28 & CD3ζ	1	PR	None
Jensen et al, 2010 (27)	Lymphoma	CD3ζ	2	2 NR	None

Abbreviations: CLL, chronic lymphocytic leukemia; DLBCL, diffuse large B-cell lymphoma; CR, complete response; CRi, complete response with incomplete count recovery; NE, not evaluable; NHL, non-Hodgkin lymphoma; NR, no objective response; PMBCL, primary mediastinal B-cell lymphoma; PR, partial response; SD, stable disease; SIRS, systemic inflammatory syndrome; SMZL, splenic marginal zone lymphoma, TLS, tumor lysis syndrome.

syndrome (MAS) may accompany CRS. Major neurological symptoms, including seizures, have occurred. The mechanism of neurological events is unclear; it may be cytokine mediated, associated with MAS, or due to direct CAR-T infiltration. Unexpectedly, CD19 CAR-T have been found in the cerebrospinal fluid of some patients without central nervous system disease (37). Cytokine-release syndrome can be managed with the anti-IL-6 antibody tocilizumab, with prompt responses in the majority of patients (37). Corticosteroids, while potentially efficacious in managing CRS/MAS, are toxic to the infused cells and may limit efficacy.

Unanticipated on-target toxicity may occur; for example, a toxic death occurred in a patient treated with a CART-T directed against Human Epidermal Growth Factor Receptor 2, or ErbB2, due to unanticipated low-level pulmonary epithelial expression (39). The inclusion of a suicide gene within the CAR, such as inducible caspase 9 (iCaspase9), which could be triggered in the event of severe toxicity, would provide an added safety measure.

Most human trials to date have focused on CD19 as a target in B-cell diseases, but a number of novel targets show potential in different diseases.

Adoptive Transfer of Natural Killer Cells to Enhance Antitumor Effect

In contrast to T and B lymphocytes, NK cells do not express rearranged, antigen-specific receptors; rather, NK effector function is dictated by the integration of signals received through germ-line-encoded receptors that can recognize ligands on their cellular targets. Functionally, NK cell receptors are classified as activating or inhibitory. Natural killer cell function, including cytotoxicity and cytokine release, is governed by a balance between inhibitory receptors, notably the killer immunoglobulin-like receptors (KIRs) and the heterodimeric C-type lectin receptor (NKG2A), and activating receptors, in particular the natural cytotoxicity receptors (NCRs) NKp46, NKp30, NKp44, and the membrane protein NKG2D ([40]). Inhibitory receptors bind to HLA class I molecules, expressed on the surface of normal cells, resulting in signals that block NK cell triggering and inhibit killing. In the setting of malignancy or viral infection, HLA class I is often downregulated or has altered peptide expression, resulting in failure of KIR-mediated recognition by the NK cell and resultant cell killing ([40]). Activating receptors, such as NKG2D, bind ligands that are induced by cellular stress (eg, viral infection and malignant transformation); binding results in NK cell activation and target lysis ([41]) (Fig. 16-3).

Early NK cell recovery (within 30 days) postallogeneic stem cell transplant has been associated with reduced rates of both relapse and aGVHD, with resultant improved survival ([42]). This dual benefit makes allogeneic NK cells an attractive option for adoptive cellular therapy peritransplant. Adoptive transfer of NK cells has previously been limited by the small numbers of circulating NK cells (5%-15% of the total lymphocytes) and consequently the low numbers obtained in an apheresis procedure ([43]).

Use of allogeneic NK cells may be more efficacious than autologous NK cells due to inhibition of autologous NK cell activity by recognition of host HLA. Adoptive transfer of ex vivo–expanded haploidentical NK cells after lympho-depleting chemotherapy is safe. High-dose, but not low-dose, chemotherapy facilitates in vivo NK cell expansion, likely due to both prevention of host T-cell-mediated rejection and reduction in competition for cytokines, particularly IL-15. Persistence for at least 4 weeks has been achieved in some patients and responses have been observed in high-risk AML without inducing GVHD ([44]). The NK cell expansion ex vivo has traditionally included culture with cytokines (IL-2 or IL-15) and cell selection (CD3 depletion) ([44]); the use of "feeder cells" (Epstein-Barr virus [EBV]–transformed lymphoblastic cell lines or gene-modified, irradiated K562 cells), and large-scale expansion flasks have dramatically increased NK cell yield and activation status. Clinically relevant NK cell numbers can be obtained from both cord blood (CB) and adult donors ([43]). The CB-derived NK cells show a similar phenotype and are similarly active against leukemic targets as PB-derived NK cells ([45]).

There are several potential limitations of NK cell adoptive transfer, particularly limited persistence and the potential for passenger lymphocyte-related complications. The NK cells may rapidly develop exhaustion in vivo after adoptive transfer, despite initial expansion and activity ([46]). In part, this may relate to NK cells' exquisite sensitivity to cytokines such as IL-2 and IL-15. In vivo use of IL-2 (which can expand NK cell numbers) can lead to severe toxicity and to T-regulatory (T-reg) expansion, which limits NK cell activation ([47]). In contrast, IL-15/IL-15Rα complexes promoted NK cell activation and enhanced function without the detrimental effects of IL-2 ([48]). Whether in vivo use of IL-15/IL-15Rα will rescue NK cells from this phenomenon is not known. Lymphocyte contamination of the infused product can be avoided by proper selection techniques. T-cell contamination should be limited to less than 1 to 5×10^5/kg ([49]) to minimize the risk of GVHD; this can be achieved by CD3 depletion ([44]). Addition of CD56$^+$ selection reduces B-cell contamination to less than 1%, minimizing passenger B-lymphocyte-mediated EBV-posttransplant lymphoproliferative disorder (PTLD) and acute hemolytic anemia ([50]).

Optimizing Natural Killer Cell Efficacy

The NK cells have a range of highly polymorphic KIRs, which are divided into inhibitory and activating subtypes. The KIRs are inherited as haplotypes (KIR-A and KIR-B). The KIR-A haplotypes, found in one-third of adult Caucasians, have one activating

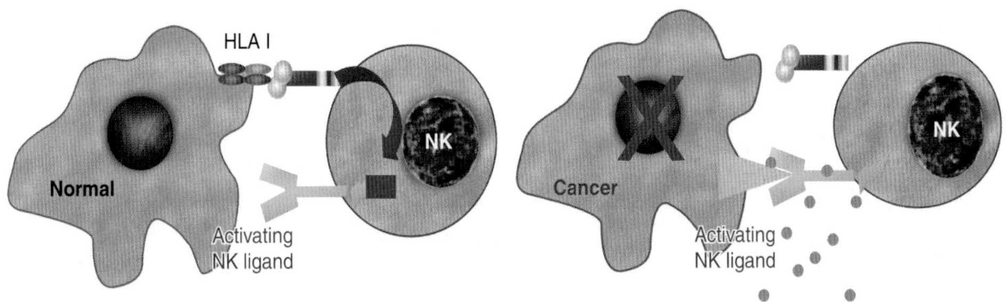

FIGURE 16-3 Selective killing of transformed cells by NK cells: In normal cells, the inhibitory signals triggered by KIR-HLA-I molecule engagement overrides activating signals. In the context of cancer, expression of stress ligands for activating receptors, in conjunction with low expression of HLA-I molecules, attenuates the triggering of inhibitory receptors and results in an activating signal.

receptor, while the KIR-B haplotypes have 2 or more. Transplantation in AML from a KIR-B haplotype donor is associated with lower relapse rates and superior survival ([51]). Donor KIR2DS1 (an activating KIR) and recipient HLA-C type influence relapse risk. The KIR2DS1-associated reduction in the rate of AML relapse is restricted to donors with HLA-C1/C1 or C1/C2, in whom KIR2DS1-expressing NK cells are presumed to be "educated," and the benefit was eliminated in transplants from donors with HLA-C2/C2, where KIR2DS1-expressing NK cells are expected to be tolerized in the setting of self HLA-C2 ([52]). Selection of adult or CB donors for ex vivo NK cell expansion based on KIR genotype may therefore enhance NK cell efficacy.

Other future strategies to enhance NK cell tumor killing include the use of immunomodulatory drugs such as lenalidomide and the use of bi-specific killer engagers (BiKEs), which consist of a single-chain Fv against CD16 and a tumor-associated antigen. A CD16x33 BiKE has been shown to have activity in refractory AML ([53]).

PD1/PDL1 Antibodies

Interaction of PD1/PDL1 induces T-cell dysfunction in CLL ([54]). Anti-PD1 antibodies are efficacious in a subset of patients with metastatic solid tumors as monotherapy and in combination with the anti-CTLA4 antibody ipilimumab ([55]). They have also shown remarkable activity in relapsed/refractory HL ([56]).

The potential importance of immune checkpoints has been demonstrated in AML. $CD8^+$ T-cell responses directed against the MiHA Liver receptor homolog-1 (LRH-1) have resulted in remission post-DLI. Despite persistence of $CD8^+$ T-memory cells specific for LRH-1, subsequent relapse with LRH-1-positive blasts occurs, unaccompanied by LRH-1-specific T-cell expansion, suggesting anergy/functional impairment. LRH-1-specific T cells from patients with relapsed AML have elevated levels of PD-1. The addition of anti-PD1 antibody to a coculture system resulted in marked LRH-1-specific T-cell expansion, IFN-γ production and cytotoxicity, suggesting a specific inhibitory effect induced by the PD-L1/PD1 interaction ([57]). Blockade of the PD-L1/PD1 axis may therefore represent an immunomodulatory target for patients with persistent/relapsed AML post-alloHCT.

REDUCING GRAFT-VERSUS-HOST DISEASE

Cellular Therapy for Prevention of Graft-Versus-Host Disease

Grades II-IV aGVHD occur in 25% to 60% of matched related donors and 45% to 70% of MUDs ([58]). Corticosteroid-based therapy for grades II-IV aGVHD is unsatisfactory, with fewer than 50% of patients showing a durable complete response ([59]). Increasing severity of aGVHD is associated with incremental TRM and inferior survival. Corticosteroid-refractory GVHD has a poor prognosis. Numerous additional agents have been studied in combination with corticosteroids or as second line therapies and showed uniformly poor response rates and numerous complications, particularly viral reactivation ([59]). Prevention of GVHD is therefore of paramount importance.

T-Cell Depletion

A T-cell-replete transplant usually contains 1 to 5×10^7 T cells/kg recipient weight ([58]). T-cell depletion is the most potent method of preventing aGVHD but is associated with increased rates of graft rejection; delayed immune reconstitution; infectious complications, including EBV-driven PTLD; and increased relapse risk ([58]). T-cell depletion can be accomplished ex vivo immunologically (T-cell antibodies, positive CD34 selection) or by the use of physical separation (eg, density gradients) or in vivo by the use of anti-T-cell antibodies such as antithymocyte globulin (ATG) or alemtuzumab. In vivo T-cell depletion with ATG reduces severe aGVHD and extensive cGVHD without increasing relapse but does not reduce TRM or improve survival ([60]), likely due to increased infection risk. Alemtuzumab-based GVHD prophylaxis achieves low rates of severe aGVHD and extensive cGVHD, but results in high rates of mixed chimerism and viral infections, particularly cytomegalovirus (CMV) reactivation ([61]).

T-Cell Depletion With Planned Postengraftment Donor Lymphocyte Infusion Utilizing a "Suicide Gene" in the Infused T Cells

Transduction of donor T cells with a "suicide gene," which can be activated in the event of developing severe aGVHD, may enhance the safety of adoptively transferred cellular therapy products. One method involves incorporating a herpes simplex virus thymidine kinase (HSV-TK) within the cellular product. Ganciclovir, a prodrug, is then administered, activated by HSV-TK and incorporated into replicating DNA, inhibiting DNA polymerase and resulting in cell death. Patients given HSV-TK-transduced DLI from haploidentical donors who developed GVHD had prompt resolution of GVHD after ganciclovir administration ([62]).

A more recent technique involves T-cell transduction with an inducible human caspase 9 protein, modified to remove its endogenous caspase activation and recruitment domain and conjugated to a sequence of human FK-binding protein, which binds to an otherwise-inert dimerizing agent, AP1903. Dimerization of the iCaspase9 protein by AP1903 activates the intrinsic apoptotic pathway and induces apoptosis. A pilot study using this technique in patients undergoing haplo-HCT showed robust in vivo expansion of gene-modified T cells and 90% and 99% killing of transduced cells within 30 minutes and 24 hours of AP1903 administration, respectively ([19, 63]). Concurrently, manifestations of aGVHD in both skin and liver rapidly resolved. Intriguingly, alloreactive T cells were preferentially eliminated by the dimerizing agent, potentially due to greater expression of the transgene in these cells. There was relative sparing of antiviral T cells, with polyclonal CD3/19⁺ transduced T cells with antiviral specificity detectable within 1 to 2 weeks postadministration of AP1903.

Adoptive Transfer of Regulatory T Cells

The level of $CD4^+CD25^+FOXP3^+$ T-reg cells in the graft and after HCT correlates inversely with aGVHD and cGVHD ([64]). Adoptive transfer of T-reg cells could therefore ameliorate GVHD.

The most efficient method for obtaining a pure T-reg population is sorting based on flow cytometry. Some effector T cells will be present in the product if $CD4^+$/$CD25^+$(high) cells are selected. Removal of CD127 (IL-7R)-positive cells, which are not expressed on T-reg cells, achieves a more purified product ([65]). Following sorting, T-reg cells can be expanded using CD3/28-coated microbeads and IL-2 and maintain suppressive function ([66, 67]). Murine xenogenic GVHD models have shown that infusion of human CB-derived T-reg cells confers protection from aGVHD and improves survival ([68]).

Potential concerns with T-reg cell infusions relate to impairment of immune reconstitution and GVT effect. However, by inhibiting GVHD-mediated thymic destruction ([69]), T-reg cells may actually facilitate functional immune reconstitution ([70]). Indeed, immune function is preserved in murine models of T-reg cell infusion ([71]). Data from mouse models regarding impairment of GVT effect is contradictory. Tumor regression after IL-2–diphtheria toxin–mediated T-reg cell depletion was seen in one model, suggesting that T-reg cells may adversely affect disease control ([72]).

In contrast, simultaneous adoptive transfer of T-reg cells and unselected donor T cells in a mismatched murine transplant model showed protection from GVHD without impairing tumor control ([73]). Timing of adoptive transfer is likely important; efficacy may be greatest if infused peritransplant to limit initial alloreactive T-cell expansion rather than if infused to treat established aGVHD ([74]). An early-phase clinical trial has shown posttransplant adoptive transfer of T-reg cells to be safe, with a reduction in risk of grades II-IV aGVHD relative to historical controls and similar disease-free survival ([75]). In this study, there did not appear to be an excess risk of disease relapse or infection.

PREVENTING AND TREATING INFECTION

Delayed recovery of cellular and humoral immunity results in morbidity and mortality from infection. Figure 16-4 shows the approximate time course of numeric recovery of immune cells post-HCT; Fig. 16-5 shows the time course of infections.

Cellular Therapy for the Prevention and Treatment of Infectious Complications Postallogeneic Stem Cell Transplantation

Viral infection is a major cause of mortality post-HCT, resulting from cellular and humoral immune deficiency; risk factors include umbilical CB transplantation, T-cell depletion, and GVHD requiring systemic immunosuppression. Viral infections of particular relevance

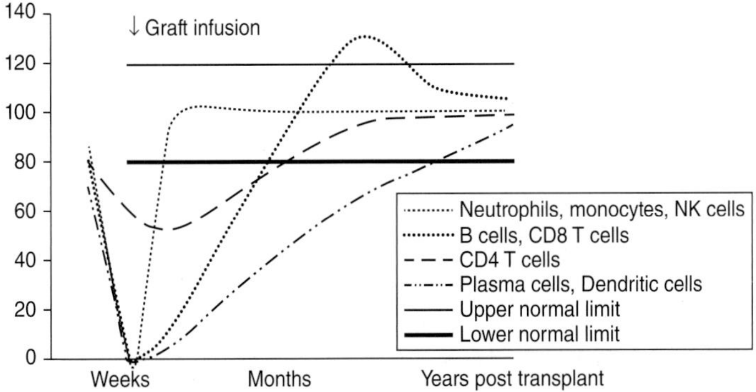

FIGURE 16-4 Time course of numeric cellular immune recovery posttransplant. [Reproduced with permission from Mackall C, Fry T, Gress R, et al. Background to hematopoietic cell transplantation, including post transplant immune recovery. *Bone Marrow Transplant.* 2009;44(8):457-462.]

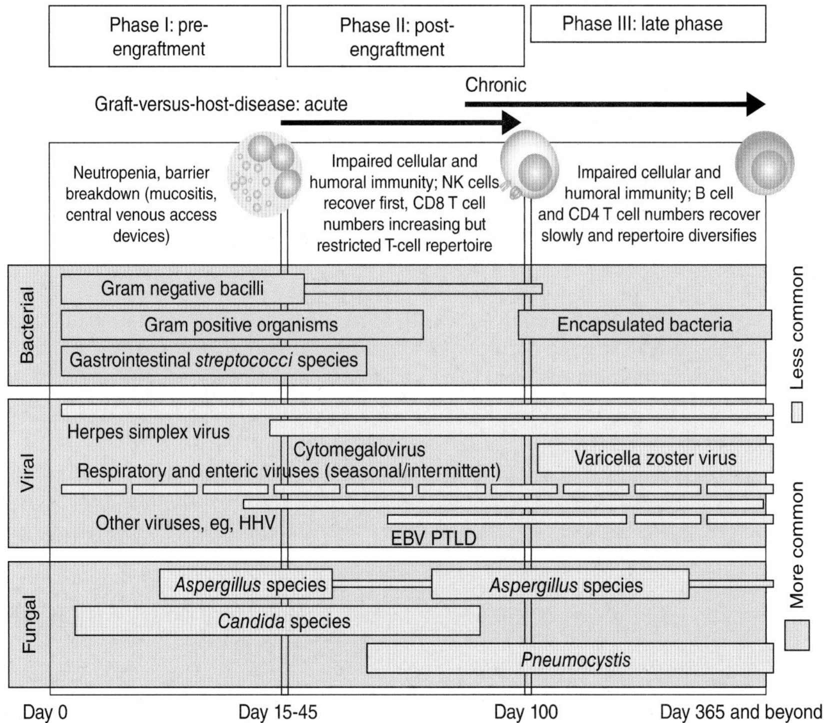

FIGURE 16-5 Time course of infections posttransplant. [Reproduced with permission from Mackall C, Fry T, Gress R, et al. Background to hematopoietic cell transplantation, including post transplant immune recovery. *Bone Marrow Transplant.* 2009;44(8):457-462.]

post-HCT are CMV, EBV, the polyoma virus BK, adenovirus (ADV), and human herpesvirus 6 (HHV-6). Pharmacotherapy for these infections has limited efficacy and substantial toxicity (76, 77). Consequently, adoptive immunotherapy for the treatment and prevention of viral reactivation/infection postallograft is attractive.

General Principles of Generating Viral-Specific T Cells

Generation of VSTs is most straightforward from an immune-experienced, adult donor who will have viral-specific memory T cells specific in their PB. The VSTs from such donors can be generated in two ways (78):

1. T-cell coculture, in the presence of specific cytokines, with an artificial APC modified to express the immunodominant antigens of the target virus and costimulatory molecules. Rapid culture techniques using overlapping peptide pools rather than live virus have shortened culture time to 7 to 14 days.
2. Rapid selection strategies without ex vivo culture. These rely on the presence of sufficient numbers of VSTs in the donor PB and hence are limited to CMV and EBV (76).

Generation of VSTs from immunologically naïve donors (eg, CB) is more challenging. However, multivirus-specific T cells against EBV, CMV, and ADV can be generated from naïve CB cells by genetically modifying EBV lymphoblastoid cell lines transduced with an adenoviral vector expressing the CMVpp65 transgene (79). These are highly active against virus, despite recognition of noncanonical CMV and EBV epitopes (79), and early clinical results are encouraging (80).

Third-party, banked VSTs from adult donors could also be used to treat viral reactivation in patients without an available adult donor or in whom rapid disease progression precludes waiting for generation of VSTs from their donor. Suitable lines (which are dependent on the recipient expressing immunodominant viral peptides on an HLA antigen shared by a donor VST line) are available in approximately 90% of patients and can be rapidly identified and made available. In an early-phase clinical trial, these VSTs demonstrated high response rates in patients with refractory CMV, ADV, and EBV-related PTLD (81). Interestingly, despite the theoretical risk of inducing GVHD due to HLA mismatch, no severe cases of de novo aGVHD were seen in initial studies, and re-treatment was successful in several cases despite initial immunologic rejection of the transferred cells (81).

Five virus-specific T cells (EBV, CMV, ADV, BK, and HHV-6) can now be produced from adult donors after culture with a peptide mix containing immunodominant antigens of the FIVE viruses (82).

Treatment of Specific Infections With Viral-Specific T Cells

Epstein-Barr Virus Reactivation and Posttransplant Lymphoproliferative Disorder

Posttransplant lymphoproliferative disorder related to EBV occurs in the setting of severe transplant-related immunosuppression when the EBV-specific T-cell response is insufficient to control latent EBV infection within recipient or donor B cells. The biology and pathology of EBV-related PTLD have been reviewed previously ([83]). Risk factors for infection predominantly relate to the degree of immunosuppression in recipients of T-cell-depleted transplants. Patients typically present with high fever and lymphadenopathy, with an elevated serum lactate dehydrogenase ([83]).

Initial therapy for EBV reactivation is reduction in immunosuppression ([83]). However, there are no randomized studies to guide the best therapy of established EBV-associated PTLD. In patients with frank PTLD, the largest study ([84]) showed a 70% CR/CRu rate with four weekly doses of rituximab monotherapy, but there were poor responses to subsequent treatment (chemotherapy, DLI, or both) in nonresponders. Chemotherapy is associated with greater toxicity in HCT recipients and may increase infection risk.

Cellular therapy shows great promise in the management of EBV-related PTLD. Unmanipulated donor T-cell infusions can control established PTLD in approximately 70% of patients but can induce severe or fatal GVHD ([85]). Therefore, when available, VSTs are preferred. The EBV-specific or polyvirus-specific cytotoxic T lymphocytes (CTLs) can be generated as described previously and have proven successful in overt PTLD in over 80% of patients, including patients with rituximab-refractory disease ([76]). Figure 16-6 demonstrates a dramatic clinical response in a patient with chemorefractory PTLD to infusion of EBV-specific CTLs.

Cytomegalovirus Infection

Risk factors for CMV reactivation and disease post-HCT include receiving umbilical CB grafts, T-cell-depleted grafts, T-cell antibody therapy for GVHD prophylaxis, or high-dose steroids ([86]). In addition, CMV-seropositive patients with seronegative donors are at particularly high risk due to the lack of memory T cells against CMV from the seronegative donor ([86]). While ganciclovir prophylaxis reduces the risk of CMV disease, it prolongs neutropenia, increases invasive bacterial and fungal infections, and does not improve survival ([86]). Close monitoring for CMV reactivation in blood, followed by preemptive therapy with ganciclovir when assays in blood become positive, reduces the incidence of CMV disease. Overall, rates of CMV disease have declined from 30% to 35% to 8% to 10% with ganciclovir prophylaxis or preemptive therapy ([86]). Gastrointestinal disease, pneumonia, and retinitis are the most common manifestations; pneumonia has a high mortality despite treatment with ganciclovir or foscarnet and CMV-immunoglobulin ([86]). Given the toxicity and expense associated with pharmacological

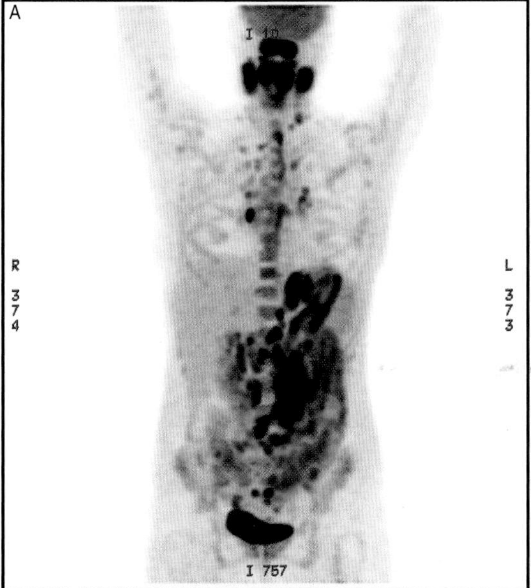

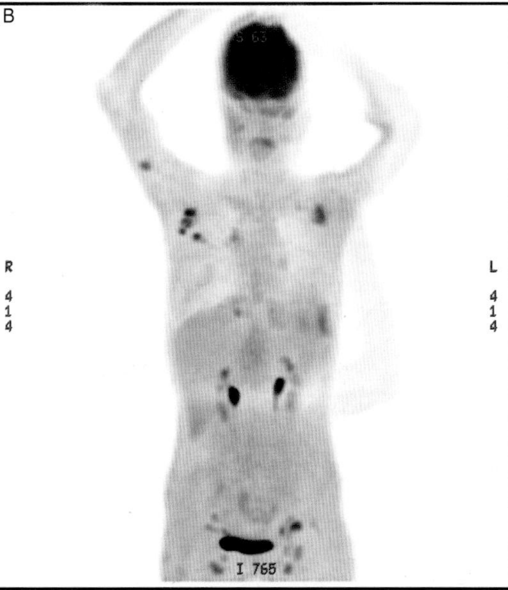

FIGURE 16-6 A patient with posttransplant EBV PTLD treated with allogeneic, most closely HLA-matched CTL against multivirus (EBV, adenovirus, CMV) ([81]). Left panel: pretreatment; right panel: posttreatment.

interventions and their imperfect efficacy, cellular therapy as treatment or prophylaxis of CMV in high-risk patients is attractive.

Adenovirus Infection

Adenovirus infection occurs in up to 21% of transplant recipients, with manifestations of adenovirus disease in 20% to 89% of infected patients ([87]). Four clinically significant syndromes are seen: pneumonitis, nephritis, hemorrhagic colitis, and hemorrhagic cystitis. Disseminated disease with multiorgan failure also occurs and has a poor outcome despite antiviral therapy; most successfully treated cases are respiratory or urinary tract infections. The ADV-specific T cells can now be generated from both CB ([79, 80]) and adult donors ([88]), with a high clinical response rate in cidofovir-refractory cases. Rapid isolation strategies are not applicable for generation of ADV-specific CTLs due to the low numbers of circulating ADV-specific T cells in donor blood.

BK Virus Infection

BK virus reactivation occurs in 5% to 68% of hematopoietic stem cell transplantation recipients. It can cause severe hematuria, urinary obstruction, renal failure, and increased mortality. It is more frequent in patients with grades III and IV aGVHD and Umbilical cord blood transplant (UCBT) recipients ([89]). Pharmacologic therapy is toxic and poorly efficacious. BK virus-specific CTLs can be generated from PB, but rapid overnight generation is not possible due to the low frequency of BK virus-specific T cells in PB; hence, culture with peptide mix or APCs is required for generation.

Human Herpes Virus 6 Infection

Infection with HHV-6 is virtually universal before age 2 years ([90]). Reactivation occurs in more than 50% of allograft recipients and can result in encephalitis, delayed engraftment, and increased rate of GVHD, with increased mortality ([90]). Production of HHV-6 VSTs using a peptide mix and 10-day culture with IL-4 and IL-7 is possible from adult donors with prior exposure ([90]). Production of HHV-6-specific VSTs has yet to be performed from CB, and rapid isolation methods are not possible given the low frequency of VSTs in blood. Clinical studies of five virus-specific CTLs (EBV, CMV, ADV, BKV, and HHV-6) are ongoing (NCT 01570283).

CONCLUSION

Allogeneic HCT, initially performed in a twin patient with leukemia by Dr. E. Donnall Thomas in the late 1950s, was one of the first elegant demonstrations of the power of cellular therapy. Much has been learned since then, and our increased understanding of the immune system has translated into exciting new therapeutic approaches, especially relevant to transplantation, leading to continued better outcomes for patients.

REFERENCES

1. Clark EA, Ledbetter JA. How B and T cells talk to each other. *Nature.* 1994;367(6462):425-428.
2. Ferrara JL, Levine JE, Reddy P, Holler E. Graft-versus-host disease. *Lancet.* 2009;373(9674):1550-1561.
3. Furst D, Muller C, Vucinic V, et al. High-resolution HLA matching in hematopoietic stem cell transplantation: a retrospective collaborative analysis. *Blood.* 2013;122(18):3220-3229.
4. Miller JS, Warren EH, van den Brink MRM, et al. NCI first international workshop on the biology, prevention, and treatment of relapse after allogeneic hematopoietic stem cell transplantation: report from the Committee on the Biology Underlying Recurrence of Malignant Disease Following Allogeneic HSCT: graft-versus-tumor/leukemia reaction. *Biol Blood Marrow Transplant.* 2001;16(5):565-586.
5. Molldrem JJ, Lee PP, Wang C, et al. Evidence that specific T lymphocytes may participate in the elimination of chronic myelogenous leukemia. *Nat Med.* 2000;6(9):1018-1023.
6. Rezvani K, Yong AS, Mielke S, et al. Leukemia-associated antigen-specific T-cell responses following combined PR1 and WT1 peptide vaccination in patients with myeloid malignancies. *Blood.* 2008;111(1):236-242.
7. Rezvani K, Yong AS, Mielke S, et al. Lymphodepletion is permissive to the development of spontaneous T-cell responses to the self-antigen PR1 early after allogeneic stem cell transplantation and in patients with acute myeloid leukemia undergoing WT1 peptide vaccination following chemotherapy. *Cancer Immunol Immunother.* 2012;61(7):1125-1136.
8. Keilholz U, Letsch A, Busse A, et al. A clinical and immunologic phase 2 trial of Wilms tumor gene product 1 (WT1) peptide vaccination in patients with AML and MDS. *Blood.* 2009;113(26):6541-6548.
9. Hirano N, Takahashi T, Takahashi T, et al. Expression of costimulatory molecules in human leukemias. *Leukemia.* 1996;10(7):1168-1176.
10. Brouwer RE, van der Heiden P, Schreuder GM, et al. Loss or downregulation of HLA class I expression at the allelic level in acute leukemia is infrequent but functionally relevant, and can be restored by interferon. *Hum Immunol.* 2002;63(3):200-210.
11. Kolb HJ. Graft-versus-leukemia effects of transplantation and donor lymphocytes. *Blood.* 2008;112(12):4371-4383.
12. Bachireddy P, Hainz U, Rooney M, et al. Reversal of in situ T-cell exhaustion during effective human antileukemia responses to donor lymphocyte infusion. *Blood.* 2014;123(9):1412-1421.
13. Peggs KS, Thomson K, Hart DP, et al. Dose-escalated donor lymphocyte infusions following reduced intensity transplantation: toxicity, chimerism, and disease responses. *Blood.* 2004;103(4):1548-1556.
14. Thomson KJ, Morris EC, Milligan D, et al. T-cell-depleted reduced-intensity transplantation followed by donor leukocyte infusions to promote graft-versus-lymphoma activity results in excellent long-term survival in patients with multiply relapsed follicular lymphoma. *J Clin Oncol.* 2010;28(23):3695-3700.
15. Kolb HJ, Schattenberg A, Goldman JM, et al. Graft-versus-leukemia effect of donor lymphocyte transfusions in marrow grafted patients. *Blood.* 1995;86(5):2041-2050.
16. Collins RH Jr, Shpilberg O, Drobyski WR, et al. Donor leukocyte infusions in 140 patients with relapsed malignancy after allogeneic bone marrow transplantation. *J Clin Oncol.* 1997;15(2):433-444.

17. Miller JS, Weisdorf DJ, Burns LJ, et al. Lymphodepletion followed by donor lymphocyte infusion (DLI) causes significantly more acute graft-versus-host disease than DLI alone. *Blood.* 2007;110(7):2761-2763.
18. Peggs KS, Kayani I, Edwards N, et al. Donor lymphocyte infusions modulate relapse risk in mixed chimeras and induce durable salvage in relapsed patients after T-cell-depleted allogeneic transplantation for Hodgkin's lymphoma. *J Clin Oncol.* 2011;29(8):971-978.
19. Di Stasi A, Tey SK, Dotti G, et al. Inducible apoptosis as a safety switch for adoptive cell therapy. *N Engl J Med.* 2011;365(18):1673-1683.
20. Fontaine P, Roy-Proulx G, Knafo L, Baron C, Roy DC, Perreault C. Adoptive transfer of minor histocompatibility antigen-specific T lymphocytes eradicates leukemia cells without causing graft-versus-host disease. *Nat Med.* 2001;7(7):789-794.
21. Dudley ME, Rosenberg SA. Adoptive-cell-transfer therapy for the treatment of patients with cancer. *Nat Rev Cancer.* 2003;3(9):666-675.
22. Keil F, Haas OA, Fritsch G, et al. Donor leukocyte infusion for leukemic relapse after allogeneic marrow transplantation: lack of residual donor hematopoiesis predicts aplasia. *Blood.* 1997;89(9):3113-3117.
23. Levine JE, Braun T, Penza SL, et al. Prospective trial of chemotherapy and donor leukocyte infusions for relapse of advanced myeloid malignancies after allogeneic stem-cell transplantation. *J Clin Oncol.* 2002;20(2):405-412.
24. Mackinnon S, Barnett L, Heller G, O'Reilly RJ. Minimal residual disease is more common in patients who have mixed T-cell chimerism after bone marrow transplantation for chronic myelogenous leukemia. *Blood.* 1994;83(11):3409-3416.
25. Topp MS, Kufer P, Gokbuget N, et al. Targeted therapy with the T-cell-engaging antibody blinatumomab of chemotherapy-refractory minimal residual disease in B-lineage acute lymphoblastic leukemia patients results in high response rate and prolonged leukemia-free survival. *J Clin Oncol.* 2011;29(18): 2493-2498.
26. Tiberghien P, Ferrand C, Lioure B, et al. Administration of herpes simplex-thymidine kinase-expressing donor T cells with a T-cell-depleted allogeneic marrow graft. *Blood.* 2001;97(1): 63-72.
27. Jensen MC, Popplewell L, Cooper LJ, et al. Antitransgene rejection responses contribute to attenuated persistence of adoptively transferred CD20/CD19-specific chimeric antigen receptor redirected T cells in humans. *Biol Blood Marrow Transplant.* 2010;16(9):1245-1256.
28. Singh H, Manuri PR, Olivares S, et al. Redirecting specificity of T-cell populations for CD19 using the Sleeping Beauty system. *Cancer Res.* 2008;68(8):2961-2971.
29. Kalamasz D, Long SA, Taniguchi R, Buckner JH, Berenson RJ, Bonyhadi M. Optimization of human T-cell expansion ex vivo using magnetic beads conjugated with anti-CD3 and Anti-CD28 antibodies. *J Immunother.* 2004;27(5):405-418.
30. Maus MV, Thomas AK, Leonard DG, et al. Ex vivo expansion of polyclonal and antigen-specific cytotoxic T lymphocytes by artificial APCs expressing ligands for the T-cell receptor, CD28 and 4-1BB. *Nat Biotechnol.* 2002;20(2):143-148.
31. Savoldo B, Ramos CA, Liu E, et al. CD28 costimulation improves expansion and persistence of chimeric antigen receptor-modified T cells in lymphoma patients. *J Clin Invest.* 2011;121(5):1822-1826.
32. Brentjens RJ, Riviere I, Park JH, et al. Safety and persistence of adoptively transferred autologous CD19-targeted T cells in patients with relapsed or chemotherapy refractory B-cell leukemias. *Blood.* 2011;118(18):4817-4828.
33. Porter DL, Levine BL, Kalos M, Bagg A, June CH. Chimeric antigen receptor-modified T cells in chronic lymphoid leukemia. *N Engl J Med.* 2011;365(8):725-733.
34. Kalos M, Frey NV, Grupp SA, et al. Chimeric antigen receptor modified T cells directed against CD19 (CTL019 cells) have long-term persistence and induce durable responses in relapsed, refractory CLL. *Blood.* 2013;122(21):4162.
35. Davila ML, Riviere I, Wang X, et al. Efficacy and toxicity management of 19-28z CAR T cell therapy in B cell acute lymphoblastic leukemia. *Sci Transl Med.* 2014;6(224):224ra225.
36. Lee DW, Kochenderfer JN, Stetler-Stevenson M, et al. T cells expressing CD19 chimeric antigen receptors for acute lymphoblastic leukaemia in children and young adults: a phase 1 dose-escalation trial. *Lancet.* 2015;385(9967):517-528.
37. Maus MV, Grupp SA, Porter DL, June CH. Antibody-modified T cells: CARs take the front seat for hematologic malignancies. *Blood.* 2014;123(17):2625-2635.
38. Kochenderfer JN, Dudley ME, Feldman SA, et al. B-cell depletion and remissions of malignancy along with cytokine-associated toxicity in a clinical trial of anti-CD19 chimeric-antigen-receptor-transduced T cells. *Blood.* 2012;119(12):2709-2720.
39. Morgan RA, Yang JC, Kitano M, Dudley ME, Laurencot CM, Rosenberg SA. Case report of a serious adverse event following the administration of T cells transduced with a chimeric antigen receptor recognizing ERBB2. *Mol Ther.* 2010;18(4):843-851.
40. Miller JS. Therapeutic applications: natural killer cells in the clinic. *Hematology Am Soc Hematol Educ Program.* 2013;2013:247-253.
41. Raulet DH. Roles of the NKG2D immunoreceptor and its ligands. *Nat Rev Immunol.* 2003;3(10):781-790.
42. Savani BN, Mielke S, Adams S, et al. Rapid natural killer cell recovery determines outcome after T-cell-depleted HLA-identical stem cell transplantation in patients with myeloid leukemias but not with acute lymphoblastic leukemia. *Leukemia.* 2007;21(10):2145-2152.
43. Childs RW, Berg M. Bringing natural killer cells to the clinic: ex vivo manipulation. *Hematology Am Soc Hematol Educ Program.* 2013;2013:234-246.
44. Miller JS, Soignier Y, Panoskaltsis-Mortari A, et al. Successful adoptive transfer and in vivo expansion of human haploidentical NK cells in patients with cancer. *Blood.* 2005;105(8):3051-3057.
45. Xing D, Ramsay AG, Gribben JG, et al. Cord blood natural killer cells exhibit impaired lytic immunological synapse formation that is reversed with IL-2 exvivo expansion. *J Immunother.* 2010;33(7):684-696.
46. Gill S, Vasey AE, De Souza A, et al. Rapid development of exhaustion and down-regulation of eomesodermin limit the antitumor activity of adoptively transferred murine natural killer cells. *Blood.* 2012;119(24):5758-5768.
47. Brandenburg S, Takahashi T, de la Rosa M, et al. IL-2 induces in vivo suppression by CD4(+)CD25(+)Foxp3(+) regulatory T cells. *Eur J Immunol.* 2008;38(6):1643-1653.
48. Huntington ND, Legrand N, Alves NL, et al. IL-15 trans-presentation promotes human NK cell development and differentiation in vivo. *J Exp Med.* 2009;206(1):25-34.
49. Curti A, Ruggeri L, D'Addio A, et al. Successful transfer of alloreactive haploidentical KIR ligand-mismatched natural killer cells after infusion in elderly high risk acute myeloid leukemia patients. *Blood.* 2011;118(12):3273-3279.
50. Berg M, Lundqvist A, McCoy P Jr, et al. Clinical-grade ex vivo-expanded human natural killer cells up-regulate activating receptors and death receptor ligands and have enhanced cytolytic activity against tumor cells. *Cytotherapy.* 2009;11(3):341-355.
51. Cooley S, Trachtenberg E, Bergemann TL, et al. Donors with group B KIR haplotypes improve relapse-free survival after unrelated hematopoietic cell transplantation for acute myelogenous leukemia. *Blood.* 2009;113(3):726-732.
52. Venstrom JM, Pittari G, Gooley TA, et al. HLA-C-dependent prevention of leukemia relapse by donor activating KIR2DS1. *N Engl J Med.* 2012;367(9):805-816.

53. Wiernik A, Foley B, Zhang B, et al. Targeting natural killer cells to acute myeloid leukemia in vitro with a CD16 x 33 bispecific killer cell engager and ADAM17 inhibition. *Clin Cancer Res.* 2013;19(14):3844-3855.
54. Ramsay AG, Clear AJ, Fatah R, Gribben JG. Multiple inhibitory ligands induce impaired T-cell immunologic synapse function in chronic lymphocytic leukemia that can be blocked with lenalidomide: establishing a reversible immune evasion mechanism in human cancer. *Blood.* 2012;120(7):1412-1421.
55. Wolchok JD, Kluger H, Callahan MK, et al. Nivolumab plus ipilimumab in advanced melanoma. *N Engl J Med.* 2013;369(2):122-133.
56. Ansell SM, Lesokhin AM, Borrello I, et al. PD-1 blockade with nivolumab in relapsed or refractory Hodgkin's lymphoma. *N Engl J Med.* 2015;372(4):311-319.
57. Norde WJ, Maas F, Hobo W, et al. PD-1/PD-L1 interactions contribute to functional T-cell impairment in patients who relapse with cancer after allogeneic stem cell transplantation. *Cancer Res.* 2011;71(15):5111-5122.
58. Ho VT, Soiffer RJ. The history and future of T-cell depletion as graft-versus-host disease prophylaxis for allogeneic hematopoietic stem cell transplantation. *Blood.* 2001;98(12):3192-3204.
59. Martin PJ, Rizzo JD, Wingard JR, et al. First- and second-line systemic treatment of acute graft-versus-host disease: recommendations of the American Society of Blood and Marrow Transplantation. *Biol Blood Marrow Transplant.* 2012;18(8):1150-1163.
60. Theurich S, Fischmann H, Shimabukuro-Vornhagen A, et al. Polyclonal anti-thymocyte globulins for the prophylaxis of graft-versus-host disease after allogeneic stem cell or bone marrow transplantation in adults. *Cochrane Database Syst Rev.* 2012;9:CD009159.
61. Chakraverty R, Orti G, Roughton M, et al. Impact of in vivo alemtuzumab dose before reduced intensity conditioning and HLA-identical sibling stem cell transplantation: pharmacokinetics, GVHD, and immune reconstitution. *Blood.* 2010;116(16):3080-3088.
62. Ciceri F, Bonini C, Stanghellini MT, et al. Infusion of suicide-gene-engineered donor lymphocytes after family haploidentical haemopoietic stem-cell transplantation for leukaemia (the TK007 trial): a non-randomised phase I-II study. *Lancet Oncol.* 2009;10(5):489-500.
63. Zhou X, Di Stasi A, Tey SK, et al. Long-term outcome after haploidentical stem cell transplant and infusion of T cells expressing the inducible caspase 9 safety transgene. *Blood.* 2014;123(25):3895-3905.
64. Rieger K, Loddenkemper C, Maul J, et al. Mucosal FOXP3+ regulatory T cells are numerically deficient in acute and chronic GvHD. *Blood.* 2006;107(4):1717-1723.
65. Trzonkowski P, Szarynska M, Mysliwska J, Mysliwski A. Ex vivo expansion of CD4(+)CD25(+) T regulatory cells for immunosuppressive therapy. *Cytometry A.* 2009;75(3):175-188.
66. Bresatz S, Sadlon T, Millard D, Zola H, Barry SC. Isolation, propagation and characterization of cord blood derived $CD4^+$ $CD25^+$ regulatory T cells. *J Immunol Methods.* 2007;327(1-2):53-62.
67. Godfrey WR, Spoden DJ, Ge YG, et al. Cord blood CD4(+) CD25(+)-derived T regulatory cell lines express FoxP3 protein and manifest potent suppressor function. *Blood.* 2005;105(2):750-758.
68. Parmar S, Liu X, Tung SS, et al. Third-party umbilical cord blood-derived regulatory T cells prevent xenogenic graft-versus-host disease. *Cytotherapy.* 2014;16(1):90-100.
69. Dong S, Maiella S, Xhaard A, et al. Multiparameter single-cell profiling of human $CD4^+FOXP3^+$ regulatory T-cell populations in homeostatic conditions and during graft-versus-host disease. *Blood.* 2013;122(10):1802-1812.
70. Nguyen VH, Shashidhar S, Chang DS, et al. The impact of regulatory T cells on T-cell immunity following hematopoietic cell transplantation. *Blood.* 2008;111(2):945-953.
71. Gaidot A, Landau DA, Martin GH, et al. Immune reconstitution is preserved in hematopoietic stem cell transplantation coadministered with regulatory T cells for GVHD prevention. *Blood.* 2011;117(10):2975-2983.
72. Zhou Q, Bucher C, Munger ME, et al. Depletion of endogenous tumor-associated regulatory T cells improves the efficacy of adoptive cytotoxic T-cell immunotherapy in murine acute myeloid leukemia. *Blood.* 2009;114(18):3793-3802.
73. Edinger M, Hoffmann P, Ermann J, et al. $CD4^+CD25^+$ regulatory T cells preserve graft-versus-tumor activity while inhibiting graft-versus-host disease after bone marrow transplantation. *Nat Med.* 2003;9(9):1144-1150.
74. Beres AJ, Drobyski WR. The role of regulatory T cells in the biology of graft versus host disease. *Front Immunol.* 2013;4:163.
75. Brunstein CG, Miller JS, Cao Q, et al. Infusion of ex vivo expanded T regulatory cells in adults transplanted with umbilical cord blood: safety profile and detection kinetics. *Blood.* 2011;117(3):1061-1070.
76. Icheva V, Kayser S, Wolff D, et al. Adoptive transfer of epstein-barr virus (EBV) nuclear antigen 1-specific t cells as treatment for EBV reactivation and lymphoproliferative disorders after allogeneic stem-cell transplantation. *J Clin Oncol.* 2013;31(1):39-48.
77. Gerdemann U, Katari UL, Papadopoulou A, et al. Safety and clinical efficacy of rapidly-generated trivirus-directed T cells as treatment for adenovirus, EBV, and CMV infections after allogeneic hematopoietic stem cell transplant. *Mol Ther.* 2013; 21(11):2113-2121.
78. Papadopoulou A, Katari UL, Gerdemann U, et al. Safety and clinical efficacy of rapidly-generated virus-specific T cells with activity against Adv, EBV, CMV, HHV6 and BK virus administered after allogeneic hematopoietic stem cell transplant. Blood. 2013;122(21):148.
79. Hanley PJ, Cruz CR, Savoldo B, et al. Functionally active virus-specific T cells that target CMV, adenovirus, and EBV can be expanded from naive T-cell populations in cord blood and will target a range of viral epitopes. *Blood.* 2009;114(9):1958-1967.
80. Hanley P, Leen A, Gee AP, et al. Multi-virus-specific T-cell therapy for patients after hematopoietic stem cell and cord blood transplantation. *Blood.* 2013;122(21):140.
81. Leen AM, Bollard CM, Mendizabal AM, et al. Multicenter study of banked third-party virus-specific T cells to treat severe viral infections after hematopoietic stem cell transplantation. *Blood.* 2013;121(26):5113-5123.
82. Papadopoulou A, Katari UL, Gerdemann U, et al. Safety and clinical efficacy of rapidly-generated virus-specific T Cells with activity against Adv, EBV, CMV, HHV6 and BK virus administered after allogeneic hematopoietic stem cell transplant. *Biol Blood Marrow Transplant.* 2014;20(2 Suppl):S48.
83. Heslop HE. How I treat EBV lymphoproliferation. *Blood.* 2009;114(19):4002-4008.
84. Fox CP, Burns D, Parker AN, et al. EBV-associated post-transplant lymphoproliferative disorder following in vivo T-cell-depleted allogeneic transplantation: clinical features, viral load correlates and prognostic factors in the rituximab era. *Bone Marrow Transplant.* 2014;49(2):280-286.
85. Heslop HE, Leen AM. T-cell therapy for viral infections. *Hematol Am Soc Hematol Educ Program.* 2013;2013:342-347.
86. Boeckh M, Ljungman P. How we treat cytomegalovirus in hematopoietic cell transplant recipients. *Blood.* 2009;113(23):5711-5719.
87. Chakrabarti S, Mautner V, Osman H, et al. Adenovirus infections following allogeneic stem cell transplantation: incidence and outcome in relation to graft manipulation, immunosuppression, and immune recovery. *Blood.* 2002;100(5):1619-1627.
88. Leen A, Gee AP, Leung K, et al. Multi-virus-specific T-cell therapy for patients after hematopoietic stem cell and cord blood transplantation. *Blood.* 2013;122(21):140.

89. Rorije NMG, Shea MM, Satyanarayana G, et al. BK virus disease after allogeneic stem cell transplantation: a cohort analysis. *Biol Blood Marrow Transplant.* 2014;20(4):564-570.
90. Gerdemann U, Keukens L, Keirnan JM, et al. Immunotherapeutic strategies to prevent and treat human herpesvirus 6 reactivation after allogeneic stem cell transplantation. *Blood.* 2013;121(1):207-218.
91. Kochenderfer JN, Dudley ME, Kassim SH, et al. Chemotherapy-refractory diffuse large B-cell lymphoma and indolent B-cell malignancies can be effectively treated with autologous T cells expressing an anti-CD19 chimeric antigen receptor. *J Clin Oncol.* 2015;33(6):540-549.
92. Kochenderfer JN, Dudley ME, Carpenter RO, et al. Donor-derived CD19-targeted T cells cause regression of malignancy persisting after allogeneic hematopoietic stem cell transplantation. *Blood.* 2013;122(25):4129-4139.
93. Brentjens RJ, Davila ML, Riviere I, et al. CD19-targeted T cells rapidly induce molecular remissions in adults with chemotherapy-refractory acute lymphoblastic leukemia. *Sci Transl Med.* 2013; 5(177):177ra138.
94. Grupp SA, Kalos M, Barrett D, et al. Chimeric antigen receptor-modified T cells for acute lymphoid leukemia. *N Engl J Med.* 2013;368(16):1509-1518.
95. Kalos M, Levine BL, Porter DL, et al. T cells with chimeric antigen receptors have potent antitumor effects and can establish memory in patients with advanced leukemia. *Sci Transl Med.* 2011;3(95):95ra73.
96. Kochenderfer JN, Wilson WH, Janik JE, et al. Eradication of B-lineage cells and regression of lymphoma in a patient treated with autologous T cells genetically engineered to recognize CD19. *Blood.* 2010;116(20):4099-4102.
97. Mackall C, Fry T, Gress R, et al. Background to hematopoietic cell transplantation, including post transplant immune recovery. *Bone Marrow Transplant.* 2009;44(8):457-462.

Section IV Lung Cancer

Section Editor: Bonnie S. Glisson

第四篇 肺癌

17 Small Cell Carcinoma of the Lung

第十七章　小细胞肺癌

Tina Cascone
Kathryn A. Gold
Bonnie S. Glisson

中文导读

小细胞肺癌近年来成为研究的热点，尤其是新的治疗手段的不断涌现使其治疗的疗效取得了进步。本章首先介绍了小细胞肺癌的流行病学特点和可能的风险因素，接着简单阐述了与预后相关的因素、病理生理学的变化以及在基因组和蛋白组学方面的相关研究结果，这可能与小细胞肺癌的发病机制有关，或许会给小细胞肺癌的治疗带来新的机会。小细胞肺癌的临床表现和最新版的TNM分期是诊断小细胞肺癌的重要手段，而分期也决定了小细胞肺癌的治疗模式。本章随之着重介绍了小细胞肺癌的治疗，内容涵盖了小细胞肺癌常用的治疗手段，如放疗、化疗、靶向治疗及免疫治疗等，对各种治疗手段的疗效、现有的临床证据及不良反应进行了分析，详细阐述了不同分期小细胞肺癌的综合治疗模式。其中对于特定的小细胞肺癌合并脑转移、合并副癌综合征、预防性脑照射等进行了探讨。本章最后简述了小细胞肺癌与相关神经内分泌肿瘤的关系。

INTRODUCTION

Small cell lung cancer (SCLC) is an aggressive bronchogenic carcinoma diagnosed in 14% of all patients with lung cancer, accounting for approximately 30,000 new cases annually in the United States ([1]). It is distinguished from non–small cell lung cancer (NSCLC) by its rapid doubling time, high proliferative fraction, and early development of metastases. Regional lymph node involvement or distant metastasis is present in 90% or more of patients at diagnosis. Historically, SCLC has been staged as limited disease (LD), which is confined to the ipsilateral thorax of origin and regional nodes, versus extensive disease (ED). The recent International Association for the Study of Lung Cancer (IASLC) staging project and American Joint Committee on Cancer/International Union Against Cancer (AJCC/UICC) seventh edition suggest use of the tumor, node, metastasis (TNM) system for the staging of SCLC ([2]). Clinically, the limited- and extensive-stage classification is practical given that most patients present with advanced disease (stages III-IV) and are only rarely candidates for resection.

Standard treatment for LD (stages I-IIIB) includes both chemotherapy and radiation; chemotherapy is the mainstay of treatment for ED (stage IV). Although a dramatic response to initial therapy is usually observed, greater than 95% of patients with ED and 80% to 90% of those with LD eventually suffer relapse and die of their disease.

Despite extensive research, no substantive advances in the systemic treatment of SCLC have been made for decades. Molecular profiling and preclinical models of SCLC have increased our understanding of the biology and genomic changes in the pathogenesis of SCLC. Translation of preclinical research to the clinical arena has resulted in recent promising data with targeted therapies, providing hope that improved outcomes for patients is on the horizon.

EPIDEMIOLOGY

Small cell lung cancer is uncommon in never smokers, who constitute only 3% to 5% of cases, and is commonly associated with intense tobacco exposure ([3]). However, transformation to SCLC has been recently documented in never smokers with epidermal growth factor receptor (*EGFR*)–mutation positive adenocarcinoma of the lung, in the setting of resistance to tyrosine kinase inhibitors ([4]). The original *EGFR* mutation is maintained in the SCLC, supporting the notion that the tumor evolved from transformation and is not a second primary cancer.

The incidence of SCLC has steadily declined, as illustrated by an analysis of the Surveillance, Epidemiology, and End Results (SEER) database ([1]), in which the proportion of SCLCs decreased from 17% in 1986 to 13% in 2002. However, this decrease was accompanied by an increase in SCLC cases arising in women (28% in 1973 vs 50% in 2002), attributed to increasing tobacco use among women starting in the 1960s. The reduced incidence may be related, in part, to changes in the pathologic criteria leading to the classification of cases as large cell neuroendocrine carcinoma (LCNEC) that would have been previously classified as SCLC.

RISK FACTORS

Of all lung cancer subtypes, SCLC shows the strongest association with tobacco exposure, which represents the most important risk factor ([3]). The risk is related to both the duration (>40 years) and intensity of tobacco use (>30 cigarettes/day). This risk is lower in former smokers versus current smokers, although the risk in former smokers still exceeds that of nonsmokers ([3]). Additional risk factors include exposure to asbestos, benzene, coal tar, and radon gas, usually as cocarcinogens with tobacco. Smoking cessation should be encouraged as a method of primary prevention. Patients with LD who continue to smoke during or after chemoradiation experience increased toxicity, have a high risk of second lung cancers, and have shorter survival than those who quit ([5]).

NATURAL HISTORY

The natural history of SCLC was documented in the placebo arm of a randomized trial from the Veterans Administration Lung Cancer Study Group (VALSG) reported in 1969, testing the effect of three doses of intravenous cyclophosphamide ([6]). In this trial, the median survival for patients in the placebo arm was 6 weeks for those with ED and 12 weeks for those with LD, based on primitive staging studies at that time. Due to stage shift with modern staging techniques, outcomes in both groups would be likely better today. Cyclophosphamide increased the median survival by 75 days in both groups, tripling the survival of patients with metastases and doubling that of patients with LD. This was the first observation foretelling the important role chemotherapy would come to play in management of SCLC.

The use of effective combination chemotherapy and, in the case of patients with tumor amenable to definitive radiation, the use of multimodality treatment have improved survival of SCLC patients. For patients with LD, 5-year survival was less than 5% in 1973 and improved to 10% in 2000. In the same period of time, 2-year survival for patients with ED improved from 1.5% to 4.6% ([1]).

PROGNOSTIC FACTORS

The most important prognostic factor for SCLC is the stage, as patients with LD have improved survival compared with those with ED ([7]). Among patients with LD, good performance status (PS), age less than 70, female gender, and normal lactate dehydrogenase (LDH) are predictive of a favorable outcome ([7]). Among these patients, a small subgroup with very LD (no mediastinal involvement) was found to have a longer median survival when treated with surgery ([8]). In patients with ED, normal LDH, multidrug regimen treatment, and a single metastasis predicted better outcomes. Liver or cerebral metastases confer significantly shorter survival compared to bone, soft tissue, or bone marrow involvement ([9]). Paraneoplastic syndromes (PNSs) may also predict outcome. Patients with the syndrome of ectopic corticotrophin (ACTH) secretion producing clinical Cushing syndrome have a dismal prognosis, with a low response to chemotherapy and poor control of hypercortisolism following treatment ([7]). Lambert-Eaton myasthenic syndrome (LEMS), an autoimmune PNS, confers a more favorable prognosis, presumably due to immunity against the cancer ([10]).

PATHOBIOLOGY

Small cell lung cancer is defined by light microscopy as a malignant epithelial tumor consisting of small cells, with round-to-fusiform shape, scant cytoplasm, finely granular nuclear chromatin, and absent or inconspicuous nucleoli ([11]). Nuclear molding and necrosis are frequent, and mitotic rates are high (Fig. 17-1). Tumors usually grow in diffuse sheets, but rosettes, peripheral palisading, organoid nesting, streams, ribbons, and rarely, tubules or ductules may be present. Typically, diagnosis is made from small biopsies and cytology specimens, as surgery is rarely performed. Due to significant crush artifact, biopsies are sometimes more problematic in diagnosis than cytology specimens.

Combined small and large cell carcinoma is histologically a tumor with a mixture of SCLC and at least 10% larger cells that morphologically fall under the definition of NSCLC. Additional variants exist, including combined SCLC with squamous cell, adenocarcinoma, spindle cell, or giant cell carcinoma. The frequency of combined SCLC varies according to tumor sample size, number of histological sections analyzed, type of specimen, and interpretation. SCLC is a "small, round, blue cell tumor" using a hematoxylin and eosin (H&E) stain, and the differential diagnosis includes other small, round, blue cell tumors, including lymphomas and small cell sarcomas. Histologically, identical tumors can arise in other organs (eg, nasopharynx, larynx, genitourinary or gastrointestinal tract, and cervix) and are termed extrapulmonary small cell carcinomas. Both pulmonary and extrapulmonary small cell carcinomas have similar biological features and clinical behavior, with high potential for widespread disease. However, malignant cells from extrapulmonary small cell carcinomas do not exhibit 3p deletions, which are common in SCLCs, indicating, at least in part, differences in carcinogenesis ([12]).

Immunohistochemical (IHC) markers are valuable in differential diagnosis of SCLC. Positive pancytokeratin (AE1/AE3) staining helps to identify the tumor as a carcinoma rather than a lymphoma or sarcoma ([11]). Neural cell adhesion molecule (CD56), chromogranin, and synaptophysin are the most useful markers. While CD56 expression is detectable in approximately 90% to 100% of cases, SCLC may be negative for expression of neuroendocrine markers, such as chromogranin and synaptophysin ([13]). Small cell lung cancer (SCLC) is a primitive undifferentiated high-grade neuroendocrine tumor (NET) and does not typically express these proteins as intensely as low-grade, well-differentiated NETs do, such as carcinoids. In 10% of cases, all neuroendocrine markers may be negative, and the diagnosis can still be established if the morphology is diagnostic. Thyroid transcriptase factor 1 (TTF-1) is expressed in 70% to 90% of SCLCs; however, this marker may also be expressed in extrapulmonary small cell carcinomas and thus does not reflect lung origin ([14]). The Ki-67 staining index, reflecting proliferation, is generally greater than 50% in SCLC and can be used to differentiate SCLC from lower-grade NETs ([15]).

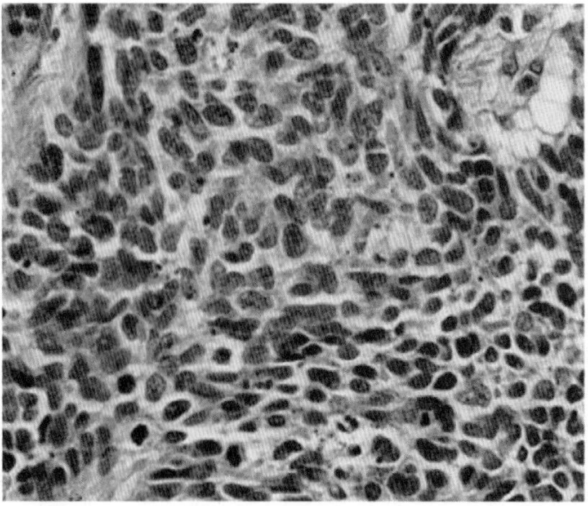

FIGURE 17-1 Light microscopic images of SCLC. Note the small, round, and spindle-shaped cells with hyperchromic nuclei and scant cytoplasm.

GENOMIC AND PROTEOMIC ALTERATIONS

Small cell lung cancer is characterized by genomic alterations, biology, and clinical behavior that are distinct from the intermediate- and low-grade pulmonary NETs. It appears that SCLC is driven more by mutations and deletions of tumor suppressor genes than by alterations in oncogenes. Loss of function of tumor protein 53 (*TP53*) occurs in 75% to 90% of SCLCs ([16]). Loss of the retinoblastoma 1 (*RB1*) gene at 13q14 occurs in virtually all patients with SCLC ([16]). Haploinsufficiency due to allele loss in multiple areas on chromosome 3p, including 3p21.3, 3p12, 3p14.2, and 3p24.4, leads to absent or lower expression of several tumor-suppressor genes in greater than 90% of SCLCs and is an early event in tumorigenesis ([12]). Deletion of the *TGFBR2* gene, encoding the transforming growth factor beta type II receptor, has been described in SCLC ([17]). The tumor suppressor gene *FUS1*, in the 3p21.3 region, was not expressed in 100% of SCLCs examined in one series ([18]). *RASSF1A* encodes a protein involved in cell cycle, apoptosis, and microtubule stability and is inactivated in 90% or more of SCLC ([19]).

Cells may acquire immortality by compensating for the loss of telomeric repeats through telomerase reactivation. Telomerase RNA subunit (hTR) and telomerase activity are upregulated in 98% or more of SCLC ([20]). Increased expression of cKit, and its ligand stem cell factor, is detected in up to 80% to 90% of SCLCs ([21]). Amplification of MYC family members (v-myc avian myelocytomatosis viral oncogene homolog, MYC, MYCL1, and MYCN) is detected in 20% of SCLCs ([16]). Loss of phosphatase and tensin homolog (PTEN) is observed in 2% to 4% of tumors ([20]); however, the Phosphoinositide 3-kinase (PTEN) pathway alteration rate(PI3K) pathway alteration rate may be overall higher and may promote SCLC tumorigenesis in preclinical models. The BCL-2 family proteins exert an antiapoptotic effect and may be upregulated in 75% to 95% of SCLC ([16]).

Two comprehensive genomic profilings of SCLC confirmed common DNA alterations and their relation with tobacco exposure ([22]) and identified novel potential therapeutic targets, including SOX2 (sex-determining region Y box 2) amplifications and RLF-MYCL1 fusions ([23]). Proteomic profiling has identified differences in protein expression between SCLC or LCNEC and other NSCLC cancers, including the DNA repair protein poly(ADP-ribose) polymerase 1 (PARP1), checkpoint kinase 1 (Chk1), and chromatin modulator enhancer of zeste 2 polycomb repressive complex 2 subunit (EZH2) ([24]). Table 17-1 describes common genomic and proteomic alterations that occur in SCLC.

Table 17-1 Representative List of Common or Potentially Targetable Genomic and Proteomic Alterations According to Percentage in Small Cell Lung Cancer

Genes	Mutation Frequency (Type of Mutation)
TP53	75-90% Loss of function (mutation, LOH, deletion)
RB1	~100% Loss of function (mutation, LOH, deletion)
PTEN	~5% Loss of function (mutation, LOH, deletion)
MYC	18-31% MYC family alterations overall Gain of function (amplification or transcrptional dysregulation)
SOX2	27% Gain of function (amplification)
FGFR1	<10% Gain of function (amplification, mutation)
CCNE1	<10% Gain of function (amplification)
EPHA7	<10% Gain of function (amplification)
PARP1	>50% (overexpression of protein target)

CCNE1, cyclin E1; EPHA7, ephrin receptor A; FGFR1, fibroblast growth factor receptor 1; MYC, v-myc avian myelocytomatosis viral oncogene homolog; PARP, poly(ADP-ripose) polymerase 1; PTEN, phosphatase and tensin homolog; RB1, retinoblastoma 1; SOX2, sex-determining region Y box 2; TP53, tumor protein 53.

CLINICAL PRESENTATION

Small cell lung cancer typically arises in the central airways and infiltrates the submucosa, with a tendency to narrow the bronchial lumen through extrinsic or endobronchial spread, in contrast to squamous cell carcinomas, where polypoid luminal occlusion is common. Rapid intrathoracic tumor growth, lymphatic and distant spread, and manifestation of PNSs can cause severe and progressive symptoms that lead to diagnosis generally within 3 months from onset. Common clinical manifestations include cough, dyspnea, weight loss, and debility. Hemoptysis and postobstructive pneumonia are relatively uncommon due to the submucosal growth pattern of the tumor. Bulky involvement of mediastinal lymph nodes is a hallmark of SCLC, and syndromes resulting from mass effects are commonly seen, including superior vena cava syndrome, hoarseness (from recurrent laryngeal nerve compression), phrenic nerve palsy, dysphagia (from esophageal compression), and stridor (from tracheal compression). Small cell lung cancer is the most common malignant cause of superior vena cava obstruction.

Radiographically, a large hilar mass with bulky mediastinal adenopathy is commonly observed (Fig. 17-2), although occasional peripheral satellite nodules may be found.

Most patients present with overt metastatic disease (60%-70%); common sites of metastasis include liver, adrenals, bone, bone marrow, and brain. Symptoms of metastatic disease can include bone or right upper quadrant abdominal pain, headache, seizures, fatigue, and anorexia. Occasionally, patients may present with PNSs, such as syndrome of inappropriate antidiuretic hormone (SIADH) or LEMS.

STAGING

The two-stage system originally proposed by the VALSG in the late 1950s and later modified by the IASLC is currently used for simplicity and practicality. Limited disease (LD) is defined as a tumor confined to one hemithorax, with involvement of regional nodes, including contralateral mediastinal or ipsilateral supraclavicular nodes, that can be included in a single tolerable radiotherapy (RT) port (TNM stages I-IIIB). Extensive disease (ED) is defined as a tumor beyond the boundaries of LD, including distant metastases, malignant pericardial or pleural effusions, and contralateral supraclavicular and contralateral hilar node involvement (TNM stage IV, any T, any N, M1a/b). More recently, IASLC proposed changes to the TNM NSCLC staging system, mainly in T and M descriptors and stage groupings. These changes have been incorporated into the AJCC seventh edition, which recommends TNM staging for SCLC and NSCLC ([2]). However, the two-stage system continues to be used in clinical practice, as most patients present with advanced disease (stages III-IV) and are only rarely candidates for surgery. This system has prognostic significance and clinical implications because patients with LD are candidates for chemoradiation with curative intent, while patients with ED receive chemotherapy alone and palliative radiation as clinically indicated. Approximately 30% to 40% of patients with SCLC present with LD; the remainder will have ED ([1]).

The initial clinical evaluation should include history and physical examination, chest radiograph, pathology review, baseline laboratory tests, including complete blood cell count, a comprehensive metabolic profile, LDH measurement, computed tomographic (CT) scans of the chest and abdomen with intravenous contrast, and brain magnetic resonance imaging (MRI) or CT scan with intravenous contrast. Brain MRI is more sensitive than CT in identifying metastases and is preferred. If LD is suspected, a positron emission tomography (PET)–CT scan may be indicated because it can identify distant disease and guide mediastinal evaluation. For most metastatic sites, a PET-CT scan is superior to other imaging modalities; however, it is inferior to MRI or CT of the brain for detection of brain metastases. Despite the fact that PET-CT may improve staging accuracy of SCLC, pathologic confirmation is still recommended for lesions depicted at PET-CT scan that may alter staging. If PET-CT scan is not available or is equivocal, bone imaging with a whole-body bone scan should be used to stage the skeleton.

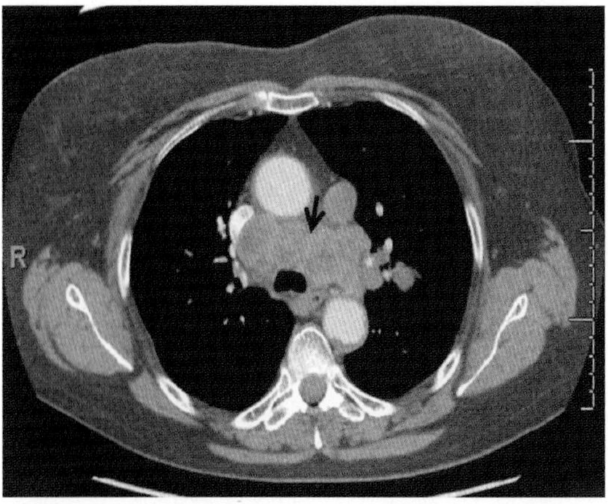

FIGURE 17-2 Bulky involvement of mediastinal adenopathy (*black arrow*) at computed tomographic scan of chest in a patient with extensive-stage SCLC.

Staging should not focus only on symptomatic sites of disease or on altered laboratory data. For example, bone scans may be positive in up to 30% of asymptomatic patients without abnormal alkaline phosphatase. The goal of complete staging is to identify those patients with LD who are candidates for definitive therapy. In the presence of obvious ED, staging may be clinically directed. Brain imaging should be obtained in all patients, given the morbidity of uncontrolled central nervous system (CNS) disease. Imaging of the CNS reveals brain metastases in 10% to 15% of patients at diagnosis, with 30% of these individuals asymptomatic.

In patients with apparent stage I disease (T1-2N0) surgical resection should be considered if mediastinal staging is negative ([8]). This can be obtained by conventional mediastinoscopy, transesophageal endoscopic ultrasound-guided fine-needle aspiration (EUS-FNA), endobronchial ultrasound-guided transbronchial needle aspiration (EBUS-TBNA), or video-assisted thoracoscopy (VATS). If a pleural effusion is present in a patient with otherwise LD, thoracentesis should be performed and fluid sent for cytology. If the fluid is exudative or if malignant cells are present, the patient should be considered to have ED (stage IV: M1a). While most pleural effusions in lung cancer are related to the malignancy, there may be a few instances in which multiple cytopathological examinations are negative for malignancy and the pleural fluid is not an exudate. When these elements and clinical judgment indicate that a pleural effusion is not malignant, the effusion should be excluded as a staging element. Pericardial effusion is classified according to the same criteria.

Sampling of cerebrospinal fluid is indicated if leptomeningeal spread is suspected. Pulmonary function tests should be performed in patients who are candidates for definitive chemoradiation therapy. Severe anemia, nucleated red blood cells on peripheral smear, neutropenia, or thrombocytopenia, in the absence of other obvious etiologies, are selection criteria for bone marrow aspiration and biopsy. The presence of tumor cells in a marrow biopsy identifies ED. Treatment should be initiated as quickly as possible after diagnosis is confirmed, given the rapid rate of progression. If the patient is significantly symptomatic or the staging evaluation prolonged, staging should be completed while chemotherapy is started.

TREATMENT

Limited Disease

Patients with SCLC rarely survive more than a few months without treatment. The disease is generally highly responsive to both chemotherapy and radiation, and patients with LD are treated with curative intent. In LD, the overall response rates (RRs) to combined chemoradiation are typically 80% to 90%, including 50% to 60% complete RRs. Median overall survival (OS) is approximately 17 months, and the 5-year survival rate is approximately 12%.

Surgery

An autopsy series on patients who died from postoperative complications revealed that 90% of patients with SCLC had mediastinal metastasis within 30 days following surgical resection ([25]). A randomized trial evaluating surgery versus thoracic RT (TRT) in patients with resectable disease revealed that the TRT group had significantly longer OS ([26]), suggesting that, even in absence of diagnosed metastases, surgery alone is an inadequate therapeutic strategy. However, surgery may play a role in multimodality therapy for those patients (5%) with early T stage and without nodal involvement (T1-T2N0M0, very LD). A 5-year survival of 48% has been reported in patients with very LD when surgery was followed by adjuvant chemotherapy ([8]). Adjuvant chemotherapy with four courses of etoposide/cisplatin (EP) should be considered for all patients with surgically resected SCLC. If nodal involvement is found at the time of surgery, chemoradiation and chemotherapy are recommended.

Combined Chemoradiation Therapy

Based on the results of a British Medical Research Council trial demonstrating surgery to be inferior to RT for the treatment of LD ([26]), TRT became standard of care for local control for these patients. Although early studies indicated that RT could increase local control compared to chemotherapy alone, these studies did not consistently show significant survival benefits to combination therapy over chemotherapy ([27]). Because of this controversy, randomized trials were performed. Two meta-analyses were performed that showed a significant 2-year survival benefit of 5.4% with the addition of RT to systemic chemotherapy for patients with LD ([27, 28]). It is noteworthy that the best outcomes from these older trials included concurrent as opposed to sequential approaches; in addition, the regimens used in this era were anthracycline- and alkylator-based therapies and were associated with excessive in-field toxicity when administered with concurrent radiation. The development of the EP regimen was critical to improving the tolerance and feasibility of concurrent chemoradiation. Etoposide/cisplatin can be given at full dose with RT, leading to improved disease control.

An anthracycline-based regimen (cyclophosphamide, epirubicin, and vincristine [CEV]) was compared in a phase III trial to EP in patients with SCLC ([29]). Patients received RT concurrently with the third cycle of chemotherapy, and prophylactic cranial irradiation (PCI) was administered to those who achieved complete remission (CR). The results showed that, in patients with LD, EP was superior to CEV for survival rates at 2 and 5 years (14% and 5% vs 6% and 2%, respectively; $P = .0001$), as well as median OS (14.5 vs 9.7 months; $P = .001$). In patients with ED, no survival difference was noted.

The addition of other cytotoxins to the EP regimen—either as a triplet with paclitaxel or alternating therapy with cyclophosphamide, doxorubicin, and vincristine—has also been studied, but to date a new standard in the treatment of LD has not emerged ([30, 31]).

Radiation Intensity

Based on the radiobiology of SCLC, the Intergroup (INT) trial 0096 studied accelerated hyperfractionated RT (AHRT) compared to conventional fractionation in a phase III trial ([32]). Over 400 patients were randomized between the two arms. All patients received four cycles of EP, and TRT was administered concurrently, starting with the first cycle of chemotherapy. All patients received 45 Gy, either in once-daily 1.8-Gy fractions for 5 weeks or twice-daily 1.5-Gy fractions for 3 weeks. Patients in the twice-daily RT group had an improved median OS (23 vs 19 months) and 5-year survival (26% vs 16%), at the cost of increased weight loss and grade 3 esophagitis (27% vs 11%). Local failure rates were lower in the twice-daily RT arm, presumably the major reason for improved survival.

Intergroup trial 0096 convincingly showed an OS benefit to concurrent chemoradiation with hyperfraction. However, because of concerns for side effects and the logistical difficulties involved in twice-daily treatment, the regimen has not been widely used in the community ([33]). The control arm of the INT 0096 study used a relatively low total RT dose, and since the results of INT 0096 have become available, conventionally fractionated radiation in higher doses has also been studied. The Cancer and Leukemia Group B (CALGB) trial tested the regimen paclitaxel and topotecan for two cycles, followed by TRT with 70 Gy in 35 daily fractions with concurrent carboplatin/etoposide (CE; total of three cycles) in a phase II study ([34]). Median OS was 22.4 months, comparable to that found with AHRT in the INT 0096 study.

Another schedule of TRT tested was concomitant boost, in which patients received once-daily radiation through most of their course, then received hyperfractionated therapy at the end of treatment, so that RT was accelerated without the need for twice-daily administration throughout the treatment course. The Radiation Therapy Oncology Group (RTOG) tested this approach in the phase II trial 0239. Patients received 61.2 Gy over 5 weeks, with twice-daily RT in the final 9 days ([35]). Radiotherapy started on day 1 of chemotherapy with four cycles of EP. Two-year survival rate was 37%, somewhat less than that found in both INT 0096 and the CALGB trial (2-year survival rates of 41% and 48%, respectively).

A prospective INT study of chemoradiation for patients with LD (RTOG 0538/CALGB 30610) is currently active. Originally, this trial included the concomitant boost regimen, but that arm has been dropped after an interim analysis. The trial currently compares 70 Gy once daily with AHRT (45 Gy twice daily) from the INT 0096 study. In both arms, concurrent EP and RT commence with the first cycle of chemotherapy (NCT [National Clinical Trial] 00632853). The primary end points are median OS and 2-year survival rates.

Timing of Chemotherapy

Sequential, concurrent, and alternating chemotherapy have all been tested with TRT. Early studies did not show a survival benefit to concurrent chemotherapy; however, this was likely due to the increased toxicity when using cyclophosphamide- or doxorubicin-based chemotherapy. Etoposide/cisplatin is far better tolerated than these earlier regimens when administered concurrently with RT.

The National Cancer Institute of Canada reported a phase III trial of alternating CAV (cyclophosphamide, anthracycline, vincristine)/EP with TRT in either the second or sixth cycle of chemotherapy ([36]). The patients receiving early RT experienced improved OS (21.2 vs 16 months). The Japan Clinical Oncology Group (JCOG) compared RT (45 Gy in twice-daily 1.5-Gy fractions) starting with either the first cycle of EP or following completion of the chemotherapy course ([37]). More myelosuppression was noted in the patients in the concurrent arm, but there was a significant reduction in risk of death for early concurrent therapy, with a hazard ratio (HR) of 0.70 ($P = .02$). Although not all trials have consistently shown a benefit for concurrent chemoradiation, the data strongly support this and its early integration in treatment when the regimen is EP, as contrasted with anthracycline- or alkylator-based regimens. Furthermore, efficacy outcomes are consistently better with EP in the treatment of LD.

Given that SCLC is such a rapidly dividing malignancy, it has been hypothesized that accelerated proliferation of tumor clonogens can affect outcome, and that treatment should be delivered in a condensed fashion ([38]). A meta-analysis examined the impact of a novel parameter, time from the start of any treatment to the end of RT, on OS in LD. A shorter SER was found to be a significant predictor of better outcome. For each week that the SER was lengthened, OS at 5 years showed an absolute decrease of almost 2% ([38]). The data from INT 0096 had a strong influence on this result.

Carboplatin is frequently used in ED due to a more favorable toxicity profile, whereas cisplatin is preferred in patients with LD with curative intent. The efficacy of cisplatin versus carboplatin regimens in LD was evaluated in a meta-analysis of four trials ([39]), which revealed no significant difference in terms of efficacy. Similar results were found in a subset analysis based on the two randomized trials conducted in patients with LD ([40, 41]), where no differences were seen in RRs or median survival time for EP versus CE, although less toxicity was reported in the carboplatin-containing arm. Nevertheless, due to its use in trials for which the best 5-year survival has been observed in LD, EP should be given unless there is a significant contraindication to cisplatin use. Notably, the dose of cisplatin in INT 0096 was only 60 mg/m^2. Figure 17-3 illustrates the treatment algorithm for management of limited-stage SCLC.

Extensive Disease

Systemic chemotherapy represents the primary therapeutic modality for patients with ED. Prophylactic cranial irradiation decreases the incidence of symptomatic brain metastases in responders to systemic chemotherapy, although its impact on OS is uncertain. Currently,

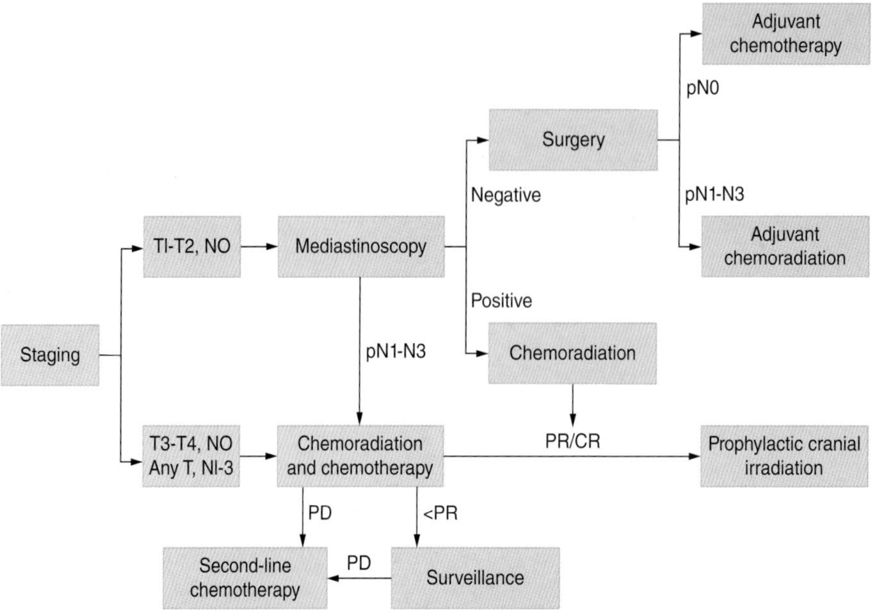

FIGURE 17-3 Treatment algorithm for management of limited-stage SCLC.

TRT is utilized for symptom palliation; however, a potential role for radiation in patients with limited systemic disease and a good response to initial therapy has been suggested. Chemotherapy prolongs survival compared with best supportive care (BSC) ([6]). From the time of diagnosis, the median OS for patients with ED is 8 to 13 months, the 5-year survival is 1% to 2%, and the 2-year survival is 4% to 5% ([1]). Figure 17-4 shows representative coronal PET-CT images in a patient with extensive-stage SCLC (ED).

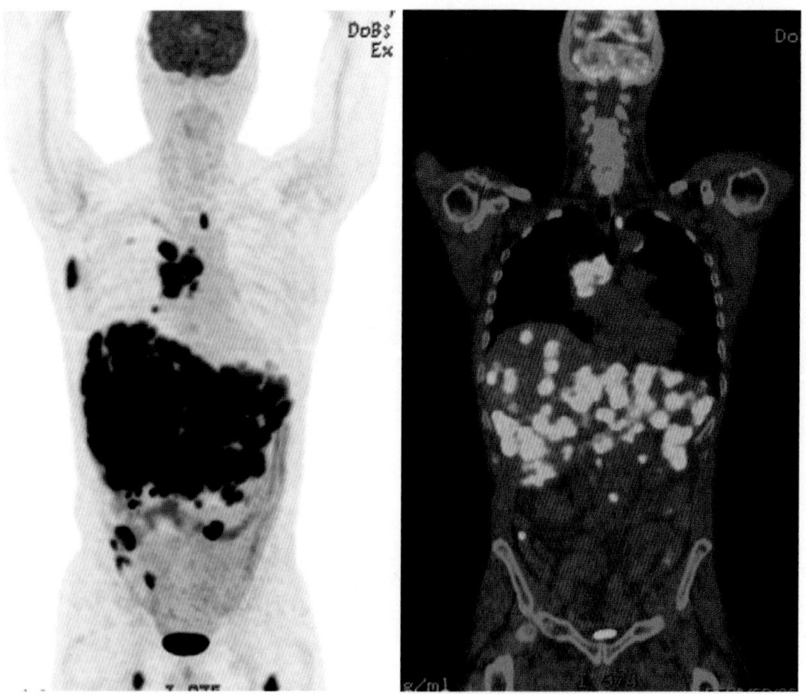

FIGURE 17-4 Representative PET-CT images in a patient with extensive-stage SCLC. Coronal PET (left panel) and fused coronal (right panel) images are shown.

Chemotherapy

In an early study, patients with SCLC had a highly significant improvement in survival with intravenous cyclophosphamide compared to placebo, increasing median survival from 12 weeks to almost 5 months [6]. As new cytotoxins became available, combination therapy was studied, and the CAV regimen became the standard of care for ED (29). Etoposide/cisplatin was initially evaluated in patients who had recurrent disease after or failed to respond to CAV, with RRs of 55% [42]. It was later evaluated as a first-line treatment in patients unable to tolerate CAV, demonstrating a median OS of 39 weeks in ED, with less toxicity [43]. In a phase III trial, the equivalent efficacy of EP and CAV was confirmed by randomizing 437 patients to receive four cycles of EP, six cycles of CAV, or alternation of these two regimens for 18 weeks (CAV/EP, three cycles each) [44]. The RRs (61%, 51%, 59%, respectively) and median OS (8.6, 8.3, and 8.1 months, respectively) were equivalent across the arms. Myelosuppression was the dose-limiting toxicity, and four cycles of EP were better tolerated. Similar results were seen in a Japanese trial [30]. Four cycles of EP became the standard of care for patients with ED [29], although it is common in practice to continue for six cycles in the face of continuing regression after four and good tolerance.

Increased Length of Induction and Maintenance Chemotherapy

A meta-analysis of 14 randomized clinical trials, including 2,550 patients with SCLC, revealed a modest reduction in both 1- and 2-year mortality with prolonged treatment, referred to as maintenance or consolidation chemotherapy [45]. Maintenance chemotherapy improved 1- and 2-year survival by 9% (from 30% to 39%, $P < .001$) and 4% (from 10% to 14%, $P < .001$), respectively. The trials in this analysis predominantly studied alkylator- or anthracycline-based regimens as induction, with one exception that studied EP with or without TRT and maintenance CAV, and failed to show a benefit for maintenance. Further, the two most positive trials studied consolidative EP following anthracycline-based chemotherapy with or without chest RT for LD patients only. The positive effect of consolidative EP in LD patients treated with anthracycline-based induction heavily contributed to the results of the meta-analysis.

Maintenance therapy with etoposide or topotecan following induction with EP has also been evaluated in ED [46, 47]. Both of these trials demonstrated a small benefit in PFS (<2 months) without improvement in OS. Thus, when EP is used as induction, maintenance therapy is not recommended.

Substitutions and Additions to Induction Therapy

Adjustments to the EP regimen have been investigated. Carboplatin is frequently used in combination with etoposide in ED because of similar efficacy to cisplatin and less toxicity. A meta-analysis of four randomized trials comparing carboplatin to cisplatin demonstrated no differences in terms of OS, PFS, and RRs (median 9.6 vs 9.4 months, 5.5 vs 5.3 months, and 67% vs 66%, respectively) [39].

Multiple-drug combinations, including variations of EP, and three- and four-drug regimens have shown higher RRs and improvement in survival without a consistent meaningful clinical benefit over EP. Based on activity of irinotecan in recurrent disease, it was combined with cisplatin in frontline therapy. Four large randomized trials have compared irinotecan/cisplatin (IP) versus EP. The multicenter phase III JCOG 9511 trial compared IP to EP in treatment-naïve patients with ED [48]. Although the projected accrual was set for 230 patients, the study was terminated early, after accrual of 154 patients, given the clear survival advantage in the IP over the EP group (median OS 12.8 vs 9.4 months, respectively; $P = .0021$). However, subsequent studies have failed to confirm the results in non-Asian populations. Two North American trials [49, 50] and one European trial [51] have not shown a significant survival benefit with IP over EP. In the Southwest Oncology Group (SWOG) S0124 trial, over 600 patients with ED received either IP or EP [50]. No significant differences were found in median PFS, OS, or overall response rates (ORRs) between the regimens (5.8 vs 5.2 months, 9.9 vs 9.1 months, and 60% vs 57%, respectively). Similarly, topotecan, given in combination with cisplatin, has failed to demonstrate a clinical advantage over EP as initial therapy for patients with ED [52].

The addition of ifosfamide to EP led to a modest survival improvement in one study (9.0 vs 7.3 months; $P = .045$); however, given the greater toxicities and minimally improved outcomes, this regimen is not commonly used [53].

In a phase III trial by the French Federation of Cancer Institutes, EP was compared to EP plus cyclophosphamide and 4′-epidoxorubicin (PCDE) in ED [54]. The four-drug regimen led to only a minimal survival improvement at the cost of increased toxicity.

Alternating or Sequential Combinations

Despite initial chemosensitivity, almost all patients will eventually relapse, due to either intrinsic multidrug resistance or development of resistance during therapy. Goldie and Coldman hypothesized that non–cross-resistant regimens could be rapidly alternated or administered sequentially to eliminate these resistant clones [55]. Several trials have evaluated alternating regimens, including EP alternating with CAV ([30]) and cyclophosphamide, doxorubicin and etoposide alternating with vincristine, carboplatin, ifosfamide, mesna ([56]), with no significant benefit in patients with ED.

Rapid sequencing of several active agents over a short period has also been evaluated. The most studied regimen comprised weekly treatments of CODE (cisplatin, vincristine, doxorubicin, etoposide). Although early studies indicated that CODE conferred a possible survival advantage to patients with ED, subsequent phase III trials did not confirm superiority to alternating traditionally scheduled CAV/EP ([57, 58]).

Altering Dose Intensity and Density

Preclinical studies of chemotherapy in SCLC have shown a dose-response relationship, leading to the evaluation of higher-dose chemotherapy in the clinical setting. A meta-analysis of 60 trials showed that increasing the dose intensity of CAV and EP did not improve survival of patients with ED ([59]). Two randomized trials comparing high-dose to standard-dose EP doublets failed to demonstrate a survival advantage ([60, 61]).

Dose-dense chemotherapy, with integration of marrow growth factors to reduce the time interval between cycles of chemotherapy, has also been studied. Several trials evaluated this approach, with conflicting results. In a randomized study, patients with LD and ED were assigned to ifosfamide, etoposide, carboplatin, and vincristine given every 3 (intensified) or 4 (standard) weeks ([62]). Patients in the dose-intense arm had a longer median survival (443 vs 351 days, respectively) and an improved 2-year survival rate (33% vs 18%, respectively; $P = .0014$). However, delivery of this regimen every 3 weeks was highly feasible and did not represent dose-dense therapy. Over 400 SCLC patients were randomized to doxorubicin, cyclophosphamide, and etoposide every 2 or 3 weeks ([63]), and only a small survival advantage was seen in the dose-dense arm (10.9 vs 11.5 months; $P = .04$). The British Medical Research Council multicenter randomized trial investigated a four-drug regimen—ifosfamide, carboplatin, etoposide, and vincristine (ICE-V)—every 4 weeks for six cycles over standard chemotherapy (according to center preference) in patients with SCLC ([64]). Prolonged OS was noted in the ICE-V group (HR 0.74, $P = .0049$), median OS was 15.6 versus 11.6 months, and 2-year survival rates were 20% versus 11%, in the ICE-V versus control groups, respectively, at the cost of increased toxicity. It is important to note that the 85% of patients enrolled had LD, and 82% of patients in the control arm were treated with non–platin-based regimens. Therefore, these results most likely reflect, again, the survival impact of platin exposure in patients with LD and do not support the ICE-V regimen.

Two randomized trials compared ICE every 4 weeks with ICE every 2 weeks with autologous stem cell support. One small trial of 83 patients stopped at interim analysis showed an OS improvement with the high-dose regimen (30.3 vs 18.5 months); however, a larger randomized phase III trial did not demonstrate a survival improvement in the high-versus standard-dose arm (14.4 vs 13.9 months, respectively) ([65, 66]).

Thoracic Radiation Therapy

Prospective trials have evaluated the role of consolidative TRT in patients with ED who initially respond to systemic chemotherapy. In a single-center study, 206 patients received three cycles of EP ([67]), and complete responders at distant sites and those with intrathoracic PR or CR (n = 109) were randomized to thoracic AHRT (54 Gy, 36 fractions over 18 days) combined with CE or four additional cycles of EP. Patients with brain metastases, stable disease, progressive disease, or only PR outside the thorax were not randomized. The addition of TRT to chemotherapy improved median OS (17 vs 11 months, 5-year survival rate 9% vs 4%, respectively; $P = .041$). There was a trend to reduced local recurrence in the radiation arm, but no difference in metastasis-free survival. Acute high-grade toxicity was higher in the chemotherapy arm.

In the phase III multicenter European CREST trial, patients with ED were initially treated with four to six cycles of platinum-based chemotherapy. Patients with any response were then randomized to TRT (30 Gy in 10 fractions) plus PCI (n = 247) or to PCI alone (n = 248) ([68]). The study did not meet the primary end point of 1-year survival improvement (33% with thoracic RT vs 28% without; $P = .07$). However, 2-year survival and PFS rates were significantly longer for those receiving TRT after prolonged follow-up (2-year OS, 13% vs 3%, $P = 0.004$; PFS, 24% vs 7%, respectively, at 6 months). The most common grade 3 toxicities in the TRT group compared with the control group were fatigue (4.5% vs 3.2%) and dyspnea (1.2% vs 1.6%). Patients most likely to benefit were those with residual disease in the thorax.

The RTOG 0937 phase II study (NCT 01055197) comparing PCI alone versus PCI with consolidative RT to residual loco-regional and metastatic disease in patients with ED who responded to platinum-based chemotherapy was closed early due to excess grade 5 toxicity in the experimental arm.

Currently, it is our practice to consider consolidative TRT in selected patients with ED with excellent control of extrathoracic disease, residual disease in the thorax, and retained PS following chemotherapy. Thoracic RT should be limited to palliative dosing and conventional fractionation, and concurrent chemotherapy should not be given.

Figure 17-5 demonstrates metabolic response on PET in a patient with ED and extensive bone metastases after four cycles of CE. Figure 17-6 shows the treatment algorithm for the management of extensive-stage SCLC.

Recurrent Disease

Despite initial response to chemoradiation, approximately 11% of patients with LD and only 1% to 2% of those with ED are alive at 5 years, with the vast majority succumbing to recurrent SCLC ([1]). Historically, recurrent disease is less responsive and survival is limited, with median survival ranging from 2 to 6 months following relapse. The response to initial treatment and the time to relapse following induction chemotherapy are both important determinants of response to second-line chemotherapy. Patients with objective response to initial treatment and PFS at least 60 to 90 days following completion of induction chemotherapy are more likely to respond to additional chemotherapy and are considered to have "sensitive"

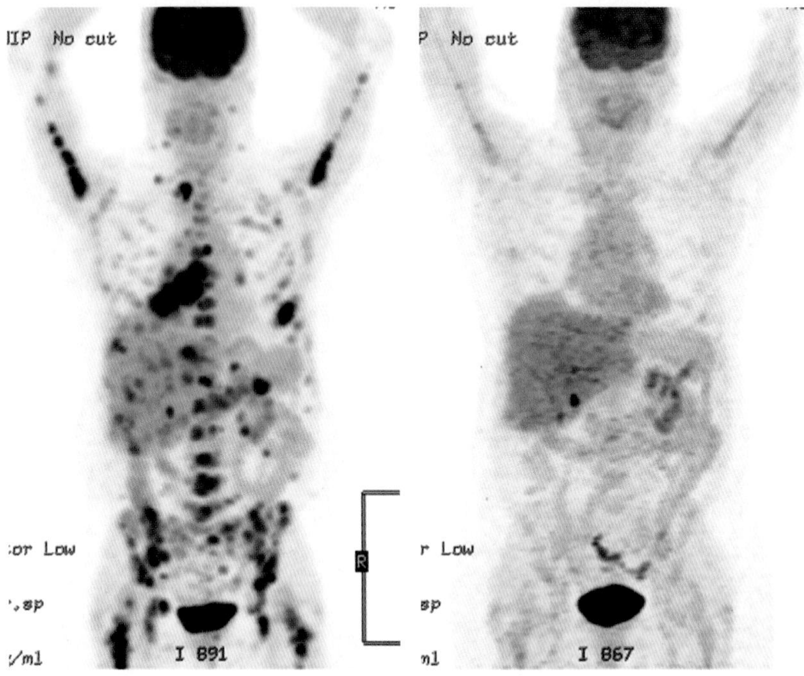

FIGURE 17-5 Response of extensive-stage SCLC following treatment with platin/etoposide at PET-CT imaging. Baseline (*left*) and restaging coronal PET (*right*) images are shown.

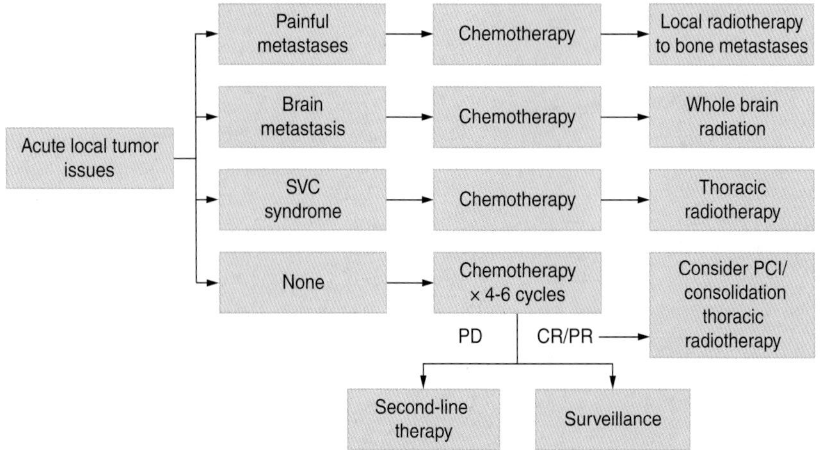

FIGURE 17-6 Treatment algorithm for management of extensive-stage SCLC.

CHAPTER 17

disease. Those who do not achieve disease regression with initial chemotherapy or with shorter duration of response after chemotherapy is discontinued are considered refractory ([69]).

Reintroduction of the chemotherapy regimen used for induction has been a therapeutic strategy for relapse in patients with prolonged PFS after first-line therapy. The first evidence to support this was suggested in a series of six patients who had achieved a greater than 2-year remission following induction chemotherapy ([70]). Five of these patients received some or all of the agents of their induction regimen, with four responses, lasting up to 18 months. Other studies also suggested responses when first-line therapy was reintroduced at relapse if patients had either a CR or a response longer than 34 weeks following induction ([71, 72]). In the modern era, when many patients receive just four courses of induction chemotherapy, re-treatment with EP could be considered if initial response was dramatic and maintained PFS for 3 months or more.

Topotecan and irinotecan have been studied in recurrent disease. Topotecan is the only drug for which there are several randomized trials in this setting and is the only agent approved by the Food and Drug Administration (FDA) for recurrent SCLC. Oral topotecan was found to have similar efficacy to intravenous topotecan, with less toxicity and ease of administration ([73]). A phase III trial showed that intravenous topotecan had similar efficacy to the CAV regimen in patients with sensitive relapse, with an RR of 24% versus 18%, with a similar median TTP (13 vs 12 weeks) and OS (25 vs 24.7 weeks) for topotecan versus CAV, respectively ([69]). The topotecan group had better symptom control, with less-severe neutropenia. The improvement in symptom control led to its FDA approval. In a phase III registration trial, oral topotecan was compared to BSC in patients who had relapsed 45 days or more after achieving a response to first-line therapy and were not candidates to receive intravenous topotecan ([74]). Topotecan significantly improved OS (25.9 vs 13.9 weeks), including significant benefit in patients who relapsed 60 days or less after initial treatment, and was associated with a slower deterioration in quality of life compared to BSC. In a phase III trial, 304 patients with sensitive relapse were randomized to oral (2.3 mg/m^2 daily for 5 days) or intravenous (1.5 mg/m^2 daily for 5 days) topotecan every 3 weeks ([73]). The RRs and the median and 1-year survival rates as well as the toxicity profiles were similar between the two arms (18% vs 22%, 33 vs 35 weeks, and 33% vs 29%, respectively). Topotecan is typically administered on days 1 to 5 of a 3-week cycle. Irinotecan has not been directly compared to topotecan, and phase III trials have not been performed; phase II studies suggested similar efficacy compared to topotecan in the recurrent setting ([75]).

Amrubicin is a novel anthracycline that showed promising activity in single-arm and randomized phase II trials for patients with recurrent SCLC in Japan ([76]). A phase III trial in North America and Europe randomized 637 patients with refractory or sensitive SCLC to amrubicin or topotecan ([77]). Median OS and PFS were 7.5 versus 7.8 months (HR 0.88; P = .17) and 4.1 versus 3.5 months (HR 0.8; P = .018) with amrubicin and topotecan, respectively. Thus, amrubicin is approved for use only in Japan.

Temozolomide is a well-tolerated oral alkylating agent with an ORR of 16% in a small phase II study ([78]). Currently, a phase II randomized trial (NCT 01638546) is evaluating the efficacy of temozolomide with or without veliparib in relapsed disease, as detailed in the experimental agents section.

BRAIN METASTASIS

The brain is a common site of metastatic spread in SCLC, with 10% of patients presenting with brain involvement at diagnosis and an additional 40% to 50% developing CNS metastasis during the course of disease.

Whole-Brain Radiation Therapy

Whole-brain radiation therapy (WBRT) rapidly resolves symptoms of brain involvement from SCLC. Radiotherapy with 30 Gy in 10 daily fractions has been shown equally effective as altered fractionation to a higher dose (54 Gy in 34 fractions) in the phase III trial RTOG 9104 ([79]), which evaluated these WBRT regimens in 429 patients with unresected brain metastases, including 39 patients with SCLC. Median OS was 4.5 months in both arms; 1-year survival was also similar, at 19% with accelerated fractionation and 16% on the control arm.

Reirradiation of the CNS may be considered (20 Gy in 10 fractions) for symptom palliation in recurrent intracranial disease ([80]). Stereotactic radiosurgery (SRS) represents a therapeutic option for progressive brain metastases following WBRT. The technique uses external irradiation beams that deliver a single, high dose of radiation to a small volume of tissue with minimal invasion of and injury to healthy tissue. Stereotactic radiosurgery for brain metastases following WBRT from SCLC (fewer than four sites) is safe and achieves 1-year local control of 60% to 90%, especially in lesions less than 2 cm ([81]); however, regional CNS recurrence risk approaches 60%.

Chemotherapy

In general, RRs to chemotherapy in brain metastases mirror those in extracranial disease sites, with higher rates in therapy-naïve patients. In a meta-analysis, a 36% RR in the CNS was revealed in the results of five trials where 135 patients with brain metastases were treated, following initial therapy, with single-agent etoposide or carboplatin. Pooled data from another five studies conducted in 64 patients with brain metastases at diagnosis treated with various combination regimens showed a RR of 66% ([82]).

In summary, for treatment-naïve patients who present with CNS involvement and are asymptomatic or minimally symptomatic, chemotherapy should be given initially, and if brain disease is controlled, WBRT may be given after completion of four cycles of chemotherapy. Brain irradiation should ultimately be administered given that it is associated with higher CR of brain metastases compared to chemotherapy alone. Symptomatic CNS involvement or progression of brain metastases during chemotherapy is an indication for WBRT. The approach of combining WBRT and induction chemotherapy must be considered in situations where brain disease is bulky and symptomatic and there is also significant extracranial disease requiring urgent treatment. Myelosuppression is increased with concurrent modalities, and this should be expectantly managed. For those patients who develop CNS involvement following initial chemotherapy, WBRT is indicated, and chemotherapy may have a palliative role in those who progress after receiving WBRT. Occasionally, previously irradiated patients with SCLC are candidates for SRS; however, the rate of brain failure is high.

PROPHYLACTIC CRANIAL IRRADIATION

Despite only 10% of patients with SCLC presenting with CNS involvement at diagnosis, there is a significant rate of occult brain disease in patients who lack neurologic symptoms; thus, staging of the brain is indicated in all patients. Approximately 15% to 20% of patients with LD SCLC who initially respond to therapy will develop brain metastases as the sole site of relapse, suggesting that brain radiation early in the treatment course might be curative in this group ([83]). The risk of developing brain disease in patients alive at 2 years after diagnosis who did not receive PCI is between 50% and 80% ([83]). Prophylactic cranial irradiation has been investigated as a means to control brain metastatic disease following chemotherapy before it becomes clinically evident, in an effort to prevent morbidity and mortality. Numerous clinical trials have established the effectiveness of PCI in decreasing the incidence of intracranial disease in patients who have responded to initial treatment for LD and ED, although its impact on survival has been variable.

Prophylactic Cranial Irradiation in Limited Disease

The PCI Overview Collaborative Group meta-analysis evaluated seven randomized trials comparing PCI (treatment group) versus no PCI (control group) in 987 patients with SCLC who achieved CR to initial therapy. Approximately 85% of the patients enrolled in both groups had LD. The PCI provided a 5.4% improvement in 3-year survival (15.3% vs 20.7% in control vs treatment group, respectively), increased disease-free survival ($P < .001$), and decreased the risk of developing brain disease (33% vs 59%, HR 0.46; $P < .001$) ([83]). A second meta-analysis evaluated 1,547 patients from 12 randomized studies, 5 of which required CR status for randomization ([84]). The results of the second analysis confirmed the reduced rate of brain metastasis for all patients, but improvement in OS only for patients in CR (HR 0.82, 95% confidence interval: 0.71-0.96). Based on these data, PCI became standard of care for patients with LD and disease control following chemoradiation.

Two large randomized trials have investigated the effect of RT doses above 25 Gy. A multinational phase III trial randomized 720 patients with LD and CR following induction therapy to receive PCI at 25 Gy in 10 fractions or 36 Gy (18 fractions of 2 Gy each or 24 fractions of 1.5 Gy twice daily) ([85]). No significant differences were noted in the 2-year incidence rates of brain metastasis, and an increased mortality was noted with higher PCI doses (2-year survival rate 37% vs 42%, HR 1.20). The phase II randomized RTOG 0212 study similarly showed no differences in the incidence of brain metastasis or OS benefit in patients with LD and CR following initial chemoradiation comparing PCI with 25 Gy to 36 Gy ([86]).

Prophylactic Cranial Irradiation in Extensive Disease

A phase III European Organization for Research and Treatment of Cancer (EORTC) study randomized patients with ED with response to initial chemotherapy to either PCI (choice of three schedules) or observation ([87]). Baseline imaging of the brain was required only for symptomatic patients. Overall, 286 patients were randomized. Patients in the PCI group had a lower risk of brain metastases (15% vs 40%, HR 0.27; $P < .001$) and a longer median OS from time of randomization versus the observation group (6.7 vs 5.4 months, respectively). It is notable that more patients in the PCI group received second-line chemotherapy (68% vs 45%), possibly accounting for the OS improvement. Fatigue was significantly worse on the PCI arm in the first 24 weeks. Global health status and cognitive functioning were assessed only up to 9 months from randomization and were a mean of 8 points less (scale of 0-100) at 6 weeks and 3 months on the PCI arm ([88]). These results are difficult to interpret given the lack of brain imaging at baseline and heterogeneity in both chemotherapy and PCI schedules. Further, the 1.3-month OS improvement could be attributed to an imbalance in subsequent chemotherapy use, which is known to influence survival.

Most recently, a Japanese trial evaluated the efficacy of PCI versus observation in 224 patients with SCLC who had response to induction chemotherapy with either etoposide or irinotecan and cisplatin ([89]). Prior to randomization, brain MRI was performed to rule out occult metastases, and patients on both arms were followed postrandomization with serial brain imaging. Prophylactic cranial irradiation was given as 25 Gy in 10 fractions. The accrual was stopped early for futility when analysis after 111 deaths revealed a trend toward shorter median survival with PCI (10.1 vs 15.1 months, HR 1.38; $P = .091$). As expected, decreased incidence of brain metastases with PCI at 1 year (32% vs 58%; $P < .001$) was observed, and fewer patients treated with PCI required RT for symptomatic brain involvement (31% vs 80%).

In summary, PCI clearly decreased the incidence of symptomatic brain disease in SCLC, but the impact on OS in patients with ED was variable. It is reasonable to discuss PCI in patients with ED who have a CR or very good PR to initial treatment and good PS. The lack of definite survival benefit and the potential for at least short-term toxicity should be discussed. It should be used with caution in the elderly and in patients with significant ischemic cerebrovascular disease due to a concern for increased acute and late brain toxicity. It is important to separate PCI from chemotherapy and to use radiation regimens that are safe in regard to late neurotoxic effects (eg, 25 Gy in 10 daily fractions).

THE ELDERLY AND INFIRM

Approximately 25% of patients with SCLC are over the age of 70 years. These patients have often been excluded from clinical trials because of concerns for greater toxicity due to lowered organ reserves, especially myelosuppression and frequently lowered functional status due to comorbidities. However, retrospective studies have shown that elderly patients with retained PS have improved outcomes with more aggressive treatment ([90]). In a Canadian analysis, elderly patients 70 years of age or older who received four or more cycles of CAV or EP had a median survival of 10.7 months; those patients who received three or fewer cycles had a median survival of 3.9 months, and untreated patients survived a median time of 1.1 months ([91]). Multivariate analysis showed that neither increasing age nor comorbidities was an adverse prognostic factor. This review reported that PS, stage, and treatment were the most important prognostic features. Additional studies have confirmed these conclusions, whereas only one retrospective Australian review reported that the complications from therapy adversely affected outcome in the elderly ([92]). In a recent retrospective cohort study examining the impact of chemotherapy on survival among patients 65 years and older with SCLC selected from the SEER database ([93]), 67% of the patients received chemotherapy, mainly EP or CE, which provided a 6.5-month improvement in median survival ($P < .001$), even in patients more than 80 years of age.

With regard to radiation tolerance in the case of LD, elderly patients have been reported to have increased toxicity. Analysis of the patients older than 70 years of age in the INT trial 0096 (EP with conventional TRT vs AHRT) showed that they experienced a higher rate of treatment-related death (>70 years vs ≤70 years: 10% vs 1%, respectively) ([94]). However, the 5-year OS rate for elderly patients was 16%, similar to that in the control arm overall. Altered fractionation did not appear to benefit the elderly subgroup.

In summary, patients with good PS and no significant organ dysfunction should receive full-dose chemotherapy and RT. Their higher risk of treatment-related death implies a need for close monitoring and intense supportive care. Patients with severe comorbidities, a worse PS prior to diagnosis, or the very elderly may require a change in strategy from standard of care. A meta-analysis of randomized trials evaluating patients with "poor-risk" SCLC (generally ED) has shown a benefit of combination chemotherapy over single-agent oral etoposide ([95]). These trials reported that intravenous combination regimens palliated symptoms better and improved median PFS and OS. Therefore, in patients with a poor PS, initial treatment should be combination chemotherapy. Etoposide/cisplatin is recommended over cyclophosphamide- or doxorubicin-based regimens in the elderly population because it is less myelosuppressive ([90]). Several studies have evaluated the CE regimen in the elderly population ([96, 97]). With the exception of the trial reported by Samantas et al, which used low doses of both agents, studies using CE have shown good RRs and tolerance in elderly patients.

In conclusion, carboplatin (area under the curve 5) and etoposide (100 mg/m^2 for 3 days) can be recommended for most patients with SCLC considered "high risk" on the basis of age, comorbidities, or reduced functional status. The time of highest risk for treatment-related mortality is in the first cycle. Prophylactic use of pegfilgrastim is recommended in this group when chemotherapy is given alone. The use of marrow growth factors is contraindicated during concurrent chemoradiation; thus, modest dose reduction and conventional fractionation should be considered. Continued research in this area, especially in the very elderly, is needed.

TARGETED AGENTS

There are no approved targeted agents for SCLC despite a plethora of trials over the past 15 years. Angiogenesis inhibitors, tyrosine kinase and other signal transduction inhibitors, as well as BH3 mimetics targeting apoptosis, have not demonstrated substantial promise in early-phase trials, and none has been validated in phase III studies ([98-101]). However, early experience with the Aurora A kinase inhibitor alisertib and inhibitors of PARP showed promise.

Aurora A Kinase Inhibitors

Data in SCLC cell lines and xenografts indicate that expression of MYC is correlated with sensitivity to Aurora A kinase inhibition ([102]). In a phase II study of alisertib (50 mg by mouth twice a day for 14 days, every 21 days) in solid tumors, a partial RR of 15% was observed in 47 patients with relapsed SCLC ([103]). A randomized phase II trial testing paclitaxel plus either alisertib or placebo in the second-line setting is ongoing (NCT 02038647). There is no molecular selection in this trial.

Poly(ADP-Ribose) Polymerase Inhibitors

Proteomic profiling of a large panel of SCLC cells showed high expression of PARP1 and other repair proteins. Several PARP inhibitors have shown single activity in in vitro and in vivo models of SCLC ([104]). BMN-673 is the most potent PARP1/2 inhibitor, inducing synthetic lethality in tumors deficient in homologous recombination. In a phase I trial of BMN-673, 2 of 11 patients with recurrent SCLC had PR ([105]). Veliparib, another PARP inhibitor, is being studied in randomized phase II trials with EP in newly diagnosed ED patients and with temozolomide in the second-/third-line setting (NCT 01642251 and NCT 01638546).

IMMUNOTHERAPY

Tumor Vaccines

The immunologic and clinical effects of a cancer vaccine consisting of dendritic cells transduced with the full-length, wild-type *p53* gene delivered via an adenoviral vector were tested in a single-arm phase study of 29 patients with ED. Most patients had disease progression to vaccination; however, retrospectively, high ORRs to chemotherapy administered post vaccination were observed (62%). This study supported the clinical use of *p53* vaccination as a chemotherapy sensitizer ([106]). However, this strategy has not been tested prospectively.

Small cell lung cancer expresses numerous gangliosides, including fucosyl monosialotetrahexosylganglioside (GM1), polysialic acid, Disialotetrahexosylganglioside (GM2), GD2, and GD3, not expressed on most normal tissues. The antiidiotypic antibody (BEC-2), which mimics GD3, failed to improve survival in a phase III trial ([107]).

Immune Checkpoint Inhibition

Experience to date with the immune checkpoint inhibitors targeting programmed death receptor 1 (PD-1) or its ligand (PD-L1) in NSCLC suggests efficacy may be directly correlated with degree of tobacco exposure and thus mutation burden and neoepitope expression. Given the strong association with tobacco, SCLC is a relevant tumor for testing. Clinical trials with the PD-1 antibody pembrolizumab planned or ongoing include maintenance following induction chemotherapy (NCT 02359019), combined with irinotecan in recurrent disease (NCT 02331251), and combined with chemoradiation for LD (NCT 02402920).

Ipilimumab, a monoclonal antibody directed against CTLA-4 (cytotoxic T lymphocyte-associated antigen 4), has been given in sequential combination with carboplatin/paclitaxel in a randomized phase II of 130 untreated patients with SCLC. There was improved PFS (HR 0.64; $P = .03$), but not OS (median 12.5 vs 9.1 months for the sequential combination vs chemotherapy alone; $P = .13$) ([108]). A phase III trial of EP with or without ipilimumab has completed accrual and results are awaited (NCT 01450761).

PARANEOPLASTIC SYNDROMES

Paraneoplastic syndromes are a complex spectrum of symptoms secondary to hormones secreted from tumor cells not related to their tissue or organ of origin or to immune-mediated tissue destruction through the production of autoantibodies against tumor cells. Small cell lung cancer is one of the most common cancer types associated with such phenomena. Ectopic hormone production has been associated with ED and a poorer outcome, whereas the antibody-mediated PNSs are associated with more favorable outcomes ([7, 10]). It is critical to recognize the manifestations of PNSs as this may lead to the diagnosis of an underlying, previously unsuspected, malignancy and be useful in monitoring the course of the underlying disease.

Endocrine Paraneoplastic Syndromes

Hyponatremia of malignancy occurs in 15% of patients with SCLC. This disorder is caused by ectopic production of antidiuretic hormone (ADH) from tumor cells, resulting in the SIADH ([109]). Fluid restriction, saline infusion with furosemide diuresis, hypertonic saline, and demeclocycline are options for acute management depending on the severity of symptoms. Chemotherapy should be started urgently.

The incidence of ectopic Cushing syndrome in SCLC is approximately 5%. Patients with SCLC with such a syndrome commonly present with signs and symptoms of rapid-onset hypercortisolism, including weight loss (83%), hypokalemia (87%), abnormal glucose tolerance (73%), and edema (58%) compared with the classic Cushingoid features of moon facies, central obesity, or hirsutism, which are more commonly seen in patients with carcinoid tumors ([109]). This may be due to the slower growth rate of carcinoids, which causes a gradual, rather than acute, increase in ACTH levels. Patients with SCLC with Cushing syndrome have higher hydroxycorticosteroid (17-OHCS) and ACTH plasma levels than those seen in the Cushing disease of pituitary origin. These patients are immunosuppressed and at high risk for opportunistic infections from hypercortisolism; therefore, cortisol-suppressing agents, such as metyrapone or ketoconazole, are recommended prior to initiating myelosuppressive antineoplastic therapy. Radiotherapy can also be used in these cases to palliate and temporize until hypercortisolism has been controlled. Endocrine syndromes parallel cancer control, subsiding with cytoreduction of tumor and recurring with progression.

Neurologic Paraneoplastic Syndromes

Neurologic PNS disorders occur as the result of onconeuronal antibodies recognizing tumor and neuronal cell antigens; thus, they are autoimmune in mechanism. Lambert-Eaton myasthenic syndrome (LEMS), seen in 1% to 3% of patients with SCLC, is caused by autoantibodies directed against P/Q-type voltage-gated calcium channels (VGCCs) on the tumor cells and at presynaptic nerve terminals. These antibodies impair acetylcholine release from the presynaptic motor terminal at the neuromuscular junction and cause transient cranial nerve palsies, upright presyncopal symptoms, proximal muscle weakness with lower extremity predominance, and depressed tendon reflexes ([10]). The electromyographic findings of decreased baseline muscle action potential that increases with repeated stimulations are characteristic and allow for clear-cut diagnosis. Lambert-Eaton myasthenic syndrome represents a favorable prognostic factor presumably based on antitumor immunity ([10]). Unfortunately, these patients frequently experience progressive neurologic decline despite tumor control with treatment due to the fact that by the time neurologic symptoms and deficits emerge, permanent neuronal damage has occurred.

Additional paraneoplastic CNS disorders are associated with inflammation and neuronal loss. The most common syndromes in this group are paraneoplastic cerebellar degeneration, limbic encephalitis, opsoclonus-myoclonus, and diffuse encephalitis with multifocal neurologic symptoms ([109]). It remains unclear whether these syndromes or the presence of antibodies can serve as predictive markers of tumor response or progression.

THE SPECTRUM OF NEUROENDOCRINE CARCINOMAS

Neuroendocrine carcinomas are a wide spectrum of diseases, including low-grade typical carcinoid (TC), intermediate-grade atypical carcinoid (AT), and high-grade neuroendocrine carcinomas (small cell carcinoma and LCNEC) ([110]). Carcinoid tumors are more often found in the gastrointestinal system than in the lungs. Behavior of these tumors is often dependent on grade of differentiation. The histopathological features of these tumors are identical regardless of their anatomic location; thus, the determination of a primary site often requires careful clinical evaluation.

Many of the same IHC markers are used to define NETs, regardless of primary site. Some IHC stains appear to be expressed in tumors in certain locations. For example, TTF-1 is commonly positive in thoracic tumors, while CDX2 is more commonly expressed in gastrointestinal tumors. On limited biopsies, definitive tumor grading may be challenging, especially in tumors of low and intermediate grade.

Pulmonary NETs comprise approximately 20% of all invasive lung malignancies. After SCLC, LCNEC accounts for 3% of resected lung cancers in surgical series, and TCs account for 1% to 2% of lung cancers. Atypical carcinoid is the rarest lung NET, as it comprises approximately 10% of all lung carcinoids, accounting for 0.1% to 0.2% of invasive lung cancers. Large cell neuroendocrine carcinoma is classified as an NSCLC but has similar biology, behavior, and natural history to SCLC ([11]). Table 17-2 shows the grading criteria and the histopathological features for pulmonary NETs ([111]). The different types of NETs possess diverse epidemiological, clinical, pathological, and molecular features ([112]).

Surgical resection is recommended for localized pulmonary NETs if pulmonary reserve is adequate. For surgically unfit patients or for exceptional low-grade cases, transbronchoscopic resection may be considered. Approximately 5% to 20% of bronchial TCs and 30% to 70% of ATs metastasize to lymph

Table 17-2 Grading Criteria and Histologic Features of Pulmonary Neuroendocrine Tumors

Grade	Histology	Conventional Nomenclature
Low grade (well-differentiated)	• < 3 mitotic figures × 10 hpf • Absent or only focal punctate necrosis • Absent or mild nuclear atypia	Carcinoid
Intermediate grade (moderately-differentiated)	• 3-10 mitotic figures × 10 hpf • Comedonecrosis present • Moderate nuclear atypia	Atypical carcinoid
High grade, poorly differentiated (small cell carcinoma)	• > 10 mitotic figures × 10 hpf • Necrosis present • Prominent nuclear atypia with or without positive NE markers	Small cell carcinoma
High grade, poorly differentiated (large cell neuroendocrine carcinoma)	• > 10 mitotic figures × 10 hpf • Necrosis present • Prominent nuclear atypia with positive NE morphologic features and positive or negative NE markers	Large cell neuroendocrine carcinoma

hpf, high-power field; NE, neuroendocrine.
Data from Moran CA, Suster S, Coppola D, et al: Neuroendocrine carcinomas of the lung: a critical analysis, *Am J Clin Pathol* 2009 Feb;131(2):206-221.

nodes; thus, a complete mediastinal lymph node sampling or dissection at the time of surgery is recommended. The 5-year survival rates of surgically resected pulmonary TCs and ATs range between 87% and 100% and 30% and 95%, respectively ([113]). Patients with TCs are unlikely to benefit from adjuvant systemic therapy, even if lymph node involvement is present. The ATs have higher recurrence rates; therefore, despite the lack of consensus, adjuvant EP with or without RT for patients with stage II or III may be considered ([112]).

Due to the rarity of LCNEC, most of the data regarding treatment are retrospective in nature. In general, there is a worse prognosis for patients with resected LCNEC compared to those with stage-matched other NSCLC. Treatment recommendations for this entity are extrapolated from treatment paradigms for SCLC. For resected stage I and II LCNEC, four cycles of adjuvant EP are recommended. For locally advanced disease (stage III), concurrent chemoradiation/chemotherapy is recommended (one or two cycles of EP concurrent with RT followed by additional chemotherapy to complete a total of four courses). For stage IV disease, four to six cycles of EP and palliative RT, if clinically indicated, are recommended. Prophylactic cranial irradiation cannot be routinely recommended due to limited data on the incidence of brain metastases in patients with LCNEC ([110]).

SUMMARY

Small cell lung cancer is a very aggressive malignancy affecting 30,000 or more individuals annually in the United States. Most patients present with widespread disease at diagnosis, and despite the initial high sensitivity to chemotherapy and RT, resistance emerges rapidly. Extensive research over the last few decades has not significantly impacted the therapeutic paradigm of SCLC. The standard of care for both LD and ED is etoposide/platin chemotherapy for a minimum of four courses. Early integration of concurrent TRT is indicated for LD. Prophylactic cranial irradiation can be offered to patients who have excellent disease control following initial therapy. Major advances in treatment will require greater understanding of the drivers of the pan-resistant phenotype that characterizes recurrent disease and development of therapy to which these cells will be vulnerable. Recent discoveries from bench research and early-phase clinical investigation fuel the hope that outcomes for patients with SCLC can be improved in the next decade.

REFERENCES

1. Govindan R, Page N, Morgensztern D, et al. Changing epidemiology of small-cell lung cancer in the United States over the last 30 years: analysis of the surveillance, epidemiologic, and end results database. *J Clin Oncol.* 2006;24(28):4539-4544. PMID: 17008692.
2. Vallieres E, Shepherd FA, Crowley J, et al. The IASLC Lung Cancer Staging Project: proposals regarding the relevance of TNM in the pathologic staging of small cell lung cancer in the forthcoming (seventh) edition of the TNM classification for lung cancer. *J Thorac Oncol.* 2009;4(9):1049-1059. PMID: 19652623.
3. Barbone F, Bovenzi M, Cavallieri F, Stanta G. Cigarette smoking and histologic type of lung cancer in men. Chest. 1997;112(6):1474-1479. PMID: 9404741.

4. Dowlati A, Wildey G. Defining subgroups of small-cell lung cancer. *J Thorac Oncol.* 2014;9(6):750-751. PMID: 24828659.
5. Videtic GM, Stitt LW, Dar AR, Kocha WI, Tomiak AT, Truong PT, et al. Continued cigarette smoking by patients receiving concurrent chemoradiotherapy for limited-stage small-cell lung cancer is associated with decreased survival. *J Clin Oncol.* 2003;21(8):1544-1549. PMID: 12697879.
6. Green RA, Humphrey E, Close H, Patno ME. Alkylating agents in bronchogenic carcinoma. *Am J Med.* 1969;46(4):516-525. PMID: 5791000.
7. Yip D, Harper PG. Predictive and prognostic factors in small cell lung cancer: current status. *Lung cancer.* 2000;28(3):173-185. PMID: 10812187.
8. Shepherd FA, Evans WK, Feld R, et al. Adjuvant chemotherapy following surgical resection for small-cell carcinoma of the lung. *J Clin Oncol.* 1988;6(5):832-838. PMID: 2835443.
9. Ihde DC, Makuch RW, Carney DN, et al. Prognostic implications of stage of disease and sites of metastases in patients with small cell carcinoma of the lung treated with intensive combination chemotherapy. *Am Rev Respir Dis.* 1981;123(5):500-507. PMID: 6263137.
10. Maddison P, Newsom-Davis J, Mills KR, Souhami RL. Favourable prognosis in Lambert-Eaton myasthenic syndrome and small-cell lung carcinoma. *Lancet.* 1999 9;353(9147):117-118. PMID: 10023900.
11. Zakowski MF. Pathology of small cell carcinoma of the lung. *Semin Oncol.* 2003;30(1):3-8. PMID: 12635085.
12. Johnson BE, Whang-Peng J, Naylor SL, et al. Retention of chromosome 3 in extrapulmonary small cell cancer shown by molecular and cytogenetic studies. *J Natl Cancer Inst.* 1989;81(16):1223-1228. PMID: 2569043.
13. Hiroshima K, Iyoda A, Shida T, et al. Distinction of pulmonary large cell neuroendocrine carcinoma from small cell lung carcinoma: a morphological, immunohistochemical, and molecular analysis. *Mod Pathol.* 2006;19(10):1358-1368. PMID: 16862075.
14. Agoff SN, Lamps LW, Philip AT, et al. Thyroid transcription factor-1 is expressed in extrapulmonary small cell carcinomas but not in other extrapulmonary neuroendocrine tumors. *Mod Pathol.* 2000;13(3):238-242. PMID: 10757334.
15. Travis WD. Update on small cell carcinoma and its differentiation from squamous cell carcinoma and other non-small cell carcinomas. *Mod Pathol.* 2012;25(Suppl 1):S18-S30. PMID: 22214967.
16. Wistuba, II, Gazdar AF, Minna JD. Molecular genetics of small cell lung carcinoma. *Semin Oncol.* 2001;28(2 Suppl 4):3-13. PMID: 11479891.
17. Hougaard S, Norgaard P, Abrahamsen N, Moses HL, Spang-Thomsen M, Skovgaard Poulsen H. Inactivation of the transforming growth factor beta type II receptor in human small cell lung cancer cell lines. *Br J Cancer.* 1999;79(7-8):1005-1011. PMID: 10098728. PMCID: 2362261.
18. Ji L, Roth JA. Tumor suppressor FUS1 signaling pathway. *J Thorac Oncol.* 2008;3(4):327-330. PMID: 18379348. PMCID: 3370667.
19. Burbee DG, Forgacs E, Zochbauer-Muller S, et al. Epigenetic inactivation of RASSF1A in lung and breast cancers and malignant phenotype suppression. *J Natl Cancer Inst.* 2001;93(9): 691-699. PMID: 11333291.
20. D'Angelo SP, Pietanza MC. The molecular pathogenesis of small cell lung cancer. *Cancer Biol Ther.* 2010;10(1):1-10. PMID: 21361067.
21. Tamborini E, Bonadiman L, Negri T, et al. Detection of overexpressed and phosphorylated wild-type kit receptor in surgical specimens of small cell lung cancer. *Clin Cancer Res.* 2004;10(24):8214-8219. PMID: 15623596.
22. Pleasance ED, Stephens PJ, O'Meara S, et al. A small-cell lung cancer genome with complex signatures of tobacco exposure. *Nature.* 2010;463(7278):184-190. PMID: 20016488. PMCID: 2880489.
23. Rudin CM, Durinck S, Stawiski EW, et al. Comprehensive genomic analysis identifies SOX2 as a frequently amplified gene in small-cell lung cancer. *Nat Genet.* 2012;44(10): 1111-1116. PMID: 22941189. PMCID: 3557461.
24. Byers LA, Rudin CM. Small cell lung cancer: Where do we go from here? *Cancer.* 2015;121(5):664-672. PMID: 25336398.
25. Matthews MJ, Kanhouwa S, Pickren J, Robinette D. Frequency of residual and metastatic tumor in patients undergoing curative surgical resection for lung cancer. Cancer chemotherapy reports Part 3. 1973;4(2):63-67. PMID: 4580861.
26. Fox W, Scadding JG. Treatment of oat-celled carcinoma of the bronchus. *Lancet.* 1973;2(7829):616-617. PMID: 4125403.
27. Warde P, Payne D. Does thoracic irradiation improve survival and local control in limited-stage small-cell carcinoma of the lung? A meta-analysis. *J Clin Oncol.* 1992;10(6):890-895. PMID: 1316951.
28. Pignon JP, Arriagada R, Ihde DC, et al. A meta-analysis of thoracic radiotherapy for small-cell lung cancer. *N Engl J Med.* 1992 3;327(23):1618-1624. PMID: 1331787.
29. Sundstrom S, Bremnes RM, Kaasa S, et al. Cisplatin and etoposide regimen is superior to cyclophosphamide, epirubicin, and vincristine regimen in small-cell lung cancer: results from a randomized phase III trial with 5 years' follow-up. *J Clin Oncol.* 2002 15;20(24):4665-4672. PMID: 12488411.
30. Fukuoka M, Furuse K, Saijo N, et al. Randomized trial of cyclophosphamide, doxorubicin, and vincristine versus cisplatin and etoposide versus alternation of these regimens in small-cell lung cancer. *J Natl Cancer Inst.* 1991 19;83(12):855-861. PMID: 1648142.
31. Levitan N, Dowlati A, Shina D, et al. Multi-institutional phase I/II trial of paclitaxel, cisplatin, and etoposide with concurrent radiation for limited-stage small-cell lung carcinoma. *J Clin Oncol.* 2000;18(5):1102-1109. PMID: 10694563.
32. Turrisi AT 3rd, Kim K, Blum R, et al. Twice-daily compared with once-daily thoracic radiotherapy in limited small-cell lung cancer treated concurrently with cisplatin and etoposide. *N Engl J Med.* 1999 28;340(4):265-271. PMID: 9920950.
33. Movsas B, Moughan J, Komaki R, et al. Radiotherapy patterns of care study in lung carcinoma. *J Clin Oncol.* 2003;21(24): 4553-4559. PMID: 14597743.
34. Bogart JA, Herndon JE 2nd, Lyss AP, et al. 70 Gy thoracic radiotherapy is feasible concurrent with chemotherapy for limited-stage small-cell lung cancer: analysis of Cancer and Leukemia Group B study 39808. *Int J Radiat Oncol Biol Phys.* 2004 1;59(2):460-8. PMID: 15145163.
35. Komaki R, Paulus R, DS E, eds. A phase II study of accelerated high-dose thoracic radiation therapy (AHTRT) with concurrent chemotherapy for limited small cell lung cancer: RTOG 0239 [Abstract 7527]. J Clin Oncol. 2009;27(Suppl):15s.
36. Murray N, Coy P, Pater JL, et al. Importance of timing for thoracic irradiation in the combined modality treatment of limited-stage small-cell lung cancer. The National Cancer Institute of Canada Clinical Trials Group. *J Clin Oncol.* 1993;11(2): 336-344. PMID: 8381164.
37. Takada M, Fukuoka M, Kawahara M, et al. Phase III study of concurrent versus sequential thoracic radiotherapy in combination with cisplatin and etoposide for limited-stage small-cell lung cancer: results of the Japan Clinical Oncology Group Study 9104. *J Clin Oncol.* 2002;20(14):3054-3060. PMID: 12118018.
38. De Ruysscher D, Pijls-Johannesma M, Bentzen SM, et al. Time between the first day of chemotherapy and the last day of chest radiation is the most important predictor of survival in limited-disease small-cell lung cancer. *J Clin Oncol.* 2006;24(7):1057-1063. PMID: 16505424.
39. Rossi A, Di Maio M, Chiodini P, et al. Carboplatin- or

cisplatin-based chemotherapy in first-line treatment of small-cell lung cancer: the COCIS meta-analysis of individual patient data. *J Clin Oncol.* 2012;30(14):1692-1698. PMID: 22473169.

40. Lee SM, James LE, Qian W, et al. Comparison of gemcitabine and carboplatin versus cisplatin and etoposide for patients with poor-prognosis small cell lung cancer. *Thorax.* 2009;64(1):75-80. PMID: 18786981.
41. Skarlos DV, Samantas E, Kosmidis P, et al. Randomized comparison of etoposide-cisplatin vs etoposide-carboplatin and irradiation in small-cell lung cancer. A Hellenic Co-operative Oncology Group study. *Ann Oncol.* 1994;5(7):601-607. PMID: 7993835.
42. Evans WK, Osoba D, Feld R, Shepherd FA, Bazos MJ, DeBoer G. Etoposide (VP-16) and cisplatin: an effective treatment for relapse in small-cell lung cancer. *J Clin Oncol.* 1985;3(1):65-71. PMID: 2981293.
43. Evans WK, Shepherd FA, Feld R, Osoba D, Dang P, Deboer G. VP-16 and cisplatin as first-line therapy for small-cell lung cancer. *J Clin Oncol.* 1985;3(11):1471-1477. PMID: 2997406.
44. Roth BJ, Johnson DH, Einhorn LH, et al. Randomized study of cyclophosphamide, doxorubicin, and vincristine versus etoposide and cisplatin versus alternation of these two regimens in extensive small-cell lung cancer: a phase III trial of the Southeastern Cancer Study Group. *J Clin Oncol.* 1992;10(2):282-291. PMID: 1310103.
45. Bozcuk H, Artac M, Ozdogan M, Savas B. Does maintenance/consolidation chemotherapy have a role in the management of small cell lung cancer (SCLC)? A metaanalysis of the published controlled trials. *Cancer.* 2005;104(12):2650-2657. PMID: 16284984.
46. Hanna NH, Sandier AB, Loehrer PJ Sr, et al. Maintenance daily oral etoposide versus no further therapy following induction chemotherapy with etoposide plus ifosfamide plus cisplatin in extensive small-cell lung cancer: a Hoosier Oncology Group randomized study. *Ann Oncol.* 2002;13(1):95-102. PMID: 11863118.
47. Schiller JH, Adak S, Cella D, DeVore RF 3rd, Johnson DH. Topotecan versus observation after cisplatin plus etoposide in extensive-stage small-cell lung cancer: E7593—a phase III trial of the Eastern Cooperative Oncology Group. *J Clin Oncol.* 2001;19(8):2114-2122. PMID: 11304763.
48. Noda K, Nishiwaki Y, Kawahara M, et al. Irinotecan plus cisplatin compared with etoposide plus cisplatin for extensive small-cell lung cancer. *N Engl J Med.* 2002;346(2):85-91. PMID: 11784874.
49. Hanna N, Bunn PA Jr, Langer C, et al. Randomized phase III trial comparing irinotecan/cisplatin with etoposide/cisplatin in patients with previously untreated extensive-stage disease small-cell lung cancer. *J Clin Oncol.* 2006;24(13):2038-2043. PMID: 16648503.
50. Lara PN Jr, Natale R, Crowley J, et al. Phase III trial of irinotecan/cisplatin compared with etoposide/cisplatin in extensive-stage small-cell lung cancer: clinical and pharmacogenomic results from SWOG S0124. *J Clin Oncol.* 2009;27(15):2530-2535. PMID: 19349543. PMCID: 2684855.
51. Zatloukal P, Cardenal F, Szczesna A, et al. A multicenter international randomized phase III study comparing cisplatin in combination with irinotecan or etoposide in previously untreated small-cell lung cancer patients with extensive disease. *Ann Oncol.* 2010;21(9):1810-1816. PMID: 20231298.
52. Eckardt JR, von Pawel J, Papai Z, et al. Open-label, multicenter, randomized, phase III study comparing oral topotecan/cisplatin versus etoposide/cisplatin as treatment for chemotherapy-naive patients with extensive-disease small-cell lung cancer. *J Clin Oncol.* 2006;24(13):2044-2051. PMID: 16648504.
53. Loehrer PJ Sr, Ansari R, Gonin R, et al. Cisplatin plus etoposide with and without ifosfamide in extensive small-cell lung cancer: a Hoosier Oncology Group study. *J Clin Oncol.* 1995;13(10):2594-2599. PMID: 7595712.
54. Pujol JL, Daures JP, Riviere A, et al. Etoposide plus cisplatin with or without the combination of 4'-epidoxorubicin plus cyclophosphamide in treatment of extensive small-cell lung cancer: a French Federation of Cancer Institutes multicenter phase III randomized study. *J Natl Cancer Inst.* 2001;93(4):300-308. PMID: 11181777.
55. Goldie JH, Coldman AJ. A mathematic model for relating the drug sensitivity of tumors to their spontaneous mutation rate. *Cancer Treat Rep.* 1979;63(11-12):1727-1733. PMID: 526911.
56. Postmus PE, Scagliotti G, Groen HJ, et al. Standard versus alternating non-cross-resistant chemotherapy in extensive small cell lung cancer: an EORTC Phase III trial. European journal of cancer. 1996;32A(9):1498-1503. PMID: 8911108.
57. Murray N, Shah A, Osoba D, et al. Intensive weekly chemotherapy for the treatment of extensive-stage small-cell lung cancer. *J Clin Oncol.* 1991;9(9):1632-1638. PMID: 1651995.
58. Furuse K, Fukuoka M, Nishiwaki Y, et al. Phase III study of intensive weekly chemotherapy with recombinant human granulocyte colony-stimulating factor versus standard chemotherapy in extensive-disease small-cell lung cancer. The Japan Clinical Oncology Group. *J Clin Oncol.* 1998;16(6):2126-2132. PMID: 9626212.
59. Klasa RJ, Murray N, Coldman AJ. Dose-intensity meta-analysis of chemotherapy regimens in small-cell carcinoma of the lung. *J Clin Oncol.* 1991;9(3):499-508. PMID: 1847968.
60. Ihde DC, Mulshine JL, Kramer BS, et al. Prospective randomized comparison of high-dose and standard-dose etoposide and cisplatin chemotherapy in patients with extensive-stage small-cell lung cancer. *J Clin Oncol.* 1994;12(10):2022-2034. PMID: 7931470.
61. Heigener DF, Manegold C, Jager E, Saal JG, Zuna I, Gatzemeier U. Multicenter randomized open-label phase III study comparing efficacy, safety, and tolerability of conventional carboplatin plus etoposide versus dose-intensified carboplatin plus etoposide plus lenograstim in small-cell lung cancer in "extensive disease" stage. *Am J Clin Oncol.* 2009;32(1):61-64. PMID: 19194127.
62. Steward WP, von Pawel J, Gatzemeier U, et al. Effects of granulocyte-macrophage colony-stimulating factor and dose intensification of V-ICE chemotherapy in small-cell lung cancer: a prospective randomized study of 300 patients. *J Clin Oncol.* 1998;16(2):642-650. PMID: 9469353.
63. Thatcher N, Girling DJ, Hopwood P, Sambrook RJ, Qian W, Stephens RJ. Improving survival without reducing quality of life in small-cell lung cancer patients by increasing the dose-intensity of chemotherapy with granulocyte colony-stimulating factor support: results of a British Medical Research Council Multicenter Randomized Trial. Medical Research Council Lung Cancer Working Party. *J Clin Oncol.* 2000;18(2):395-404. PMID: 10637255.
64. Thatcher N, Qian W, Clark PI, et al. Ifosfamide, carboplatin, and etoposide with midcycle vincristine versus standard chemotherapy in patients with small-cell lung cancer and good performance status: clinical and quality-of-life results of the British Medical Research Council multicenter randomized LU21 trial. *J Clin Oncol.* 2005;23(33):8371-8379. PMID: 16293867.
65. Lorigan P, Woll PJ, O'Brien ME, Ashcroft LF, Sampson MR, Thatcher N. Randomized phase III trial of dose-dense chemotherapy supported by whole-blood hematopoietic progenitors in better-prognosis small-cell lung cancer. *J Natl Cancer Inst.* 2005;97(9):666-674. PMID: 15870437.
66. Buchholz E, Manegold C, Pilz L, Thatcher N, Drings P. Standard versus dose-intensified chemotherapy with sequential reinfusion of hematopoietic progenitor cells in small cell lung cancer patients with favorable prognosis. *J Thorac Oncol.*

2007;2(1):51-58. PMID: 17410010.

67. Jeremic B, Shibamoto Y, Nikolic N, et al. Role of radiation therapy in the combined-modality treatment of patients with extensive disease small-cell lung cancer: a randomized study. *J Clin Oncol.* 1999;17(7):2092-2099. PMID: 10561263.
68. Slotman BJ, van Tinteren H, Praag JO, et al. Use of thoracic radiotherapy for extensive stage small-cell lung cancer: a phase 3 randomised controlled trial. *Lancet.* 2014;385(9962):36-42. PMID: 25230595.
69. von Pawel J, Schiller JH, Shepherd FA, et al. Topotecan versus cyclophosphamide, doxorubicin, and vincristine for the treatment of recurrent small-cell lung cancer. *J Clin Oncol.* 1999;17(2):658-667. PMID: 10080612.
70. Batist G, Ihde DC, Zabell A, et al. Small-cell carcinoma of lung: reinduction therapy after late relapse. *Ann Intern Med.* 1983;98(4):472-474. PMID: 6301321.
71. Giaccone G, Ferrati P, Donadio M, Testore F, Calciati A. Reinduction chemotherapy in small cell lung cancer. *Eur J Cancer Clin Oncol.* 1987;23(11):1697-9. PMID: 2828074.
72. Vincent M, Evans B, Smith I. First-line chemotherapy rechallenge after relapse in small cell lung cancer. Cancer Chemother Pharmacol. 1988;21(1):45-48. PMID: 2830043.
73. Eckardt JR, von Pawel J, Pujol JL, et al. Phase III study of oral compared with intravenous topotecan as second-line therapy in small-cell lung cancer. *J Clin Oncol.* 2007;25(15):2086-2092. PMID: 17513814.
74. O'Brien ME, Ciuleanu TE, Tsekov H, et al. Phase III trial comparing supportive care alone with supportive care with oral topotecan in patients with relapsed small-cell lung cancer. *J Clin Oncol.* 2006;24(34):5441-5447. PMID: 17135646.
75. Masuda N, Fukuoka M, Kusunoki Y, et al. CPT-11: a new derivative of camptothecin for the treatment of refractory or relapsed small-cell lung cancer. *J Clin Oncol.* 1992;10(8):1225-1229. PMID: 1321891.
76. Jotte R, Conkling P, Reynolds C, et al. Randomized phase II trial of single-agent amrubicin or topotecan as second-line treatment in patients with small-cell lung cancer sensitive to first-line platinum-based chemotherapy. *J Clin Oncol.* 2011;29(3):287-293. PMID: 21135284.
77. von Pawel J, Jotte R, Spigel DR, et al. Randomized phase III trial of amrubicin versus topotecan as second-line treatment for patients with small-cell lung cancer. *J Clin Oncol.* 2014;32(35):4012-4019. PMID: 25385727.
78. Pietanza MC, Kadota K, Huberman K, et al. Phase II trial of temozolomide in patients with relapsed sensitive or refractory small cell lung cancer, with assessment of methylguanine-DNA methyltransferase as a potential biomarker. *Clin Cancer Res.* 2012;18(4):1138-1145. PMID: 22228633.
79. Murray KJ, Scott C, Greenberg HM, et al. A randomized phase III study of accelerated hyperfractionation versus standard in patients with unresected brain metastases: a report of the Radiation Therapy Oncology Group (RTOG) 9104. *Int J Radiat Oncol Biol Phys.* 1997;39(3):571-574. PMID: 9336134.
80. Imanaka K, Sugimoto K, Obayashi Y, Tada K, Sakurai T, Iwasaki H. Reirradiation therapy for brain metastases from small cell lung cancer. Radiation medicine. 1998;16(2):153-156. PMID: 9650907.
81. Sneed PK, Suh JH, Goetsch SJ, et al. A multi-institutional review of radiosurgery alone vs radiosurgery with whole brain radiotherapy as the initial management of brain metastases. *Int J Radiat Oncol Biol Phys.* 2002;53(3):519-526. PMID: 12062592.
82. Grossi F, Scolaro T, Tixi L, Loprevite M, Ardizzoni A. The role of systemic chemotherapy in the treatment of brain metastases from small-cell lung cancer. *Crit Rev Oncol/Hematol.* 2001;37(1):61-67. PMID: 11164720.
83. Auperin A, Arriagada R, Pignon JP, et al. Prophylactic cranial irradiation for patients with small-cell lung cancer in complete remission. Prophylactic Cranial Irradiation Overview Collaborative Group. *N Engl J Med.* 1999 12;341(7):476-484. PMID: 10441603.
84. Meert AP, Paesmans M, Berghmans T, et al. Prophylactic cranial irradiation in small cell lung cancer: a systematic review of the literature with meta-analysis. *BMC Cancer.* 2001;1:5. PMID: 11432756. PMCID: 34096.
85. Le Pechoux C, Dunant A, Senan S, et al. Standard-dose versus higher-dose prophylactic cranial irradiation (PCI) in patients with limited-stage small-cell lung cancer in complete remission after chemotherapy and thoracic radiotherapy (PCI 99-01, EORTC 22003-08004, RTOG 0212, and IFCT 99-01): a randomised clinical trial. The *Lancet Oncol.* 2009;10(5):467-474. PMID: 19386548.
86. Wolfson AH, Bae K, Komaki R, et al. Primary analysis of a phase II randomized trial Radiation Therapy Oncology Group (RTOG) 0212: impact of different total doses and schedules of prophylactic cranial irradiation on chronic neurotoxicity and quality of life for patients with limited-disease small-cell lung cancer. *Int J Radiat Oncol Biol Phys.* 2011;81(1):77-84. PMID: 20800380. PMCID: 3024447.
87. Slotman B, Faivre-Finn C, Kramer G, et al. Prophylactic cranial irradiation in extensive small-cell lung cancer. *N Engl J Med.* 2007;357(7):664-672. PMID: 17699816.
88. Slotman BJ, Mauer ME, Bottomley A, et al. Prophylactic cranial irradiation in extensive disease small-cell lung cancer: short-term health-related quality of life and patient reported symptoms: results of an international Phase III randomized controlled trial by the EORTC Radiation Oncology and Lung Cancer Groups. *J Clin Oncol.* 2009;27(1):78-84. PMID: 19047288. PMCID: 2645093.
89. Seto T, Takahashi T, Yamanaka T, et al., eds. Prophylactic cranial irradiation (PCI) has a detrimental effect on the overall survival (OS) of patients (pts) with extensive disease small cell lung cancer (ED-SCLC): Results of a Japanese randomized phase III trial [Abstract 7503]. American Society of Medical Oncology (ASCO) Annual Meeting; 2014. J Clin Oncol. 2014;32(Suppl):5s.
90. Johnson DH. Small cell lung cancer in the elderly patient. *Semin Oncol.* 1997;24(4):484-491.
91. Shepherd FA, Amdemichael E, Evans WK, et al. Treatment of small cell lung cancer in the elderly. *J Am Geriatr Soc.* 1994;42(1):64-70. PMID: 8277118.
92. Findlay MP, Griffin AM, Raghavan D, et al. Retrospective review of chemotherapy for small cell lung cancer in the elderly: does the end justify the means? *Eur J Cancer.* 1991;27(12):1597-1601. PMID: 1664217.
93. Caprario LC, Kent DM, Strauss GM. Effects of chemotherapy on survival of elderly patients with small-cell lung cancer: analysis of the SEER-medicare database. *J Thorac Oncol.* 2013;8(10):1272-1281. PMID: 24457238. PMCID: 3901951.
94. Yuen AR, Zou G, Turrisi AT, et al. Similar outcome of elderly patients in intergroup trial 0096: cisplatin, etoposide, and thoracic radiotherapy administered once or twice daily in limited stage small cell lung carcinoma. *Cancer.* 2000;89(9):1953-1960. PMID: 11064352.
95. Girling DJ. Comparison of oral etoposide and standard intravenous multidrug chemotherapy for small-cell lung cancer: a stopped multicentre randomised trial. Medical Research Council Lung Cancer Working Party. *Lancet.* 1996;348(9027):563-566. PMID: 8774567.
96. Samantas E, Skarlos DV, Pectasides D, et al. Combination chemotherapy with low doses of weekly carboplatin and oral etoposide in poor risk small cell lung cancer. *Lung Cancer.* 1999;23(2):159-168. PMID: 10217620.
97. Okamoto H, Watanabe K, Nishiwaki Y, et al. Phase II study of area under the plasma-concentration-versus-time curve-based carboplatin plus standard-dose intravenous etoposide in elderly patients with small-cell lung cancer. *J Clin Oncol.*

1999;17(11):3540-3545. PMID: 10550152.

98. Pujol JL, Lavole A, Quoix E, et al. Randomized phase II-III study of bevacizumab in combination with chemotherapy in previously untreated extensive small-cell lung cancer: results from the IFCT-0802 trialdagger. *Ann Oncol.* 2015;26(5):908-914. PMID: 25688059.
99. Pujol JL, Breton JL, Gervais R, et al. Phase III double-blind, placebo-controlled study of thalidomide in extensive-disease small-cell lung cancer after response to chemotherapy: an intergroup study FNCLCC cleo04 IFCT 00-01. *J Clin Oncol.* 2007;25(25):3945-3951. PMID: 17761978. Epub 2007/09/01. eng.
100. Rudin CM, Salgia R, Wang X, et al. Randomized phase II Study of carboplatin and etoposide with or without the bcl-2 antisense oligonucleotide oblimersen for extensive-stage small-cell lung cancer: CALGB 30103. *J Clin Oncol.* 2008;26(6):870-876. PMID: 18281659. PMCID: 3715075.
101. Dy GK, Miller AA, Mandrekar SJ, et al. A phase II trial of imatinib (ST1571) in patients with c-kit expressing relapsed small-cell lung cancer: a CALGB and NCCTG study. *Ann Oncol.* 2005;16(11):1811-1816. PMID: 16087693.
102. Hook KE, Garza SJ, Lira ME, et al. An integrated genomic approach to identify predictive biomarkers of response to the aurora kinase inhibitor PF-03814735. *Mol Cancer Ther.* 2012;11(3):710-719. PMID: 22222631.
103. Melichar B, Adenis A, Havel L, et al. Phase (Ph) I/II study of investigational Aurora A kinase (AAK) inhibitor MLN8237 (alisertib): updated ph II results in patients (pts) with small cell lung cancer (SCLC), non-SCLC (NSCLC), breast cancer (BrC), head and neck squamous cell carcinoma (HNSCC), and gastroesophageal cancer (GE) [Abstract]. 2013 ASCO Annual Meeting. *J Clin Oncol.* 2013;13(suppl).
104. Byers LA, Wang J, Nilsson MB, et al. Proteomic profiling identifies dysregulated pathways in small cell lung cancer and novel therapeutic targets including PARP1. *Cancer Discov.* 2012;2(9):798-811. PMID: 22961666. PMCID: 3567922.
105. Wainberg Z, Rafii S, Ramanathan R, et al. Safety and antitumor activity of the PARP inhibitor BMN673 in a phase 1 trial recruiting metastatic small-cell lung cancer (SCLC) and germline BRCAmutation carrier cancer patients [Abstract 7522]. American Association of Clinical Oncology 2014 Annual Meeting. *J Clin Oncol.* 2014;32(suppl):5s.
106. Antonia SJ, Mirza N, Fricke I, et al. Combination of p53 cancer vaccine with chemotherapy in patients with extensive stage small cell lung cancer. *Clin Cancer Res.* 2006;12(3 Pt 1):878-887. PMID: 16467102.
107. Giaccone G, Debruyne C, Felip E, et al. Phase III study of adjuvant vaccination with Bec2/bacille Calmette-Guerin in responding patients with limited-disease small-cell lung cancer (European Organisation for Research and Treatment of Cancer 08971-08971B; Silva Study). *J Clin Oncol.* 2005;23(28):6854-6864. PMID: 16192577.
108. Reck M, Bondarenko I, Luft A, et al. Ipilimumab in combination with paclitaxel and carboplatin as first-line therapy in extensive-disease-small-cell lung cancer: results from a randomized, double-blind, multicenter phase 2 trial. *Ann Oncol.* 2013;24(1):75-83. PMID: 22858559.
109. Gandhi L, Johnson BE. Paraneoplastic syndromes associated with small cell lung cancer. *J Natl Compr Cancer Netw.* 2006;4(6):631-638. PMID: 16813730.
110. Glisson BS, Moran CA. Large-cell neuroendocrine carcinoma: controversies in diagnosis and treatment. *J Natl Compr Cancer Netw.* 2011;9(10):1122-1129. PMID: 21975912.
111. Moran CA, Suster S, Coppola D, Wick MR. Neuroendocrine carcinomas of the lung: a critical analysis. *Am J Clin Pathol.* 2009;131(2):206-221. PMID: 19141381.
112. Kunz PL. Carcinoid and neuroendocrine tumors: building on success. *J Clin Oncol.* 2015;33(16):1855-1863. PMID: 25918282.
113. Ferguson MK, Landreneau RJ, Hazelrigg SR, et al. Long-term outcome after resection for bronchial carcinoid tumors. *Eur J Cardiothorac Surg.* 2000;18(2):156-161. PMID: 10925223.

18

Non-Small Cell Lung Cancer

第十八章　非小细胞肺癌

Diogo Bugano Diniz Gomes
Kathryn A. Gold
Don L. Gibbons
Commentary: George A. Eapen

中文导读

肺癌是目前死亡率和确诊率最高的恶性肿瘤之一，其中非小细胞肺癌一直是肿瘤学研究中的重点。本章首先从非小细胞肺癌的流行病学展开叙述，接着指出已开展的关于肺癌的病因研究已取得了显著的成效，吸烟与肺癌的因果关系已经得到证实。在病因学理论的基础上，本章进一步提出了非小细胞肺癌的预防策略。近年来，随着实验技术的迅速发展，非小细胞肺癌的组织学和分子病理学研究成为新的热点，肺癌的分型也逐渐细化，新的分子分型不断被发现，这也影响了非小细胞肺癌的治疗。在介绍了临床表现和诊断要点之后，本章对非小细胞肺癌的治疗方法进行了详述。除了常规的手术和放疗、化疗外，靶向药物和免疫治疗在非小细胞肺癌治疗中发挥的作用已成为新的研究热点。本章对相关药物的临床试验进行了汇总，并指导不同分期、分型的患者如何选择最佳治疗方案，并在最后指出这一命题仍有广阔的研究前景。

INTRODUCTION

Lung cancer is the third most commonly diagnosed cancer, after breast and prostate cancers, but it is the most common cause of cancer-related death ([1]). Every year, 1.5 million patients die of lung cancer worldwide ([1]). About 70% of patients will be diagnosed with advanced stages that are not amenable to curative therapies. Only 15% of all patients diagnosed with lung cancer are alive 5 years after diagnosis.

Lung cancer is broadly divided into small cell lung cancer (SCLC) and non–small cell lung cancer (NSCLC). Approximately 85% of lung cancer is NSCLC. This chapter briefly describes the epidemiology, etiology, histology, prevention, and molecular biology of NSCLC. The major focus will be clinical presentation, diagnosis, staging, and treatment based on current clinical knowledge, with an emphasis on our approach at the University of Texas MD Anderson Cancer Center (MDACC).

EPIDEMIOLOGY

Lung cancer is rarely diagnosed in people younger than 35 years old. Incidence and death rates rise exponentially until age 75, when a plateau is reached. Non–small cell lung cancer accounts for the greatest number of deaths from cancer in both men and women over age 60.

The geographic, social, and temporal trends of the incidence of NSCLC are closely related to tobacco consumption. In developed Western countries, the incidence of NSCLC has been declining; however, it has been increasing in Asia, Eastern Europe, and developing countries ([1]).

Worldwide, NSCLC is more common in men, and this difference has been attributed to higher tobacco consumption. In some regions, like Eastern Europe and South America, there was an uptake of smoking by women in the 1980s, and these areas are currently experiencing a rise in NSCLC cases in women. In the United States, the incidence has been declining for both men and women as tobacco use declines; the male-to-female ratio from 2007 to 2011 was 1.4:1 ([2]).

There is some evidence that African Americans might be more susceptible to the carcinogenic effects of tobacco smoke ([3]); however, smoking behaviors might also account for socioeconomic and racial differences in lung cancer incidence.

ETIOLOGY

Smoking

The causal relationship between tobacco smoke and lung cancer was established in the 1950s in case-control and cohort studies. This led to the 1964 report of the US Surgeon General, concluding that smoking can cause lung cancer. Currently, it is estimated that 85% to 90% of lung cancers are due to smoking. Nonsmokers who are exposed to secondhand smoke are also at an increased risk. There is a dose-response relationship between smoking and lung cancer risk, and smoking cessation leads to a significant risk reduction (Table 18-1) ([4]).

Tobacco smoke is a complex mixture of chemicals that includes multiple carcinogens, most importantly the *N*-nitrosamines (nicotine-derived nitrosamino ketone [NNK] and N'-nitrosonornicotine [NNN]) and polycyclic aromatic hydrocarbons [benzo(a)pyrene and dimethylbenz(a)anthracene]. They are activated

Table 18-1 Approximate 10-Year Risk of Developing Lung Cancer[a]

	Duration of Smoking					
	25 Years		40 Years		50 Years	
Age (years)	Quit (%)	Still Smoking (%)	Quit (%)	Still Smoking (%)	Quit (%)	Still Smoking (%)
One-pack-per-day smokers						
55	<1	1	3	5	NA	NA
65	<1	2	4	7	7	10
75	1	2	5	8	8	11
Two-packs-per-day smokers						
55	<1	2	4	7	NA	NA
65	1	3	6	9	10	14
75	2	3	7	10	11	15

NA, not available.

[a]This table assumes that people who have quit smoking will continue to abstain for the next 10 years and those who are still smoking will keep smoking the same amount for the next 10 years.

Adapted, with permission, from Bach PB, Kattan MW, Thornquist MD, et al. Variations in lung cancer risk among smokers. *Cancer.* 2003;95(1):470-478.

through hydroxylation by the P450 enzyme system and exert their action through the formation of DNA adducts.

Smokeless tobacco is frequently advocated as a safer alternative. There has not been a clear association between smokeless tobacco and lung cancer; however, it increases the risk of head and neck, pancreatic, and gastric cancer. E-cigarettes deliver water vapor with scents and different amounts of nicotine containing lower amounts of nitrosamines. However, they still contain high levels of propylene glycol and glycerin, and their long-term effects on health are unknown. Their use should not be recommended to nonsmokers, and use as part of a smoking cessation approach needs further study.

Approximately 10% to 15% of cases of NSCLC occur in never smokers, corresponding to approximately 20,000 deaths annually. In addition to secondhand smoke exposure, several other agents have also been linked to the development of lung cancer (Table 18-2).

Asbestos

Asbestos exists in many natural forms. The silicate fiber has been implicated in carcinogenesis, is chemically inert, and can remain in a person's lungs for a lifetime. Epidemiologic studies have confirmed the association between asbestos exposure and certain lung diseases, such as pulmonary fibrosis, mesothelioma, and lung cancer ([5]). Most exposure occurs in the workplace. When smoking is combined with asbestos exposure, the relative risk of lung cancer is strikingly increased ([5]).

Radon

Radon is a naturally occurring decay product of uranium. It is a colorless, odorless, chemically inert gas that can penetrate the earth's crust and accumulates in buildings. It emits heavy ionizing alpha particles, which may damage DNA. It was shown that many households in Europe, Canada, and the United States have some degree of radon radiation that may increase NSCLC risk among smokers and nonsmokers ([6]).

Table 18-2 Relative Risk Of Developing Lung Cancer

Risk Factor	Relative Risk	Reference
Cigarette smoking in males	17.4	8
Cigarette smoking in females	10.8	8
Passive smoking	1.5	4
Asbestos	1.2-2.6	9, 18
Asbestos and smoking	28.8	19
Mining	3-8	4, 21
Radon (residential)	1.1-2	4

Diet

The majority of studies that have examined vegetable consumption in relation to lung cancer have shown a protective effect (reviewed in Alberg and Samet [[7]]), but there are inherent biases in these population studies. There is also epidemiologic evidence that dietary intake of certain vitamins decreases lung cancer risk; however, trials of vitamin supplementation for cancer prevention have ultimately been unsuccessful (see later "Chemoprevention" section).

Other Factors

Environmental or industrial exposure to arsenic, chromium, chloromethyl ether, vinyl chloride, and polycyclic aromatic hydrocarbons increases lung cancer risk (reviewed by Field and Withers [[8]]). Preexisting lung disease such as tuberculosis, silicosis, pulmonary fibrosis, and chronic obstructive pulmonary disease are also associated with an increased lung cancer incidence even when correcting for the degree of cigarette consumption. This suggests that common pathways to these conditions, such as chronic inflammation, may drive the tumorigenic process.

Genetic Predisposition

Family history of lung cancer is associated with a two- to three-fold increase in lung cancer risk, even after correction for smoking, and this risk seems to be inherited in a Mendelian co-dominant fashion ([9]).

Many studies describe weak but consistent associations between some polymorphisms and lung cancer risk. The cytochrome P450 (CYP) family is responsible for the metabolism of tobacco smoke, and the polymorphism CYP1A1 Ile^{462}Val is associated with a higher risk in Asians (odds ratio [OR], 1.61) ([10]). The glutathione *S*-transferase (GST) enzyme prevents oxidative damage, and the polymorphism GSTM1 increases risk in Asians (OR, 1.17) ([11]). Finally, individuals with impaired DNA repair capacity are at higher risk for developing lung cancer, even if they are nonsmokers, and the polymorphism Lys^{751}Gln in the DNA-repairing enzyme ERCC2 was associated with lung cancer (OR, 1.15) ([12]).

Large genome-wide association studies (GWAS) ([13]) have identified three loci strongly associated with lung cancer risk in different populations: 15q25, 5p15, and 6p21. The 15q25 susceptibility region encodes three cholinergic nicotine receptor genes (*CHRNA3*, *CHRNA5*, *CHRNB4*), and alterations in those regions have been associated with a higher risk for nicotine dependence and higher smoking burden. In nonsmokers, they have also been associated with impaired healing of the respiratory mucosa, suggesting a higher sensitivity to toxin-induced airway damage. The 5p15 region encodes the *TERT* gene, responsible for telomerase function, which is frequently altered in many cancers.

PREVENTION OF LUNG CANCER

Smoking Cessation and Prevention

The most effective method of preventing lung cancer is reducing tobacco exposure, either through encouraging smoking cessation or preventing young people from starting to smoke. In the United States, campaigns to reduce smoking rates have been successful. The estimated percentage of Americans who actively smoke decreased from 42.4% in 1965 to 25% in 1990 and to 18.1% in 2012. However, former smokers retain an increased risk of lung cancer, and there are still a considerable number of smokers, highlighting the need for better education and prevention strategies, especially those targeted to youths.

Early Detection and Screening

Previous studies examined the role of chest x-ray, with or without cytologic analysis of sputum, to screen for lung cancer, and none showed a clear benefit. Most of them were confounded by lead time, length time, and overdiagnosis biases.

Spiral computed tomography (CT)—also called helical CT or low-dose CT—is much more sensitive to detect early NSCLC than chest x-ray. In 2011, the results of the National Lung Screening Trial (NLST) were published ([14]). In this trial, 53,454 current or former smokers age 55 to 74 years old with at least a 30-pack-year smoking history and no symptoms that could be related to lung cancer were randomized to undergo yearly chest x-rays or low-dose CT for 3 years. After a median follow-up of 6.5 years, the low-dose CT group had a 20% reduction in the rate of lung cancer–specific mortality, from 309 to 247 per 100,000 person-years, as well as a 6.7% reduction in overall mortality. In the CT group, 39% of patients had suspicious lung nodules (vs 16% in the control arm), and the majority of these (96%) were considered false-positive results. Sensitivity and specificity of low-dose CT were 93.8% and 73.4%, respectively, compared to 73.5% and 91.3% for chest radiography. Cost-effectiveness analysis showed a median cost of $43,000 per quality-adjusted life-year gained for current smokers assigned to the low-dose CT group. Based on these results, the US Preventive Services Task Force currently recommends lung cancer screening with yearly low-dose CT for current or past smokers, age 55 to 80, with a smoking history of at least 30 pack-years. Screening should be discontinued once a person has not smoked for 15 years. Another trial is currently being conducted in Belgium and the Netherlands (the NELSON study) looking at the 10-year impact of lung cancer screening using low-dose CT scan.

Despite recent developments, low-dose CT screening still has significant limitations, including high false-positive ratios and the development of interval lung cancers, which can be aggressive. Positron emission tomography (PET)-CT scan, epigenetic markers, and cell-free tumor DNA are additional approaches under investigation, which are only recommended in the setting of a clinical trial.

Chemoprevention

Cigarette smoking has an effect of field cancerization, with the accumulation of genetic mutations and other premalignant changes throughout the lungs and the aerodigestive tract. Patients treated and cured of early-stage lung cancer have a high risk of developing second primary tumors. Therefore, a series of chemoprevention trials has focused on smokers and survivors of lung and head and neck cancers.

Multiple studies evaluated supplementation with vitamins and oligo-elements, but none showed a benefit to supplementation, and several studies showed risk, with increased lung cancer incidence and mortality (Table 18-3) ([15–21]).

Given the potential connection between inflammation and tumorigenesis, phase II studies have used anti-inflammatory agents, such as celecoxib, and prostaglandin analogues, such as iloprost. These agents have been able to reduce proliferation and dysplasia of oral and bronchial epithelium in smokers and former smokers, but their benefit in cancer prevention remains to be proven. There are currently no proven agents for the chemoprevention of lung cancer.

HISTOLOGY AND MOLECULAR PATHOLOGY

Most lung tumors arise from epithelial cells and are called bronchogenic carcinomas. Neuroendocrine tumors also arise in the lung and can appear as SCLC, carcinoids, or large cell neuroendocrine carcinomas. Bronchogenic carcinomas include NSCLCs, a category comprising three major types: adenocarcinoma, squamous cell carcinoma (SCC), and large cell carcinoma.

The most current histologic classification of NSCLC was proposed by the International Association for the

Table 18-3 Large Randomized Lung Cancer Chemoprevention Trials

Study	Intervention	Population	Size	End Point	Outcome
ATBC ([15])	β-Carotene; α-tocopherol	Male smokers	29,133	Lung cancer incidence	Harmful
CARET ([16])	β-Carotene; retinol	Current and former smokers	18,314	Lung cancer incidence	Harmful
Intergroup Lung Trial ([17])	Isotretinoin	Resected NSCLC	1,166	Second malignancies	Harmful
Euroscan ([18])	Retinol, *N*-acetylcysteine	Resected NSCLC and head and neck cancer	2,592	Second malignancies	Negative
ECOG 5597 ([19])	Selenium	Resected NSCLC	1,772	Second malignancies	Negative
Physicians' Health Study II ([20])	Vitamin C and vitamin E	Healthy male physicians	14,641	Cancer incidence	Negative
NORVIT and WENBIT ([21])	Vitamin B_{12} and folic acid	Patients with ischemic heart disease	6,845	Cancer incidence	Harmful

NSCLC, non–small cell lung cancer.

Study of Lung Cancer/American Thoracic Society/European Respiratory Society in 2011 ([22]) and uses immunohistochemistry to identify subgroups with different molecular profiles and clinical behaviors (Tables 18-4 and 18-5). Adenocarcinomas usually stain positive for cytokeratin 7, thyroid transcription factor 1 (TTF-1), and surfactant apoprotein A and are negative for cytokeratin 20. Metastatic adenocarcinomas from other sites except the thyroid stain negative for TTF-1. All carcinoids and most SCLCs stain positive for chromogranin and synaptophysin, whereas NSCLC is usually negative for these two markers. Mesothelioma is distinguished from adenocarcinoma by the presence of calretinin and cytokeratin 5/6 and the absence of carcinoembryonic antigen (CEA), B72.3, Ber-EP4, and MOC-31.

Adenocarcinoma

Adenocarcinoma is the most common subtype of NSCLC in the United States, representing 40% of cases in men and 50% in women. It is predominant in nonsmokers, and its incidence has been rising. These tumors are classically peripheral and, on histologic examination, demonstrate gland formation, papillary structures, or mucin production (Fig. 18-1).

Non–small cell lung cancer is one of the cancer types with the highest mutation burden, with an average of 360 exonic mutations per sample ([23]). However, the patterns of mutations are different for adenocarcinomas and SCCs.

About 75% of lung adenocarcinomas have alterations in driver genes that activate intracellular pathways leading to proliferation, cell survival, and oxidative stress response ([24]) (Fig. 18-2). Up to 79% of those alterations are in the RTK/RAS/RAF pathway, including mutations in the ErbB family member *EGFR* (ErbB1).

The prevalence of *EGFR* mutations ranges from 5% to 10% in smokers to 40% to 50% in nonsmokers in the Western population ([25]). The alterations are usually in the tyrosine kinase domain of the gene within exons 18 to 24, most specifically in the intracellular adenosine triphosphate (ATP)-binding domain (Table 18-6) ([25–27]).

Frequencies of *EGFR*, *KRAS*, *ALK*, *ROS1*, and other driver genetic alterations commonly found in lung adenocarcinoma samples are listed in Table 18-7 ([24, 25, 28–32]). This is a rapidly changing landscape that is defining the many molecular subsets of this heterogeneous disease.

Squamous Cell Carcinoma

Squamous cell carcinoma is now the second most frequent histology, accounting for 30% of NSCLC in men and 20% in women. This tumor arises most frequently in the proximal bronchi and has the strongest association with smoking. Pathologically, it is characterized by visible keratinization, with prominent desmosomes and intercellular bridges (Fig. 18-3).

Squamous cell carcinomas frequently have amplifications in chromosome 3q, which contains genes involved in squamous differentiation (*SOX2* and *TP53*) and cell proliferation (*PI3K*). About 81% to 90% of patients with SCCs have *TP53* mutations, and 47% have alterations in the PI3K/AKT/mTOR pathway, whereas only 26% of SCCs have activations of the RTK/RAS/RAF pathway ([23]). The prevalence of *EGFR* mutations is 1% to 3%, 6% of patients have *EGFR* amplifications, and 1% to 6% have *KRAS* mutations ([23]) (Fig. 18-4).

Large Cell Carcinoma

The least common subtype of NSCLC, large cell carcinoma, accounts for approximately 8% of all NSCLCs (Fig. 18-5). Refinements in histopathologic techniques

Table 18-4 The 2011 International Association for the Study of Lung Cancer/American Thoracic Society/European Respiratory Society Histologic Classification of Invasive Malignant Epithelial Tumors

Squamous cell carcinoma
Small cell carcinoma
Adenocarcinoma Lepidic predominant (formerly nonmucinous bronchoalveolar carcinoma pattern, with >5 mm invasion) Acinar predominant Papillary predominant Micropapillary predominant Solid predominant with mucin production
Variants of invasive adenocarcinoma Invasive mucinous adenocarcinoma (formerly mucinous bronchoalveolar carcinoma) Colloid Fetal (low and high grade) Enteric
Large cell carcinoma Variants: large cell neuroendocrine (NSCLC NOS); large cell neuroendocrine (NE) carcinoma (positive NE markers); large cell carcinoma with NE morphology (morphology suggestive of NE carcinoma, but negative stains)
Adenosquamous carcinoma/NSCLC with squamous cell and adenocarcinoma patterns
Carcinomas with pleomorphic, sarcomatoid, or sarcomatous elements Carcinoma with spindle and/or giant cells Pleomorphic carcinoma Spindle cell carcinoma Giant cell carcinoma
Carcinosarcoma Blastoma (pulmonary blastoma) Others
Carcinoid tumor Typical carcinoid Atypical carcinoid
Carcinomas of salivary gland type Mucoepidermoid carcinoma Adenocystic carcinoma, others
Unclassified carcinoma

NOS, not otherwise specified; NSCLC, non–small cell lung cancer.
Adapted with permission from Travis WD, Brambilla E, Noguchi M, et al. International Association for the Study of Lung Cancer/American Thoracic Society/European Respiratory Society international multidisciplinary classification of lung adenocarcinoma, *J Thorac Oncol* 2011 Feb;6(2):244-285.

have led to the diagnosis of adenocarcinoma or SCC in cases previously diagnosed as undifferentiated large cell carcinoma.

CLINICAL PRESENTATION

Non–small cell lung cancer is often asymptomatic at diagnosis and may be found incidentally on imaging performed for other reasons. If symptoms are present, they are often related to the specific locations of tumor masses and the occurrence of paraneoplastic syndromes. The symptoms of centrally located lesions include cough, hemoptysis, wheezing, stridor, dyspnea, and postobstructive pneumonia. Peripheral lesions can cause pain due to pleural or chest wall invasion, cough, or restrictive dyspnea.

The involvement of thoracic and cervical structures can also lead to classical clinical presentations:

- Pancoast syndrome: Shoulder pain radiating to the arm in an ulnar distribution caused by invasion of the eighth cervical and first thoracic nerves in the superior sulcus.
- Horner syndrome: Enophthalmos, ptosis, miosis, and ipsilateral dyshidrosis caused by involvement of the paravertebral sympathetic nerves.
- Hoarseness: Involvement of the left recurrent laryngeal nerve as it passes through the aortopulmonary window.
- Elevation of the hemidiaphragm: Involvement of phrenic nerve at the mediastinum.
- Superior vena cava syndrome: Swelling of the face and arm and superficial venous engorgement caused by compression of the superior vena cava.

The production of hormones or hormone-like substances can lead to paraneoplastic syndromes:

- Cancer cachexia: The most common paraneoplastic syndrome, characterized by weight loss, impaired immune function, and weakness that are not completely explained by poor oral intake. The exact mechanism for development of cachexia is unknown, but tumor-elaborated cytokines have been implicated.
- Hypercalcemia: The second most common paraneoplastic syndrome in NSCLC, hypercalcemia is caused by ectopic production of a parathyroid hormone-related protein (PTHrP) or bone metastases. It is more common in the squamous cell subtype.
- Hypertrophic pulmonary osteoarthropathy: Arthropathy and clubbing of the fingers and toes with evidence of periostitis of the long bones (Fig. 18-6). Its etiology is unknown, and it is more common in adenocarcinomas and large cell carcinoma.

Non–small cell lung cancer is frequently metastatic, and symptoms secondary to metastases are common. The most common sites for metastases are

Table 18-5 Adenocarcinoma Histologic Subtypes and Molecular and Radiologic Associations

Predominant Histologic Subtype	Molecular Features	Computed Tomography Scan Appearance	Relative Risk of Recurrence After Resection
Lepidic	TTF-1 positive: 100% *EGFR* amplification: 20%-50% *EGFR* mutation (nonsmokers): 10%-30% *KRAS* mutations (smokers): 10% *BRAF* mutations: 5%	Ground glass or solid nodule	1.0
Papillary	TTF-1 positive: 90%-100% *EGFR* amplification: 20%-60% *EGFR* mutation: 10%-30% *KRAS* mutations: 3% *BRAF* mutations: 5% *ERBB2* mutations: 3% *P53* mutations: 30%	Solid nodule	2.7 (95% CI, 1.1-6.8)
Acinar	TTF-1 positive or negative *EGFR* amplification: 10% *EGFR* mutation (non-smokers): <10% *KRAS* mutation (smokers): 20% *P53* mutation: 40% *EML4/ALK* translocation: >5%	Solid nodule	2.3 (95% CI, 0.9-5.7)
Micropapillary	*EGFR* mutation: 20% *KRAS* mutation: 33% *BRAF* mutation: 20%	Unknown	4.4 (95% CI, 1.8-11.2)
Solid	TTF-1 positive: 70% MUC1 positive *EGFR* amplification: 20%-50% *EGFR* mutation (nonsmokers): 10%-30% *KRAS* mutation (smokers): 10%-30% *EML4/ALK* translocations: >5% *P53* mutations: 50% *LRP1B* mutations *INHBA* mutations	Solid nodule	5.7 (95% CI, 2.2-14.7)
Invasive mucinous adenocarcinoma	TTF-1 negative (0%-33% positive) No *EGFR* mutation *KRAS* mutation: 80%-100% MUC5, MUC6, MUC2, CK20 positive	Consolidation; air bronchograms	Unknown

CI, confidence interval.
Adapted with permission from Travis WD, Brambilla E, Noguchi M, et al. International Association for the Study of Lung Cancer/American Thoracic Society/European Respiratory Society international multidisciplinary classification of lung adenocarcinoma, *J Thorac Oncol* 2011 Feb;6(2):244-285.

intrathoracic nodes, pleura, contralateral lung, liver, adrenal glands, bone, and brain.

DIAGNOSIS

Solitary Pulmonary Nodule

A solitary pulmonary nodule is a single asymptomatic mass that is surrounded by lung tissue, is well circumscribed, measures less than 3 cm, and does not show evidence of mediastinal or hilar adenopathy. The differential diagnosis includes primary cancer, metastatic cancer, infection, benign tumors (eg, hamartomas), vascular abnormalities, and inflammation

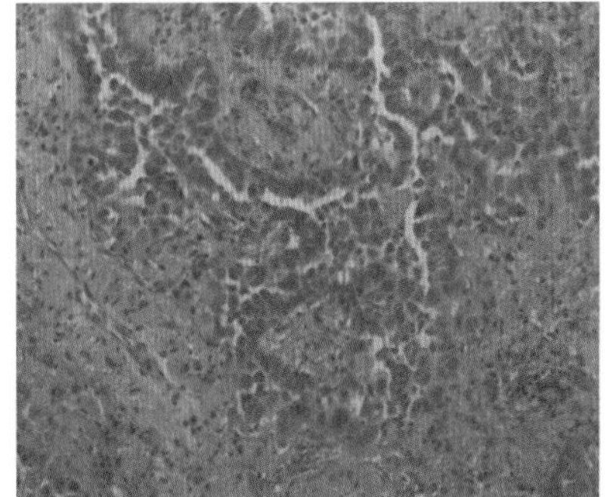

FIGURE 18-1 Adenocarcinoma. Photomicrograph of adenocarcinoma of the lung stained with hematoxylin and eosin. (Used with permission from Cesar Moran, MD.)

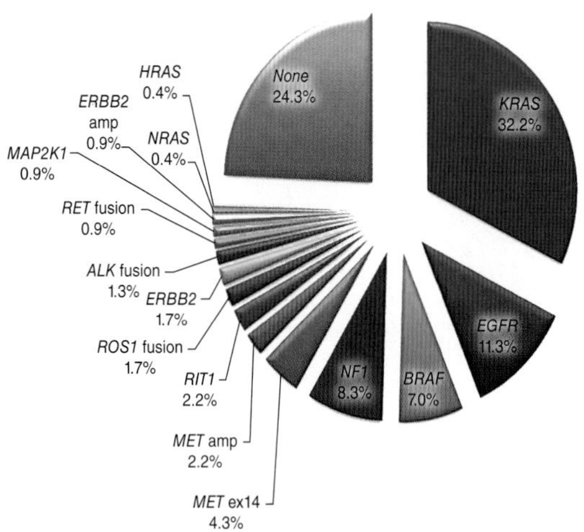

FIGURE 18-2 Somatic alterations in the RTK/RAS/RAF pathway in lung adenocarcinoma. (Adapted with permission from Collisson EA, Campbell JD, Brooks AN, et al. Comprehensive molecular profiling of lung adenocarcinoma, *Nature* 2014 Jul 31;511(7511):543-550.)

Table 18-6 Most Common *EGFR* Mutations in Lung Adenocarcinomas

Mutation	Prevalence in Treatment-Naïve *EGFR*-Mutant Tumors	Sensitivity to Erlotinib/Gefitinib
Exon 19 deletion (del19)	45%-50% ([25])	Sensitive
Exon 21 Leu858Arg insertion (L858R)	40%-45% ([25])	Sensitive
Exon 20 insertions	5% ([26])	Resistant
Exon 12 and 18 insertions	2%-3% ([26])	Unknown
Exon 20 T790M	1%-5% ([27])	Resistant

Table 18-7 Common Driver Genes Altered in Lung Adenocarcinoma

Name	Alteration	Main Effects	Incidence
KRAS mutations	Multiple, usually in codons 12 and 13; most common G12D (nonsmokers) and G12C (smokers)	Activation of RAS/RAF/MEK/ERK pathway	30%-35% (mostly in smokers) ([25])
EGFR mutations	Several alterations in the ATP-binding domain of the receptor	Activation of RAS/RAF/MEK and PI3K/AKT/mTOR pathways	10%-15% (40%-50% in nonsmokers) ([28])
BRAF mutations	About 50% are the V600E mutation also described in other cancers	Activation of RAS/RAF/MEK/ERK pathway	7%-10% ([24])
MET mutations	Exon 14 skipping; can occur with or without *MET* amplification	Activation of MET	7% ([24])
PIK3CA	Many activating mutations	AKT, TSC, and mTOR	7% ([24])
EML4/ALK and other *ALK* translocations	Inversion within chromosome 2p	Constitutively activates the anaplastic lymphoma kinase (*ALK*) gene leading to downstream activation of RAS and PI3K	1%-4% ([29, 30])
ROS1 fusions	Multiple rearrangements of the *ROS1* gene with different genes	Related to the ALK protein, also activates RAS and PIK3CA	1%-2% ([29])
RET fusions	Multiple rearrangements of the *RET* gene with different genes	Activation of the *RET* proto-oncogene and RAS pathway	1% ([31])
ERBB2 (*HER2*) mutations	Various mutations; in about 50% of cases co-occurrence with *HER2* amplification	Activation of RAS/RAF/MEK and PI3K/AKT/mTOR pathways	2%-4% ([32])

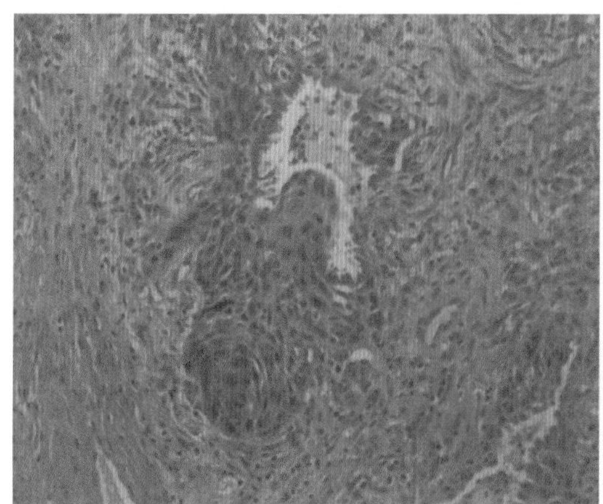

FIGURE 18-3 Squamous cell carcinoma. Photomicrograph of squamous cell carcinoma of the lung stained with hematoxylin and eosin. (Used with permission from Cesar Moran, MD.)

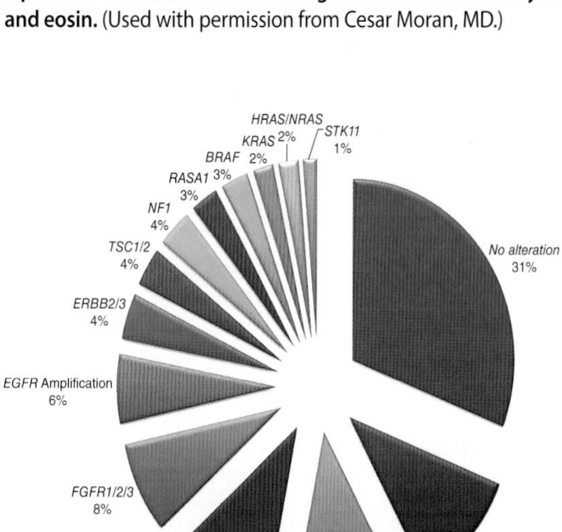

FIGURE 18-4 Somatic alterations in the RTK/RAS/RAF and PIK3CA/AKT/mTOR pathways in lung squamous cell carcinoma. [Data from the Cancer Genome Atlas Research Network. Comprehensive genomic characterization of squamous cell lung cancers. *Nature*. 2012;489(7417):519-525.]

(eg, granulomatous disease). The American College of Chest Physicians has issued guidelines on the evaluation of solitary lung nodules, based on their size (≤ or >8 mm), the clinical probability of malignancy, and the patient's surgical risk ([33]) (Table 18-8 and Fig. 18-7).

The management of small nodules (<8 mm) is less clear. Lesions that are too small to be biopsied (<5 mm) should be followed with CT scans in 6 months (any risk factors for lung cancer) or 12 months (no risk factors for lung cancer). For lesions 5 to 8 mm, some recommend close follow-up with CT scans in 3, 6, and 12 months, and others recommend nonsurgical biopsies ([33]).

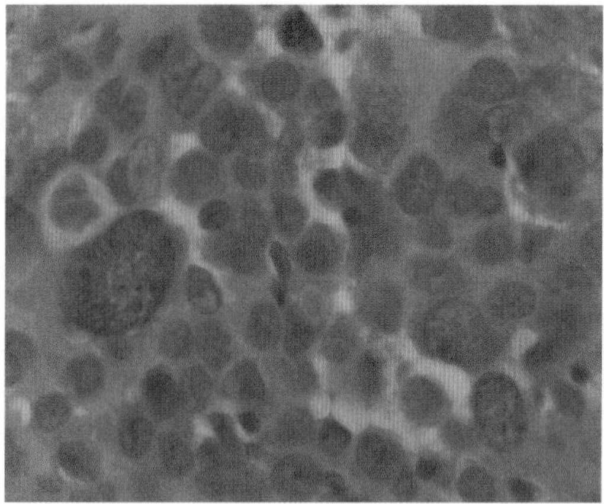

FIGURE 18-5 Large cell carcinoma. Photomicrograph of large cell carcinoma of the lung stained with hematoxylin and eosin. (Used with permission from Cesar Moran, MD.)

Pulmonary Mass

Lesions that are large (>3 cm), multiple, or with enlarged hilar, mediastinal, and/or supraclavicular lymph nodes should undergo complete lung cancer staging and a nonsurgical biopsy. Fiberoptic bronchoscopy is appropriate for central lesions and is able to establish the diagnosis in 97% of cases. For peripheral lesions, the diagnostic yield of bronchoscopy is only 55%, and percutaneous transthoracic biopsies can be considered. Because of the tissue requirements for immunohistochemistry and molecular marker testing of lung cancers, at MDACC, we usually perform an image-guided core-needle biopsy. Mediastinoscopy or endobronchial ultrasound (EBUS) can be used to obtain biopsy samples from mediastinal nodes.

Staging

Once the histologic diagnosis of NSCLC has been established, the extent of disease must be determined (Fig. 18-8).

The stage of disease will dictate therapy. All patients must undergo a complete history and physical examination, chest x-ray, CT scan of the chest and upper abdomen (to include the adrenal glands), a complete blood count, and blood chemistry tests that include electrolyte and liver enzyme studies. All patients with stage II to IV disease should have evaluation of the brain, with magnetic resonance imaging (MRI) if possible. Central nervous system (CNS) imaging may be considered for patients with stage I disease. For stage I to III NSCLC, ^{18}F-fluorodeoxyglucose (FDG)-PET should be performed to evaluate mediastinal nodes and for distant metastases. Because the involvement of mediastinal lymph

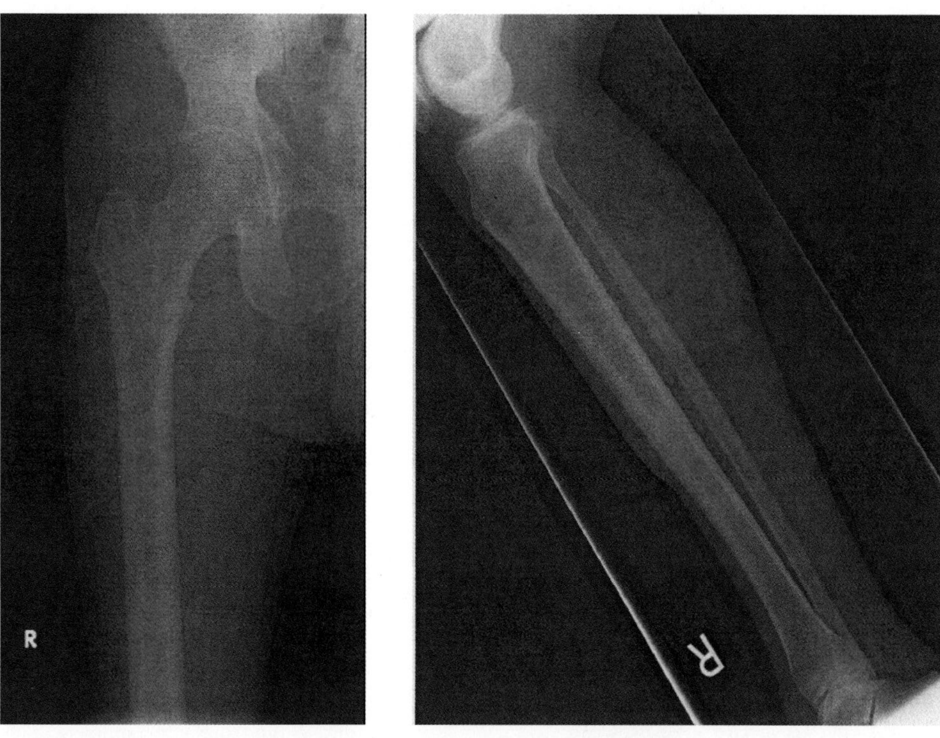

FIGURE 18-6 Hypertrophic pulmonary osteoarthropathy (HPO). This 62-year-old man with non–small cell lung cancer reported a 1-month history of finger clubbing and arthritic lower extremity pain. The plain radiographs of the lower extremities show periosteal reaction in both femora as well as in bilateral tibias/fibulas that is consistent with HPO.

Table 18-8 Clinical Probability of Malignancy of Solitary Lung Nodules

	Low Probability (<5%)	Intermediate Probability (6-65%)	High Probability (>65%)
Patient	Young, low smoking burden, no previous history of cancer	Mixture of low- and high-probability features	Older, heavy smoker, previous cancer
Nodule (CT scan)	Small, regular margins, non–upper lobe location, enhancement <15 HU in the contrast phase	Mixture of low- and high-probability features	Large, irregular/spiculated, upper lobe location; enhancement >15 HU in the contrast phase
FDG-PET results	Low or moderate clinical probability with low PET probability	Weak or moderate PET activity	Intense hypermetabolic nodule
Nonsurgical biopsy results (bronchoscopy or transthoracic biopsy)	Specific benign diagnostic	Nondiagnostic	Suspicious for malignancy
Behavior on CT surveillance	Progressive decrease in size or resolution; no growth over ≥2 years (solid nodules) or over ≥3 years (semi-solid nodules)	NA	Clear evidence of growth

CT, computed tomography; FDG-PET, ^{18}F-fluorodeoxyglucose–positron emission tomography; NA, not applicable.

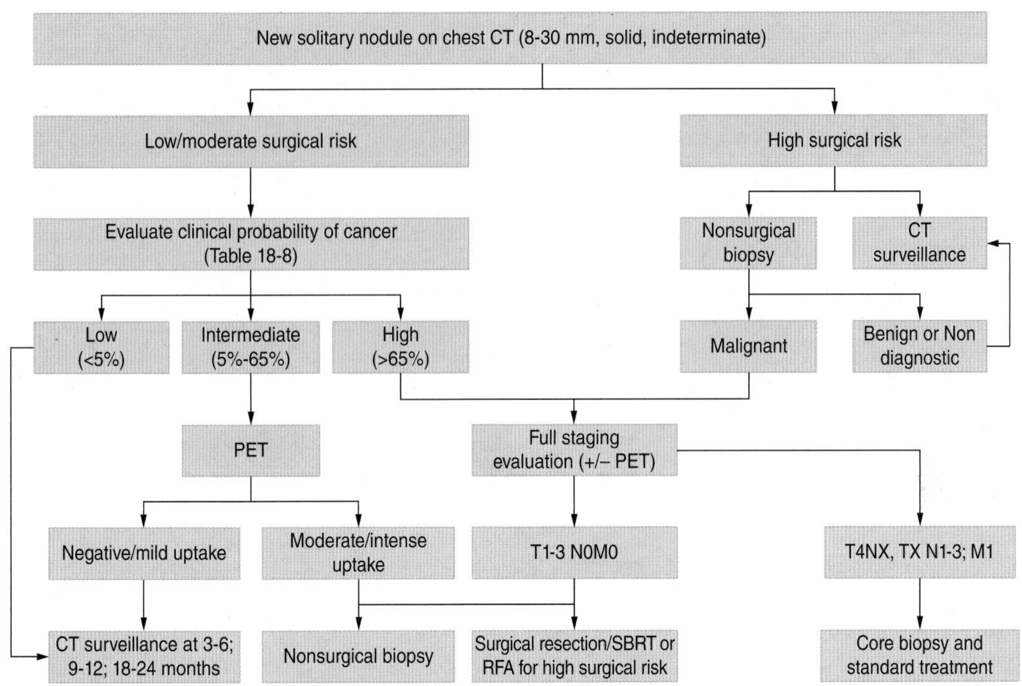

FIGURE 18-7 Management algorithm for individuals with solitary nodules (8-30 mm). CT, computed tomography; PET, positron emission tomography; RFA, radiofrequency ablation; SBRT, stereotactic body radiotherapy. [Adapted with permission from Gould MK, Donington J, Lynch WR, et al. Evaluation of individuals with pulmonary nodules: when is it lung cancer? Diagnosis and management of lung cancer, 3rd ed: American College of Chest Physicians evidence-based clinical practice guidelines, *Chest* 2013 May;143(5 Suppl):e93S-120S.]

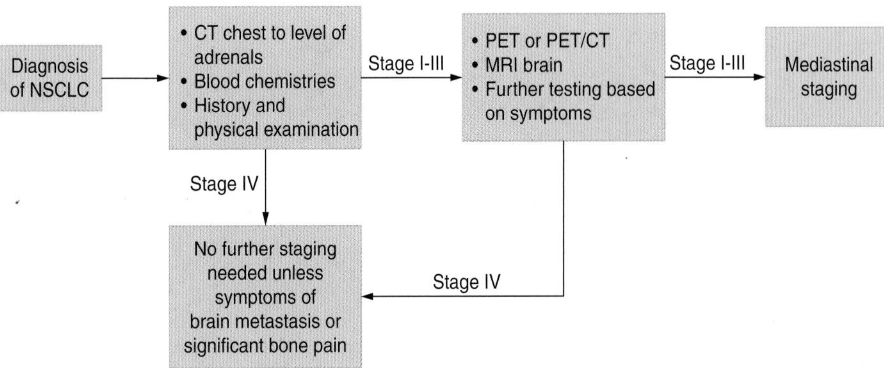

FIGURE 18-8 Staging algorithm for non–small cell lung cancer (NSCLC). CT, computed tomography; MRI, magnetic resonance imaging; PET, positron emission tomography. See text for details.

nodes will influence surgical decisions (see section "Treatment"), the presence of FDG-avid mediastinal lymph nodes in a PET-CT scan should be confirmed with either mediastinoscopy or EBUS (see "Commentary"). Routine use of mediastinoscopy or EBUS in patients with a normal-appearing mediastinum on PET-CT scans is controversial.

After the completion of staging evaluation, the disease is assigned a TNM stage (Figs. 18-9 to 18-17; Tables 18-10 and 18-11). The TNM staging for NSCLC was revised and updated in 2009 in the seventh edition of the American Joint Committee on Cancer/International Union Against Cancer staging system ([34]).

Clinical staging has inherent inaccuracies and therefore typically underestimates the true extent of disease. In patients who undergo surgical tumor resection, surgical/pathologic staging should be done to predict recurrence and to evaluate the need for adjuvant therapy. Patients' 5-year survival rates by tumor stage are shown in Table 18-11.

TREATMENT

Stages I and II Disease

Surgery

Surgery is standard treatment for stages I and II NSCLC (Figs. 18-18 and 18-19).

The extent of lung resection will be dictated by the size and location of the tumor. The entire tumor must be removed, with margins negative for cancer. Wedge resection and segmentectomy are associated with higher rates of local recurrence than lobectomy and pneumonectomy and are not considered standard of care, although they may be an option for patients who cannot tolerate a larger surgery due to poor pulmonary function ([35]). All patients should also undergo complete ipsilateral mediastinal lymph node dissection or systematic mediastinal sampling for accurate staging ([36]).

Any patient who is being considered for surgery must undergo pulmonary function tests to assess the ability to withstand pulmonary resection. Split-lung function studies can further help to predict lung function after the planned resection. There is no single accepted value, criterion, or cutoff for pulmonary resection. Published criteria that have been shown to predict high risk for lung resection include estimated posttreatment forced vital capacity <2 L, forced expiratory volume in 1 second <1 L, and diffusing capacity of the lungs for carbon dioxide <40% to 60% ([37]).

Commentary: Mediastinal Lymph Node Sampling Using Endobronchial Ultrasound and Transbronchial Needle Aspiration

Accurate mediastinal lymph node staging is a critical aspect of non–small cell lung cancer (NSCLC) management. Non- invasive staging typically relies on a combination of computed tomography (CT) and ^{18}F-fluorodeoxyglucose (FDG)– positron emission tomography (PET) data to detect mediastinal metastases. Lymph nodes are considered abnormal by CT criteria if the short-axis diameter is >10 mm; however, both false negatives and false positives are possible. FluorodeoxyglucoseFDG-PET scanning has been a welcome addition to the staging armamentarium and increases diagnostic accuracy. However, limitations of non-invasive staging modalities remain, and current guidelines recommend tissue sampling by invasive means to improve diagnostic accuracy among patients whose subsequent therapy is contingent on mediastinal involvement.

Multiple modalities are available for sampling mediastinal and hilar lymph nodes. These range from minimally invasive approaches such as endobronchial ultrasound–guided transbronchial needle aspiration (EBUS-TBNA), endoscopic ultrasound guided–fine-needle aspiration (EUS-FNA), and CT-guided needle aspiration to surgical approaches such as mediastinoscopy and thoracotomy.

Endobronchial ultrasound–guided transbronchial needle aspiration EBUS-TBNA is a technology that ustilizes an integrated ultrasonic bronchoscope to obtain real- time image–guided transbronchial needle aspiration biopsy of lymph nodes in proximity to the central airways and. EBUS-TBNA is currently our preferred method for assessing mediastinal lymph node involvement. It is a minimally invasive procedure that is typically performed on an outpatient basis and often utilizes only moderate sedation. Biopsies can be taken at all lymph node stations adjacent to a major airway, and as such, EBUS-TBNA can sample more lymph nodes in a single procedure than any other invasive mediastinal tissue sampling technique. Furthermore, rather than merely confirming malignancy in an enlarged or FDG-avid lymph node, true lymph node mapping can be carried out using this technology. It can be safely performed in most patients, including those that who have undergone prior surgical or radiation therapy to the thorax. The risk profile is minimal and similar to the risks of standard bronchoscopy. Numerous studies have documented the safety and diagnostic accuracy of EBUS-TBNA in staging lung cancer. Samples obtained have also been shown to be adequate for molecular testing. Importantly, EBUS-TBNA has shown significant utility even in patients with radiologically normal mediastinum.

AlthoughWhile cervical mediastinoscopy was traditionally considered the reference standard for invasive mediastinal lymph node sampling, it is difficult to repeat, is more invasive, and has higher associated morbidity and mortality than EBUS-TBNA, and increasing evidence suggests diagnostic equivalence. Current American College of Clinical Pharmacy ACCP guidelines recommend a needle biopsy technique such as EBUS- TBNA as the initial invasive mediastinal staging technique of choice for lung cancer with the caveat that negative biopsies may need surgical confirmation. In summary, EBUS-TBNA provides a safe, minimally invasive, and highly accurate method of mediastinal lymph node sampling and has rapidly become part of our standard practice in the mediastinal staging of NSCLC.

George A. Eapen

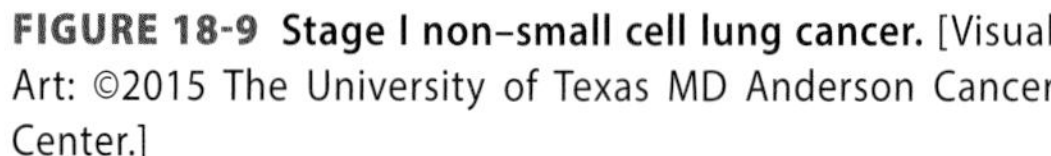

FIGURE 18-9 Stage I non–small cell lung cancer. [Visual Art: ©2015 The University of Texas MD Anderson Cancer Center.]

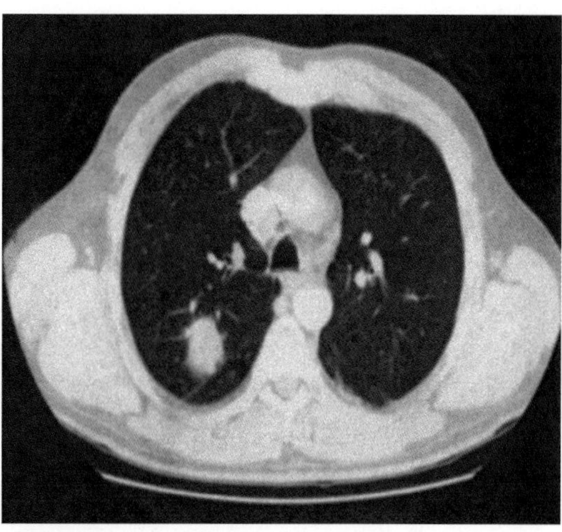

FIGURE 18-10 Stage I non–small cell lung cancer. This T2N0M0 NSCLC was an incidental finding when the patient presented with an unrelated medical illness. The computed tomography of the chest revealed a 3.8- by 3.1-cm right-upper-lobe mass with no hilar or mediastinal adenopathy. Pathologic staging after a right upper lobectomy and mediastinal lymph node dissection confirmed the clinical stage.

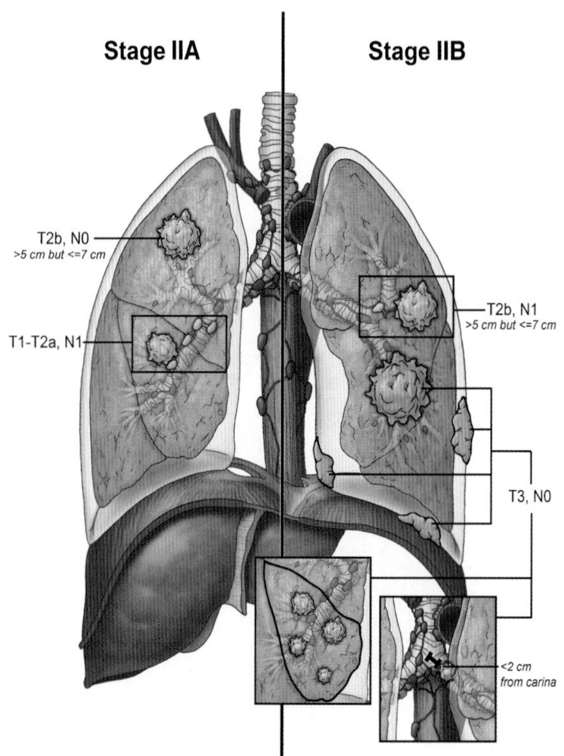

FIGURE 18-11 Stage II non–small cell lung cancer. [Visual Art: ©2015 The University of Texas MD Anderson Cancer Center.]

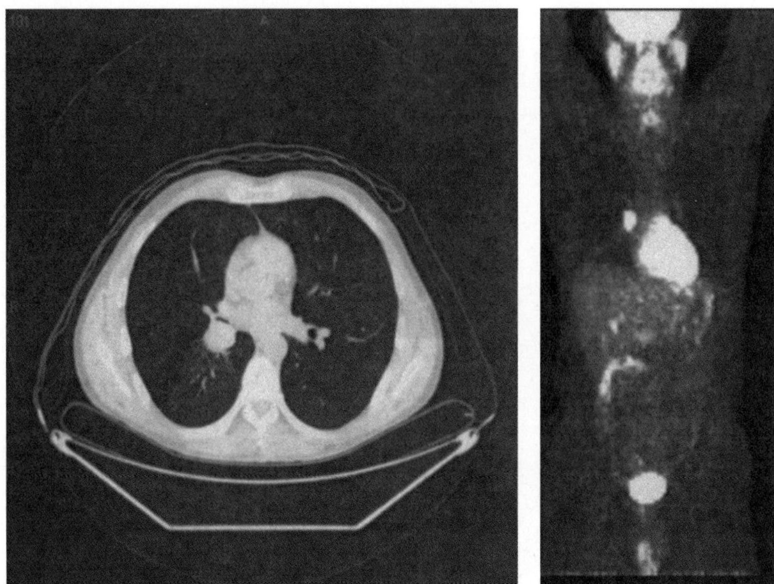

FIGURE 18-12 Stage II non–small cell lung cancer. This patient presented with symptoms of pneumonia and was found to have a right hilar mass impinging on the right-lower-lobe bronchus and a right-lower-lobe infiltrate by computed tomography scan. Positron emission tomography scan showed increased uptake in the hilar mass and physiologic uptake. Staging evaluation showed no distant metastatic disease. He underwent a right middle and lower lobectomy with a mediastinal lymph node dissection. This revealed a 3.1-cm primary squamous cell carcinoma with two positive hilar nodes and no involved mediastinal nodes (T2N1M0).

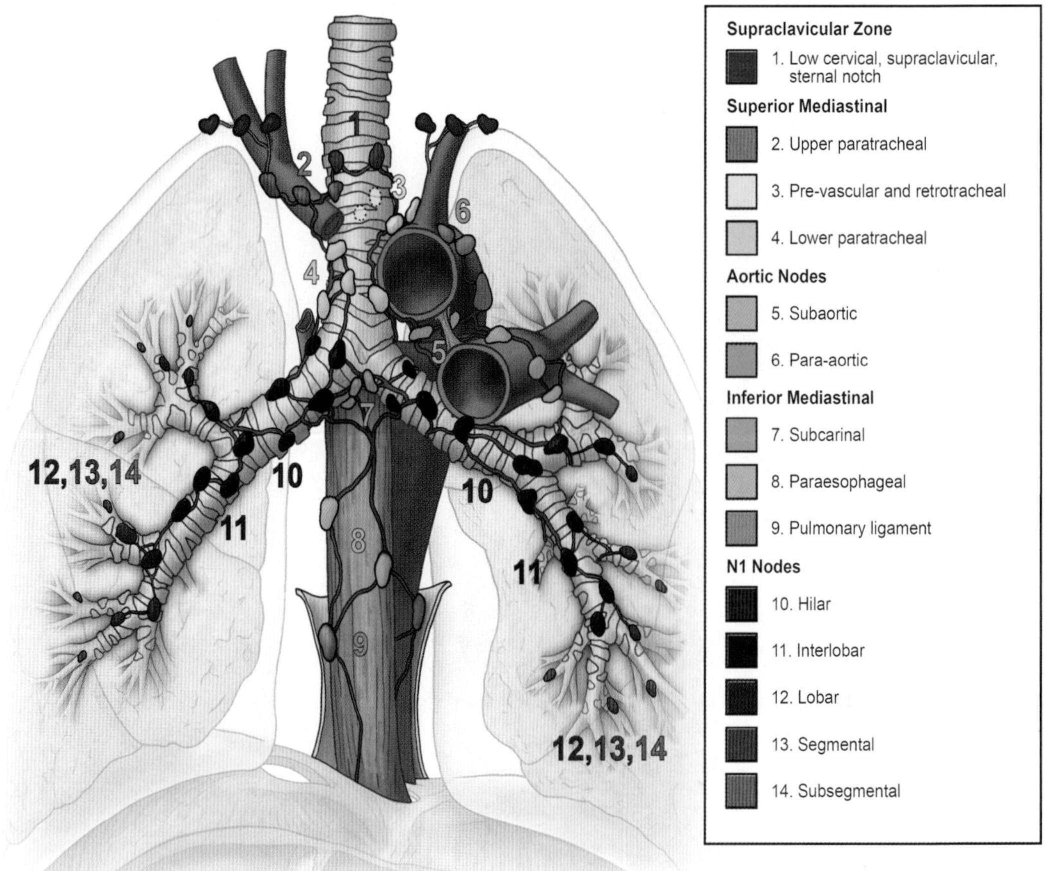

FIGURE 18-13 Classification of regional lymph nodes. [Visual Art: ©2015 The University of Texas MD Anderson Cancer Center.]

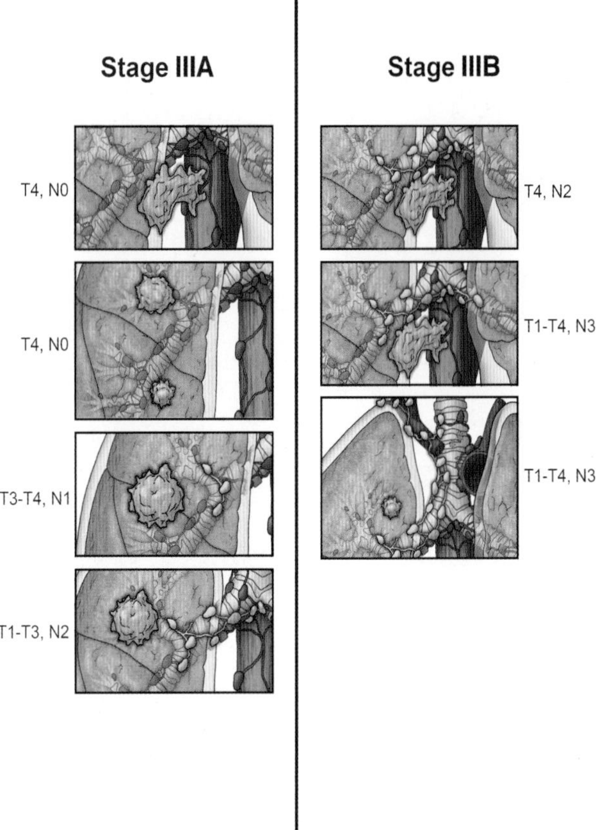

FIGURE 18-14 **Stage III non–small cell lung cancer.** [Visual Art: ©2015 The University of Texas MD Anderson Cancer Center.]

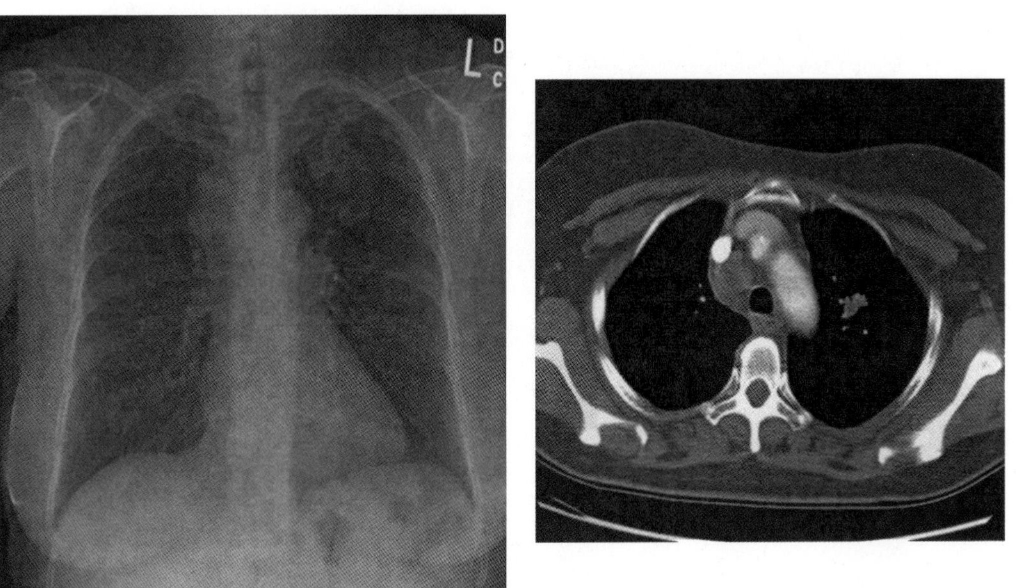

FIGURE 18-15 **Stage IIIB non–small cell lung cancer (NSCLC). This patient presented with chest pain, and the chest x-ray (*left*) showed an approximately 4.0- by 3.0-cm mass in the left upper lobe and an additional mass in the right mediastinum. Initial computed tomography (CT) revealed a 4.5-cm mass in the left upper lobe and a 5-cm mass in the paratracheal region. Biopsy confirmed NSCLC. Staging evaluation showed no distant metastatic disease (T2N3M0). The patient was treated with concurrent chemotherapy and radiotherapy. The posttreatment CT (*right*) showed significant therapeutic response.**

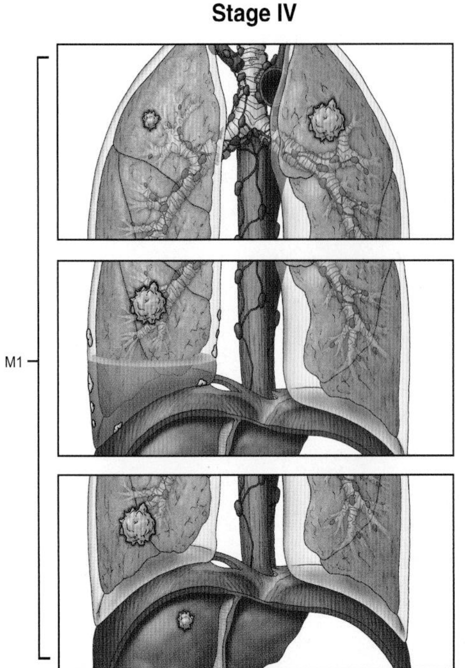

FIGURE 18-16 Stage IV non–small cell lung cancer. [Visual Art: ©2015 The University of Texas MD Anderson Cancer Center.]

Radiation Therapy

For patients with early-stage lung cancer who cannot undergo surgery because of poor pulmonary reserve or medical comorbidities, stereotactic radiosurgery is a feasible option with local control rates of 90% and cancer-specific survival of 88% at 3 years ([38]).

There is controversy regarding whether stereotactic radiosurgery should be considered in patients who are candidates for surgery and who have small primary tumors and no lymph node involvement. Retrospective series suggest that outcomes with radiation may be similar to those of surgery ([38]). Surgery, however, remains the standard of care for patients who can tolerate it.

Adjuvant Chemotherapy

Even after complete resection, rates of recurrence of NSCLC are high, prompting the study of adjuvant chemotherapy in this disease. The potential benefit of adjuvant chemotherapy is the eradication of micrometastatic disease before it becomes clinically evident, thus potentially increasing cure rates. For patients with completely resected stage II or III NSCLC, multiple meta-analyses demonstrate that adjuvant platinum-based chemotherapy is associated with an absolute

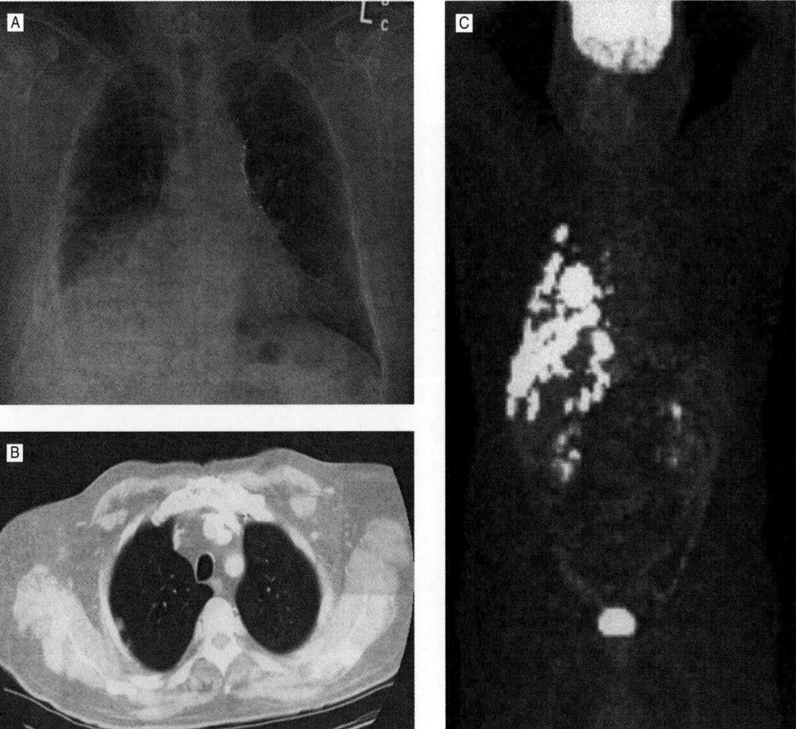

FIGURE 18-17 Stage IV non–small cell lung cancer (NSCLC). Upon evaluation for back pain, this patient was found to have a pleural effusion (**A, B**), and biopsy revealed NSCLC. Positron emission tomography/computed tomography (**C**) revealed a 5.4- by 3.6-cm hypermetabolic mass in the right middle lobe, many small satellite fluorodeoxyglucose (FDG)-avid right lung nodules, and extensive FDG-avid pleural-based masses on the right (T4N0M1). No disease was found outside the chest.

Table 18-9 Definitions for T, N, and M Descriptors

Descriptors	Definitions	Subgroups[a]
T	**Primary tumor**	
T0	No primary tumor	
T1	Tumor ≤3 cm,[b] surrounded by lung or visceral pleura, not more proximal than the lobar bronchus	
T1a	Tumor ≤2 cm[b]	T1a
T1b	Tumor >2 but ≤3 cm[b]	T1b
T2	Tumor >3 but ≤7 cm[b] or tumor with any of the following[c]:	
	Invades visceral pleura, involves main bronchus ≥2 cm distal to the carina, atelectasis/obstructive pneumonia extending to hilum but not involving the entire lung	
T2a	Tumor >3 but ≤5 cm[b]	T2a
T2b	Tumor >5 but ≤7 cm[b]	T2b
T3	Tumor >7 cm;	$T3_{>7}$
	or directly invading chest wall, diaphragm, phrenic nerve, mediastinal pleura, or parietal pericardium;	$T3_{inv}$
	or tumor in the main bronchus <2 cm distal to the carina[d];	$T3_{center}$
	or atelectasis/obstructive pneumonitis of entire lung;	$T3_{center}$
	or separate tumor nodules in the same lobe	$T3_{satell}$
T4	Tumor of any size with invasion of heart, great vessels, trachea, recurrent laryngeal nerve, esophagus, vertebral body, or carina;	$T4_{inv}$
	or separate tumor nodules in a different ipsilateral lobe	$T4_{ipsi\ nod}$
N	**Regional lymph nodes**	
N0	No regional node metastasis	
N1	Metastasis in ipsilateral peribronchial and/or perihilar lymph nodes and intrapulmonary nodes, including involvement by direct extension	
N2	Metastasis in ipsilateral mediastinal and/or subcarinal lymph nodes	
N3	Metastasis in contralateral mediastinal, contralateral hilar, ipsilateral or contralateral scalene, or supraclavicular lymph nodes	
M	**Distant metastasis**	
M0	No distant metastasis	
M1a	Separate tumor nodules in a contralateral lobe;	$M1a_{contr\ Nod}$
	or tumor with pleural nodules or malignant pleural dissemination[e]	$M1a_{p1\ Dissem}$
M1b	Distant metastasis	M1b
Special situations		
TX, NX, MX	T, N, or M status not able to be assessed	
Tis	Focus of in situ cancer	Tis
T1[d]	Superficial spreading tumor of any size but confined to the wall of the trachea or mainstem bronchus	$T1_{ss}$

[a]These subgroups labels are not defined in the International Association for the Study of Lung Cancer publications but are added here to facilitate a clear discussion.
[b]In the greatest dimension.
[c]T2 tumors with these features are classified as T2a if ≤5 cm.
[d]The uncommon superficial spreading tumor in central airways is classified as T1.
[e]Pleural effusions are excluded that are cytologically negative, nonbloody, transudative, and clinically judged not to be due to cancer.
Reproduced with permission from from Detterbeck, FC, Boffa DJ, Tanoue LT. The new lung cancer staging system. *Chest*. 2009;136(1):260-271.

Table 18-10 7th Edition American Joint Committee On Cancer TNM Staging System for Non–Small Cell Lung Cancer

T/M Stage	N0	N1	N2	N3
T1	Ia	IIa	IIIa	IIIb
T2a	Ib	IIa	IIIa	IIIb
T2b	IIa	IIb	IIIa	IIIb
T3	IIb	IIIa	IIIa	IIIb
T4	IIIa	IIIa	IIIb	IIIb
M1	IV	IV	IV	IV

Adapted with permission from Detterbeck, FC, Boffa DJ, Tanoue LT. The new lung cancer staging system. *Chest.* 2009;136(1):260-271.

Table 18-11 Five-Year Survival for Non–Small Cell Lung Cancer by Pathologic and Clinical Stage

Stage	Clinical	Pathologic
Ia	50%	73%
Ib	43%	58%
IIa	36%	46%
IIb	25%	36%
IIIa	19%	24%
IIIb	7%	9%
IV	2%	13%

Data from Detterbeck, FC, Boffa DJ, Tanoue LT. The new lung cancer staging system. *Chest.* 2009;136(1):260-271.

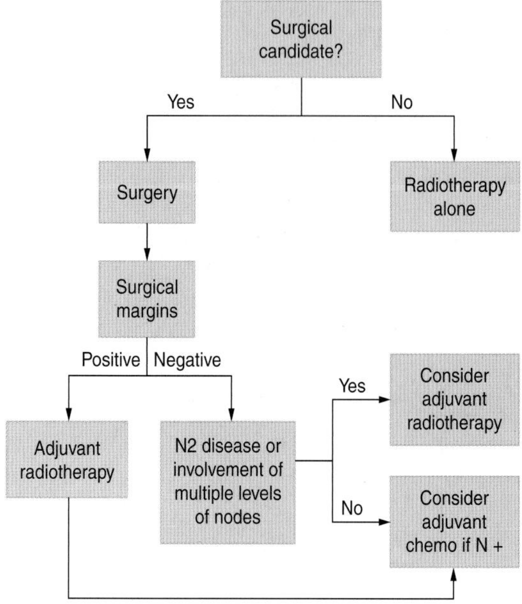

FIGURE 18-18 Treatment algorithm for stage I non–small cell lung cancer. See text for details.

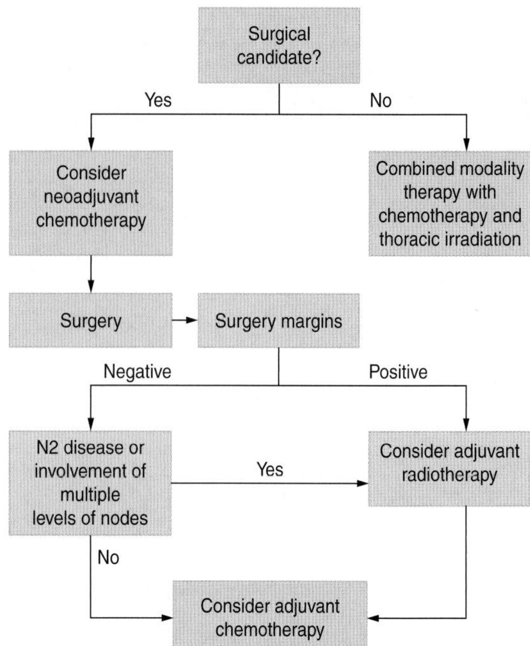

FIGURE 18-19 Treatment algorithm for stage II non–small cell lung cancer. See text for details.

benefit in 5-year survival of about 5% ([39]) and should be offered to all patients with good performance status (Table 18-12) ([40–44]). For patients with no lymph node involvement and a primary tumor smaller than 4 cm, adjuvant chemotherapy is not recommended. For node-negative tumors larger than 4 cm, the Cancer and Leukemia Group B 9633 trial suggested a benefit of adjuvant platinum-based chemotherapy, and it should be considered ([40]) (see Table 18-12).

Cisplatin-vinorelbine is the most studied regimen for adjuvant chemotherapy; in practice, other cisplatin-based doublets are frequently used. Acceptable second agents include pemetrexed (for nonsquamous NSCLC), docetaxel, etoposide, and gemcitabine. Cisplatin is preferred over carboplatin, but if cisplatin is not feasible, carboplatin/paclitaxel is an appropriate alternative ([40]). There is no evidence that targeted agents such as bevacizumab, erlotinib, and crizotinib are effective in the adjuvant setting, although the National Cancer Institute ALCHEMIST trial will assess the benefit for specific molecular subsets of patients.

Neoadjuvant chemotherapy offers several real and theoretical advantages over postoperative therapy: better patient compliance, improved tumor resectability, earlier treatment of micrometastatic disease, and earlier assessment of clinical and pathologic response. There has been one randomized trial and one meta-analysis ([45]) that suggest the equivalence of the neoadjuvant and adjuvant approaches. Adjuvant treatment is the standard of care, but neoadjuvant chemotherapy could be considered in special situations, such as for stage III

Table 18-12 Chemotherapy Regimens for Adjuvant Treatment of NSCLC

Trial	Regimen
IALT ([41])	Cisplatin 80-120 mg/m^2 every 3 of 4 weeks, for 3-4 cycles, with:
	Vinorelbine 30 mg/m^2 weekly; or
	Vinblastine 4 mg/m^2 every week for 5 weeks, then every 2 weeks; or
	Etoposide 100 mg/m^2, days 1-3, with each cisplatin
ANITA ([42])	Cisplatin 100 mg/m^2, day 1, every 4 weeks and vinorelbine 30 mg/m^2 weekly for 4 cycles
NCIC-CTG JBR.10 ([43])	Cisplatin 50 mg/m^2, days 1 and 8, every 4 weeks for 4 cycles; vinorelbine 25 mg/m^2 every week for 16 cycles
TREAT ([44]) (nonsquamous histology)	Cisplatin 75 mg/m^2 and pemetrexed 500 mg/m^2 every 3 weeks for 4 cycles
CALGB 9633 ([40])	Carboplatin AUC 6 and paclitaxel 200 mg/m^2 every 3 weeks for 4 cycles
Others	Cisplatin 75 mg/m^2 and docetaxel 75 mg/m^2, day 1, every 3 weeks for 4 cycles Cisplatin 75-80 mg/m^2, day 1; vinorelbine 25-30 mg/m^2, days 1 and 8, every 3 weeks for 4 cycles Cisplatin 75 mg/m^2, day 1, and gemcitabine 1,250 mg/m^2, days 1 and 8, every 3 weeks for 4 cycles Carboplatin AUC 6 and pemetrexed 500 mg/m^2 every 3 weeks for 4 cycles (nonsquamous histology)

AUC, area under the curve; NSCLC, non–small cell lung cancer.

disease when response to chemotherapy may help to determine whether a patient should undergo surgery or chemoradiation.

Adjuvant radiation or chemoradiation for resected stage I and II NSCLC has been shown to be detrimental and should not be recommended ([46]).

Stage III Disease

Patients with stage III disease have better outcomes with multimodality rather than single-modality therapy, and their care should be managed by a multidisciplinary team. For patients with stage IIIB disease, chemoradiation represents the standard of care. Chemoradiation is often used for patients with stage IIIA disease as well, but surgery with adjuvant treatment can be considered for carefully selected patients.

In a randomized trial of chemoradiation alone versus chemoradiation followed by resection, the patients who benefited from the surgical approach were those with stage IIIA disease who had limited involvement of mediastinal lymph nodes and who underwent lobectomy (as opposed to pneumectomy) ([47]). Neoadjuvant chemoradiation followed by surgery has been compared to neoadjuvant chemotherapy followed by surgery and adjuvant radiation ([48]) and was associated with more toxicity with no survival benefit. At MDACC, we consider surgical treatment in patients with stage IIIA disease with good performance status and without multistation mediastinal adenopathy. These patients are typically treated with neoadjuvant chemotherapy followed by consideration of surgery. Adjuvant radiation therapy is typically given if there is evidence of mediastinal node involvement based on assessment of surgical pathology (Fig. 18-20).

Patients with stage IIIA disease and extensive mediastinal involvement or IIIB disease should be treated with concurrent chemoradiation. When compared with sequential radiotherapy and chemotherapy, this approach is associated with higher survival rates (23.8% vs 18.1% at 3 years; hazard ratio [HR], 0.84; $P = .004$) but increased toxicity (acute esophageal toxicity, 18% vs 4%; relative risk [RR], 4.9; $P = .001$) ([49]).

Standard radiotherapy for stage III NSCLC consists of radiation given once daily for 6 weeks (30 fractions) to a total dose of 60 Gy. All attempts to increase efficacy through hyperfractionation, acceleration, or increased radiation dose have failed ([50]). In the recent Radiation Therapy Oncology Group 0617 trial, patients receiving high-dose radiation (74 Gy) had higher rates of locoregional failure (44% vs 35.3%; $P = .04$) and worse median survival (19.5 vs 28.7 months; $P = .0007$) than those receiving standard-dose radiation (60 Gy) ([51]). Proton therapy is a newer technique that is able to deliver a higher dose to the tumor while delivering lower doses to normal surrounding tissue; it is currently being compared to standard radiation in a randomized phase III trial (NCT00915005).

Multiple concurrent chemotherapy regimens have been tested against radiation alone with proven benefit ([52]); however, these regimens have not been directly compared to each other, and multiple regimens are considered acceptable (Table 18-13). At MDACC, many physicians favor carboplatin and paclitaxel because retrospective data suggest that this regimen is less toxic than cisplatin and etoposide ([53]).

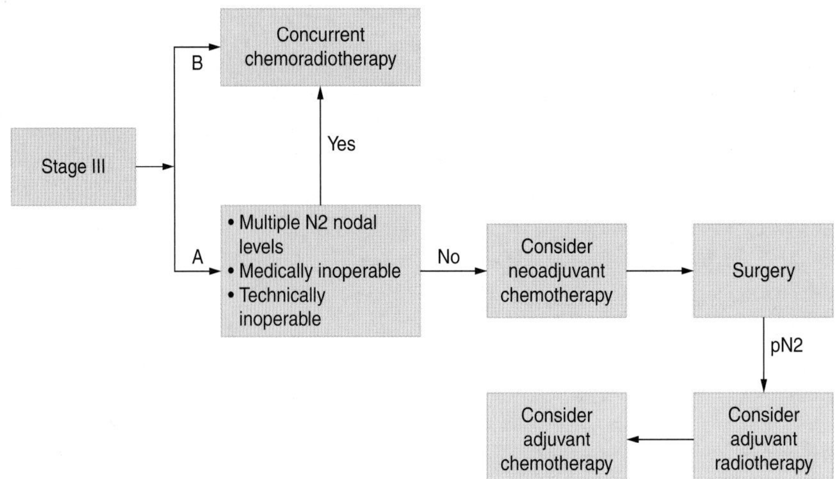

FIGURE 18-20 Treatment algorithm for stage III non–small cell lung cancer. See text for details.

Table 18-13 Chemoradiation Regimens for Stage III NSCLC

Regimen	Histology	Doses	Adjuvant Treatment After the Completion of Chemoradiation
Cisplatin + etoposide	All NSCLC	Cisplatin 50 mg/m^2 days 1, 8, 29, 36 Etoposide 50 mg/m^2 days 1-5, 29-33	No
Cisplatin + vinblastine	All NSCLC	Cisplatin 100 mg/m2 days 1 and 29 Vinblastine 5 mg/m^2 weekly × 5	No
Carboplatin + pemetrexed	Adenocarcinoma	Carboplatin AUC 5 day 1 every 21 days × 4 Pemetrexed 500 mg/m^2 day 1 every 21 days × 4	Yes; continue carboplatin + pemetrexed to a total of 4 cycles
Cisplatin + pemetrexed	Adenocarcinoma	Cisplatin 75 mg/m^2 day 1 every 21 days × 3 Pemetrexed 500 mg/m^2 day 1 every 21 days × 3	Yes; continue cisplatin + pemetrexed to a total of 3 cycles
Carboplatin + paclitaxel	All NSCLC	Carboplatin AUC 2 weekly during radiation Paclitaxel 45-50 mg/m^2 weekly during radiation	Yes; 2 cycles of carboplatin AUC 6 + paclitaxel 200 mg/m^2 every 21 days after the completion of chemoradiation

AUC, area under the curve; NSCLC, non–small cell lung cancer.

The use of consolidation docetaxel after concurrent chemoradiation with cisplatin and etoposide was detrimental in the phase III Hoosier Oncology Group LUN 01-24 trial ([54]). However, most studies with carboplatin/cisplatin and pemetrexed or carboplatin and paclitaxel included consolidation chemotherapy after radiation. It is reasonable to consider consolidation chemotherapy for patients who received those regimens and have a good performance status at the end of concurrent therapy.

There are no definitive data on adjuvant anti-EGFR tyrosine kinase inhibitors (TKIs) in stage III NSCLC patients with activating *EGFR* mutations. In a population not selected for *EGFR* mutations, adjuvant gefitinib was detrimental ([55]). There is no proven benefit for any targeted therapies in combination with chemoradiation for locally advanced lung cancer, although this is an active area of investigation.

Tumors in the lung apex invading apical structures, termed Pancoast tumors (Fig. 18-21), are challenging. Tumors that are N0 to N1 should undergo preoperative concurrent chemoradiation followed by resection. For these patients, 5-year disease-free survival rates are 40% to 50% ([56]). Patients with N2 to N3 disease should be treated with concurrent chemoradiation alone.

Stage IV Disease

Stage IV NSCLC remains an incurable disease, and management should include adequate palliation of symptoms. Patients with symptomatic brain or spinal cord metastases, hemoptysis, postobstructive pneumonia,

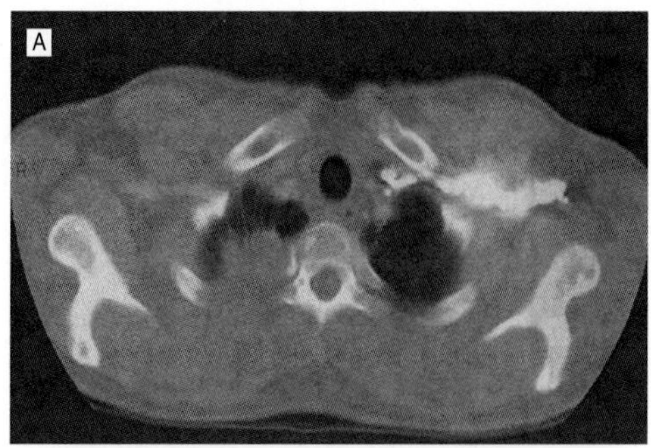

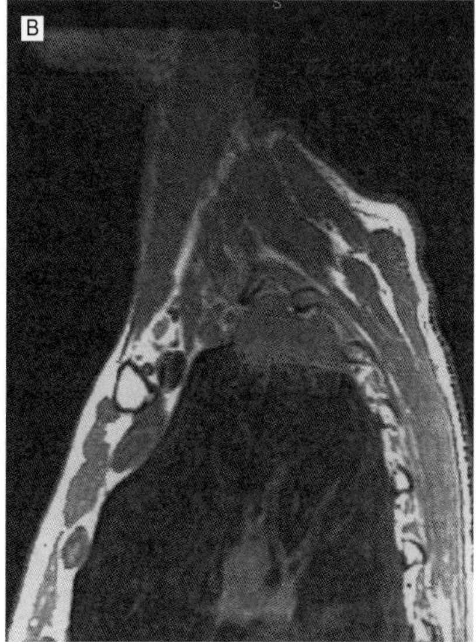

FIGURE 18-21 A. Pancoast tumor. B. By magnetic resonance imaging, this non–small cell lung cancer tumor at the right lung apex invades the second right rib and extends apically into right apical fat, with a loss of the fat plane between the tumor and the T1 nerve. The T2 nerve is also involved by the mass.

or painful bone metastases should receive radiotherapy before any consideration for systemic therapy. Early referral to specialized palliative care services has also been shown to improve overall survival ([57]).

Decisions about systemic therapy demand the classification into SCC versus nonsquamous carcinoma and the testing of adenocarcinoma cases for actionable alterations (eg, *EGFR* mutations, *ALK* and *ROS1* rearrangements). The most recent guidelines ([58]) recommend that all adenocarcinomas, mixed adenosquamous carcinomas, and NSCLCs not otherwise specified should undergo evaluation for *EGFR* mutations using polymerase chain reaction–based tests and testing for *ALK* and *ROS1* translocations using fluorescent in situ hybridization. Often, in practice, more complete molecular profiling is being performed, which also includes testing for less common alterations such as *BRAF* and *HER2* mutations and *RET* fusions. Pure SCC with no immunohistochemistry markers of adenocarcinoma should not undergo molecular testing. Because of the importance of molecular testing, attempts should be made to obtain core biopsies rather than fine-needle aspirations to ensure sufficient tissue for profiling.

Epidermal Growth Factor Receptor Tyrosine Kinase Inhibitors for EGFR Mutant Lung Adenocarcinoma

Epidermal growth factor receptor (EGFR) TKIs should be considered first-line therapy in patients with metastatic lung adenocarcinoma with *EGFR* exon 19 deletion or L858R mutation. Exon 20 mutations (including T790M), which are found in 5% of cases at diagnosis, have an intrinsic resistance to EGFR-TKIs ([27]) and should be treated with standard chemotherapy.

The EGFR-TKIs erlotinib, afatinib, and gefitinib have been tested against standard chemotherapy as first-line agents in patients with NSCLC with *EGFR*-activating mutations and showed improvement in response rates (70% vs 33%, $P < .001$), progression-free survival (PFS) (9.5 to 13.1 months vs 4.1 to 6.3 months, $P < .0001$), and quality of life ([59–61]). No benefit in overall survival (OS) has been detected because most trials allowed for cross-over after progression (Table 18-14) ([59–65]). Gefitinib is not available in the United States, so either erlotinib or afatinib can be used in the frontline setting. There are no head-to-head data comparing erlotinib to afatinib, and afatinib has higher reported rates of toxicity. There is some evidence that combining EGFR-TKIs with the anti–vascular endothelial growth factor (VEGF) monoclonal antibody bevacizumab improves response rates and PFS ([66]), but benefits in OS have not been confirmed.

Acquired Resistance to Epidermal Growth Factor Receptor Tyrosine Kinase Inhibitors

Patients with activating *EGFR* mutations who progress on EGFR-TKIs and those with unknown mutation status who have a prolonged response to EGFR TKIs (>6 months) and then progress are classified as having acquired resistance to EGFR-TKIs. For these patients, a postprogression biopsy is recommended to identify the mechanisms of resistance ([67, 68]) (Fig. 18-22).

In about half of cases, the mechanism of resistance is the development of an acquired exon 20 T790M mutation, which occurs at the binding site of the TKI to EGFR, displacing the TKI. The growth of those tumors still shows EGFR dependence, and multiple trials are currently evaluating the effects of third-generation TKIs (eg, AZD9291 and CO-1686) with specific affinity for *EGFR* with T790M mutation. Early data look promising, and these agents may receive regulatory approval in the near future. There are also phase I/II data on using the

Table 18-14 Summary of Selected Trials of TKIs in Lung Adenocarcinoma

Drug	Pivotal Trial	Dose	Response Rate	Progression-Free Survival	Grade 3-4 Side Effects of TKIs
EGFR exon 19 del and L875R					
Gefitinib	IPASS ([60])	Gefitinib 250 mg once daily	71%	9.5 months	Rash 3.1%; diarrhea 3.8%
		Carboplatin AUC 5 + paclitaxel 200 mg/m^2 every 3 weeks	47%	6.3 months	
Erlotinib	EURTAC ([59])	Erlotinib 150 mg once daily	58%	9.7 months	Rash 13%; diarrhea 5%
		Cisplatin 75 mg/m^2 or carboplatin AUC 6 + docetaxel 75 mg/m^2 every 3 weeks	15%	5.2 months	
Afatinib	LUX-Lung 3 ([61])	Afatinib 40 mg once daily	56%	11.1 months	Rash 14%; diarrhea 16%
		Cisplatin 75 mg/m^2 + pemetrexed 500 mg/m^2	23%	6.9 months	
EML4-ALK translocation					
Crizotinib	PROFILE 1014 ([62])	Crizotinib 250 mg twice daily	74%	10.9 months	Elevated AST/ALT 14%; neutropenia 11%; vision disorder 1%
		Cisplatin 75 mg/m^2 or Carboplatin AUC 5-6 and pemetrexed 500 mg/m^2 every 3 weeks	45%	7.0 months	
Ceritinib	Second-line after crizotinib failure ([63])	Ceritinib 750 mg once daily	58%	6.9 months	Elevated AST/ALT 23%; elevated lipase 10%
Alectinib	Second-line after crizotinib failure ([64])	Alectinib 300-900 mg twice daily	55%	Not reported	Edema 2%; neutropenia 4%; elevated liver enzymes 4%
ROS1 fusions					
Crizotinib	Second-line after platinum chemotherapy ([65])	Crizotinib 250 mg twice daily	72%	19.2 months	Elevated AST/ALT 4%; hypophosphatemia 10%; neutropenia 10%

ALT, alanine aminotransferase; AST, aspartate aminotransferase; AUC, area under the curve; TKI, tyrosine kinase inhibitor.

combination of afatinib with the anti-EGFR monoclonal antibody cetuximab in patients with acquired EGFR resistance (response rate, 29%; PFS, 4.7 months) ([69]). Interestingly, efficacy was similar in patients with and without T790M mutations. Currently, however, there are no approved targeted agents for patients with resistance to first-line TKIs.

About 5% of patients experience small cell transformation. These patients should be treated similarly to de novo SCLC with combination chemotherapy such as platinum-etoposide (see Chapter 17 on SCLC for further details on SCLC chemotherapy regimens) ([67]).

Because erlotinib has poor penetration through the blood-brain barrier, patients with controlled extracranial disease who are progressing in the CNS may benefit from pulsatile high-dose erlotinib (1,500 mg once a week), with response rates in the CNS of 67% and median time to CNS progression of 2.7 months ([70]). This approach is also being further studied in clinical trials. Another option is treating the brain metastases with radiation and continuing with erlotinib ([71]).

Outside of clinical trials, patients with resistance to frontline TKIs should receive standard chemotherapy (see below). Postprogression continuation of EGFR-TKIs in combination with chemotherapy has recently been addressed with two clinical trials. The data demonstrate that despite increases in response rates compared to chemotherapy alone, PFS and OS are not improved ([72]).

ALK Inhibitors for Patients With Adenocarcinomas With ALK Translocations or ROS1 Fusions

Approximately 5% of patients with adenocarcinoma have tumors harboring an *ALK* fusion, and another 1%

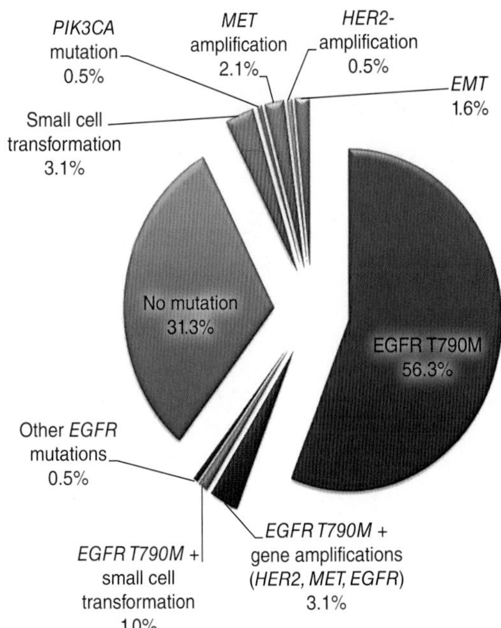

FIGURE 18-22 Most common acquired alterations in patients with *EGFR*-mutant tumors and acquired resistance to epidermal growth factor receptor tyrosine kinase inhibitors.

to 2% of patients have a *ROS1* fusion. For patients with an *ALK* translocation, treatment with crizotinib is associated with response rates greater than 60% and median PFS around 8 months ([62]). Crizotinib is similarly effective in patients with *ROS1* translocations, with response rates over 70% and median PFS over 19 months ([65]). Crizotinib is the standard first-line therapy in patients with advanced lung adenocarcinoma with *EML4-ALK* translocations or *ROS1* fusions (see Table 18-14).

The mechanisms of resistance to crizotinib therapy have been studied. About 46% of patients develop further alterations in the *ALK* gene (28% secondary *ALK* mutations, 18% *ALK* copy number gains), 8% develop *EGFR* mutations, and 18% develop *KRAS* mutations ([73]). The most common resistance mutations are L1196M and G1269A, which occur at the crizotinib binding site. Another proposed mechanism of resistance is the overexpression of insulin-like growth factor receptor 1 (IGF-1), which activates the same downstream pathways as ALK.

Regardless of the mechanism of resistance, patients with acquired resistance to crizotinib should receive second-line treatment with one of the second-generation ALK inhibitors. Ceritinib has shown promising results in a large phase I trial and is US Food and Drug Administration (FDA) approved for ALK-positive patients following progression on crizotinib ([63]). Other second-generation ALK inhibitors, including alectinib, AP26113, and X-396, are currently in clinical development (see Table 18-14).

Frontline Chemotherapy for Advanced Non–Small Cell Lung Cancer

Most patients with lung cancer do not have a tumor that is targetable with an approved therapy. For these patients, as well as for patients with *EGFR* mutation or *ALK* or *ROS1* fusions progressing on targeted therapies, cytotoxic chemotherapy represents the standard of care.

When compared to best supportive care, chemotherapy is associated with a modest improvement in median OS (1.5 months) and significant gains in symptom control ([74]). Multiple platinum-based doublets are equally effective with response rates around 18% to 35%, PFS of 3 to 6 months, and OS of 8 to 12 months ([75-79]) (Table 18-15). Acceptable agents to combine with platinum include paclitaxel ([75]), docetaxel ([75]), pemetrexed ([76, 77]) (nonsquamous only), gemcitabine ([75]), and nab-paclitaxel ([78]). One trial showed that cisplatin-pemetrexed is superior to cisplatin-gemcitabine in patients with adenocarcinoma but inferior in patients with SCC ([76,77]). Because this combination is relatively well tolerated and has a convenient once every 3 weeks dosing schedule, it is often used as first-line therapy in patients with adenocarcinoma.

In the past, trials suggested that cisplatin was associated with better response rates and PFS than carboplatin, but a meta-analysis focusing only on modern regimens (docetaxel, paclitaxel, vinorelbine, or gemcitabine combined with platinum) ([80]) showed that carboplatin and cisplatin lead to similar outcomes. The toxicity profile is different, and cisplatin has a higher risk for nausea, whereas carboplatin has higher rates of myelosuppression.

The addition of the VEGF monoclonal antibody bevacizumab to carboplatin/paclitaxel can be considered in patients with adenocarcinomas. The phase III Eastern Cooperative Oncology Group (ECOG) 4599 trial ([79]) randomized patients with nonsquamous NSCLC to carboplatin and paclitaxel with or without bevacizumab. The bevacizumab-containing arm had better response rates (35% vs 15%, $P < .001$), PFS (6.2 vs 4.5 months, $P < .001$), and OS (12.3 vs 10.3 months, $P = .003$), although there were higher rates of adverse events, including a higher risk of severe bleeding (4.4% vs 0.7%, $P < .001$). Patients with squamous histology, hemoptysis, or uncontrolled hypertension and those older than 70 are at higher risk for bleeding with bevacizumab and are not candidates for this therapy.

Maintenance Chemotherapy

For patients who do not progress after four to six cycles of therapy with a platinum doublet, multiple trials have studied maintenance therapy—either continuation

Table 18-15 Summary of First-Line Chemotherapy Trials in NSCLC

Pivotal Trial	Histology	Drug	Response Rate	PFS (months)	OS (months)	Trial Interpretation
ECOG 1594, 2002 ([75])	All NSCLC	Cisplatin 75 mg/m^2 D1 + paclitaxel 135 mg/m^2 over 24 h D2 every 3 weeks	21%	3.4	7.8	No significant difference between the 4 drug regimens
		Cisplatin 100 mg/m^2 D1 + gemcitabine 1,000 mg/m^2 D1, D8 every 4 weeks	22%	4.2	8.1	
		Cisplatin 75 mg/m^2 + docetaxel 75 mg/m^2 every 3 weeks	17%	3.7	7.4	
		Carboplatin AUC 6 + paclitaxel 225 mg/m^2 every 3 weeks	19%	3.1	8.1	
Socinski et al, 2012 ([78])	All NSCLC	Carboplatin AUC 6 D1 + nab-paclitaxel 100 mg/m^2 D1, 8, 15 every 3 weeks	33%	6.3	12.1	Similar efficacy; nab-paclitaxel associated with more neutropenia and less neuropathy
		Carboplatin AUC 6 + paclitaxel 200 mg/m^2 every 3 weeks	25%	5.8	11.2	
ECOG 4599, 2006 ([79])	Nonsquamous	Carboplatin AUC 6 + paclitaxel 200 mg/m^2 + bevacizumab 15 mg/kg every 3 weeks × 6 then maintenance bevacizumab every 3 weeks	35%	6.2	12.3	Benefit of adding bevacizumab to the induction and maintenance phases; high risk of bleeding in squamous histology
		Carboplatin AUC 6 + paclitaxel 200 mg/m^2 every 3 weeks × 6	15%	4.5	10.3	
Scagliotti et al, 2008 ([76,77])	Nonsquamous	Cisplatin 75 mg/m^2 + pemetrexed 500 mg/m^2 every 3 weeks	29%	5.5	12.6	Benefit of pemetrexed in nonsquamous histology
		Cisplatin 75 mg/m^2 + gemcitabine 1,250 mg/m^2 D1, D8 every 3 weeks	22%	5.0	10.9	
	Squamous	Cisplatin 75 mg/m^2 + pemetrexed 500 mg/m^2 every 3 weeks	23%	4.4	9.4	Benefit of gemcitabine in squamous NSCLC
		Cisplatin 75 mg/m^2 + gemcitabine 1,250 mg/m^2 D1, D8 every 3 weeks	31%	5.5	10.8	

AUC, area under the curve; D, day; NSCLC, non–small cell lung cancer; OS, overall survival; PFS, progression-free survival.

maintenance (continuing the same nonplatinum drug) or switch maintenance (initiating a non-cross-resistant nonplatinum drug) (Table 18-16) ([81–87]).

Patients receiving either pemetrexed or bevacizumab as part of their initial therapy should continue these drugs as long as tolerated or until progression ([79, 85, 86]). For patients who are treated with other frontline regimens, maintenance therapy is more controversial. Switch maintenance to either pemetrexed (for nonsquamous NSCLC) ([82]) or docetaxel ([81]) is associated with benefits in PFS, although effects on OS are unclear, particularly for patients who go on to receive second-line therapy. Maintenance pemetrexed in patients with SCC has been shown to be associated with shorter PFS ([82]) than observation alone; based on these data and the other data described earlier, pemetrexed should not be used for patients with NSCLC with predominantly squamous histology.

Chemotherapy for Patients With Platinum-Refractory Disease

Patients with disease progression after platinum-based therapy who maintain good performance status are candidates for second-line therapy. The agents with proven efficacy in this setting are single-agent docetaxel, pemetrexed (in nonsquamous NSCLC only), and ramucirumab in combination with docetaxel (Table 18-17) ([77, 88–95]). Second-line pemetrexed is equivalent to docetaxel in nonsquamous histologies (response rate, 12.8% vs 9.9%; OS, 9 vs 9.2 months) but inferior in squamous NSCLC (response rate, 2.8% vs 8.1%; OS, 6.2 vs 7.4 months; $P = .018$).

Reexposure to platinum in second-line therapy increases response rates, but not PFS or OS, even in patients with long (>6 months) platinum-free intervals ([91]) and is not frequently used. The only combination therapy approved in the second-line setting is docetaxel with the anti-VEGF receptor 2 (anti-VEGFR2) monoclonal antibody ramucirumab ([92]). In the pivotal REVEL trial comparing docetaxel alone to docetaxel plus ramucirumab in patients with NSCLC of any histology, the combination arm had better PFS (4.5 vs 3 months, $P < .0001$) and OS (10.5 vs 9.1 months, $P = .023$) with no increased risk of severe bleeding. It is important to highlight that only 14% of patients enrolled in REVEL had received prior bevacizumab, making it difficult to draw conclusions about this group. Also, unlike the phase III bevacizumab trials that excluded patients with SCC, 25% of patients on this trial had squamous histology, and there was no increased risk of bleeding seen in this group.

For patients with wild-type EGFR, docetaxel and pemetrexed appear to be better second-line options than erlotinib ([93, 95]), although erlotinib remains an FDA-approved option for third-line therapy ([94]).

Treatment of Stage IV Non–Small Cell Lung Cancer in the Elderly

Treatment of advanced NSCLC in the elderly has been addressed in several prospective studies and retrospective analyses, and the International Society of Geriatric Oncology (SIOG) has issued clear guidelines ([96]). Basically, patients older than age 70 years should undergo functional evaluation, and those with good functionality should receive standard therapy.

For lung adenocarcinomas with actionable mutations, TKIs should be recommended. For patients without actionable mutations, platinum-based doublets should be offered. In the IFCT-0501 trial ([97]), patients older than age 70 were randomized to carboplatin-paclitaxel or single-agent therapy with vinorelbine or gemcitabine. The combination arm had a significant improvement in OS (10.3 vs 6.2 months, $P < .0001$) and better pain control rates with a small increase in the rates of toxic death (4.4% vs 1.3%). Based on the subgroup analysis from ECOG 4599 ([98]) and on other trials, bevacizumab should not be added to chemotherapy in elderly patients because of lack of benefit and increased risk of severe side effects.

Immunotherapy in Advanced Non–Small Cell Lung Cancer

Immunotherapy has recently achieved significant outcomes in the treatment of metastatic melanoma, leading to the approval of immune checkpoint inhibitors such as anti-PD-1/PD-L1 and anti-CTLA4 antibodies (see chapter on cancer immunotherapy). Lung cancers are among the malignancies with the highest mutation burden, averaging 360 exonic mutations per sample ([23]). Many of those mutations generate neoantigens potentially able to stimulate effector $CD8^+$ T cells. It has also been shown that NSCLC with high tumor-infiltrating lymphocytes have better outcomes after resection and in the metastatic setting ([99]), suggesting lung cancers as good candidates for the investigational use of immunotherapies.

Previous trials focused on cancer vaccines in NSCLC, which were shown to induce tumor-specific immune responses but failed to improve survival ([100]). The development of immune checkpoint inhibitors has renewed the interest in immunotherapy approaches for NSCLC (Table 18-18) ([101–106]).

Table 18-16 Summary of Maintenance Chemotherapy Trials in NSCLC

Trial	Histology	Drug	Response Rate	PFS (months)	OS (months)	Trial Interpretation
Fidias et al, 2009 ([81])	All NSCLC	Maintenance docetaxel 75 mg/m^2 every 3 weeks × 6 after 4 cycles of carboplatin + gemcitabine	41.4%	5.7	12.3	Better PFS with switch maintenance. No OS benefit.
		No maintenance; docetaxel at time of progression	NA	2.7	9.7	
Ciuleanu et al, 2009 ([82])	Nonsquamous	Maintenance pemetrexed 500 mg/m^2 every 3 weeks after 4 cycles of platinum doublet	58%	4.4	15.5	Benefit of switch maintenance with pemetrexed.
		No maintenance	NA	1.8	10.3	
SATURN, 2010 ([83])	*EGFR*-mutant	Erlotinib 150 mg/day maintenance after 4 cycles of platinum-based chemotherapy	NA	11	NA	Benefit of switch maintenance with erlotinib in *EGFR*-mutant patients.
	NSCLC	No maintenance	NA	3	NA	
	EGFR WT	Erlotinib 150 mg/day maintenance after 4 cycles of platinum-based chemotherapy	11.9%	3.07	12	
	NSCLC	No maintenance	5.4%	2.7	11	
IFCT-GFPC 0502, 2012 ([84])	All NSCLC (mostly *EGFR* WT)	Erlotinib 150 mg/day maintenance after cisplatin-gemcitabine × 4	NA	2.9	11.4	No benefit of switch maintenance with erlotinib or maintenance with gemcitabine in *EGFR* WT patients.
		Gemcitabine 1,250 mg/m^2 D1, D8 maintenance	NA	3.8	12.1	
		No maintenance	NA	1.9	10.8	
PARAMOUNT, 2013 ([85])	Nonsquamous	Maintenance pemetrexed 500 mg/m^2 every 3 weeks after 4 cycles of cisplatin + pemetrexed	NA	4.4	13.9	Benefit of continuation maintenance with pemetrexed.
		No maintenance	NA	2.8	11	
AVAPERL, 2012 ([86])	Nonsquamous	Carboplatin AUC 6 + pemetrexed 500 mg/m^2 + bevacizumab 15 mg/kg ever 3 weeks × 4 then maintenance pemetrexed 500 mg/m^2 + bevacizumab 15 mg/kg every 3 weeks	NA	7.4	Not reached	PFS benefit of adding pemetrexed to maintenance bevacizumab after cisplatin-pemetrexed induction.
		Carboplatin AUC 6 + pemetrexed 500 mg/m^2 + bevacizumab 15 mg/kg every 3 weeks × 4 then bevacizumab 15 mg/kg every 3 weeks	NA	3.7	12.8	
PointBreak, 2013 ([87])	Nonsquamous	Carboplatin AUC 6 + pemetrexed 500 mg/m^2 + bevacizumab 15 mg/kg every 3 weeks × 4 then maintenance pemetrexed 500 mg/m^2 + bevacizumab 15 mg/kg every 3 weeks	34%	6	12.6	No difference between the 2 treatment strategies.
		Carboplatin AUC 6 + paclitaxel 200 mg/m^2 + bevacizumab 15 mg/kg every 3 weeks × 4 then maintenance bevacizumab 15 mg/kg every 3 weeks	33%	5.6	13.4	

AUC, area under the curve; D, day; NA, not applicable; NSCLC, non–small cell lung cancer; OS, overall survival; PFS, progression-free survival; WT, wild type.

Table 18-17 Summary of Second- and Third-Line Chemotherapy Trials in NSCLC

Pivotal Trial	Histology	Drug	Response Rate	PFS (months)	OS (months)	Trial Interpretation
Second line						
TAX 317, 2000 ([88])	All NSCLC	Docetaxel 75 mg/m^2 every 3 weeks	7.1%	2.65	7	Benefit of second-line docetaxel
		Best supportive care	0%	1.67	4.6	
TAX 320, 2000 ([89])	All NSCLC	Docetaxel 75 mg/m^2 every 3 weeks	6.7%	2.1	5.7	Benefit of docetaxel over vinorelbine (less toxicity, same PFS/OS)
		Vinorelbine 30 mg/m^2 weekly or ifosfamide 2 mg/m^2/day D1-3 every 3 weeks	0.8%	1.9	5.6	
Hanna et al, 2004 ([77,90])	Nonsquamous	Pemetrexed 500 mg/m^2 every 3 weeks	12.8%	3.5	9	Benefit of pemetrexed over docetaxel in nonsquamous histologies
		Docetaxel 75 mg/m^2 every 3 weeks	9.9%	3.5	9.2	
	Squamous	Pemetrexed 500 mg/m^2 every 3 weeks	2.8%	2.3	6.2	Benefit of docetaxel over pemetrexed in squamous NSCLC
		Docetaxel 75 mg/m^2 every 3 weeks	8.1%	2.7	7.4	
GOIRC 02-2006/NVALT-7, 2012 ([91])	All NSCLC	Carboplatin AUC 5 + pemetrexed 500 mg/m^2 every 3 weeks	15%	3.6	8.7	No benefit of platinum doublets over nonplatinum single-agent second-line therapy
		Pemetrexed 500 mg/m^2 every 3 weeks	9%	3.5	8.2	
REVEL, 2014 ([92])	All NSCLC	Docetaxel 75 mg/m^2 + ramucirumab 10 mg/kg every 3 weeks	23%	4.5	10.5	Benefit of ramucirumab when added to docetaxel in second line
		Docetaxel 75 mg/m^2 every 3 weeks	14%	3.0	9.1	
TAILOR, 2013 ([93])	*EGFR* wild-type NSCLC	Erlotinib 150 mg/day	3%	2.4	5.4	No benefit of second-line erlotinib in *EGFR* wild-type NSCLC
		Docetaxel 75 mg/m^2 every 3 weeks	15%	2.9	8.2	
Third line						
BR.21, 2005 ([94])	All NSCLC (*EGFR* status unknown)	Erlotinib 150 mg/day	8.9%	2.2	6.7	Third-line erlotinib can prolong survival in patients with NSCLC and unknown *EGFR* status
		Placebo	<1%	1.8	4.7	
DELTA, 2014 ([95])	*EGFR* wild-type NSCLC	Erlotinib 150 mg/day	17%	1.3	9	Docetaxel is superior to erlotinib as second- or third-line therapy in patients with no activating *EGFR* mutations
		Docetaxel 60 mg/m^2 every 3 weeks	17%	2.9	10.1	

AUC, area under the curve; D, day; NSCLC, non–small cell lung cancer; OS, overall survival; PFS, progression-free survival.

Table 18-18 Summary of the Larger Trials of Immune Checkpoint Inhibitors in Stage IV NSCLC

Trial Sample size	Design and Treatment Line	Drug and Dose	Response Rate	Outcomes	Conclusion
Anti-CTLA4 antibodies					
Lynch et al, 2012 ([101]) (204 patients)	Phase II First line	Carboplatin + paclitaxel every 3 weeks × 6 cycles	18%	PFS 4.2 mo OS: 8.3 mo	Nonsignificant improvement in OS; suggests more benefit in squamous histology
		Ipilimumab 10 mg/kg every 3 weeks added to cycles 1-4	21%	PFS 4.1 mo OS: 9.7 mo	
		Ipilimumab 10 mg/kg every 3 weeks added to cycles 3-6	32%	PFS 5.1 mo OS: 12.2 mo	
Anti-PD-1 antibodies					
Topalian et al, 2012 ([102]) (76 patients)	Phase I Second/third line	Nivolumab 1-10 mg/kg every 2 weeks	18%	26% progression free at 6 mo	First signal of activity of nivolumab
Antonia et al, 2014 ([103]) (56 patients)	Phase II First line	Nivolumab 10 mg/kg every 2 weeks + paclitaxel/carboplatin (any histology)	47%	38% progression free at 6 mo 59% alive at 12 mo	Good tolerability of combination nivolumab + chemotherapy; signal of activity in first line
		Nivolumab 10 mg/kg every 2 weeks + pemetrexed/cisplatin (nonsquamous)	47%	71% progression free at 6 mo 87% alive at 12 mo	
		Nivolumab 10 mg/kg every 2 weeks + gemcitabine and cisplatin (squamous)	33%	36% progression free at 6 mo 59% alive at 12 mo	
CheckMate – 063, 2015 ([104]) (117 patients)	Phase II Third-line	Nivolumab 3 mg/kg every 3 weeks (squamous cell only)	14.5%	OS 8.2 mo 41% alive at 12 mo	Confirms activity seen in previous trials
KEYNOTE-001 ([105]) (282 patients, ongoing)	Phase II First line	Pembrolizumab 10 mg/kg every 2 weeks or every 3 weeks	26%	PFS 6.7 mo OS not reached 86% alive at 6 mo	Only patients with PD-L1 expression were included; no difference between every 2 weeks and every 3 weeks dose or squamous vs nonsquamous carcinoma
	Phase II Second line	Pembrolizumab 10 mg/kg every 2 weeks or every 3 weeks	20%	PFS 2.2 mo OS 8.2 mo 57% alive at 6 mo	
Anti-PD-L1 antibodies					
Herbst et al, 2014 ([106]) (85 patients)	Phase I Second/third line	MDPL3280A 10, 15, or 20 mg/kg every 3 weeks	26%	PFS 3.75 mo	More benefit in cases with high expression of PD-L1 in TILs
				44% alive at 6 mo	

NSCLC, non–small cell lung cancer; OS, overall survival; PD-1, programmed cell death protein 1; PD-L1, programmed cell death ligand 1; PFS, progression-free survival; TILs, tumor-infiltrating lymphocytes.

The CTLA4 receptor on T cells interacts with the B7-1 and B7-2 proteins on antigen-presenting cells and downregulates the T-cell response to tumor-related antigens. There are two anti-CTLA4 antibodies currently approved for the treatment of melanoma: ipilimumab and tremelimumab. In a randomized phase II trial for NSCLC patients ([101]), the addition of ipilimumab during cycles 3 to 6 of first-line chemotherapy with carboplatin and paclitaxel was associated with better response rates and a nonsignificant increase in OS. There are multiple trials under way to investigate how best to use these agents in patients with metastatic disease (eg, alone or in combination, timing in combinations, incorporation of molecular markers for selection), such as the randomized trial with carboplatin/paclitaxel with or without ipilimumab for patients with squamous histology (NCT01285609).

PD-1 is another receptor expressed on T cells that, upon interaction with its ligand, PD-L1, suppresses immune cell activation. Expression of PD-L1 on antigen-presenting cells and on tumor cells is believed to be a key player in local tumor microenvironment-mediated immunosuppression. Approximately 35% to 50% of stage IV NSCLC patients have moderate to high staining of PD-1 or PD-L1 depending on the methodology for staining and scoring.

Two anti-PD-1 antibodies have been studied in phase I and II trials of NSCLC: nivolumab and pembrolizumab (see Table 18-18). In general, the response rates have been 15% to 25% both in the first- and second-line settings, and the OS has been around 8 to 10 months, with no difference between adenocarcinoma and SCC. However, some responders have prolonged disease control, sometimes for more than 12 months. No predictor of response has been validated yet, but it appears that tumors with higher expression of PD-L1 ([105]) and those with PD-L1–positive tumor-infiltrating lymphocytes ([106]) have better outcomes when treated with anti-PD-1/PD-L1 agents. There are also data emerging from several groups on regulation of the dynamic PD-L1 expression of tumor cells, including the effect of epithelial-to-mesenchymal transition to drive $CD8^+$ T-cell suppression through PD-L1 activation ([107]).

The use of anti-PD-1/anti-PD-L1 therapy currently remains investigational, but the pending results of phase II and III trials of pembrolizumab and nivolumab in metastatic NSCLC could substantially change the landscape of treatments options in the near future.

Other Therapies for Advanced Disease and Management of Oligometastatic Disease

Radiotherapy and surgery may be helpful in managing selected patients with stage IV NSCLC. Radiotherapy can be used to palliate pain or to manage hemoptysis and obstructive symptoms in large primary tumors.

In patients with solitary brain metastasis as their only site of metastatic disease, resection or stereotactic radiation of the brain lesion followed by definitive therapy to the primary tumor (resection or radiation) is associated with significant improvement in median OS (26 months vs 13 months in patients who do not undergo therapy to the primary tumor), and 5-year survival rates are 34% versus 0% ([108]).

In patients with solitary adrenal metastasis, adrenalectomy associated with definitive therapy to the primary tumor also has good outcomes, with a median OS of 26 months and 5-year survival rates of 30%, which has been consistent in multiple studies ([109]). Patients who develop isolated adrenal metastasis more than 6 months after the resection of the primary tumor are the ones with the most benefit.

Patients with oligometastatic disease (one to five lesions) should undergo extensive workup including PET-CT scan and brain MRI. They can then be classified into three subgroups ([110]):

- Low risk: Development of oligometastatic disease more than 2 months after resection of the primary tumor (5-year OS, 47.8%).
- Intermediate risk: Synchronous metastases (at presentation or within 2 months of the resection of the primary) and no lymph node involvement (N0) disease (5-year OS, 36.2%).
- High risk: Synchronous metastases and N1/N2 disease (5-year OS, 13.8%).

There is currently one randomized trial ongoing evaluating the effect of definitive treatment (surgery or radiation) for oligometastatic disease (NCT01725165). However, observational studies have shown that, in patients who received two cycles of systemic therapy and did not have progression, definitive therapy to oligometastasis was associated with improvements in OS (27 vs 13 months; HR, 0.37; 95% confidence interval [CI], 0.2-0.7; $P < .01$) ([111]). There are also data suggesting that, for patients with oligometastatic disease receiving chemotherapy, radiation therapy to the primary tumor is associated with improved OS (HR, 0.65; 95% CI, 0.43-0.93; $P = .019$) ([112]).

FUTURE DIRECTIONS

The treatment for NSCLC, especially in the metastatic setting, has witnessed remarkably rapid change over the last 10 years. This change has been driven primarily by the recognition of the significant molecular heterogeneity of the disease and identification of targetable genetic changes defining the many subgroups. We expect that this trend will continue to facilitate the successful application of targeted agents, especially for the squamous cell histology where there are still no approved targeted agents. Examples of molecular alterations under investigation are *BRAF*, *MEK*, *MET*, *mTOR*, and *HER2*, as well as new approaches to target *KRAS* mutant disease. There is also continued research on new-generation TKIs able to overcome acquired resistance to erlotinib and crizotinib. Because the molecular profile of tumors is dynamic, with variability at each tumor site and varying over time at any one site, the need for repeat biopsies has become increasingly accepted and therapeutic options are more frequently based on the changing genetics of an individual patient's tumor. In the future, this personalized evaluation of mutations in circulating tumor cells or circulating cell-free tumor DNA might be an important tool in the process.

For patients with early-stage disease, large centralized trials like ALCHEMIST have been developed to evaluate molecular testing and the application of targeted agents in the adjuvant setting. The hope is to achieve more cures and/or produce longer periods of disease-free recurrence in this group of patients who have undergone curative-intent therapy.

Certainly the future of oncology and lung cancer, in particular, will be substantially impacted by the incorporation of immunotherapies. However, it is difficult to predict how this landscape might emerge as the currently available agents and new agents are developed. The investigation of single-agent immune checkpoint molecule (PD-1 and CTLA4) inhibitors in the refractory metastatic setting is moving very rapidly, with the expectation that one or more of the PD-1/PD-L1 axis inhibitors will be approved soon. Research is also focusing on evaluating combination strategies and on moving their use to the frontline and adjuvant settings. As with all other therapies, one particularly challenging aspect of applying immunotherapies to the clinic is the determination of which biomarkers are useful to select patients more or less likely to respond and to monitor response. However, given the complexity of the immune system and our limited experience in developing drugs of this type, the technical and conceptual challenges of marker development may lag behind the efficacy trials. It is hard to understate the current excitement around the immunotherapy agents, and it will be intriguing to see how they finally find their proper role in the treatment of patients with NSCLC.

CONCLUSIONS

Non–small cell lung cancer remains one of the most devastating illnesses in the United States and worldwide in terms of incidence and overall mortality rates. Primary prevention by smoking cessation and secondary prevention with screening have managed to reduce the incidence of NSCLC and NSCLC-related deaths in some areas of the world, but the incidence of lung cancers not related to smoking is still rising. Surgery and chemoradiation offer a potential for long-term survival in patients with localized disease, but metastatic disease remains lethal. In recent years, the evolving understanding of the molecular pathology of NSCLC has produced effective targeted agents, with high response rates and low toxicity, but resistance is still an issue. The development of new targeted agents able to overcome resistance and the effective implementation of cancer immunotherapy have the potential to further improve outcomes for patients with NSCLC.

REFERENCES

1. Ferlay J, Soerjomataram I I, Dikshit R, et al. Cancer incidence and mortality worldwide: sources, methods and major patterns in GLOBOCAN 2012. *Int J Cancer*. 2015;136:E359–E386. doi:10.1002/ijc.29210.
2. Edwards BK, Noone A-M, Mariotto AB, et al. Annual Report to the Nation on the status of cancer, 1975-2010, featuring prevalence of comorbidity and impact on survival among persons with lung, colorectal, breast, or prostate cancer. *Cancer*. 2014;120(9):1290–1314. doi:10.1002/cncr.28509.
3. Haiman CA, Stram DO, Wilkens LR, et al. Ethnic and racial differences in the smoking-related risk of lung cancer. *N Engl J Med*. 2006;354:333–342. doi:10.1056/NEJMoa033250.
4. Bach PB, Kattan MW, Thornquist MD, et al. Variations in lung cancer risk among smokers. *J Natl Cancer Inst*. 2003;95(6):470–478. doi:10.1093/jnci/95.6.470.
5. Markowitz SB, Levin SM, Miller A, Morabia A. Asbestos, asbestosis, smoking, and lung cancer. New findings from the North American insulator cohort. *Am J Respir Crit Care Med*. 2013;188(1):90–96. doi:10.1164/rccm.201302-0257OC.
6. Torres-Durán M, Ruano-Ravina A, Parente-Lamelas I, et al. Lung cancer in never-smokers: a case-control study in a radon-prone area (Galicia, Spain). *Eur Respir J*. 2014;44(4):994–1001. doi:10.1183/09031936.00017114.
7. Alberg AJ, Samet JM. Epidemiology of lung cancer. *Chest*. 2003;123(1 Suppl):21S–49S.
8. Field RW, Withers BL. Occupational and environmental causes of lung cancer. *Clin Chest Med*. 2012;33(4):681–703. doi:10.1016/j.ccm.2012.07.001.
9. Sellers TA, Chen PL, Potter JD, Bailey-Wilson JE, Rothschild H, Elston RC. Segregation analysis of smoking-associated malignancies: evidence for Mendelian inheritance. *Am J Med Genet*. 1994;52(3):308–314. doi:10.1002/ajmg.1320520311.
10. Wang J-J, Zheng Y, Sun L, et al. CYP1A1 Ile462Val polymorphism and susceptibility to lung cancer: a meta-analysis based on 32 studies. *Eur J Cancer Prev*. 2011;20(6):445–452. doi:10.1097/CEJ.0b013e328345f937.
11. Langevin SM, Ioannidis JP, Vineis P, Taioli E. Assessment of cumulative evidence for the association between glutathione S-transferase polymorphisms and lung cancer: application of the Venice interim guidelines. *Pharmacogenet Genomics*. 2010;20(10):586–597. doi:10.1097/FPC.0b013e32833c3892.
12. Li W, Li K, Zhao L, Zou H. DNA repair pathway genes and lung cancer susceptibility: a meta-analysis. *Gene*. 2014;538(2):361–365. doi:10.1016/j.gene.2013.12.028.

13. Brennan P, Hainaut P, Boffetta P. Genetics of lung-cancer susceptibility. *Lancet Oncol.* 2011;12(4):399–408. doi:10.1016/S1470-2045(10)70126-1.
14. Aberle DR, Adams AM, Berg CD, et al. Reduced lung-cancer mortality with low-dose computed tomographic screening. *N Engl J Med.* 2011;365(5):395–409. doi:10.1056/NEJMoa1102873.
15. The effect of vitamin E and beta carotene on the incidence of lung cancer and other cancers in male smokers. The Alpha-Tocopherol, Beta Carotene Cancer Prevention Study Group. *N Engl J Med.* 1994;330(15):1029–1035. doi:10.1056/NEJM199404143301501.
16. Omenn GS, Goodman GE, Thornquist MD, et al. Effects of a combination of beta carotene and vitamin A on lung cancer and cardiovascular disease. *N Engl J Med.* 1996;334(18):1150–1155. doi:10.1056/NEJM199605023341802.
17. Lippman SM, Lee JJ, Karp DD, et al. Randomized phase III intergroup trial of isotretinoin to prevent second primary tumors in stage I non-small-cell lung cancer. *J Natl Cancer Inst.* 2001;93(8):605–618.
18. Khuri FR, Lee JJ, Lippman SM, et al. Randomized phase III trial of low-dose isotretinoin for prevention of second primary tumors in stage I and II head and neck cancer patients. *J Natl Cancer Inst.* 2006;98(7):441–450. doi:10.1093/jnci/djj091.
19. Karp DD, Lee SJ, Keller SM, et al. Randomized, double-blind, placebo-controlled, phase III chemoprevention trial of selenium supplementation in patients with resected stage I non-small-cell lung cancer: ECOG 5597. *J Clin Oncol.* 2013;31(33):4179–4187. doi:10.1200/JCO.2013.49.2173.
20. Gaziano JM, Glynn RJ, Christen WG, et al. Vitamins E and C in the prevention of prostate and total cancer in men: the Physicians' Health Study II randomized controlled trial. *JAMA.* 2009;301(1):52–62. doi:10.1001/jama.2008.862.
21. Ebbing M, Bønaa KH, Nygård O, et al. Cancer incidence and mortality after treatment with folic acid and vitamin B12. *JAMA.* 2009;302(19):2119–2126. doi:10.1001/jama.2009.1622.
22. Travis WD, Brambilla E, Noguchi M, et al. International Association for the Study of Lung Cancer/American Thoracic Society/European Respiratory Society international multidisciplinary classification of lung adenocarcinoma. *J Thorac Oncol.* 2011;6(2):244–285. doi:10.1097/JTO.0b013e318206a221.
23. The Cancer Genome Atlas Research Network. Comprehensive genomic characterization of squamous cell lung cancers. *Nature.* 2012;489(7417):519–525. doi:10.1038/nature11404.
24. Collisson EA, Campbell JD, Brooks AN, et al. Comprehensive molecular profiling of lung adenocarcinoma. *Nature.* 2014;511:543–550. doi:10.1038/nature13385.
25. Dogan S, Shen R, Ang DC, et al. Molecular epidemiology of EGFR and KRAS mutations in 3,026 lung adenocarcinomas: higher susceptibility of women to smoking-related KRAS-mutant cancers. *Clin Cancer Res.* 2012;18(22):6169–6177. doi:10.1158/1078-0432.CCR-11-3265.
26. Beau-Faller M, Prim N, Ruppert A-M, et al. Rare EGFR exon 18 and exon 20 mutations in non-small-cell lung cancer on 10 117 patients: a multicentre observational study by the French ERMETIC-IFCT network. *Ann Oncol.* 2014;25(1):126–131. doi:10.1093/annonc/mdt418.
27. Arcila ME, Nafa K, Chaft JE, et al. EGFR exon 20 insertion mutations in lung adenocarcinomas: prevalence, molecular heterogeneity, and clinicopathologic characteristics. *Mol Cancer Ther.* 2013;12(2):220–229. doi:10.1158/1535-7163.MCT-12-0620.
28. D'Angelo SP, Pietanza MC, Johnson ML, et al. Incidence of EGFR exon 19 deletions and L858R in tumor specimens from men and cigarette smokers with lung adenocarcinomas. *J Clin Oncol.* 2011;29(15):2066–2070. doi:10.1200/JCO.2010.32.6181.
29. Pan Y, Zhang Y, Li Y, et al. ALK, ROS1 and RET fusions in 1139 lung adenocarcinomas: a comprehensive study of common and fusion pattern-specific clinicopathologic, histologic and cytologic features. *Lung Cancer.* 2014;84(2):121–126. doi:10.1016/j.lungcan.2014.02.007.
30. Gainor JF, Varghese AM, Ou S-HI, et al. ALK rearrangements are mutually exclusive with mutations in EGFR or KRAS: an analysis of 1,683 patients with non-small cell lung cancer. *Clin Cancer Res.* 2013;19(15):4273–4281. doi:10.1158/1078-0432.CCR-13-0318.
31. Tsuta K, Kohno T, Yoshida A, et al. RET-rearranged non-small-cell lung carcinoma: a clinicopathological and molecular analysis. *Br J Cancer.* 2014;110(6):1571–1578. doi:10.1038/bjc.2014.36.
32. Arcila ME, Chaft JE, Nafa K, et al. Prevalence, clinicopathologic associations, and molecular spectrum of ERBB2 (HER2) tyrosine kinase mutations in lung adenocarcinomas. *Clin Cancer Res.* 2012;18(18):4910–4918. doi:10.1158/1078-0432.CCR-12-0912.
33. Gould MK, Donington J, Lynch WR, et al. Evaluation of individuals with pulmonary nodules: when is it lung cancer? Diagnosis and management of lung cancer, 3rd ed: American College of Chest Physicians evidence-based clinical practice guidelines. *Chest.* 2013;143(5 Suppl):e93S–120S. doi:10.1378/chest.12-2351.
34. Detterbeck FC, Boffa DJ, Tanoue LT. The new lung cancer staging system. *Chest.* 2009;136(1):260–271. doi:10.1378/chest.08-0978.
35. Landreneau RJ, Normolle DP, Christie NA, et al. Recurrence and survival outcomes after anatomic segmentectomy versus lobectomy for clinical stage I non-small-cell lung cancer: a propensity-matched analysis. *J Clin Oncol.* 2014;32(23):2449–2455. doi:10.1200/JCO.2013.50.8762.
36. Darling GE, Allen MS, Decker PA, et al. Randomized trial of mediastinal lymph node sampling versus complete lymphadenectomy during pulmonary resection in the patient with N0 or N1 (less than hilar) non-small cell carcinoma: results of the American College of Surgery Oncology Group Z0030 Trial. *J Thorac Cardiovasc Surg.* 2011;141(3):662–670. doi:10.1016/j.jtcvs.2010.11.008.
37. Brunelli A, Kim AW, Berger KI, Addrizzo-Harris DJ. Physiologic evaluation of the patient with lung cancer being considered for resectional surgery: Diagnosis and management of lung cancer, 3rd ed: American College of Chest Physicians evidence-based clinical practice guidelines. *Chest.* 2013;143(5 Suppl):e166S–190S. doi:10.1378/chest.12-2395.
38. Onishi H, Araki T, Shirato H, et al. Stereotactic hypofractionated high-dose irradiation for stage I nonsmall cell lung carcinoma: clinical outcomes in 245 subjects in a Japanese multiinstitutional study. *Cancer.* 2004;101:1623–1631. doi:10.1002/cncr.20539.
39. Arriagada R, Auperin A, Burdett S, et al. Adjuvant chemotherapy, with or without postoperative radiotherapy, in operable non-small-cell lung cancer: two meta-analyses of individual patient data. *Lancet.* 2010;375(9722):1267–1277. doi:10.1016/S0140-6736(10)60059-1.
40. Strauss GM, Herndon JE, Maddaus MA, et al. Adjuvant paclitaxel plus carboplatin compared with observation in stage IB non-small-cell lung cancer: CALGB 9633 with the Cancer and Leukemia Group B, Radiation Therapy Oncology Group, and North Central Cancer Treatment Group Study Groups. *J Clin Oncol.* 2008;26(31):5043–5051. doi:10.1200/JCO.2008.16.4855.
41. Arriagada R, Bergman B, Dunant A, Le Chevalier T, Pignon J-P, Vansteenkiste J. Cisplatin-based adjuvant chemotherapy in patients with completely resected non-small-cell lung cancer. *N Engl J Med.* 2004;350(4):351–60.doi:10.1056/NEJMoa031644.
42. Douillard JY, Rosell R, De Lena M, et al. Adjuvant vinorelbine plus cisplatin versus observation in patients with completely resected stage IB-IIIA non-small-cell lung cancer (Adjuvant Navelbine International Trialist Association [ANITA]): a

randomised controlled trial. *Lancet Oncol.* 2006;7:719–727. doi:10.1016/S1470-2045(06)70804-X.
43. Winton T, Livingston R, Johnson D, et al. Vinorelbine plus cisplatin vs. observation in resected non-small-cell lung cancer. *N Engl J Med.* 2005;352:2589–2597. doi:10.1056/NEJMoa043623.
44. Kreuter M, Vansteenkiste J, Fischer JR, et al. Randomized phase 2 trial on refinement of early-stage NSCLC adjuvant chemotherapy with cisplatin and pemetrexed versus cisplatin and vinorelbine: the TREAT study. *Ann Oncol.* 2013;24:986–992. doi:10.1093/annonc/mds578.
45. Lim E, Harris G, Patel A, Adachi I, Edmonds L, Song F. Preoperative versus postoperative chemotherapy in patients with resectable non-small cell lung cancer: systematic review and indirect comparison meta-analysis of randomized trials. *J Thorac Oncol.* 2009;4(11):1380–1388. doi:10.1097/JTO.0b013e3181b9ecca.
46. PORT Meta-analysis Trialists Group. Postoperative radiotherapy for non-small cell lung cancer. *Cochrane Database Syst Rev.* 2005;2:CD002142. doi:10.1002/14651858.CD002142.pub2.
47. Albain KS, Swann RS, Rusch VW, et al. Radiotherapy plus chemotherapy with or without surgical resection for stage III non-small-cell lung cancer: a phase III randomised controlled trial. *Lancet.* 2009;374(9687):379–386. doi:10.1016/S0140-6736(09)60737-6.
48. Thomas M, Rübe C, Hoffknecht P, et al. Effect of preoperative chemoradiation in addition to preoperative chemotherapy: a randomised trial in stage III non-small-cell lung cancer. *Lancet Oncol.* 2008;9(7):636–648. doi:10.1016/S1470-2045(08)70156-6.
49. Aupérin A, Le Péchoux C, Rolland E, et al. Meta-analysis of concomitant versus sequential radiochemotherapy in locally advanced non-small-cell lung cancer. *J Clin Oncol.* 2010;28(13):2181–2190. doi:10.1200/JCO.2009.26.2543.
50. Mauguen A, Le Péchoux C, Saunders MI, et al. Hyperfractionated or accelerated radiotherapy in lung cancer: an individual patient data meta-analysis. *J Clin Oncol.* 2012;30(22): 2788–2797. doi:10.1200/JCO.2012.41.6677.
51. Bradley J, Paulus R, Komaki R, et al. An intergroup randomized phase III comparison of standard-dose (60 Gy) versus high-dose (74 Gy) chemoradiotherapy (CRT) +/- cetuximab (cetux) for stage III non-small cell lung cancer (NSCLC): results on cetux from RTOG 0617 [abstract]. *Proceedings of the 15th World Conference on Lung Cancer.* 2013;8:S3.
52. O'Rourke N, Roqué I, Figuls M, Farré Bernadó N, Macbeth F. Concurrent chemoradiotherapy in non-small cell lung cancer. *Cochrane Database Syst Rev.* 2010;6:CD002140. doi:10.1002/14651858.CD002140.pub3.
53. Santana-Davila R, Devisetty K, Szabo A, et al. Cisplatin and etoposide versus carboplatin and paclitaxel with concurrent radiotherapy for stage III non-small-cell lung cancer: an analysis of Veterans Health Administration Data. *J Clin Oncol.* 2015;33(6):567–574. doi:10.1200/JCO.2014.56.2587.
54. Jalal SI, Riggs HD, Melnyk A, et al. Updated survival and outcomes for older adults with inoperable stage III non-small-cell lung cancer treated with cisplatin, etoposide, and concurrent chest radiation with or without consolidation docetaxel: analysis of a phase III trial from the Hoosier Oncology Group (HOG) and US Oncology. *Ann Oncol.* 2012;23(7):1730–1738. doi:10.1093/annonc/mdr565.
55. Kelly K, Chansky K, Gaspar LE, et al. Phase III trial of maintenance gefitinib or placebo after concurrent chemoradiotherapy and docetaxel consolidation in inoperable stage III non-small-cell lung cancer: SWOG S0023. *J Clin Oncol.* 2008;26(15): 2450–2456. doi:10.1200/JCO.2007.14.4824.
56. Kunitoh H, Kato H, Tsuboi M, et al. Phase II trial of preoperative chemoradiotherapy followed by surgical resection in patients with superior sulcus non-small-cell lung cancers: report of Japan Clinical Oncology Group trial 9806. *J Clin Oncol.* 2008;26(4):644–649. doi:10.1200/JCO.2007.14.1911.
57. Temel JS, Greer JA, Muzikansky A, et al. Early palliative care for patients with metastatic non-small-cell lung cancer. *N Engl J Med.* 2010;363(8):733–742. doi:10.1056/NEJMoa1000678.
58. Leighl NB, Rekhtman N, Biermann WA, et al. Molecular testing for selection of patients with lung cancer for epidermal growth factor receptor and anaplastic lymphoma kinase tyrosine kinase inhibitors: American Society of Clinical Oncology Endorsement of the College of American Pathologists/International Association for the Study of Lung Cancer/Association for Molecular Pathology Guideline. *J Clin Oncol.* 2014;32(32): 3673–3679. doi:10.1200/JCO.2014.57.3055.
59. Rosell R, Carcereny E, Gervais R, et al. Erlotinib versus standard chemotherapy as first-line treatment for European patients with advanced EGFR mutation-positive non-small-cell lung cancer (EURTAC): a multicentre, open-label, randomised phase 3 trial. *Lancet Oncol.* 2012;13(3):239–246. doi:10.1016/S1470-2045(11)70393-X.
60. Mok TS, Wu Y, Thongprasert S, et al. Gefitinib or carboplatin-paclitaxel in pulmonary adenocarcinoma. *N Engl J Med.* 2009;361(10):947–957. doi:10.1056/NEJMoa0810699.
61. Sequist LV, Yang JC-H, Yamamoto N, et al. Phase III study of afatinib or cisplatin plus pemetrexed in patients with metastatic lung adenocarcinoma with EGFR mutations. *J Clin Oncol.* 2013;31(27):3327–3334. doi:10.1200/JCO.2012.44.2806.
62. Solomon BJ, Mok T, Kim D-W, et al. First-line crizotinib versus chemotherapy in ALK-positive lung cancer. *N Engl J Med.* 2014;371(23):2167–2177. doi:10.1056/NEJMoa1408440.
63. Shaw AT, Kim D-W, Mehra R, et al. Ceritinib in ALK-rearranged non-small-cell lung cancer. *N Engl J Med.* 2014;370(13): 1189–1197. doi:10.1056/NEJMoa1311107.
64. Gadgeel SM, Gandhi L, Riely GJ, et al. Safety and activity of alectinib against systemic disease and brain metastases in patients with crizotinib-resistant ALK-rearranged non-small-cell lung cancer (AF-002JG): results from the dose-finding portion of a phase 1/2 study. *Lancet Oncol.* 2014;15(10):1119–1128. doi:10.1016/S1470-2045(14)70362-6.
65. Shaw AT, Ou S-HI, Bang Y-J, et al. Crizotinib in ROS1-rearranged non–small-cell lung cancer. *N Engl J Med.* 2014;371(21):1963–1971. doi:10.1056/NEJMoa1406766.
66. Seto T, Kato T, Nishio M, et al. Erlotinib alone or with bevacizumab as first-line therapy in patients with advanced non-squamous non-small-cell lung cancer harbouring EGFR mutations (JO25567): an open-label, randomised, multicentre, phase 2 study. *Lancet Oncol.* 2014;15(11):1236–1244. doi:10.1016/S1470-2045(14)70381-X.
67. Sequist LV, Waltman BA, Dias-Santagata D, et al. Genotypic and histological evolution of lung cancers acquiring resistance to EGFR inhibitors. *Sci Transl Med.* 2011;3(75):75ra26. doi:10.1126/scitranslmed.3002003.
68. Yu HA, Arcila ME, Rekhtman N, et al. Analysis of tumor specimens at the time of acquired resistance to EGFR-TKI therapy in 155 patients with EGFR-mutant lung cancers. *Clin Cancer Res.* 2013;19(8):2240–2247. doi:10.1158/1078-0432.CCR-12-2246.
69. Janjigian YY, Smit EF, Groen HJM, et al. Dual inhibition of EGFR with afatinib and cetuximab in kinase inhibitor-resistant EGFR-mutant lung cancer with and without T790M mutations. *Cancer Discov.* 2014;4(9):1036–1045. doi:10.1158/2159-8290.CD-14-0326.
70. Grommes C, Oxnard GR, Kris MG, et al. "Pulsatile" high-dose weekly erlotinib for CNS metastases from EGFR mutant non-small cell lung cancer. *Neuro Oncol.* 2011;13(12):1364–1369. doi:10.1093/neuonc/nor121.
71. Welsh JW, Komaki R, Amini A, et al. Phase II trial of erlotinib plus concurrent whole-brain radiation therapy for patients with brain metastases from non-small-cell lung cancer. *J Clin Oncol.* 2013;31(7):895–902. doi:10.1200/JCO.2011.40.1174.

72. Mok T, Nakagawa K, Yang J, Wang J, Ponce S, Jiang H. Gefitinib/chemotherapy vs chemotherapy in epidermal growth factor receptor (EGFR) mutation-positive non-small-cell lung cancer (NSCLC) after progression on first-line gefitinib: the phase III randomised IMPRESS study [abstract]. *2014 ESMO Annual Conference*. 2014;25:1–41.
73. Doebele RC, Pilling AB, Aisner DL, et al. Mechanisms of resistance to crizotinib in patients with ALK gene rearranged non-small cell lung cancer. *Clin Cancer Res*. 2012;18(5):1472–1482. doi:10.1158/1078-0432.CCR-11-2906.
74. NSCLC Meta-analyses Collaborative. Chemotherapy in addition to supportive care improves survival in advanced non-small-cell lung cancer: a systematic review and meta-analysis of individual patient data from 16 randomized controlled trials. *J Clin Oncol*. 2008;26(28):4617–4625. doi:10.1200/JCO.2008.17.7162.
75. Schiller JH, Harrington D, Belani CP, et al. Comparison of four chemotherapy regimens for advanced non-small-cell lung cancer. *N Engl J Med*. 2002;346(2):92–98. doi:10.1056/NEJMoa011954.
76. Scagliotti GV, Parikh P, von Pawel J, et al. Phase III study comparing cisplatin plus gemcitabine with cisplatin plus pemetrexed in chemotherapy-naive patients with advanced-stage non-small-cell lung cancer. *J Clin Oncol*. 2008;26(21):3543–3551. doi:10.1200/JCO.2007.15.0375.
77. Scagliotti G, Hanna N, Fossella F, et al. The differential efficacy of pemetrexed according to NSCLC histology: a review of two phase III studies. *Oncologist*. 2009;14(3):253–263. doi:10.1634/theoncologist.2008-0232.
78. Socinski MA, Bondarenko I, Karaseva NA, et al. Weekly nab-paclitaxel in combination with carboplatin versus solvent-based paclitaxel plus carboplatin as first-line therapy in patients with advanced non-small-cell lung cancer: final results of a phase III trial. *J Clin Oncol*. 2012;30(17):2055–2062. doi:10.1200/JCO.2011.39.5848.
79. Sandler A, Gray R, Perry MC, et al. Paclitaxel-carboplatin alone or with bevacizumab for non-small-cell lung cancer. *N Engl J Med*. 2006;355(24):2542–2550. doi:10.1056/NEJMoa061884.
80. De Castria TB, da Silva EMK, Gois AFT, Riera R. Cisplatin versus carboplatin in combination with third-generation drugs for advanced non-small cell lung cancer. *Cochrane Database Syst Rev*. 2013;8(8):CD009256. doi:10.1002/14651858.CD009256.pub2.
81. Fidias PM, Dakhil SR, Lyss AP, et al. Phase III study of immediate compared with delayed docetaxel after front-line therapy with gemcitabine plus carboplatin in advanced non-small-cell lung cancer. *J Clin Oncol*. 2009;27(4):591–598. doi:10.1200/JCO.2008.17.1405.
82. Ciuleanu T, Brodowicz T, Zielinski C, et al. Maintenance pemetrexed plus best supportive care versus placebo plus best supportive care for non-small-cell lung cancer: a randomised, double-blind, phase 3 study. *Lancet*. 2009;374(9699):1432–1440. doi:10.1016/S0140-6736(09)61497-5.
83. Cappuzzo F, Ciuleanu T, Stelmakh L, et al. Erlotinib as maintenance treatment in advanced non-small-cell lung cancer: a multicentre, randomised, placebo-controlled phase 3 study. *Lancet Oncol*. 2010;11(6):521–529. doi:10.1016/S1470-2045(10)70112-1.
84. Pérol M, Chouaid C, Pérol D, et al. Randomized, phase III study of gemcitabine or erlotinib maintenance therapy versus observation, with predefined second-line treatment, after cisplatin-gemcitabine induction chemotherapy in advanced non-small-cell lung cancer. *J Clin Oncol*. 2012;30(28):3516–3524. doi:10.1200/JCO.2011.39.9782.
85. Paz-Ares LG, de Marinis F, Dediu M, et al. PARAMOUNT: final overall survival results of the phase III study of maintenance pemetrexed versus placebo immediately after induction treatment with pemetrexed plus cisplatin for advanced nonsquamous non-small-cell lung cancer. *J Clin Oncol*. 2013;31(23):2895–2902. doi:10.1200/JCO.2012.47.1102.
86. Barlesi F, Scherpereel A, Rittmeyer A, et al. Randomized phase III trial of maintenance bevacizumab with or without pemetrexed after first-line induction with bevacizumab, cisplatin, and pemetrexed in advanced nonsquamous non-small-cell lung cancer: AVAPERL (MO22089). *J Clin Oncol*. 2013;31(24):3004–3011. doi:10.1200/JCO.2012.42.3749.
87. Patel JD, Socinski MA, Garon EB, et al. PointBreak: a randomized phase III study of pemetrexed plus carboplatin and bevacizumab followed by maintenance pemetrexed and bevacizumab versus paclitaxel plus carboplatin and bevacizumab followed by maintenance bevacizumab in patients with stage IIIB or IV nonsquamous non-small-cell lung cancer. *J Clin Oncol*. 2013;31(34):4349–4357. doi:10.1200/JCO.2012.47.9626.
88. Shepherd FA, Dancey J, Ramlau R, et al. Prospective randomized trial of docetaxel versus best supportive care in patients with non-small-cell lung cancer previously treated with platinum-based chemotherapy. *J Clin Oncol*. 2000;18(10):2095-2103.
89. Fossella FV, DeVore R, Kerr RN, et al. Randomized phase III trial of docetaxel versus vinorelbine or ifosfamide in patients with advanced non-small-cell lung cancer previously treated with platinum-containing chemotherapy regimens. The TAX 320 Non-Small Cell Lung Cancer Study Group. *J Clin Oncol*. 2000;18(12):2354–2362.
90. Hanna N, Shepherd FA, Fossella FV, et al. Randomized phase III trial of pemetrexed versus docetaxel in patients with non-small-cell lung cancer previously treated with chemotherapy. *J Clin Oncol*. 2004;22(9):1589–1597. doi:10.1200/JCO.2004.08.163.
91. Ardizzoni A, Tiseo M, Boni L, et al. Pemetrexed versus pemetrexed and carboplatin as second-line chemotherapy in advanced non-small-cell lung cancer: results of the GOIRC 02-2006 randomized phase II study and pooled analysis with the NVALT7 trial. *J Clin Oncol*. 2012;30(36):4501–4507. doi:10.1200/JCO.2012.43.6758.
92. Garon EB, Ciuleanu T-E, Arrieta O, et al. Ramucirumab plus docetaxel versus placebo plus docetaxel for second-line treatment of stage IV non-small-cell lung cancer after disease progression on platinum-based therapy (REVEL): a multicentre, double-blind, randomised phase 3 trial. *Lancet*. 2014;384(9944):665–673. doi:10.1016/S0140-6736(14)60845-X.
93. Garassino MC, Martelli O, Broggini M, et al. Erlotinib versus docetaxel as second-line treatment of patients with advanced non-small-cell lung cancer and wild-type EGFR tumours (TAILOR): a randomised controlled trial. *Lancet Oncol*. 2013;14(10):981–988. doi:10.1016/S1470-2045(13)70310-3.
94. Shepherd FA, Rodrigues Pereira J, Ciuleanu T, et al. Erlotinib in previously treated non-small-cell lung cancer. *N Engl J Med*. 2005;353(2):123–132. doi:10.1056/NEJMoa050753.
95. Kawaguchi T, Ando M, Asami K, et al. Randomized phase III trial of erlotinib versus docetaxel as second- or third-line therapy in patients with advanced non-small-cell lung cancer: Docetaxel and Erlotinib Lung Cancer Trial (DELTA). *J Clin Oncol*. 2014;32(18):1902–1908. doi:10.1200/JCO.2013.52.4694.
96. Pallis AG, Gridelli C, Wedding U, et al. Management of elderly patients with NSCLC; updated expert's opinion paper: EORTC Elderly Task Force, Lung Cancer Group and International Society for Geriatric Oncology. *Ann Oncol*. 2014;25(7):1270–1283. doi:10.1093/annonc/mdu022.
97. Quoix E, Zalcman G, Oster J-P, et al. Carboplatin and weekly paclitaxel doublet chemotherapy compared with monotherapy in elderly patients with advanced non-small-cell lung cancer: IFCT-0501 randomised, phase 3 trial. *Lancet*. 2011;378(9796):1079–1088. doi:10.1016/S0140-6736(11)60780-0.
98. Ramalingam SS, Dahlberg SE, Langer CJ, et al. Outcomes for elderly, advanced-stage non small-cell lung cancer patients

treated with bevacizumab in combination with carboplatin and paclitaxel: analysis of Eastern Cooperative Oncology Group Trial 4599. *J Clin Oncol.* 2008;26(1):60–65. doi:10.1200/JCO.2007.13.1144.

99. Kawai O, Ishii G, Kubota K, et al. Predominant infiltration of macrophages and CD8(+) T cells in cancer nests is a significant predictor of survival in stage IV nonsmall cell lung cancer. *Cancer.* 2008;113(6):1387–1395. doi:10.1002/cncr.23712.
100. Vansteenkiste J, Cho B, De Pas T, Jassem J. MAGRIT, a double-blind randomized, placebo-controlled phase III study to assess the efficacy of the recMAGE-A3+AS15 cancer immunotherapy as adjuvant therapy in patients with resected MAGE-A3-positive NSCLC [abstract]. *2014 ESMO Annual Conference.* 2014:11730.
101. Lynch TJ, Bondarenko I, Luft A, et al. Ipilimumab in combination with paclitaxel and carboplatin as first-line treatment in stage IIIB/IV non-small-cell lung cancer: results from a randomized, double-blind, multicenter phase II study. *J Clin Oncol.* 2012;30(17):2046–2054. doi:10.1200/JCO.2011.38.4032.
102. Topalian SL, Hodi FS, Brahmer JR, et al. Safety, activity, and immune correlates of anti-PD-1 antibody in cancer. *N Engl J Med.* 2012;366(26):2443–2454. doi:10.1056/NEJMoa1200690.
103. Antonia S, Brahmenr J, Gettinger S, Chow L, Juergens R. Nivolumab (antiPD1; BMS936558, ONO4538) in combination with platinumbased doublet chemotherapy (PTDC) in advanced nonsmall cell lung cancer (NSCLC) [abstract]. *J Clin Oncol.* 2014;32(5s):8113.
104. Rizvi NA, Mazières J, Planchard D, et al. Activity and safety of nivolumab, an anti-PD-1 immune checkpoint inhibitor, for patients with advanced, refractory squamous non-small-cell lung cancer (CheckMate 063): a phase 2, single-arm trial. *Lancet Oncol.* 2015;63:257–265. doi:10.1016/S1470-2045(15)70054-9.
105. Garon E, Rizvi N, Balmanoukian A, Patnaik A, Blumenshein G. Antitumor activity of pembrolizumab (Pembro; MK-3475) and correlation with programmed death ligand 1 (PD-L1) expression in a pooled analysis of patients (pts) with advanced non-small cell lung carcinoma (NSCLC) [abstract]. *2014 ESMO Annual Conference.* 2014;25:LBA43.
106. Herbst RS, Soria J-C, Kowanetz M, et al. Predictive correlates of response to the anti-PD-L1 antibody MPDL3280A in cancer patients. *Nature.* 2014;515(7528):563–567. doi:10.1038/nature14011.
107. Chen L, Gibbons DL, Goswami S, et al. Metastasis is regulated via microRNA-200/ZEB1 axis control of tumour cell PD-L1 expression and intratumoral immunosuppression. *Nat Commun.* 2014;5:1–12. doi:10.1038/ncomms6241.
108. Flannery TW, Suntharalingam M, Regine WF, et al. Long-term survival in patients with synchronous, solitary brain metastasis from non-small-cell lung cancer treated with radiosurgery. *Int J Radiat Oncol Biol Phys.* 2008;72(1):19–23. doi:10.1016/j.ijrobp.2007.12.031.
109. Moreno P, de la Quintana Basarrate A, Musholt TJ, et al. Adrenalectomy for solid tumor metastases: results of a multicenter European study. *Surgery.* 2013;154(6):1215–1222; discussion 1222-1223. doi:10.1016/j.surg.2013.06.021.
110. Ashworth AB, Senan S, Palma DA, et al. An individual patient data metaanalysis of outcomes and prognostic factors after treatment of oligometastatic non-small-cell lung cancer. *Clin Lung Cancer.* 2014;15(5):346–355. doi:10.1016/j.cllc.2014.04.003.
111. Sheu T, Heymach JV, Swisher SG, et al. Propensity score-matched analysis of comprehensive local therapy for oligometastatic non-small cell lung cancer that did not progress after front-line chemotherapy. *Int J Radiat Oncol Biol Phys.* 2014;90(4):850–857. doi:10.1016/j.ijrobp.2014.07.012.
112. Parikh RB, Cronin AM, Kozono DE, et al. Definitive primary therapy in patients presenting with oligometastatic non-small cell lung cancer. *Int J Radiat Oncol Biol Phys.* 2014;89(4):880–887. doi:10.1016/j.ijrobp.2014.04.007.

SECTION V Head and Neck Cancer

Section Editor: Bonnie S. Glisson

第五篇 头颈部肿瘤

19

Head and Neck Cancer

第十九章　头颈部肿瘤

Jennifer L. McQuade
G. Brandon Gunn
William N. William Jr.
Merrill S. Kies

中文导读

头颈部肿瘤是一组疾病，每一种肿瘤均具有不同的流行病学、解剖学和病理特征，自然病史与治疗方式迥异。本章重点是头颈部鳞状细胞癌的一级管理。首先介绍了头颈部鳞状细胞癌的流行病学特征，尤其是其与人乳头状瘤病毒的关系。接下来，结合头颈部鳞状细胞癌的分子病理学特征、体格检查、影像学及解剖特征阐述了头颈部肿瘤的诊断及分期。治疗方面，首先按不同发病部位介绍了疾病的自然病史及治疗选择，包括：鼻咽部肿瘤、口咽部肿瘤、口腔肿瘤、下咽癌、喉癌和唾液腺癌。随后又按治疗策略及其适应证对各种治疗方式进行了介绍，包括：诱导化疗，序贯放疗、化疗，辅助放疗、化疗。在整体治疗策略中特别强调了器官保护的重要性，对头颈部肿瘤患者来说，追求疗效与功能保护的平衡较难达到。对晚期头颈部肿瘤，本章总结了化疗、靶向治疗及免疫治疗在整体治疗策略中的地位及应用。本章最后探讨了化学预防的问题：如视黄酸、厄洛替尼等药物对癌前病变恶化的预防效果。

Head and neck cancers are a diverse group of diseases, each with distinct epidemiologic, anatomic, and pathologic features. The natural history and treatment considerations may vary widely. In this chapter, our focus is on the primary management of squamous cell carcinomas (SCCs) of the head and neck (HNSCC). In recent years, we have observed significant advances in diagnosis and treatment and recognition of the human papillomavirus (HPV) as a significant causative agent and prognostic factor for cancers of the oropharynx. Tumor imaging is increasingly precise. Primary therapy eradicates disease in a majority of patients with early-stage HNSCC, and the long-term management of these patients currently involves an emphasis on general medical care, avoiding known carcinogens such as alcohol and tobacco, and participation in chemoprevention strategies to reduce the risk of second primary tumors. Therapy for patients with locally advanced disease is multimodal, and success has been achieved in improving local tumor control, disease remission, organ preservation, and overall survival. The integration of chemotherapy and novel "targeting" systemic treatment approaches with surgery and/or radiotherapy is under study and discussed.

EPIDEMIOLOGY

In the United States, HNSCC is estimated to represent approximately 3% (46,000) of new cancer cases and 2% (9,000) of cancer deaths in 2015 ([1]). However, the disease is more common in many developing countries, with a worldwide annual incidence of more than 500,000 ([2]).

The risk of developing head and neck cancer increases with age; most patients are older than age 50. There has been a clearly demonstrated association with tobacco and alcohol use. Molecular studies provide evidence that carcinogens found in these substances have a causal role. The prevalence and spectrum of *p53* mutations are prominent in cancers of patients with a history of tobacco and alcohol use ([3]). Cancers of the oral cavity, larynx, and hypopharynx are uncommon in persons with no smoking history.

Human papillomavirus infection is now widely accepted as another etiologic factor for HNSCC. In the United States, more than 50% of cancers arising in the oropharynx, particularly in the palatine tonsils and tongue base, harbor oncogenic HPV ([4]). The incidence of oropharyngeal cancer in the United States is increasing, primarily due to HPV-associated cases in men ([5]). It appears that the HPV-positive oropharyngeal malignancy represents a distinct clinical and pathologic subgroup of HNSCC, with poorly differentiated basaloid histopathology ([6]) and marked tumor responsiveness to radiation and chemotherapy. Moreover, HNSCCs with transcriptionally active HPV-16 DNA are characterized by occasional chromosomal loss, whereas those lacking HPV DNA typically have gross deletions, involving chromosomal arms known to be abnormal in HNSCC ([7]). Thus, HPV-16 infection may be an early carcinogenic event. Patients with HPV DNA–positive tumors, particularly those associated with E6 and E7 proteins, have improved survival after chemoradiotherapy when compared to patients with HPV-negative tumors ([8, 9]). A recent case-control study reported that HPV-16–positive HNSCCs were independently associated with several measures of sexual behavior and exposure to marijuana but not with cumulative measures of tobacco smoking, alcohol use, or poor oral hygiene ([10]). These findings indicate that HPV-16–positive HNSCC and HPV-16–negative HNSCC have different risk factor profiles. In addition to detection of oncogenic HPV DNA by in situ hybridization, tumor overexpression of p16 by immunohistochemistry serves as a surrogate for HPV association in oropharyngeal cancer with prognostic implications, particularly when coupled with patient smoking status ([8]). In addition, HNSCC patients with heavy tobacco and alcohol exposures are at high risk of developing multiple cancers, with "field cancerization" throughout the upper aerodigestive tract and bladder. The observation that treated head and neck cancer patients may have a high risk (estimated to be 3%-4% per year) of metachronous tumors has driven chemoprevention trials designed to reduce the risk of second primary tumors.

MOLECULAR PATHOGENESIS

The progression of HNSCC is thought to involve multiple stepwise alterations of molecular pathways in the squamous epithelium ([11]). Aberrations in the p53 and Rb tumor suppressor pathways are the most common molecular events, resulting in uncontrolled cell proliferation. Approximately 50% to 80% of HPV-negative tumor samples harbor a *p53* mutation ([12, 13]). The Rb pathway can be disrupted either through inactivation of the *CDKN2A* gene, which encodes p16, an inhibitor of cyclin-dependent kinase, or amplification or the *CCND1* gene encoding cyclin D1 ([14–16]).

The epidermal growth factor receptor (*EGFR*) is overexpressed in invasive HNSCC in a majority of sample tumors ([17]). Binding to *EGFR* by its natural ligands, mainly epidermal growth factor or transforming growth factor α (TGF-α), prompts a conformational change in the receptor through dimerization, which results in subsequent autoactivation of the tyrosine kinase from the intracellular domain of the receptor. This process activates an intracellular signaling pathway, leading to the inhibition of apoptosis, activation of cell proliferation and angiogenesis, and an increase in metastatic spread potential ([18]).

In 2011, Stransky et al performed whole exome sequencing on 74 HNSCC tumor specimens ([19]). Not surprisingly, the mutational landscape of the disease is quite complex, and smoking-related HNSCC specimens had a mutation rate approximately twice that of HPV-positive HNSCC. Mutations in genes previously implicated in HNSCC were detected at a high rate, including *TP53*, *CDKN2A*, *PTEN*, *PIK3CA*, and *HRAS*, validating this approach. However, this unbiased approach also identified a high rate of mutations in numerous genes not previously linked to HNSCC. In approximately 30% of cases, mutations were identified in genes that regulate squamous differentiation, such as *NOTCH1*, *IRF6*, and *TP63*. Mutations in genes regulating apoptosis were also frequent events. These novel findings have provided the rationale for testing novel therapeutic targets such as NOTCH inhibitors.

There are numerous challenges to the development of molecularly targeted therapies in HNSCC, including frequent tumor suppressor loss and difficulty in identification of true driver mutations within a complex mutational landscape. However, an improved understanding of the molecular biology of this disease should facilitate discovery of new prognostic markers and therapeutic targets.

DIAGNOSIS AND STAGING

Optimal therapy and treatment outcomes depend on the precise identification of the primary tumor (Fig. 19-1) as well as the local, regional, and distant extent of disease.

Patients with early-stage disease may present with vague symptoms and minimal physical findings, which is why a high index of suspicion for early diagnosis is needed, especially for tobacco users. A majority of patients will present with signs and symptoms of locally advanced disease, which vary according to the subsite in the head and neck. Sinusitis, unilateral nasal airway obstruction, and epistaxis may be early signs of cancers of the nasal cavity or paranasal sinuses. Otitis media that is recurrent or is refractory to antibiotics is an indication for a complete ear, nose, and throat

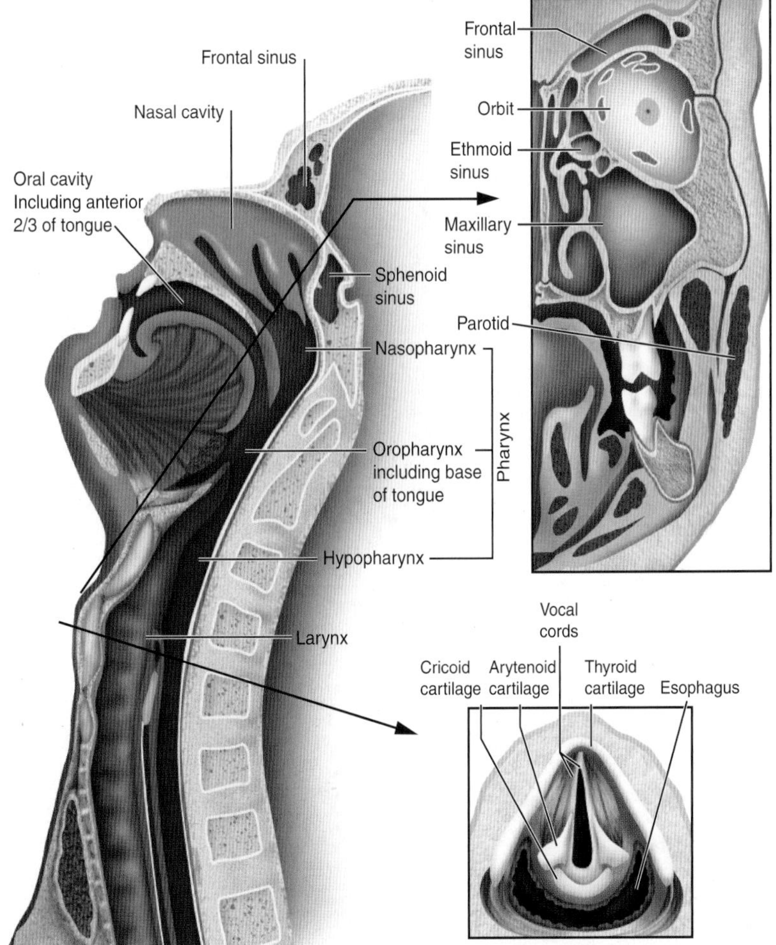

FIGURE 19-1 Head and neck anatomy.

evaluation to rule out a nasopharyngeal neoplasm. Chronic otalgia, dysphagia, odynophagia, and throat soreness lasting weeks may be the presenting symptoms of oropharyngeal or hypopharyngeal cancer. However, many patients with HPV-associated oropharyngeal cancer present with an otherwise asymptomatic neck mass and may have limited or no smoking history. Persistent hoarseness demands visualization of the larynx. Supraglottic laryngeal neoplasms do not usually present early, and a neck mass may be the presenting sign. Careful examination of lymph nodes in the facial, cervical, and supraclavicular regions is important because the anatomic patterns of lymphatic drainage may reflect the specific subsite of a head and neck primary tumor (Fig. 19-2) ([20]). Level 2/3 adenopathy, for example, suggests a primary cancer of the oral tongue or oropharynx, and posterior cervical adenopathy is frequently a result of regional spread of a nasopharyngeal tumor.

Physical examination should include careful inspection of the skin and oral/oropharyngeal mucosal surfaces; palpation of the tongue, floor of the mouth, and oropharynx; and systematic palpation of the neck. A complete examination also requires an indirect mirror examination of the oropharynx, hypopharynx, and larynx, complemented by fiberoptic endoscopy ([21]). Leukoplakia (white mucosal patches that cannot be removed by scraping) and higher risk erythroplakia (red or mixed red-white patches) are the most common premalignant lesions in the head and neck. Any suspicious surface in the oral mucosa should undergo biopsy.

Three-dimensional imaging with computed tomography (CT), magnetic resonance imaging (MRI), and/or ultrasonography is also needed to evaluate the extent of disease and to complete staging. Magnetic resonance imaging is the preferred local imaging modality for nasopharyngeal cancer. Because the lungs are the most common sites of distant metastases, a chest x-ray should be performed as well. Computed tomography scanning of the chest should be performed for symptomatic or high-risk patients. This would include patients with nasopharyngeal cancer or those with primary tumors of other sites presenting with N2b or greater nodal disease and low neck or supraclavicular metastases. Circulating tumor markers that would be reliable in early detection of HNSCC have not yet been identified.

Patients who present with a suspicious neck mass and no obvious primary mucosal lesion should undergo a systematic examination of the head and neck. Head and neck imaging may be helpful. If no obvious primary site is found, fine-needle aspiration of the mass may establish a diagnosis of cancer. Detection of HPV or Epstein-Barr virus DNA in a lymph node suggests a tumor of oropharyngeal or nasopharyngeal origin, respectively. If metastatic SCC is demonstrated, examination under anesthesia is often performed. Suspicious lesions are biopsied, and consideration is given to tonsillectomy and blind biopsies of the nasopharynx, base of the tongue, and hypopharynx, depending on the pattern of lymphadenopathy. Open biopsy of the neck mass may be performed if fine-needle aspiration biopsy and panendoscopy have failed to yield a

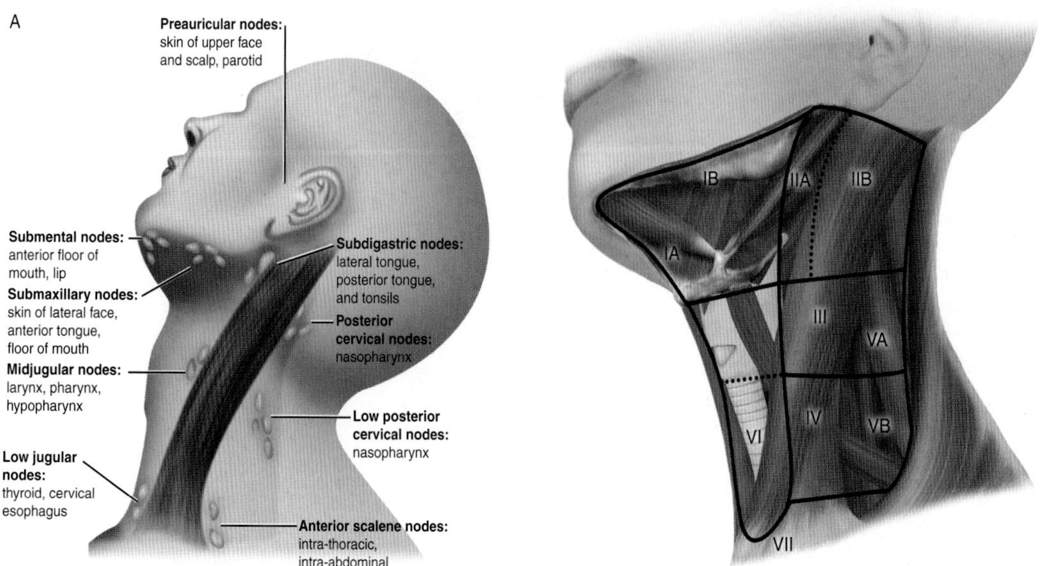

FIGURE 19-2 A. Nodal drainage. B. Nodal levels in the head and neck. (Reproduced with permission from Hong WK, Bast RB Jr, Hait WN, et al: *Cancer Medicine*. 8th ed. Shelton, CT: BC Decker—People's Medical Publishing House-USA; 2010: 959-998.)

Table 19-1A TNM Staging for the Oral Cavity and Oropharynx

Primary Tumor (T)	
TX	Primary tumor cannot be assessed.
T0	No evidence of primary tumor.
Tis	Carcinoma in situ.
T1	Tumor ≤2 cm in greatest dimension.
T2	Tumor >2 cm but not >4 cm in greatest dimension.
T3	Tumor >4 cm in greatest dimension.
T4(lip)	Tumor invades through cortical bone, inferior alveolar nerve, floor of mouth, or skin of face, ie, chin or nose.
T4a	Tumor invades structures adjacent to the oral cavity (eg, through cortical bone, into deep [extrinsic] muscle of tongue [genioglossus, hyoglossus, palatoglossus, and styloglossus], maxillary sinus, skin of face).
T4b	Tumor invades masticator space, pterygoid plates, or skull base and/or encases internal carotid artery.
Note: Superficial erosion alone of bone/tooth socket by gingival primary tumor is not sufficient to classify a tumor as T4.	
Regional Lymph Nodes (N)	
NX	Regional lymph nodes cannot be assessed.
N0	No regional node metastases.
N1	Metastasis to a single ipsilateral lymph node ≤3 cm in greatest dimension.
N2	Metastasis to a single ipsilateral lymph node >3 cm but not >6 cm in greatest dimension, or to multiple ipsilateral lymph nodes none >6 cm in greatest dimension, or to bilateral or contralateral lymph nodes none >6 cm in greatest dimension.
N2a	Metastasis to a single ipsilateral lymph node >3 cm but not >6 cm in greatest dimension.
N2b	Metastasis to multiple ipsilateral lymph nodes >3 cm but not >6 cm in greatest dimension.
N2c	Metastases to bilateral or contralateral lymph nodes none >6 cm in greatest dimension.
N3	Metastasis in a lymph node >6 cm in greatest dimension.
Distant Metastasis (M)	
MX	Presence of distant metastasis cannot be assessed.
M0	No evidence of distant metastasis.
M1	Distant metastasis.

diagnosis or in patients suspected of having an alternative process (eg, lymphoma). An experienced head and neck surgeon may be prepared to proceed with selective neck dissection if SCC of unknown head and neck primary origin is determined.

Staging criteria for head and neck cancers are based on the American Joint Committee on Cancer TNM staging system, which classifies tumors according to anatomic site and extent of disease ([22]). Head and neck primary tumor (T) staging is complex, varying with the primary subsite in the head and neck region. Classifications for lymph node (N) and distant metastases (M) are uniform for sites (Table 19-1) other than nasopharynx ([22a]).

NATURAL HISTORY AND IMPLICATIONS FOR THERAPY

Two-thirds of patients with HNSCC will present with stage III or IV disease. For patients with T1/2 disease

Table 19-1B Stage Grouping

Stage 0	Tis	N0	M0
Stage I	T1	N0	M0
Stage II	T2	N0	M0
Stage III	T3	N0	M0
	T1	N1	M0
	T2	N1	M0
	T3	N1	M0
Stage IVA	T4a	N0	M0
	T4a	N1	M0
	T1	N2	M0
	T2	N2	M0
	T3	N2	M0
	T4a	N2	M0
Stage IVB	Any T	N3	M0
	T4b	Any N	M0
Stage IVC	Any T	Any N	M1

CHAPTER 19

(stage I/II), surgery or radiotherapy as a single modality is most often applicable and effective. Depending on the precise primary site and stage, a curative outcome will be achieved in 70% to 95% of cases. In patients with intermediate and locally advanced disease at diagnosis, combined treatment strategies have become the standard of care. Multimodal treatment plans are designed to balance competing goals of tumor eradication and organ preservation ([11, 23, 24]). Despite optimal local therapy, 30% to 50% of patients may develop local or regional recurrence, and nearly 20% to 30% are at risk for distant metastases depending on the primary site and staging.

Nasopharynx

Over 95% of endemic nasopharyngeal carcinomas (NPCs) are associated with EBV. Nasopharyngeal carcinoma tends to occur in younger persons and is not associated with tobacco use. Nasopharyngeal carcinoma is an aggressive neoplasm with cervical lymph node metastases present in 60% to 90% of patients at diagnosis. Because of unique anatomic, biologic, and clinical characteristics, therapy for NPC is distinctive. Radiotherapy is the mainstay of local treatment. The anatomy of the nasopharynx and tumor sensitivity to radiotherapy limit the role of surgery to obtaining the initial biopsy and, for selected patients, resection of residual lymphadenopathy after radiotherapy. Nasopharyngeal carcinomas are highly sensitive to chemoradiotherapy. Because of the proximity of the nasopharynx to normal critical structures of the central nervous system and given the propensity of NPC for skull base invasion, intensity-modulated radiation therapy (IMRT) is the usual radiation therapy technique for NPC, which improves tumor coverage, reduces xerostomia, and improves patient quality of life compared to traditional techniques ([25, 26]). Locoregional tumor control following chemoradiotherapy approaches 90%.

For stages III and IV, concomitant chemotherapy and radiotherapy followed by adjuvant chemotherapy is the accepted standard of care based on the Head and Neck Intergroup NPC 0099 trial ([27]). Compared to radiation alone, chemoradiation with cisplatin (100 mg/m^2 on days 1, 22, and 43), followed by adjuvant chemotherapy with cisplatin and 5-fluorouracil (5-FU) demonstrated significant improvement in 3-year survival (78% vs 47%). Chan et al ([28]) have also demonstrated the efficacy of concomitant radiation and weekly cisplatin 40 mg/m^2. Phase III studies investigating the value of induction chemotherapy are under way. The NRG-HN001 study is an ongoing phase II/III study investigating the value of measuring plasma EBV DNA as a marker of the efficacy of concomitant chemoradiotherapy. With undetectable DNA, patients are randomized to observation or adjuvant chemotherapy. Patients with detectable DNA after chemoradiotherapy receive additional treatment, testing an alternative regimen consisting of paclitaxel and gemcitabine versus cisplatin and 5-FU.

Oral Cavity

The majority of oral cavity neoplasms occur in the anterior two-thirds of the tongue (oral tongue) and the floor of the mouth. Surgical resection, often with postoperative radiotherapy, is the most common and effective local treatment approach ([11, 24]). Depending on site and tumor volume, early cancers should be resected but may be treated with radiotherapy. Local tumor control rates of patients with stage I and II tumors are 80% to 90% and 50% to 80%, respectively ([29]). For deeply invasive T1/2 disease, we favor surgical resection and neck dissection with postoperative concomitant chemoradiotherapy for selected patients with narrow margins or nodal metastases, particularly if there is extracapsular spread. Perineural invasion is also a significant negative prognostic sign. Forty percent of patients present with clinically evident lymph nodes, and bilateral nodal involvement is not uncommon. Although primary surgical approaches are preferred at our center, interstitial radiotherapy (brachytherapy) has been used in combination with external-beam therapy for selected cases to achieve higher control rates than external radiation alone.

For patients with locally more advanced disease (Fig. 19-3 shows an example of a patient with a retromolar trigone primary tumor invading bone, T4), surgery followed by radiation therapy (or chemoradiotherapy) is the most widely accepted approach. At the University of Texas MD Anderson Cancer Center (MDACC), selective neck dissections are routinely performed for patients with stages II to IVa disease.

Oropharynx

The most common cancers of the oropharynx are of the base of tongue and tonsils, and an increasing percentage of these are HPV associated, with an improved prognosis. In an unplanned, post hoc analysis of RTOG 0129, Ang et al classified oropharyngeal cancer patients treated with concurrent chemoradiotherapy in to three risk-of-death groups using recursive partition analysis. The "low-risk" group were those with p16 positive tumors and minimal smoking history (94% 3-year overall survival). Conversely, the "high-risk" group were those characterized mostly by p16 negative tumors and greater smoking intensity (42% 3-year overall survival) ([8]). Radiation therapy serves as the principal treatment modality for the majority of oropharyngeal malignancies and is used as a single modality for T1 and many T2 tumors. Local control is obtained in over 90% of patients ([30]). Regional lymph nodes are treated in all cases, and unilateral neck

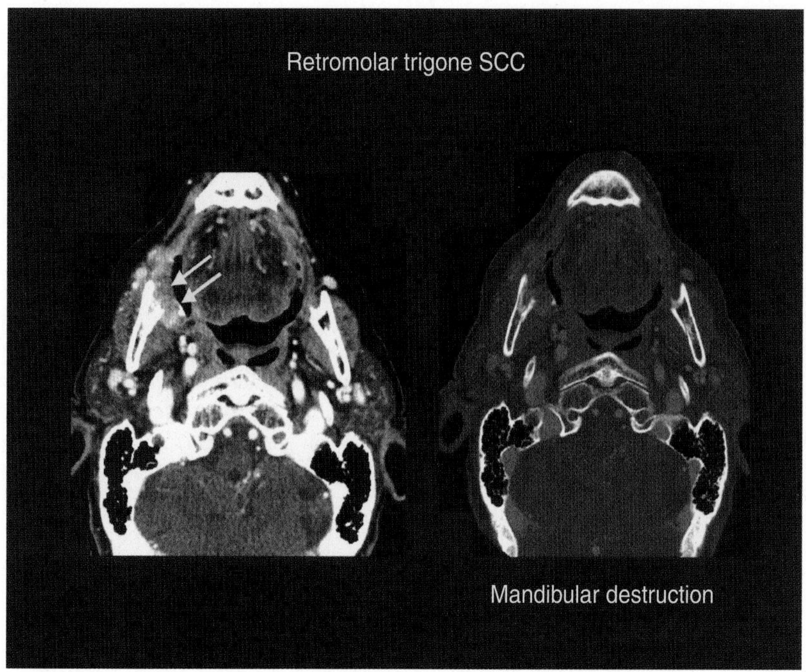

FIGURE 19-3 Retromolar trigone squamous cell carcinoma (SCC) with mandibular destruction.

radiation is considered for well-lateralized earlier-stage tonsillar primaries, which reduces greatly the radiation dose to the contralateral parotid gland and key swallowing structures. Given recent technical advances and the popularity of minimally invasive transoral approaches, surgical resection for oropharyngeal cancer is being performed more frequently at many centers, and this approach is currently under study (Eastern Cooperative Oncology Group [ECOG] 3311). However, adjuvant radiation or chemoradiation may also be required, depending on the surgical pathology findings.

Concomitant chemoradiotherapy using IMRT is the current standard of care for patients with locally advanced disease. Under study, protons have unique physical properties compared with x-rays or photons due to the Bragg peak, where most of the proton dose is delivered at a finite depth, thus reducing dose to certain nontarget structures. Investigators at MDACC are currently conducting a phase II/III randomized trial of concomitant chemotherapy with intensity-modulated proton therapy vs IMRT for stage III/IV oropharyngeal cancer. Objectives are to compare tumor control and long-term toxicity.

Hypopharynx

With 75% of lesions occurring in the pyriform sinus, carcinoma of the hypopharynx is relatively uncommon but virulent (Fig. 19-4). Small-volume disease may be treated with surgery or radiation, but later-stage disease requires multimodal therapy. At presentation, more than 75% of patients have advanced disease (T3 or T4). The overall 5-year survival rate is lower than 30%. For many patients, surgical treatment also requires removal of the larynx. The European Organization for Research and Treatment of Cancer (EORTC), in a phase III trial, demonstrated that laryngeal preservation with sequential chemoradiotherapy is a feasible alternative to radical surgery for many patients with locally advanced disease ([31]). In a more recent trial of patients with resectable advanced SCC of the larynx or hypopharynx, Lefebvre et al ([32]) compared sequential treatment with two cycles of cisplatin and 5-FU followed by radiotherapy with an arm of four cycles of cisplatin and 5-FU administered during weeks 1, 4, 7, and 10, alternating with radiotherapy. Survival with a functional larynx was similar in both arms, as was overall survival (median, 4.4 vs 5.1 years, respectively). Please see the "Organ Preservation" section for further discussion.

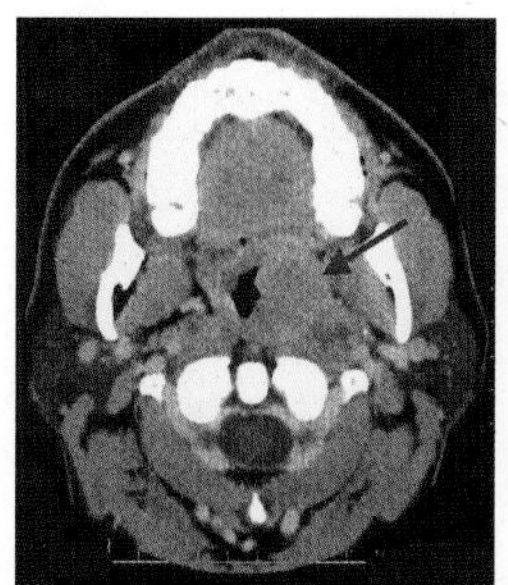
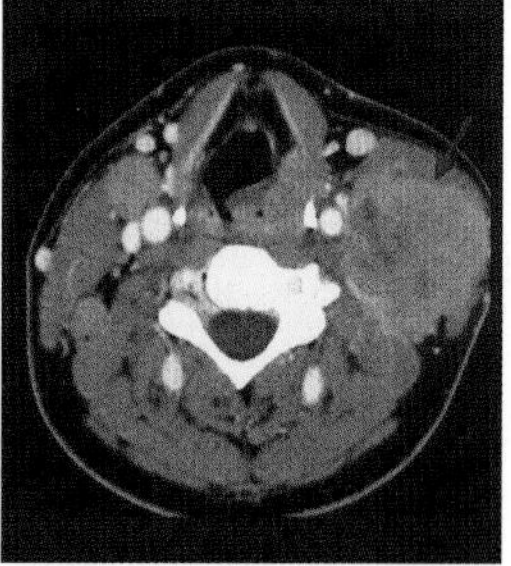

FIGURE 19-4 Axial computed tomography of advanced squamous carcinoma of the pyriform sinus, T3N3N0.

Larynx

Given the critical role of the larynx in communication, swallowing, respiration, and airway protection, organ preservation to maintain functional status and quality of life has been the focus of laryngeal cancer treatment since the 1970s. The most widely used treatment of T1 and T2 cancers of the larynx is radiotherapy, which has demonstrated control rates greater than 90% for T1 disease and approximately 70% to 80% for T2 tumors ([33]). For carefully selected patients with intermediate-stage disease, sequential chemotherapy followed by radiation and surgical salvage, if needed, showed equivalent survival outcomes compared with surgery in the Veterans Affairs (VA) laryngeal study ([34]). Although the rate of local failure is higher with organ preservation approaches, salvage surgery is effective, and this approach allows 60% of patients to preserve organ function ([35]). Larynx cancer treatment strategies are discussed in detail in the "Organ Preservation" section.

Salivary Gland Cancers

Tumors of the salivary glands are uncommon, with approximately 5,000 cases per year in the United States. Histologies are diverse, and risk factors are poorly defined, although radiotherapy may be causative. The age range of patients affected is broad. Many salivary neoplasms are benign, often involving the parotid gland, accounting for approximately 80% of parotid tumors, 50% of tumors arising in submandibular glands, and 25% of tumors arising in minor salivary glands.

Table 19-2 lists primary salivary malignancies.

Primary treatment depends on tumor extent and histology. Notably, parotid lymphadenopathy may reflect metastatic involvement by squamous cancers of the scalp or melanomas, and this must be borne in mind when evaluating these patients. Following a complete head and neck evaluation, consideration may be given to CT imaging of chest and a bone scan because these are common metastatic sites.

Surgical resection is the fundamental primary treatment for most patients, and the approach will be influenced by the primary histology ([36]). Adenoid cystic carcinoma (ACC) tends to track along nerves and may involve structures of the skull base, an important consideration in surgical and radiation therapy planning. C-kit is overexpressed in ACC ([37]). Lymph node metastases are uncommon. Low-grade mucoepidermoid carcinomas tend to be localized and are most often treated by surgery alone. High-grade mucoepidermoid carcinomas carry a much higher risk of lymph node and distant metastases. Salivary ductal carcinomas may be high grade and share biomarker characteristics, such as estrogen or progesterone receptor and HER2/neu overexpression, with breast cancer.

As a generalization, large tumors or those with close surgical margins will require postoperative radiotherapy. Postoperative concomitant chemoradiation is now under study (Radiation Therapy Oncology Group [RTOG] 1008) in a randomized trial of high-risk patients and is a consideration for patients with good performance status with locally advanced resectable disease.

For the palliative treatment of patients with recurrent disease not amenable to further local treatment or those with distant metastases, treatment with systemic chemotherapy, most often with a platinum-based combination, is an option ([38]). Cisplatin, 5-FU, cyclophosphamide, and doxorubicin are active compounds. The taxanes also have activity, although not demonstrated in patients with ACC. Combinations may be more effective, with response rates ranging from 20% to 30%. Salivary ductal cancers are much more sensitive to chemotherapy than ACC.

Treatment goals in the setting of distant metastatic disease are palliative because there has not been an overall survival advantage with chemotherapy. See Table 19-3 for a listing of tumor markers in salivary cancer that have prompted clinical trials. *EGFR*, KIT, HER2, and AR are prospective targets for systematic study. Fibroblast growth factor receptor (FGFR) expression ([39]) and *MYB-NFIB* fusion oncogene ([40]) have been identified in subsets of ACC. In a phase II trial, lapatinib, a dual inhibitor of *EGFR* and erbB2 tyrosine kinase activity, showed biologic activity in ACC ([41]).

Some patients with advanced salivary tumors will have a protracted and indolent clinical course. This has been frequently observed in patients with metastatic ACC involving lung, so it is important to assess the pace of the disease before committing a patient to systemic therapy.

Table 19-2 Selected Salivary Gland Cancers

Frequently Observed
Adenoid cystic carcinoma
Adenocarcinoma not otherwise specified
Mucoepidermoid carcinoma (well vs poorly differentiated)
Less Common
Salivary ductal carcinoma
Acinic cell carcinoma
Squamous cell carcinoma

COMBINED-MODALITY THERAPY

For patients with locally or regionally advanced SCC, much effort has been directed toward improvements

Table 19-3 Molecular Tumor Markers in Salivary Gland Carcinomas

Histology	*EGFR* Expression	*EGFR* Mutation	HER2 Expression	*HER2* Amplification	c-kit Expression	Androgen Receptor Expression
Adenoid cystic cancer	Yes	Rare	Rare	No	Yes	Rare
Mucoepidermoid cancer	Yes	No	Yes	Uncommon	Rare	Uncommon
Adenocarcinoma	Yes	—	Yes	Uncommon	Rare	Uncommon
Salivary duct cancer	Yes	—	Yes	Yes	Rare	Yes

Modified with permission from Andry G, Hamoir M, Locati LD, Licitra L, Langendijk JA. Management of salivary gland tumors, *Expert Rev Anticancer Ther* 2012 Sep;12(9):1161-1168.

in primary management with the addition of chemotherapy to surgery, radiotherapy, or both. Toward this end, three general strategies have been undertaken: (1) induction, also known as neoadjuvant therapy, with chemotherapy given before surgery or radiation; (2) concomitant chemoradiation, with chemotherapy given simultaneously with radiation to enhance its effect; and (3) adjuvant therapy, where chemotherapy is given after surgery or radiation in an effort to decrease microscopic metastatic disease burden.

Induction Chemotherapy

Induction chemotherapy has been investigated as an approach to improve outcomes in terms of overall survival and tumor control in patients with stage III/IV disease undergoing definitive local therapy. Theoretical advantages to this approach include reducing the risk of distant disease recurrence, enhancing organ preservation, improving response to definitive radiotherapy by reducing tumor bulk, and modification of subsequent local therapy to response.

This approach was first investigated in the 1970s after the cisplatin and 5-FU regimen proved to be highly active in metastatic disease. Trials over the next three decades investigated the role of chemotherapy added to local therapy in locally advanced disease. In the 2009 meta-analysis that established concomitant chemoradiation as a standard of care for nonsurgical management of stage III/IV SCC, direct comparisons of concomitant chemoradiation and induction chemotherapy indicated that although concomitant chemoradiation was superior to induction chemotherapy followed by radiation for local control and survival, induction chemotherapy was more effective at decreasing distant failure ([42]). This conclusion lent credence to contemporaneous trials investigating induction chemotherapy followed by chemoradiation.

Following demonstration of the activity of taxanes in head and neck cancer, a series of trials investigated the combination of three-drug regimens with a platinum, taxane, and 5-FU. In 2007, two multicenter phase III trials, the European TAX 323 ([43]) and the North American TAX 324 ([44]), demonstrated the superiority of induction TPF (docetaxel, cisplatin, 5-FU) over PF (cisplatin, 5-FU). In TAX 323, a total of 358 patients with untreated, unresectable, and locally advanced tumors were randomized to receive either docetaxel 75 mg/m^2, cisplatin 75 mg/m^2, and 5-FU 750 mg/m^2/d for 5 days (TPF) or cisplatin 100 mg/m^2 and 5-FU 1,000 mg/m^2/d for 5 days (PF), followed by radiotherapy alone. The primary end point, median progression-free survival, was 11.0 months in the TPF group and 8.2 months in the PF group (hazard ratio [HR], 0.72; P = .007), and median overall survival was 18.8 months versus 14.5 months. The TAX 324 trial also compared TPF to PF, but in that study, the doses in the TPF arm were docetaxel 75 mg/m^2, cisplatin 100 mg/m^2, and 5-FU 1,000 mg/m^2/d for 4 days. Both induction regimens were followed by concomitant chemoradiotherapy with weekly carboplatin area under the curve (AUC) of 1.5. The median overall survival was 71 months in the TPF group and 30 months in the PF group (P = .006). Notably, there was better locoregional control in the TPF group than in the PF group (P = .04). Rates of neutropenia and febrile neutropenia were significantly higher in the TPF group in both studies.

These two phase III trials led to US Food and Drug Administration (FDA) approval of induction chemotherapy TPF for patients with locally advanced HNSCC in 2007. Despite the impressive results of TAX 324, the value of adding induction chemotherapy to chemoradiation remained an unanswered question given the lack of definitive randomized trials comparing this approach to upfront chemoradiation. A randomized phase II trial by Paccagnella et al of induction TPF followed by chemoradiation versus chemoradiation alone reported a higher radiologic clinical response and a trend toward improved progression-free survival and overall survival ([45]).

Two recent phase III trials, PARADIGM ([46]) and DeCIDE ([47]), were designed to test the hypothesis that induction chemotherapy followed by chemoradiation would confer a survival benefit over chemoradiation alone. These studies failed to meet their accrual targets and were therefore underpowered. The PARADIGM trial enrolled previously untreated patients with SCC of the oral cavity, oropharynx, hypopharynx, or larynx, patients with tumors deemed to be either unresectable or of low surgical curability on the basis of T stage (T3 or T4) and/or nodal status (N2 or N3), or patients who were candidates for organ preservation. The concomitant chemoradiation alone control group received cisplatin 100 mg/m^2 on days 1 and 22, and radiotherapy was given as an accelerated concomitant boost over 6 weeks for a total of 72 Gy in 1.8-/1.5-Gy fractions. Induction TPF was given as per TAX 324, and subsequent chemoradiation was adapted to response. Partial and complete responders received weekly carboplatin at AUC 1.5 for 7 weeks and 70 Gy of radiotherapy over 7 weeks in 2-Gy fractions. Patients who responded poorly were treated with an intensified regimen of weekly docetaxel 20 mg/m^2 for 4 weeks and 6 weeks of radiation to 72 Gy. The trial was powered to detect an improvement in 3-year survival from 55% in the control group (based on historical controls) to 70% in the induction group. However, due to slow accrual, the trial closed with 145 patients enrolled, less than half of the planned enrollment. Overall 3-year survival was 73% (95% confidence interval [CI], 60%-82%) in the induction TPF followed by chemoradiation group versus 78% in the chemoradiation alone group ([46]).

The DeCIDE trial ([47]) randomized patients with N2/3 M0 disease to either two cycles of induction TPF followed by chemoradiation or chemoradiation alone. Chemoradiation was given as DFHX (docetaxel, 5-FU, and hydroxyurea) with concurrent twice-daily radiotherapy or IMRT. Radiation doses were adaptive, with 74 to 75 Gy given to gross disease, 54 Gy to high-risk microscopic disease, and 39 Gy to low-risk microscopic disease. This study was similarly powered to detect an improvement in 3-year survival from 50% in the control group to 65% in the induction group. However, this trial also failed to accrue well, enrolling 280 patients versus the planned 400 patients. There were no statistically significant differences in overall survival (HR, 0.91; 95% CI, 0.59-1.41) or relapse-free survival. In competing risk analysis, there was a statistically significant reduction in risk of distant relapse without locoregional recurrence in the induction arm (P = .043).

Given that both studies failed to show survival benefit, but were ultimately underpowered to do so, the role of induction chemotherapy remains controversial. Importantly, in both studies, the 3-year overall survival rate of 70% to 78% in the chemoradiation alone arm was significantly higher than the historical control of 50% to 55% used in the pretreatment power calculations. This improvement in survival is likely multifactorial—a result of improved supportive care, technical advances in radiotherapy, and a shift in the biology of the disease the incidence as smoking-induced cancers declines and HPV-associated HNSCCs increases. Although the PARADIGM trial did not test for HPV, in DeCIDE, the HPV-positive rate of the 31% of patients tested was over 80%, and HPV-associated disease is known to have higher survival rates.

The Gruppo di Studio Tumori della Testa e del Collo (GSTCC) trial presented by Ghi and colleagues at the 2014 American Society of Clinical Oncology (ASCO) annual meeting, but not yet published, is a 2 × 2 factorial design of induction TPF versus no induction followed by chemoradiation with either cetuximab or PF in 415 patients. This trial showed a survival benefit of 53.7 months in the induction arm versus 30.3 months in the upfront chemoradiation arm (HR, 0.72; 95% CI, 0.55-0.96; P = .025) and additionally showed a reduction in distant metastases. The difference in outcomes observed in this trial versus the DeCIDE and PARADIGM trials is likely due to different patient populations and inclusion criteria.

Induction chemotherapy may also have value as a component of a sequential approach in which chemotherapy is followed by radiotherapy as a single modality in select locally advanced patients, thus sparing some of the toxicity of concomitant chemoradiation. In our center, a phase II trial with 47 patients investigated the efficacy of combining cetuximab with paclitaxel and carboplatin in a 6-week induction regimen followed by risk-based local therapy (radiation, concomitant chemoradiotherapy, or surgery) based on tumor stage and site at diagnosis. Inclusion criteria were stage IV M0 with nodal staging of N2b/c/N3. Of note, local therapy was determined at diagnosis and was not adapted to response. After induction chemotherapy, 9 patients (19%) achieved a clinically complete response, and 36 patients (77%) achieved a partial response. Local therapy consisted of concomitant chemoradiotherapy in 23 patients, radiotherapy alone in 23 patients, and surgery in 1 patient. The 3-year progression-free survival and overall survival rates were 87% and 91%, respectively ([48]). A recent update to this trial reported a 5-year overall survival rate of 89% and very favorable long-term speech and swallow functions ([49]). This strategy is undergoing further testing. At the ASCO 2014 annual meeting, Cmelak et al ([50]) presented preliminary results of E2399. Patients with locally advanced HPV-positive disease responding to induction chemotherapy with paclitaxel, cisplatin, and cetuximab were effectively treated with a reduced-dose cetuximab-IMRT regimen, 54 Gy, if they achieved a clinical complete response to the induction chemotherapy. An early outcomes analysis showed 84% progression-free-survival and 95% overall survival at 2 years.

Concomitant Radiotherapy and Chemotherapy

In patients with locally advanced but M0 disease, the strategy of concomitant radiotherapy and chemotherapy has led to improved local and regional tumor control compared to radiotherapy alone ([42]). Synergy between chemotherapy and radiation is based on several mechanisms, including (1) inhibition of DNA repair; (2) redistribution of cells to sensitive phases of the cell cycle; and (3) promoting oxygenation of anoxic tissues. The net effect is to improve cellular cytotoxicity ([51–53]). However, combined therapy also enhances acute mucocutaneous toxicity, which may prompt subsequent dose reductions and treatment interruptions in radiotherapy. Thus, in combining these two treatment modalities, it is essential that toxicity not preclude the delivery of therapy in an effective schedule to avoid compromise of efficacy.

In a landmark phase II trial in 1987, the RTOG administered cisplatin (100 mg/m^2) every 3 weeks to 124 patients with locally advanced unresectable head and neck cancer ([54]). Sixty percent of patients completed the combined treatment per protocol, and 69% of all patients achieved a complete response. A comparison to RTOG patients treated with radiotherapy alone suggested improvement in survival time for the combined treatment.

The use of concomitant combination chemotherapy and radiation has long been under intense study ([55]). Meta-analysis ([42]) of prospective clinical trials demonstrates an enhancement of local tumor control and improvement of survival with combined therapy over radiation treatment alone, and chemoradiation is the standard of care in locally advanced non-surgical disease.

Combining several drugs with radiation will enhance acute toxicity, which may be severe. Therefore, investigators have piloted trials designed with split-course radiation to allow for healthy tissue recovery. Most of these studies have been limited to patients with stage III or IV locally advanced SCC, with local control and improved survival time as the primary objectives. These regimens alternate chemotherapy and radiotherapy or use split-course radiotherapy to maximize tumor cell kill and minimize tissue toxicity. However, protracted radiation treatment times may result in decreased local control rates because of accelerated repopulation of cancer stem cells ([56, 57]). The strategy of alternating non–cross-resistant agents may potentially eliminate not only tumor cell repopulation but also primary drug resistance.

Brizel et al ([58]) compared a hyperfractionated radiotherapy arm to total dose of 75 Gy versus concomitant PF and hyperfractionated radiation to 70 Gy followed by two cycles of adjuvant chemotherapy. There was a statistically significant improvement in local disease control and a strong trend toward improved overall survival for the combined-modality arm. In this trial, neck dissection was recommended in patients with N2/3 disease. Clayman et al ([59]) have reviewed the MDACC experience, examining the indication for neck dissection in this patient population. Their report suggests that neck dissections are required only when there is radiographic evidence of residual disease 6 to 8 weeks following the completion of definitive chemoradiation. Wendt et al ([60]) reported a statistically significant 3-year survival advantage after the concomitant use of cisplatin, 5-FU, and leucovorin with split-course radiotherapy versus radiotherapy given as a single therapeutic modality. Calais et al ([61]) compared a more standard once-daily fractionation radiation schedule with the same radiotherapy and concomitant carboplatin and 5-FU, demonstrating a statistically significant advantage in locoregional tumor control and overall survival at 3 years. Jeremic et al ([62]) also investigated the value of adding cisplatin given daily to a hyperfractionated radiation therapy program versus the same radiation schedule given alone in patients with locally advanced HNSCC. In this report, locoregional and distant disease control and overall survival were improved at 5 years. Adelstein et al ([63]) compared standard daily radiotherapy with two schedules of concomitant chemoradiotherapy in a large intergroup study. The addition of high-dose cisplatin to conventional single daily dose radiotherapy improved survival from 23% to 37% at 3 years. The clearest benefit in these studies was an improvement in locoregional control, which translated into a survival advantage. Acute toxicity was increased, especially mucositis and hematologic effects, but there was no obvious escalation of long-term sequelae. However, this may need further investigation. In aggregate, overall 3-year survival exceeded 50% in these experimental programs, underscoring the potential therapeutic efficacy of concomitant chemotherapy and radiation in patients with advanced head and neck cancers.

Cetuximab, a monoclonal antibody, is approved for use in combination with radiation in previously untreated patients. In a landmark study, patients with locoregionally advanced head and neck cancer were randomly assigned to receive either high-dose radiotherapy alone (213 patients) or high-dose radiotherapy plus weekly cetuximab (211 patients) at an initial dose of 400 mg/m^2 of body surface area, followed by 250 mg/m^2 weekly for the duration of radiotherapy ([64]). The primary end point, median duration of locoregional control, was 24.4 months among patients treated with cetuximab plus radiotherapy and 14.9 months among patients given radiotherapy alone (HR, 0.68; $P = .005$). The median duration of overall survival was 49.0 months among patients treated with combined therapy and 29.3 months among patients treated

CHAPTER 19

with radiotherapy alone (HR for death, 0.74; $P = .03$). However, the rates of distant metastases at 1 and 2 years were similar in both groups. With the exception of acneiform rash and infusion reactions, the incidence of grade 3 or greater toxic effects, including mucositis, did not differ significantly between the two groups.

Cetuximab plus radiotherapy is directly compared to chemoradiation for patients with HPV-associated oropharyngeal cancer in a phase III randomized trial (RTOG 1016), but results from this trial are not yet available. This trial represents the recent trend in investigational treatment strategies undertaken by clinical trial cooperative groups that have focused on treatment "de-intensification" for selected patients (namely those with HPV-associated oropharyngeal cancer), with the goals of maintaining or improving established cure rates but reducing treatment-related toxicity.

There has been a series of trials investigating the use of *EGFR* antibodies with chemoradiation. The phase III RTOG 0522 trial randomized 940 patients to high-dose cisplatin-based chemoradiotherapy with or without cetuximab ([65]). The combined biochemoradiotherapy failed to meet the primary end point of improving progression-free survival, with a 3-year rate of 61.2% versus 58.9% with cetuximab, and demonstrated a trend toward worse locoregional control. This trend was likely the result of significantly increased toxicities that led to radiation interruptions in 26.9% of patients. There was also a significant difference in treatment-related deaths (10 vs 3; $P = .05$). The CONCERT-1 and -2 trials have further explored bioradiotherapy with panitumumab (Table 19-4) ([66, 67]), showing no overall survival or local disease control advantage after matching chemoradiotherapy with the addition of the antibody.

The aggregate results of these trials indicate that improved disease-free and overall survival times have been obtained for patients with locally advanced HNSCC using concomitant chemotherapy and radiotherapy rather than radiotherapy as a single treatment modality. Combination chemotherapy with radiotherapy may increase response but causes increased toxicity. Well-designed clinical trials are still needed to determine optimal chemotherapy and radiotherapy schedules.

Table 19-4 *EGFR*-Based Bioradiotherapy With Panitumumab

	No.	2-Year LRC (%)
CONCERT-1		
CT-RT	63	68
CT-RT + P	87	61
CONCERT-2		
CT-RT	61	61
P-RT	90	51

CT, chemotherapy; LRC, locoregional control; P, panitumumab; RT, radiotherapy.

Adjuvant Chemoradiotherapy

Adjuvant chemotherapy is indicated in patients at high risk of recurrence after surgical resection, generally defined as having narrow or involved margins at the primary site, multiple nodal metastases, or extracapsular spread (Table 19-5) ([68–70]).

Two large phase III studies, RTOG 9501 ([69]) and EORTC 22931 ([70]), tested cisplatin-based concomitant chemoradiotherapy in the adjuvant setting. Although with some variations between the studies, patients with high-risk features (positive margin, extracapsular spread, lymphovascular invasion, perineural invasion, and multiple positive lymph nodes) were randomly assigned to receive either radiotherapy alone or radiotherapy plus cisplatin at 100 mg/m^2 every 3 weeks for three cycles. In RTOG 9501, concomitant chemoradiotherapy significantly reduced the risk of locoregional recurrence compared with radiotherapy alone (HR for local or regional recurrence, 0.61; $P = .01$). However, no survival benefit was observed. In addition, the incidence of grade 3 or greater adverse effects was 34% in the radiotherapy group and 77% in the combined-therapy group ($P < .001$). In EORTC 22931, both the progression-free survival (HR, 0.75; $P = .04$) and overall survival (HR, 0.70; $P = .02$) rates were significantly

Table 19-5 Postoperative Chemoradiation: Randomized Trials

Study	Eligibility	Experimental Arms	Outcome
Bachaud et al ([68]), 1996	Nodal ECS	RT + weekly cisplatin (n = 39)	DFS ($P < .02$) and OS ($P < .01$) better
RTOG 9501 ([69]), 2004	Multiple nodal metastases, ECS, or positive margins	RT + cisplatin days 1, 22, 43 (n = 228)	2-y LRC (82% vs 72%; $P = .01$) + PFS ($P = .04$) better
EORTC 22931 ([70]), 2004	Stage III/IV	RT + cisplatin days 1, 22, 43 (n = 167)	PFS ($P = .04$) + OS ($P = .02$) better

DFS, disease-free survival; ECS, extracapsular spread; EORTC, European Organization for Research and Treatment; LRC, local and regional control; OS, overall survival; PFS, progression-free survival; RT, radiotherapy; RTOG, Radiation Therapy Oncology Group.

higher in the combined-therapy group than in the radiotherapy group. Severe acute adverse effects were more frequent after combined therapy (41%) than in the radiotherapy group (21%).

More recently, based on the benefit of cetuximab bioradiotherapy in the definitive setting and the additive benefit of cetuximab to chemotherapy in the metastatic setting ([71]), RTOG 0234 explored the incorporation of cetuximab into adjuvant chemoradiation ([72]). This phase II trial compared two biochemoradiotherapy regimens to historical high-dose cisplatin-based chemoradiotherapy in RTOG 9501 with the intent to select a regimen for further testing against standard high-dose cisplatin-based chemoradiotherapy in a phase III trial. Both docetaxel (15 mg/m^2)/radiation/cetuximab and weekly cisplatin (30 mg/m^2)/radiation/cetuximab outperformed the historical control with 2-year overall survival rates of 79% and 69% and 2-year disease-free survival rates of 66% and 57%, respectively (HR, 0.69 for the docetaxel arm vs control, P = .01; and HR, 0.76 for the cisplatin arm vs control, P = .05). Grade 3 or 4 myelosuppression was observed in 28% of patients in the cisplatin arm and 14% of patients in the docetaxel arm, and mucositis was observed in 56% and 54% of patients, respectively. Although these results are promising, as has been noted previously, comparison with historical controls is problematic given the shifting epidemiology from smoking-related cancer to better prognosis HPV-related cancers, which has likely contributed to the improvements in survival rates of the control arms seen in the recent induction trials ([46, 47]). RTOG 1216 is an ongoing phase II/III trial of surgery and postoperative radiation delivered with concurrent cisplatin versus docetaxel versus docetaxel and cetuximab for high-risk HNSCC.

Although adjuvant concomitant chemoradiotherapy has been demonstrated to be more effective than radiotherapy, there is significant associated toxicity. The two risk factors most associated with benefit from concomitant chemoradiotherapy are extracapsular extension and positive surgical margins ([73]).

ORGAN PRESERVATION

Many HNSCCs are diagnosed at a late stage. Stages III and IV tumors often necessitate extensive or radical surgery, which may alter organ function. Problems with radical surgery include loss of speech, loss of swallowing function, or disfigurement without a concomitant improvement in survival time. Therefore, preservation of function became one of the major challenges. This approach was first explored in laryngeal cancer given the high morbidity associated with laryngectomy.

The landmark VA study published in 1991 randomized 332 patients with stage III or IV SCC of the larynx to receive either induction chemotherapy consisting of PF followed by radiotherapy or surgery and postoperative radiotherapy ([34]). Patients who experienced no tumor response to chemotherapy or those who had locally persistent or recurrent cancer underwent salvage laryngectomy. Two-year survival for both treatment groups was 68%, and 41% of patients randomly assigned to the experimental arm were alive with a functional larynx at 2 years. Thus, the efficacy of chemotherapy followed by radiotherapy (with surgical salvage) was similar to that of surgery followed by radiotherapy and established organ preservation as a realistic goal of nonsurgical treatment administered with curative intent. Patterns of failure differed, with patients in the chemotherapy arm more likely to have locoregional recurrence and distant recurrence more common in the surgical arm. Lefebvre et al ([31]) later reported that sequential chemotherapy and radiation could also be effective in selected patients with cancers of the hypopharynx.

The VA larynx study prompted further investigations of chemotherapy and radiotherapy for the treatment of larynx cancer using the sequential administration of induction chemotherapy, consisting of PF, followed by radiotherapy versus concomitant cisplatin-radiotherapy versus radiotherapy administered as a single treatment modality in RTOG 91-11 ([74]). For all groups, totaling 547 patients, surgical salvage was reserved for patients with persistent or locally recurrent disease. Both chemotherapy groups demonstrated improved laryngectomy-free survival (the composite primary end point) compared to radiotherapy alone. The results indicated a significant advantage for concomitant cisplatin treatment, with preservation of the larynx in 88% of patients treated in the concomitant arm. In the recently published 10-year update ([75]), locoregional control and larynx preservation were significantly improved with concomitant chemoradiotherapy compared with the induction arm RT (HR, 0.58; 95% CI, 0.37-0.89; P = .005), whereas the induction chemotherapy group showed a nonsignificant trend toward improved overall survival (HR, 1.25; 95% CI, 0.98-1.61; P = .08). This difference in survival was driven by non–cancer-related deaths, the cause of which remains unexplained.

Organ preservation has also been studied in hypopharyngeal cancer given that laryngectomy is often part of the surgical treatment of this disease. Similar to the VA study, the EORTC study compared induction chemotherapy with PF followed by radiation versus conventional surgery plus postoperative radiation. As in the VA study, survival between the two arms did not differ, and patients in the chemotherapy arm had a high rate of larynx preservation.

As with TAX 323 and TAX 324, TPF was also explored in locally advanced but resectable SCC of the larynx or hypopharynx ([76]). Compared to PF, TPF was shown to increase tumor responsiveness and lead to improved larynx preservation (70% vs 58% in the PF arm), with no compromise in overall survival. The efficacy of induction TPF versus concurrent chemoradiation has not been explored. The concurrent approach tends to be favored in the United States, whereas Europeans tend to prefer induction.

These trials indicate that for patients with intermediate-stage SCC of the larynx, a combined treatment program with the objectives of tumor eradication and laryngeal preservation is appropriate. It is also important to recognize that patients with locally advanced, destructive primary laryngeal cancers were not included in the more recent multigroup trial. These patients may require total laryngectomy for optimal tumor control and preservation of function.

It should be noted, however, that nonsurgical treatment also carries risk of morbidity and functional impact. Radiation produces tissue changes that can result in immediate and long-term alterations in speech and swallowing. The adverse impact of radiation may equal or exceed that associated with surgery, depending on the treatment dose and volume, and the sequelae of treatment may manifest or increase in severity years after the completion of treatment. Fibrosis may reduce the range of motion of the tongue and jaw and diminish pharyngeal wall motion. Historically, 20% to 40% of patients receiving chemoradiotherapy for SCC of the oropharynx and hypopharynx may require long-term gastrostomy tube feedings. However, the long-term gastrostomy rate for patients with oropharynx cancer treated with modern radiation therapy approaches (eg, IMRT) is less than 10% ([77]). Radiation to the larynx often results in swallowing problems related to pharyngeal transport. To counteract the deleterious effects of radiation and chemoradiotherapy, there are rehabilitative options, which are best administered by a qualified speech pathologist.

RECURRENT OR METASTATIC DISEASE

Patients with tumor recurrence after primary treatment who are not candidates for surgical salvage may be offered palliative cytotoxic chemotherapy or investigational therapy. Methotrexate, cisplatin, carboplatin, bleomycin, 5-FU, and the taxanes are drugs with single-agent activity in the range of 15% to 25%. Previous studies have consistently demonstrated response rates of 30% to 40% for combination chemotherapy, usually cisplatin based, with a median survival of 6 to 9 months. There has been no clear demonstration of a survival advantage over single-agent treatment or even best supportive care. However, in the appropriate context with the goal of reducing symptoms, combination chemotherapy with PF or a platinum-taxane combination has become a frequently exercised practice in the care of patients with incurable HNSCC, and a fraction of patients treated with these combinations have extended survival.

Current investigations are under way in an attempt to develop effective targeted treatment approaches. Epidermal growth factor receptor is overexpressed in a majority of invasive HNSCCs. The small-molecule inhibitors gefitinib (500 mg/d) and erlotinib (150 mg/d) downregulate the phosphorylation of tyrosine kinase residues in the cytoplasmic domain of *EGFR* and have demonstrated single-agent activity in 11% and 5% of patients, respectively, with advanced disease ([78–80]). Cetuximab is a chimeric murine-human monoclonal antibody directed against the extracellular domain of *EGFR*. Burtness et al ([81]) conducted a prospective randomized trial in patients with recurrent HNSCC and demonstrated responses in 26% of patients treated with cetuximab and cisplatin versus 10% of patients treated with cisplatin alone. However, the primary end point, progression-free survival, was not significantly different. Cetuximab was tested in a phase II trial as monotherapy in 103 patients with recurrent or metastatic HNSCC refractory to platinum-based therapy ([82]). The response rate was 13%, disease control rate (complete response/partial response/stable disease) was 46%, and median time to progression was 70 days. There appeared to be no benefit in adding cisplatin to these patients. Afatinib is a small-molecule tyrosine kinase inhibitor that targets *EGFR* and HER2. This compound is under study in ECOG 1311 as an adjuvant systemic therapy after definitive chemoradiation and neck dissection for high-risk patients.

In a major phase III trial, cetuximab in combination with chemotherapy was investigated in patients with untreated recurrent or metastatic HNSCC ([71]). In this trial, 442 patients were randomized to receive either cisplatin or carboplatin plus 5-FU, with or without cetuximab. The cetuximab group had longer overall survival (10.1 vs 7.4 months) and median progression-free survival (5.6 vs 3.3 months). Thus, cetuximab plus PF chemotherapy improved overall survival when given as first-line treatment in patients with recurrent or metastatic HNSCC.

Further study of molecular biomarkers and selection of targeted therapies for trials both in definitive and palliative treatment settings is receiving much emphasis. Activation of the PI3k/Akt signaling pathway is under study in HNSCC, and phase I/II trials with PI3K inhibition are ongoing ([83]). One of the more exciting agents currently under investigation is

MK-3475, a PD-1 antibody that acts as an immune checkpoint inhibitor. This type of immunotherapy has been approved in melanoma and lung cancer and is being investigated in multiple tumor types with promising results. A phase Ib study presented by Seiwert et al ([84]) at ASCO 2014 enrolled 61 patients with metastatic HNSCC, 36 HPV-negative patients and 23 HPV-positive patients. The response rate was 19.6%, and an additional eight patients experienced stable disease for over 6 months. Response was correlated with programmed death ligand 1 (PD-L1) expression. There was no difference in response between HPV-negative and HPV-positive disease. A phase III study is planned.

CHEMOPREVENTION

The decades-long history of clinical and translational study of retinoids in oral premalignant lesions, or intraepithelial neoplasia (IEN), has advanced our understanding of the biology of carcinogenesis and molecular-targeted drug development, even though definitive clinical testing has not shown that retinoids can prevent oral cancer ([85]). One early trial in 1986 tested a high dose of the retinoid 13-*cis*-retinoic acid (13cRA) against placebo in 44 evaluable oral IEN patients for only 3 months ([86]). The complete plus partial clinical response rate in the retinoid arm was 67% (vs 10% in the placebo arm) ($P = .0002$). Histopathologic responses also favored the 13cRA arm. Over half of the responders in the 13cRA arm, however, recurred or developed new lesions within 3 months of stopping the intervention. This high-dose, short-term trial led to another early trial in oral IEN patients, which was designed to reduce the toxicity of and prolong the response to 13cRA. A short-term (3-month) course of high-dose 13cRA (1.5 mg/kg/d) was followed by a 9-month maintenance course with low-dose 13cRA (0.5 mg/kg/d) or β-carotene (30 mg/d) in IEN patients who responded to or were stable after the induction phase ([87]). The maintenance-phase progression rates were 8% in the 13cRA group and 55% in the β-carotene group ($P < .001$). Nonetheless, on long-term follow-up (median of 66 months), the incidence of in situ or invasive cancer was not different between the two arms (23% for low-dose 13cRA vs 27% for β-carotene) ([88]).

To address the short-lived chemopreventive effects of 13cRA, Papadimitrakopoulou et al designed a follow-up study comparing an extended, 3-year treatment period with 13cRA at lower doses (0.5 mg/kg/d for 1 year followed by 0.25 mg/kg/d orally for 2 years; control arm) to β-carotene (50 mg/d) plus vitamin A (ie, retinyl palmitate 25,000 IU/d; experimental arm) in 162 patients with leukoplakia, using a noninferiority design ([89]). During the study, β-carotene had to be dropped from the experimental arm due to emerging data demonstrating an increased risk of lung cancer incidence and mortality in other ongoing chemoprevention trials at that time. The study showed an inferior 3-month response rate in the vitamin A alone arm, lower tolerance to treatment with 13cRA, a lack of statistical significance in the test for noninferiority between the control and the experimental arm(s), and, more importantly, a similar oral cancer–free survival across all groups. This study, which is one of the longest term performed to date in patients with leukoplakia, demonstrated that 13cRA is still not well tolerated for long-term treatment, even at reduced doses and that less toxic regimens (ie, vitamin A alone) are ineffective. Furthermore, an impact on oral cancer incidence has yet to be demonstrated with any of these regimens. In addition to trials involving oral IEN, retinoids have also been studied for prevention of second primary head and neck cancers. A randomized, placebo-controlled study of high-dose 13cRA (50–100 mg/m^2/d for 12 months) in definitively resected head and neck cancer patients demonstrated a lack of effect of the retinoid on distant, nodal, or local recurrence rates, but there was a statistically significant decrease in the incidence of second primary tumors (4% vs 24%, $P = .005$) that persisted on long-term follow-up ([90, 91]). Unfortunately, a follow-up trial of a tolerable low dose of 13cRA (30 mg/d for 3 years) in 1,190 early-stage patients did not prevent second primary tumors ([92]). Randomized studies in this setting with the second-generation retinoid etretinate (n = 316 patients) ([93]), vitamin A and/or *N*-acetylcysteine (n = 2,592) ([94]), β-carotene (n = 264) ([95]), and α-tocopherol plus β-carotene (n = 540) ([96]) also did not demonstrate any clinical benefit in terms of prevention of second primary tumors.

Although the randomized retinoid trials failed to produce a chemoprevention strategy that could be considered standard of care, they were embedded with translational studies that helped to advance the overall understanding of the biology of intraepithelial carcinogenesis, molecular markers—for example, retinoic acid receptor (RAR) β, *p53*, *p16*, *EGFR*, and genetic instability—for developing drugs, monitoring interventions, and assessing cancer risk and pharmacogenomics.

In terms of cancer risk assessment, cyclin D1 genotype ([97, 98]) and loss of heterozygosity at certain chromosomal sites ([99, 100]) have emerged in multiple studies as prognostic factors that could be potentially useful in the clinic. Building on these data, investigators at MDACC led a clinical study evaluating the effects of erlotinib (150 mg/d for 1 year) on the incidence of invasive cancer in patients with oral premalignant lesions (with or without a prior history of oral cancer) selected for high risk based on loss of heterozygosity testing—the Erlotinib Prevention of Oral Cancer (EPOC) study ([101, 102]). This was the first large-scale study in oral IEN that used molecular risk assessment as part of the inclusion criteria, thus bringing the concept of precision medicine to the chemoprevention field. Loss of heterozygosity high-risk profiles were indeed associated with increased oral cancer incidence on long term follow-up and are now considered the most robust molecular markers of cancer risk in oral IEN. Erlotinib, however, did not improve oral cancer-free survival in this high-risk population.

As the role of HPV-16 in the pathogenesis of a subgroup of HNSCC becomes substantiated, preventive strategies targeting this infectious agent could be explored as well. Human papillomavirus vaccination is already being used to prevent cervical cancer. Human papillomavirus vaccine has been shown to reduce the prevalence of oral HPV infections, but its impact on incidence of HNSCC is yet to be determined ([103]). One anticipates, though, that widespread HPV vaccination may contribute to reducing the burden of HPV-induced HNSCC in the coming decades.

SUMMARY

Head and neck SCC is a major international health problem. General public health strategies such as reducing tobacco usage and increasing awareness of associated risks are of primary importance.

The demonstration of HPV as a causative agent for oropharyngeal cancers is of great importance because this will carry implications for prevention and also will influence decision making in treatment planning as well as the conduct of clinical trials.

The optimal care and treatment of head and neck cancer patients are multidisciplinary. Surgical resection and/or radiotherapy are powerful local modalities and the care of treatment for most patients. Emerging data support the administration of chemotherapy as a component of combined-modality treatments, especially in patients with advanced HNSCC. For patients with locally recurrent or metastatic disease, combination chemotherapy may produce response rates of 30% to 40%. However, responses tend to be brief, lasting a median of 3 to 6 months, and are associated with only a modest prolongation of survival. Thus, chemotherapy for these patients is palliative. An exception to this is for patients with NPC, with higher response rates and a small proportion of long-term disease-free survivors. For patients with metastatic HNSCC of any primary site, the addition of cetuximab to platinum–5-FU appears to improve tumor responses and overall survival. Targeted agents are currently under investigation. Prognostic and predictive markers are needed to improve selection of patients who are most likely to benefit from palliative treatment. Enrolling in investigational studies is strongly supported.

In the newly diagnosed patient with locally advanced disease, high response rates have been observed with induction chemotherapy. The addition of a taxane to the more traditional PF platform has increased overall activity, but the use of induction treatment for most patients remains an investigational endeavor. The potential for augmentation of local control with a substantial response to chemotherapy followed by definitive surgery or radiation is also under investigation. Three large multicenter randomized trials have been successfully conducted in larynx cancer with preservation of function in subsets of patients.

Chemotherapy administered concomitantly with radiotherapy has improved local control and survival in a sequence of studies and is recognized as the standard of care for nonsurgical therapy of patients with locally advanced squamous cancers of the pharynx and larynx. The increase in toxicity associated with these regimens should be carefully considered in selecting patients for combined treatment.

Patients with earlier-stage disease (ie, stage I or II) generally should receive therapy with either surgery or radiotherapy or both. Patients with locally advanced M0 (stage III/IVA/B) disease may be considered for nonsurgical therapy, most often with chemotherapy and radiation, or entered into a combined chemoradiation treatment protocol. Patients with "resectable" disease can be further divided by site. Patients with primary oral cavity tumors are best served with surgery followed by radiotherapy (or chemoradiotherapy if there are high-risk pathologic features), whereas those with oropharyngeal, hypopharyngeal, or laryngeal tumors are often treated with radiation, with or without chemotherapy, depending on precise site and stage.

Basic and translational chemoprevention research in head and neck carcinogenesis is advancing our understanding of the molecular characteristics of carcinogenesis and cancer risk. We have studied *EGFR* inhibition in a prospective, controlled trial in high-risk patients. This project illustrates the convergence of prevention and therapy, whereby a molecularly targeted agent known to have efficacy in the setting of invasive cancer is brought into the premalignant space.

The management of head and neck cancer is a multidisciplinary activity. The identification of effective chemotherapeutic agents and their integration into the initial therapy of head and neck cancer have the potential to improve survival time and preserve organ function. Moreover, studies are under way to reduce treatment intensity and thereby long-term toxicity. Through well-designed and executed clinical trials, coupled with basic research of the biology of upper aerodigestive tract tumors, further advances in the management and prevention of these cancers can be achieved.

REFERENCES

1. Siegel RL, Miller KD, Jemal A. Cancer statistics, 2015. *CA Cancer J Clin.* 2015;65(1):5-29.
2. Parkin DM, Bray F, Ferlay J, Pisani P. Global cancer statistics, 2002. *CA Cancer J Clin.* 2005;55(2):74-108.
3. Brennan JA, Boyle JO, Koch WM, et al. Association between cigarette smoking and mutation of the p53 gene in squamous-cell carcinoma of the head and neck. *N Engl J Med.* 1995; 332(11):712-717.
4. Gillison ML, Koch WM, Capone RB, et al. Evidence for a causal association between human papillomavirus and a subset of head and neck cancers. *J Natl Cancer Inst.* 2000;92(9):709-720.
5. Chaturvedi AK, Engels EA, Pfeiffer RM, et al. Human papillomavirus and rising oropharyngeal cancer incidence in the United States. *J Clin Oncol.* 2011;29(32):4294-4301.
6. Gillison ML. Human papillomavirus-associated head and neck cancer is a distinct epidemiologic, clinical, and molecular entity. *Semin Oncol.* 2004;31(6):744-754.
7. Braakhuis BJ, Snijders PJ, Keune WJ, et al. Genetic patterns in head and neck cancers that contain or lack transcriptionally active human papillomavirus. *J Natl Cancer Inst.* 2004;96(13):998-1006.
8. Ang KK, Harris J, Wheeler R, et al. Human papillomavirus and survival of patients with oropharyngeal cancer. *N Engl J Med.* 2010;363(1):24-35.
9. Fakhry C, Westra WH, Li S, et al. Improved survival of patients with human papillomavirus-positive head and neck squamous cell carcinoma in a prospective clinical trial. *J Natl Cancer Inst.* 2008;100(4):261-269.
10. Gillison ML, D'Souza G, Westra W, et al. Distinct risk factor profiles for human papillomavirus type 16-positive and human papillomavirus type 16-negative head and neck cancers. *J Natl Cancer Inst.* 2008;100(6):407-420.
11. Haddad RI, Shin DM. Recent advances in head and neck cancer. *N Engl J Med.* 2008;359(11):1143-1154.
12. Poeta ML, Manola J, Goldwasser MA, et al. TP53 mutations and survival in squamous-cell carcinoma of the head and neck. *N Engl J Med.* 2007; 357(25):2552-2561.
13. Kandoth C, McLellan MD, Vandin F, et al. Mutational landscape and significance across 12 major cancer types. *Nature.* 2013;502(7471):333-339.
14. Callender T, el-Naggar AK, Lee MS, Frankenthaler R, Luna MA, Batsakis JG. PRAD-1 (CCND1)/cyclin D1 oncogene amplification in primary head and neck squamous cell carcinoma. *Cancer.* 1994;74(1):152-158.
15. Papadimitrakopoulou VA, Izzo J, Mao L, et al. Cyclin D1 and p16 alterations in advanced premalignant lesions of the upper aerodigestive tract: role in response to chemoprevention and cancer development. *Clin Cancer Res.* 2001;7(10):3127-3134.
16. Gasco M, Crook T. The p53 network in head and neck cancer. *Oral Oncol.* 2003;39(3):222-231.
17. Grandis JR, Tweardy DJ. Elevated levels of transforming growth factor alpha and epidermal growth factor receptor messenger RNA are early markers of carcinogenesis in head and neck cancer. *Cancer Res.* 1993;53(15):3579-3584.
18. Roskoski R Jr. The ErbB/HER receptor protein-tyrosine kinases and cancer. *Biochem Biophys Res Commun.* 2004;319(1):1-11.
19. Stransky N, Egloff AM, Tward AD, et al. The mutational landscape of head and neck squamous cell carcinoma. *Science.* 2011;333(6046):1157-1160.
20. Kupferman ME, Sturgis EM, Schwartz DL, Garden A, Kies MS. Neoplasms of the head and neck. In: Hong WK, Bast Jr RB, Hait WN, et al., eds. *Cancer Medicine.* 8th ed. Shelton, CT: BC Decker - People's Medical Publishing House-USA; 2010: 959-998.
21. Holsinger FC, Kies MS, Weinstock YE, et al. Videos in clinical medicine. Examination of the larynx and pharynx. *N Engl J Med.* 2008;358(3):e2.
22. Greene FL, Sobin LH. A worldwide approach to the TNM staging system: collaborative efforts of the AJCC and UICC. *J Surg Oncol.* 2009;99(5):269-272.

22a. Sobin L, Gospodarowicz M, Whittekind C. UICC (International Union Against Cancer): TNM - Classification of Malignant Tumours. West Sussex, UK: Wiley-Blackwell, Seventh Edition, 2009.

23. Vokes EE, Weichselbaum RR, Lippman SM, Hong WK. Head and neck cancer. *N Engl J Med.* 1993;328(3):184-194.
24. Forastiere A, Koch W, Trotti A, Sidransky D. Head and neck cancer. *N Engl J Med.* 2001;345(26):1890-1900.
25. Pow EH, Kwong DL, McMillan AS, et al. Xerostomia and quality of life after intensity-modulated radiotherapy vs. conventional radiotherapy for early-stage nasopharyngeal carcinoma: initial report on a randomized controlled clinical trial. *Int J Radiat Oncol Biol Phys.* 2006;66(4):981-991.
26. Hu K, Chan ATC, Costantino P. Cancer of the nasopharynx. In: Harrison LB, Sessions RB, Kies MS, eds. *Head and Neck Cancer: A Multidisciplinary Approach.* 4th ed. Philadelphia, PA: Lippincott Williams & Wilkins; 2014: 588634.
27. Al-Sarraf M, LeBlanc M, Giri PG, et al. Chemoradiotherapy versus radiotherapy in patients with advanced nasopharyngeal cancer: phase III randomized Intergroup study 0099. *J Clin Oncol.* 1998;16(4):1310-1317.
28. Chan AT, Leung SF, Ngan RK, et al. Overall survival after concurrent cisplatin-radiotherapy compared with radiotherapy alone in locoregionally advanced nasopharyngeal carcinoma. *J Natl Cancer Inst.* 2005;97(7):536-539.
29. Koch WA, Stafford E, Bajaj G. Head and neck cancer. In: Harrison LB, Sessions RB, Hong WK, eds. *Cancer of the Oral Cavity, General Principles and Management.* 3rd ed. Philadelphia, PA: Lippincott Williams & Wilkins; 2009.
30. Garden AS, Asper JA, Morrison WH, et al. Is concurrent chemoradiation the treatment of choice for all patients with stage III or IV head and neck carcinoma? *Cancer.* 2004;100(6):1171-1178.
31. Lefebvre JL, Chevalier D, Luboinski B, Kirkpatrick A, Collette L, Sahmoud T. Larynx preservation in pyriform sinus cancer: preliminary results of a European Organization for Research and Treatment of Cancer phase III trial. EORTC Head and Neck Cancer Cooperative Group. *J Natl Cancer Inst.* 1996;88(13):890-899.
32. Lefebvre JL, Rolland F, Tesselaar M, et al. Phase 3 randomized trial on larynx preservation comparing sequential vs alternating chemotherapy and radiotherapy. *J Natl Cancer Inst.* 2009;101(3):142-152.
33. Mendenhall WM, Werning JW. Cancer of the larynx. In: Harrison LB, Sessions RB, Kies MS, eds. *Head and Neck Cancer: A Multidisciplinary Approach.* 4th ed. Philadelphhia, PA: Lippincott Williams & Wilkins; 2014: 441-481.
34. Induction chemotherapy plus radiation compared with surgery plus radiation in patients with advanced laryngeal cancer. The Department of Veterans Affairs Laryngeal Cancer Study Group. *N Engl J Med.* 1991;324(24):1685-1690.
35. Weber RS, Berkey BA, Forastiere A, et al. Outcome of salvage total laryngectomy following organ preservation therapy: the Radiation Therapy Oncology Group trial 91-11. *Arch Otolaryngol Head Neck Surg.* 2003;129(1):44-49.
36. Eisele D, Kleinberg L. Management of malignant salivary gland tumors. In: Harrison LB, Sessions RB, Hong WK, eds. *Head and Neck Cancer: A Multidisciplinary Approach.* 2nd ed. Philadelphia, PA: Lippincott Williams & Wilkins; 2004.
37. Jeng YM, Lin CY, Hsu HC. Expression of the c-kit protein is associated with certain subtypes of salivary gland carcinoma. *Cancer Lett.* 2000;154(1):107-111.
38. Andry G, Hamoir M, Locati LD, Licitra L, Langendijk JA. Management of salivary gland tumors. *Expert Rev Anticancer Ther.*

2012;12(9):1161-1168.

39. Vekony H, Ylstra B, Wilting SM, et al. DNA copy number gains at loci of growth factors and their receptors in salivary gland adenoid cystic carcinoma. *Clin Cancer Res.* 2007;13(11):3133-3139.
40. Mitani Y, Li J, Rao PH, et al. Comprehensive analysis of the MYB-NFIB gene fusion in salivary adenoid cystic carcinoma: incidence, variability, and clinicopathologic significance. *Clin Cancer Res.* 2010;16(19):4722-4731.
41. Agulnik M, Cohen EW, Cohen RB, et al. Phase II study of lapatinib in recurrent or metastatic epidermal growth factor receptor and/or erbB2 expressing adenoid cystic carcinoma and non adenoid cystic carcinoma malignant tumors of the salivary glands. *J Clin Oncol.* 2007;25(25):3978-3984.
42. Pignon JP, le Maitre A, Maillard E, Bourhis J, MACH-NC Collaborative Group. Meta-analysis of chemotherapy in head and neck cancer (MACH-NC): an update on 93 randomised trials and 17,346 patients. *Radiother Oncol.* 2009;92(1):4-14.
43. Vermorken JB, Remenar E, van Herpen C, et al. Cisplatin, fluorouracil, and docetaxel in unresectable head and neck cancer. *N Engl J Med.* 2007;357(17):1695-1704.
44. Posner MR, Hershock DM, Blajman CR, et al. Cisplatin and fluorouracil alone or with docetaxel in head and neck cancer. *N Engl J Med.* 2007;357(17):1705-1715.
45. Paccagnella A, Ghi MG, Loreggian L, et al. Concomitant chemoradiotherapy versus induction docetaxel, cisplatin and 5 fluorouracil (TPF) followed by concomitant chemoradiotherapy in locally advanced head and neck cancer: a phase II randomized study. *Ann Oncol.* 2010;21(7):1515-1522.
46. Haddad R, O'Neill A, Rabinowits G, et al. Induction chemotherapy followed by concurrent chemoradiotherapy (sequential chemoradiotherapy) versus concurrent chemoradiotherapy alone in locally advanced head and neck cancer (PARADIGM): a randomised phase 3 trial. *Lancet Oncol.* 2013;14(3):257-264.
47. Cohen EE, Karrison TG, Kocherginsky M, et al. Phase III randomized trial of induction chemotherapy in patients with N2 or N3 locally advanced head and neck cancer. *J Clin Oncol.* 2014;32(25):2735-2743.
48. Kies MS, Holsinger FC, Lee JJ, et al. Induction chemotherapy and cetuximab for locally advanced squamous cell carcinoma of the head and neck: results from a phase II prospective trial. *J Clin Oncol.* 2010;28(1):8-14.
49. Hutcheson KA, Lewin JS, Holsinger FC, et al. Long-term functional and survival outcomes after induction chemotherapy and risk-based definitive therapy for locally advanced squamous cell carcinoma of the head and neck. *Head Neck.* 2014;36(4):474-480.
50. Cmelak A, Li S, Marur S, et al. E1308: reduced-dose IMRT in human papilloma virus (HPV)-associated resectable oropharyngeal squamous carcinomas (OPSCC) after clinical complete response (cCR) to induction chemotherapy (IC) [abstract]. *J Clin Oncol.* 2014;32:LBA6006.
51. Seiwert TY, Salama JK, Vokes EE. The chemoradiation paradigm in head and neck cancer. *Nat Clin Pract Oncol.* 2007;4(3):156-171.
52. Seiwert TY, Salama JK, Vokes EE. The concurrent chemoradiation paradigm—general principles. *Nat Clin Pract Oncol.* 2007;4(2):86-100.
53. Vokes EE, Schilsky RL, Weichselbaum RR, Kozloff MF, Panje WR. Induction chemotherapy with cisplatin, fluorouracil, and high-dose leucovorin for locally advanced head and neck cancer: a clinical and pharmacologic analysis. *J Clin Oncol.* 1990;8(2):241-247.
54. Al-Sarraf M, Pajak TF, Marcial VA, et al. Concurrent radiotherapy and chemotherapy with cisplatin in inoperable squamous cell carcinoma of the head and neck. An RTOG Study. *Cancer.* 1987;59(2):259-265.
55. Kies MS, Bennett CL, Vokes EE. Locally advanced head and neck cancer. *Curr Treat Options Oncol.* 2001;2(1):7-13.
56. Amdur RJ, Parsons JT, Mendenhall WM, Million RR, Cassisi NJ. Split-course versus continuous-course irradiation in the postoperative setting for squamous cell carcinoma of the head and neck. *Int J Radiat Oncol Biol Phys.* 1989;17(2):279-285.
57. Pajak TF, Laramore GE, Marcial VA, et al. Elapsed treatment days—a critical item for radiotherapy quality control review in head and neck trials: RTOG report. *Int J Radiat Oncol Biol Phys.* 1991;20(1):13-20.
58. Brizel DM, Albers ME, Fisher SR, et al. Hyperfractionated irradiation with or without concurrent chemotherapy for locally advanced head and neck cancer. *N Engl J Med.* 1998;338(25):1798-1804.
59. Clayman GL, Johnson CJ 2nd, Morrison W, Ginsberg L, Lippman SM. The role of neck dissection after chemoradiotherapy for oropharyngeal cancer with advanced nodal disease. *Arch Otolaryngol Head Neck Surg.* 2001;127(2):135-139.
60. Wendt TG, Grabenbauer GG, Rodel CM, et al. Simultaneous radiochemotherapy versus radiotherapy alone in advanced head and neck cancer: a randomized multicenter study. *J Clin Oncol.* 1998;16(4):1318-1324.
61. Calais G, Alfonsi M, Bardet E, et al. Randomized trial of radiation therapy versus concomitant chemotherapy and radiation therapy for advanced-stage oropharynx carcinoma. *J Natl Cancer Inst.* 1999;91(24):2081-2086.
62. Jeremic B, Shibamoto Y, Milicic B, et al. Hyperfractionated radiation therapy with or without concurrent low-dose daily cisplatin in locally advanced squamous cell carcinoma of the head and neck: a prospective randomized trial. *J Clin Oncol.* 2000;18(7):1458-1464.
63. Adelstein DJ, Li Y, Adams GL, et al. An intergroup phase III comparison of standard radiation therapy and two schedules of concurrent chemoradiotherapy in patients with unresectable squamous cell head and neck cancer. *J Clin Oncol.* 2003;21(1):92-98.
64. Bonner JA, Harari PM, Giralt J, et al. Radiotherapy plus cetuximab for squamous-cell carcinoma of the head and neck. *N Engl J Med.* 2006;354(6):567-578.
65. Ang KK, Zhang Q, Rosenthal DI, et al. Randomized phase III trial of concurrent accelerated radiation plus cisplatin with or without cetuximab for stage III to IV head and neck carcinoma: RTOG 0522. *J Clin Oncol.* 2014;32(27):2940-2950.
66. Mesia R, Henke M, Fortin A, et al. Chemoradiotherapy with or without panitumumab in patients with unresected, locally advanced squamous-cell carcinoma of the head and neck (CONCERT-1): a randomised, controlled, open-label phase 2 trial. *Lancet Oncol.* 2015;16(2):208-220.
67. Giralt J, Trigo J, Nuyts S, et al. Panitumumab plus radiotherapy versus chemoradiotherapy in patients with unresected, locally advanced squamous-cell carcinoma of the head and neck (CONCERT-2): a randomised, controlled, open-label phase 2 trial. *Lancet Oncol.* 2015;16(2):221-232.
68. Bachaud JM, Cohen-Jonathan E, Alzieu C, David JM, Serrano E, Daly-Schveitzer N. Combined postoperative radiotherapy and weekly cisplatin infusion for locally advanced head and neck carcinoma: final report of a randomized trial. *Int J Radiat Oncol Biol Phys.* 1996;36(5):999-1004.
69. Cooper JS, Pajak TF, Forastiere AA, et al. Postoperative concurrent radiotherapy and chemotherapy for high-risk squamous-cell carcinoma of the head and neck. *N Engl J Med.* 2004;350(19):1937-1944.
70. Bernier J, Domenge C, Ozsahin M, et al. Postoperative irradiation with or without concomitant chemotherapy for locally advanced head and neck cancer. *N Engl J Med.* 2004;350(19):1945-1952.
71. Vermorken JB, Mesia R, Rivera F, et al. Platinum-based

chemotherapy plus cetuximab in head and neck cancer. *N Engl J Med.* 2008;359(11):1116-1127.
72. Harari PM, Harris J, Kies MS, et al. Postoperative chemoradiotherapy and cetuximab for high-risk squamous cell carcinoma of the head and neck: Radiation Therapy Oncology Group RTOG-0234. *J Clin Oncol.* 2014;32(23):2486-2495.
73. Bernier J, Cooper JS, Pajak TF, et al. Defining risk levels in locally advanced head and neck cancers: a comparative analysis of concurrent postoperative radiation plus chemotherapy trials of the EORTC (#22931) and RTOG (# 9501). *Head Neck.* 2005;27(10):843-850.
74. Forastiere AA, Goepfert H, Maor M, et al. Concurrent chemotherapy and radiotherapy for organ preservation in advanced laryngeal cancer. *N Engl J Med.* 2003;349(22):2091-2098.
75. Forastiere AA, Adelstein DJ, Manola J. Induction chemotherapy meta-analysis in head and neck cancer: right answer, wrong question. *J Clin Oncol.* 2013;31(23):2844-2846.
76. Pointreau Y, Garaud P, Chapet S, et al. Randomized trial of induction chemotherapy with cisplatin and 5-fluorouracil with or without docetaxel for larynx preservation. *J Natl Cancer Inst.* 2009;101(7):498-506.
77. Setton J, Lee NY, Riaz N, et al. A multi-institution pooled analysis of gastrostomy tube dependence in patients with oropharyngeal cancer treated with definitive intensity-modulated radiotherapy. *Cancer.* 2015;121(2):294-301.
78. Cohen EE, Rosen F, Stadler WM, et al. Phase II trial of ZD1839 in recurrent or metastatic squamous cell carcinoma of the head and neck. *J Clin Oncol.* 2003;21(10):1980-1987.
79. Cohen EE, Lingen MW, Vokes EE. The expanding role of systemic therapy in head and neck cancer. *J Clin Oncol.* 2004;22(9):1743-1752.
80. Soulieres D, Senzer NN, Vokes EE, Hidalgo M, Agarwala SS, Siu LL. Multicenter phase II study of erlotinib, an oral epidermal growth factor receptor tyrosine kinase inhibitor, in patients with recurrent or metastatic squamous cell cancer of the head and neck. *J Clin Oncol.* 2004;22(1):77-85.
81. Burtness B, Goldwasser MA, Flood W, Mattar B, Forastiere AA, Eastern Cooperative Oncology Group. Phase III randomized trial of cisplatin plus placebo compared with cisplatin plus cetuximab in metastatic/recurrent head and neck cancer: an Eastern Cooperative Oncology Group study. *J Clin Oncol.* 2005;23(34):8646-8654.
82. Vermorken JB, Trigo J, Hitt R, et al. Open-label, uncontrolled, multicenter phase II study to evaluate the efficacy and toxicity of cetuximab as a single agent in patients with recurrent and/or metastatic squamous cell carcinoma of the head and neck who failed to respond to platinum-based therapy. *J Clin Oncol.* 2007;25(16):2171-2177.
83. Wen Y, Grandis JR. Emerging drugs for head and neck cancer. *Expert Opin Emerg Drugs.* 2015;20:313-329.
84. Seiwert TY, Burtness B, Weiss J, et al. A phase Ib study of MK-3475 in patients with human papillomavirus (HPV)-associated and non-HPV-associated head and neck (H/N) cancer [abstract]. *J Clin Oncol.* 2014;32:6011.
85. Hong WK, Endicott J, Itri LM, et al. 13-cis-retinoic acid in the treatment of oral leukoplakia. *N Engl J Med.* 1986;315(24):1501-1505.
86. Lippman SM, Batsakis JG, Toth BB, et al. Comparison of low-dose isotretinoin with beta carotene to prevent oral carcinogenesis. *N Engl J Med.* 1993;328(1):15-20.
87. Lotan R, Xu XC, Lippman SM, et al. Suppression of retinoic acid receptor-beta in premalignant oral lesions and its up-regulation by isotretinoin. *N Engl J Med.* 1995;332(21):1405-1410.
88. Papadimitrakopoulou VA, Hong WK, Lee JS, et al. Low-dose isotretinoin versus beta-carotene to prevent oral carcinogenesis: long-term follow-up. *J Natl Cancer Inst.* 1997;89(3):257-258.
89. Papadimitrakopoulou VA, Lee JJ, William WN Jr, et al. Randomized trial of 13-cis retinoic acid compared with retinyl palmitate with or without beta-carotene in oral premalignancy. *J Clin Oncol.* 2009;27(4):599-604.
90. Hong WK, Lippman SM, Itri LM, et al. Prevention of second primary tumors with isotretinoin in squamous-cell carcinoma of the head and neck. *N Engl J Med.* 1990;323(12):795-801.
91. Benner SE, Pajak TF, Lippman SM, Earley C, Hong WK. Prevention of second primary tumors with isotretinoin in patients with squamous cell carcinoma of the head and neck: long-term follow-up. *J Natl Cancer Inst.* 1994;86(2):140-141.
92. Dannenberg AJ, Lippman SM, Mann JR, Subbaramaiah K, DuBois RN. Cyclooxygenase-2 and epidermal growth factor receptor: pharmacologic targets for chemoprevention. *J Clin Oncol.* 2005;23(2):254-266.
93. Bolla M, Lefur R, Ton Van J, et al. Prevention of second primary tumours with etretinate in squamous cell carcinoma of the oral cavity and oropharynx. Results of a multicentric double-blind randomised study. *Eur J Cancer.* 1994;30A(6):767-772.
94. van Zandwijk N, Dalesio O, Pastorino U, de Vries N, van Tinteren H. EUROSCAN, a randomized trial of vitamin A and N-acetylcysteine in patients with head and neck cancer or lung cancer. For the European Organization for Research and Treatment of Cancer Head and Neck and Lung Cancer Cooperative Groups. *J Natl Cancer Inst.* 2000;92(12):977-986.
95. Mayne ST, Cartmel B, Baum M, et al. Randomized trial of supplemental beta-carotene to prevent second head and neck cancer. *Cancer Res.* 2001;61(4):1457-1463.
96. Bairati I, Meyer F, Gelinas M, et al. A randomized trial of antioxidant vitamins to prevent second primary cancers in head and neck cancer patients. *J Natl Cancer Inst.* 2005;97(7):481-488.
97. Izzo JG, Papadimitrakopoulou VA, Liu DD, et al. Cyclin D1 genotype, response to biochemoprevention, and progression rate to upper aerodigestive tract cancer. *J Natl Cancer Inst.* 2003;95(3):198-205.
98. Papadimitrakopoulou V, Izzo JG, Liu DD, et al. Cyclin D1 and cancer development in laryngeal premalignancy patients. *Cancer Prev Res (Phila).* 2009;2(1):14-21.
99. Mao L, Lee JS, Fan YH, et al. Frequent microsatellite alterations at chromosomes 9p21 and 3p14 in oral premalignant lesions and their value in cancer risk assessment. *Nat Med.* 1996;2(6):682-685.
100. Rosin MP, Cheng X, Poh C, et al. Use of allelic loss to predict malignant risk for low-grade oral epithelial dysplasia. *Clin Cancer Res.* 2000;6(2):357-362.
101. William WN Jr, Heymach JV, Kim ES, Lippman SM. Molecular targets for cancer chemoprevention. *Nat Rev Drug Discov.* 2009;8(3):213-225.
102. William WN, Papadimitrakopoulou V, Lee JJ, et al. Randomized placebo-controlled trial (RCT) of erlotinib for prevention of oral cancer (EPOC) [abstract]. *J Clin Oncol.* 2014;32:6007.
103. Herrero R, Quint W, Hildesheim A, et al. Reduced prevalence of oral human papillomavirus (HPV) 4 years after bivalent HPV vaccination in a randomized clinical trial in Costa Rica. *PLoS One.* 2013;8(7):e68329.

Section VI

Gastrointestinal Cancers

Section Editor: Robert A. Wolff

第六篇 胃肠道肿瘤

20

Gastric, Gastroesophageal Junction, and Esophageal Cancers

第二十章　胃、胃食管结合部及食管癌

Elena Elimova
Roopma Wadhwa
Nikolaos Charalampakis
Alexandria T. Phan
Prajnam Das
M. Blum Murphy

中文导读

本章主要分为胃癌和胃食管结合部及食管癌两部分。首先分别介绍了两类疾病的流行病学、病原学特征和危险因素，在胃癌部分还专门针对幽门螺杆菌感染的预防和治疗的重要性进行了阐释。接下来由首发症状开始，结合病理及分子特征、内镜下及影像学（CT/MRI/PET-CT等）表现等讲解了疾病的诊断、分期及预后。治疗方面先分别对可切除性的肿瘤进行介绍，包括：手术，围手术期化疗，围手术期放疗、化疗，围手术期放疗、化疗对比围手术期化疗的疗效以及术后化疗。在胃食管结合部及食管癌的治疗中，还介绍了根治性放疗、化疗，根治性放疗、化疗与根治性放疗、化疗联合手术的疗效对比。本章接着对转移性胃癌和胃食管结合部及食管癌的治疗进行了统一的介绍，详述了一、二、三线治疗方案的选择和MD安德森癌症中心在晚期上消化道肿瘤治疗的研究进展。最后本章介绍了最佳支持治疗对这类患者治疗的重要性。

GASTRIC CANCER

Epidemiologic Characteristics

The incidence of gastric cancer varies widely worldwide. The highest incidence (>20 per 100,000 in men) is seen in Japan, China, Eastern Europe, and South America, while the lowest incidence (<10 per 100,000 in men) is seen in Northern America, parts of Africa, and Northern Europe ([1]). In the United States, 24,590 new cases of gastric cancer are estimated in 2015, with 10,720 deaths ([2]). Gastric cancers occur at a median age of 69 years for men and 73 years for women ([3]). African Americans, Hispanic Americans, and Native Americans are 1.5 to 2.5 times more likely to develop gastric cancer than whites ([3]). In the United States, there are changing epidemiologic patterns regarding the anatomic location of esophagogastric cancers, with a trend of decreased occurrence of distal or noncardia gastric cancers ([4]). The reason for the decline is not known but may be related to change in dietary habits and food preservation. However, an increase in the incidence of gastric cardia cancers has been observed, from 2.4 cases per 100,000 individuals (1977-1981) to 2.9 cases per 100,000 individuals (2001-2006) in the white population ([4]). Similarly, the Surveillance, Epidemiology, and End Results (SEER) cancer registry program in the United States shows an approximate 2.5-fold increase in the incidence of gastroesophageal junction (GEJ) adenocarcinomas from 1973 to 1992, from 1.22 cases per 100,000 individuals (1973-1978) to 2.00 cases per 100,000 individuals (1985-1990), with rates stabilizing in the last two decades, with an incidence of 1.94 cases per 100,000 individuals (2003-2008) ([3,5]).

Population studies suggest that proximal cancers have a different pathogenesis than distal cancers ([6]). Potential causes of distal gastric cancers include *Helicobacter pylori* infection or E-cadherin expression loss, whereas proximal gastric cancers may behave similarly to distal esophageal and GEJ cancers, which progress from Barrett metaplasia to dysplasia to invasive adenocarcinoma. Only 26% of newly diagnosed gastric cancers are localized. The 5-year overall survival (OS) rate is 28.3%, which has not changed significantly over the past 30 to 40 years ([1]). Surgery is still the only chance for cure, and survival can be improved with multimodality therapy. The 5-year OS rate of patients with advanced disease remains dismal at less than 5%. Thus, despite decreasing incidence, gastric cancer remains a public health concern in the United States because of its high fatality rate.

Etiologic Characteristics and Risk Factors

The most frequent type of gastric cancer is adenocarcinoma, which consists of two main histologic variants: intestinal and diffuse. Intestinal-type gastric adenocarcinoma likely begins with an *H pylori* infection that leads to multistep progression (chronic active nonatrophic gastritis, multifocal atrophic gastritis, intestinal metaplasia, dysplasia, and invasive adenocarcinoma) ([7]). More than 40% to 50% of distal gastric adenocarcinomas are associated with *H pylori* infection ([6]). Other environmental risk factors and inflammatory cytokines may influence and contribute to this multistep progression.

Population studies have identified certain environmental risk factors associated with gastric cancer. Low consumption of fruits and vegetables, high intake of N-nitroso compounds in salted and preserved foods, and occupational exposure in coal mining and nickel, rubber and timber processing are commonly described risk factors. Long-standing chronic superficial gastritis caused by a high-salt diet and conditions such as pernicious anemia eventually leads to chronic atrophic gastritis and intestinal metaplasia ([7]). Additional notable risk factors include meat consumption ([8]), smoking ([9]), gastric surgery ([10]), and reproductive hormones ([11]).

Overall, the pathogenesis of intestinal-type gastric adenocarcinomas involves a series of events. This sequence of events—increased cell proliferation due to the promotional effects of hypergastrinemia or bile reflux, increased luminal levels of mutagens (eg, N-nitroso compounds and free radicals), and decreased luminal levels of protective factors (eg, vitamin C)—provides an ideal milieu for carcinogenesis in susceptible hosts ([7]).

In contrast to intestinal-type gastric cancer, diffuse-type gastric adenocarcinoma results from defective intracellular adhesion molecules, which is the consequence of loss of E-cadherin protein expression, which is encoded by the cadherin 1 (*CDH1*) gene. This can occur through germline or somatic mutation, loss of heterozygosity, or epigenetic silencing of gene transcription through aberrant methylation of the *CDH1* promoter. A study by Zheng et al showed a positive rate of E-cadherin promoter methylation in dysplasia, early cancer, and advanced cancer ([12]). Furthermore, 30% of hereditary diffuse gastric cancer (HDGC) families show *CDH1* germline mutations, whereas the rest remain genetically unexplained ([13]). Currently, many families with HDGC have *CDH1* germline mutations. Inheritance is dominant. The lifetime cumulative risk for advanced gastric cancer has been estimated to be 40% to 67% in men and 60% to 83% in women ([14]). Women in affected families are also at high risk for developing lobular breast cancer, with a cumulative risk of 52% ([14]). A germline mutation in *TP53* is associated with familial gastric cancer ([13]), which includes Li-Fraumeni syndrome. Another familial cancer syndrome associated with gastric cancer is hereditary nonpolyposis colorectal cancer, resulting from defects of DNA mismatch repair genes (*hMLH1* and *hMSH2*, more frequent) ([13]) (Table 20-1).

Epstein-Barr virus (EBV)–associated gastric cancers have distinct clinicopathologic characteristics, including male predominance, preferential location in the gastric cardia or postsurgical gastric stump, lymphocytic infiltration, and a more favorable prognosis ([15, 16]).

Despite recent progress, the precise etiologic characteristics of gastric cancer and the relationship between the environment and host are unknown. Ongoing research promises to better elucidate the tumorigenesis of gastric cancer.

Table 20-1 Summary of Selected Recurrent Cytogenetic Abnormalities and Frequent Molecular Changes Associated With Gastric Cancer

Conventional Cytogenetics	Simple Karyotypes	Complex Karyotypes
	+X, +8, +9, +19, del(7q), i(8q)	1, 3, 6, 7, 8, 11, 13, 17, 19
Molecular Cytogenetics	**Gains**	**Loss**
	3q, 7p, 7q, 8q, 13q, 17q, 20p, 20q	4q, 9p, 17p, 18q
Genes	**Abnormalities**	**Clinical Association**
c-met	Amplification	Tumor invasion, lymph node metastasis, poor prognosis
K-sam	Amplification	Advanced tumor stage/poor prognosis
c-erbB2	Amplification	Advanced tumor stage, lymph node and liver metastases, poor prognosis
c-myc	Amplification	Poor clinical course/predictor of aggressiveness
TP53	Loss of heterozygosity	Proliferative rate/lymph node metastasis/ shortened survival
	Mutation	
	Hypermethylation	
BCL-2	Loss of heterozygosity	Depth of invasion, lymph node metastasis and survival
RUNX3	Deletion	Metastasis
	Hypermethylation	
	Loss of expression	
PTEN	Loss of heterozygosity	Advanced tumor stage/metastasis
	Mutation	
E-cadherin (*CDH1*)	Loss of heterozygosity	Tumor metastatic ability and poor prognosis
	Mutation	
	Hypermethylation	
	Reduced expression	
Cyclin E	Amplification	Disease aggressiveness/lymph node metastasis
p27	Reduced expression	Advanced tumor stage/depth of invasion/lymph node metastasis
p16	Reduced expression	Tumor invasion/metastasis
DNA repair genes/ microsatellite instability	Mutation	Age/low prevalence of lymph node metastasis/ prolonged survival
	Hypermethylation	
	Reduced expression	
Syndecan-1	Reduce expression	Tumor differentiation
β-catenin	Amplification	Lymph node metastasis
CD44s and *CD44v6*	Amplification	Lymph node metastasis
Sp1	Amplification	Cancer angiogenic potential, poor prognosis

Prevention

Results from a number of population studies have demonstrated an increased likelihood of *H pylori* infection in patients with gastric cancer, particularly cancer of the distal stomach ([17, 18]). However, gastric cancer does not occur in most patients infected with *H pylori*. Although the role of *H pylori* in gastric cancer pathogenesis is well defined, currently there is no definitive evidence showing that mass eradication could reduce the incidence of gastric cancer ([19]). A large Chinese study of 1,630 patients showed no benefit in the prevention of gastric cancer with the eradication of *H pylori* ([20]). However, in a subgroup of patients with no precancerous lesions on presentation, no patient developed gastric cancer during a follow-up of 7.5 years after *H pylori* eradication treatment compared with six patients who received placebo ($P = .02$) ([20]). In another large study, short-term treatment with amoxicillin and omeprazole statistically significantly reduced gastric cancer incidence by 39% during the period extending 14.7 years after *H pylori* treatment ([21]). A meta-analysis suggested that eradication could reduce the risk of gastric cancer; however, this meta-analysis was criticized for methodologic issues ([22]). At present, the treatment of this infection should be confined to patients with peptic ulcer disease, patients with mucosa-associated lymphoid tissue lymphoma, and after endoscopic resection for esophagogastric cancer; a role for a broad prevention strategy has yet to be defined. Applicable to distal gastric cancer and *H pylori*, vaccination may be relevant as a preventive measure against development of *H pylori*.

CHAPTER 20

Clinical Presentation

At presentation, most symptomatic patients will likely have advanced gastric cancer. Symptoms can be constitutional such as night sweats and unintentional weight loss, as well as vague, such as early satiety, abdominal pain, and nausea. Dysphagia is more common in patients with cancer originating in the gastric cardia or GEJ. Occult gastrointestinal (GI) bleeding is also common, whereas overt bleeding is observed in only 20% of cases.

Pathologic and Molecular Characteristics

More than 95% of gastric cancers are adenocarcinoma. The remaining 5% include neuroendocrine tumor, lymphoma, squamous cell cancer, and sarcoma.

The Cancer Genome Atlas (TCGA) Research Network has classified gastric cancer into four subtypes based on the molecular characterization of 295 primary adenocarcinomas in a way that can ultimately guide patient therapy ([23]). They clearly converged on four major genomic subtypes of gastric cancer with distinct features and classes of molecular alterations:

- Tumors containing EBV, along with recurrent mutations in the *PIK3CA* gene pathway, extreme DNA hypermethylation, amplification of Janus kinase 2 (*JAK2*), and extra copies of programmed death ligand 1 (*PD-L1*) and *PD-L2* genes, which are suppressors of immune response. This group made up about 10% of the cancers, with nearly 80% harboring a protein-changing alteration in *PIK3CA*.
- Tumors showing microsatellite instability, in which malfunctioning DNA repair mechanisms cause a high rate of mutations, including mutations of genes encoding targetable oncogenic signaling proteins. About 20% of tumors fell into this subtype.
- The largest category of tumors, making up about half of the cancer specimens, was termed *chromosomally unstable*. These contained a jumble of extra or missing pieces of genes and chromosomes (aneuploidy) and have a striking number of genomic amplifications of key receptor tyrosine kinases. This subtype of tumor is frequently found in the junction between the stomach and the esophagus, a type of gastric cancer that has been dramatically increasing in the United States.
- The fourth group was termed *genomically stable* because they lacked the molecular features of the other three types. These tumors, making up 20% of the specimens, were largely those of a specific class of gastric cancer enriched for the diffuse-type histologic variant, with approximately 30% of these tumors having genomic alterations in the Ras homolog gene family, member A (*RHOA*) signaling pathway. These tumors were characterized by the lack of high levels of aneuploidy and high metastatic potential.

This classification may serve as a valuable adjunct to histopathology and provides patient stratification as a guide to targeted agents.

Staging and Prognosis

Upper GI series with barium swallow and upper esophagogastroduodenoscopy (EGD) are mainstays for diagnosing gastric cancer and provide complementary diagnostic information. Esophagogastroduodenoscopy is more sensitive and specific to obtain tissue diagnosis. A single biopsy has 70% sensitivity for diagnosing gastric cancer; performing seven biopsies from the ulcer margin and base increases the sensitivity to >98% [24]. In contrast, barium swallow with upper GI series can identify both malignant gastric ulcers and infiltrating lesions, including some early gastric cancers. However, the false-negative rate with barium swallow can be as high as 50% [25] and may be even higher for early gastric cancer, and sensitivity can be as low as 14% [25].

Cancer staging is important because treatment is based on the pathology and the stage of disease at diagnosis, according to the TNM (tumor, node, metastasis) system of the American Joint Committee on Cancer (AJCC). Version 7 is the most current [26] (Table 20-2). In this newest version, GEJ and proximal gastric cancers <5 cm from the GEJ are now included in the esophageal cancer staging system. The T classification has been modified to harmonize with the new esophageal T classification. T1 and T4 have been further subdivided. Positive peritoneal cytologic results are classified as M1. Because of its noninvasive nature, computed tomography (CT) has become the cornerstone of gastric cancer staging, although it is not sensitive at detecting the tumor invasion depth and local and regional lymph node involvement. Currently, CT is used in conjunction with endoscopic ultrasonography (EUS) of the primary site, which provides the most accurate data for depth of tumor invasion and locoregional lymph node involvement. Endoscopic ultrasonography has an accuracy of 77% (vs 40%-50% with CT) for staging depth and 69% for staging nodes [27]. Limitations of EUS include understaging nodal disease and its short field of vision (5-7 cm). The availability of EUS-guided biopsy of suspicious local and regional lymph nodes has circumvented its former limitation (Figs. 20-1 and 20-2). Laparoscopy is more invasive than CT or EUS, but it has the advantage of directly visualizing the liver surface, peritoneum, and local lymph nodes. It is sensitive at diagnosing liver metastases and peritoneal metastases in up to 23% of patients in whom no such involvement was seen on CT [28]. Diagnostic laparoscopy is usually performed when all noninvasive studies (CT and EUS) demonstrate localized or potentially resectable disease in patients with >T1b disease on EUS.

The effectiveness of fluorodeoxyglucose (FDG) positron emission tomography (PET) at diagnosing gastric cancer is uncertain because as many as 50% of primary tumors are FDG negative, particularly early gastric cancers [29]. Insufficient FDG uptake is mostly associated with diffuse-type gastric cancer with signet ring cells and mucinous content [30]. Currently, FDG-PET has no role in the primary detection of gastric cancer because of its low sensitivity. On the other hand, FDG-PET shows better results in the evaluation of lymph node metastases in gastric cancer compared with CT and could thus have a role in preoperative staging. For patients with FDG-positive disease, FDG-PET can be used to predict histologic response and survival outcomes [31], similar to results seen among patients with distal esophageal and GEJ adenocarcinoma [32–34]. The addition of FDG-PET to CT increases diagnostic accuracy for recurrent gastric cancer because PET/CT is as sensitive and specific as contrast CT at detecting recurrent disease, except peritoneal seeding [35].

Among gastric cancer patients who had surgery, status of nodal involvement is perhaps the most powerful prognostic factor for them. Additionally, after curative resection, other factors affecting gastric cancer prognosis include tumor location, histologic grade, and lymphovascular invasion [26]. Patients with proximal gastric cancer have poorer prognosis than those with distal gastric cancer, at 28.5 versus 58.6 months ($P < .02$) [36]. Although associations have been found between molecular genetic changes and pathologic features and biologic behavior and prognosis, the clinical significance of these genetic changes has not yet been established. In other words, these genetic parameters have been unable to translate into meaningful clinical diagnostic, predictive, or prognostic biomarkers. Therefore, the putative biomarker screening method for gastric cancer also remains elusive. However, with better appreciation of the complex interplay between environment and host factors leading to gastric tumorigenesis, researchers hope to produce more effective screening methods for high-risk patients, better prognostic and predictive biomarkers, and superior therapeutic indices of cancer drugs. The recent comprehensive molecular characterization of gastric adenocarcinoma by the TCGA project is an approach toward this goal.

Treatment

Gastric cancer is treated according to the cancer stage at presentation. Reflecting the newest changes in the AJCC staging system, treatment for GEJ and proximal gastric adenocarcinoma <5 cm from the GEJ is discussed in the esophageal cancer section. Treatment for patients with locally advanced gastric cancer is dichotomized into resectable and unresectable disease. Surgery remains the best chance for long-term survival, but 5-year survival rates after surgery alone are 20% to 50%, and adjunctive therapy, such as chemotherapy or chemoradiotherapy, must be offered. Localized gastric cancer can be classified as clinical T1 disease or higher with or without involved regional lymph nodes. A minimum of

Table 20-2 American Joint Cancer Committee TNM Staging System for Gastric Cancer

Primary Tumor (T)				
Tx	Primary tumor cannot be assessed			
T0	No evidence of primary tumor			
Tis	Carcinoma in situ: intraepithelial tumor with invasion of the lamina propria			
T1	Tumor invades muscularis propria or submucosa			
T1a	Tumor invades lamina propria, muscularis mucosae, or submucosa			
T1b	Tumor invades submucosa			
T2	Tumor invades muscularis propria			
T3	Tumor penetrates the subserosal connective tissue without invasion of visceral peritoneum or adjacent structures			
T4	Tumor invades serosa (visceral peritoneum) or adjacent structures			
T4a	Tumor invades serosa (visceral peritoneum)			
T4b	Tumor invades adjacent structures			
Regional Lymph Nodes (N)				
Nx	Regional lymph node(s) cannot be assessed			
N0	No regional lymph node metastasis			
N1	Metastasis in 1-2 regional lymph nodes			
N2	Metastasis in 3-6 regional lymph nodes			
N3	Metastasis in ≥7 regional lymph nodes			
N3a	Metastasis in 7-15 regional lymph nodes			
N3b	Metastasis in ≥16 regional lymph nodes			
Distant Metastases (M)				
Mx	Distant metastasis cannot be assessed			
M0	No distant metastases			
M1	Distant metastases			
Stage Grouping				**5-Year Survival Rates (%)**
Stage 0 (in situ)	Tis	N0	M0	>90
Stage IA	T1	N0	M0	71
Stage IB	T1	N1	M0	57
	T2	N0	M0	
Stage IIA	T1	N2	M0	46
	T2	N1	M0	
Stage IIB	T3	N0	M0	
	T1	N3	M0	33
	T2	N2	M0	
	T3	N1	M0	
	T4a	N0	M0	
Stage IIIA	T2	N3	M0	20
	T3	N2	M0	
	T4a	N1	M0	
Stage IIIB	T3	N3	M0	14
	T4a	N2	M0	
	T4b	N1	M0	
	T4b	N0	M0	
Stage IIIC	T4a	N3	M0	9
	T4b	N3	M0	
	T4b	N2	M0	
Stage IV	Any T	Any N	M1	4

Reproduced with permission from Edge SB, Byrd DR, Compton CC (eds): *AJCC Cancer Staging Manuarl*, 7th ed. New York, NY: Springer; 2010.

CHAPTER 20

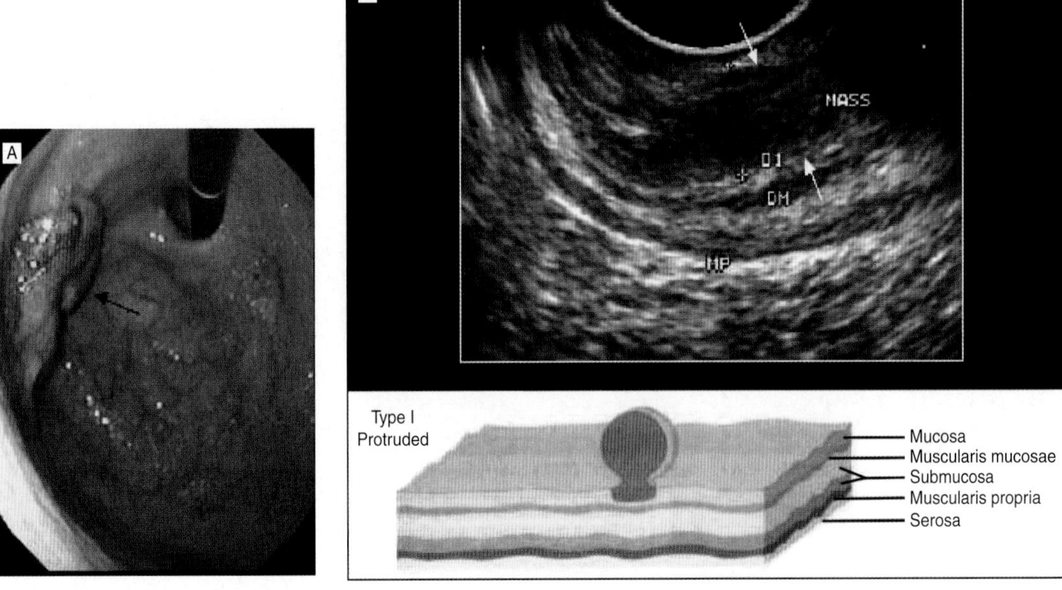

FIGURE 20-1 Gastric cancer: T1 lesion. A. Endoscopic view. B. Endoscopic ultrasound view. (Reproduced, with permission, from http://www.massgeneral.org/gastro/endo_homepage.htm.)

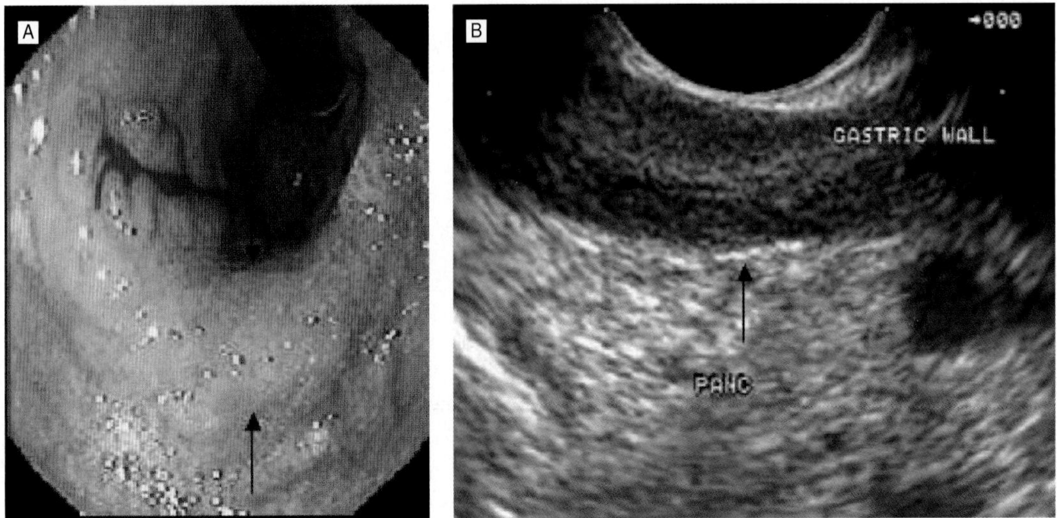

FIGURE 20-2 Gastric cancer: T2N1 lesion. A. Endoscopic view. B. Endoscopic ultrasound view. (Reproduced, with permission, from http://www.massgeneral. org/gastro/endo_homepage.htm.)

15 examined lymph nodes is recommended for adequate surgical staging ([37]). The adjunctive therapy used for the treatment of localized gastric cancer in addition to surgery depends on geographic location in the world. In North America and Europe, results from the Intergroup INT-0116 ([38]) (the adjuvant chemoradiotherapy approach) and Medical Research Council Adjuvant Infusional Chemotherapy (MAGIC) ([39]) (the perioperative chemotherapy approach) trials have established the standard of care in the early 2000s. In Asia, however, adjuvant chemotherapy following a D2 nodal dissection is considered the gold standard ([40, 41]).

Unfortunately, the main therapeutic goal in patients with unresectable locally advanced disease remains symptom palliation. The treatment of unresectable locally advanced and metastatic gastric cancers is discussed in two separate subsections: Unresectable Locally Advanced Gastric, Gastroesophageal Junction, and Esophageal Cancers; and Advanced and Metastatic Gastric, Gastroesophageal Junction, and Esophageal Cancers.

Resectable Disease

Surgery

Surgical resection offers the best chance for long-term survival in patients with localized disease, particularly in combination with postoperative (adjuvant) chemoradiotherapy ([38]) or perioperative chemotherapy ([39]). Even with newer staging modalities, the major barrier to accurately identify patients with potentially resectable disease is the ability to accurately stage disease. In the United States, 67% of patients present with stage III or IV disease, and only 10% present with stage I disease ([42]).

By definition, curative resection (also referred to as R0 resection) involves removal of the primary cancer and regional lymph nodes with free margins. The goals of surgery are twofold: (1) local control and hopefully eradication of gastric cancer and (2) attainment of accurate pathologic staging. Considerations for surgical management of gastric cancer are the (1) extent of luminal resection (total vs partial gastrectomy) and (2) extent of lymph node dissection. Total gastrectomy is mainly reserved for proximal gastric cancer and large midgastric tumors or linitis plastica (wherein a large region of the stomach is extensively infiltrated by cancer, resulting in a rigid, thickened fold), whereas partial gastrectomy may be used in distal gastric tumors. Two randomized control trials have demonstrated similar survival outcomes for total and partial gastrectomy for distal gastric cancer ([43, 44]). Overall survival rates improved from 5% for R2 (surgical resection with gross residual disease) to 50% for R0 ([45]).

Japanese surgeons routinely perform extended lymphadenectomy, whereas in the United States, 54% of primary gastrectomy patients undergo less than a D1 lymphadenectomy ([38]). A D1 lymphadenectomy refers to a limited dissection of the perigastric lymph nodes, whereas D2 refers to the removal of nodes along the hepatic, left gastric, celiac, and splenic arteries, as well as those in the splenic hilum. A D3 lymph node dissection includes lymph nodes located within the porta hepatis and periaortic regions.

Proponents of extended lymphadenectomy argue that only with extended dissection can accurate staging be guaranteed, which also implies accurate prediction of stage-specific survival. Furthermore, with extensive nodal dissection, locoregional relapse rates are lower. Using SEER Project data from 1973 to 2000, Schwarz and Smith[46] evaluated 1,377 patients with locally advanced gastric cancer (stages IIIA, IIIB, and IV, M0). The total lymph node (LN) count (or number of negative LNs examined; $P < .0001$) and number of positive LNs ($P < .0001$) were independent prognostic survival predictors. Furthermore, the stage-based survival prediction depended on the total LN number and number of negative LNs. In their earlier analysis of SEER data from 1973 to 1999, these same investigators demonstrated that for every 10 extra LNs dissected, survival improved by 7.6% (T1/2N0), 5.7% (T1/2N1), 11% (T3N0), or 7% (T3N1) ([47]). The results of this analysis demonstrated that for all T stages, extensive nodal dissection affects survival outcomes. Similarly, a 5-year survival benefit was reported for patients with D2 and D3 dissections compared with D1 lymphadenectomy (60% vs 54%, $P = .041$) in a Taiwanese study involving 221 patients with resectable gastric cancer ([48]).

Despite this evidence, prospective studies performed in non-Asian countries were unable to confirm these findings ([37, 49–51]). The Medical Research Council (MRC) randomly assigned 400 patients with resectable gastric cancer to D1 or D2 nodal dissection. Postoperative morbidity and mortality rates were higher for D2 (46% and 13%) than for D1 (28% and 6%) dissection ([51]). Both the initial and long-term follow-up results in the Dutch Gastric Cancer Group (DGCG) study demonstrated a significant increase in morbidity and mortality, with no survival difference between D1 and D2 dissections ([37, 50]). Although these large prospective studies performed in non-Asian countries could not confirm the initial findings, they went on to suggest that extended lymphadenectomy carries increased rates of morbidity and mortality, with a negligible change in survival.

Despite some disagreement about the benefits of D2 dissection, most experts agree that localized gastric cancer with clinical stage >T1b is best treated with multidisciplinary approaches and at high-volume centers, particularly by high-volume surgeons ([52, 53]). There is great value of thorough LN dissection along with gastrectomy ([54]). We acknowledge that the literature lacks convincing results in favor of D2 dissection in randomized studies to date that have compared D1 versus D2 dissections; however, the pendulum is swinging in favor of a more thorough nodal dissection by experienced surgeons. A nodal dissection approaching D2 can have the following advantages: accurate nodal staging and removal of more uninvolved nodes that is associated with prolonged survival ([50, 51, 55]). A 15-year update of the Dutch trial showed benefit in the D2 group in terms of the hazard ratio (HR) for gastric cancer–related death (0.74; 95% confidence interval [CI], 0.59-0.93; $P = .01$); however, only a few patients were at risk ([56]).

Perioperative Chemotherapy

This approach is based on the assumption that neoadjuvant systemic therapy can lead to tumor downstaging, leading to an improved R0 resection rate. This is particularly significant in Western patients in whom the tumors are usually bulky at diagnosis ([57]). The MAGIC trial has established level 1 evidence for this approach ([39]). It enrolled 503 patients with gastric, GEJ, and esophageal adenocarcinoma ([39]). These patients were randomized to receive three cycles of perioperative chemotherapy consisting of epirubicin, cisplatin, and infusional 5-fluorouracil (5-FU) (ECF) followed by surgery, followed by three more cycles of ECF, or undergo surgery followed by observation. In this trial, postoperative chemotherapy proved hard to deliver, with only 34% of patients receiving this treatment, and only 68% of patients underwent a curative resection. Despite this, both progression-free survival (PFS) and OS were improved in the group receiving ECF (HR for progression, 0.66; 95% CI, 0.53-0.81; $P < .001$; HR for death, 0.75; 95% CI, 0.60-0.93; $P = .009$). Five-year survival rates were 36.3% (95% CI, 29.5%-43.0%) among patients in the perioperative chemotherapy group and 23.0% (95% CI, 16.6%-29.4%) among those in the surgery group ([39]). Taken together, this suggests that the majority of the benefit may in fact come from the preoperative portion of the chemotherapy.

A second, French study supports the findings of the MAGIC trial. The Fédération Nationale des Centres de Lutte Contre le Cancer (FNCLCC) and the Fédération Francophone de Cancérologie Digestive (FFCD) multicenter phase III trial was terminated prematurely for poor accrual and is therefore not adequately powered ([58]). Overall, 224 patients with resectable adenocarcinoma of the lower esophagus, GEJ, or stomach (only 25%) were randomly assigned to either perioperative chemotherapy (with cisplatin and 5-FU) and surgery followed by three to four cycles of cisplatin and 5-FU or surgery alone. Only approximately 50% of patients received any postoperative chemotherapy. Despite these issues, the chemotherapy and surgery group had a significantly higher OS (HR for death, 0.69; 95% CI, 0.50-0.95; $P = .02$) and disease-free survival (DFS; HR for recurrence or death, 0.65; 95% CI, 0.48-0.89; $P = .003$). Five-year survival rates were 38% (95% CI, 29%-47%) in the chemotherapy and surgery group compared to 24% (95% CI, 17%-33%) in the surgery group. These results are quite similar to those of the MAGIC trial and bring into question the usefulness of the addition of epirubicin to cisplatin and 5-FU.

In contrast, a study by the European Organization for Research and Treatment of Cancer (EORTC 40954) did not demonstrate a benefit from the addition of perioperative chemotherapy ([59]). This trial showed a significantly increased R0 resection rate but failed to demonstrate a survival benefit for the addition of chemotherapy; however, it was not sufficiently powered to demonstrate a difference, given its premature termination due to poor accrual. An ongoing Japanese Clinical Oncology Group (JCOG 0501) trial is attempting to answer the question of whether perioperative chemotherapy with cisplatin and S-1 (an oral fluoropyrimidine) adds anything to their standard of care, which is surgery followed by adjuvant S-1 chemotherapy. The results of this trial are awaited; however, they are unlikely to be generalizable to the North American population because of different tumor biology. Meanwhile, other researchers in the United Kingdom are evaluating the addition of targeted therapy to perioperative chemotherapy in the localized gastric cancer setting. The MAGIC B/ST03 trial will determine whether the addition of bevacizumab to perioperative epirubicin plus cisplatin and capecitabine improves survival ([60]). This trial is expected to enroll 1,100 patients.

Postoperative Chemoradiotherapy

The indication of adjuvant chemoradiotherapy comes from level 1 evidence of its benefit from the Intergroup INT-0116 trial that showed a significant improvement in OS in the group of patients treated with adjuvant chemoradiotherapy ([38, 61]). In this trial, 559 patients with stage IB to IV disease were randomized to chemoradiotherapy following surgery or surgery alone. The chemoradiotherapy group received chemotherapy consisting of one 5-day cycle of 5-FU and leucovorin (LV) starting on day 1, followed by chemoradiotherapy beginning 28 days after the start of the initial cycle of chemotherapy. Chemoradiotherapy consisted of 45 Gy of radiation at 1.8 Gy/d 5 days per week for 5 weeks, with 5-FU (400 mg/m^2/d) and LV (20 mg/m^2/d) on the first 4 and the last 3 days of radiotherapy. One month after the completion of radiotherapy, two 5-day cycles of 5-FU (425 mg/m^2/d) plus LV (20 mg/m^2/d) were given 1 month apart. The 3-year survival rates were 50% in the chemoradiotherapy group and 41% in the surgery-only group. The HR for death in the surgery-only group, as compared with the chemoradiotherapy group, was 1.35 (95% CI, 1.09-1.66; $P = .005$). The HR for relapse in the surgery-only group, as compared with the chemoradiotherapy group, was 1.52 (95% CI, 1.23-1.86; $P < .001$) ([38]). Recently updated results of this study continue to demonstrate a benefit in terms of both OS and recurrence-free survival (RFS) ([61]). The major issue of this study was that the majority of patients did not receive an adequate LN dissection. Although a D1 resection was mandated per protocol, more than 50% of patients underwent a D0 resection, and only 10% of patients underwent a D2 nodal dissection. Therefore, it is questioned whether the survival difference occurred because of inadequate surgery rather than a true benefit of chemoradiotherapy.

Cancer and Leukemia Group B (CALGB) 80101, a US intergroup study, was designed to evaluate postoperative bolus 5-FU and LV with 5-FU plus concurrent radiation (an INT0116 trial treatment regimen) versus postoperative ECF (the MAGIC trial regimen) before and after 5-FU plus concurrent radiation in 546 patients with gastric or GEJ tumors after curative resection ([62]). In a preliminary report presented at the 2011 American Society of Clinical Oncology annual meeting, patients receiving ECF had lower rates of diarrhea, mucositis, and grade 4 or worse neutropenia. Overall survival, the primary end point, was not significantly better with ECF (3-year OS, 52% vs 50% for ECF and 5-FU/LV, respectively), regardless of the location of the primary tumor.

The Adjuvant Chemoradiation Therapy in Stomach Cancer (ARTIST) trial compared adjuvant chemoradiotherapy with adjuvant chemotherapy after an R0 resection with D2 dissection in 458 patients ([63]). The ARTIST trial was a negative study because its primary end point, 3-year DFS rate, was not statistically different between the two groups. In subgroup analyses, patients with node-positive disease in the adjuvant chemoradiotherapy group had a significantly improved 3-year DFS rate than those in the adjuvant chemotherapy group. Patients on the adjuvant chemoradiotherapy group were treated with two courses of postoperative capecitabine plus cisplatin (XP) followed by concurrent chemoradiotherapy with capecitabine and two additional courses of XP, whereas those on the adjuvant chemotherapy group were treated with six courses of postoperative XP without radiotherapy. The improved DFS among patients with node-positive disease was later confirmed in the recently published update; however, there was no improved OS despite the prolonged follow-up interval ([64]). This improved DFS finding may suggest that compared to adjuvant chemotherapy, adjuvant chemoradiotherapy may be beneficial among node-positive resectable gastric cancer patients, a theory currently being tested in the ARTIST-2 trial. Different from INT0116, all patients in ARTIST-2 trial are required to have a D2 nodal dissection, and the chemotherapy administered to all patients consists of S-1 versus S-1 and oxaliplatin with or without radiotherapy. Hence, ARTIST-2 was designed to evaluate the benefit of chemoradiotherapy after a D2 nodal dissection.

The results of two trials, Chemoradiotherapy After Induction Chemotherapy in Cancer of the Stomach (CRITICS) and Trial of Preoperative Therapy for Gastric and Esophagogastric Junction Adenocarcinoma (TOPGEAR), are expected to determine the benefit and indication of chemoradiotherapy ([65, 66]). In the Dutch CRITICS trial, all patients receive induction chemotherapy followed by surgery and are randomized to postoperative chemotherapy versus chemoradiotherapy. The TOPGEAR trial, which is under way in Australia, Europe, and Canada, directly compares preoperative chemotherapy alone (ECF) versus chemoradiotherapy (two cycles of ECF followed by concurrent fluoropyrimidine-based chemoradiotherapy) in patients with resectable adenocarcinoma of the stomach and GEJ; both groups will receive three further cycles of ECF postoperatively.

Postoperative Chemotherapy

The benefits of adjuvant chemotherapy after a D2 nodal dissection were initially demonstrated in Japan, and the chemotherapy used was S-1 ([40]). The Adjuvant Chemotherapy Trial of S-1 for Gastric Cancer (ACTS-GC) trial randomized 1,059 patients to 1 year of S-1 or observation. The updated analysis after 5 years of follow-up has demonstrated consistent results ([67]). The OS rate at 5 years was 71.7% in the S-1 group and 61.1% in the surgery-only group (HR, 0.669; 95% CI, 0.540-0.828). The RFS rate at 5 years was 65.4% in the S-1 group and 53.1% in the surgery-alone group (HR, 0.653; 95% CI, 0.537-0.793).

A second Asian study, the Capecitabine and Oxaliplatin Adjuvant Study in Stomach Cancer (CLASSIC) trial, randomized 1,035 patients who had undergone D2 gastrectomy to capecitabine plus oxaliplatin for 6 months or observation ([41]). The study demonstrated a benefit in patients treated with capecitabine and oxaliplatin for the primary end point of DFS (at 3 years; HR, 0.56; 95% CI, 0.44-0.72; $P < .0001$) at the prespecified interim analysis. After this analysis, the trial was stopped after a recommendation by the data monitoring committee. The mature OS data were recently published in *The Lancet Oncology* ([64]). By the clinical cutoff date, 103 patients (20%) had died in the adjuvant capecitabine and oxaliplatin group versus 141 patients (27%) in the observation group (stratified HR, 0.66; 95% CI, 0.51-0.85, $P = .0015$). Estimated 5-year OS was 78% (95% CI, 74%-82%) in the adjuvant capecitabine and oxaliplatin group versus 69% (95% CI, 64%-73%) in the observation group.

A phase III randomized clinical trial, the Stomach Cancer Adjuvant Multi-institutional Group Trial (SAMIT), of adjuvant paclitaxel followed by oral fluoropyrimidines for locally advanced gastric cancer brought into question the sequential administration of chemotherapy compared to 5-FU/LV ([68]). Although the 2 × 2 factorial design was not optimal to compare sequences, the study did not achieve its primary end point (3-year DFS: 57.2% vs 54%), showing no benefit with a sequential regimen compared to 5-FU/LV, which was consistent with previous studies (HR, 0.92; 95% CI, 0.80-1.07; $P = .273$).

All major phase III trials in localized gastric cancer and the most important ongoing studies in this setting are summarized in Tables 20-3 and 20-4. Given the variability in outcomes in many phase III trials, several meta-analyses have been undertaken (Table 20-5), all of which support a significant survival benefit for perioperative or adjuvant chemotherapy with somewhat better prognosis shown in Asian compared to Western populations ([69–71]), including one that was limited to trials from Western (non-Asian) countries ([72]). One of the most recent of these analyses evaluated data from 34 randomized trials comparing adjuvant systemic chemotherapy versus surgery alone, conducted in both Asian and Western populations ([69]). The risk of death in patients receiving adjuvant chemotherapy was reduced by 15% (HR for death, 0.85; 95% CI, 0.80-0.90).

Table 20-3 Major Phase III Trials for Gastric Cancer in the Localized Setting

Trial	No. of Patients	Treatment Arms	HR for OS (*P* value)	Primary End Point Comparison in Months (survival rates in %)
Perioperative chemotherapy				
Cunningham et al (MAGIC) ([39])	503	ECF → surgery → ECF vs surgery	0.75 (.009)	5-year OS: 36.3% vs 23%
Ychou et al (FNLCC/FFCP) ([58])	224	CF → surgery → CF vs surgery	0.69 (.02)	5-year OS: 38% vs 24%
Schuhmacher et al (EORTC 40954) ([59])	144	CFL → surgery vs surgery (only preoperative CT)	0.16	Underpowered to demonstrate a survival end point due to limited accrual (144/360 patients)
Postoperative chemoradiotherapy				
Macdonald et al ([38]) (INT-0116)	556	Surgery → FL/CTRT (45 Gy + FL)/FL vs surgery	1.32 (.004)	OS: 36 vs 27
Fuchs et al ([62]) (CALGB 80101)	546	Surgery → ECF/CTRT+FL/ECF vs surgery → FL/CTRT+FL/FL	1.03 (.80)	OS: 38 vs 37
Park et al ([64]) (ARTIST)	458	Surgery → XP/XRT/XP vs surgery → XP	1.130 (.5272); N+ patients: HR for DFS, 0.70 (.04)	5-year OS: 75% vs 73%; N+ patients: 3-year DFS: 76% vs 72%
Postoperative chemotherapy				
Sakuramoto et al ([40]) (ACTS- GC)	1,059	Surgery → S-1 vs surgery	0.68 (.003); HR at 5 years: 0.669	3-year OS: 80.1% vs 70.1%; 3-year RFS: 72.2% vs 59.6%
Bang et al ([41]) (CLASSIC)	1,035	Surgery → CapeOx vs surgery	0.56 (< .0001)	3-year DFS: 74% vs 59%
Tsuburaya et al ([68]) (SAMIT), 2 × 2 factorial design	1,495	Surgery → UFT vs surgery → S-1 vs surgery → paclitaxel + UFT vs surgery → paclitaxel + S-1	HR for DFS 0.81 (.0048) for monotherapy (0.151 for noninferiority of UFT), 0.92 (.273) for monotherapy vs sequential	3-year DFS: 53% vs 58.2% (UFT vs S-1), 54% vs 57.2% (monotherapy vs sequential)

CapeOx, capecitabine and oxaliplatin; CF, cisplatin and 5-fluorouracil; CFL, cisplatin, 5-fluorouracil, and leucovorin; CT, chemotherapy; CTRT, chemoradiotherapy; DFS, disease-free survival; ECF, epirubicin, cisplatin, and 5-fluorouracil; FL, 5-fluorouracil and leucovorin; HR, hazard ratio; OS, overall survival; RFS, recurrence-free survival; UFT, tegafur and uracil; XP, capecitabine and cisplatin; XRT, capecitabine and radiotherapy.

Table 20-4 List of Ongoing Phase III Trials in Localized Gastric Cancer

Trials	No. of Patients	Treatment Arms	Control Arm	Status
Perioperative chemotherapy				
Ychou et al (FNLCC 94012-FFCD 9703)	250	CF → surgery (Only neoadjuvant CT)	Surgery	Active, not recruiting
JCOG 0501	316	Cisplatin + S-1 → surgery → S-1	Surgery → S-1	Recruiting
Okines et al (MAGIC B/ST03)	1,103	ECX + bevacizumab → surgery → ECX + bevacizumab → maintenance bevacizumab	ECX → Surgery → ECX	Recruiting
Postoperative + preoperative chemoradiotherapy				
ARTIST-2	1,000	Surgery → S-1 Ox → CTRT + S-1 → S-1 Ox	Surgery → S-1 Ox	Recruiting
Dikken et al (CRITICS)	788	ECX → Surgery → CTRT + CX	ECX → Surgery → ECX	Recruiting
Leong et al (TOPGEAR)	752	ECF → CTRT + 5-FU–based CT → Surgery → ECF	ECF → Surgery → ECF	Recruiting

CF, cisplatin and 5-fluorouracil; CT, chemotherapy; CTRT, chemoradiotherapy; CX, cisplatin and capecitabine; ECF, epirubicin, cisplatin, and 5-fluorouracil; ECX, epirubicin, cisplatin, and capecitabine; 5-FU, 5-fluorouracil; S-1 Ox, S-1 and oxaliplatin.

Table 20-5 Perioperative or Postoperative Therapy for Localized Gastric Cancer: Results of Meta-Analyses

Reference	No. of Studies	No. of Patients	HR for OS	Treatment
Diaz-Nieto et al ([69])	34	7,824	0.85	Postoperative chemotherapy
Ronellenfitsch et al ([70])	14	2,422	0.81	Perioperative chemo(radio)therapy
Oba et al ([71])	14	3,288	DFS: 0.92	Postoperative chemotherapy
Earle et al ([72])	13	NR (non-Asian patients)	0.80	Postoperative chemotherapy

DFS, disease-free survival; HR, hazard ratio; NR, not reported yet; OS, overall survival.

Based on the previously mentioned trials and meta-analyses, postoperative chemoradiotherapy (United States), perioperative chemotherapy (Europe), and adjuvant chemotherapy after a D2 nodal dissection (Asia) can all be regarded as standards of care in the management of localized gastric cancer.

The University of Texas MD Anderson Cancer Center Approach to Resectable Gastric Cancer

All patients with newly diagnosed gastric cancer undergo a complete staging workup. Patients with resectable gastric cancer are evaluated by a multidisciplinary team that consists of surgeons, radiation oncologists, and medical oncologists. Treatment recommendations are made in multidisciplinary conferences. Both standard-of-care treatment options and clinical trials are discussed with our patients. Patients' treatment plans are individualized to optimize outcomes for each patient. For decades, the University of Texas MD Anderson Cancer Center (MDACC) has been developing the practice of multimodality management in a multidisciplinary setting for all patients, but it is especially useful for those with resectable disease. Arguments for front-loading therapy before surgery include poor tolerance and compliance to postoperative therapy, early initiation of therapy, early palliation of symptoms, and opportunity for cancer downstaging, enhanced surgical resectability, and higher rates of pathologic complete remission (pathCR).

Preoperative trimodality therapy consisting of induction chemotherapy followed by chemoradiotherapy and then surgical resection has been tested and evolved at MDACC over many years. Since the mid-1990s, it has been clinically recognized that preoperative trimodality therapy does not increase morbidity or mortality rates of subsequent surgery and can improve pathologic response. Ajani et al ([73]) reported the results of several phase II studies that demonstrated the feasibility and effectiveness of a three-step strategy. Thirty-seven patients with locally advanced resectable gastric cancer were treated with trimodality therapy on a phase II clinical trial. Chemotherapy consisted of infusional 5-FU, cisplatin, and paclitaxel (FPT); 45 Gy of radiotherapy was administered concurrently with FPT. R0 and pathCR rates were 95% and 30%, respectively. Fourteen percent of patients had only microscopic residual disease. Patients who achieved pathCR or pathologic partial response after preoperative chemoradiotherapy had significantly longer median survival durations than those who did not (63.9 vs 12.6 months; $P = .03$).

As a result of the MDACC's single-institution success with preoperative trimodality therapy, the Radiation Therapy Oncology Group (RTOG) sponsored a multi-institution cooperative study, RTOG 9904. The primary end point was pathCR rate. Forty-nine patients with localized resectable gastric cancer from 20 institutions received 5-FU, LV, and cisplatin (FLP) as induction chemotherapy, followed by concurrent chemoradiotherapy with 5-FU and weekly paclitaxel. The pathCR and R0 resection rates were 26% and 77%, respectively. At 1 year, more patients who had achieved pathCR (82%) were alive than those who did not (69%) ([74]). A D2 dissection was performed in 50% of patients. The heterogeneity of different treating institutions minimized the selection bias typical of single-institution results. Outcomes in RTOG 9904 were no better or worse than those of more recent studies, particularly the pathCR and D2 lymphadenectomy rates. Figure 20-3A summarizes the MDACC's approach to localized gastroesophageal cancer.

ESOPHAGEAL AND GASTROESOPHAGEAL JUNCTION CANCERS

Esophageal cancer is estimated to be the eighth most common cause of cancer death among men in the United States and the fifth most common cause of cancer death worldwide ([75]). In 2015, the estimated numbers of new cases and deaths from esophageal cancer in the United States are 16,980 and 15,590, respectively ([2]). Esophageal cancer is three to four times more common in men than in women ([76]), with a mean age of 67 years ([77]). Lifetime risk of developing esophageal cancer is 1 in 125 for men and 1 in 435 for women ([76]). For classification purposes (AJCC staging version 7), primary tumors of the GEJ and proximal gastric cancer extending 5 cm into the stomach are included with

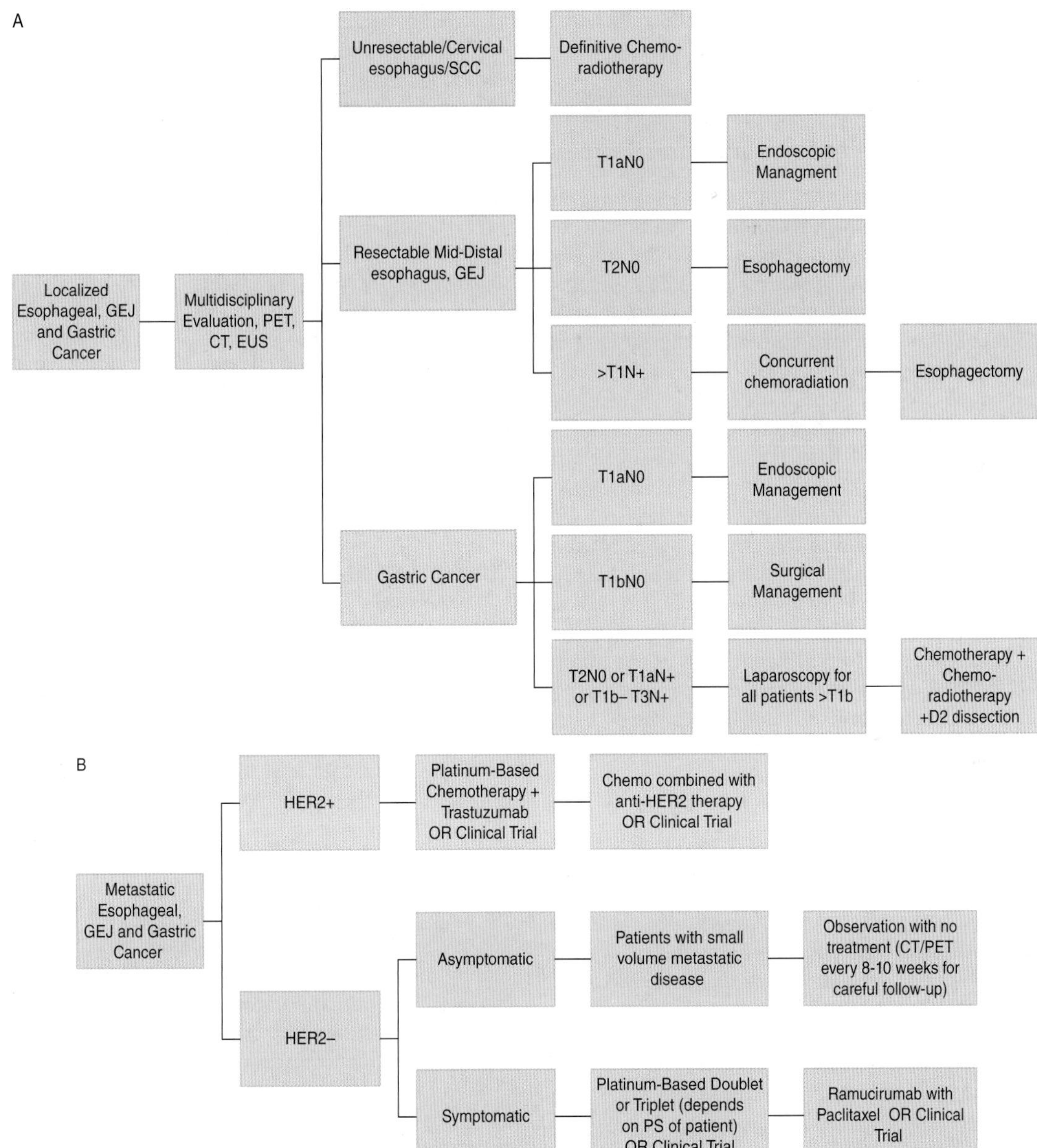

FIGURE 20-3 The University of Texas MD Anderson Cancer Center Treatment algorithms for (A) localized gastroesophageal cancer and (B) metastatic gastroesophageal cancer. CT, computed tomography; EUS, endoscopic ultrasound; GEJ, gastroesophageal junction; HER2, human epidermal growth factor receptor 2; PET, positron emission tomography; PS, performance status; SCC, squamous cell carcinoma.

esophageal cancers. The incidence of GEJ cancer has continued to increase over the last several decades. In recent years, this trend reached a new plateau, coinciding with the increased incidence of distal esophageal adenocarcinoma since the mid-1990s, a phenomenon confined to North America and other non-Asian countries. Overall, the prognosis of patients with esophageal/GEJ cancer remains poor. Histologic type makes a difference, because squamous cell cancer has a poorer prognosis than adenocarcinoma. Surgery is still the only chance for cure, and survival can be improved with multimodality therapy.

Epidemiologic Characteristics

Although squamous cell cancer is the most common histologic type in many parts of the world, it is relatively uncommon outside of Asian and middle-Eastern countries. Squamous cell cancer is 20 times more common in China than in the United States ([78]).

Esophageal cancer has a poor survival rate; only 17.5% of patients in the United States ([3]) and 10% of patients in Europe ([79]) survive at 5 years.

Etiologic Characteristics and Risk Factors

The most significant risk factors associated with almost 90% of esophageal squamous cell cancers are tobacco use, alcohol use, and a diet low in fruits and vegetables ([9, 80]). Smoking and alcohol can synergistically increase the risk of esophageal squamous cell cancer. Dietary associations with esophageal squamous cell cancer, such as foods containing N-nitroso compounds, have long been implicated ([81]). Betel nut chewing, widespread in certain regions of Asia ([82]), and the ingestion of hot foods and beverages (such as tea) ([83]) in other endemic regions, such as Iran, Russia, and South Africa, have been associated with esophageal squamous cell cancer. Long-standing achalasia increases the risk of squamous cell cancer by 16 times ([84]). On average, squamous cell cancer develops 41 years after ingestion of lye. Tylosis, a rare disease associated with hyperkeratosis of the palms of the hands and soles of the feet, is associated with a high rate of esophageal squamous cell cancer ([85]).

Unlike squamous cell cancer, the risk factors for esophageal adenocarcinoma remain elusive. The strongest and most consistent risk factors include gastroesophageal reflux disease (GERD), smoking, obesity ([86]), and dietary exposure to nitrosamines; these are found in almost 80% of cases in the United States ([87]). According to a Denmark study, more than 50% of esophageal adenocarcinoma cases were found to have no history of symptomatic reflux disease ([88]). However, a large study conducted in Sweden demonstrated an association between reflux symptoms and esophageal adenocarcinoma (odds ratio, 7.7) and adenocarcinoma of gastric cardia (odds ratio, 2.0) ([89]). A high-fat, low-protein, high-calorie diet can also increase the risk. Some data have suggested that interactions between risk factors may be more important than individual risk factors. A study was performed on 305 esophageal adenocarcinoma patients and 339 age- and sex-matched controls; the strongest individual risk factor identified was reflux ([90]).

Barrett esophagus (BE) is generally believed to be a consequence of severe and chronic GERD. The presence of BE is associated with an increased risk of esophageal adenocarcinoma. The median age of BE diagnosis is 40 to 55 years, and it is most common in men ([91]).

Clinical Presentation

The presenting symptoms of esophageal cancer usually include dysphagia, weight loss, bleeding, throat pain, and hoarseness. Early symptoms are usually nonspecific, and the patient may present with subtle symptoms, for example, food "sticking" transiently and reflux/regurgitation of food or saliva. This may precede frank dysphagia, which by all accounts is the most common complaint and becomes apparent when the esophageal lumen is narrowed to one-third of its normal diameter. For proximal esophageal tumors, increasing cough may be a sign of tracheoesophageal fistula. Chronic GI blood loss resulting from esophageal cancer may result in iron deficiency anemia.

Pathologic Characteristics

Esophageal cancer includes adenocarcinoma, squamous cell cancer, mucoepidermoid carcinoma, small cell cancer, sarcoma, adenoid cystic carcinoma, and primary lymphoma. Adenocarcinoma is now more prevalent than squamous cell cancer in non-Asian countries and mostly develops in the distal esophagus ([92]). In general, squamous cell cancer is found in the upper half of the esophagus, whereas adenocarcinoma predominates closer to the GEJ. This chapter will focus on carcinomas of the esophagus/GEJ, whereas other chapters in this book will be dedicated to other types of malignancy of the esophagus/GEJ.

Staging and Prognosis

Esophageal cancer is a treatable disease but is rarely curable. Since the mid-1990s, the histologic type and location of cancer of the upper GI tract have changed. The incidences of proximal gastric, GEJ, and distal esophageal adenocarcinomas have steadily increased up until the last several years, where it now appears to have reached a steady state. The most current version of the AJCC TNM staging (version 7, Table 20-6) now includes primary tumors of the GEJ or proximal gastric cancer extending 5 cm into the stomach as part of esophageal cancer staging ([26]).

Clinical staging uses EGD with EUS, CT, and FDG-PET. In patients with proximal esophageal cancer, additional bronchoscopy is recommended to evaluate potential tracheal invasion or document and palliate tracheoesophageal fistula. Among patients with disease extending into the gastric cardia, most experts agree that laparoscopic peritoneal staging is also necessary to evaluate occult peritoneal seeding that is not well visualized with noninvasive modalities (Figs. 20-4 to 20-9).

In various studies, FDG-PET has been consistently shown to have better specificity than CT at diagnosing metastatic disease and LN status. Positron emission tomography serves the primary purpose of detecting occult metastases that are present in 15% to 20% of newly diagnosed esophageal cancer patients ([93, 94]). Multiple studies have been performed in esophageal cancer patients after preoperative treatment, with PET being examined for predicting prognosis ([93, 95]) and

Table 20-6 American Joint Cancer Committee TNM Staging System for Gastroesophageal Junction and Esophageal Cancers

Primary Tumor (T)	
TX	Primary tumor cannot be assessed
T0	No evidence of primary tumor
Tis	High-grade dysplasia
T1	Tumor invades lamina propria, muscularis mucosae, or submucosa
T1a	Tumor invades lamina propria or muscularis mucosae
T1b	Tumor invades submucosa
T2	Tumor invades muscularis propria
T3	Tumor invades adventitia
T4	Tumor invades adjacent structures
T4a	Resectable tumor invading pleura, pericardium, or diaphragm
T4b	Unresectable tumor invading other adjacent structures, such as aorta, vertebral body, trachea, etc.
Regional Lymph Nodes (N)	
Nx	Regional nodes cannot be assessed
N0	No regional nodal metastasis
N1	Metastasis in 1-2 regional lymph nodes
N2	Metastasis in 3-6 regional lymph nodes
N3	Metastasis in ≥7 regional lymph nodes
Distant Metastases (M)	
M0	No distant metastases
M1	Distant metastases
Grade (G)	
GX	Grade cannot be assessed—stage grouping as G1
G1	Well differentiated
G2	Moderately differentiated
G3	Poorly differentiated
G4	Undifferentiated—stage group as G3 squamous
Location	
Upper	15 to <20 cm
Middle	25 to <30 cm
Lower	30-45 cm

Squamous Cell Cancer Stage Grouping

Stage	T	N	M	Grade	Tumor Location	5-Year Survival Rates (%)
0	Tis	N0	M0	1, X	Any	>80
IA	T1	N0	M0	1, X	Any	>80
IB	T1	N0	M0	2-3	Any	60
	T2-3	N0	M0	1, X	Lower, X	
IIA	T2-3	N0	M0	1, X	Upper, middle	53
	T2-3	N0	M0	2-3	Lower, X	
IIB	T1-2	N1	M0	Any	Any	40
	T2-3	N0	M0	2-3	Upper, middle	
IIIA	T1-2	N2	M0	Any	Any	25
	T3	N1	M0	Any	Any	
	T4a	N0	M0	Any	Any	

(Continued)

Table 20-6 American Joint Cancer Committee TNM Staging System for Gastroesophageal Junction and Esophageal Cancers (*Continued*)

Squamous Cell Cancer Stage Grouping						
Stage	T	N	M	Grade	Tumor Location	5-Year Survival Rates (%)
IIIB	T3	N2	M0	Any	Any	17
IIIC	T4a	N1-2	M0	Any	Any	13
	T4b	Any	M0	Any	Any	
	Any	N3	M0	Any	Any	
IV	Any	Any	M1	Any	Any	5
0	Tis	N0	M0	1, X	83	
IA	T1	N0	M0	1-2, X	77	
IB	T1	N0	M0	3	65	
	T2	N0	M0	1-2, X		
IIA	T2	N0	M0	3	50	
IIB	T1-2	N1	M0	Any	40	
	T3	N0	M0	Any		
IIIA	T1-2	N2	M0	Any	25	
	T3	N1	M0	Any		
	T4a	N0	M0	Any		
IIIB	T3	N2	M0	Any	17	
IIIC	T4a	N1-2	M0	Any	15	
	T4b	Any	M0	Any		
	Any	N3	M0	Any		
IV	Any	Any	M1	Any	<5	

Reproduced with permission from Edge SB, Byrd DR, Compton CC (eds): *AJCC Cancer Staging Manuarl*, 7th ed. New York, NY: Springer; 2010.

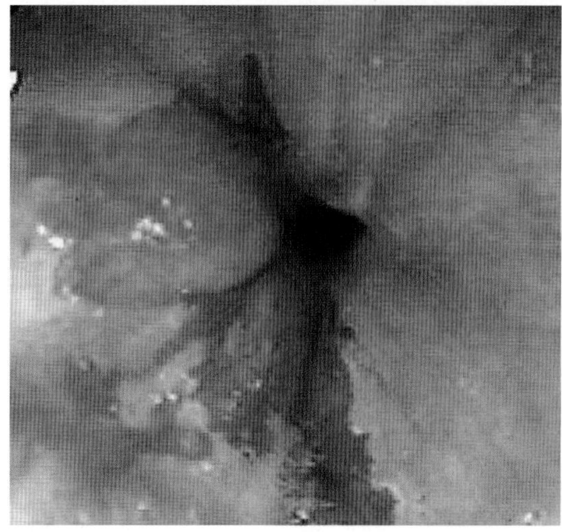

FIGURE 20-4 Barrett esophagus, endoscopic view. (Used with permission from Klaus Monkemuller, MD, University of Alabama at Birmingham, Birmingham, AL.)

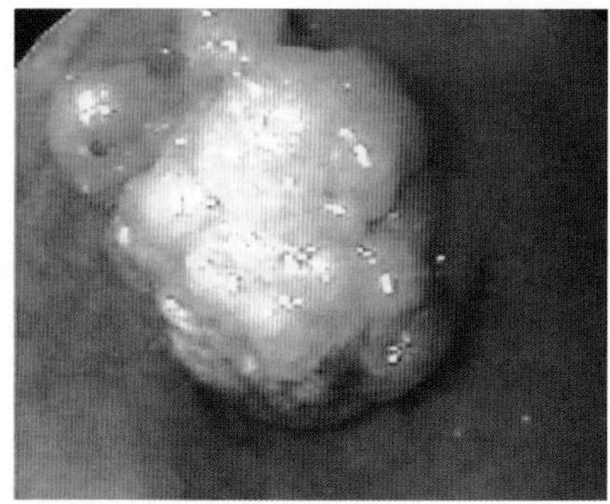

FIGURE 20-5 Esophageal mass, endoscopic view. (Used with permission from Klaus Monkemuller, MD, University of Alabama at Birmingham, Birmingham, AL.)

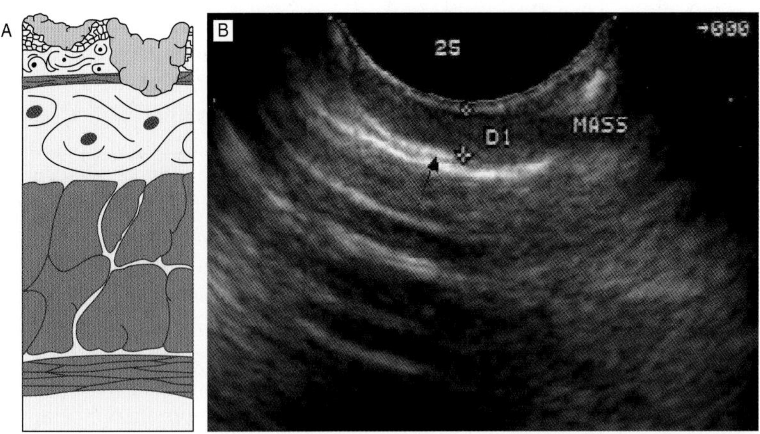

FIGURE 20-6 A. Schematic representation of esophagus layers showing depth of tumor invasion. **B.** Endoscopic ultrasound image of T1 esophageal cancer. (Reproduced, with permission, from http://www.massgeneral.org/gastro/endo_ homepage.htm.)

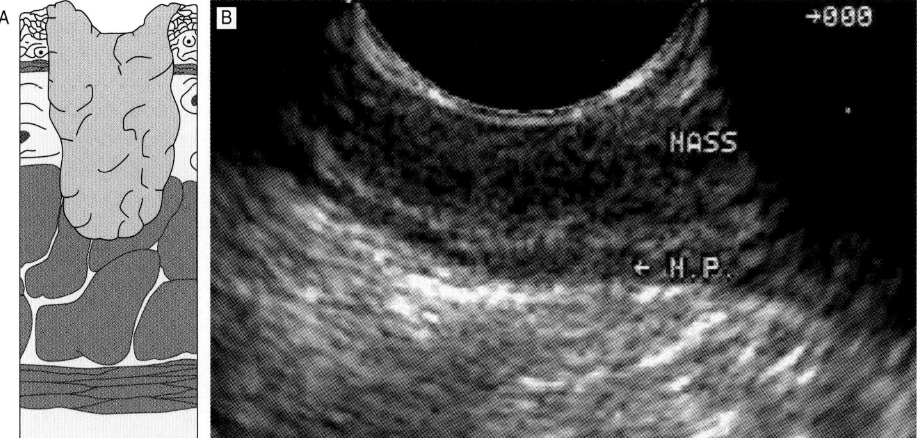

FIGURE 20-7 A. Schematic representation of esophagus layers showing depth of tumor invasion. **B.** Endoscopic ultrasound image of T2 esophageal cancer. (Reproduced, with permission, from http://www.massgeneral.org/gastro/endo_ homepage.htm.)

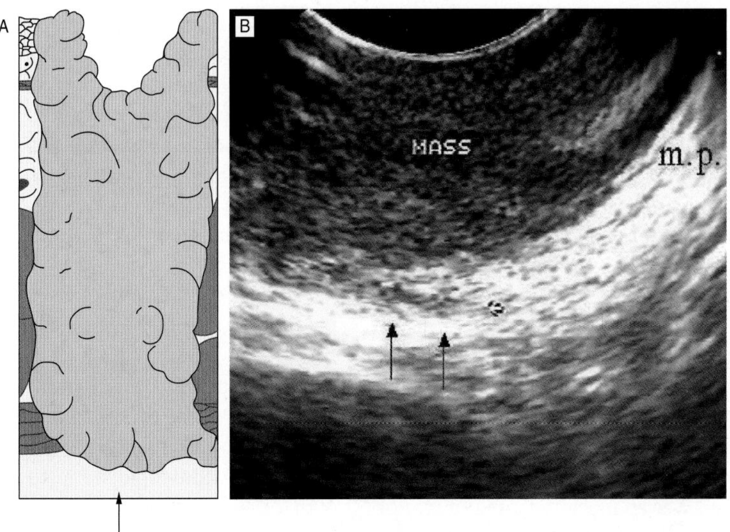

FIGURE 20-8 A. Schematic representation of esophagus layers showing depth of tumor invasion. **B.** Endoscopic ultrasound image of T3 esophageal cancer. (Reproduced, with permission, from http://www.massgeneral.org/gastro/endo_ homepage.htm.)

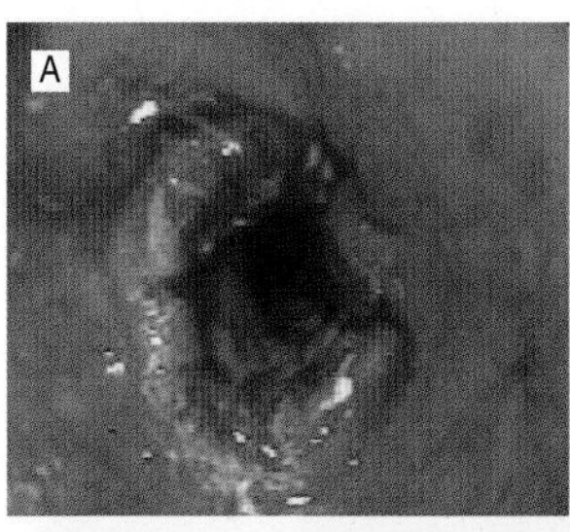

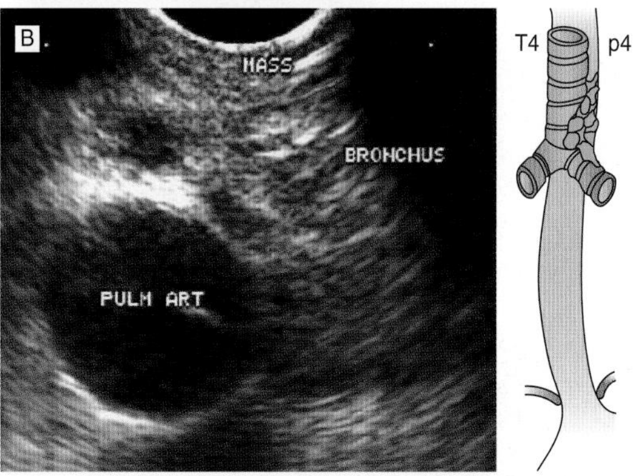

FIGURE 20-9 A. Endoscopic image of T4 esophageal cancer. B. Endoscopic ultrasound image of the same tumor. (Reproduced, with permission, from http://www.massgeneral.org/gastro/endo_homepage.htm.)

treatment response ([96]). Other studies have shown conflicting results. For example, one study showed that complete response by PET was prognostic of the outcomes of patients receiving definitive chemoradiotherapy ([97]); however, another study found no correlation of posttreatment PET with survival or pathologic response ([98]). Fluorodeoxyglucose PET can better reveal bone metastasis than bone scans ([99]) and commonly reflects images of multiple foci of intense uptake. Studies have shown significant correlations between FDG uptake and tumor invasion depth and LN metastasis and survival rates, with a high degree of accuracy in the neck and upper thoracic and abdominal regions ([100]). Unlike with gastric cancer, FDG-PET results have been found to be important predictors of response and prognosis. In a retrospective analysis, Swisher et al reported the results of FDG-PET use in 103 consecutive patients with locally advanced esophageal cancer who underwent preoperative chemoradiotherapy ([101]). At surgery, 58 patients (56%) had experienced a pathologic response to chemoradiotherapy (surgical pathologic results ≤10% viable residual cancer cells). Pathologic response was associated with FDG-PET standardized uptake value (SUV) (3.1 vs 5.8, *P* = .01). A postchemoradiotherapy FDG-PET SUV ≥4 had the highest accuracy and was an independent predictor of survival (HR, 3.5; *P* = .04) on multivariate analysis ([101]).

Perhaps the strongest endorsement for using FDG-PET as predictor of response came from the Metabolic Response Evaluation for Individualization of Neoadjuvant Chemotherapy in Esophageal and Esophagogastric Adenocarcinoma (MUNICON-1) trial. Lordick et al ([34]) evaluated the feasibility and applicability of FDG-PET in clinical practice in 110 evaluable patients with locally advanced esophageal adenocarcinoma. Patients with adenocarcinoma of the esophagogastric junction types I and II (tumors extending to the esophagus 5 cm above and 2 cm below the GEJ) underwent 2 weeks of induction chemotherapy with FLP. Fluorodeoxyglucose PET scans were obtained for all patients at baseline and after induction chemotherapy. Metabolic response was defined as an SUV decrease by ≥35%. Responders underwent more chemotherapy with FLP or folinic acid, 5-FU, and oxaliplatin (FOLFOX) for 12 weeks followed by surgery. Nonresponders discontinued further chemotherapy after the 2 weeks of initial induction chemotherapy and underwent surgery. In this study, there were 54 responders (metabolic response rate, 49%). One hundred four patients (54 responders and 50 nonresponders) underwent surgery. At 2.3 years of follow-up, the median OS was not reached for responders and was 25.8 months (HR, 2.13; *P* = .015) for nonresponders. The median event-free survival durations for responders and nonresponders were 29.7 months and 14.1 months, respectively (HR, 2.18; *P* = .002). Major pathologic remissions (<10% residual tumor) were noted in 58% of responders and 0% of nonresponders ([34]). In the MUNICON-1 study, the response to induction therapy was valuable for stratifying patients to appropriate therapy, further establishing the clinical utility of FDG-PET in limiting exposure to unnecessary toxicity and maximizing therapeutic benefits. The MUNICON-2 and -3 trial results might be useful in establishing the role of PET in restaging esophageal cancer patients undergoing induction therapy ([102]).

The role of tumor markers (N-cadherin [[103]], activin A, nuclear factor-κB [[104]]) and cytogenetics in esophageal cancer staging and prognosis is another subject of active investigation. Esophageal cancer has certain molecular markers that may be predictive. Large population-based studies to validate these preliminary results remain incomplete. Until then, the clinical interpretation of currently available data should be done with caution.

Treatment

The gold standard for treating high-grade dysplasia (HGD) and early or superficial esophageal cancer is esophagectomy. However, endoscopic mucosal resection (EMR)/endoscopic submucosal dissection (ESMD), with or without photodynamic therapy (PDT), has become a popular alternative to surgery for early esophageal disease. Despite the recognized epidemiologic and clinical differences between esophageal squamous cell cancer and adenocarcinomas, there is still inadequate evidence that treatment for esophageal cancer should be based on histologic type. Locally advanced cervical esophageal cancer is preferably managed with definitive chemoradiotherapy. For all other esophageal cancers, current evidence supports the use of preoperative chemoradiotherapy to enhance surgical survival outcome in patients with locally advanced resectable disease. Surgery remains the best chance for long-term survival. Ongoing international clinical research with novel cytotoxic and targeted agents will continue to further define and improve survival outcomes of patients with locally advanced curable esophageal and GEJ cancers. Unfortunately, the main therapeutic goal is symptom palliation in patients with locally advanced, unresectable disease.

Endoscopic mucosal resection has gained popularity in Asia for the treatment of superficial or early esophageal cancer as well as BE with HGD. By providing large tissue specimens that can be examined to determine the characteristics and extent of the lesion and the adequacy of resection, EMR is both therapeutic and diagnostic. Endoscopic mucosal resection has been reported in several small prospective case series to be effective, with an initial complete remission (CR) rate of 59% to 99% ([105, 106]). The ideal clinical characteristics for EMR are small (<2 cm diameter), solitary, flat lesions that are confined to the mucosa (T1a). Because EMR has a relatively high recurrence rate, it is recommended that BE and HGD or early esophageal cancer patients be followed up endoscopically every 3 months during the first year and annually thereafter. Complications associated with EMR are bleeding (4%-46%), perforation (1%), and stricture (20%) ([107]).

Resectable Disease

Surgery

Only 23% of patients with esophageal cancer present with clinically resectable localized disease ([108]). Surgical resection is the mainstay of treatment for these patients ([109]) and should only be recommended as upfront treatment in T1b/T2 tumors without nodal involvement by EUS. Recent data indicate that the overall 5-year survival rate of esophageal cancer patients after curative surgery is about 25% ([38, 39, 110]). Therefore, preoperative chemotherapy or preoperative chemoradiotherapy have become the mainstay strategies for treatment to improve surgical outcome, whereas definitive chemoradiotherapy has been recommended for patients with cervical tumors or unresectable disease.

Cancers of middle or lower third of the esophagus (squamous cell carcinoma or esophageal adenocarcinoma, except GEJ cancers) generally require total esophagectomy, which is a challenging procedure with a high complication rate. No uniform surgical approaches to curative resection exist, but the most common procedures in North America include transhiatal, transthoracic (Ivor-Lewis), and tri-incisional esophagectomy. Transhiatal esophagectomy involves anastomosis of the stomach to the cervical esophagus ([111]). Ivor-Lewis transthoracic esophagectomy involves abdominal mobilization of the stomach and transthoracic excision of the esophagus, with anastomosis of the stomach to the upper thoracic or cervical esophagus. Limitations of the Ivor-Lewis procedure include a limited proximal resection margin and a higher risk of bile reflux because of the intrathoracic location of the anastomosis ([112]). The modified Ivor-Lewis procedure involves a left thoracoabdominal incision with a gastric pull-up into the left chest ([113]). Another surgical approach is tri-incisional esophagectomy in which transhiatal and transthoracic approaches are combined, allowing for transthoracic esophagectomy with node dissection and cervical esophagogastric anastomosis ([114]). For patients with potentially resectable disease, R0 resection is generally believed to be necessary to achieve durable survival ([115]). R0 resection is defined as resection of the primary tumor with negative proximal, distal, and circumferential margins. In one retrospective case-control analysis, 220 patients underwent limited transhiatal or extensive mediastinal lymphadenectomy with transthoracic esophagectomy. At a median of 4.7 years of follow-up, there was a trend toward higher DFS (39% vs 27%) and OS (39% vs 29%) rates in patients with more extensive nodal dissection ([39, 116]). Despite a lack of prospective randomized studies, there is a growing consensus that more extensive nodal dissection is needed; including the removal of all cancerous tissue from the mediastinum improves DFS and OS durations through better control of locoregional recurrence. Also, aggressive lymphadenectomy is generally recommended to increase the accuracy of pathologic staging. In the latest version of the AJCC staging manual, an adequate number of LNs is required for defining stage of disease. In the United States, en bloc resection of the mediastinal and upper abdominal LNs is considered standard for transthoracic esophagectomy, and three-field lymphadenectomy is not considered a standard treatment for patients with esophageal cancer.

Preoperative Chemotherapy

Preoperative chemotherapy theoretically increases the curative resection rates by downsizing and downstaging the primary tumor and LN metastases, reducing the local and distant relapse rates through suppression and elimination of micrometastases, improving tumor-related symptoms with early initiation of antineoplastic therapy, and appraising in vivo the chemosensitivity of the primary tumor that will influence the choice of chemotherapy in the adjuvant setting.

Preoperative therapy is hypothesized to result in tumor downstaging, which allows for higher R0 resection and pathCR rates ([117]).

The two largest studies evaluating the role of preoperative chemotherapy were the US Intergroup trial (INT0113) ([118, 119]) and UK Marsden Royal College (MRC)-OEO-2 randomized controlled trials ([120]). Both studies determined the survival benefit of preoperative chemotherapy compared with surgery alone in patients with resectable esophageal squamous cell cancer and adenocarcinoma. Cisplatin plus 5-FU (CF) was administered in both studies. The two studies had completely divergent findings. INT0113 found no clinical/pathologic benefit or survival improvement with preoperative chemotherapy followed by surgery compared with surgery alone ([118]). The median survival was 14.9 months for patients who received preoperative chemotherapy and16.1 months for those who underwent immediate surgery (*P* = .53). The recent updated analysis of INT0113 confirmed the lack of benefit of preoperative chemotherapy ([119]). The MRC-OEO-2 trial, however, reported a statistically significant improved R0 resection rate (78% vs 70%) and median OS time (17.2 vs 13.3 months) in patients who underwent preoperative chemotherapy ([120]). Results of both INT0113 and OEO-2 studies did not help determine the role of preoperative chemotherapy in patients with resectable esophageal cancer. In the United Kingdom and other countries in Europe, preoperative chemotherapy has become the acceptable standard of care.

The two most recent randomized studies of preoperative and perioperative chemotherapy, the French Actions Concertées dans les Cancer Colorectaux et Digestifs (ACCORD) 7 ([58]) and UK MAGIC trials ([39]), are the strongest validations of the benefits of preoperative and perioperative chemotherapy. These two studies are described in detail in the "Gastric Cancer" section of this chapter. In addition to the MAGIC and FRENCH trials, a third Japanese trial on squamous cell carcinoma patients (JCOG 9907) deserves mention because it was positive. Patients were given two cycles of CF preoperatively. Postoperatively, CF was administered to node-positive patients only. Of the above mentioned three trials, this one showed the highest 5-year survival rate in both arms ([121]).

Investigators at MRC are currently conducting two large phase III randomized controlled studies. MRC-OEO-5 is evaluating the use of preoperative chemotherapy, comparing two preoperative chemotherapy regimens, CF versus ECX (epirubicin, cisplatin, and capecitabine) ([122]). Meanwhile, other researchers in the United Kingdom are evaluating the addition of targeted therapy to perioperative chemotherapy. The MRC ST03 trial will determine whether the addition of bevacizumab to perioperative ECX improves survival. Table 20-7 lists the ongoing studies of locally advanced resectable gastric, GEJ, and distal esophageal adenocarcinomas.

Preoperative Radiation

Preoperative radiotherapy was studied in the early 1980s. However, in several phase III studies, a benefit similar to that of surgery alone was not shown. In a recent quantitative meta-analysis comprising five randomized trials and 1,147 patients, it was again demonstrated that there is no improvement in survival with preoperative radiotherapy alone in potentially resectable esophageal cancer ([123, 124]).

Preoperative Chemoradiotherapy

In the United States, pre- or perioperative chemotherapy is not as common as preoperative chemoradiotherapy for locally advanced esophageal and GEJ cancer. Preoperative chemoradiotherapy has the goal to improve pathCR rate, locoregional control, and survival.

The CALGB 9781 trial provided additional support for preoperative chemoradiotherapy, although it was stopped early because of a slow accrual rate. Fifty-six patients were randomly assigned to surgery alone (n = 26) or CF chemotherapy and concurrent radiotherapy (n = 30). At a median follow-up of 6 years, an intent-to-treat analysis showed a median OS duration of 4.5 versus 1.8 years (*P* = .002) in favor of trimodality therapy. The 5-year OS rates were 39% (95% CI, 21%-57%) versus 16% (95% CI, 5%-33%) in favor of trimodality therapy ([125]). Gebski et al ([126]) reported improved survival with preoperative chemotherapy and chemoradiotherapy. The HR for all-cause mortality with preoperative chemoradiotherapy versus surgery alone was 0.81 (95% CI, 0.70-0.93; *P* = .002), corresponding to a 13% absolute difference in survival at 2 years, with similar results for different histologic tumor types (squamous cell cancer: HR, 0.84, *P* = .04; adenocarcinomas: HR, 0.75, *P* = .02). The HR for preoperative chemotherapy was 0.90 (95% CI, 0.81-1.00; *P* = .05), which indicates a 2-year absolute survival benefit of 7%. There was no significant effect on all-cause mortality for preoperative chemotherapy in squamous cell cancer (HR, 0.88; *P* = .12), but there was a benefit in adenocarcinoma (HR, 0.78; *P* = .014) ([126]). With chemoradiotherapy, evidence seems to suggest that treating physicians can expect a pathCR rate of 20% to 30%, a median OS duration of 16 to 24 months, and a therapy-related mortality rate of 5% to 10%.

The Chemoradiotherapy for Oesophageal Cancer Followed by Surgery Study (CROSS) trial was a well-executed study that established level 1 evidence for preoperative chemoradiotherapy. Three hundred sixty-eight localized esophageal cancer (adenocarcinoma or squamous) patients were randomly assigned to receive either preoperative paclitaxel and carboplatin with concurrent radiation 41.4 Gy (n = 178)

Table 20-7 Key Esophageal Cancer Trials

Study	No. of Patients	Treatment Arm Control Arm	HR for OS (*P* value)	OS (%)
Pre- and perioperative chemotherapy				
Kelsen et al ([119]) (INT-113)	467	3 × CF → S S	0.75 (NR)	5-year OS: 36% vs 23%
Allum et al ([120]) (MRC-OEO-2)	802	2 × CF → S S	0.84 (.03)	5-year OS: 23% vs 17.1%
Ychou et al ([58]) (ACCORD 7)	169	2/3 × CF → S S	0.69 (.02)	5-year OS: 38% vs 24%
Cunningham et al ([122]) (MRC-OEO-5)	897	2 × CF → S 4 × ECX → S	Survival data not mature	
MRC ST-03 (NCT00450203)	1,100	3 × ECX → S ECX, B → S	Survival data not mature	
Ando et al ([121]) (JCOG 9907)	380	S → 2 × CF 2 × CF → S	0.73 (.04)	5-year OS: 43% vs 55%
Preoperative chemoradiotherapy				
Tepper et al ([125]) (CALGB 9781)	56	2 × CF; 50.4 Gy → S S	1.46-5.69 (NR)	5-year OS: 39% vs 16%
van Hagen et al ([127]) (CROSS)	366	5 × carboplatin/paclitaxel; 41.4 Gy → S S	0.657 (.003)	5-year OS: 47% vs 34%
Preoperative CT vs preoperative CRT				
Stahl et al ([131]) (POET)	119	2.5 × CF, Leu → S 2 × CF, Leu → CE 30 Gy → S	0.67 (.07)	3-year OS: 27.7% vs 47.4%
Postoperative CT				
Ando et al ([134]) (JCOG 9204)	242	S S → 2 × CF	(.13)	5-year OS: 52% vs 61%

B, bevacizumab; CE, cisplatin and etoposide; CF, cisplatin and 5-fluorouracil; CRT, chemoradiotherapy; CT, chemotherapy; ECX, epirubicin, cisplatin, and capecitabine; HR, hazard ratio; Leu, leucovorin; NR, not reported; OS, overall survival, S; surgery.

or surgery alone (n = 188). With a median follow-up time of 45.4 months, the median OS for preoperative chemoradiotherapy group was 49.4 months versus 24.0 months for the surgery-alone group (HR, 0.657; 95% CI, 0.495-0.871; $P = .003$). Five-year OS was again in favor of the chemoradiotherapy group (47%) versus the surgery-alone group (34%) ([127]). The complete resection rate was higher in the chemoradiotherapy group (92%) versus the surgery-alone group (69%), and 29% of patients in the chemoradiotherapy group had pathCR. In a subgroup analysis, the patients with squamous cancer demonstrated the best outcomes (HR was 0.453 for squamous cancer vs 0.732 for adenocarcinoma) ([127, 128]).

Preoperative Chemotherapy Versus Preoperative Chemoradiotherapy

Meta-analyses have been performed to further support the available evidence for preoperative therapy ([126, 129, 130]). Cumulatively, these three meta-analyses determined that the most consistent significant survival benefit resulted from the combination of surgery and preoperative chemoradiotherapy and, to a lesser extent, preoperative chemotherapy.

Since these studies, results from the Preoperative Chemotherapy or Radiochemotherapy in Esophagogastric Adenocarcinoma (POET) trial, presented by Stahl et al ([131]), have provided further support for three-step preoperative therapy, although the study was closed prematurely because of slow accrual. The POET trial was designed to evaluate the survival outcomes of patients treated with preoperative chemotherapy compared with preoperative chemoradiotherapy. One hundred nineteen patients were randomly assigned to chemotherapy followed by chemoradiotherapy and surgery (n = 59) or chemotherapy followed by surgery (n = 60); the R0 resection rates were 72% and 70% (P = not significant), the pathCR rates were 16% and 2% ($P < .001$), and the N0 rates were 64% and 38% ($P < .001$), respectively. The 3-year OS rate trended toward improvement with induction chemotherapy, chemoradiotherapy, and surgery (47% vs 28% with chemotherapy and surgery; P = .07) ([131]). Patients in the chemoradiotherapy arm had a significantly higher probability of a pathCR (15.6% vs 2.0%). Postoperative mortality rates did not differ between the chemoradiotherapy and chemotherapy arms (10% vs 4%; P = .26). These results suggest that preoperative chemoradiotherapy confers a survival advantage over preoperative chemotherapy in distal esophageal and GEJ adenocarcinoma. Maximizing duration and amount of therapy before surgery theoretically could improve the ability to deliver all planned effective therapies and initiate palliative therapy early and improve pathCR, local control, cure, and survival rates.

The use of induction chemotherapy before chemoradiotherapy and surgery has been evaluated in several phase II studies. Ajani et al ([73]) performed a feasibility study of preoperative induction combination chemotherapy with chemoradiotherapy to improve curative resection, local control, and survival in 2001. Thirty-seven potentially resectable cancers of the esophagus and GEJ were treated with induction chemotherapy followed by chemoradiotherapy and curative surgery. Induction chemotherapy consisted of two cycles of CF plus paclitaxel (CFP). After chemoradiotherapy, consisting of 45 Gy of radiation and concurrent CF, patients underwent surgery. Thirty-five (95%) of the 37 patients underwent surgery (R0 resection). The pathCR rate was 30% (11 of 37 patients); an additional five patients (14%) had only microscopic cancer. Downstaging was significant; the rates of T3 before surgery and at surgery were 89% and 9%, respectively (P = .01), and the rates of N1 were 66% and 20%, respectively (P = .01) ([73]). Patient selection is important because the current three-step strategy exchanges moderate toxicity for modest survival improvement.

In Europe and the United Kingdom, the treatment approach varies accordingly to tumor histology. For resectable squamous cell carcinoma, patients are commonly treated with preoperative chemoradiotherapy ([132]), whereas for resectable adenocarcinomas, either preoperative CRT or perioperative chemotherapy is administered. In the United States, preoperative chemoradiotherapy is the standard of care irrespective of histology.

Postoperative Therapy

Few studies have been performed to evaluate postoperative chemotherapy versus surgery alone. Reflecting the incidence of esophageal cancer during the 1980s and 1990s, these studies included more patients with squamous cell cancer than with adenocarcinoma; this is a shortcoming of these early studies. In a study by Pouliquen et al, no survival improvement was found in the patients who were administered postoperative chemotherapy (CF) ([133]).

The second study, a randomized trial, JCOG 9204, compared the outcomes of patients who underwent surgery alone versus patients who underwent surgery followed by adjuvant CF. The 5-year DFS rates favored the postoperative chemotherapy group (55% vs 45%; P = .037). However, the difference in the 5-year OS rate was not statistically significant (61% vs 52%; P = .13). The duration of adjuvant therapy was suboptimal, and approximately 25% of patients assigned to the postoperative chemotherapy group failed to receive the full course of therapy ([134]).

Another retrospective case-control study was designed to evaluate the effect of postoperative chemotherapy in 211 patients who underwent R0 esophagectomy with radical lymphadenectomy. Of 211 patients, 94 received postoperative chemotherapy, whereas the other 117 patients received surgery alone. The OS was compared between the two groups after they were stratified by the numbers of metastasis-positive LNs. In the subgroup of patients with more than eight positive LNs, postoperative chemotherapy significantly improved the OS compared with surgery alone. Therefore, the authors suggested that postoperative chemotherapy was beneficial only in patients with more than eight metastatic LNs ([135]), reducing the risk of relapse. However, postoperative chemotherapy did not improve the OS compared with surgery alone.

Many studies have been performed to evaluate the role of postoperative radiotherapy versus surgery alone. In two studies, conducted by Teniere et al ([136]) and postoperative radiotherapy did not improve survival. Results from two other randomized studies revealed conflicting findings. Xiao et al ([137]) demonstrated that postoperative radiotherapy improved the 5-year OS in esophageal cancer patients with stage III disease. In contrast, Fok et al found shorter survival durations in patients who underwent postoperative radiotherapy as a direct result of irradiation-related death and the early appearance of metastatic disease ([138]). Thus, the utility of postoperative radiotherapy may be limited. Of these studies, only the one by Zieren et al evaluated quality of life, which was found to be better in the surgery-alone group.

Malthaner et al ([139]) performed a meta-analysis of 34 randomized controlled trials and six meta-analyses in which patients with locally advanced esophageal cancer underwent pre- or postoperative chemotherapy, radiotherapy, or chemoradiotherapy. No significant difference in survival was observed in the postoperative radiotherapy group.

The available evidence suggests that postoperative chemotherapy or radiotherapy does not result in a benefit. However, few randomized comparisons have been performed with surgery alone versus surgery and postoperative treatment. In the INT-0116 study ([38]), 556 patients with resected GEJ and gastric adenocarcinoma were randomly assigned to surgery plus postoperative chemoradiotherapy or surgery alone. Adjuvant treatment consisted of 5-FU plus LV for 5 days, followed by 45 Gy of radiation with modified doses of 5-FU/LV on the first 4 and the last 3 days of radiotherapy. One month after radiotherapy, two 5-day cycles of 5-FU/LV were given 1 month apart. The median OS improved with postoperative chemoradiotherapy from 27 to 36 months (HR, 1.35; 95% CI, 1.09-1.66; $P = .005$), and the HR for relapse was 1.52 (95% CI, 1.23-1.86; $P < .001$). INT-0116 included 111 patients (20%) with GEJ or lower esophageal adenocarcinoma ([38]). Extrapolation of these results as supporting evidence for postoperative chemoradiotherapy in esophageal cancer should be performed with caution.

On the basis of the available evidence, patients with esophageal cancer gain limited survival benefit with postoperative chemotherapy and chemoradiotherapy after R0 resection. The limited contribution of postoperative therapy is probably due to the moderate toxicity, which leads to treatment-related complications or an inability to complete therapy.

The limited ability to deliver therapy after surgery, as demonstrated by results from both the INT-0116 and MAGIC studies ([38, 39]), suggests that all effective therapy should be administered before surgery.

Definitive Chemoradiotherapy

The potential activity of chemotherapy against micrometastases and its ability to act as a radiotherapy-sensitizing agent formed the basis for combining chemotherapy and radiotherapy to treat locally advanced cancer. In the RTOG 85-01 study, patients with locally advanced esophageal adenocarcinoma or squamous cell cancer were randomly assigned to chemoradiotherapy with CF or radiotherapy alone. The 5-year OS rates were 0% and 26% for radiotherapy and chemoradiotherapy, respectively ([140]).

A comprehensive review of the pattern of care for esophageal cancer in the United States from 1992 to 1994 surveyed 400 patients with locally advanced esophageal cancer treated at 63 institutions ([141]). The study confirmed that using combined concurrent chemoradiotherapy as a nonoperative strategy to achieve superior survival and local tumor control was better than radiotherapy alone ([141]). The report also suggested a trend toward survival improvement with chemoradiotherapy before surgery compared with chemoradiotherapy or surgery alone.

In the INT-0123 (RTOG 94-05) study, patients (n = 236) were administered concurrent CF (similar to RTOG 85-01) but were assigned randomly to different radiation doses, either 50.4 or 64.8 Gy. No association was found between higher radiation doses and higher median survival (13 vs 18 months for 50.4 vs 64.8 Gy, respectively) or 2-year survival (31% vs 40%, respectively). Higher radiation dose was also more toxic ([142]). The reason for the failure of the higher radiation dose to improve survival is unclear.

The multi-institutional RTOG 0113 trial evaluated induction chemotherapy followed by definitive chemoradiotherapy in patients with localized unresectable esophageal cancer. The primary goal was to determine whether any approach would result in a >78% 1-year OS, surpassing the historical 66% rate from RTOG 94-05. Seventy-two evaluable patients were randomly assigned to induction with CFP followed by CFP and 50.4 Gy of radiation (CFP arm, n = 37) or induction with paclitaxel plus cisplatin (PP) followed by PP and 50.4 Gy of radiation (PP arm, n = 35). The median OS durations for the CFP and PP arms were 28.7 and 14.9 months, respectively (18.8 months in RTOG 9405). The study did not reach its preset objective because the 1-year OS rates of the CFP and PP arms did not meet or surpass 78% (CFP 1-year OS, 76%). The 2-year OS rates for the CFP and PP arms were 56% and 37%, respectively. Toxicity was quite high in both arms (43% to 54% and 27% to 40% of patients experienced grade 3 and 4 toxicities, respectively). Therefore, neither combination (CFP or PP) was recommended for further evaluation ([143]).

CHAPTER 20

Definitive Chemoradiotherapy Versus Chemoradiotherapy Plus Surgery

Stahl et al ([131]) performed a randomized comparison of chemotherapy followed by chemoradiotherapy and then surgery (surgical arm, n = 86) and chemotherapy followed by chemoradiotherapy and no surgery (nonoperative arm, n = 86) in 172 patients with locally advanced esophageal squamous cell cancer. The median follow-up duration was 6 years. The OS rates were similar for the surgical and nonsurgical arms ($P < .05$). The 2-year local PFS rate was higher in the surgical arm than the nonsurgical arm (64% vs 41%; HR, 2.1; 95% CI, 1.3-3.5; $P = .003$). The treatment-related mortality rate was significantly higher in the surgical arm (12.8% vs 3.5%; $P = .03$). The clinical tumor response to induction chemotherapy was the only independent prognostic factor for OS (HR, 0.30; 95% CI, 0.19-0.47; $P < .0001$). The results of this study suggested that adding surgery to chemoradiotherapy improves local tumor control but not survival in patients with locally advanced esophageal squamous cell cancer. Tumor response to induction chemotherapy is associated with a favorable prognostic group in these high-risk patients, regardless of treatment. Of course, the difficulty of incorporating these results into clinical practice is detecting residual disease or response after preoperative therapy.

Another randomized comparison in only responders to chemoradiotherapy (45 Gy conventional or 60 Gy split-course radiation) was conducted by Bedenne et al ([144]). Patients with resectable esophageal squamous cell cancer were treated with two cycles of CF along with concurrent radiotherapy (conventional/split course). Patients who experienced a response (n = 259) were then randomly assigned to surgery or more chemoradiotherapy. The 2-year OS rates were 34% and 40% (HR, 0.90; $P = .44$), the median OS durations were 18 and 19 months (P = not significant), the 2-year local control rates were 66% and 57% ($P < .01$), and the 3-month mortality rates were 9.3% and 0.8% ($P = .002$), respectively. The authors concluded that in patients who experience a response to chemoradiotherapy, surgery after chemoradiotherapy results in no added benefit over continued chemoradiotherapy ([144]).

Most data are not yet sufficiently mature to allow conclusions about optimal therapy for locally advanced squamous cell cancer of the noncervical esophagus. In a phase III study by the Chinese University Research Group for Esophageal Cancer (CURE), investigators from China are comparing the survival benefits of esophagectomy versus chemoradiotherapy. From 2000 to 2004, 80 patients were randomly assigned to esophagectomy (n = 44) or chemoradiotherapy (n = 36). A two- or three-stage esophagectomy with two-field lymphadenectomy was performed. Chemoradiotherapy consisted of CF and concurrent 50 to 60 Gy of radiation. Tumor response was assessed by EGD, EUS, and CT. Salvage esophagectomies were performed for incomplete response or recurrence. The median follow-up time was 1.4 years. No difference in the early cumulative survival rate was found between the two groups (Relative risk, 0.89; 95% CI, 0.37-2.17; $P = .45$), nor was there a difference in DFS. Patients treated with surgery only had a slightly higher recurrence rate in the mediastinum, whereas those treated with chemoradiotherapy had a higher rate in the cervical or abdominal region ([145]).

Surgery is the foundation of treatment for locally advanced resectable esophageal cancer. Early results from European studies suggested that patients with esophageal squamous cell cancer will not benefit from surgery after chemoradiotherapy ([146]). The caveat of the nonsurgical approach to solid tumors is detecting minimal residual disease. Therefore, until more confirmatory evidence and clinical tools become available for detecting minimal residual disease or molecular or imaging predictive markers in patients who require surgery after preoperative therapy, the treatments for squamous cell cancer and adenocarcinoma will remain similar.

The University of Texas MD Anderson Cancer Center Approach to Resectable Esophageal and Gastroesophageal Junction Cancers

All patients with newly diagnosed invasive cancer undergo careful staging, which includes endoscopic assessment of the location and size of the primary tumor and EUS staging, CT, and PET/CT. Patients with cervical or proximal esophageal cancer also undergo bronchoscopy as part of a recommended staging workup. For distal esophageal disease or gastric cardia cancer, staging laparoscopy is performed in some patients, but the decision is made on a case-by-case basis. Again, as in locally advanced gastric cancer, all patients with only localized disease are further evaluated by a multidisciplinary team that includes thoracic surgeons and radiation oncologists. Furthermore, patients with localized disease are discussed at the weekly Esophageal Multidisciplinary Tumor Board.

Currently, at the MDACC, treatment modalities for locally advanced resectable esophageal cancer include chemoradiotherapy and then surgery. For GEJ adenocarcinoma, postoperative chemoradiotherapy and perioperative chemotherapy are additional options available to patients. Patients with locally advanced cervical esophageal cancer are treated with primary definitive chemoradiotherapy, even those with resectable disease. Salvage surgery is considered only in patients with persistent or locally recurrent disease. Results from the RTOG 85-01 and 94-05 studies established that adding chemotherapy to radiotherapy improved survival and local relapse rates and that the optimal radiation dosage is 50.4 Gy in 28 fractions. With the results of the CROSS trial, we now recognize that a minimum dose of 41.4 Gy may be sufficient in the preoperative setting, although our preference is to use a higher dose. If at all possible, all locally advanced resectable esophageal cancers are treated on protocol at the MDACC or with preoperative chemoradiotherapy followed by surgical resection. Figure 20-3A summarizes the MDACC approach to resectable gastroesophageal cancer.

Advanced and Metastatic Gastric, Gastroesophageal Junction, and Esophageal Cancers

The prognosis of patients with advanced or metastatic gastric, GEJ, and esophageal cancers is poor; thus, clinicians should be cognizant of the patient's quality of life and weigh the risks and benefits of therapy. The overall 5-year survival rate of upper GI cancer patients is less than 5%. The standard of care for advanced disease is chemotherapy. Many frontline combination chemotherapy regimens are available, but no head-to-head comparison has been performed for most of these; thus, the optimal choice is not obvious, and treatment remains regionally variable. However, with the advent of molecular targeted therapy, it may be possible to select therapy based on the disease's molecular characteristics. The results of the Trastuzumab in Gastric Cancer (ToGA) study ([147]) raised the exciting possibility of personalized treatment for upper GI cancers; however, other results have since been disappointing. Until more specific and accurate molecular markers of response and prognosis become available, patient outcome with systemic therapy is best predicted by clinical characteristics, such as performance status.

The medical treatment of metastatic gastric cancer is primarily palliative and confers a modest effect on OS. Multiple agents are active in the treatment of gastric cancer, including fluoropyrimidines (5-FU, capecitabine, and S-1), anthracyclines, platinum agents, taxanes, irinotecan, and some targeted therapies such as trastuzumab for human epidermal growth factor receptor 2 (HER2)-overexpressing gastric cancers. Combination regimens are associated with higher response rates and, according to one meta-analysis, are also associated with increased survival when compared with single-agent chemotherapies ([148]). By and large, the trials addressing the value of targeted therapies, for example targeting epidermal growth factor receptor (*EGFR*) and vascular endothelial growth factor (VEGF), were done in unselected (not biomarker enriched) populations and have, not surprisingly, yielded disappointing results.

First-Line Therapy

Only a minor amount of level 1 evidence exists for the treatment of gastric cancer in the first-line setting. In fact, only docetaxel ([149]), cisplatin/oxaliplatin ([150]), and trastuzumab ([147]) are supported by high level evidence.

A phase III trial involving 445 patients with metastatic cancer randomized patients to receive CF or CF plus docetaxel. The investigators found that the addition of docetaxel was superior in terms of response rate (37% vs 25%; $P = .01$), time to tumor progression (5.6 vs 3.7 months; $P < .001$), and OS (9.2 vs 8.6 months; $P = .02$) ([149]). One could question the clinical significance of a less than 1 month absolute improvement in OS, particularly in the context of significant toxicities, most notably a high rate of febrile neutropenia (30%). Importantly, this regimen should not be used in patients who have a reduced performance status.

Another randomized phase III trial including 1,002 patients tried to improve on the regimen of ECF by substituting oral capecitabine for infusional 5-FU and by using the nonnephrotoxic oxaliplatin rather than cisplatin. The combination of epirubicin/oxaliplatin/capecitabine (EOX) was found to be less toxic and at least as effective as ECF. The median survival times in the ECF (control), ECX, EOF (epirubicin/oxaliplatin/5-FU), and EOX arms were 9.9, 9.9, 9.3, and 11.2 months, respectively. The 1-year survival rates were 37.7%, 40.8%, 40.4%, and 46.8%, respectively. In the secondary analysis, OS was longer with EOX than with ECF, with an HR for death of 0.80 in the EOX group (95% CI, 0.66-0.97; $P = .02$). Progression-free survival and response rates did not differ significantly among the regimens ([150]).

The third randomized phase III trial enrolled 305 patients in Japan to either S-1 alone or S-1 and cisplatin. Median OS was significantly longer in patients assigned to S-1 plus cisplatin (13.0 months) than in those assigned to S-1 alone (11.0 months; HR for death, 0.77; 95% CI, 0.61-0.98; $P = .04$). Progression-free survival was significantly longer in patients assigned to S-1 plus cisplatin than in those assigned to S-1 alone (median PFS, 6.0 vs 4.0 months; $P < .0001$) ([151]). This trial provided evidence for the superiority of the addition of cisplatin when compared to a fluoropyrimidine alone and established the use of a fluoropyrimidine in addition to a platinum as a reasonable treatment option.

Trastuzumab was the first targeted agent with documented clinical activity in the advanced gastric and gastroesophageal cancer setting. This treatment is useful in the HER2-enriched population; however, approximately 20% of gastric cancers and 30% of gastroesophageal cancers overexpress HER2, so that a relatively small proportion of patients benefit from the treatment. The ToGA trial randomized 584 patients whose tumors overexpressed HER2 by immunohistochemistry (IHC) or fluorescence in situ hybridization (FISH) to receive a fluoropyrimidine (5-FU or capecitabine) plus cisplatin with or without trastuzumab. The chemotherapy was administered every 3 weeks for six cycles, and trastuzumab was administered every 3 weeks until disease progression ([147]). The investigators found that the addition of trastuzumab to chemotherapy increased OS from 11.1 to 13.8 months (HR, 0.74; 95% CI, 0.60-0.91; $P = .0046$). The secondary end points of PFS (6.7 vs 5.5 months; $P = .0002$) and response rate (47.3% vs 34.5%; $P = .0017$) were also improved. On extended follow-up, the HR of OS for the addition of trastuzumab has decreased to 0.80 ([152]), indicating that although real, the response to trastuzumab may be short lived. The difference in median OS was reduced from 2.7 months to merely 1.4 months, representing an approximate 50% decrease in the effect of trastuzumab, which suggests that only a few patients benefit. Based on this trial, the combination of trastuzumab and chemotherapy has become the standard of care in patients whose tumors overexpress HER2.

In contrast to the positive results with trastuzumab in HER2-overexpressing gastroesophageal cancers, bevacizumab failed to demonstrate an OS benefit when it was added to a combination of cisplatin and fluoropyrimidine in patients with advanced gastric and GEJ adenocarcinoma ([153]). A total of 774 patients were randomized, and the median OS was 12.1 months with bevacizumab plus fluoropyrimidine-cisplatin and 10.1 months with placebo plus fluoropyrimidine-cisplatin

(HR, 0.87; 95% CI, 0.73-1.03; P = .1002). Both median PFS (6.7 vs 5.3 months; HR, 0.80; 95% CI, 0.68-0.93; P = .0037) and overall response rate (46.0% vs 37.4%; P = .0315) were significantly improved with bevacizumab versus placebo ([153]). In a preplanned subgroup analysis, the investigators were able to show that a benefit in terms of OS existed for "Pan-American" patients but not for European and Asian patients. This might point to differences in tumor biology, but is also dependent on other factors. A subsequent retrospective biomarker analysis of the AVAGAST trial showed that patients with high baseline plasma VEGF-A levels and low baseline expression of neuropilin-1 seemed to have an improved OS. For both biomarkers, subgroup analyses demonstrated significance only in patients from non-Asian regions ([154]). It is important to note that neither of these biomarkers has been validated. Unlike the ToGA trial, the AVAGAST trial did not use a biomarker-enriched patient population, underscoring the importance of appropriate patient selection in randomized controlled trials and the use of predictive biomarkers to direct care. Similarly, the AVATAR trial, which included an all Asian patient population, did not show any survival benefit of adding bevacizumab to the cisplatin-capecitabine combination ([155]).

Equally disappointing results were also reported from two *EGFR*-targeting trials: the Erbitux (cetuximab) in Combination with Xeloda (capecitabine) and Cisplatin in Advanced Esophagogastric Cancer (EXPAND) and Revised European American Lymphoma (REAL-3) trials ([156, 157]). The EXPAND trial randomized 904 patients to receive capecitabine and cisplatin, with or without cetuximab. This study did not achieve its primary end point, with the median PFS for 455 patients allocated to capecitabine-cisplatin plus cetuximab being 4.4 months compared to 5.6 months for 449 patients who were allocated to receive capecitabine-cisplatin alone (HR, 1.09; 95% CI, 0.92-1.29; P = .32) ([156]). The REAL-3 study was terminated prematurely because a statistically significant lower OS was noted in patients treated with modified epirubicin/oxaliplatin/capecitabine (EOC) and panitumumab. The final analysis of this study, which randomized patients with advanced gastroesophageal adenocarcinoma, was published ([157]). Median OS of patients allocated to EOC was 11.3 months (95% CI, 9.6-13.0 months) compared with 8.8 months (95% CI, 7.7-9.8 months) in 278 patients allocated to modified EOC and panitumumab (HR, 1.37; 95% CI, 1.07-1.76; P = .013). There was a nonsignificant trend to worse outcomes in patients treated with panitumumab, again highlighting the importance of patient selection in randomized controlled trials. A biomarker analysis of the REAL-3 trial did not identify any biomarkers whose presence predicted resistance to modified EOC and panitumumab; however, only a few biomarkers were evaluated in this study ([158]).

The role of lapatinib, a dual *EGFR* and HER2 tyrosine kinase inhibitor (TKI), was investigated in combination with capecitabine plus oxaliplatin (CapeOx) in 545 patients with HER2-positive advanced/metastatic gastroesophageal adenocarcinomas in the TRIO-013/LOGiC trial. The addition of lapatinib to CapeOx did not improve efficacy (OS and PFS) among untreated HER2-positive metastatic gastric cancer patients ([159]).

In summary, the standard of care in the first-line setting remains a combination of fluoropyrimidine and platinum-containing chemotherapy, with the addition of trastuzumab in the HER2-enriched population. The results of targeted therapy trials have mostly been disappointing, but none of these trials looked at an appropriately biomarker-enriched population.

Second-Line Therapy

The validity of the use of second-line chemotherapy and its benefit in gastric cancer has long been questioned; however, all recently published trials demonstrated an OS prolongation, albeit very modest, when chemotherapy was compared to best supportive care (BSC) ([160–163]). Arbeitsgemeinschaft Internistische Onkologie (AIO), a small German phase III study, compared the efficacy of irinotecan plus BSC to BSC alone in patients with advanced gastric or GEJ adenocarcinoma ([161]). Only 40 patients were randomized, and the study closed early due to poor accrual. The HR for death was 0.48, with a 95% CI of 0.25 to 0.92, favoring the active treatment with irinotecan (P = .023). The median survival time was 4.0 months (95% CI, 3.6-7.5 months) in the irinotecan arm and 2.4 months (95% CI, 1.7-4.9 months) in the BSC arm ([161]). There were no documented responses to irinotecan in this trial.

The second trial, COUGAR-02, randomized 186 patients to docetaxel plus BSC versus BSC alone. Docetaxel significantly improved OS compared with BSC alone, with a median OS of 5.2 months (95% CI, 4.1-5.9 months) for docetaxel and 3.6 months (95% CI, 3.3-4.4 months) for BSC (HR, 0.67; 95% CI, 0.49-0.92; P = .01) ([162]).

The role of angiogenesis inhibition as a target in gastric cancer was investigated in the Ramucirumab Monotherapy for Previously Treated Advanced Gastric or Gastro-Oesophageal Junction Adenocarcinoma (REGARD) trial, which randomized 355 patients to receive ramucirumab or placebo ([160]). This study demonstrated a marginal improvement in median OS (5.2 months in patients in the ramucirumab group and 3.8 months in patients in the placebo group; HR, 0.776; 95% CI, 0.603-0.998; P = .047). Interestingly, the average patient on study treated with ramucirumab received treatments for 2 weeks longer than the average patient on placebo. In the recently published Ramucirumab in Metastatic Gastric Adenocarcinoma

(RAINBOW) trial, ramucirumab was added to weekly paclitaxel as a second-line therapy in 665 patients with advanced or metastatic gastric cancer, demonstrating a significant improvement in both PFS and OS over paclitaxel alone ([163]). A statistically significant prolongation of OS was demonstrated (HR, 0.81; 95% CI, 0.68-0.96; $P = .017$). Median OS times were 9.6 and 7.4 months in the ramucirumab-plus-paclitaxel arm and placebo-plus-paclitaxel arm, respectively. The PFS was also significantly longer for patients receiving ramucirumab plus paclitaxel (HR, 0.64; 95% CI, 0.54-0.75; $P < .001$) with an overall good safety profile, further supporting its role in combination with chemotherapy.

Another study that demonstrated an OS benefit for patients treated with chemotherapy (either docetaxel or irinotecan) versus BSC was published by Kang et al ([164]). Median OS was 5.3 months among 133 patients in the chemotherapy arm and 3.8 months among 69 patients in the BSC arm (HR, 0.657; 95% CI, 0.485-0.891; one-sided $P = .007$). There was no median OS difference between docetaxel and irinotecan (5.2 vs 6.5 months; $P = .116$).

In the randomized phase III Taiwan Cooperative Oncology Group (TCOG) GI-0801/Biweekly Irinotecan Plus Cisplatin (BIRIP) trial, BIRIP was compared to irinotecan alone after S1-based chemotherapy failure in patients with advanced gastric cancer ([165]). Significant PFS improvement was demonstrated (primary end point met) with cisplatin added to irinotecan as second-line treatment of advanced gastric cancer in 130 patients, providing the first evidence supporting combination chemotherapy in the second-line setting (median PFS, 3.8 vs 2.8 months, $P = .04$; disease control rate, 75.0% vs 54.0%; $P = .02$).

In the second-line setting, targeted HER2 therapy with TKIs has been a failure ([166, 167]). Lapatinib has been investigated in a large 420-patient study (TyTAN trial), which randomized HER2-positive patients to lapatinib plus paclitaxel (L+P) versus paclitaxel alone. Median OS was 11.0 months for L+P and 8.9 months for paclitaxel alone in the intent-to-treat population (HR, 0.84; $P = .2088$). In a preplanned subgroup analysis, median OS in the HER2 IHC 3+ subgroup was 14.0 months for the combination therapy and 7.6 months for paclitaxel alone (HR, 0.59; $P = .0176$) ([167]). Interestingly, it has recently been demonstrated that although the study mandated IHC HER2 positivity, 35% of patients in TyTAN had tumors classified as IHC 0/1 ([167]).

Equally disappointing, the most recent UK Gefitinib for Oesophageal Cancer Progressing After Chemotherapy (COG) trial in patients with adenocarcinoma of the esophagogastric junction types I/II (tumors extending to the esophagus 5 cm above and 2 cm below the GEJ) in the second-line setting ([168]) randomized 449 patients to receive gefitinib or placebo. The primary end point was OS. Secondary end points were PFS and quality-of-life outcomes. However, the median OS was 3.73 months for patients who received gefitinib and 3.63 months for those who received placebo (HR, 0.9; $P = .29$). There was a minor prolongation of PFS by 0.4 months for patients who received gefitinib compared to those who received placebo (HR, 0.80; $P = .02$).

Multiple studies highlight the importance of identification and targeting of driver mutations and their usefulness in the creation of appropriate biomarkers to direct care ([169, 170]). *MET* amplification and/or overexpression of its protein product has long been implicated in the pathogenesis of gastric cancer, supporting its role as a poor prognostic factor ([41]). This has been studied in two phase II trials using the monoclonal antibodies rilotumumab and onartuzumab. Rilotumumab demonstrated prolonged PFS for patients whose tumors had high total c-MET expression ([171]), whereas onartuzumab failed to prolong PFS in patients with MET-positive tumors ([172]). Recently, the investigational oral MET TKI AMG 337 trial is generating excitement based on early-phase results, where 8 of 13 patients who were found to have *MET*-amplified gastroesophageal adenocarcinomas showed partial to near-complete responses to the small-molecule inhibitor AMG-337 ([173]).

The role of poly (ADP-ribose) polymerase (PARP) inhibitors in gastric cancer was investigated in a phase II study where 124 patients who progressed on fluoropyrimidines (second-line metastatic setting) were randomized to olaparib plus paclitaxel versus paclitaxel alone ([174]). There was no improvement in PFS, but the addition of olaparib significantly improved OS (HR, 0.56; 95% CI, 0.35-0.87; $P = .010$). A phase III trial is ongoing.

Third-Line Therapy

Apatinib is a small-molecule multitargeted TKI with activity against VEGF receptor (VEGFR). After showing improved PFS and OS in heavily pretreated metastatic gastric cancer patients in a phase II trial ([175]), apatinib was evaluated in a phase III trial in 271 patients with advanced gastric cancer ([176]). Patients had prior failure to second-line chemotherapy and were stratified according to the number of metastatic sites (≤ or >2 sites). This trial met its primary end point, showing significant improvement in OS and PFS. The median OS time was 6.5 months for apatinib and 4.7 months for placebo (HR, 0.71; 95% CI, 0.54-0.94; $P = 0.015$), and the median PFS was 2.6 months for apatinib and 1.8 months for placebo (HR, 0.44; 95% CI, 0.33-0.61; $P < .0001$). This is the first phase III evidence for efficacy of a third-line therapy in advanced gastric cancer and further supports the angiogenesis inhibition as a target in this disease.

CHAPTER 20

The role of mammalian target of rapamycin (mTOR) inhibitor everolimus was investigated in heavily pretreated metastatic gastric cancer patients with disappointing results. The RAD001 (Everolimus) Monotherapy Plus Best Supportive Care in Patients With Advanced Gastric Cancer (GRANITE-1) study randomized 656 patients to everolimus plus BSC versus placebo plus BSC. Unfortunately, this study did not achieve its primary OS end point (5.4 months with everolimus and 4.3 months with placebo; HR, 0.90; 95% CI, 0.75-1.08; *P* = .124) ([166]). Notably, the estimated percentage of patients remaining progression free at 6 months was higher with everolimus (12.0% vs 4.3%), as were the disease control rate (43.3% vs 22.0%) and the tumor shrinkage rate (37.8% vs 12.3%). These results suggest everolimus has activity in this heavily pretreated population. Identification of specific biomarkers for various patient subpopulations with advanced gastric cancer may help define those patients who would receive the most benefit from everolimus treatment ([166]).

Table 20-8 lists major phase III trials for advanced/metastatic esophageal, GEJ, and gastric cancer involving chemotherapy agents, and Table 20-9 lists trials involving targeted agents in the first-, second-, and third-line settings.

The University of Texas MD Anderson Cancer Center Approach to Advanced Gastric, Gastroesophageal Junction and Esophageal Cancers

In terms of our approach to metastatic gastric, GEJ, or esophageal cancer, clearly in the context that this is no longer a curative situation, our approach is to provide palliation of symptoms and prolongation of life. In a select subgroup of patients who have small-volume disease and who are asymptomatic, it is reasonable to take a careful watch-and-wait strategy as long as the patient is comfortable with this approach. Otherwise, we would treat differently based on HER2 status. Clearly, in HER2-positive gastric cancer, there is an OS benefit with the addition of anti-HER2 therapy to first-line chemotherapy. It is our practice to typically use trastuzumab and not lapatinib because of the negative results of the lapatinib trial in combination with platinum-based doublet. Although no convincing data exist as to the benefit of the addition of HER2 therapy in gastric cancer, we extrapolate from the breast cancer trials and continue anti-HER2 therapy beyond progression, typically switching to an alternative agent. In the context of HER2-negative metastatic disease, our options continue to be limited. A reasonable option

Table 20-8 Major Phase III Gastric Cancer Trials Involving Chemotherapy Agents in the Advanced/Metastatic Setting

Trials	No. of Patients	Treatment Arms	HR for OS (*P* value)	Primary End Point Comparison in Months
Advanced gastric cancer: first line				
Van Cutsem et al ([149]) (V325 study group)	445	DCF vs CF	TTP: 1.47 (<.001) OS: 1.29 (.02)	TTP: 5.6 vs 3.7 OS: 9.2 vs 8.6
Cunningham et al ([150])	1,002	ECF vs ECX vs EOF vs EOX	0.80 (.02)	OS: 9.9 vs 9.9 vs 9.3 vs 11.2
Koizumi et al ([151]) (SPIRITS)	305	S-1 + cisplatin vs S-1	0.77 (.04)	OS: 13.0 vs 11.0
Ajani et al ([178]) (FLAGS)	1,053	Cisplatin + S-1 vs cisplatin + 5-FU	0.92 (.20)	OS: 8.6 vs 7.9
Advanced gastric cancer: second line				
Thuss-Patience et al ([161]) (AIO)	40	Irinotecan + BSC vs BSC	0.48 (.012)	OS: 4.0 vs 2.4
Cook et al ([162]) (COUGAR-02)	168	Docetaxel + ASC vs ASC	0.67 (.01)	OS: 5.2 vs 3.6
Kang et al ([164])	202	Docetaxel or irinotecan vs BSC	0.657 (.007)	OS: 5.3 vs 3.8
Higuchi et al ([165]) (TCOG GI-0801/BIRIP)	130	Biweekly irinotecan + cisplatin vs irinotecan	1.00 (.9823)	PFS: 3.8 vs 2.8 OS: 10.7 vs 10.1

ASC, active symptom control; BSC, best supportive care; CF, cisplatin and 5-fluorouracil; DCF, docetaxel, cisplatin, and 5-fluorouracil; ECF, epirubicin, cisplatin, and 5-fluorouracil; ECX, epirubicin, cisplatin, and capecitabine; EOF, epirubicin, oxaliplatin, and 5-fluorouracil; EOX, epirubicin, oxaliplatin, and capecitabine; 5-FU, 5-fluorouracil; HR, hazard ratio; OS, overall survival; PFS, progression-free survival; TTP, time to progression.

Table 20-9 Major Phase III Gastric Cancer Trials Involving Targeted Agents in the Advanced/ Metastatic Setting

Trials	No. of Patients	Treatment Arms	HR for OS (*P* value)	Primary End Point Comparison in Months
Advanced gastric cancer: first Line				
Bang et al ([147]) (ToGA)[a]	584	CX/CF + trastuzumab vs CX/CF	0.74 (.0046)	OS: 13.8 vs 11.1
Ohtsu et al ([153]) (AVAGAST)	774	CF + bevacizumab vs CF	0.87 (.1002)	OS: 12.1 vs 10.1 PFS: 6.7 vs 5.3
Lordick et al ([156]) (EXPAND)	904	CX + cetuximab vs CX	1.004 (.9547)	OS: 9.4 vs 10.7
Waddell et al ([157]) (REAL -3)	553	mEOC + panitumumab vs EOC	1.37 (.013)	OS: 8.8 vs 11.3
Hecht et al ([159]) (TRIO – 013 / LOGiC)	545	CapeOx + lapatinib vs CapeOx + placebo	0.91 (.35)	OS: 12.2 vs 10.5
Advanced gastric cancer: second line				
Fuchs et al ([160]) (REGARD)	355	Ramucirumab + BSC vs BSC	0.776 (.0473)	OS: 5.2 vs 3.8
Wilke et al ([163]) (RAINBOW)	665	Paclitaxel + ramucirumab vs paclitaxel	0.81 (.017)	OS: 9.6 vs 7.4
Ohtsu et al ([166]) (GRANITE-1)	656	Everolimus + BSC vs placebo + BSC	0.90 (.1244)	OS: 5.4 vs 4.3
Bang et al ([167]) (TyTAN)	261	Lapatinib + paclitaxel vs paclitaxel	0.84 (.2088)	OS: 11.0 vs 8.9
Dutton et al ([168]) (COG)	449	Gefitinib vs placebo	0.90 (.29)	OS: 3.73 vs 3.63
Advanced gastric cancer: third line				
Qin et al ([176]) (apatinib)	271	Apatinib + BSC vs BSC	0.71 (.015)	OS: 6.5 vs 4.7 PFS: 2.6 vs 1.8
Ohtsu et al ([166]) (GRANITE-1)	656	Everolimus + BSC vs placebo + BSC	0.90 (.1244)	OS: 5.4 vs 4.3

[a] HR reduced to 0.8 on follow-up analysis.
BSC, best supportive care; CapeOx, capecitabine and oxaliplatin; CF, cisplatin and 5-fluorouracil; CX, cisplatin and capecitabine; EOC, epirubicin, oxaliplatin, and capecitabine; HR, hazard ratio; mEOC, modified epirubicin, oxaliplatin, and capecitabine; OS, overall survival; PFS, progression-free survival.

in the first-line setting is a platinum-based doublet with the addition of docetaxel or epirubicin depending on the performance status of the patient. In the second line, we use ramucirumab combined with a second chemotherapy agent. Figure 20-3B summarizes the MDACC approach to advanced gastric, GEJ, and esophageal cancer.

Although genetic profiling of tumors is becoming a more widely used tool in the treatment of gastric, GEJ, and esophageal cancer, patients are often found to have multiple and nontargetable mutations. Even when a potentially targetable mutation is found and the patient is treated with a given drug, we have found that responses are rare, likely because of our poor knowledge of driver mutations. Therefore, we do not consider genetic evaluation as a critical part of treatment, but rather emphasize the enrollment of patients into available clinical trials.

Supportive Measures for Advanced Gastric, Gastroesophageal Junction, and Esophageal Cancers

For patients with advanced gastric, GEJ, and esophageal cancers, the most important objective is symptom palliation rather than cure. The goal of symptom palliation is to optimize quality of life. Current or potential signs or symptoms that affect quality of life should be assessed during the initial evaluation of patients with unresectable disease. Available treatment options include external-beam radiotherapy without concurrent chemotherapy ([177]); chemotherapy; endoscopic palliation with luminal dilation, stents, or laser or chemical ablation; and palliative surgery. Palliative surgery is rarely performed because it is rare that the potential benefits clearly outweigh the risks of surgery. Several special issues to consider in this group

CHAPTER 20

of patients include (1) problems specifically associated with local disease, (2) nutrition, (3) diagnosis and treatment of tracheoesophageal fistulas, and (4) management of oral secretions.

All patients, especially those who present with more than 15% weight loss from their normal baseline, should undergo formal nutritional evaluation, and alternative nutritional support methods should be considered. Adequate nutrition and hydration are crucial to ensure that patients complete the full course of therapy. Jejunostomy feeding tubes (J-tubes), which are inserted primarily via a surgical procedure, can be considered in patients with gastric and GEJ cancer; they can be placed during the initial laparoscopic evaluation. Percutaneous gastrostomy feeding tubes, placed by endoscopic (percutaneous endoscopic gastrostomy) or radiologic (G-tube) guidance, can be considered for esophageal cancer. The continued use of jejunostomy, gastrostomy, or nasogastric feeding tubes is considered the first choice if nutrition cannot be supported orally.

All patients with advanced gastric, GEJ, and esophageal cancers are candidates for definitive chemoradiotherapy. Chemotherapy agents used in combination with radiotherapy include cisplatin, paclitaxel, carboplatin, or 5-FU. Patients with borderline performance status may not be candidates for definitive chemoradiotherapy, even with consistent nutritional support via feeding tubes. Therapy should be based on the patient's most pressing symptoms. Malnutrition should be addressed, whenever feasible, with gastrostomy or a jejunostomy tube. Upper GI bleeding and pain can be palliated with radiotherapy, alone or with endoscopic cauterization. Finally, effective chemotherapy can directly improve symptoms such as dysphagia and pain, as well as indirectly improve nutrition and minimize bleeding risk and aspiration.

SUMMARY

Gastric cancer remains the third most common cause of cancer-related death worldwide. Its incidence in the United States is decreasing, resulting in a significant increase in distal esophageal and GEJ adenocarcinoma. In fact, according to the current version of the AJCC TNM staging manual, esophageal cancer now includes GEJ to 5 cm below the gastric cardia.

Two different pathogeneses of gastric cancer have been proposed, correlating to two histologic types, intestinal and diffuse. *H pylori* infection, chronic inflammatory state, cytokines, and host response, leading to acquisition of different genetic mutations and abnormalities, are the likely steps leading to intestinal-type invasive adenocarcinoma. On the other hand, diffuse-type gastric cancer may result from defective intracellular adhesion molecules, which is the consequence of loss of E-cadherin protein expression in gastric cancer.

Most patients with newly diagnosed gastric cancer have distant or locally advanced disease; hence, curative resection may not be possible. Because of mass screening programs in high-risk countries such as Japan, more cases of early gastric cancer are being identified. Gastric cancer treatment is based on disease stage. Early gastric cancer is cured by gastrectomy with lymphadenectomy, but similar outcomes have been reported for EMR/ESMD, which is gaining popularity in Japan and other Asian countries. Although surgery is the only chance for durable survival from gastric cancer, by itself, it is not adequate.

The results of two pivotal trials have shaped the current practice of resectable gastric cancer treatment. The INT-0116 study was the first to establish postoperative chemoradiotherapy as standard practice in the United States, whereas MRC ST02/MAGIC led to the use of perioperative chemotherapy. Postoperative chemotherapy alone after R0 resection is more widely accepted in the United States. Many ongoing large international clinical trials will likely answer some of the questions regarding the role of postoperative versus preoperative therapy.

The focus of future research is on optimizing the chemotherapy regimen, defining the role of radiation therapy, and exploring the effect of treatment timing (preoperative, postoperative, or both). Neoadjuvant therapy is under study in a European trial comparing preoperative 5-FU and cisplatin versus surgery alone. In the United Kingdom, the MAGIC B/ST03 study is exploring ECX with or without bevacizumab followed by surgery and adjuvant ECX with and without maintenance bevacizumab. The Korean ARTIST-2 trial will shed light on whether postoperative chemotherapy (S-1 versus S-1/oxaliplatin) with or without radiotherapy contributes to improved outcomes after surgery. Similarly, a Japanese study is evaluating preoperative cisplatin plus S-1 followed by surgery and postoperative S-1 versus surgery and postoperative S-1 alone (KYUH-UHA-GC04-03). In the Dutch CRITICS study, all patients receive induction chemotherapy followed by surgery, and randomization will compare postoperative chemoradiotherapy and perioperative chemotherapy. Most interesting of all is the TOPGEAR trial, which is under way in Europe and Canada and directly compares preoperative chemotherapy alone (ECF) versus chemoradiotherapy (two cycles of ECF followed by concurrent fluoropyrimidine-based chemoradiotherapy) in patients with resectable adenocarcinoma of the stomach and GEJ; both groups will receive three further cycles of ECF postoperatively.

Only 30% to 40% of patients with esophageal cancer have potentially resectable disease at presentation, and in many series, only 5% to 20% of those undergoing surgery alone for clinically localized disease are alive at 3 to 5 years. The last AJCC TNM staging system (7th edition) for esophageal cancer introduced several important changes: (1) disease extending approximately 5 cm into the gastric cardia is now part of esophageal cancer staging, (2) the grade and number of LNs involved are important in surgical staging, and (3) esophageal squamous cell cancer and adenocarcinoma have their own staging groups.

Barrett esophagus-dysplasia-cancer is the favored mechanism of esophageal tumorigenesis. Both long-segment Barrett esophagus and short-segment Barrett esophagus are treated by treating GERD, which is frequently associated with Barrett esophagus, with a proton pump inhibitor, careful surveillance and monitoring (the frequency of monitoring should be based on the presence of high-risk characteristics), and therapy for any high-grade dysplasia or invasive cancer. High-grade dysplasia and early esophageal cancer are not common in the United States but are treated with esophagectomy or EMR/ESMD (commonly used in high-risk countries such as Japan and Korea). Although no large randomized controlled prospective studies have compared EMR/ESMD with primary esophagectomy, the results of a retrospective case-control series suggest that the initial curative resection rates are similar. Endoscopic therapy is most effective when used to treat small (<2 cm diameter), solitary, flat lesions that are confined to mucosa (T1a).

The use of EMR for diagnosis and therapy has been validated in many studies. Endoscopic mucosal resection combined with PDT is the most popular treatment for patients with early esophageal cancer who are not surgical candidates because of comorbidity or who decline surgery. However, surgery remains the best chance for durable survival for patients with locally advanced esophageal and GEJ cancers. After multidisciplinary evaluation, patients with locally advanced disease that is deemed potentially resectable should be considered for combined-modality therapy. Evidence from several small randomized controlled studies and meta-analyses suggest that pre- or perioperative chemotherapy or preoperative chemoradiotherapy can improve surgical survival outcomes.

The results of the RTOG 85-01 trial established that chemoradiotherapy is more effective at reducing local recurrence and improving survival than radiotherapy alone. In addition, the results of the RTOG 9405 trial established a standard dose of radiation of 50.4 Gy. The POET study concluded that the addition of preoperative chemoradiotherapy improves pathCR rates and hence survival. Moreover, the results of the CROSS trial also emphasized the beneficial role of chemoradiotherapy before surgery, which led to a significant increase in OS irrespective of tumor histology.

Cervical esophageal cancer staging should include bronchoscopy. Because surgery for cervical esophageal cancer includes removal of portions of several neck organs, including the voice box, most patients with localized disease undergo definitive chemoradiotherapy. The results of several randomized studies from Europe suggest that esophageal squamous cell cancer be treated differently than adenocarcinoma. However, as of this writing, esophageal squamous cell cancer and adenocarcinoma treatments remain the same. The incidence of distal esophageal, GEJ, and proximal gastric adenocarcinoma was on a steep increase until recently. Stage for stage, esophageal cancer has a poorer prognosis than gastric cancer. Therefore, it is important that all patients with localized esophageal cancer be accurately staged and that management decisions be made by a multidisciplinary panel. Ongoing international and national randomized studies will further elucidate the role of adjuvant therapy in esophageal squamous cell cancer.

In summary, complete surgical resection of the tumor provides the best chance for cure; however, only a minority of patients present with resectable disease. We strongly believe that a multidisciplinary approach and preoperative therapy are the cornerstones of management in the West. Gastrectomy is the recommended treatment in relatively early localized gastric cancer (T1b); however, in more advanced gastric cancers (T2N0, T1aN+, or T1b-T3N+), adjunctive therapy besides gastrectomy is recommended. The evidence-based approach should include perioperative chemotherapy or postoperative chemoradiotherapy for selected patients. All patients should be encouraged to enroll in clinical trials. Similarly, for resectable esophageal and GEJ cancers, preoperative chemoradiotherapy will enhance surgical outcomes and improve the pathCR rate.

The development of response or survival biomarkers appears to be more advanced for esophageal cancer. Positron emission tomography after induction therapy and pathCR are solid predictors of response and prognosis, respectively. Advanced or metastatic gastric, GEJ, and esophageal cancers are treated similarly. More than 60% of patients who present with newly diagnosed gastric, GEJ, and esophageal cancers will have advanced unresectable or metastatic disease. Although a cure is not possible, systemic therapy can prolong survival compared with BSC. In recent decades, advances have been made in the treatment of gastric cancer, with expansion of effective agents in several cytotoxic classes—docetaxel, oxaliplatin, capecitabine, and S-1. So far, the only targeted therapy that has demonstrated a survival benefit is trastuzumab in patients with HER2-positive disease.

Over the last 5 to 7 years, more chemotherapy combinations have been introduced for frontline treatment, including ECF and its derivatives (ECX, EOF, and EOX), DCF (docetaxel, cisplatin, and 5-FU) and its less toxic modifications (mDCX [modified] and mDX [modified], CF and its modern derivatives (XP and FLO [5-FU, leucovorin, and oxaliplatin]), and S-1 plus cisplatin. On the basis of the results of the FLAGS study ([178]), S-1 is not in use in Western countries. Unfortunately, despite the wealth of chemotherapy regimens, no clear consensus exists as to which chemotherapy regimen is best. Currently, patients in the United States are likely to undergo frontline therapy with platinum-, fluoropyrimidine-, or taxane-based chemotherapy regimens. Meanwhile, patients in Europe are likely to receive ECF or its derivatives and taxane-based chemotherapy regimens. The positive results of the ToGA trial have likely transformed frontline therapy for patients with HER2-positive metastatic gastric, GEJ, and esophageal cancers. However, only 20% of gastric, GEJ, and esophageal cancer patients have HER2 overexpression. In hopes of improving outcomes, biologic therapies have been introduced targeting markers shown to be prognostic in gastric cancer. The results of ongoing randomized controlled phase III trials using targeted agents, in combination and alone, could transform the treatment of patients with advanced disease. Unfortunately, none of the trials have been done in a biomarker-enriched population.

Despite the rarity of upper GI cancers in the United States, they are common in many other countries. Both gastric and esophageal cancers carry an ominous prognosis; thus, they are still considered a major public health problem. Advancements have been made in the areas of surgery and radiotherapy that have improved the mortality rates of upper GI cancer patients. Many more reference chemotherapy regimens are available for the treatment of advanced disease. The recent TCGA analysis has uncovered four genotypes of gastric cancer; however, it is not sufficient to change our treatment strategies, and more work needs to be done. A multimodality approach to therapy will be the cornerstone to screening, diagnosing, staging, treating, and supporting patients with upper GI cancers. Figures 20-3A and 20-3B summarize the MDACC approach to gastric, GEJ, and esophageal cancers.

Surgery remains the treatment modality of choice for stage I and II cancers. Treatment consisting of definitive chemoradiotherapy can also be considered for selected patients. Metastatic gastric, GEJ, and esophageal cancers (stage IV) are not curable, but survival and cancer-related symptom control can be improved with systemic chemotherapy. Effective palliation may be achieved with various combinations of chemotherapy, radiotherapy, and therapeutic endoscopy. In particular, systemic chemotherapy can result in temporary palliation. Objective response rates of 30% to 50% and a median survival duration of <1 year have been reported for platinum-based combination regimens with 5-FU, a taxane, or a topoisomerase inhibitor. The search for new classes of cytotoxics has almost stopped, but it is clear that cytotoxic therapy continues to contribute and it is here to stay. The incorporation of biologic agents that modulate the immune system of the host and the uncovering of true driver mutations of gastric cancer in individual patients appear promising, along with many other biologics that can potentially inhibit signaling pathways. Therefore, all patients should be offered the opportunity to participate in clinical trials.

REFERENCES

1. Ferlay J, Soerjomataram I, Dikshit R, et al. Cancer incidence and mortality worldwide: sources, methods and major patterns in GLOBOCAN 2012. *Int J Cancer.* 2015;136(5):E359-E386.
2. American Cancer Society. Cancer Facts & Figures. Atlanta, GA: American Cancer Society; 2015.
3. National Cancer Institute Surveillance, Epidemiology, and End Results. SEER Stats Facts Sheet. http://seer.cancer.gov/statfacts/. Accessed December 4, 2014.
4. The University of Texas MD Anderson Cancer Center, Camargo MC, Fraumeni JF Jr, Correa P, Rosenberg PS, Rabkin CS. Age-specific trends in incidence of noncardia gastric cancer in US adults. *JAMA.* 2010;303:1723-1728.
5. Buas MF, Vaughan TL. Epidemiology and risk factors for gastroesophageal junction tumors: understanding the rising incidence of this disease. *Semin Radiat Oncol.* 2013;23:3-9.
6. Alexander GA, Brawley OW. Association of *Helicobacter pylori* infection with gastric cancer. *Mil Med.* 2000;165: 21–27.
7. Correa P. Human gastric carcinogenesis: a multistep and multifactorial process—First American Cancer Society Award Lecture on Cancer Epidemiology and Prevention. *Cancer Res.* 1992;52:6735-6740.
8. Larsson SC, Orsini N, Wolk A. Processed meat consumption and stomach cancer risk: a meta-analysis. *J Natl Cancer Inst.* 2006;98:1078-1087.
9. Freedman ND, Abnet CC, Leitzmann MF, et al. A prospective study of tobacco, alcohol, and the risk of esophageal and gastric cancer subtypes. *Am J Epidemiol.* 2007;165:1424-1433.
10. Stalnikowicz R, Benbassat J. Risk of gastric cancer after gastric surgery for benign disorders. *Arch Intern Med.* 1990;150: 2022–2026.
11. Freedman ND, Chow WH, Gao YT, et al. Menstrual and reproductive factors and gastric cancer risk in a large prospective study of women. *Gut.* 2007;56:1671-1677.
12. Zheng ZH, Sun XJ, Ma MC, Hao DM, Liu YH, Sun KL. [Studies of promoter methylation status and protein expression of E-cadherin gene in associated progression stages of gastric cancer]. *Yi Chuan Xue Bao.* 2003;30:103-108.
13. Oliveira C, Ferreira P, Nabais S, et al. E-Cadherin (CDH1) and p53 rather than SMAD4 and Caspase-10 germline mutations contribute to genetic predisposition in Portuguese gastric cancer patients. *Eur J Cancer.* 2004;40:1897-1903.
14. Kaurah P, MacMillan A, Boyd N, et al. Founder and recurrent CDH1 mutations in families with hereditary diffuse gastric cancer. *JAMA.* 2007;297:2360-2372.
15. Murphy G, Pfeiffer R, Camargo MC, Rabkin CS. Meta-analysis shows that prevalence of Epstein-Barr virus-positive gastric cancer differs based on sex and anatomic location. *Gastroenterology.* 2009;137:824-833.

CHAPTER 20

16. Kusano M, Toyota M, Suzuki H, et al. Genetic, epigenetic, and clinicopathologic features of gastric carcinomas with the CpG island methylator phenotype and an association with Epstein-Barr virus. *Cancer*. 2006;106:1467-1479.
17. Eslick GD, Lim LL, Byles JE, Xia HH, Talley NJ. Association of *Helicobacter pylori* infection with gastric carcinoma: a meta-analysis. *Am J Gastroenterol*. 1999;94:2373-2379.
18. Huang JQ, Sridhar S, Chen Y, Hunt RH. Meta-analysis of the relationship between *Helicobacter pylori* seropositivity and gastric cancer. *Gastroenterology*. 1998;114:1169-1179.
19. Parsonnet J, Forman D. *Helicobacter pylori* infection and gastric cancer: for want of more outcomes. *JAMA*. 2004;291:244-245.
20. Wong BC, Lam SK, Wong WM, et al. *Helicobacter pylori* eradication to prevent gastric cancer in a high-risk region of China: a randomized controlled trial. *JAMA*. 2004;291:187-194.
21. Ma JL, Zhang L, Brown LM, et al. Fifteen-year effects of *Helicobacter pylori*, garlic, and vitamin treatments on gastric cancer incidence and mortality. *J Natl Cancer Inst*. 2012;104:488-492.
22. Fuccio L, Zagari RM, Eusebi LH, et al. Meta-analysis: can *Helicobacter pylori* eradication treatment reduce the risk for gastric cancer? *Ann Intern Med*. 2009;151:121-128.
23. Comprehensive molecular characterization of gastric adenocarcinoma. *Nature*. 2014;513:202-209.
24. Graham DY, Schwartz JT, Cain GD, Gyorkey F. Prospective evaluation of biopsy number in the diagnosis of esophageal and gastric carcinoma. *Gastroenterology*. 1982;82:228-231.
25. Moss AA, Schnyder P, Marks W, Margulis AR. Gastric adenocarcinoma: a comparison of the accuracy and economics of staging by computed tomography and surgery. *Gastroenterology*. 1981;80:45-50.
26. Edge SB, Compton CC. The American Joint Committee on Cancer: the 7th edition of the AJCC cancer staging manual and the future of TNM. *Ann Surg Oncol*. 2010;17:1471-1474.
27. Rosch T, Lorenz R, Zenker K, et al. Local staging and assessment of resectability in carcinoma of the esophagus, stomach, and duodenum by endoscopic ultrasonography. *Gastrointest Endosc*. 1992;38:460-467.
28. Conlon KC, Karpeh MS Jr. Laparoscopy and laparoscopic ultrasound in the staging of gastric cancer. *Semin Oncol*. 1996;23:347-351.
29. Sun L, Su XH, Guan YS, et al. Clinical role of 18F-fluorodeoxyglucose positron emission tomography/computed tomography in post-operative follow up of gastric cancer: initial results. *World J Gastroenterol*. 2008;14:4627-4632.
30. Ott K, Lordick F, Herrmann K, Krause BJ, Schuhmacher C, Siewert JR. The new credo: induction chemotherapy in locally advanced gastric cancer: consequences for surgical strategies. *Gastric Cancer*. 2008;11:1-9.
31. Ott K, Herrmann K, Lordick F, et al. Early metabolic response evaluation by fluorine-18 fluorodeoxyglucose positron emission tomography allows in vivo testing of chemosensitivity in gastric cancer: long-term results of a prospective study. *Clin Cancer Res*. 2008;14:2012-2018.
32. Javeri H, Xiao L, Rohren E, et al. The higher the decrease in the standardized uptake value of positron emission tomography after chemoradiation, the better the survival of patients with gastroesophageal adenocarcinoma. *Cancer*. 2009;115:5184-5192.
33. Swisher SG, Erasmus J, Maish M, et al. 2-Fluoro-2-deoxy-D-glucose positron emission tomography imaging is predictive of pathologic response and survival after preoperative chemoradiation in patients with esophageal carcinoma. *Cancer*. 2004;101:1776-1785.
34. Lordick F, Ott K, Krause BJ, et al. PET to assess early metabolic response and to guide treatment of adenocarcinoma of the oesophagogastric junction: the MUNICON phase II trial. *Lancet Oncol*. 2007;8:797-805.
35. Sim SH, Kim YJ, Oh DY, et al. The role of PET/CT in detection of gastric cancer recurrence. *BMC Cancer*. 2009;9:73.
36. Talamonti MS, Kim SP, Yao KA, et al. Surgical outcomes of patients with gastric carcinoma: the importance of primary tumor location and microvessel invasion. *Surgery*. 2003;134:720–727; discussion 727-729.
37. Bonenkamp JJ, Hermans J, Sasako M, et al. Extended lymph-node dissection for gastric cancer. *N Engl J Med*. 1999;340:908-914.
38. Macdonald JS, Smalley SR, Benedetti J, et al. Chemoradiotherapy after surgery compared with surgery alone for adenocarcinoma of the stomach or gastroesophageal junction. *N Engl J Med*. 2001;345:725-730.
39. Cunningham D, Allum WH, Stenning SP, et al. Perioperative chemotherapy versus surgery alone for resectable gastroesophageal cancer. *N Engl J Med*. 2006;355:11-20.
40. Sakuramoto S, Sasako M, Yamaguchi T, et al. Adjuvant chemotherapy for gastric cancer with S-1, an oral fluoropyrimidine. *N Engl J Med*. 2007;357:1810-1820.
41. Bang YJ, Kim YW, Yang HK, et al. Adjuvant capecitabine and oxaliplatin for gastric cancer after D2 gastrectomy (CLASSIC): a phase 3 open-label, randomised controlled trial. *Lancet*. 2012;379:315-321.
42. Wanebo HJ, Kennedy BJ, Chmiel J, Steele G Jr, Winchester D, Osteen R. Cancer of the stomach. A patient care study by the American College of Surgeons. *Ann Surg*. 1993;218:583-592.
43. Bozzetti F, Marubini E, Bonfanti G, Miceli R, Piano C, Gennari L. Subtotal versus total gastrectomy for gastric cancer: five-year survival rates in a multicenter randomized Italian trial. Italian Gastrointestinal Tumor Study Group. *Ann Surg*. 1999;230:170-178.
44. Gouzi JL, Huguier M, Fagniez PL, et al. Total versus subtotal gastrectomy for adenocarcinoma of the gastric antrum. A French prospective controlled study. *Ann Surg*. 1989;209:162-166.
45. Martin RC 2nd, Jaques DP, Brennan MF, Karpeh M. Extended local resection for advanced gastric cancer: increased survival versus increased morbidity. *Ann Surg*. 2002;236:159-165.
46. Schwarz RE, Smith DD. Clinical impact of lymphadenectomy extent in resectable gastric cancer of advanced stage. *Ann Surg Oncol*. 2007;14:317-328.
47. Smith DD, Schwarz RR, Schwarz RE. Impact of total lymph node count on staging and survival after gastrectomy for gastric cancer: data from a large US-population database. *J Clin Oncol*. 2005;23:7114-7124.
48. Wu CW, Hsiung CA, Lo SS, et al. Nodal dissection for patients with gastric cancer: a randomised controlled trial. *Lancet Oncol*. 2006;7:309-315.
49. Danielson H, Kokkola A, Kiviluoto T, et al. Clinical outcome after D1 vs D2-3 gastrectomy for treatment of gastric cancer. *Scand J Surg*. 2007;96:35-40.
50. Hartgrink HH, van de Velde CJ, Putter H, et al. Extended lymph node dissection for gastric cancer: who may benefit? Final results of the randomized Dutch gastric cancer group trial. *J Clin Oncol*. 2004;22:2069-2077.
51. Cuschieri A, Weeden S, Fielding J, et al. Patient survival after D1 and D2 resections for gastric cancer: long-term results of the MRC randomized surgical trial. Surgical Co-operative Group. *Br J Cancer*. 1999;79:1522-1530.
52. Coupland VH, Lagergren J, Luchtenborg M, et al. Hospital volume, proportion resected and mortality from oesophageal and gastric cancer: a population-based study in England, 2004-2008. *Gut*. 2013;62:961-966.
53. Dikken JL, Dassen AE, Lemmens VE, et al. Effect of hospital volume on postoperative mortality and survival after oesophageal and gastric cancer surgery in the Netherlands between 1989 and 2009. *Eur J Cancer*. 2012;48:1004-1013.
54. Ajani JA, Bentrem DJ, Besh S, et al. Gastric cancer, version 2.2013: featured updates to the NCCN Guidelines. *J Natl Compr Canc Netw*. 2013;11:531-546.

55. Degiuli M, Calvo F. Survival of early gastric cancer in a specialized European center. Which lymphadenectomy is necessary? *World J Surg.* 2006;30: 2193–2203.
56. Songun I, Putter H, Kranenbarg EM, Sasako M, van de Velde CJ. Surgical treatment of gastric cancer: 15-year follow-up results of the randomised nationwide Dutch D1D2 trial. *Lancet Oncol.* 2010;11:439-449.
57. Okines A, Verheij M, Allum W, Cunningham D, Cervantes A. Gastric cancer: ESMO Clinical Practice Guidelines for diagnosis, treatment and follow-up. *Ann Oncol.* 2010;21(suppl 5): v50-54.
58. Ychou M, Boige V, Pignon JP, et al. Perioperative chemotherapy compared with surgery alone for resectable gastroesophageal adenocarcinoma: an FNCLCC and FFCD multicenter phase III trial. *J Clin Oncol.* 2011;29:1715-1721.
59. Schuhmacher C, Gretschel S, Lordick F, et al. Neoadjuvant chemotherapy compared with surgery alone for locally advanced cancer of the stomach and cardia: European Organisation for Research and Treatment of Cancer randomized trial 40954. *J Clin Oncol.* 2010;28:5210-5218.
60. Okines AF, Langley RE, Thompson LC, et al. Bevacizumab with peri-operative epirubicin, cisplatin and capecitabine (ECX) in localised gastro-oesophageal adenocarcinoma: a safety report. *Ann Oncol.* 2013;24:702-709.
61. Smalley SR, Benedetti JK, Haller DG, et al. Updated analysis of SWOG-directed intergroup study 0116: a phase III trial of adjuvant radiochemotherapy versus observation after curative gastric cancer resection. *J Clin Oncol.* 2012;30:2327-2333.
62. Fuchs JET, Niedwiecki D, Hollis D, et al. Postoperative adjuvant chemoradiation for gastric or gastroesophageal adenocarcinoma using epirubicin, cisplatin, and infusional (CI) 5-FU (ECF) before and after CI 5-FU and radiotherapy (RT): interim toxicity results from Intergroup trial CALGB 80101 [abstract]. *J Clin Oncol.* 2011;29:4003.
63. Lee J, Lim do H, Kim S, et al. Phase III trial comparing capecitabine plus cisplatin versus capecitabine plus cisplatin with concurrent capecitabine radiotherapy in completely resected gastric cancer with D2 lymph node dissection: the ARTIST trial. *J Clin Oncol.* 2012;30:268-273.
64. Park SH, Sohn TS, Lee J, et al. Phase III trial to compare adjuvant chemotherapy with capecitabine and cisplatin versus concurrent chemoradiotherapy in gastric cancer: final report of the adjuvant chemoradiotherapy in stomach tumors trial, including survival and subset analyses. J Clin Oncol. 2015. *J Clin Oncol.* 2015 January 5. pii: JCO.2014.58.3930.
65. Dikken JL, van Sandick JW, Maurits Swellengrebel HA, et al. Neo-adjuvant chemotherapy followed by surgery and chemotherapy or by surgery and chemoradiotherapy for patients with resectable gastric cancer (CRITICS). *BMC Cancer.* 2011; 11:329.
66. Leong T, Michael M, Gebski V, et al. TOPGEAR: an international randomized phase III trial of preoperative chemoradiotherapy versus preoperative chemotherapy for resectable gastric cancer (AGITG/TROG/EORTC/NCIC CTG) [abstract]. *J Clin Oncol.* 2012;30:TPS4141.
67. Sasako M, Sakuramoto S, Katai H, et al. Five-year outcomes of a randomized phase III trial comparing adjuvant chemotherapy with S-1 versus surgery alone in stage II or III gastric cancer. *J Clin Oncol.* 2011;29:4387-4393.
68. Tsuburaya A, Yoshida K, Kobayashi M, et al. Sequential paclitaxel followed by tegafur and uracil (UFT) or S-1 versus UFT or S-1 monotherapy as adjuvant chemotherapy for T4a/b gastric cancer (SAMIT): a phase 3 factorial randomised controlled trial. *Lancet Oncol.* 2014;15:886-893.
69. Diaz-Nieto R, Orti-Rodriguez R, Winslet M. Post-surgical chemotherapy versus surgery alone for resectable gastric cancer. *Cochrane Database Syst Rev.* 2013;9:CD008415.
70. Ronellenfitsch U, Schwarzbach M, Hofheinz R, et al. Perioperative chemo(radio)therapy versus primary surgery for resectable adenocarcinoma of the stomach, gastroesophageal junction, and lower esophagus. *Cochrane Database Syst Rev.* 2013;5:CD008107.
71. Oba K, Paoletti X, Alberts S, et al. Disease-free survival as a surrogate for overall survival in adjuvant trials of gastric cancer: a meta-analysis. *J Natl Cancer Inst.* 2013;105:1600-1607.
72. Earle CC, Maroun JA. Adjuvant chemotherapy after curative resection for gastric cancer in non-Asian patients: revisiting a meta-analysis of randomised trials. *Eur J Cancer.* 1999;35:1059-1064.
73. Ajani JA, Komaki R, Putnam JB, et al. A three-step strategy of induction chemotherapy then chemoradiation followed by surgery in patients with potentially resectable carcinoma of the esophagus or gastroesophageal junction. *Cancer.* 2001;92:279-286.
74. Ajani JA, Winter K, Okawara GS, et al. Phase II trial of preoperative chemoradiation in patients with localized gastric adenocarcinoma (RTOG 9904): quality of combined modality therapy and pathologic response. *J Clin Oncol.* 2006;24:3953-3958.
75. Jemal A, Bray F, Center MM, Ferlay J, Ward E, Forman D. Global cancer statistics. *CA Cancer J Clin.* 2011;61:69-90.
76. Boslaugh SE. *American Cancer Society. Encyclopedia of Cancer and Society.* Thousand Oaks, CA: SAGE Publications; 2007.
77. Cummings LC, Cooper GS. Descriptive epidemiology of esophageal carcinoma in the Ohio Cancer Registry. *Cancer Detect Prev.* 2008;32:87-92.
78. Parkin DM, Bray F, Ferlay J, Pisani P. Global cancer statistics, 2002. *CA Cancer J Clin.* 2005;55:74-108.
79. Sant M, Aareleid T, Berrino F, et al. EUROCARE-3: survival of cancer patients diagnosed 1990-94—results and commentary. *Ann Oncol.* 2003;14(suppl 5):v61-118.
80. Chen ZM, Xu Z, Collins R, Li WX, Peto R. Early health effects of the emerging tobacco epidemic in China. A 16-year prospective study. *JAMA.* 1997;278:1500-1504.
81. Keszei AP, Goldbohm RA, Schouten LJ, Jakszyn P, van den Brandt PA. Dietary N-nitroso compounds, endogenous nitrosation, and the risk of esophageal and gastric cancer subtypes in the Netherlands Cohort Study. *Am J Clin Nutr.* 2013;97:135-146.
82. Wu CM, Lee YS, Wang TH, et al. Identification of differential gene expression between intestinal and diffuse gastric cancer using cDNA microarray. *Oncol Rep.* 2006;15:57-64.
83. Islami F, Pourshams A, Nasrollahzadeh D, et al. Tea drinking habits and oesophageal cancer in a high risk area in northern Iran: population based case-control study. *BMJ.* 2009;338:b929.
84. Rios-Galvez S, Meixueiro-Daza A, Remes-Troche JM. Achalasia: a risk factor that must not be forgotten for esophageal squamous cell carcinoma. *BMJ Case Rep.* 2015;2015.
85. Ribeiro U Jr, Posner MC, Safatle-Ribeiro AV, Reynolds JC. Risk factors for squamous cell carcinoma of the oesophagus. *Br J Surg.* 1996;83:1174-1185.
86. Lindkvist B, Johansen D, Stocks T, et al. Metabolic risk factors for esophageal squamous cell carcinoma and adenocarcinoma: a prospective study of 580,000 subjects within the Me-Can project. *BMC Cancer.* 2014;14:103.
87. Engel LS, Chow WH, Vaughan TL, et al. Population attributable risks of esophageal and gastric cancers. *J Natl Cancer Inst.* 2003;95:1404-1413.
88. Bytzer P, Christensen PB, Damkier P, Vinding K, Seersholm N. Adenocarcinoma of the esophagus and Barrett's esophagus: a population-based study. *Am J Gastroenterol.* 1999;94:86-91.
89. Lagergren J, Bergstrom R, Lindgren A, Nyren O. Symptomatic gastroesophageal reflux as a risk factor for esophageal adenocarcinoma. *N Engl J Med.* 1999;340:825-831.
90. Zhai R, Chen F, Liu G, et al. Interactions among genetic variants in apoptosis pathway genes, reflux symptoms, body mass index, and smoking indicate two distinct etiologic patterns of

esophageal adenocarcinoma. *J Clin Oncol.* 2010;28:2445-2451.
91. Cook MB, Wild CP, Forman D. A systematic review and meta-analysis of the sex ratio for Barrett's esophagus, erosive reflux disease, and nonerosive reflux disease. *Am J Epidemiol.* 2005;162:1050-1061.
92. Brown LM, Devesa SS, Chow WH. Incidence of adenocarcinoma of the esophagus among white Americans by sex, stage, and age. *J Natl Cancer Inst.* 2008;100:1184-1187.
93. Downey RJ, Akhurst T, Ilson D, et al. Whole body 18FDG-PET and the response of esophageal cancer to induction therapy: results of a prospective trial. *J Clin Oncol.* 2003;21:428-432.
94. Kato H, Nakajima M, Sohda M, et al. The clinical application of 18F-fluorodeoxyglucose positron emission tomography to predict survival in patients with operable esophageal cancer. *Cancer.* 2009;115:3196-3203.
95. Skinner HD, McCurdy MR, Echeverria AE, et al. Metformin use and improved response to therapy in esophageal adenocarcinoma. *Acta Oncologica.* 2013;52:1002-1009.
96. Suzuki A, Xiao L, Taketa T, et al. Results of the baseline positron emission tomography can customize therapy of localized esophageal adenocarcinoma patients who achieve a clinical complete response after chemoradiation. *Ann Oncol.* 2013;24:2854-2859.
97. Monjazeb AM, Riedlinger G, Aklilu M, et al. Outcomes of patients with esophageal cancer staged with [(1)(8)F]fluorodeoxyglucose positron emission tomography (FDG-PET): can postchemoradiotherapy FDG-PET predict the utility of resection? *J Clin Oncol.* 2010;28:4714-4721.
98. Vallbohmer D, Holscher AH, Dietlein M, et al. [18F]-Fluorodeoxyglucose-positron emission tomography for the assessment of histopathologic response and prognosis after completion of neoadjuvant chemoradiation in esophageal cancer. *Ann Surg.* 2009;250:888-894.
99. Nakamoto Y, Osman M, Wahl RL. Prevalence and patterns of bone metastases detected with positron emission tomography using F-18 FDG. *Clin Nucl Med.* 2003;28:302-307.
100. Kato H, Kuwano H, Nakajima M, et al. Comparison between positron emission tomography and computed tomography in the use of the assessment of esophageal carcinoma. *Cancer.* 2002;94:921-928.
101. Swisher SG, Maish M, Erasmus JJ, et al. Utility of PET, CT, and EUS to identify pathologic responders in esophageal cancer. *Ann Thorac Surg.* 2004;78:1152–1160; discussion 1152-1160.
102. Klaeser B, Nitzsche E, Schuller JC, et al. Limited predictive value of FDG-PET for response assessment in the preoperative treatment of esophageal cancer: results of a prospective multicenter trial (SAKK 75/02). *Onkologie.* 2009;32:724-730.
103. Yoshinaga K, Inoue H, Utsunomiya T, et al. N-cadherin is regulated by activin A and associated with tumor aggressiveness in esophageal carcinoma. *Clin Cancer Res.* 2004;10:5702-5707.
104. Abdel-Latif MM, O'Riordan J, Windle HJ, et al. NF-kappaB activation in esophageal adenocarcinoma: relationship to Barrett's metaplasia, survival, and response to neoadjuvant chemoradiotherapy. *Ann Surg.* 2004;239:491-500.
105. Prasad GA, Wu TT, Wigle DA, et al. Endoscopic and surgical treatment of mucosal (T1a) esophageal adenocarcinoma in Barrett's esophagus. *Gastroenterology.* 2009;137:815-823.
106. Ciocirlan M, Lapalus MG, Hervieu V, et al. Endoscopic mucosal resection for squamous premalignant and early malignant lesions of the esophagus. *Endoscopy.* 2007;39:24-29.
107. Soetikno RM, Gotoda T, Nakanishi Y, Soehendra N. Endoscopic mucosal resection. *Gastrointest Endosc.* 2003;57:567-579.
108. Siersema PD, van Hillegersberg R. Treatment of locally advanced esophageal cancer with surgery and chemoradiation. *Curr Opin Gastroenterol.* 2008;24:535-540.
109. Hirst J, Smithers BM, Gotley DC, Thomas J, Barbour A. Defining cure for esophageal cancer: analysis of actual 5-year survivors following esophagectomy. *Ann Surg Oncol.* 2011;18:1766-1774.
110. Hofstetter W, Swisher SG, Correa AM, et al. Treatment outcomes of resected esophageal cancer. *Ann Surg.* 2002;236: 376–384; discussion 384-375.
111. Ellis FH Jr, Gibb SP, Watkins E Jr. Esophagogastrectomy. A safe, widely applicable, and expeditious form of palliation for patients with carcinoma of the esophagus and cardia. *Ann Surg.* 1983;198:531-540.
112. Baba M, Aikou T, Natsugoe S, et al. Appraisal of ten-year survival following esophagectomy for carcinoma of the esophagus with emphasis on quality of life. *World J Surg.* 1997;21:282–285; discussion 286.
113. Krasna MJ. Left transthoracic esophagectomy. *Chest Surg Clin N Am.* 1995;5:543-554.
114. Swanson SJ, Batirel HF, Bueno R, et al. Transthoracic esophagectomy with radical mediastinal and abdominal lymph node dissection and cervical esophagogastrostomy for esophageal carcinoma. *Ann Thorac Surg.* 2001;72:1918–1924; discussion 1924-1925.
115. Rudiger Siewert J, Feith M, Werner M, Stein HJ. Adenocarcinoma of the esophagogastric junction: results of surgical therapy based on anatomical/topographic classification in 1,002 consecutive patients. *Ann Surg.* 2000;232:353-361.
116. Lerut T, Coosemans W, De Leyn P, Van Raemdonck D, Deneffe G, Decker G. Treatment of esophageal carcinoma. *Chest.* 1999;116:463S-465S.
117. Parker EF, Reed CE, Marks RD, Kratz JM, Connolly M. Chemotherapy, radiation therapy, and resection for carcinoma of the esophagus. Long-term results. *J Thorac Cardiovasc Surg.* 1989;98:1037-1042.
118. Kelsen DP, Ginsberg R, Pajak TF, et al. Chemotherapy followed by surgery compared with surgery alone for localized esophageal cancer. *N Engl J Med.* 1998;339:1979-1984.
119. Kelsen DP, Winter KA, Gunderson LL, et al. Long-term results of RTOG trial 8911 (USA Intergroup 113): a random assignment trial comparison of chemotherapy followed by surgery compared with surgery alone for esophageal cancer. *J Clin Oncol.* 2007;25:3719-3725.
120. Allum WH, Stenning SP, Bancewicz J, Clark PI, Langley RE. Long-term results of a randomized trial of surgery with or without preoperative chemotherapy in esophageal cancer. *J Clin Oncol.* 2009;27:5062-5067.
121. Ando N, Kato H, Igaki H, et al. A randomized trial comparing postoperative adjuvant chemotherapy with cisplatin and 5-fluorouracil versus preoperative chemotherapy for localized advanced squamous cell carcinoma of the thoracic esophagus (JCOG9907). *Ann Surg Oncol.* 2012;19:68-74.
122. Cunningham DA, Nankivell MG, Stenning SP, et al. Toxicity, surgical complications, and short-term mortality in a randomized trial of neoadjuvant cisplatin/5FU versus epirubicin/cisplatin and capecitabine prior to resection of lower esophageal/gastroesophageal junction (GOJ) adenocarcinoma (MRC OEO5, ISRCTN01852072, CRUK 02/010) [abstract]. *J Clin Oncol.* 32;2014:4014.
123. Gignoux M, Roussel A, Paillot B, et al. The value of preoperative radiotherapy in esophageal cancer: results of a study by the EORTC. *Recent Results Cancer Res.* 1988;110:1-13.
124. Arnott SJ, Duncan W, Gignoux M, et al. Preoperative radiotherapy for esophageal carcinoma. *Cochrane Database Syst Rev.* 2005;4:CD001799.
125. Tepper J, Krasna MJ, Niedzwiecki D, et al. Phase III trial of trimodality therapy with cisplatin, fluorouracil, radiotherapy, and surgery compared with surgery alone for esophageal cancer: CALGB 9781. *J Clin Oncol.* 2008;26:1086-1092.
126. Gebski V, Burmeister B, Smithers BM, Foo K, Zalcberg J, Simes J. Survival benefits from neoadjuvant chemoradiotherapy or chemotherapy in oesophageal carcinoma: a meta-analysis. *Lancet Oncol.* 2007;8:226-234.
127. van Hagen P, Hulshof MCCM, van Lanschot JJB, et al.

Preoperative chemoradiotherapy for esophageal or junctional cancer. *N Engl J Med*. 2012;366:2074-2084.

128. Oppedijk V, van der Gaast A, van Lanschot JJ, et al. Patterns of recurrence after surgery alone versus preoperative chemoradiotherapy and surgery in the CROSS trials. *J Clin Oncol*. 2014;32:385-391.
129. Urschel JD, Vasan H. A meta-analysis of randomized controlled trials that compared neoadjuvant chemoradiation and surgery to surgery alone for resectable esophageal cancer. *Am J Surg*. 2003;185:538-543.
130. Malthaner RA, Wong RK, Rumble RB, Zuraw L. Neoadjuvant or adjuvant therapy for resectable esophageal cancer: a systematic review and meta-analysis. *BMC Med*. 2004;2:35.
131. Stahl M, Walz MK, Stuschke M, et al. Phase III comparison of preoperative chemotherapy compared with chemoradiotherapy in patients with locally advanced adenocarcinoma of the esophagogastric junction. *J Clin Oncol*. 2009;27:851-856.
132. Stahl M, Mariette C, Haustermans K, Cervantes A, Arnold D. Oesophageal cancer: ESMO Clinical Practice Guidelines for diagnosis, treatment and follow-up. *Ann Oncol*. 2013;24(suppl 6):vi51-56.
133. Pouliquen X, Levard H, Hay JM, McGee K, Fingerhut A, Langlois-Zantin O. 5-Fluorouracil and cisplatin therapy after palliative surgical resection of squamous cell carcinoma of the esophagus. A multicenter randomized trial. French Associations for Surgical Research. *Ann Surg*. 1996;223:127-133.
134. Ando N, Iizuka T, Ide H, et al. Surgery plus chemotherapy compared with surgery alone for localized squamous cell carcinoma of the thoracic esophagus: a Japan Clinical Oncology Group Study—JCOG9204. *J Clin Oncol*. 2003;21:4592-4596.
135. Heroor A, Fujita H, Sueyoshi S, et al. Adjuvant chemotherapy after radical resection of squamous cell carcinoma in the thoracic esophagus: who benefits? A retrospective study. *Dig Surg*. 2003;20:229-235.
136. Teniere P, Hay JM, Fingerhut A, Fagniez PL. Postoperative radiation therapy does not increase survival after curative resection for squamous cell carcinoma of the middle and lower esophagus as shown by a multicenter controlled trial. French University Association for Surgical Research. *Surg Gynecol Obstet*. 1991;173:123-130.
137. Xiao ZF, Yang ZY, Liang J, et al. Value of radiotherapy after radical surgery for esophageal carcinoma: a report of 495 patients. *Ann Thorac Surg*. 2003;75:331-336.
138. Fok M, Sham JS, Choy D, Cheng SW, Wong J. Postoperative radiotherapy for carcinoma of the esophagus: a prospective, randomized controlled study. *Surgery*. 1993;113:138-147.
139. Malthaner RA, Wong RK, Rumble RB, Zuraw L. Neoadjuvant or adjuvant therapy for resectable esophageal cancer: a clinical practice guideline. *BMC Cancer*. 2004;4:67.
140. Cooper JS, Guo MD, Herskovic A, et al. Chemoradiotherapy of locally advanced esophageal cancer: long-term follow-up of a prospective randomized trial (RTOG 85-01). Radiation Therapy Oncology Group. *JAMA*. 1999;281:1623-1627.
141. Coia LR, Minsky BD, Berkey BA, et al. Outcome of patients receiving radiation for cancer of the esophagus: results of the 1992-1994 Patterns of Care Study. *J Clin Oncol*. 2000;18:455-462.
142. Minsky BD, Pajak TF, Ginsberg RJ, et al. INT 0123 (Radiation Therapy Oncology Group 94-05) phase III trial of combined-modality therapy for esophageal cancer: high-dose versus standard-dose radiation therapy. *J Clin Oncol*. 2002;20:1167-1174.
143. Ajani JA, Winter K, Komaki R, et al. Phase II randomized trial of two nonoperative regimens of induction chemotherapy followed by chemoradiation in patients with localized carcinoma of the esophagus: RTOG 0113. *J Clin Oncol*. 2008;26:4551-4556.
144. Bedenne L, Michel P, Bouche O, et al. Chemoradiation followed by surgery compared with chemoradiation alone in squamous cancer of the esophagus: FFCD 9102. *J Clin Oncol*. 2007;25:1160-1168.
145. Chiu PW, Chan AC, Leung SF, et al. Multicenter prospective randomized trial comparing standard esophagectomy with chemoradiotherapy for treatment of squamous esophageal cancer: early results from the Chinese University Research Group for Esophageal Cancer (CURE). *J Gastrointest Surg*. 2005;9:794-802.
146. Stahl M. Is there any role for surgery in the multidisciplinary treatment of esophageal cancer? *Ann Oncol*. 2010;21(suppl 7): vii283-285.
147. Bang YJ, Van Cutsem E, Feyereislova A, et al. Trastuzumab in combination with chemotherapy versus chemotherapy alone for treatment of HER2-positive advanced gastric or gastro-oesophageal junction cancer (ToGA): a phase 3, open-label, randomised controlled trial. *Lancet*. 2010;376:687-697.
148. Wagner AD, Grothe W, Haerting J, Kleber G, Grothey A, Fleig WE. Chemotherapy in advanced gastric cancer: a systematic review and meta-analysis based on aggregate data. *J Clin Oncol*. 2006;24:2903-2909.
149. Van Cutsem E, Moiseyenko VM, Tjulandin S, et al. Phase III study of docetaxel and cisplatin plus fluorouracil compared with cisplatin and fluorouracil as first-line therapy for advanced gastric cancer: a report of the V325 Study Group. *J Clin Oncol*. 2006;24:4991-4997.
150. Cunningham D, Starling N, Rao S, et al. Capecitabine and oxaliplatin for advanced esophagogastric cancer. *N Engl J Med*. 2008;358:36-46.
151. Koizumi W, Narahara H, Hara T, et al. S-1 plus cisplatin versus S-1 alone for first-line treatment of advanced gastric cancer (SPIRITS trial): a phase III trial. *Lancet Oncol*. 2008;9:215-221.
152. US Food and Drug Administration. Trastuzumab. Office of Medical Products and Tobacco. http://www.fda.gov/AboutFDA/CentersOffices/OfficeofMedicalProductsandTobacco/CDER/ucm230418.htm. Accessed September 21, 2015.
153. Ohtsu A, Shah MA, Van Cutsem E, et al. Bevacizumab in combination with chemotherapy as first-line therapy in advanced gastric cancer: a randomized, double-blind, placebo-controlled phase III study. *J Clin Oncol*. 2011;29:3968-3976.
154. Van Cutsem E, de Haas S, Kang YK, et al. Bevacizumab in combination with chemotherapy as first-line therapy in advanced gastric cancer: a biomarker evaluation from the AVAGAST randomized phase III trial. *J Clin Oncol*. 2012;30:2119-2127.
155. Shen L, Li J, Xu J, et al. Bevacizumab plus capecitabine and cisplatin in Chinese patients with inoperable locally advanced or metastatic gastric or gastroesophageal junction cancer: randomized, double-blind, phase III study (AVATAR study). *Gastric Cancer*. 2015;18:168-176.
156. Lordick F, Kang YK, Chung HC, et al. Capecitabine and cisplatin with or without cetuximab for patients with previously untreated advanced gastric cancer (EXPAND): a randomised, open-label phase 3 trial. *Lancet Oncol*. 2013;14:490-499.
157. Waddell T, Chau I, Cunningham D, et al. Epirubicin, oxaliplatin, and capecitabine with or without panitumumab for patients with previously untreated advanced oesophagogastric cancer (REAL3): a randomised, open-label phase 3 trial. *Lancet Oncol*. 2013;14:481-489.
158. Okines AF, Gonzalez de Castro D, Cunningham D, et al. Biomarker analysis in oesophagogastric cancer: Results from the REAL3 and TransMAGIC trials. *Eur J Cancer*. 2013;49(9):2116-2125.
159. Hecht JR, Qin S, Chung HC, et al. Lapatinib in combination with capecitabine plus oxaliplatin (CapeOx) in HER2-positive advanced or metastatic gastric, esophageal, or gastroesophageal adenocarcinoma (AC): the TRIO-013/LOGiC Trial [abstract]. *J Clin Oncol*. 2013;31:LBA4001.
160. Fuchs CS, Tomasek J, Yong CJ, et al. Ramucirumab monotherapy for previously treated advanced gastric or gastro-oesophageal junction adenocarcinoma (REGARD): an international,

randomised, multicentre, placebo-controlled, phase 3 trial. *Lancet.* 2014;383(9911):31-39.

161. Thuss-Patience PC, Kretzschmar A, Bichev D, et al. Survival advantage for irinotecan versus best supportive care as second-line chemotherapy in gastric cancer: a randomised phase III study of the Arbeitsgemeinschaft Internistische Onkologie (AIO). *Eur J Cancer.* 2011;47:2306-2314.
162. Cook N, Marshall A, Blazeby JM, et al. Cougar-02: a randomized phase III study of docetaxel versus active symptom control in patients with relapsed esophago-gastric adenocarcinoma [abstract]. *J Clin Oncol.* 2013;31:4023.
163. Wilke H, Muro K, Van Cutsem E, et al. Ramucirumab plus paclitaxel versus placebo plus paclitaxel in patients with previously treated advanced gastric or gastro-oesophageal junction adenocarcinoma (RAINBOW): a double-blind, randomised phase 3 trial. *Lancet Oncol.* 2014;15:1224-1235.
164. Kang JH, Lee SI, Lim do H, et al. Salvage chemotherapy for pretreated gastric cancer: a randomized phase III trial comparing chemotherapy plus best supportive care with best supportive care alone. *J Clin Oncol.* 2012;30:1513-1518.
165. Higuchi K, Tanabe S, Shimada K, et al. Biweekly irinotecan plus cisplatin versus irinotecan alone as second-line treatment for advanced gastric cancer: a randomised phase III trial (TCOG GI-0801/BIRIP trial). *Eur J Cancer.* 2014;50:1437-1445.
166. Ohtsu A, Ajani JA, Bai YX, et al. Everolimus for previously treated advanced gastric cancer: results of the randomized, double-blind, phase III GRANITE-1 study. *J Clin Oncol.* 2013;31:3935-3943.
167. Bang Y-J. A randomized, open-label, phase III study of lapatinib in combination with weekly paclitaxel versus weekly paclitaxel alone in the second-line treatment of HER2 amplified advanced gastric cancer (AGC) in Asian population: Tytan study [abstract]. *J Clin Oncol.* 2013;31:11.
168. Dutton SJ, Ferry DR, Blazeby JM, et al. Gefitinib for oesophageal cancer progressing after chemotherapy (COG): a phase 3, multicentre, double-blind, placebo-controlled randomised trial. *Lancet Oncol.* 2014;15:894-904.
169. Lennerz JK, Kwak EL, Ackerman A, et al. MET amplification identifies a small and aggressive subgroup of esophagogastric adenocarcinoma with evidence of responsiveness to crizotinib. *J Clin Oncol.* 2011;29:4803-4810.
170. Oliner KS, Abraham RT, Lan T, et al. Evaluation of MET pathway biomarkers in a phase II study of rilotumumab (R, AMG 102) or placebo (P) in combination with epirubicin, cisplatin, and capecitabine (ECX) in patients (pts) with locally advanced or metastatic gastric (G) or esophagogastric junction (EGJ) cancer [abstract]. *J Clin Oncol.* 2012;30:4005.
171. Iveson T, Donehower RC, Davidenko I, et al. Rilotumumab in combination with epirubicin, cisplatin, and capecitabine as first-line treatment for gastric or oesophagogastric junction adenocarcinoma: an open-label, dose de-escalation phase 1b study and a double-blind, randomised phase 2 study. *Lancet Oncol.* 2014;15:1007-1018.
172. Manish A, Shah JYC, Huat ITB, et al. Randomized phase II study of FOLFOX +/- MET inhibitor, onartuzumab (O), in advanced gastroesophageal adenocarcinoma (GEC) [abstract]. *J Clin Oncol.* 2015;33(suppl 3):2.
173. Kwak EL, Hamid O, Janku F, et al. Clinical activity of AMG 337, an oral MET kinase inhibitor, in adult patients (pts) with MET-amplified gastroesophageal junction (GEJ), gastric (G), or esophageal (E) cancer [abstract]. *J Clin Oncol.* 2015;33(suppl 3):1.
174. Bang YJ, Lee KW, Cho JY, et al. Olaparib plus paclitaxel in patients with recurrent or metastatic gastric cancer: a randomized, double-blind phase II study [abstract]. *J Clin Oncol.* 2013;31(suppl):4013.
175. Li J, Qin S, Xu J, et al. Apatinib for chemotherapy-refractory advanced metastatic gastric cancer: results from a randomized, placebo-controlled, parallel-arm, phase II trial. *J Clin Oncol.* 2013;31:3219-3225.
176. Qin S. Phase III study of apatinib in advanced gastric cancer: a randomized, double-blind, placebo-controlled trial [abstract]. *J Clin Oncol.* 2014;32:4003.
177. Penniment MG. Full report of the TROG 03.01, NCIC CTG ES2 multinational phase III study in advanced esophageal cancer comparing palliation of dysphagia and quality of life in patients treated with radiotherapy or chemoradiotherapy [abstract]. *J Clin Oncol.* 2015;33:6.
178. Ajani JA, Rodriguez W, Bodoky G, et al. Multicenter phase III comparison of cisplatin/S-1 with cisplatin/infusional fluorouracil in advanced gastric or gastroesophageal adenocarcinoma study: the FLAGS trial. *J Clin Oncol.* 2010;28:1547-1553.

21 Pancreatic Cancer

第二十一章　胰腺癌

Jennifer B. Goldstein
Rachna T. Shroff
Robert A. Wolff
Milind M. Javle

中文导读

胰腺癌是当今肿瘤学家面临的最具挑战性的恶性肿瘤之一。胰腺癌预后差，与癌症相关死亡仅次于肺癌、结直肠癌和乳腺癌。低效的筛查策略、高难度及创伤的手术策略，以及化疗、放疗效果不佳等是胰腺癌患者的存活率低的原因。本章从流行病学、危险因素、肿瘤发生的分子机制、病理学、临床表现、诊断和分期以及临床治疗策略等方面详细讲解了对胰腺癌的认识。本章着重介绍了针对可切除胰腺癌和转移性胰腺癌在MD安德森癌症中心多学科团队分别采取的不同治疗策略和流程。最后，本文展望了分子靶向治疗、抗血管治疗、间质改造和免疫治疗等在胰腺癌治疗中的发展前景。

PANCREATIC CANCER

When clinicians use the term *pancreatic cancer,* they refer to adenocarcinoma of the pancreas, one of the most challenging malignancies facing oncologists today. This disease is characterized by significant morbidity and poor prognosis.

At the University of Texas MD Anderson Cancer Center (MDACC), we manage patients with pancreatic cancer with a multidisciplinary team and view palliation as the primary goal. However, for patients with potentially resectable disease, we take an aggressive approach whenever appropriate. In the setting of advanced disease, cure is not possible, but as our understanding of carcinogenesis, invasion, and metastasis expands, more effective therapeutic strategies are expected to emerge. This chapter reviews our current knowledge about pancreatic cancer, including its epidemiology, risk factors, molecular biology, diagnosis and staging, and clinical strategies for therapy.

HARD FACTS ABOUT PANCREATIC CANCER

Pancreatic cancer, the most common pancreatic neoplasm, is an aggressive and often rapidly fatal malignancy. In the United States, it represents 2% of all cancer cases but accounts for 5% of all cancer deaths ([1]). Currently, it is the fourth leading cause of cancer death, ranking behind lung, colorectal, and breast cancer. While evidence suggests marginal improvements in 5-year survival rates over the last 25 years (2% in 1974-1976, 3% in 1983-1985, and 4% in 1992-1997), life expectancy remains short and is generally measured in months ([2]). By 2030, deaths due to pancreas cancer are projected to increase dramatically and will become the second leading cause of cancer-related death ([3]). Significant improvements in survival have been hampered by a number of factors, including inefficient screening strategies, technically challenging and often debilitating surgery, and minimally effective chemotherapy and radiotherapy.

Pancreatic cancer is a dynamic disease, and sudden changes in clinical status occur frequently. Patients may rapidly develop worsening pain, biliary obstruction, or stent occlusion with cholangitis, thromboembolism, peritoneal carcinomatosis, or intractable ascites. Any of these problems may preclude the timely delivery of cytotoxic therapy and limit survival. Therefore, most efforts should focus on symptom control, but for patients with adequate performance status (PS), treatment is encouraged.

EPIDEMIOLOGY

There are approximately 45,000 new cases of pancreatic cancer each year in the United States and 330,000 cases worldwide. Incidence rates are highest in industrialized societies and Western countries. Of note, the risk of pancreatic cancer among African Americans, in whom pancreatic cancer mortality rates are higher than most other ethnic groups in the United States, is considerably higher than the rates for African blacks ([4]). These observations implicate environmental factors conspiring with genetic background as causes of the increased risk.

The risk of developing pancreatic cancer is low in the first three to four decades of life but increases sharply after the age of 50. Average age at the time of diagnosis is 72 years. Pancreatic cancer is uncommon in patients under 40. In the past, pancreatic cancer occurred more frequently in men, but now the disease is becoming more common in women, probably secondary to the increased use of tobacco by women.

RISK FACTORS FOR PANCREATIC CANCER

Surprisingly, relatively little is known about the risk factors for the development of pancreatic cancer. Table 21-1 summarizes genetic and environmental factors associated with an increased risk.

Tobacco

Aside from age, the only consistently reported risk factor for pancreatic cancer is cigarette smoking. Cigarette smoking is estimated to account for roughly 30% of pancreatic cancer mortality ([5]). Experimental models have demonstrated that nitrosamines found in tobacco smoke are carcinogenic for the pancreas. Research performed at MDACC has shown that smoking-related aromatic DNA adducts and other types of DNA damage may be critical in carcinogenesis.

Diabetes Mellitus

Diabetes has been implicated both as an early manifestation of pancreatic cancer and as a predisposing factor. A meta-analysis published between 1975 and 1994 showed that pancreatic cancer occurred with increased frequency in patients with long-standing diabetes (diagnosed at least 5 years prior to the diagnosis or death due to pancreatic cancer) ([6]). It is believed that insulin resistance and secondary hyperinsulinism may be involved in pancreatic carcinogenesis.

Table 21-1 Acquired and Genetic Risks Factors Associated With Pancreatic Cancer

Acquired Risk Factors	Relative Risk	Comments
Tobacco smoking	2-5	Risk increases with increasing exposure
Diabetes mellitus	2	Not all authorities concur; many patients have altered glucose metabolism on presentation
High body mass index	2	
Chronic pancreatitis	13-18	Not all authorities concur with this degree of increased risk
Inherited Disorders	**Relative Risk**	**Known Defects**
Hereditary pancreatitis	10-53	PRSS1
FAMMM syndrome	22	p16INK/CDKN2
HNPCC	8	MLH1, MSH2, MSH6
Peutz-Jeghers syndrome	13-30	LBK1/STK11
Familial adenomatous polyposis	4-5	APC
Li-Fraumeni syndrome	?	p53
Familial breast and ovarian cancer	3-5	DNA repair pathways, BRCA2

FAMMM, familial atypical mole and melanoma; HNPCC, hereditary nonpolyposis colon cancer.

Chronic Pancreatitis

Early clinical studies have suggested an association between chronic pancreatitis and pancreatic cancer. In a study of 715 patients with chronic pancreatitis diagnosed between 1971 and 1995, there was a 13- to 18-fold increase in pancreatic cancer rates ([7]).

Studies have suggested that hereditary pancreatitis, in particular, may affect the risk. Lowenfels and Maisonneuve studied 246 patients with hereditary pancreatitis from 10 countries. The estimated cumulative risk of pancreatic cancer by age 70 was approximately 40%, with a mean age at diagnosis of 57 years ([8]). Molecular data strongly suggested that mutations in the trypsinogen gene *PRSS1* play an important role in hereditary and possibly acquired forms of pancreatitis ([9]).

Diet

Positive associations have been discovered between pancreatic cancer and meat and carbohydrate intake. However, there is no consensus on the contribution of dietary fat. Epidemiologic studies of pancreatic cancer have shown a protective role for high fruit and vegetable intake. This effect may be related to dietary folate and other methyl donor groups.

Body Mass Index

Epidemiologic studies have also implicated a high body mass index as increasing risk for pancreatic cancer. This may be explained by relative hyperinsulinemia thought to promote pancreatic carcinogenesis ([10]).

Familial Pancreatic Cancer and Other Genetic Syndromes

Patients with pancreatic cancer who have two first-degree relatives with a history of pancreatic cancer are defined as having familial pancreatic cancer. The estimated relative risk for other family members is increased 10- to 20-fold over the general population. In addition, hereditary nonpolyposis colorectal cancer, ataxia-telangiectasia, Peutz-Jeghers syndrome, familial breast and ovarian cancer, and familial atypical multiple-mole melanoma are all associated with increased risk of pancreatic cancer ([11]).

The familial breast and ovarian cancer syndrome, associated with mutations in the *BRCA* genes, accounts for 17% of cases ([12]). The BRCA1 and BRCA2 proteins are key components of homologous recombination through the repair of DNA double-strand breaks. Cells deficient in these proteins demonstrate genomic instability and a tendency toward malignant transformation ([13]). The poly(ADP-ribose) polymerase (PARP) enzyme is integral for single-stranded DNA repair, and inhibition results in DNA breaks that require intact BRCA proteins for repair. In the presence of mutant BRCA proteins, PARP inhibition results in synthetic lethality ([14]).

Preclinical work has demonstrated the sensitivity of *BRCA* mutated pancreatic cancer cell lines to cross-linking chemotherapeutic agents, such as mitomycin-c and cisplatin ([15]). This finding has translated clinically as studies have shown superior overall survival and response in patients with advanced pancreatic cancer with *BRCA* mutations treated with platinum ([13]).

Furthermore, studies with PARP inhibitors have shown promise either alone or in combination with cytotoxic chemotherapy ([16]). Currently, an ongoing study is investigating the efficacy of a single-agent PARP inhibitor, rucaparib, in patients with advanced pancreatic cancer with known *BRCA* mutations.

Occupational Exposures

Exposure to carcinogens in the workplace has been implicated in pancreatic cancer, but with the possible exception of formaldehyde, the available evidence is insufficient to identify any specific exposure to increase the risk.

Prior Gastrointestinal Surgery

Surgical procedures such as gastrectomy and cholecystectomy have been reported to increase risk and are possibly linked to elevated levels of cholecystokinin and hypergastrinemia. However, other studies have not demonstrated such an association ([17]).

MOLECULAR EVENTS IN HUMAN PANCREATIC CARCINOGENESIS

The molecular events leading to pancreatic cancer have not been fully elucidated, but mutations in a few oncogenes and tumor suppressors appear critical for carcinogenesis. Investigators from Johns Hopkins performed a comprehensive genomic analysis of pancreatic cancer reported in the journal *Science*. They noted an average of 63 alterations, the majority of which were point mutations. These alterations defined a core set of 12 cellular signaling pathways and processes that were altered in the majority of pancreatic cancers. These included the K-*ras*, *wnt/notch*, hedgehog, *TGF-β*, integrin, and JNK signaling pathways ([18]). Recently, Waddell et al characterized pancreatic cancer into four subtypes termed stable, locally rearranged, scattered, and unstable ([19]).

Oncogene Mutation: The ras Oncogene

Pancreatic cancer has the highest frequency of K-*ras* mutation among all human cancers. Greater than 85% of cases have an activating point mutation in the K-*ras* gene, most commonly a G-to-T transversion at codon 12 ([20]). This leads to constitutive activation of RAS, leading to growth-promoting signal cascades via the mitogen-activated protein (MAP) kinase pathway. Preclinical models have implicated this mutation as a very early event in carcinogenesis. The *ras* oncogene mutations were also retrospectively seen in pancreatic juice collected 3.5 years prior to a patient's diagnosis of pancreatic cancer ([21]).

Tumor Suppressor Gene Mutation and Inactivation

The *p16* tumor suppressor gene is inactivated in approximately 95% of pancreatic cancers; this typically occurs later in carcinogenesis. The second most frequently inactivated tumor suppressor gene, *p53*, located on chromosome 17p, also appears to be a late event in tumorigenesis. The *DPC4* gene (SMAD4) is inactivated in 55% of pancreatic adenocarcinomas and, like *p53*, is a relatively late event in tumorigenesis. In a comprehensive mutational analysis of 42 pancreatic ductal cancers, Rozenblum and colleagues found individual mutational frequencies of tumor suppressor genes *p16*, *p53*, *DPC4*, and *BRCA2* were 82%, 76%, 53%, and 10%, respectively ([21]).

The Multistep Sequence of Pancreatic Carcinogenesis

Current data suggest a temporal sequence of molecular events in pancreatic carcinogenesis leading from an "adenomatous" or proliferative ductal cell phenotype to pancreatic intraepithelial neoplasia (Pan-IN) and finally to invasive cancer. This theory has been supported by the recognition of noninvasive proliferative ductal lesions (Pan-IN1) that demonstrate mutations commonly found in pancreatic cancer. Growing evidence suggests that the gradual accumulation of genetic and biochemical alterations in early lesions causes progression to higher levels of dysplasia (Pan-IN2 and Pan-IN3) and ultimately to cancer.

Other Molecular Events in Pancreatic Carcinogenesis, Invasion, and Metastasis

The overexpression of epidermal growth factor receptor (*EGFR*), vascular endothelial growth factor (VEGF), matrix metalloproteinases, cyclooxygenase 2 (COX-2), hedgehog signaling, and insulinlike growth factor type 1 (IGF-1) pathways have been implicated in pancreatic cancer. Studies conducted at MDACC have also demonstrated that the nuclear transcription factor–κB (NF-κB) is commonly activated in pancreatic cancer ([22]).

Hedgehog Signaling Pathway

Hedgehog signaling is an essential pathway during embryogenesis of the normal pancreas, and its dysregulation has been reported in precancerous PanIN-1 and -2 as well as in primary and metastatic pancreatic adenocarcinomas. Inhibition of hedgehog signaling by cyclopamine-induced apoptosis and blocked proliferation in vitro and in vivo ([23]). Although debatable, hedgehog inhibition also depletes tumor-associated stroma and may play a role in the delivery of chemotherapeutic agents like gemcitabine [24]. Clinical trials of hedgehog inhibitors have failed to create a meaningful impact in this disease. Recent data indicated that stromal depletion may actually be deleterious, suggesting a critical need for accurate interpretation of preclinical data before incorporation into the clinical trial setting [25].

Insulinlike Growth Factor Type 1 Pathway

Insulinlike growth factor type 1 upregulates cell proliferation and invasiveness through activation of the phosphoinositide 3-kinase (PI3K)/Akt signaling pathway and downregulates the tumor suppressor chromosome 10 (PTEN). Akt mediates the gemcitabine and erlotinib resistance mechanisms. At MDACC, we recently concluded a clinical trial with dalotuzumab (MK-0646), which targets the IGF-1 pathway.

Targeted therapy has been a major focus of clinical research, taking priority over the study of more conventional cytotoxic agents. Preliminary studies with agents designed to abrogate RAS function have been disappointing [26]. Likewise, administration of inhibitors of matrix metalloproteinases has failed to demonstrate a meaningful clinical impact [27]. Recent studies of *EGFR*, VEGF, NF-kB, or COX-2 inhibitors are discussed in further detail in this chapter. Immune therapies may have a significant impact as well.

PATHOLOGY

Pancreatic acinar cells account for approximately 80% of the cell number and volume of the gland, with islet cells accounting for 1% to 2%. The ductal system is made up of single-layer, cuboidal epithelial cells comprising 10% to 15% of the gland's structure, with a sparse interlacing network of blood vessels, lymphatics, nerves, and collagenous stroma. In carcinoma, this architecture is markedly altered: The predominant histologic feature is a dense collagenous stroma with atrophic acini, remarkably preserved islet cell clusters, and a slight-to-moderate increase in the number of normal-appearing and cancerous ducts (Fig. 21-1). The diagnosis of ductal adenocarcinoma rests on the identification of mitoses, nuclear and cellular pleomorphism, discontinuity of ductal epithelium, and evidence of perineural, vascular, or lymphatic invasion.

Almost all malignant neoplasms of pancreatic origin (95%) arise from the exocrine portion of the gland. Tumors arising from the islets of Langerhans (endocrine) cells are much more infrequent, and primary nonepithelial tumors (eg, lymphomas or sarcomas) are extremely rare. The histologic classification of exocrine pancreatic neoplasms is presented in Table 21-2.

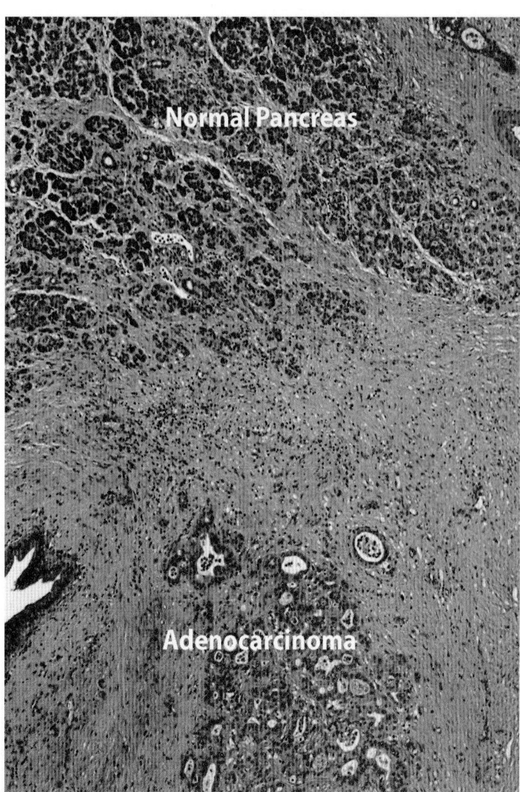

FIGURE 21-1 Photomicrograph of ductal adenocarcinoma of the pancreas with well-preserved islet cells and pancreatic architecture above and infiltrating tumor with poorly formed glandular structures below.

Table 21-2 Histologic Classification of Primary Exocrine Pancreatic Tumors

Malignant
Ductal adenocarcinoma
Mucinous cystadenocarcinoma
Acinar carcinoma
Unclassified large cell carcinoma
Small cell carcinoma
Pancreatoblastoma
Benign
Serous cystadenoma
Variable malignant potential
Intraductal papillary mucinous tumor
Mucinous cystadenoma
Papillary cystic neoplasm

CLINICAL PRESENTATION

The clinical presentation of pancreatic cancer is primarily dependent on the location of the tumor within the pancreas. The majority (85%) develop within the pancreatic head. About 10% are located in the pancreatic body and 5% in the tail. Nonspecific, poorly localized, epigastric or back pain is the most common initial presentation. It is usually caused by invasion or compression of the celiac, splanchnic, or mesenteric plexi. Tumors in the head or neck typically cause pain in the epigastric area or in the right upper quadrant of the abdomen. Cancers of the body may cause unremitting, severe back pain, and tumors in the pancreatic tail are associated with left upper quadrant pain.

Painless jaundice, another common presentation, is generally associated with tumors in the pancreatic head or uncinate process. When the tumor does not arise in proximity to the intrapancreatic portion of the bile duct, diagnosis may be delayed and characterized by abdominal pain or back pain without jaundice.

Acute pancreatitis, while uncommon, can be caused by a ductal adenocarcinoma; in patients with no other reason for acute pancreatitis (lack of gallstones, no history of alcohol or precipitating drugs) ([28]). Symptoms of chronic pancreatitis are relatively common, including diarrhea, bloating or constipation, abdominal distention, and weight loss. Patients with tail lesions often present with signs or symptoms of metastatic disease.

DIAGNOSIS AND STAGING OF PANCREATIC CANCER

Pancreatic cancer can be difficult to diagnose, particularly in patients with nonspecific complaints. Therefore, patients who present to the oncologist for treatment recommendations may harbor feelings of frustration and anger, having endured a significant delay from the onset of symptoms to diagnosis. Upper endoscopy may have been performed to rule out peptic ulcer disease or other pathology. Endoscopy is seldom helpful unless the pancreatic tumor has invaded the adjacent gastric or duodenal mucosa, leading to ulceration. In this uncommon situation, biopsies may demonstrate adenocarcinoma, and subsequent cross-sectional body imaging reveals an underlying pancreatic mass. Even more rarely, extrinsic compression on the gastric or duodenal wall may be appreciated endoscopically. Unfortunately, upper endoscopy may be misleading and demonstrate mild esophagitis, gastritis, or duodenitis, with or without evidence of *Helicobacter pylori*. Alternatively, patients complaining of right upper quadrant pain may undergo ultrasonography, potentially revealing gallstones, prompting cholecystectomy. This procedure is usually of temporary benefit and delays the discovery of a pancreatic tumor until pain returns. Last, for patients presenting with complaints of back pain, a musculoskeletal evaluation commonly ensues, with the procurement of plain x-rays, myelograms, or magnetic resonance imaging (MRI) of the spine.

For those patients who present with obstructive jaundice, suspicion of pancreatic cancer is sufficiently high that the diagnostic workup usually proceeds in an orderly fashion with directed imaging studies. These usually include an abdominal ultrasound, computed tomographic (CT) scan of the abdomen, or both. In some centers, discovery of a mass in the head of the pancreas without obvious metastatic disease or evidence for unresectability will prompt an exploratory laparotomy prior to biopsy confirmation of malignancy. This approach is not embraced at MDACC for reasons outlined further in this chapter.

Tissue Acquisition

With rare exception, all patients seen at MDACC are advised to undergo tissue confirmation. Cross-sectional imaging (multidetector CT) should always be performed before interventional endoscopic or radiologic procedures to prevent procedure-related inflammatory changes from confounding assessment. For patients presenting with obstructive jaundice, tissue may be obtained at the time of endoscopic retrograde cholangiopancreatography (ERCP) via brushings of the bile duct at the level of stricture. If brushings are nondiagnostic and CT or MRI suggests that the tumor may be nonmetastatic, we advise endoscopic ultrasound (EUS) with EUS-guided fine-needle aspiration (FNA) ([29]). This can be performed by experienced operators with minimal risk of duodenal perforation. Moreover, it is thought to decrease the risk of peritoneal or needle-track seeding, which has been reported among patients undergoing transcutaneous ultrasound- or CT-directed biopsies ([30]). Alternatively, when CT or MRI clearly demonstrates an unresectable, locally advanced cancer, CT- or ultrasound-guided transcutaneous biopsy may substitute for EUS-guided aspiration. If a patient presents with obstructive jaundice and biliary stricture without radiographic evidence of a pancreatic mass, EUS examination is also advised.

When there is radiographic evidence of metastatic disease and an obvious pancreatic mass, we recommend biopsy of a metastatic site, such as the liver. This confirms both the diagnosis and the presence of metastatic disease with one procedure.

Misdiagnosis of Pancreatic Cancer

It is not uncommon for patients to be misdiagnosed with pancreatic cancer. The most common mistake we see is in the setting of bulky peripancreatic adenopathy without a parenchymal pancreatic mass. Adenocarcinomas of the pancreas do metastasize to regional lymph nodes, but lymph nodes are typically small to medium in size. Bulky lymph nodes are seen in other gastrointestinal (GI) malignancies, such as tumors of the esophagus, stomach, duodenum, and occasionally, colon. Lymphoma, non–small cell lung cancer, and carcinomas of unknown primary origin may also lead to bulky peripancreatic lymphadenopathy, thus mimicking a primary pancreatic neoplasm. Thin-cut, dynamic-phase, contrast-enhanced CT will usually rule out the presence of a primary mass in the pancreas in this setting. Another helpful radiographic finding may be the presence or absence of atrophy of the pancreatic body and tail. Although commonly seen in adenocarcinomas originating in the head of the pancreas, this finding is usually absent in the setting of bulky peripancreatic adenopathy, neuroendocrine tumors, and acinar cell tumors. Importantly, patients with neuroendocrine tumors of the pancreas are sometimes misdiagnosed as having a poorly differentiated carcinoma of the pancreas.

High-Quality Computed Tomographic Imaging

The single most important imaging modality is multidetector (multislice) CT. This technique is used to objectively define (anatomically) potentially resectable disease. For optimal pretreatment staging, a CT report in a patient with suspected pancreatic cancer should include the following:

1. The presence or absence of a primary tumor in the pancreas or periampullary region
2. The presence or absence of peritoneal and hepatic metastases
3. Description of the patency of the superior mesenteric vein (SMV) and portal vein (PV) and the relationship of these veins to the tumor
4. Description of the relationship of the tumor to the superior mesenteric artery (SMA), celiac axis, and hepatic artery

Objective radiographic criteria can be used to define a potentially resectable primary tumor of the pancreatic head or uncinate process (Fig. 21-2). The MDACC criteria include: (1) no extrapancreatic disease; (2) a patent SMV and PV (assuming the technical ability to resect and reconstruct this venous confluence); and (3) a definable tissue plane between the tumor and regional arterial structures, including the celiac axis and SMA. Using CT staging and objective criteria for assessment of resectability, many centers have reported resectability rates as high as 75% to 80% ([31]). Of note, CT of the chest is not routinely part of our staging workup. However, if either plain chest x-rays or CT images of the lung bases reveal pulmonary nodules or other suspicious findings, a dedicated CT scan of the chest is obtained. Bone scans and brain imaging are rarely indicated and should not be part of routine staging.

Positron Emission Tomography

Positron emission tomographic (PET) scans are occasionally obtained in the setting of equivocal radiographic findings, such as indeterminate lesions in the liver or lungs. Lesions may be subcentimeter in size, and ^{18}F-fluorodeoxyglucose negative, even when metastatic disease is present ([32]). Scanning by PET is commonly considered when a patient has undergone previous resection and subsequently develops a rising CA19-9 and soft tissue changes in the surgical bed with no other evidence of relapse.

Serum CA19-9 Determinations

CA19-9 measures the specific carbohydrate moiety of the mucin MUC-1 ([33]). This is the most commonly elevated tumor marker in pancreatic cancer, but it is not specific and may be elevated in other GI tumors. Whether it should be measured prior to surgery as an independent predictor of resectability or as an adjunct to other clinical staging has not been rigorously studied. Most retrospective analyses generally suggested that a high preoperative CA19-9 level (>500-1,000 IU/mL) implies more advanced disease that is not amenable to resection. We retrospectively analyzed pretreatment CA19-9 levels obtained from 79 patients enrolled in a trial of gemcitabine-based preoperative chemoradiation. All patients had radiographically defined, biopsy-proven, resectable cancer without evidence of metastatic disease. It was found that serum levels greater than 668 IU/mL predicted either the development of overt metastatic disease prior to surgery or early relapse after surgical resection ([34]). Presently,

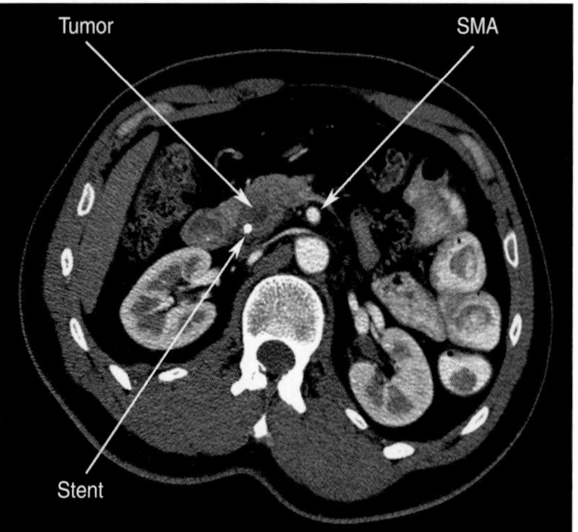

FIGURE 21-2 Computed tomographic image of tumor within the pancreatic head. Note the stent in the bile duct and the subtle low-density mass within the head. The superior mesenteric artery (SMA) has a fat plane completely surrounding it. This defines a potentially resectable tumor.

serum CA19-9 measurements are obtained at presentation to MDACC. When postoperative CA19-9 levels do not normalize within this time frame, it portends early relapse ([35]). Patients clinically staged as having locally advanced disease but with markedly elevated CA19-9 levels (>5,000) are suspected of having occult metastatic disease. These patients are usually advised to undergo a trial of systemic therapy with serial measurements of CA19-9 levels prior to considering chemoradiation. Improvement of CA19-9 of 50% has been correlated with an improved survival ([36]).

The Role of Laparoscopy

For patients with potentially resectable disease, some have advocated laparoscopy with biopsies and peritoneal washings as part of routine staging ([37, 38]). In our experience, fewer than 20% of patients with tumors in the head of the pancreas will have occult metastatic disease when laparoscopy is performed. Given the expense and expected negative findings for 80% of patients, our approach has been to limit this procedure to patients with indeterminate findings on CT ([39]). An exception applies to the small subset of patients who present with radiographically resectable tumors in the body or tail of the pancreas who are more likely to have occult metastatic disease. The chance of a visible peritoneal metastasis or positive cytology on peritoneal washing is sufficiently high to justify laparoscopy as part of staging ([40]).

The TNM System Versus Clinically Oriented Staging

The TNM (tumor, node, metastasis) staging system for pancreatic cancer is outlined in Table 21-3. For patients undergoing resection, the TNM system is somewhat useful in providing prognostic information and, to a lesser degree, in guiding adjuvant therapy. Generally, patients are staged as having potentially resectable disease, locally advanced unresectable disease, or metastatic disease. For patients with resectable disease who are able to tolerate it, surgery is indicated. Surgery can be preceded by preoperative or adjuvant therapy. Patients with metastatic disease and adequate PS usually receive systemic therapy. For patients presenting with locally advanced disease, treatment should be individualized and may initially involve either chemoradiation or systemic therapy.

Table 21-3 TNM Criteria for Pancreatic Adenocarcinoma TNM Definitions

Tx:	Primary tumor cannot be assessed
T0:	No evidence of primary tumor
Tis	Carcinoma in situ
T1:	Tumor <2 cm in greatest dimension
T2:	Tumor >2 cm in greatest dimension
T3:	Tumor extends beyond the pancreas but without involvement of the celiac axis or the superior mesenteric artery
T4:	Tumor involves the celiac axis or the superior mesenteric artery (unresectable primary tumor)
Nx:	Regional lymph node status cannot be assessed
N0:	No regional lymph node metastasis
N1:	Positive regional lymph node metastasis
Mx:	Distant metastasis cannot be assessed
M0:	No distant metastasis
M1:	Distant metastasis

Staging Classification

Stage	T	N	M
0	Tis	N0	M0
IA	T1	N0	M0
IB	T2	N0	M0
IIA	T3	N0	M0
IIB	T1-T3	N1	M0
III	T4	Any N	M0
IV	Any T	Any N	M1

Reproduced with permission from Edge SB, Byrd DR, Compton CC (eds): *AJCC Cancer Staging Manuarl*, 7th ed. New York, NY: Springer; 2010.

TREATMENT STRATEGIES FOR PANCREATIC CANCER

Resectable Pancreatic Cancer

It is widely known that surgery holds the only hope of cure for patients with pancreatic cancer. With some exceptions, resectable pancreatic cancers are limited to small tumors in the head of the pancreas. These are removed with a Whipple procedure ([41]), more appropriately described as a pancreaticoduodenectomy. Caution is advised when considering a resection of a tail neoplasm; even when these tumors appear localized, they are associated with a higher likelihood of peritoneal seeding compared to a head lesion. Body lesions are almost never amenable to resection.

Unfortunately, there are potential drawbacks associated with up-front surgery:

1. *Surgical morbidity and mortality are inversely correlated to experience with the procedure.* Several studies have confirmed significant differences in the risk of major perioperative complications and death between hospitals that perform the operation frequently and those that do not ([42, 43]). Moreover, long-term survival after pancreaticoduodenectomy is improved when performed at a high-volume center ([44]). This

is likely attributable to a combination of decreased operative mortality and superior patient selection.

2. *Positive surgical margins are associated with a very poor prognosis* (see Table 21-4). Surgical margins after pancreaticoduodenectomy can be either microscopically positive (R1 resection) or grossly positive (R2). Median survivals with a positive surgical margin usually range between 6 and 12 months, similar to, if not worse than, the survival of patients with locally advanced disease ([45, 46]). Many patients undergo laparotomy without adequate preoperative assessment. Some will be found to have unresectable tumors intraoperatively or be left with a grossly positive surgical margin when it might have been possible to predict this prior to surgery. Patients may therefore have a delay in chemoradiation or systemic therapy while the patient recovers. With the exception of patients who present with gastric outlet obstruction or biliary obstruction not amenable to endoscopic or percutaneous stenting, we discourage surgical intervention without high-quality radiographic evidence of resectability. If the surgeon has failed to perform a complete resection, surgery may even be deleterious and compromise the patient's survival.
3. *A substantial proportion of patients do not recover sufficiently to receive postoperative adjuvant therapy*. Pancreaticoduodenectomy is a major surgical procedure with removal of portions of the stomach, duodenum, pancreas, and bile duct requiring extensive reconstruction of the upper alimentary canal. Pancreatic anastomotic leaks and delayed gastric emptying are common complications. Retrospective analyses and prospective clinical trials of adjuvant therapy demonstrated that a significant percentage of people do not adequately recover to receive postoperative therapy. For example, Johns Hopkins University demonstrated that of 870 patients who underwent resection for pancreatic cancer with curative intent between 1993 and 2005, only 53% received adjuvant therapy ([47]). Furthermore, analyses of Medicare-eligible patients suggested that among patients 65 years of age or older, fewer than half receive adjuvant therapy ([48]). It is reasonable to assume that a substantial proportion of elderly patients have sufficient difficulty recovering from surgery and this has an impact on adjuvant therapy.
4. *Surgically resected patients remain at risk for local failure and metastatic disease*. Approximately 80% of resected patients will ultimately relapse and die of disease recurrence. The high risk of relapse stems from an inability to prevent locoregional failure and to eradicate microscopic metastatic disease. Factors predisposing to local recurrence have not been fully elucidated, but recent evidence implicated perineural invasion as an important mediating process. Invasion of nerve sheaths may occur as a pervasive superficial infiltration that cannot be appreciated intraoperatively, even by the most experienced surgeons.

Table 21-4 Median Survival Rates of Patients With a Gross (R2) or Microscopic (R1) Surgical Margin at the Time of Resection

Author	Number of Patients	Margin Status	Median Survival (Months)
Sohn	184	R1/R2	12
Neoptolemos	101	R1	11
Nishimura	70	R1/R2	6
Millikan	22	R1	8
Richter	72	R1/R2	12
Kuhlman	80	R1/R2	16
Takai	42	R1/R2	8

Once patients relapse with distant disease or local failure, no curative strategy is available. Adjuvant therapy, while tending to improve median survival, has not made any significant advances over the past 20 years.

The Role of Adjuvant Therapy

Since the mid-1980s, efforts have been directed toward improving outcomes for patients with resected disease by delivering postoperative adjuvant therapy intended to reduce the risk of relapse and improve long-term survival. Early retrospective analyses of resected patients suggested local failure rates as high as 50% to 80%, which prompted many centers to advocate radiotherapy as a component of adjuvant therapy. The first randomized trial, performed by the Gastrointestinal Tumor Study Group (GITSG), demonstrated a significant survival advantage with chemoradiation based on 5-fluorouracil (5-FU) compared with resection alone (21 vs 11 months) ([49]). The 5-year survival rates were 18% versus 8%, respectively. The European Organization for Research and Treatment of Cancer (EORTC) 40891 trial produced conflicting results 15 years later. In this case, 218 patients receiving 5-FU chemoradiation did not demonstrate a survival advantage over those on observation, although this population was more heterogeneous than that of GITSG because patients with periampullary cancer and those with an R1 resection were included ([50]).

Large randomized adjuvant trials were conducted by the European Study Group for Pancreatic Cancer (ESPAC). In the ESPAC-1 trial, 289 patients were randomized to observation, chemotherapy, chemoradiation, or chemoradiation followed by chemotherapy ([51]).

Interestingly, chemoradiation was found to have a deleterious effect on survival (median survival 15.9 vs 17.9 months, respectively, $P = .05$). On the other hand, chemotherapy appeared beneficial over observation, with a median survival of 20.1 months versus 15.5 months ($P = .009$). As a result of these studies, the role of radiation in adjuvant therapy became controversial. Radiation has been abandoned in the adjuvant setting in many European centers.

After gemcitabine showed superiority to 5-FU in advanced disease, a number of randomized trials tested its role in the adjuvant setting. The Radiation Therapy Oncology Group (RTOG) 9704 trial compared gemcitabine with 5-FU given before and after 5-FU–based chemoradiation. Gemcitabine demonstrated a modest, but not significant, improvement in survival over 5-FU (20.5 months compared to 16.9 months, $P = .09$) ([52]).

The benefit of adjuvant gemcitabine was further confirmed with the long-term data from the CONKO 001 trial. Investigators showed a significant improvement in disease-free survival and overall survival with the use of gemcitabine postoperatively (13 and 22.8 months, respectively) compared to surgery alone (6.9 and 20.2 months) ([53]). ESPAC-3 further compared postoperative gemcitabine to 5-FU ([54]). No statistical difference in survival was noted after a median follow-up of 34 months, although gemcitabine appeared to be better tolerated.

Picozzi and colleagues reported their findings of a phase II study involving adjuvant interferon alpha-2b (IFN-α2b), cisplatin, and continuous infusion 5-FU given concurrently with external beam radiation ([55]). In this study, 89 patients with R0 or R1 resections received IFN-α2b on days 1, 3, and 5 each week for 5½ weeks, cisplatin weekly for 6 weeks, and infusional 5-FU for 38 days with radiation dosed to 50.4 Gy. Overall survival at 18 months was 69% with a median disease-free survival of 14.1 months and overall survival of 25.4 months. Of the patients, 95% experienced grade 3 or greater toxicity. Additional combination trials, however, did not show an improvement in survival compared to 5-FU monotherapy ([56]). Table 21-5 summarizes the adjuvant trials.

Preoperative Therapy for Potentially Resectable Disease

Sadly, there has been no significant progress in adjuvant therapy since the GITSG study was first reported in 1985. More recent studies have been fairly consistent with the GITSG findings: Median survival for resected patients treated with postoperative therapy hovers around 20 months and remains at 12 months for patients undergoing surgery alone. Of the patients who undergo potentially curative surgery, up to 50% do not recuperate enough to begin postoperative

Table 21-5 Summary of Randomized and Nonrandomized Adjuvant Trials

Study Year	Number of Patients	Patients With R1 Resection (%)	Treatment A Median Survival (Months)	Treatment B Median Survival (Months)	*P* Value	Local Failure Rate (%)
GITSG 1985	49	0	5-FU/XRT + 5-FU	Observation	.035	NR
			21.0	10.9		
EORTC 1999	114	19	5-FU/XRT	Observation	.099	34
			17.1	12.6		
ESPAC-1 2004	289	18	5-FU/LV	No 5-FU/LV	.009	60
			20.1	15.5		
			5-FU/XRT	No 5-FU/XRT	.05	
			15.9	17.9		
RTOG 9704 2008	368	>35	Gem + 5-FU/XRT	5-FU + 5-FU/XRT	.09	34
			20.5	16.9		
CONKO 001 2008	388	19	Gem	Observation	.005	25
			22.8	20.2		
ESPAC-1/ESPAC-3 2009	458	25	5-FU/LV	Observation	.003	NR
			23.2	16.8		
ESPAC-3 (v2) 2009	1,088	35	Gem	5-FU/LV	.39	NR
			23.6	23.0		

5-FU, 5-fluorouracil; Gem, gemcitabine; LV, leucovorin; NR, not reported; XRT, radiation.

chemoradiation or require prolonged recovery to consider treatment. Moreover, rapid disease progression with early systemic relapse is not uncommon after surgery. Therefore, neoadjuvant therapy followed by surgery offers some theoretical advantages over immediate surgery.

Patients who present with potentially resectable disease are generally physiologically fit and make attractive candidates for neoadjuvant therapy. Preoperative therapy allows delivery of chemotherapy or chemoradiation to a relatively well-perfused tumor bed and provides early treatment to microscopic metastases. Positive surgical margins are commonly reported after up-front resection; this is associated with poor prognosis, suggesting that surgery alone provides inadequate local control. Preoperative therapy may provide for sufficient tumor destruction, particularly at the periphery, to increase the chances of a margin-negative resection. Preoperative therapy also allows for observation of the tumor's underlying biology, and those with aggressive disease are spared a major surgical procedure.

Five preoperative trials have been completed at MDACC (Table 21-6) ([57–61]). These trials, performed in sequence, have had nearly identical inclusion criteria, with standardized radiographic criteria for resectability, surgical technique, and assessment of resection margins. Our data demonstrated that preoperative therapy is associated with a relatively low local failure rate compared to adjuvant therapy and, over time, modest improvements in overall survival, especially with the use of gemcitabine over 5-FU or paclitaxel-based chemoradiation.

In the work of Evans et al, a total of 86 patients received gemcitabine followed by chemoradiation, and 74% of them were able to undergo pancreaticoduodenectomy ([57]). The median survival was 34 months compared to 7 months for those who did not receive resection. The pattern of failure favored distant metastases; thus, a second trial was designed to increase the amount of systemic therapy. This trial enrolled 90 patients to receive gemcitabine with cisplatin followed by chemoradiation, and 66% underwent resection. The addition of cisplatin did not improve survival beyond gemcitabine alone (31 vs 34 months). While these studies were not designed to be compared to adjuvant trials, the median survival in both preoperative studies was notably better than that seen in the adjuvant data we have to date. In the gemcitabine-based chemoradiation trial, complete pathologic responses were observed in two surgical specimens. While preoperative chemoradiation has not been established as a standard approach, by using preoperative therapy, negative surgical margins are more frequently reported. While these are probably not sufficient to ensure cure, they are likely to be necessary for extended survival (Fig. 21-3).

MDACC Approach to Adjuvant Therapy

At MDACC, adjuvant therapy is delivered with the following principles:

1. Patients must demonstrate adequate recovery from surgery to be considered for further treatment. This includes ample oral caloric intake and no significant impairment of the alimentary tract (delayed gastric emptying, dumping syndrome, uncontrolled pancreatic exocrine insufficiency). Adequate wound healing and absence of infection are also required. Patients should have a PS of 0 to 1.
2. Patients must have adequate hepatic and renal function with sufficient hematologic parameters to undergo cytotoxic therapy.
3. Restaging CT scans are obtained just prior to initiation of adjuvant therapy generally performed 6 to 10 weeks postoperatively. A serum CA19-9 level twice the upper limit of normal precludes patients from enrollment on adjuvant therapy on in-house protocols. Recent retrospective analysis suggested that 5% to 10% of patients who undergo surgery at MDACC will have early radiographic or serologic evidence of relapsing disease prior to initiation of adjuvant therapy. When this occurs, any further therapy is not considered adjuvant.

Table 21-6 Summary of Preoperative Trials Performed at MDACC

Author, Year	Number of Patients	Preoperative Regimen	Resection Rate (%)	% R1	Median Survival Resected Patients	Local Recurrence Rate (%)
Evans, 1992	28	5-FU + XRT 50.4 Gy	61		18	
Pisters, 1998	35	5-FU + XRT 30 Gy	57	10	25	10
Pisters, 2002	37	Paclitaxel + XRT 30 Gy	54	32	19	NR
Evans, 2008	86	Gem + XRT 30 Gy	75	12	34	11
Varadhachary, 2008	90	Gem/Cis then Gem + XRT 30 Gy	58	4	31	25

5-FU, 5-fluorouracil; Gem, gemcitabine; XRT, radiotherapy.

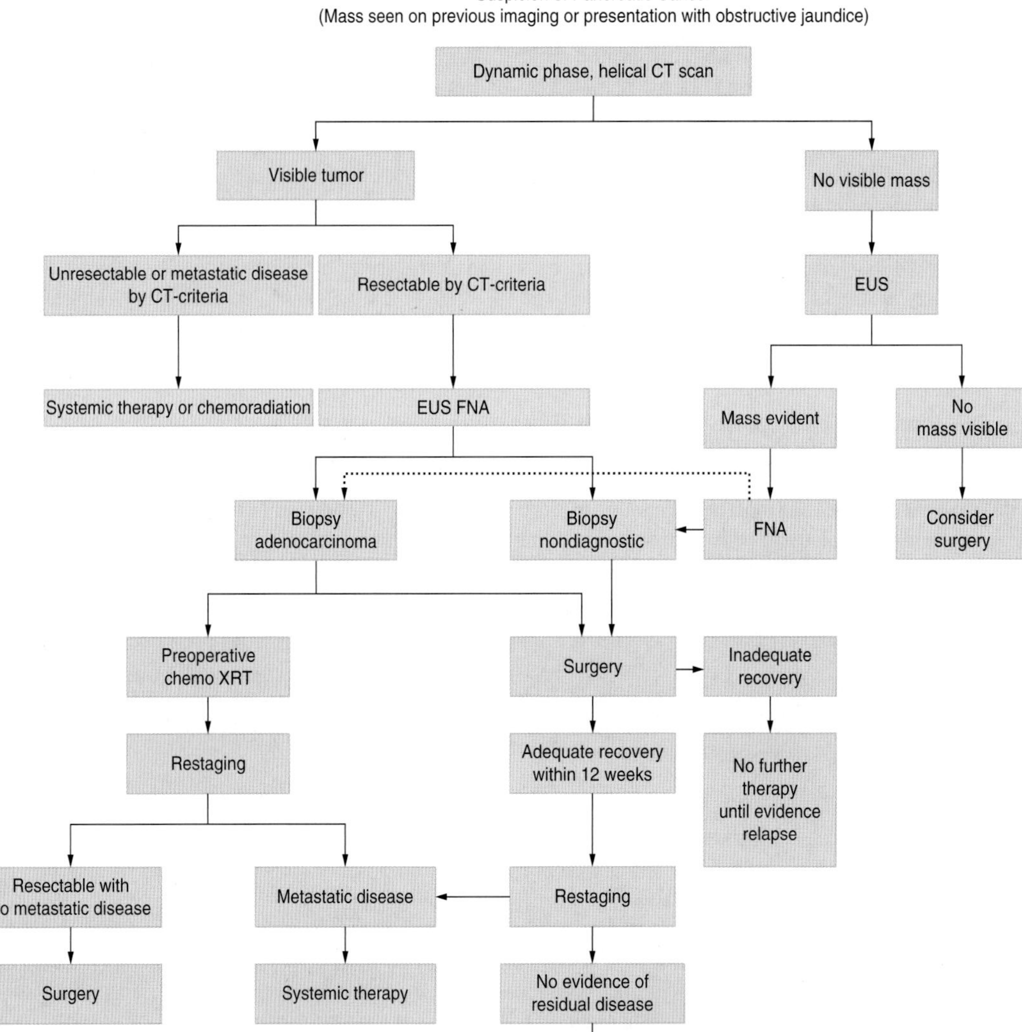

FIGURE 21-3 General algorithm for diagnostic workup and management of newly diagnosed pancreatic cancer.

4. Chemotherapy plus or minus chemoradiation remains the foundation of adjuvant therapy.

At MDACC, patients are encouraged to enroll in postoperative trials of adjuvant therapy. To extrapolate from the experience in locally advanced unresectable disease, patients benefiting from chemoradiation are those who have experienced stable disease with induction chemotherapy. Therefore, our approach at this time includes induction chemotherapy with gemcitabine or a gemcitabine-based doublet for 3 months followed by restaging scans. If no radiographic or serologic evidence of relapse is present at that time, chemoradiation with 5-FU or capecitabine is advised. Radiation is administered in a dose of 50.4 Gy in 28 fractions.

Once postoperative therapy has been completed, patients are followed with restaging CT scans, chest x-ray, physical examination, and standard laboratory tests, including CA19-9 every 6 months for the first 5 years and annually thereafter. A rising CA19-9 after adjuvant therapy does not trigger further systemic therapy until clear evidence of relapse based on physical examination or radiographic studies. Scanning by PET is considered in this situation.

MDACC Approach to Preoperative Therapy

Patients with clinical and radiographic evidence of potentially resectable disease are generally advised to receive protocol-based preoperative therapy, which typically involves chemoradiation. Chemoradiation regimens have varied, and our most encouraging results have been achieved with our gemcitabine-based regimen. After chemoradiation is completed, patients are allowed to recover over 4 to 5 weeks prior to restaging studies. For patients with no clinical or radiographic evidence of metastatic disease and no contraindications to surgery, laparotomy proceeds. At the time of exploration, when no visible evidence of distant disease is encountered, pancreaticoduodenectomy is performed. Postoperatively, further chemotherapy or radiation may be delivered based on the final pathology and the consensus of the multidisciplinary group. Patients are then followed expectantly with periodic restaging studies as outlined previously. Patients who relapse with adequate PS are offered further systemic therapy on or off protocol.

It is important to emphasize that we do not deliver preoperative therapy as a means of staging the primary tumor downward. The medical literature has scattered reports of neoadjuvant therapy being used to successfully stage down patients with locally advanced disease to the point of resectability ([62]). Caution is advised in interpreting these results because we believe it is possible to stage down patients with borderline or marginally resectable tumors (tumors that abut but do not encase the celiac artery or SMA). These tumors represent a discrete subset; their management, while similar, is more tailored. Figure 21-4 displays an algorithmic approach for resectable pancreatic cancer.

MDACC Approach to Patients With Borderline Resectable Pancreatic Cancer

As high-quality, dynamic-phase, helical CT scanning has developed, an appreciation for the existence of a distinct subset of tumors best described as borderline resectable or marginally resectable has emerged. In this situation, some authorities believe that up-front surgery is more likely to lead to an R1 or R2 rather than an R0 resection. This entity is defined as ≤180 tumor abutment of the SMA or celiac axis, short segment abutment or encasement of the common hepatic artery that is amenable to segmental resection and reconstruction, or short segment occlusion of the SMV, PV, or SMV-PV confluence with a normal SMV below and PV above the tumor to allow for reconstruction ([63]). Up to 40% of patients with borderline resectable disease have been seen at MDACC, and these patients have a median survival of more than 40 months.

At MDACC, patients with marginally resectable tumors are typically treated with gemcitabine-based chemotherapy for an indefinite period of time, with

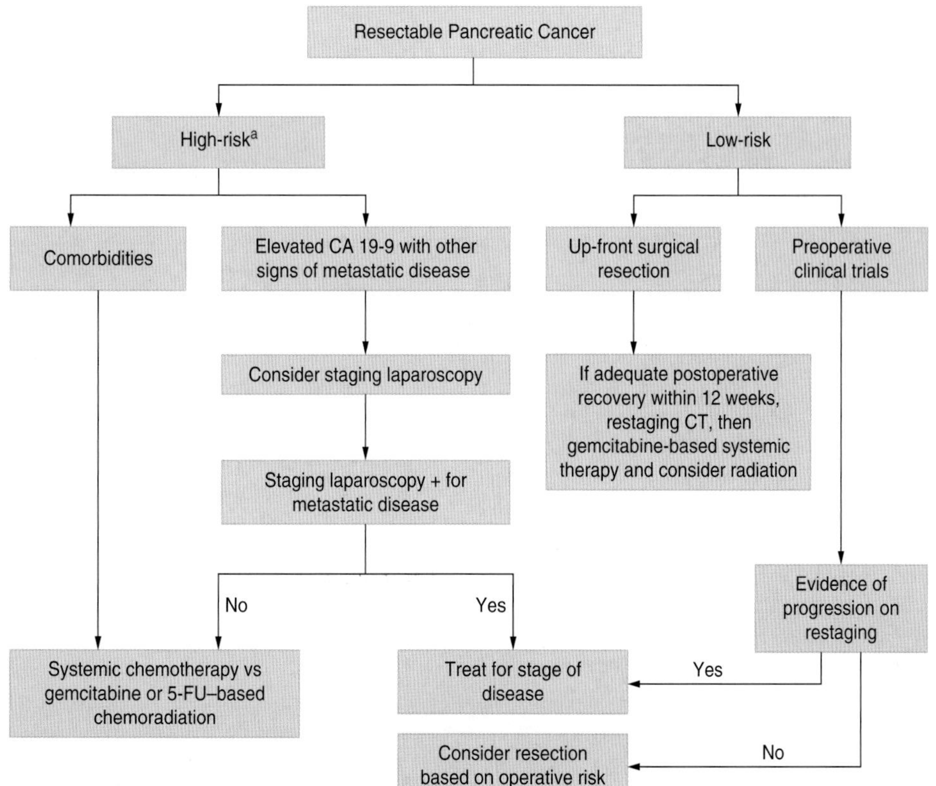

FIGURE 21-4 Treatment algorithm for the management of resectable pancreatic cancer. [a]High-risk clinical features: suspicion of metastatic disease; CA19-9 >1,000 with normal bilirubin; comorbidities suggesting high operative risk.

restaging studies every 2 months. Treatment is continued to maximum benefit, as defined by a nadir in the CA19-9 level or best radiographic response. Thereafter, chemoradiation is delivered, and subsequent restaging studies are performed about 4 to 6 weeks after treatment is complete. Surgery will proceed if there has been some evidence of tumor response, and if no interval development of metastatic disease is apparent, an attempt at surgery will proceed. It remains unclear whether the staging of such tumors downward to technical resectability is of biological significance; therefore, at least 6 months generally elapse at MDACC prior to the contemplation of surgery.

Management of Patients With Locally Advanced Disease

Patients are defined as having locally advanced pancreatic cancer when there is radiographic evidence of SMA or celiac artery encasement, occlusion of the SMV-PV confluence, or significant involvement of the common hepatic artery originating from the celiac trunk. There should be no clinical or radiographic evidence of metastatic disease. Currently, roughly half of all patients present with locally advanced disease. As with resectable pancreatic cancer, an understanding of certain principles will aid in decision making.

1. Locally advanced pancreatic cancer typically progresses over the course of some months. Local tumor progression with worsening pain, new or recurrent biliary obstruction, and gastric outlet obstruction represent difficult management problems. Development of metastatic disease is usually associated with worsening functional status and, unless preceded by a long progression-free interval, is rarely responsive to further therapy.
2. Assessment of response to therapy can be challenging. These tumors may be composed of small nests of adenocarcinoma surrounded by large areas of desmoplasia (Fig. 21-5). Even when cytotoxic therapy is effective, the desmoplastic component of the residual mass may not regress, and the overall tumor mass may appear unchanged. Furthermore, distinguishing the primary tumor mass from surrounding inflammatory changes can complicate the reliable measurement of tumors.
3. All surgical interventions should be considered carefully and be based on PS and life expectancy. Palliative nonsurgical procedures may produce results similar to those of aggressive surgery.
4. One of the primary reasons for considering chemoradiation for patients with locally advanced disease is palliation of pain. However, the clinical benefit associated with chemoradiation has not been rigorously studied. Minsky et al reported significant variations in the estimation of pain relief, with 31% to 77% of patients having improvement in pain after receiving chemoradiation for unresectable disease ([64]).

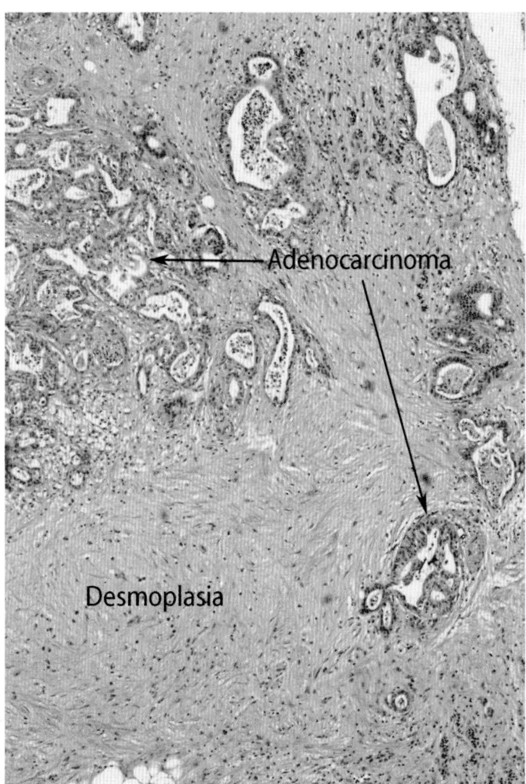

FIGURE 21-5 Photomicrograph of ductal adenocarcinoma of the pancreas with intense desmoplastic reaction. Even if the tumor cells regress in response to therapy, a residual fibrotic mass may remain. This confounds assessment of response to therapy using standard radiographic criteria.

Data Regarding Chemoradiation Based on 5-Fluoruracil

Support for chemoradiation originates from studies performed by the GITSG. In the original study, patients with locally advanced pancreatic cancer were randomly assigned to receive 40 Gy of radiation plus 5-FU, 60 Gy plus 5-FU, or 60 Gy alone. The median survival was 10 months in each of the chemoradiation groups and 6 months for patients who received 60 Gy without 5-FU ([65]). Of note, these patients had undergone laparotomy and were surgically staged. Only those patients with disease confined to the pancreas and peripancreatic organs, regional lymph nodes, or regional peritoneum were eligible for the study. While this made for a more uniform study population, it also introduced significant selection bias: Enrollment was limited to rapidly recovering patients. In subsequent GITSG studies, neither doxorubicin used as a radiation sensitizer nor multidrug chemotherapy with streptozocin, mitomycin, and 5-FU (SMF) alone or continued after chemoradiation was found to be superior to 5-FU–based chemoradiation ([66]). Additional chemotherapy after 5-FU–based chemoradiation increased toxicity without apparent therapeutic benefit.

In contrast to the results from the GITSG, an ECOG study suggested no benefit of chemoradiation over 5-FU alone ([67]). The ECOG study randomly assigned patients with locally advanced or incompletely resected pancreatic adenocarcinoma to receive chemoradiation (40 Gy and 600 mg/m^2/d 5-FU for 3 days) or 5-FU alone (600 mg/m^2/week). As in the GITSG studies, all patients were surgically staged and entered in the study within 6 weeks of surgery. The median survival was 8.3 months in the group that received chemoradiation and 8.2 months in the group that received 5-FU alone.

More recent trials of chemoradiation for locally advanced pancreatic cancer have investigated continuous infusion 5-FU in combination with EBRT (external beam radiation). The ECOG performed a phase I study to determine the maximal tolerated dose (MTD) of prolonged infusional 5-FU when combined with EBRT to 59.4 Gy. The MTD of 5-FU was 250 mg/m^2/d, with GI toxicity the dose-limiting factor ([68]). A subsequent study conducted in Japan demonstrated the feasibility of utilizing low-dose continuous infusion 5-FU (200 mg/m^2/d) over 5.5 weeks combined with a single course of EBRT to 50.4 Gy. This was followed by weekly 5-FU treatments until disease progression. The median survival of treated patients was 10 months, similar to that of patients treated with bolus 5-FU and EBRT in the GITSG trials ([69]). Thus, while infusional 5-FU may provide greater radiosensitivity than bolus 5-FU, no clear survival advantage has been established. In general, for selected patients, treatment programs consisting of EBRT and chemotherapy may result in median survivals of approximately 10 to 12 months and a 2-year survival rate of 20%. Long-term survivors are rare.

Concurrent Chemoradiation Versus Systemic Chemotherapy

Chemoradiotherapy was compared with chemotherapy in a randomized trial by the French Fédération Francophone de Cancérologie Digestive (FFCD) group. In this study, chemoradiotherapy was administered in a dose of 60 Gy concurrently with cisplatin and 5-FU (continuous infusion at 300 mg/m^2/d). The chemotherapy arm consisted of gemcitabine (1,000 mg/m^2/week). Surprisingly, the overall survival was shorter in the chemoradiotherapy arm ([70]). Higher grade 3 to 4 toxicity rates were observed in the chemoradiotherapy arm compared with the chemotherapy arm (66% vs 40%, respectively), which may partially account for the worse survival.

In 2008, ECOG 4201 compared chemoradiotherapy and chemotherapy alone in a phase III trial. Patients with locally unresectable disease were randomly assigned between chemoradiotherapy with concurrent gemcitabine followed by gemcitabine and gemcitabine alone. In the chemoradiotherapy arm, the total radiotherapy dose was 50.4 Gy with concurrent gemcitabine (600 mg/m^2/week). The inclusion of 316 patients was planned, but the study closed after the inclusion of 74 patients because of low accrual. Median overall survival was slightly better in the chemoradiotherapy arm (11 vs 9.2 months, P = .044) ([71]). These results should be considered cautiously because of the limited number of patients included. A literature-based meta-analysis concluded that overall survival was not significantly different after chemoradiotherapy or chemotherapy ([72]).

At the 2013 annual American Society of Clinical Oncology (ASCO) conference, Hammel and colleagues presented the final results of the phase III international LAP 07 study ([73]). The objective was to determine whether consolidative chemoradiotherapy affected overall survival in patients with inoperable locally advanced pancreatic cancer when tumors were controlled after 4 months of induction gemcitabine-based chemotherapy. Patients were randomly assigned to gemcitabine (1,000 mg/m^2/week × 3) or gemcitabine plus erlotinib (100 mg/d) for 4 months. Participants with controlled disease were subsequently randomly assigned to further chemotherapy or chemoradiation (54 Gy [5 × 1.8 Gy/d] and capecitabine 1,600 mg/m^2/d). Of the 442 patients initially randomly assigned, 269 patients (61%) entered the second-round randomization phase. A planned interim analysis was conducted after a median follow-up of 36 months and 221 deaths. Median overall survival in the chemotherapy arm was 16.4 months compared with 15.2 months for the chemoradiation group (hazard ratio [HR] 1.03, 95% CI, 0.79-1.34, P = .8295). It appeared neither radiation nor erlotinib improved survival in this population ([73]). However, administration of radiation did delay the institution of second-line chemotherapy for progressive disease, which had an impact on quality of life.

Integration of Novel Agents Into Concurrent Chemoradiation Strategies

Given the limited benefit noted with 5-FU–based chemoradiation, there has been an effort to incorporate alternative agents into concurrent therapies, including gemcitabine, paclitaxel, capecitabine, and targeted agents, including bevacizumab, cetuximab, and erlotinib. Because of its role in metastatic disease, gemcitabine with EBRT has been extensively investigated for patients with localized cancer. Currently, there is no compelling evidence to suggest improved survival using gemcitabine-based chemoradiation over 5-FU for patients with locally advanced disease. Li et al conducted a small randomized trial that directly compared 5-FU–based chemoradiation with gemcitabine-based chemoradiation. Median survival for the 18 patients randomized to receive gemcitabine with EBRT was 14.5 months, compared with 6.7 months in 16 patients treated with 5-FU. This trial should be interpreted with caution, given the small sample size and poor outcome of patients treated with 5-FU and EBRT ([74]). Another prospective study compared FU with cisplatin-gemcitabine–based chemoradiation and did not demonstrate any difference in overall survival ([75]).

At present, there is no standard approach, dose, or schedule for gemcitabine combined with radiation. Based on completed phase I and II studies, we have defined the MTD of gemcitabine, associated toxicity, and the size of radiation port ([76]). 5-Fluorouracil or capecitabine-based chemoradiation is now standard at MDACC for locally advanced pancreatic cancer.

At MDACC, investigations of novel agents used after chemoradiation have been conducted. In RTOG 0411, patients with locally advanced pancreatic cancer were treated with capecitabine, bevacizumab, and radiation followed by maintenance with capecitabine and bevacizumab. The overall median survival reported was 11 months, which is similar to previous RTOG trials that did not include bevacizumab ([77]).

Systemic chemotherapy alone may improve both pain control and PS and avoids the GI toxicity associated with chemoradiation. For those patients with stable or responding disease after 4 to 6 months of treatment, chemoradiation is often delivered to maximize locoregional tumor control. Chemoradiation is applied only to the patients most likely to benefit as defined by the absence of disease progression during systemic therapy. This strategy was validated by the Groupe Cooperateur Multidisciplinaire en Oncologie (GERCOR) group, who performed a retrospective analysis of patients with locally advanced cancer who received chemoradiation. Investigators noted that 30% of patients developed metastatic disease after induction chemotherapy and were not candidates for radiation. The remaining 70% received continued chemotherapy or consolidative chemoradiation. The overall survival in the two groups was 12 and 15 months ($P = .0009$) and the progression-free survival was 7 and 11 months, respectively. These data support the strategy of consolidative chemoradiation following induction chemotherapy in patients with locally advanced disease ([78]). Retrospective data from MDACC also strongly suggested that patients who have received induction chemotherapy have a better outcome than those receiving primary chemoradiation ([79]).

MDACC Approach to Locally Advanced Pancreatic Cancer

For patients who have poor PS, supportive care is encouraged, and radiation is contraindicated. In the subgroup of patients with significant pain related to the primary tumor, aggressive use of narcotics is initiated. For patients with poor tolerance of narcotics or inadequate pain control with their administration, celiac or splanchnic nerve block is recommended. Once pain control has improved, therapeutic options are discussed. In our institution, consolidative chemoradiation continues to be used in select cases after an informative discussion with the patient regarding the issues mentioned. When so chosen, at least 3 to 4 months of induction chemotherapy with a gemcitabine-based regimen followed by capecitabine or 5-FU and radiation is the favored approach. Figure 21-6 shows the MDACC protocol for treatment of patients with locally advanced disease.

Management of Metastatic Disease

Compared with patients having other common malignancies, such as cancer of the colon or breast, patients with advanced pancreatic cancer are often much more debilitated. Palliation remains the primary goal of therapy. Management of metastatic disease should be guided by the following principles:

1. The disease course may be quite dynamic, and the clinical status of a patient can change quickly. Patients therefore require frequent reassessment, whether or not they are undergoing cytotoxic therapy.
2. Pancreatic cancer is quite resistant to systemic therapy, and responses to therapy are rarely observed in patients with poor PS or high tumor burden.
3. Peritoneal disease is usually not responsive to chemotherapy and carries a particularly poor prognosis. Metastatic disease predominantly located in the liver or lung is more likely to be responsive to systemic therapy. When the disease is metastatic to the lung only, its course may be somewhat more indolent.
4. Improvement in the treatment for pancreatic cancer is desperately needed, and patients with good PS should be encouraged to participate in clinical trials.

Systemic Therapy for Metastatic Disease—Lessons From the Past

Early published data frequently reported response rates to chemotherapy exceeding 20%. However, with the advent of high-quality CT and MRI, substantially lower response rates have been reported. Importantly, cooperative group studies dating to the 1980s have not

CHAPTER 21

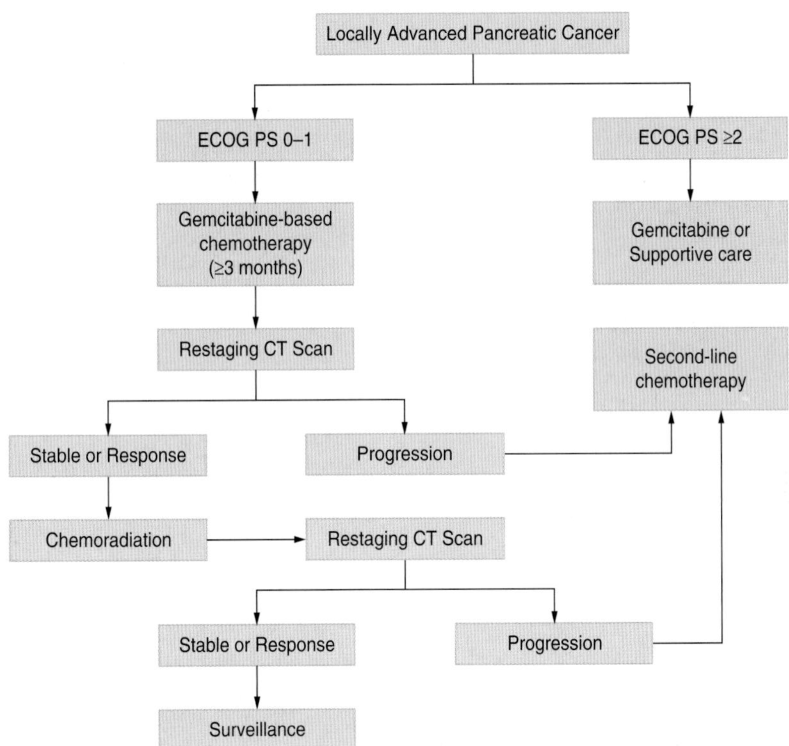

FIGURE 21-6 Treatment algorithm applied to the management of patients with locally advanced pancreatic cancer.

clearly demonstrated meaningful survival advantage for patients treated with single-agent chemotherapy compared with 5-FU combinations or even best supportive care. Thus, for many years, no standard drug or drug regimen had emerged as an accepted frontline therapy for metastatic pancreatic cancer.

Gemcitabine for Metastatic Pancreatic Cancer

Chemotherapy for pancreatic cancer changed with the advent of gemcitabine, which was developed in the 1990s. In an early multicenter trial of gemcitabine in 44 patients, 5 objective responses (11%) were documented ([80]). In another study, gemcitabine again led to few objective responses (2 of 32 patients), but symptomatic improvement was also reported ([81]). Based on these observations, two subsequent trials of gemcitabine for advanced pancreatic cancer were completed. In the randomized trial that led to gemcitabine's approval in the United States, weekly gemcitabine was compared to bolus weekly 5-FU in previously untreated patients ([82]). Patients treated with gemcitabine achieved a higher response rate (5.4% vs 0%) and a statistically significant improvement in median survival compared to those treated with 5-FU (5.65 vs 4.41 months, $P = .0025$). The 1-year survival rate for gemcitabine-treated patients was 18%, compared to 2% for those treated with 5-FU. Importantly, more clinically meaningful effects on disease-related symptoms were recorded with gemcitabine. This trial enrolled a heterogeneous patient population, with patients having either locally advanced, unresectable disease or metastatic disease. About 70% of the treated patients had metastatic pancreatic cancer, and this is the basis for its use as frontline therapy in patients with disseminated disease.

Fixed-Dose-Rate Gemcitabine

Gemcitabine is a prodrug that is phosphorylated to its active metabolites gemcitabine diphosphate and triphosphate. Gemcitabine diphosphate inhibits ribonucleotide reductase, thereby depleting intracellular pools of the triphosphate nucleotides. Gemcitabine triphosphate can incorporate into an elongating chain of DNA and lead to premature chain termination and cell death. Gemcitabine triphosphate may also inhibit normal DNA repair mechanisms. This may explain its potent radiosensitizing properties and synergy with other DNA-damaging cytotoxic agents.

Once phosphorylated intracellular concentrations are highest when the drug is given at a fixed-dose rate (FDR) of 10 mg/m²/min. A randomized phase II trial in metastatic pancreatic cancer demonstrated that gemcitabine given at 2,300 mg/m² over 30 min compared to 1,500 mg/m² delivered over 150 min (10 mg/m²/min) led to a higher objective response rate (16.2 vs 2.7%) and a trend toward improved survival (6.1 vs 4.7 months) ([83]). Therefore, when used off protocol, it is administered at an FDR.

Gemcitabine Combinations: Cytotoxic Agents

In an effort to build on gemcitabine for advanced cancer, one approach has been to combine gemcitabine with other cytotoxic drugs. In addition, regimens using two to four other drugs with gemcitabine are reported in the literature. These include combinations of gemcitabine, capecitabine, and docetaxel (GTX) and gemcitabine, 5-FU, leucovorin, irinotecan, and cisplatin (G-FLIP). Randomized trials of gemcitabine versus gemcitabine-based doublets of cytotoxic therapy have shown no statistically significant survival advantage (Table 21-7). However, gemcitabine combined with a platinum does appear to have some benefit in patients with good PS ([84]).

CHAPTER 21

Recent Trials Evaluating Combination Therapy

Cancer and Leukemia Group B (CALGB) 89904 was a four-arm phase II study comparing FDR gemcitabine with the gemcitabine doublets cisplatin, docetaxel, and irinotecan. Six-month survival, the primary end point, did not differ significantly between the four arms (range 53%-57%) ([85]). Overall survival was also similar across groups. A phase III trial combining gemcitabine and cisplatin had a non–statistically significant improvement in progression-free and median survival over single-agent gemcitabine (median survival 7.5 vs 6.0 months, $P = .15$) ([86]). Similarly, a phase III trial evaluating the combination of gemcitabine and irinotecan versus gemcitabine alone failed to demonstrate a survival advantage over gemcitabine ([87]).

Previously, the GERCOR/GISCAD (Italian Group for the Study of Digestive Tract Cancer) phase III trial with FDR gemcitabine and oxaliplatin demonstrated a statistically significant higher response rate and progression-free survival in patients with locally advanced and metastatic disease; however, overall survival did not reach statistical significance (9.0 vs 7.1 months, $P = .13$) ([88]). ECOG 6201 enrolled 832 patients in three arms: gemcitabine in a 30-minute infusion, FDR gemcitabine, and FDR gemcitabine with oxaliplatin. Overall survival was not statistically different between the three groups: 4.9, 6.2, and 5.7 months, respectively ([89]).

It was not until September 2013 when the Food and Drug Administration (FDA) first approved a gemcitabine-based combination chemotherapy regimen with nab-paclitaxel. This was based on a follow-up phase III study published in the *New England Journal of Medicine* that showed an overall survival advantage of gemcitabine plus nab-paclitaxel over gemcitabine alone (8.5 months vs 6.7 months, HR for death, 0.72; 95% CI, 0.62 to 0.83; $P < .001$). The 1-year survival rates were 35% versus 22%, respectively. The response rate according to independent review was 23% versus 7% in the two groups ($P < .001$). The combination arm did have increased neutropenia, fatigue, and neuropathy ([90]).

Capecitabine, the orally bioavailable fluorinated pyrimidine, when combined with gemcitabine, demonstrated a modest clinical benefit over gemcitabine alone and appeared to improve median overall survival in patients with good PS ([91]). In a phase III trial, Cunningham and colleagues randomized patients to receive gemcitabine versus gemcitabine plus capecitabine (gemcitabine 1,000 mg/m^2 IV weekly × 3 every 4 weeks; capecitabine 1,660 mg/m^2/d by mouth

Table 21-7 Summary of Trials Combining Gemcitabine With a Second Cytotoxic Agent

Author, Year	Number of Patients	% of Patients With Metastatic Disease	Control Arm Median Survival (Months)	Combination Therapy Median Survival (Months)	P Value
Berlin, 2002	322	90	Gem 5.4	Gem/5-FU 6.7	.09
Colucci, 2002	107	58	Gem 5.4	Gem/cisplatin 7.0	.43
Heinemann, 2006	195	80	Gem 6.0	Gem/cisplatin 7.5	.12
Rocha-Lima, 2004	342	80	Gem 6.6	Gem/irinotecan 6.3	NS
Louvet, 2004	313	70	Gem 7.0	Gem/oxaliplatin 9.0	.13
Poplin, 2006	555	88	Gem 4.9	Gem/oxaliplatin 5.9	.16
Abou-Alfa, 2006	349	78	Gem 6.2	Gem/exactecan 6.7	.52
Hermann, 2007	319	80	Gem 7.2	Gem/capecitabine 8.4	.23
Cunningham, 2009	533	71	Gem 6.2	Gem/capecitabine 7.1	.08

5-FU, 5-fluorouracil; Gem, gemcitabine.

for 3 weeks and 1 week's rest) ([92]). The addition of capecitabine to gemcitabine significantly improved overall response rate and progression-free survival ($P = .03$ and .004, respectively) and trended toward an improved overall survival ($P = .08$).

Based on preclinical data showing effectiveness of combination chemotherapy in solid tumors, investigators tested a combination chemotherapy regimen consisting of oxaliplatin, irinotecan, fluorouracil, and leucovorin (FOLFIRINOX) as compared with gemcitabine. There was random assignment of 342 patients with an ECOG PS of 0 or 1 to receive FOLFIRINOX (oxaliplatin, 85 mg/m^2 body surface area; irinotecan, 180 mg/m^2; leucovorin, 400 mg/m^2; and fluorouracil, 400 mg/m^2 given as a bolus followed by 2,400 mg/m^2 given as a 46-hour continuous infusion every 2 weeks) or gemcitabine at a dose of 1,000 mg/m^2 weekly for 7 of 8 weeks and then weekly for 3 of 4 weeks. The primary end point was overall survival. The median overall survival was 11.1 months in the FOLFIRINOX group as compared to 6.8 months in the gemcitabine group (HR for death, 0.57; 95% CI, 0.45 to 0.73; $P < .001$). The objective response rate was also improved in the FOLFIRINOX group, 31.6% versus 9.4% ($P < .001$). More adverse events were noted in the FOLFIRINOX group. At 6 months, 31% versus 66% of patients in the FOLFIRINOX versus gemcitabine group had a definitive degradation of the quality of life (HR, 0.47; 95% CI, 0.30 to 0.70; $P < .001$) ([93]).

FUTURE DIRECTIONS OF CHEMOTHERAPY IN PANCREATIC CANCER

Molecular Therapeutics for Pancreatic Cancer

While other cytotoxic drugs may provide some survival benefit when combined with gemcitabine, patient outcomes are predicted to be relatively small. Therefore, the investigation of targeted molecular therapies should be given priority. Treatment strategies being developed include interruption or modulation of known growth factors and signal transduction pathways involved with cell growth, invasion, and angiogenesis.

Epidermal Growth Factor Receptor Inhibition

Antibodies to the *EGFR* have been shown to compete with the growth-stimulatory ligands for binding to this receptor. Small molecular inhibitors of the tyrosine kinase activity of the *EGFR* have also been developed in a variety of solid tumors, including pancreatic cancer. In a large international phase III trial, erlotinib, an oral small molecule inhibitor of *EGFR*, in combination with gemcitabine led to a slightly longer median survival compared to gemcitabine alone (6.24 vs 5.91 months, $P = .038$) ([94]). Importantly, treatment-related toxicities were not significantly worse for the patients receiving the combination compared to monotherapy. This trial resulted in FDA approval for erlotinib in metastatic pancreatic cancer; it remains the only targeted agent approved for this disease to date. Subsequent studies combining the anti-*EGFR* antibody cetuximab have been less successful. Southwest Oncology Group (SWOG) S0205, a phase III trial evaluating gemcitabine with cetuximab, reported an overall survival of 6 months for gemcitabine versus 6.5 months for the combination ($P = .14$). Progression-free survival and response rates were similar between the arms ([95]).

Antiangiogenic Agents

Tumor angiogenesis is important in the establishment and progression of metastatic implants. It is now generally accepted that inhibition of these factors represents a feasible approach to impeding metastasis. One cytokine believed to be central to angiogenesis is VEGF, which is often overexpressed in pancreatic cancer. Inhibition of VEGF may have two roles: blocking VEGF receptors to inhibit tumor growth and impeding angiogenesis.

Bevacizumab, an anti-VEGF antibody, has been investigated in patients with advanced pancreatic cancer. Phase II data demonstrated promising response rates ranging from 11% to 24% and overall survivals of 8.1 to 9.8 months ([96]). Unfortunately, a randomized phase III trial, CALGB 80303, did not mirror these results. Patients were assigned to receive gemcitabine alone versus gemcitabine plus bevacizumab (10 mg/kg). Median overall survival was similar (5.2 vs 5.8 months), with no significant improvement in response rate or progression-free survival ([97]). More recently, a multicenter randomized phase III trial with gemcitabine, bevacizumab, and erlotinib was reported and also did not show a significant improvement in survival when compared to gemcitabine, erlotinib, and placebo (7.1 vs 6.0 months; HR 0.89; 95% CI, 0.74-1.07; $P = .2087$) ([98]). There was, however, a significant improvement in progression-free survival (4.6 vs 3.6 months; HR, 0.73; 95% CI, 0.61-0.86; $P = .0002$).

Insulinlike Growth Factor Type 1 Targeted Therapies

The IGF-1 clinical trial with ganitumab showed a trend toward improved 6-month and overall survival when combined with gemcitabine as compared with gemcitabine plus placebo ([99]). On the other hand, the addition of cixitumumab to gemcitabine plus erlotinib did not improve survival when compared with gemcitabine and erlotinib ([100]). Our randomized phase II study of dalotuzumab showed promising activity when combined with gemcitabine as compared with gemcitabine plus erlotinib. Final analysis of correlative studies from this trial is under way.

Stromal Reengineering and Targeted Therapy

The traditional view of pancreatic cancer stroma has been as a hindrance to delivery of chemotherapy and accounting for the adverse prognosis associated with this cancer. Hedgehog inhibitors were particularly effective in causing stromal depletion ([101]). This theory, however, was disproven in the clinical setting, with randomized trials of two hedgehog inhibitors, IPI-926 and vismodegib, failing to improve survival when added to gemcitabine as compared with gemcitabine alone. Kalluri et al, from MDACC, recently showed that stromal depletion in genetic engineered mouse models resulted in accelerated tumor growth. In addition, they showed that stromal-depleted pancreatic cancers were sensitive to the CTLA-4 (cytotoxic T lymphocyte-associated antigen 4) antibody ipilimumab ([102]). Similar findings were reported by Rhim et al, who demonstrated that stroma is protective in pancreatic cancer, and deletion of sonic hedgehog accelerated tumor growth; this effect was again reproduced by treatment with smoothened inhibitor ([23]). Stroma as a target for therapy continues to be investigated in the clinic.

A recently investigated stromal component is the extracellular matrix component hyaluronan. Enzymatic depletion of hyaluronan by the pegylated hyaluronidase (PEGPH20) resulted in inhibition of cancer growth and prolonged survival when combined with gemcitabine in preclinical studies ([103]). Currently, PEGPH20 is at an advanced stage of clinical development in combination with gemcitabine and nab-paclitaxel.

Second-Line Therapy for Pancreatic Cancer

There is an increasing recognition that second-line therapies have been inadequately researched in pancreatic cancer, representing an important avenue for drug development. Irinotecan liposome injection (MM-398) is a nanoliposomal encapsulation of irinotecan that has been successfully combined with 5-FU in a phase III study (NAPOLI-1) in the second-line setting for pancreatic cancer. The MM-398 with 5-FU and leucovorin achieved an overall survival of 6.1 months compared to 4.2 months' survival with 5-FU and leucovorin in those who progressed on gemcitabine (HR = 0.67, P = .012) ([104]).

Another exciting development in second-line therapy is with ruxolitinib, a JAK1/2 inhibitor that is approved for the treatment of myelofibrosis. In the randomized phase II trial, patients with metastatic pancreatic cancer who had progressed on first-line gemcitabine received capecitabine with ruxolitinib or placebo ([105]). On subgroup analysis, patients with a high C-reactive protein level—who represented 50% of the total patient population—had a 6-month survival rate of 42% compared with 11% with placebo (HR = 0.47; P = .005). Interestingly, patients on ruxolitinib also experienced improved weight gain.

Immunotherapy for Pancreatic Cancer

Immune therapy has finally come of age, and immune targeting is rapidly changing the course of multiple cancers. Both innate and adaptive immune systems are involved in the immunosurveillance mechanisms, which include cytotoxic CD8 T cells, T helper 1 (Th1) cells, dendritic cells, tissue macrophages (M1), and natural killer cells. Cancers must escape these surveillance mechanisms to grow and have a clinically significant impact ([106]). Preclinical models of pancreatic cancer have informed us that immunosuppressive tumor-associated macrophages (TAMs), Treg cells, along with scarce effector (CD8) T cells occur at even the earliest preinvasive stages and persist through the development of invasive cancer. High concentrations of CD8 T cells, when infrequently present in pancreas cancer, are associated with a good prognosis ([107]).

Current immunotherapy approaches for pancreatic cancer have yielded promising results that are being investigated in clinical trials. These approaches include checkpoint inhibitors, pancreatic cancer vaccines, adoptive T-cell transfer, monoclonal antibodies acting at the immune checkpoint level, cytokines, and Treg depletion. Immune checkpoint targeting has the potential of changing the treatment paradigm for melanoma, non–small cell lung cancer, and gastric cancer. These agents either alone or in combination are currently in clinical trials.

In regard to checkpoint inhibitors, ipilimumab has been investigated in 27 cases of pancreatic adenocarcinoma, and one delayed response occurred. The PD1 antibody was studied in an expansion cohort of pancreatic cases (n = 14) without any therapeutic responses ([106]). These data, while discouraging, have highlighted the fact that predictive criteria for checkpoint inhibitors are needed. The CD40 agonist was combined with gemcitabine in a study, with four objective responses seen (of the 22 patients treated), and a greater number had metabolic responses on FDG-PET imaging ([108]). Anti-OX40 antibodies and IDO inhibitors are currently undergoing testing as well.

Algenpantucel-L, also known as hyperacute pancreatic adenocarcinoma vaccine, is a composite of two irradiated, live, human allogeneic pancreatic cancer cell lines that express murine α-1,3-galactosyl transferase. This results in α-galactosylated epitopes on cell surface proteins, which result in an immune response. A phase II study of this agent, in combination with gemcitabine and radiotherapy, for resected pancreatic cancer resulted in a 1-year overall survival of 86% and disease-free survival of 62% ([109]). An increased anti–calreticulin antibody (anti-CALR Ab) level following algenpantucel-L treatment correlated with a statistically significant improvement in overall survival (35.8 months in patients with elevated levels of anti-CALR Ab vs 19.2 months in patients without elevated levels; P = .03). The addition of algenpantucel-L to standard adjuvant therapy for resected patients has been investigated in a phase III clinical study, and the results are anticipated.

Immunotherapy agent GVAX is composed of two irradiated, granulocyte-macrophage colony-stimulating factor (GM-CSF)–secreting allogeneic pancreatic cancer cell lines administered after treatment with low-dose cyclophosphamide (Cy/GVAX) to inhibit Treg cells. The GVAX induces T cells against numerous cancer antigens, including mesothelin-specific T-cell responses. CRS-207 is recombinant live-attenuated *Listeria monocytogenes* engineered to secrete mesothelin into antigen-presenting cells. These vaccines demonstrated synergistic activity in both antigen-specific T-cell induction and antitumor activity in preclinical models. These two vaccines were investigated in a randomized phase II trial for previously treated patients. This randomized study demonstrated that Cy/GVAX followed by CRS-207 significantly improved overall survival as compared with Cy/GVAX alone in patients with metastatic pancreatic cancer (6.1 months with Cy/GVAX followed by CRS-207 vs 3.9 months with Cy/GVAX alone [HR, 0.59; P = .02]) ([110]). In this study, mesothelin-specific T-cell immune responses correlated with improved survival. This strategy is now being investigated in a phase III randomized study.

Bruton tyrosine kinase (Btk) is a nonreceptor enzyme of the Tec kinase family that is expressed in B cells, myeloid cells, and mast cells, where it regulates cellular proliferation, differentiation, apoptosis, and cell migration. Inhibition of Btk leads to preferential differentiation of macrophages into M1 instead of immunosuppressive M2 macrophages; Btk inhibition thus decreases the TAMs that promote tumor invasion and metastasis. The BTK inhibitor ibrutinib results in stromal suppression and inhibition of pancreatic tumor growth in preclinical models ([111]). Based on this rationale, the BTK inhibitor, ACP-196, is being investigated in the clinical setting for first- and second-line therapy at MDACC.

MDACC APPROACH TO THE PATIENT WITH METASTATIC DISEASE

Metastatic pancreatic cancer is a disease characterized by anorexia, cachexia, and pain. Therefore, palliation must always be the primary goal for this group of patients and is facilitated by a multidisciplinary approach. Symptomatic relief of biliary obstruction and pain should be addressed prior to consideration of systemic therapy. If pain is not well controlled with oral or transdermal narcotics or if these agents are poorly tolerated, patients should undergo an evaluation with an anesthesiologist or neurologist to consider ablation of the celiac or splanchnic plexus. In addition to aggressive pain control efforts, other supportive measures should be considered, including appetite enhancers, antidepressants, and central nervous system stimulants.

Biliary obstruction should be relieved by nonsurgical means whenever possible, and we advocate the insertion of expandable metal stents rather than polyethylene biliary stents. On occasion, percutaneous biliary drainage may be required in the setting of extrahepatic biliary obstruction.

When a patient develops gastric outlet obstruction, we try to estimate the prognosis at that juncture. If life expectancy is greater than 12 weeks, surgical intervention for definitive gastric bypass is considered. For patients with end-stage metastatic disease, the use of duodenal stents is encouraged. For patients with intractable symptomatic ascites, it is important to realize that this may not be caused by carcinomatosis and frequently results from PV or SMV thrombosis. Ascites secondary to portal hypertension will respond to diuretics, including spironolactone, whereas malignant ascites requires repeated paracentesis or an indwelling peritoneal catheter. Gastroparesis is another commonly occurring problem that requires promotility agents and dietary and behavioral modification.

MDACC Approach to Systemic Therapy for Advanced Pancreatic Cancer

Systemic therapy for metastatic disease should be actively discouraged in patients with poor PS (ECOG >2) or significant metastatic burden. End-of-life discussions are appropriate at the time of diagnosis.

Whenever possible, patients with good PS should be treated with systemic therapy in a clinical trial. The current trial includes the addition of the Btk inhibitor ACP-196 to gemcitabine and nab-paclitaxel for the first-line treatment. In the second-line setting, we are

CHAPTER 21

initiating studies with ACP-196, an orally bioavailable, small molecule inhibitor of Btk in combination with the PD1 antibody pembrolizumab.

In terms of nonclinical trial options, after progression on FOLFIRINOX, gemcitabine-based regimens like gemcitabine plus nab-paclitaxel are considered. After gemcitabine and nab-paclitaxel, FOLFOX or single-agent capecitabine are preferred. Patients who have experienced disease stability or response with gemcitabine-based first-line therapy can be considered for second-line therapy with gemcitabine-based combinations (such as gemcitabine, docetaxel, and capecitabine [GTX]) ([112]).

For patients who are not candidates for multiagent chemotherapy, gemcitabine as first-line therapy is reasonable. At MDACC, our off-protocol approach is to deliver FDR gemcitabine (600-1,000 mg/m^2) at rate of 10 mg/m^2/min) weekly. The utility of erlotinib has significantly declined at this time but is a consideration in the first- or second-line setting in combination with gemcitabine. When an objective response or stable disease is observed, chemotherapy is usually continued until there is radiographic or clinical evidence of disease progression, with restaging studies generally performed every 8 to 12 weeks. Gemcitabine-platinum doublets are offered only to those patients with excellent PS and those with BRCA-associated pancreatic cancer.

In summary, clinically meaningful advances in the treatment of metastatic pancreatic cancer have occurred in the past 5 years. These developments have changed the treatment paradigm for patients experiencing modest but significantly improved survival and quality of life. Continued efforts to enroll patients with advanced disease into well-designed clinical trials should remain a high priority for oncologists.

REFERENCES

1. Jemal A, Siegel R, Ward E, et al. Cancer statistics, 2009. *CA Cancer J Clin.* 2009;59:225-249.
2. Konner J, O'Reilly E. Pancreatic cancer: Epidemiology, genetics, and approaches to screening. *Oncology (Williston Park).* 2002;16:1615-1622.
3. Rahid L, Smith BD, Aizenberg R, et al. Projecting cancer incidence and deaths to 2030: the unexpected burden of thyroid, liver, and pancreas cancers in the United States. *Cancer Res.* 2014;74:2913-2921.
4. Villeneuve PJ, Johnson KC, Mao Y, et al. Environmental tobacco smoke and the risk of pancreatic cancer: findings from a Canadian population-based case-control study. *Can J Public Health.* 2004;95:32-37.
5. Hassan MM, Abbruzzese JL, Bondy ML, et al. Passive smoking and the use of noncigarette tobacco products in association with risk for pancreatic cancer: a case-control study. *Cancer.* 2007;109:2547-2556.
6. Everhart J, Wright D. Diabetes mellitus as a risk factor for pancreatic cancer: a meta-analysis. *JAMA.* 1995;273:1605-1609.
7. Talamini G, Falconi M, Bassi C, et al. Incidence of cancer in the course of chronic pancreatitis. *Am J Gastroenterol.* 1999;94:1253-1260.
8. Lowenfels AB, Maisonneuve P. Epidemiologic and etiologic factors of pancreatic cancer. *Hematol Oncol Clin North Am.* 2002;16:1-16.
9. Felderbauer P, Stricker I, Schnekenburger J, et al. Histopathological features of patients with chronic pancreatitis due to mutations in the PRSS1 gene: evaluation of BRAF and KRAS2 mutations. *Digestion.* 2008;78:60-65.
10. Hanley AJ, Johnson KC, Villeneuve PJ, et al. Physical activity, anthropometric factors and risk of pancreatic cancer: results from the Canadian enhanced cancer surveillance system. *Int J Cancer.* 2001;94:140-147.
11. Hruban RH, Canto MI, Yeo CJ. Prevention of pancreatic cancer and strategies for management of familial pancreatic cancer. *Dig Dis.* 2001;19:76-84.
12. Murphy KM, Brune, KA, Griffin C, et al. Evaluation of candidate genes MAP2K4, MADH4, ACVR1B, and BRCA2 in familial pancreatic cancer: deleterious BRCA2 mutation in 17%. *Cancer Res.* 2002;62:3789-3793.
13. Golan T, Kanji ZS, Epelbaum R, et al, Overall survival and clinical characteristics of pancreatic cancer in BRCA mutation carriers. *Br J Cancer.* 2014;111:132-138.
14. Bryant HE, Schultz N, Thomas HD, et al. Specific killing of BRCA2-deficient tumours with inhibitors of poly(ADP-ribose) polymerase. *Nature.* 2005;434:913-917.
15. van der Heijden MS, Brody JR, Dezentje DA, et al. In vivo therapeutic responses contingent on Fanconi anemia/BRCA2 status of the tumor. *Clin Cancer Res.* 2005;11:7508-7515.
16. Bhalla A, Saif MW. PARP-inhibitors in BRCA-associated pancreatic cancer. *JOP.* 2014;15:340-343.
17. Guo YS, Townsend CM Jr. Roles of gastrointestinal hormones in pancreatic cancer. *J Hepatobiliary Pancreat Surg.* 2000;7:276-285.
18. Jones S, Zhang X, Parsons DW, et al. Core signaling pathways in human pancreatic cancers revealed by global genomic analyses. *Science.* 2008;321:1801-1806.
19. Waddell N, Pajic M, Patch A, et al. Whole genomes redefine the mutational landscape of pancreatic cancer. *Nature.* 2015;518:495-501.
20. Grunewald K, Lyons J, Frohlich A, et al. High frequency of Kiras codon 12 mutations in pancreatic adenocarcinomas. *Int J Cancer.* 1989;43:1037-1041.
21. Rozenblum E, Schutte M, Goggins M, et al. Tumor-suppressive pathways in pancreatic carcinoma. *Cancer Res.* 1997;57:1731-1734.
22. Wang W, Abbruzzese JL, Evans DB, et al. The nuclear factor-kappa B RelA transcription factor is constitutively activated in human pancreatic adenocarcinoma cells. *Clin Cancer Res.* 1999;5:119-127.
23. Feldmann G, Habbe N, Dhara S, et al. Hedgehog inhibition prolongs survival in a genetically engineered mouse model of pancreatic cancer. *Gut.* 2008;57:1420-1430.
24. Olive KP, Jacobetz MA, Davidson CJ, et al. Inhibition of Hedgehog signaling enhances delivery of chemotherapy in a mouse model of pancreatic cancer. *Science.* 2009;324:1457-1461.
25. Rhim AD, Oberstein PE, Thomas DH, et al. Stromal elements act to restrain, rather than support, pancreatic ductal adenocarcinoma. *Cancer Cell.* 2014;25(6):735-747.
26. Van CE, van de VH, Karasek P, et al. Phase III trial of gemcitabine plus tipifarnib compared with gemcitabine plus placebo in advanced pancreatic cancer. *J Clin Oncol.* 2004;22:1430-1438.
27. Bramhall SR, Schulz J, Nemunaitis J, et al. A double-blind placebo-controlled, randomised study comparing gemcitabine and marimastat with gemcitabine and placebo as first line therapy in patients with advanced pancreatic cancer. *Br J Cancer.* 2002;87:161-167.
28. Mujica VR, Barkin JS, Go VL. Acute pancreatitis secondary

to pancreatic carcinoma. Study Group Participants. *Pancreas.* 2000;21:329-332.

29. Raut CP, Grau AM, Staerkel GA, et al. Diagnostic accuracy of endoscopic ultrasound-guided fine-needle aspiration in patients with presumed pancreatic cancer. *J Gastrointest Surg.* 2003;7:118-126.
30. Rashleigh-Belcher HJ, Russell RC, Lees WR. Cutaneous seeding of pancreatic carcinoma by fine-needle aspiration biopsy. *Br J Radiol.* 1986;59:182-183.
31. Tamm EP, Loyer EM, Faria S, et al. Staging of pancreatic cancer with multidetector CT in the setting of preoperative chemoradiation therapy. *Abdom Imaging.* 2006;31:568-574.
32. Kalady MF, Clary BM, Clark LA, et al. Clinical utility of positron emission tomography in the diagnosis and management of periampullary neoplasms. *Ann Surg Oncol.* 2002;9:799-806.
33. Pleskow DK, Berger HJ, Gyves J, et al. Evaluation of a serologic marker, CA19-9, in the diagnosis of pancreatic cancer. *Ann Intern Med.* 1989;110:704-709.
34. Fogelman DR, Pathak P, Qiao W, et al. Serum CA 19-9 level as a surrogate marker for prognosis in locally advanced pancreatic cancer (LAPC). *J Clin Oncol (Meeting Abstracts).* 2008;26:15514.
35. van den Bosch RP, van Eijck CH, Mulder PG, et al. Serum CA19-9 determination in the management of pancreatic cancer. *Hepatogastroenterology.* 1996;43:710-713.
36. Ko AH, Hwang J, Venook AP, et al. Serum CA19-9 response as a surrogate for clinical outcome in patients receiving fixed-dose rate gemcitabine for advanced pancreatic cancer. *Br J Cancer.* 2005;93:195-199.
37. Warshaw AL, Tepper JE, Shipley WU. Laparoscopy in the staging and planning of therapy for pancreatic cancer. *Am J Surg.* 1986;151:76-80.
38. Fernandez-del Castillo CL, Warshaw AL. Pancreatic cancer. Laparoscopic staging and peritoneal cytology. *Surg Oncol Clin N Am.* 1998;7:135-142.
39. Pisters PW, Lee JE, Vauthey JN, et al. Laparoscopy in the staging of pancreatic cancer. *Br J Surg.* 2001;88:325-337.
40. Warshaw AL. Implications of peritoneal cytology for staging of early pancreatic cancer. *Am J Surg.* 1991;161:26-29.
41. Whipple AO. The rationale of radical surgery for cancer of the pancreas and ampullary region. *Ann Surg.* 1941;114:612-615.
42. Wade TP, Virgo KS, Johnson FE. Distal pancreatectomy for cancer: results in US Department of Veterans Affairs hospitals, 1987-1991. *Pancreas.* 1995;11:341-344.
43. Birkmeyer JD, Siewers AE, Finlayson EV, et al. Hospital volume and surgical mortality in the United States. *N Engl J Med.* 2002;346:1128-1137.
44. Birkmeyer JD, Warshaw AL, Finlayson SR, et al. Relationship between hospital volume and late survival after pancreaticoduodenectomy. *Surgery.* 1999;126:178-183.
45. Chang DK, Johns AL, Merrett ND, et al. Margin clearance and outcome in resected pancreatic cancer. *J Clin Oncol.* 2009;27:2855-2862.
46. Neoptolemos JP, Stocken DD, Dunn JA, et al. Influence of resection margins on survival for patients with pancreatic cancer treated by adjuvant chemoradiation and/or chemotherapy in the ESPAC-1 randomized controlled trial. *Ann Surg.* 2001;234:758-768.
47. Herman JM, Swartz MJ, Hsu CC, et al. Analysis of fluorouracil-based adjuvant chemotherapy and radiation after pancreaticoduodenectomy for ductal adenocarcinoma of the pancreas: Results of a large, prospectively collected database at the Johns Hopkins Hospital. *J Clin Oncol.* 2008;26:3503-3510.
48. Lim JE, Chien MW, Earle CC. Prognostic factors following curative resection for pancreatic adenocarcinoma: a population-based, linked database analysis of 396 patients. *Ann Surg.* 2003;237:74-85.
49. Kalser MH, Ellenberg SS. Pancreatic cancer. Adjuvant combined radiation and chemotherapy following curative resection. *Arch Surg.* 1985;120:899-903.
50. Smeenk HG, van Eijck CH, Hop WC, et al. Long-term survival and metastatic pattern of pancreatic and periampullary cancer after adjuvant chemoradiation or observation: long-term results of EORTC trial 40891. *Ann Surg.* 2007;246: 734-740.
51. Neoptolemos JP, Stocken DD, Friess H, et al. A randomized trial of chemoradiotherapy and chemotherapy after resection of pancreatic cancer. *N Engl J Med.* 2004;350:1200-1210.
52. Regine WF, Winter KA, Abrams RA, et al. Fluorouracil vs gemcitabine chemotherapy before and after fluorouracil-based chemoradiation following resection of pancreatic adenocarcinoma: a randomized controlled trial. *JAMA.* 2008;299:1019-1026.
53. Javle M, Hsueh CT. Updates in gastrointestinal oncology—insights from the 2008 44th annual meeting of the American Society of Clinical Oncology. *J Hematol Oncol.* 2009;2:9.
54. Neoptolemos J, Buchler M, Stocken DD, et al. ESPAC-3(v2): a multicenter, international, open-label, randomized, controlled phase III trial of adjuvant 5-fluorouracil/folinic acid (5-FU/FA) versus gemcitabine (GEM) in patients with resected pancreatic ductal adenocarcinoma. *J Clin Oncol (Meeting Abstracts).* 2009;27:LBA4505.
55. Picozzi VJ, Abrams RA, Decker PA, et al. Multicenter phase II trial of adjuvant therapy for resected pancreatic cancer using cisplatin, 5-fluorouracil, and interferon-alfa-2b-based chemoradiation: ACOSOG Trial Z05031. *Ann Oncol.* 2011;22:348-54.
56. Schmidt J, Patrut JM, Ma J, et al. Open-label, multicenter, randomized phase III trial of adjuvant chemoradiation plus interferon alfa-2b versus fluorouracil and folinic acid for patients with resected pancreatic adenocarcinoma. *J Clin Oncol.* 2012;30:4077-4083.
57. Evans DB, Varadhachary GR, Crane CH, et al. Preoperative gemcitabine-based chemoradiation for patients with resectable adenocarcinoma of the pancreatic head. *J Clin Oncol.* 2008; 26:3496-3502.
58. Pisters PW, Wolff RA, Janjan NA, et al. Preoperative paclitaxel and concurrent rapid-fractionation radiation for resectable pancreatic adenocarcinoma: toxicities, histologic response rates, and event-free outcome. *J Clin Oncol.* 2002;20:2537-2544.
59. Varadhachary GR, Wolff RA, Crane CH, et al. Preoperative gemcitabine and cisplatin followed by gemcitabine-based chemoradiation for resectable adenocarcinoma of the pancreatic head. *J Clin Oncol.* 2008;26:3487-3495.
60. Pisters PW, Abbruzzese JL, Janjan NA, et al. Rapid-fractionation preoperative chemoradiation, pancreaticoduodenectomy, and intraoperative radiation therapy for resectable pancreatic adenocarcinoma. *J Clin Oncol.* 1998;16:3843-3850.
61. Crane CH, Ellis LM, Abbruzzese JL, et al. Phase I trial evaluating the safety of bevacizumab with concurrent radiotherapy and capecitabine in locally advanced pancreatic cancer. *J Clin Oncol.* 2006;24:1145-1151.
62. Todd KE, Gloor B, Lane JS, et al. Resection of locally advanced pancreatic cancer after downstaging with continuous-infusion 5-fluorouracil, mitomycin-C, leucovorin, and dipyridamole. *J Gastrointest Surg.* 1998;2:159-166.
63. Varadhachary GR, Tamm EP, Abbruzzese JL, et al. Borderline resectable pancreatic cancer: Definitions, management, and role of preoperative therapy. *Ann Surg Oncol.* 2006;13:1035-1046.
64. Minsky BD, Hilaris B, Fuks Z. The role of radiation therapy in the control of pain from pancreatic carcinoma. *J Pain Symptom Manage.* 1988;3:199-205.
65. Moertel CG, Frytak S, Hahn RG, et al. Therapy of locally unresectable pancreatic carcinoma: a randomized comparison of high dose (6000 rads) radiation alone, moderate dose radiation (4000 rads + 5-fluorouracil), and high dose radiation + 5-fluorouracil: the Gastrointestinal Tumor Study Group. *Cancer.* 1981;48:1705-1710.
66. The concept of locally advanced gastric cancer. Effect of treatment on outcome. The Gastrointestinal Tumor Study Group.

Cancer. 1990;66:2324-2330.
67. Klaassen DJ, MacIntyre JM, Catton GE, et al. Treatment of locally unresectable cancer of the stomach and pancreas: a randomized comparison of 5-fluorouracil alone with radiation plus concurrent and maintenance 5-fluorouracil—an Eastern Cooperative Oncology Group study. *J Clin Oncol.* 1985;3:373-378.
68. Whittington R, Neuberg D, Tester WJ, et al. Protracted intravenous fluorouracil infusion with radiation therapy in the management of localized pancreaticobiliary carcinoma: a phase I Eastern Cooperative Oncology Group Trial. *J Clin Oncol.* 1995;13:227-232.
69. Ishii H, Okada S, Tokuuye K et al. Protracted 5-fluorouracil infusion with concurrent radiotherapy as a treatment for locally advanced pancreatic carcinoma. *Cancer.* 1997;79:1516-1520.
70. Chauffert B, Mornex F, Bonnetain F et al. Phase III trial comparing intensive induction chemoradiotherapy (60 Gy, infusional 5-FU and intermittent cisplatin) followed by maintenance gemcitabine with gemcitabine alone for locally advanced unresectable pancreatic cancer. Definitive results of the 2000-01 FFCD/SFRO study. *Ann Oncol.* 2008;19:1592-1599.
71. Cardenes HR, Powell M, Loehrer PJ, et al. E4201: randomized phase II study of gemcitabine in combination with radiation therapy versus gemcitabine alone in patients with locally advanced, unresectable, pancreatic cancer (LAPC): quality-of-life (QOL) analysis. *J Clin Oncol (Meeting Abstracts).* 2009;27:4627.
72. Sultana A, Tudur SC, Cunningham D, et al. Systematic review, including meta-analyses, on the management of locally advanced pancreatic cancer using radiation/combined modality therapy. *Br J Cancer.* 2007;96:1183-1190.
73. Hammel P, Hugeut F, Van Laethem JL, et al. Comparison of chemoradiotherapy (CRT) and chemotherapy (CT) in patients with a locally advanced pancreatic cancer (LAPC) controlled after 4 months of gemcitabine with or without erlotinib: final results of the international phase III LAP 07 study. *J Clin Oncol (Meeting Abstracts).* 2013;31:4003.
74. Li CP, Chao Y, Chi KH, et al. Concurrent chemoradiotherapy treatment of locally advanced pancreatic cancer: gemcitabine versus 5-fluorouracil, a randomized controlled study. *Int J Radiat Oncol Biol Phys.* 2003;57:98-104.
75. Huguet F, Girard N, Guerche CS-E, et al. Chemoradiotherapy in the management of locally advanced pancreatic carcinoma: a qualitative systematic review. *J Clin Oncol.* 2009;27:2269-2277.
76. Crane CH, Wolff RA, Abbruzzese JL, et al. Combining gemcitabine with radiation in pancreatic cancer: understanding important variables influencing the therapeutic index. *Semin Oncol.* 2001;28:25-33.
77. Crane CH, Winter K, Regine WF, et al. Phase II study of bevacizumab with concurrent capecitabine and radiation followed by maintenance gemcitabine and bevacizumab for locally advanced pancreatic cancer: Radiation Therapy Oncology Group RTOG 0411. *J Clin Oncol.* 2009;27:4096-4102.
78. Huguet F, Andre T, Hammel P, et al. Impact of chemoradiotherapy after disease control with chemotherapy in locally advanced pancreatic adenocarcinoma in GERCOR phase II and III studies. *J Clin Oncol.* 2007;25:326-331.
79. Krishnan S, Rana V, Janjan NA, et al. Induction chemotherapy selects patients with locally advanced, unresectable pancreatic cancer for optimal benefit from consolidative chemoradiation therapy. *Cancer.* 2007;110:47-55.
80. Casper ES, Green MR, Kelsen DP, et al. Phase II trial of gemcitabine (2,2′-difluorodeoxycytidine) in patients with adenocarcinoma of the pancreas. *Invest New Drugs.* 1994;12:29-34.
81. Carmichael J, Fink U, Russell RC, et al. Phase II study of gemcitabine in patients with advanced pancreatic cancer. *Br J Cancer.* 1996;73:101-105.
82. Burris HA III, Moore MJ, Andersen J, et al. Improvements in survival and clinical benefit with gemcitabine as first-line therapy for patients with advanced pancreas cancer: a randomized trial. *J Clin Oncol.* 1997;15:2403-2413.
83. Tempero M, Plunkett W, Ruiz VHV, et al. Randomized phase II comparison of dose-intense gemcitabine: thirty-minute infusion and fixed dose rate infusion in patients with pancreatic adenocarcinoma. *J Clin Oncol.* 2003;21:3402-3408.
84. Heinemann V, Boeck S, Hinke A, et al. Meta-analysis of randomized trials: evaluation of benefit from gemcitabine-based combination chemotherapy applied in advanced pancreatic cancer. *BMC Cancer.* 2008;8:82.
85. Kulke MH, Tempero MA, Niedzwiecki D, et al. Randomized phase II study of gemcitabine administered at a fixed dose rate or in combination with cisplatin, docetaxel, or irinotecan in patients with metastatic pancreatic cancer: CALGB 89904. *J Clin Oncol.* 2009;27:5506-5512.
86. Heinemann V, Quietzsch D, Gieseler F, et al. Randomized phase III trial of gemcitabine plus cisplatin compared with gemcitabine alone in advanced pancreatic cancer. *J Clin Oncol.* 2006;24:3946-3952.
87. Rocha Lima CM, Green MR, Rotche R, et al. Irinotecan plus gemcitabine results in no survival advantage compared with gemcitabine monotherapy in patients with locally advanced or metastatic pancreatic cancer despite increased tumor response rate. *J Clin Oncol.* 2004;22:3776-3783.
88. Heinemann V, Labianca R, Hinke A, et al. Increased survival using platinum analog combined with gemcitabine as compared to single-agent gemcitabine in advanced pancreatic cancer: Pooled analysis of two randomized trials, the GERCOR/GISCAD intergroup study and a German multicenter study. *Ann Oncol.* 2007;18:1652-1659.
89. Poplin E, Feng Y, Berlin J, et al. Phase III, randomized study of gemcitabine and oxaliplatin versus gemcitabine (fixed-dose rate infusion) compared with gemcitabine (30-minute infusion) in patients with pancreatic carcinoma E6201: a trial of the Eastern Cooperative Oncology Group. *J Clin Oncol.* 2009;27:3778-3785.
90. Von Hoff DD, Ervin T, Arena FP, et al. Increased survival in pancreatic cancer with nab-paclitaxel plus gemcitabine. *N Engl J Med.* 2013;369(18):1691-703.
91. Herrmann R, Bodoky G, Ruhstaller T, et al. Gemcitabine plus capecitabine compared with gemcitabine alone in advanced pancreatic cancer: a randomized, multicenter, phase III trial of the Swiss Group for Clinical Cancer Research and the Central European Cooperative Oncology Group. *J Clin Oncol.* 2007;25:2212-2217.
92. Cunningham D, Chau I, Stocken DD, et al. Phase III randomized comparison of gemcitabine versus gemcitabine plus capecitabine in patients with advanced pancreatic cancer. *J Clin Oncol.* 2009;27:5513-5518.
93. Conroy T, Desseigne F, Ychou M, et al. Groupe Tumeurs Digestives of Unicancer; PRODIGE Intergroup. FOLFIRINOX versus gemcitabine for metastatic pancreatic cancer. *N Engl J Med.* 2011;364(19):1817-1825.
94. Moore MJ, Goldstein D, Hamm J, et al. Erlotinib plus gemcitabine compared with gemcitabine alone in patients with advanced pancreatic cancer: a phase III trial of the National Cancer Institute of Canada Clinical Trials Group. *J Clin Oncol.* 2007;25:1960-1966.
95. Philip PA, Benedetti J, Corless CL, et al. Phase III study comparing gemcitabine plus cetuximab versus gemcitabine in patients with advanced pancreatic adenocarcinoma: Southwest Oncology Group-Directed Intergroup Trial S0205. *J Clin Oncol.* 2010;28:3605-3610.
96. Kindler HL, Friberg G, Singh DA, et al. Phase II trial of bevacizumab plus gemcitabine in patients with advanced pancreatic cancer. *J Clin Oncol.* 2005;23:8033-8040.
97. Kindler HL, Niedzwiecki D, Hollis D, et al. A double-blind,

placebo-controlled, randomized phase III trial of gemcitabine (G) plus bevacizumab (B) versus gemcitabine plus placebo (P) in patients (pts) with advanced pancreatic cancer (PC): a preliminary analysis of Cancer and Leukemia Group B (CALGB). *J Clin Oncol (Meeting Abstracts)*. 2007;25:4508.

98. Van Cutsem E, Vervenne WL, Bennouna J, et al. Phase III trial of bevacizumab in combination with gemcitabine and erlotinib in patients with metastatic pancreatic cancer. *J Clin Oncol.* 2009;27:2231-2237.
99. Kindler HL, Richards DA, Garbo LE, et al. A randomized, placebo-controlled phase 2 study of ganitumab (AMG 479) or conatumumab (AMG 655) in combination with gemcitabine in patients with metastatic pancreatic cancer. *Ann Oncol.* 2012;23(11):2834-2842.
100. Philip PA, Goldman B, Ramanathan RK, et al. Dual blockade of epidermal growth factor receptor and insulin-like growth factor receptor-1 signaling in metastatic pancreatic cancer: phase Ib and randomized phase II trial of gemcitabine, erlotinib, and cixutumumab versus gemcitabine plus erlotinib (SWOG S0727). *Cancer.* 2014;120(19):2980-2985.
101. Olive KP, Jacobetz MA, Davidson CJ, et al. Inhibition of Hedgehog signaling enhances delivery of chemotherapy in a mouse model of pancreatic cancer. *Science.* 2009;324 (5933):1457-1461.
102. Ozdemir BC, Pentcheva-Hoang T, Carstens JL, et al. Depletion of carcinoma-associated fibroblasts and fibrosis induces immunosuppression and accelerates pancreas cancer with reduced survival. *Cancer Cell.* 2014;25(6):719-734.
103. Jacobetz MA, Chan DS, Neesse A, et al. Hyaluronan impairs vascular function and drug delivery in a mouse model of pancreatic cancer. *Gut.* 2013;62(1):112-120.
104. Chen L-T, Von Hoff DD, Li C-P, et al. Expanded analyses of napoli-1: phase 3 study of MM-398 (nal-IRI), with or without 5-fluorouracil and leucovorin, versus 5-fluorouracil and leucovorin, in metastatic pancreatic cancer (mPAC) previously treated with gemcitabine-based therapy. *ASCO Meeting Abstracts.* 2015;33(3, suppl):234.
105. O'Reilly EM, Walker C, Clark J, Brill KJ, Dawkins FW, Bendell JC. JANUS 2: a phase III study of survival, tumor response, and symptom response with ruxolitinib plus capecitabine or placebo plus capecitabine in patients with advanced or metastatic pancreatic cancer (mPC) who failed or were intolerant to first-line chemotherapy. *ASCO Meeting Abstracts.* 2015;33(15, suppl):TPS4146.
106. Sideras K, Braat H, Kwekkeboom J, et al. Role of the immune system in pancreatic cancer progression and immune modulating treatment strategies. *Cancer Treat Rev.* 2014;40(4):513-522.
107. Fukunaga A, Miyamoto M, Cho Y, et al. $CD8^+$ tumor-infiltrating lymphocytes together with $CD4^+$ tumor-infiltrating lymphocytes and dendritic cells improve the prognosis of patients with pancreatic adenocarcinoma. *Pancreas.* 2004;28(1):e26-e31.
108. Vonderheide RH, Bajor DL, Winograd R, Evans RA, Bayne LJ, Beatty GL. CD40 immunotherapy for pancreatic cancer. *Cancer Immunol Immunother CII.* 2013;62(5):949-954.
109. Hardacre JM, Mulcahy M, Small W, et al. Addition of algenpantucel-L immunotherapy to standard adjuvant therapy for pancreatic cancer: a phase 2 study. *J Gastrointest Surg.* 2013;17(1):94-100; discussion 100-101.
110. Le DT, Wang-Gillam A, Picozzi V, et al. Safety and survival with GVAX pancreas prime and *Listeria monocytogenes*-expressing mesothelin (CRS-207) boost vaccines for metastatic pancreatic cancer. *J Clin Oncol.* 2015;33(12):1325-1333.
111. Masso-Valles D, Jauset T, Serrano E, et al. Ibrutinib exerts potent antifibrotic and antitumor activities in mouse models of pancreatic adenocarcinoma. *Cancer Res.* 2015;75(8):1675-1681.
112. Fine RL, Fogelman DR, Schreibman SM, et al. The gemcitabine, docetaxel, and capecitabine (GTX) regimen for metastatic pancreatic cancer: a retrospective analysis. *Cancer Chemother Pharmacol.* 2008;61:167-175.

22 Hepatocellular Carcinoma

第二十二章　肝细胞肝癌

Marc Uemura
Sunil Krishnan
Ahmed O. Kaseb
Nishin A. Bhadkamkar
Milind M. Javle
Rony Avritscher

中文导读

本章首先介绍了肝恶性肿瘤的类型，包括肝细胞肝癌、胆管细胞癌、胆管癌、胆囊癌以及少见肿瘤类型如肉瘤、血管肉瘤、肝母细胞瘤等，其中重点阐述了肝细胞肝癌和胆管细胞癌的相关内容。本章从发病概况、流行病学、病因学、临床表现、病理学、诊断分期和治疗等几个方面进行详述。在大致阐述了肝细胞肝癌在全球及美国的发病概况后，详细介绍了肝细胞肝癌的流行病学内容。病因学内容主要包括：慢性病毒性肝炎、乙醇及肝硬化、代谢障碍、其他环境因素等，尤其提到了黄曲霉菌、避孕药以及砷剂等环境因素的作用。临床症状部分则从早期较为隐匿，到中晚期出现右上腹疼痛以及各种伴随症状分阶段作了详细讲解。病理类型结合大体病理及镜下病理进行了详尽说明，并作了相应的鉴别诊断。诊断分期部分包括实验室检查、影像检查（包括超声、CT、MRI、PET等）、AJCC分期系统，并以流程图的形式详细阐述了不同分期肝癌的诊断方法、治疗策略和随访计划。其中以表格形式列出了AJCC分期、ECOG评分系统、CLIP评分、Child-Pugh分级等。肝细胞肝癌治疗内容包括肝移植、手术切除、局部治疗（包括TACE、射频消融等）、系统性全身化疗、内分泌治疗、靶向治疗、放疗等，这部分详尽地介绍了不同治疗策略的优劣以及5年生存率差异。最后本章简单总结了MD安德森癌症中心对肝细胞肝癌治疗的总体策略。

Hepatobiliary malignancies comprise a diverse group of tumors, including hepatocellular carcinoma (HCC), variants such as fibrolamellar HCC (FLHCC) and cholangiocellular carcinoma, cholangiocarcinoma, carcinoma of the gallbladder, and rare cancers such as sarcoma, angiosarcoma, and hepatoblastoma. The relative frequency of these tumors is shown in Table 22-1. The estimated new cases and deaths from liver and intrahepatic bile duct cancer in the United States in 2014 totaled 33,190 and 23,000, respectively ([1]).

The majority of primary liver tumors are HCC or cholangiocarcinoma. These tumor types have different etiologies, epidemiology, clinical presentations, and treatment options. Thus, they are discussed separately.

HEPATOCELLULAR CARCINOMA

Hepatocellular carcinoma is a malignancy of worldwide significance and has become increasingly important in the United States. It is the most common primary liver malignancy, the sixth most common cancer, and the third most common cause of cancer-related deaths worldwide ([2]). Eighty percent of new cases occur in developing countries, but the incidence is rising in economically developed regions, including Japan, Western Europe, and the United States ([3–6]). The worldwide distribution of HCC and its associated etiologies are summarized in Table 22-2. Liver cirrhosis is the seventh leading cause of death in the world, the tenth most common cause of death in the United States, and acknowledged as a premalignant condition for developing HCC ([7–9]).

In the United States, hepatitis C virus (HCV), alcohol use, and nonalcoholic fatty liver disease (NAFLD) are the most common causes of cirrhosis ([9]). The incidence of HCC doubled during the period 1975 to 1995 and continued to rise through 1998 ([10, 11]). This trend was previously expected to continue due to the estimated 4 million US individuals who are hepatitis C seropositive and the known latency of HCC development from the initial HCV infection, which may take two to three decades ([11]). However, given the improved treatment regimens now available for patients with chronic hepatitis C, HCV-related HCC incidence may decrease in the next few years ([12]). It is also known that NAFLD-associated cirrhosis is on the rise in the United States ([13–15]). A majority of patients present with advanced disease that is not amenable to curative procedures. Overall, HCC has a very poor prognosis, with a 5-year survival rate of 5%.

Table 22-1 Relative Frequency of Hepatobiliary Tumors Diagnosed in the United States

Subtype of Hepatobiliary Cancer	Frequency (%)
Hepatocellular	84
Cholangiocarcinoma	13
Cholangiocellular and fibrolamellar	2
Angiosarcoma, sarcoma, hepatoblastoma	1

EPIDEMIOLOGY

As shown in Table 22-1, HCC represents approximately 85% of all primary liver cancers ([16]). The distribution of HCC varies significantly by geography; it is endemic in parts of the world where hepatitis B virus (HBV) is also endemic. In Western countries, HCV infection and alcoholic cirrhosis are the principal risk factors for HCC. Due to rising incidence of HCV infection in American subpopulations, the incidence

Table 22-2 Incidence of Hepatocellular Carcinoma Worldwide

	Incidence[a]			
Region	Men	Women	Number of Cases	Principal Associations
Asia, sub-Saharan Africa	30-120	9-30	>500,000 cases per year	HBV, aflatoxin exposure
Japan	10-30	3-9		HCV
Southern Europe, Argentina, Switzerland	5-10	2-5		HCV
Western Europe	<5	<3		HCV
United States	<5	<3	19,000 predicted for 2004	HCV, alcohol

HBV, hepatitis B virus; HCV, hepatitis C virus.
[a]Cases per 100,000 population.

of HCC is projected to increase fourfold by 2015 ([11]). Moreover, HCC incidence increases with age, with the age of peak incidence varying somewhat with population. The median age group of HCC is between the fifth and sixth decades. The disease is also seen in children and young adults in areas where HBV is endemic, and most of these infections occur perinatally. In all populations worldwide, there is a strong male predominance in HCC incidence. In the United States, the male-to-female ratio is 2.7 to 1, and HCC incidence rates are higher among African Americans than Caucasians (6.1 vs 2.8 per 100,000 in men). Hispanics, Asians, Pacific Islanders, and Native Americans have a much higher HCC frequency. Independent of HBV status, a family history of HCC in first-degree relatives carries a relative risk (RR) of 2.4 and overall risk (OR) of 2.9 ([17]). Familial aggregation and germline mutations of the *APC* (adenomatous polyposis coli) gene have been reported in hepatoblastoma ([18]).

ETIOLOGY AND RISK FACTORS

Hepatocellular carcinoma develops commonly, but not exclusively, in a setting of liver cell injury, which leads to inflammation, hepatocyte regeneration, liver matrix remodeling, fibrosis, and ultimately cirrhosis. The major etiologies of liver cirrhosis are diverse and include chronic HBV and HCV infection, alcohol consumption, certain medications or toxic exposures, and genetic metabolic diseases. The mechanisms by which these varied etiologies lead to HCC are not fully elucidated. The principal risk factors that have been associated with cirrhosis and HCC are listed in Table 22-3.

Chronic Viral Hepatitis

Chronic hepatitis B or C viral infection is the most important risk factor for developing HCC. Alone, HCV causes about 40% of HCCs in the United States.

Table 22-3 Etiologic Factors Associated With an Increased Risk of Cirrhosis and Hepatocellular Carcinoma

Category	Specific Etiology	Comment
Infectious (77% of cases of HCC worldwide attributed to viral hepatitis)	Hepatitis B virus	Underlying etiology in a significant majority of HCC cases worldwide, primarily in Asia, sub-Saharan Africa
	Hepatitis C virus	Principal underlying etiology in Japan, the United States, Western Europe, Mediterranean basin countries; may account for 20%-25% HCC cases worldwide
Metabolic disorders deficiency	Hemachromatosis a_1 antitrypsin	
	Wilson disease	
	Porphyria cutanea tarda	
	Glycogen storage disease	
	Citrullinemia	
	Familial cholestatic cirrhosis	
Other	Alcohol	Significant cause of liver cirrhosis; cofactor with HCV
	Aflatoxin B	Cofactor with HBV that increases risk of developing HCC
		Relative risk varies from two- to fourfold in nonendemic regions
	Androgenic steroids	Some association reported, primarily case reports and small series
	Oral contraceptives	
	Autoimmune hepatitis	
	Nonalcoholic steatohepatitis (NASH)	Increasing evidence for association with HCC with or without cirrhosis; incidence of NAFLD is rising in the United States
	Tobacco	Weak association suggested that it is independent of HBV infection, alcohol

Chronic HBV or HCV carriers usually take 10 to 20 years to develop hepatic cirrhosis and 30 to 40 years to develop HCC. Hepatitis B virus is a DNA virus that commonly integrates into the host hepatocyte genome and may play a direct procarcinogenic role. Hepatitis C virus is an RNA virus with no insertional mutagenesis. Although HBV and HCV contain no known viral oncogene to immortalize hepatocytes, hepatitis Bx antigen may inactivate p53 protein and downregulate DNA repair ability ([19, 20]). Some of the principal differences between HBV- and HCV-associated HCC are listed in Table 22-4.

Alcohol and Cirrhosis

Excessive alcohol consumption can lead to hepatic cirrhosis and thus is a risk factor for HCC. The autopsies of patients with alcoholic cirrhosis have reported up to 10% undiagnosed HCC. In the United States, alcoholic cirrhosis is associated with about 15% of HCC and cholangiocarcinoma ([21, 22]). In HCV carriers, alcohol increases circulating HCV viral titer and HCC risk. Other types of cirrhosis and parenchymal liver diseases—such as primary biliary cirrhosis, hemochromatosis, Wilson disease, alpha-1 antitrypsin deficiency, and glycogen storage disease—significantly increase HCC risks when alcohol is a cofactor.

Aflatoxin

Food contaminated with aflatoxin, a mycotoxin found in grains, can induce HCC in animals. There is also a strong association between aflatoxin exposure and HBV carrier status. Relative risks of HCC are 3-fold for aflatoxin, 9-fold for chronic HBV infection, and 59-fold for concurrent aflatoxin and chronic HBV infection. The underlying mechanism is polymorphism variants of glutathione-S-transferase M1 and epoxide hydrolase genes and G-to-T point mutation of the *p53* gene ([20]).

Other Environmental Factors

The use of oral contraceptive pills (OCPs) significantly increases the incidence of benign hepatic adenomas. There is some evidence that OCPs also increase HCC risk. Multiple studies of tobacco smoking and HCC risk have yielded mixed conclusions. Occupational exposure to arsenic or vinyl chloride significantly increases the risk of liver angiosarcoma. Exposure to the x-ray contrast medium thorium dioxide from 1930 to 1955 is associated with an extremely high risk of hemangiosarcoma, cholangiocarcinoma, and HCC.

CLINICAL PRESENTATION

Most cases of HCC are identified incidentally or through screening programs of high-risk individuals. It is common for patients to be asymptomatic until their disease is very far advanced; fewer than 30% of patients are candidates for surgery or other liver-directed therapy at presentation. Many patients present with symptoms of advanced liver dysfunction from both cirrhosis and HCC. The most common initial symptom is right upper quadrant abdominal pain. Anorexia or early satiety with weight loss is the second most common symptom. Also, HCC may present with various paraneoplastic symptoms through the secretion of numerous hormones. Late-stage symptoms include jaundice, tumor fever, bone pain due to metastatic lesions, and complications from portal venous hypertension, such as esophagogastric varices, hypoalbuminemia, ascites, thrombocytopenia, and coagulopathy.

On physical examination, hepatomegaly is present in over 90% of patients. A hepatic arterial bruit or a friction rub, ascites, splenomegaly, and jaundice are found in up to 50% of patients. Muscle wasting, fever, and dilated abdominal veins are also common. The Budd-Chiari syndrome is caused by malignant invasion and occlusion

Table 22-4 Comparison Between Hepatitis B Viral Infection and Hepatitis C Infection and Hepatocellular Carcinoma

Factor	HBV	HCV
Mean age	52-56 (20-80)	62
Highest incidence	400 million carriers in Asia and Africa	170 million infected worldwide; accounts for 50% of HCC cases in Japan, the United States, and Western Europe
Cirrhosis	25%-50%	>75%
Morphology	Solitary lesions	Multifocal lesions, more severe inflammation
Rate of progression to HCC	10-30 years	>30 years
Percentage likely to develop HCC	4% per year	1%-7% per year

of the hepatic veins. The HCC marker alpha-fetoprotein (AFP) is often elevated to above 400 ng/mL.

PATHOLOGY

Based on the growth pattern, HCC may be classified into four major gross anatomic types: spreading, multifocal, encapsulated, and combined patterns ([23]). Normal liver parenchyma is shown in Fig. 22-1. The spreading type of HCC grows in nodular, pseudolobular, or invasive patterns with poorly defined margins, occurs in the setting of hepatic cirrhosis, and accounts for nearly 50% of cases in the United States. The multifocal type has numerous tumors of similar size that make it difficult to determine whether the lesions are intrahepatic metastases or second primary tumors (Figs. 22-2A and 22-2B). The encapsulated type of tumor grows by expanding, compressing, and distorting the surrounding liver tissue. Satellite or metastatic lesions are seen in late-stage disease. This type is most common in Asia and Africa but seen in only 13% of cases in the United States. The combined patterns of the three are seen in up to 25% of cases. Figure 22-3 shows an HCC histopathology specimen.

Approximately 60% to 70% of Caucasian and 80% to 90% of Asian HCC cases show elevated AFP, which is the most useful marker for HCC. Originally, AFP is produced by the fetal liver and yolk sac but falls to below 10 ng/mL in adult serum. A transient elevation of AFP to 20 to 400 ng/mL may occur when there is hepatocyte regeneration, as in cirrhosis, active hepatitis, or partial hepatectomy. The HCC positive predictive value of an AFP level of 400 ng/mL is over 95%, and normal AFP levels may exist in patients with low tumor burden. The lectin-reactive isoenzyme of AFP (AFP-L3) has shown increased sensitivity. Other markers, such as gamma-glutamyl transferase isoenzymes,

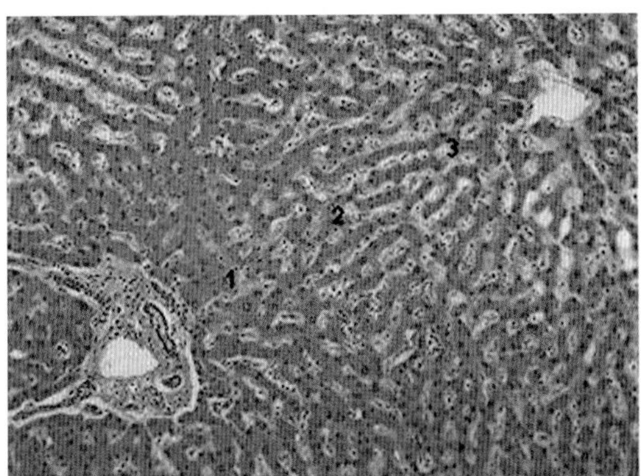

FIGURE 22-1 Photomicrograph of normal parenchyma.

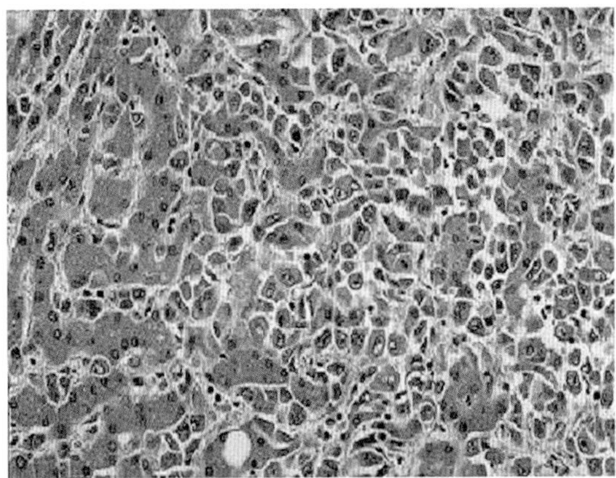

FIGURE 22-3 Photomicrograph with standard hematoxylin and eosin stain of hepatocellular carcinoma cells in hepatic parenchyma.

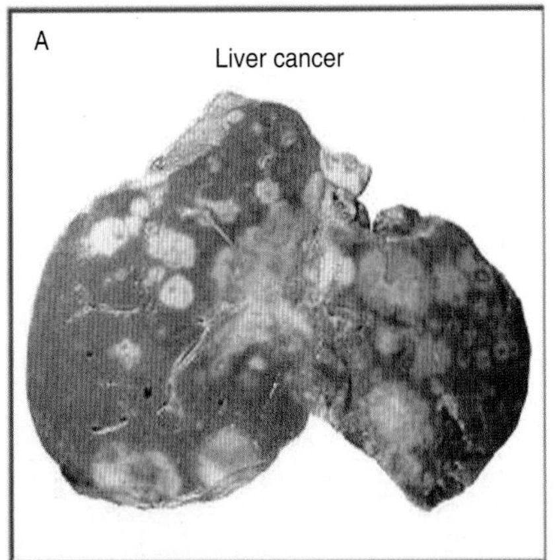

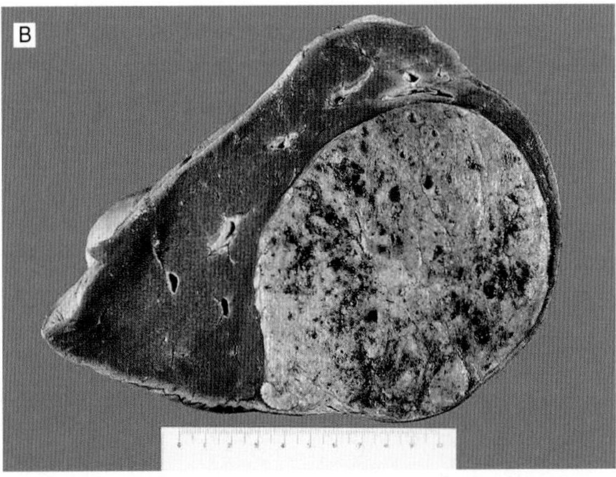

FIGURE 22-2 A. Gross pathologic specimens of multifocal hepatocellular carcinoma. B. Gross appearance of liver cell carcinoma. Courtesy of Dr RA Cooke, Brisbane, Australia. Reproduced with permission from Cooke RA, Stewart B: *Colour Atlas of Anatomical Pathology*, 3rd ed. Edinburgh, Churchill Livingstone, 2004.

alkaline phosphatase, isoferritins, and monoclonal antibodies are not more useful than AFP ([24]). Currently, serum AFP level and ultrasonography are the "gold standard" for HCC screening in high-risk populations ([24]).

Variants of Hepatocellular Carcinoma

There are five HCC variants: HCC with biliary differentiation, clear cell HCC, cholangiocellular carcinoma (CCC), FLHCC, and focal nodular hyperplasia (FNH). Cholangiocellular carcinoma is a combination of cholangiocarcinoma and HCC. It occurs in the noncirrhotic liver and behaves like a cholangiocarcinoma; it has a predominance for men. The outcome of patients with CCC is uniformly fatal.

Fibrolamellar HCC is predominantly seen in the right hepatic lobe, accounts for 2% to 4% of HCC, and occurs equally in men and women. It typically occurs in adolescents and young adults; the etiology is unknown. It is characterized by fibrosis arranged in lamellar fashion around HCC cells. Fibrolamellar HCC consists of well-circumscribed, large, solitary lesions without hepatic cirrhosis or elevated AFP ([25]). The imaging studies often show a heterogeneous mass with a central scar that is similar to FNH. In comparison to classic HCC, FLHCC demonstrates a higher resection rate and better survival, with a 3-year survival of almost 100%.

Focal nodular hyperplasia occurs predominantly in young women. Liver function studies and the serum AFP level are normal. A technetium sulfur colloid radioisotope scan of the liver shows increased radioisotope uptake in FNH compared with hepatic adenomas or carcinomas. The prognosis is excellent.

Clear cell HCC has a distinguishing appearance and better prognosis. Hepatocellular carcinoma with biliary differentiation has a much poorer prognosis because of its rapid growth, decreased vascularity, and resistance to embolic therapy.

Rare primary liver neoplasms include hepatoblastoma, sarcoma, angiosarcoma, rhabdomyosarcoma, and epithelioid hemangioendothelioma. Patients may present with fatigue, anorexia, weight loss, and abdominal pain. Hemorrhagic ascites is common, and AFP level is normal. Angiography and contrast-enhanced computed tomography (CT) of the liver are the best diagnostic tools. Open or percutaneous liver biopsy is needed for diagnosis. Surgical resection is still the principal means of therapy if tumors are diagnosed at relatively early stages. They are often resistant to chemotherapy and radiotherapy (RT), and the overall prognosis is poor.

Benign Liver Tumors

Hemangiomas are the most common benign tumors of the liver. Their size ranges from a few millimeters to 25 cm. They appear as calcified solitary lesions in up to 7% of the general population. Magnetic resonance imaging (MRI) is much better than CT in distinguishing HCC from hemangioma on heavily T2-weighted images. Surgical resection is used for symptomatic lesions or when malignancy cannot be excluded. Hepatic artery ligation is an alternative for large cavernous hemangiomas. Hepatic adenoma is another common benign solitary tumor seen in women who have used OCPs for more than 10 years. It is composed of sinusoids, central veins, and arteries without well-defined portal tracts or bile ducts. Hepatic angiography is the most valuable diagnostic tool. Small adenomas usually regress when OCPs are discontinued. Symptomatic lesions are treated with resection.

DIAGNOSTIC EVALUATION, STAGING, AND PROGNOSIS

In addition to performing a complete medical history and physical examination, the diagnostic workup for a patient suspected of having HCC should include serum for complete blood cell count, electrolytes, liver function tests (LFTs), albumin, prothrombin time, hepatitis B and C serologies, and tumor markers (AFP, CA19-9, CA125). The medical history should include a thorough review of potential HCC risk factors: transfusions, tattoos, intravenous drug abuse, high-risk sexual practices, familial syndromes, OCP or hormone replacement use, androgenic steroid use, and chemical exposures.

Several radiographic imaging modalities are useful in evaluating a patient with HCC. Ultrasound often serves as the initial screening modality, followed by triple-phase CT scan or MRI. Randomized studies have shown that hepatic ultrasonography has 78% sensitivity and 93% specificity to detect HCC in high-risk populations, especially for patients with normal AFP levels ([26, 27]). Color-flow Doppler can assist preoperative assessment and planning.

Abdominal CT has relatively higher sensitivity and specificity than ultrasonography. With special arterial- and venous-phase scans, CT also makes it possible to evaluate the blood supply of the normal liver parenchyma (portal vein) and neoplastic lesions (hepatic artery). Magnetic resonance imaging is useful in distinguishing benign lesions from malignant tumors by the combination of T2-weighted phase contrast and spin echo sequences. Also, MRI can demonstrate fatty degeneration of tumor and vascular invasion ([28]).

Hepatic radionuclide imaging has low spatial resolution and is only about 70% sensitive in demonstrating neoplasms. Using the glucose metabolic difference between neoplastic and normal cells, positron emission tomography (PET) differentiates benign lesions from malignant tumors, detects extrahepatic metastasis, and evaluates response to therapy.

In summary, ultrasonography is the most cost-effective HCC screening test in high-risk populations. Abdominal CT with liver protocol is the most helpful in accurately staging patients prior to surgery. No single diagnostic modality has greater than 50% to 60% sensitivity in detecting lesions less than 1 cm in size. The combination of AFP level, ultrasonography, and CT provides the best hope of early diagnosis.

A variety of staging and prognostic systems has been developed to evaluate patients with HCC. Four staging systems (Okuda; CLIP, Cancer of the Liver Italian Program; CUPI, Chinese University Prognostic Index; and American Joint Committee on Cancer [AJCC] TNM) have evolved since the 1980s. Currently, we use a combined AJCC-TNM staging system at MD Anderson Cancer Center (MDACC) (Table 22-5) ([25]). The Child-Pugh Classification System (Fig. 22-4 and its Appendix C) provides an estimate of a patient's functional liver reserve and is used principally to assist in evaluating a patient's suitability for hepatic resection.

Based on a review of the database developed at MDACC, patients with HCC had an overall 3-year survival rate of 10% and a median survival time of 7.8 months. Favorable prognostic factors are female gender, absence of cirrhosis, and resection of the tumor; these factors correlated with longer survival, especially if the tumors were located in the left hepatic lobe. For patients with unresectable HCC, systemic chemotherapy or supportive care yielded a 44% 1-year survival rate, and no patient survived for 3 years. The size and number of nodules were not determinants of survival. Poor prognostic factors included advanced stage, unresectability associated with cirrhosis, and vascular invasion.

TREATMENT

The current treatment options for HCC are summarized in Table 22-6. At present, liver transplantation is considered the only potentially "curative" treatment. The current 1- and 5-year survival rates for patients with HCC undergoing orthotopic liver transplantation are 77.0% and 61.1%, respectively. The 5-year survival rate has steadily improved, from 25.3% in 1987 to 61.1% in the most recent period studied (1996-2001) ([29]). The authors attributed this improvement to the incorporation of the "Milan" criteria as guidelines for patient selection at most US liver transplantation centers. These criteria, as published by Mazzaferro et al, suggest that long-term survival after liver transplantation is highest in patients with HCC with either a single lesion 5 cm or smaller or three lesions 3 cm or smaller each and no evidence of gross vascular invasion ([30]). A large number of liver transplant candidates remain on the waiting list until they die of tumor progression or cirrhosis-related complications. Partial hepatectomy is the current standard treatment for localized T1 to T3, N0, M0 HCC. Resectability is determined by the extent of liver cirrhosis, the future liver remnant (FLR), and an adequate surgical margin. An FLR of 35% to 40% is considered the minimal cutoff for a safe liver remnant. Patients of Child-Pugh class B and C or with significant signs of portal hypertension are not surgical candidates.

Minor or major resection is based on the following criteria: (1) minor resection: Child A, normal LFTs (bilirubin ≤1.0 mg/dL), absence of ascites, and platelet count above 100,000/mm; and (2) major resection: minor criteria as in criterion 1, absence of portal hypertension, and portal vein embolization for a small future remnant ([31]). The perioperative mortality has decreased from 20% in the 1980s to less than 5% at present ([31]).

Table 22-5 Combined AJCC-TNM Staging System for Hepatocellular Carcinoma

Stage Group	TNM	Scheme
Stage I	T1N0M0	Single tumor <2 cm without vascular invasion
Stage II	T2N0M0	Single tumor <2 cm with vascular invasion or multiple tumors <2 cm in one lobe or single tumor 2 cm without vascular invasion
Stage IIIA	T3N0M0	Multiple tumors in one lobe ± vascular invasion or any tumor >5 cm or single tumor >2 cm with vascular invasion
Stage IIIB	T1-T3N1M0	Positive regional lymph node
Stage IVA	T4N0-N1M0	Multiple tumor in 2+ lobes or tumors involving major portal or hepatic vein
Stage IVB	T1-T4N0-N1M1	Remote metastasis
Fibrosis score		0-4, none to moderate; 5-6, severe fibrosis/cirrhosis

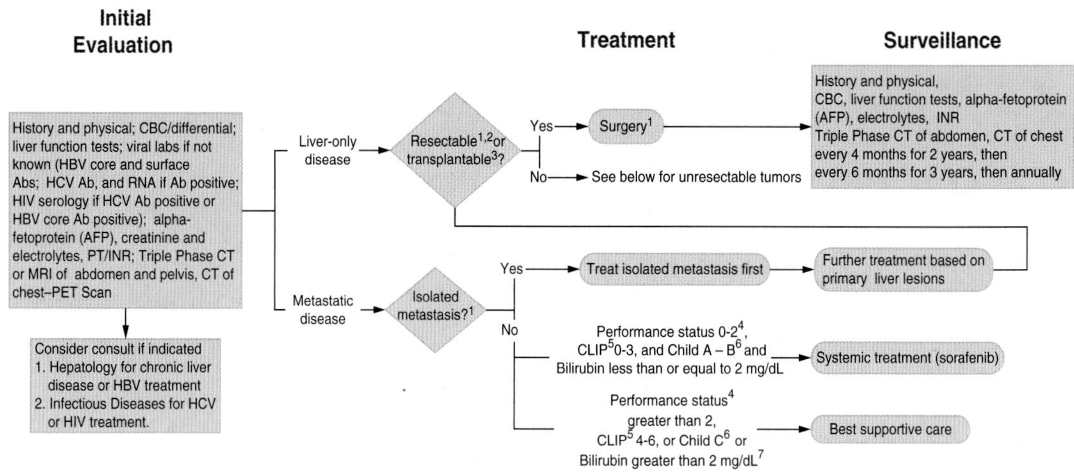

[1] Consider biomarkers (See Appendix A for MDA approved hepatocellular biomarkers)
[2] Minor or Major Resection based on:
• Minor Resection: Child-Pugh A, normal liver function tests (bilirubin less than or equal 1.0 mg%), absence of ascites, and platelet count greater than 100,000/mm^3
• Major Resection: Same as minor resection plus absence of portal hypertension, portal vein embolization (PVE) for a small future liver remnant
[3] Milan criteria; criteria for eligibility for liver transplantation for patients with hepatocellular carcinoma and cirrhosis: the presence of a tumor 5 cm or less in diameter in patients with single hepatocellular carcinomas, or no more than three tumor nodules, each 3 cm or less in diameter, in patients with multiple tumors, and without macrovascular invasion per imaging studies
[4] See Appendix B for ECOG performance status
[5] CLIP—refer to Appendix C for determination of CLIP score
[6] Child-Pugh—refer to Appendix D for Child-Pugh scores
[7] Treatment may be considered in select cases with bilirubin 2-3 mg/dL

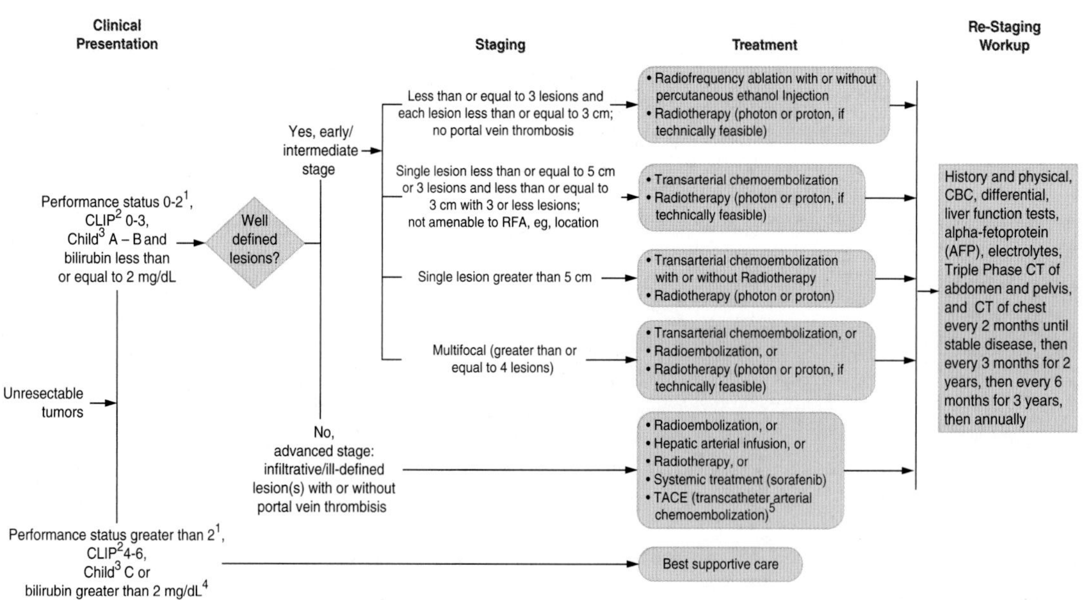

[1] See Appendix A for ECOG performance status
[2] CLIP—refer to Appendix B for determination of CLIP score
[3] Child-Pugh—refer to Appendix C for Child-Pugh scores
[4] Treatment may be considered in select cases with bilirubin 2-3 mg/dL
[5] TACE is a relative contraindication in the presence of portal vein thrombosis

Appendix A: Hepatocellular Carcinoma Molecular Markers, MD Anderson Approved[1]

		Biomarker		
Disease Site	Cell Type	FISH	Immunohistochemistry	Molecular
GI	Hepatocellular	MET	MET	

[1] Literature support for MD Anderson approved biomarkers is available and can be found under Clinical Management Algorithms→"Biomarkers –MD Anderson Approved"

FIGURE 22-4 MDACC approach to HCC treatment.

CHAPTER 22

Appendix B: Eastern Cooperative Oncology Group (ECOG) Performance Status Criteria

Grade	Scale
0	Fully active, able to carry on all pre-disease performance without restriction (Karnofsky 90-100)
1	Restricted in physically strenuous activity but ambulatory and able to carry out work of a light or sedentary nature, i.e., light housework, office work (Karnofsky 70-80)
2	Ambulatory and capable of all self-care but unable to carry out any work activities. Up and about more than 50% of waking hours (Karnofsky 50-60)
3	Capable of only limited self-care, confined to bed or chair more than 50% of waking hours (Karnofsky 30-40)
4	Completely disabled. Cannot carry out any self-care. Totally confined to bed or chair (Karnofsky 10-20)
5	Dead

Appendix C: CLIP Scoring System

Variables	0	1	2
Child-Pugh Stage	A	B	C
Tumor morphology	Uninodular and extension less than or equal to 50%	Multinodular and extension less than or equal to 50%	Massive or Greater than 50%
AFP	Less than 400 ng/dL	Greater than or equal to 400 ng/dL	
Portal vein thrombosis	No	Yes	

Appendix D: Child-Pugh Scale

Chemical and Biochemical Parameters	Scores (Points) for Increasing Abnomality		
	1	2	3
Encephalopathy	None	1-2	3-4
Ascites	None	Slight	Moderate
Albumin	Greater than 3.5 g/dL	2.8-3.5 g/dL	Less than 2.8 g/dL
Prothrombin time prolonged	1-4 seconds	4-6 seconds	Greater than 6 seconds
Bilirubin For primary biliary cirrhosis	1-2 mg/dL 1-4 mg/dL	2-3 mg/dL 4-10 mg/dL	Greater than 3 md/dL Greater than 10 mg/dL

Class A = 5 to 6 points
Class B = 7 to 9 points
Class C = 10 to 15 points

FIGURE 22-4 *Continued*

CHAPTER 22

Table 22-6 Treatment Options for Management of Hepatocellular Carcinoma

Treatment Option	Comments
Liver transplantation	Historically low survival rates (20%-36%).
	Recent improvement (61.1%, 1996-2001), likely related to adoption of "Milan" criteria at US transplant centers.
	Currently HCC represents 20% or more of liver transplants performed annually in the United States.
Surgical resection	Historic 5-year survival rates 30%-40%.
	Recent series indicated 5-year progression-free survival as high as 48%. A majority of patients develop recurrence or second primary tumors.
	Resection in cirrhotic patients carries high morbidity and mortality.
Transarterial embolization/ chemoembolization (TACE)	Multiple trials showed objective tumor responses and "slowed" tumor progression but questionable survival benefit compared to supportive care. Greatest benefit seen in patients with preserved liver function, absence of vascular invasion, and smallest tumors.
	Modest survival benefit demonstrated for repeated TACE (82% 1-year survival) versus supportive care (63%) in patients with preserved liver function, PS 0, small tumor burden.
	Improvement in 1-year survival from 32% in control (supportive care) to 57% for TACE shown in randomized study of 279 primarily HBV+ patients with tumors <7 cm.
Percutaneous treatments (ethanol injection, thermal ablation, cryoablation, hypertonic saline injection)	PEI well tolerated, high RR in small (<3 cm) solitary tumors. No randomized trial comparing resection to percutaneous treatments. Recurrence rates similar to postresection.
Hormonal therapy	Antiestrogen therapy with tamoxifen studied in several trials; mixed results across studies, but generally considered ineffective.
	Octreotide (somatostatin analogue) showed 13-month MS versus 4-month MS in untreated patients in a small randomized study.
Chemotherapy	*Adjuvant:* No randomized trials showing benefit of neoadjuvant or adjuvant systemic therapy in HCC. Single trial showed decrease in new tumors in patients receiving oral synthetic retinoid for 12 months after resection/ablation. Results not reproduced.
	Palliative: Regimens including as single agents or combinations of doxorubicin, cisplatin, 5-fluorouracil, interferon, epirubicin, and paclitaxel have not shown any survival benefit; RR ranged from 0%–25%. A few isolated major responses allowed patients to undergo partial hepatectomy. No published results from any randomized trial of systemic chemotherapy.

PEI, Percutaneous Ethanol Injection.

The median disease-free survival after partial hepatectomy is about 2 years. Tumor size less than 5.0 cm (0.6 RR) was associated with improved survival, while the presence of vascular invasion, AFP greater than 2,000 mg/mL, and advanced Child-Pugh classification was associated with worse outcome. Patients with cirrhosis generally are not considered good candidates for surgical resection due to the high morbidity and mortality associated with cirrhosis and its complications. For those who do undergo resection, recurrence rates are among the highest of any solid tumor and approach 75% to 100% at 5 years. Estimated 5-year survival rates are in the range of 26% to 50%, and disease-free survival is 13% to 29% ([32]).

Locoregional Therapy for Hepatocellular Carcinoma

Hepatocellular carcinoma derives its blood supply almost exclusively from the hepatic artery. This important anatomic feature offers unique advantages for catheter-based therapies because arterial embolization interrupts blood flow to the tumor while preserving the portal vein and normal liver parenchyma. The combination of tissue ischemia with highly concentrated chemotherapy delivered into the hepatic artery enhances tumor necrosis. Transarterial chemoembolization (TACE) was first described by Yamada and incorporates these concepts ([33]). It has since become one of the most commonly utilized procedures in interventional radiology practice.

Landmark prospective randomized clinical trials published in 2002 validated the use of chemoembolization for unresectable advanced HCC. In the multicenter study by Llovet et al including 112 patients, when compared to bland embolization or best supportive therapy, patients who underwent TACE with a combination of doxorubicin and iodized oil followed by gelatin sponge demonstrated a clear survival advantage, leading to premature stoppage of the trial ([34]). Survival in the chemoembolization group at 1 and 2 years was 82% and 63%, respectively. Survival in the bland embolization group was 75% and 50%, respectively; in the best supportive care group, survival was 63% and 27%, respectively, and reached statistical significance.

Lo et al conducted a single-center study comparing 80 patients with unresectable HCC randomized to TACE with cisplatin and iodized oil followed by gelatin sponge or best supportive care ([35]). Survival in the chemoembolization group at 1 and 2 years was 57% and 31%, respectively. Survival for the patients randomized to the supportive care group was 32% and 11%, respectively, also reaching statistical significance. The difference in survival rates between the Llovet and Lo studies can be attributed to the inclusion of a larger proportion of patients with more advanced stages of underlying chronic liver disease in the latter study. Chemoembolization is contraindicated in patients with overt signs of portal hypertension and advanced underlying liver disease.

An important limitation of conventional chemoembolization using iodized oil lies in the uncontrolled washout of the cytotoxic drugs into the systemic circulation. Recently, a drug-eluting bead that allows controlled and sustained release of chemotherapeutic agents into the surrounding tumor was made available. This device enables delivery of a higher concentration of drugs with low systemic toxicity. Initial studies demonstrated that chemoembolization using drug-eluting beads is safe, with potentially increased effectiveness for patients with more advanced disease ([36–38]).

At MD Anderson, TACE is routinely utilized for patients with HCC with more than three lesions measuring up to 3 cm each or a single lesion greater than 5 cm. In patients with portal vein thrombosis, infiltrative disease, or more than four lesions, radio embolization with yttrium-90 microspheres is well tolerated and has been shown to improve outcomes. A recent study assessing the use of radio embolization in HCC showed response rates of 42% based on World Health Organization criteria ([39]).

Radiofrequency ablation causes tissue necrosis by controlled deposition of thermal energy. This technique is highly effective in the treatment of small and early HCC, with outcomes similar to surgical resection ([40]). Radiofrequency ablation is limited by lesion proximity to adjacent structures such as colon, gallbladder, and diaphragm. In addition, vascular structures adjacent to the target lesion steal heat from the area and decrease effectiveness of the ablation. The combination of chemoembolization followed by radiofrequency ablation may improve cell death because occlusion of blood flow leads to larger ablation zones ([41, 42]).

Systemic Chemotherapy and Hormonal Therapy

A majority (>80%) of patients diagnosed with HCC have advanced disease at presentation and—based on the number, size, and location of lesions, as well as the severity of the underlying cirrhosis—are not candidates for transplantation, surgical resection, or liver-directed therapies. At present, systemic chemotherapy is ineffective in HCC, as evidenced by low response rates and no demonstrated survival benefit (see Table 22-6). HCCs are inherently chemotherapy resistant ([43]) and known to express the multidrug-resistance gene *MDR-1* ([44, 45]).

Few well-controlled, randomized chemotherapy trials have been published regarding HCC. That being said, we conducted a retrospective analysis of patients with unresectable HCC at MD Anderson who received either a conventional or a modified neoadjuvant PIAF chemotherapy regimen, consisting of cisplatin, interferon a-2b, doxorubicin, and 5-fluorouracil (5-FU). We found that select patients with HCC (patients who are noncirrhotic and without hepatitis B with good performance status [PS]) benefit from neoadjuvant-modified PIAF chemotherapy with improved response rates, resectability, and survival ([46]). Therefore, we consider this regimen in the neoadjuvant setting in select patients with unresectable tumors as bridge to surgery. Unfortunately, the ability to conduct controlled clinical trials of systemic regimens in patients with HCC has been hampered by many factors, including the multiple comorbidities of cirrhosis (Table 22-7), the advanced nature of HCC at presentation, rapid disease progression in many instances, and the distribution of patients primarily in developing nations, where multidisciplinary treatment of HCC may not be available.

Approximately 15% to 40% of HCCs are estrogen receptor positive. Hormonal therapy with tamoxifen or octreotide analogues has demonstrated some survival benefit ([47]); however, the results of other studies are conflicting.

Clinical Trials of Antiangiogenesis Agents

Several systemic targeted agents have recently been tested in clinical trials for patients with advanced

Table 22-7 Medical Comorbidities Complicating Hepatocellular Carcinoma

Problem	Intervention
Esophageal, gastric varices	Beta blockade for portal HTN for primary prophylaxis of GI bleeding
	Endoscopic variceal banding for clinically significant GI bleeding
Thrombocytopenia	Splenic artery embolization
Hypoalbuminemia	Nutrition, caution with protein-bound medications
Ascites	K^+-sparing diuretics, fluid restriction
Chronic active hepatitis	HCV: IFN/ribavirin have antiviral, antifibrotic effects. HBV: lamivudine, ±IFN
Coagulopathy	PT most sensitive indicator of liver dysfunction

GI, gastrointestinal; HBV, hepatitis B virus; HCV, hepatitis C virus; HTN, hypertension; IFN, interferon; K, potassium; PT, protime.

CHAPTER 22

HCC, including agents targeting the vascular endothelial growth factor (VEGF) pathway, either alone ([48–60]) or in combination with other systemic therapies ([61–68]). The cancer cell has been the only target of anticancer systemic therapy for more than 50 years. However, the cancer cell is genetically unstable, leading to accumulation of mutations. On the other hand, antiangiogenic therapy agents target endothelial cells that are genetically stable. Interestingly, the mechanism of action of thalidomide was thought to be partly based on its antiangiogenic effects. Nevertheless, several clinical trials of thalidomide showed rare responses, ranging from 0% to 6.3% ([58, 59]).

Newer agents that target this antiangiogenic mechanism include sunitinib and sorafenib. Sunitinib is an oral multikinase inhibitor that exerts its antiangiogenic effects by targeting VEGF receptor (VEGFR) and platelet-derived growth factor receptor (PDGFR) tyrosine kinases. Sorafenib, another oral multikinase inhibitor, exerts its antitumor effect by targeting Raf/MEK/ERK signaling at the level of Raf kinase and possesses an antiangiogenic effect by targeting VEGFR-2/-3. Recently, two phase III trials of sorafenib have been reported ([48, 60]). The pivotal randomized, placebo-controlled phase III trial of sorafenib in patients with advanced HCC (SHARP trial [Sorafenib Hepatocellular Carcinoma Assessment Randomized Protocol Study group trial]) reported modest activity with a 2.8-month improvement in median overall survival (OS) (P = .0006). In addition, it demonstrated an increased time to progression and disease control rate while showing a response rate of 2.3% as defined by RECIST criteria ([48]). This led to Food and Drug Administration (FDA) approval of sorafenib for advanced HCC in 2007, and it remains the only FDA-approved drug for this indication.

Other agents that target antiangiogenesis include bevacizumab and erlotinib. Bevacizumab is a recombinant, humanized monoclonal antibody that exerts its antitumor activity by targeting VEGF and may augment chemotherapy administration by making tumor vasculature less permeable, which decreases the elevated tumor interstitial pressure. Erlotinib is an oral tyrosine kinase inhibitor that blocks phosphorylation at the intracellular domain level of the *EGFR*. Most recently, we reported a phase II single-arm, open-label trial of bevacizumab and erlotinib that showed improved response rate, median OS, and progression-free survival ([53]).

Collectively, application of antiangiogenesis agents to patients with advanced HCC has eventually led to improved survival despite surprisingly low response rates. Notably, there is a poor correlation between survival benefit and conventional methods of response assessment, namely, RECIST. This poses questions regarding how best to evaluate response to antiangiogenic agents and quantify efficacy of antiangiogenic agents. Despite tumors increasing in size sometimes, the observation of tumor necrosis in many studies is intriguing. Therefore, in 2000, a panel of experts recommended that the response criteria be amended to take into account tumor necrosis induced by targeted agent therapy ([69]). Although its utility in assessing efficacy of anticancer agents in HCC needs to be established, tumor necrosis is a potentially significant clinical end point that warrants further investigation in future studies.

Targeted Therapies in Hepatocellular Carcinoma: Beyond Sorafenib

Given the paucity of available FDA-approved medications for advanced HCC, a number of other targeted agents have been tested in clinical trials in the adjuvant and advanced/metastatic setting. In the adjuvant setting, sorafenib did not show improved OS versus placebo in patients with previously resected or ablated HCC ([70]). Similar results were seen for orantinib, a multireceptor tyrosine kinase inhibitor of VEGFR2, PDGFR, and fibroblast growth factor receptor (FGFR), in patients who received previous transcatheter arterial embolization ([71]).

In the advanced, unresectable or metastatic setting, first-line therapy with linifanib (VEGFR and PDGFR tyrosine kinase inhibitor), sunitinib (VEGFR and PDGFR), and brivanib (VEGFR and FGFR) have all been tested in phase III trials against sorafenib with no improvement in OS ([72–74]). In the second-line setting, brivanib, everolimus (mTOR pathway inhibitor), and ramicirumab (fully human immunoglobulin G1 monoclonal antibody against VEGFR2) have all been tested versus placebo in patients who have either progressed on or were intolerant to sorafenib. None of these trials showed any significant improvement in OS ([75–77]). Two other agents, tivantinib (MET inhibitor) and cabozantinib (MET, RET, and VEGFR tyrosine kinase inhibitor) are currently being studied in clinical trials for patients in the second-line setting described. Enrollment in these trials is ongoing, and results are incomplete ([78, 79]). At present, no therapy has better proven efficacy than sorafenib in the advanced, unresectable, or metastatic setting. Table 22-8 is a summary of targeted therapies in HCC.

Radiation

Advances in our understanding of partial liver tolerance of RT, ability to visualize target tumors during respiration, and radiation planning and delivery techniques have permitted us to escalate the dose of radiation to focal HCCs without dose-limiting toxicity. This improved ability to deliver tumoricidal doses of RT safely has led to a resurgence of interest in treatment of HCC using RT. Promising clinical data from multiple studies suggested that HCCs are indeed radiosensitive. Sustained local control rates ranging from 71% to 100% have been reported following 30 to 90 Gy delivered over 1 to 8 weeks ([80, 81]).

Investigators from Michigan have used conformal RT (1.5 Gy twice daily over 6-8 weeks) with concurrent hepatic arterial fluorodeoxyuridine to treat HCCs safely to doses as high as 90 Gy and achieved a median survival duration of 15.2 months ([82]). Analysis of these data suggested that doses greater than 75 Gy resulted in more durable in-field local control than lower doses.

A prospective French phase II trial administered 66 Gy in 33 fractions to HCCs ineligible for curative therapies and noted 92% tumor responses and 78% 1-year local control rates ([83]). Using higher doses and fewer fractions (hypofractionated RT), Canadian researchers have noted excellent local control rates ranging from 70% to 90% when the radiation beam can be directed from multiple planes (stereotactic RT) converging on the tumor; the majority of the liver can be spared from irradiation, and treatment is image guided ([81, 84, 85]).

In contrast to photon irradiation, for which the dose delivered to the tumor is limited by the entrance and exit doses that can potentially harm normal tissues, accelerated proton beams deposit a dose within the tumor without exiting through normal tissues beyond the tumor ([86]). Japanese investigators have reported mature results of the treatment of 162 patients with 192 unresectable HCCs with 72 Gy in 16 fractions of proton beam therapy ([87]). The 5-year local control rate of 87% and OS rate of 23.5% in the absence of significant toxicity are clinically noteworthy. Furthermore, an impressive 5-year survival rate of 53.5% was

Table 22-8 Targeted Therapies in HCC

Trial	Drug	Primary End Point	Median (Months) (Drug vs Placebo)	Median (Months) (Drug vs Sorafenib)
Adjuvant trials				
STORM	NEXAVAR® (sorafenib)	RFS	33.4 vs 33.8	–
ORIENTAL	TSU-68 (orantinib)	OS	Unknown, terminated	–
First-line trials				
NCT01009593	ABT-869 (linifanib)	OS	–	9.1 vs 9.8
NCT00699374	Sutent® (sunitinib)	OS	–	7.9 vs 10.2
BRISK-FL	Brivanib	OS	–	9.5 vs 9.9
Second-line trials				
BRISK-PS	Brivanib	OS	9.4 vs 8.2	–
EVOLVE-1	Affinitor® (everolimus)	OS	7.6 vs 7.3	–
REACH	Cyramza® (ramucirumab)	OS	9.2 vs 7.6	–
METIV-HCC	Tivantinib	OS	Ongoing	–
CELESTIAL	XL184 (cabozantinib)	OS	Ongoing	–

OS, overall survival; RFS, relapse-free survival.

CHAPTER 22

achieved in a subset of 50 patients with solitary tumors and Child-Pugh Class A cirrhosis.

Our own experience reflects these observations that higher doses are associated with better overall, in-field progression-free and biochemical progression-free survival ([88]). Across all partial liver radiation paradigms, the most common site of first recurrence is intrahepatic but outside the high-dose irradiated volume, and toxicities are more common in Child-Pugh class B patients.

Given the excellent local control rate as noted with RT alone, RT has been combined with TACE to overcome treatment resistance. Korean researchers initially noted more than 60% response rates and a significant drop in tumor marker levels using this combination treatment strategy ([89, 90]). It was reported that TACE followed by RT improved OS over TACE alone in a retrospective analysis of this experience. Similar results have been reported by other groups as well ([91–93]).

For the treatment of unfavorable tumors, multiple groups have reported favorable outcomes in patients with portal venous tumor thrombus (PVTT) treated with RT ([94–103]). Response rates ranged from 37.5% to 100%, and median survival durations ranged from 3.8 to 10.7 months.

Taken together, these advances have permitted the escalation of radiation dose to unresectable HCCs without causing undue toxicity. Strategies that combine RT with other therapies merit continued evaluation to maximize the relative benefits of each approach.

MDACC APPROACH TO HEPATOCELLULAR CARCINOMA

Hepatocellular carcinoma and other primary liver tumors require multidisciplinary input, and patients benefit from clinical care that integrates the expertise of surgical oncology, liver transplantation, diagnostic and interventional radiology, gastroenterology and hepatology, radiation oncology, and medical oncology. New cases of HCC are reviewed at a weekly multidisciplinary liver tumor conference to develop a consensus approach to each patient's case. Careful attention is paid to precise tumor staging, histopathologic diagnosis, and each patient's PS.

Patients with HCC who meet current United Network for Organ Sharing (UNOS) criteria are offered liver transplantation or resection if they are highly likely to benefit. Liver-directed therapies, principally RFA and TACE, are commonly employed in patients who are not candidates for surgical intervention. In addition, select patients who present with unresectable tumors are considered for neoadjuvant chemotherapy as a bridge to surgery. Patients with good PS with advanced HCC are encouraged to participate in a clinical trial of systemic therapy. Figure 22-4 depicts the general approach followed by the multidisciplinary hepatobiliary team in managing patients with HCC evaluated at MDACC.

REFERENCES

1. Siegel R, et al. Cancer statistics, 2014. *CA Cancer J Clin.* 2014; 64(1):9-29.
2. World Health Organization. Mortality Database. WHO Statistical Information System. http://www.who.int/whosis.
3. Taylor-Robinson, S.D., et al. Increase in primary liver cancer in the UK, 1979-94. *Lancet.* 1997;350(9085):1142-1143.
4. Deuffic, S., et al. Trends in primary liver cancer. *Lancet.* 1998; 351(9097):214-215.
5. Davis, GL, et al. Projecting future complications of chronic hepatitis C in the United States. *Liver Transpl.* 2003;9(4):331-338.
6. Parkin DM, Bray FI, Devesa SS. Cancer burden in the year 2000. The global picture. *Eur J Cancer.* 2001;37(Suppl 8):S4-S66.
7. Smart RG, Mann RE, Suurvali H. Changes in liver cirrhosis death rates in different countries in relation to per capita alcohol consumption and Alcoholics Anonymous membership. *J Stud Alcohol.* 1998;59(3):245-249.
8. Wong JB, et al. Estimating future hepatitis C morbidity, mortality, and costs in the United States. *Am J Public Health.* 2000;90(10):1562-1569.
9. *National Vital Statistics Report.* 2002;50;28-31.
10. El-Serag HB, et al. The continuing increase in the incidence of hepatocellular carcinoma in the United States: an update. *Ann Intern Med.* 2003;139(10):817-823.
11. El-Serag HB, Mason AC. Rising incidence of hepatocellular carcinoma in the United States. *N Engl J Med.* 1999;340(10):745-750.
12. Kohli A, et al. Treatment of hepatitis C: a systematic review. *JAMA.* 2014;312(6):631-640.
13. Loguercio, C., et al. Non-alcoholic fatty liver disease: a multicentre clinical study by the Italian Association for the Study of the Liver. *Dig Liver Dis.* 2004;36(6):398-405.
14. McCullough AJ. The clinical features, diagnosis and natural history of nonalcoholic fatty liver disease. *Clin Liver Dis.* 2004; 8(3):521-533, viii.
15. Ruhl CE, Everhart JE. Epidemiology of nonalcoholic fatty liver. *Clin Liver Dis.* 2004;8(3):501-519, vii.
16. Parkin DM. The global burden of cancer. *Semin Cancer Biol.* 1998; 8(4):219-235.
17. Shen FM, et al. Complex segregation analysis of primary hepatocellular carcinoma in Chinese families: interaction of inherited susceptibility and hepatitis B viral infection. *Am J Hum Genet.* 1991;49(1):88-93.
18. Giardiello FM. et al. Hepatoblastoma and APC gene mutation in familial adenomatous polyposis. *Gut.* 1996;39(6):867-869.
19. Jia L, Wang XW, Harris CC. Hepatitis B virus X protein inhibits nucleotide excision repair. *Int J Cancer.* 1999;80(6):875-879.
20. Groisman IJ, et al. Downregulation of DNA excision repair by the hepatitis B virus-x protein occurs in p53-proficient and p53-deficient cells. *Carcinogenesis.* 1999;20(3):479-483.
21. Sorensen HT, et al. Risk of liver and other types of cancer in patients with cirrhosis: a nationwide cohort study in Denmark. *Hepatology.* 1998;28(4):921-925.
22. Di Bisceglie AM, et al. NIH conference. Hepatocellular carcinoma. *Ann Intern Med.* 1988;108(3):390-401.
23. Fong Y, et al. An analysis of 412 cases of hepatocellular carcinoma at a Western center. *Ann Surg.* 1999;229(6):790-799; discussion 799-800.
24. Sutton FM, et al. Factors affecting the prognosis of primary liver carcinoma. *J Clin Oncol.* 1988. 6(2):321-8.

25. Vauthey JN, et al. Simplified staging for hepatocellular carcinoma. *J Clin Oncol.* 2002;20(6):1527-1536.
26. Pateron D, et al. Prospective study of screening for hepatocellular carcinoma in Caucasian patients with cirrhosis. *J Hepatol.* 1994;20(1):65-71.
27. Fong Y, Kemeny N, Lawrence TS. Cancer of the liver and biliary tract. In: DeVita VT, Hellman H, Rosenberg SA, eds. *Cancer: Principles and Practice of Oncology*. Philadelphia, PA: Lippincott, Williams & Wilkins; 2001:1162-1203.
28. Rummeny, E., et al. Primary liver tumors: diagnosis by MR imaging. *AJR Am J Roentgenol.* 1989;152(1):63-72.
29. Yoo HY, et al. The outcome of liver transplantation in patients with hepatocellular carcinoma in the United States between 1988 and 2001: 5-year survival has improved significantly with time. *J Clin Oncol.* 2003;21(23):4329-4335.
30. Mazzaferro V, et al. Liver transplantation for the treatment of small hepatocellular carcinomas in patients with cirrhosis. *N Engl J Med.* 1996;334(11):693-699.
31. Pawlik TM, et al. Critical appraisal of the clinical and pathologic predictors of survival after resection of large hepatocellular carcinoma. *Arch Surg.* 2005;140(5):450-457; discussion 457-458.
32. Poon RT, et al. Clinicopathologic features of long-term survivors and disease-free survivors after resection of hepatocellular carcinoma: a study of a prospective cohort. *J Clin Oncol.* 2001;19(12):3037-3044.
33. Yamada R, et al. Hepatic artery embolization in 32 patients with unresectable hepatoma. *Osaka City Med J.* 1980; 26(2):81-96.
34. Llovet JM, et al. Arterial embolisation or chemoembolisation versus symptomatic treatment in patients with unresectable hepatocellular carcinoma: a randomised controlled trial. *Lancet.* 2002;359(9319):1734-1739.
35. Lo CM, et al. Randomized controlled trial of transarterial lipiodol chemoembolization for unresectable hepatocellular carcinoma. *Hepatology.* 2002;35(5):1164-1171.
36. Lammer J, et al. Prospective randomized study of doxorubicin-eluting-bead embolization in the treatment of hepatocellular carcinoma: results of the PRECISION V study. *Cardiovasc Intervent Radiol.* 2010;33(1):41-52.
37. Reyes DK, et al. Single-center phase II trial of transarterial chemoembolization with drug-eluting beads for patients with unresectable hepatocellular carcinoma: initial experience in the United States. *Cancer J.* 2009;15(6):526-532.
38. Poon RT, et al. A phase I/II trial of chemoembolization for hepatocellular carcinoma using a novel intra-arterial drug-eluting bead. *Clin Gastroenterol Hepatol.* 2007;5(9):1100-1108.
39. Salem R, et al. Radioembolization for hepatocellular carcinoma using yttrium-90 microspheres: a comprehensive report of long-term outcomes. *Gastroenterology.* 2010;138(1):52-64.
40. Chen MS, et al. A prospective randomized trial comparing percutaneous local ablative therapy and partial hepatectomy for small hepatocellular carcinoma. *Ann Surg.* 2006;243(3):321-328.
41. Veltri A, Moretto P, Doriguzzi A, et al. Radiofrequency thermal ablation (RFA) after transarterial chemoembolization (TACE) as a combined therapy for unresectable non-early hepatocellular carcinoma (HCC). *Eur Radiol.* 2006;16(3): 661-669.
42. Marelli L, et al. Treatment outcomes for hepatocellular carcinoma using chemoembolization in combination with other therapies. *Cancer Treat Rev.* 2006;32(8):594-606.
43. Huang M, Liu G. The study of innate drug resistance of human hepatocellular carcinoma Bel7402 cell line. *Cancer Lett.* 1999;135(1):97-105.
44. Kato A, Miyazaki M, Ambiru S, et al. Multidrug resistance gene (MDR-1) expression as a useful prognostic factor in patients with human hepatocellular carcinoma after surgical resection. *J Surg Oncol.* 2001;78:110-115.
45. Kuo MT, et al. Activation of multidrug resistance (P-glycoprotein) mdr3/mdr1a gene during the development of hepatocellular carcinoma in hepatitis B virus transgenic mice. *Cell Growth Differ.* 1992;3(8):531-540.
46. Kaseb AO, et al. Modified cisplatin/interferon alpha-2b/doxorubicin/5-fluorouracil (PIAF) chemotherapy in patients with no hepatitis or cirrhosis is associated with improved response rate, resectability, and survival of initially unresectable hepatocellular carcinoma. *Cancer.* 2013;119(18):3334-3342.
47. Kouroumalis E, et al. Treatment of hepatocellular carcinoma with octreotide: a randomised controlled study. *Gut.* 1998; 42(3):442-447.
48. Llovet JM, et al. Sorafenib in advanced hepatocellular carcinoma. *N Engl J Med.* 2008;359(4):378-390.
49. Gruenwald V, Wilkens L, Gebel M, et al. A phase II open-label study of cetuximab in unresectable hepatocellular carcinoma. *J Clin Oncol.* 2006;24(18S):14079.
50. O'Dwyer PJ, Giantonio B, Levy DE, et al. Gefitinib in advanced unresectable hepatocellular carcinoma: results from the Eastern Cooperative Oncology Group's Study E1203. *J Clin Oncol.* 2006;24(18S):4143.
51. Abou-Alfa GK, et al. Phase II study of sorafenib in patients with advanced hepatocellular carcinoma. *J Clin Oncol.* 2006;24(26): 4293-4300.
52. Siegel AB, et al. Phase II trial evaluating the clinical and biologic effects of bevacizumab in unresectable hepatocellular carcinoma. *J Clin Oncol.* 2008;26(18):2992-2998.
53. Thomas MB, et al. Phase 2 study of erlotinib in patients with unresectable hepatocellular carcinoma. *Cancer.* 2007; 110(5):1059-1067.
54. Ramanathan RK, Belani C, Singh DA, et al. Phase II study of lapatinib, a dual inhibitor of epidermal growth factor receptor (EGFR) tyrosine kinase 1 and 2 (Her2/Neu) in patients (pts) with advanced biliary tree cancer (BTC) or hepatocellular cancer (HCC). A California Consortium (CCC-P) Trial. *J Clin Oncol.* 2006;24(18S):4010.
55. Philip PA, et al. Phase II study of erlotinib (OSI-774) in patients with advanced hepatocellular cancer. *J Clin Oncol.* 2005;23(27):6657-6663.
56. Zhu AX, Sahani D, di Tomaso E, et al. A phase II study of sunitinib in patients with advanced hepatocellular carcinoma. *J Clin Oncol.* 2007;25(18S):4637.
57. Zhu AX, B.L., Enzinger PC, et al. Phase II study of cetuximab in patients with unresectable or metastatic hepatocellular carcinoma. *J Clin Oncol.* 2006;24(18S):14096.
58. Patt YZ, et al. Thalidomide in the treatment of patients with hepatocellular carcinoma: a phase II trial. *Cancer.* 2005;103(4): 749-755.
59. Schwartz JD, et al. Thalidomide in advanced hepatocellular carcinoma with optional low-dose interferon-alpha2a upon progression. *Oncologist.* 2005;10(9):718-727.
60. Cheng A, K.Y., Chen Z, et al. Randomized phase III trial of sorafenib versus placebo in Asian patients with advanced hepatocellular carcinoma. *J Clin Oncol.* 2008;26(15S):4509.
61. Thomas MB, et al. Phase II trial of the combination of bevacizumab and erlotinib in patients who have advanced hepatocellular carcinoma. *J Clin Oncol.* 2009;27(6):843-850.
62. Sun W, HD, Mykulowycz K, et al. Combination of capecitabine, oxaliplatin with bevacizumab in treatment of advanced hepatocellular carcinoma (HCC): a phase II study. *J Clin Oncol.* 2007;25(18S):4574.
63. Zhu AX, et al. Phase II study of gemcitabine and oxaliplatin in combination with bevacizumab in patients with advanced hepatocellular carcinoma. *J Clin Oncol.* 2006;24(12):1898-1903.
64. Louafi S, et al. Gemcitabine plus oxaliplatin (GEMOX) in patients with advanced hepatocellular carcinoma (HCC): results of a phase II study. *Cancer.* 2007;109(7):1384-1390.
65. O'Neil BH, B.S., Goldberg RM, et al. Phase II study of

oxaliplatin, capecitabine, and cetuximab in advanced hepatocellular carcinoma. *J Clin Oncol.* 2008;26(15S):4604.
66. Abou-Alfa GK, Johnson P, Knox J, et al. Final results from a phase II (PhII), randomized, double-blind study of sorafenib plus doxorubicin (S+D) versus placebo plus doxorubicin (P+D) in patients (pts) with advanced hepatocellular carcinoma (AHCC). Paper presented at the 2008 Gastrointestinal Cancers Symposium Proceedings; January 25-27, 2008; Orlando, FL. Abstract 128.
67. Hsu C, YT, Hsu C, et al. Phase II study of bevacizumab (A) plus capecitabine (X) in patients (pts) with advanced/metastatic hepatocellular carcinoma (HCC): Final report. *J Clin Oncol.* 2008;26(15S):4603.
68. Shen Y SY, Hsu C. Phase II study of sorafenib plus tegafur/ uracil (UFT) in patients with advanced hepatocellular carcinoma (HCC). *J Clin Oncol.* 2008;26(15S):15664.
69. Bruix J, et al. Clinical management of hepatocellular carcinoma. Conclusions of the Barcelona-2000 EASL conference. European Association for the Study of the Liver. *J Hepatol.* 2001;35(3):421-430.
70. Bruix J, Takayama T, Mazzaferro V, et al. STORM: A phase III randomized, double-blind, placebo-controlled trial of adjuvant sorafenib after resection or ablation to prevent recurrence of hepatocellular carcinoma (HCC) (abstract 4006). *J Clin Oncol.* 2014;32(suppl):5s).
71. Taiho Pharma website. http://www.taiho.co.jp/english/news/20140731.html. Accessed December 19.
72. Cainap C, Qin Shukui Q, Wen-Tsung H, et al. Phase III trial of linifanib versus sorafenib in patients with advanced hepatocellular carcinoma (HCC). *J Clin Oncol* 31, 2013 (suppl 4; abstr 249).
73. Cheng AL, et al. Sunitinib versus sorafenib in advanced hepatocellular cancer: results of a randomized phase III trial. *J Clin Oncol.* 2013; 31(32):4067-4075.
74. Johnson PJ, et al. Brivanib versus sorafenib as first-line therapy in patients with unresectable, advanced hepatocellular carcinoma: results from the randomized phase III BRISK-FL study. *J Clin Oncol.* 2013;31(28):3517-3524.
75. Llovet JM, et al. Brivanib in patients with advanced hepatocellular carcinoma who were intolerant to sorafenib or for whom sorafenib failed: results from the randomized phase III BRISK-PS study. *J Clin Oncol.* 2013;31(28):3509-3516.
76. Zhu AX, et al. Effect of everolimus on survival in advanced hepatocellular carcinoma after failure of sorafenib: the EVOLVE-1 randomized clinical trial. *JAMA.* 2014;312(1):57-67.
77. Zhu AX, Park JO, Ryoo BY, et al. Ramucirumab versus placebo as second-line treatment in patients with advanced hepatocellular carcinoma following first-line therapy with sorafenib (REACH): a randomised, double-blind, multicentre, phase 3 trial. *Lancet Oncol.* 2015 Jul;16(7):859-70.
78. Santoro A, Porta C, Rimassa L, et al. Metiv-HCC: A phase III clinical trial evaluating tivantinib (ARQ 197), a MET inhibitor, versus placebo as second-line in patients (pts) with MET-high inoperable hepatocellular carcinoma (HCC) (abstract TPS4159. *J Clin Oncol.* 2013;(suppl):31.
79. Ghassan K Abou-Alfa, e.a.P.r., double-blind, controlled study of cabozantinib (XL184) versus placebo in subjects with hepatocellular carcinoma who have received prior sorafenib (CELESTIAL; NCT01908426) (abstract TPS4150). *J Clin Oncol.* 2014; 32(suppl):5s.
80. Krishnan S, et al. Radiotherapy for hepatocellular carcinoma: an overview. *Ann Surg Oncol.* 2008;15(4):1015-1024.
81. Hawkins MA, Dawson LA. Radiation therapy for hepatocellular carcinoma: from palliation to cure. *Cancer.* 2006;106(8):1653-1663.
82. Ben-Josef E, et al. Phase II trial of high-dose conformal radiation therapy with concurrent hepatic artery floxuridine for unresectable intrahepatic malignancies. *J Clin Oncol.* 2005; 23(34):8739-8747.
83. Mornex F, G.N., Beziat C, et al. Feasibility and efficacy of high-dose three-dimensional-conformal radiotherapy in cirrhotic patients with small-size hepatocellular carcinoma non-eligible for curative therapies-mature results of the French Phase II RTF-1 trial. *Int J Radiat Oncol Biol Phys.* 2006;66:1152-1158.
84. Mendez Romero A, et al. Stereotactic body radiation therapy for primary and metastatic liver tumors: a single institution phase i-ii study. *Acta Oncol.* 2006;45(7):831-837.
85. Dawson LA, Eccles C, Craig T. Individualized image guided iso-NTCP based liver cancer SBRT. *Acta Oncol.* 2006;45(7):856-864.
86. Skinner HD, Hong TS, Krishnan S. Charged-particle therapy for hepatocellular carcinoma. *Semin Radiat Oncol.* 2011;21(4): 278-286.
87. Chiba T, et al. Proton beam therapy for hepatocellular carcinoma: a retrospective review of 162 patients. *Clin Cancer Res.* 2005;11(10):3799-3805.
88. Skinner HD, et al. Radiation treatment outcomes for unresectable hepatocellular carcinoma. *Acta Oncol.* 2011;50(8):1191-1198.
89. Seong J, et al. Combined transcatheter arterial chemoembolization and local radiotherapy of unresectable hepatocellular carcinoma. *Int J Radiat Oncol Biol Phys.* 1999;43(2):393-397.
90. Seong J, et al. Local radiotherapy for unresectable hepatocellular carcinoma patients who failed with transcatheter arterial chemoembolization. *Int J Radiat Oncol Biol Phys.* 2000;47(5):1331-1335.
91. Yasuda S, et al. Radiotherapy for large hepatocellular carcinoma combined with transcatheter arterial embolization and percutaneous ethanol injection therapy. *Int J Oncol.* 1999;15(3):467-473.
92. Guo WJ, Yu EX. Evaluation of combined therapy with chemoembolization and irradiation for large hepatocellular carcinoma. *Br J Radiol.* 2000;73(874):1091-1097.
93. Chia-Hsien Cheng J, et al. Unresectable hepatocellular carcinoma treated with radiotherapy and/or chemoembolization. *Int J Cancer.* 2001;96(4):243-252.
94. Tazawa J, et al. Radiation therapy in combination with transcatheter arterial chemoembolization for hepatocellular carcinoma with extensive portal vein involvement. *J Gastroenterol Hepatol.* 2001;16(6):660-665.
95. Yamada K, et al. Prospective trial of combined transcatheter arterial chemoembolization and three-dimensional conformal radiotherapy for portal vein tumor thrombus in patients with unresectable hepatocellular carcinoma. *Int J Radiat Oncol Biol Phys.* 2003;57(1):113-119.
96. Ishikura S, et al. Radiotherapy after transcatheter arterial chemoembolization for patients with hepatocellular carcinoma and portal vein tumor thrombus. *Am J Clin Oncol.* 2002;25(2):189-193.
97. Yamada K, et al. Pilot study of local radiotherapy for portal vein tumor thrombus in patients with unresectable hepatocellular carcinoma. *Jpn J Clin Oncol.* 2001;31(4):147-152.
98. Nakagawa, K., et al. Radiation therapy for portal venous invasion by hepatocellular carcinoma. *World J Gastroenterol.* 2005;11(46):7237-7241.
99. Zeng ZC, et al. A comparison of treatment combinations with and without radiotherapy for hepatocellular carcinoma with portal vein and/or inferior vena cava tumor thrombus. *Int J Radiat Oncol Biol Phys.* 2005;61(2):432-443.
100. Lin CS, et al. Treatment of portal vein tumor thrombosis of hepatoma patients with either stereotactic radiotherapy or three-dimensional conformal radiotherapy. *Jpn J Clin Oncol.* 2006;36(4):212-217.
101. Hsu WC, et al. Results of three-dimensional conformal radiotherapy and thalidomide for advanced hepatocellular carcinoma. *Jpn J Clin Oncol.* 2006;36(2):93-99.

102. Kim DY, et al. Three-dimensional conformal radiotherapy for portal vein thrombosis of hepatocellular carcinoma. *Cancer.* 2005;103(11):2419-2426.

103. Minagawa M, Makuuchi M. Treatment of hepatocellular carcinoma accompanied by portal vein tumor thrombus. *World J Gastroenterol.* 2006;12(47):7561-7567.

23

Small Bowel Cancer and Appendiceal Tumors

第二十三章　小肠恶性肿瘤和阑尾肿瘤

Michael J. Overman
Kanwal Raghav
Christopher H. Lieu
Commentary: Keith F. Fournier

中文导读

小肠恶性肿瘤和阑尾肿瘤发病率均较低，本章分别介绍了小肠恶性肿瘤和阑尾肿瘤的相关内容。第一部分回顾了小肠类癌和腺癌，小肠腺癌的病因与大肠癌相似，这部分在环境和饮食因素、遗传性肿瘤和炎症性肠病等方面进行了相关分析。接着进一步描述了小肠恶性肿瘤的临床表现、诊断、TNM分期和预后。治疗方面介绍了外科治疗、复发类型和辅助治疗，并重点介绍了MD安德森癌症中心关于转移性和非转移性小肠肿瘤的治疗方法，同时绘制了详细的小肠腺癌治疗标准流程图。本章第二部分主要介绍了阑尾肿瘤的发病率、临床表现和预后。根据肿瘤病理类型分别介绍了阑尾类癌和阑尾上皮肿瘤的治疗。重点阐述了阑尾上皮肿瘤分子图谱，主要包括KRAS、GNAS、AKT、MET、PIK3CA和TP53，和组织病理亚型，主要包括：腹膜假性黏液瘤、弥散性腹膜黏液蛋白病、腹膜黏液癌和非黏液性/结肠型腺癌。治疗方面介绍了减瘤手术、腹腔热灌注化疗和全身化疗，并重点介绍了MD安德森癌症中心治疗阑尾上皮肿瘤的经验和方法。

PART A: SMALL BOWEL CANCER

Small bowel cancer is a rare malignancy representing approximately 3% of gastrointestinal neoplasms ([1]). In 2014, it was estimated that 9,160 new cases of small bowel cancer and 1,210 small bowel cancer–related deaths would occur ([1]). The two most common histologies seen in cancers of the small intestine are carcinoids and adenocarcinomas ([2]). Because of the nonspecific clinical presentation of small bowel adenocarcinoma and the difficulty in imaging the small bowel, most patients with small bowel adenocarcinoma present with lymph node involvement or distant metastases. Even in patients with localized disease who undergo resection with curative intent, the prognosis is poor, and no studies have yet demonstrated a clear benefit from adjuvant therapy. However, there have been some recent advances in the use of chemotherapy as palliative treatment. In this chapter, the epidemiology, diagnosis, and treatment of small bowel cancers, in particular small bowel adenocarcinoma, are reviewed.

Epidemiology

Based on an analysis of the Surveillance, Epidemiology, and End Results (SEER) database, the age-adjusted incidence rate for small bowel cancers has slowly increased from 0.9 per 100,000 persons in the years 1973 to 1982 to 1.8 per 100,000 persons in the years 2000 to 2004 ([3,4]). The majority of this increase has been attributed to an increase in the incidence of carcinoid tumors. A recent analyses of 67,643 patients with small bowel malignancies between 1973 and 2004 using the National Cancer Data Base and SEER showed carcinoids to be dominant with 37.4% cases compared to 36.9% cases of adenocarcinomas ([5]). The incidence of histologic subtypes varies in the different sections of the small intestine, with adenocarcinomas representing 80% of duodenal cancers and carcinoids representing 60% of ileal cancers.

The incidence of small bowel adenocarcinoma peaks in the seventh and eighth decades of life, with a mean age at diagnosis of 65 years. A slightly increased incidence is seen in men and blacks ([6]).

One of the more interesting aspects of small bowel adenocarcinoma is its rarity in comparison to large intestine adenocarcinoma. Even though the small intestine represents approximately 70% to 80% of the length and over 90% of the surface area of the alimentary tract, the incidence of small bowel adenocarcinoma is 30-fold less than the incidence of colon adenocarcinoma. Numerous theories have been proposed to explain the small intestine's relative protection from the development of carcinoma. Proposed protective factors have centered on two concepts. First, the rapid turnover time of small intestinal cells results in epithelial cell shedding prior to the necessary acquisition of multiple genetic defects. Second, the small bowel's exposure to the carcinogenic components of our diet are limited due to rapid small bowel transit time, the lack of bacterial degradation activity that occurs in the small bowel, and the relatively dilute, alkaline environment of the small bowel. In a population-based comparison of adenocarcinomas of the large (n = 261,521) and small (n = 4,518) intestine identified from the SEER registry, small bowel adenocarcinomas demonstrated a distinctly worse stage-adjusted cancer-specific survival compared to colorectal adenocarcinomas ([7]).

Anatomy

The small intestine is divided into three sections. The duodenum represents the first 25 cm of the small intestine and is subdivided into four anatomic segments. The proximal portion of the first (ascending) segment of the duodenum is intraperitoneal, and then the distal portion, as well as the rest of the duodenum, becomes retroperitoneal. The second (descending) segment of the duodenum contains the ampulla of Vater, through which the pancreatic and biliary secretions exit. The third (horizontal) segment of the duodenum is the longest, and as it crosses the left border of the aorta, the fourth (ascending) segment of the duodenum begins. The duodenal-jejunal junction is characterized by the attachment of the suspensory ligament of Treitz. The next segment of the small bowel, the jejunum, is approximately 2.5 m long, and the final segment, the ileum, is approximately 3.5 m long.

Etiology

Little is known about the etiology of small bowel adenocarcinoma. As seen in colorectal adenocarcinomas, adenocarcinomas of the small intestine undergo a similar phenotypic adenoma-carcinoma transformation ([8–10]). An increase in the size of small bowel adenomas and the presence of a villous histology are risk factors for the development of invasive adenocarcinoma.

Common underlying genetic or environmental factors of both large and small intestine adenocarcinomas have been suggested by studies that have demonstrated an increased risk of small bowel adenocarcinoma in patients with colon adenocarcinoma and vice versa ([11]). In small bowel adenocarcinoma, microsatellite instability occurs at a similar rate to that seen in colorectal cancer (CRC). In a study of 89 patients with small bowel adenocarcinoma identified from a Swedish population-based cancer registry, the rate of microsatellite instability was 18% ([12]). This result along with the known clinical association between hereditary nonpolyposis colorectal cancer (HNPCC) syndrome and small bowel adenocarcinoma indicate that in a subset of patients with small bowel adenocarcinoma, a germline mutation in one of the mismatch repair proteins contributes to carcinogenesis.

The possible role of pancreaticobiliary secretions in the development of adenocarcinoma of the duodenum has been suggested by the anatomic clustering of duodenal carcinomas in the periampullary area. For example, in patients with familial adenomatous polyposis (FAP), 80% of small intestinal adenocarcinomas will occur in the second portion of the duodenum. One study evaluating 213 cases of duodenal carcinomas identified from the Los Angeles County tumor registry determined that 57% of the cases originated in the second part of the duodenum ([13]).

Environment and Dietary Risk Factors

A number of case-control studies have analyzed associations between environmental and dietary factors and the development of small bowel adenocarcinoma. Two studies have demonstrated that there is an association between the ingestion of smoked or salt-cured foods and the development of small bowel adenocarcinoma ([14, 15]). An association between tobacco use and cancer risk has been inconsistently demonstrated. Case-control studies have demonstrated an association between an increased risk of small bowel adenocarcinoma and high alcohol intake, high sugar intake, high red meat intake, low fiber intake, celiac disease, peptic ulcer disease, and prior cholecystectomy ([14–18]). Studies of the relationship with obesity have been conflicting, although a recent case-cohort study of 500,000 subjects with 134 incident cases of small bowel cancer showed a statistically nonsignificant trend toward increased risk in subjects with high body mass index (BMI) (hazard ratio [HR] 1.5 [95% CI, 0.76-2.96] for BMI >27.5 kg/m^2 compared with 22.6-25.0 kg/m^2) ([19]).

Genetic Cancer Syndromes

The genetic cancer syndromes HNPCC, FAP, and Peutz-Jeghers syndrome (PJS) are all associated with small bowel adenocarcinoma. The estimated lifetime risk for small bowel adenocarcinoma is 1% to 4% in patients with HNPCC, 5% in those with FAP, and 13% in those with PJS ([20–23]). Patients with HNPCC develop small bowel adenocarcinoma at a younger age, with a median age at diagnosis of 49 years. Patients with PJS, an autosomal dominant polyposis disorder characterized by multiple hamartomatous polyps throughout the intestinal tract, have a markedly increased risk for small bowel adenocarcinoma, with one meta-analysis demonstrating a 520-fold increased relative risk ([24]). Duodenal adenomas are seen in approximately 80% of patients with FAP, and regular endoscopic screening for the development of adenocarcinoma is required for these patients. The optimal frequency of endoscopic screening depends on a number of factors, such as the number of polyps, polyp size, polyp histology, and amount of dysplasia present ([20]). With the early use of colectomy in patients with FAP, duodenal adenocarcinomas and desmoid tumors are now a more common cause of death in this population than cancer arising from the colorectum.

Inflammatory Bowel Disease

Inflammatory bowel disease, particularly Crohn disease, is associated with the development of small bowel adenocarcinoma. The increase in risk varies depending on both the extent and duration of small bowel involvement. In one study, the cumulative risk of small bowel adenocarcinoma in patients with Crohn disease was 0.2% at 10 years and 2.2% at 25 years ([25]). Because Crohn disease frequently involves the ileum, 70% of the small bowel cancers in patients with Crohn disease will occur in the ileum. Patients with Crohn disease who develop small bowel adenocarcinoma appear to have a worse prognosis, with one study of 37 patients with small bowel adenocarcinoma demonstrating significantly shorter overall survival (OS) in the patients with Crohn disease ([26]).

Molecular Profile

Early limited data has begun to accumulate regarding molecular characterization of small bowel adenocarcinomas. Accumulation of genetic defects such as loss of e-cadherin and smad4 and mutations in *KRAS*, *P53*, and *SMAD4* have been implicated in the adenoma-dysplasia-carcinoma sequence of small bowel adenocarcinomas ([2]). In a pivotal study comparing chromosomal copy number aberrations in 85 gastric, colorectal, and small bowel adenocarcinomas, hierarchical clustering revealed a substantial overlap of sba copy number profiles with matched colorectal adenocarcinomas but less overlap with profiles of gastric adenocarcinomas, indicating a genetic profile similar to CRC ([27]). Large screening of somatic mutations in 83 patients revealed *KRAS*, *TP53*, *APC*, *SMAD4*, *PIK3CA*, erbb2, braf, and fbxw7 mutations in >5% of small bowel adenocarcinomas ([24]). Understanding the biology of small bowel adenocarcinomas may lead to the possibility of developing targeted therapy in this rare cancer.

Presentation and Diagnosis

Clinical Presentation

The symptoms associated with small bowel adenocarcinoma are nonspecific and frequently do not occur until advanced disease is present. The most commonly reported symptoms are abdominal pain (45%-76% of patients), nausea and vomiting (31%-52%), weight loss (22%-29%), and gastrointestinal bleeding (8%-34%). Delays in diagnosis are common, with one retrospective study reporting a mean delay of 7.8 months from the time of initial physician evaluation until a final diagnosis was made ([28]). According to the National Cancer Database, 39% of patients present with stage I/II disease, 26% present with stage III disease, and 32% present with stage IV disease ([29]).

Diagnosis

Given the nonspecific presenting symptoms, a high index of suspicion is a crucial first step in diagnosis. Because imaging of the small intestine is difficult, multiple tests may be needed. However, with the availability of wireless capsule endoscopy, the need for older small bowel imaging techniques has declined.

A barium small bowel follow-through study has been the radiographic gold standard for small bowel evaluation. In patients with advanced-stage disease, this technique has a sensitivity of approximately 60% for diagnosing small bowel tumors. Enteroclysis, in which contrast material is infused directly into the small intestine through a nasogastric tube, provides a slightly higher sensitivity than small bowel follow-through. Endoscopic evaluation of the small intestine, or enteroscopy, requires expertise and is frequently unable to evaluate the entire small intestine.

The incorporation of wireless capsule endoscopy, which was approved by the US Food and Drug Administration in 2001, has allowed a much simpler and improved method for evaluating the lumen of the small intestine. This technique has primarily been applied to the evaluation of obscure gastrointestinal bleeding, for which it has shown superiority over other imaging and endoscopy techniques ([30]). In one study evaluating capsule endoscopy in 60 patients with suspected small bowel pathology but without gastrointestinal bleeding, the overall diagnostic yield of capsule endoscopy was 62% ([31]). In that study, all patients had undergone upper and lower gastrointestinal endoscopy, and many had undergone enteroclysis, small bowel follow-through, push enteroscopy, and abdominal computed tomography (CT). In a large single-center retrospective review of 562 patients who underwent capsule endoscopy, small bowel tumors were found in 8.9% of cases ([32]). The major limitations of capsule endoscopy are that no tissue sampling can be conducted and that the patients cannot have bowel obstruction, which could result in the capsule's becoming trapped in the bowel.

Three-dimensional imaging with either CT or magnetic resonance imaging (MRI) is useful in identifying locoregional lymph node involvement and the presence of distant metastatic disease. For tumors of the duodenum, endoscopic ultrasonography can be useful in assessing both the tumor and nodal status. Although not directly studied for duodenal adenocarcinomas, endoscopic ultrasonography has been demonstrated to improve staging accuracy for both ampullary and pancreatic cancers.

Staging and Prognosis

The TNM (tumor, node, metastasis) staging system for small bowel adenocarcinoma is shown in Table 23-1 ([33]). In a study of 4,995 patients who were diagnosed with small bowel adenocarcinoma between 1985 and 1995 (identified in the National Cancer Database), the 5-year disease-specific survival (DSS) rate was 65% for patients with stage I disease, 48% for patients with stage II disease, 35% for patients with stage III disease, and 4% for patients with stage IV disease ([29]). A multivariate analysis from this study identified age >75 years, primary duodenal tumor site, non–cancer-directed surgery, and higher-stage disease as poor prognostic factors. Though significant on a univariate analysis, a poorly differentiated histology was not a significant prognostic factor on multivariate analysis (P = .089). In other studies, the histopathologic factors reported to be correlated with poor survival were poorly differentiated histology, positive margins, lymphovascular invasion, lymph node involvement, and T4 tumor stage ([26, 34-36]). The 5-year OS rates from various single-institution studies for resected small bowel adenocarcinoma are presented in Table 23-2.

Treatment

Surgical Management

For patients with localized disease, complete removal of the tumor with negative surgical margins and local lymph node removal are critical for a potentially curative resection. For jejunal and ileal lesions, an oncologically successful resection requires a wide local excision with lymphadenectomy. Lesions located in the duodenum generally require a pancreaticoduodenectomy; however, for small distal lesions in the third and fourth portions of the duodenum, a wide local excision may be an option. In a surgical series of 68 patients with duodenal adenocarcinoma, no differences in the 5-year OS rates, local recurrence rates, or margin-negative resection rates were seen between the 50 patients who underwent pancreatic resections and the 18 patients who underwent distal duodenal segmental resections ([37]). The presence of locoregional lymph node involvement should not deter surgical intervention because well over one-third of patients will survive long

Table 23-1 TNM Staging for Adenocarcinoma of the Small Intestine

Primary Tumor (T)			
TX	Primary tumor cannot be assessed		
T0	No evidence of primary tumor		
Tis	Carcinoma in situ		
T1a	Tumor invades lamina propria		
T1b	Tumor invades submucosa		
T2	Tumor invades muscularis propria		
T3	Tumor invades through the muscularis propria into the subserosa or into the nonperitonealized perimuscular tissue (mesentery or retroperitoneum) with extension 2 cm or less[a]		
T4	Tumor perforates the visceral peritoneum or directly invades other organs or structures (includes other loops of small intestine, mesentery, or retroperitoneum >2 cm and abdominal wall by way of serosa; for duodenum only, invasion of pancreas or bile bile duct)		
Regional Lymph Nodes (N)			
NX	Regional lymph nodes cannot be assessed		
N0	No regional lymph node metastasis		
N1	Metastasis in 1-3 regional lymph nodes		
N2	Metastasis in 4 or more regional lymph nodes		
Distant Metastasis (M)			
M0	No distant metastasis		
M1	Distant metastasis		
Stage Grouping			
Stage 0	Tis	N0	M0
Stage I	T1	N0	M0
	T2	N0	M0
Stage IIA	T3	N0	M0
Stage IIB	T4	N0	M0
Stage IIIA	Any T	N1	M0
Stage IIIB	Any T	N2	M0
Stage IV	Any T	Any N	M1

[a]The nonperitonealized perimuscular tissue is for the jejunum and ileum, part of the mesentery; and for duodenum in areas where serosa is lacking, part of the interface with the pancreas.

Reproduced with permission from Edge SB, Byrd DR, Compton CC (eds): *AJCC Cancer Staging Manuarl*, 7th ed. New York, NY: Springer; 2010.

Table 23-2 Reported Overall Survival of Patients With Curatively Resected Small Bowel Adenocarcinoma

First Author	Period	Tumor Location	Number of Patients	Overall Survival	
				Median (Months)	5 Year (%)
Agarawal	1971-2005	Small intestine	30	56	45
Kelsey	1975-2005	Duodenum	25	NR	64
Wu	1983-2003	Small intestine	45	NR	27
Swartz	1994-2003	Duodenum	14	41	44
Dabaja	1978-1998	Small intestine	142	36	29
Czaykowski	1990-2000	Small intestine	19	39	NR
Talamonti	1977-2000	Small intestine	26	40	42
Abrahams	1978-1999	Small intestine	37	NR	52
Brucher	1985-1998	Small intestine	22	NR	45
Bakaeen	1976-1996	Duodenum	68	NR	54
Rose	1983-1994	Duodenum	42	NR	60
Cunningham	1970-1991	Small intestine	19	23	32
Frost	1960-1989	Small intestine	22	NR	32

NR, not reported.

term ([29, 38]). This is in contrast to patients with lymph node–positive pancreatic cancer, of whom only 7% survive 5 years ([39]). As is seen with colon cancer, the total lymph nodes (TLNs) assessed during surgery and the number of positive lymph nodes (PLNs) have prognostic implications in small bowel adenocarcinomas. In a SEER registry retrospective review of 1,991 patients, the 5-year DSS for patients with stage II disease appeared to be associated with the TLNs assessed (44%, 69%, and 83% for 0 TLNs, 1 to 7 TLNs, and >7 TLNs, respectively) ([40]). Furthermore, the 5-year DSS with stage III disease was associated with the number of PLNs (58% and 37% for <3 PLNs and ≥3 PLNs, respectively) ([40]).

Patterns of Recurrence

Recurrence after potentially curative resection of small bowel adenocarcinoma occurs most commonly at distant sites. In a series of 146 patients who underwent resection for small bowel adenocarcinoma, 56 patients relapsed at a median of 25 months, with the sites of relapse reported as distant in 59%, peritoneum in 20%, abdominal wall in 7%, and local in 18% ([41]). In a second study of 30 patients who underwent potentially curative resection for small bowel adenocarcinoma, 21 patients experienced a relapse, with the sites of relapse being the liver in 67% of the patients, lung in 38%, retroperitoneum in 29%, and peritoneum in 25% ([34]).

Patients with duodenal adenocarcinoma have a higher rate of locoregional failure than for jejunal and ileal adenocarcinoma, with one study reporting a 39% rate of locoregional failure among 31 patients after curative resection of duodenal adenocarcinoma ([42]). In that study, positive margin status was the strongest predictor of local recurrence, with 4 of the 5 patients who had a margin positive resection developing a local recurrence. However, distant recurrences are still predominant, with a retrospective review of recurrence patterns in 67 patients with resected duodenal adenocarcinoma revealing local recurrences in 33% of the patients and distant recurrences in 67% ([43]).

Adjuvant Therapy

Currently, there is no evidence demonstrating a benefit from adjuvant therapy in patients with small bowel adenocarcinoma who undergo potentially curative resection. However, owing to the rarity of small bowel adenocarcinoma, only a limited number of primarily small retrospective studies have been conducted (Table 23-3). Selection bias is the major limitation of these retrospective studies because the patients selected to receive adjuvant therapy were the patients believed to be at highest risk for disease recurrence. One prospective phase III study conducted by the European Organization for Research and Treatment of Cancer randomized 93 eligible patients with periampullary carcinoma (defined as adenocarcinoma of the distal common bile duct, ampulla of Vater, or duodenum) to receive either no adjuvant therapy or concurrent 5-fluorouracil (5-FU) and radiation therapy ([44]). The 5-year OS rates were similar in the two groups, but 30% of the patients assigned to receive adjuvant therapy did not actually receive it, and no description of the results in the duodenal adenocarcinoma subgroup were reported.

In a series by Kelsey et al, no differences in the 5-year OS rates were seen between the patients who did or did not receive adjuvant therapy after resection of duodenal adenocarcinoma. However, in the subgroup of patients who had undergone a margin-negative resection, the 5-year OS rate was 53% in the patients who underwent resection only and 83% in the patients who had resection and adjuvant chemoradiation therapy ($P = .07$) ([42]). A trend toward improvement of disease-free survival and OS was seen in patients receiving adjuvant therapy in a retrospective series at MD Anderson Cancer Center (n = 54) ([45]). However, in the subgroup analyses in patients with high-risk disease, defined by a lymph node ratio ≥10%, adjuvant therapy was associated with significant improvement in OS ([45]). In contrast, in a single-institution retrospective review at Mayo Clinic, no benefit of adjuvant chemotherapy or chemoradiotherapy was seen in patients with resected small bowel adenocarcinoma ([46]).

Limited data are available regarding a neoadjuvant (preoperative) treatment approach for duodenal adenocarcinoma. In one report in which 11 patients underwent neoadjuvant chemoradiation therapy followed by resection for duodenal adenocarcinoma, a complete pathologic response was seen in 2 patients, and none of the 11 patients had histopathologic nodal involvement at the time of surgery ([42]).

The MD Anderson Approach to Nonmetastatic Disease

At the University of Texas MD Anderson Cancer Center, patients with high-risk, resected small bowel adenocarcinoma are typically offered postoperative adjuvant chemotherapy. In general, patients who are considered to be at high risk are those with lymph node involvement and positive resection margins. The lack of proven benefit from adjuvant chemotherapy for this tumor type must be discussed with the patient. However, the rationale for considering adjuvant chemotherapy is based on

1. The known poor prognosis of patients with high-risk disease
2. The predominantly systemic relapse pattern for small intestinal adenocarcinoma

Table 23-3 Reported Overall Survival of Patients Who Received Adjuvant Therapy After Resection of Small Bowel Adenocarcinoma

					Number of Patients			Median Overall Survival (Months)		
First Author	Time Period	Study Type	Tumor Location	Type of Adjuvant Therapy	Total	No Adjuvant Therapy	Adjuvant Therapy	No Adjuvant Therapy	Adjuvant Therapy	*P* Value
Agrawal	1971-2005	Retrospective review	Small bowel	Not specified	30	19	11	41	56	NR
Kelsey	1975-2005	Retrospective review	Duodenum	5-FU/radiation	32	16	16	44%[a]	57%[a]	0.42
Fishman	1986-2004	Retrospective review	Small bowel	Not specified	60	45	15	28	22	NR
Dabaja	1978-1998	Retrospective review	Small bowel	Not specified	120	62	58	36	19	0.49
Klinkenbiji	1987-1995	Randomized phase III trial	Periampullary	5-FU/radiation	93	49	44	40	40	0.74
Sohn	1984-1996	Retrospective review	Duodenum	5-FU/radiation	48	37	11	35	27	0.73
Overman	1990-2008	Retrospective review	Small Bowel	Chemo/radiation	54	24	30	NR	NR	0.84
Halfdanarson	1970-2005	Retrospective review	Small Bowel	Chemo/radiation	58	60	45	26.5	30.2	0.36

5-FU, 5-fluorouracil; NR, not reported.
[a]Five-year overall survival rate.

3. The proven activity of chemotherapy in the treatment of metastatic small intestinal adenocarcinoma
4. The known benefit of adjuvant chemotherapy in large intestinal adenocarcinoma, which appears to have a number of similarities to small intestinal adenocarcinoma
5. The extremely limited amount of high-quality data to support or refute the role of adjuvant therapy for small bowel adenocarcinoma

Based on the substantial activity of a 5-FU and platinum combination in the metastatic disease setting, we generally utilize the combination of capecitabine and oxaliplatin (CAPOX) as adjuvant therapy for nonmetastatic small bowel adenocarcinoma. In addition to systemic chemotherapy, radiation therapy is considered for patients with duodenal adenocarcinoma who are at high risk for a local recurrence based on the presence of positive margins or T4 disease.

Metastatic Disease

In general, chemotherapy for metastatic small bowel adenocarcinoma has been based on the principles used for treating colon cancer. Several single-institution retrospective series have demonstrated a survival benefit in patients with metastatic or unresectable small bowel adenocarcinoma who received chemotherapy when compared to patients who did not receive chemotherapy ([41, 47]).

Most of the studies evaluating chemotherapy for small bowel adenocarcinoma have been retrospective, with only four prospective phase II studies reported (Table 23-4). One multicenter study conducted by the

CHAPTER 23

Table 23-4 Reported Response and Overall Survival for Patients Treated With Systemic Chemotherapy for Metastatic Small Bowel Adenocarcinoma

First Author	Year	Study Type	Disease Status	Number of Patients	Type of Chemotherapy	Overall Response Rate (%)	Median Overall Survival (Months)
McWilliams	2012	Prospective phase II trial	Metastatic	23	CAPOXIRI	39	12.7
Xiang	2012	Prospective phase II trial	Metastatic	33	FOLFOX	49	15.2
Zaanan	2010	Retrospective review	Metastatic	93	5-FU–based therapy	26	17.8
Overman	2009	Prospective phase II trial	Metastatic, LAD	30	CAPOX	50	20.3
Overman	2008	Retrospective review	Metastatic	29	5-FU + platinum	41	14.8
				51	Various agents	16	12.0
Fishman	2007	Retrospective review	Metastatic, LAD	44	Various agents	29	18.6
Locher	2005	Retrospective review	Metastatic, LAD	20	5-FU + platinum	21	14.0
Gibson	2005	Prospective phase II trial	Metastatic	38	FAM	18	8
Enzinger	2005	Prospective phase I trial	Metastatic	4	5-FU + cisplatin + irinotecan	50	NS
Czaykowski	2007	Retrospective review	Metastatic, LAD	16	5-FU–based therapy	6	15.6
Goetz	2003	Prospective phase I trial	Metastatic, LAD	5	5-FU + oxaliplatin + irinotecan	40	NS
Polyzos	2003	Case series	Metastatic	3	Irinotecan	0	NS
Crawley	1998	Retrospective review	Metastatic, LAD	8	ECF +5-FU–based	37	13
Jigyasu	1984	Retrospective review	Metastatic	14	5-FU–based therapy	7	9
Ouriel	1984	Retrospective review	Metastatic	14	5-FU–based therapy	NS	10.7
Morgan	1977	Retrospective review	Metastatic	7	5-FU–based therapy	0	NS
Rochlin	1965	Retrospective review	NS	11	5-FU	36	NS

CAPOX, capecitabine and oxaliplatin; CAPOXIRI, capecitabine, oxaliplatin, and irinotecan; ECF, 5-FU, epirubicin, and cisplatin; FAM, 5-FU, doxorubicin, and mitomycin C; FOLFOX, 5-fluorouracil and oxaliplatin; 5-FU, 5-fluorouracil; LAD, locally advanced, unresectable disease; NS, not significant.

Eastern Cooperative Oncology Group reported on the combination of 5-FU, doxorubicin, and mitomycin C (FAM) in 39 patients with adenocarcinomas of the duodenum, jejunum, ileum, or ampulla of Vater. The overall response rate was 18%, with a median OS time of 8 months ([48]). A single-institution study conducted at MD Anderson evaluated CAPOX in 30 patients with metastatic or locally advanced small bowel or ampullary adenocarcinomas. The overall response rate was 50%, with a median time to progression of 9.8 months and an OS time of 20.3 months ([49]). An example of a response to CAPOX chemotherapy in a patient treated in that study is shown in Fig. 23-1. In 33 patients treated with continuous infusional 5-FU and leucovorin in combination oxaliplatin (modified 5-FU and oxaliplatin [FOLFOX] regimen), the objective response rate was 48.5%, and the median OS was 15.2 months ([50]). Another prospective, multicenter, first-line study (n = 23) using CAPOXIRI (capecitabine, oxaliplatin, and irinotecan) showed a response rate of 39% and a median survival of 12.7 months ([51]).

Several retrospective studies have confirmed the substantial activity of 5-FU combined with a platinum agent for metastatic small bowel adenocarcinoma, with response rates of 18%-46% ([52–55]). In one of the largest retrospective studies to date, a total of 80 patients with metastatic small bowel adenocarcinoma were treated with various regimens: 29 received 5-FU with a platinum (19 received cisplatin, 4 received carboplatin, and 6 received oxaliplatin); 41 received 5-FU–based therapy without a platinum (32 received 5-FU alone, 3 received FAM, 3 received 5-FU and mitomycin, and 3 received other 5-FU combinations); and 10 received non-platinum–based and non-5-FU–based therapy ([55]). Patients who received 5-FU combined with a platinum agent had a higher overall response rate (46% vs 16%; $P < .01$) and longer median progression-free survival (PFS) time (8.7 vs 3.9 months; $P < .01$) than patients who received other chemotherapy regimens. Although not statistically significant, there was also a trend toward improved median OS times in patients who received 5-FU plus a platinum agent (14.8 vs 12.0 months; $P = .1$). A French multicenter study in SBA receiving frontline chemotherapy with LV5FU2 (n = 10), FOLFOX (n = 48), FOLFIRI (n = 19), and LV5FU2-cisplatin (n = 16) demonstrated a median PFS of 7.7, 6.9, 6.0, and 4.8 months, respectively ([47]). The corresponding median OS was 13.5, 17.8, 10.6, and 9.3 months, respectively ([47]). In the subgroup analysis, patients treated with LV5FU2-cisplatin had poorer PFS ($P < .01$) and OS ($P = .02$) compared with oxaliplatin-based chemotherapy ([47]).

Irinotecan-based chemotherapy is also active against metastatic small bowel adenocarcinoma. One retrospective study reported that 5 of 12 patients responded to irinotecan-based therapy (3 patients responded to 5-FU plus irinotecan, 1 responded to capecitabine plus irinotecan, and 1 responded to single-agent irinotecan) ([53]). A second study of salvage therapy with irinotecan in the second-line setting noted stable disease in 4 of 8 treated patients ([54]). Among the 19 patients in the AGEO study treated with 5-FU plus irinotecan, 1 had a partial

CHAPTER 23

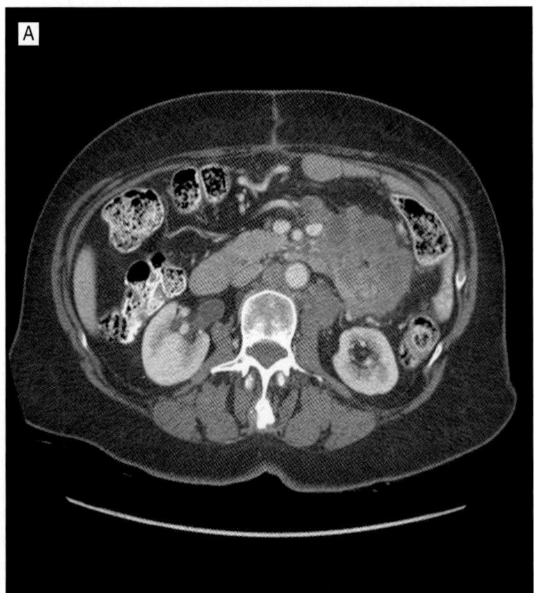

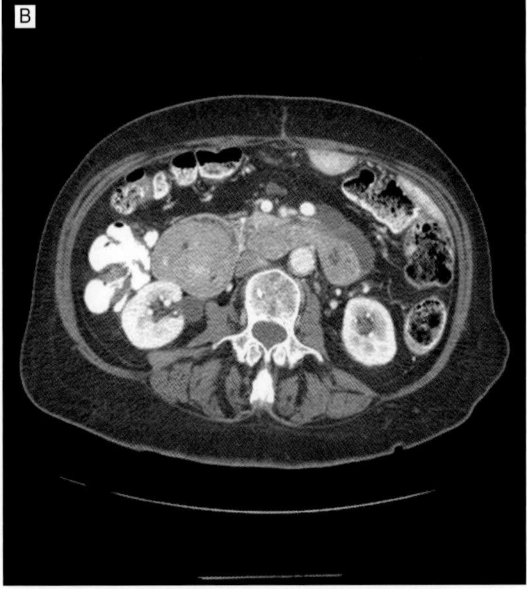

FIGURE 23-1 Radiographic response to capecitabine and oxaliplatin (CAPOX) chemotherapy in a patient with locally advanced small bowel adenocarcinoma. Pretreatment (**A**) and posttreatment (**B**) computed tomographic scans shown.

response, and stable disease was seen in 7 patients ([47]). Responses to gemcitabine-based therapy have also been noted, although the number of patients treated has been small. The role of targeted therapies against the vascular endothelial growth factor (VEGF) or epidermal growth factor receptors (*EGFRs*) has not been studied in small bowel adenocarcinoma.

The MD Anderson Approach to Metastatic Disease

The substantial response rates and prolonged OS times recently reported with modern-day chemotherapy combinations in small bowel adenocarcinomas strongly argue for an aggressive approach in treating patients with metastatic small bowel adenocarcinoma. Given the extremely encouraging results with CAPOX and FOLFOX for metastatic small bowel adenocarcinoma, we generally recommend these regimens at MD Anderson. Following frontline CAPOX or FOLFOX chemotherapy, patients are then treated with an irinotecan-based regimen. In addition, patients with limited metastatic disease who respond to initial chemotherapy are considered for surgical resection if all disease sites can be successfully excised. Investigations are ongoing at MD Anderson to evaluate the role of *EGFR* inhibition in addition to CAPOX chemotherapy for small bowel adenocarcinoma. More effective treatments for small bowel adenocarcinoma remain needed, and participation in clinical trials for this rare tumor type is strongly encouraged. A proposed treatment algorithm for small bowel adenocarcinoma is presented in Fig. 23-2.

PART B: APPENDICEAL TUMORS

Appendiceal tumors encompass a rare and diverse group of neoplasms. With an age-adjusted incidence of about 0.12 cases per 1 million individuals per year, appendiceal tumors represent only 1% of all CRCs diagnosed each year in the United States ([56,57]). Historically, appendiceal tumors have been grouped together with CRCs. However, appendiceal tumors, in which outcomes are strongly determined by histologic subtype, tend to have a biology very different from that of CRC. Appendiceal tumors comprise two types: appendiceal carcinoid tumors and appendiceal epithelial tumors. Appendiceal carcinoid tumors account for approximately 50% of all appendiceal neoplasms, and appendiceal epithelial tumors represent the remaining 50% ([58]). This chapter on appendiceal tumors discusses the management of these two tumor types (carcinoid and epithelial) and, in particular, the unusual clinical syndrome of pseudomyxoma peritonei (PMP).

Incidence

Data derived from the SEER database of the National Cancer Institute between 1973 and 1998 revealed that the most common histologic subtypes of malignant tumors of the appendix were adenocarcinomas (67%) and carcinoids (33%) ([56]). However, this analysis captured neither adenomatous tumors nor benign carcinoids. The subtypes of adenocarcinoma were mucinous type (56%), nonmucinous intestinal type (38%), and signet ring cell type (6%). Alternatively, in a separate study of 7,970 appendectomy specimens, tumors were identified in 1% of specimens, with carcinoids representing 57% of all tumors identified ([58]). Adenomas and adenocarcinomas represented 18% and 11% of the identified tumors, respectively.

Presentation and Prognosis

The majority of appendiceal tumors are identified incidentally at the time of pathological review of appendectomy specimens. Symptoms of appendicitis are most often the presenting symptom, especially with tumors located at the base of the appendix, where obstruction is more likely to occur. Other symptoms seen with more advanced appendiceal disease can reflect the nonspecific abdominal symptoms associated with peritoneal involvement: abdominal pain and distention, altered bowel motility, and early satiety. Metastatic carcinoid tumors may also present with symptoms related to the carcinoid syndrome, with episodic flushing, wheezing, and diarrhea. Patient age at presentation differs depending on histologic subtype of the tumor, with the mean age of 38 years for patients with carcinoid tumors and the mean age of 60 years for those with adenocarcinomas ([56]).

Prognosis for appendiceal cancer is strongly dependent on the histopathologic subtype of the tumor, with patients who have carcinoids having a significantly better survival than do patients with adenocarcinomas (Fig. 23-3) ([56]). In addition, patients with early-stage tumors identified incidentally at the time of appendectomy have a better prognosis than patients who are diagnosed once symptoms develop.

Prognosis for patients with epithelial tumors is also strongly dependent on histopathology of the tumor. Staging for appendiceal carcinomas is based on the TNM) seventh edition staging system and incorporates histological grade in the differentiation between stage IVA and IVB (Table 23-5) ([33]).

For metastatic epithelial tumors of the appendix, prognosis is excellent for those with low-grade mucinous tumors, termed disseminated peritoneal adenomucinosis (DPAM), whereas appendiceal adenocarcinomas with high-grade histological features such as poor differentiation or signet ring cell morphology have a much poorer survival. Presence of lymph node

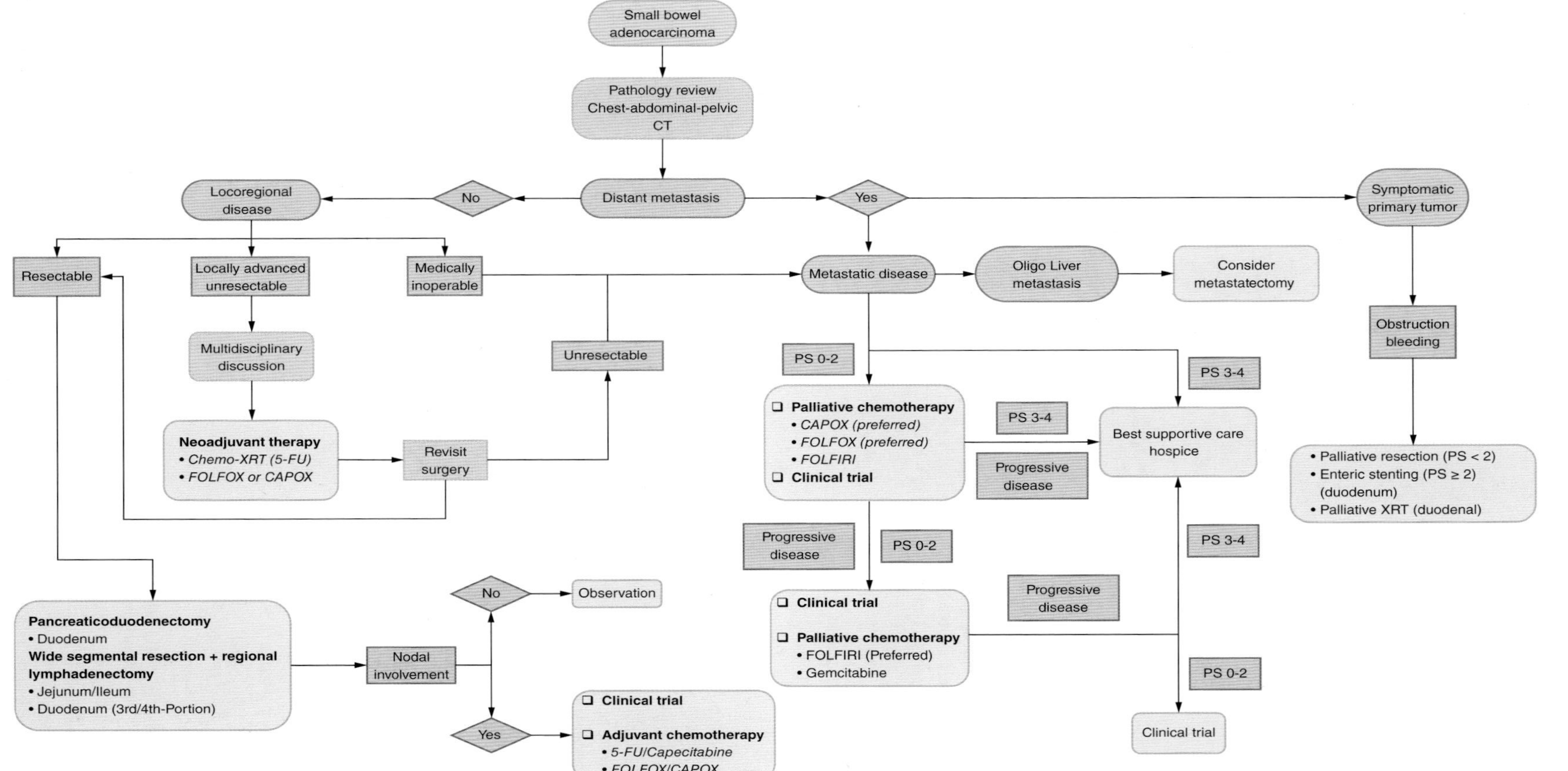

FIGURE 23-2 Treatment algorithm for small bowel adenocarcinoma. (Reproduced with permission from Raghav K. and Overman M. J. Small bowel adenocarcinomas—existing evidence and evolving paradigms. *Nat Rev Clin Oncol*. 2013;10:534.)

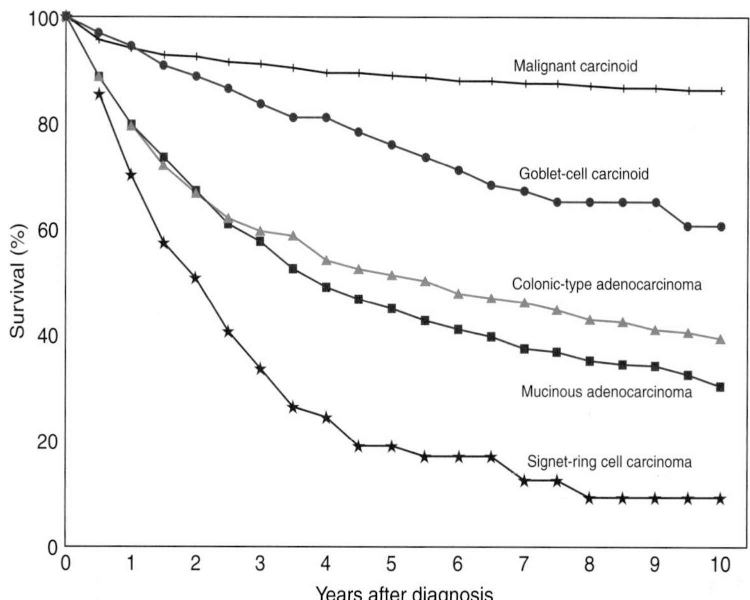

FIGURE 23-3 Overall survival of malignant appendiceal cancers according to the Surveillance, Epidemiology and End Results registry (SEER), stratified by histological subtype. (Reproduced with permission from McCusker ME, Coté TR, Clegg LX, et al. Primary malignant neoplasms of the appendix. *Cancer*. 2002;94:3307-3312.)

metastases is a predictor of recurrence in early-stage tumors ([59]). Stage IV mucinous appendiceal adenocarcinomas are categorized as either mucinous low grade (well differentiated) or mucinous high grade (moderate and poor differentiation) by the American Joint Committee on Cancer (AJCC) seventh edition. However, recent population-based efforts utilizing the SEER database have demonstrated that mucinous moderate-differentiated adenocarcinomas appear to have a prognosis more akin to mucinous well-differentiated carcinomas as opposed to mucinous poorly differentiated carcinomas ([59]).

Appendiceal Carcinoid Tumors

Similar to other intestinal carcinoid tumors, appendiceal carcinoid tumors arise from neuroendocrine cells within the lamina propria and submucosa. Appendiceal carcinoid tumors can secrete serotonin and vasoactive substances responsible for the carcinoid syndrome, although this is rarely seen in patients in the absence of extensive liver metastases. Appendiceal carcinoid tumors are usually seen in young patients and are seen slightly more often in women ([60, 61]).

A rare histological variant of carcinoid tumors, termed goblet cell carcinoids or adenocarcinoids, is characterized by malignant cells that demonstrate both exocrine and neuroendocrine characteristics. This histological subtype has outcomes in between that of a carcinoid and that of an adenocarcinoma (see Fig. 23-3).

Management of Appendiceal Carcinoids

As most appendiceal carcinoid tumors are discovered incidentally from an appendectomy specimen, a critical and somewhat-controversial oncologic question relates to the need for performing a more complete surgical staging procedure. For appendiceal cancers, a complete surgical staging procedure would entail a right hemicolectomy with complete removal of the base of the appendix, mesoappendix, and draining lymph nodes.

The most useful criteria for determining the need for a complete right hemicolectomy are tumor size (≥2 cm in diameter) or mesoappendix involvement ([62]). In a retrospective study of appendiceal carcinoids, Moertel et al reported no metastases in 127 patients with tumors <2 cm, whereas metastatic disease was seen in 3 of the 14 patients with tumors 2 to 3 cm and 4 of the 9 patients with tumors ≥3 cm ([63]). Patients with an adenocarcinoid histological variant are generally treated as having an appendiceal adenocarcinoma.

For patients with metastatic disease, the use of somatostatin analogues can alleviate the symptoms of the carcinoid syndrome but rarely causes objective tumor regression. Given the slow-growing nature of appendiceal carcinoid tumors, local modality therapies such as hepatic embolization or surgical resection may also be beneficial in selected patients with metastatic disease. For additional information on management of this type of tumor, please refer to Chapter 23.

Table 23-5 TNM Staging for Appendiceal Carcinomas

	Primary Tumor (T)			
TX	Primary tumor cannot be assessed			
T0	No evidence of primary tumor			
Tis	Carcinoma in situ			
T1	Tumor invades submucosa			
T2	Tumor invades muscularis propria			
T3	Tumor invades through muscularis propria into subserosa or into mesoappendix			
T4	Tumor penetrates visceral peritoneum, including mucinous peritoneal tumor within the right lower quadrant and/or directly invades other organs or structures			
T4a	Tumor penetrates visceral peritoneum, including mucinous peritoneal tumor within the right lower quadrant			
T4b	Tumor directly invades other organs or structures			
	Regional Lymph Nodes (N)			
NX	Regional lymph nodes cannot be assessed			
N0	No regional lymph node metastasis			
N1	Metastasis in 1-3 regional lymph nodes			
N2	Metastasis in 4 or more regional lymph nodes			
	Distant Metastasis (M)			
M0	No distant metastasis			
M1	Distant metastasis			
M1a	Intraperitoneal metastasis beyond the right lower quadrant, including pseudomyxoma peritonei			
M1b	Nonperitoneal metastasis			
	Histologic Grade (G)			
GX	Grade cannot be assessed			
G1	Well differentiated	Mucinous low grade		
G2	Moderately differentiated	Mucinous high grade		
G3	Poorly differentiated	Mucinous high grade		
G4	Undifferentiated			
	Stage Grouping			
Stage 0	Tis	N0	M0	
Stage I	T1	N0	M0	
	T2	N0	M0	
Stage IIA	T3	N0	M0	
Stage IIB	T4a	N0	M0	
Stage IIC	T4b	N0	M0	
Stage IIIA	T1	N1	M0	
	T2	N1	M0	
Stage IIIB	T3	N1	M0	
	T4	N1	M0	
Stage IIIC	Any T	N2	M0	
Stage IVA	Any T	N0	M1a	G1
Stage IVB	Any T	N0	M1a	G2, 3
	Any T	N1	M1a	Any G
	Any T	N2	M1a	Any G
Stage IVC	Any T	Any N	M1b	Any G

Reproduced with permission from Edge SB, Byrd DR, Compton CC (eds): *AJCC Cancer Staging Manuarl*, 7th ed. New York, NY: Springer; 2010.

CHAPTER 23

Appendiceal Epithelial Tumors

Little is known about the risk factors or etiology of epithelial tumors of the appendix. Although generally viewed as a subset of CRC, most epithelial tumors of the appendix have a markedly different biology and natural history than do adenocarcinomas of the colorectum. In particular, a subset of appendiceal epithelial tumors that have disseminated peritoneal mucinous deposits derived from a ruptured appendiceal mucinous adenoma can demonstrate excellent long-term survival with aggressive cytoreductive surgery (CRS) and hyperthermic intraperitoneal chemotherapy (HIPEC) ([64,65]).

Most appendiceal epithelial tumors begin as a mucinous adenoma with appendiceal distention caused by excessive mucin production. On gross inspection or radiographic evaluation, this dilated mucin-filled appendix is frequently referred to as a mucocele. With progressive growth, the appendiceal lumen can become obstructed and result in increased intraluminal pressure within the appendix, which can cause the appendix to rupture. Appendiceal rupture represents the critical step in the dissemination of the mucinous appendiceal tumor to the peritoneal cavity. For this reason, it is critical that care is taken when surgically removing an appendiceal mucocele to prevent rupture and peritoneal seeding during a routine appendectomy ([66]). When resecting an appendiceal mucocele, the peritoneum should be inspected closely to evaluate any evidence of dissemination to the peritoneal cavity. During pathological examination of the appendix, any fluid or mucus in the peritoneal spaces surrounding the appendix should undergo cytologic examination ([62]). In patients with localized disease, the presence of carcinoma requires a completion right hemicolectomy for oncologic staging.

Molecular Profile

The molecular characterization of appendiceal adenocarcinomas is limited. Mutations are frequently seen in these tumors and include *KRAS, GNAS, AKT, MET, PIK3CA,* and *TP53* genes ([67–70]). In a cohort of 149 patients with appendiceal adenocarcinomas at MD Anderson Cancer Center, *KRAS, PIK3CA,* and *BRAF* mutations were seen in 55%, 17%, and 4% of patients, respectively ([71]). The study also demonstrated that well- and moderately differentiated appendiceal adenocarcinomas were molecularly distinct from poorly differentiated appendiceal adenocarcinomas ([71]).

Pseudomyxoma Peritonei

Pseudomyxoma peritonei, or false mucinous tumor, is a term originally described by Werth in 1884, who described the pathological findings in a patient with a ruptured ovarian cystadenoma who had copious gelatinous intraperitoneal ascites (Fig. 23-4) ([72]). This term has been applied broadly to include any mucinous tumor type involving the peritoneal cavity with any histologic grade of differentiation. However, this imprecise definition has resulted in the grouping of patients with dramatically different outcomes and has generated considerable confusion for patients and even among clinicians. A better understanding of disease biology has shown that this clinical term is most appropriately applied to the pathological subtype of appendiceal tumors called disseminated peritoneal adenomucinosis ([73]).

However, the term *PMP* is frequently utilized to refer to the clinical syndrome of mucinous peritoneal deposits resulting from any mucinous appendiceal tumor. When used in this fashion, this term encompasses both DPAM and the appendiceal epithelial tumor subtype termed peritoneal mucinous carcinomatosis (PMCA). However, the inclusion of these two histological subtypes combines two appendiceal epithelial tumor types with markedly different OSs (Table 23-6) ([73,74]).

Histopathologic Subtypes of Epithelial Appendiceal Tumors

Disseminated Peritoneal Adenomucinosis

Disseminated peritoneal adenomucinosis is characterized by peritoneal lesions composed of abundant extracellular, mucin-containing, scant, simple to focally

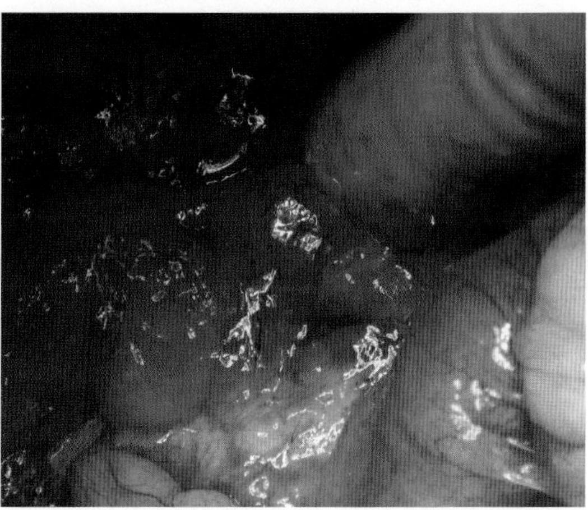

FIGURE 23-4 Peritoneal mucin in a patient undergoing surgical cytoreduction for peritoneal mucinous carcinomatosis (PMCA). (Reproduced with permission from Ronnett BM, Zahn CM, Kurman RJ, et al. Disseminated peritoneal adenomucinosis and peritoneal mucinous carcinomatosis. A clinicopathologic analysis of 109 cases with emphasis on distinguishing pathologic features, site of origin, prognosis, and relationship to "pseudomyxoma peritonei." *Am J Surg Pathol.* 1995;19:1390-408.)

Table 23-6 Overall Survival for Appendiceal Epithelial Tumors Stratified by Histology Subtype of Disseminated Peritoneal Adenomucinosis (DPAM) or Peritoneal Mucinous Carcinomatosis (PMCA)

			DPAM			PMCA		
Author	Year	Study	No. of Pts.	5-Year OS	10-Year OS	No. of Pts.	5-Year OS	10-Year OS
Miner	2005	Retrospective, MSKCC	42	85%	70%	46	40%	12%
Sugarbaker	1999	Retrospective, Washington Cancer Institute	224	80%		161	28%	
Stewart	2006	Retrospective, Wake Forest University	55	68%		29	35%	
Ronnett	2001	Retrospective, Washington Cancer Institute	65	75%	68%	43	26%	9%
Smeenk[a]	2007	Retrospective, Netherlands Cancer Institute	66	73%[a]		7	0%[a]	

MSKCC, Memorial Sloan Kettering Cancer Center; No. of Pts., number of patients; OS, overall survival.
[a]Disease-specific survival.

proliferative mucinous epithelium with little cytologic atypia or mitotic activity, with or without an associated appendiceal mucinous adenoma ([73]). In essence, the underlying epithelium in DPAM may have low-grade adenomatous changes but may not have any evidence of invasion or carcinoma. This subgroup of tumors (DPAMs) demonstrates the classic PMP clinical syndrome of massive amounts of benign-appearing mucinous ascites that over time slowly fill the entire peritoneal cavity (Fig. 23-5). Although spread to the peritoneal cavity is present, these tumors do not metastasize to regional lymph nodes or via hematogenous spread to the liver or other distant sites.

Patients with DPAM typically present with gradually increasing abdominal girth. For women, DPAM may present as a new ovarian mass, and for men it may present as a new-onset hernia. In women, secondary involvement of the ovaries is common, and because histopathological features of DPAM from a primary ovarian tumor are extremely rare, a thorough pathological examination of the appendix should be conducted ([75]). When molecular and immunohistochemical evaluations have been performed on cases with both appendix and ovarian involvement, these evaluations have uniformly demonstrated the primary site of disease as the appendix ([76–78]).

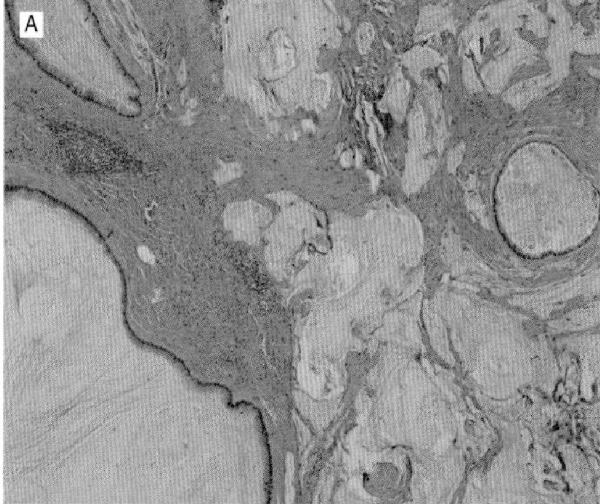

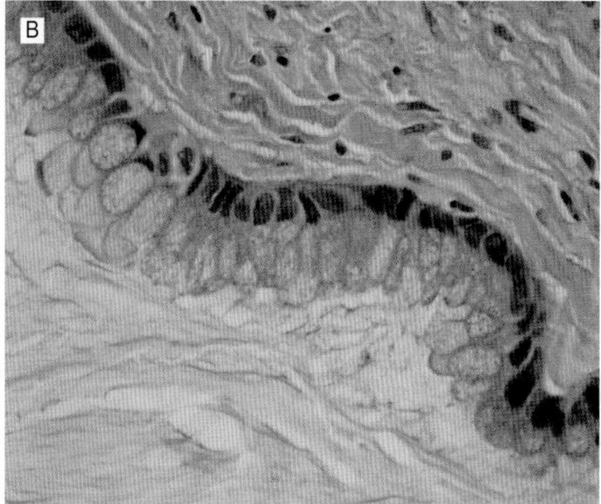

FIGURE 23-5 Histology from a patient with disseminated peritoneal adenomucinosis (DPAM) and the clinical syndrome of pseudomyxoma peritonei (PMP): (**A**) adenoma-like epithelium with acellular mucin pools dissecting through the fibrous stroma with chronic inflammation, ×40; (**B**) adenoma-like epithelium with abundant acellular mucin, ×400.

Peritoneal Mucinous Carcinomatosis

If evidence of invasion and carcinoma is present, then the pathological diagnosis of PMCA should be used ([73]). Peritoneal mucinous carcinomatosis is characterized by peritoneal lesions composed of more abundant mucinous epithelium with the architectural and cytologic features of carcinoma, with or without an associated primary mucinous adenocarcinoma. A subset of PMCA tumors that demonstrate features of both DPAM and PMCA have been termed PMCA with intermediate or discordant features (PMCA-I/D) ([73]). In an analysis of 109 patients with clinical features of PMP, 60% were classified as DPAM, 27% were classified as PMCA, and 13% were classified as PMCA-I/D ([73,79]). In this study, the 5- and 10-year survival rates for patients with DPAM were 75% and 68%, respectively. This was significantly higher than patients with PMCA, who demonstrated 5- and 10-year survival rates of 14% and 3%. Those patients with PMCA-I/D had survival more closely associated with that of PMCA patients (Fig. 23-6).

Although appendiceal PMCAs are invasive tumors with distant metastatic potential, the majority of these tumors will remain localized to the peritoneal cavity. Even in the subset of patients with very aggressive-appearing histologies, the rate of distant hematogenous metastases remains low. In one retrospective study of 90 appendiceal adenocarcinomas with either poor differentiation or signet ring cell morphology, the rate of extraperitoneal metastases was only 17% ([80]).

Nonmucinous/Colonic-Type Adenocarcinoma

Occurring less frequently, nonmucinous or colonic-type adenocarcinomas of the appendix demonstrate a different tumor biology than mucinous appendiceal tumors. These cancers are more aggressive and appear to behave more like colonic adenocarcinomas. In a study by Kabbani et al, 43% of patients with nonmucinous appendiceal adenocarcinoma had evidence of extraperitoneal metastases ([81]). The patients with nonmucinous carcinomas in this study had a significantly worse OS and disease-free survival than those with mucinous carcinomas.

Treatment

Cytoreductive Surgery

Because of the relative rarity of this disease, prospective randomized clinical trials studying the treatment of appendiceal epithelial tumors are lacking. The majority of data evaluating the various treatment modalities in this disease have been derived from retrospective, single-institution studies. Surgical cytoreduction has been the primary mode of therapy for these tumors based on the following factors:

1. Lack of extraperitoneal disease spread
2. Primarily mucinous nature of peritoneal deposits
3. Indolent growth rate
4. Limited activity of systemic chemotherapy
5. Lack of an effective systemic mucolytic agent

The goal of surgical cytoreduction is complete tumor removal from the peritoneal cavity. Because of the large surface area of the peritoneum, surgical cytoreduction to remove all visible sites of disease can be challenging. Optimal CRS may involve removal of the appendix, right colon, intraperitoneal tumor debulking, resection of multiple abdominal and pelvic organs with peritoneal tumor studding, and stripping of all involved parietal peritoneum ([82]). Following successful surgical cytoreduction, patients with the DPAM or PMCA tumors can experience reaccumulation of

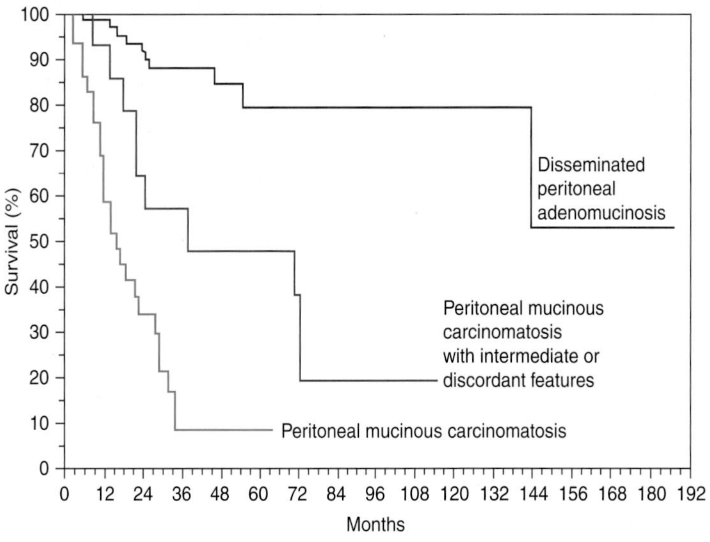

FIGURE 23-6 Overall survival for 109 cases with the clinical syndrome of pseudomyxoma peritonei (PMP) according to histological subtype.

mucinous peritoneal implants, which may be complicated by fibrosis from prior surgery, requiring repeated surgical cytoreductive procedures.

In a 97-patient series from Memorial Sloan Kettering Cancer Center, in which surgical resection alone represented the primary treatment modality in over two-thirds of the patients, the 5-year OS rate was 90% for patients with DPAM and 50% for patients with PMCA ([64]). In the 55% of patients who underwent a complete cytoreduction of all visible tumors, 91% had recurrent disease. The average number of surgical cytoreductions that patients underwent in this study was 2.2, with a range of 1 to 6 ([64]). In patients who develop recurrence after CRS, repeat CRS should be attempted because survival in these patients is prolonged with repeat CRS ([83]).

Hyperthermic Intraperitoneal Chemotherapy

In an attempt to diminish the rate of disease recurrence following CRS, the administration of intraperitoneal chemotherapy following a surgical cytoreduction has been used to try to treat any residual microscopic disease in the peritoneal cavity. Historically, a number of methods of delivering intraperitoneal chemotherapy have been utilized, although the most commonly utilized method is HIPEC administered at the time of cytoreduction.

At MD Anderson, following complete CRS, administration of heated mitomycin C at a dose of 25 mg/m^2 for patients who are chemonaïve or 20 mg/m^2 for patients who have received previous chemotherapy in a volume of 5 to 6.5 L of electrolyte solution at a flow rate of 3 to 3.5 L/min. Intraoperative hemodynamic monitoring and thermal monitoring are essential for optimal outcomes in these patients. The HIPEC is continued for 90 minutes with vigorous shaking of the closed abdomen. On completion of HIPEC, necessary bowel anastomoses are performed, and gastrostomy and jejunostomy tubes are placed for postoperative management of nutritional deficiencies and prolonged gastric ileus.

Intraperitoneal administration of chemotherapy offers an advantage of providing high concentrations of drug directly to the target, while hyperthermia provides a synergistic antitumor effect when combined with chemotherapy ([84]). However, as a locally applied modality, the maximum penetration into tumor tissue is usually limited to 2 to 5 mm from the surface ([85]). At present, no randomized study has compared the benefit of adding HIPEC to surgical cytoreduction, although single-institution series have indirectly suggested a benefit when disease-free survival rates of patients treated with surgical cytoreduction and HIPEC (37%-57%) ([74, 76]) are compared with the historical rates of surgical cytoreduction alone (9%-12%) ([64, 77]).

Cytoreductive surgery with HIPEC represents an aggressive treatment requiring significant surgical expertise and should only be conducted at centers experienced in performing peritoneal cytoreduction. Operation time is approximately 8 to 12 h, with an average hospital stay of 20 to 25 days. The 30-day postoperative mortality and morbidity range from 0% to 12% and 12% to 56%, respectively ([76, 78]).

In one of the largest retrospective multi-institutional registry-based study of 2,298 patients with PMP originating from an appendiceal mucinous neoplasm undergoing CRS, the reported median OS was 16.3 years, with a 10-year survival rate of 63% ([86]). The treatment-related mortality was 2%, and major operative complications occurred in 24% of cases ([86]). A high PCI, lack of complete cytoreduction, and lack of HIPEC were associated with poorer PFS and OS ([86]).

Prognosis for patients undergoing CRS with HIPEC is primarily dependent on two critical factors: histologic classification and completeness of surgical resection. A quantitative score, the completeness of cytoreduction score proposed by Sugarbaker and colleagues, categorizes the completeness of cytoreduction (CC) based on the size of nodules remaining at the end of surgery: CC-0 (no visible disease), CC-1 (nodules <0.25 cm), CC-2 (nodules 0.25 to <2.5 cm), and CC-3 (nodules ≥2.5 cm) ([65]). In an analysis of 224 patients with DPAM histology, Sugarbaker et al found that patients with complete cytoreduction (CC-0 or CC-1) had a 5-year OS rate of 86%, whereas patients with incomplete cytoreduction (CC-2 or CC-3) had a 5-year OS rate of 20% ($P < .0001$) (Fig. 23-7) ([65]). The importance of completeness of cytoreduction has been confirmed by other authors, although various methods of categorizing a complete cytoreduction have been used ([74, 76]).

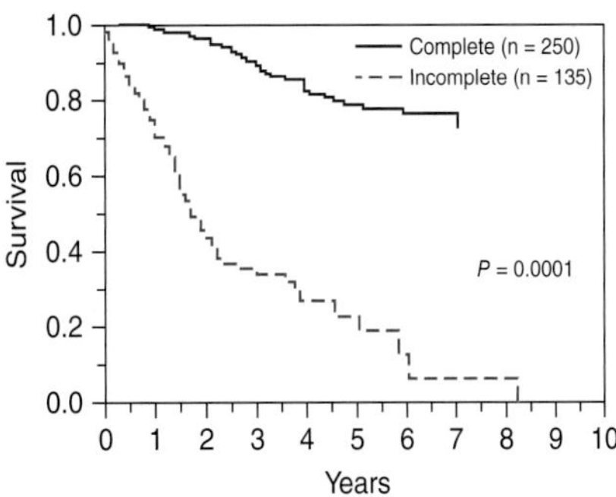

FIGURE 23-7 Overall survival for 385 cases with the mucinous epithelial tumors of the appendix (disseminated peritoneal adenomucinosis and peritoneal mucinous carcinomatosis) according to completeness of surgical cytoreduction. Complete cytoreduction defined as a completeness of cytoreduction score (CC) of CC-0 or CC-1, and an incomplete cytoreduction defined as a score of CC-2 or CC-3. [Reproduced with permission from Sugarbaker PH. Results of treatment of 385 patients with peritoneal surface spread of appendiceal malignancy. *Ann Surg Oncol.* 1999;6(8).]

CHAPTER 23

Additional prognostic measures include the peritoneal cancer index (PCI), a quantitative measure of the size and distribution of nodules on the peritoneal surface; the previous surgical score (PSS), a measure of the extent of prior cytoreduction; and the extent of disease on the small bowel and small bowel mesentery ([64, 65, 87, 88]). The prognostic value of these different factors relates primarily to their ability to predict the likelihood of obtaining a complete cytoreduction.

For patients who cannot undergo complete CRS, the benefit obtained from an incomplete cytoreduction remains unknown. If complete CRS cannot be performed, a surgical cytoreduction is generally considered only if there are particular symptoms that can be palliated by tumor debulking. Given that HIPEC has limited tumor penetration, use of HIPEC should be limited to patients with a complete or near-complete CRS.

Systemic Chemotherapy

The role of systemic chemotherapy has not been well delineated in appendiceal epithelial tumors and has generally been utilized in patients who are not candidates for surgical cytoreduction ([82]). The challenges of using systemic chemotherapy to treat appendiceal tumors relate to the slow-growing nature of the disease, the primarily mucinous component of the tumors, and the challenges in radiographically measuring disease response.

Traditionally, PMP has been considered resistant to systemic chemotherapy, although a recently completed phase II study evaluating the use of concurrent mitomycin C and capecitabine in patients with advanced, unresectable DPAM or PMCA has suggested a role for systemic chemotherapy ([89]). In this study of 39 patients,

Commentary: Surgical Perspectives in Appendiceal Carcinoma

Once the diagnosis of appendiceal carcinoma has been established, a thorough evaluation must be performed, including CT imaging, colonoscopy, laboratory studies, and a complete medical history to determine the potential resectability of the tumor and the appropriateness and fitness of the patient for aggressive treatment.

In our experience, patients over the age of 70 must be approached with caution because the potential risks of CRS and HIPEC may be greater than the potential benefits. A number of studies have also identified an Eastern Cooperative Oncology Group (ECOG) status of <2 as essential for patients to tolerate CRS/HIPEC. Similarly, because of the sensitivity of the liver to hyperthermia, patients with evidence of cirrhosis are not offered HIPEC. Likewise, patients with renal insufficiency may prove difficult to manage postoperatively because of significant fluid shifts associated with surgery and HIPEC. Previous surgical procedures and obesity offer the same challenges as in other complex operations but are not contraindications to surgery.

To determine the extent of the tumor and potential for complete cytoreduction, CT scans of the chest, abdomen, and pelvis appear to be the most useful. We do not use MRI or positron emission tomographic scanning routinely as these offer little advantage over CT alone. Imaging findings suggestive of an inability to completely cytoreduce the tumor include a large volume of disease involving the porta hepatis and the retrohepatic vena cava, large volume of tumor involving the small bowel mesentery with a gathering together of this mesentery termed *cauliflowering*, obstruction of more than one segment of small bowel, and evidence for retroperitoneal organ involvement. In these patients, consideration for systemic chemotherapy should be given with surgery limited to palliation of symptoms.

At MD Anderson, we often see patients who have been evaluated and treated at outside institutions. Many patients have undergone an incomplete cytoreduction or combinations of therapy that we would not consider standard. The approach to these patients begins with an evaluation of the pathology, review of all operative notes to assess the amount of disease present at the time of surgery, and extent of disease left behind at the completion of surgery. Repeat imaging is obtained as necessary. On completion of the workup, an individualized plan is developed. If the patient had what was described as a complete cytoreduction, and CT imaging demonstrates no evidence of disease, repeat imaging is performed at 6-month intervals and consideration is given to diagnostic laparoscopy at the 1-year anniversary of the original surgery. If there is disease identified during these steps, CRS/HIPEC is offered if the patient meets the selection criteria previously outlined.

In patients who have clearly had an incomplete cytoreduction or have evidence of disease on baseline imaging, if the pathology is low- or moderate-grade appendiceal adenocarcinoma, we offer CRS/HIPEC. In the setting of high-grade/signet ring cell appendiceal adenocarcinoma, we typically have the patient evaluated for systemic chemotherapy. If after completing systemic chemotherapy there is stability of disease and the disease is potentially resectable based on imaging studies, we may offer CRS/HIPEC in selected cases.

Keith F. Fournier

a clinical benefit rate of 38% was determined based on the definition of either semiquantitative reductions in mucinous deposition or stabilization of previously progressive disease ([89]). In this study, the 2-year cancer-related mortality rate was 39%. Elevations in tumor markers (CEA, CA 19-9, or CA-125) occurred in all patients, and a 50% reduction in one of these markers occurred in 51% of patients ([89]). Although limited by the small sample size, tumor marker response did not appear to correlate with radiographically assessed clinical benefit rate ([89]).

In an additional study supporting the role of systemic chemotherapy in patients with PMCA, Shapiro et al retrospectively reviewed data collected from 54 patients who were suboptimal surgical cytoreductive candidates ([82]). Systemic chemotherapy in this report consisted of a fluoropyrimidine with or without a platinum agent in 69% of patients. Radiographic stabilization or response to therapy was noted in 55% of patients, median PFS was 7.6 months, and median OS was 56 months ([82]). In this study, poorly differentiated histology and signet ring histology were both negative prognostic indicators for OS. Systemic chemotherapy may play a role in the management of poorly differentiated and signet ring cell adenocarcinomas of the appendix. In a retrospective review of 142 patients with these tumors, systemic chemotherapy resulted in a response rate of 44%, a median PFS of 6.9 months, and a median OS of 1.7 years ([90]). Patients with response to chemotherapy and complete CRS were associated with improved PFS and OS ([90]). Although data regarding role of targeted therapy is limited in appendix cancers, retrospective data suggest that combining bevacizumab with chemotherapy may improve survival outcomes in surgically unresectable appendiceal epithelial neoplasms ([71, 91]).

The studies discussed in this section suggest a role for chemotherapy in patients who are suboptimal candidates for CRS, but further prospective randomized clinical trials will be needed before any definitive statement regarding the exact benefit and timing of chemotherapy use can be made.

The MD Anderson Approach to Epithelial Appendiceal Tumors

Unlike CRC, appendiceal epithelial malignancies have a more indolent natural history that is determined by their underlying histopathology. At MD Anderson, patients with DPAM and well-to-moderately differentiated PMCA tumors are evaluated initially for CRS. Patients with a complete cytoreduction (CC-0 or CC-1) are treated with HIPEC utilizing intraperitoneal mitomycin at 42°C. If a complete CRS is not obtained, if radiographic imaging indicates that obtaining a complete cytoreduction is highly unlikely, or if medical comorbidities preclude a surgical procedure, then patients are considered for systemic chemotherapy. Also, HIPEC is utilized at MD Anderson for the control of refractory ascites. We have found that the use of HIPEC in patients who have undergone an incomplete CRS can provide long-term control of ascites and should be considered in patients with refractory ascites.

Given the indolent nature of well-to-moderately differentiated PMCA tumors, systemic chemotherapy is generally reserved for patients who either have clear evidence of disease progression on radiographic imaging or have significant tumor-related symptoms. Front-line chemotherapy is fluoropyrimidine based, and additional agents may be added based on the perceived tolerance of more aggressive combinations. Given the general good prognosis of these patients, it is critical that treatment is closely aligned with quality of life and that cumulative toxicities are kept to a minimum.

The use of multiagent systemic chemotherapy, as administered in CRC, is the treatment of choice for patients who have signet ring cells, poorly differentiated tumors, or nonmucinous tumors. Because patients with poorly differentiated or signet ring cell appendiceal adenocarcinomas have consistently shown worse outcomes following aggressive CRS, our approach has been only to consider surgical cytoreduction in these patients following initial treatment with systemic chemotherapy. In a recent retrospective study from MD Anderson, Lieu et al showed that patients with stage IV poorly differentiated or signet ring cell morphology appendiceal adenocarcinomas had a median OS of 24 months, which appears similar to the known OS for metastatic CRC ([80]).

Although trials evaluating the benefit of VEGF inhibitors or *EGFR* inhibitors in appendiceal epithelial tumors are lacking, their effectiveness in CRC suggests a possible role for these agents in appendiceal epithelial tumors. Expression of VEGF has been demonstrated in appendiceal adenocarcinomas, and high levels of expression have been correlated with poor outcome ([92]). Although not well studied, it appears that mutations in the *K*-ras oncogene are common, with 22 of 31 tested samples demonstrating an activating mutation in *K*-ras ([93]).

Due to the rarity of appendiceal tumors, our understanding of these tumors is limited, and further research into the molecular characteristics of these tumors is needed. The role of CRS is well established for appendiceal epithelial tumors. The use of systemic chemotherapy in appendiceal epithelial tumors needs further study; in particular, the role of newer targeted therapies needs to be determined.

CHAPTER 23

REFERENCES

1. Siegel R, Ma J, Zou Z, Jemal A. Cancer statistics, 2014. *CA Cancer J Clin.* 2014;64:9.
2. Raghav K, Overman MJ. Small bowel adenocarcinomas—existing evidence and evolving paradigms. *Nat Rev Clin Oncol.* 2013;10:534.
3. Key C, Meisner A. Cancers of the esophagus, stomach, and small intestine. In Ries LAG, et al, eds., *SEER Survival Monograph: Cancer Survival Among Adults: U.S. SEER Program, 1988-2001, Patient and Tumor Characteristics.* Bethesda, MD: National Cancer Institute, SEER Program; 2007. NIH Pub. No. 07-6215.
4. Weiss NS, Yang CP. Incidence of histologic types of cancer of the small intestine. *J Natl Cancer Inst.* 1987;78:653.
5. Bilimoria KY, et al. Small bowel cancer in the United States: changes in epidemiology, treatment, and survival over the last 20 years. *Ann Surg.* 2009;249:63.
6. Scelo G, Boffetta P, Hemminki K, et al. Associations between small intestine cancer and other primary cancers: an international population-based study. *Int J Cancer.* 2006;118:189-196.
7. Overman MJ et al. A population-based comparison of adenocarcinoma of the large and small intestine: insights into a rare disease. *Ann Surg Oncol.* 2012;19:1439.
8. Sellner F. Investigations on the significance of the adenoma-carcinoma sequence in the small bowel. *Cancer.* 1990;66:702.
9. Ryan DP, Schapiro RH, Warshaw AL. Villous tumors of the duodenum. *Ann Surg.* 1986;203:301.
10. Joesting DR, Beart RW Jr, van Heerden JA, Weiland LH. Improving survival in adenocarcinoma of the duodenum. *Am J Surg.* 1981;141:228.
11. Neugut A, Santos J. The association between cancers of the small and large bowel. *Cancer Epidemiol Biomarkers Prev.* 1993;2:551-553.
12. Planck M, et al. Microsatellite instability and expression of MLH1 and MSH2 in carcinomas of the small intestine. *Cancer.* 2003;97:1551.
13. Ross, RK, Hartnett NM, Bernstein L, Henderson BE. Epidemiology of adenocarcinomas of the small intestine: is bile a small bowel carcinogen? *Br J Cancer.* 1991;63:143.
14. Wu AH, Yu MC, Mack TM. Smoking, alcohol use, dietary factors and risk of small intestinal adenocarcinoma. *Int J Cancer.* 1997;70:512.
15. Chow W, Linet MS, McLaughlin JK, Hsing AW, Chien HT, Blot WJ. Risk factors for small intestine cancer. *Cancer Causes Control.* 1993;4:163-169.
16. Neugut AI, Jacobson JS, Suh S, Mukherjee R, Arber N. The epidemiology of cancer of the small bowel. *Cancer Epidemiol Biomarkers Prev.* 1998;7:243.
17. Schatzkin A, Park Y, Leitzmann MF, Hollenbeck AR, Cross AJ. Prospective study of dietary fiber, whole grain foods, and small intestinal cancer. *Gastroenterology.* 135, 1163.
18. Delaunoit T, Neczyporenko F, Limburg PJ, Erlichman C. Pathogenesis and risk factors of small bowel adenocarcinoma: a colorectal cancer sibling? *Am J Gastroenterol.* 2005;100:703.
19. Boffetta P, Hazelton WD, Chen Y, et al. Body mass, tobacco smoking, alcohol drinking and risk of cancer of the small intestine—a pooled analysis of over 500,000 subjects in the Asia Cohort Consortium. *Ann Oncol.* 2012;23:1894-1898.
20. Groves CJ, Saunders BP, Spigelman AD, Phillips RK. Duodenal cancer in patients with familial adenomatous polyposis (FAP): results of a 10 year prospective study. *Gut.* 2002;50:636.
21. Giardiello FM, et al. Very high risk of cancer in familial Peutz-Jeghers syndrome. *Gastroenterology.* 2000;119:1447.
22. Aarnio M, Mecklin JP, Aaltonen LA, Nystrom-Lahti M, Jarvinen HJ. Life-time risk of different cancers in hereditary non-polyposis colorectal cancer (HNPCC) syndrome. *Int J Cancer.* 1995;64:430.
23. Vasen HF, et al. Cancer risk in families with hereditary nonpolyposis colorectal cancer diagnosed by mutation analysis. *Gastroenterology.* 1996;110:1020.
24. Laforest A, et al. ERBB2 gene as a potential therapeutic target in small bowel adenocarcinoma. *Eur J Cancer.* 2014;50:1740.
25. Palascak-Juif V. et al. Small bowel adenocarcinoma in patients with Crohn's disease compared with small bowel adenocarcinoma de novo. *Inflamm Bowel Dis.* 2005;11:828.
26. Abrahams NA, Halverson A, Fazio VW, Rybicki LA, Goldblum JR. Adenocarcinoma of the small bowel: a study of 37 cases with emphasis on histologic prognostic factors. *Dis Colon Rectum.* 2002;45:1496.
27. Haan JC, et al. Small bowel adenocarcinoma copy number profiles are more closely related to colorectal than to gastric cancers. *Ann Oncol.* 2012;23:367.
28. Maglinte DD, O'Connor K, Bessette J, Chernish SM, Kelvin FM. The role of the physician in the late diagnosis of primary malignant tumors of the small intestine. *Am J Gastroenterol.* 1991;86:304.
29. Howe JR, Karnell LH, Menck HR, Scott-Conner C. The American College of Surgeons Commission on Cancer and the American Cancer Society. Adenocarcinoma of the small bowel: review of the National Cancer Data Base, 1985-1995. *Cancer.* 1999;86:2693.
30. Lewis BS, Eisen GM, Friedman S. A pooled analysis to evaluate results of capsule endoscopy trials. *Endoscopy* 2005;37:960.
31. Sturniolo GC, Di Leo V, Vettorato MG, D'Inca R. Clinical relevance of small-bowel findings detected by wireless capsule endoscopy. *Scand J Gastroenterol.* 2005;40:725.
32. Cobrin, G. M., Pittman, R. H. & Lewis, B. S. *Increased diagnostic yield of small bowel tumors with capsule endoscopy.* Cancer 107, 22-27. (2006).
33. Greene FL, Page DL, Fleming ID, et al. *AJCC Cancer Staging Manual.* 6th ed. New York, NY: Springer; 2005.
34. Agrawal S, et al. Surgical management and outcome in primary adenocarcinoma of the small bowel. *Ann Surg Oncol.* 2007;14:2263.
35. Talamonti MS, Goetz LH, Rao S, Joehl RJ. Primary cancers of the small bowel: analysis of prognostic factors and results of surgical management. *Arch Surg.* 2002;137:564.
36. Wu TJ, Yeh CN, Chao TC, Jan YY, Chen MF. Prognostic factors of primary small bowel adenocarcinoma: univariate and multivariate analysis. *World J Surg.* 2006;30:391.
37. Bakaeen FG, et al. What prognostic factors are important in duodenal adenocarcinoma? *Arch Surg.* 2000;135:635.
38. Sohn TA, et al. Adenocarcinoma of the duodenum: factors influencing long-term survival. *J Gastrointest Surg.* 1998;2:79.
39. Jemal A, et al. Cancer statistics, 2008. *CA Cancer J Clin.* 2008;58:71.
40. Overman MJ, Hu CY, Wolff RA, Chang GJ. Prognostic value of lymph node evaluation in small bowel adenocarcinoma: analysis of the surveillance, epidemiology, and end results database. *Cancer.* 2010;116:5374.
41. Dabaja BS, Suki D, Pro B, Bonnen M, Ajani J. Adenocarcinoma of the small bowel: presentation, prognostic factors, and outcome of 217 patients. *Cancer.* 2004;101:518.
42. Kelsey CR, et al. Duodenal adenocarcinoma: patterns of failure after resection and the role of chemoradiotherapy. *Int J Radiat Oncol Biol Phys.* 2007;69:1436.
43. Barnes G Jr, Romero L, Hess KR, Curley SA. Primary adenocarcinoma of the duodenum: management and survival in 67 patients. *Ann Surg Oncol.* 1994;1:73.
44. Klinkenbijl JH, et al. Adjuvant radiotherapy and 5-fluorouracil after curative resection of cancer of the pancreas and periampullary region: phase III trial of the EORTC gastrointestinal tract cancer cooperative group. *Ann Surg.* 1999;230:776.

45. Overman MJ, Kopetz S, Lin E, Abbruzzese JL, Wolff RA. Is there a role for adjuvant therapy in resected adenocarcinoma of the small intestine. *Acta Oncol.* 2010;49:474.
46. Halfdanarson TR, McWilliams RR, Donohue JH, Quevedo JF. A single-institution experience with 491 cases of small bowel adenocarcinoma. *Am J Surg.* 2010;199:797.
47. Zaanan A, et al. Chemotherapy of advanced small-bowel adenocarcinoma: a multicenter AGEO study. *Ann Oncol.* 2010;21:1786.
48. Gibson MK, Holcroft CA, Kvols LK, Haller D. Phase II study of 5-fluorouracil, doxorubicin, and mitomycin C for metastatic small bowel adenocarcinoma. *Oncologist.* 2005;10:132.
49. Overman MJ, et al. Phase II study of capecitabine and oxaliplatin for advanced adenocarcinoma of the small bowel and ampulla of Vater. *J Clin Oncol.* 2009;27:2598.
50. Xiang XJ, et al. A phase II study of modified FOLFOX as first-line chemotherapy in advanced small bowel adenocarcinoma. *Anticancer Drugs.* 2012;23:561.
51. McWilliams, Pharmacogenetic dosing by UGT1A1 genotype as first-line therapy for advanced small-bowel adenocarcinoma: a North Central Cancer Treatment Group (NCCTG) trial (abstract 314). *J Clin Oncol.* 2012;30(suppl 4).
52. Crawley C, Ross P, Norman A, Hill A, Cunningham D. The Royal Marsden experience of a small bowel adenocarcinoma treated with protracted venous infusion 5-fluorouracil. *Br J Cancer.* 1998;78:508.
53. Fishman PN, et al. Natural history and chemotherapy effectiveness for advanced adenocarcinoma of the small bowel: a retrospective review of 113 cases. *Am J Clin Oncol.* 2006;29:225.
54. Locher C, et al. Combination chemotherapy in advanced small bowel adenocarcinoma. *Oncology.* 2005;69:290.
55. Overman MJ, et al. Chemotherapy with 5-fluorouracil and a platinum compound improves outcomes in metastatic small bowel adenocarcinoma. *Cancer.* 2008;113:2038.
56. McCusker ME, Coté TR, Clegg LX, Sobin LH. Primary malignant neoplasms of the appendix. *Cancer.* 2002;94:3307.
57. Fann J, Vierra M, Fisher D, Oberhelman HA Jr, Cobb L. Pseudomyxoma peritonei. *Surg Gynecol Obstet.* 1993;177:441.
58. Connor SJ, Hanna GB, Frizelle FA. Appendiceal tumors: retrospective clinicopathologic analysis of appendiceal tumors from 7,970 appendectomies. *Dis Colon Rectum.* 1998;41:75.
59. Overman MJ, et al. Improving the AJCC/TNM staging for adenocarcinomas of the appendix: the prognostic impact of histological grade. *Ann Surg.* 2013;257:1072.
60. Irvin MM, Kevin DL, Mark K. A 5-decade analysis of 13,715 carcinoid tumors. *Cancer.* 2003;97:934.
61. Sandor A, Modlin I. A retrospective analysis of 1570 appendiceal carcinoids. *Am J Gastroenterol.* 1998;93:422.
62. Sugarbaker. Epithelial appendiceal neoplasms. *SO Cancer J.* 2009;15:225.
63. Moertel C, Weiland L, Nagorney D, Dockerty M. Carcinoid tumor of the appendix: treatment and prognosis. *N Engl J Med.* 1987;317:1699.
64. Miner TJ, et al. Long-term survival following treatment of pseudomyxoma peritonei: an analysis of surgical therapy. *Ann Surg.* 2005;241:300.
65. Sugarbaker PH, Chang D. Results of treatment of 385 patients with peritoneal surface spread of appendiceal malignancy. *Ann Surg Oncol.* 1999;6:727.
66. Misdraji J, Yantiss RK, Graeme-Cook FM, Balis UJ, Young RH. Appendiceal mucinous neoplasms: a clinicopathologic analysis of 107 cases. *Am J Surg Pathol.* 2003;27:1089.
67. Liu X, et al. Molecular profiling of appendiceal epithelial tumors using massively parallel sequencing to identify somatic mutations. *Clin Chem.* 2014;60:1004.
68. Nummela P, et al. Genomic profile of pseudomyxoma peritonei analyzed using next-generation sequencing and immunohistochemistry. *Int J Cancer.* 2015;136:E282.
69. Singhi AD, et al. GNAS is frequently mutated in both low-grade and high-grade disseminated appendiceal mucinous neoplasms but does not affect survival. *Hum Pathol.* 2014;45:1737.
70. Alakus H, et al. Genome-wide mutational landscape of mucinous carcinomatosis peritonei of appendiceal origin. *Genome Med.* 2014;6:43.
71. Raghav KP, et al. Impact of molecular alterations and targeted therapy in appendiceal adenocarcinomas. *Oncologist.* 2013;18:1270.
72. Werth R. Klinische and anatomische Unteruschungen Zur Lehre Von den Bauchgeschwilsten und der Laparotomie. *Arch Gynecol Obstet.* 1884;42:100-118.
73. Ronnett BM, et al. Disseminated peritoneal adenomucinosis and peritoneal mucinous carcinomatosis. A clinicopathologic analysis of 109 cases with emphasis on distinguishing pathologic features, site of origin, prognosis, and relationship to "pseudomyxoma peritonei." *Am J Surg Pathol.* 1995;19:1390.
74. Smeenk RM, Verwaal VJ, Antonini N, Zoetmulder FA. Survival analysis of pseudomyxoma peritonei patients treated by cytoreductive surgery and hyperthermic intraperitoneal chemotherapy. *Ann Surg.* 2007;245:104.
75. Ronnett BM, et al. Pseudomyxoma peritonei in women: a clinicopathologic analysis of 30 cases with emphasis on site of origin, prognosis, and relationship to ovarian mucinous tumors of low malignant potential. *Hum Pathol.* 1995;26:509.
76. Stewart JHt, et al. Appendiceal neoplasms with peritoneal dissemination: outcomes after cytoreductive surgery and intraperitoneal hyperthermic chemotherapy. *Ann Surg Oncol.* 2006;13:624.
77. Gough DB, et al. Pseudomyxoma peritonei. Long-term patient survival with an aggressive regional approach. *Ann Surg.* 1994;219:112.
78. Sugarbaker PH, et al. Prospective morbidity and mortality assessment of cytoreductive surgery plus perioperative intraperitoneal chemotherapy to treat peritoneal dissemination of appendiceal mucinous malignancy. *Ann Surg Oncol.* 2006;13:635.
79. Ronnett BM, et al. Patients with pseudomyxoma peritonei associated with disseminated peritoneal adenomucinosis have a significantly more favorable prognosis than patients with peritoneal mucinous carcinomatosis. *Cancer.* 2001;92:85.
80. Lieu C, Lambert L, Wolff R, Eng C, et al. The role of surgical cytoreduction and systemic chemotherapy in metastatic poorly differentiated or signet ring cell adenocarcinomas of the appendix. Paper resented at the ASCO GI Symposium 2010; January 2010; Orlando, FL. #479.
81. Kabbani W, Houlihan PS, Luthra R, Hamilton SR, Rashid A. Mucinous and nonmucinous appendiceal adenocarcinomas: different clinicopathological features but similar genetic alterations. *Mod Pathol.* 2002;15:599.
82. Shapiro JF, Chase JL, Wolff RA, et al. Modern systemic chemotherapy in surgically unresectable neoplasms of appendiceal origin: a single-institution experience. *Cancer.* 2010; 116(2):316-322.
83. Lord AC, et al. Recurrence and outcome after complete tumour removal and hyperthermic intraperitoneal chemotherapy in 512 patients with pseudomyxoma peritonei from perforated appendiceal mucinous tumours. *Eur J Surg Oncol.* 2015;41:396.
84. Witkamp AJ, de Bree E, Van Goethem R, Zoetmulder FA. Rationale and techniques of intra-operative hyperthermic intraperitoneal chemotherapy. *Cancer Treat Rev.* 2001;27:365.
85. Los G, Verdegaal E, Mutsaers P, McVie J. Penetration of carboplatin and cisplatin into rat peritoneal tumor nodules after intraperitoneal chemotherapy. *Cancer Chemother Pharmacol.* 1991;28:159.
86. Chua TC, et al. Early- and long-term outcome data of patients with pseudomyxoma peritonei from appendiceal origin treated by a strategy of cytoreductive surgery and hyperthermic intraperitoneal chemotherapy. *J Clin Oncol.* 2012;30:2449.
87. Glehen O, Mohamed F, Sugarbaker PH. Incomplete

cytoreduction in 174 patients with peritoneal carcinomatosis from appendiceal malignancy. *Ann Surg.* 2004;240:278.
88. Yan TD, Bijelic L, Sugarbaker PH. Critical analysis of treatment failure after complete cytoreductive surgery and perioperative intraperitoneal chemotherapy for peritoneal dissemination from appendiceal mucinous neoplasms. *Ann Surg Oncol.* 2007;14:2289.
89. Farquharson AL, et al. A phase II study evaluating the use of concurrent mitomycin C and capecitabine in patients with advanced unresectable pseudomyxoma peritonei. *Br J Cancer.* 2008;99:591.
90. Lieu CH, et al. Systemic chemotherapy and surgical cytoreduction for poorly differentiated and signet ring cell adenocarcinomas of the appendix. *Ann Oncol.* March 2012;652.
91. Choe JH, et al. Improved survival with anti-VEGF therapy in the treatment of unresectable appendiceal epithelial neoplasms. *Ann Surg Oncol.* 2015;8:2578.
92. Logan-Collins J, et al. VEGF expression predicts survival in patients with peritoneal surface metastases from mucinous adenocarcinoma of the appendix and colon. *Ann Surg Oncol.* 2008;15:738.
93. Catalogue of somatic mutations in cancer. http://www.sanger.ac.uk/genetics/CGP/cosmic/. February 1, 2010.

24

Colorectal Cancer

第二十四章　结直肠癌

Van Morris
Ishwaria M. Subbiah
Scott Kopetz
Cathy Eng

中文导读

结直肠癌是全球范围内常见的肿瘤之一。目前，其为美国发病率第三高的癌症，约占所有癌症相关的死亡的8.5%。本章回顾了结直肠癌的流行病学和病因学特点，阐述了发病的危险因素，包括饮食、肥胖、腺瘤性息肉、炎症性肠病和家族综合征。接着阐述了结直肠癌的筛查手段，详细介绍了大便隐血试验、空气对比钡灌肠、电子肠镜、CT以及遗传学检查和咨询，提供了非甾体类抗炎药的一级预防以及相关二级预防的措施。随后，本章大篇幅介绍了结直肠癌的诊断和分期、临床表现、术前分期以及PET/CT在诊断中的运用，描述了病理诊断，包括病理分期以及淋巴结检出的重要性。详细解读了结直肠癌的治疗方法和策略。① 结肠癌局部与区域控制策略：包括外科处理原则、新辅助治疗的证据；② 直肠癌的治疗策略：包括局部外科治疗、放疗、术前治疗以及辅助治疗、MD安德森癌症中心的临床路径以及术后随访监测。并重点介绍了晚期结直肠癌的治疗，局部复发的治疗手段以及转移性结直肠癌系统性治疗的策略，包括传统细胞毒药物以及靶向治疗的进展、晚期患者外科手术的选择等。最后，本章提出了恶性息肉、不全肠梗阻和伴有神经内分泌功能肿瘤等临床治疗的挑战。

Colorectal cancer is a major cause of cancer-related mortality in the world. It is currently the third-most-common cancer in incidence in the United States and accounts for about 8.5% of all cancer-related mortality (nearly 136,000 new cases and 50,000 deaths each year) ([1]). This chapter reviews our current understanding of colorectal cancer, describes the known genetic mutations and risk factors, and outlines emerging screening, prevention, and therapeutic strategies, with particular emphasis on the approach taken at MD Anderson Cancer Center (MDACC).

EPIDEMIOLOGY AND ETIOLOGY OF COLORECTAL NEOPLASIA

Carcinogenesis: The Adenoma–Adenocarcinoma Sequence

Colorectal neoplasia results from accumulation of alterations over years, ultimately transforming normal epithelium to intraepithelial neoplasia (dysplasia) and then malignant epithelium. Three different pathways driving carcinogenesis include chromosomal instability, microsatellite instability (MSI), and CpG island methylation. The chromosomal instability pathway identifies early mutations in genes such as the tumor suppressor *APC* and the K-*ras* proto-oncogene and later genetic events, including mutations in the deleted in colon cancer (*DCC*) gene and the tumor suppressor gene *p53*.

Risk Factors

Genetic predisposition and acquired risk factors progress stepwise from normal colonic mucosa to adenomatous polyps to invasive adenocarcinoma in individuals with acquired (somatic) or inherited genetic (germline) mutations, with further environmental, dietary, or other less-well-understood factors. Personal or family histories of colorectal cancer or polyps, older age, and inflammatory bowel disease (IBD) have all been associated with an increased risk of colorectal cancer (Table 24-1).

Table 24-1 Lifetime Risks of Colorectal Cancer

Characteristic	Incidence
General population	5%
Personal history of colorectal cancer	15%-20%
Inflammatory bowel disease	15%-40%
Adenomatous polyps: personal	Variable
Hereditary nonpolyposis colorectal cancer mutation	70%-80%
Familial adenomatous polyposis	>95%

Diet

A "Western" diet rich in saturated fat has been associated with an increased risk of colon cancer. Fiber may decrease the fecal carcinogen concentration and transit time, thus reducing the period of exposure to colonic mucosa. However, the prospective Nurses Health Study of 88,757 women aged 34 to 59 years found no association between fiber intake and the risk of colorectal cancer after a median follow-up of 16 years ([2]).

Obesity

Increased body mass index (BMI), and central obesity are emerging as risk factors for colorectal cancer. The Framingham Study found that a BMI >30 increased the risk of colon cancer by 50% among middle-aged (30-54 years) individuals and by 2.4-fold for those aged 55 to 79 years, and waist circumference was a stronger predictor than BMI ([3]).

Adenomatous Polyps

Carcinoma is present in 5% of adenomas, where the potential for malignant transformation is 8 to 10 times higher for villous and tubulovillous adenomas than tubular adenomas. Just over 1% of adenomatous polyps less than 1 cm in size are malignant, whereas up to 40% of adenomas larger than 2 cm are malignant ([4]).

Inflammatory Bowel Disease

Patients with IBD (ulcerative colitis or Crohn disease) are at increased risk of developing colorectal carcinoma based on the duration and extent of active disease, colitis, and mucosal dysplasia ([5]). Recognizing the increased risk of colorectal cancer for patients with IBD, appropriate screening should be instituted as detailed in Table 24-2.

Familial Syndromes

About 20% of all colorectal cancer cases are attributed to inherited autosomal dominant syndromes, including familial adenomatous polyposis (FAP), Gardner syndrome, and hereditary nonpolyposis colorectal cancer (HNPCC) (Table 24-1). Most genetic abnormalities involve deletion of fragments of chromosomes, known as allelic loss or loss of heterozygosity (LOH), or errors in DNA mismatch repair.

Familial Adenomatous Polyposis

Familial adenomatous polyposis is caused by a mutation of *APC* leading to the functional loss of both *APC* alleles, one inherited as a germline mutation and the other mutated in early childhood. Familial adenomatous polyposis has high penetrance, manifesting as thousands of adenomatous polyps—some invariably progress to cancer, thereby warranting a prophylactic colorectal resection. The onset of malignancy in untreated patients occurs at about 42 years, with invasive cancer developing 20 to 30 years later.

Hereditary Nonpolyposis Colorectal Cancer

The genetic penetrance of HNPCC (also known as Lynch syndrome) is caused by defects in DNA mismatch repair through germline mutations in the repair genes. Additional mutations involving tumor suppressor genes and oncogenes rapidly accumulate within these DNA repair–deficient cells, leading to malignant transformation in only 3 to 5 years.

MUTYH-Associated Polyposis

MutY Homolog-associated polyposis is caused by biallelic mutation in the base excision repair gene *MUTYH*. Patients with the syndrome are characterized by oligopolyposis, usually more than 15 but fewer than 100 polyps. The onset of adenomas is older than in classic FAP, but similar to attenuated adenomatous polyposis (45-55 years of age).

SCREENING FOR COLORECTAL NEOPLASIA

Researchers have attempted to identify individuals at greatest risk of developing colorectal cancer who would benefit most from screening (see Table 24-2). Despite the benefits associated with screening, the majority of colon cancers continue to be diagnosed in symptomatic patients.

Detection Methods

Fecal Occult Blood Testing

Meta-analysis of four randomized trials investigating the role of fetal occult blood testing (FOBT) demonstrated an increased percentage of early-stage colorectal cancers discovered through FOBT and a reduction in mortality from colorectal cancer ([6]). The current recommendation of the US Preventative Services Task Force is to screen using FOBT, sigmoidoscopy, or colonoscopy in adults from age 50 to 75 years ([7]).

CHAPTER 24

Table 24-2 Current Recommendations for Colorectal Cancer Screening

Patient Populations	Screening Tests
General population *AND*	FOBT annually and sigmoidoscopy every 3-5 years or colonoscopy every 10 years, beginning at age 50
Patient with any distant relative with CRC or polyps	
Patient with first-degree relative with CRC	FOBT annually and sigmoidoscopy every 3-5 years or colonoscopy every 10 years; begin at age 40
Moderate-risk patients	Polyp removal; repeat colonoscopy at 3 years; if normal, extend interval to 5 years
Patient with two first-degree relatives with CRC	Colonoscopy every 3-5 years
	Begin screening at age 40 or 10 years younger than youngest affected relative
OR	
Patient with one first-degree relative with colorectal cancer diagnosed at 50 years of age or younger	
Patient with HNPCC risk	Colonoscopy every 2 years, then yearly after age 40; begin screening at age 25 or 10 years younger than the youngest affected relative; consider genetic counseling and testing
Patient with FAP risk	Sigmoidoscopy every 1-2 years; begin screening at age 12 years; genetic counseling and testing
Patient with personal history of CRC	Total colon examination (TCE: ACBE or colonoscopy) within 1 year after resection; repeat at 3 years; repeat at 5 years if normal
Patient with personal history of adenoma	Polyp removal; repeat at 3 years; repeat at 5 years if normal

ACBE, air contrast barium enema; CRC, colorectal cancer; FAP, familial adenomatous polyposis; FOBT, fecal occult blood test; HNPCC, hereditary nonpolyposis colon cancer.

Air Contrast Barium Enema

High-quality air contrast barium enema (ACBE) plus flexible sigmoidoscopy was considered in lieu of a full colonoscopy but has fallen out of favor due to its lack of sensitivity for small polyps (<1 cm), its highly operator-dependent nature, and reliance on the patient's mobility to optimize imaging.

Sigmoidoscopy

Flexible sigmoidoscopy is a relatively safe and inexpensive procedure that may be suitable for screening large populations at low risk, in combination with FOBT. However, adenomas in the distal colon are not indicative of proximal lesions, and sigmoidoscopy may miss nearly 50% of all colonic lesions ([8]). Patients with adenomas in the distal colon detected by flexible sigmoidoscopy should have a full colonoscopy.

Computed Tomographic Colonography (Virtual Colonoscopy)

Virtual colonoscopy (VC) involves reconstruction of three-dimensional images of the colon from the two-dimensional data obtained by a spiral CT scanner. Bowel preparation is required, but the technique is less invasive and does not require sedation. However, VC lacks the advantage of a colonoscopy for direct access to colonic tissue for biopsies.

Colonoscopy

Colonoscopy not only enables full visualization of the entire colon but also allows for biopsy or removal of any suspicious lesions. In one retrospective study, 1,994 patients were examined to determine whether the size and histologic features of distal lesions are predictive of proximal lesions, as identification of these factors would help determine who should undergo full colonoscopy after sigmoidoscopic screening. The findings in the distal and proximal colon are shown in Table 24-3 ([9]).

Despite widespread use, the colonoscopy for the purposes of cancer screening has not been studied in a randomized prospective trial until the Nordic-European Initiative on Colorectal Cancer (NordICC) study. This multinational trial randomizes patients aged 55 to 64 years to either once-only screening colonoscopy with removal of all lesions or no screening, which is the standard of care in those trial countries ([10]). After a 15-year follow-up, the primary end points of cumulative colorectal cancer–specific death and incidence will be evaluated. Results are anticipated beyond 2020, given that the study began accrual in 2009.

Genetic Testing and Counseling

Genetic testing for *APC* mutations, *MUTYH* mutations, and DNA mismatch repair gene mutations are now available to identify carriers. A patient with classic FAP or with oligopolyposis but negative *APC* mutation testing should undergo *MUTYH* mutation testing given the incidence (7%-29%) of biallelic *MUTYH* in patients with polyposis with negative *APC* testing ([11]). At MD Anderson, suspected FAP patients are referred to a genetic counselor to discuss screening recommendations, genetic testing, and intervention for themselves and family members.

All patients with colorectal cancer at MD Anderson are screened for HNPCC. Table 24-4 summarizes the Amsterdam Criteria (both original and modified) to assess the risk of HNPCC ([12]). Microsatellite instability, which is a hallmark of HNPCC, also occurs in about 15% of spontaneous colon cancers. Histology that suggests an MSI tumor may include mucinous features, poor differentiation, or the presence of tumor-infiltrating lymphocytes (Fig. 24-1). In female patients less than 50 years of age with proximal tumors, poorly differentiated histology, or mucinous tumors, HNPCC should be considered even when the patient's family history is not suggestive.

Immunohistochemical (IHC) stains done on sections from the diagnostic biopsy assess tumors for loss of heterozygosity in hMSH2, hMSH6, or hMLH1 gene loci. At MD Anderson, we test all patients with surgically resection for MSI status as a predictive and prognostic marker. Further testing for germline mutations may follow an uninformative IHC stain. In particular, the absence of the MLH1 protein on IHC staining

Table 24-3 Findings in the Distal and Proximal Colon in Cohort of 1,994 Patients

	Distal Colon		Proximal Colon	
Finding	No.	%	No.	%
No polyp	1,564	78.4	1,686	84.6
Hyperplastic polyp	201	10.1	72	3.6
Tubular adenoma	168	8.4	186	9.3
Advanced neoplasm	61	3.1	50	2.5

Table 24-4 Original and Revised ICG-HNPCC Criteria ("Amsterdam" Criteria I and II)

Original Criteria (Amsterdam Criteria I)	Revised Criteria (Amsterdam Criteria II)
There should be at least three relatives with colorectal cancer; all the following criteria should be present:	There should be at least three relatives with an HNPCC-associated cancer (colorectal cancer; cancer of endometrium, small bowel, ureter, or renal pelvis):
One should be a first-degree relative of the other two.	One should be a first-degree relative of the other two.
At least two successive generations should be affected.	At least two successive generations should be affected.
At least one colorectal cancer should be diagnosed before age of 50.	At least one should be diagnosed before age of 50.
Familial adenomatous polyposis should be excluded.	Familial adenomatous polyposis should be excluded in the colorectal in cancer case(s) if any.
Tumors should be verified by pathological examination.	Tumors should be verified by pathological examination.

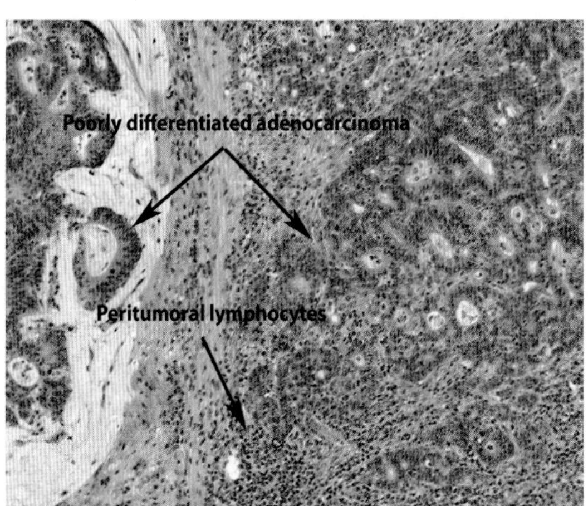

FIGURE 24-1 Photomicrograph of a tumor with microsatellite instability. ***Upper arrows*** **point to poorly differentiated malignant cells with some glandular differentiation and mucin.** ***Lower arrow*** **shows peritumoral lymphocytes clustering near areas of malignant cells and permeating the local stroma.**

calls for the testing of the *BRAF* gene, where a *BRAF* mutation signifies the downregulation of *MLH1* gene expression not through a germline mutation, but rather somatic promoter hypermethylation ([13]). Furthermore, 10% to 15% of all MSIs are not detected through conventional IHC methods, highlighting standardized MSI testing by polymerase chain reaction (PCR) as is done at MD Anderson ([14]). Thus, genetic counseling and testing are strongly recommended.

PREVENTION STRATEGIES

Primary Prevention

Prevention of colorectal neoplasia is usually considered primary or secondary. In primary prevention, broad-based interventions may decrease the risk of colorectal cancer for those at average risk. Americans currently have a 1-in-20 lifetime risk of developing colorectal cancer. Consequently, primary preventive strategies may have a significant impact on the overall incidence of colorectal cancer.

Nonsteroidal Anti-Inflammatory Drugs

For over 20 years, data suggested that nonsteroidal anti-inflammatory agents such as sulindac slow or prevent the formation of adenomatous polyps, particularly in patients with FAP ([15]). Prostaglandin E_2 (PGE_2), an important modulator of cell proliferation and malignant transformation, is formed by the catalytic activity of two predominant isoforms of cyclooxygenase. Cyclooxygenase 1 (COX-1) is constitutively active and widely expressed; it appears to regulate tissue repair and homeostasis. Cyclooxygenase 2 is an inducible enzyme that appears to play a role in inflammation and tumor promotion. In a study of patients with FAP, the selective COX-2 inhibitor celecoxib at a higher dose significantly reduced the number of adenomas when compared with placebo or a lower dose of celecoxib ([16]).

However, the increased incidence of stroke and myocardial infarctions make the use of COX-2 inhibitors as primary chemoprevention unclear ([17]). Aspirin has primary chemopreventive properties, with the risk of colorectal cancer substantially reduced among women who were regular users of aspirin for at least 20 years ([18]). An additional prospective cohort study of male physicians followed over 4 years showed that regular users of aspirin (≥2 times per week) had a lower risk of developing colorectal cancer during the study period (RR = 0.68; 95% CI, 0.52-0.92) ([19]).

Secondary Prevention

Outside the clinical trial setting, patients with FAP are treated with celecoxib 400 mg twice daily. Recognizing the cardiovascular risk associated with COX-2 inhibitors, patients with cardiovascular disease or risk

CHAPTER 24

factors need aggressive risk management (eg, hypertension, diabetes, hyperlipidemia) or forgo therapy with celecoxib.

Aspirin also has secondary chemopreventive benefits. In a large randomized, placebo-controlled trial, aspirin demonstrated a benefit for patients with a prior history of colorectal cancer, showing a significantly reduced risk of developing adenomatous polyps compared to the placebo group (RR = 0.65; 95% CI, 0.46-0.91) ([20]). In a separate study, 1,121 patients with recent adenomatous polyp removal were randomized to receive aspirin 81 mg daily, aspirin 325 mg daily, or a placebo. Both groups receiving aspirin had a reduced risk of subsequent colorectal adenomas, with the 81-mg dose superior to the 325-mg dose ([21]). In a prospective cohort study of 1,279 patients with stage I to III colorectal cancer, after a median follow-up of 11.8 years, participants who regularly used aspirin had lower colorectal cancer–specific mortality, including those who initiated aspirin after diagnosis.

DIAGNOSTIC EVALUATION AND STAGING

Clinical Presentation

Colonic lesions in any location can cause change in bowel habits and bleeding, which may manifest as melena, hematochezia, a positive hemoccult test, or iron deficiency anemia in addition to weight loss, anorexia, and other constitutional symptoms. Unexplained iron deficiency anemia warrants an evaluation of the gastrointestinal tract.

Staging Studies

Preoperative evaluation is not always possible, particularly in the setting of acute bowel obstruction, and the staging evaluation in these cases should be completed within several weeks of surgery. Accurate postoperative staging may be confounded by the preceding surgery and therefore should not be obtained for at least 3 to 6 weeks after the operative procedure. Patients at MD Anderson are advised to wait a minimum of 4 weeks after surgery before undergoing imaging and a colonoscopy to allow wound healing and minimize risk to the surgical anastomosis.

Preoperative Staging for Colonic Neoplasms

In patients found to have a colonic neoplasm not requiring urgent surgery, a complete history, physical exam, and full colonoscopy with biopsies should be performed. Laboratory evaluation should include a complete blood cell count with differential, electrolytes, liver function studies, carcinoembryonic antigen (CEA) level, serum urea nitrogen (BUN), and creatinine. Imaging studies should include CT of the chest and CT scan or magnetic resonance imaging (MRI) of the abdomen/pelvis.

Rectal Cancer Staging

Patients with newly diagnosed rectal cancer at MD Anderson are staged with an endorectal ultrasound (EUS) or pelvic MRI. The EUS is more accurate than CT for assessing the depth of tumor invasion into the bowel wall and perirectal lymph node involvement. A pelvic MRI to evaluate the mesorectal planes and perirectal lymph nodes allows improved accuracy of preoperative staging. At MD Anderson, all patients with rectal cancer are staged with a CT scan of the chest and abdomen, with a dedicated MRI of the pelvis in the preoperative setting.

The Role of Positron Emission Tomography in Staging Cancers of the Colon and Rectum

Positron emission tomographic (PET) scanning using (^{18}F)-fluorodeoxyglucose (FDG-PET) is obtained in patients with a rising CEA without clinical or radiographic evidence of disease or in the setting of equivocal CT findings. However, inflammation may increase ^{18}FDG uptake, thus confounding accurate assessment. At MD Anderson, FDG-PET is not part of routine staging for newly diagnosed colon or rectal cancer.

Pathology

More than 95% of all colorectal malignancies are adenocarcinomas that are well differentiated, moderately differentiated, poorly differentiated, and undifferentiated. Other subtypes include mucinous and signet ring cell, which confer a poorer prognosis. These tumors are more likely to be present in younger patients and more commonly spread to the peritoneum. Treatment, however, does not differ from the more typical adenocarcinoma subtypes.

Pathologic Staging

Currently, the widely accepted system is the American Joint Committee on Cancer (AJCC) TNM classification system (Table 24-5) to guide treatment.

Importance of Lymph Node Dissection and Sampling

At the time of resection, tumor removal should involve segmental resection of the involved colon or rectum along the appropriate vascular pedicles with careful

Table 24-5 TNM Staging of Colorectal Cancer

TNM Stage	Primary Tumor	Lymph Metastasis	Distant Metastasis
0	Tis	N0	M0
I	T1	N0	M0
	T2	N0	M0
II	T3	N0	M0
	T4	N0	M0
IIIA	T1, T2	N1	M0
IIIB	T3, T4	N1	M0
IIIC	Any T	N2	M0
IV	Any T	Any N	M1

M1, any distant metastatic site; N1, metastases to 1-3 regional lymph nodes; N2, metastases in 4 or more regional lymph nodes; Tis, tumor in situ; T1, tumor invades submucosa; T2, tumor invades muscularis propria; T3, tumor invades through muscularis mucosa to subserosa or periolic or perirectal tissues; T4, tumor perforates the visceral peritoneum or directly invades other organs.

Reproduced with permission from Edge SB, Byrd DR, Compton CC (eds): *AJCC Cancer Staging Manuarl*, 7th ed. New York, NY: Springer; 2010.

removal of all regional lymph nodes. Failing to do so may lead to relapse in lymph nodes draining the affected segment of bowel, as shown in Fig. 24-2. Therefore, tumors are considered high-risk stage II (T3N0M0 or T4N0M0) unless at least 12 lymph nodes are negative for metastatic disease ([22]).

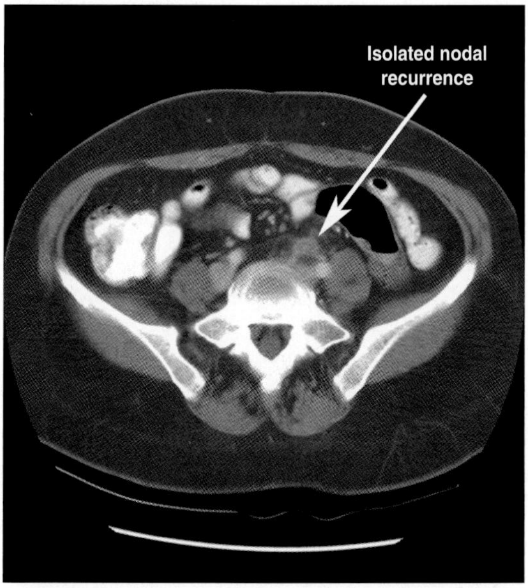

FIGURE 24-2 Computed tomographic image of a 54-year-old woman with a history of T3N0M0 adenocarcinoma of the sigmoid colon found incidentally at the time of hysterectomy for benign disease. Surgical resection of the sigmoid mass was performed by her gynecologist. The patient received adjuvant therapy for 6 months but subsequently developed a rising serum CEA level and a nodal mass at the base of the inferior mesenteric artery (IMA). After a course of chemotherapy for metastatic disease, she underwent repeat laparotomy with the finding of an isolated nodal mass, which was removed and was positive for adenocarcinoma. In retrospect, inadequate resection of the sigmoid mesentery to the level of the IMA was thought to explain the recurrence.

THERAPEUTIC APPROACHES

Local and Regional Control

Almost half of the patients undergoing curative resection will ultimately die of metastatic disease as a result of residual microscopic disease not evident at the time of surgery. Patients with stage II colon cancer at high risk of relapse have been defined by the National Comprehensive Cancer Network (NCCN) as those individuals with T4 tumors (stage IIB/IIC); poorly differentiated history (excluding MSI-H cancers); lymphovascular invasion; perineural invasion; bowel obstruction; localized perforation; margins that are close, indeterminate, or positive; and inadequate sampling of lymph nodes (<12 nodes examined) ([23]).

Surgical Management of Colon Cancer

Resection for localized colon cancer removes the affected segment of bowel, the adjacent mesentery, and the draining lymph nodes. Asymptomatic patients with stage IV disease with their primary malignancy intact do not require surgical resection of their primary except for impending bowel obstruction. Laparoscopic colectomy was noninferior to an open colectomy in several prospective randomized studies, with the laparoscopic surgery group having a shorter perioperative recovery, hospital stay, duration of parenteral narcotic use and oral analgesics, as well as comparable intraoperative complications and postoperative mortality ([24]).

Evidence Regarding Adjuvant Therapy for Colon Cancer

Patients with stages II and III colon cancer have a risk of relapse after surgical resection of macroscopic disease. Systemic chemotherapy has been employed to eradicate micrometastases. Currently, patients with stage III colon cancer (node positive without clinically detectable metastases) receive 6 months of adjuvant chemotherapy. The MOSAIC (Multicenter International Study of Oxaliplatin/5-Fluorouracil/Leucovorin in the Adjuvant Treatment of Colon Cancer) trial demonstrated an improved 5-year disease-free survival (DFS) from 67% to 73% for patients receiving FOLFOX (5-fluorouracil [5-FU], leucovorin calcium, and oxaliplatin) versus 5-FU and leucovorin alone ([25]) with the DFS and overall survival (OS) benefits achieving statistical significance in patients with stage III disease.

The evidence for adjuvant therapy for stage II disease is less robust. To date, the largest study of patients with stage II disease, QUASAR (Quick and Simple and Reliable), showed a modest survival benefit of 3.6% in patients receiving adjuvant 5-FU versus observation following surgical resection ([26]). The 2012 subset analysis of the 889 patients with stage II disease in the MOSAIC (Multicenter International Study of Oxaliplatin/5FU-LV in the Adjuvant Treatment of Colon Cancer) trial showed no statistically significant benefit in either OS or DFS with the addition of oxaliplatin to 5-FU in the adjuvant setting for stage II ([27]). Furthermore, the analysis of the patients with low- and high-risk stage II demonstrated that neither subgroup unequivocally derived benefit from the addition of oxaliplatin.

Multigene assays have been in development for prognostic and predictive value in patients with stage II colon cancer. Among the assays furthest along in development is the Oncotype Dx colon cancer assay (Genomic Health, Inc.), which provides a prognostic classification of low, intermediate, or high risk of recurrence based on the expression of seven recurrence risk genes and five reference genes. In two large trials, QUASAR and NSABP C-07, of patients with stage II and III disease, this score was validated as prognostic for recurrence, DFS, and OS but not predictive of benefit from chemotherapy ([28]).

A second assay, ColoPrint (Agendia), identifies the expression of 18 genes and produces one of two recurrence risk categories, high or low. Although it was studied in stages I-IV, it has emerged to be of the most value in patients with stage II in identifying the risk of recurrence between high- and low-risk groups (hazard ratio [HR] 3.34, P = .017) ([29]). It is currently being prospectively validated in patients with stage II in the PARSC trial, which will predict the 3-year recurrence-free survival using ColoPrint and clinical factors ([30]). Both assays share limitations particularly the inability to predict clinical benefit from chemotherapy.

Irinotecan has no established role in the adjuvant setting. Three randomized phase III trials failed to show an improvement in DFS or OS in the adjuvant setting ([31–33]). An exploratory analysis of CALGB 89803 (IFL versus bolus 5-FU/LV) indicates that patients with MSI-H may have an improved DFS from irinotecan-based therapy (HR 0.76; 95% CI, 0.64-0.88; P = .03). However, the PETACC 3 study confirmed that while patients with stage II disease with MSI-H tumors have a survival advantage over MSS patients with a 5-FU-based treatment, the addition of irinotecan produced no additive benefit, affirming the overall consensus against using an irinotecan-based regimen in the adjuvant setting ([34]).

Furthermore, data have not supported the addition of bevacizumab, cetuximab, or panitumumab in the adjuvant setting. The NSABP trial C-08 showed no improvement in DFS or OS with the addition of bevacizumab to adjuvant FOLFOX6 in stage II and III colon cancer ([35]). A second phase III randomized controlled study, the bevacizumab plus oxaliplatin-based chemotherapy as adjuvant treatment for colon cancer (AVANT) trial of resected stage III or high-risk stage II colon cancer ([36]) also failed to show any improvement in DFS and, in fact, suggested a poorer OS with the addition of bevacizumab.

The IDEA (International Duration Evaluation of Adjuvant Chemotherapy) Collaboration is a prospective combined analysis of phase III trials investigating duration of adjuvant chemotherapy (3 vs 6 months) for stage III colon cancer ([37]). The ongoing US CALGB/SWOG 80702 colon trial, which is among the six trials that are part of the IDEA collaboration, further randomizes patients beyond the duration of adjuvant therapy to 3 years of celecoxib versus placebo ([37]). Overall, few therapeutic changes appear to be on the horizon for the treatment of adjuvant colon cancer.

The MDACC Approach to Nonmetastatic Colon Cancer

When patients present to MDACC with a diagnosis of colon cancer, a detailed history, including family history; routine laboratory tests, including CEA level; and imaging (CT chest, CT or MRI abdomen, pelvis) are obtained. Previous endoscopic findings and pathology are reviewed and are tested for MSI by IHC or by PCR. Patients without metastatic disease or contraindications to surgery should undergo primary resection with curative intent (Fig. 24-3). If there is an obstruction, colonoscopy is usually performed. Surgery may consist of segmental resection or subtotal colectomy, depending on the underlying colonic pathology

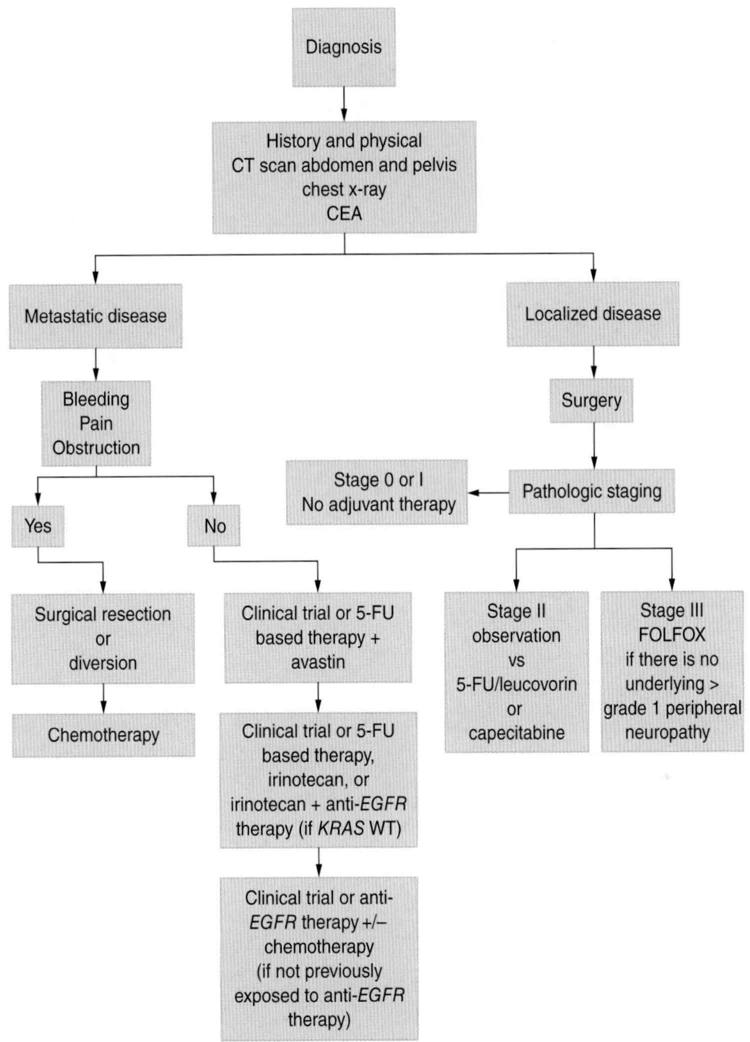

FIGURE 24-3 Diagnostic and therapeutic algorithm for colon cancer.

(multifocal cancer, FAP, HNPCC, etc.); pathologic staging is then determined from the surgical specimens, which is the standard for all such resections at MD Anderson irrespective of age. Patients with stage 0 or I tumors are placed on surveillance only. Patients with stage II colon cancer have a 75% to 80% chance of long-term DFS with surgical resection alone. Patients with stage II colon cancer are referred for discussion of adjuvant chemotherapy with full consideration provided to all patients with stage III disease.

Our current approach favors FOLFOX or XELOX (Table 24-6) for 6 months for all stage III patients unless chemotherapy is contraindicated. Those who are better candidates for a single-agent fluoropyrimidine are offered capecitabine over intravenous 5-FU. Adjuvant therapy should begin within 4 to 8 weeks after surgery, unless postoperative complications warrant a delay.

Surveillance for Patients With Resected Colon Cancer

Once active therapy is completed, patients undergo clinical evaluations every 3 to 4 months for the first 3 years during the period of highest risk of recurrence, then every 6 months for the following 2 years, and annually thereafter. Of all recurrences, 80% occur within the first 3 years following surgical resection ([38]). Colonoscopy is recommended 1 year after surgery and every 3 years thereafter at a minimum. Laboratory studies, including CEA level, are checked every 3 to 6 months; abdominopelvic CT or MRI and a chest x-ray/CT of the chest are obtained at 12 months. At 5 years, patients are followed with surveillance colonoscopy (every 3 years), annual physical examination, and CEA level.

Table 24-6 Summary of Common Chemotherapy Regimens Used at MDACC for Colorectal Cancer

Adjuvant Chemotherapy
Capecitabine: 1,000 mg/m² by mouth twice daily on days 1-14 (3-week cycle, total 8 cycles)
5-Fluorouracil/leucovorin: Leucovorin 400 mg/m² IV on day 1; 5-fluorouracil 400 mg/m² IV bolus on day 1, followed by 5-fluorouracil 2,400 mg/m² IV continuous infusion over 46 hours (2-week cycle, total 12 cycles)
Modified FOLFOX 6: Oxaliplatin 85 mg/m² IV on day 1; leucovorin 400 mg/m² IV on day 1; 5-fluorouracil 400 mg/m² IV bolus on day 1, followed by 5-fluorouracil 2,400 mg/m² IV continuous infusion over 46 hours (2-week cycle, total 12 cycles)
XELOX: Oxaliplatin 130 mg/m² on day 1; capecitabine 850 mg/m² by mouth twice a day on days 1-14 (3-week cycle, total 8 cycles)
Therapy for Metastatic Disease
Capecitabine: 1,000 mg/m² by mouth twice a day on days 1-14 (3-week cycle)
• With or without bevacizumab (7.5 mg/kg IV every 3 weeks)
5-Fluorouracil/leucovorin: Leucovorin 400 mg/m² IV on day 1; 5-fluorouracil 400 mg/m² IV bolus on day 1, followed by 5-fluorouracil 2,400 mg/m² IV continuous infusion over 46 hours (2-week cycle)
With or without bevacizumab (5 mg/kg IV every 2 weeks)
Modified FOLFOX 6: Oxaliplatin 85 mg/m² IV on day 1; leucovorin 400 mg/m² IV on day 1; 5-fluorouracil 400 mg/m² IV bolus on day 1, followed by 5-fluorouracil 2,400 mg/m² IV continuous infusion over 46 hours (2-week cycle)
• With or without bevacizumab (5 mg/kg IV every 2 weeks)
• With or without cetuximab[a] (400 mg/m² IV first infusion followed by 250 mg/m² IV weekly or 500 mg/m² IV every 2 weeks) or panitumumab[a] (6 mg/kg IV every 2 weeks)
XELOX: Oxaliplatin 130 mg/m² on day 1; capecitabine 850 mg/m² by mouth twice a day on days 1-14 (3-week cycle)
With or without bevacizumab (7.5 mg/kg IV every 3 weeks)
• With or without cetuximab[a] (400 mg/m² IV first infusion followed by 250 mg/m² IV weekly or 500 mg/m² IV every 2 weeks) or panitumumab[a] (9 mg/kg IV every 3 weeks)
Modified FOLFIRI: Irinotecan 180 mg/m² IV on day 1; leucovorin 400 mg/m² IV on day 1; 5-fluorouracil 400 mg/m² IV bolus on day 1, followed by 5-fluorouracil 2,400 mg/m² IV continuous infusion over 46 hours (2-week cycle)
• With or without bevacizumab (5 mg/kg IV every 2 weeks)
• With or without cetuximab[a] (400 mg/m² IV first infusion followed by 250 mg/m² IV weekly) or panitumumab[a] (6 mg/kg IV every 2 weeks)
Irinotecan: 180 mg/m² IV on day 1 (2-week cycle) or 300-350 mg/m² IV on day 1 (3-week cycle)
Cetuximab[a]/Irinotecan:
• Cetuximab[a] 400 mg/m² IV first infusion followed by 250 mg/m² IV weekly + irinotecan 350 mg/m² IV on day 1 (3-week cycle) or 180 mg/m² IV on day 1 (2-week cycle)
• Cetuximab[a] 500 mg/m² IV every 2 weeks ± irinotecan 180 mg/m² IV every 2 weeks
Panitumumab[a]: 6 mg/kg IV every 2 weeks or 9 mg/kg IV every 3 weeks

[a]Cetuximab and panitumumab are indicated only in patients with *KRAS* wild-type tumors.
Concurrent chemotherapy and radiation therapy (rectal cancer)
Continuous infusion 5-fluorouracil: 250-300 mg/m² IV daily (Monday-Friday on days of radiation therapy only)
Capecitabine: 825 mg/m² by mouth twice a day (Monday-Friday on days of radiation therapy only)

Local Therapy for Rectal Cancer

In general, over two-thirds of the patients with rectal cancer will be able to have a sphincter-saving procedure whether it is a low anterior resection or a proctectomy with a coloanal anastomosis (CAA). An abdominoperineal resection (APR), which includes removal of the rectum, anus, sphincter muscles, and a permanent colostomy is reserved for patients with tumor involvement of sphincter muscles or with poor preoperative sphincter function. A sharp mesorectal excision should be performed; there is no role for blunt dissection in the pelvis in rectal cancer surgery.

Radiotherapy

Radiotherapy improves survival in patients with locally advanced rectal cancer. Standard radiotherapy doses are 45 Gy in 25 fractions, followed by a 5.4-Gy boost. Concurrent protracted venous infusional (PVI) 5-FU provides similar efficacy with lower gastrointestinal and hematologic toxicity rates than bolus 5-FU or a high-dose infusion of 5-FU ([39]). A phase III intergroup trial demonstrated inferiority for bolus 5-FU during radiation therapy versus prolonged infusional 5-FU and resulted in higher OS rates ($P = .005$) ([22]).

CHAPTER 24

Preoperative Therapy for Rectal Cancer

Two European studies have supported the use of preoperative therapy for resectable rectal cancer. The German Arbeitsgemeinschaft Internistische Onkologie (AIO) trial comparing preoperative and postoperative chemoradiation in T3 or T4 tumors showed a lower pelvic recurrence rate in the preoperative chemoradiation arm (6% vs 13% postoperative, respectively, $P = .0006$) ([40]). In patients who, based on pretreatment clinical evaluation, were believed to require APR, chemoradiation also led to increased sphincter preservation rates (39% vs 19%, $P = .004$). Only 54% of patients in the postoperative arm received the full radiation dose, and 50% received full-dose chemotherapy, compared with 92% and 89%, respectively, in the preoperative arm ($P < .001$).

Neoadjuvant chemotherapy with concurrent radiotherapy has been extensively studied. NSABP R-04, a four-arm phase III trial of 5-FU, capecitabine, 5-FU/oxaliplatin, and XELOX showed no improvement in locoregional recurrence, DFS, or OS with the addition of oxaliplatin ([41]). Two phase III trials (Studio Terapia Adiuvante Retto and Action Clinique Coordonnées en cancérologie Digestive [STAR and ACCORD, respectively] 12) did not have higher rates of pCR with the addition of weekly oxaliplatin ([42, 43]).

Another treatment principle under investigation is *induction chemotherapy*, defined as administration of chemotherapy prior to chemoradiotherapy and surgery in resectable stage II or III rectal cancer. One small study out of the United Kingdom evaluated neoadjuvant capecitabine and oxaliplatin followed by synchronous chemoradiation and total mesorectal excision in patients with MRI-defined poor-risk rectal cancer ([44]). Overall, 77 patients received neoadjuvant capecitabine and oxaliplatin, with 88% demonstrating a radiologic response and 86% a symptomatic response after just one cycle of therapy. The response rates increased to 97% on completion of chemoradiation. Then, 66 of 67 patients who then underwent a TME had R0 resection, with a pathologic complete response seen in 16 patients and only microscopic disease noted in 32 patients (48%).

To investigate the sequence of therapies, the randomized phase II study from Spain, the Grupo cancer de recto 3 (GCR-3) study, randomized 108 patients into two arms: arm A for preoperative concurrent chemoradiation with capecitabine and oxaliplatin followed by surgery and four cycles of adjuvant capecitabine and oxaliplatin or arm B for induction capecitabine and oxaliplatin followed by chemoradiation and surgery ([45]). Rates of pathologic complete response, which was the study's primary end point, were not significantly different in the arms; however, patients who received induction capecitabine/oxaliplatin combination had fewer grade 3 or 4 adverse events occur during the induction period when compared to those in the adjuvant chemotherapy arm.

The addition of the neoadjuvant bevacizumab was also investigated in a randomized, noncomparative phase II study in locally advanced T3 resectable rectal cancer ([46]). Arm A incorporated bevacizumab plus FOLFOX4 as induction prior to bevacizumab–5-FU–RT and then TME; arm B did not have the induction component but did include bevacizumab–5-FU–RT prior to surgery. While the pathologic CR end point was not met in arm B, arm A did show a statistically significant improvement in pathologic CR (23.5%; 95% CI, 12.1% to 39.5%) when compared to a defined standard rate of 10% ($P = .015$).

In studies incorporating cetuximab, the EXPERT-C trial was a multicenter randomized phase II clinical trial comparing neoadjuvant oxaliplatin, capecitabine, and preoperative radiotherapy with or without cetuximab followed by total mesorectal excision in high-risk rectal cancer, with high risk defined by the high-resolution, thin-slice MRI (3 mm) finding of tumor within 1 mm of mesorectal fascia, T3 tumor at or below levators, extramural extension of 5 mm or greater, T4 tumor, or presence of extramural venous invasion ([47, 48]). This study showed higher response rates and OS with cetuximab in KRAS/BRAF wild-type (WT) rectal cancer; however, the primary end point of improved pathologic or radiologic complete response was not met.

A potentially pivotal ongoing study led by the Alliance (N0148) is a phase II/III trial that evaluates the need for chemoradiation therapy versus induction FOLFOX in patients with mid–high-lying rectal cancers (NCT01515787).

Adjuvant Therapy for Rectal Cancer

Since the mid-1970s, studies have shown that combined-modality therapy offers a clear benefit for patients with stage II or III rectal cancer. The Gastrointestinal Tumor Study Group (GITSG) performed a randomized trial in patients with rectal cancer undergoing surgery with curative intent. Patients were randomized to four arms: observation, chemotherapy alone, radiotherapy alone, or chemoradiotherapy. The rates of DFS and OS were higher in the combined-modality therapy group than in the other arms ([49]). Currently, standard adjuvant therapy for patients with stage II or III rectal cancer should consist of fluoropyrimidine-based chemotherapy and external-beam radiotherapy of the pelvis.

The MDACC Approach to Nonmetastatic Rectal Cancer

Preoperative Chemoradiation

The approach to rectal cancer is outlined in Fig. 24-4. At MD Anderson, patients see a multidisciplinary team of radiation, medical, and surgical oncology specialists for a thorough history, including family cancer history,

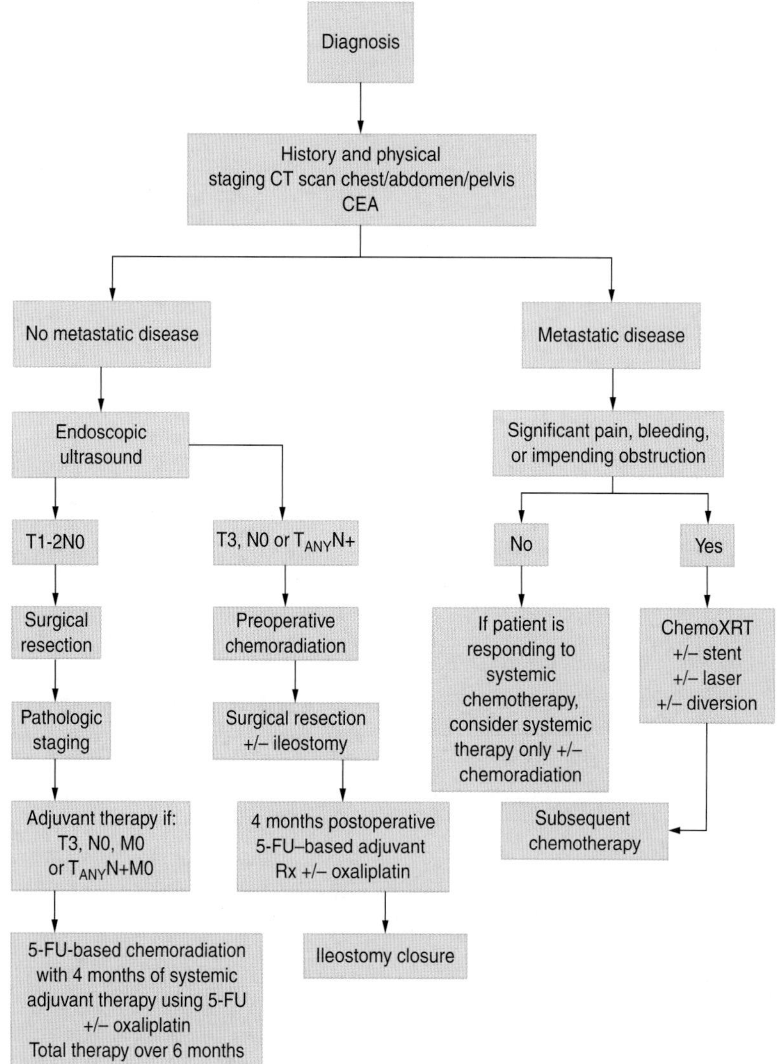

FIGURE 24-4 Diagnostic and therapeutic algorithm for rectal cancer.

physical exam with a digital rectal exam, inguinal lymph node exam, rigid proctoscopy, and staging studies. The patency of the colonic lumen is evaluated by proctoscopy, flexible sigmoidoscopy, or colonoscopy before starting systemic chemotherapy.

For patients with nonmetastatic disease, EUS and MRI of the pelvis are obtained as pretreatment staging. Capecitabine is given as the radiation sensitizer (825 mg/m^2 twice daily, Monday-Friday, on days of radiation therapy only). Bowel exclusion techniques during simulation minimize the small bowel in the field. We conduct a toxicity evaluation every 1 to 2 weeks during radiation to ensure symptom control. Electrolytes, renal function, and hematologic parameters are checked weekly. Topical barrier creams are prescribed for grades 1 to 3 perineal radiation dermatitis. Should grade 2 or higher nonhematologic toxicity develop (excluding radiation dermatitis), concurrent chemotherapy is held until resolution but radiation is continued.

After chemoradiation, perianal pain and ulceration, anorexia, and diarrhea typically subside within 2 to 3 weeks. Approximately 6 weeks after completion, patients undergo repeat physical examination with proctoscopy and then surgical resection. We recommend reversal of the diverting ileostomy after the completion of adjuvant chemotherapy due to erratic bowel managements. For those patients who recover fully from surgery, postoperative chemotherapy is delivered for a total of 4 months.

In the adjuvant setting, patients with stage III rectal cancer and no contraindication to oxaliplatin are advised to receive it as a component of FOLFOX or XELOX. In select cases, a patient with a pCR after preoperative 5-FU–based chemoradiation may receive single-agent 5-FU–based adjuvant therapy rather than FOLFOX. The choice of adjuvant therapy may vary based on degree of response to single-agent fluoropyrimidine-based therapy and the patient's underlying comorbidities.

Postoperative Chemoradiation

Patients who have undergone surgery as their initial intervention may require postoperative chemoradiation and systemic therapy when they present to MD Anderson after surgery. For patients with T3N0M0 or T2N1 disease, radiotherapy is often omitted if the tumor was located in the high pelvis (>10 cm from the anal verge), there is good nodal sampling (>12 lymph nodes) ([50]), and the radial margin is negative (>2 mm) because pelvic tumor control is excellent without the use of chemoradiation ([51]). In all other stage II and III rectal cancer cases, local failure is high enough to warrant the use of chemoradiation. In addition, 4 months of systemic therapy with either capecitabine or 5-FU/leucovorin is typically integrated with chemoradiation. Patients at higher risk of distant metastasis often receive chemotherapy first with FOLFOX.

Surveillance for Patients With Resected Rectal Cancer

Follow-up for patients with resected rectal cancer is very similar to that for colon cancer. Patients with a sphincter-preserving procedure also require periodic proctoscopies for local relapses and anastomotic strictures. A rising CEA without other clinical or CT evidence of relapse prompts a pelvic MRI or PET/CT particularly for local recurrence.

Patterns of Spread and Recurrence After Primary Therapy

Among patients who undergo surgical resection, at least 25% will have a recurrence, with most (60%) relapsing at multiple sites; the remaining relapse in the liver (15%), lung (4%), and locally (21%) ([52]). Relapse in multiple sites is generally managed with palliative systemic chemotherapy, while surgery can be considered for oligometastatic disease.

Management of Locally Recurrent Disease

Locally recurrent rectal cancer presents a therapeutic challenge for which salvage surgery may not be feasible. The collective experience at MD Anderson suggests that systemic therapy has limited activity against locally recurrent disease with few durable responses. Palliative radiation is delivered as external-beam radiotherapy or brachytherapy catheters. Aggressive use of narcotics and intrathecal analgesics or neurolytic blocks is employed for pain control concurrently with aggressive bowel management.

For the subset of patients who may be surgical candidates, treatment planning is vetted in the weekly multidisciplinary conference at MD Anderson. In our experience, pelvic MRI is superior to CT for distinguishing posttreatment changes from viable tumor while identify resectable disease. Biopsy confirmation of recurrence is always recommended; EUS has not been particularly useful with locally recurrent rectal tumors.

Prior to salvage surgery, additional chemoradiation may be considered using a hypofractionated schedule to a total dose of 39 Gy (if at least 1 year has elapsed since prior pelvic radiation). Radiosensitization with 5-FU or capecitabine is also considered. Approximately 6 to 8 weeks after completion of chemoradiation, a final decision about surgery is made. In most cases, the operative strategy may also include intraoperative radiotherapy or insertion of brachytherapy catheters for high-dose afterloading. Postoperative chemotherapy after aggressive preoperative chemoradiation is at the discretion of the treating physician. However, there is broad agreement that surgery for locally recurrent disease is not indicated in those patients with unresectable metastatic disease, given the overall poor prognosis, significant morbidity, and prolonged recovery associated with this complex pelvic surgery.

Systemic Therapy for Metastatic Disease: A Rapidly Changing Therapeutic Landscape

Since the late 1950s, systemic chemotherapy with 5-FU has been the mainstay of palliative treatment for patients with metastatic disease not amenable to surgical intervention. During the ensuing decades, a variety of 5-FU schedules have been employed, including bolus injections administered either weekly (Roswell Park regimen) or daily for 5 days (Mayo regimen) and continuous infusion given via central catheter and portable pump. Objective response rates have ranged from 15% to 25% with these schedules. When 5-FU is administered as a bolus injection, leucovorin is often added to enhance binding of 5-FU to its target, thymidylate synthase. After a long period of uncertainty regarding the optimal dose and schedule of 5-FU with leucovorin, infusional 5-FU regimens have been recognized as superior to bolus regimens. However, prior to the advent of irinotecan and oxaliplatin, while infusional delivery of 5-FU led to better response rates compared with bolus therapy, no clear survival advantage was ever demonstrated. Given the barriers to delivery of infusional 5-FU, including the need for a central venous catheter and its associated risks, bolus 5-FU with leucovorin was widely accepted in the United States as frontline therapy for metastatic colorectal cancer well into the 1990s.

Since that time, therapeutic options for metastatic disease have been rapidly evolving, and oncologists now have access to several drugs with activity in the first-, second-, and even third-line settings. In addition to cytotoxic drugs, the targeted agents cetuximab, panitumumab, and bevacizumab have emerged as clinically relevant components of systemic therapy for advanced disease. It is important for oncologists to have a general understanding of these drugs and their roles in the treatment of metastatic disease.

Capecitabine: An Orally Bioavailable Fluoropyrimidine

Capecitabine is an oral fluoropyrimidine that is converted to 5-FU primarily in tumor tissues. It passes through the intestinal mucosa essentially unchanged and is subsequently metabolized by a sequential three-enzyme pathway ([53]). First, capecitabine is converted to 5′-deoxy-5-fluorocytidine (5′-DFCR) by carboxylesterase (primarily in the liver). The 5′-DFCR is then converted to 5′-deoxy-5-fluorouridine (5′-DFUR) by cytidine deaminase, which is found in both the liver and tumor tissues. The metabolism of 5′-DFUR to the pharmacologically active agent 5-FU is mediated by thymidine phosphorylase (TP), also known as platelet-derived endothelial cell growth factor. Concentrations of TP are relatively higher in tumor tissue than normal tissue, which accounts for the preferential intratumoral release of 5-FU. Two large phase III trials compared capecitabine with a bolus regimen of 5-FU ([54, 55]), and the results were subsequently pooled. The response rates were superior with capecitabine, and the median survival was equivalent, with less neutropenia and mucositis among those patients receiving capecitabine.

In patients with contraindications to combination chemotherapy, capecitabine monotherapy is a reasonable alternative to 5-FU and leucovorin in the metastatic setting.

Irinotecan

Irinotecan, an inhibitor of topoisomerase I, was originally developed as second-line chemotherapy for patients in whom 5-FU was ineffective ([56–58]). In phase II trials of irinotecan performed in the United States, response rates in patients refractory for 5-FU were approximately 15% superior to those reported prior to the advent of irinotecan; this led the Food and Drug Administration (FDA) to approve the drug as a second-line therapy in patients with advanced 5-FU-refractory disease ([59]). The survival benefit of second-line irinotecan was subsequently verified in a European trial, in which patients who had been previously treated with 5-FU were randomized to receive irinotecan every 3 weeks or best supportive care (BSC) ([60]). Patients randomized to BSC were allowed to receive infusional 5-FU. This trial demonstrated a survival advantage for patients in the irinotecan arm compared to those in the BSC arm (9.2 vs 6.5 months; $P = .0001$).

Shortly thereafter, studies were performed to investigate the potential benefit of irinotecan as a component of frontline therapy in patients with metastatic colorectal cancer. Two large, randomized trials were conducted in the United States and Europe comparing 5-FU and leucovorin with 5-FU, leucovorin, and irinotecan as first-line treatment of metastatic colorectal cancer ([61, 62]). Both studies demonstrated that the response and OS rates for the group treated with triple-drug therapy were superior to those for the group treated with 5-FU and leucovorin. The response rates for the triple-drug combination ranged from 35% to 40%, the median time to disease progression was 7 months, and median survival was prolonged by 2 months. These results prompted the FDA in 2000 to approve the use of these irinotecan-based combinations for first-line treatment of colorectal cancer. For a brief period of time, the IFL regimen (bolus 5-FU at 500 mg/m^2, leucovorin 20 mg/m^2, and irinotecan 125 mg/m^2, administered weekly for 4 weeks on a 6-week cycle) became standard first-line therapy for patients with metastatic colon cancer in the United States. However, as these studies were being performed, a novel platinum analog, oxaliplatin, was also showing impressive activity in combination with 5-FU and leucovorin, generating great interest in the drug.

Oxaliplatin

Oxaliplatin is a third-generation platinum derivative that has shown additive or synergistic antitumor activity in combination with a variety of standard antineoplastic agents, including 5-FU; oxaliplatin is ineffective without 5-FU ([63]). While irinotecan was being studied in the United States, oxaliplatin was already approved in Europe. In 2000, de Gramont and colleagues reported the results of a phase III trial of infusional 5-FU/leucovorin and oxaliplatin (FOLFOX4), versus 5-FU/leucovorin alone, as first-line treatment in advanced colorectal cancer ([64]). Four hundred twenty patients were randomized to the study, and progression-free survival (PFS) was the primary end point. Progression-free survival and response rates were significantly better for the FOLFOX arm compared to the 5-FU/leucovorin arm (9.0 months and 50% vs 6.2 months and 22%, respectively). Even though the FOLFOX arm experienced more grade 3 and 4 neutropenia, diarrhea, and neurosensory toxicity, this did not impair quality of life. The primary objective of median OS was not met (14.7 months for the 5-FU/leucovorin arm and 16.2 months for the FOLFOX arm, *P* = .12); consequently, initial approval by the FDA failed.

Goldberg and associates subsequently compared the activity and toxicity of three different drug combinations in untreated patients with metastatic colorectal cancer. Seven hundred ninety-five patients were randomized to receive IFL, FOLFOX, or IROX (irinotecan + oxaliplatin) ([65]). The results favored FOLFOX for all end points, including time to progression, response rate, and OS. Median survival in the FOLFOX, IFL, and IROX groups was 19.5, 15.0, and 17.4 months, respectively. The authors concluded that FOLFOX should be considered a standard first-line regimen for advanced colorectal cancer. A limitation of this study was that 60% of the patients treated with oxaliplatin received irinotecan in the second-line setting, but only 24% of patients in the IFL arm could get oxaliplatin as second-line treatment because it was not approved in the United States at the time of the study.

Tournigand and colleagues answered the important question of how to sequence these regimens. They reported the results of a phase III study investigating 5-FU, leucovorin, and irinotecan (FOLFIRI), followed by FOLFOX6 (see Table 24-6) on progression of disease, versus the opposite sequence (FOLFOX6 followed by FOLFIRI) ([66]). The two sequences were equivalent in terms of progression-free and OS, although the toxicity profiles were different. Median survival was 21.5 months in the FOLFIRI-FOLFOX arm (109 patients) and 20.6 months in the FOLFOX-FOLFIRI arm (111 patients) (*P* = .99).

An aggressive approach is the combination of oxaliplatin, irinotecan, and 5-FU/leucovorin (FOLFOXIRI) ([67]). An impressive response rate of 66% was noted in a phase III trial of FOLFOXIRI versus FOLFIRI, fulfilling the primary end point of PFS. However, a serious adverse toxicity reaction associated with this regimen is severe myelosuppression. Concerns about this regimen are largely due to discussion of limited options for second-line therapy if the patient's disease should progress. Furthermore, an earlier phase III Greek trial failed to note an improvement in OS, perhaps due to the limited second-line chemotherapy options for patients treated with FOLFOXIRI ([68]). Common chemotherapy regimens for both colon and rectal carcinoma are listed in Table 24-6.

Monoclonal Antibodies

Therapeutic use of the immune system against cancer has been studied for decades but remained elusive until recently due to technical difficulties. The fact that tumor cells are recognized as a part of the normal host makes the development of vaccines difficult, and the logical alternative would involve development of foreign antibodies that could be delivered to the patient. The development of those antibodies was not possible until 1975, when the hybridoma technique was perfected by Kohler and others, allowing the development of specific antibodies against antigens restricted to, or overexpressed in, tumor cells ([69]). Initially, the development of these antibodies was proposed as a direct immunologic and cytotoxic approach for treatment of malignant disease. While such efforts continue, this strategy has been refined to include the development of antibodies that target specific proteins critical to intracellular signaling, tumor cell function, or the host-tumor interface. Three new monoclonal antibodies have been recently approved in the United States for treatment of metastatic colorectal cancer.

Cetuximab

Cetuximab is a chimeric immunoglobulin G1 (IgG1) monoclonal antibody directed against the epidermal growth factor receptor (*EGFR*), also known as ErbB-1 ([70]). In the colorectal cancer arena, it was primarily studied in previously treated patients. Cetuximab monotherapy yielded a response rate of 9% and median survival of 6.4 months in a small group of irinotecan-refractory patients ([71]). When compared to BSC in a treatment-refractory patient population, single-agent cetuximab resulted in superior OS (6.1 vs 4.6 months) and quality of life. Two phase III randomized trials (Bowel Oncology and *Cetuximab* Antibody, Erbitux Plus Irinotecan for Metastatic Colorectal Cancer [BOND, EPIC]) subsequently confirmed the efficacy of cetuximab in combination with irinotecan in previously treated patients ([72, 73]), with response rates of approximately 20%. Improvement in OS versus BSC has since been validated in heavily pretreated patients ([74]). The reason for the apparent synergy between cetuximab and irinotecan is not well understood; it is known that *EGFR* mediates not only proliferation signals but also a number of other processes whose inhibition may render cells more sensitive to apoptotic stimuli, such as chemotherapy.

The *EGFR* inhibition is fraught with potential treatment-related toxicities, including a pustular acneiform rash of the upper torso and scalp. Hence, identification of a predictive marker for efficacy of anti-*EGFR* therapy would decrease unnecessary drug exposure and financial burden. It is now recognized that *EGFR* expression does not correlate with efficacy of therapy ([75]). However, mutation of the *KRAS* oncogene is present in 35% to 50% of all patients with colorectal cancer and has an early role in the transition of adenoma to carcinoma, with reported concordance between the primary and the metastatic site ([76]).

CHAPTER 24

The mutations are commonly G>A transitions and G>T transversions; codons 12 and 13 are the most frequently affected and rarely codons 61 and 146. In addition to *KRAS*, mutations in *NRAS* have been recently identified as a potential predictive indicator of anti-*EGFR* efficacy. The *NRAS* mutation may be present in 10% of patients and was also associated with reduced response to panitumumab ([77]). Patients with *KRAS* WT and *NRAS* WT tumors had improved PFS (HR = 0.39, 95% CI = 0.27, 0.56) compared with those receiving BSC, whereas those with *NRAS* mutant tumors did not appear to benefit from panitumumab (HR = 1.94, 95% CI = 0.44, 8.44).

The Cetuximab Combined With Irinotecan in First-Line Therapy for Metastatic Colorectal (CRYSTAL) phase III trial randomized nearly 1,200 patients with untreated metastatic colorectal cancer to FOLFIRI with or without cetuximab. Median PFS (8.9 vs 8.0 months) and response rate (47% vs 39%) were modestly improved with cetuximab. Most important, however, investigators later discovered in an unplanned retrospective analysis that clinical benefit was limited to those patients with *KRAS* WT tumors. In this group of patients, the findings were impressive; cetuximab improved the response rate from 43% to 59% and median PFS from 8.7 months to 9.9 months ([78]). Updated results of the CRYSTAL trial were recently presented, indicating an OS advantage for FOLFIRI and cetuximab in the *KRAS* WT group (23.5 vs 20.0 months) ([79]). This is the first trial to demonstrate an improvement in OS with cetuximab in combination with chemotherapy in treatment-naïve patients. In addition, OPUS, a randomized phase II trial in treatment-naïve patients, compared FOLFOX4 plus cetuximab to FOLFOX4 alone and also showed improvement in response rate and PFS with cetuximab. Once again, analysis revealed that this benefit was restricted to patients without *KRAS* mutations ([80]). Neither study has indicated what percentage of specimens analyzed was from the primary versus the metastatic site and if true concordance existed. Despite the current evidence supporting *KRAS* testing, the FDA delayed mandating *KRAS* testing largely due to the retrospective unplanned analyses. Soon after, the American Society of Clinical Oncology (ASCO) released a provisional clinical opinion advising against use of *EGFR* monoclonal antibodies in colorectal cancer patients with *KRAS* mutant tumors ([81]); subsequently, the FDA revised the label of cetuximab and panitumumab in July 2009.

The most significant toxicities associated with cetuximab include diarrhea, hypomagnesemia, hypocalcemia, and an acneiform rash. Traditionally, the risk of an allergic hypersensitivity reaction is reported to be <5%. However, life-threatening anaphylactic hypersensitivity reactions have been reported in up to 30% of patients residing in select geographic locations ([82]). Immunoglobulin E antibodies against cetuximab have been discovered and may allow screening for patients at risk for this reaction.

Development of the skin rash appears to be a clinical predictor of response and survival, but the mechanisms involved in this process are poorly understood ([83]). The Dose-Escalation Study of Cetuximab for Metastatic Colorectal Cancer (EVEREST), which was undertaken to address the association between skin rash and clinical response to cetuximab, stratified patients with no or mild rash to standard-dose or dose-escalated cetuximab. Dose escalation increased the response rate from 13% to 30%. Although these results are intriguing, firm conclusions about the dose–response relationship with cetuximab cannot be drawn from this small phase II trial, and the final results have not been reported. Recent data support that the pharmacokinetics of cetuximab is not compromised with administration every 2 weeks rather than weekly ([82]). Furthermore, a small phase II trial indicated that preemptive dermatological care may improve patient outcome when using *EGFR* inhibitors ([84]).

Cetuximab is currently FDA approved as monotherapy for patients with metastatic colorectal cancer who are intolerant of irinotecan-based regimens or in combination with irinotecan after progression of disease. The findings of the CRYSTAL trial will likely result in an FDA application for approval for cetuximab in the frontline setting.

Panitumumab

Panitumumab is a fully human IgG2 monoclonal antibody directed against the *EGFR*. In a randomized phase III trial, patients with refractory metastatic disease received BSC with or without panitumumab. The response rate and stable disease rate with panitumumab were 10% and 27%, respectively, compared to 0% and 10%, respectively, with BSC alone. An OS difference could not be demonstrated in this trial, likely due to crossover from the BSC group ([85]). Subsequent analysis revealed that only patients with *KRAS* WT tumors benefited from panitumumab ([86]). Although cetuximab and panitumumab have not been compared head to head, they appear to have similar efficacy and toxicity in patients. Infusion reactions are uncommon with panitumumab because it is a fully human monoclonal antibody. It is now FDA approved as a single agent for patients failing irinotecan- and oxaliplatin-based chemotherapy. Two phase III trials have recently been reported of FOLFOX or FOLFIRI with or without panitumumab for both treatment-naïve and previously treated patients, respectively ([87, 88]). Both studies reported superior response and PFS for the combination and will likely also result in an application for approval in combination with chemotherapy in the front- and second-line setting.

Bevacizumab

In studies dating back more than 40 years, Dr. Judah Folkman demonstrated that tumors cannot grow beyond 1 mm without creating new vessels to deliver oxygen and nutrients. He therefore predicted that a drug capable of blocking angiogenesis would be able to arrest the growth of tumors ([89]). Among the several angiogenic factors isolated to date, vascular endothelial growth factor (VEGF) seems to be particularly important, with elevated circulating levels associated with poor prognosis in patients with colorectal cancer ([90, 91]). Bevacizumab is a humanized monoclonal antibody that binds all isoforms of circulating VEGF, thereby inhibiting permeability and angiogenesis mediated by this factor ([92]).

Bevacizumab is currently FDA approved in multiple tumor types, including lung, breast, and colorectal cancer. A randomized phase II trial compared weekly 5-FU/leucovorin with the same chemotherapy combined with either 5 mg/kg or 10 mg/kg of bevacizumab. Both experimental arms performed better than the control 5-FU/leucovorin arm ([93]). However, the best results were seen with the lower dose of bevacizumab, leading the investigators to recommend a dose of 5 mg/kg for a phase III trial in colorectal cancer.

The phase III trial compared the IFL regimen, which was considered the standard regimen for metastatic colorectal cancer at that time, with IFL plus bevacizumab (5 mg/kg) ([94]). A third arm with 5-FU/leucovorin plus bevacizumab was added as a precaution, but it was dropped after the first 100 patients were treated safely. Patients on the exploratory arm were allowed to continue bevacizumab with their second-line chemotherapy regimen following progression of disease. When compared to IFL alone, the addition of bevacizumab resulted in a 10% increase in overall response rate (35%-45%). More important, patients randomized to IFL plus bevacizumab had a median survival of 20.3 months, while patients randomized to IFL alone had a median survival of 15.6 months ($P < .0004$). The absolute improvement in OS was superior to any incremental survival advantage observed using conventional combination chemotherapy alone. As a result, bevacizumab became the first drug of its class to receive FDA approval for colorectal cancer.

These promising results in the frontline setting have been confirmed in other trials. In the phase II TREE-2 study, Hochster and colleagues demonstrated the safety and efficacy of bevacizumab in combination with oxaliplatin-based chemotherapy (mFOLFOX6, bFOL, or XELOX) ([95]). This trial was not powered for direct comparisons among the three arms, but time to progression (9.9 and 10.3 months, respectively) and OS (26.1 and 24.6 months, respectively) were virtually identical in the mFOLFOX6 and XELOX arms. In the NO16966 trial, untreated patients were randomized in a 2 × 2 design to FOLFOX4 or XELOX (noninferiority) with or without bevacizumab ([96]). The pooled analysis revealed superior median PFS (9.4 vs 8.0 months, $P = .002$) in the bevacizumab-containing groups, but a difference in response and OS did not achieve statistical significance. Surprisingly, when PFS was stratified by chemotherapy regimen, the XELOX regimen fared better. In both of these trials, bevacizumab did not increase the toxicities of chemotherapy. However, it may exist when bevacizumab is combined with an oxaliplatin-based regimen, and the use of antiangiogenic therapy in conjunction with oxaliplatin-based chemotherapy is not well understood as originally believed. The most significant adverse events associated with bevacizumab were hypertension, proteinuria, thrombosis, and rare instances of bleeding (mostly epistaxis), delayed wound healing, and gastrointestinal perforation.

The Bolus, Infusional, or Capecitabine With Camptosar-Celecoxib (BICC) trial was a phase III trial that evaluated the role of bevacizumab in combination with irinotecan-based regimens (IFL, FOLFIRI, and CapeIri). During patient enrollment, bevacizumab was subsequently approved, requiring an amendment to the trial design. An expanded cohort of 117 patients randomized to IFL or FOLFIRI plus bevacizumab was created. No statistical difference in PFS or response was noted, but an impressive median OS was reported for the FOLFIRI plus bevacizumab arm (28.0 vs 19.2 months, $P = .037$).

The efficacy of bevacizumab as an adjunct to chemotherapy has been validated in the second-line setting as well. ECOG 3200 randomized over 800 patients with metastatic colorectal cancer previously treated with 5-FU and irinotecan (but not oxaliplatin or bevacizumab) to one of three arms: FOLFOX4, bevacizumab, or the combination. The arm receiving bevacizumab as monotherapy was closed to accrual after an interim analysis revealed inferior outcomes compared to the other two arms. Ultimately, the addition of bevacizumab to chemotherapy resulted in improved PFS (median 7.3 vs 4.7 months, $P < .0001$) and OS (median 12.9 vs 10.8 months, $P = .0011$) ([97]).

A recent large patient registry trial (Bevacizumab Regimens: Investigation of Treatment Effects and Safety [BRiTE]) suggested that continuation of bevacizumab following first-line progression of disease will have a positive impact on patient outcome versus no therapy or continuing second-line chemotherapy without continuing bevacizumab ([98]). These data are intriguing but were not collected in a prospective randomized fashion. Regardless, ongoing clinical trials have adopted this methodology of bevacizumab as the control arm. Admittedly in the patient with *KRAS* MT tumor, consideration of continuing bevacizumab is an option given the limitations of biologic therapy in a *KRAS* MT tumor–type patient, but it should be considered with a note of caution given the lack of evidence-based medicine and potential toxicities associated with bevacizumab.

The role of bevacizumab in the adjuvant setting is questionable at this time. A large phase III trial (NSABP C-08) was completed in patients with both stage II and III ([99]). Patients were randomized to FOLFOX (6 months) versus FOLFOX plus bevacizumab (5 mg/kg × 12 months). After a median follow-up of 35.6 months, the investigators failed to meet their primary end point of DFS (HR = 0.89, *P* = .15). The AVANT trial is a three-arm randomized study of FOLFOX4 (6 months) versus FOLFOX4 plus bevacizumab (5 mg/kg × 12 months) versus XELOX plus bevacizumab (7.5 mg/kg × 12 months) in the adjuvant treatment of patients with stage III or high-risk stage II colon cancer. Preliminary toxicity results have been reported with final efficacy results pending ([100]).

Unlike the *EGFR* inhibitors, predictive markers for the efficacy of initial anti-VEGF therapy have not been identified. Intriguing data from a phase II study of bevacizumab in treatment-naïve patients has noted a possible correlation with levels of basic fibroblast growth factor ([101]).

Bevacizumab represents a significant step for the use of antiangiogenesis agents in the treatment of colorectal cancer. It was FDA approved for use in combination with fluorouracil-based regimens as a first- or second-line treatment for metastatic colorectal cancer. Because bevacizumab has essentially no clinical activity as monotherapy in colorectal cancer, it cannot be recommended as a single agent in colorectal cancer and should not be considered for adjuvant therapy outside a clinical trial.

Dual Antibody Anti–Vascular Endothelial Growth Factor and Anti-Epidermal Growth Factor Receptor Therapy

Based on compelling preclinical data suggesting additive antitumor efficacy, the concept of dual inhibition of VEGF and *EGFR* has been investigated in several clinical studies. The BOND-2 trial randomized 83 irinotecan-refractory, bevacizumab-naïve patients to cetuximab plus bevacizumab with or without irinotecan (CB vs CBI). The CBI arm showed a better response rate (37% vs 20%) and time to progression (7.3 vs 4.9 months). In addition, the concurrent use of monoclonal antibodies did not result in any unexpected safety signals. These encouraging data prompted two large phase III trials (Capecitabine, Irinotecan, Oxaliplatin 2 [CAIRO2], Panitumumab Advanced Colorectal Cancer Evaluation [PACCE]) to examine the efficacy of dual biologic therapy in metastatic colorectal cancer. The CAIRO2 trial randomized 755 untreated patients to XELOX/bevacizumab with or without cetuximab. Unexpectedly, the patients receiving cetuximab experienced shorter PFS (9.4 vs 10.7 months, *P* = .01). Furthermore, in subgroup analyses, cetuximab-treated patients with *KRAS* mutant tumors had significantly inferior PFS (8.1 vs 12.5 months, *P* = .003) and OS (17.2 vs 24.9 months, *P* = .03) compared to patients with *KRAS* mutant tumors who did not receive cetuximab. Even in the subset of *KRAS* WT patients, the addition of cetuximab did not produce a PFS benefit ([102]).

The PACCE trial investigated dual biologic therapy in the first-line setting by randomizing patients receiving oxaliplatin- or irinotecan-based chemotherapy (investigator's discretion) to bevacizumab plus or minus panitumumab ([103]). The panitumumab arms were discontinued after a planned interim analysis of patients in the oxaliplatin cohort revealed inferior PFS (8.8 vs 10.5 months, *P* = .04) with the addition of panitumumab. The final results showed worse OS (19.4 vs 24.5 months) and significant excess toxicity with dual-antibody therapy. The negative clinical impact of panitumumab was seen irrespective of *KRAS* status. In light of the data from PACCE and CAIRO2, dual VEGF and *EGFR* inhibition currently has no role in the treatment of patients with colorectal cancer and should not be pursued outside a clinical trial.

Decision Making for Potential Surgical Resection in Patients With Metastatic Colorectal Cancer

Despite therapeutic advances, the estimated 5-year OS for a patient unable to be surgically resected will remain at 11%. Therefore, when surgical resection with curative intent is a possibility for a patient with metastatic colorectal cancer, it is best to initiate discussion with your colleagues in the other disciplines. It is imperative discussion regarding each individual patient is initiated early if there is a potential for surgical resection with curative intent to optimize patient outcomes. Maximizing diagnostic imaging capabilities has an important role when considering surgical resection, such as MRI, PET/CT, and volumetric imaging. The use, choice, and duration of neoadjuvant chemotherapy should be determined by the treating medical oncologist and surgeon in a multidisciplinary fashion. Prior studies indicated that patients who have a partial response or stable disease to neoadjuvant therapy will fare better than those with progression of disease ([104]). Prior studies have indicated a trend in DFS and OS for adjuvant single-agent 5-FU–based chemotherapy versus observation following hepatic resection ([105]). Hence, clinical trials are under way to modify the neoadjuvant and adjuvant approach for candidates of hepatic resection. Challenges remain in the setting of a patient with a primary rectal cancer and the timing and role of radiotherapy.

In general, it is recommended that patients have

KRAS testing completed early on in preparation for both immediate and subsequent chemotherapy treatment planning. When considering hepatic resection, it is crucial that patients are not treated until the point of radiographic CR. It is well known that a radiographic CR harbors microscopic disease that is only appreciated on the tissue specimen once surgically resected ([106]). Furthermore, if patients are not surgically resected following path CR or near-path CR, progression of disease will develop. In addition, prolonged chemotherapy may have a negative impact on surgical mortality ([107]).

Follow-Up for Patients With Resected Metastatic Colorectal Cancer

Following metastasectomy, patients are followed closely with physician visits, CEA level analysis, and diagnostic imaging. Patients undergo clinical evaluations every 3 to 4 months for the first 3 years, every 6 months for the following 2 years, and annually thereafter. Colonoscopy will continue to be completed every 3 years thereafter (some patients require more frequent examinations based on endoscopic findings or high-risk status). Computed tomography of chest, abdomen, and pelvis (or MRI) is the standard recommended cross-sectional imaging modality. Use of PET/CT is completed only if inconclusive findings are noted on CT/MRI or if a rising CEA is noted without measurable disease on CT/MRI. All patients are encouraged to maintain a relationship with a primary care physician for optimal surveillance and health care.

The MDACC Approach to Patients With Metastatic Disease

It is difficult to articulate a general treatment algorithm for patients with metastatic disease, but individual consideration of each patient's case is always taken into account. For the majority of patients with metastatic colorectal cancer, surgical resection of metastatic disease will not be technically possible or clinically appropriate. Whenever possible, patients with good performance status and no significant problems related to local tumor are offered therapy as part of a clinical trial.

Once patients fail frontline therapy, a period of observation may ensue, or second-line therapy may be instituted. Previous analyses have suggested a survival advantage for patients treated with all three active conventional cytotoxic agents (5-FU, irinotecan, and oxaliplatin) during the course of their treatment ([108]), but the precise order of targeted agents in the therapeutic sequence has yet to be fully elucidated. However, *KRAS* tumor mutation status has become a core part of treatment decision making.

Broad principles have emerged as the foundation for therapeutic decisions at MDACC:

1. *Asymptomatic patients with metastatic disease are usually offered systemic chemotherapy treatment.* Systemic chemotherapy has served an integral role in our care of patients with metastatic disease with regard to quality of life, palliation of pain, and improvement in OS. A multidisciplinary approach is always considered when the primary malignancy remains in place. Evaluation of lumen patency is completed before initiating systemic chemotherapy. With the advent of newer agents such as irinotecan, oxaliplatin, and the monoclonal antibodies, OS of patients with metastatic disease has been steadily improving over the last several years. Moreover, frontline therapy is better tolerated and more likely to be beneficial in asymptomatic patients with good performance status. An exception to this principle applies to those patients with known metastatic disease that is either not evaluable or extremely low volume. In these cases, close follow-up with frequent cross-sectional imaging may be an appropriate initial strategy. Therapy is then initiated once measurable disease is evident or, in the oncologist's judgment, further expectant follow-up is likely to lead to symptoms. Patients with a rising serum CEA level are usually not recommended to undergo treatment in the absence of clear clinical or radiographic evidence of metastatic disease and are followed closely. When deciding between an oxaliplatin- or irinotecan-containing regimen, the choice of chemotherapy is largely based on the objectives of treatment: surgical intent, borderline resectable, and unresectable for palliation. FOLFIRI and FOLFOX are comparable in terms of efficacy, but toxicities are distinctly different. When considering systemic chemotherapy for an unresectable patient, FOLFIRI is commonly selected at our institution given its lack of dose-limiting toxicities.
2. *The initial treatment for metastatic disease may depend on the timing and residual toxicities of prior adjuvant therapy.* Many patients who develop metastatic disease have received prior adjuvant therapy consisting of oxaliplatin, 5-FU, and leucovorin. When patients relapse, they should be considered refractory to this combination if fewer than 12 months have elapsed since the completion of adjuvant therapy. Irinotecan often becomes the primary cytotoxic agent in the treatment of relapsed disease after recent adjuvant therapy.
3. *Patients should be treated to maximal benefit or until therapy becomes intolerable.* When patients are receiving systemic therapy for metastatic disease, we usually continue treatment until the tumor becomes refractory to the regimen, toxicity dictates discontinuation, or patient deferment of therapy. Patients receiving oxaliplatin in conjunction with capecitabine

or 5-FU, as part of a FOLFOX or XELOX regimen, may develop unacceptable peripheral neuropathy. A study performed in France suggested that there is no disadvantage to discontinuation of oxaliplatin, provided maintenance therapy with 5-FU and leucovorin continues. Oxaliplatin may be reintroduced as a component of the regimen once neuropathic symptoms subside or the tumor starts to progress ([109]).

This concept was analyzed in a prospective trial, Optimized 5-FU and Oxaliplatin Study (OPTIMOX1). It demonstrated that switching to a nonoxaliplatin maintenance regimen (5-FU/ leucovorin) after 6 cycles of FOLFOX, with reintroduction of oxaliplatin after 12 cycles of maintenance therapy or at disease progression, did not worsen clinical outcomes when compared to continuous FOLFOX until disease progression. In fact, patients on the maintenance arm experienced less grade 3 and 4 toxicities after the initial six cycles of treatment ([110]). A subsequent trial (OPTIMOX2) randomized patients to maintenance therapy (as in OPTIMOX1) or a chemotherapy holiday after six cycles of FOLFOX, with similar rules for oxaliplatin reintroduction. The maintenance arm showed superior median PFS (8.6 vs 6.6 months, $P = .0017$) and duration of disease control (13.1 vs 9.2 months, $P = .046$), with a trend toward improved overall ([111]). In clinical practice, however, the benefit of maintenance therapy must be weighed against potential toxicity, and patient preference must be considered as well. Therefore, a chemotherapy treatment holiday may be appropriate for patients after prolonged response or stability of disease.

4. *Once frontline therapy has been exhausted, a period of observation may be advantageous.* With newer drugs and combinations creating significant inroads as debulking agents, metastatic colorectal cancer can be viewed as a chronic illness for some patients, rather than a suddenly life-threatening disease. Therefore, immediate initiation of second- or third-line therapy after failing frontline treatment is not always necessary, and punctuating regimens with periods of observation has at least two advantages. First, it provides patients with a chemotherapy holiday, which may improve overall quality of life; second, it allows for more robust physiologic and hematopoietic recovery after prior treatment. Therefore, once a decision is made to restart cytotoxic therapy, timely delivery of full-dose therapy is more likely to proceed without interruption. As described previously, when we follow patients expectantly, restaging studies are performed every 8 to 12 weeks unless the clinical situation requires restaging sooner.
5. *The need for local control should always be considered.* Some patients with metastatic disease may also have intact primary tumors or locally recurrent disease. Recent experience with combination therapies suggested that the primary tumor may respond well to systemic therapy in some cases, obviating the need for local therapies. As a general rule, however, locally recurrent tumor at a site of previous surgery or radiotherapy is not particularly responsive to systemic therapy. Therefore, oncologists must continuously reassess whether local tumor control should take priority over treatment for disseminated disease. Such decisions are usually made with input from a multidisciplinary team, which may include radiotherapists, surgical oncologists, and gastroenterologists.

Challenging Clinical Management Problems

The Malignant Polyp

On occasion, an endoscopically removed polyp may demonstrate invasive adenocarcinoma within a villous or tubular adenoma. Treatment recommendations in this situation should be individualized based on features, including negative margins, no evidence of invasion beyond the submucosa, well- or moderately differentiated adenocarcinoma, and no evidence of lymphatic or vascular invasion. In this setting, the risk of lymph node metastases is low (5%), and follow-up with periodic colonoscopic examinations is reasonable ([4]). Unfortunately, retrieval of a sessile or bulky polyp distorts the depth of invasion or margin status. Furthermore, if pathology demonstrates poor differentiation, invasion into the muscularis, or lymphovascular invasion, surgical resection is advised. In particular, T2 tumors have a 20% likelihood of lymph node metastases, so continued endoscopic follow-up without further surgical intervention is not appropriate.

A malignant polyp in the distal or midrectum is often not amenable to further local staging because endoscopic rectal polypectomy leads to unreliable EUS imaging. Definitive surgical resection should be considered for a resected rectal polyp without clear margins or with adverse pathologic features. If margins are equivocal without muscle invasion, transanal excision may be feasible. Even when laparotomy is considered, a sphincter-preserving procedure is usually possible. Occasionally, an adequately informed patient will refuse surgery, or medical comorbidities preclude surgery as an option. In these special circumstances, nonstandard combined-modality chemoradiation is an alternative to definitive resection.

Nonsurgical Options for Partially Obstructing Tumors

The clinical diagnosis of bowel obstruction usually is based on an endoscopy or CT that may show obstructing mass(es). However, clinically significant bowel obstruction may not be present without proximal colonic dilation or evidence of perforation.

Bowel resection or diverting ostomy may be appropriate, but in patients with poor performance status, nonsurgical management should be considered, which includes expandable metal stents, especially in the rectosigmoid region. Obstructing sites higher in the colon can pose technical barriers to stent insertion. An endoscopically placed colonic decompression tube *proximal* to the obstruction may provide temporary relief. Endoscopic electrosurgical procedures, including argon plasma coagulation may recanalize the lumen. External-beam radiotherapy may then prevent complete obstruction while alleviating partial obstruction. Radiotherapy in rectal primaries may also relieve sacral plexus pain syndromes. Patients with impending bowel obstruction are hospitalized for bowel rest, nasogastric tube decompression, and intravenous hydration, followed by multidisciplinary evaluation by a gastroenterologist, surgical oncologist, medical oncologist, and radiotherapist. While stent insertion, photocoagulation of intraluminal disease, or radiotherapy may all rapidly reverse impending bowel obstruction, the use of systemic therapy in a patient with tenuous bowel patency should be discouraged.

Multidisciplinary Management of Poor Bowel Function After Curative Treatment

Segmental bowel resections particularly for rectal cancer lead to permanent alterations in the frequency and character of bowel movements. Loss of the rectal vault and subsequent radiotherapy lead to compromised stool storage and stricture formation at the anastomotic site, while sphincter function may not return to baseline, leading to functional and mechanical dysfunction manifesting as small, frequent bowel movements, with episodic fecal incontinence.

In general, patients are advised that bowel habits may improve for up to 1 year from the time of surgery or up to 6 months after completion of all adjuvant therapy. For patients with more chronic and severe problems (innumerable small bowel movements or fecal incontinence), a multidisciplinary team of surgeons, gastroenterologists, and enterostomal nursing staff recommends a personalized detailed bowel regimen that, with adequate adherence, can improve quality of life and satisfaction with sphincter preservation. On rare occasions, when a sphincter-preserving procedure leads to unbearable dissatisfaction with bowel function, a colostomy or ileostomy may be recommended to improve functional status and quality of life.

Carcinoma With Neuroendocrine Features

Histologically, a colorectal carcinoma may demonstrate neuroendocrine differentiation, which should be readily distinguished from small cell carcinomas or high-grade neuroendocrine tumors by additional stains for chromogranin and synaptophysin. Metastatic gastrointestinal neuroendocrine carcinomas have been treated with irinotecan/cisplatin or irinotecan/oxaliplatin at MDACC, with observed partial responses, but durable responses remain uncommon. Individuals with adenocarcinoma with focal neuroendocrine features are offered standard colorectal cancer chemotherapy.

SUMMARY

Advances in pathogenesis and management of colorectal cancer contribute to continued reduction in mortality as biologic agents are under investigation in the advanced disease setting (Table 24-7). Many of these trials include correlatives to identify predictors of clinical benefit to ultimately aid in patient selection.

Table 24-7 Targeted Therapies in Development for Advanced Colorectal Cancer

Mechanism of Action	Example of Agents	Phase of Study[a]
PI3K/Akt/mTOR inhibition	Perifosine, RAD001, MK-2206, GSK690693	Phase III
FGFR inhibition	Brivanib, AZD-4547	Phase III
cMET/HGF inhibition	ARQ-197, AMG-102	Randomized phase II
Apo2L/TRAIL inhibition	AMG-655, CS-1008	Randomized phase II
MEK/BRAF inhibition	AS703026, selumetinib, PLX-4032, XL281	Randomized phase II
IGFR inhibition	MK-0646, AMG-479	Randomized phase II
PARP inhibition	Olaparib, ABT-888	Phase II
Demethylating agent	Decitabine, azacitadine	Phase II
Histone deacetylase	Vorinostat, entinostat	Phase II
Notch/_γ secretase inhibition	RO4929097	Phase II
PPAR-γ inhibition	CS7017	Phase II
PDGFR inhibition	Imatinib	Phase II
Src inhibition	Dasatinib	Phase II
Integrin inhibition	EMD 525797	Phase II

[a]For most advanced agent in development.

CHAPTER 24

Hence, patient enrollment in clinical trials is highly encouraged.

REFERENCES

1. Siegel R, Ma J, Zou Z, Jemal A. Cancer statistics, 2014. *CA Cancer J Clin.* 2014;64(64):9-29.
2. Fuchs CS, Giovannucci EL, Colditz GA, et al. Dietary fiber and the risk of colorectal cancer and adenoma in women. *N Engl J Med.* 1999;340(340):169-176.
3. Moore LL, Bradlee ML, Singer MR, et al. BMI and waist circumference as predictors of lifetime colon cancer risk in Framingham Study adults. *Int J Obes.* 2004;28(28):559-567.
4. Skibber J, Minsky B, Hoff P. Cancer of the colon and rectum. In: DeVita VT Jr, Hellmann S, Rosenberg SA, eds. *Cancer: Principles and Practice of Oncology*. 6th ed. Philadelphia, PA: Lippincott Willams & Wilkins; 2001:1216-1271.
5. Itzkowitz S. Colon carcinogenesis in inflammatory bowel disease: applying molecular genetics to clinical practice. *J Clin Gastroenterol.* 2003;36(suppl 5):S70-S74.
6. Towler B, Irwig L, Glasziou P, Kewenter J, Weller D, Silagy C. A systematic review of the effects of screening for colorectal cancer using the faecal occult blood test, hemoccult. *BMJ.* 1998;317(317):559-565.
7. Calonge N, Petitti DB, DeWitt TG, et al. Screening for colorectal cancer: US Preventive Services Task Force recommendation statement. *Ann Intern Med.* 2008;149(149):627-637.
8. Lieberman DA, Weiss DG, Bond JH, Ahnen DJ, Garewal H, Chejfec G. Use of colonoscopy to screen asymptomatic adults for colorectal cancer. Veterans Affairs Cooperative Study Group 380. *N Engl J Med.* 2000;343(343):162-168.
9. Imperiali G, Minoli G. Colonic neoplasm in asymptomatic patients with family history of colon cancer: results of a colonoscopic prospective and controlled study. Results of a pilot study of endoscopic screening of first degree relatives of colorectal cancer patients in Italy. *Gastrointest Endosc.* 1999;49(49):132-133.
10. Kaminski MF, Bretthauer M, Zauber AG, et al. The NordICC Study: rationale and design of a randomized trial on colonoscopy screening for colorectal cancer. *Endoscopy.* 2012;44(44):695-702.
11. Lindor NM. Hereditary colorectal cancer: MYH-associated polyposis and other newly identified disorders. *Best Pract Res Clin Gastroenterol.* 2009;23(23):75-87.
12. Vasen HF, Watson P, Mecklin JP, Lynch HT. New clinical criteria for hereditary nonpolyposis colorectal cancer (HNPCC, Lynch syndrome) proposed by the International Collaborative group on HNPCC. *Gastroenterology.* 1999;116(116):1453-1456.
13. Poeggel G, Bernstein HG, Rechardt L, Brandt H, Luppa H. Second messenger enzymes in glial cells: a cytochemical point of view. *Acta Histochem.* 1991;91(91):147-155.
14. Xicola RM, Llor X, Pons E, et al. Performance of different microsatellite marker panels for detection of mismatch repair-deficient colorectal tumors. *J Natl Cancer Inst.* 2007;99(99):244-252.
15. Giardiello FM, Hamilton SR, Krush AJ, et al. Treatment of colonic and rectal adenomas with sulindac in familial adenomatous polyposis. *N Engl J Med.* 1993;328(328):1313-1316.
16. Steinbach G, Lynch PM, Phillips RK, et al. The effect of celecoxib, a cyclooxygenase-2 inhibitor, in familial adenomatous polyposis. *N Engl J Med.* 2000;342(342):1946-1952.
17. Solomon SD, McMurray JJ, Pfeffer MA, et al. Cardiovascular risk associated with celecoxib in a clinical trial for colorectal adenoma prevention. *N Engl J Med.* 2005;352(352):1071-1080.
18. Giovannucci E, Egan KM, Hunter DJ, et al. Aspirin and the risk of colorectal cancer in women. *N Engl J Med.* 1995;333(333):609-614.
19. Giovannucci E, Rimm EB, Stampfer MJ, Colditz GA, Ascherio A, Willett WC. Aspirin use and the risk for colorectal cancer and adenoma in male health professionals. *Ann Intern Med.* 1994;121(121):241-246.
20. Sandler RS, Halabi S, Baron JA, et al. A randomized trial of aspirin to prevent colorectal adenomas in patients with previous colorectal cancer. *N Engl J Med.* 2003;348(348):883-890.
21. Baron JA, Cole BF, Sandler RS, et al. A randomized trial of aspirin to prevent colorectal adenomas. *N Engl J Med.* 2003;348(348):891-899.
22. Benson III AB, Schrag D, R. SM, et al. American Society of Clinical Oncology recommendations on adjuvant chemotherapy for stage II colon cancer. *J Clin Oncol.* 2004;22(22):3408-3419.
23. National Comprehensive Cancer Network. Colon Cancer. *Clinical Practice Guidelines in Oncology (NCCN Guidelines).* 2015. http://www.nccn.org/professionals/physician_gls/pdf/colon.pdf. Accessed May 1, 2015.
24. Fleshman J, Sargent DJ, Green E, et al. Laparoscopic colectomy for cancer is not inferior to open surgery based on 5-year data from the COST Study Group trial. *Ann Surg.* 2007;246(246):655-664.
25. Andre T, Boni C, Mounediji-Boudiaf L, et al. Oxaliplatin, fluorouracil, and leucovorin as adjuvant treatment for colon cancer. *N Engl J Med.* 2004;350(350):2342-2341.
26. Group QC, Gray R, Barnwell J, et al. Adjuvant chemotherapy versus observation in patients with colorectal cancer: a randomised study. *Lancet.* 2007;370(370):2020-2029.
27. Tournigand C, André T, Bonnetain F, et al. Adjuvant therapy with fluorouracil and oxaliplatin in stage II and elderly patients (between ages 70 and 75 years) with colon cancer: subgroup analyses of the Multicenter International Study of Oxaliplatin, Fluorouracil, and Leucovorin in the Adjuvant Treatment of Colon Cancer trial. *J Clin Oncol.* 2012;30(30):3353-3360.
28. Gray RG, Quirke P, Handley K, et al. Validation study of a quantitative multigene reverse transcriptase-polymerase chain reaction assay for assessment of recurrence risk in patients with stage II colon cancer. *J Clin Oncol.* 2011;29(29):4611-4619.
29. Salazar R, Roepman P, Capella G, et al. Gene expression signature to improve prognosis prediction of stage II and III colorectal cancer. *J Clin Oncol.* 2011;29(29):17-24.
30. Salazar R, Rosenberg R, Lutke Holzik M, et al. The PARSC trial, a prospective study for the assessment of recurrence risk in stage II colon cancer (CC) patients using ColoPrint. *J Clin Oncol.* 2011;29(suppl; abstr TPS167).
31. Saltz LB, Niedzwiecki D, Hollis D, et al. Irinotecan fluorouracil plus leucovorin is not superior to fluorouracil plus leucovorin alone as adjuvant treatment for stage III colon cancer: results of CALGB 89803. *J Clin Oncol.* 2007;25(25):3456-3461.
32. Van Cutsem E, Labianca R, Bodoky G, et al. Randomized phase III trial comparing biweekly infusional fluorouracil/leucovorin alone or with irinotecan in the adjuvant treatment of stage III colon cancer: PETACC-3. *J Clin Oncol.* 2009;27(27):3117-3125.
33. Ychou M, Raoul JL, Doulliard JY, et al. A phase III randomised trial of LV5FU2 + irinotecan versus LV5FU2 alone in adjuvant high-risk colon cancer (FNCLCC Accord02/FFCD9802). *Ann Oncol.* 2009;20(20):674-680.
34. Klingbiel D, Saridaki Z, Roth AD, Bosman FT, Delorenzi M, Teipar S. Prognosis of stage II and III colon cancer treated with adjuvant 5-fluorouracil or FOLFIRI in relation to microsatellite status: results of the PETACC-3 trial. *Ann Oncol.* 2015;26(26):126-132.
35. Allegra CJ, Yothers G, O'Connell MJ, et al. Bevacizumab in stage II-III colon cancer: 5-year update of the National Surgical Adjuvant Breast and Bowel Project C-08 trial. *J Clin Oncol.* 2013;31(31):359-364.
36. de Gramont A, Van Cutsem E, Schmoll HJ, et al. Bevacizumab

plus oxaliplatin-based chemotherapy as adjuvant treatment for colon cancer (AVANT): a phase 3 randomised controlled trial. *Lancet Oncol.* 2012;13(13):1225-1233.

37. André T, Iveson T, Labianca R, et al. The IDEA (International Duration Evaluation of Adjuvant Chemotherapy) Collaboration: prospective combined analysis of phase III trials investigating duration of adjuvant therapy with the FOLFOX (FOLFOX4 or Modified FOLFOX6) or XELOX (3 versus 6 months) regimen for patients with stage III colon cancer: trial design and current status. *Curr Colorectal Cancer Rep.* 2013;9:261-269.
38. Renfro LA, Shah MA, Allegra CJ, et al. Time-dependent patterns of recurrence and death in resected colon cancer (CC): pooled analysis of 12,223 patients from modern trials in the ACCENT database containing oxaliplatin. *J Clin Oncol.* 2015;33(suppl; abstr 3593).
39. Smalley SR, Benedetti J, Williamson SK, et al. Phase III trial of fluorouracil-based chemotherapy regimens plus radiotherapy in postoperative adjuvant rectal cancer: GI INT 0144. *J Clin Oncol.* 2006;24(24):3542-3547.
40. Sauer R, Becker H, Hohenberger W, et al. Preoperative versus postoperative chemoradiotherapy for rectal cancer. *N Engl J Med.* 2004;351(351):1731-1740.
41. O'Connell MJ, Colangelo LH, Beart RW, et al. Capecitabine and oxaliplatin in the preoperative multimodality treatment of rectal cancer: surgical end points from National Surgical Adjuvant Breast and Bowel Project trial R-04. *J Clin Oncol.* 2014;32(32):1927-1934.
42. Gerard J, Azria D, Gourgou-Bourgade S, et al. Randomized multicenter phase III trial comparing two neoadjuvant chemoradiotherapy (CT-RT) regimens (RT45-Cap versus RT50-Capox) in patients (pts) with locally advanced rectal cancer (LARC): Results of the ACCORD 12/0405 PRODIGE 2. *J Clin Oncol.* 2009;27(18).
43. Aschele C, Pinto C, Cordio S, et al. Preoperative FU-based chemoradiation with or without weekly oxaliplatin in locally advanced rectal cancer: preliminary safety findings of the STAR (Studio Terapia Adiuvante Retto)-01 randomized trial. *J Clin Oncol.* 2007;25(18S, suppl):4040.
44. Chua YJ, Barbachano Y, Cunningham D, et al. Neoadjuvant capecitabine and oxaliplatin before chemoradiotherapy and total mesorectal excision in MRI-defined poor-risk rectal cancer: a phase 2 trial. *Lancet Oncol.* 2010;11(11):241-248.
45. Fernández-Martos C, Pericay C, Aparicio J, et al. Phase II, randomized study of concomitant chemoradiotherapy followed by surgery and adjuvant capecitabine plus oxaliplatin (CAPOX) compared with induction CAPOX followed by concomitant chemoradiotherapy and surgery in magnetic resonance imaging-defined, locally advanced rectal cancer: Grupo cancer de recto 3 study. *J Clin Oncol.* 2010;28(28):859-865.
46. Borg C, André T, Mantion G, et al. Pathological response and safety of two neoadjuvant strategies with bevacizumab in MRI-defined locally advanced T3 resectable rectal cancer: a randomized, noncomparative phase II study. *Ann Oncol.* 2014;25(25):2205-2210.
47. Dewdney A, Cunningham D, Tabernero J, et al. Multicenter randomized phase II clinical trial comparing neoadjuvant oxaliplatin, capecitabine, and preoperative radiotherapy with or without cetuximab followed by total mesorectal excision in patients with high-risk rectal cancer (EXPERT-C). *J Clin Oncol.* 2012;30(30):1620-1627.
48. Smith NJ, Barbachano Y, Norman AR, Swift RI, Abulafi AM, Brown G. Prognostic significance of magnetic resonance imaging-detected extramural vascular invasion in rectal cancer. *Br J Surg.* 2008;95(95):229-236.
49. Prolongation of the disease-free interval in surgically treated rectal carcinoma. Gastrointestinal Tumor Study Group. *N Engl J Med.* 1985;312(312):1465-1472.
50. Tepper JE, O'Connell MJ, Niedzwiecki D, et al. Impact of number of nodes retrieved on outcome in patients with rectal cancer. *J Clin Oncol.* 2001;19(19):157-163.
51. Kapiteijn E, Marijnen CA, Nagtegaal ID, et al. Preoperative radiotherapy combined with total mesorectal excision for resectable rectal cancer. *N Engl J Med.* 2001;345(345):638-646.
52. August DA, Ottow RT, Sugarbaker PH. Clinical perspective of human colorectal cancer metastasis. *Cancer Metastasis Rev.* 1984;3(3):303-324.
53. Eng C, Kindler HL, Schilsky RL. Oral fluoropyrimidine treatment of colorectal cancer. *Clin Colorectal Cancer.* 2001;1(1):95-103.
54. Hoff PM, Ansari R, Batist G, et al. Comparison of oral capecitabine versus intravenous fluorouracil plus leucovorin as first-line treatment in 605 patients with metastatic colorectal cancer: results of a randomized phase III study. *J Clin Oncol.* 2001;18(18):2282-2292.
55. Van Cutsem E, Twelves C, Cassidy J, et al. Oral capecitabine compared with intravenous fluorouracil plus leucovorin in patients with metastatic colorectal cancer: results of a large phase III study. *J Clin Oncol.* 2001;19(19):4097-4106.
56. Van Cutsem E, Cunningham D, Ten Bokkel Huinink WW, et al. Clinical activity and benefit of irinotecan (CPT-11) in patients with colorectal cancer truly resistant to 5-fluorouracil (5-FU). *Eur J Cancer.* 1999;35(35):54-59.
57. Rothenberg ML, Cox JV, Devore RF, et al. A multicenter, phase II trial of weekly irinotecan (CPT-11) in patients with previously treated colorectal carcinoma. *Cancer.* 2000;85(85):786-795.
58. Rothenberg ML, Eckardt JR, Kuhn JG, et al. Phase II trial of irinotecan in patients with progressive or rapidly recurrent colorectal cancer. *J Clin Oncol.* 1996;14(14):1128-1135.
59. Rougier P, Bugat R, Doulliard JY, et al. Phase II study of irinotecan in the treatment of advanced colorectal cancer in chemotherapy-naive patients and patients pretreated with fluorouracil-based chemotherapy. *J Clin Oncol.* 1997;15(15):251-260.
60. Cunningham D, Pyrhonen S, James RD, et al. Randomised trial of irinotecan plus supportive care versus supportive care alone after fluorouracil failure for patients with metastatic colorectal cancer. *Lancet.* 1998;352(352):1413-1418.
61. Saltz LB, Cox JV, Blanke C, et al. Irinotecan plus fluorouracil and leucovorin for metastatic colorectal cancer. Irinotecan Study Group. *N Engl J Med.* 2000;343(343):905-914.
62. Douillard JY, Cunningham D, Roth AD, et al. Irinotecan combined with fluorouracil compared with fluorouracil alone as first-line treatment for metastatic colorectal cancer: a multicentre randomised trial. *Lancet.* 2000;355(355):1041-1047.
63. Rothenberg ML, Oza AM, Bigelow RH, et al. Superiority of oxaliplatin and fluorouracil-leucovorin compared with either therapy alone in patients with progressive colorectal cancer after irinotecan and fluorouracil-leucovorin: interim results of a phase III trial. *J Clin Oncol.* 2003;21(21):2059-2069.
64. de Gramont A, Figer A, Seymour M, et al. Leucovorin and fluorouracil with or without oxaliplatin as first-line treatment in advanced colorectal cancer. *J Clin Oncol.* 2000;18(18):2938-2947.
65. Goldberg RM, Sargent D, Morton RF, et al. A randomized controlled trial of fluorouracil plus leucovorin, irinotecan, and oxaliplatin combinations in patients with previously untreated metastatic colorectal cancer. *J Clin Oncol.* 2004;22(22):23-30.
66. Tournigand C, Andre T, Achille E, et al. FOLFIRI followed by FOLFOX6 or the reverse sequence in advanced colorectal cancer: a randomized GERCOR study. *J Clin Oncol.* 2004;22(22):229-237.
67. Falcone A, Ricci S, Brunetti I, et al. Phase III trial of infusional fluorouracil, leucovorin, oxaliplatin, and irinotecan (FOLFOXIRI) compared with infusional fluorouracil, leucovorin, and irinotecan (FOLFIRI) as first-line treatment for metastatic colorectal cancer: the Gruppo Oncologico Nord Ovest. *J Clin*

Oncol. 2007;25(25):1670-1676.
68. Souglakos J, Androulakis N, Syrigos K, et al. FOLFOXIRI (folinic acid, 5-fluorouracil, oxaliplatin and irinotecan) vs FOLFIRI (folinic acid, 5-fluorouracil and irinotecan) as first-line treatment in metastatic colorectal cancer (MCC): a multicentre randomised phase III trial from the Hellenic Oncology Research Group (HORG). *Br J Cancer.* 2006;94(94):798-805.
69. Kohler G, Milstein C. Continuous cultures of fused cells secreting antibody of predefined specificity. *Nature.* 1975;256(256):495-497.
70. Baselga J. The EGFR as a target for anticancer therapy—focus on cetuximab. *Eur J Cancer.* 2001;37(37):16-22.
71. Saltz LB, Meropol NJ, Loehrer PJ Jr, Needle MN, Kopit J, Mayer RJ. Phase II trial of cetuximab in patients with refractory colorectal cancer that expresses the epidermal growth factor receptor. *J Clin Oncol.* 2004;22(22):1201-1208.
72. Sobrero AF, Maurel J, Fehrenbacher L, et al. EPIC: phase III trial of cetuximab plus irinotecan after fluoropyrimidine and oxaliplatin failure in patients with metastatic colorectal cancer. *J Clin Oncol.* 2008;26(26):2311-2319.
73. Cunningham D, Humblet Y, Siena S, et al. Cetuximab monotherapy and cetuximab plus irinotecan in irinotecan-refractory metastatic colorectal cancer. *N Engl J Med.* 2004;351(351):337-345.
74. Jonker DJ, O'Callaghan CJ, Karapetis CS, et al. Cetuximab for the treatment of colorectal cancer. *N Engl J Med.* 2007;357(357):2040-2048.
75. Chung KY, Shia J, Kemeny NE, et al. Cetuximab shows activity in colorectal cancer patients with tumors that do not express the epidermal growth factor receptor by immunohistochemistry. *J Clin Oncol.* 2005;23(23):1803-1810.
76. Santini D, Loupakis F, Vincenzi B, et al. High concordance of KRAS status between primary colorectal tumors and related metastatic sites: implications for clinical practice. *Oncologist.* 2008;13(13):1270-1275.
77. Peeters M, Oliner KS, Parker A, et al. Use of massively parallel, next-generation sequencing to identify gene mutations beyond KRAS that predict response to panitumumab in a randomized, phase 3, monotherapy study of metastatic colorectal cancer (mCRC). In: Proceedings of the 101st Annual Meeting of the American Association for Cancer Research; April 17-21, 2010; Washington, DC. Abstract LB-174.
78. Van Cutsem E, Kohne CH, Hitre E, et al. Cetuximab and chemotherapy as initial treatment for metastatic colorectal cancer. *N Engl J Med.* 2009;360(360):1408-1417.
79. Van Cutsem E, Lang G, Folprecht M, et al. Cetuximab plus FOLFIRI in the treatment of metastatic colorectal cancer (mCRC): the influence of KRAS and BRAF biomarkers on outcome: updated data from the CRYSTAL trial. In: 2010 Gastrointestinal Cancers Symposium; January 22-24, 2010; Orlando, FL. Abstract 281.
80. Bokemeyer C, Bondarenko I, Makhson A, et al. Fluorouracil, leucovorin, and oxaliplatin with and without cetuximab in the first-line treatment of metastatic colorectal cancer. *J Clin Oncol.* 2009;27(27):663-671.
81. Allegra CJ, Jessup JM, Somerfield MR, et al. American Society of Clinical Oncology provisional clinical opinion: testing for KRAS gene mutations in patients with metastatic colorectal carcinoma to predict response to anti-epidermal growth factor receptor monoclonal antibody therapy. *J Clin Oncol.* 2009;27(27):2091-2096.
82. Chung CH, Mirakhur B, Chan E, et al. Cetuximab-induced anaphylaxis and IgE specific for galactose-alpha-1,3-galactose. *N Engl J Med.* 2008;358(358):1109-1117.
83. Susman E. Rash correlates with tumour response after cetuximab. *Lancet Oncol.* 2004;5(11):647.
84. Lacouture ME, Mitchell EP, Piperdi B, et al. Skin toxicity evaluation protocol with panitumumab (STEPP), a phase II, open-label, randomized trial evaluating the impact of a pre-emptive skin treatment regimen on skin toxicities and quality of life in patients with metastatic colorectal cancer. *J Clin Oncol.* 2010;28(28):1351-1357.
85. Van Cutsem E, Peeters M, Siena S, et al. Open-label phase III trial of panitumumab plus best supportive care compared with best supportive care alone in patients with chemotherapy-refractory metastatic colorectal cancer. *J Clin Oncol.* 2007;25(25):1658-1664.
86. Amado RG, Wolf M, Peeters M, et al. Wild-type KRAS is required for panitumumab efficacy in patients with metastatic colorectal cancer. *J Clin Oncol.* 2008;26(26):1626-1634.
87. Peeters M, Price TJ, Hotko YS, et al. Randomized phase III study of panitumumab (pmab) with FOLFIRI versus FOLFIRI alone as second-line treatment (tx) in patients (pts) with metastatic colorectal cancer (mCRC): Patient-reported outcomes (PRO). In: 2010 Gastrointestinal Cancers Symposium; January 22-24, 2010; Orlando, FL. Abstract 282.
88. Douillard JY, Siena S, Cassidy J, et al. Randomized phase 3 study of panitumumab with FOLFOX4 compared to FOLFOX4 alone as 1st-line treatment (tx) for metastatic colorectal cancer (mCRC): The PRIME trial. *Gastrointest Cancer Res.* 2010(suppl 1):S32-S33.
89. Folkman J. Tumor angiogenesis: a possible control point in tumor growth. *Ann Intern Med.* 1975;82(82):96-100.
90. Werther K, Christensen IJ, Brünner N, Nielsen HJ. Soluble vascular endothelial growth factor levels in patients with primary colorectal carcinoma. The Danish RANX05 Colorectal Cancer Study Group. *Eur J Surg Oncol.* 2000;26(26):657-662.
91. De Vita F, Orditura M, Lieto E, et al. Elevated perioperative serum vascular endothelial growth factor levels in patients with colon carcinoma. *Cancer.* 2004;100(100):270-278.
92. Salgaller ML. Technology evaluation: bevacizumab, Genentech/Roche. *Curr Opin Mol Ther.* 2003;5(5):657-667.
93. Kabbinavar F, Hurwitz HI, Fehrenbacher L, et al. Phase II, randomized trial comparing bevacizumab plus fluorouracil (FU)/leucovorin (LV) with FU/LV alone in patients with metastatic colorectal cancer. *J Clin Oncol.* 2003;21(21):60-65.
94. Hurwitz H, Fehrenbacher L, Novotny W, et al. Bevacizumab plus irinotecan, fluorouracil, and leucovorin for metastatic colorectal cancer. *N Engl J Med.* 2004;350(350):2335-2342.
95. Hochster HS, Hart LL, Ramanathan RK, et al. Safety and efficacy of oxaliplatin and fluoropyrimidine regimens with or without bevacizumab as first-line treatment of metastatic colorectal cancer: results of the TREE study. *J Clin Oncol.* 2008;26(26):3523-3529.
96. Saltz LB, Clarke S, Díaz-Rubio E, et al. Bevacizumab in combination with oxaliplatin-based chemotherapy as first-line therapy in metastatic colorectal cancer: a randomized phase III study. *J Clin Oncol.* 2008;26(26):2013-2019.
97. Giantonio BJ, Catalano PJ, Meropol NJ, et al. Bevacizumab in combination with oxaliplatin, fluorouracil, and leucovorin (FOLFOX4) for previously treated metastatic colorectal cancer: results from the Eastern Cooperative Oncology Group Study E3200. *J Clin Oncol.* 2007;25(25):1539-1544.
98. Grothey A, Sugrue MM, Purdie DM, et al. Bevacizumab beyond first progression is associated with prolonged overall survival in metastatic colorectal cancer: results from a large observational cohort study (BRiTE). *J Clin Oncol.* 2008;26(26):5326-5334.
99. Wolmark N, Yothers G, O'Connell MJ, et al. A phase III trial comparing mFOLFOX6 to mFOLFOX6 plus bevacizumab in stage II or III carcinoma of the colon: results of NSABP Protocol C-08. *J Clin Oncol.* 2009;27(18s):LBA4.
100. Hoff PM, Clarke S, Cunningham D, et al. A three-arm phase III randomized trial of FOLFOX-4 vs. FOLFOX-4 plus bevacizumab vs. XELOX plus bevacizumab in the adjuvant treatment of patients with stage III or high-risk stage II colon cancer:

Results of the interim safety analysis of the AVANT trial. *Eur J Cancer.* 2009;7(suppl):324.

101. Kopetz S, Hoff PM, Morris JS, et al. Phase II trial of infusional fluorouracil, irinotecan, and bevacizumab for metastatic colorectal cancer: efficacy and circulating angiogenic biomarkers associated with therapeutic resistance. *J Clin Oncol.* 2010;28(28):453-459.
102. Tol J, Koopman M, Cats A, et al. Chemotherapy, bevacizumab, and cetuximab in metastatic colorectal cancer. *N Engl J Med.* 2009;360(360):563-572.
103. Hecht JR, Mitchell E, Chidiac T, et al. A randomized phase IIIB trial of chemotherapy, bevacizumab, and panitumumab compared with chemotherapy and bevacizumab alone for metastatic colorectal cancer. *J Clin Oncol.* 2009;27(27):672-680.
104. Adam R, Pascal G, Castaing D, et al. Tumor progression while on chemotherapy: a contraindication to liver resection for multiple colorectal metastases? *Ann Surg.* 2004;240(6):1052-1061; discussion 1061-1064.
105. Mitry E, Fields AL, Bleiberg H, et al. Adjuvant chemotherapy after potentially curative resection of metastases from colorectal cancer: a pooled analysis of two randomized trials. *J Clin Oncol.* 2008;26(26):4906-4911.
106. Benoist S, Brouguet A, Penna C, et al. Complete response of colorectal liver metastases after chemotherapy: does it mean cure? *J Clin Oncol.* 2006;24(24):3939-3945.
107. Vauthey JN, Pawlik TM, Ribero D, et al. Chemotherapy regimen predicts steatohepatitis and an increase in 90-day mortality after surgery for hepatic colorectal metastases. *J Clin Oncol.* 2006;24(24):2065-2072.
108. Grothey A, Sargent D, Goldberg RM, Schmoll HJ. Survival of patients with advanced colorectal cancer improves with the availability of fluorouracil-leucovorin, irinotecan, and oxaliplatin in the course of treatment. *J Clin Oncol.* 2004;22(22):1209-1214.
109. Maindrault-Goebel F, Tournigand C, André T, et al. Oxaliplatin reintroduction in patients previously treated with leucovorin, fluorouracil and oxaliplatin for metastatic colorectal cancer. *Ann Oncol.* 2004;15(15):1210-1214.
110. Tournigand C, Cervantes A, Figer A, et al. OPTIMOX1: a randomized study of FOLFOX4 or FOLFOX7 with oxaliplatin in a stop-and-Go fashion in advanced colorectal cancer—a GERCOR study. *J Clin Oncol.* 2006;24(24):394-400.
111. Chibaudel B, Maindrault-Goebel F, Lledo G, et al. Can chemotherapy be discontinued in unresectable metastatic colorectal cancer? The GERCOR OPTIMOX2 Study. *J Clin Oncol.* 2009;27(27):5727-5733.

25 Anal Cancer

第二十五章　肛管癌

Van Morris
Christopher H. Crane
Cathy Eng

中文导读

肛管癌是一类罕见肿瘤，约占所有消化道肿瘤的2.5%，近年来肛管癌的发病率有稳步上升的趋势。本章重点关注肛管鳞癌的治疗。首先，本章介绍了肛管癌的解剖和组织病理，同时，系统性阐述了肛管癌的潜在病因，包括性行为、人乳头状瘤病毒、人类免疫缺陷病毒、慢性免疫抑制和吸烟。接下来，本章介绍了肛管癌的临床表现、诊断、分期和预后。然后本章重点阐述了肛管癌的治疗。治疗部分包括放疗、化疗，放疗对比放疗、化疗，放疗技术的发展，疗效评估以及复发性疾病的处理等。在放疗、化疗部分，详细介绍了里程碑式的临床研究及治疗进展，包括确立NIGRO方案、丝裂霉素、顺铂等药物引入的研究，如UKCCCR研究、ECOG 4292研究、ACCORD 03研究、RTOG 98-11研究等。疗效评价部分主要介绍了CT和MRI的应用。本章还介绍了相对罕见的肛管腺癌、转移性肛管癌的挽救处理及患者的随访。最后，本章展望了肛管癌未来的发展方向和未来的挑战，如生物制剂的应用等。

Carcinoma of the anal canal is a rare malignancy representing approximately 2.5% of all gastrointestinal malignancies. It is estimated in 2015 that over 7,200 patients will be diagnosed with carcinoma of the anal canal in the United States, resulting in greater than 1,000 deaths ([1]). The incidence of this disease continues to rise steadily. A practicing oncologist will evaluate and treat less than one such patient per year. The majority of anal carcinoma arises within the mucosa of the anus and is of squamous cell histology ([2]). Traditionally, 74% to 90% of carcinomas of the anal canal are cured with the combined modalities of chemoradiation, reserving an abdominoperineal resection (APR) for salvage therapy of persistent or recurrent disease ([3]). This chapter focuses on treatment of squamous cell carcinoma of the anal canal and the potential innovative strategies that lie ahead.

ANATOMY/HISTOLOGY

The anal canal is approximately 4 cm wide and is composed of the region extending from the proximal anorectal ring to the distal anal verge (margin) (Fig. 25-1). Because various definitions of the normal anal canal anatomy exist, classifying these tumors by a histologic definition based on the lining mucosa offers a more consistent approach to guide diagnosis and treatment ([2]).

Malignancies of the anal margin are treated as primary skin cancers and are often surgically excised. The rectal mucosa adjacent to the anorectal ring is composed of columnar epithelium. A transition zone of both cuboidal and columnar epithelium (6-12 mm in length) extends from the distal rectum to the dentate line. The dentate line separates the columnar epithelium (columns of Morgagni) of the proximal anal canal and the squamous epithelium of the distal canal, which extends to the anal verge. The anal verge is the convergence of squamous epithelium and the anal margin. The anal margin comprises the dermis, located within 5 cm of the anal verge.

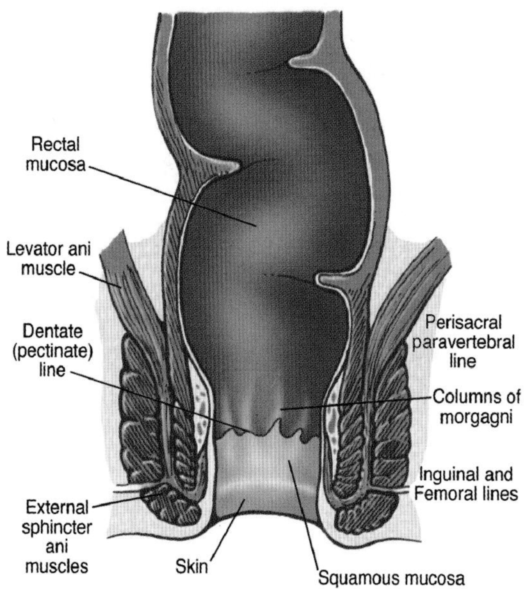

FIGURE 25-1 Anatomy of the anal canal.

The mucosa of the transition zone, formally referred to as the cloacogenic mucosa, represents 66% of the lesions now commonly referred to as nonkeratinizing squamous cell carcinoma (SCC) (Figs. 25-2 and 25-3) ([4]). Tumors distal to the dentate line are usually keratinizing SCC (Figs. 25-4 and 25-5).

The vascular supply of the anal canal consists of the superior, middle, and inferior rectal vessels that originate from the inferior mesenteric, internal iliac, and internal pudendal arteries, respectively. Lymphatic drainage superior to the dentate line is identical to rectal carcinomas flowing to the perirectal and paravertebral nodes. Tumors located inferior to the dentate

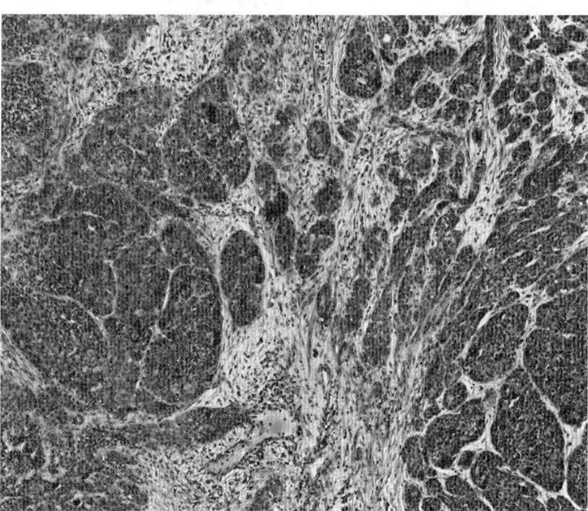

FIGURE 25-2 Nonkeratinized squamous cell carcinoma of the anal canal.

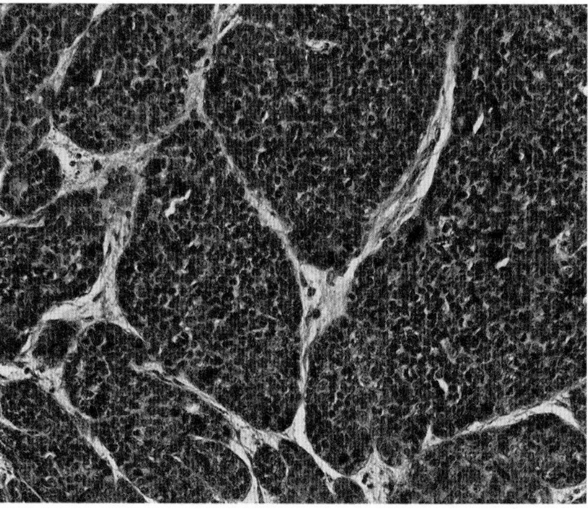

FIGURE 25-3 Magnified view of nonkeratinized squamous cell carcinoma of the anal canal.

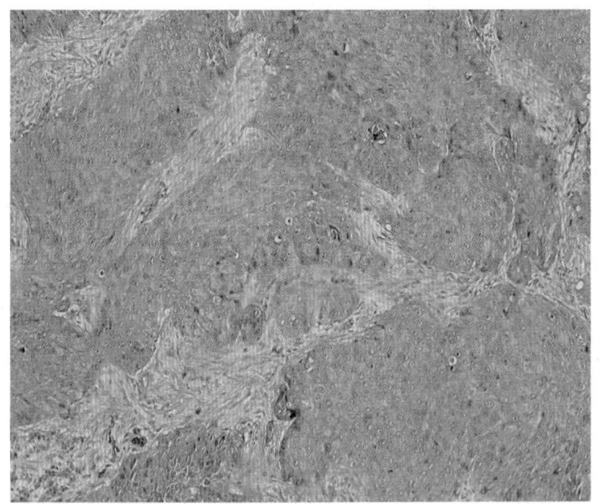

FIGURE 25-4 Keratinized squamous cell carcinoma of the anal canal.

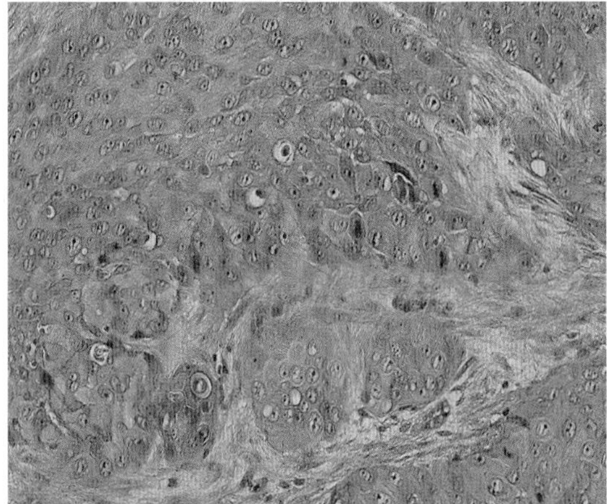

FIGURE 25-5 Magnified view of keratinized squamous cell carcinoma of the anal canal.

line drain to the inguinal and femoral lymph nodes. A complete physical examination should include examination of the lymph nodes of the groin.

ETIOLOGY

Multiple risk factors have been associated with the development of carcinoma of the anal canal. Benign conditions such as hemorrhoids, fissures, and anal fistulas have not been determined to be causal factors ([5]). Rather, it has been postulated that these benign conditions may instead represent the initial symptoms of anal cancer ([5]).

Sexual Activity

The pathogenesis of developing anal cancer is largely related to infection with specific subtypes of human papillomavirus (HPV), most commonly with HPV-16 or HPV-18. Common risk factors associated with anal cancer include a history of more than 10 sexual partners; receptive anal intercourse before the age of 30; and sexually transmitted diseases, including condyloma acuminata (genital warts, attributed to HPV), gonorrhea, herpes virus, hepatitis, *Chlamydia trachomatis*, or a history of infection with human immunodeficiency virus (HIV) ([6-8]). Women with a history of cervical, vaginal, or vulvar cancer are three to five times more likely to develop anal cancer as opposed to stomach or colon cancer, demonstrating the link between sexual activity and likely field cancerization effects from prior high-risk HPV infection ([9]).

Human Papillomavirus

Human papillomavirus is the most common sexually transmitted disease in the United States and has been strongly associated with the development of anal carcinoma ([10]). It is estimated that 75% of men and women of reproductive age have been infected with genital HPV.

High-risk subtypes HPV-16 and HPV-18 are associated with anal cancer—and also cervical dysplasia—and may result in anal intraepithelial neoplasia (AIN). Human papillomavirus subtype 16 reportedly results in a greater incidence of high-grade AIN ([11]). However, unlike cervical dysplasia, AIN is a premalignant condition for which standard screening methods currently have not been universally recommended and have been limited to select high-risk individuals.

A systematic literature review on HPV type distribution in anal cancer showed a combined prevalence of HPV-16 and/or HPV-18 of 72% in invasive anal cancer, with the prevalence of HPV-16 being the highest in these cases, as in cervical cancer ([12]). A cohort of patients with metastatic SCC of the anal canal at the University of Texas MD Anderson Cancer Center (MDACC) revealed the presence of HPV, via detectable HPV DNA and/or expression of the protein p16, in 68 (95%) of 72 tumor samples analyzed ([13]). Therefore, HPV appears to be found in the vast majority of anal cancers.

The presence of HPV also has been reported to be a positive prognostic biomarker for patients with nonmetastatic SCC of the anal canal. In one study of patients with stages I to III anal cancer, HPV was detected in 120 (88%) of 137 tumors analyzed. In a multivariate analysis, p16 expression was determined to be associated with an improvement both in overall survival and disease-specific survival relative to patients with HPV-negative tumors ([14]).

Introduction in 2006 and 2009 of the prophylactic vaccines Gardasil and Cervarix, respectively, directed against primary infection by HPV has demonstrated efficacy in reducing precancerous anogenital lesions caused by the targeted subtypes 6, 11, 16, and 18 [15-17]. In late 2014, the US Food and Drug Administration (FDA) approved the introduction of a nonavalent vaccine targeting nine HPV subtypes (6, 11, 16, 18, 31, 33, 45, 52, and 58). A large, double-blind placebo-controlled study of men who have sex with men between 16 and 26 years of age demonstrated that the use of a quadrivalent vaccine against HPV not only was safe and well tolerated but also decreased the incidence of precancerous AIN [18]. These findings generate early optimism that this preventative approach may decrease the incidence of this disease in the future. Even though initially approved for the vaccination of adolescent females, Gardasil has subsequently received extended FDA approval for males of the same age category after it was shown to be efficacious and may offer a promising primary prevention strategy in both genders [19].

Human Immunodeficiency Virus

Although a direct relationship between HIV and carcinoma of the anal canal has not been clearly established, a strong correlation exists between HIV and HPV. Compared with HIV-negative patients, HIV-positive patients are two to six times more likely to be diagnosed with HPV regardless of sexual practices and are also more likely to have a persistent infection [20, 21]. Human immunodeficiency virus–positive men and women exposed to HIV are less likely to clear the virus and become HPV negative [21, 22]. For patients who are infected with HIV, the prevalence of anal carcinoma is greater and cancer presents at a younger age of onset than in HIV-negative patients [23].

Chronic Immunosuppression

Solid organ transplantation has been associated with a 10-fold increased risk of developing anal cancer and a 20-fold increased risk for vulvar and vaginal cancers [24]. A recent population-based cohort study conducted using the Danish National Patient Registry and the Danish Cancer Registry (DCR) from 1978 to 2005 found that HIV infection, solid organ transplantation, hematologic malignancies, and a range of specific autoimmune diseases were strongly associated with increased risk of anal SCC [25].

Tobacco Use

Prior case-control studies have indicated that chronic tobacco use may result in a two- to five-fold increased likelihood of developing anal cancer [26]. Moreover, tobacco smoking appears to be associated with recurrence of anal carcinoma and is related to increased mortality; thus, smoking cessation should be encouraged once a diagnosis of anal carcinoma is made [27].

PRESENTATION AND DIAGNOSIS

The mean age of diagnosis is approximately 62 years [28]. The most common presenting complaint is rectal bleeding. Other symptoms may include tenesmus, pain, local irritation, discharge, or a change in bowel habits. Clinically enlarged lymph nodes are present in 15% to 25% of patients at presentation [29]. Extreme case presentations may include a fungating perianal mass or a verrucous mass, as seen in Figs. 25-6 and 25-7.

A diagnostic evaluation should consist of a complete physical examination including examination of the inguinal lymph nodes, a digital rectal examination (DRE), and evaluation of the surrounding mucosa of the anus. Diagnostic studies should include proctosigmoidoscopy or anoscopy, chest x-ray, and computed tomography (CT) of the chest, abdomen, or pelvis or magnetic resonance imaging (MRI) of the abdomen and

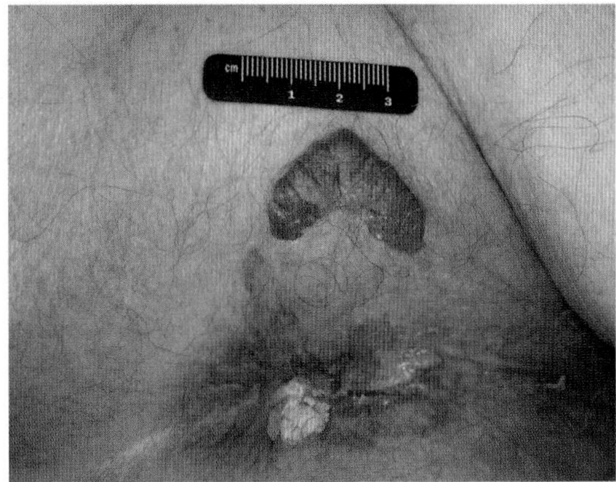

FIGURE 25-6 Perianal mass.

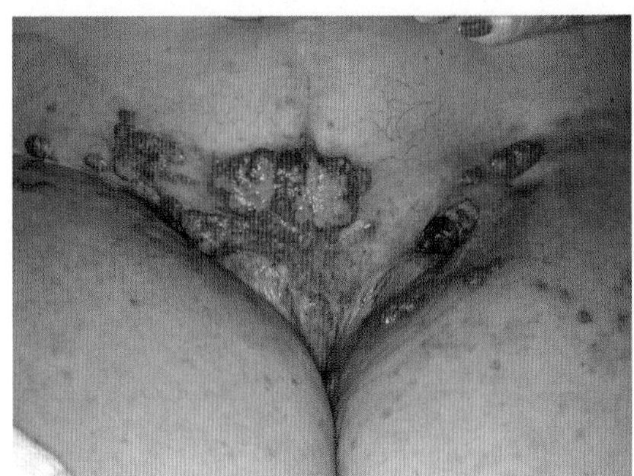

FIGURE 25-7 Multiple verrucous lesions originating from squamous cell carcinoma of the anal canal.

pelvis to rule out distant disease. A transrectal or transvaginal ultrasound may be of added benefit in accurate disease staging ([30-33]). Histologic confirmation is recommended, with a tissue biopsy of the suspected area and/or fine-needle aspiration of any palpable inguinal lymph nodes because this may impact the radiation fields. An HIV test should be considered in all patients, and a one-time test for hepatitis C infection may also be considered for patients born before the year 1965 given the disproportionately high risk of incidence of viral infection for patients in this age range ([34]).

STAGING AND PROGNOSIS

The staging classification system for anal cancer was adopted by the American Joint Committee on Cancer. The T stage, unlike most gastrointestinal malignancies, is not dependent on the degree of tumor tissue penetration but rather on the size of the primary tumor site.

Carcinomas of the anal margin are commonly excised with complete resolution of the tumor. Independent poor prognostic features include tumor size (T stage) with a clear distinction in prognosis between T2 and T3 tumors ([23, 35, 36]). Patients with T1 to T2 tumors have an expected 5-year survival of 80%, whereas patient with T3 to T4 tumors have an expected median 5-year survival of <20% ([28]). Inguinal lymph node involvement may reduce the cure rate by 50%, with increased nodal stage also being a significant prognostic factor ([37-40]). Multivariate analysis of the results from the Radiation Therapy Oncology Group (RTOG) 98-11 trial indicates that tumor-related prognosticators for poorer overall survival included node-positive status (hazard ratio [HR], 1.88), large tumor diameter >5 cm (HR, 1.30), and male sex (HR, 1.38; $P = .031$) ([41]).

CHEMORADIATION—NIGRO REGIMEN

A pivotal approach led to the anecdotal finding that surgery may not be necessary for curative intent in the treatment of SCC of the anal canal ([42]). The benefits of combined chemoradiation in other gastrointestinal malignancies prompted Nigro and colleagues to consider the use of chemotherapy as a radiation sensitizer. Patients received concomitant 5-fluorouracil (5-FU) and mitomycin C, which was administered along with external beam radiation therapy (EBRT) (30 Gy). The pathologic specimens in three of three patients failed to demonstrate any viable tumor. This observation culminated in the use of chemoradiation as the primary treatment modality for the treatment of anal cancer and revolutionized the approach to its treatment. The Nigro approach of chemoradiation has subsequently been evaluated in several other small phase II studies with radiation doses ranging from 30 to 60 Gy.

A retrospective analysis from the Princess Margaret Hospital reviewed the outcomes of patients who had been treated with (1) radiation alone, (2) 5-FU/mitomycin C, (3) split-course 5-FU/mitomycin C, or (4) split-course 5-FU ([43]). The 5-year disease-free survival (DFS) was significantly improved in the 5-FU/mitomycin C arms versus 5-FU alone (76% vs 64%). Although the combination of 5-FU/mitomycin C was superior in locoregional control (LRC) with the addition of mitomycin C (86% vs 60%), the use of split-course radiation resulted in decreased morbidity, notably acute skin toxicities.

RADIATION VERSUS CHEMORADIATION: THE ROLE OF MITOMYCIN C

United Kingdom Coordinating Committee on Cancer Research

The UK Coordinating Committee on Cancer Research (UKCCCR) created the phase III anal cancer trial (ACT I). Patients were randomized to radiation alone (45 Gy) versus continuous infusion 5-FU (1,000 mg/m^2 on days 1-4 or 750 mg/m^2 on days 1-5) during the first and last weeks of radiation (45 Gy) with mitomycin C (12 mg/m^2 on day 1) ([44]). After a median follow-up time of 42 months, the 3-year local failure rate was significantly reduced in the chemoradiation arm versus the radiation-alone arm (39% vs 61%, $P < .0001$; Table 25-1).

Notably, the 3-year mortality rate in the radiation-only arm was greater than that of the chemoradiation arm (39% vs 28%). Twenty patients (3%) required a palliative colostomy or anorectal excision due to treatment-related morbidities. Early morbidity was significant in the chemoradiation arm. Subsequently, dose reduction of mitomycin C was recommended if the patient was ≥70 years old or if deemed medically necessary. The authors concluded that chemoradiation provided a 46% reduction in local recurrence compared with radiation alone.

European Organization for Research and Treatment of Cancer

A smaller study completed by the European Organization for Research and Treatment of Cancer (EORTC) explored the role of chemoradiation and its potential benefit in LRC and colostomy-free interval ([45]). A total of 110 patients were randomized to radiation (45 Gy) with or without continuous infusion 5-FU (750 mg/m^2

CHAPTER 25

Table 25-1 Randomized Phase III Studies of Radiation Therapy Versus Chemoradiation

	Radiation	Chemoradiation
UKCCCR	n = 285	n = 292
Complete response	76 (30%)	100 (39%)
Partial response (>50%)	157 (62%)	138 (53%)
Minimal response (<50%)	22 (9%)	21 (8%)
Three-year local failure	164 (61%)	101 (39%)
Three-year overall survival	58%	65%, *P* = .25
EORTC	n = 52	n = 51
Complete response	54%	80%
Five-year locoregional control	—	*P* = .02
Five-year colostomy-free interval	—	*P* = .002
Three-year overall survival	65%	72% (*P* = .17)

EORTC, European Organization for Research and Treatment of Cancer; UKCCCR, UK Coordinating Committee on Cancer Research.
Data from UK Coordinating Committee on Cancer Research. Epidermoid anal cancer: results from the UKCCCR randomised trial of radiotherapy alone versus radiotherapy, 5-fluorouracil, and mitomycin. UKCCCR Anal Cancer Trial Working Party. UK Coordinating Committee on Cancer Research. *Lancet.* 1996;348:1049-1054. Bartelink H, Roelofsen F, Eschwege F, et al. Concomitant radiotherapy and chemotherapy is superior to radiotherapy alone in the treatment of locally advanced anal cancer: results of a phase III randomized trial of the European Organization for Research and Treatment of Cancer Radiotherapy and Gastrointestinal Cooperative Groups. *J Clin Oncol.* 1997;15:2040-2049.

on days 1-5 and 29-33) and mitomycin C (15 mg/m^2 on day 1).

Event-free survival was superior in the combined-modality arm (P = .03). The overall 5-year survival was 56% in this patient population. In contrast to the UKCCCR study, this clinical trial was limited to T3 to T4 or node-positive tumors. Chemoradiation contributed 18% actuarial improvement in 5-year LRC and an increase in colostomy-free survival (CFS) (36%). In summary, the phase III UKCCCR and EORTC studies established combined chemoradiation as superior to radiation alone for LRC and CFS.

THE INTRODUCTION OF CISPLATIN

Despite the evident benefits of mitomycin C in the treatment of anal cancer, potential treatment-related toxicities may include leukopenia, thrombocytopenia, and, rarely, hemolytic uremic syndrome (HUS) and leukemia. Although a review of prior 5-FU/mitomycin C clinical trials in SCC of the anal canal suggests the potential for superior results, these often come at the cost of treatment-related morbidity and mortality. Therefore, other agents that may reduce treatment-related toxicities without compromising efficacy would be preferable.

The Eastern Cooperative Group (ECOG) 4292 trial attempted to evaluate the combination of 5-FU/cisplatin (Table 25-2) ([46]). The overall response rate was 95%. Thirteen patients (68%) were determined to have a complete response (CR), and five patients (26%) had partial response. Fifteen patients (79%) experienced grade ≥3 toxicities. Locoregional control could not be achieved in approximately one-third of patients accrued. This treatment schedule with split-course radiation was identical to that reported in

Table 25-2 RTOG Study of 5-FU/Radiation Versus 5-FU/Mitomycin C/Radiation

	5-FU/Radiation (n = 145)	5-FU/Mitomycin C/Radiation (n = 146)	*P* Value
Complete response	115 (86)	119 (92)	.135
Tumor size >5 cm	42 (81)	42 (86)	.02
Tumor size <5 cm	73 (90)	77 (96)	.002
Time to colostomy (4 years)	32 (22)	13 (9)	.002
Colostomy-free survival	89 (61)	109 (75)	.014
Four-year DFS	71 (51)	98 (73)	.0003
Four-year OS	42 (29)	32 (22)	.31

5-FU, 5-fluorouracil; DFS, disease-free survival; OS, overall response; RTOG, Radiation Therapy Oncology Group.
Data from Flam M, John M, Pajak TF, et al. Role of mitomycin in combination with fluorouracil and radiotherapy, and of salvage chemoradiation in the definitive nonsurgical treatment of epidermoid carcinoma of the anal canal: results of a phase III randomized intergroup study. *J Clin Oncol.* 1996;14:2527-2539.

CHAPTER 25

RTOG 92-08. The authors concluded that the delay in radiation treatment likely accounted for the inferior LRC rate and recommended examining this combination further.

A retrospective analysis in 197 patients with TxNxM0 SCC of the anal canal was completed at MDACC ([47]). Patients received continuous infusion of 5-FU and cisplatin for the duration of radiation therapy (55 Gy), and median follow-up was 8.6 years. Complete responses after chemoradiation were observed in 185 patients (94%). The local recurrence rate was 11% with the use of 5-FU and cisplatin, and all patients with a local recurrence underwent salvage APR or diverting colostomies. Only 16 patients (8%) developed distant metastases. Overall survival at 5 years was 86%. Grade 4 acute toxicities (diarrhea, dehydration, and skin ulceration) were infrequent. These studies suggest that the use of cisplatin and 5-FU with concurrent radiation is safe and effective in patients with locally advanced anal cancer and may be an acceptable alternative to the traditional 5-FU/mitomycin C regimen.

Neoadjuvant (Induction) Chemotherapy

In place of standard chemoradiation therapy, could the addition of systemic induction treatment provide an improvement in overall survival and decrease the risk of distant disease development?

The phase III Intergroup/ACCORD 03 trial created a 2 × 2 factorial design to compare standard-dose (45 Gy/25 fractions + boost of 15 Gy) versus high-dose radiation therapy (boost of 20-25 Gy) and the potential benefits of induction chemotherapy with 5-FU (800 mg/m^2 on days 1-4) and cisplatin (80 mg/m^2 on day 1) for two cycles in locally advanced SCC of the anal canal ([48]). Patients were required to have T2 >4 cm or node-positive disease. Three hundred six patients were allocated to one of four treatment arms: (1) induction with standard-dose radiation therapy, (2) induction with high-dose radiation therapy, (3) control arm of 5-FU/cisplatin plus standard boost, and (4) control arm of 5-FU/cisplatin plus high-dose boost. The results were compared in terms of CFS. After a median follow-up of 43 months, no difference in CFS was noted for the induction arm (P = not significant) or the higher dose radiation therapy arm ($P = .67$) versus the control arm. Overall, no statistical differences were noted across all arms for local control, CFS, event-free survival, or overall survival.

Radiation Therapy Oncology Group 98-11

The RTOG 98-11 trial was a large phase III multi-institutional randomized trial for locally advanced SCC of the anal canal ([41]) that randomized 682 patients with T2 to T4 tumors and any nodal status to receive 5-FU/mitomycin C and concurrent radiation (control arm) or induction 5-FU/cisplatin followed by concurrent 5-FU/cisplatin and radiation. All patients received 45 to 50 Gy of radiation, with an additional 10 to 14 Gy in 2-Gy fractions given to patients with residual evidence of disease, tumors >5 cm, or tumor invasion of adjacent organs. From a recent long-term update, improved outcomes were noted in the group randomized to 5-FU/mitomycin C and concurrent radiation. Five-year DFS was better in this group (68% vs 58%, $P = .026$) when compared to those receiving induction 5-FU/cisplatin followed by concurrent 5-FU/cisplatin and radiation, as was 5-year overall survival (78% vs 71%, $P = .026$). Trends in CFS, locoregional failure, and colostomy failure all favored the 5-FU/mitomycin C arm as well, although none reached statistical significance. Grade 3 or 4 hematologic toxicity was observed more frequently in patients randomized to the 5-FU/mitomycin C arm (62% vs 42%, $P < .0001$).

Despite the initial appearance that 5-FU/mitomycin C treatment is superior for patients with nonmetastatic SCC of the anal cancer, these findings must be interpreted with caution. This study has since been criticized for the inequality of the two treatment schedules, making a direct comparison of mitomycin C and cisplatin difficult due to the confounding factor of induction chemotherapy in the investigational arm ([49]). Additionally, administration of induction chemotherapy delayed the time to initiation of curative chemoradiation and thereby prolonged the overall treatment time, a metric that, when extended, has been associated with worse clinical outcomes in clinical trials for anal cancer. Nonetheless, induction chemotherapy in patients with early-stage SCC of the anal canal is not routinely administered, based on these findings, at MDACC.

Mitomycin Versus Cisplatin and the Role of Adjuvant Therapy

The UK ACT II trial is the largest phase III trial conducted in SCC of the anal cancer and is the first direct analysis of 5-FU/mitomycin C versus 5-FU/cisplatin with concurrent radiation therapy. The ACT II trial also evaluated whether maintenance (adjuvant) chemotherapy following completion of chemoradiotherapy reduces recurrence-free survival (RFS) ([50]). Using a 2 × 2 factorial design, 940 patients with T1 to T4 node-negative and -positive disease were randomly assigned to either 5-FU/mitomycin C or 5-FU/cisplatin administered concurrently with continuous radiotherapy of 50.4 Gy. The second randomization was to two courses of 5-FU/cisplatin (same schedule) consolidation chemotherapy or no further treatment. There was a greater incidence of acute grade 3 or 4 hematologic toxicity on the mitomycin C arm (26% vs 16%, $P = .001$) but no statistical differences in grade 3 or 4 nonhematologic toxicities. Results after a median follow-up of 5 years demonstrated no statistically significant difference for the end point of 6-month CR rate for concurrent chemoradiation with 5-FU/mitomycin C versus 5-FU/cisplatin (90.5% vs 89.6%, respectively), no difference in RFS, and no difference in CFS, respectively. The role of maintenance (adjuvant) 5-FU/cisplatin chemotherapy showed no added benefit for RFS or overall survival.

Although the investigators failed to fulfill the primary end point of superiority for the cisplatin-based regimen, the final results indicate that 5-FU/cisplatin is noninferior to 5-FU/mitomycin C in achieving a CR and is associated with fewer significant hematologic toxicities. Based on these findings, at MDACC, 5-FU/cisplatin remains our preferred regimen due to its efficacy and decreased myelosuppression relative to 5-FU/mitomycin C. This also allows for safer treatment of immunocompromised and elderly patients who otherwise might not tolerate myelosuppressive combinations.

RADIATION TECHNIQUE

Currently, the most commonly used approach in the combined-modality treatment of carcinoma of the anal canal is continuous-course radiation (45 Gy in 1.8-Gy fractions using opposed anterior and posterior treatment fields with a boost to the primary tumor to 5.4 Gy) plus two cycles of concurrent continuous infusion 5-FU plus mitomycin C. This regimen is considered by most to be the standard of care. Review of the literature has shown the gradual increase in radiation from 30 to 59.4 Gy in recent studies. Prior studies have indicated that there is a dose-response relationship between treatment and outcome. An analysis completed at MDACC from 1979 to 1987 revealed a dramatic difference in LRC for patients who received 45 to 49 Gy (50%) versus ≥55 Gy (90%) ([51]).

At MDACC, our initial experience of 55 Gy for all patients indicated that the local failure rate was 25% to 30% in patients with T3-4 tumors ([52]). In 1999, based on this data, the dose was increased to 59 Gy for T3-4 tumors. Definitive evidence that the higher dose improves local tumor control will eventually be determined. It should be noted that radiation dosages >60 Gy result in an unacceptably high risk of anal canal and urethral stricture, ulceration, and fistula formation.

EVALUATION OF RESPONSE

Studies using CT imaging are often relatively insensitive for detecting the total burden of disease in patients during evaluation for anal cancer, and traditionally evaluation for response following definitive treatment for nonmetastatic anal cancer has been based on clinical assessment. Although the literature is scant regarding use of MRI in evaluation of response to anal cancer, MRI may be used to evaluate a concerning lesion of interest noted on CT with relation to the adjacent anatomic structures.

The question arises regarding the duration of time to wait for a complete clinical response before referral to a surgeon for APR. Review of outcomes from ACT II revealed that 29% of patients without CR by week 11 following completion of definitive chemoradiation did achieve a CR by week 26 ([53]). Based on these findings, in the presence of improving symptoms and/or continued tumor regression on evaluation, at MDACC patients are allowed 26 weeks to achieve a CR before referral for APR. Should clinical progression become apparent prior to this point, then patients are sent promptly for salvage evaluation. Response is largely based on clinical examination. A tissue biopsy should only be pursued if there is clinical evidence of progression or significant residual disease despite an adequate surveillance period. Because anal cancer tends to remain locoregionally confined, the opportunity will not typically be missed for salvage APR with curative intent even if a clinically concerning area is followed closely without biopsy. Treatment guidelines suggest that a tumor biopsy be performed only if recurrent or persistent disease is suspected after serial DRE (Fig. 25-8) ([54]).

RECURRENT DISEASE

Salvage of Recurrent Disease

Abdominoperineal resection is the only effective treatment option for localized recurrent or residual primary disease following chemoradiation for SCC of the anal canal. Fifty to 70% of patients are cured who undergo APR for recurrence at the primary site ([55,56]). There is no role for definitive reirradiation for an in-field recurrence, but neoadjuvant chemoradiation (39 Gy in 26 fractions twice daily with chemotherapy) may be used in cases where there are concerns about the radial margin.

The management of nodal recurrences should be individualized based on the extent of disease, prior radiation delivered to the area of recurrence, and performance status of the patient. In cases where patients have been referred to MDACC with nodal recurrence outside of or at the margin of a prior radiation field, salvage chemoradiation has been effective provided that a full dose of reirradiation is possible. For in-field nodal recurrences, we typically use preoperative chemoradiation to 39 Gy in 26 fractions twice daily followed by surgical resection.

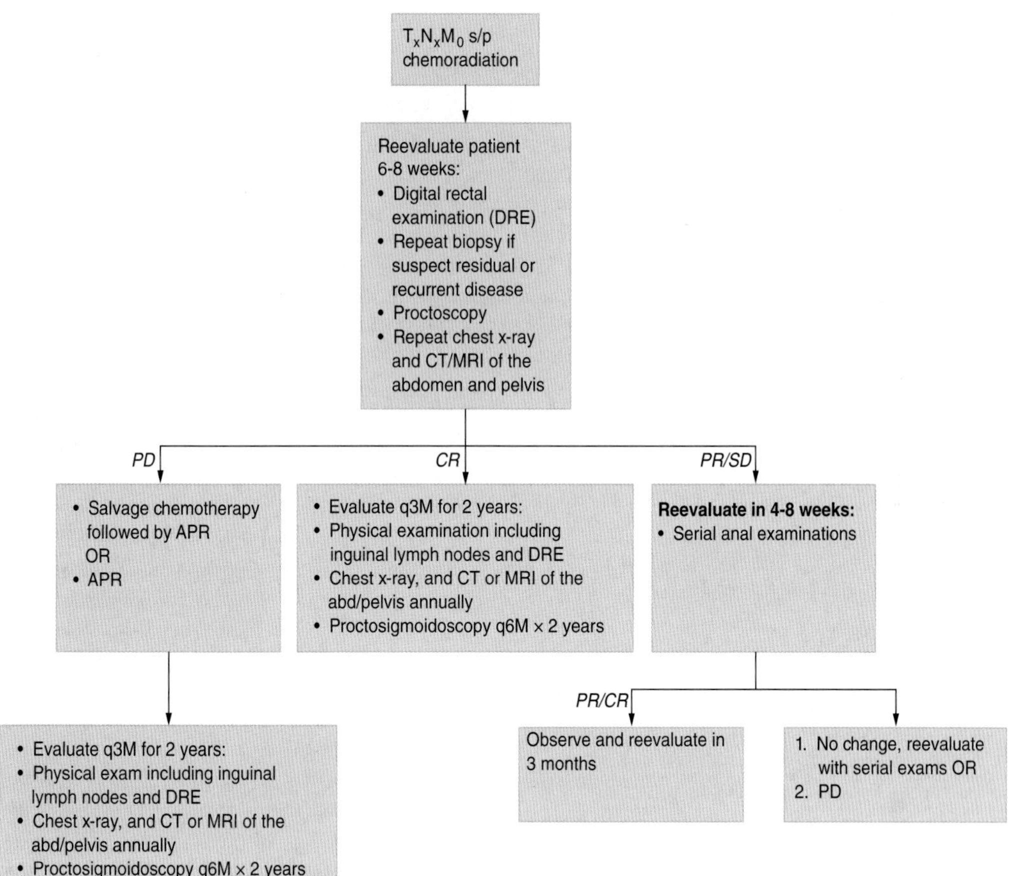

FIGURE 25-8 Postchemoradiation evaluation and surveillance APR, abdominoperineal resection; CR, complete response; CT, computed tomography; MRI, magnetic resonance imaging; PD, progressive disease; PR, partial response; SD, stable disease.

ADENOCARCINOMA OF THE ANAL CANAL

Adenocarcinomas of the anal canal occur less frequently than SCCs ([28]). Nonetheless, most of the reports overestimate the incidence of adenocarcinoma of the anal canal because they do not exclude contamination by the more common distal rectal cancer. The true incidence is likely less than 10%. Its etiology remains unclear, but like its squamous cell counterpart, it has been linked in the past to chronic inflammatory conditions and HPV ([37, 55]). The most appropriate management remains to be defined, with no large prospective studies completed to date. The most striking difference between adenocarcinoma and SCC of the anal canal is the high distant metastasis rate, which tends to undermine the impact of local tumor control. Retrospective analysis from the MDACC experience with adenocarcinoma of the anal canal has suggested a benefit of neoadjuvant chemoradiation followed by APR with the consideration of adjuvant chemotherapy analogous to the treatment of rectal cancer ([57]).

METASTATIC ANAL CARCINOMA

Although the majority of patients with SCC of the anal canal will be cured with chemoradiation, a minority of patients will develop distant metastatic disease. Overall, 5% of patients initially present with extrapelvic metastases, and 10% to 20% of patients treated with curative intent will develop metastatic disease. Due to the rarity of this disease, a universally accepted treatment paradigm has not been established, with choice and duration of therapy largely based on individual case studies and small case series ([58]).

One recent retrospective analysis of our experience at MDACC, the largest series published to date of 72 patients with metastatic anal cancer treated between 2000 and 2012, demonstrated that the majority of patients (55%) with metastatic anal carcinoma receive a 5-FU– and cisplatin-based regimen as first-line therapy ([59]). Patients received a median of two lines of cytotoxic chemotherapy, with carboplatin and paclitaxel being the most popular second-line treatment for patients still able to tolerate further therapy following progression on frontline chemotherapy. With a median follow-up period of 42 months, the median overall survival was 22 months. Systemic treatment should be considered in any patient demonstrating a good performance status, with duration of therapy continued indefinitely for maximal outcome if tolerated well. A subset of patients in this cohort (43%) with oligometastatic disease was able to proceed to surgical resection of distant metastases or chemoradiation to affected regions that had not received prior radiotherapy. For these patients, overall survival was prolonged (53 months vs 17 months, $P < .001$), which was likely a reflection of a lower total burden of disease and favorable clinical characteristics that enabled this group to withstand multidisciplinary management of their metastatic disease. Consideration of surgical resection with curative intent should be encouraged for patients if surgically resectable or borderline resectable.

SURVEILLANCE

When patients are treated with chemoradiation therapy with curative intent, patients should be evaluated every 6 to 8 weeks until a maximal clinical response is achieved. Biopsy should not be performed before 26 weeks following chemoradiation therapy unless there is clear evidence of residual disease or progression is suspected. If clinical CR is achieved, then patients should be evaluated every 3 months for 2 years after diagnosis. Physical examination must include a DRE and assessment for any palpable inguinal lymph nodes. Vaginal dilators may be used three times a week if needed. The critical time for the prevention of vaginal stenosis is 3 to 6 months following completion of chemoradiation therapy. Vaginal hormonal creams and suppositories are also useful for treatment of vaginal dryness and dyspareunia. Proctosigmoidoscopy should be performed biannually following a CR for 2 years. Chest x-ray and CT of the chest, abdomen, and pelvis or MRI of the abdomen and pelvis should be completed annually for 2 years. Pap smears should continue to be performed annually.

FUTURE DIRECTIONS AND CHALLENGES

It is likely that additional chemotherapy agents other than 5-FU, mitomycin C, and cisplatin may provide benefit to patients with SCC of the anal canal. A prospective, randomized trial (InterAACT) comparing cisplatin/5-FU with carboplatin/paclitaxel as frontline therapy for patients with metastatic anal cancer is currently under way and will elucidate the optimal choice of cytotoxic agents to be used in patients with nonresectable disease. Given the tight association between HPV infection and anal cancer, there is interest that these immune checkpoint blockade agents may have efficacy for this virally associated tumor. A phase II trial of nivolumab, a monoclonal antibody against PD-1, is under way for patients with refractory metastatic anal cancer, and these results will be important in understanding the safety and efficacy of this class of agents in patients with metastatic disease.

Biologic Agents

The role of the anti–vascular endothelial growth factor (VEGF) agent bevacizumab in SCC of the anal canal has not been well defined. However, although this drug has received recent approval by the FDA in combination with paclitaxel and either cisplatin or topotecan in patients with recurrent/metastatic cervical cancer ([60]), further investigation in the coming years will clarify the benefit of this anti-VEGF agent in advanced anal cancer.

Anti–epidermal growth factor receptor monoclonal antibodies such as cetuximab have demonstrated efficacy in patients with *KRAS* wild-type metastatic colorectal cancer ([61, 62]). This oncogene appears to be mutated infrequently in anal cancer. Data published from the ACCORD 16 phase II trial studying cetuximab in combination with cisplatin/5-FU in patients receiving concomitant radiation for locally advanced anal cancer revealed an unacceptably high frequency of significant adverse events ([63]).

CONCLUSION

Carcinoma of the anal canal is a unique malignancy where chemoradiation therapy is provided with curative intent or failure to respond to therapy will result in an APR. Hence, it is recommended that all patients diagnosed be initially evaluated at a tertiary cancer center or the equivalent given the rarity of the disease and the potential for permanent loss of sphincter preservation. We highly recommend a multidisciplinary team discussion with significant expertise for the most appropriate treatment in this rare malignancy.

ACKNOWLEDGMENTS

The authors would like to acknowledge Amir Mehdizadeh for editorial input and Dr. Stanley Hamilton and the anal carcinoma patients at the University of Texas MD Anderson Cancer Center who allowed their photographs to be taken as a contribution to this chapter.

REFERENCES

1. Tabaries S, Ouellet V, Hsu BE, et al. Granulocytic immune infiltrates are essential for the efficient formation of breast cancer liver metastases. *Breast Cancer Res*. 2015;17(1):45.
2. Rickert RR, Compton CC. Protocol for the examination of specimens from patients with carcinomas of the anus and anal canal: a basis for checklists. Cancer Committee of the College of American Pathologists. *Arch Pathol Lab Med*. 2000;124(1):21-25.
3. Bendell JC, Ryan DP. Current perspectives on anal cancer. *Oncology (Williston Park)*. 2003;17(4):492-497, 502-503; discussion 503, 507-509.
4. Gervasoni JE, Wanebo HJ. Cancers of the anal canal and anal margin. *Cancer Invest*. 2003;21(3):452-464.
5. Frisch M, Olsen JH, Bautz A, Melbye M. Benign anal lesions and the risk of anal cancer. *N Engl J Med*. 1994;331:300-302.
6. Frisch M, Glimelius B, Van Den Brule AJ, et al. Sexually transmitted infection as a cause of anal cancer. *N Engl J Med*. 1997;337(19):1350-1358.
7. Patel P, Hanson DL, Sullivan PS, et al. Incidence of types of cancer among HIV-infected persons compared with the general population in the United States, 1992-2003. *Ann Intern Med*. 2008;148(10):728-736.
8. Daling JR, Madeleine MM, Johnson LG, et al. Human papillomavirus, smoking, and sexual practices in the etiology of anal cancer. *Cancer*. 2004;101(2):270-280.
9. Melbye M, Sprogel P. Aetiological parallel between anal cancer and cervical cancer. *Lancet*. 1991;338(8768):657-659.
10. Naomi J, Moscicki A. *Human Papilloma Virus Infection in Women*. San Diego, CA: Academic Press; 2000.
11. Critchlow CW, Surawicz CM, Holmes KK, et al. Prospective study of high grade anal squamous intraepithelial neoplasia in a cohort of homosexual men: influence of HIV infection, immunosuppression and human papillomavirus infection. *AIDS*. 1995;9(11):1255-1262.
12. Hoots BE, Palefsky JM, Pimenta JM, Smith JS. Human papillomavirus type distribution in anal cancer and anal intraepithelial lesions. *Int J Cancer*. 2009;124(10):2375-2383.
13. Morris VK, Rashid A, Rodriguez-Bigas M, et al. Association of human papillomavirus with unique clinicopathologic features in patients with metastatic squamous cell carcinoma of the anal canal [abstract]. *J Clin Oncol*. 2014;32:479.
14. Serup-Hansen E, Linnemann D, Skovrider-Ruminski W, Høgdall E, Geertsen PF, Havsteen H. Human papillomavirus genotyping and p16 expression as prognostic factors for patients with American Joint Committee on Cancer stages I to III carcinoma of the anal canal. *J Clin Oncol*. 2014;32(17):1812-1817.
15. Kahn JA. HPV vaccination for the prevention of cervical intraepithelial neoplasia. *N Engl J Med*. 2009;361(3):271-278.
16. Garland SM, Hernandez-Avila M, Wheeler CM, et al. Quadrivalent vaccine against human papillomavirus to prevent anogenital diseases. *N Engl J Med*. 2007;356(19):1928-1943.
17. US Food and Drug Administration. Approval Letter: Cervarix. http://www.fda.gov/BiologicsBloodVaccines/Vaccines/ApprovedProducts/ucm186959.htm. Accessed November 30, 2009.
18. Palefsky JM, Giuliano AR, Goldstone S, et al. HPV vaccine against anal HPV infection and anal intraepithelial neoplasia. *N Engl J Med*. 2011;365:1576-1585.
19. US Food and Drug Administration. Approval Letter: Gardasil. http://www.fda.gov/BiologicsBloodVaccines/Vaccines/ApprovedProducts/ucm186991.htm. Accessed November 30, 2009.
20. Piketty C, Darragh TM, DaCosta MM, et al. High prevalence of anal human papillomavirus infection and anal cancer precursors among HIV-infected persons in the absence of anal intercourse. *Ann Intern Med*. 2003;138(6):453-459.
21. Sun XW, Kuhn L, Ellerbrock TV, Chiasson MA, Bush TJ, Wright TCJ. Human papillomavirus infection in women infected with the human immunodeficiency virus. *N Engl J Med*. 1997;337(19):1343-1349.
22. Critchlow CW, Hawes SE, Kuypers JM, et al. Effect of HIV infection on the natural history of anal human papillomavirus infection. *AIDS*. 1998;12(10):1177-1184.
23. Sobhani I, Vuagnat A, Walker F, et al. Prevalence of high-grade dysplasia and cancer in the anal canal in human papillomavirus-infected individuals. *Gastroenterology*. 2001;120(4):857-866.
24. Adami J, Gäbel H, Lindelöf B, et al. Cancer risk following organ transplantation: a nationwide cohort study in Sweden. *Br J Cancer*. 2003;89(7):1221-1227.
25. Sunesen KG, Nørgaard M, Thorlacius-Ussing O, Laurberg S. Immunosuppressive disorders and risk of anal squamous cell carcinoma: a nationwide cohort study in Denmark, 1978-2005. *Int J Cancer*. 2010;127(3):675-684.
26. Daling JR, Sherman KJ, Hislop TG, et al. Cigarette smoking and the risk of anogenital cancer. *Am J Epidemiol*. 1992;135(2):180-189.
27. Ramamoorthy S, Luo L, Luo E, Carethers JM. Tobacco smoking and risk of recurrence for squamous cell cancer of the anus. *Cancer Detect Prev*. 2008;32(2):116-120.
28. Myerson RJ, Karnell LH, Menck HR. The National Cancer Data Base report on carcinoma of the anus. *Cancer*. 1997;80(4):805-815.
29. Khatri VP, Chopra S. Clinical presentation, imaging, and staging of anal cancer. *Surg Oncol Clin N Am*. 2004;13(2):295-308.
30. Cotter SE, Grigsby PW, Siegel BA, et al. FDG-PET/CT in the evaluation of anal carcinoma. *Int J Radiat Oncol Biol Phys*. 2006;65(3):720-725.
31. Mackay SG, Pager CK, Joseph D, Stewart PJ, Solomon MJ. Assessment of the accuracy of transrectal ultrasonography in anorectal neoplasia. *Br J Cancer*. 2003;90(3):346-350.
32. Tarantino D, Bernstein MA. Endoanal ultrasound in the staging and management of squamous-cell carcinoma of the anal canal: potential implications of a new ultrasound staging system. *Dis Colon Rectum*. 2002;45(1):16-22.
33. Berton F, Gola G, Wilson SR. Perspective on the role of transrectal and transvaginal sonography of tumors of the rectum and anal canal. *Am J Roentgenol*. 2008;190(6):1495-1504.
34. Smith BD, Morgan RL, Beckett GA, et al. Recommendations for the identification of chronic hepatitis C virus infection among persons born during 1945-1965. *MMWR Recomm Rep*. 2012;61(RR-4):1-32.
35. Ferenczy A, Coutlée F, Franco E, Hankins C. Human papillomavirus and HIV coinfection and the risk of neoplasias of the lower genital tract: a review of recent developments. *CMAJ*. 2003;169(5):431-434.
36. D'Souza G, Wiley DJ, Li X, et al. Incidence and epidemiology of anal cancer in the multicenter AIDS cohort study. *J Acquir Immune Defic Syndr*. 2008;48(4):491-499.
37. Belkacémi Y, Berger C, Poortmans P, et al. Management of primary anal canal adenocarcinoma: a large retrospective study from the Rare Cancer Network. *Int J Radiat Oncol Biol Phys*. 2003;56(5):1274-1283.
38. Touboul E, Schlienger M, Buffat L, et al. Epidermoid carcinoma of the anal canal. Results of curative-intent radiation therapy in a series of 270 patients. *Cancer*. 1994;73(6):1569-1579.
39. Esiashvili N, Landry J, Matthews RH. Carcinoma of the anus: strategies in management. *Oncologist*. 2002;7(3):188-199.
40. Hill J, Meadows H, Haboubi N, Talbot IC, Northover JMA. Pathological staging of epidermoid anal carcinoma for the new era. *Colorectal Dis*. 2003;5(3):206-213.
41. Gunderson LL, Winter KA, Ajani JA, et al. Long-term update of US GI Intergroup RTOG 98-11 phase III trial for anal carcinoma: survival, relapse, and colostomy failure with concurrent chemoradiation involving fluorouracil/mitomycin versus fluorouracil/

cisplatin. *J Clin Oncol*. 2012;30(35):4344-4351.

42. Nigro ND, Vaitkevicius VK, Considine BJ. Combined therapy for cancer of the anal canal: a preliminary report. *Dis Colon Rectum*.1974;17(3):354-356.
43. Cummings BJ, Keane TJ, O'Sullivan B, Wong CS, Catton CN. Epidermoid anal cancer: treatment by radiation alone or by radiation and 5-fluorouracil with and without mitomycin C. *Int J Radiat Oncol Biol Phys*. 1991;21(5):1115-1125.
44. KCCCR Anal Cancer Trial Working Party. Epidermoid anal cancer: results from the UKCCCR randomised trial of radiotherapy alone versus radiotherapy, 5-fluorouracil, and mitomycin. UKCCCR Anal Cancer Trial Working Party. UK Co-ordinating Committee on Cancer Research. *Lancet*. 1996;348(9034):1049-1054.
45. Bartelink H, Roelofsen F, Eschwege F, et al. Concomitant radiotherapy and chemotherapy is superior to radiotherapy alone in the treatment of locally advanced anal cancer: results of a phase III randomized trial of the European Organization for Research and Treatment of Cancer Radiotherapy and Gastrointestinal Cooperative Groups. *J Clin Oncol*. 1997;15(5):2040-2049.
46. Martenson JAJ, Lipsitz SR, Wagner HJ, et al. Initial results of a phase II trial of high dose radiation therapy, 5-fluorouracil, and cisplatin for patients with anal cancer (E4292): an Eastern Cooperative Oncology Group study. *Int J Radiat Oncol Biol Phys*. 1996;35(4):745-749.
47. Eng C, Chang GJ, You YN, et al. Long-term results of weekly/daily cisplatin-based chemoradiation for locally advanced squamous cell carcinoma of the anal canal. *Cancer*. 2013;119(21):3769-3775.
48. Conroy T, Ducreux M, Lemanski C, et al. Treatment intensification by induction chemotherapy (ICT) and radiation dose escalation in locally advanced squamous cell anal canal carcinoma (LAAC): definitive analysis of the intergroup ACCORD 03 trial [abstract]. *J Clin Oncol*. 2009;27(15s):4033.
49. Glynne-Jones R, Mawdsley S. Anal cancer: the end of the road for neoadjuvant chemoradiotherapy? *J Clin Oncol*. 2008;26(22):3669-3671.
50. James RD, Glynne-Jones R, Meadows HM, et al. Mitomycin or cisplatin chemoradiation with or without maintenance chemotherapy for treatment of squamous-cell carcinoma of the anus (ACT II): a randomised, phase 3, open-label, 2 × 2 factorial trial. *Lancet Oncol*. 2013;14(6):516-524.
51. Hughes LL, Rich TA, Delclos L, Ajani JA, Martin RG. Radiotherapy for anal cancer: experience from 1979-1987. *Int J Radiat Oncol Biol Phys*. 1989;17(6):1153-1160.
52. Hung A, Crane C, Delclos M, et al. Cisplatin-based combined modality therapy for anal carcinoma: a wider therapeutic index. *Cancer*. 2003;97(5):1195-1202.
53. Glynne-Jones R, James R, Meadows H, et al. Optimum time to assess complete clinical response (CR) following chemoradiation (CRT) using mitomycin (MMC) or cisplatin (CisP), with or without maintenance CisP/5FU in squamous cell carcinoma of the anus: results of ACT II [abstract]. *J Clin Oncol*. 2012;30:4004.
54. National Comprehensive Cancer Network. The NCCN Clinical Practice Guidelines in Oncology - Anal Carcinoma (Version V.II.2015). 2015. www.NCCN.org. Accessed February 5, 2015.
55. Nilsson PJ, Svensson C, Goldman S, Glimelius B. Salvage abdominoperineal resection in anal epidermoid cancer. *Br J Cancer*. 2002;89(11):1425-1429.
56. Tarazi R, Nelson RL. Anal adenocarcinoma: a comprehensive review. *Semin Surg Oncol*. 1994;10(3):235-240.
57. Chang GJ, Gonzalez RJ, Skibber JM, Eng C, Das P, Rodriguez-Bigas MA. A twenty-year experience with adenocarcinoma of the anal canal. *Dis Colon Rectum*. 2009;52(8):1375-1380.
58. Eng C, Pathak P. Treatment options in metastatic squamous cell carcinoma of the anal canal. *Curr Treat Options Oncol*. 2008;9(4-6):400-407.
59. Eng C, Chang GJ, You YN, et al. The role of systemic chemotherapy and multidisciplinary management in improving the overall survival of patients with metastatic squamous cell carcinoma of the anal canal. *Oncotarget*. 2014;5(22):11133-11142.
60. Tewari KS, Sill MW, Long HJ, et al. Improved survival with bevacizumab in advanced cervical cancer. *N Engl J Med*. 2014;370:734-743.
61. Vale CL, Tierney JF, Fisher D, et al. Does anti-EGFR therapy improve outcome in advanced colorectal cancer? A systematic review and meta-analysis. *Cancer Treat Rev*. 2012;38(6):618-625.
62. Karapetis CS, Khambata-Ford S, Jonker DJ, et al. K-ras mutations and benefit from cetuximab in advanced colorectal cancer. *N Engl J Med*. 2008;359:1757-1765.
63. Deutsch E, Lemanski C, Pignon JP, et al. Unexpected toxicity of cetuximab combined with conventional chemoradiotherapy in patients with locally advanced anal cancer: results of the UNICANCER ACCORD 16 phase II trial. *Ann Oncol*. 2013;24(11):2834-2838.

26 Neuroendocrine Tumors

第二十六章　神经内分泌肿瘤

Daniel M. Halperin
James C. Yao

中文导读

神经内分泌肿瘤来自分布于全身的肠嗜铬细胞。尽管神经内分泌肿瘤这一术语还包括了小细胞癌、甲状腺髓样癌、神经母细胞瘤和Merkel细胞瘤等，但本章着重介绍低—中级别的胃肠胰神经内分泌肿瘤。本章首先介绍了神经内分泌肿瘤的流行病学、预后、发病机制和分子改变。接着本章介绍了神经内分泌肿瘤的病理学特征，以及用于诊断的免疫组化标志物。根据神经内分泌肿瘤的病理特征决定肿瘤分级至关重要，主要依据的是肿瘤细胞有丝分裂计数或Ki-67增殖指数不同肿瘤分级，能够用来预测神经内分泌肿瘤的临床特点，为后续的治疗决策提供依据。本章随后介绍了该病的临床表现、分子诊断、影像学诊断及临床分期。根据肿瘤部位，分别介绍了包括胃、小肠、阑尾、直肠和胰腺神经内分泌肿瘤的临床表现和预后，并介绍了类癌综合征、心脏损害和类癌危象的具体临床表现。最后，本章介绍了神经内分泌肿瘤的总体治疗原则，并强调需要发挥MDT团队的作用。对于低—中级别的神经内分泌肿瘤，手术切除是治疗局部疾病的方法。对于不可切除或转移性疾病长效生长抑素类似物可改善患者的生活质量和无进展生存期。靶向治疗如依维莫司和舒尼替尼，及烷化剂化疗如链脲菌素和替莫唑胺等，也是可选药物。针对肝转移灶，可进行局部治疗。放射性核素肽受体介导治疗（PRRT）也可应用于转移性神经内分泌肿瘤的治疗。

INTRODUCTION

Neuroendocrine tumors (NETs) originate from enterochromaffin cells distributed throughout the body. This chapter focuses on low- to intermediate-grade gastroenteropancreatic NETs (GEP-NETs), although the term *neuroendocrine tumor* also denotes diseases such as small cell carcinoma, medullary thyroid carcinoma, neuroblastoma, and Merkel cell tumor. Pancreatic NETs (PNETs), previously known as islet cell carcinomas, arise from pancreatic ductal progenitors. Extrapancreatic low- to intermediate-grade NETs are generally called carcinoids and most often originate along the aerodigestive tract. These tumors share the capacity for hormone production and usually have an indolent clinical course. Presenting symptoms are caused by secreted hormones, local tumor growth, and/or metastasis. Surgical resection is the curative approach for localized disease. In unresectable or metastatic disease, long-acting somatostatin analogues improve quality of life and progression-free survival. In PNETs, recent randomized studies support the use of targeted therapies such as everolimus and sunitinib, with older prospective and retrospective data supporting the use of alkylating chemotherapy such as streptozocin and temozolomide. This chapter presents a comprehensive overview of the diagnosis and management of pancreatic and extrapancreatic NETs.

EPIDEMIOLOGY

The overall incidence of NETs in the United States is rising and presently estimated at 5.25 cases per 100,000 ([1]). Most NETs progress slowly and may remain undiagnosed for years or even a person's entire natural life. Small bowel NETs are found in 0.65% to 1.2% of patients during unselected necropsy ([2, 3]). These tumors are usually diagnosed in the sixth and seventh decades of life ([1, 4]). The gastrointestinal tract is the most common primary site of NETs, accounting for 58% of NETs ([1]). The distribution of NETs is illustrated in Table 26-1.

PROGNOSIS

The prognosis for patients with NETs varies by histologic grade, stage, and primary site. High-grade NETs demonstrate similar biology and prognosis to small cell lung carcinoma. Low- to intermediate-grade NETs have a more favorable prognosis. The median overall survival of patients with localized low- to intermediate-grade NET is 223 months, according to a recent analysis of the Surveillance, Epidemiology, and End Results (SEER) database of patients registered from 1973 to 2004. For patients with regional disease, defined as involvement of regional lymph nodes, extension to adjacent tissue, or both, the median overall survival is 111 months. For metastatic disease, the median overall survival is 33 months ([1]). The prognoses of NETs by anatomic site are discussed subsequently.

Table 26-1 Organ Distribution of Neuroendocrine Tumors (Carcinoids and Pancreatic Neuroendocrine Tumors)

Organ Site	Distribution (%)
Pulmonary	27
Gastrointestinal	58
Stomach	6
Small intestine	17
Appendix	3
Colon	4
Rectum	17
Pancreas	6
Unknown/other	15

Data from analysis of Surveillance, Epidemiology, and End Results 17 Registry, 2000 to 2004 ([1]).

PATHOGENESIS AND MOLECULAR BIOLOGY

Sporadic and hereditary tumors have yielded insights into NET biology. The *MEN1* gene, mutated in *mul*tiple *e*ndocrine *n*eoplasia, type 1, was mutated in 44% of patients with resected sporadic PNETs in a recent exome sequencing study, with 43% having mutations in the *DAXX/ATRX* complex and 14% harboring mutations in the mammalian target of rapamycin (mTOR) pathway ([5]). Menin, the protein product of the *MEN1* gene, suppresses tumorigenesis by multiple mechanisms, including transcription regulation via interaction with histone methyltransferases, direct cell cycle regulation via interaction with the genetic loci of cyclin dependent kinase inhibitors, and facilitation of apoptosis by increased caspase 8 production ([6]). Genomic analyses of small intestinal NETs revealed rare mutation events, with alterations in *CDKN2B* observed in nearly 10% of cases ([7]). Multiple older techniques, such as comparative genomic hybridization ([8]) and single-nucleotide polymorphism–based array technology ([9]), have confirmed chromosome 18 loss in up to 43% of midgut NETs. Therefore, the somatic genomic alterations in pancreatic and extrapancreatic NETs are qualitatively and quantitatively different, aligning their genetic and clinical heterogeneity. By immunohistochemistry, vascular endothelial growth factor (VEGF) has been associated with poorer clinical outcomes in

GEP-NETs [10], generating significant interest in antiangiogenic therapies, as discussed later.

A significant minority of NETs (5%-10%) occur in the context of multiple endocrine neoplasia, type 1 (MEN1), an autosomal dominant disorder characterized by pituitary tumors, hyperparathyroidism, and PNETs. Neuroendocrine tumors related to MEN1 demonstrate a unique pattern of symptomatic and asymptomatic lesions. Duodenal gastrinomas, causing the Zollinger-Ellison syndrome of peptic ulcers, gastroesophageal reflux, and diarrhea, afflict nearly 60% of MEN1 patients. Characteristic asymptomatic lesions include small duodenal foci of somatostatin expression and pancreatic adenomas secreting glucagon or pancreatic polypeptide. Roughly 20% of MEN1-associated pancreatic macroadenomas are "insulinomas," causing hyperinsulinemic hypoglycemic syndrome. Notably, approximately 10% of PNETs are associated with MEN1 syndrome [11]. Neurofibromatosis type 1, von Hippel-Lindau syndrome, and tuberous sclerosis complex 2 also predispose to NETs, but with very low penetrance, and these diseases account for far fewer NETs than MEN1 [11].

PATHOLOGIC CLASSIFICATION

NETs are characterized by monotonous sheets of small round cells with uniform nuclei and cytoplasm (Fig. 26-1). Neuroendocrine cells store secreted substances in membrane-bound vesicles. Malignant neuroendocrine cells have minimal mitotic activity, cytologic atypia, or nuclear polymorphism. Immunohistochemical markers used to confirm a NET diagnosis include neuron-specific enolase, CD56, chromogranin A (CgA), and synaptophysin (Table 26-2).

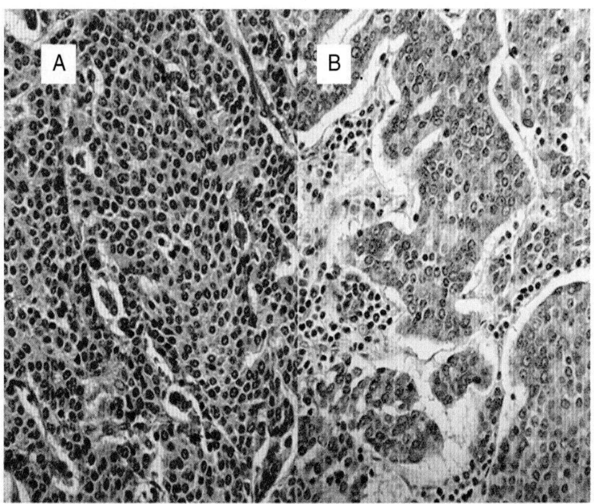

FIGURE 26-1 Histologic appearance of neuroendocrine tumors (NETs). Microscopic appearance of low-grade NET. A. Standard microscopy showing few mitoses, no necrosis, and large numbers of tumor vessels. B. Immunohistochemical staining for chromogranin A.

Assessing tumor grade is critical in all NETs. Modern grading schemes distinguish principally between high-grade (grade 3) tumors, with mitotic count >20/10 high-powered fields or Ki-67 proliferation index >20%, and low- or intermediate-grade (grade 1-2) tumors. Clinical behavior and therapy are largely determined by this distinction [12]. However, a large retrospective analysis revealed a Ki-67 index of 55% or greater to better predict responsiveness to the platinum-based chemotherapy recommended for high-grade NETs [13]. Therefore, it is likely that grading systems will evolve with our biological understanding and therapeutic options.

CLINICAL PRESENTATION, DIAGNOSTIC WORKUP, AND CLINICAL STAGING

Although NETs are well known for their hormonal syndromes, many malignant PNETs are nonfunctional, and carcinoid syndrome is typically present only in the setting of metastases. Symptoms can be insidious and present for years before diagnosis. Symptoms of local and regional extrapancreatic and nonfunctional pancreatic NETs are often vague, relating to obstruction, mesenteric fibrosis, or vascular compromise.

Neuroendocrine Tumor Laboratory Tests and Markers

Although general serum and urine biomarkers are useful for tumor monitoring, they are insufficient for NET diagnosis, which requires pathologic evaluation. Frequently measured tumor markers in carcinoid disease

Table 26-2 Immunohistochemical Markers of Neuroendocrine Tumors

Marker	Significance
Neuron-specific enolase	Cytoplasmic glycolytic enzyme, a less specific neuroendocrine marker
Synaptophysin	Presynaptic vesicle membrane glycoprotein, present on normal and neoplastic neuroendocrine cells
Chromogranin A	Acidic protein, universal marker for neuroendocrine tissue
CD56	Neural adhesion molecule
Cytokeratin(s)	Lack of cytokeratin expression suggests the tumor is either an anaplastic neoplasm or may not be a carcinoma

include serum CgA and 5-hydroxyindoleacetic acid (5-HIAA) levels in a 24-hour urine sample. False-positive results occur with consumption of tryptophan- or serotonin-rich foods (bananas, butternuts, kiwis, mockernuts, pecans, pineapples, plantains, plums, shagbark, sweet pignuts, tomatoes, and walnuts). Common medications affecting urinary 5-HIAA levels include guaifenesin, acetaminophen, and salicylates. Serum CgA level is a sensitive, but nonspecific, marker for NETs, and is elevated among patients receiving proton pump inhibitors or with impaired renal, hepatic, or cardiac function.

In addition to CgA and 5-HIAA, NETs can synthesize other bioactive amines and peptides including 5-hydroxytryptamine (5-HTP), 5-hydroxytryptophan (5-HT), serotonin, insulin, gastrin, glucagon, somatostatin, vasoactive intestinal polypeptide (VIP), adrenocorticotropic hormone, melanocyte-stimulating hormone, pancreatic polypeptide, and pancreastatin ([14]).

Imaging

Endoscopy

Endoscopic techniques localize tumors and facilitate biopsy. Esophagogastroduodenoscopy (EGD) can often locate gastric and duodenal NETs. Colonoscopy can identify colorectal NETs. Double-balloon enteroscopy and capsule endoscopy may assist in localizing small bowel NETs. Disadvantages of endoscopy include the requirement for patient sedation and the difficulty in visualizing small submucosal lesions. Endoscopic ultrasound is useful in the assessment, visualization, and biopsy of pancreatic and some small duodenal NETs.

Computed Tomography and Magnetic Resonance Imaging

Computed tomography (CT) and magnetic resonance imaging (MRI) are the preferred initial imaging studies for localizing NETs. However, the utility of cross-sectional imaging for diagnosing typical small bowel NETs is limited; usually their presence must be inferred from luminal narrowing, adenopathy, and mesenteric fibrosis. Computed tomography and MRI technologies are far more useful in detection of hepatic metastases, which frequently present convenient sites for diagnostic biopsy. Computed tomography and MRI are helpful in the detection of PNETs, for which the sensitivities of CT and MRI are up to 82% and 100%, respectively ([15]).

Somatostatin Receptor Scintigraphy

Somatostatin receptor scintigraphy (SRS) has improved the visualization of NETs. Somatostatin receptor scintigraphy uses a somatostatin analogue, ^{111}In-labeled diethylenetriamine penta-acetic acid octreotide (DTPA-D-Phe^{1}-octreotide), to visualize tumors expressing somatostatin receptors 2 and 5. Compared with CT or MRI, SRS detects additional metastases in about one-third of patients. Moreover, SRS may help to identify small tumors when conventional scans are unrevealing. The overall sensitivity of SRS is 80% to 90% ([16]).

Positron Emission Tomography

Because ^{18}F-fluorodeoxyglucose (FDG) positron emission tomography (PET) identifies tumors with significant proliferative activity, it is unreliable in NETs. Gallium-68 (^{68}Ga)-DOTA-NOC PET, which uses labeled octreotide to detect somatostatin-avid tumors, had a sensitivity of 78.3% and a specificity of 92.5% in an initial study ([17]). Ongoing studies are evaluating alternative ^{68}Ga-labelled somatostatin analogues, and this technology may emerge as more convenient than SRS, with potentially improved test characteristics.

Other Nuclear Scintigraphy Techniques

Metaiodobenzylguanidine (MIBG) is absorbed by carcinoid tumor cells. Iodine-131-labeled MIBG (^{131}I-MIBG) has an overall sensitivity of 55% to 70% in detecting NETs ([18]). Although ^{131}I-MIBG is less sensitive than SRS, it may be used in patients receiving long-acting octreotide, which competitively inhibits uptake of radiolabeled somatostatin analogues.

Clinical Staging

The American Joint Committee on Cancer (AJCC) has proposed site-specific staging systems for grade 1 to 2 NETs using the TNM system ([19]). The details vary, particularly with respect to the T stage, which can depend on depth of invasion or involvement of critical structures. This staging is prognostic, but not predictive of the benefit with any therapy. The relevant distinction is therefore between resectable and unresectable/metastatic disease. High-grade NETs are described with a TNM stage according to guidelines for carcinomas of the primary site but are summarized as limited stage or extensive stage disease, defined by the ability of the cancer to be treated in a single radiation port, based on the staging of the biologically analogous small cell lung cancer ([20]).

CARCINOID CLINICAL BEHAVIOR BY SITE

Gastric Carcinoid

Gastric carcinoid tumors are divided into three types. Type 1 (75%) is associated with chronic atrophic gastritis, type 2 (5%-10%) is associated with with Zollinger-Ellison syndrome, and type 3 (15%-25%) is sporadic ([21]). Conceptually, type 1 and 2 gastric carcinoids arise as a physiologic response to excessive gastrin secretion, with the gastrin being physiologic in type 1 gastric carcinoids and pathologic in type 2 gastric carcinoids. Because they are independent of known stimuli, type 3 gastric carcinoids have the worst prognosis, frequently presenting with metastatic disease. A SEER analysis revealed a median overall survival of 13 months for patients with metastatic gastric carcinoid ([1]). Clinical features of the three groups of gastric carcinoid are summarized in Table 26-3.

Small Intestine Carcinoid

Small intestine NETs, most frequently associated with carcinoid syndrome, are often found in the distal ileum within 60 cm of the ileocecal valve. At diagnosis, multiple putative "primary" lesions may be present. Analysis of SEER data from 1973 to 2004 demonstrates that jejunum and ileum NETs (30%) were far more likely than duodenal (9%), rectal (5%), or appendiceal (9%) lesions to be metastatic at diagnosis. The median overall survival times of patients with duodenal and jejunum/ileum carcinoids were 107 and 111 months, respectively, for localized disease and 57 and 56 months, respectively, for metastatic disease ([1]).

Appendiceal Carcinoid

Neuroendocrine tumors are found incidentally in 1 of 200 to 300 appendectomies in young adults. For appendiceal NETs under 1 cm in diameter, surgical resection is sufficient. For tumors over 2 cm, the risk of metastasis is significantly higher, and a right hemicolectomy is recommended ([22]). Histologic subtype also influences surgical management; right hemicolectomy is recommended for goblet cell (including signet ring) NETs, regardless of size, because of their aggressiveness ([22]). The median overall survival of patients with NET restricted to the appendix is over 360 months. In contrast, individuals with metastatic disease at diagnosis have a median overall survival of 27 months ([1]).

Rectal Carcinoid

Rectal NETs occur most frequently in middle-aged adults. They are found incidentally in approximately 1 in 2,500 proctoscopies as a small yellow-gray submucosal nodule in the rectal wall. Most rectal NETs are under 1 cm in diameter and rarely metastasize, whereas 60% to 80% of lesions over 2 cm metastasize. Local excision is adequate for rectal NETs smaller than 1 cm. Lesions measuring 1 to 1.9 cm without evidence of high-risk features such as muscularis, lymphovascular, or perineural invasion can be excised locally ([23]). A tumor displaying any of these high-risk features should prompt consideration of a more aggressive segmental rectal resection, preferably sphincter sparing. In patients with metastatic disease at diagnosis, palliative excision may still be required. The median overall survival of patients with metastatic rectal NET is 22 months ([1]).

CLINICAL FEATURES OF PANCREATIC NEUROENDOCRINE TUMORS

Insulinoma

Insulinoma is the most common type of PNET. The incidence of insulinoma peaks in patients between 30 and 60 years of age and is more frequent in women. Insulinoma is usually benign (90%), intrapancreatic (nearly 100%), solitary, and small (<2 cm). About 5% of insulinomas are associated with the MEN1 syndrome; screening of family members of an MEN1 index case should be considered ([24]). Hyperinsulinemia causes a classic "Whipple triad" of hypoglycemia, neuroglycopenic symptoms, and resolution with eating.

The insulinoma diagnosis is made by detection of inappropriately high serum concentrations of insulin and C-peptide at a symptomatic blood glucose

Table 26-3 The Clinical Features of Gastric Carcinoid by Group

Group	Clinical Feature	Tumor Size	Metastasis	Prognosis
Group 1	Chronic gastritis	<1 cm	10%	Good
Group 2	ZES, gastrinoma	<1.5 cm	25%	Intermediate
Group 3	Atypical	>1 cm	Frequent	Poor

ZES, Zollinger-Ellison syndrome.

level <50 mg/dL. Although single imaging modalities fail to localize an insulinoma in about 40% of cases, over 90% sensitivity can be achieved with combinations of MRI, pancreatic protocol CT scan, and endoscopic ultrasound. Somatostatin receptor scintigraphy is another noninvasive modality available to assist in localization. Portal venous sampling and arterial calcium stimulation are technically demanding, invasive procedures that are not widely available. When preoperative studies cannot definitively localize the insulinoma, surgical exploration with intraoperative ultrasonography can be considered ([25]). At some institutions, radiologic innovations have eliminated blind surgical exploration.

Gastrinoma

Gastrinoma causes Zollinger-Ellison syndrome, marked by multiple recurrent peptic ulcers. Most gastrinomas are located in the "gastrinoma triangle," encompassing the duodenum, pancreatic head, and hepatoduodenal ligament. Duodenal gastrinoma is often submucosal and difficult to visualize during routine EGD; gastrinoma of the pancreas can exceed 1 cm in size ([26]).

The diagnostic workup for gastrinoma often involves two steps. Elevated fasting serum gastrin and increased basal gastric acid output (>15 mEq/h) suggest hypergastrinemia, with a secretin stimulation test differentiating gastrinoma from other causes. Somatostatin receptor scintigraphy has 77% sensitivity for gastrinoma. Sixty percent of gastrinomas are malignant, and 50% of those have metastases at diagnosis. The median survival of patients with gastrinoma is 3 to 6 years. Roughly one-fifth of gastrinomas occur in the context of MEN1 syndrome ([26]).

Glucagonoma

Glucagonoma is a rare α-cell tumor that typically occurs in people age 50 to 70 years. These tumors are located primarily within the pancreas; most are malignant. Symptoms may not appear until the tumor is over 5 cm in diameter. At diagnosis, up to 80% of these tumors have metastasized. Serum glucagon levels are usually elevated (>1,000 pg/mL; normal range, 150-200 pg/mL), assisting in diagnosis.

Mild glucose intolerance is the most common clinical feature of glucagonoma. A characteristic red-brown maculopapular skin rash of the face, abdomen, perineum, or extremities called necrolytic migratory erythema may precede the diagnosis by up to 5 years. The erythematous areas form bullae that eventually break and encrust. Thromboembolic disease and psychiatric disturbances are also seen. Anticoagulation therapy is recommended ([27]).

Somatostatinoma

Somatostatinoma is very rare. Most occur in the pancreas or duodenum. Patients often present with diabetes mellitus, cholelithiasis, steatorrhea, hypochlorhydria, anemia, and/or weight loss. These tumors are typically metastatic at diagnosis ([27]).

VIPoma

VIPoma is characterized by watery diarrhea (>3 L/d), mediated by vasoactive intestinal peptide (VIP) and other tumor-secreted peptides. VIPomas are located in the pancreas in adults. They are often metastatic at diagnosis. Their syndrome, known as "pancreatic cholera," manifests as secretory diarrhea with potassium and bicarbonate wasting, causing hypokalemia and metabolic acidosis. Diagnosis is made from the typical clinical presentation, the presence of a large pancreatic mass on imaging, and the elevated plasma VIP levels. Somatostatin analogues can effectively control the hormonal syndrome ([27]).

Pancreatic Polypeptidoma

Pancreatic polypeptide is synthesized and released from pancreatic polypeptide cells in the normal pancreas. Pancreatic polypeptidoma is often found unexpectedly in patients with symptoms produced by metastases ([28]).

CARCINOID SYNDROME, HEART DISEASE, AND CRISIS

Carcinoid Syndrome

Carcinoid syndrome often occurs with metastatic disease or when the primary tumor site allows secreted amines to escape the enterohepatic circulation (Table 26-4). Common symptoms include flushing, diarrhea, abdominal cramping, and, less frequently, wheezing, heart valve dysfunction, and pellagra, resulting from 5-HTP metabolites, kinins, and prostaglandins. The incidence of carcinoid syndrome ranges from 10% in localized carcinoid to 50% in advanced tumors. Somatostatin analogues are the mainstay of medical therapy.

Carcinoid Heart Disease

Carcinoid heart disease is due to right heart endocardial fibrosis, occasionally causing tricuspid regurgitation and right heart failure. However, the relationship between carcinoid heart disease and frank heart failure

Table 26-4 Symptoms of Carcinoid Syndrome

Symptom	Frequency (%)	Characteristics	Involved Mediators
Flushing	85-90	Foregut: long-lasting, purple	Kallikrein, 5-HTP
			Histamine, substance P
		Midgut: short-lasting, pink	PGs
Diarrhea	70	Secretory	Gastrin, 5-HTP, histamine, PGs, VIP
Abdominal pain	35	Progressive	Small bowel obstruction, hepatomegaly, ischemia
Telangiectasia	25	Face	Unknown
Bronchospasm	15	Wheezing	Histamine, 5-HTP
Pellagra	5	Dermatitis, diarrhea, dementia	Niacin deficiency

5-HTP, 5-hydroxytryptophan; PGs, prostaglandins; VIPs, vasoactive intestinal peptide.

in the somatostatin analogue era is unclear. A study of 150 patients with carcinoid syndrome described a 20% prevalence of carcinoid valvulopathy on echocardiography. Of those with valvulopathy, 53% had minimally symptomatic heart failure. Over 70% of the patients received a somatostatin analogue, but no relationship was demonstrated between somatostatin analogue use and carcinoid heart disease or heart failure. Patients with carcinoid heart disease exhibited increased urine 5-HIAA and serum CgA levels ([29]). Currently, echocardiography is recommended for patients with carcinoid syndrome and clinical evidence of heart failure or in whom major surgery is planned ([30]).

Carcinoid Crisis

Carcinoid crisis is caused by a massive release of bioactive products to the systemic circulation and is characterized by hypotension, diarrhea, and abdominal cramps. Carcinoid crisis is often precipitated by a procedure; treatment consists of prompt initiation of octreotide infusion, typically beginning at 50 to 100 μg/h. Premedication of carcinoid patients with octreotide in subcutaneous or intravenous form is often used as prophylaxis against periprocedural carcinoid crisis ([31]).

GENERAL APPROACH TO TREATMENT

Treatment is largely dependent on the tumor grade and the primary site. Grade 3 NETs are treated similarly to small cell lung cancer, with platinum-based chemotherapy or chemoradiotherapy, depending on the disease stage. For grade 1 or 2 NETs, surgical removal of all gross disease is advocated whenever feasible. For advanced grade 1 or 2 NETs, regional therapeutic options are largely similar, whereas systemic therapies diverge for pancreatic and extrapancreatic NETs.

Somatostatin analogues are the primary medical treatment for advanced NETs. When carcinoid syndrome persists despite somatostatin analogue or mass effect symptoms worsen, debulking surgery can provide effective palliation. Liver-directed therapy, such as hepatic artery embolization and radiofrequency ablation, should be considered for bulky disease, progression, or symptom palliation. Targeted therapies, such as everolimus and sunitinib, as well as alkylating chemotherapy, such as streptozocin and temozolomide, are also options for systemic therapy in PNETs, with our preference being to use chemotherapy when cytoreduction of larger-volume disease is desired. A general approach to the therapy of advanced disease is depicted in Fig. 26-2.

TREATMENT OF RESECTABLE NEUROENDOCRINE TUMORS

Surgery offers the only potential cure for NETs. Principal considerations include the site and histology of the primary tumor, the extent of detectable disease, and the clinical presentation. Types I and II gastric carcinoids under 2 cm can be removed endoscopically, whereas partial gastrectomy should be considered for larger tumors. Type III gastric carcinoids are more aggressive, requiring excision even when small. Small bowel NET should be managed with resection of the intestinal segment and its associated mesentery because of the risk of nodal involvement. The rest of the intestinal tract should be examined carefully because 20% of tumors are accompanied by a second primary malignancy ([32]). Low-risk appendiceal NETs under 2 cm can be treated with appendectomy; larger and high-risk lesions are treated with right hemicolectomy. Colorectal NETs

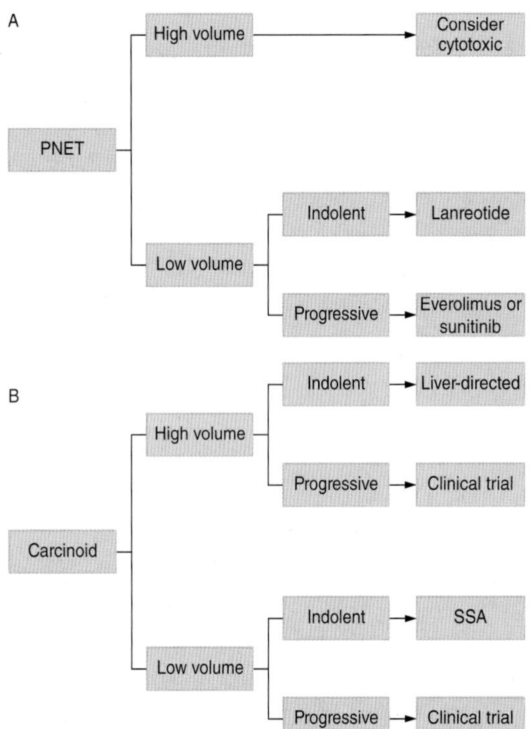

FIGURE 26-2 Approach to therapy for advanced neuroendocrine tumors. A. Approach to initial therapy for advanced pancreatic neuroendocrine tumors. PNET, pancreatic neuroendocrine tumor. B. Approach to initial therapy for advanced extrapancreatic neuroendocrine tumors. SSA, somatostatin analogue. (Modified with permission from Halperin DM, Kulke MH, Yao JC. A tale of two tumors: treating pancreatic and extrapancreatic neuroendocrine tumors. *Ann Rev Med*. 2015;66:1-16.)

are successfully treated with formal hemicolectomy, adhering to the usual techniques of mesenteric lymphadenectomy as with colon adenocarcinoma. Grade 3 NETs are rare and aggressive, seldom benefit from resection, and are usually treated with chemotherapy.

TREATMENT OF ADVANCED NEUROENDOCRINE TUMORS

The current goal of treatment of advanced unresectable NET is improvement of symptoms and survival. Tumor burden reduction is desirable insofar as it is subsumed in these goals. The current standard of care for hormone-related symptom control remains a somatostatin analogue. Other therapies, including surgical resection of hepatic metastases, hepatic artery embolization/chemoembolization, and peptide receptor radionuclide therapy, are useful adjuncts. For PNETs, additional systemic treatment options are also available.

Somatostatin Analogues

Somatostatin analogues such as octreotide and lanreotide are the primary medications for control of symptoms from hormonally active NETs. Octreotide is an intermediate-acting somatostatin analogue that can be administered subcutaneously every 6 to 12 hours. It provides complete or partial relief of flushing or diarrhea in about 85% of patients with carcinoid syndrome and produces a biochemical response rate of up to 72% [33]. The dose of octreotide varies from 50 to 500 μg.

Long-acting somatostatin analogues have obviated the need for multiple daily injections in most patients. Depot octreotide (10, 20, or 30 mg) is given intramuscularly once a month [34]. An intermediate-acting somatostatin analogue should be used to supplement long-acting agents until steady state is reached. Rarely, somatostatin analogue can cause sinus bradycardia or cardiac conduction abnormalities. Caution is advised in patients with preexisting cardiac disease. Cholelithiasis may develop with long-term use of somatostatin analogues. Hypoglycemia or, more commonly, hyperglycemia may occur, especially among patients with brittle diabetes. Steatorrhea may occur but can be managed with pancreatic enzymes. Lanreotide is an alternative somatostatin analogue and, in extended release form, is administered subcutaneously monthly in doses of 60, 90, or 120 mg.

Somatostatin analogues also have anticancer activity. Interim analysis of the phase III randomized trial of depot octreotide 30 mg monthly in untreated metastatic midgut NET (PROMID) demonstrated a significantly longer time to progression with octreotide compared with placebo (14.3 vs 6 months, $P < .001$) [35]. An international, double-blind, placebo-controlled, phase III trial of lanreotide (120 mg every 28 days) in patients with a nonfunctioning NET (CLARINET) also demonstrated significantly improved progression-free survival with lanreotide compared with placebo (median, not reached vs 18 months, $P < .001$) [36].

Surgical Resection of Hepatic Metastases

Liver metastases are generally resectable if: (1) all tumors in the liver can be completely resected and (2) an adequate volume of liver (20% of the standardized total liver volume) with adequate biliary drainage, arterial inflow, and venous outflow can be preserved. If the locoregional and hepatic tumor burden is completely resectable, then this is the preferred management of metastatic NETs, whether functional or nonfunctional. Hepatic resection is most effective for low-grade NETs [37]. Debulking at least 90% of the hepatic tumor burden in patients with functional metastases improves endocrine symptoms and may prolong survival [38].

Radiofrequency Ablation

Local ablative therapies such as radiofrequency ablation (RFA) are being used increasingly for treatment of liver tumors. Radiofrequency ablation involves placing a probe in the liver tumor percutaneously or intraoperatively using image-guidance techniques. The radiofrequency waves increase the intratumoral temperature, resulting in tumor destruction.

Radiofrequency ablation has been used for the treatment of hormone-related symptoms in selected patients with NET liver metastases, alleviating symptoms in up to 80% of cases ([39]). Furthermore, RFA may achieve local control of liver metastases in up to 74% of patients. The use of RFA is generally limited to patients with five or fewer lesions in the liver, with each tumor measuring less than 3 cm in size. The largest reported series using RFA in NET patients with liver metastases included 34 patients with 234 tumors treated in 42 sessions with laparoscopic RFA. "Complete" or "significant" symptom relief was achieved in 80% of the symptomatic patients and lasted an average of 10 months (range, 6-24 months) ([39]).

Hepatic Arterial Embolization and Chemoembolization

Liver metastases from NETs are hypervascular, receiving over 80% of their blood supply via the hepatic artery, whereas liver parenchyma receives 60% to 70% of its perfusion from the portal vein. Thus, embolizing the hepatic artery targets tumor metastases while leaving parenchyma relatively unharmed. The addition of a chemotherapeutic agent to the embolic material, also known as transcatheter arterial chemoembolization (TACE), allows delivery of relatively larger doses of chemotherapy to the tumor, combining local cytotoxicity and ischemia. The most frequently used chemotherapeutic agents for NET TACE include doxorubicin, cisplatin, mitomycin C, and streptozocin ([40, 41]).

Potential benefits include symptom relief, slowing progression, and reducing tumor burden before resection or ablation. Many retrospective reports in markedly heterogeneous populations have shown that either technique can reduce tumor burden, hormone levels, and symptoms in NET patients. No study has clearly demonstrated one technique to be superior. The primary risk is postembolization syndrome, which is typically self-limited and characterized by gastrointestinal distress, fever, leukocytosis, and transaminitis. Major complications such as liver and/or renal failure, gallbladder perforation, cholangitis, peptic ulcer hemorrhage, and abscess formation are rare ([42]). Embolization can occasionally precipitate carcinoid crisis as well.

In patients with extensive liver tumor burden, multiple embolization sessions may be required, starting with the hepatic lobe with greatest tumor burden. Embolization of the whole liver in one session runs the risk of prolonged postembolization syndrome or liver failure. The timing of subsequent embolizations is determined primarily by symptoms, tumor behavior, and patient tolerance.

The timing of embolizations in the disease course remains controversial. Although some investigators advocate early embolization to reduce tumor burden before initiating systemic therapy, late embolization can also be effective. In a randomized study, NET patients treated with initial liver embolization followed by interferon therapy had a higher objective response rate after 1 year (86%) than patients who received interferon only (42%), without altering survival ([43]). In contrast, when embolization or chemoembolization was performed at a median of 37 months after diagnosis, the median survival after embolization was 80 months, indicating that later embolization is still effective ([44]).

CHAPTER 26

Selective Internal Radiation Therapy

Intra-arterial radioembolization with yttrium-90 (^{90}Y) microspheres is an emerging technique being used increasingly in patients with unresectable liver lesions. Yttrium-90 is a pure β emitter with a mean soft tissue penetration of 2.5 mm and a maximal depth of 1.1 cm. Radioembolization with ^{90}Y has a significantly lower incidence of postembolization syndrome than embolization or chemoembolization, allowing it to be performed as an outpatient procedure. However, great care must be taken with ^{90}Y radioembolization to avoid nontarget delivery of radioactive microspheres to organs, making an angiogram with selective embolization of all extrahepatic arteries essential before treatment.

There is limited literature on the use of radioembolization for treatment of neuroendocrine liver metastases. In a retrospective review of 148 patients with NET liver metastases treated with 185 separate ^{90}Y radioembolization procedures, complete response was observed in 3% of patients, and a partial response was observed in 66.7%. The median survival duration was 70 months ([45]). Further investigation, long-term follow-up, and prospective clinical trials are warranted to determine the exact role of this treatment method in the management of NET.

Peptide Receptor Radionuclide Therapy

Radiolabeled somatostatin analogues have also been developed. A prospective study of ^{90}Y-DOTA-Tyr^{3}-

octreotide in 90 patients with metastatic, symptomatic carcinoid tumors refractory to octreotide treated showed subjective improvement in over 50% of patients and objective radiologic responses in 4% of patients ([46]). In another report of 310 patients treated with ^{177}Lu-DOTA-Tyr^3-octreotate, the reported radiologic response rate was 30%, but without intent-to-treat analysis incorporating the additional 194 patients accrued to the protocol, meaningful interpretation is challenging ([47]). The ongoing phase III NETTER-1 study, comparing ^{177}Lu-DOTA-Tyr^3-octreotate to high-dose octreotide long-acting release (60 mg intramuscularly every 28 days) in patients with advanced small bowel NETs should allow clearer conclusions to be drawn.

Chemotherapy

High-grade NETs are responsive to platinum-based chemotherapy ([13]). Well-differentiated extrapancreatic NETs respond poorly to cytotoxic chemotherapy. Pancreatic NETs respond better. The authors' group noted radiographic response rates of 39% in a series of 84 PNET patients using a regimen of 5-fluorouracil, doxorubicin, and streptozocin (FAS) ([41]). This regimen is derived from prior streptozocin-based chemotherapy regimens observed in randomized studies to achieve biochemical responses ([48, 49]).

Targeted Therapy

The NET field has made significant progress over the past 5 years, principally in the area of targeted therapy. Building on the observation that increased VEGF portends poor survival in NET patients, the VEGF receptor (VEGFR) inhibitor sunitinib was tested in a phase III study ([50]). An interim analysis demonstrated a hazard ratio for progression or death of 0.42 favoring sunitinib over placebo ($P < .001$) in 154 PNET patients with advanced and progressive disease. This resulted in the regulatory approval of sunitinib for the indication. Simultaneously, the mTOR inhibitor everolimus was studied in RADIANT-3. This randomized phase III trial investigated everolimus versus placebo in 410 patients with advanced, progressive PNET. The hazard ratio for progression or death was 0.35 ($P < .001$) favoring everolimus over placebo ([51]).

The phase II study of sunitinib showed limited evidence of benefit in extrapancreatic NET patients ([52]). The RADIANT-2 study of everolimus in extrapancreatic NET patients, although limited by randomization imbalance and informative censoring in central radiology review, also failed to demonstrate statistically significant benefit ([53]). It is hoped that RADIANT-4, a randomized study of everolimus in nonfunctional extrapancreatic NET patients buttressed against informative censoring, will convincingly answer the question of whether mTOR inhibition has a role in a broader range of NETs.

Additional Symptom Control Methods

Carcinoid symptoms can be exacerbated by epinephrine, exercise, emotions, eating tryptophan-rich foods, and ethanol and may be controlled through modulating these factors or supplementing dietary nicotinamide. Medical management of carcinoid symptoms can include a bronchodilator for bronchospasm, loperamide or diphenoxylate for diarrhea, and diuretics for fluid overload secondary to valvular dysfunction. A proton pump inhibitor can manage gastric hypersecretion in gastrinoma patients. Since our initial report, multiple groups have confirmed the efficacy of everolimus for the management of malignant hypoglycemia due to insulinoma ([54]).

CONCLUSION

Multidisciplinary diagnosis and management of NETs is mandatory. For localized disease, clear communication between the surgeon and the pathologist is required for appropriate prognostication and treatment. Advanced NETs present different challenges, and surgeons, interventional radiologists, medical oncologists, and endocrinologists may all play roles in improving the quality and quantity of life for the patient. Despite recent advances in targeted therapy for PNET, extrapancreatic NETs remain challenging to treat, and NETs remain life-limiting diseases for many patients. Ongoing studies of targeted agents, peptide receptor radionuclide therapy, and immunotherapy will hopefully continue to advance our understanding of the biology of these diverse diseases while bringing needed therapies to this growing patient population.

REFERENCES

1. Yao JC, Hassan M, Phan A, et al. One hundred years after "carcinoid": epidemiology of and prognostic factors for neuroendocrine tumors in 35,825 cases in the United States. *J Clin Oncol.* 2008;26:3063-3072.
2. Moertel CG, Sauer WG, Dockerty MB, Baggenstoss AH. Life history of the carcinoid tumor of the small intestine. *Cancer.* 1961;14:901-912.
3. Berge T, Linell F. Carcinoid tumours. Frequency in a defined population during a 12-year period. *Acta Pathol Microbiol Scand A.* 1976;84(4):322-30. Epub 1976/07/01.

4. Modlin IM, Lye KD, Kidd M. A 5-decade analysis of 13,715 carcinoid tumors. *Cancer*. 2003;97:934-959.
5. Jiao Y, Shi C, Edil BH, et al. DAXX/ATRX, MEN1, and mTOR pathway genes are frequently altered in pancreatic neuroendocrine tumors. *Science*. 2011;331(6021):1199-1203.
6. Yang Y, Hua X. In search of tumor suppressing functions of menin. *Mol Cell Endocrinol*. 2007;265-266:34-41.
7. Francis JM, Kiezun A, Ramos AH, et al. Somatic mutation of CDKN1B in small intestine neuroendocrine tumors. *Nat Genet*. 2013;45(12):1483-1486.
8. Kytola S, Hoog A, Nord B, et al. Comparative genomic hybridization identifies loss of 18q22-qter as an early and specific event in tumorigenesis of midgut carcinoids. *Am J Pathol*. 2001;158(5):1803-1808.
9. Kim Do H, Nagano Y, Choi IS, White JA, Yao JC, Rashid A. Allelic alterations in well-differentiated neuroendocrine tumors (carcinoid tumors) identified by genome-wide single nucleotide polymorphism analysis and comparison with pancreatic endocrine tumors. *Genes Chromosomes Cancer*. 2008;47(1):84-92.
10. Zhang J, Jia Z, Li Q, et al. Elevated expression of vascular endothelial growth factor correlates with increased angiogenesis and decreased progression-free survival among patients with low-grade neuroendocrine tumors. *Cancer*. 2007;109(8):1478-1486.
11. Anlauf M, Garbrecht N, Bauersfeld J, et al. Hereditary neuroendocrine tumors of the gastroenteropancreatic system. *Virchows Arch*. 2007;451(Suppl 1):S29-S38.
12. Kulke MH, Siu LL, Tepper JE, et al. Future directions in the treatment of neuroendocrine tumors: consensus report of the National Cancer Institute Neuroendocrine Tumor clinical trials planning meeting. *J Clin Oncol*. 2011;29:934-943.
13. Sorbye H, Welin S, Langer SW, et al. Predictive and prognostic factors for treatment and survival in 305 patients with advanced gastrointestinal neuroendocrine carcinoma (WHO G3): the NORDIC NEC study. *Ann Oncol*. 2013;24(1):152-160.
14. Halperin DM, Kulke MH, Yao JC. A tale of two tumors: treating pancreatic and extrapancreatic neuroendocrine tumors. *Ann Rev Med*. 2015;66:1-16.
15. Tamm EP, Kim EE, Ng CS. Imaging of neuroendocrine tumors. *Hematol Oncol Clin North Am*. 2007;21(3):409-432.
16. Krenning EP, Kooij PP, Bakker WH, et al. Radiotherapy with a radiolabeled somatostatin analogue, [111In-DTPA-D-Phe1]-octreotide. A case history. *Ann N Y Acad Sci*. 1994;733:496-506.
17. Naswa N, Sharma P, Kumar A, et al. Gallium-68-DOTA-NOC PET/CT of patients with gastroenteropancreatic neuroendocrine tumors: a prospective single-center study. *AJR Am J Roentgenol*. 2011;197(5):1221-1228.
18. Hanson MW, Feldman JM, Blinder RA, et al. Carcinoid tumors: iodine-131 MIBG scintigraphy. *Radiology*. 1989;172(3):699-703.
19. Edge SB, Byrd DR, Compton CC, Fritz AG, Greene FL, Trotti A. *AJCC Cancer Staging Manual*. 7th ed. New York: Springer; 2010.
20. Kalemkerian GP, Gadgeel SM. Modern staging of small cell lung cancer. *J Natl Compr Canc Netw*. 2013;11(1):99-104.
21. Kulke MH, Anthony LB, Bushnell DL, et al. NANETS treatment guidelines: well-differentiated neuroendocrine tumors of the stomach and pancreas. *Pancreas*. 2010;39(6):735-752.
22. Boudreaux JP, Klimstra DS, Hassan MM, et al. The NANETS consensus guideline for the diagnosis and management of neuroendocrine tumors: well-differentiated neuroendocrine tumors of the jejunum, ileum, appendix, and cecum. *Pancreas*. 2010;39(6):753-766.
23. Kwaan MR, Goldberg JE, Bleday R. Rectal carcinoid tumors: review of results after endoscopic and surgical therapy. *Arch Surg*. 2008;143(5):471-475.
24. Toumpanakis CG, Caplin ME. Molecular genetics of gastroenteropancreatic neuroendocrine tumors. *Am J Gastroenterol*. 2008;103(3):729-732.
25. Tucker ON, Crotty PL, Conlon KC. The management of insulinoma. *Br J Surg*. 2006;93(3):264-275.
26. Fendrich V, Langer P, Waldmann J, Bartsch DK, Rothmund M. Management of sporadic and multiple endocrine neoplasia type 1 gastrinomas. *Br J Surg*. 2007;94(11):1331-1341.
27. Halperin DM, Kulke MH. Management of pancreatic neuroendocrine tumors. *Gastroenterol Clin North Am*. 2012;41(1):119-131.
28. Sakai H, Kodaira S, Ono K, et al. Disseminated pancreatic polypeptidioma. *Intern Med*. 1993;32(9):737-741.
29. Bhattacharyya S, Toumpanakis C, Caplin ME, Davar J. Analysis of 150 patients with carcinoid syndrome seen in a single year at one institution in the first decade of the twenty-first century. *Am J Cardiol*. 2008;101(3):378-381.
30. Kulke MH, Benson AB 3rd, Bergsland E, et al. Neuroendocrine tumors. *J Natl Compr Canc Netw*. 2012;10(6):724-64. Epub 2012/06/09.
31. Dierdorf SF. Carcinoid tumor and carcinoid syndrome. *Curr Opin Anaesthesiol*. 2003;16(3):343-347.
32. Memon MA, Nelson H. Gastrointestinal carcinoid tumors: current management strategies. *Dis Colon Rectum*. 1997;40(9):1101-1118.
33. Schnirer, II, Yao JC, Ajani JA. Carcinoid—a comprehensive review. *Acta Oncol*. 2003;42(7):672-692.
34. Rubin J, Ajani J, Schirmer W, et al. Octreotide acetate long-acting formulation versus open-label subcutaneous octreotide acetate in malignant carcinoid syndrome. *J Clin Oncol*. 1999;17(2):600-606.
35. Rinke A, Müller H-H, Schade-Brittinger C, et al. Placebo-controlled, double-blind, prospective, randomized study on the effect of octreotide LAR in the control of tumor growth in patients with metastatic neuroendocrine midgut tumors: a report from the PROMID Study Group. *J Clin Oncol*. 2009;27:4656-4663.
36. Caplin ME, Pavel M, Cwikla JB, et al. Lanreotide in metastatic enteropancreatic neuroendocrine tumors. *N Engl J Med*. 2014;371(3):224-233.
37. Cho CS, Labow DM, Tang L, et al. Histologic grade is correlated with outcome after resection of hepatic neuroendocrine neoplasms. *Cancer*. 2008;113(1):126-134.
38. Que FG, Nagorney DM, Batts KP, Linz LJ, Kvols LK. Hepatic resection for metastatic neuroendocrine carcinomas. *Am J Surg*. 1995;169(1):36-42.
39. Berber E, Flesher N, Siperstein AE. Laparoscopic radiofrequency ablation of neuroendocrine liver metastases. *World J Surg*. 2002;26(8):985-990.
40. Hajarizadeh H, Ivancev K, Mueller CR, Fletcher WS, Woltering EA. Effective palliative treatment of metastatic carcinoid tumors with intra-arterial chemotherapy/chemoembolization combined with octreotide acetate. *Am J Surg*. 1992;163(5):479-483.
41. Kim YH, Ajani JA, Carrasco CH, et al. Selective hepatic arterial chemoembolization for liver metastases in patients with carcinoid tumor or islet cell carcinoma. *Cancer Invest*. 1999;17(7):474-478.
42. O'Toole D, Ruszniewski P. Chemoembolization and other ablative therapies for liver metastases of gastrointestinal endocrine tumours. *Best Pract Res Clin Gastroenterol*. 2005;19(4):585-594.
43. Hanssen LE, Schrumpf E, Kolbenstvedt AN, Tausjo J, Dolva LO. Treatment of malignant metastatic midgut carcinoid tumours with recombinant human alpha2b interferon with or without prior hepatic artery embolization. *Scand J Gastroenterol*. 1989;24(7):787-795.
44. Eriksson BK, Larsson EG, Skogseid BM, Lofberg AM, Lorelius LE, Oberg KE. Liver embolizations of patients with malignant neuroendocrine gastrointestinal tumors. *Cancer*. 1998;83(11):2293-2301.
45. Kennedy AS, Dezarn WA, McNeillie P, et al. Radioembolization for unresectable neuroendocrine hepatic metastases using resin 90Y-microspheres: early results in 148 patients. *Am J Clin Oncol*.

2008;31(3):271-279.
46. Bushnell DL Jr, O'Dorisio TM, O'Dorisio MS, et al. 90Y-edotreotide for metastatic carcinoid refractory to octreotide. *J Clin Oncol*. 2010;28(10):1652-1659.
47. Kwekkeboom DJ, de Herder WW, Kam BL, et al. Treatment with the radiolabeled somatostatin analog [177 Lu-DOTA 0,Tyr3]octreotate: toxicity, efficacy, and survival. *J Clin Oncol*. 2008;26(13):2124-2130.
48. Moertel CG, Lefkopoulo M, Lipsitz S, Hahn RG, Klaassen D. Streptozocin-doxorubicin, streptozocin-fluorouracil or chlorozotocin in the treatment of advanced islet-cell carcinoma. *N Engl J Med*. 1992;326:519-523.
49. Moertel CG, Hanley JA, Johnson LA. Streptozocin alone compared with streptozocin plus fluorouracil in the treatment of advanced islet-cell carcinoma. *N Engl J Med*. 1980;303:1189-1194.
50. Raymond E, Dahan L, Raoul J-L, et al. Sunitinib malate for the treatment of pancreatic neuroendocrine tumors. *N Engl J Med*. 2011;364:501-513.
51. Yao JC, Shah MH, Ito T, et al. Everolimus for advanced pancreatic neuroendocrine tumors. *N Engl J Med*. 2011;364(6):514-523.
52. Kulke MH, Lenz H-J, Meropol NJ, et al. Activity of sunitinib in patients with advanced neuroendocrine tumors. *J Clin Oncol*. 2008;26:3403-3410.
53. Pavel ME, Hainsworth JD, Baudin E, et al. Everolimus plus octreotide long-acting repeatable for the treatment of advanced neuroendocrine tumours associated with carcinoid syndrome (RADIANT-2): a randomised, placebo-controlled, phase 3 study. *Lancet*. 2011;378(9808):2005-2012.
54. Kulke MH, Bergsland EK, Yao JC. Glycemic control in patients with insulinoma treated with everolimus. *N Engl J Med*. 2009;360:195-197.

Section VII

Breast Cancer

Section Editor: Gabriel N. Hortobagyi

第七篇 乳腺癌

27

Early-Stage and Locally Advanced Breast Cancer

第二十七章　早期和局部进展期乳腺癌

Aron S. Rosenstock
Gabriel N. Hortobagyi

中文导读

本章首先介绍了乳腺癌的流行病学特点，从发病率和死亡率阐述近年来全球变化的趋势。接着介绍了影响乳腺癌发生的危险因素，包括遗传性因素（家族史、基因突变）、乳腺疾病、自身激素状况（月经初潮、初次妊娠、绝经年龄、妊娠）以及外源性激素使用等。乳腺癌的分期参照2010年第7版AJCC的TNM分期。本章随之阐述了乳腺癌的预后因素，包括与病理因素相关的腋窝淋巴结、细胞核分级、激素受体状态、增殖指数、HER2过表达等。关于辅助治疗以及新辅助治疗，本章均分别从化疗、内分泌治疗以及抗HER2靶向治疗这3个方面讲述，并回顾了重要的临床试验结果。本章最后分别从早期乳腺癌（Ⅰ期、Ⅱ期）以及局部进展期乳腺癌（Ⅲ期）的手术、辅助治疗、放疗以及新辅助治疗等方面阐述了MD安德森癌症中心的诊治策略。

EPIDEMIOLOGY

Incidence

Breast cancer is the second most common cause of death for women and is the most common cause of death for women age 45 to 55. In 2015, it is estimated that 231,840 American women would be diagnosed with breast cancer and that 40,290 would die from this disease, making breast cancer the second most common cause of cancer-related morality in the United States, with lung cancer being the most common ([1]).

In the early 1980s, the rates of breast cancer diagnosis rose sharply, likely related to increased mammographic screening, because it was the incidence of stage 0 and I carcinomas that rose most sharply. Data from the Surveillance, Epidemiology, and End Results (SEER) program of the National Cancer Institute demonstrate that although the incidence of breast cancer has been stable since the late 1980s, there has been an increase in the percentage of breast cancers that are hormone receptor positive, which is thought to be due either changes in receptor assays or an increased use of hormone replacement therapy by women ([2, 3]). The incidence of primary breast cancer then decreased around 2003, shortly after the publication of the Women's Health Initiative (WHI) results, which prompted many healthy postmenopausal women to stop using hormone replacement therapy ([4]).

Worldwide Trends

Breast cancer incidence has long varied in different regions of the world. Incidence is highest in Northern Europe and North America and lowest in Asia and Africa. Data suggest that this variability is due not only to environmental factors but also to lifestyle. This is supported by the observation that breast cancer incidence is higher in second-generation Asian immigrants in the United States ([5]).

Mortality

Breast cancer overall mortality rates had been stable for more than 50 years prior to 1989. Starting in the 1990s, there has been a steady decrease in breast cancer deaths every year. Mortality rates declined by 1.4% per year from 1989 to 1995 and by 3.2% per year thereafter. This is thought to be due in part to increased use of mammography, resulting in earlier diagnosis, and the use of effective treatments. Mortality rates continue to be higher for African American women. This is due in part to disparities in health care access that exist both for diagnosis as well as treatment ([6]).

RISK FACTORS

Hereditary

Family History

Although it is known that family history is an important risk factor for breast cancer, only 25% of newly diagnosed patients have a positive family history. The Gail model was the first to incorporate the number of first-degree relatives into a comprehensive model of breast cancer risk assessment ([7]). Claus then assessed the estimated risk of breast cancer based on the number of familial cases and their ages of diagnosis ([8]). It is now well known that the risk for each patient with a positive family history is affected by the age of the family member at diagnosis, the total number of first-degree relatives affected, and the patient's age. Based on data from a large meta-analysis, the risk of breast cancer for a patient with one affected first-degree relative increased 1.80-fold; if there were two affected first-degree relatives, that risk increased 2.93-fold. This risk was then further modified by the age of the patient, such that a woman's risk of breast cancer prior to age 40 was increased to 5.7-fold if one relative was diagnosed prior to age 40 ([9]).

Genetic Mutations

The overall prevalence of specific genetic mutations accounting for breast cancer is rare, accounting for only 5% to 10% of all cases. Risk can be further subdivided based on a patient's history. The most commonly studied mutations are on the *BRCA1* and *BRCA2* genes, although multiple other mutations exist on genes such as *p53*, *ATM*, *CHEK2*, *PTEN*, *MLH1*, *MSH2*, and *PALB2* ([10]). In a study that analyzed 10,000 individuals, excluding those with Ashkenazi ancestry, the prevalence of *BRCA1* and *BRCA2* mutations varied, with a low of 2.9% if the patient and all first- or second-degree relatives had no prior history of breast cancer or ovarian cancer at less than 50 years of age. A maximum prevalence of 81.3% was noted if the patient and any first- or second-degree relative had breast cancer diagnosed at less than 50 years of age and ovarian cancer at any age ([11]). Because genetic testing often leads to complicated medical decisions both for the patient and other family members, it is important to determine whom it is most appropriate to screen by taking into account population-dependent positive and negative predictive values of the test, using statistical models.

Conditions of the Breast

Ductal Carcinoma In Situ and Lobular Carcinoma In Situ

There has been a rapid increase in the literature concerning the epidemiology, natural history, and treatment of ductal carcinoma in situ (DCIS) and lobular carcinoma in situ (LCIS). (See detailed information in Chapter 30).

With DCIS, the 10-year risk of invasive breast cancer is 5% in the contralateral breast. Lobular carcinoma in situ has been regarded as a risk factor for ipsilateral and contralateral breast cancer. Recent research supports that LCIS is a direct precursor of both invasive lobular and ductal carcinoma. For patients diagnosed with LCIS, the risk of developing breast cancer in either breast is 1% a year ([12]).

Natural Hormonal Factors

Age at Menarche

A later age of menarche is protective. One study has reported that for every 2-year delay in menarche, there was a 10% reduction in breast cancer risk ([13]).

Age at First Pregnancy

There is a favorable risk reduction associated with earlier age of pregnancy. Women who give birth for the first time at age 35 have a 1.6-fold higher risk of breast cancer compared with women who were 26 to 27 at time of first birth. Women who are over age 30 at the time of first birth are at higher risk than nulliparous women ([14]).

Age at Menopause

Late menopause is associated with a higher risk of breast cancer. Oophorectomy before age 40 will decrease the lifetime risk of breast cancer by 50% ([15]).

Pregnancy

Breast cancer is the second most common cancer associated with pregnancy, with its incidence being 1 in 3,000. The incidence of pregnancy-associated breast cancer is likely related to the delay of childbirth until after age 30. There are controversial data from two reports suggesting that pregnancy might cause a transient rise in breast cancer risk. However, a clearly documented decreased risk of breast cancer occurs 10 to 15 years after childbirth ([16]). (See detailed information in Chapter 30.)

Exogenous Hormonal Use

Oral Contraceptives

Most studies have not shown an increased risk of breast cancer with oral contraceptive use ([17, 18]). However, a meta-analysis showed a significant but small increase in relative risk of breast cancer ([19]). A concern about the meta-analysis is that follow-up was limited.

Hormone Replacement Therapy

The WHI showed that the relative risk of breast cancer was increased to 1.26 for women who took combined treatment with estrogen and progesterone for a mean of 5.2 years as compared to placebo ([20]). Although long-term hormone replacement therapy was associated with a higher risk of breast cancer, short-term use did not seem to significantly increase the risk of breast cancer.

STAGING OF BREAST CANCER

2010 TNM Revisions

The 2010 seventh edition of the *Cancer Staging Manual* published by the American Joint Committee on Cancer (AJCC) was modified from the prior staging criteria, published in 2002 (Tables 27-1 and 27-2) ([21]).

The changes were based on continuing developments in breast cancer diagnosis and management. Specifically, isolated tumor cells and micrometastases in axillary lymph node staging and M0(i+) for tumor cells in circulation and bone marrow were added. The AJCC also recommended that all specimens have a histologic tumor grade and description of estrogen receptor (ER), progesterone receptor (PR), and human epidermal growth factor receptor 2 (HER2) status.

PROGNOSTIC FACTORS

There is interest in the assessment of prognostic factors in breast cancer. About 30% of patients with node-negative disease will die from a breast cancer–related cause. Thus, there is a great thrust of research to determine markers that could further identify which patients would benefit most from available adjuvant treatment.

Predictive Versus Prognostic Factors

With the growing array of articles in this field, it is important to distinguish predictive prognostic factors. A predictive factor is one that can provide information on the likelihood of response to a given therapeutic intervention. A prognostic factor is one that can provide information on outcome at the time of diagnosis, independent of treatment ([22]). Lymph node status is an example of a prognostic factor; ER status is an example of a prognostic and predictive factor.

Pathologic Factors

Prognosis is still determined in large part by histopathology. Multiple studies showed that the most powerful prognostic factor is the extent of disease in the

Table 27-1 TNM Staging System for Breast Cancer

Primary Tumor (T)		
TX		Primary tumor cannot be assessed
T0		No evidence of primary tumor
Tis		Carcinoma in situ
	Tis (DCIS)	Ductal carcinoma in situ
	Tis (LCIS)	Lobular carcinoma in situ
	Tis (Paget)	Paget disease of the nipple with no tumor
		Note: Paget disease associated with a tumor is classified according to the size of the tumor.
T1		Tumor ≤20 mm in greatest dimension
	T1mi	Microinvasion ≤1 mm in greatest dimension
	T1a	Tumor >1 mm but ≤5 mm in greatest dimension
	T1b	Tumor >5 mm but ≤10 mm in greatest dimension
	T1c	Tumor >10 mm but ≤20 mm in greatest dimension
T2		Tumor >20 mm but ≤50 mm in greatest dimension
T3		Tumor >50 mm in greatest dimension
T4		Tumor of any size with direct extension to
		(a) chest wall or
		(b) skin, only as described below
	T4a	Extension to chest wall, not including pectoralis muscle adherence/invasion
	T4b	Ulceration and/or ipsilateral satellite nodules and/or edema (including peau d'orange) of the skin, which do not meet the criteria for inflammatory carcinoma
	T4c	Both T4a and T4b
	T4d	Inflammatory carcinoma with typical skin changes involving a third or more of the skin of the breast
Regional Lymph Nodes (N)		
NX		Regional lymph nodes cannot be assessed (eg, previously removed)
N0		No regional lymph node metastases
N1		Metastases in movable ipsilateral axillary level I, II axillary lymph node(s)
N2		Metastases in ipsilateral level I, II axillary lymph nodes that are clinically fixed or matted; or in clinically detected ipsilateral internal mammary nodes in the absence of clinically evident axillary lymph node metastases
	N2a	Metastases in ipsilateral level I, II axillary lymph nodes fixed to one another (matted) or to other structures
	N2b	Metastases only in clinically detected ipsilateral internal mammary nodes and in the absence of clinically evident level I, II axillary lymph node metastases
N3		Metastases in ipsilateral infraclavicular (level III axillary) lymph node(s) with or without level I, II axillary lymph node involvement; or in clinically detected[a] ipsilateral internal mammary lymph node(s) with clinically evident level I, II axillary lymph node metastases; or metastases in ipsilateral supraclavicular lymph node(s) with or without axillary or internal mammary lymph node involvement
	N3a	Metastases in ipsilateral infraclavicular lymph node(s)
	N3b	Metastases in ipsilateral internal mammary lymph node(s) and axillary lymph node(s)
	N3c	Metastases in ipsilateral supraclavicular lymph node(s)
Regional Lymph Nodes (pN)		
pNX		Regional lymph nodes cannot be assessed (eg, previously removed or not removed for pathologic study)
pN0		No regional lymph node metastases histologically Note: Isolated tumor cell clusters (ITC) are defined as small clusters of cells not greater than 0.2 mm, or single tumor cells, or a cluster of fewer than 200 cells in a single histologic cross-section. ITCs may be detected by routine histology or by IHC methods. Nodes containing only ITCs are excluded from the total positive node count for purposes of N classification but should be included in the total number of nodes evaluate
	pN0(i–)	No regional lymph node metastases histologically, negative IHC

(Continued)

Table 27-1 TNM Staging System for Breast Cancer (*Continued*)

Regional Lymph Nodes (pN) (cont.)	
pN0(i+)	Malignant cells in regional lymph node(s) no greater than 0.2 mm (detected by H&E or IHC including ITC)
pN0(mol−)	No regional lymph node metastases histologically, negative molecular findings (RT-PCR)
pN0(mol+)	No regional lymph node metastases histologically, positive molecular findings (RT-PCR)
pN1	Micrometastases; or metastases in 1–3 axillary lymph nodes; and/or in internal mammary nodes with metastases detected by sentinel lymph node biopsy but not clinically detected
pN1mi	Micrometastases (>0.2 mm and/or >200 cells, but none >2.0 mm)
pN1a	Metastases in 1–3 axillary lymph nodes, at least one metastasis greater than 2.0 mm
pN1b	Metastases in internal mammary nodes with micrometastases or macrometastases detected by sentinel lymph node biopsy but not clinically detected[a]
pN1c	Metastases in 1–3 axillary lymph nodes and in internal mammary lymph nodes with micrometastases or macrometastases detected by sentinel lymph node biopsy but not clinically detected
pN2	Metastases in 4–9 axillary lymph nodes; or in clinically detected[b] internal mammary lymph nodes in the absence of axillary lymph node metastases
pN2a	Metastases in 4–9 axillary lymph nodes (at least one tumor deposit >2.0 mm)
pN2b	Metastases in clinically detected[b] internal mammary lymph nodes in the absence of axillary lymph node metastases
pN3	Metastases in 10 or more axillary lymph nodes; or in infraclavicular (level III axillary) lymph nodes; or in clinically detected ipsilateral internal mammary lymph nodes in the presence of one or more positive level I, II axillary lymph nodes; or in more than three axillary lymph nodes and in internal mammary lymph nodes with micrometastases or macrometastases detected by sentinel lymph node biopsy but not clinically detected, or in ipsilateral supraclavicular lymph nodes
pN3a	Metastases in 10 or more axillary lymph nodes (at least one tumor deposit >2.0 mm); or metastases to the infraclavicular (level III axillary lymph) nodes
pN3b	Metastases in clinically detected[b] ipsilateral internal mammary lymph nodes in the presence of one or more positive axillary lymph nodes; or in more than three axillary lymph nodes and in internal mammary lymph nodes with micrometastases or macrometastases detected by sentinel lymph node biopsy but not clinically detected
pN3c	Metastases in ipsilateral supraclavicular lymph nodes
Distant Metastases (M)	
M0	No clinical or radiographic evidence of distant metastases
cM0(i+)	No clinical or radiographic evidence of distant metastases, but deposits of molecularly or microscopically detected tumor cells in circulating blood, bone marrow, or other nonregional nodal tissue that are no larger than 0.2 mm in a patient without symptoms or signs of metastases
M1	Distant detectable metastases as determined by classic clinical and radiographic means and/or histologically proven larger than 0.2 mm

H&E, hematoxylin and eosin; IHC, immunohistochemistry; RT-PCR, reverse transcription polymerase chain reaction.
[a]Not clinically detected is defined as not detected by imaging studies (excluding lymphoscintigraphy) or not detected by clinical examination.
[b]Clinically detected is defined as detected by imaging studies (excluding lymphoscintigraphy) or by clinical examination or presumed pathologic macrometastasis based on fine needle aspiration biopsy with cytologic examination.
Reproduced with permission from Edge SB, Byrd DR, Compton CC (eds): *AJCC Cancer Staging Manuarl*, 7th ed. New York, NY: Springer; 2010.

axillary lymph nodes ([23, 24]). Other important pathologic factors are hormone receptor status, HER2 status, histologic grade, tumor type, and lymphovascular invasion.

Axillary Lymph Nodes

More than 30 years ago, it was established that the number of involved lymph nodes could be used to predict disease-free survival (DFS) and overall survival (OS). The 5-year DFS was 62% with 1 to 3 positive axillary lymph nodes, 58% for 4 to 9 positive lymph nodes, and 29% for ≥10 positive lymph nodes ([24]).

Nuclear Grade

Nuclear or histologic grade describes the degree of tumor differentiation and is based on a pathologist's assessment of nuclear size and shape, number of mitoses, and degree of tubule formation. Although a nuclear grade of 1 (most differentiated) to 3 (least differentiated)

CHAPTER 27

Table 27-2 TNM Stage Grouping for Breast Cancer

Stage Grouping			
0	Tis	N0	M0
IA	T1[a]	N0	M0
IB	T0	N1mi	M0
	T1[a]	N1mi	M0
IIA	T0	N1	M0
	T1[a]	N1	M0
	T2	N0	M0
IIB	T2	N1	M0
	T3	N0	M0
IIIA	T0	N2	M0
	T1[a]	N2	M0
	T2	N2	M0
	T3	N1	M0
	T3	N2	M0
IIIB	T4	N0	M0
	T4	N1	M0
	T4	N2	M0
IIIC	Any T	N3	M0
IV	Any T	Any N	M1

[a]T1 includes T1mi.
Reproduced with permission from Edge SB, Byrd DR, Compton CC (eds): *AJCC Cancer Staging Manuarl*, 7th ed. New York, NY: Springer; 2010.

is reported with every breast cancer pathology report, its use in predicting outcome is still debated ([25]). This is in part secondary to interobserver variation in the classification of differentiation. The Nottingham combined grading system seems to be most useful because of its semiquantitative approach and is currently recommended by the College of American Pathologists.

Hormone Receptor Status

Estrogen receptor and PR positivity correlate with prolonged DFS and OS. The importance of hormone receptor status has been documented more consistently in node-positive than in node-negative disease. Immunohistochemical assays have now become the favored approach because they can be used with a variety of specimens. A "positive" specimen is defined as at least 1% of positive cells ([26]).

Proliferative Rate

This can be evaluated by a variety of methods including mitotic figure count, S-phase fraction (the fraction of cells synthesizing DNA) as determined by flow cytometry, thymidine labeling index, and monoclonal antibodies to antigens in proliferating cells. A high S-phase fraction is usually associated with poor differentiation and lack of ER positivity. Antibodies to Ki-67 can be used to determine a proliferative rate that corresponds with the S-phase fraction. A recent meta-analysis showed a positive correlation between high Ki-67 and poor prognosis ([27]).

HER2/neu Overexpression

The *HER2/neu* oncogene codes for a 185-kDa transmembrane glycoprotein that has intracellular tyrosine kinase activity and is a member of the family of epidermal growth factor receptors. This group of receptors has an important role in the activation of epidermal signal transduction pathways controlling for epithelial growth and differentiation. Overexpression of the *HER2/neu* oncogene is present in up to 30% of invasive breast cancers.

The current standard is to perform either fluorescence in situ hybridization (FISH) by single or dual probe or immunohistochemistry (IHC). Breast cancer is defined as HER2-positive overexpressed if IHC is noted to be 3+, which is defined as >10% of membrane staining. By FISH, for single probe, the average copy number is ≥6.0 signals per cell. For dual probe, the *HER2*/CEP17 ratio should be ≥2.0 or if *HER2* copy number is ≥6.0 signals/cell regardless of *HER2*/CEP17 ratio. Equivocal results include IHC 2+ or dual probe FISH *HER2*/CEP17 ratio <2.0 and an *HER2* copy number between 4.0 and 6.0 signals/cell. These results should be confirmed with the other approved diagnostic tests. If results continue to be equivocal, repeat testing or a new biopsy should be considered ([28]).

Prior to the introduction of HER2-targeted therapy, overexpression of *HER2/neu* was associated with shorter DFS and OS ([29]). A large single-institution study reviewed all women with T1a and T1b disease diagnosed between 1990 and 2002. Multivariate analysis of 965 patients showed that patients with HER2-positive tumors had 5.09 times the rate of recurrence and 7.81 times the rate of distant recurrence at 5 years compared to patients with hormone receptor–positive, HER2-negative tumors ([30]). The predictive response with HER2 has been demonstrated in prospective randomized controlled trials (discussed later in the "Adjuvant Therapy" section) ([31, 32]).

Future Thoughts

DNA microarrays classify breast cancer into five major subtypes defined as luminal A, luminal B, basal, HER2 positive, and normal-appearing breast tissue. In a retrospective analysis, these subtypes were associated with differing prognoses ([33]). At present, microarrays for these classifications are too expensive to be performed routinely. Cheaper and more cost-effective diagnostics may change the approach.

ADJUVANT THERAPY

After definitive local therapy is completed, it is important to plan for adjuvant systemic therapy. The use of chemotherapy, hormonal therapy, and targeted therapy before or after definitive local therapy has had a significant effect on the management and outcomes of breast cancers. All women with node-positive disease and a significant percentage of node-negative women with tumors that are hormone receptor negative or >1 cm in size benefit from chemotherapy. The choice of agents to be used for chemotherapy and hormonal therapy should be guided by the patient's age, concomitant medical issues, positive or negative axillary lymph node involvement, and the status of the hormone receptors and HER2. Estimation of risk of recurrence and death should be assessed. Adjuvant! Online is a validated model that estimates DFS and OS based on age, comorbidity, tumor size and grade, hormone receptor status, and number of involved lymph nodes ([34]). Additionally, Onco*type* Dx, Mammaprint, and other assays can help stratify risk for hormone receptor–positive, node-negative patients ([35]).

Chemotherapy

Historical Perspective

Studies in the 1960s and 1970s evaluated whether single-agent chemotherapy after local therapy had any benefit compared with observation alone. The single agents studied included cyclophosphamide, thiotepa, and melphalan. Most reports documented that single agents have modest or no effect on DFS. Subsequently, the focus shifted to polychemotherapy, with most trials evaluating variations of the three-drug regimen of cyclophosphamide, methotrexate, and 5-fluorouracil (CMF) or similar anthracycline-containing regimens ([36, 37]).

These polychemotherapy regimens clearly showed a greater benefit in DFS and OS, but it was often unclear to clinicians which regimens were superior or equivalent. The Oxford Overview in 1998 helped clarity this issue by reviewing data from about 18,000 women in 47 trials that compared polychemotherapy or no chemotherapy, about 6,000 women in 11 trials that compared longer versus shorter polychemotherapy, and about 6,000 women in 11 trials of anthracycline-containing regimens versus CMF ([38]). The final interpretation concluded that adjuvant polychemotherapy for patients under 50 years of age resulted in an absolute improvement in 10-year survival of 7% to 11%, whereas the overall 10-year survival benefit was 2% to 3% for patients age 50 to 69 years.

Anthracyclines

The 1998 Oxford Overview further demonstrated that anthracycline-containing regimens were superior to CMF. There was a statistically significant 12% reduction in risk of recurrence for anthracycline-containing regimens, a 2.7% decrease in mortality, and a 3.2% decrease in relapse. The information gained from this important systematic analysis began a shift toward administration of anthracycline-based regimens for adjuvant therapy of breast cancer.

Official recommendations have been made based on the above data. These were presented at the National Institutes of Health Consensus Development Conference in 2000 and suggested an anthracycline be included as part of breast cancer adjuvant therapy. Several studies have investigated the role of *HER2/neu* in the positive response to anthracyclines. Both the Cancer and Leukemia Group B (CALGB) 8082 and National Surgical Adjuvant Breast and Bowel Project (NSABP) B-11 studies have shown a benefit in DFS in patients who overexpressed *HER2/neu* and received anthracycline therapy ([39, 40]).

Evaluation of 5-fluorouracil, doxorubicin, and cyclophosphamide (FAC) began in 1974 at the University of Texas MD Anderson Cancer Center (MDACC). For 1,107 women with node-positive disease, the results were favorable. The 10-year DFS was 72% for patients with 1 to 3 positive nodes, 55% for patients with 4 to 10 positive nodes, and 36% for those with >10 positive nodes ([41]).

Investigations addressing accelerating the delivery of anthracyclines in a dose-dense manner are discussed later.

Taxanes

The role of taxanes for breast cancer treatment was first investigated in metastatic disease. In randomized trials, paclitaxel and docetaxel improved response rates, duration of response, and OS ([42]). These positive results prompted their investigation in early-stage breast cancer. Several major studies contributed to the current use of taxanes in the adjuvant setting. The CALGB 9344 study evaluated the addition of paclitaxel to doxorubicin and cyclophosphamide (AC) and showed improvements versus placebo in DFS and OS at 69 months of 70% versus 65% and 80% versus 77%, respectively.

The use of docetaxel was evaluated by the Breast Cancer International Research Group (BCIRG) 001 trial, which compared TAC (docetaxel plus AC) versus FAC for the adjuvant treatment of node-positive breast cancer. There was a significant difference in DFS and a trend in OS suggesting docetaxel could reduce the risk of recurrence of breast cancer in the adjuvant setting compared to the standard FAC regimen. However, with the higher rates of myelosuppression and febrile neutropenia seen with TAC, the use of this regimen requires extensive supportive care, including utilization of granulocyte colony-stimulating growth factor ([43, 44])

The Eastern Cooperative Oncology Group (ECOG) E1199 trial attempted to define the more effective adjuvant taxane and the optimal schedule of administration ([45]). All patients received a standard dose and schedule of doxorubicin and cyclophosphamide and were randomized to receive paclitaxel (175 mg/m^2) every 3 weeks for four cycles, paclitaxel (80 mg/m^2) every week for 12 doses, docetaxel (100 mg/m^2) every 3 weeks for four cycles, or docetaxel (35 mg/m^2) every week for 12 doses. Weekly paclitaxel compared to every 3 weeks was better, with an odds ratio of 1.27 for DFS (P = .006) and 1.32 for OS (P = .01). No significant difference existed between paclitaxel and docetaxel. Paclitaxel every 3 weeks was no longer recommended after this trial (Fig. 27-1).

The US09735 trial was a randomized study that compared four cycles of standard-dose AC with four cycles of docetaxel (75 mg/m^2) and cyclophosphamide (TC) (600 mg/m^2). Most patients (84.3%) were younger than 65 years old, and 48% were node negative. At a median follow-up of 7 years, there was a significant difference in DFS between TC and AC (81% vs 75%; hazard ratio, 0.74). Additionally, there was a significant difference in OS (87% vs 82%). Febrile neutropenia in older patients was 8% with TC and 4% with AC ([46]). This indicates that TC is

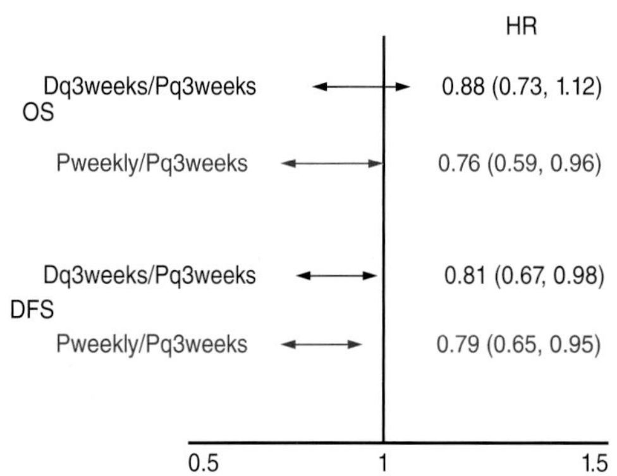

FIGURE 27-1 Results of Eastern Cooperative Oncology Group E1199: Optimal adjuvant taxane and optimal schedule of administration. D, docetaxel; DFS, disease-free survival; HR, hazard ratio; OS, overall survival; P, paclitaxel. (Data from Sparano JA, Wang M, Martino S, et al. Weekly paclitaxel in the adjuvant treatment of breast cancer. *N Engl J Med*. 2008;358:1663-1671.)

a treatment option but should be used with caution in higher risk cancers given the large percentage of young node-negative patients in the study.

Endocrine Therapy

The correlation between the endocrine system and breast cancer was first recognized more than 100 years ago. Beatson first described bilateral oophorectomy in treating inoperable cases of breast cancer ([47]). However, the true understanding of the biological mechanisms that cause estrogen to stimulate the growth of hormone receptor–positive tumors is more recent. Jensen first identified the ER and led subsequent cloning of ER and PR. This knowledge has enabled the development of multiple therapies. Many of these therapies have varying mechanisms of action, but all have the common goal of decreasing estrogen availability for hormone receptor–positive malignancies.

Tamoxifen

Monotherapy

In the late 1970s, tamoxifen was shown to be effective for the treatment of metastatic breast cancer. This form of treatment was well received, because data from trials showed that patients experienced fewer side effects than they did with traditional chemotherapy or with old fashioned endocrine therapy (high-dose estrogens, androgens, adrenalectomy, or hypophysectomy). The proven efficacy of tamoxifen in the metastatic setting enabled its study for adjuvant use.

Tamoxifen was the first targeted drug to be used as an endocrine treatment for early breast cancer. An early placebo-controlled trial of tamoxifen as adjuvant therapy for early breast cancer, NATO, showed that 2 years of tamoxifen treatment reduced treatment failure at 21 months compared with control (14.2% vs 20.5%, respectively) ([48]). Since then, the efficacy of tamoxifen in the adjuvant treatment of primary breast cancer has been demonstrated repeatedly.

Since tamoxifen became available over 35 years ago, a large number of trials investigated its efficacy and tolerability in the treatment of primary breast cancer. Although some individual trials are too small to justify firm conclusions, a meta-analysis has increased confidence in the effectiveness of tamoxifen in improving DFS and OS. Additionally, large cooperative group (NSABP B-14) and international randomized trials (Stockholm and Scottish trials) of tamoxifen versus placebo have demonstrated a clear benefit in DFS and OS ([49-51]).

An overview of 55 trials studying adjuvant tamoxifen for 1, 2, or 5 years versus no treatment in patients with primary breast cancer showed that tamoxifen treatment produced highly significant benefits in terms of both recurrence of first events and mortality in the hormone receptor–positive population. The reductions in recurrence were 21%, 28%, and 50%, and the reductions in death rate were 14%, 18%, and 28% for 1, 2, and 5 years of tamoxifen treatment, respectively ($P < .00001$ for each). Tamoxifen treatment for 1, 2, and 5 years also reduced the incidence of contralateral breast cancer by 13%, 26%, and 47%, respectively ([52]). The benefits occurred almost exclusively in the hormone receptor–positive population. Tamoxifen improves the 10-year survival of women who have ER-positive or ER-unknown tumors.

Further clarification of the optimal treatment duration of tamoxifen was investigated in two large trials: ATTOM (Adjuvant Tamoxifen Treatment Offers More) and ATLAS (Adjuvant Tamoxifen—Longer Against Shorter).

The ATLAS trial enrolled women with early breast cancer who had completed 5 years of tamoxifen and randomly assigned the women to either continue tamoxifen for 10 years or stop at 5 years ([53]). The risk of recurrence during years 5 to 14 was 21.4% versus 25.1% for women who continued tamoxifen versus those who did not. Breast cancer mortality during years 5 to 14 for women who continued tamoxifen versus the control group was 12.2% and 15.0%, respectively. Pulmonary embolus and endometrial cancer occurred significantly more frequently in the extended tamoxifen group (Fig. 27-2).

The ATTOM trial had a similar design to ATLAS ([54]). Women randomized to continue tamoxifen, versus those who stopped tamoxifen, had significantly less breast cancer recurrence (580 of 3,468 patients vs 672 of 3,485 patients, $P = .003$) and significantly decreased breast cancer mortality (392 of 3,468 patients vs 443 of 3,485 patients, $P = .050$). Combining the two trials strengthens the statistical significance of recurrence ($P < .0001$), breast cancer mortality ($P = .002$), and OS ($P = .005$).

With Chemotherapy

The addition of chemotherapy in intermediate- or high-risk groups is recommended ([55]). The Early Breast Cancer Trialists' Collaborative Group (EBCTCG) overviews in 1990 showed that chemotherapy in combination with tamoxifen had a beneficial effect in premenopausal women. The 1998 EBCTCG overview ([52]) showed that the benefits of chemotherapy combined with tamoxifen in patients with ER-positive disease occurred irrespective of age or menopausal status. The benefits of chemotherapy in terms of contralateral breast cancer and improved survival also occurred irrespective of age or menopausal status.

It was not until recently that the appropriate sequence of chemotherapy and hormonal therapy was definitively documented. One difficulty was that evidence had existed in experimental systems that tamoxifen could antagonize the cytotoxic effects of particular chemotherapeutic agents.

One particular study was designed to address the specific timing of tamoxifen therapy ([56]). Patients were divided among three groups: tamoxifen alone, FAC chemotherapy followed by tamoxifen, and concomitant

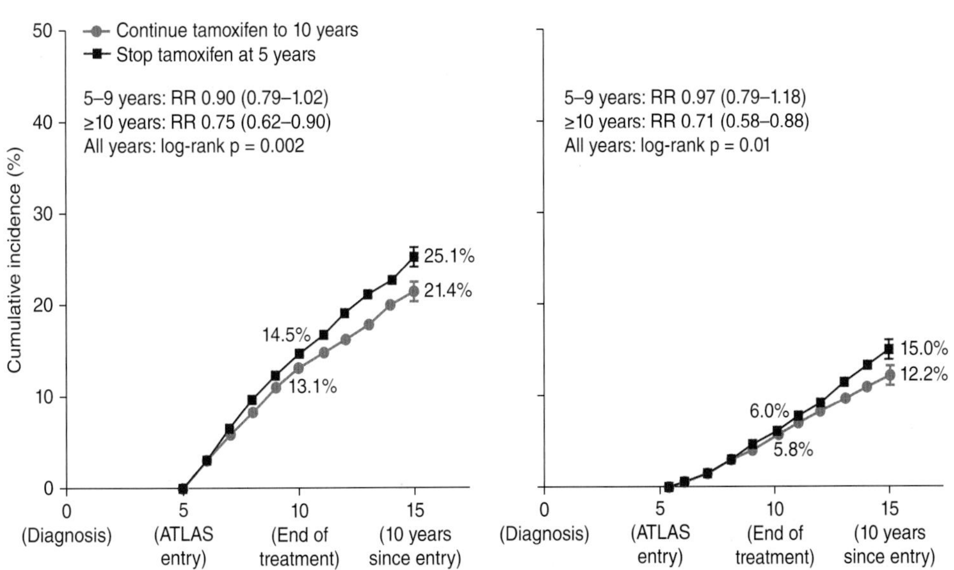

FIGURE 27-2 ATLAS trial studying 5 years versus 10 years of tamoxifen with respect to recurrence (left) and breast cancer mortality (right). RR, relative risk. (Reproduced with permission from Davies C, Pan H, Godwin J, et al. Long-term effects of continuing adjuvant tamoxifen to 10 years versus stopping at 5 years after diagnosis of oestrogen receptor-positive breast cancer: ATLAS, a randomised trial. *Lancet*. 2013 Mar 9;381(9869):805-816.)

FAC and tamoxifen. Patients were followed up for a median of 8.5 years. The estimated DFS was 67% in the sequential treatment group compared with 62% in the concurrent treatment group.

Aromatase Inhibitors

First Line

Although tamoxifen has proven efficacy for the treatment of hormone receptor–positive breast cancer both alone and in combination with chemotherapy, its usefulness is in part curtailed by its partial estrogen agonist activity. The documented negative secondary effects of tamoxifen include an increased incidence of endometrial cancer, uterine sarcoma, and thromboembolic disease. Thus, there is great interest in exploring other endocrine therapies.

In women whose ovarian function has ceased, the primary remaining estrogen source is the conversion of adrenal androgens to estrogens in peripheral tissues by the cytochrome P450 enzyme aromatase. Aromatase inhibitors (AIs) reduce the availability of estrogen by inhibiting the aromatase enzyme and are indicated for the treatment of breast cancer in postmenopausal women whose ovarian function has ceased ([57]). The first-generation AI aminoglutethimide became available 25 years ago but was limited by excessive toxicity. Newer generation selective AIs, including anastrozole, letrozole, fadrozole, and exemestane, are now available for the treatment of metastatic breast cancer and in the adjuvant setting. Common side effects of all AIs include hot flashes, osteoporosis, arthritis, and joint and muscle pains.

Based on the antitumor activity of the third-generation AIs in the setting of metastatic disease, these drugs were evaluated in the adjuvant setting. The ATAC (Arimidex [anastrozole], Tamoxifen, Alone or in Combination) trial was a double-blind, multicenter study of postmenopausal women with invasive operable breast cancer who had completed primary therapy and were eligible for adjuvant treatment. They were randomized to tamoxifen, anastrozole, or a combination of the two ([58]). Time to recurrence was significantly longer with anastrozole versus tamoxifen in the overall population, with a larger benefit seen in the hormone receptor–positive population. A reduction in the incidence of contralateral breast cancers favored anastrozole, with statistical significance in the hormone receptor–positive population. The DFS estimates at 4 years were 86.9% and 84.5% for anastrozole and tamoxifen, respectively ([59]).

Anastrozole was associated with significantly fewer withdrawals from treatment than tamoxifen (21.9% vs 26.0%, $P = .0002$) and significantly fewer withdrawals due to adverse events (7.8% vs 11.1%, $P < .0001$). Anastrozole also resulted in a lower incidence of hot flashes, vaginal discharge, and vaginal bleeding ($P < .0001$ for each), of ischemic cerebrovascular events and thromboembolic events ($P = .0006$ for each), including deep venous thrombosis ($P = .02$), and of endometrial cancer ($P = .02$). Tamoxifen resulted in a lower incidence of musculoskeletal disorders (including myalgias and arthralgias) and fractures ($P < .0001$ for both). The tolerability results in the updated analysis showed no major difference from those seen in the first analysis ([60]).

A meta-analysis published in 2010 reviewed the use of AIs versus tamoxifen in postmenopausal women with ER-positive tumors. This review compared AIs as initial monotherapy to tamoxifen monotherapy or as a hormone switch after 2 to 3 years of tamoxifen for a total of 5 years. The conclusion was that AI therapy was associated with a lower rate of recurrence when used as an initial monotherapy or after 2 to 3 years of tamoxifen when compared to tamoxifen monotherapy ([61]).

Following Tamoxifen

It is postulated that tamoxifen might stop being effective because breast cancer cells develop resistance to tamoxifen, dependence on tamoxifen, or great sensitivity to circulating estrogen. Consequently, the use AIs after tamoxifen was investigated. The MA-17 trial showed that the addition of letrozole after 5 years of tamoxifen resulted in a significant improvement in DFS ([62]).

The Breast International Group (BIG) 1-98 trial compared letrozole versus tamoxifen in postmenopausal hormone receptor–positive women and was later amended to include two sequential strategies using letrozole either before or after tamoxifen for a total of 5 years. The results showed that upfront AI reduced the risk of recurrence and improved DFS better than upfront tamoxifen and better than either switching strategy ([63, 64]).

Another double-blind randomized trial investigated the use of exemestane to complete the 5 years of adjuvant endocrine treatment after 2 to 3 years of tamoxifen in postmenopausal women with primary breast cancer ([65]). The results showed that exemestane improved the absolute benefit in DFS by 4.7% Thus, exemestane therapy following 2 to 3 years of tamoxifen significantly improved DFS.

The above data for therapy beyond 5 years of tamoxifen is becoming more convincing, and AIs should be considered as extended therapy for high-risk postmenopausal patients. In general, outcomes with antiestrogen therapies are hindered by noncompliance, with 20% to 50% nonadherence rates. This is the same difficulty faced in other disease states, and a cancer diagnosis does not necessarily command optimal compliance with oral therapy. Many barriers influence compliance including medication cost, access to mail-order pharmacies, and a lack of understanding of the benefits of such medicine. A population-based study performed in British Columbia noted that adherence was still difficult even when these oral agents were given free of charge in a country with a national formulary system. Patients who are on oral medication should be followed regularly, and compliance should be reinforced as highly important, as shown in multiple studies, even when drug cost is not a barrier ([66]).

Ovarian Ablation and Suppression

The use of oophorectomy or ovarian irradiation to cause ovarian ablation is an efficacious method for treating early-stage disease in premenopausal patients. The 1996 meta-analysis by the EBCTCG demonstrated that for women below age 50 there was a distinct advantage in OS and DFS when they were treated with ovarian ablation versus no adjuvant therapy. In addition, the outcomes for these patients were similar to those who received the CMF regimen. The ZEBRA trial displayed similar results in hormone receptor–positive patients when comparing a luteinizing hormone–releasing hormone (LH-RH) analog, goserelin, to CMF ([67]).

The TEXT and SOFT trials were designed to determine the value of the addition of adjuvant ovarian suppression to tamoxifen or exemestane in premenopausal hormone receptor–positive breast cancer patients. The patients were randomized to receive tamoxifen, tamoxifen plus ovarian suppression, or exemestane plus ovarian suppression for 5 years. In the total population, the addition of ovarian suppression to tamoxifen did not produce a significant benefit. However, in the high-risk cohort who received chemotherapy, ovarian suppression plus tamoxifen improved outcomes when compared to tamoxifen alone. The combined analysis also showed that 5-year DFS with adjuvant endocrine therapy with exemestane was significantly more effective than tamoxifen when ovarian suppression was added. Longer follow-up is needed to evaluate survival data ([68, 69]).

Ovarian suppression does come at significant costs because the adverse effects are not trivial. In these trials, women receiving ovarian suppression developed significant hot flashes, vaginal dryness, depression, and possible long-term health implications like hypertension, diabetes, and osteoporosis.

HER2 Targeted Therapy

Trastuzumab is a high-affinity humanized monoclonal antibody that recognizes the *HER2/neu* receptor and is a targeted therapeutic for tumors that overexpress this growth factor receptor. Trastuzumab has been evaluated extensively in the *HER2/neu*-overexpressing metastatic setting and has been shown to be effective as a single agent both before ([70]) and after chemotherap, ([71]) and in combination with multiple agents ([72]). One notable side effect has been a high rate of cardiotoxicity, particularly when trastuzumab is combined with anthracycline-based chemotherapy. This is due in part to overlapping toxicities and the long half-life of trastuzumab (up to 32 days). The toxicity rarely occurs in patients without a history of cardiac disease and not previously or simultaneously exposed to chemotherapy, especially anthracyclines ([73]).

Therefore trastuzumab was an accepted and standard therapy for metastatic breast cancer that overexpresses *HER2/neu*. The safety and efficacy of trastuzumab-based therapy were then established for earlier stage breast cancer with the NSABP B-31 and North Central Cancer Treatment Group (NCCTG) N9831 trials, where patients received AC plus paclitaxel with the addition of trastuzumab versus placebo.

The joint analysis of these trials showed an absolute difference in DFS of 12% at 3 years and a 33% reduction in the risk of death ($P = .015$) ([74]). An updated analysis with a mean time of 8.4 years on study showed a 37% relative improvement in OS (95% confidence interval [CI], 0.54-0.73; $P < .001$) and an increase in 10-year OS from 75.2% to 84% ([75]).

The BCIRG 006 trial was designed to evaluate the efficacy and safety of docetaxel and carboplatin plus 52 weeks of trastuzumab (TCH) ([32]). Patients were randomly assigned to standard doses of doxorubicin and cyclophosphamide followed by docetaxel (100 mg/m^2) every 3 weeks (AC-T), the same regimen plus 52 weeks

Table 27-3 Five-Year Rates of Recurrence of Patients in SOFT and TEXT Stratified by Chemotherapy Use

	No Chemotherapy			Previous Chemotherapy		
	E + OS	T + OS	T	E + OS	T + OS	T
5-Year Rate, %	(n = 470)	(n = 473)	(n = 476)	(n = 544)	(n = 542)	(n = 542)
FBC	97.1	95.1	95.8	85.7	82.5	78
FDR	99.3	98.7	98.6	87.8	84.8	83.6

E, exemestane; FBC, freedom from breast cancer; FDR free from distant recurrence; OS, ovarian suppression; T, tamoxifen.
Data from Francis PA, Regan MM, Fleming G, et al. Adjuvant ovarian suppression in premenopausal breast cancer. *N Engl J Med*. 2015;372(5):436-446.

CHAPTER 27

of trastuzumab (AC-TH), or docetaxel (75 mg/m^2) and carboplatin (area under the curve [AUC] 6 mg/mL/min) plus 52 weeks of trastuzumab (TCH). At a median follow-up of 65 months, the 5-year estimated DFS was 75% for patients receiving AC-T, 84% with AC-T, and 81% with TCH. Estimated rates of OS were 87%, 92%, and 91%, respectively. All trastuzumab regimens were statistically superior for DFS and OS to nontrastuzumab regimens. There were significant difference in both DFS and OS between AC-TH and TCH. Rates of cardiac dysfunction were significantly higher with AC-TH compared with TCH ($P = .001$).

The PHARE trial attempted to answer the appropriate duration for trastuzumab by comparing 6 versus 12 months of adjuvant therapy. After a median follow-up of 42.5 months, the 2-year DFS rate was 93.8% for the 12-month group versus 91.1% for the 6-month group, with a hazard ratio of 1.28 (95% CI, 1.05-1.56). These results support continuing with the standard of care of 1 year of trastuzumab ([76]).

The HERA trial was also designed to answer the question regarding the optimal duration of trastuzumab. Patients were assigned to observation or 1 or 2 years of trastuzumab. Patients were allowed a variety of standard neoadjuvant or adjuvant chemotherapies and had node-positive or high-risk node-negative disease. A recent update includes mature data from patients receiving trastuzumab for 2 years. Comparing 1 year of trastuzumab versus observation revealed a hazard ratio of 0.76 (95% CI, 0.67-0.86; $P < .0001$) for DFS and 0.76 (95% CI, 0.65-0.88; $P = .0005$) for OS despite significant (52%) crossover. No significant differences in DFS or OS were noted between the 1- and 2-year groups ([31]).

NEOADJUVANT THERAPY

Chemotherapy

The concept of giving chemotherapy in the preoperative setting was first evaluated more than 30 years ago for the treatment of locally advanced and inoperable breast cancer. There are multiple possible benefits. One is the ability to downstage a tumor, which would result in making an unresectable tumor operable or enable breast-conserving surgery or segmental mastectomies to be offered to a greater number of patients with operable breast cancer. In addition, there are biological advantages, such as the ability to assess response or resistance to chemotherapy early, delivering the chemotherapy prior to surgical alterations to the vasculature, and using molecular profiling in conjunction with pathologic response to predict outcomes for patients.

In 1978, a study was published that addressed whether there was a benefit for patients with inoperable breast cancer treated with neoadjuvant chemotherapy. A total of 110 patients were enrolled and were treated with doxorubicin and vincristine. Complete response was seen in 16% of patients, and partial response was seen in 55% of patients. All patients also received standard radiation therapy. The 36-month survival rates were 53% for the study group and 41% for the historical controls. The positive results of this study led to other trials ([77]).

The NSABP B-18 trial was the largest to date to investigate neoadjuvant chemotherapy. A total of 1,523 patients with T1 to T3 and N0 to N1 disease were randomized to receive preoperative versus postoperative AC for four cycles ([78]). Results showed a significant increase in lumpectomies in the neoadjuvant group. Final comparison of the two groups showed no difference in DFS or OS at 5 years. This was true for all groups including tumors larger than 5 cm.

Another trial investigated downstaging of axillary nodal metastases after primary chemotherapy ([79]). From Cox regression analysis, it was shown that one of the parameters associated with poor distant disease–free survival was persistent nodal involvement after neoadjuvant therapy. Thus, it was concluded that the response of the axillary nodes to neoadjuvant chemotherapy was a better predictor than the response of the primary tumor.

In general, neoadjuvant therapy with either anthracycline- or taxane-containing regimens has been shown in multiple trials to result in an increase in the number of women able to undergo breast-conserving surgery. Studies have also shown that the use of neoadjuvant therapy, especially with taxanes, can lead to pathologic complete responses (pCRs) as well as clinical responses ([80]). These responses have been well correlated to DFS and OS, making response to preoperative chemotherapy a novel prognostic factor in the treatment of early and locally advanced breast cancer. At this time, the majority of neoadjuvant studies have not yet shown an increase in OS for patients treated with this approach. Preoperative chemotherapy is especially clinically warranted for patients with tumors greater than 3 cm and for axillary node disease.

Endocrine Therapy

Most studies have investigated the potential of using this approach for patients with locally advanced disease rather than early-stage disease. It is a treatment option for women with tumors expressing ER, PR, or both and for patients with low histologic grade tumors.

At this time, neoadjuvant hormonal therapy based on trial results seems to be best suited to women who have locally advanced breast cancer who are otherwise thought to be not suitable for neoadjuvant chemotherapy or whose tumors are noted to be low-grade with expression of ER or PR ([81, 82]). However, the standard neoadjuvant approach for node-positive or locally advanced breast cancer remains chemotherapy.

HER2 Targeted Therapy

The addition of trastuzumab to standard chemotherapy when given neoadjuvantly has been shown to have improved pathologic responses ([83]). Additionally, neoadjuvant therapy has helped accelerate approval of promising drugs because clinical and pathologic responses can be quickly obtained.

Dual blockade of the HER2 signaling is currently under investigation. Lapatinib, a tyrosine kinase inhibitor that blocks both HER2 and *EGFR*, improved progression-free survival when given with capecitabine in the metastatic setting ([84]). In the NeoALTTO trial, trastuzumab and lapatinib (1,000 mg PO daily) were investigated in the neoadjuvant setting. The pCR was significantly higher with both medications (51.3%) versus trastuzumab alone (29.5%; difference 21.1%, 9.1-34.2%, $P = .0001$) ([85]).

The interest in lapatinib was blunted by the first results from the ALTTO trial presented at the American Society of Clinical Oncology (ASCO) annual conference in Chicago in 2014 ([86]). The four-arm trial compared 1 year of lapatinib alone, trastuzumab alone, or both agents in sequence or in combination. After 4.5 years of follow up, DFS was not significantly different between the patients receiving trastuzumab alone versus the patients receiving the combination. This was surprising given the doubling of the pCR rate seen in NeoALTTO. Additional follow-up is necessary for both trials.

Pertuzumab is a monoclonal antibody that inhibits dimerization with other HER receptors, notably HER3, and binds to an independent domain from trastuzumab. With impressive results in the metastatic setting ([87]), pertuzumab was studied in the neoadjuvant setting.

The NeoSphere trial was designed to evaluate the safety and efficacy of pertuzumab along with trastuzumab in locally advanced, inflammatory, and early HER2-positive breast cancer ([88]). The phase II study randomly assigned patients to four treatment groups: trastuzumab plus docetaxel (75 mg/m^2, escalating if tolerated to 100 mg/m^2, every 3 weeks); pertuzumab (loading dose of 840 mg, followed by 420 mg every 3 weeks) and trastuzumab plus docetaxel; pertuzumab plus trastuzumab; or pertuzumab plus docetaxel. After completing this regimen, all patients underwent surgery and then received 5-fluorouracil (600 mg/m^2), epirubicin (90 mg/m^2) and cyclophosphamide 600 mg/m^2) (FEC) every 3 weeks. The results were that 45.8% (95% CI, 36.1%-55.7%) of patients receiving dual HER2-targeted therapy with docetaxel achieved a pCR compared with 29.0% (95% CI, 20.6%-38.5%) of patients receiving trastuzumab and docetaxel alone (Fig. 27-3).

The TRYPHAENA trial was a phase II that explored the tolerability and efficiency of pertuzumab and trastuzumab given with three different chemotherapy regimens ([89]). All patients had HER2-positive node-positive or node-negative disease but at least a total of T2. Two hundred twenty-five patients were randomized to receive one of the following regimens FEC (doses of 500 mg/m^2, 100 mg/m^2, 600 mg/m^2 respectively) with trastuzumab and pertuzumab followed by docetaxel (FEC+H+P × 3 → T+H+P × 3; arm A); FEC followed by docetaxel plus pertuzumab and trastuzumab all at same dose and schedule as (FEC → T+H+P × 3; arm B); or carboplatin (AUC6) and docetaxel plus pertuzumab and trastuzumab (TCHP × 6; arm CC). Upon completion of chemotherapy, all patients underwent surgery and then received adjuvant trastuzumab to complete 1 full year. The majority of patients achieved pCR in the breast (61.6% in arm A, 57.3% in arm B, and 66.2% in arm C), with pCR including lymph nodes in 50.7% (arm A), 45.3% (arm B), and 51.9% of patients (arm C). Eleven patients had declines in left ventricular ejection fraction to less than 50%, and diarrhea was the most common adverse event (Fig. 27-4).

Given the results of these phase II trials, the US Food and Drug Administration granted accelerated approval of pertuzumab in combination with docetaxel for neoadjuvant therapy for node-positive or greater than T2 HER2-positive breast cancer.

OTHER SYSTEMIC THERAPY TOPICS

Dose Density

One approach to increase response rate to chemotherapy is dose density. This term refers to the

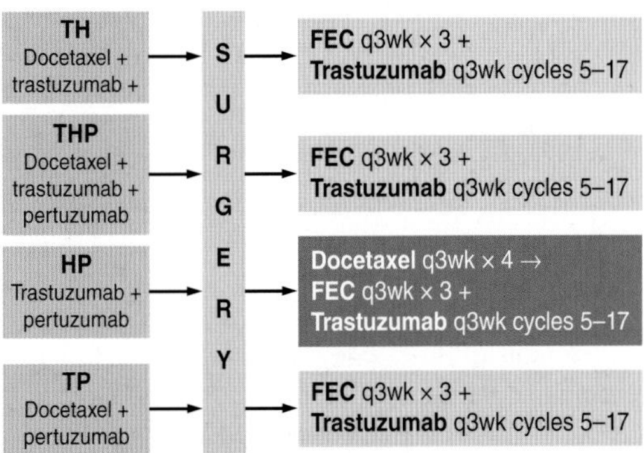

FIGURE 27-3 NeoSphere study design. FEC, 5-fluorouracil, epirubicin, and cyclophosphamide. (Data from Gianni L, Pienkowski T, Im YH, et al. Efficacy and safety of neoadjuvant pertuzumab and trastuzumab in women with locally advanced, inflammatory, or early HER2-positive breast cancer (NeoSphere): a randomised multicentre, open-label, phase 2 trial. *Lancet Oncol.* 2012;13:25-32.)

CHAPTER 27

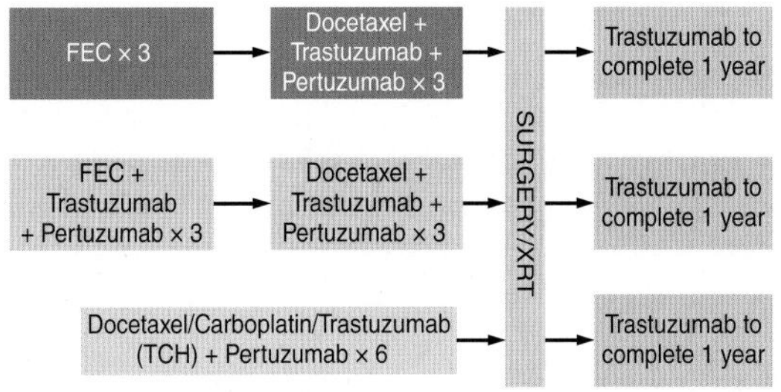

FIGURE 27-4 TRYPHAENA study design. FEC, 5-fluorouracil, epirubicin, and cyclophosphamide; XRT, radiotherapy. (Data from Schneeweiss A, Chia S, Hickish T, et al. Pertuzumab plus trastuzumab in combination with standard neoadjuvant anthracycline-containing and anthracycline-free chemotherapy regimens in patients with HER2-positive early breast cancer: a randomized phase II cardiac safety study (TRYPHAENA). *Ann Oncol*. 2013;24:2278-2284.)

administration of chemotherapeutic agents with a shortened interval between treatments, based on the knowledge that a given dose always kills a particular fraction of cancer cells. More frequent administration of cytotoxic therapy may thus be more efficacious than dose escalation to reduce tumor burden. Several recently published trials have explored dose-density regimens.

The CALGB 9741 trial explored the possible superiority of dose-dense over conventional scheduling of adjuvant chemotherapy for node-positive breast cancer ([90]). Patients were randomly assigned to receive doxorubicin, cyclophosphamide, and paclitaxel (175 mg/m^2) either in 2-week or 3-week schedules, with growth factor support provided to the dose-dense schedule. At a median follow-up of 36 months, dose-dense treatment improved DFS to 82% (every 2 weeks) versus 75% (every 3 weeks) (P = .01). OS was also improved (92% with every 2 weeks vs 90% with every 3 weeks; P = .013). There was no difference between OS or DFS between the sequential and concurrent schedules.

As noted in the "Taxanes" section, E1199 demonstrated a significant improvement of weekly paclitaxel over paclitaxel every 3 weeks ([45]). It is not clear whether the benefit demonstrated in CALGB 9741 is from the dose-dense nature of the anthracycline or the schedule of the taxane. Additionally, NSABP B-38 found no significant difference in outcomes between TAC for 6 cycles and dose-dense AC with weekly paclitaxel ([91]).

Lastly, the Southwest Oncology Group (SWOG) S0221 trial compared weekly paclitaxel (80 mg/m^2) versus dose-dense paclitaxel (175 mg/m^2) in node-positive breast cancer patients who had already received AC ([92]). The results showed equivalent 5-year PFS between the weekly (82%) and biweekly regimens (81%). The weekly schedule was less toxic and did not require growth factor supplementation.

Oncotype DX

Recent efforts have identified multigene assays that can help quantify a patient's risk of breast cancer recurrence ([35]). Onco*type* DX is a commercially available, validated laboratory test performed on a tumor specimen that analyzes 21 genes associated with receptor expression, proliferation, invasion, and other factors. Calculations based on the expression of these 21 genes result in a recurrence score that relays the likelihood of breast cancer recurrence in the first 10 years after diagnosis ([93]). These studies found that patients with a low recurrence score derive little benefit from chemotherapy, whereas those with a high recurrence score are likely to benefit from chemotherapy. For women with an intermediate recurrence score, the benefit of chemotherapy was uncertain. To elucidate the benefit of systemic cytotoxic therapy for this middle group, ECOG has designed a trial known at TAILORx, the Trial Assigning Individualized Options for Treatment ([94]). This study randomly assigned node-negative, HER2/neu-negative, hormone receptor–positive women with early breast cancer with a mid-range recurrence score to treatment with either hormonal therapy or chemotherapy followed by hormonal therapy. Disease-free survival, recurrence-free interval, and OS will be compared in these large cohorts.

Data are emerging that perhaps analysis of 21 genes is not better than immunohistochemical analysis of receptor status and Ki-67 percentage. A prognostic score based on staining of ER, PR, HER2/neu, and Ki-67, known collectively as IHC4, correlated with the prognostic information provided by the Onco*type* DX score ([95]). This may scale back the elaborate, costly, and time-consuming testing that currently accompanies the evaluation of early-stage breast cancer. The observation regarding IHC4 is based on a single-institution report and requires validation.

The use of a genomic-derived recurrence score helps predict recurrences in patients with node-negative, hormone receptor–positive early breast cancer. However, the details regarding which assay will emerge as most useful, innovative, and cost-effective remain to be seen. The important question is how to manage intermediate-risk patients in terms of adjuvant therapy. Today, intermediate-risk patients should be counseled regarding the uncertainty of their benefit with chemotherapy and encouraged to enroll on clinical trials.

MD ANDERSON CANCER CENTER MANAGEMENT STRATEGIES

Early-Stage Breast Cancer (Stages I and II)

At MDACC, every effort is made to integrate clinical information with imaging, pathologic staging, and molecular characteristics to optimize treatment efficacy and, whenever possible, perform breast-conserving surgery. A multidisciplinary approach is of upmost importance, especially with regard to planning and combined-modality therapy. Stage I breast cancer includes primary malignancies ≤2 cm in greatest dimension that do not involve the lymph nodes and microinvasive tumors that are ≤0.1 cm in greatest dimension. Stage II breast cancer encompasses primary tumors of 2 to 5 cm that can involve ipsilateral axillary lymph nodes and tumors >5 cm without lymph node involvement. All patients at MDACC (including those with DCIS) undergo receptor testing for hormone receptor status for ER and PR. In addition, patients are tested for *HER2/neu* status by IHC, and 2+ results are confirmed by FISH.

Stage I

Breast-Conserving Therapy

Breast-conserving surgery (BCS), or segmental resection, has revolutionized patient care for breast cancer over the last two decades. Women are able to preserve their breasts without a negative effect on survival. Breast-conserving therapy involves the surgical removal of tumor followed by radiation therapy to the breast. Multiple studies have shown that patients with stage I breast cancer treated with BCS have DFS and OS rates similar to patients treated with modified radical mastectomies ([96]).

There are only a few true absolute contraindications to BCS, including persistently positive resection margins, multicentric disease, diffuse malignant-appearing microcalcifications, a history of prior radiation to the breast or mantle region (for Hodgkin disease), and pregnancy, although it might be possible to perform BCS in the third trimester. Relative contraindications include a history of connective tissue disease suggesting that radiation would be poorly tolerated, centrally located tumors involving the nipple-areolar complex, and a large tumor in a small breast that might lead to a poor cosmetic result. Although the final decision about whether to offer BCS is left to the discretion of surgical colleagues, most patients who do not meet one of the absolute or relative contraindications are offered this surgical approach.

Risk Factors for Ipsilateral Recurrence With Breast-Conserving Surgery

The risk of ipsilateral tumor recurrence ranges from 0.5% to 2.0% per year. Risk factors include age <35 years, an extensive intraductal component, major lymphocytic stromal reaction, peritumoral invasion, positive margins of resection, and presence of tumor necrosis.

Axillary Lymph Node Dissection

Sentinel lymph node biopsy is the standard of care for patients with clinically negative axilla. In accordance with the American College of Surgeons Oncology Group (ACOSOG) Z0011 trial, patients undergoing BCS with T1 or T2 tumors with less than three positive sentinel nodes can forgo complete axillary dissection if they are treated with whole-breast irradiation. Otherwise, if a positive sentinel node is identified, complete axillary node dissection should be performed ([97]).

Radiation Therapy After Breast-Conserving Surgery

Patients with node-negative disease are treated to achieve a total dose of 50 Gy with an approximate dose of 2 Gy/d on a schedule of 5 days per week for a total of 5 weeks. A boost of radiation to the tumor bed is standard. Regional nodal irradiation is no longer used for negative axillary lymph nodes. Radiation is usually begun after chemotherapy is completed, but it can be given concomitantly with hormone-based therapy.

Adjuvant Therapy

HER2-Negative Tumors

Based on data detailed in the earlier section on adjuvant therapy, both pre- and postmenopausal women are offered chemotherapy. We do not routinely give chemotherapy to patients with node-negative breast tumors that are ER positive and/or PR positive and HER2/neu negative. For these patients, we are incorporating the use of the Onco*type* DX test for an estimation of the risk of recurrence (see the "Other Systemic Therapy Topics" section). Patients with a low recurrence score are recommended for adjuvant endocrine therapy. Patients with a high recurrence score are counseled for chemotherapy followed by endocrine therapy. Patients with a mid-range recurrence score are offered a choice of either therapy. Our current standard chemotherapy is either dose-dense AC for four cycles followed by weekly paclitaxel for 12 weeks or FAC for 4 weeks preceded by weekly paclitaxel for 12 weeks.

Chemotherapy is usually initiated 2 to 4 weeks after surgery. Studies have shown that delaying chemotherapy for up to 8 to 10 weeks does not have a negative effect on the development of metastasis or survival.

Chemotherapy is administered if the absolute neutrophil count is ≥1,000/μL and platelets are ≥100,000/μL. A complete blood count with differential is checked prior to each chemotherapy cycle and weekly after the first cycle. Growth factor support is always given for dose-dense AC plus paclitaxel and TAC but otherwise is not routinely used. If both chemotherapy and endocrine therapy are used, we give chemotherapy first followed by endocrine therapy. If indicated, radiotherapy follows chemotherapy.

Endocrine Therapy

Estrogen Receptor– and/or Progesterone Receptor–Positive Tumors

Our standard approach, based on previously described information, is to treat receptor-positive stage I disease using a hormonal treatment regimen. Based on the ATAC trial data discussed previously, tamoxifen is given to premenopausal women and AI to postmenopausal women. The ATLAS and ATTOM trials suggest extending tamoxifen to 10 years, which is now recommended. Postmenopausal patients are recommended to receive 5 years of an AI. Endocrine therapies are begun after completion of chemotherapy but can be given concomitantly with radiation therapy (Table 27-4). Given the results of the TEXT and SOFT trials, ovarian suppression therapy is now discussed with premenopausal patients, particularly the younger higher risk patients who received chemotherapy.

HER2-Positive Tumors

Patients with HER2-positive tumors benefit significantly from trastuzumab addition to chemotherapy. For node-negative patients with tumors less than 2.0 cm, the standard of care is AC for four cycles followed by trastuzumab and paclitaxel for 12 weeks or paclitaxel, carboplatin, and trastuzumab for six cycles. Trastuzumab is then given alone to complete 1 full year. If the tumor is hormone receptor–positive, patients are recommended to initiate their antiestrogen therapy once chemotherapy has been completed.

Table 27-4 Adjuvant Endocrine Treatment Regimens Commonly Used at the MD Anderson Cancer Center[a]

Premenopausal	Postmenopausal
Tamoxifen 20 mg PO daily for 10 years	Anastrozole 1 mg PO daily for 5 years
or	or
Goserelin 3.6 mg SC every 4 weeks + anastrozole 1 mg PO daily for 5 years (high-risk patients)	Tamoxifen 20 mg PO daily for 10 years

[a]Based on ATAC, ATLAS, TEXT, and SOFT data in women PO, oral; SC, subcutaneous.

Stage II

Surgery

As with stage I disease, multiple studies of stage II patients treated with either BCS or modified radical mastectomy have documented similar long-term outcomes. Patients with tumors >4 to 5 cm are often not considered to be ideal candidates for BCS because of the potential for residual tumor and poor cosmetic result. These patients are usually treated with neoadjuvant systemic therapy. Patients with strongly ER-positive, PR-positive, HER2-negative, low-grade or low Ki-67 tumors would either have a mastectomy or be offered neoadjuvant endocrine therapy.

Radiation Therapy

After Breast-Conserving Surgery

Radiation of the breast after this form of surgery is similar in terms of area treated and dose given to the treatment of stage I. Regional nodal irradiation to negative axillary lymph nodes is not routinely given. Some groups recommend irradiation of the supraclavicular fossa or internal mammary chain for those with positive lymph nodes.

After Mastectomy

Postmastectomy irradiation should be considered for patients with positive postmastectomy margins, primary tumors >5 cm, or four or more positive lymph nodes. The ASCO clinical care guidelines recommend the routine use of postmastectomy radiation for women with stage III or T3 disease or those with four or more positive lymph nodes ([98]).

According to current recommendations, the dose to be delivered ranges from 45 to 50 Gy. Electron boosts to doses of 60 Gy can be considered if there is gross residual disease or positive margins. Treatment of the axilla in the absence of gross residual disease, even for patients with multiple positive lymph nodes, is not routinely recommended.

Neoadjuvant Therapy

Neoadjuvant therapy is typically given to patients with positive axillary nodal involvement. These institutional guidelines are based on information previously discussed under the sections "Neoadjuvant Therapy" and "Dose Density." Neoadjuvant therapy for HER2-negative patients uses the same regimens discussed in the adjuvant section. Patients with HER2-positive, node-positive disease or T2 tumors are strongly advised to receive neoadjuvant therapy in order to receive pertuzumab. The regimens offered are those used in the NeoSphere or TRYPHAENA (see Figs. 27-5 and 27-6) clinical trials, while substituting epirubicin for doxorubicin. Following surgery, patients complete a full year of trastuzumab.

Clinical response is documented by serial imaging examinations, usually ultrasound or magnetic resonance imaging. If there is evidence of a level of response that could possibly lead to a tumor pCR, a marker is placed in the breast to identify the primary tumor site. This is done to guide resection, so that if a pCR has occurred, the "scar" tissue from the prior tumor can be resected.

Adjuvant Therapy

Chemotherapy

Patients who do not meet the criteria for neoadjuvant therapy or those who prefer upfront surgery are treated with adjuvant chemotherapy in a fashion similar to those with stage I breast cancer. Data are lacking for pertuzumab in the adjuvant setting. Consequently, patients with HER2-positive breast cancer receive adjuvant chemotherapy regimens with trastuzumab alone.

Endocrine Therapy

Whether patients are treated with neoadjuvant or adjuvant therapy, those with hormone receptor–positive tumors are treated with hormone-based therapy in a similar fashion to those with stage I breast cancer.

Locally Advanced Breast Cancer (Stage III)

About 10% of new patients present with locally advanced breast cancer. These patients usually have easily palpable tumors with large breast masses and/or axillary nodal disease. Inflammatory breast cancer is also included in locally advanced disease and represents 1% to 3% of diagnosed breast cancers. Patients with this very aggressive form of breast cancer can present without a discrete mass and only erythema and edema.

One challenging issue about this group of patients is the heterogeneous nature of their disease, with multiple different subgroups including tumors >5 cm, those with extensive regional lymph node involvement, direct involvement of the skin or chest wall, tumors that have no metastases but are still inoperable, and inflammatory breast cancer. The majority of patients with locally advanced breast cancers will have involved lymph nodes at diagnosis; 50% will have four or more lymph nodes involved. The DFS rates are variable. The most common cause of treatment failure is distant metastases, usually occurring within 2 years of diagnosis. Both locally advanced breast cancer and inflammatory breast cancer can be divided into the same molecular subtypes as operable breast cancer: luminal A and B, HER2, basal-like, etc. Systemic therapy is selected on that basis.

The importance of a multimodality approach cannot be stressed enough. Previously, women with locally advanced disease were classified as being inoperable. Patients who were treated with a single modality of therapy with surgery or radiation had 5-year survival rates of less than 20%. Chemotherapy was first introduced into the treatment algorithm for this subset of breast cancer in the 1970s ([99]). The EBCTCG review noted a modest benefit in survival for patients treated with postoperative chemotherapy ([38]). The righ risk of developing metastatic disease faced by these patients led to the use of neoadjuvant therapy as part of a multimodality approach.

Neoadjuvant-Based Therapy

Neoadjuvant-based therapy offers many important benefits, including direct in vivo measurement of sensitivity of tumor cells to chemotherapy, which allows for early discontinuation of ineffective therapy. Also, treatment prior to surgical intervention allows the delivery of the chemotherapy through an intact vasculature and thus possibly decreases the probability of developing resistant tumor cells.

Patients with locally advanced disease receive the same chemotherapy as stage II patients. Clinical response is documented by serial physical examinations, mammograms, and ultrasounds of the breast and nodal regions. If there is evidence of response that could possibly lead to a tumor pCR, a radiopaque marker is placed in the breast. Overall, the response to neoadjuvant therapy regimens depends on the patient's tumors characteristics and the treatment. The tumor effect on the axillary lymph nodes, rather than the response of the primary tumor itself, may be more important in predicting long-term outcome ([100]).

Surgery

The historical surgical procedure for locally advanced disease is mastectomy. Clinical trials using neoadjuvant chemotherapy have noted that 50% or more of women with locally advanced breast cancer can be treated with BCS after neoadjuvant therapy ([101]). One concern is that women who need to be downstaged with preoperative chemotherapy to be eligible for segmental mastectomy have a higher local failure rate ([102]). This can be improved through accurate localization of the tumor using a radiopaque clip, so that the appropriate area of tumor involvement can be resected, even if a complete or near-complete response is achieved with neoadjuvant therapy.

Radiation Therapy

Radiation treatment guidelines recommend that patients with a pathologic response in the primary tumor and axillary lymph nodes, whether they undergo lumpectomy or mastectomy, should receive radiation to the breast and/or chest wall and/or internal mammary lymph nodes to a total dose of 50 to 60 Gy. Patients who achieve a partial response in the primary tumor and have residual nodal disease should have radiation in a comprehensive fashion, including the axillary field.

Adjuvant Therapy

Endocrine Therapy

As in stage I and stage II disease, our standard approach is to treat receptor-positive stage I disease using a hormonal treatment regimen. Based on the ATAC trial data discussed previously, tamoxifen is given to premenopausal women; postmenopausal women receive an AI. The ATLAS and ATTOM trials suggest extending tamoxifen to 10 years. An AI along with ovarian suppression should be considered for this population. Postmenopausal patients are recommended to receive 5 years of an AI. Endocrine therapies are started after completion of chemotherapy but can be given concomitantly with radiation therapy.

Prognosis

Clinical end points have been shown to improve with neoadjuvant therapy involving a combined-modality approach. Patients who are treated with a multimodality treatment approach can achieve long-term survival of 50%. Those who do not respond to neoadjuvant therapy have poorer outcomes. Women who fail to respond to neoadjuvant anthracycline-based therapy remain free of distant disease in only 30% of cases ([103]).

CONCLUSION

Treatment of breast cancer has evolved from single-agent therapies to more contemporary combinations. Combined-modality approaches with refinement in local therapies (surgery, irradiation) have resulted in progressive improvement in survival in this disease. This is reflected in a single-center series of breast cancer patients treated from diagnosis at our institution from the 1940s to the present (Fig. 27-5).

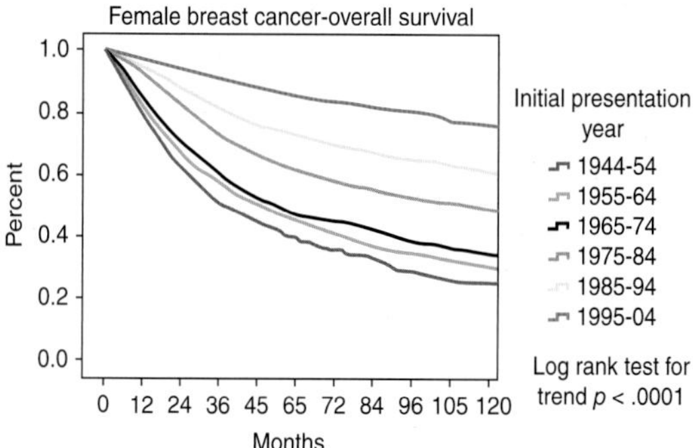

FIGURE 27-5 Survival of breast cancer patients treated at MD Anderson Cancer Center by decades.

Over the past six decades, there have been significant advances in the care of early-stage, locally advanced breast cancer. Between 1991 and 2005, the rate of death from breast cancer decreased by 37% in the United States ([1]). The use of optimal stage- and hormone receptor–specific therapy is of utmost importance, and can significantly affect the risk of recurrence and death from breast cancer. Outcomes have improved with the addition of neoadjuvant therapy, taxanes, hormonal therapy, and HER2-targeted therapy.

REFERENCES

1. National Cancer Institute. SEER Cancer Statistics Factsheets: Breast Cancer. Bethesda, MD: National Cancer Institute; 2015. http://seer.cancer.gov/statfacts/html/breast.html.
2. Chu KC, Tarone RE, Kessler LG, et al. Recent trends in U.S. breast cancer incidence, survival, and mortality rates. *J Natl Cancer Inst.* 1996;88(21):1571-1679. PMID: 8901855.
3. Li CI, Daling JR, Malone KE. Incidence of invasive breast cancer by hormone receptor status from 1992 to 1998. *J Clin Oncol.* 2003;21(1):28-34. PMID: 12506166.
4. Ravdin PM, Cronin KA, Howlader N, et al. The decrease in breast-cancer incidence in 2003 in the United States. *N Engl J Med.* 2007;356(16):1670-1674. PMID: 17442911.
5. Willett WC RB, Hankinson SE, Hunter DJ, Colditz GA. Epidemiology and Nongenetic Causes of Breast Cancer. Diseases of the Breast. 2nd ed. Philadelphia, PA: Lippincott Williams & Wilkins; 2000:175-220.
6. Fedewa SA, Ward EM, Stewart AK, Edge SB. Delays in adjuvant chemotherapy treatment among patients with breast cancer are more likely in African American and Hispanic populations: a national cohort study 2004-2006. *J Clin Oncol.* 2010;28(27):4135-4141. PMID: 20697082.
7. Gail MH, Brinton LA, Byar DP, et al. Projecting individualized probabilities of developing breast cancer for white females who are being examined annually. *J Natl Cancer Inst.* 1989;81(24):1879-1886. PMID: 2593165.
8. Claus EB, Risch N, Thompson WD. Genetic analysis of breast cancer in the cancer and steroid hormone study. *Am J Hum Genet.* 1991;48(2):232-242. PMID: 1990835.
9. Collaborative Group on Hormonal Factors in Breast Cancer. Familial breast cancer: collaborative reanalysis of individual data from 52 epidemiological studies including 58,209 women

with breast cancer and 101,986 women without the disease. *Lancet*. 2001;358(9291):1389-1399. PMID: 11705483.

10. Antoniou AC, Casadei S, Heikkinen T, et al. Breast-cancer risk in families with mutations in PALB2. *N Engl J Med*. 2014;371:497-506. PMID: 25099575.
11. Frank TS, Deffenbaugh AM, Reid JE, et al. Clinical characteristics of individuals with germline mutations in BRCA1 and BRCA2: analysis of 10,000 individuals. *J Clin Oncol*. 2002;20(6):1480-1490. PMID: 11896095.
12. Fisher B, Dignam J, Wolmark N, et al. Tamoxifen in treatment of intraductal breast cancer: National Surgical Adjuvant Breast and Bowel Project B-24 randomised controlled trial. *Lancet*. 1999;353(9169):1993-2000. PMID: 10376613.
13. Hsieh CC, Trichopoulos D, Katsouyanni K, Yuasa S. Age at menarche, age at menopause, height and obesity as risk factors for breast cancer: associations and interactions in an international case-control study. *Int J Cancer*. 1990;46(5):796-800. PMID: 2228308.
14. Layde PM, Webster LA, Baughman AL, Wingo PA, Rubin GL, Ory HW. The independent associations of parity, age at first full term pregnancy, and duration of breastfeeding with the risk of breast cancer. Cancer and Steroid Hormone Study Group. *J Clin Epidemiol*. 1989;42(10):963-973. PMID: 2681548.
15. Brinton LA, Schairer C, Hoover RN, Fraumeni JF Jr. Menstrual factors and risk of breast cancer. *Cancer Invest*. 1988;6(3):245-254. PMID: 3167610.
16. Bruzzi P, Negri E, La Vecchia C, et al. Short term increase in risk of breast cancer after full term pregnancy. *BMJ*. 1988;297(6656):1096-1098. PMID: 3143438.
17. Hankinson SE, Colditz GA, Manson JE, et al. A prospective study of oral contraceptive use and risk of breast cancer (Nurses' Health Study, United States). *Cancer Causes Control*. 1997;8(1):65-72. PMID: 9051324.
18. Marchbanks PA, McDonald JA, Wilson HG, et al. Oral contraceptives and the risk of breast cancer. *N Engl J Med*. 2002;346(26):2025-2032. PMID: 12087137.
19. Collaborative Group on Hormonal Factors in Breast Cancer. Breast cancer and hormonal contraceptives: collaborative reanalysis of individual data on 53 297 women with breast cancer and 100 239 women without breast cancer from 54 epidemiological studies. *Lancet*. 1996;347(9017):1713-1727. PMID: 8656904.
20. Rossouw JE, Anderson GL, Prentice RL, et al. Risks and benefits of estrogen plus progestin in healthy postmenopausal women: principal results from the Women's Health Initiative randomized controlled trial. *JAMA*. 2002;288(3):321-333. PMID: 12117397.
21. Edge SB, Compton CC. The American Joint Committee on Cancer: the 7th edition of the AJCC cancer staging manual and the future of TNM. *Ann Surg Oncol*. 2010;17(6):1471-1474. PMID: 20180029.
22. Gasparini G, Pozza F, Harris AL. Evaluating the potential usefulness of new prognostic and predictive indicators in node-negative breast cancer patients. *J Natl Cancer Inst*. 1993;85(15):1206-1219. PMID: 8331681.
23. Weiss RB, Woolf SH, Demakos E, et al. Natural history of more than 20 years of node-positive primary breast carcinoma treated with cyclophosphamide, methotrexate, and fluorouracil-based adjuvant chemotherapy: a study by the Cancer and Leukemia Group B. *J Clin Oncol*. 2003;21(9):1825-1835. PMID: 12721260.
24. Nemoto T, Vana J, Bedwani RN, Baker HW, McGregor FH, Murphy GP. Management and survival of female breast cancer: results of a national survey by the American College of Surgeons. *Cancer*. 1980;45(12):2917-2924. PMID: 7388735.
25. Elston CW, Ellis IO. Pathological prognostic factors in breast cancer. I. The value of histological grade in breast cancer: experience from a large study with long-term follow-up. *Histopathology*. 1991;19(5):403-410. PMID: 1757079.
26. Hammond MEH, Hayes DF, Dowsett M, et al. American Society of Clinical Oncology/College of American Pathologists guideline recommendations for immunohistochemical testing of estrogen and progesterone receptors in breast cancer. *J Clin Oncol*. 2010;28(16):2784-2795. PMID: 20404251.
27. Kontzoglou K, Palla V, Karaolanis G, et al. Correlation between Ki67 and breast cancer prognosis. *Oncology*. 2013;84(4):219-225. PMID: 23364275.
28. Wolff AC, Hammond ME, Hicks DG, et al. Recommendations for human epidermal growth factor receptor 2 testing in breast cancer: American Society of Clinical Oncology/College of American Pathologists clinical practice guideline update. *J Clin Oncol*. 2013;31(31):3997-4013. PMID: 24101045.
29. Tandon AK, Clark GM, Chamness GC, Ullrich A, McGuire WL. HER-2/neu oncogene protein and prognosis in breast cancer. *J Clin Oncol*. 1989;7(8):1120-1128. PMID: 2569032.
30. Gonzalez-Angulo AM, Litton JK, Broglio KR, et al. High risk of recurrence for patients with breast cancer who have human epidermal growth factor receptor 2-positive, node-negative tumors 1 cm or smaller. *J Clin Oncol*. 2009;27(34):5700-5706. PMID: 19884543.
31. Goldhirsch A, Gelber RD, Piccart-Gebhart MJ, et al. 2 years versus 1 year of adjuvant trastuzumab for HER2-positive breast cancer (HERA): an open-label, randomised controlled trial. *Lancet*. 2013;382(9897):1021-1028. PMID: 23871490.
32. Slamon D, Eiermann W, Robert N, et al. Adjuvant trastuzumab in HER2-positive breast cancer. *N Engl J Med*. 2011;365(14):1273-1283. PMID: 21991949.
33. Sorlie T, Perou CM, Tibshirani R, et al. Gene expression patterns of breast carcinomas distinguish tumor subclasses with clinical implications. *Proc Natl Acad Sci USA*. 2001;98(19):10869-10874. PMID: 11553815.
34. Ravdin PM, Siminoff LA, Davis GJ, et al. Computer program to assist in making decisions about adjuvant therapy for women with early breast cancer. *J Clin Oncol*. 2001;19(4):980-991. PMID: 11181660.
35. Paik S, Shak S, Tang G, et al. A multigene assay to predict recurrence of tamoxifen-treated, node-negative breast cancer. *N Engl J Med*. 2004;351(27):2817-2826. PMID: 15591335.
36. Fisher B, Ravdin RG, Ausman RK, Slack NH, Moore GE, Noer RJ. Surgical adjuvant chemotherapy in cancer of the breast: results of a decade of cooperative investigation. *Ann Surg*. 1968;168(3):337-356. PMID: 4970947.
37. Nissen-Meyer R, Kjellgren K, Mansson B. Preliminary report from the Scandinavian adjuvant chemotherapy study group. *Cancer Chemother Rep*. 1971;55(5):561-566. PMID: 4946080.
38. Polychemotherapy for early breast cancer: an overview of the randomised trials. Early Breast Cancer Trialists' Collaborative Group. *Lancet*. 1998;352(9132):930-942. PMID: 9752815.
39. Paik S, Bryant J, Tan-Chiu E, et al. HER2 and choice of adjuvant chemotherapy for invasive breast cancer: National Surgical Adjuvant Breast and Bowel Project Protocol B-15. *J Natl Cancer Inst*. 2000;92(24):1991-1998. PMID: 11121461.
40. Thor AD, Berry DA, Budman DR, et al. erbB-2, p53, and efficacy of adjuvant therapy in lymph node-positive breast cancer. *J Natl Cancer Inst*. 1998;90(18):1346-1360. PMID: 9747866.
41. Buzdar AU, Hortobagyi GN, Singletary SE, et al. *Adjuvant Adjuvant Therapy of Cancer VIII*. Philadelphia, PA: Lippincott-Raven; 1997:93-100.
42. Bishop JF, Dewar J, Toner GC, et al. Initial paclitaxel improves outcome compared with CMFP combination chemotherapy as front-line therapy in untreated metastatic breast cancer. *J Clin Oncol*. 1999;17(8):2355-2364. PMID: 10561297.
43. Martin M, Pienkowski T, Mackey J, et al. Adjuvant docetaxel for node-positive breast cancer. *N Engl J Med*. 2005;352(22):2302-2313. PMID: 15930421.

44. Nabholtz JM, Senn HJ, Bezwoda WR, et al. Prospective randomized trial of docetaxel versus mitomycin plus vinblastine in patients with metastatic breast cancer progressing despite previous anthracycline-containing chemotherapy. 304 Study Group. *J Clin Oncol.* 1999;17(5):1413-1424. PMID: 10334526.
45. Sparano JA, Wang M, Martino S, et al. Weekly paclitaxel in the adjuvant treatment of breast cancer. *N Engl J Med.* 2008;358(16):1663-1671. PMID: 18420499.
46. Jones S, Holmes FA, O'Shaughnessy J, et al. Docetaxel with cyclophosphamide is associated with an overall survival benefit compared with doxorubicin and cyclophosphamide: 7-year follow-up of US Oncology Research Trial 9735. *J Clin Oncol.* 2009;27(8):1177-1183. PMID: 19204201.
47. Beatson GT. On the treatment of inoperable cases of carcinoma of the mamma: suggestions for a new method of treatment with illustrative cases. *Lancet.* 1896;2(3803):104-107.
48. Controlled trial of tamoxifen as adjuvant agent in management of early breast cancer. Interim analysis at four years by Nolvadex Adjuvant Trial Organisation. *Lancet.* 1983;1(8319):257-261. PMID: 6130291.
49. Fisher B, Costantino J, Redmond C, et al. A randomized clinical trial evaluating tamoxifen in the treatment of patients with node-negative breast cancer who have estrogen-receptor-positive tumors. *N Engl J Med.* 1989;320(8):479-484. PMID: 2644532.
50. Rutqvist LE, Cedermark B, Glas U, et al. Randomized trial of adjuvant tamoxifen in node negative postmenopausal breast cancer. Stockholm Breast Cancer Study Group. *Acta Oncologica.* 1992;31(2):265-270. PMID: 1622644.
51. Stewart HJ. The Scottish trial of adjuvant tamoxifen in node-negative breast cancer. Scottish Cancer Trials Breast Group. J Natl Cancer Inst Monogr. 1992;11:117-120. PMID: 1320920.
52. Tamoxifen for early breast cancer: an overview of the randomised trials. Early Breast Cancer Trialists' Collaborative Group. *Lancet.* 1998;351(9114):1451-1467. PMID: 9605801.
53. Davies C, Pan H, Godwin J, et al. Long-term effects of continuing adjuvant tamoxifen to 10 years versus stopping at 5 years after diagnosis of oestrogen receptor-positive breast cancer: ATLAS, a randomised trial. *Lancet.* 2013;381(9869):805-816. PMID: 23219286.
54. Gray RG, Rea D, Handley SJB, et al. aTTom: long term effects of continuing adjuvant tamoxifen to 10 years versus stopping at 6 years in 6,953 women with early breast cancer [abstract]. *J Clin Oncol.* 2013;31:5.
55. Goldhirsch A, Glick JH, Gelber RD, Senn HJ. Meeting highlights: International Consensus Panel on the Treatment of Primary Breast Cancer. *J Natl Cancer Inst.* 1998;90(21):1601-1608. PMID: 9811309.
56. Albain KS, Barlow WE, Ravdin PM, et al. Adjuvant chemotherapy and timing of tamoxifen in postmenopausal patients with endocrine-responsive, node-positive breast cancer: a phase 3, open-label, randomised controlled trial. *Lancet.* 2009;374(9707):2055-2063. PMID: 20004966.
57. Brodie AM, Njar VC. Aromatase inhibitors and their application in breast cancer treatment. *Steroids.* 2000;65(4):171-179. PMID: 10713305.
58. Baum M, Buzdar A, Cuzick J, et al. Anastrozole alone or in combination with tamoxifen versus tamoxifen alone for adjuvant treatment of postmenopausal women with early-stage breast cancer: results of the ATAC (Arimidex, Tamoxifen Alone or in Combination) trial efficacy and safety update analyses. *Cancer.* 2003;98(9):1802-1810. PMID: 14584060.
59. Buzdar AU, ATAC Trialists' Group. Arimidex (anastrozole) versus tamoxifen as adjuvant therapy in postmenopausal women with early breast cancer—efficacy overview. *J Steroid Biochem Mol Biol.* 2003;86(3-5):399-403. PMID: 14623537.
60. Sainsbury R. Beneficial side-effect profile of anastrozole compared with tamoxifen confirmed by additional 7 months of exposure data: a safety update from the Arimidex, Tamoxifen, Alone or in Combination (ATAC) trial. *Breast Cancer Res Treat.* 2002;76:S156.
61. Dowsett M, Cuzick J, Ingle J, et al. Meta-analysis of breast cancer outcomes in adjuvant trials of aromatase inhibitors versus tamoxifen. *J Clin Oncol.* 2010;28(3):509-518. PMID: 19949017.
62. Goss PE, Ingle JN, Martino S, et al. A randomized trial of letrozole in postmenopausal women after five years of tamoxifen therapy for early-stage breast cancer. *N Engl J Med.* 2003;349(19):1793-1802. PMID: 14551341.
63. Breast International Group 1-98 Collaborative Group, Thurlimann B, Keshaviah A, et al. A comparison of letrozole and tamoxifen in postmenopausal women with early breast cancer. *N Engl J Med.* 2005;353(26):2747-2757. PMID: 16382061.
64. Breast International Group 1-98 Collaborative Group, Mouridsen H, Giobbie-Hurder A, et al. Letrozole therapy alone or in sequence with tamoxifen in women with breast cancer. *N Engl J Med.* 2009;361(8):766-776. PMID: 19692688.
65. Coombes RC, Hall E, Gibson LJ, et al. A randomized trial of exemestane after two to three years of tamoxifen therapy in postmenopausal women with primary breast cancer. *N Engl J Med.* 2004;350(11):1081-1092. PMID: 15014181.
66. Chan A, Speers C, O'Reilly S, et al. Adherence of adjuvant hormonal therapies in post-menopausal hormone receptor positive (HR+) early stage breast cancer: a population based study from British Columbia [abstract]. *Cancer Res.* 2009;69:36.
67. Jonat W, Kaufmann M, Sauerbrei W, et al. Goserelin versus cyclophosphamide, methotrexate, and fluorouracil as adjuvant therapy in premenopausal patients with node-positive breast cancer: the Zoladex Early Breast Cancer Research Association Study. *J Clin Oncol.* 2002;20(24):4628-4635. PMID: 12488406.
68. Chlebowski RT, Pan K. Exemestane with ovarian suppression in premenopausal breast cancer. *N Engl J Med.* 2014;371(14):1358. PMID: 25271612.
69. Francis PA, Regan MM, Fleming GF, et al. Adjuvant ovarian suppression in premenopausal breast cancer. *N Engl J Med.* 2015;372(5):436-446. PMID: 25495490.
70. Vogel CL, Cobleigh MA, Tripathy D, et al. Efficacy and safety of trastuzumab as a single agent in first-line treatment of HER2-overexpressing metastatic breast cancer. *J Clin Oncol.* 2002;20(3):719-726. PMID: 11821453.
71. Cobleigh MA, Vogel CL, Tripathy D, et al. Multinational study of the efficacy and safety of humanized anti-HER2 monoclonal antibody in women who have HER2-overexpressing metastatic breast cancer that has progressed after chemotherapy for metastatic disease. *J Clin Oncol.* 1999;17(9):2639-2648. PMID: 10561337.
72. Slamon DJ, Leyland-Jones B, Shak S, et al. Use of chemotherapy plus a monoclonal antibody against HER2 for metastatic breast cancer that overexpresses HER2. *N Engl J Med.* 2001;344(11):783-792. PMID: 11248153.
73. Perez EA. Cardiac toxicity of ErbB2-targeted therapies: what do we know? *Clin Breast Cancer.* 2008;8(Suppl 3):S114-S120. PMID: 18777950.
74. Perez EA, Romond EH, Suman VJ, et al. Four-year follow-up of trastuzumab plus adjuvant chemotherapy for operable human epidermal growth factor receptor 2-positive breast cancer: joint analysis of data from NCCTG N9831 and NSABP B-31. *J Clin Oncol.* 2011;29(25):3366-3373. PMID: 21768458.
75. Perez EA, Romond EH, Suman VJ, et al. Trastuzumab plus adjuvant chemotherapy for human epidermal growth factor receptor 2-positive breast cancer: planned joint analysis of overall survival from NSABP B-31 and NCCTG N9831. *J Clin Oncol.* 2014;32(33):3744-3752. PMID: 25332249.
76. Pivot X, Romieu G, Debled M, et al. 6 months versus 12 months

of adjuvant trastuzumab for patients with HER2-positive early breast cancer (PHARE): a randomised phase 3 trial. *Lancet Oncol.* 2013;14(8):741-748. PMID: 23764181.

77. De Lena M, Zucali R, Viganotti G, Valagussa P, Bonadonna G. Combined chemotherapy-radiotherapy approach in locally advanced (T3b-T4) breast cancer. *Cancer Chemother Pharmacol.* 1978;1(1):53-59. PMID: 373908.
78. Fisher B, Brown A, Mamounas E, et al. Effect of preoperative chemotherapy on local-regional disease in women with operable breast cancer: findings from National Surgical Adjuvant Breast and Bowel Project B-18. *J Clin Oncol.* 1997;15(7):2483-2493. PMID: 9215816.
79. Rouzier R, Extra JM, Klijanienko J, et al. Incidence and prognostic significance of complete axillary downstaging after primary chemotherapy in breast cancer patients with T1 to T3 tumors and cytologically proven axillary metastatic lymph nodes. *J Clin Oncol.* 2002;20(5):1304-1310. PMID: 11870173.
80. Green MC, Buzdar AU, Smith T, et al. Weekly paclitaxel improves pathologic complete remission in operable breast cancer when compared with paclitaxel once every 3 weeks. *J Clin Oncol.* 2005;23(25):5983-5992. PMID: 16087943.
81. Hoff PM, Valero V, Buzdar AU, et al. Combined modality treatment of locally advanced breast carcinoma in elderly patients or patients with severe comorbid conditions using tamoxifen as the primary therapy. *Cancer.* 2000;88(9):2054-2060. PMID: 10813717.
82. Veronesi A, Frustaci S, Tirelli U, et al. Tamoxifen therapy in postmenopausal advanced breast cancer: efficacy at the primary tumor site in 46 evaluable patients. *Tumori.* 1981;67(3):235-238. PMID: 7281242.
83. Buzdar AU, Ibrahim NK, Francis D, et al. Significantly higher pathologic complete remission rate after neoadjuvant therapy with trastuzumab, paclitaxel, and epirubicin chemotherapy: results of a randomized trial in human epidermal growth factor receptor 2-positive operable breast cancer. *J Clin Oncol.* 2005;23(16):3676-3685. PMID: 15738535.
84. Geyer CE, Forster J, Lindquist D, et al. Lapatinib plus capecitabine for HER2-positive advanced breast cancer. *N Engl J Med.* 2006;355(26):2733-2743. PMID: 17192538.
85. Baselga J, Bradbury I, Eidtmann H, et al. Lapatinib with trastuzumab for HER2-positive early breast cancer (NeoALTTO): a randomised, open-label, multicentre, phase 3 trial. *Lancet.* 2012;379(9816):633-640. PMID: 22257673.
86. Piccart MJ, Holmes AP, Baselga J, et al. First results from the phase III ALTTO trial (BIG 2-06; NCCTG [Alliance] N063D) comparing one year of anti-HER2 therapy with lapatinib alone (L), trastuzumab alone (T), their sequence (T→L), or their combination (T+L) in the adjuvant treatment of HER2-positive early breast cancer (EBC) [abstract]. *J Clin Oncol.* 2014;32:LBA4.
87. Baselga J, Cortes J, Kim SB, et al. Pertuzumab plus trastuzumab plus docetaxel for metastatic breast cancer. *N Engl J Med.* 2012;366(2):109-119. PMID: 22149875.
88. Gianni L, Pienkowski T, Im YH, et al. Efficacy and safety of neoadjuvant pertuzumab and trastuzumab in women with locally advanced, inflammatory, or early HER2-positive breast cancer (NeoSphere): a randomised multicentre, open-label, phase 2 trial. *Lancet Oncol.* 2012;13(1):25-32. PMID: 22153890.
89. Schneeweiss A, Chia S, Hickish T, et al. Pertuzumab plus trastuzumab in combination with standard neoadjuvant anthracycline-containing and anthracycline-free chemotherapy regimens in patients with HER2-positive early breast cancer: a randomized phase II cardiac safety study (TRYPHAENA). *Ann Oncol.* 2013;24(9):2278-2284. PMID: 23704196.
90. Citron ML, Berry DA, Cirrincione C, et al. Randomized trial of dose-dense versus conventionally scheduled and sequential versus concurrent combination chemotherapy as postoperative adjuvant treatment of node-positive primary breast cancer: first report of Intergroup Trial C9741/Cancer and Leukemia Group B Trial 9741. *J Clin Oncol.* 2003;21(8):1431-1439. PMID: 12668651.
91. Swain SM, Tang G, Geyer CE Jr, et al. Definitive results of a phase III adjuvant trial comparing three chemotherapy regimens in women with operable, node-positive breast cancer: the NSABP B-38 trial. *J Clin Oncol.* 2013;31(26):3197-3204. PMID: 23940225.
92. Budd GT, Barlow WE, Moore HC, et al. SWOG S0221: a phase III trial comparing chemotherapy schedules in high-risk early-stage breast cancer. *J Clin Oncol.* 2015;33(1):58-64. PMID: 25422488.
93. Paik S, Tang G, Shak S, et al. Gene expression and benefit of chemotherapy in women with node-negative, estrogen receptor-positive breast cancer. *J Clin Oncol.* 2006;24(23):3726-3734. PMID: 16720680.
94. Sparano JA. TAILORx: trial assigning individualized options for treatment (Rx). *Clin Breast Cancer.* 2006;7(4):347-350. PMID: 17092406.
95. Cuzick J, Dowsett M, Pineda S, et al. Prognostic value of a combined estrogen receptor, progesterone receptor, Ki-67, and human epidermal growth factor receptor 2 immunohistochemical score and comparison with the Genomic Health recurrence score in early breast cancer. *J Clin Oncol.* 2011;29(32):4273-4278. PMID: 21990413.
96. Fisher B, Anderson S, Bryant J, et al. Twenty-year follow-up of a randomized trial comparing total mastectomy, lumpectomy, and lumpectomy plus irradiation for the treatment of invasive breast cancer. *N Engl J Med.* 2002;347(16):1233-1241. PMID: 12393820.
97. Olson JA Jr, McCall LM, Beitsch P, et al. Impact of immediate versus delayed axillary node dissection on surgical outcomes in breast cancer patients with positive sentinel nodes: results from American College of Surgeons Oncology Group Trials Z0010 and Z0011. *J Clin Oncol.* 2008;26(21):3530-3535. PMID: 18640934.
98. Recht A, Edge SB. Evidence-based indications for postmastectomy irradiation. *Surg Clin North Am.* 2003;83(4):995-1013. PMID: 12875606.
99. Grohn P, Heinonen E, Klefstrom P, Tarkkanen J. Adjuvant postoperative radiotherapy, chemotherapy, and immunotherapy in stage III breast cancer. *Cancer.* 1984;54(4):670-674. PMID: 6744203.
100. McCready DR, Hortobagyi GN, Kau SW, Smith TL, Buzdar AU, Balch CM. The prognostic significance of lymph node metastases after preoperative chemotherapy for locally advanced breast cancer. *Arch Surg.* 1989;124(1):21-25. PMID: 2910244.
101. Veronesi U, Bonadonna G, Zurrida S, et al. Conservation surgery after primary chemotherapy in large carcinomas of the breast. *Ann Surg.* 1995;222(5):612-618. PMID: 7487207.
102. Rouzier R, Extra JM, Carton M, et al. Primary chemotherapy for operable breast cancer: incidence and prognostic significance of ipsilateral breast tumor recurrence after breast-conserving surgery. *J Clin Oncol.* 2001;19(18):3828-3835. PMID: 11559720.
103. Huang E, McNeese MD, Strom EA, et al. Locoregional treatment outcomes for inoperable anthracycline-resistant breast cancer. *Int J Radiat Oncol Biol Phys.* 2002;53(5):1225-1233. PMID: 12128124.

28 Metastatic Breast Cancer

第二十八章　转移性乳腺癌

Meghan Karuturi
Vicente Valero
Mariana Chavez-MacGregor

中文导读

本章主要概述转移性乳腺癌的标准治疗方法，同时介绍了MD安德森癌症中心特有的诊治手段。首先，阐述了转移性乳腺癌的诊断流程。其次，介绍了转移性乳腺癌患者制定治疗策略需考虑患者激素受体状态、HER2状态以及疾病负荷，主要的治疗手段包括内分泌治疗、抗HER2靶向治疗以及化疗。在内分泌治疗部分，分别阐述了卵巢去势（手术、放疗）、功能性卵巢抑制（促黄体激素释放激素类似物）、选择性雌激素受体调节剂、选择性雌激素受体调节剂、非甾体类和甾体类选择性芳香化酶抑制剂、雌激素、孕激素、雄激素等在转移性乳腺癌中的应用。在化疗部分，分别从方案的选择、治疗维持时间、单药化疗方案、联合化疗方案4个方面详细介绍。在靶向治疗部分，主要介绍了转移性乳腺癌抗HER2靶向治疗的4个药物的重要临床试验，包括曲妥珠单抗、帕妥珠单抗、T-DM1、拉帕替尼。另外介绍了抗血管内皮生长因子的靶向药物、骨修复药物等其他治疗方案。尽管目前在治疗方面取得了诸多进展，但转移性乳腺癌患者的预后仍然不理想，因此，本章也介绍了正在进行临床试验的一些新靶点及其药物。本章的最后阐述了局部治疗在转移性乳腺癌中的应用，但尚需要更多的合作与讨论。

Breast cancer is a significant cause of morbidity and mortality among women. In the United States, it is the most common malignancy among women. It is estimated that approximately 231,840 new cases of invasive breast cancer will have occurred in the United States in 2015 ([1, 2]). Although lung cancer has surpassed breast cancer as the leading cause of cancer death among women, nearly 39,620 deaths were estimated to occur from breast cancer alone in 2013 ([1]).

Since the 1970s, advances in combined-modality therapies have substantially improved the outcomes of patients with breast cancer. Still, approximately 10% to 60% of patients with initial localized breast cancer will suffer a systemic relapse. Metastatic disease is diagnosed at the time of presentation in 3% to 12% of patients depending on the series ([1, 3]). Bone is the most common site of first distant relapse; other common sites of metastases include lymph nodes, lung, liver, and, less frequently, brain. The 5-year survival rate for localized breast cancer is 99%; for metastatic disease, this rate is only 17% to 28% ([1-3]). As is true with cancers in general, the clinical course for patients with metastatic breast cancer (MBC) varies, but as a group, patients with MBC have a median survival of 2 years ([4]). Patients with bone-only disease tend to live longer than patients with visceral involvement. Untreated patients with MBC have a median overall survival time of 9 to 12 months. With systemic therapy, the mean survival time is 21 months for patients with visceral disease and as long as 60 months for patients with bone-only disease. Survival and response to therapy are affected by several factors, including estrogen receptor (ER), progesterone receptor (PR), and *HER2*/neu receptor status; performance status; site of disease; number of disease sites; and duration of disease-free interval (DFI).

The therapeutic objectives and approach to patients with advanced breast cancer is distinct from that of patients with early-stage disease. Treatment for MBC is triaged to endocrine therapy, biological therapy, or chemotherapy, depending on the hormonal and *HER2*/neu receptor status of the tumor, the severity of symptoms, and the site and extent of disease. Generally, breast cancer can be classified as three molecularly and clinically different syndromes: hormone-receptor positive/*HER2*/neu negative, *Her-2*/neu positive (hormone-receptor negative or positive) and triple negative breast cancer. They have different clinical courses, prognoses, metastatic patterns, and responsiveness to available therapies. Systemic treatment prolongs survival, provides palliation of symptoms, and enhances quality of life but, in general, is not considered curative. Therefore, a discussion regarding goals of care is imperative between the patient and treating oncologist. Cure in MBC is rare; less than 2% of patients with MBC may remain disease free after anthracycline-containing therapy. The overall survival of patients has improved in the last few decades due to more effective therapies. This chapter reviews standard care for patients with MBC and discusses some unique approaches used at the University of Texas MD Anderson Cancer Center (MDACC).

DIAGNOSTIC WORKUP

Once metastatic disease is suspected, careful evaluation of the primary disease history, current symptoms, and existing comorbid diseases is essential. The history of the primary disease should include a review of the initial presentation, stage of disease, histology, hormone receptor and *HER2*/neu status, nuclear grade, and treatment modalities employed. Knowledge of the initial tumor type may yield clues about the sites of disease as well as its biology. For instance, infiltrating ductal carcinoma most commonly involve the lungs, pleura, liver, and brain. Infiltrating lobular carcinoma may metastasize to unusual sites such as the bone marrow, meninges, peritoneum, and retroperitoneal structures, such as the ureters ([5]).

If possible, a biopsy of the metastatic or recurrence site is required to confirm the histologic type, as well as ER, PR, and *HER2*/neu status, because there is some evidence of significant discordance in the receptor status between the time of diagnosis of the primary tumor and the time of diagnosis of metastasis ([6, 7]). Changes in ER status occur in 14.5% to 40% of cases, whereas changes in *HER2* expression/amplification range from 0% to 37% ([8]). Pathologic confirmation is also essential in patients suspected of having metastases if the clinical presentation or course is not typical. Such relapse scenarios include single-lesion metastasis, unusual metastatic sites, and long DFI. Solitary lesions should always be biopsied because of the possibility that the lesion may not be not malignant or may be caused by a second different primary malignancy. This occurs in up to 10% of patients with solitary lesions and would have a direct impact on the treatment selection.

In addition to a comprehensive physical examination, basic laboratory evaluation should include a complete blood count with differential, liver and renal function tests, and serum calcium determination. In addition, CA 15-3 and CA 27-29 are potentially helpful in monitoring response to therapy. The CA 15-3 test is a combination of two monoclonal antibodies bearing two reactive determinants directed against DF3 and MAM-6 antigens expressed on mammary epithelial cells ([9, 10]). CA 15-3 and CA 27-29, which are more sensitive than CEA, are elevated in approximately 70% of patients with MBC, but they lack sensitivity and specificity for breast cancer progression. Therefore, their prognostic significance remains indeterminate ([9]). Carcinoembryonic antigen (CEA) is elevated in 40% to 50% of patients with metastatic disease ([10, 11]). Current recommendations from the American Society of Clinical Oncology are that tumor markers can be used in conjunction with diagnostic imaging, history, and physical examination to monitor patients with metastatic disease during active therapy; however, data are insufficient to recommend their use alone to monitor response to treatment ([12]). Caution should be used when interpreting tumor marker levels during the first 4 to 12 weeks of a new therapy, because spurious early rises may occur ([9, 12]). Furthermore, the absolute value of a tumor marker measurement does not represent the extent of disease, and no therapeutic decision should be based on a single tumor marker measurement. However, trends over time are helpful to monitor clinical course. In monitoring treatment, the physician should be aware of the coefficient of variation of the assays used for CA 15-3 and CA 27-29: changes <10% fall within the accepted intra-assay variability and do not represent real change. The measurement of circulating tumor cells (CTCs) has been studied in patients with MBC. Several studies showed that high levels of CTCs (>5 cells/75 mL of blood) are correlated with poor survival in MBC and with decreased response to treatment ([13, 14]). However, based on current recommendations, the measurement of CTCs should not be used to make the diagnosis of breast cancer or to influence any treatment decisions. Similarly, the use of the US Food and Drug Administration (FDA)-cleared test for CTCs (CellSearch Assay) in patients with MBC cannot be recommended for routine use until further validation confirms its clinical value. An intergroup trial is under way to determine the implication of changing treatment based on the CTC level ([12]).

In most cases, we perform a baseline evaluation that also includes a computed tomography (CT) of the chest and abdomen (ultrasonography is less accurate for the chest and abdomen and would be indicated only in patients who cannot have CT or magnetic resonance imaging [MRI]), but occasionally, MRI of the abdomen may be indicated ([15]). The presence of bone metastases should be evaluated, and in general, we recommend a bone scan to determine the presence and extent of bone metastasis. Only 30% to 60% of patients with true-positive bone scans have increased levels of alkaline phosphatase ([16, 17]). Conversely, only 20% of patients with elevated levels of alkaline phosphatase are disease free ([17]). Impending fractures in the weight-bearing bones, such as the femur, and an unstable spine must be ruled out. The preferred test for spinal evaluation for metastases is MRI. Monitoring of bone metastases is best done with serial MRI or CT scans. Radiographic evaluations of the brain, leptomeninges, and spinal cord have low yield unless the patient is symptomatic or has abnormal neurologic findings ([15]). Current guidelines discourage the use of positron emission tomography (PET)/CT except in situations where other staging studies are equivocal or suspicious ([15]).

TREATMENT

General Considerations

The decision whether to use chemotherapy or biological or hormonal therapy for the initial treatment of MBC should be guided by several factors including hormone receptor and *HER2*/neu status and the presence of symptomatic visceral disease or life-threatening disease (Fig. 28-1). Patients with moderately symptomatic visceral disease or life-threatening disease should be considered for treatment with systemic chemotherapy regardless of hormone receptor status because systemic therapy offers faster palliation of symptoms. Among women who do not have life-threatening or symptomatic visceral disease, those whose tumors are negative for ER and PR should be also considered for systemic chemotherapy. Those whose tumors are positive for ER or PR should be treated with hormonal therapy. Since the discovery of the importance of *HER2* gene amplification in breast cancer and the development of anti-HER2 therapies, patients with tumors positive for *HER2*/neu overexpression or gene amplification should be treated with anti-HER2 therapy in combination with chemotherapy because this provides a significant survival advantage.

Multiple agents are active against hormone-responsive tumors. Endocrine therapy tends to be associated with fewer side effects and helps maintain quality of life for many patients. If the tumor does not respond to endocrine therapy or becomes unresponsive to hormonal therapy, systemic chemotherapy should be initiated. For patients with hormone receptor–positive breast cancer, endocrine therapy is at least as effective as chemotherapy.

Currently, the primary goals of chemotherapy for MBC should be palliation of symptoms attributable to cancer and prolongation of life. It is the physician's duty to balance the benefits of therapy with possible toxic effects and to fully discuss therapeutic options with patients. The patient's multiple previous therapies, decline in performance status, comorbid conditions, and organ function should be taken into consideration in the treatment decision. The MDACC treatment algorithm of patients with MBC is illustrated in Fig. 28-2.

Patients presenting with solitary metastases or oligometastases represent a unique subset of patients who are potentially curable and should be approached with combined-modality therapy, including surgical resection of the metastases (or radiotherapy at curative doses), combination chemotherapy before or after local treatment, anti-HER2 agents for HER2-positive MBC, and endocrine therapy for hormone receptor–positive MBC. Such patients have a 20% to 25% probability of long-term cure after such treatment.

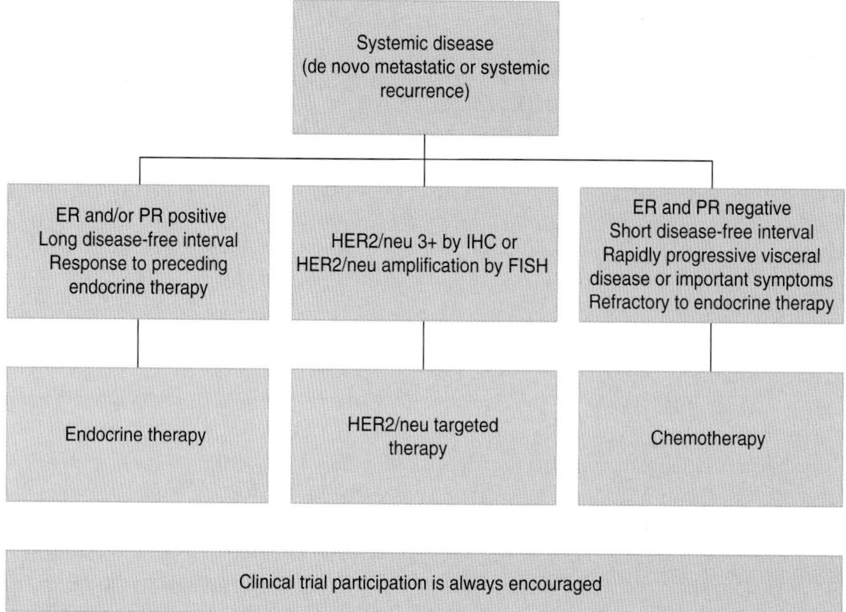

FIGURE 28-1 Principles of treatment selection in patients with metastatic breast cancer. ER, estrogen receptor; FISH, fluorescence in situ hybridization; IHC, immunohistochemistry; PR, progesterone receptor.

Stage IV breast cancer

Determination of tumor subtype

HER2 negative

ER/PR

Postmenopausal

- Tamoxifen (if none prior) +/– ovarian suppression
- Ovarian ablation/suppression + postmenopausal treatment

Postmenopausal

- Prior aromatase inhibitor: steroidal AI +/– everolimus, fulvestrant, tamoxifen
- No prior treatment: nonsteroidal aromatase inhibitor + fulvestrant as first-line, tamoxifen, AI, steroidal AI +/– everolimus, fulvestrant,

ER/PR+ and extensive symptomatic disease or ER/PR–

Need rapid response: could use combination chemotherapy (eg, FAC, AC, EC, docetaxel/capecitabine, gemcitabine/paclitaxel, carboplatin/paclitaxel, ixabepilone/capecitabine, gemcitabine/carboplatin)

Need rapid response or has exhausted endocrine therapy: Sequential single agents (selected after evaluation of prior regimen and comorbidities)
- Paclitaxel, docetaxel
- Doxil
- Capecitabine
- Ixabepilone
- Eribulin
- Gemcitabine
- Vinorelbine

No response to several lines of therapy or ECOG >3

Consider best supportive care alone and no further systemic therapy

HER2 positive

1st line therapy: Trastuzumab + pertuzumab + taxane

- 2nd line: T-DM1

- 3rd line and beyond:
- Lapatinib + capecitabine
- Trastuzumab + lapatinib
- Trastuzumab + other chemotherapy agent

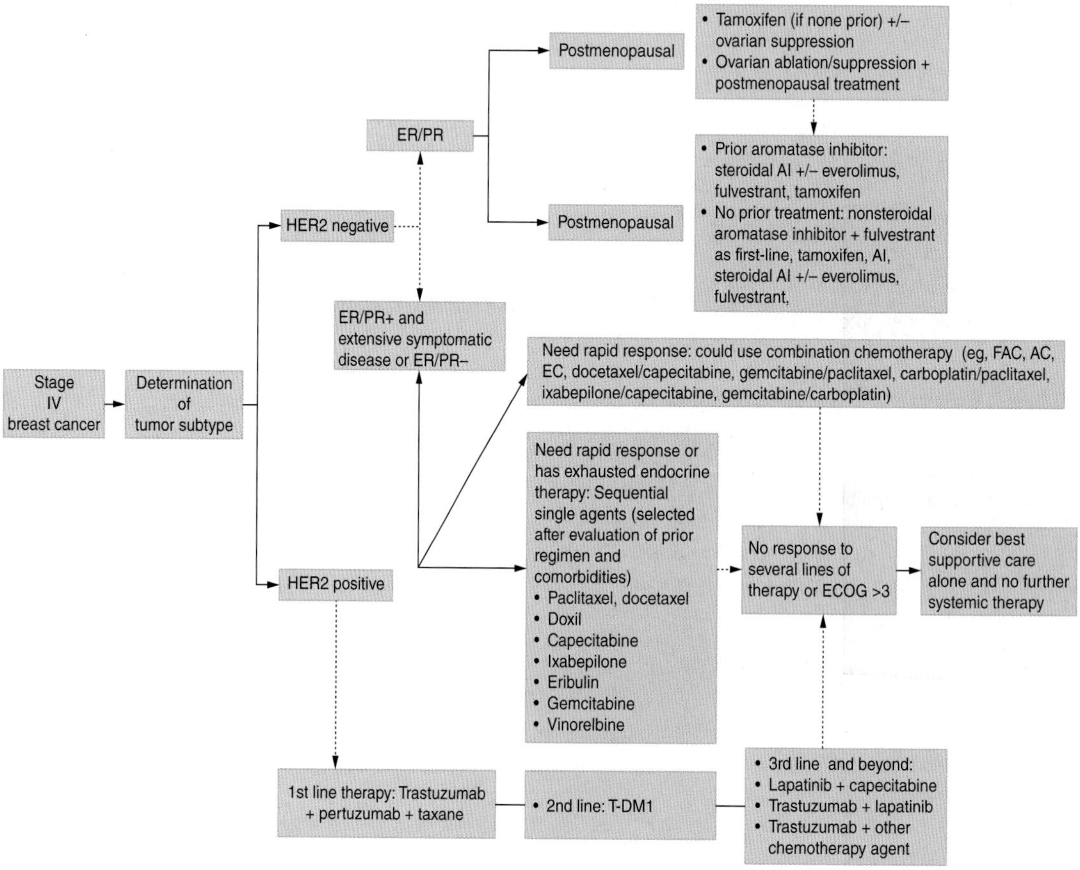

FIGURE 28-2 Algorithm for the treatment of metastatic breast cancer. AC, doxorubicin and cyclophosphamide; AI, aromatase inhibitor; EC, epirubicin and cyclophosphamide; ECOG, Eastern Cooperative Oncology Group performance status; ER, estrogen receptor; FAC, 5-fluorouracil, doxorubicin, and cyclophosphamide; PR, progesterone receptor.

ENDOCRINE THERAPY

Endocrine therapy has dramatically improved outcomes in patients with hormone receptor–positive breast cancer. It can result in significant palliation of symptoms and improvement in quality of life in patients with hormone receptor–positive MBC. Manipulation of the endocrine system as a treatment for MBC was introduced in 1896, when Beatson demonstrated objective regression of breast cancer after oophorectomy. Today, a number of endocrine therapies are used in patients with hormone-sensitive MBC; most therapies are directed at reducing the synthesis of estrogen or blocking ERs in hormone-dependent tumors.

Tumors that are positive for ER and/or PR expression do not respond to endocrine therapy, and these patients should be offered endocrine therapy ([18, 19]). Patients who have tumors that are both ER and PR positive have a 50% to 70% probability of receiving clinical benefit from endocrine therapy. Patients with either ER-positive or PR-positive tumors have a 30% probability of receiving clinical benefit from endocrine therapy. Of patients with a prior history of hormonal response in the metastatic setting, 30% to 50% will have a response or clinical benefit from another hormonal regimen. Patients with low-volume disease and better performance status generally have higher response rates. The duration of first response is usually 9 to 12 months, similar to that with chemotherapy. The selection of endocrine therapy depends on the menopausal status of the patient: tamoxifen and/or ovarian suppression/ablation for premenopausal women and aromatase inhibitors or selective ER downregulators (SERDs) for postmenopausal women. The side effect profile also aids in the determination of which hormonal therapy to use, because the efficacy of all agents is nearly equal ([20]). A substantial minority of patients with hormone receptor–positive MBC will benefit from sequential single-agent endocrine therapy. Some patients might benefit from three or four lines of endocrine therapy, and a few will continue to respond to multiple lines and for many years. Additionally, for patients whose tumors are unusually sensitive to hormonal manipulation, repeated treatment with a previously effective agent may again be effective if a long interval has elapsed since it was discontinued.

The clinical criteria used to determine eligibility for endocrine therapy are longer DFI, no involvement of vital organs, no major dysfunction of the organs involved by the disease, minimal or moderate visceral involvement, and metastases confined to the soft tissue or bone.

Several types of endocrine therapy are available in managing MBC (Table 28-1). They include ovarian

Table 28-1 Types of Endocrine Therapy for Metastatic Breast Cancer

Type of Therapy	Examples
Ovarian ablation	Surgery, radiation therapy, pharmacologic interventions
LHRH agonists	Goserelin acetate
Selective estrogen receptor modulators	Tamoxifen
	Toremifene
	Raloxifene
	Arzoxifene hydrochloride
Selective estrogen receptor downregulators	Fulvestrant
Selective aromatase inhibitors	Anastrozole
	Letrozole
	Exemestane
	Fadrozole
	Formestane
Nonselective aromatase inhibitors	Testolactone
	Aminoglutethimide
Estrogens	Diethylstilbestrol Estradiol Megestrol acetate
Progestins	Medroxyprogesterone acetate
Androgens	Fluoxymesterone Danazol

LHRH, luteinizing hormone–releasing hormone.

ablation (oophorectomy, ovarian radiation), functional suppression (luteinizing hormone–releasing hormone [LHRH] agonists), selective ER modulators (SERMs), ER downregulators, progestins, androgens, estrogens, and nonsteroidal and steroidal selective aromatase inhibitors (AIs). Medical ovarian castration obviates surgery as a first choice. There is no current indication for adrenalectomy or hypophysectomy. There are no conclusive data to support combined hormonal therapies in postmenopausal breast cancer, aside from the use of fulvestrant with AIs in the first-line setting based on a recent trial noting clinical benefit. In most trials of combinations, some minimal increases in response rates were seen, but without a significant improvement in survival. Additional toxicities are usually observed ([21, 22]). As the understanding of the mechanisms of resistance to endocrine-based therapies has improved, the addition of therapies targeting these pathways has resulted in improved clinical outcomes. SERMs (tamoxifen and toremifene) are effective in pre- and postmenopausal patients with breast cancer. The LHRH agonists are effective in premenopausal women only ([23]), and the combination of tamoxifen and ovarian ablation is superior to ovarian ablation alone ([20, 23]). Estrogen biosynthesis is reduced by inhibiting the aromatase enzyme, which catalyzes the final step in estrogen production in humans. This does not completely block ovarian estrogen production in premenopausal women, and there is concern that the use of an AI as a single agent in this patient population may cause a reflex increase in gonadotropin levels and result in ovarian hyperstimulation. Thus, AIs must be used only in postmenopausal women; they are not effective in premenopausal women ([15, 24-26]). The AIs can broadly be categorized as selective and nonselective. The nonselective AIs block not only aromatase but also other enzymes in the cytochrome P450 family. Thus, they alter other steroid hormone levels and are associated with more side effects. Therefore, they are not frequently used.

Endocrine therapy is better tolerated than cytotoxic chemotherapy. However, several unique complications of endocrine therapy should be anticipated. One such complication, flare, is defined clinically by an abrupt, diffuse onset of musculoskeletal pain, increased size of skin lesions, or erythema surrounding the skin lesion within the first month of endocrine therapy. Flare may also be characterized as the worsening of bone lesions on bone scan, the reason for which bone scans may make assessing response to endocrine therapy difficult. The most serious manifestation of flare is hypercalcemia, which can be seen with several hormonal therapies except AIs and surgical castration. Hypercalcemia usually occurs in patients with bone metastases and manifests itself within the first 2 weeks after treatment. The underlying mechanism is the predominating early agonist effect of hormonal agents. Low doses of prednisone (10-30 mg/d) may abrogate the initial flare of bone pain.

Side effects of endocrine therapy, such as hot flashes and mood disturbances, are related to estrogen deprivation and are common with tamoxifen and AIs, reflecting the mechanism of action of these drugs. Tamoxifen has estrogenic effects that are beneficial in some tissues; it lowers serum cholesterol levels and protects against bone loss and cardiovascular disease but is also associated with potentially life-threatening side effects, such as endometrial cancer and thromboembolic events. AIs are associated with musculoskeletal side effects, such as arthralgias, myalgias, and bone loss. Weight gain is clearly associated with estrogens, androgens, corticosteroids, and progestins. Randomized trials of tamoxifen do not support an association with weight gain because patients on placebo experienced the same degree of weight gain as those on tamoxifen. This side effect is most common with progestins, which can cause both a true increase in weight from their anabolic effect and fluid retention secondary to their glucocorticoid effect. Progestins are the drugs most likely to cause thromboembolism; tamoxifen is the next most likely drug to cause this complication.

The preferred agent for endocrine therapy depends on the menopausal status of the patient. In premenopausal women, tamoxifen is recommended as the initial therapy, although ovarian suppression with an LHRH agonist alone or with tamoxifen can also be used. In patients who are within 1 year of antiestrogen exposure, the preferred second-line therapy is surgical oophorectomy or an LHRH agonist with endocrine therapy ([15]). In postmenopausal women who are antiestrogen naïve or who are more than 1 year from previous antiestrogen therapy, an AI is recommended as initial first-line therapy, but tamoxifen or the combination of fulvestrant with an anastrozole can be considered. Aromatase inhibitors appear to have superior outcome compared with tamoxifen, but differences are modest ([27, 28]). The use of anastrozole or letrozole as initial therapy in postmenopausal women with ER-positive tumors results in increased response rates and longer disease control ([29]). Patients who respond to initial therapy have a higher probability of response to second- and third-line endocrine therapies. There is a partial lack of cross-resistance between steroidal and nonsteroidal AIs. These agents may provide palliation of disease if used sequentially in patients with hormone receptor–positive tumors. There is evidence that a steroidal AI (exemestane) is effective in patients who have disease progression after a nonsteroidal AI. Most patients with hormone-responsive breast cancer benefit from the sequential use of endocrine therapies at the time of disease progression. Patients who respond to endocrine therapy with tumor shrinkage or long-term disease stabilization should receive additional endocrine therapy at the time of disease progression ([15]).

Fulvestrant is an ER antagonist that downregulates ER and has no agonist effects. It was compared with tamoxifen in a large randomized trial involving 587 postmenopausal women with advanced breast cancer or MBC who had not previously been treated with endocrine therapy. Patients were given either fulvestrant 250 mg intramurally monthly or tamoxifen 20 mg orally (PO) daily. At a median follow-up of 14.5 months, there was no significant difference between fulvestrant and tamoxifen in time to progression (TTP; median, 6.8 vs 8.3 months, respectively) ([30]). Fulvestrant also appears to be as effective as anastrozole in patients whose disease progressed on tamoxifen ([31, 32]). The clinical benefit rates of exemestane and fulvestrant observed in a phase III trial of postmenopausal women with hormone receptor–positive breast cancer who experienced disease progression on prior nonsteroidal AIs were comparable (32.2% vs 31.5%) ([33]). The CONFIRM trial (n = 736) compared fulvestrant at different doses (250 and 500 mg) in postmenopausal women with advanced disease recurring or progressing after prior endocrine therapy. Response rates were similar in both groups (13.8% vs 14.6%), but TTP and overall survival (OS) were significantly longer for the patients who received 500 mg (hazard ratio [HR], 0.80; 95% confidence interval [CI], 0.68-0.94) ([33, 34]).

Based on preclinical studies suggesting that the combination of fulvestrant and an AI was superior compared with either agent alone, three prospective clinical trials evaluated this approach in postmenopausal women with hormone receptor–positive MBC. In the Southwest Oncology Group SO226 trial, postmenopausal women (n = 707) with previously untreated metastatic disease were randomized to anastrozole versus anastrozole and fulvestrant, with crossover to fulvestrant encouraged ([35]). Median progression-free survival (PFS) and OS were significantly improved with the combination (median OS, 41.3 months with anastrozole vs 47.7 months with the combination; HR, 0.81; 95% CI, 0.65-1), despite the fact that 41% of patients receiving anastrozole crossed over to fulvestrant. Subgroup analysis revealed that those deriving the greatest benefit were patients who received no prior tamoxifen. The other two studies showed equivalent outcomes in patients receiving the combination. In a randomized phase III trial, Johnston et al reported that patients with hormone receptor–positive MBC who relapsed or progressed while receiving a nonsteroidal AIs had similar PFS when treated with fulvestrant plus anastrozole, fulvestrant plus anastrozole-matched placebo, or exemestane ([36]). Another phase III trial showed no advantages in clinical efficacy for the combination of anastrozole and fulvestrant compared to treatment with anastrozole alone as first-line treatment in postmenopausal women with hormone receptor–positive MBC ([37]). One possible reason for the difference in outcomes of the three studies is a potential imbalance in the prognostic subgroups in the SWOG study ([38]). Given the positive phase III findings and especially the significant prolongation in OS, the combination can still be considered, especially in patients who have never received tamoxifen.

De novo and acquired resistance is a known phenomenon. Options in this setting include changing the class of AI or using a drug with a different mechanism of action, such as fulvestrant or tamoxifen. Another approach is the addition of a mammalian target of rapamycin (mTOR) inhibitor, such as everolimus. Activation of the PI3K/Akt/mTOR pathway in breast cancer has been implicated as a mechanism of resistance to endocrine therapy. Preclinical research has evaluated the molecular basis of resistance to endocrine therapy, combatting resistance by incorporating inhibitors of this pathway ([39]). A phase II study demonstrated similar efficacy and safety with the use of everolimus in combination with tamoxifen in the treatment of of 111 patients with hormone receptor–positive, HER2-negative MBC with prior exposure to AI treatment either in the adjuvant and/or metastatic setting ([40]). The study fulfilled its primary end point, with a clinical benefit rate at 6 months of 61.1% with everolimus plus tamoxifen versus 42% with tamoxifen alone (P = .045). There was a delay in time to disease progression with the combination; the TTP was 8.6 months in patients treated with everolimus plus tamoxifen versus 4.5 months in those treated with tamoxifen alone, resulting in a significant reduction in the risk of disease progression (HR, 0.54; 95% CI, 0.35-0.81; P = .002).

The BOLERO-2 study, a randomized, phase III, double-blind, placebo-controlled, multicenter trial ([41]), randomized 724 patients with hormone receptor–positive advanced breast cancer who had recurrence or progression after receiving previous nonsteroidal AIs to receive either exemestane or exemestane plus everolimus. The combination arm resulted in an improvement in the primary end point of PFS (10.6 vs 4.1 months; P < .001). Adverse effects of everolimus reported to affect 30% of more of patients included stomatitis, infections, rash, fatigue, diarrhea, and reduced appetite. The most common grade 3 to 4 adverse reactions affecting 2% or more of patients included infections, hyperglycemia, fatigue, stomatitis, diarrhea, dyspnea, and pneumonitis. In 2012, everolimus in combination with exemestane was approved by the FDA for the treatment of postmenopausal women with recurrent or progressive hormone receptor–positive, HER2/neu-negative disease after failure of therapy with either letrozole or anastrozole.

Enticing new options in the treatment of hormone receptor–positive, HER2-negative MBC are cyclin-dependent kinase (CDK) 4/6 inhibitors ([42, 43]). Together with cyclin D1, CDK4 and CDK5 are kinases that facilitate the transition of dividing cells from the G_1 phase of the cell cycle to the S phase. Preclinical studies have demonstrated that breast cancer cells rely on both CDK4 and CDK6 for division and cell growth. Inhibition of these pathways leads to cell cycle arrest at the G_1/S phase checkpoint ([43]). Palbociclib, LEE011 (ribociclib), and LY2835219 (abemaciclib) are three selective CDK inhibitors presently under evaluation for the treatment of hormone receptor–positive MBC. In a phase I trial of LY2835219, 132 patients with five different tumor types, including MBC, received 150- to 200-mg doses of oral drug every 12 hours ([44]). The overall disease control rate for the 36 patients with hormone receptor–positive breast cancer was 81%, with a median PFS of 9.1 months. Common adverse events included diarrhea, nausea, vomiting, fatigue, and neutropenia. In a phase II trial, the oral CDK4/6 inhibitor, palbociclib, resulted in a near doubling of the primary end point of PFS as compared to control in the first-line treatment of 165 postmenopausal women with hormone receptor–positive MBC ([45]). Those receiving the combination of palbociclib in addition to letrozole had an objective response rate of 43% compared to 33%, with a PFS of 20.2 months versus 10.2 months (HR, 0.488; $P = .0004$). Common adverse events included leukopenia, neutropenia, and fatigue. The CDK inhibitors are being studied in phase III trials. The PALOMA-2 trial is testing the combination of palbociclib with letrozole in MBC in the frontline setting, and PALOMA-3 (NCT01740427) is evaluating the combination with fulvestrant in patients who have failed previous endocrine therapy. The MONALEESA-2 study is evaluating the efficacy and safety of the selective CDK inhibitor LEE011 in combination with letrozole in postmenopausal women with hormone receptor–positive MBC who have received no prior treatment for advanced disease (NCT01958021).

After third-line endocrine therapy, little high-level evidence exists to help select the optimal sequence of endocrine therapy. There are other hormonal agents available; progestins, for example, are synthetic derivatives of progesterone that have a progesterone agonist effect. Progestins such as megestrol acetate and medroxyprogesterone acetate are effective in treating MBC. These drugs are thought to have antiestrogenic properties and may result in interruption of the pituitary-ovarian axis. Androgens (eg, fluoxymesterone, danazol) have been evaluated and used in patients with MBC treated with multiple endocrine agents who still have hormone-dependent disease. Prior to the identification of hormone receptors or the development of SERMs, high-dose estrogens were commonly used to treat MBC. Their efficacy is similar to that of tamoxifen, although high-dose estrogens (eg, diethylstilbestrol, ethinyl estradiol) are associated with more severe side effects. Recent data suggest that the use of estrogens can be beneficial for patients with AI-resistant breast cancer ([46]). In a phase II study, 66 patients with AI-resistant MBC were randomized to receive 6 versus 30 mg of estradiol. The clinical benefit rates were 25% with 30 mg and 29% with 6 mg. The authors concluded that 6 mg of estradiol was as effective as 30 mg with greater safety and that this regimen could be a palliative therapeutic strategy in MBC progressing after other endocrine therapies ([46]). The treatment algorithm for treating patients with MBC at MDACC is illustrated Fig. 28-2.

CHEMOTHERAPY

No predictive test for response to chemotherapy has been sufficiently validated to use in a standard clinical setting. For patients with MBC not previously treated with chemotherapy, the response rates are 30% to 75%. Predictors of response to chemotherapy include DFI, sites of disease, organ function, and performance status, among others. Different biomarkers have been studied; some correlate with treatment response, but none is sufficiently accurate to help make a decision to treat or withhold therapy ([47]).

Selection of Agents/Regimen

In deciding which cytotoxic regimen to use in the setting of negative ER/PR and *HER2* status or in patients who have progressive disease after endocrine therapy, consideration should be given to the previous therapies, organ function, and comorbid conditions. Typically, chemotherapy within the conventional range of doses is associated with higher response rates than "low-dose chemotherapy." As in the setting of adjuvant therapy, high-dose chemotherapy with peripheral blood/bone marrow stem cell transplantation has not been found to be of clinical benefit in randomized trials ([48]).

The choice between sequential single agents and combination chemotherapy is controversial. The principle of nonoverlapping mechanisms of resistance and toxicities has been the basis of combination chemotherapy. Multiple randomized trials involving single-agent versus multiple-agent regimens in MBC have generally demonstrated that combination chemotherapy has improved response rates and TTP, but OS is not improved. Fossati et al ([49]), in a systematic review that included 31,510 patients, estimated that the proportional reduction in overall mortality for combinations versus single-agent regimens is only 18%, translating to an absolute benefit in survival of 9% at

1 year, 5% at 2 years, and only 3% after 5 years. More toxicity was associated with combination therapy. In two randomized trials of combination versus single-agent therapy in MBC, formal quality-of-life analyses favored the single-agent arms, even though response rates were slightly lower ([50, 51]).

A Cochrane review ([52]) including 28 trials and 5,707 patients with MBC randomly assigned to receive single-agent or combination chemotherapy found that combination therapy was associated with a higher response rate (odds ratio, 1.28; 95% CI, 1.15-1.42), longer TTP (HR, 0.78; 95% CI, 0.73-0.83), and longer OS (HR, 0.88; 95% CI, 0.83-0.94) than single-agent therapy. Most trials included in the Cochrane review did not specifically investigate the combination versus the sequential use of the single agents, and few studies reported the rate of "crossover" to an additional therapy following progression in the monotherapy arm. Therefore, the studies included evaluated the value of the use of two agents versus a single agent and do not address whether a simultaneous combination or a sequential monotherapy strategy should be pursued.

In the absence of strong evidence to guide the decision, and in agreement with different oncologic societies ([53]), we believe that use of single-agent therapy is preferable in the absence of rapid clinical progression, life-threatening visceral metastases, or the need for rapid symptom or disease control. Ultimately the choice of the use of sequential versus combination chemotherapy depends on a careful evaluation of risks and benefits for individual patients. The other major indication for combination therapy, as in the adjuvant setting, is the treatment of oligometastases.

Duration of Chemotherapy

The optimal duration of chemotherapy for MBC is controversial. Several studies have compared continuous (maintenance) chemotherapy with intermittent therapy. Several studies found that continuous therapy was associated with a longer time to relapse ([54-58]) but with worse side effects ([57]). None of the individual studies comparing continuous and intermittent therapy showed prolongation of life with continuous therapy. However, a recent meta-analysis of these data showed a statistically significant improvement in survival for patients receiving chemotherapy for a longer versus a shorter time ([58]). Some regimens, such as anthracycline-containing treatments, have inherent dose-limiting toxic effects that prohibit prolonged use. Other agents, such as trastuzumab, capecitabine, and, possibly taxanes given weekly, lend themselves to prolonged continued therapy. In an unplanned interim analysis, the recently presented Italian MANTA trial found no PFS or OS benefits for maintenance treatment with paclitaxel (175 mg/m^2 every 3 weeks for eight cycles) after first-line chemotherapy for MBC with an anthracycline/taxane-containing regimen (six to eight cycles) ([59]). Many trials are designed to treat patients until they have progression of disease or for two to three cycles after maximum benefits. Currently, the optimal treatment duration is unknown. The practice at MDACC is to treat patients with MBC with continuous chemotherapy unless unacceptable toxicity arises, at least until a third-line or fourth-line regimen comes into play and/or Eastern Cooperative Oncology Group (ECOG) performance status is ≥3 in patients with MBC.

Single-Agent Chemotherapy

Anthracyclines

The introduction of anthracyclines (doxorubicin and epirubicin) in the 1970s represented a significant advance in the treatment of advanced breast cancer. In patients with MBC, response rates to single-agent doxorubicin (25-75 mg/m^2 every 3 weeks) ranged from 25% to 60% and were heavily influenced by patient characteristics such as prior chemotherapy exposure, performance status, and extent and sites of disease ([60-64]). At MDACC, doxorubicin-containing regimens have historically been the initial treatment of choice for MBC treated previously with non–anthracycline-containing chemotherapy. Patients who received anthracyclines and had a prolonged DFI before the development of metastatic disease occasionally benefit from repeat administration of doxorubicin. However, given the increasing number of active agents available to treat MBC, repeat management with anthracyclines should be reserved for patients in whom other treatments have failed, given the potential risk of heart failure.

Epirubicin is a doxorubicin analog that has been shown to have similar efficacy and somewhat less toxicity than doxorubicin at equimolar doses. Although not designed to perform a head-to-head comparison, results from a randomized trial suggested that epirubicin might be as efficacious as doxorubicin. A formal comparison of two different anthracyclines in combination (5-fluorouracil, doxorubicin, and cyclophosphamide [FAC] vs 5-fluorouracil, epirubicin, and cyclophosphamide [FEC]) at equimolar doses found both regimens to be equally effective in terms of response rate, TTP, and survival. The FEC regimen was associated with less gastrointestinal, hematologic, and cardiac toxicity ([65]).

Efforts to improve the safety profile of doxorubicin while preserving efficacy have resulted in liposomal formulations of doxorubicin. Response rates with these products appear comparable to those seen in other multicenter trials using conventional single-agent doxorubicin. In a phase III clinical trial, O'Brien et al compared the efficacy and safety of pegylated liposomal doxorubicin with those of conventional doxorubicin as first-line therapy in patients with MBC ([66]). A total of 509 women received a 1-hour infusion of pegylated liposomal doxorubicin (50 mg/m^2 once every 4 weeks) or conventional doxorubicin (60 mg/m^2 once every 3 weeks). The median PFS and OS were similar in both treatment groups (6.9 vs 7.8 months and 20.1 vs 22.0 months, respectively). The rates of alopecia, myelosuppression, nausea, and vomiting were lower with pegylated liposomal doxorubicin than with conventional doxorubicin. Perhaps most notably, pegylated liposomal doxorubicin was associated with a significantly lower incidence of cardiotoxicity, even at higher cumulative doses ($P < .001$) ([66]). The most important dose-limiting toxicity of pegylated liposomal doxorubicin is palmar-plantar erythrodysesthesia, which is both dose and duration related. The polyethylene glycol coating results in preferential concentration of the drug in the skin; this explains why small amounts of the drug can leak from capillaries in the palms and soles, resulting in redness, tenderness, and peeling of the skin that can be uncomfortable and even painful. As with all liposomal drug delivery systems, there is a low incidence of hypersensitivity reactions.

Taxanes

Taxanes (paclitaxel, docetaxel, and the nanoparticle albumin-bound [nab]-paclitaxel) are among of the most active classes of cytotoxic drugs available today for the treatment of breast cancer. They rival the anthracyclines in terms of response rates and positive impact on TTP. Taxanes are frequently used as first-line chemotherapy for treatment-naive MBC and also in MBC treated with anthracyclines or if anthracyclines are contraindicated. Response rates with paclitaxel range from 21% to 62%; in anthracycline-resistant breast cancer, response rates are 40%.

Two trials have directly compared doxorubicin and paclitaxel, using different dosing and administration schedules. In the Intergroup E1193 study ([67]), similar response rates and TTP were demonstrated with doxorubicin administered at 60 mg/m^2 and paclitaxel at 175 mg/m^2 over 24 hours. Thus, paclitaxel may be as effective as doxorubicin when administered as a single agent. The dose and administration schedule may influence the response to paclitaxel. The use of weekly paclitaxel has recently become very popular due to the improvement in the toxicity profile and the ability to deliver a more dose-intensive regimen. At MDACC, the most popular taxane regimen is weekly paclitaxel 80 mg/m^2, commonly in a "3 weeks on, 1 week off" or "2 weeks on, 1 week off" schedule.

Docetaxel is a semisynthetic taxane with several preclinical, pharmacokinetic, biological, and clinical differences in comparison to paclitaxel. It has demonstrated a 37% to 57% response rate in patients with anthracycline-resistant tumors and was initially FDA approved for this indication at a dose of 60 to 100 mg/m^2 every 3 weeks. At this dose, hematologic toxicity is the greatest and the rates of neutropenia are similar to those seen when paclitaxel is given every 3 weeks. In a large clinical trial, 527 patients were randomized to receive docetaxel 60, 75, or 100 mg/m^2 every 3 weeks. A relationship between increasing dose of docetaxel and increased tumor response was observed, but toxicities were also related to increasing doses ([68]). Docetaxel every 3 weeks at doses between 75 and 100 mg/m^2 are appropriate choices as first-line therapy for MBC; in most cases at MDACC, we use 75 mg/m^2. Compared to every-3-week paclitaxel, docetaxel 100 mg/m^2 was associated with longer TTP (HR, 1.64; 95% CI, 1.33-2.02) and improved OS (HR, 1.64; 95% CI, 1.33-2.02), but also greater incidence of treatment-related toxicities ([69]). To place these data in context, it is important to remember that paclitaxel has greater activity when given on a weekly schedule, yet it is not clear whether docetaxel or paclitaxel provides superior outcomes when each agent is administered at its optimal dose and schedule. In patients who had received paclitaxel previously, docetaxel administration was associated with response rates of 18% to 21%, demonstrating a lack of cross-resistance between the two agents ([70]).

Moderate nail changes and fatigue are commonly seen with weekly paclitaxel and docetaxel; excessive tearing due to partial or complete canalicular stenosis is seen with weekly docetaxel. Diarrhea, stomatitis, and neutropenia and its complications are uncommon with weekly taxane administration. Fluid retention is seen in patients who receive a docetaxel cumulative dose greater than 300 mg/m^2. Premedication with steroids greatly reduces the magnitude of fluid retention; the optimal doses and schedules for steroid administration are not well established. At MDACC, we routinely prescribe dexamethasone 4 mg PO twice a day for 3 days beginning the day before chemotherapy administration.

Nab-paclitaxel is a nanoparticle albumin-bound paclitaxel (Abraxane) that has been investigated in the treatment of MBC. In different comparisons, it has proven to be better, or at least as effective, as the other taxanes ([71, 72]), with the advantage that it does not require Cremophor for solubility and therefore is associated with less hypersensitivity reactions. In a phase III study, 454 patients were randomly assigned to 3-week cycles of nab-paclitaxel 260 mg/m^2 or paclitaxel 175 mg/m^2. Nab-paclitaxel demonstrated significantly higher response rates compared with paclitaxel (33% vs 19%, $P = .001$) and longer TTP (23.0 vs 16.9 weeks, $P = .006$). Grade 3 sensory neuropathy was more common with nab-paclitaxel, the incidence of grade 4 neutropenia was significantly lower with nab-paclitaxel, but the rate of febrile neutropenia was similar in both groups. A phase II four-arm study compared nab-paclitaxel (300 mg/m^2 every 3 weeks, 100 mg/m^2 weekly, or 150 mg/m^2 weekly) and docetaxel (100 mg/m^2 every 3 weeks). The weekly dose of 150 mg/m^2 of nab-paclitaxel demonstrated longer PFS than docetaxel (12.9 vs 7.5 months, P = .006), but no differences in PFS or response rates were seen when comparing docetaxel and the 3-week schedule of nab-paclitaxel. Grade 3 or 4 fatigue, neutropenia, and febrile neutropenia were less frequent in all nab-paclitaxel arms, but the frequency and grade of peripheral neuropathy were similar in all groups ([71]). At MDACC, nab-paclitaxel is frequently used as first- or second-line therapy administered in a weekly schedule, and it is preferred to paclitaxel for patients with contraindications to steroid use.

Antimetabolites

Capecitabine

Capecitabine (Xeloda) is an oral fluoropyrimidine approved by the FDA in April 1998 as single-agent therapy for the treatment of MBC resistant to anthracyclines and taxanes. In September 2001, capecitabine was approved for use in combination with docetaxel in MBC previously treated with an anthracycline. The first phase II study of capecitabine in breast cancer involved 162 patients previously treated with paclitaxel for MBC ([73]). The majority of patients had also received previous anthracycline therapy. Capecitabine was administered at 2,500 mg/m^2/d in two divided doses for 14 days, followed by 1 week of rest. Twenty-seven (20%) of 135 women with measurable disease demonstrated complete or partial responses. The median duration of response was 8.1 months, and the median survival was 12.8 months. In a phase II trial, O'Shaughnessy et al randomized patients to receive cyclophosphamide, methotrexate and 5-fluorouracil (CMF) or capecitabine in the frontline setting ([74]). The overall response rate was 30% for capecitabine and 16% for CMF; no differences in TTP were seen. Similar levels of nausea, vomiting, and stomatitis were observed in both groups. More cases of grade 3 or 4 diarrhea (8%), fatigue (5%), and hand-foot syndrome (15%) were noted with capecitabine.

Capecitabine is active in the treatment of MBC, and significant response rates can be achieved in women previously treated with an anthracycline and a taxane. However, patients with triple-negative tumors do not benefit from it. The FDA-approved dose and schedule are 2,500 mg/m^2/d given orally in two divided doses for 14 days, followed by 1 week of rest. Retrospective studies suggest that a lower starting dose (2,000 mg/m^2/d) is better tolerated, with preserved efficacy. Capecitabine as first-line therapy for MBC results in response rates of 30% to 58%, and it is a reasonable option for some patients. At MDACC, it is often used as first-line therapy for patients who have been previously treated with anthracyclines and/or taxanes in the adjuvant or neoadjuvant setting.

Gemcitabine

Gemcitabine (Gemzar), a nucleoside analog, was approved by the FDA in April 2004 for the first-line treatment of MBC in the United States. In patients with MBC, single-agent response rates have ranged from 14% to 37% ([75-77]). These were small trials, and the disparate results may be due to dosing differences. Generally, chemotherapy-naive patients tolerate doses of 1,000 to 1,250 mg/m^2/wk on days 1, 8, and 15 every 28 days. Omitting the day 15 dose or reducing the dose in subsequent cycles of chemotherapy may improve the patient's ability to tolerate therapy beyond the initial cycles. Pretreated patients may require dose reductions in order to decrease the risk of thrombocytopenia. Gemcitabine has been investigated in many different doublet and triplet combinations; it is a promising agent for its efficacy as a single drug, but also due to its ability to readily combine with paclitaxel, vinorelbine, docetaxel, or cisplatin/carboplatin as first- or second-line therapy. At present, gemcitabine is appropriate treatment for patients with MBC after treatment failure with standard regimens.

Other Agents

Vinorelbine

Vinorelbine (Navelbine) is a semisynthetic vinca alkaloid that interferes with microtubule assembly and is an important active agent in the treatment of MBC. Phase II trials investigating its efficacy in pretreated MBC have demonstrated response rates ranging from 25% to 47% ([78-80]). The primary side effects are neutropenia, pain with infusion, flu-like symptoms, and gastrointestinal symptoms such as nausea or constipation. Vinorelbine is appropriate third-line (or later) therapy for patients with MBC. At MDACC, it is usually given at a dose of 25 mg/m^2 on days 1, 8, and 15 of 21-day cycles.

Ixabepilone

Ixabepilone (Ixempra) is an epothilone B analog that binds to microtubules and causes microtubule stabilization and mitotic arrest. It was approved by the FDA in October 2007 (alone or in combination with capecitabine) for the treatment of patients with MBC resistant to treatment with an anthracycline and a taxane or whose cancer is taxane resistant and for whom further anthracycline therapy is contraindicated. As a single agent, it is also indicated for patients with tumors resistant or refractory to capecitabine.

Ixabepilone monotherapy was evaluated in a single-arm trial in 126 patients who had previously received an anthracycline, a taxane, and capecitabine ([81]). The objective response rate was 11.5%, the median response duration was 5.7 months, and the median OS was 8.6 months. Grade 3 or 4 neutropenia was seen in 54% of patients, and grade 3 or 4 peripheral neuropathy was seen in 14%. When used as first-line therapy in patients with MBC who received anthracycline-based chemotherapy in the adjuvant setting, the response rates was 41.5%, with a median duration of response of 8.2 months and a median survival of 22 months ([82]). At MDACC, we frequently use it in patients who have received anthracyclines, taxanes, and capecitabine. Ixabepilone is given at 40 mg/m^2, but based on toxicities and tolerance, it is not uncommon to reduce the dose to 32 mg/m^2.

Eribulin

Eribulin mesylate is a synthetic analog, a novel microtubule modulator that induces a conformational change that suppresses microtubule growth and sequestration of tubulin into nonfunctional aggregates. In the phase III study that led to its approval, 762 heavily pretreated women with locally or recurrent MBC were randomized to receive eribulin or physicians' treatment of choice. Patients treated with eribulin had an improvement in OS (13.1 vs 10.6 months; HR, 0.81; 95% CI, 0.66-0.99) ([83]). Asthenia, fatigue, and neutropenia were the most common side effects associated with eribulin. Peripheral neuropathy led to discontinuation of treatment in 5% of patients. Recently, a phase II study evaluated the efficacy and safety of eribulin in the treatment of HER2-negative MBC in the first-line setting ([84]). Fifty-six patients were treated, with the majority having received anthracycline- and/or taxane-containing chemotherapy in the adjuvant setting. The objective response rate was 29% (95% CI, 17.3%-42.2%), the clinical benefit rate was 52%, the median response duration was 5.8 months, and the median PFS was 6.8 months.

Combination Chemotherapy

Anthracycline-Based Combination Regimens

Doxorubicin-containing combinations result in overall response rates ranging from 50% to 80%, with response durations of 8 to 15 months. The median survival with doxorubicin–alkylating agent combinations was 17 to 25 months. Although doxorubicin-containing regimens are more efficacious in the metastatic setting than are non-doxorubicin-containing combinations, anthracycline-based combinations are not commonly used because of the associated side effects.

As was discussed previously, the issue of whether combination chemotherapy is superior to single-agent chemotherapy in the treatment for MBC continues to be debated. For patients with rapidly progressing disease, treatment regimens most likely to produce an objective tumor response are highly desirable; therefore, there is still an important role for the use of combination chemotherapy. For many years, FAC (500/50/500 mg/m^2) was the standard regimen for patients with MBC treated at MDACC. Several randomized clinical trials have compared different anthracycline-based chemotherapy regimens in patients with MBC. Nabholtz et al ([85, 86]) compared the use of docetaxel/doxorubicin/cyclophosphamide (TAC; 75/50/500 mg/m^2) with FAC as first-line therapy for MBC (n = 484). The objective response rate was 55% with TAC and 44% with FAC (P = .02; HR, 1.5; 95% CI, 1.1-2.2). There was no significant difference in TTP or OS between treatment arms. Febrile neutropenia occurred more frequently with TAC than FAC (29% vs 5%), but similar rates of infection were seen. Carmichael et al reported the results of a trial comparing epirubicin and cyclophosphamide (EC) with epirubicin and paclitaxel (EP) in patients with MBC ([87]). A total of 705 patients received up to six cycles of therapy. The objective response rate was higher with EP (67%) than with EC (56%). However, the TTP and OS were similar between the treatment arms. Doxorubicin and cyclophosphamide (AC) were compared to doxorubicin and docetaxel (AT) in 429 patients with MBC ([88]). The AT regimen significantly improved the TTP (37.9 vs 31.9 weeks, P = .014) and overall response rate (59% vs 47%, P = .008) compared with AC, but there was no difference in OS. The AT regimen is a valid option for the treatment of MBC.

Platinum-Based Combination Regimens

As single agents, the platinum salts (primarily cisplatin and carboplatin) have had relatively limited use in the treatment of MBC. Platinum compounds have been reserved for third-line therapy or beyond. Objective responses in this setting are less than 10% ([89]). In a limited number of trials of cisplatin or carboplatin first-line chemotherapy for MBC, objective responses were up to 50% ([89]). The availability of many active chemotherapeutic regimens and the significant toxicities associated with platinum compounds resulted in their being largely used in the salvage setting. With the introduction of newer cytotoxic agents and preclinical data demonstrating their synergy with platinum compounds, there is renewed interest in incorporating the platinum compounds into regimens for MBC. The major reason for the revival of interest in platinum compounds is a greater understanding of the sensitivity of cells with homologous recombination deficiency, especially those with *BRCA* mutations, to platinum. Platinum monotherapy or platinum-based combinations are being widely tested in primary breast cancer and MBC in *BRCA* mutation carriers. By extrapolation, there is also much interest in testing platinum-based therapies in patients with triple-negative breast cancer and in those with HER+ tumors because in vitro synergy has been shown with anti-HER2 therapy in experimental models.

Phase II trials have been reported with the combination of paclitaxel and cisplatin. As first-line therapy for MBC, overall response rates have ranged from 50% to 90%. Trials evaluating this combination as second- or third-line therapy reported response rates of 30% to 50% [89]. These results suggest that the combination of cisplatin and paclitaxel produces response rates higher than those expected with paclitaxel alone. Perez et al reported on the combination of paclitaxel (200 mg/m^2) and carboplatin (area under the curve [AUC] 6 every 3 weeks) as first-line treatment of MBC [90]. In 53 patients, an overall response rate of 62% was observed, including a complete response rate of 16%. The median TTP was 7.3 months, with a 1-year survival rate of 72%. A similar trial combining paclitaxel (175 mg/m^2) and carboplatin (AUC 6) administered every 3 weeks [91] reported an objective response rate of 43% (14% complete response rate); the objective response rate was higher among patients who had received prior adjuvant therapy (76% vs 45%). A phase II study examined the combination of a platinum compound and docetaxel [92]. Among this previously treated group of patients, the overall response rate was 61%, the median duration of response was 8 months, and the median TTP was 10 months.

The activity of the cisplatin/gemcitabine combination in MBC had been explored with promising results. In one trial, patients previously treated with an anthracycline and/or taxane received cisplatin (30 mg/m^2) plus gemcitabine (750 or 1,000 mg/m^2) on days 1, 8, and 15 of 21-day cycles. The objective response rate was 50%, with 10% of patients attaining a complete response. The most common toxicities were peripheral neuropathy, nausea/vomiting, and hematologic toxicities (neutropenia, thrombocytopenia, and anemia) [93]. In a trial evaluating cisplatin 25 mg/m^2 on days 1 through 4 and gemcitabine 1,000 mg/m^2 on days 2 and 8 of a 21-day cycle, patients (n = 136) were divided in two cohorts according to prior treatments (heavily pretreated and not heavily pretreated). The response rate for both of the cohorts was 26%, and the median durations of response were 5.3 and 5.9 months, respectively [94].

Platinum agents may prove to have a specific role in the treatment of triple-negative breast cancers, particularly in tumors harboring *BRCA* dysfunction. In preclinical and clinical studies, mutations in *BRCA* have greater sensitivity to DNA-damaging chemotherapeutic agents, such as platinum agents. Several studies are evaluating the safety and efficacy of platinum-based chemotherapy in combination with novel agents, particularly poly(ADP-ribose)polymerase (PARP) inhibitors. Given the similarities between triple-negative tumors and tumors harboring *BRCA1* mutations, a large phase III study evaluated the combination of gemcitabine and carboplatin versus gemcitabine, carboplatin, and iniparib. The overall response rate for 258 patients treated with gemcitabine plus carboplatin was 33.7%, with a median PFS of 4.1 months and median OS of 11.1 months [95]. Unfortunately, iniparib was not an active PARP inhibitor, and the trial did not meet its primary end point. A recent meta-analysis evaluated four studies of platinum-based combination chemotherapy in the metastatic setting [96]. The overall response rates were comparable, but patients with triple-negative breast cancer treated with platinum agents had longer PFS. At present, we believe there may be a benefit in the use of platinum-based chemotherapy in all patients with triple-negative breast cancer regardless of *BRCA* status. Ongoing clinical trials will help clarify whether the majority of the benefit is derived from the efficacy of the platinum agents among *BRCA* mutation carriers.

Gemcitabine in Combination With Other Agents

Several phase II trials have investigated salvage therapy with docetaxel/gemcitabine combinations in MBC. Drug doses and schedules varied. Among previously treated patients, the objective response rates ranged from 36% to 79%. In a phase III study, the combination of gemcitabine (1,250 mg/m^2 on days 1 and 8) and paclitaxel (175 mg/m^2 on day 1) was associated with an improvement in response rate and TTP compared with paclitaxel alone (39.3% vs 25.6% and 5.4 vs 3.5 months, respectively) as first-line therapy for MBC [97]. Median OS was also significantly improved with the combination (18.6 vs 15.8 months; HR, 0.77; 95% CI, 0.62-0.95). There was more frequent grade 4 hematologic toxicity with the combination. Of note, most patients randomized to paclitaxel alone did not receive subsequent gemcitabine.

A phase III European trial found no difference between gemcitabine-docetaxel (1,000 mg/m^2 on days 1 and 8 and 75 mg/m^2 on day 1) and capecitabine-docetaxel (1,250 mg/m^2 twice a day on days 1-14 and 75 mg/m^2 on day 1) [98]. Similar PFS, OS, and response rates were seen. The toxicity profile for the gemcitabine-docetaxel combination was better.

Vinorelbine-Based Combination Regimens

A trial of single-agent doxorubicin compared to doxorubicin plus vinorelbine failed to demonstrate a superior response rate with the combination ([99]). Vinorelbine has been successfully combined with taxanes. There are no phase III trials to confirm that these combinations are better than either single agent. Phase II studies combining vinorelbine and paclitaxel in MBC have been reported ([100]). The overall response rates with first-line vinorelbine/paclitaxel are 49% to 60%. The overall response rates for second-line vinorelbine/paclitaxel and vinorelbine/docetaxel are 46% to 56% and 37% to 59%, respectively. Toxicities associated with vinorelbine/taxane combinations were myelosuppression and mild neurotoxicity ([100]).

Capecitabine Combination Regimens

In September 2001, the FDA approved capecitabine in combination with docetaxel for patients with MBC previously treated with an anthracycline. This was based on the results of a multinational phase III trial that randomized 511 anthracycline-refractory patients to receive docetaxel 100 mg/m^2 or capecitabine 1,250 mg/m^2 twice daily for 14 days plus docetaxel 75 mg/m^2 intravenously every 3 weeks ([101]). The response rates for the single-agent and combination regimens were 30% and 42%, respectively (*P* =.006). The TTP was 4.2 and 6.1 months, respectively (*P* = .0001). The OS was significantly superior with the combination (HR, 0.775; 95% CI, 0.63-0.94). This is one of the few randomized trials that reported a survival benefit of one treatment over the other, but the design of the trial does not confirm that the combination is better than the sequential administration of single-agent docetaxel followed by capecitabine, or vice versa. Grade 3 treatment-related adverse events were more common with the combination versus docetaxel alone (71% vs 49%, respectively), but overall, the incidence of treatment-related adverse events was similar between the two groups (98% vs 94%, respectively).

Capecitabine in combination with ixabepilone has been approved for the management of resistant MBC or MBC progressing after anthracyclines and taxanes. The trial that led to the approval of this combination randomized 752 patients to ixabepilone (40 mg/m^2 intravenously every 3 weeks) plus capecitabine (2,000 mg/m^2 on days 1-14 of a 21-day cycle) or capecitabine alone (2,500 mg/m^2 on the same day schedule) ([102]). Patients receiving the combination had a 25% reduction in the estimated risk of disease progression (HR, 0.75; 95% CI, 0.64-0.88). Median PFS (5.8 vs 4.2 months) and response rate (35% vs 14%) were also higher with the combination. Grade 3 or 4 treatment-related sensory neuropathy, fatigue, and neutropenia were more frequent with combination therapy, as was the rate of death as a result of toxicity (3% vs 1%). Patients with liver dysfunction were at higher risk of complications and therefore should not be treated with this regimen. Despite its toxicity, this combination represents a good alternative for patients with resistant disease previously treated with anthracyclines and taxanes and in whom a fast response is needed.

TARGETED THERAPIES

HER2/neu-Targeted Therapies

Since the introduction on anti-HER2 therapies to the treatment armamentarium of breast cancer, the outcome of patients with HER2-positive breast cancers has dramatically changed. The use of these therapies is now an integral part of the standard treatment of this subset of patients. For many years, the use of trastuzumab and a taxane was considered as the optimal first-line therapy among patients with MBC. In the past 2 years, the treatment algorithm of patients with HER2-positive MBC has dramatically changed as a result of the introduction of pertuzumab and T-DM1. In the following sections, we will review the most relevant data associated with the different anti-HER2 therapies. At MDACC, the use of trastuzumab, pertuzumab, and a taxane is considered the best regimen, and we use it as first-line therapy, followed by T-DM1 at the time of progression. For third- or fourth-line treatment, a number of different agents can be used. Commonly, we use trastuzumab and lapatinib, lapatinib and capecitabine, or another single chemotherapeutic agent in combination with trastuzumab.

Trastuzumab

The HER2/neu protein, a receptor tyrosine kinase, is overexpressed in 25% to 30% of human breast cancers and plays an important role in tumor development and progression. Trastuzumab (Herceptin) is a murine-human chimeric monoclonal antibody targeted against the HER protein. Trastuzumab was evaluated in two pivotal trials in women with HER2/neu-overexpressed MBC. In one trial, trastuzumab (4 mg/kg loading dose, then 2 mg/kg weekly) was evaluated as a single agent in 222 heavily pretreated women with MBC ([103]). Nine (4%) of 213 treated patients achieved complete response, and 37 (17%) achieved partial response. The median duration of response was 9.1 months. For all treated patients, the median TTP was 3.1 months, and the median OS was 13 months. The most clinically significant adverse event was cardiac dysfunction, which occurred in 10 patients (4.7%), nine of whom had received prior anthracycline therapy. This trial demonstrated that trastuzumab can induce durable objective responses and is associated with an acceptable toxicity profile. The second pivotal trial evaluated the use of chemotherapy with or without trastuzumab in 469 patients who had not received prior chemotherapy for metastatic disease ([104]). Women who had received an anthracycline in the adjuvant setting received paclitaxel 175 mg/m^2 every 3 weeks. All of the other patients received doxorubicin 60 mg/m^2 or epirubicin 75 mg/m^2 plus cyclophosphamide 600 mg/m^2 every 3 weeks. Trastuzumab 2 mg/kg (after a 4 mg/kg loading dose) was administered weekly until disease progression. The combination of chemotherapy plus trastuzumab resulted in a significantly higher objective response rate than chemotherapy alone (50% vs 32%). Women in the chemotherapy plus trastuzumab arm also had a significantly longer TTP and OS than those treated with chemotherapy alone. Symptomatic or asymptomatic cardiac dysfunction was seen in 27% of women treated with concurrent anthracycline/cyclophosphamide and trastuzumab. Based on the results of this trial, the FDA approved the combination of paclitaxel and trastuzumab as first-line therapy for HER2-overexpressed MBC.

The combination of trastuzumab and docetaxel has a high level of activity and an acceptable toxicity profile ([105, 106]). When docetaxel (100 mg/m^2 every 3 weeks) with or without trastuzumab (4 mg/kg loading dose followed by 2 mg/kg weekly) was evaluated, the combination was significantly superior to docetaxel alone in terms of overall response rate (61% vs 34%; $P = .0002$), OS (31.2 vs 22.7 months; $P = .032$), TTP (11.7 vs 6.1 months; $P = .0001$), and duration of response (11.7 vs 5.7 months; $P = .009$). There was little difference in the number and severity of adverse events between the arms.

Given the success of the trastuzumab and paclitaxel combination, trastuzumab has been combined with other active agents against breast cancer ([107]). A multicenter phase III study comparing trastuzumab/vinorelbine to trastuzumab/taxane (TRAVIOTA study) randomized 81 patients to receive trastuzumab with weekly vinorelbine or weekly taxane therapy (paclitaxel or docetaxel at the investigator's choice) ([108]). Response rates were 51% and 40% for the vinorelbine/trastuzumab arm and the taxane/trastuzumab arm, respectively. The median times to disease progression were 8.5 and 6.0 months, respectively ($P = .09$). Treatment with either regimen was well tolerated. Trastuzumab has also been safely combined with other agents. The trastuzumab/gemcitabine combination provides response rates of 30% to 44% in heavily pretreated patients. For patients who had disease progression on anthracyclines, taxanes, and vinorelbine, the combination of capecitabine (1,250 mg/m^2 divided twice a day for 14 days) and trastuzumab was shown to be very effective ([109, 110]). In different trials, the response rates were between 20% and 45% with clinical benefit rates of 70% to 85%. The safety profile of the combination was favorable and predictable, with a low incidence of grade 3 or 4 adverse events. This supports the use of the combination of capecitabine and trastuzumab in heavily pretreated MBC patients with tumors that have *HER2* overexpression.

A number of trials evaluated triplet combinations. A phase III clinical trial evaluated the combination of trastuzumab/paclitaxel/carboplatin (TPC; trastuzumab 4 mg/kg loading dose followed by 2 mg/kg weekly, paclitaxel 175 mg/m^2, and carboplatin AUC 6 every 21 days) versus trastuzumab/paclitaxel. The triple combination arm had statistically significant improved response rates and PFS. Both treatments were well tolerated, but more cases of grade 4 neutropenia were seen in the triple combination arm ([111]).

Pertuzumab

Pertuzumab is a humanized anti-HER2 monoclonal antibody approved by the FDA in 2012 for the treatment of advanced or late-stage (metastatic) HER2-positive breast cancer. Compared with trastuzumab, pertuzumab binds to a different extracellular dimerization subdomain of the *HER2* receptor to inhibit signaling, thereby resulting in the reduction of tumor cell proliferation, invasiveness, and survival. The combination of pertuzumab, trastuzumab, and docetaxel was shown to have efficacy in the first-line treatment of HER2-positive MBC in a randomized trial known as the CLEOPATRA study ([112]). In this study of 800 patients, the addition of pertuzumab resulted in a PFS benefit of 18.5 months versus 12.4 months for the control group (HR, 0.62; 95% CI, 0.51-0.75; $P < .001$). At a median follow-up of 50 months, the addition of pertuzumab significantly improved median OS by 15.7 months (40.8 vs 56.5 months; HR, 0.68; 95% CI, 0.56-0.84; $P = .0002$), with a benefit consistently seen across all subgroups. The side effects profile was comparable between the two groups, although the rates of febrile neutropenia and diarrhea of grade ≥3 were higher in the pertuzumab arm. The combination of pertuzumab and trastuzumab was evaluated in a phase II study of 66 patients with progressive metastatic disease in the setting of prior trastuzumab exposure ([113]). The overall response rate was 24.2% and PFS was 5.5 months, with 17 patients experiencing stable disease for greater than 6 months. An ongoing study is evaluating the role of pertuzumab in patients with disease progression on trastuzumab, through a randomized phase II trial of trastuzumab/capecitabine alone or with pertuzumab for HER2-positive MBC progressing during or after trastuzumab-based first-line therapy ([114]). A nonrandomized phase II study is evaluating the efficacy of pertuzumab in combination with paclitaxel and trastuzumab in patients treated with up to one prior regimen for MBC, allowing for prior trastuzumab either in the metastatic or adjuvant setting (NCT01276041)

T-DM1

Ado-trastuzumab emtansine (T-DM1; Kadcyla) is the first HER2-antibody drug conjugate, combining trastuzumab with a linked antimicrotubule drug, maytansine (DM1). The FDA approved it in 2013 for the treatment of patients with metastatic HER2-positive breast cancer previously treated with trastuzumab and taxanes. The initial phase I study conducted in heavily pretreated patients with *HER2* overexpression showed clinical activity, leading to a single-arm phase II study in 112 patients who progressed on trastuzumab, lapatinib, or both. A response rate of 25.9%, clinical benefit rate of 34%, and PFS of 4.6 months were observed ([115]). Hypokalemia (8.9%), thrombocytopenia (8%), and fatigue (4.5%) were the most common grade 3 or 4 toxicities. The EMILIA trial was an open-label, phase III study comparing T-DM1 versus capecitabine/lapatinib in trastuzumab pretreated HER2-positive patients with advanced/metastatic breast cancer (n = 980) ([116]). A significant improvement in PFS was observed with T-DM1 (9.6 vs 6.4 months; HR, 0.650; 95% CI, 0.549-0.771; $P < .0001$). The OS at 2 years was 65.4% with T-DM1 compared to 47.5% with capecitabine/lapatinib. An added benefit is the favorable safety profile of T-DM1 and the potential role of T-DM1 in treating brain metastasis. A phase II trial evaluated the role of treatment with T-DM1 in the first-line setting as compared to trastuzumab and docetaxel, resulting in an improvement in PFS ([117]). At a median follow-up of 14 months, the median PFS was 9.2 months with trastuzumab plus docetaxel and 14.2 months with T-DM1 (HR, 0.59; 95% CI, 0.36-0.97). The overall response rate with T-DM1 was 64.2% (95% CI, 51.8%-74.8%) versus 58% (95% CI, 45.5%-69.2%) with trastuzumab plus docetaxel. In the TH3RESA trial, 602 patients previously treated with two or more HER2-directed therapies were randomized to receive T-DM1 or treatment of physician's choice ([118]). The PFS was significantly improved with T-DM1 compared with physician's choice (median, 6.2 vs 3.3 months; HR, 0.528; 95% CI, 0.422-0.661; $P < .0001$). An interim OS analysis showed a trend favoring T-DM1. A lower incidence of grade 3 or worse adverse events was reported with T-DM1 than with physician's choice treatment.

The MARIANNE trial is a phase III randomized trial evaluating the efficacy of T-DM1 with or without pertuzumab compared with trastuzumab plus taxane for first-line treatment of HER2-positive MBC (NCT01120184). A second phase III trial is seeking to compare T-DM1 to physician's choice of treatment in patients with HER2-positive unresectable locally advanced or metastatic breast cancer treated with at least two prior anti-HER2 regimens (NCT01419197). Finally, a phase IB/II trial is evaluating the role of T-DM1 in combination with pertuzumab in patients with HER2-positive advanced breast cancer previously treated with trastuzumab ([119]).

Lapatinib

Lapatinib (Tykerb) is a selective, reversible dual EGFR-HER2 inhibitor. Phase II trials of single-agent lapatinib have shown modest clinical benefit in patients with HER2-positive breast cancer. Lapatinib in combination with capecitabine was approved by the FDA in 2007 for the treatment of advanced or HER2-overexpressing MBC previously treated with an anthracycline, a taxane, and trastuzumab. The trial that led to the approval showed that patients treated with lapatinib and capecitabine had a significant increase in PFS compared to capecitabine alone ([120]). The study was closed prematurely because the first interim analysis showed that the addition of lapatinib was associated with a 51% reduction in the risk of disease progression. The median TTP for patients treated with lapatinib plus capecitabine compared with capecitabine plus placebo was 8.4 versus 4.4 months (HR, 0.49; 95% CI, 0.34-0.71). In a phase II study of patients with HER2-positive breast cancer and brain metastasis treated with lapatinib, 6% of patients had an objective response, defined as ≥50% volumetric reduction of the brain metastasis ([121]), suggesting that lapatinib could be of help in the treatment of patients with central nervous system metastasis.

Preclinical studies have shown a synergistic interaction between trastuzumab and lapatinib in HER2-overexpressing breast cancer cell lines and tumor xenografts. Results of a randomized phase III trial combining lapatinib with trastuzumab compared with lapatinib alone in heavily pretreated HER2-positive MBC (n = 296) demonstrated synergy and improved response rates and PFS in the combination arm. Despite a high crossover rate, there was a significant improvement in OS with the lapatinib and trastuzumab combination (HR, 0.71; 95% CI, 0.54-0.93) ([122]).

Table 28-2 Clinical Predictors of Improved Response to Chemotherapy for Metastatic Breast Cancer

- Low tumor burden
- Normal organ function
- Normal blood count
- Good performance status
- No recent weight loss
- No prior chemotherapy or radiation therapy
- Softtissue metastases
- Premenopausal status
- Prolonged disease-free interval after adjuvant chemotherapy
- Negative estrogen receptor

Lapatinib has also been combined with hormonal agents. In a preclinical model, lapatinib restored tamoxifen sensitivity in tamoxifen-resistant breast cancer ([123]). The EGF3008 trial, a phase III study combining letrozole plus lapatinib versus letrozole, demonstrated a 29% reduction in risk of disease progression and an improvement in median PFS ([124]). A summary of some of the trials evaluating different anti-HER2 therapies is shown in Table 28-3.

OTHER AGENTS

Vascular Endothelial Growth Factor–Targeted Therapies

Bevacizumab

Bevacizumab (Avastin), a monoclonal antibody against all vascular endothelial growth factor (VEGF)-A isoforms has single-agent response rates of 9% in patients with refractory MBC. In a randomized phase III trial comparing capecitabine with or without bevacizumab in patients previously treated with an anthracycline and a taxane, the addition of bevacizumab produced a significant increase in response rates but no improvement in in PFS or OS ([125]).

The ECOG 2108 trial randomized 680 patients with previously untreated locally recurrent breast cancer or MBC to receive weekly paclitaxel (90 mg/m^2 on days 1, 8, and 15) with or without bevacizumab (10 mg/kg on days 1 and 15) in 4-week cycles until progression ([125]). The overall response rate (29.9% vs 13.8%, $P = .0001$) and the PFS (11.4 vs 6.11 months; HR, 0.51; 95% CI, 0.43-0.62) were significantly better with combination therapy; no OS differences were seen. Based on this trial, the combination of bevacizumab and paclitaxel was approved for first-line therapy of MBC. Several phase III studies using bevacizumab combined with different chemotherapy agents have shown improvements in PFS but failed to demonstrate a survival benefit with the addition of bevacizumab. Based on these studies, the FDA revoked the indication of bevacizumab in breast cancer. At MDACC, we have occasionally continued to use bevacizumab in addition to paclitaxel in very selected patients who need to achieve a rapid response and in whom the benefits associated with bevacizumab use outweigh the risks.

Bone Agents

Bisphosphonates are analogs of pyrophosphates that bind to hydroxyapatite crystals and inhibit bone resorption by osteoclasts. They are widely used to prevent skeletal complications in patients with bone metastases. Clinical trials have shown that the use of pamidronate or zoledronic acid is associated with fewer skeletal-related events and pathologic fractures and less need for radiation therapy and surgery to treat bone pain, with some suggesting that zoledronic acid is superior ([126]). During bisphosphonate treatment, monitoring of renal function is needed. Physicians should also be aware of the risk of developing osteonecrosis of the jaw, a rare but serious complication of bisphosphonate therapy. Trial results support the use of bisphosphonates for 2 years, but there are limited long-term safety data. The OPTOMIZE-2 trial evaluated the frequency of zoledronic acid administration in 403 women with bone metastasis who previously received at least nine doses of intravenous bisphosphonate. The study showed that giving zoledronic acid 4 mg intravenously every 3 months was as effective as giving it monthly, with a rate of skeletal-related events of 22% in the monthly group versus 23.2% in the every-3-months group. The less frequent dosing corresponded to lower rates of renal failure and osteonecrosis of the jaw ([127]).

Denosumab is a fully human monoclonal antibody that targets RANK ligand, a protein that acts as the primary signal to promote bone removal. Denosumab is being used in the treatment of osteoporosis, treatment-induced bone loss, and bone metastases. A large (n = 2,033), randomized, placebo-controlled trial evaluated denosumab (120 mg subcutaneously) versus zoledronic acid (4 mg intravenously) in patients with MBC and bone metastases ([128]). Denosumab was superior to zoledronic acid in delaying or preventing skeletal-related events and delayed or prevented hypercalcemia, radiation to bone, and bone pain, suggesting that monthly denosumab is a viable option for the management of bone metastases. An advantage of denosumab therapy is that it is given as a subcutaneous injection. At MDACC, all patients with MBC and bone metastasis who do not have a contraindication to receive bone agents are treated with zoledronic acid or denosumab.

INVESTIGATIONAL THERAPY

Despite therapeutic advances, the prognosis for many women with breast cancer is still poor. Investigational therapies for MBC include new molecules and agents with novel mechanisms of action.

In breast cancer, epidermal growth factor receptor (*EGFR*) plays a major role in promoting cell proliferation and malignant growth. Multiple studies evaluating the use of tyrosine kinase (TK) inhibitors in MBC are ongoing. Phase II studies of gefitinib (Iressa) used as a single agent or in combination with chemotherapy or endocrine therapy have been completed. Single-agent gefitinib showed minimal clinical benefit; no improvement in response rates was seen when it was used in

Table 28-3 Phase II and III Trials of HER2/neu-Targeted Therapies for Treatment of Metastatic Breast Cancer

Trial	No. of Patients	Patient Population	Regimen	Response	Patient Outcome
Trastuzumab					
Slamon ([125a]) et al (H0648g) Phase III	469	HER2+, first-line setting	1. Trastuzumab/paclitaxel 2. Paclitaxel 3. Trastuzumab/AC 4. AC	ORR = 50% (chemotherapy + trastuzumab)	Addition of trastuzumab to chemotherapy was associated with a longer time to disease progression (median, 7.4 vs 4.6 mo; $P < .001$), longer duration of response (median, 9.1 vs 6.1 mo; $P < .001$), higher rate of objective response (50% vs 32%; $P < .001$), lower rate of death at 1 yr (22% vs 33%; $P = .008$), longer survival (median, 25.1 vs 20.3 mo; $P = .046$), and 20% reduction in risk of death. Most important adverse event was cardiac dysfunction, occurring in 27% of the group given AC/trastuzumab, 8% of group given AC, 13% of group given paclitaxel/trastuzumab, and 1% of group given paclitaxel alone.
Andersson (HERNATA) Phase III	141	HER2+, first-line setting, included if completed adjuvant/neoadjuvant therapy at least 12 mo prior to diagnosis (accepted if included trastuzumab)	1. Trastuzumab/vinorelbine 2. Trastuzumab/docetaxel	PR = 48.3% CR = 11% ORR = 50.3% (trastuzumab/vinorelbine)	The PFS for trastuzumab/docetaxel vs trastuzumab/vinorelbine was 12.4 vs 15.3 mo (HR, 0.94; 95% CI, 0.71-1.25; $P = .67$).
Inoue Phase III	107	HER2+, first-line setting	1. Trastuzumab/docetaxel 2. Trastuzumab followed by trastuzumab/docetaxel	PR = 35% CR = 1% ORR = 36% (trastuzumab/docetaxel)	The PFS of trastuzumab followed by trastuzumab/docetaxel vs trastuzumab/docetaxel was 3.7 vs 14.6 mo (HR, 4.24; 95% CI, 2.48-7.24; $P < .01$). OS was significantly longer in the trastuzumab/docetaxel group (HR, 2.72; $P = .04$). Study was terminated early given significant benefit in the trastuzumab/docetaxel group.

(*Continued*)

Table 28-3 Phase II and III Trials of HER2/neu-Targeted Therapies for Treatment of Metastatic Breast Cancer (*Continued*)

Trial	No. of Patients	Patient Population	Regimen	Response	Patient Outcome
Kaufman (TAnDEM) Phase III	207	Postmenopausal, HER2+, ER positive and/or progesterone receptor positive, first-line setting, accepted if previously treated with tamoxifen as adjuvant therapy for hormonal therapy (completed >6 mo from diagnosis), with anastrozoleinitiated up to 4 wk prior to assignment	1. Trastuzumab/anastrozole 2. Anastrozole	PR = 15% CR = 0%, ORR = 73% (trastuzumab/vinorelbine)	The PFS for trastuzumab/anastrozole vs anastrozole was 5.6 vs 3.9 mo (HR, 0.62; 95% CI, 3.8-8.3; *P* = .006), with a TTP of 4.8 vs 2.4 mo (HR, 0.63; 95% CI, 95% CI 0.47-0.84). There was a higher incidence of grade 3 or 4 AEs in the trastuzumab/anastrozole arm (23% vs 5%). However, no specific grade 3 or 4 AEs occurred in more than three patient in the trastuzumab/anastrozole arm. Grade 4 AEs included hypercalcemia, dyspnea, lower respiratory tract infarction, and myocardial ischemia.
Pertuzumab					
Baselga (CLEOPATRA) Phase III	808	HER2+, first-line setting, included if completed adjuvant/neoadjuvant therapy at least 12 mo prior to diagnosis (accepted if included trastuzumab)	1. Pertuzumab/trastuzumab/docetaxel 2. Trastuzumab/docetaxel/placebo	PR = 65.2% CR = 4.2% ORR = 69.3% (pertuzumab/trastuzumab/docetaxel)	The PFS for pertuzumab/trastuzumab/docetaxel vs trastuzumab/docetaxel/placebo was 18.5 vs 12.4 mo (HR, 0.62; 95% CI, 0.51-0.75; *P* < .001), with an improvement in OS of 15.7 mo (56.5 vs 40.8 mo; HR, 0.68; 95% CI, 0.56-0.84; *P* = .0002). The safety profile was generally similar in the two groups with no increase in left ventricular systolic dysfunction. The rates of febrile neutropenia (56% vs 30%) and diarrhea (32% vs 20%) of grade ≥3 were higher in the pertuzumab group than in the control group.

(*Continued*)

Table 28-3 Phase II and III Trials of HER2/neu-Targeted Therapies for Treatment of Metastatic Breast Cancer (*Continued*)

Trial	No. of Patients	Patient Population	Regimen	Response	Patient Outcome
T-DM1					
Verma (EMILIA) Phase III	991	HER2+, previous progression on taxane and trastuzumab	1. T-DM1 2. Lapatinib/ capecitabine	1. PR = 42.6% 2. CR = 4% 3. ORR = 43.6% (T-DM1)	The PFS for T-DM1 vs lapatinib/capecitabine was 0.4 vs 5.8 mo (HR, 0.66; 95% CI, 0.56-0.77;*P*<.001). The incidence rates of AEs of grade ≥3 were higher in the lapatinib/capecitabine group than in the T-DM1 group (57% vs 40.8%). Diarrhea and palmar-plantar erythrodysesthesia were the most commonly reported grade 3 or 4 events in the lapatinib/capecitabine group (20.7% and 16.4%, respectively). The most commonly reported grade 3 or 4 events with T-DM1 were thrombocytopenia (12.9%) and elevated AST/ ALT (4.3% and 2.9%, respectively).
Lapatinib					
Johnston Phase III	1,286	HR+/HER2−or HR+/ HER2+	1. Lapatinib/ letrozole 2. Letrozole/ placebo	ORR = 48% (lapatinib/letrozole)	HR+/HER2−: no significant treatment benefit on PFS (HR, 0.90; 95% CI, 0.77-1.05). Subgroup analysis of patients with HER2− and lower expression of ER had significant improvement in median PFS (13.6 vs 6.6 mo; HR, 0.65; 95% CI, 0.47-0.9) when treated with combination therapy. HR+/HER2+: The PFS was 8.2 for the letrozole/lapatinib arm versus 3 months for the letrozole alone arm versus 3 months for the lapatinib arm. Significant improvement in clinical benefit rate for the combination arm.
Blackwell Phase III	296	HER2+; anthracycline, taxane, capecitabine, trastuzumab refractory	1. Lapatinib/ trastuzumab 2. Lapatinib	PR = 10.3% ORR = 24.7% (lapatinib/trastuzumab)	PFS in the combination arm versus lapatinib arm was 12.0 vs 8.1 mo (HR, 0.73;95% CI, 0.57-0.93); OS was also improved (14.0 vs 9.5 mo; HR, 0.74; 95% CI, 0.57-0.97).

AC, doxorubicin and cyclophosphamide; AE, adverse event; ALT, alanine aminotransferase; AST, aspartate aminotransferase; CI, confidence interval; CR, complete response; ER, estrogen receptor; HER2, human epidermal growth factor receptor; HR, hormone receptor; ORR, overall response rate; OS, overall survival; PFS, progression-free survival; PR, partial response; TTP, time to progression.

combination. An exploratory analysis of two randomized phase II trials compared anastrozole or tamoxifen plus gefitinib versus single-agent anastrozole or tamoxifen plus placebo ([129]). In both trials, among endocrine-naïve patients, gefitinib was associated with improved PFS when combined with hormonal therapy compared to anastrozole or tamoxifen alone. Erlotinib (Tarceva) is a small molecule that reversibly inhibits the *EGFR* TK and prevents receptor autophosphorylation. Combinations of erlotinib with drugs known to be active in breast cancer have been conducted. In a dose-escalation study of capecitabine, docetaxel, and erlotinib in patients with MBC, the overall response rate was 67% ([130]). The regimen was well tolerated; manageable skin and gastrointestinal problems were the most common treatment-related adverse effects.

Multikinase inhibitors that inhibit VEGF receptors are under investigation. Sunitinib malate (Sutent) is an oral TK inhibitor that targets several receptor TKs, including VEGFR-1, -2, and -3. In a phase II trial in MBC previously treated with anthracyclines and taxanes (n = 64), sunitinib was associated with a clinical benefit rate of 16% ([131]). In a phase II randomized study, 46 patients with HER2-negative MBC were randomized to receive paclitaxel (90 mg/m^2 weekly), bevacizumab (10 mg/kg every 2 weeks), and sunitinib (25 mg daily for 21 days) as first-line chemotherapy. High rates of dose modification and treatment discontinuation due to toxic effects were seen, leading to the study closure. In previously treated MBC patients, sunitinib (37.5 mg PO daily dose) was compared to capecitabine (n = 482); no differences in PFS or OS were seen, and capecitabine was better tolerated.

Sorafenib (Nexavar) has been evaluated in patients with MBC refractory to anthracyclines and taxanes. Results from the SOLTI-0701 trial evaluated the combination of sorafenib (400 mg PO bid) and capecitabine (1,000 mg/m^2 on days 1-14 of a 21-day cycle) versus capecitabine and placebo in HER2-negative MBC ([132]). Similar response rates were seen (38.3% vs 30.7%), but improved PFS (6.4 vs 4.1 months, $P < .001$) was observed with sorafenib and capecitabine. The combination treatment was associated with a 45% rate of grade 3 hand-foot syndrome. The Trials to Investigate the Effects of Sorafenib in Breast Cancer program evaluated the combination of sorafenib and paclitaxel versus paclitaxel and placebo in the frontline setting. The TTP and overall response rate, but not PFS, were improved with the combination. There was also an increase in cases of grade 3 toxicities and an imbalance in the number of deaths due to unusual causes in the paclitaxel and sorafenib group. Other VEGF TK inhibitors such as vandetanib (Zactima), valatinib, and axitinib are currently being tested.

Ongoing research is evaluating insulin-like growth factor inhibitors (CP-751, 856, AMG-479, IMC-A12), RAS/MEK/ERK (tipifarnib), and PI3K/AKT/mTOR pathway inhibitors. The PARP inhibitors are agents that have shown promise, particularly in the setting of metastatic triple-negative breast cancer associated with *BRCA* mutations; PARP-1 is a critical enzyme of cell proliferation and DNA repair. In addition, PARP-1 and -2 are fundamental in the repair of single-stranded DNA breaks ([133]). Olaparib, a PARP inhibitor, has shown single-agent activity in patients with *BRCA1/2* mutations, with little activity in sporadic breast cancer. Single-agent response rate was 41% in the phase I trial, with a median TTP of 5.7 months. Higher doses of 400 mg twice daily correlated with higher response rates. In a phase II randomized study of triple-negative MBC (n = 123), BSI-201 (iniparib) added to gemcitabine plus carboplatin showed significantly higher objective response rates and survival ([134]). However, the phase III trial revealed modest improvement in PFS/OS that was not statistically significant. The phase III study (n = 519) compared chemotherapy alone versus chemotherapy plus iniparib in the treatment of triple-negative MBC ([95]). Several studies of PARP inhibitors in the setting of *BRCA*-associated MBC are under way. At MDACC, we offer such patients clinical trials that include new and promising molecules.

LOCAL THERAPY

Retrospective studies have suggested a potential survival benefit from complete tumor excision in selected patients with MBC. Substantial selection biases exist in all of these reports that likely confound the results. Recently, two trials evaluated the role of locoregional therapies in women with MBC. In a trial by Indian investigators, 350 patients with MBC and intact primary tumor were randomized to mastectomy followed by complete axillary dissection and radiation therapy versus no locoregional treatment ([135]). All patients received anthracyclines with or without taxanes, with stratification by hormone receptor status, metastatic site, and number of metastases. No difference in OS was noted in the surgical versus nonsurgical group at 72 months. Although the local PFS was better in the surgical group, distant PFS was worse. In a second trial conducted by Turkish investigators, no difference in OS at 40 months was noted between patients with MBC randomized to upfront surgery followed by chemotherapy and patients assigned to chemotherapy alone ([136]). A subgroup analysis identified an apparent survival benefit in women with solitary bone metastases. In the United States, ECOG 2108 is a randomized phase III trial presently evaluating early local therapy for the intact primary tumor in patients with MBC (NCT01242800). According to the most recent guidelines, patients with MBC and an intact primary should be treated systemically. Consideration for surgery for palliation is indicated in women with impending complications that may compromise quality of life such as skin ulceration, bleeding, fungation, and pain. Surgery in such cases should be performed only if complete local tumor resection can be achieved and if other disease sites are not immediately life threatening. Such surgery requires the collaboration between the breast surgeon and the reconstructive surgeon to provide optimal cancer control and wound closure. Alternatively, radiation therapy may be considered.

SUMMARY

Despite great advances in the treatment of MBC, this conditions remains largely incurable, with a median survival of 2 to 3 years. The therapeutic concepts in MBC have changed with the realization that breast cancer is a conglomerate of several molecularly defined subtypes, each with a distinct prognosis, clinical course, and sensitivity to existing therapeutics. Treatment for MBC has dramatically evolved, incorporating new hormonal therapies, cytotoxic agents, and monoclonal antibodies. Refinements of chemotherapy with different combinations of newer agents along with modulating agents and growth factor support have allowed further advancement in the treatment of MBC. Despite great enthusiasm for targeted therapies, these agents have exhibited modest activity when used as single agents. A better understanding of the molecular biology of signaling pathways and the discovery of new biomarkers will help select patients who benefit from specific treatments.

CHAPTER 28

REFERENCES

1. American Cancer Society. *Breast Cancer Facts and Figures 2013-2014*. Atlanta, GA: American Cancer Society; 2014.
2. American Cancer Society. *Cancer Treatment and Survivorship Facts and Figures*. Atlanta, GA: American Cancer Society; 2014-2015.
3. National Cancer Institute. SEER Cancer Statistics Review 1975-2006. Cancer Staistics Branch, Released May 2009. http://www.seer.cancer.gov. Accessed October 5, 2015.
4. Dawood S, Broglio K, Gonzalez-Angulo AM, et al. Trends in survival over the past two decades among white and black patients with newly diagnosed stage IV breast cancer. *J Clin Oncol*. 2008;26:4891-4898.
5. Jain S, Fisher C, Smith P, et al. Patterns of metastatic breast cancer in relation to histological type. *Eur J Cancer*. 1993;29A:2155-2157.
6. Amir E, Ooi WS, Simmons C, et al. Discordance between receptor status in primary and metastatic breast cancer: an exploratory study of bone and bone marrow biopsies. *Clin Oncol (R Coll Radiol)*. 2008;20:763-768.
7. Broom RJ, Tang PA, Simmons C, et al. Changes in estrogen receptor, progesterone receptor and Her-2/neu status with time: discordance rates between primary and metastatic breast cancer. *Anticancer Res*. 2009;29:1557-1562.
8. Foukakis T, Åström G, Lindström L, et al. When to order a biopsy to characterise a metastatic relapse in breast cancer. *Ann Oncol*. 2012;23(Suppl 10):349-353.
9. Saad A, Abraham J. Role of tumor markers and circulating tumors cells in the management of breast cancer. *Oncology (Williston Park)*. 2008;22:726-731; discussion 734, 739, 743-744.
10. Tondini C, Hayes DF, Gelman R, et al. Comparison of CA15-3 and carcinoembryonic antigen in monitoring the clinical course of patients with metastatic breast cancer. *Cancer Res*. 1988;48:4107-4112.
11. Tormey DC, Waalkes TP. Clinical correlation between CEA and breast cancer. *Cancer*. 1978;42(3 Suppl):1507-1511.
12. Harris L, Fritsche H, Mennel R, et al. American Society of Clinical Oncology 2007 update of recommendations for the use of tumor markers in breast cancer. *J Clin Oncol*. 2007;25(33):5287-5312.
13. Cristofanilli M, Budd GT, Ellis MJ, et al. Circulating tumor cells, disease progression, and survival in metastatic breast cancer. *N Engl J Med*. 2004;351(8):781-791.
14. Hayes DF, Cristofanilli M, Budd GT, et al. Circulating tumor cells at each follow-up time point during therapy of metastatic breast cancer patients predict progression-free and overall survival. *Clin Cancer Res*. 2006;12:4218-4224.
15. Carlson RW, Allred DC, Anderson BO, et al. Metastatic breast cancer, version 1.2012: featured updates to the NCCN guidelines. *J Natl Compr Canc Netw*. 2012;10(7):821-829.
16. Khansur T, Haick A, Patel B, et al. Evaluation of bone scan as a screening work-up in primary and local-regional recurrence of breast cancer. *Am J Clin Oncol*. 1987;10:167-170.
17. White DR, Maloney JJ, 3rd, Muss HB, et al. Serum alkaline phosphatase determination. Value in the staging of advanced breast cancer. *JAMA*. 1979;242:1147-1149.
18. Allegra JC, Lippman ME. Estrogen receptor status and the disease-free interval in breast cancer. *Recent Results Cancer Res*. 1980;71:20-25.
19. Allegra JC, Lippman ME, Thompson EB, et al. Estrogen receptor status: an important variable in predicting response to endocrine therapy in metastatic breast cancer. *Eur J Cancer*. 1980;16:323-331.
20. Buzdar AU. Current status of endocrine treatment of carcinoma of the breast. *Semin Surg Oncol*. 1990;6(2):77-82.
21. Ingle JN, Ahmann DL, Green SJ, et al. Randomized clinical trial of megestrol acetate versus tamoxifen in paramenopausal or castrated women with advanced breast cancer. *Am J Clin Oncol*. 1982;5:155-160.
22. Smith IE, Harris AL, Stuart-Harris R, et al. Combination treatment with tamoxifen and aminoglutethimide in advanced breast cancer. *Br Med J (Clin Res Ed)*. 1983;286:1615-1616.
23. Saphner T, Troxel AB, Tormey DC, et al. Phase II study of goserelin for patients with postmenopausal metastatic breast cancer. *J Clin Oncol*. 1993;11:1529-1535.
24. Come SE, Buzdar AU, Ingle JN, et al. Endocrine and targeted manipulation of breast cancer: summary statement for the Sixth Cambridge Conference. *Cancer*. 2008;112:673-678.
25. Goss PE, Gwyn KM. Current perspectives on aromatase inhibitors in breast cancer. *J Clin Oncol*. 1994;12(11):2460-2470.
26. Klijn JG, Blamey RW, Boccardo F, et al. Combined tamoxifen and luteinizing hormone-releasing hormone (LHRH) agonist versus LHRH agonist alone in premenopausal advanced breast cancer: a meta-analysis of four randomized trials. *J Clin Oncol*. 2001;19:343-353.
27. Bonneterre J, Thurlimann B, Robertson JF, et al. Anastrozole versus tamoxifen as first-line therapy for advanced breast cancer in 668 postmenopausal women: results of the Tamoxifen or Arimidex Randomized Group Efficacy and Tolerability study. *J*

Clin Oncol. 2000;18:3748-3757.

28. Nabholtz JM, Buzdar A, Pollak M, et al. Anastrozole is superior to tamoxifen as first-line therapy for advanced breast cancer in postmenopausal women: results of a North American multicenter randomized trial. Arimidex Study Group. *J Clin Oncol*. 2000;18:3758-3767.
29. Mouridsen H, Gershanovich M, Sun Y, et al. Phase III study of letrozole versus tamoxifen as first-line therapy of advanced breast cancer in postmenopausal women: analysis of survival and update of efficacy from the International Letrozole Breast Cancer Group. *J Clin Oncol*. 2003;21:2101-2109.
30. Howell A, Robertson JF, Abram P, et al. Comparison of fulvestrant versus tamoxifen for the treatment of advanced breast cancer in postmenopausal women previously untreated with endocrine therapy: a multinational, double-blind, randomized trial. *J Clin Oncol*. 2004; 22:1605-1613.
31. Osborne CK, Pippen J, Jones SE, et al. Double-blind, randomized trial comparing the efficacy and tolerability of fulvestrant versus anastrozole in postmenopausal women with advanced breast cancer progressing on prior endocrine therapy: results of a North American trial. *J Clin Oncol*. 2002;20:3386-3395.
32. Robertson JF, Osborne CK, Howell A, et al. Fulvestrant versus anastrozole for the treatment of advanced breast carcinoma in postmenopausal women: a prospective combined analysis of two multicenter trials. *Cancer*. 2003;98:229-238.
33. Di Leo A, Jerusalem G, Petruzelka L, et al. Results of the CONFIRM phase III trial comparing fulvestrant 250 mg with fulvestrant 500 mg in postmenopausal women with estrogen receptor-positive advanced breast cancer. *J Clin Oncol*. 2010;28(30):4594-4600.
34. Di Leo A, Jerusalem G, Petruzelka L, et al. Final overall survival: fulvestrant 500 mg vs 250 mg in the randomized CONFIRM trial. *J Natl Cancer Inst*. 2014;106(1):djt337.
35. Mehta RS, Barlow WE, Albain KS, et al. Combination anastrozole and fulvestrant in metastatic breast cancer. *N Engl J Med*. 2012;367(5):435-444.
36. Johnston SR, Kilburn LS, Ellis P, et al. Fulvestrant plus anastrozole or placebo versus exemestane alone after progression on non-steroidal aromatase inhibitors in postmenopausal patients with hormone-receptor-positive locally advanced or metastatic breast cancer (SoFEA): a composite, multicentre, phase 3 randomised trial. *Lancet Oncol*. 2013;14(10):989-998.
37. Bergh J, Jönsson PE, Lidbrink EK, et al. FACT: an open-label randomized phase III study of fulvestrant and anastrozole in combination compared with anastrozole alone as first-line therapy for patients with receptor-positive postmenopausal breast cancer. *J Clin Oncol*. 2012;30(16):1919-1925.
38. Buzdar AU. Combination endocrine treatments unproven in breast cancer. *Lancet Oncol*. 2013;14(10):917-918.
39. Beeram M, Tan QT, Tekmal RR, et al. Akt-induced endocrine therapy resistance is reversed by inhibition of mTOR signaling. *Ann Oncol*. 2007;18(8):1323-1328.
40. Bachelot T, Bourgier C, Cropet C, et al. Randomized phase II trial of everolimus in combination with tamoxifen in patients with hormone receptor-positive, human epidermal growth factor receptor 2-negative metastatic breast cancer with prior exposure to aromatase inhibitors: a GINECO study. *J Clin Oncol*. 2012;30(22):2718-2724.
41. Baselga J, Campone M, Piccart M, et al. Everolimus in postmenopausal hormone-receptor-positive advanced breast cancer. *N Engl J Med*. 2012;366(6):520-529.
42. Finn RS, Dering J, Conklin D, et al. PD 0332991, a selective cyclin D kinase 4/6 inhibitor, preferentially inhibits proliferation of luminal estrogen receptor-positive human breast cancer cell lines in vitro. *Breast Cancer Res*. 2009;11(5):R77.
43. Arnold A, Papanikolaou A. Cyclin D1 in breast cancer pathogenesis. *J Clin Oncol*. 2005;23(18):4215-4224.
44. Patnaik A, Rosen LS, Tolaney SM, et al. Clinical activity of LY2835219, a novel cell cycle inhibitor selective for CDK4 and CDK6, in patients with metastatic breast cancer [abstract]. *Cancer Res*. 2014;74:CT232.
45. Finn RS, Crown J, Lang I, et al. The cyclin-dependent kinase 4/6 inhibitor palbociclib in combination with letrozole versus letrozole alone as first-line treatment of oestrogen receptor-positive, HER2-negative, advanced breast cancer (PALOMA-1/TRIO-18): a randomised phase 2 study. *Lancet Oncol*. 2015;16(1):25-35.
46. Ellis MJ, Dehdahti F, Jamalabadi-Majidi S, et al. A randomized phase 2 trial of low dose (6 mg daily) versus high dose (30 mg daily) estradiol for patients with estrogen receptor positive aromatase inhibitor resistant advanced breast cancer [abstract]. *Cancer Res*. 2009;69:16.
47. Burstein HJ, Mangu PB, Somerfield MR, et al. American Society of Clinical Oncology clinical practice guideline update on the use of chemotherapy sensitivity and resistance assays. *J Clin Oncol*. 2011;29(24):3328-3330.
48. Berry DA, Ueno NT, Johnson MM, et al. High-dose chemotherapy with autologous hematopoietic stem-cell transplantation in metastatic breast cancer: overview of six randomized trials. *J Clin Oncol*. 2011;29(24):3224-3231.
49. Fossati R, Confalonieri C, Torri V, et al. Cytotoxic and hormonal treatment for metastatic breast cancer: a systematic review of published randomized trials involving 31,510 women. *J Clin Oncol*. 1998;16:3439-3460.
50. Bishop JF, Dewar J, Toner GC, et al. Initial paclitaxel improves outcome compared with CMFP combination chemotherapy as front-line therapy in untreated metastatic breast cancer. *J Clin Oncol*. 1999;17:2355-2364.
51. Joensuu H, Holli K, Heikkinen M, et al. Combination chemotherapy versus single-agent therapy as first- and second-line treatment in metastatic breast cancer: a prospective randomized trial. *J Clin Oncol*. 1998;16:3720-3730.
52. Carrick S, Parker S, Wilcken N, et al. Single agent versus combination chemotherapy for metastatic breast cancer. *Cochrane Database Syst Rev*. 2005;2:CD003372.
53. Cardoso F, Bedard PL, Winer EP, et al. International guidelines for management of metastatic breast cancer: combination vs sequential single-agent chemotherapy. *J Natl Cancer Inst*. 2009;101:1174-1181.
54. Coates A, Gebski V, Bishop JF, et al. Improving the quality of life during chemotherapy for advanced breast cancer. A comparison of intermittent and continuous treatment strategies. *N Engl J Med*. 1987;317:1490-1495.
55. Ejlertsen B, Pfeiffer P, Pedersen D, et al. Decreased efficacy of cyclophosphamide, epirubicin and 5-fluorouracil in metastatic breast cancer when reducing treatment duration from 18 to 6 months. *Eur J Cancer*. 1993;29A:527-531.
56. Falkson G, Gelman RS, Pandya KJ, et al. Eastern Cooperative Oncology Group randomized trials of observation versus maintenance therapy for patients with metastatic breast cancer in complete remission following induction treatment. *J Clin Oncol*. 1998;16:1669-1676.
57. Muss HB, Case LD, Richards F 2nd, et al. Interrupted versus continuous chemotherapy in patients with metastatic breast cancer. The Piedmont Oncology Association. *N Engl J Med*. 1991;325:1342-1348.
58. Stockler M, Wilcken N, Coates A. Chemotherapy for metastatic breast cancer–when is enough enough? *Eur J Cancer*. 1997;33:2147-2148.
59. Gennari A, Conte P, Nanni O, et al. Multicenter randomized trial of paclitaxel (P) for maintenance chemotherapy (CT) versus control in metastatic breast cancer (MBC) patients achieving a response or stable disease to first-line CT including anthracyclines and paclitaxel: final results from the Italian

MANTA study [abstract]. *J Clin Oncol*. 2005;23(s16):522.
60. Weiss RB. The anthracyclines: will we ever find a better doxorubicin? *Semin Oncol*. 1992;19:670-686.
61. Hoogstraten B, George SL, Samal B, et al. Combination chemotherapy and adriamycin in patients with advanced breast cancer. A Southwest Oncology Group study. *Cancer*. 1976;38:13-20.
62. Jain KK, Casper ES, Geller NL, et al. A prospective randomized comparison of epirubicin and doxorubicin in patients with advanced breast cancer. *J Clin Oncol*. 1985;3:818-826.
63. Lawton PA, Spittle MF, Ostrowski MJ, et al. A comparison of doxorubicin, epirubicin and mitozantrone as single agents in advanced breast carcinoma. *Clin Oncol (R Coll Radiol)*. 1993;5:80-84.
64. Van Oosterom AT, Mouridsen HT, Wildiers J, et al. Carminomycin versus doxorubicin in advanced breast cancer, a randomized phase II study of the E.O.R.T.C. Breast Cancer Cooperative Group. *Eur J Cancer Clin Oncol*. 1986;22:601-605.
65. A prospective randomized phase III trial comparing combination chemotherapy with cyclophosphamide, fluorouracil, and either doxorubicin or epirubicin. French Epirubicin Study Group. *J Clin Oncol*. 1988;6(4):679-688.
66. O'Brien ME, Wigler N, Inbar M, et al. Reduced cardiotoxicity and comparable efficacy in a phase III trial of pegylated liposomal doxorubicin HCl (CAELYX/Doxil) versus conventional doxorubicin for first-line treatment of metastatic breast cancer. *Ann Oncol*. 2004;15:440-449.
67. Sledge GW, Neuberg D, Bernardo P, et al. Phase III trial of doxorubicin, paclitaxel, and the combination of doxorubicin and paclitaxel as front-line chemotherapy for metastatic breast cancer: an intergroup trial (E1193). *J Clin Oncol*. 2003;21(4):588-592.
68. Harvey V, Mouridsen H, Semiglazov V, et al. Phase III trial comparing three doses of docetaxel for second-line treatment of advanced breast cancer. *J Clin Oncol*. 2006;24:4963-4970.
69. Jones SE, Erban J, Overmoyer B, et al. Randomized phase III study of docetaxel compared with paclitaxel in metastatic breast cancer. *J Clin Oncol*. 2005;23:5542-5551.
70. Valero V, Jones SE, Von Hoff DD, et al. A phase II study of docetaxel in patients with paclitaxel-resistant metastatic breast cancer. *J Clin Oncol*. 1998;16(10):3362-3368.
71. Gradishar WJ, Krasnojon D, Cheporov S, et al. Significantly longer progression-free survival with nab-paclitaxel compared with docetaxel as first-line therapy for metastatic breast cancer. *J Clin Oncol*. 2009;27:3611-3619.
72. Gradishar WJ, Tjulandin S, Davidson N, et al. Phase III trial of nanoparticle albumin-bound paclitaxel compared with polyethylated castor oil-based paclitaxel in women with breast cancer. *J Clin Oncol*. 2005;23:7794-7803.
73. Blum JL, Jones SE, Buzdar AU, et al. Multicenter phase II study of capecitabine in paclitaxel-refractory metastatic breast cancer. *J Clin Oncol*. 1999;17(2):485-493.
74. O'Shaughnessy JA, Blum J, Moiseyenko V, et al. Randomized, open-label, phase II trial of oral capecitabine (Xeloda) vs. a reference arm of intravenous CMF (cyclophosphamide, methotrexate and 5-fluorouracil) as first-line therapy for advanced/metastatic breast cancer. *Ann Oncol*. 2001;12(9):1247-1254.
75. Blackstein M, Vogel CL, Ambinder R, et al. Gemcitabine as first-line therapy in patients with metastatic breast cancer: a phase II trial. *Oncology*. 2002;62(1):2-8.
76. Possinger K, Kaufmann M, Coleman R, et al. Phase II study of gemcitabine as first-line chemotherapy in patients with advanced or metastatic breast cancer. *Anticancer Drugs*. 1999;10:155-162.
77. Carmichael J, Possinger K, Phillip P, et al. Advanced breast cancer: a phase II trial with gemcitabine. *J Clin Oncol*. 1995;13:2731-2736.
78. Canobbio L, Boccardo F, Pastorino G, et al. Phase-II study of navelbine in advanced breast cancer. *Semin Oncol*. 1989;16:33-36.
79. Jones S, Winer E, Vogel C, et al. Randomized comparison of vinorelbine and melphalan in anthracycline-refractory advanced breast cancer. *J Clin Oncol*. 1995;13:2567-2574.
80. Livingston RB, Ellis GK, Gralow JR, et al. Dose-intensive vinorelbine with concurrent granulocyte colony-stimulating factor support in paclitaxel-refractory metastatic breast cancer. *J Clin Oncol*. 1997;15:1395-1400.
81. Perez EA, Lerzo G, Pivot X, et al. Efficacy and safety of ixabepilone (BMS-247550) in a phase II study of patients with advanced breast cancer resistant to an anthracycline, a taxane, and capecitabine. *J Clin Oncol*. 2007;25(23):3407-3714.
82. Roche H, Yelle L, Cognetti F, et al. Phase II clinical trial of ixabepilone (BMS-247550), an epothilone B analog, as first-line therapy in patients with metastatic breast cancer previously treated with anthracycline chemotherapy. *J Clin Oncol*. 2007;25(23):3415-3420.
83. Cortes J, O'Shaughnessy J, Loesch D, et al. Eribulin monotherapy versus treatment of physician's choice in patients with metastatic breast cancer (EMBRACE): a phase 3 open-label randomised study. *Lancet*. 2011;377(9769):914-923.
84. McIntyre K, O'Shaughnessy J, Schwartzberg L, et al. Phase 2 study of eribulin mesylate as first-line therapy for locally recurrent or metastatic human epidermal growth factor receptor 2-negative breast cancer. *Breast Cancer Res Treat*. 2014;146(2):321-328.
85. Nabholtz J, Paterson A, Dirix L, et al. A phase III randomized trial comparing docetaxel (T), doxorubicin (A) and cyclophosphamide (C) (TAC) to FAC as first line chemotherapy (CT) for patients (Pts) with metastatic breast cancer (MBC) [abstract]. *J Clin Oncol*. 2001;20:83.
86. Mackey J, Paterson A, Dirix L, et al. Final results of the phase III randomized trial comparing docetaxel (T), doxorubicin (A) and cyclophosphamide (C) to FAC as first line chemotherapy (CT) for patients (pts) with metastatic breast cancer (MBC) [abstract]. *J Clin Oncol*. 2002;21:137.
87. Carmichael J. UKCCCR trial of epirubicin and cyclophosphamide (EC) vs. epirubicin and taxol (ET) in the first line treatment of women with metastatic breast cancer (MBC) [abstract]. *J Clin Oncol*. 2001;20:84.
88. Nabholtz JM, Falkson C, Campos D, et al. Docetaxel and doxorubicin compared with doxorubicin and cyclophosphamide as first-line chemotherapy for metastatic breast cancer: results of a randomized, multicenter, phase III trial. *J Clin Oncol*. 2003;21(6):968-975.
89. Martin M. Platinum compounds in the treatment of advanced breast cancer. *Clin Breast Cancer*. 2001;2(3):190-208; discussion 209.
90. Perez EA, Hillman DW, Stella PJ, et al. A phase II study of paclitaxel plus carboplatin as first-line chemotherapy for women with metastatic breast carcinoma. *Cancer*. 2000;88:124-131.
91. Fountzilas G, Athanassiadis A, Kalogera-Fountzila A, et al. Paclitaxel by 3-h infusion and carboplatin in anthracyclineresistant advanced breast cancer. A phase II study conducted by the Hellenic Cooperative Oncology Group. *Eur J Cancer*. 1997;33:1893-1895.
92. Mavroudis D, Alexopoulos A, Malamos N, et al. Salvage treatment of metastatic breast cancer with docetaxel and carboplatin. A multicenter phase II trial. *Oncology*. 2003;64:207-212.
93. Nagourney RA, Link JS, Blitzer JB, et al. Gemcitabine plus cisplatin repeating doublet therapy in previously treated, relapsed breast cancer patients. *J Clin Oncol*. 2000;18(11):2245-2249.
94. Chew HK, Doroshow JH, Frankel P, et al. Phase II studies of gemcitabine and cisplatin in heavily and minimally pretreated metastatic breast cancer. *J Clin Oncol*. 2009;27(13):2163-2169.
95. O'Shaughnessy J, Schwartzberg L, Danso MA, et al. Phase III study of iniparib plus gemcitabine and carboplatin versus

gemcitabine and carboplatin in patients with metastatic triple-negative breast cancer. *J Clin Oncol.* 2014;32(34):3840-3847.

96. Liu M, Mo QG, Wei CY, et al. Platinum-based chemotherapy in triple-negative breast cancer: a meta-analysis. *Oncol Lett.* 2013;5(3):983-991.
97. Albain KS, Nag SM, Calderillo-Ruiz G, et al. Gemcitabine plus paclitaxel versus paclitaxel monotherapy in patients with metastatic breast cancer and prior anthracycline treatment. *J Clin Oncol.* 2008;26(24):3950-3957.
98. Chan S, Romieu G, Huober J, et al. Phase III study of gemcitabine plus docetaxel compared with capecitabine plus docetaxel for anthracycline-pretreated patients with metastatic breast cancer. *J Clin Oncol.* 2009;27(11):1753-1760.
99. Norris B, Pritchard KI, James K, et al. Phase III comparative study of vinorelbine combined with doxorubicin versus doxorubicin alone in disseminated metastatic/recurrent breast cancer: National Cancer Institute of Canada Clinical Trials Group Study MA8. *J Clin Oncol.* 2000;18(12):2385-2394.
100. Domenech GH, Vogel CL. A review of vinorelbine in the treatment of breast cancer. *Clin Breast Cancer.* 2001;2(2):113-128.
101. O'Shaughnessy J, Miles D, Vukelja S, et al. Superior survival with capecitabine plus docetaxel combination therapy in anthracycline-pretreated patients with advanced breast cancer: phase III trial results. *J Clin Oncol.* 2002;20:2812-2823.
102. Thomas ES, Miles D, Vukelja S, et al. Ixabepilone plus capecitabine for metastatic breast cancer progressing after anthracycline and taxane treatment. *J Clin Oncol.* 2007;25(33): 5210-5217.
103. Cobleigh MA, Vogel CL, Tripathy D, et al. Multinational study of the efficacy and safety of humanized anti-HER2 monoclonal antibody in women who have HER2-overexpressing metastatic breast cancer that has progressed after chemotherapy for metastatic disease. *J Clin Oncol.* 1999;17(9):2639-2648.
104. Slamon DJ, Leyland-Jones B, Shak S, et al. Use of chemotherapy plus a monoclonal antibody against HER2 for metastatic breast cancer that overexpresses HER2. *N Engl J Med.* 2001;344(11):783-792.
105. Esteva FJ, Valero V, Booser D, et al. Phase II study of weekly docetaxel and trastuzumab for patients with HER-2-overexpressing metastatic breast cancer. *J Clin Oncol.* 2002; 20(7):1800-1808.
106. Montemurro F, Choa G, Faggiuolo R, et al. Safety and activity of docetaxel and trastuzumab in HER2 overexpressing metastatic breast cancer: a pilot phase II study. *Am J Clin Oncol.* 2003;26(1):95-97.
107. Pegram MD, Lopez A, Konecny G, Slamon DJ. Trastuzumab and chemotherapeutics: drug interactions and synergies. *Semin Oncol.* 2000;27(6 Suppl 11):21-5; discussion 92-100.
108. Burstein HJ, Keshaviah A, Baron AD, et al. Trastuzumab plus vinorelbine or taxane chemotherapy for HER2-overexpressing metastatic breast cancer: the trastuzumab and vinorelbine or taxane study. *Cancer.* 2007;110(5):965-972.
109. Bartsch R, Wenzel C, Altorjai G, et al. Capecitabine and trastuzumab in heavily pretreated metastatic breast cancer. *J Clin Oncol.* 2007;25(25):3853-3858.
110. Schaller G, Fuchs I, Gonsch T, et al. Phase II study of capecitabine plus trastuzumab in human epidermal growth factor receptor 2 overexpressing metastatic breast cancer pretreated with anthracyclines or taxanes. *J Clin Oncol.* 2007;25(22):3246-3250.
111. Robert N, Leyland-Jones B, Asmar L, et al. Randomized phase III study of trastuzumab, paclitaxel, and carboplatin compared with trastuzumab and paclitaxel in women with HER-2-overexpressing metastatic breast cancer. *J Clin Oncol.* 2006;24(18):2786-2792.
112. Baselga J, Cortés J, Kim SB, et al. Pertuzumab plus trastuzumab plus docetaxel for metastatic breast cancer. *N Engl J Med.* 2012;366(2):109-119.
113. Baselga J, Gelmon KA, Verma S, et al. Phase II trial of pertuzumab and trastuzumab in patients with human epidermal growth factor receptor 2-positive metastatic breast cancer that progressed during prior trastuzumab therapy. *J Clin Oncol.* 2010;28(7):1138-1144.
114. Munoz-Mateu M, Urruticoechea A, Separovic R, et al. Trastuzumab plus capecitabine with or without pertuzumab in patients with HER2-positive MBC whose disease has progressed during or following trastuzumab-based therapy for first-line metastatic disease: a multicenter, randomized, two-arm, phase II study (PHEREXA) [abstract]. *J Clin Oncol.* 2011;29:TPS118.
115. Burris HA 3rd, Rugo HS, Vukelja SJ, et al. Phase II study of the antibody drug conjugate trastuzumab-DM1 for the treatment of human epidermal growth factor receptor 2 (HER2)-positive breast cancer after prior HER2-directed therapy. *J Clin Oncol.* 2011;29(4):398-405.
116. Verma S, Miles D, Gianni L, et al. Trastuzumab emtansine for HER2-positive advanced breast cancer. *N Engl J Med.* 2012;367(19):1783-1791.
117. Hurvitz SA, Dirix L, Kocsis J, et al. Phase II randomized study of trastuzumab emtansine versus trastuzumab plus docetaxel in patients with human epidermal growth factor receptor 2-positive metastatic breast cancer. *J Clin Oncol.* 2013;31(9):1157-1163.
118. Krop IE, Kim SB, González-Martín A, et al. Trastuzumab emtansine versus treatment of physician's choice for pretreated HER2-positive advanced breast cancer (TH3RESA): a randomised, open-label, phase 3 trial. *Lancet Oncol.* 2014;15(7):689-699.
119. Miller K, Gianni L, Andre F, et al. A phase Ib/II trial of trastuzumab-DM1 (T-DM1) with pertuzumab (P) for women with HER2-positive, locally advanced or metastatic breast cancer (BC) who were previously treated with trastuzumab (T) [abstract]. *J Clin Oncol.* 2010;28:1012.
120. Geyer CE, Forster J, Lindquist D, et al. Lapatinib plus capecitabine for HER2-positive advanced breast cancer. *N Engl J Med.* 2006;355(26):2733-2743.
121. Lin NU, Diéras V, Paul D, et al. Multicenter phase II study of lapatinib in patients with brain metastases from HER2-positive breast cancer. *Clin Cancer Res.* 2009;15(4):1452-1459.
122. Blackwell KL, Pegram MD, Tan-Chiu E, et al. Single-agent lapatinib for HER2-overexpressing advanced or metastatic breast cancer that progressed on first- or second-line trastuzumab-containing regimens. *Ann Oncol.* 2009;20(6):1026-1031.
123. Chu I, Blackwell K, Chen S, Slingerland J. The dual ErbB1/ErbB2 inhibitor, lapatinib (GW572016), cooperates with tamoxifen to inhibit both cell proliferation- and estrogen-dependent gene expression in antiestrogen-resistant breast cancer. *Cancer Res.* 2005;65(1):18-25.
124. Johnston S, Pegram M, Press M, et al. Lapatinib combined with letrozole vs. letrozole alone for front line postmenopausal hormone receptor positive metastatic breast cancer: first results from the EGF30008 trial [abstract]. *Breast Cancer Res Treat.* 2008;102:46.
125. Miller KD, Chap LI, Holmes FA, et al. Randomized phase III trial of capecitabine compared with bevacizumab plus capecitabine in patients with previously treated metastatic breast cancer. *J Clin Oncol.* 2005;23(4):792-799.

125a. Slamon DJ, Leyland-Jones B, Shak S, et al: Use of chemotherapy plus a monoclonal antibody against HER2 for metastatic breast cancer that overexpresses HER2. *N Engl J Med* 344:783-792, 2001

126. Theriault RL, Lipton A, Hortobagyi GN, et al. Pamidronate reduces skeletal morbidity in women with advanced breast cancer and lytic bone lesions: a randomized, placebo-controlled trial. Protocol 18 Aredia Breast Cancer Study Group.

J Clin Oncol. 1999;17(3):846-854.

127. Hortobagyi GN, Lipton A, Chew HK, et al. Efficacy and safety of continue zolendroinic acid every 4 weeks versus every 12 weeks in women with bone metastasis from breast cancer: results of the OPTIMIZE-2 trial [abstract]. *J Clin Oncol.* 2014;32:LBA9500.
128. Stopeck AT, Lipton A, Body JJ, et al. Denosumab compared with zoledronic acid for the treatment of bone metastases in patients with advanced breast cancer: a randomized, double-blind study. *J Clin Oncol.* 2010;28(35):5132-5139.
129. Cristofanilli M, Schiff R, Valero V. Exploratory subset analysis according to prior endocrine treatment of two randomized phase II trials comparing gefitinib with placebo in combination with tamoxifen or anastrozole in hormone receptor-positive metastatic breast cancer [abstract]. *J Clin Oncol.* 2009;27:1014.
130. Twelves C, Trigo JM, Jones R, et al. Erlotinib in combination with capecitabine and docetaxel in patients with metastatic breast cancer: a dose-escalation study. *Eur J Cancer.* 2008;44(3):419-426.
131. Burstein HJ, Elias AD, Rugo HS, et al. Phase II study of sunitinib malate, an oral multitargeted tyrosine kinase inhibitor, in patients with metastatic breast cancer previously treated with an anthracycline and a taxane. *J Clin Oncol.* 2008;26(11):1810-1816.
132. Baselga J, Segalla JG, Roché H, et al. Sorafenib in combination with capecitabine: an oral regimen for patients with HER2-negative locally advanced or metastatic breast cancer. *J Clin Oncol.* 2012;30(13):1484-1491.
133. Tutt A, Robson M, Garber JE, et al. Oral poly(ADP-ribose) polymerase inhibitor olaparib in patients with BRCA1 or BRCA2 mutations and advanced breast cancer: a proof-of-concept trial. *Lancet.* 2010;376(9737):235-244.
134. O'Shaugnessy J, Schwartzberg LS, Danso MA, et al. A randomized phase III study of iniparib in combination with gemcitabine/carboplatin in metastatic triple negative breast cancer [abstract]. *J Clin Oncol.* 2011;29:1007.
135. Badwe R, Parmar V, Hawaldar R, et al. Surgical removal of primary tumor and axillary lymph nodes in women metastatic breast cancer at first presentation: a randomized controlled trial. San Antonio Breast Cancer Symposium [abstract]. *Breast Cancer Res Treat.* 2013;2:S2-02.
136. Soran A. Early follow-up of a randomized trial evaluating resection of the primary beast tumor in women presenting with de novo stage IV breast cancer; Turkish study (protocol MF07-01). San Antonio Breast Cancer Symposium 2013. Abstract S2-03.

29

Inflammatory Breast Cancer

第二十九章　炎性乳腺癌

Tamer M. Fouad
Vincente Valero
Naoto T. Ueno

中文导读

炎性乳腺癌是一种恶性程度高，疾病进展快的特殊类型乳腺癌。本章首先分别从发病率和死亡率的情况介绍了炎性乳腺癌的流行病学特征。随之从患病年龄、种族、BMI指数、地理位置、社会经济地位、生育史、家族史等因素展开叙述炎性乳腺癌的易感因素。在分子发病机制部分，阐述了基因表达谱、E-钙黏蛋白过表达、p53基因突变、血管生成、炎症、肿瘤干细胞等在炎性乳腺癌发病中可能的作用。在临床表现部分，着重介绍了该疾病的临床诊断标准和鉴别诊断，并简单描述了炎性乳腺癌的预后。在病理学方面，着重介绍了炎性乳腺癌的组织学特点。在影像学方面，分别阐述了钼靶、超声、磁共振、CT和PET/CT用于诊断炎性乳腺癌的价值。分期主要参考TNM分期，并详述了炎性乳腺癌的诊断标准。治疗方面，炎性乳腺癌应结合多学科治疗，本章阐述了手术、放疗、新辅助治疗、内分泌治疗等方法。此外，介绍了Ⅳ期炎性乳腺癌的临床诊疗策略以及炎性乳腺癌相关 的试验药物。本章最后介绍了当前MD安德森癌症中心对于炎性乳腺癌的治疗策略，分别从诊断和分期、多学科治疗、辅助治疗、术后监测随访以及入组临床试验这些方面详细阐述。

Inflammatory breast carcinoma (IBC) is a very aggressive disease and accounts for less than 6% of all breast cancers in the United States. It is characterized by a rapidly progressive clinical course and diagnosed on the basis of distinct skin manifestations that are often confused with inflammation, hence its name. These manifestations include erythema, edema, skin nodules, and nipple retraction. A characteristic infiltration of the dermal lymphatics with tumor emboli is often seen by pathology but is not required to establish a diagnosis.

Although clinically more than 50% of patients do not have a detectable breast mass at the time of diagnosis, up to 85% have already metastasized disease that has spread to the regional lymph nodes, while more than 30% present with gross distant metastasis ([1]). Not surprisingly, owing to its high metastatic potential, IBC is associated with a 5-year overall survival (OS) rate of no more than 55% ([2, 3]). Multimodality treatment in the form of neoadjuvant chemotherapy, surgery, and radiation aims to prevent metastatic failure as well as achieve local control.

EPIDEMIOLOGIC CHARACTERISTICS

The epidemiology of IBC has been a challenging area to study due to a number of factors. The rarity of the disease combined with its rapid progression and short OS mean that there are few single centers able to recruit an adequate sample of patients for investigation. In addition, confusion about its clinical definition has led to difficulties in comparing the results of different studies. As a result, the primary source of epidemiologic data comes from large national registries, which are limited by nonuniform data collection, inability to capture comprehensive details on risk factors, and in the case of IBC, varying case definitions.

To address these issues, the Morgan Welch Inflammatory Breast Cancer Research Program and Clinic at the University of Texas, MD Anderson Cancer Center (MDACC) spearheaded the development of an international IBC Registry. The IBC Registry prospectively collects tissue, serum, plasma, whole blood, imaging, clinical, and epidemiological data from patients with IBC, allowing a more comprehensive examination of the underlying mechanisms associated with the development of this lethal disease.

Incidence

The incidence of IBC is reported to range from 1% to 6% of all breast cancers diagnosed in the United States ([4]). Higher proportions have been reported in North Africa, specifically in Tunisia and Egypt, where IBC accounts for 6% and 10% of all breast cancers, respectively ([5-7]). Data from the National Cancer Institute's Surveillance, Epidemiology, and End Results (SEER) program have demonstrated a rise in the incidence of IBC over time, although this trend seems to be slowing. Between 1973 and 2002, the incidence of IBC is reported to have increased at an annual rate that ranged from 1.23% to 4.35% per year, depending on the specific database analyzed and the case definition used ([4, 8, 9]). In comparison, during the same time period, breast cancer as a whole saw a slower rise of 0.42% per year (95% CI, 0.14% to 0.71%) ([9]).

Mortality

Inflammatory breast carcinoma is commonly lethal and associated with a high risk of early recurrence ([10]). Women diagnosed with IBC have a statistically significant poorer survival than women with noninflammatory locally advanced breast cancer (LABC) ($P < .001$), with a median OS of 2.9 years and a 5-year survival rate of 30% to 40% ([4, 11]). This was also true for patients presenting with stage IV disease. Patients with stage IV IBC had a shorter median OS than stage IV non-IBC (2.3 vs 3.4 years, $P = .004$) ([12]). Also, although IBC accounted for only 2.5% of all breast cancer cases in the period 1988 to 2000, it led to 7% of all breast cancer–specific deaths ([4]).

Higher mortality rates were reported for African American women, according to data from SEER, with a median survival of 2.0 versus 2.9 years when compared with Caucasians ($P < .001$) ([4, 13]). The early age at diagnosis and poor survival outcomes observed among African American patients with IBC suggests epidemiological differences between different ethnic groups that could involve an interplay of genetic, environmental, and lifestyle risk factors.

Earlier reports suggested a trend for a modest improvement in mortality rates for IBC ([4]). This trend was compared to a similar improvement seen in non-IBC and attributed to improvements in multidisciplinary treatment, the effect of new therapies, and an increasing awareness of IBC. However, more recently, this trend toward improved survival was not supported by retrospective data at our institution ([11]). The authors looked at the survival of 398 women with IBC treated over a period of 30 years (between January 1974 and April 2005). After adjusting for patient and disease characteristics, Cox proportional hazards models did not show an association between year of diagnosis and the risk of recurrence or death.

RISK FACTORS

While clearly established risk factors have been associated with the development of non-IBC, this is not the case with IBC, which is much rarer and not consistently defined. For example, while family history, menopausal status, and age at menarche are important risk factors for the development of non-IBC, they have not been confirmed as risk factors for IBC. Despite these limitations, several important epidemiologic factors appear to be consistently associated with IBC (Table 29-1).

Age of Diagnosis

According to an analysis of breast cancer cases diagnosed in the SEER 9 Registries between 1988 and 2000 (n = 180,224), IBC developed at a younger age (median 57 years) when compared with non-IBC (61.9 years) ([9]). Young age at diagnosis was also seen in earlier population-based studies ([8, 14, 15]). In addition, these studies found that age of onset varied according to ethnicity, with African American women presenting at a younger age than Caucasians ([15]). Age at diagnosis also varied between genders, and men usually were diagnosed 10 years later than women (median 66.5 vs 57 years, $P < .001$) ([9]).

Ethnicity

African Americans have at least a 50% higher incidence of IBC than whites in the United States (3.1 vs 2.2 per 100,000 woman-years, $p < .001$) ([4]). The higher incidence of IBC in African Americans has been confirmed in four different population-based studies ([4, 8, 14, 15]). Three of these studies used the SEER dataset to cover different time periods; the fourth used the North American Association of Central Cancer Registries (NAACCR) database.

Moreover, African Americans were diagnosed at a younger age (median 55.2 vs 58.1 years) and had a poorer prognosis when compared with Caucasians. Of note, Hispanic women have the youngest mean age of onset of the disease (median 50.5 years) ([15]).

A recent SEER study that examined patients with breast cancer (IBC and non-IBC) diagnosed between 1990 and 2000 suggested that the inferior outcome seen in African American women was independent of stage or inflammatory status ([13]).

Table 29-1 Risk Factors Associated With the Development of Inflammatory Breast Cancer

Risk Factor	Degree of Association
• Younger age at diagnosis	+++
• African American ethnicity	+++
• Increased body mass index (≥30)	+++
• North Africa	++
• Ever pregnant	+
• Younger age at live first birth	+
• Duration of breast feeding	+

Body Mass Index

One of the most consistent risk factors associated with IBC is a high body mass index (BMI). In contrast to non-IBC, for which elevated BMI is a risk factor in postmenopausal patients only, high BMI is associated with IBC in both pre- and postmenopausal patients. In a case-comparison study conducted at MDACC, patients with IBC weighed more (median weight 77.6 kg) than those with non-IBC (70.0 kg) or those with history of other cancers (68.0 kg) ([8]). After adjusting for other factors, women with the highest BMI (>26 kg/m^2) had an increased risk for development of IBC compared to those with non-IBC (odds ratio 2.54). This was irrespective of menopausal status, age at menarche, or family history of breast cancer.

In the largest case-control study to evaluate the association between risk factors for breast cancer and the development of IBC, Schairer et al compared 617 patients with IBC to three reference groups: LABC (n = 7,600), noninflammatory breast cancer not involving the chest wall or skin (n = 1,151), and healthy controls (n = 93,654). They found that high BMI at diagnosis was associated with an increased risk of IBC irrespective of menopausal status or hormone receptor expression ([16]).

The impact of obesity and menopausal status on IBC survival was also evaluated in a cohort of 177 women patients with IBC seen at MDACC between 1974 and1993. After adjusting for axillary lymph node involvement and chemotherapy protocol, premenopausal obese women had significantly worse survival compared to postmenopausal obese women (hazard ratio [HR] 1.51) ([17]). After stratifying by menopausal status, postmenopausal obese women had significantly worse survival than those who were not obese (HR 1.86). These findings suggest that factors associated with a higher BMI at diagnosis may contribute to shorter IBC survival among postmenopausal women but not premenopausal women, who were found to have poorer survival regardless of body size.

Finally, the prognostic value of BMI at diagnosis was evaluated in a retrospective study of 602 patients with LABC, which included a subset of patients with IBC (18%). Obese patients were more commonly associated with a diagnosis of IBC compared with overweight and normal or underweight groups ($p = .01$) ([18]). Patients with LABC who were obese or overweight had a significantly worse OS and relapse-free survival (RFS) and a higher incidence of visceral recurrence compared with normal/underweight patients.

Overall, these results are of great importance for IBC because obesity is a modifiable risk factor, and preventive strategies aimed at reducing obesity may yield significant rewards.

Geographic Location

The incidence of IBC has been observed to vary according to geographic location. Using the SEER program registries from 1992 to 2002, rates ranged from 2.064 per 100,000 woman-years in San Jose-Monterey (California) up to 3.042 cases per 100,000 in Los Angeles ([9]). Similarly, reports have suggested that North Africa is associated with the highest rates in the world, with countries such as Tunisia and Egypt reporting proportions of 6% and 10% of all breast cancers, respectively ([5-7]). These variations are currently under study and may suggest underlying differences in environmental and lifestyle or genetic risk factors. Alternatively, differences in case definitions and the lack of specificity associated with clinical identification of IBC have somewhat limited the value of these comparisons.

Socioeconomic Position

Data suggest that socioeconomic position (SEP) can affect both the incidence and the outcome of IBC. Whereas the incidence of breast cancer overall has been associated with higher SEP, several studies have suggested a higher incidence rate of IBC among patients with lower SEP ([13, 16]). Likewise, in a large, nested case-control study of patients identified from the Breast Cancer Surveillance Consortium database (1994-2009), the risk of developing IBC gradually decreased with increasing level of education ([16]).

On the other hand, differences in SEP are associated with different exposure patterns to risk factors and with differences in disease awareness and access to health care, leading to diagnostic delays, mismanagement, and potentially worse OS. This may explain why the association between lower SEP and poorer survival was not significant for IBC after adjustment for other prognostic factors ([16]).

Reproductive History

Although IBC is diagnosed at a younger age than non-IBC, there does not appear to be a consistent association between IBC and premenopausal status. Of the patients evaluated at MDACC, 49% of patients with IBC were premenopausal compared to 39% of non-IBC patients ([8]). Similarly, while patients with IBC presented with earlier age at menarche than patients with non-IBC (12.2 vs 12.7 years), this difference was not statistically significant. A study conducted in Pakistan did not show a significant difference in menopausal status among the various comparison groups, including IBC ([19]). Larger studies are required to establish relationships between IBC and menstrual history.

Early age at first birth has also been associated with the development of IBC. Women with aggressive breast cancer, including IBC, are more likely to have their first child before the age of 20 when compared to patients with nonaggressive breast cancer ([9]). A later age at first birth was associated with a reduced risk of developing IBC that was estrogen receptor (ER) negative compared to locally advanced and early breast cancer ([16]).

An association with pregnancy or lactation has been suggested in earlier reports ([20]). In a study by Bonnier et al, IBC accounted for approximately 21% to 26% of breast cancer tumors in patients who developed breast cancer during or after pregnancy ([21]). Later studies reported that the risk of pregnancy seen with IBC was not different from the risk seen in non-IBC ([22]). Results from our group suggest that lack of breast-feeding history maybe associated with the development of specific IBC subtypes (ER+, triple negative). No association between oral contraceptive use and development of IBC has been found ([8]).

Family History

Approximately 15% of women with breast cancer have a positive family history of breast cancer in a first-degree relative, while 5% to 10% of breast cancers are directly attributed to heredity. In a study comparing 68 patients with IBC and 143 patients with non-IBC seen at MDACC, 13% of patients with IBC reported a positive family history of breast cancer, compared with 8% of patients with non-IBC; this was not statistically significant ([23]). However, in a study conducted in Pakistan, 20% of patients with IBC reported a positive family history of breast cancer, compared to 5% in the non-IBC group, which was statistically significant ([19]).

Using data from the Breast Cancer Surveillance Consortium database (1994-2009), Schairer et al also found that the presence of a first-degree family history of breast cancer was associated with increased risk of developing IBC (HR 1.6; 95% CI, 1.1 to 2.2) ([16]).

Other Risk Factors

A host of other risk factors have been explored in IBC, including blood type and area of residence. A higher proportion of Tunisian patients with IBC have blood type A. In addition, a larger proportion of patients lived in rural locations ([20]). Smoking and alcohol use were not associated with a risk of developing IBC ([23]). Other studies have suggested a link between IBC and a variant of mouse mammary tumor virus ([24]). This relationship remains under investigation.

MOLECULAR PATHOGENESIS

Attempts to distinguish between IBC and non-IBC at the molecular level have so far not been successful. Inflammatory breast carcinoma shares some of the molecular characteristics associated with breast cancer in general, as well as some important differences.

Gene expression profiles: There has been no shortage of gene expression studies aimed at distinguishing IBC from non-IBC at the genomic level ([25-27]). Although several gene expression studies of IBC tumors have revealed useful and promising results, none has yielded an IBC-specific signature.

In breast cancer, the success associated with the identification of several gene expression subtypes of prognostic significance has led to their incorporation in the treatment strategy for women with nonmetastatic breast cancer ([28]). These molecular subtypes are classified into luminal (ER-related genes), *HER2* (*HER2*-related genes), and basal subtypes. Despite differences in their relative frequency, the molecular subtypes of IBC are similar to those expressed in non-IBC ([26, 29]). Likewise, there are no unique differences between triple-negative IBC and non-IBC at the messenger RNA gene expression level ([30]).

RhoC GTPase overexpression/loss of WNT1 Inducible Signaling Pathway Protein 3 (WISP3): The transforming oncogene *RhoC* GTPase (guanosine triphosphatase) is one of the most upregulated genes in IBC and is found in 91% of IBC tumors compared to 38% in non-IBC tumors in some studies ([31]). *RhoC* GTPase overexpression is thought to be involved in tumor invasion and increased expression of cyclin D1, vascular endothelin growth factor (VEGF), fibronectin, and caveolin-2 ([31]). The overexpression of *RhoC* GTPase, combined with the loss of the tumor suppressor gene *WISP3/WINT-1*, was found to characterize the IBC cell line SUM149 and is believed to be partially responsible for the aggressive phenotype of IBC tumors ([32, 33]).

E-cadherin overexpression: E-cadherin is a cell adhesion molecule that is lost in malignant progression and is thought to promote tumor cell metastasis. Loss of E-cadherin is considered to be a fundamental event in epithelial-mesenchymal transition (EMT) that is associated with tumor metastasis and stem cell–like phenotypes. Paradoxically, E-cadherin is overexpressed in IBC and appears to be necessary for tumor emboli formation by enhancing tumor cell–cell contact ([34]).

Increased expression of E-cadherin and nonsialylated mucin-1 (MUC1) has been identified in up to 100% of IBC tumors compared to 68% of non-IBC tumors in one study ([35]). In another study using a xenograft model, a 10- to 20-fold increased expression of E-cadherin and MUC1 was noted and thought to contribute to the passive dissemination of tumor emboli in IBC ([36]). Dual overexpression of these two proteins in IBC is thought to play a role in the aggressive, invasive nature of IBC ([37]).

p53 mutation: In breast cancer, studies have linked p53 mutation to worse prognosis ([38]). In a study performed at MDACC, p53 overexpression was noted in up to 58% of IBC tumors and was independent of histologic grade ([39]). Patients with p53 overexpression were younger (median age 45.2 vs 52.2 years; $P = .02$) and had lower 5-year progression-free survival rates (35% vs 55%; $P = .03$) and 5-year OS rates (44% vs 54%; $P = .4$). Patients with tumors overexpressing p53 had an 8.6-fold higher risk of death in multivariate analysis. These results were in line with previous studies ([40]).

Angiogenesis: Inflammatory breast carcinoma is a vascular tumor with overexpression of lymphangiogenic factors such as VEGF and Flt-4 ([34, 41]). A significantly higher intratumoral microvessel density has been reported in IBC tumors compared to non-IBC tumors ([42]). Evidence also suggests that IBC tumors exhibit the phenomenon of vasculogenic mimicry, by which tumors form vessel-like structures in the absence of endothelial cells. These structures act as a supplementary blood supply by which tumor tissue is able to nourish itself. Both the WIBC-9 and the Mary-X xenograft models have demonstrated a role for vasculogenic mimicry in IBC ([43]).

Inflammation: The degree to which inflammation plays a role in inflammatory breast cancer remains largely unknown. Recent evidence comes from the constitutive activation of major inflammatory signaling pathways (nuclear factor kappa B [NF-κB], cyclooxygenase 2 [COX-2], and JAK/STAT [Janus kinase/signal transducer and activator of transcription]) as well as in vitro, in vivo, and patient studies ([44]). Similarly, inflammatory cytokines and chemokines such as interleukin 6, transforming growth factor beta, tumor necrosis factor alpha (TNF-α), and gamma interferon are involved in all steps of tumorigenesis in IBC. These findings have prompted the testing of several compounds for their anti-inflammatory activity, with the aim of developing therapeutic or prevention strategies for IBC ([44]).

Cancer stem cells: Some evidence suggests that IBC cells have characteristics similar to cancer stem cells ([45, 46]). The IBC tumors as well as the SUM149 IBC cell line and the Mary-X preclinical model of IBC have all been shown to express stem cell surface markers (CD44+/CD24⁻/low and aldehyde dehydrogenase 1 [ALDH-1] enzyme production) as assessed by the ALDEFLUOR assay ([46, 47]). Expression of ALDH-1 in samples from patients diagnosed with IBC was associated with poor prognosis ([47]). Using microarray analysis, IBC was found to express genes known to be associated with breast cancer stem cells ([48]). A study using a xenograft model of IBC has demonstrated the potential to reverse the EMT process by which epithelial cells are thought to acquire stem cell–like properties ([49]).

Other molecular mechanisms: Overexpression of epidermal growth factor receptor (*EGFR*) is observed in more than 30% of patients with IBC. Patients with *EGFR*-positive tumors have an increased risk of recurrence and worse 5-year OS rates [50]. Elevated levels of extracellular signal-regulated kinase (ERK) have been reported in both SUM149 and KPL-4 IBC cell lines [49]. Dual blockade of *EGFR* and ERK1/2 phosphorylation in SUM19 cells was associated with decreased mitogen-activated protein kinase (MAPK) signaling and induced apoptosis [51].

On the other hand, WISP3 was able to modulate insulinlike growth factor (IGF) signaling in SUM149 cells, which may be an effective therapeutic target for IBC [32, 52].

The expanded knowledge gained from preclinical studies has resulted in several promising molecular targets for directed therapy (Table 29-2).

CLINICAL PRESENTATION

The clinical identification of IBC is frequently confused with more common benign diseases and requires a high index of suspicion on the part of the diagnosing physician. On suspicion, the physician must obtain pathologic evidence of breast carcinoma to establish the presence of malignancy. Once evidence of breast carcinoma is obtained, the presence of dermal lymphatic invasion helps to confirm the diagnosis but is neither required nor sufficient to make the diagnosis [53].

Table 29-2 Summary of Potential Biological Targets in the Treatment of Inflammatory Breast Cancer

Category	Molecular Marker	Pharmacologic Class
Oncogenes	Her-2/neu	mAbs, TKIs
	RhoC GTPase	FTIs
Tumor suppressor genes	p53	Gene therapy, p53-stabilizing agents
	PTEN	Proteasome inhibitors, PI3K inhibitors
Angiogenesis modulators	Tie-2	Tie-2 kinase inhibitor
	VEGF	TKIs, mAbs
	Flt-1/Flk-1	TKIs, mAbs
	E-cadherin	E-cadherin inhibitors
	MUC1	MUC1 inhibitors, PIAS
	RhoC GTPase	FTIs

FTIs, farnesyltransferase inhibitors; mAbs, monoclonal antibodies; MUC-1, mucin 1; PIAS, protein inhibitor of activated signal transducer and activator of transcription; PI3K, phosphatidylinositol-3-kinase; TKIs, tyrosine kinase inhibitors; VEGF, vascular endothelial growth factor.

The affected breast typically presents with a rapid onset of erythema, tenderness, edema, and swelling, accompanied by an enlargement of the draining lymph nodes, frequently in the absence of a breast mass. This clinical picture closely mimics common inflammatory conditions of the breast, such as simple bacterial mastitis [54]. As a result, many patients with IBC unnecessarily undergo repeated courses of antibiotics before a diagnosis is made.

On the other hand, in the presence of a breast mass, these symptoms are often confused with LABC with secondary erythematous skin involvement. The lack of specific pathologic or molecular characteristics for IBC means that the distinction between IBC and non-IBC is based mainly on clinical grounds.

The confusing clinical presentation of IBC often leads to unnecessary delays in diagnosis and treatment. Haagensen reported that the median duration of symptoms before diagnosis was 2.5 months compared to 5 months for non-IBC [55]. However, a recent study examining the impact of delayed diagnosis, defined as more than 60 days from the time of first contact with a physician, found no effect on patient outcome [56].

Clinical Criteria

Inflammatory breast carcinoma commonly presents unilaterally, although bilateral disease can occur [57]. Haagensen's original description of IBC outlined a list of characteristic symptoms and their corresponding frequencies [55]. The author's criteria included breast mass (57%), redness of the skin (57%), breast enlargement (48%), pain in breast or nipple (29%), breast tenderness (16%), generalized breast hardness (16%), nipple retraction (13%), edema of the skin (13%), axillary mass (9%), and warmness of the skin (8%).

One of the defining characteristics of IBC is the **rapid onset** of skin changes. Patients with primary IBC exhibit symptoms characterized by rapid onset erythema occurring less than 6 months from the diagnosis of breast cancer [58]. In contrast, those presenting with delayed erythema occurring more than 6 months after breast cancer diagnosis are considered to have neglected breast cancer with secondary erythematous changes.

Skin changes, in the form of erythema and edema, are a distinguishing feature of IBC and should involve at least one-third of the skin overlying the breast to establish the diagnosis. Patients who present with skin changes involving less than one-third of the skin should not be classified as having IBC.

Erythema tends to be one of the earliest manifestations and typically presents with a mottled pink discoloration of the skin in the affected breast, which may be associated with a sensation of heat. Comparison with the contralateral, unaffected breast helps to identify erythema (Figs. 29-1A, 29-1B). During the course of its evolution, the degree of erythema may change from a flush of pink to red to bronze; it even may briefly fade and give the misleading picture of disease regression ([54]). In more severe cases, skin discoloration involves the entire breast and may change to dark red or purple. These manifestations can vary in African American women, for whom skin erythema is not the predominant symptom, leading to more difficulties in diagnosis. In these cases, peau d'orange changes may be easier to identify (Fig. 29-1C).

On the other hand, edema of the skin results from blockage of the draining lymphatics. This also leads to swelling of the breast and exaggeration of pits around hair follicles, giving the characteristic **peau d'orange** (orange peel) appearance. This can cause generalized breast induration as well as wheals and ridging ([59]).

Rapid **swelling of the breast** results from breast edema and in some cases can increase in size two- to threefold in a period of a few weeks.

At the time of diagnosis, almost all patients present with **lymph node metastasis**, and up to 30% also have distant metastasis at presentation ([1]). The ipsilateral axillary lymph nodes are the most common areas of spread, followed by ipsilateral supraclavicular lymph nodes. Contralateral and distant lymph node spread are also common, especially in more advanced and neglected cases ([1]). On physical examination, lymph nodes are usually enlarged, palpable, and fixed and in extreme cases may be accompanied with arm lymphedema.

Other clinical features not considered diagnostic of IBC include **nipple involvement**, itching, and axillary pain. The nipple may be flattened and retracted and appear blistered or associated with an area of crusting ([1]). Ulceration is not a common feature of IBC and generally suggests neglected LABC.

Secondary IBC

A distinction must be made between primary IBC and secondary IBC, which is the development of inflammatory changes in a breast or chest wall after a history of non-IBC in either the same or opposite breast. The outcomes from these disease entities are likely very different. In a recent review of eight patients with secondary IBC identified from the Inflammatory

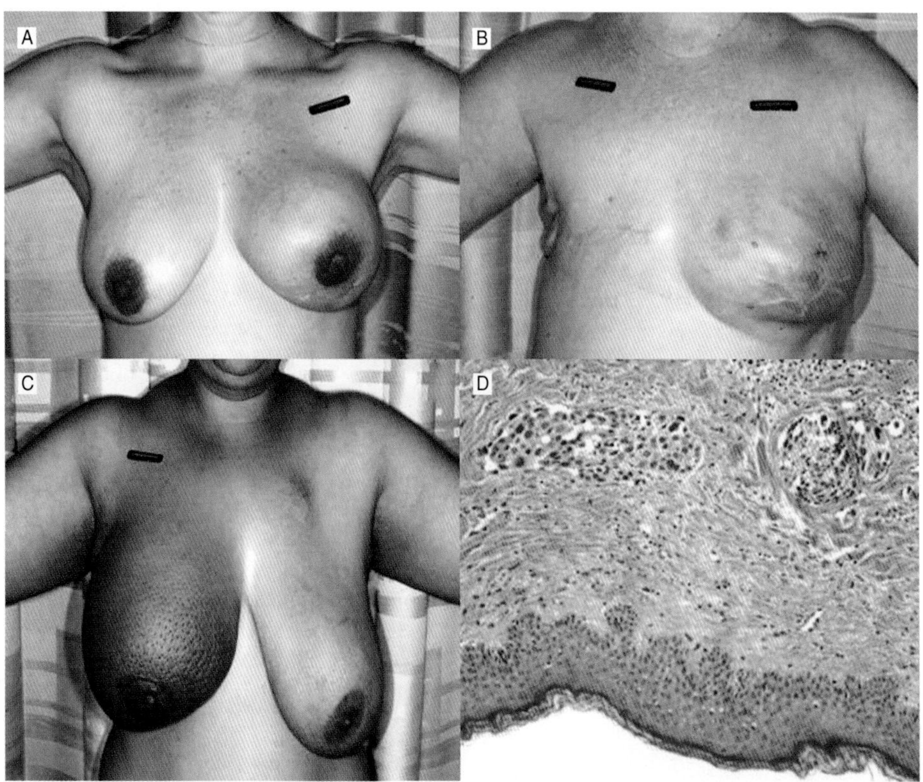

FIGURE 29-1 Clinical appearance of inflammatory breast cancer. **A.** Erythema and enlargement noted when compared to normal breast. **B.** Diffuse erythema of the left breast in a woman with prior history of right breast cancer. **C.** Peau d'orange appearance of the skin of the right breast. **D.** Photomicrograph of breast biopsy from a woman with inflammatory breast cancer showing normal-appearing epidermis (*bottom of figure*) with tumor cells infiltrating the lymphatic channels of the dermis.

Breast Cancer Registry database, patients commonly presented with redness at the surgical scar site, peau d'orange, a diffuse rash, or chest wall nodules, which, unlike primary IBC, can become ulcerated ([59, 60]). An early study at MDACC identified 96 patients with secondary IBC diagnosed between 1954 and 1981 and suggested there were no major differences in clinical course or outcome between primary and secondary IBC ([61]). This conclusion should be interpreted cautiously. In view of the recent progress achieved in the treatment of non-IBC, secondary IBC is likely to have a different outcome compared to primary IBC, and the two entities should be clearly distinguished.

Differential Diagnosis

Inflammatory breast carcinoma is often misdiagnosed as an infection of the breast, such as cellulitis, bacterial mastitis, or breast abscess, which are treated with repeated courses of anti-inflammatory or antibiotic treatment ([54]). A high degree of suspicion and the absence of fever, pain, leukocytosis, or other symptoms and signs associated with inflammation help distinguish IBC from breast infection. Acute bacterial mastitis commonly occurs during lactation and resolves in several days. Other infectious entities that can mimic IBC include erysipelas, which is usually caused by group A streptococcus.

Inflammatory breast cancer is also commonly confused with locally advanced neglected breast cancer with secondary erythematous changes. This condition presents with delayed erythema occurring more than 6 months after the initial diagnosis of breast cancer ([58]).

Paget disease of the nipple can also mimic IBC but generally develops more slowly and is usually associated with destruction of the nipple ([54]). Radiation dermatitis, in its acute phase, may also appear to be IBC; however, desquamation of the skin usually occurs with resolution of skin changes in 2 to 3 weeks.

Other less-common conditions that may be confused with IBC include rare breast malignancies such as sarcoma, inflammatory metastatic melanoma, or breast lymphoma; distant breast metastasis from another primary cancer may also produce a similar clinical picture (Table 29-3).

Table 29-3 Differential Diagnosis of Inflammatory Breast Cancer

Infectious conditions:
• Lactational mastitis • Breast abscess • Other infections: erysipelas, tuberculosis, syphilis
Benign (noninfectious) conditions:
• Dermatitis • Duct ectasia
Malignant conditions:
• Locally advanced neglected breast cancer with secondary erythematous changes • Radiation dermatitis • Rare malignancies of the breast: leukemia, breast lymphoma, sarcoma, inflammatory metastatic melanoma, distant breast metastasis from another primary cancer

Natural History of Inflammatory Breast Carcinoma

Inflammatory breast carcinoma is a rapidly progressive disease and is characterized by high rates of locoregional and distant recurrence. In a pooled analysis of 10 clinical trials conducted at MDACC, patterns of recurrence in 240 patients with IBC were compared to 831 patients with stage-matched non-IBC ([10]). All patients were reported to have received similar multidisciplinary treatment. Patients with IBC had a higher cumulative incidence of recurrence at 5 years compared to individuals with non-IBC (64.8% vs 43.4%; $P < .0001$) and a lower 5-year OS rate (40.5% vs 63.2%; $P < .0001$). Inflammatory breast carcinoma was associated with significantly higher rates of soft tissue recurrence (skin and lymph nodes) both locoregionally and at distant sites. There was no difference between IBC and non-IBC in terms of distant recurrence to the bone or viscera.

Using data from the SEER registries, Schairer et al compared the risk of contralateral breast cancer in 5,631 patients with IBC versus and 174,634 patients with comparably staged non-IBC among women diagnosed with first breast cancer between 1973 and 2006 ([62]). Contralateral breast cancer was further divided into recurrent/metastatic (occurring between 2 and 23 months of diagnosis) and independent second primary breast cancer (occurring in the opposite breast 2 or more years after the first diagnosis). Absolute risk of contralateral breast cancer was higher in IBC (4.9% vs 1.1% at 2 years), irrespective of age or hormonal status. The majority of IBC events occurred within 2 to 23 months from the first diagnosis, reflecting a higher risk of recurrence compared to non-IBC. The risk of contralateral breast cancer continued to be higher for those with IBC, up to 15 years from the time of first diagnosis.

PATHOLOGY

Obtaining a core biopsy with evidence of malignancy is considered the cornerstone of diagnosing IBC. Two additional skin punch biopsies are strongly recommended to detect dermal lymphatic tumor emboli and confirm the diagnosis.

CHAPTER 29

It should be emphasized that IBC is not a true inflammatory process and does not demonstrate any of the pathologic hallmarks of inflammation, such as the presence of inflammatory cells or pus formation.

One of the most striking gross features of IBC is that it commonly presents in the absence of a dominant mass. The cancer usually presents as clumps of tumor cells within the lymphovascular spaces of the skin. These microscopic lesions are known as lymphovascular tumor emboli and represent the pathologic hallmark of the disease as well as explain most of its clinical manifestations. As a result, IBC often presents with multicentric disease, in some cases bilaterally, and has a high propensity to spread to the regional lymph nodes and the distant organs.

Otherwise, the gross pathology of IBC tends to correspond with its clinical characteristics and includes erythema, thickening of the skin, and generalized enlargement of the breast due to edema.

Histologic Examination

In conjunction with the clinical features associated with IBC, several histopathological features have also been identified. Histologically, IBC tumors are characterized as being of higher tumor grade, with small areas of invasive carcinoma and extensive vascular tumor emboli associated with large tumor-free skip areas (Fig. 29-1D).

Histologic type: Inflammatory breast carcinoma may be associated with any of the invasive subtypes of breast cancer. Invasive ductal carcinoma of no special type or not otherwise specified (NST or NOS, respectively) is the most frequently identified histologic subtype associated with IBC. Other subtypes include lobular, medullary, papillary, mucinous, comedo carcinoma, or Paget disease (rare). An in situ component may be present but is usually minimal. There are no known precursor lesions for IBC.

Histologic grade, proliferative rate: Inflammatory breast carcinoma is an aggressive phenotype of breast cancer that is associated with a high histologic grade ([63]). It is also associated with higher proliferative rates, manifested by higher mitotic index and higher Ki-67 values when compared to non-IBC. These values have also been shown to be prognostic.

Pathology of lymphovascular tumor emboli: Tumor emboli are considered a hallmark of IBC and result from the pathologic plugging of dermal lymphatics by clumps of tumor cells. These clumps ultimately lead to lymphatic obstruction and are responsible for most of the clinical manifestations of IBC. Lymphovascular tumor emboli usually appear early in the disease and migrate readily to distant organs.

Despite being a defining signature, the presence of lymphovascular emboli is inconsistent and hence not required for the diagnosis of IBC. Even with adequate skin samples and tissue sections, dermal lymphatic tumor emboli are found in only 75% of patients with IBC. This is not only partly because IBC is characterized by the presence of large areas of tumor-free skip areas but also also because of sampling error. Dermal lymphatic tumor emboli are also present in other malignancies, such as non-IBC and breast lymphoma. As a result, they are useful only in confirming the diagnosis of patients with positive clinical criteria for IBC ([64]).

Although the metastatic potential of IBC has been attributed to the presence of tumor emboli, the prognostic significance of dermal lymphatic invasion remains an area of controversy.

Molecular subtypes: Breast cancer is classified into distinct molecular subtypes based on gene expression profiling or immunohistochemistry ([28]). When compared to non-IBC, IBC tumors have a tendency toward more aggressive subtypes. In a retrospective study conducted at MD Anderson, patients with IBC were assigned according to ER and *HER2* status into four subgroups: ER positive (33%), ER positive/*HER2* positive (12%), *HER2* positive (26%), and triple negative (29%) ([65]).

1. *Hormone receptor status*: In contrast to non-IBC, the majority of patients with IBC present with hormone receptor–negative tumors, which are known to be associated with a poorer prognosis than receptor-positive tumors ([3, 4]). Data from several studies have suggested that patients with hormone receptor–positive IBC is less frequently associated with favorable subtypes, such as luminal A tumors, when compared to non-IBC ([3]).
2. HER2 *overexpression*: On the other hand, IBC tumors are associated with a higher incidence of *HER2* overexpression (36% to 60%) compared to non-IBC. Unlike non-IBC, the prognostic relevance of *HER2* overexpression in IBC is currently unknown, although it plays a predictive role in determining which patients will benefit from *HER2*-directed therapy. A population-based study using data from the California Cancer Registry found a borderline significant difference in breast cancer–specific survival (BCS) favoring patients with *HER2*-positive IBC (HR 0.82; CI, 0.68-0.99) ([66]).
3. *Triple-negative IBC*: Approximately 29% of patients with IBC present with triple-negative tumors, which are associated with the poorest outcome when compared to other subtypes ([65]). The 5-year OS rates for triple-negative disease was 42.7%, compared to 69.7% for ER-positive, 73.5% for ER-positive/*HER2*-positive, and 54% for *HER2*-positive disease ($P < .0001$). Similarly, both the 5-year locoregional relapse rate (38.6%) and the distant relapse rate (56.7%) were significantly worse when compared to other subtypes ($P < .001$).

CHAPTER 29

IMAGING MODALITIES

Imaging modalities play a key role in the diagnosis and staging of IBC. In the absence of a dominant mass, it is often challenging to define with precision the correct area for biopsy without image guidance. In addition, imaging plays a crucial role in disease staging as well as assessment of treatment response.

Mammography

Because IBC commonly presents with lymphovascular tumor emboli and not with a breast mass, early detection strategies, such as breast self-examination, physical exams, and mammographic screening, are of little use.

In a retrospective analysis of various imaging modalities in the diagnosis of IBC, mammography was the least sensitive, detecting a mere 43% of primary breast parenchymal lesions ([67]). Most readings are negative for malignancy, with thickening of the skin as the most common finding suggestive of IBC (Fig. 29-2) ([68]). Other radiological findings include increased breast tissue density, trabecular and stromal thickening, breast swelling, axillary lymphadenopathy, and nipple retraction. These findings are usually subtle and can only be detected by comparison to the contralateral breast ([67]). Focal asymmetry and architectural distortion are not frequent findings in IBC. In addition, calcification is less common than in non-IBC and was detectable in only 41% of patients in one study ([67]).

Ultrasound

As with non-IBC, ultrasound is useful in localizing sites for biopsy in patients with masses. In a series evaluating 142 women with histologically proven IBC, in contrast to mammography, ultrasound was able to detect an additional 24 masses (18%) obscured by edema, when compared to mammogram alone ([69]). The greatest benefit of ultrasound may be its potential to provide comprehensive evaluation of the nodal stations and pectoral muscle invasion. In this same series, ultrasound was able to detect axillary lymphadenopathy in the majority (73%) of patients and pectoral muscle invasion in 10%. These findings have been confirmed in a series at MDACC, in which sonography found a parenchymal breast lesion and skin thickening in 95% of patients and regional axillary nodal disease in 93% of cases (Fig. 29-3) ([68]).

Magnetic Resonance Imaging

Magnetic resonance imaging has superior sensitivity in diagnosing breast cancer without the disadvantages of ionizing radiation. It is able to detect skin thickening in more than 90% of patients with IBC and axillary lymphadenopathy in up to 75% ([68, 70]). A discrete mass could also be seen in 38% of cases ([71, 72]). In a recent study, MRI was shown to detect the primary breast

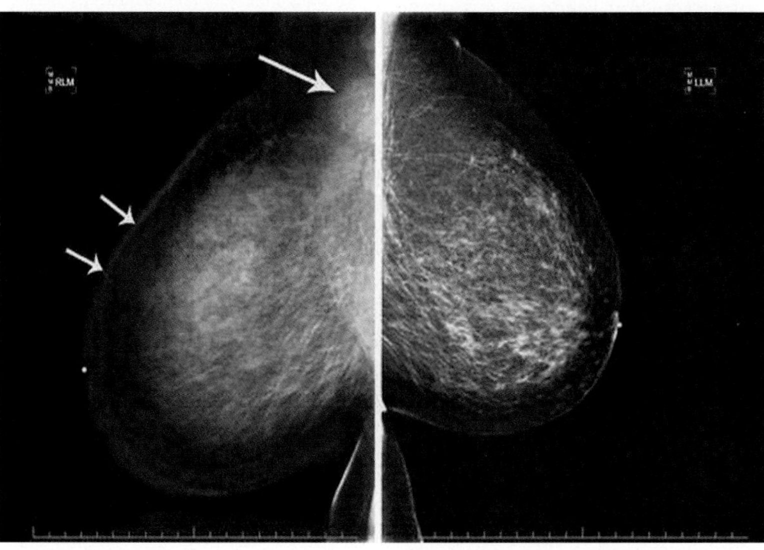

FIGURE 29-2 Bilateral mediolateral oblique mammograms in a 54-year-old woman show global skin and trabecular thickening (*short arrows*) of the right breast with associated right axillary adenopathy (*long arrow*). No visible primary breast parenchymal lesion is noted in the right breast. (Reproduced with permission from Yang WT, Le-Petross HT, Macapinlac H, et al. Inflammatory breast cancer: PET/CT, MRI, mammography, and sonography findings. *Breast Cancer Res Treat* 2008;109:417-426.)

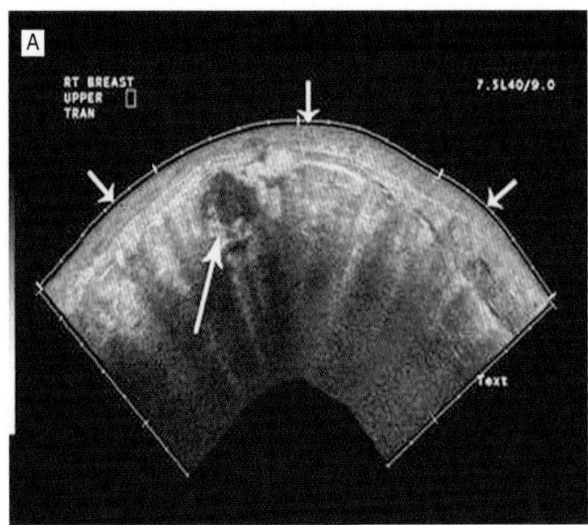

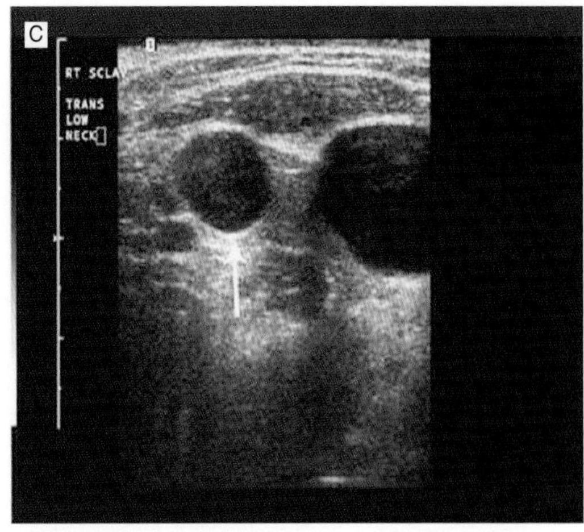

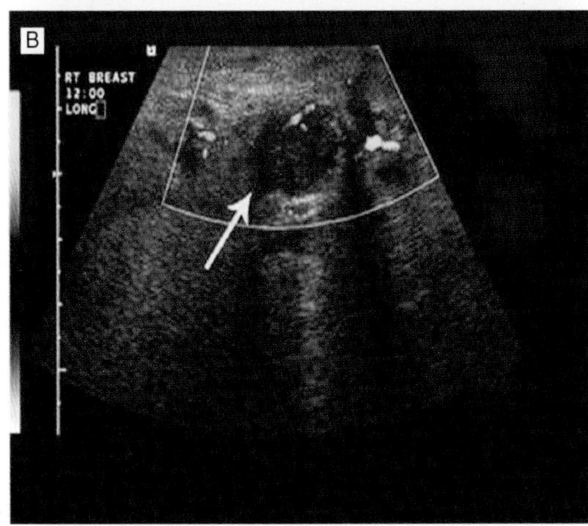

FIGURE 29-3 Ultrasound images of the right breast from patient described in Fig. 29-2. A. Extended-field-of-view ultrasound of the right breast in the patient of Fig. 29-2 showing marked diffuse skin thickening and subcutaneous edema (*short arrows*) and a focal solid hypoechoic mass (*long arrow*) representing primary breast parenchymal lesion. B. Transverse ultrasound with power Doppler imaging of the primary mass in the right breast shows marked internal hypervascularity. C. Transverse ultrasound of the right supraclavicular region shows a solid hypoechoic node that showed metastatic carcinoma on biopsy. (Reproduced with permission from Yang WT, Le-Petross HT, Macapinlac H, et al. Inflammatory breast cancer: PET/CT, MRI, mammography, and sonography findings. *Breast Cancer Res Treat* 2008;109:417-426.)

lesion in 98% of patients with IBC compared to 68% with mammography ($P < .0001$) ([73]). The majority of masses detected (83%) were multiple, small, and confluent. These findings make MRI the imaging modality of choice in the detection of IBC for many clinicians (Fig. 29-4).

Moreover, MRI is useful in differentiating between acute mastitis and IBC ([72,74]). In a study evaluating 90 patients (48 with IBC and 42 with acute mastitis), MRIs were able to statistically detect more T2-hypodense masses, infiltration of pectoralis major muscle, and pectoralis edema ([74]). In addition, MRI has been useful in follow-up of acute mastitis by evaluating the success of antibiotic treatment and diagnosis of coexisting or confounding inflammatory carcinoma ([72]).

The utility of breast MRI has also been evaluated in monitoring response to therapy ([75,76]). In a study by Chen et al, the accuracy of complete clinical response on MRI to predict pathological complete response (pCR) was 69% (11 of 16), with a sensitivity of 58% (7 of 12), specificity of 92% (11 of 12), and a false-negative rate of 21% (5 of 24) ([77]). These results suggest that treatment decisions based on MRI findings should be done with extreme caution, especially in cases where no discrete mass was identified.

Computerized Tomography

The utility of helical computerized tomography (CT), which provides high-resolution thin cuts, was also investigated in the diagnosis of IBC. Helical CT was able to detect skin thickening in 100% of the patients with IBC (Fig. 29-5). Axillary lymphadenopathy was found in 82% of patients and distant metastases in 64% in a small cohort of 11 patients ([78]).

Helical CT has also been evaluated for its role in monitoring response to therapy for IBC. Compared to clinical examination and mammography, breast helical CT was useful in the quantitative assessment of response to neoadjuvant chemotherapy and preoperative determination of residual tumor volume in patients with round opacities (correlation coefficients of 0.97) ([79]). However, it was not as reliable for tumors

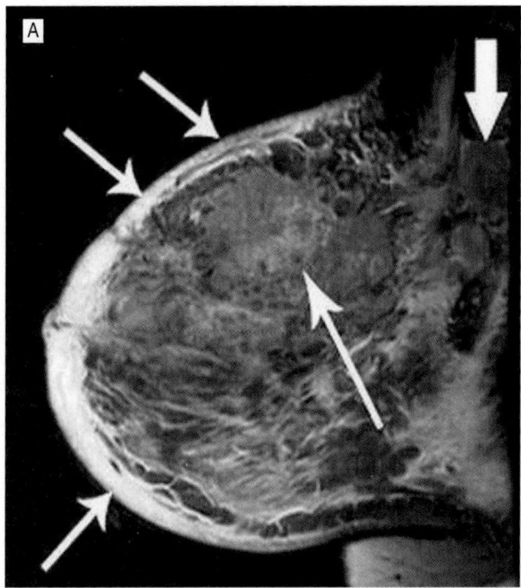

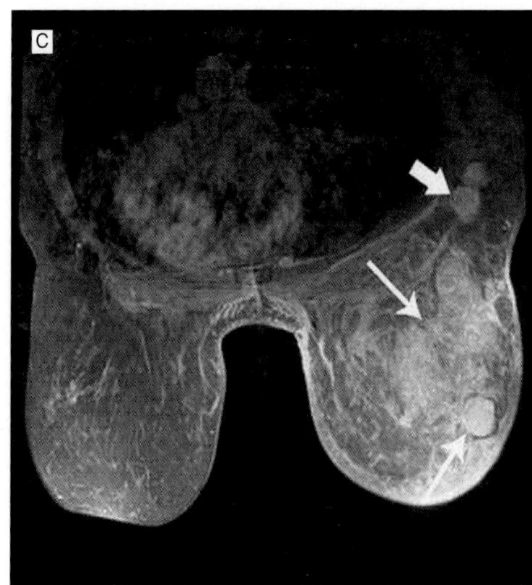

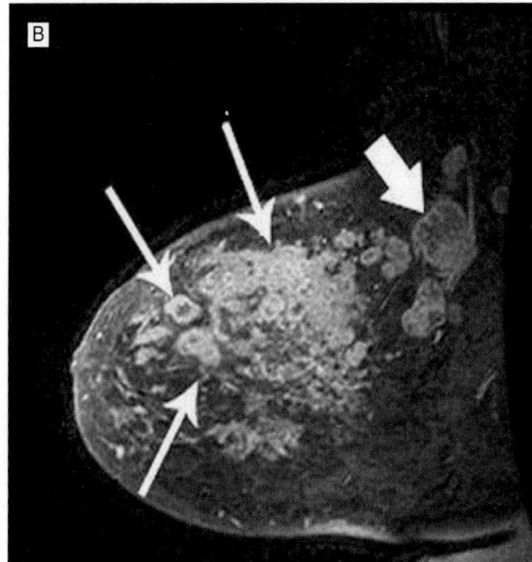

FIGURE 29-4 A. Sagittal T2-weighted fast spin-echo image with fat suppression shows a dominant heterogeneous mass in the superior right breast (*long arrow*), global skin and subcutaneous edema (*medium arrows*), and right axillary adenopathy (*broad arrow*). **B.** Sagittal fat-suppressed three-dimensional spoiled gradient-recalled-echo sequence with parallel imaging at 2 minutes postcontrast administration demonstrates multiple rim-enhancing tumor masses (*arrows*) in the right breast and malignant-appearing necrotic right axillary lymph nodes (*broad arrow*). **C.** Delayed axial fat-suppressed, contrast-enhanced three-dimensional fast spoiled gradient-recalled-echo MRI reveals multiple heterogeneously enhancing masses in the central and lateral right breast (*arrows*) and right axillary adenopathy (*broad arrow*). (Reproduced with permission from Yang WT, Le-Petross HT, Macapinlac H, et al. Inflammatory breast cancer: PET/CT, MRI, mammography, and sonography findings. *Breast Cancer Res Treat* 2008;109:417-426.)

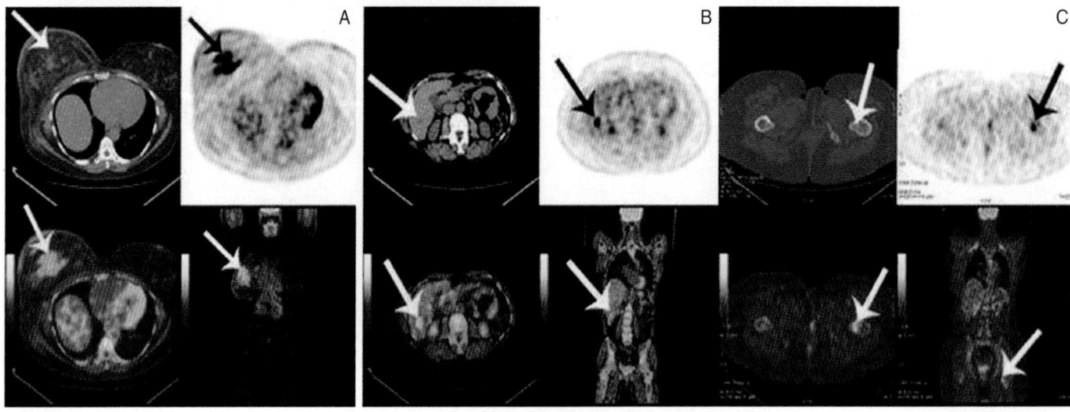

FIGURE 29-5 A. PET/CT shows multicentric hypermetabolism in the right breast (*arrow*) associated with hypermetabolic diffuse skin thickening. **B.** PET/CT shows a solitary focal hypermetabolic focus in the right lobe of the liver (*arrows*) that showed a maximum SUV of 5.7. Corresponding CT of the liver shows a focal hypoechoic mass with indistinct margins. **C.** PET/CT shows a solitary focal hypermetabolic focus in the left proximal femur (*arrows*) that showed a maximum SUV of 7.7. Corresponding CT of the proximal femur shows this area of hypermetabolism to be within the marrow (whole body bone imaging was negative in this patient). (Reproduced with permission from Yang WT, Le-Petross HT, Macapinlac H, et al. Inflammatory breast cancer: PET/CT, MRI, mammography, and sonography findings. *Breast Cancer Res Treat* 2008;109:417-426.)

with diffuse, scattered, or multinodular opacities (correlation coefficient 0.60). As with MRI, these results have led many to advise caution in the interpretation of helical CT in this setting ([80]).

Positron Emission Tomography

Data regarding the role of positron emission tomography (PET) in the diagnosis of IBC is limited. In one study that evaluated PET in seven patients with IBC, skin enhancement was noted in 100% of the patients, axillary lymphadenopathy in 85%, and skeletal metastases in 14% (Fig. 29-5) ([68]).

On the other hand, its role in staging is clearer, and it is recommended as an option in the staging workup for breast cancer ([81]). Its role may even be more relevant in the staging of IBC tumors with their penchant for distant spread. Use of PET/CT can also aid in treatment planning for radiotherapy by determining the extent of skin and nodal involvement.

The prognostic impact of using PET/CT scans in the staging of LABC (IBC and non-IBC) was evaluated in a retrospective study of 935 patients diagnosed with stage III breast cancer between 2000 and 2009 ([82]). The RFS and OS times were compared between patients staged with conventional imaging alone and those staged using conventional imaging plus PET/CT. Relapse-free survival was significantly improved in the subgroup of women with IBC who underwent PET/CT compared to those who did not (HR 0.33; $P = .004$). Although there was a trend for better OS in women with IBC who underwent PET/CT, these results were not statistically significant.

The role of PET/CT in assessment of response to neoadjuvant therapy is another promising area under study. A decrease in SUVmax by PET/CT was an independent predictor of survival in patients with IBC undergoing neoadjuvant chemotherapy ([83]). Further studies are needed to determine the cost-benefit utility of this diagnostic modality.

DIAGNOSIS AND STAGING

Inflammatory breast cancer has had its share of numerous and often-conflicting diagnostic criteria ever since Haagensen's original description in 1956. This has severely limited our ability to compare research across different IBC studies ([84]).

Tumor-Node-Metastases System

The diagnosis of IBC has been recognized since the first edition of the American Joint Committee on Cancer (AJCC) manual as a separate clinicopathological entity: inflammatory carcinoma" and classifed as T4d within the Tumor-Node-Metastasis (TNM) staging system. The diagnosis required the pathological presence of microscopic dermal lymphatic permeation to exclude "inflamed cancers due to inflammation, infection or necrosis." With the arrival of the third edition in 1989, patients presenting with specific inflammatory criteria, including diffuse erythema and edema involving a third or more of the skin of the breast, were designated T4d status. This meant that patients with IBC will have at least stage IIIB disease.

The current TNM classification (seventh edition) defines IBC as "a clinicopathological entity characterized by diffuse erythema and edema of the breast, often without an underlying palpable mass" ([64]). The diagnosis is determined clinically, while pathologic evidence of lymphatic emboli is used for confirmation (see Table 29-4).

Other definitions such as the Poussée Évolutive (PEV) system were commonly used in Europe and North Africa and have led to confusion ([7]). Under the PEV system, PEV3 (inflammatory signs involving more than half the breast) would coincide with IBC as defined by the AJCC system. However, PEV2 (inflammatory signs involving less than half the breast) includes patients who would not be classified as having IBC in the AJCC system (inflammatory signs involving less than a third of the breast).

Diagnostic Criteria

In an effort aimed at standardizing the definition of IBC, an international panel of experts agreed on a minimal set of criteria required for diagnosis. The consensus statement endorsed the criteria established by the AJCC and addressed issues of ambiguity, such as the rapidity of disease onset ([58]).

Table 29-4 TNM Staging System for Breast Cancer

Tumor Classification	Definition
T4	Any size tumor growing into the chest wall or affecting the skin
T4a	Extension of tumor to the chest wall
T4b	Edema (including peau d'orange), ulceration of the skin, or satellite skin nodules confined to the same breast
T4c	Both 4a and 4b
T4d	Inflammatory breast carcinoma

CHAPTER 29

Table 29-5 shows a summary of the clinical criteria and workup required to establish the diagnosis of IBC.

MULTIDISCIPLINARY TREATMENT

Inflammatory breast carcinoma presents with advanced locoregional disease and extensive skin involvement that precludes certain therapeutic procedures. Treatment with up-front surgery is not an option, and patients without metastasis are treated with a multimodality approach similar to that used in LABC. This includes tumor downstaging with primary systemic chemotherapy followed by definitive surgery and radiation therapy. The use of *HER2*-targeting therapy (trastuzumab) is indicated for *HER2*-positive cancer. This multidisciplinary approach has dramatically altered the survival outcomes for women with IBC over the last 40 years, with improved 5-year OS rates ranging between 30% and 70% ([11]).

Surgery

Historically, the efficacy of surgery alone in the treatment of IBC was associated with a median survival of 19.8 months, with a 5-year OS less than 5% ([85]).

Table 29-5 Diagnostic Criteria for Inflammatory Breast Cancer and Imaging Workup

Medical history:
• Rapid onset of skin changes in the breast including erythema, edema (peau d'orange), tender/painful and/or warm breast. • Duration of history of no more than 6 months.
Physical examination:
• Erythema and edema occupying at least one-third of the breast. • Presence of mass (absent in more than 50% of patients). • Presence of palpable locoregional lymph nodes.
Pathology:
• Core biopsy to establish the presence of invasive carcinoma. • At least two skin punch biopsies are strongly recommended to detect dermal lymphatic (used to confirm the diagnosis). • All tumor tissue should be evaluated for ER and *HER2* status.
Imaging and staging workup:
• Diagnostic bilateral mammography with ultrasonography of the regional lymph nodes. • Breast MRI is used when breast parenchymal lesions are not detected by mammography/ultrasound. • Staging with PET/CT is optional. Otherwise, chest, abdomen, and pelvis CT and bone scan.

Up-front surgery for IBC also provided poor local control, with a local recurrence rate around 50%.

The addition of mastectomy to a combination of chemotherapy plus radiotherapy improved local control in patients with IBC as well as distant disease-free survival (DFS) and OS in patients with a complete or partial response to induction chemotherapy ([86]).

Procedure: For patients with complete resolution of inflammatory skin changes following neoadjuvant chemotherapy, the recommended surgical procedure is a modified radical mastectomy with complete axillary lymph node dissection. Conservative surgery as well as skin-sparing mastectomies are not recommended in IBC due to widespread dermal lymphatic involvement ([87]). Because the majority of patients present with lymphatic spread at diagnosis, sentinel lymph node biopsies are not recommended in the management of women with IBC ([88, 89]).

The goal of surgery is complete resection of the primary tumor and the axillary lymph nodes with negative safety margins and no gross residual disease ([90]). Patients who achieve a complete pathological response after chemotherapy and surgery have an improved outcome ([91]).

Breast reconstruction: Despite reports of reasonable success, the international expert panel on IBC recommends against immediate breast reconstruction following surgery ([58]). Breast reconstruction conducted immediately after mastectomy for women with IBC can limit radiation coverage and therefore compromise locoregional disease control in this highly aggressive disease ([92]). In addition, the radiation given after reconstruction is associated with poor cosmetic outcomes. The optimal timing of reconstruction is not known and should be determined after completion of preoperative chemotherapy by a multidisciplinary team based on the aggressiveness and course of the disease.

Radiotherapy

The standard approach is to provide locoregional control for IBC in the form of a combination of modified radical mastectomy followed by radiation therapy in patients who respond adequately to neoadjuvant chemotherapy. This approach does not have an impact on OS but results in optimal local control ([93]).

Historically, local control with radiotherapy alone was given to the breast and draining lymphatics but was associated with a high locoregional recurrence rate ([14, 93, 94]).

The dose and fractionation used for postmastectomy radiotherapy at our institution has changed over time ([90]). The standard postmastectomy radiation dose in non-IBC (60 Gy) is composed of 50 Gy given in 2-Gy fractions delivered once a day to the chest wall and draining lymph nodes (axillary, infra- and supraclavicular, as well as internal mammary lymph nodes), followed by an additional boost of 10 Gy to the chest wall and any undissected regional nodes that were involved at diagnosis.

Several retrospective studies have suggested that dose escalation (from 60 to 66 Gy) with accelerated fractionation (1.5 Gy given twice daily) schedules may improve locoregional control in patients with IBC ([93]). However, this approach was associated with significant delayed skin toxicity (29% vs 15%). As a result, the hyperfractionated regimen is recommended for patients with a high risk of recurrence. This includes women less than 45 years old, those who responded poorly to neoadjuvant chemotherapy, as well as those with positive, close, or unknown surgical margin status ([90]). At MDACC, patients with IBC who do not present with these high risk criteria are offered a once a day dose similar to the standard regimen used in non-IBC (50 Gy), albeit with 16 Gy boost (total 66Gy). This provides dose escalation with a less aggressive regimen. Generous coverage of the chest wall is essential to ensure treatment of dermal lymphatic infiltration.

Complications: Acute radiation complications include radiation skin changes such as moist desquamation. Late complications such as pneumonitis, lymphedema, chest wall fibrosis, rib fractures, and brachial plexopathies are less common ([93]). Operative complications were found to be higher in women who received preoperative radiotherapy.

Neoadjuvant Systemic Therapy

Preoperative systemic chemotherapy is recommended, with the dual objective of downstaging of the primary tumor as well as reducing the risks of distant metastasis, given the high propensity of IBC for distant recurrence. The rarity and poor prognosis associated with IBC often resulted in these patients being excluded from most clinical trials. As a result, treatment recommendations are based mainly on retrospective IBC studies and extrapolation from the results of large prospective trials that recruited patients with non-IBC.

Neoadjuvant chemotherapy has transformed a disease that was once considered uniformly fatal with a 5-year survival rate of less than 5% after locoregional strategies alone.

Anthracyclines

Anthracycline-based chemotherapy regimens have been the cornerstone of systemic treatment of IBC since 1974 at our institution ([95]). The standard regimen consisted of three to four cycles of 5-fluorouracil, doxorubicin, and cyclophosphamide (FAC). Over the years, additional agents, such as vincristine, methotrexate, and vinblastine, were added but failed to improve the outcome of anthracycline-based regimens, with the exception of taxanes (discussed in the next section).

A pooled analysis of four prospective trials conducted at MD Anderson and covering a 20-year period examined the outcome of induction chemotherapy followed by local radiation with or without mastectomy. Patients who received anthracycline-based regimens had an overall response rate of 71% and 5- and 10-year OS rates of 40% and 33%, respectively ([96]). The combined-modality approach resulted in a long-term DFS of 28% at 15 years.

Similar results were seen in a cohort of 68 patients with IBC who received three courses of neoadjuvant therapy in the form of cyclophosphamide, 5-fluorouracil, and an anthracycline (doxorubicin or epirubicin) followed by surgery, adjuvant therapy, and radiation therapy. The 5- and 10- year OS rates were 44% and 32%, respectively ([86]).

In a prospective trial conducted by the National Cancer Institute, pCR rates of 33% were observed in a subgroup of patients with IBC (n = 46) who received neoadjuvant CAFM. The 10-year OS was 26.7% ([97]).

These findings have helped establish combined-modality treatment (anthracycline-based neoadjuvant chemotherapy, then mastectomy, then adjuvant chemotherapy and radiotherapy) as the standard of care for the treatment of IBC.

Taxanes

Taxanes were introduced at MDACC in the treatment of IBC in 1994. Initial small studies examining the addition of paclitaxel showed promising results, with improvements in clinical response rates and OS ([98]). A pooled analysis of patients treated with these protocols stratified patients based on whether they had received paclitaxel as part of either induction or adjuvant chemotherapy. A subset analysis of patients with ER-negative tumors revealed a significantly higher 3-year OS (54 vs 32 months, $P = .03$) and PFS (27 vs 18 months, $P = .04$) in those receiving the paclitaxel regimens compared with anthracycline-based therapy without paclitaxel ([98]). The addition of paclitaxel was also associated with higher pCR rates compared with treatment using FAC alone (25% vs 10%, $P = .012$) ([91]).

A large, multicenter, randomized trial (GeparTrio) prospectively examined the benefit of neoadjuvant docetaxel-/anthracycline-containing regimens by comparing the outcome of patients with IBC (n = 93) or LABC (n = 194) to the outcome of patients with operable breast cancer (n = 1,777) ([99]). Patients received four or six cycles of docetaxel/doxorubicin/cyclophosphamide (TAC) or four cycles of TAC and four cycles of vinorelbine/capecitabine, depending on their initial response to two cycles of TAC. Although pathological response rates were higher for patients in the operable breast cancer group, tumor stage (including IBC status) was not an independent predictor for pCR in multivariate

CHAPTER 29

analysis (odds ratio 1.51; 95% CI, 0.88 to 2.59; $P = .13$).

Using data from the SEER registry, Dawood et al found that women with stage III IBC continued to have a poorer outcome than those with stage III non-IBC in the era of multidisciplinary management and anthracycline-/taxane-based polychemotherapy ([100]). The authors examined women diagnosed between 2004 and 2007 who had received surgery and radiotherapy under the assumption that the majority of patients would have received the indicated form of treatment. The 2-year BCS was shorter for IBC compared to non-IBC, 84% (95% CI, 80%-87%) and 91% (95% CI, 90%-91%), respectively. Patients with IBC had a 43% increased risk of death from breast cancer compared with patients with stage III non-IBC.

In an analysis of 398 patients with IBC diagnosed at MDACC between 1974 and 2005, patients who received taxanes had an improved median survival of 6.3 years compared to 3.8 years for those who did not ([11]). A similar improvement was seen in patients who underwent surgery or achieved pCR. Despite the clear advantages of taxanes in this study, the survival trends did not differ over four decade groups. The authors attributed this to changes in diagnostic and treatment criteria, as well as patient and tumor characteristics over time.

Similarly, an analysis of 104 patients with nonmetastatic IBC diagnosed between 2000 and 2009 aimed to examine contemporary outcomes in the era of trastuzumab and taxane-based chemotherapy. The 5-year OS and distant metastasis-free survival were 46% and 44%, respectively, despite excellent locoregional control (83% at 5 years) ([101]).

Taken together, these results establish the role of anthracyclines and taxanes as the most effective chemotherapeutic agents in the treatment of IBC.

HER2-TARGETED THERAPY

Up to 40% of IBC tumors overexpress *HER2/neu* compared to approximately 25% in non-IBC ([102]). These patients should receive *HER2*-targeted therapy in the form of trastuzumab in combination with preoperative systemic therapy and trastuzumab continued postoperatively for 1 year ([58]).

Early studies have shown that the addition of trastuzumab contributed to higher rates of pCR in patients with *HER2*-positive IBC ([92]). This was also confirmed in the NOAH trial, which randomized women with LABC (including IBC) to neoadjuvant chemotherapy with trastuzumab followed by 1 year of adjuvant trastuzumab versus neoadjuvant alone. The addition of trastuzumab was associated with improved pCR rates and event-free survival ([103]).

In a retrospective review of 260 patients with newly diagnosed stage III IBC at MDACC, the inclusion of neoadjuvant *HER2*-directed therapy was associated with improved survival in multivariate analysis (HR 0.38; 95% CI, 0.17-0.84; $P = 0.02$) ([102]).

Treatment with preoperative trastuzumab in 16 patients with newly diagnosed *HER2/neu*-positive IBC at MDACC was associated with a complete pathological response in 10 patients (62.5%). Despite the high pCR rate, three patients developed brain metastasis (of four patients who experienced disease progression). Brain metastasis was associated with a high expression of CXCR4 ([104]).

Recently, the US Food and Drug Administration granted accelerated approval to the combination of pertuzumab, trastuzumab, and docetaxel for the neoadjuvant treatment of patients with *HER2*-positive, locally advanced, inflammatory, or early-stage breast cancer (either greater than 2 cm in diameter or node positive). This combination is designed to overcome trastuzumab resistance due to the formation of *HER2:HER3* heterodimers. The approval was based on the higher pCR rates obtained from two studies (NeoSphere and TRYPHAENA). As a result, patients with *HER2*-positive tumors can now be offered one of two neoadjuvant combinations: (a) pertuzumab, trastuzumab, and docetaxel followed by adjuvant FEC, FAC, or AC or (b) trastuzumab, pertuzumab, docetaxel, and carboplatin for six cycles (see Table 29-6).

Endocrine Therapy

There is little evidence to suggest a role for preoperative endocrine therapy in the treatment of IBC, and this option is not encouraged in light of studies suggesting hormone receptor–positive IBC may be more endocrine resistant. Despite this, adjuvant endocrine therapy should be offered to all women with hormone receptor–positive tumors, with similar duration and indications as in non-IBC. Ongoing breast cancer studies exploring the combination of endocrine therapy plus molecular targeted agents (eg, everolimus, entinostat) provide promising options for overcoming endocrine resistance in IBC.

Underutilization of Multimodality Treatment

A recent study found evidence of continued underutilization of trimodality therapy (neoadjuvant chemotherapy, surgery, and postoperative radiation) in community practice ([2]). Using data from National Cancer Database, the researchers identified 10,197 patients with stage III IBC who underwent surgery between 1998 and 2010. The use of trimodality therapy ranged from 58.4% to 73.4% annually. Five- and 10-year survival rates were significantly lower among those who did not receive all three treatment modalities compared to those who did. This may explain in part the

Table 29-6 Trimodality Therapy for Inflammatory Breast Cancer at MDACC

A. Neoadjuvant Systemic Chemotherapy	
• Weekly paclitaxel followed by FEC/FAC/AC	Weekly paclitaxel (80 mg/m^2) for 12 weeks (In TN-IBC*: consider adding carboplatin AUC 5-6 every 3 weeks for 4 cycles) FEC: Fluorouracil (500 mg/m^2), epirubicin (100 mg/m^2), cyclophosphamide (500 mg/m^2) every 3 weeks for 4 cycles FAC: Fluorouracil (500 mg/m^2), doxorubicin (50 mg/m^2), cyclophosphamide (500 mg/m^2) every 3 weeks for 4 cycles AC: Doxorubicin (60 mg/m^2), cyclophosphamide (600 mg/m^2) every 3 weeks for 4 cycles
• Docetaxel + trastuzumab/pertuzumab with or without carboplatin followed by FEC/FAC/AC – Prior to surgery:	Pertuzumab 840 mg loading dose, 420 mg for subsequent 3 cycles Trastuzumab 8 mg/kg loading dose, 6 mg/kg for subsequent 3 cycles; docetaxel 75 mg/m^2 every 3 weeks for 4 cycles Carboplatin AUC 5-6. FEC/FAC/AC (see above) every 3 weeks for 4 cycles.
– Following surgery:	Trastuzumab every 3 weeks to complete 1 year of therapy exposure
• Dose dense AC-T – Prior to surgery:	AC: doxorubicin (60 mg/m^2), and cyclophosphamide (600 mg/m^2) every 2 weeks for 4 cycles" "Paclitaxel (175 mg/m^2) every 2 weeks for 4 cycles
B. Surgery	
• Procedure	Modified radical mastectomy with complete axillary lymph node dissection
• Safety margin	Adequate margins are defined as more than or equal to 2 mm
C. Radiation Therapy	
Postmastectomy radiation • Standard schedule	Initial dose of 50 Gy is given in fractions of 2 Gy delivered once a day to the locoregional areas followed by a boost to the chest wall of 16 Gy (total dose up to 66 Gy. Regional nodes are also boosted if involved at presentation.)
• Accelerated hyperfractionated schedule	Initial dose of 51 Gy is delivered in 34 fractions of 1.5 Gy, given twice daily at least 6 hours apart This is followed by boost of 15 Gy to the chest wall administered in twice-daily fractions of 1.5 Gy (5 days) Regional nodes are also boosted if involved at presentation
Preoperative radiation	Personalized

*TN-IBC, Triple-negative IBC

poor outcome seen in women with stage III IBC in the SEER study ([100]).

MANAGEMENT OF STAGE IV

Up to 30% of patients with IBC present with metastasis at diagnosis, compared to 6% to 10% in non-IBC ([15,105,106]). The most common sites of distant metastasis at presentation include bone and visceral metastasis, especially to the lung ([105, 106]). There is no specific treatment for patients with metastatic IBC. Current regimens are based on the most active therapeutic agents discussed in the nonmetastatic setting as well as the molecular subtype of IBC ([59]). Enrollment in clinical trials is highly recommended whenever possible. In patients with IBC who present with de novo metastasis, chemotherapy alone results in a 5-year OS rate of less than 10% ([107]).

Using data from SEER, the outcome of 1,085 patients with stage IV IBC was compared to the outcome of 4,441 patients with stage IV non-IBC, diagnosed between 1990 and 2008. The median BCS was significantly lower for stage IV IBC than stage IV non-IBC (1.75 years, range 0–15.7 vs 2.3 years, range 0–18.9, respectively; $P < .0001$) ([13]).

We compared the outcome of 218 patients with stage IV IBC to 1,454 patients with stage IV non-IBC diagnosed at our institution between 1986 and 2012. The median OS was shorter in IBC versus non-IBC (2.3 vs 3.4 years, $p = .004$). The diagnosis of IBC was associated with poorer OS (HR 1.33; 95% CI 1.05-1.69) ([12]).

The success of multimodality therapy in nonmetastatic IBC has encouraged exploring its use in the metastatic setting. In a review of the SEER database, patients with IBC who presented with metastatic disease in the era of multimodality therapy had a 40% 2-year OS ([108]). To evaluate the role of multimodality therapy, the outcomes of 172 patients with metastatic IBC were retrospectively reviewed. Response to chemotherapy and treatment with surgery and radiotherapy were independent predictors of better OS and progression-free survival. These results suggest that in select patients with metastatic IBC, multimodality treatment, including surgery, may offer better local control and OS.

The role of definitive locoregional surgery in patients with breast cancer presenting with metastatic disease remains controversial. Benefit in this situation may reflect a selection bias for patients who present with less-advanced tumors, better performance status, or higher chemosensitivity. A randomized, controlled trial is needed to validate the findings.

INVESTIGATIONAL THERAPY

Despite advances in systemic and locoregional therapy, the prognosis of IBC has not improved since the introduction of multidisciplinary management ([11]). Therefore, it is important to explore different treatment approaches and new molecular targets in IBC and to investigate the impact of novel agents.

Despite several encouraging studies, the use of **high-dose chemotherapy** (HDCT) with stem cell support remains controversial. Small phase II trials have reported 3- to 4-year OS rates of 52% to 89% and DFS rates of 45% to 65%, which were favorable compared to historical survival data with standard-dose chemotherapy ([109]). In the absence of definitive prospective, randomized trials, the use of HDCT remains investigational ([110]).

Novel *HER2*-targeting agents include **tyrosine kinase inhibitors**, lapatinib and neratinib; the **monoclonal antibody** pertuzumab; as well as ado-trastuzumab emtansine (TDM-1). Lapatinib is a dual-action *HER1* and *HER2* tyrosine kinase inhibitor currently being investigated in the treatment of *HER2*-positive IBC. The combination of neoadjuvant lapatinib and paclitaxel was evaluated in a phase II, open-label, multicenter study and resulted in clinical response rates of 78.6% and pCR rates of 18.2% (95% CI, 5.2% to 40.3%) ([111]). The combination of trastuzumab and lapatinib, with or without concurrent chemotherapy, is considered investigational in the neoadjuvant setting and should not be offered in routine clinical practice.

Angiogenesis inhibitors could potentially target lymphangiogenesis and vasculogenesis, which play an important role in the pathogenesis of IBC. In a study including 21 patients with inflammatory and LABC, bevacizumab reduced angiogenesis in posttreatment tumor biopsies and dynamic contrast-enhanced MRI ([112]). Likewise, some clinical activity was observed in a phase I trial of semaxanib (SU5416), a potent tyrosine kinase inhibitor that targets the VEGF pathway ([113]).

Farnesyl transferase inhibitors (FTIs) inhibit RhoC proteins, which are overexpressed in IBC. An example is tipifarnib, which has entered phase II trials in combination with neoadjuvant chemotherapy for IBC ([114]).

Several agents that target the inflammatory pathways have been explored in the preclinical and clinical settings in IBC ([44]). These include chemokine receptor antagonists, prostanoid receptors (EP4) antagonists, novel selective COX inhibitors (apricoxib, tranilast), as well as others.

Inflammatory breast carcinoma has been an appealing target for **immunotherapy**. Numerous trials have aimed at improving the outcome of IBC by combining immunotherapy with chemotherapy and radiation. Ongoing studies aim to explore the immunogenic effects of standard therapy (eg, taxanes and trastuzumab) with the addition of breast cancer vaccines to multimodality regimens.

Personalized molecular medicine based on the genotypic characteristics of individual patients is promising owing to the heterogeneous and complex biology of IBC. The recent integration of genomic medicine in the clinical practice and management of patients with breast cancer and advances in genotypic testing and next-generation sequencing have prompted the search for specific IBC gene expression signatures ([29]). Other potential agents in preclinical phase are shown in Table 29-2.

CURRENT MANAGEMENT STRATEGIES AT MD ANDERSON CANCER CENTER

All patients who present at MDACC with IBC are referred to a specialized IBC clinic and simultaneously enrolled in the MDACC IBC Registry. In addition to samples collected for diagnosis, the IBC Registry prospectively collects additional blood or tissue specimens for translational research. The recommended schema for multimodality treatment of IBC at MDACC is presented in Fig. 29-6.

Diagnosis and Staging

The diagnosis of IBC relies heavily on the medical history and physical examination to establish the presence of minimal diagnostic criteria (see Table 29-5). These include the presence of skin changes in the form of erythema, edema, or peau d'orange occupying

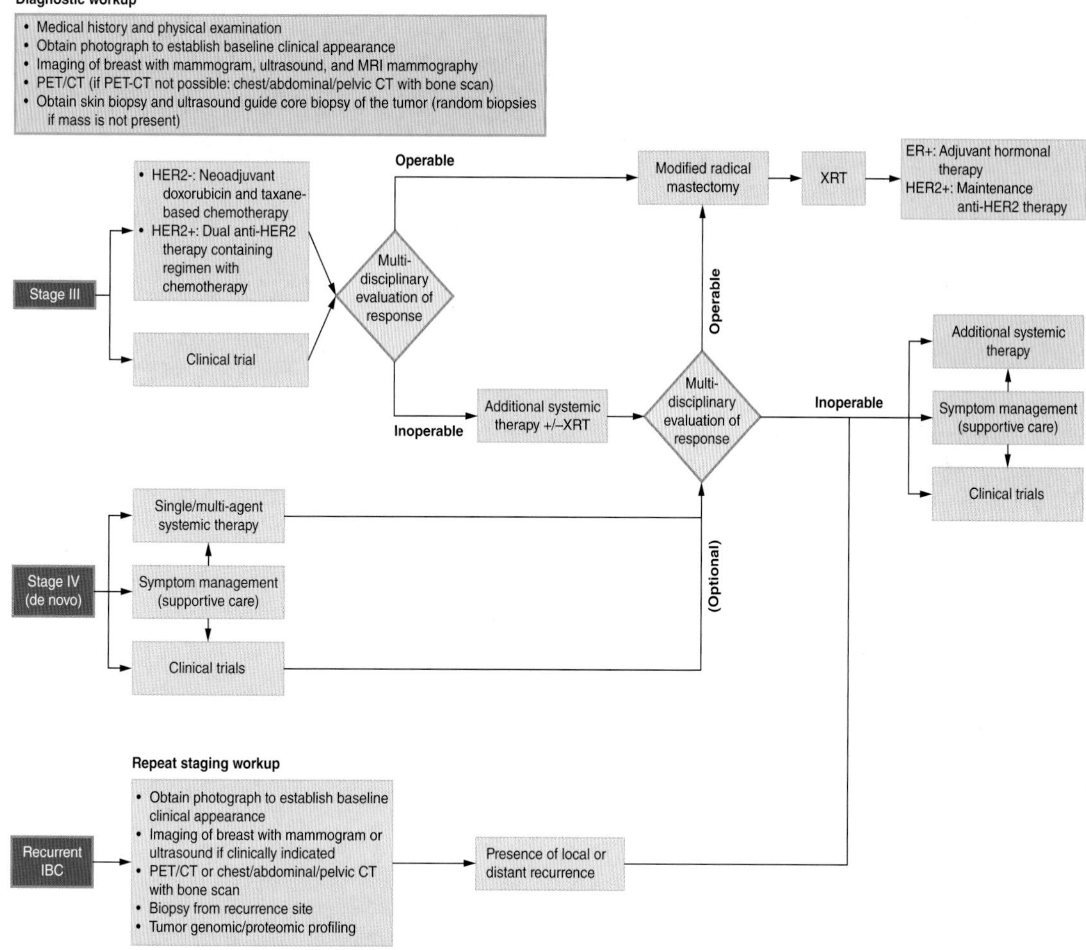

FIGURE 29-6 Diagnostic workup. XRT, x-ray therapy.

at least one-third of the skin overlying the affected breast. The duration of these symptoms should not be longer than 6 months ([58]). Baseline medical photography is extremely important for assessment of response to treatment and for monitoring the reduction in erythema and edema ([1]).

Patients who present with a clinical picture suggestive of IBC should undergo baseline bilateral mammography with ultrasonography of the regional lymph nodes. Breast MRI is recommended when breast parenchymal lesions are not detected by mammography/ultrasound. All women should undergo staging with CT and bone scan. Use of PET or PET/CT is optional ([53]).

Patients should also undergo a core biopsy to establish the presence of invasive carcinoma. At least two skin punch biopsies are highly recommended to detect dermal lymphatic invasion and confirm the diagnosis of IBC. All tumor tissue is evaluated for ER and *HER2* status. If the workup, including core biopsies, is negative, a trial of antibiotics is initiated. If after 2 weeks there is no evidence of resolution, the workup is repeated.

Multimodality Management

At MDACC, the multidisciplinary treatment of IBC was first evaluated in 1974 and has since become the standard of care ([95]). Patients receive neoadjuvant systemic chemotherapy followed by definitive surgery and radiation therapy. The *HER2*-targeting therapy (trastuzumab) is indicated for *HER2*-positive cancer (see Table 29-6).

Neoadjuvant Systemic Chemotherapy

Patients receiving chemotherapy should have an Eastern Cooperative Oncology Group performance status equal to 0 or 1 and adequate cardiac function. Pretreatment blood tests include routine blood counts and renal and hepatic function tests.

Anthracyclines (epirubicin or doxorubicin) and taxanes (paclitaxel or docetaxel) are the most effective cytotoxic agents. The most commonly used regimens at MDACC are listed in Table 29-6 and consist of paclitaxel

80 mg/m² weekly (12 weeks) followed by four cycles of either (a) FEC-100, (b) FAC or (c) AC. Patients with triple-negative IBC may benefit from the addition of carboplatin to paclitaxel. Patients with *HER2*-positive tumors should preferably receive neoadjuvant chemotherapy plus dual-target therapy in the form of pertuzumab, trastuzumab, and docetaxel with or without carboplatin followed by adjuvant FEC, FAC, or AC.

Assessment of Treatment Toxicity and Response

Toxicity from chemotherapy is monitored after each cycle and graded according to the National Cancer Institute's Common Terminology Criteria for Adverse Events version 4.0 (NCI-CTCAE v4.0). Cardiac monitoring should be performed at baseline and 3, 6, and 9 months to detect evidence of cardiac toxicity. Depending on the toxicity, dose reduction or treatment modification may be needed.

Response to primary systemic therapy is monitored every 6 to 9 weeks by physical examination and by radiological assessment at the end of therapy to compare with baseline images. Clinical response to chemotherapy is evaluated according to the RECIST response criteria. Comparison with medical photographs taken at baseline can help make a more accurate assessment of response. Patients with adequate response, including complete resolution of inflammatory skin changes, are treated surgically and their pathological response to chemotherapy is evaluated.

Approximately, 20% of patients with IBC fail to respond to neoadjuvant chemotherapy. For these patients, the options include preoperative radiotherapy or radiotherapy alone ([90]).

Surgery

The recommended surgical procedure is a modified radical mastectomy with complete axillary lymph node dissection. Conservative surgery and skin-sparing mastectomies as well as sentinel lymph node evaluation of lymph nodes are not recommended in the management of women with IBC ([87-89]).

The goal of surgery is complete resection of the primary tumor and the axillary lymph nodes with negative safety margins and no gross residual ([90]). Adequate margins are defined as more than or equal to 2 mm; those with resection margins less than 2 mm are considered positive ([90]).

Assessment of Pathological Response

Pathological complete response is defined as no evidence of invasive carcinoma in the breast and the axillary lymph nodes at the time of surgery. Patients who achieve pCR after chemotherapy and surgery have an improved outcome ([91]).

Reconstruction: Immediate breast reconstruction following surgery is not recommended ([58]).

Postoperative Radiation

Postoperative radiation therapy delivered to the chest wall and draining lymph nodes (axillary, infra- and supraclavicular, internal mammary lymph nodes) improves local control.

The standard fractionation schedule is an initial dose of 50 Gy given in fractions of 2 Gy delivered once a day to the locoregional areas followed by a boost to the chest wall and any undissected involved regional nodes (ie N3b or N3c) of 16 Gy (total dose equals 66 Gy and represents a 10% escalation over the standard dose for non-IBC). The standard fractionation schedule is indicated in patients above the age of 45 years and those who have achieved pathological CR in response to neoadjuvant chemotherapy.

At MDACC, we prescribe an accelerated hyper fractionation schedule for patients at higher risk of recurrence with a total dose of 66 Gy ([90]). A dose of 51 Gy is delivered in 34 fractions of 1.5 Gy, given twice daily at least 6 hours apart to the chest wall and undissected draining lymphatics. This is followed by a boost of 15 Gy to the chest wall and any clinically involved undissected regional nodes, administered in twice-daily fractions of 1.5 Gy (5 days).

Preoperative radiation: Those who remain inoperable after neoadjuvant chemotherapy may benefit from preoperative radiotherapy ([58, 106]). The schedule and doses for patients who require preoperative radiation and personalized.

Adjuvant therapy

There is currently no evidence of benefit from adding chemotherapy postoperatively for patients who have already completed four to six cycles of neoadjuvant anthracycline- and taxane-based regimens.

Treatment with trastuzumab is resumed postoperatively in patients with *HER2*-positive IBC until completion of 1 year of treatment. Adjuvant endocrine therapy should be offered to all women with hormone receptor–positive IBC, with similar duration and indications as in non-IBC.

Posttherapy Surveillance and Follow-up

Following completion of trimodality therapy, patients should be evaluated by clinical examination every 3 to 6 months for 5 years and thereafter every year. Mammograms to the contralateral breast should be performed on an annual basis. Additional investigation may be requested according to clinical indication.

Enrollment in Clinical Trials

It is strongly recommended to enroll patients with IBC in clinical trials, including phase I trials when possible. This is particularly important for patients who relapse after trimodality therapy or those who have metastatic disease at presentation.

CONCLUSION

Inflammatory breast carcinoma remains one of the most lethal forms of breast cancer. Despite promising advances in the diagnosis and treatment of IBC over the past several decades, patients continue to have a poor outcome. Survival has not improved since the introduction of multidisciplinary management.

Epidemiological studies suggested several important risk associations but have yet to identify a risk model for IBC. Progress in imaging modalities such as MRI and PET/CT continues to enhance the precision of biopsy site identification as well as improve disease staging and assessment of response to treatment.

Advances in molecular biology have unveiled the heterogeneous nature of IBC, and new technologies, such as next-generation sequencing, could help identify new molecular targets and biomarkers. The approval of new target therapies such as pertuzumab as well as a large number of new drugs currently under development may help improve survival of this lethal disease.

Acknowledgments: We (the current authors) would like to thank and acknowledge the significant contribution of the previous authors of this chapter, Drs. Windy Marie Dean and Massimo Cristofanilli. This edition is a revision and update of the original authors' work.

REFERENCES

1. Walshe JM, Swain SM. Clinical aspects of inflammatory breast cancer. *Breast Disease*. 2005;22:35-44.
2. Rueth NM, Lin HY, Bedrosian I, et al. Underuse of trimodality treatment affects survival for patients with inflammatory breast cancer: an analysis of treatment and survival trends from the National Cancer Database. *J Clin Oncol*. 2014;32(19):2018-2024.
3. Masuda H, Brewer TM, Liu DD, et al. Long-term treatment efficacy in primary inflammatory breast cancer by hormonal receptor- and HER2-defined subtypes. *Ann Oncol*. 2014;25(2):384-391.
4. Hance KW, Anderson WF, Devesa SS, Young HA, Levine PH. Trends in inflammatory breast carcinoma incidence and survival: the surveillance, epidemiology, and end results program at the National Cancer Institute. *J Natl Cancer Inst*. 2005;97(13):966-975.
5. Soliman AS, Banerjee M, Lo AC, et al. High proportion of inflammatory breast cancer in the Population-Based Cancer Registry of Gharbiah, Egypt. *Breast J*. 2009;15(4):432-434.
6. Schairer C, Soliman AS, Omar S, et al. Assessment of diagnosis of inflammatory breast cancer cases at two cancer centers in Egypt and Tunisia. *Cancer Med*. 2013;2(2):178-184.
7. Boussen H, Bouzaiene H, Ben Hassouna J, Gamoudi A, Benna F, Rahal K. Inflammatory breast cancer in Tunisia: reassessment of incidence and clinicopathological features. *Semin Oncol*. 2008;35(1):17-24.
8. Chang S, Parker SL, Pham T, Buzdar AU, Hursting SD. Inflammatory breast carcinoma incidence and survival: the surveillance, epidemiology, and end results program of the National Cancer Institute, 1975-1992. *Cancer*. 1998;82(12):2366-2372.
9. Anderson WF, Schairer C, Chen BE, Hance KW, Levine PH. Epidemiology of inflammatory breast cancer (IBC). *Breast Dis*. 2005;22:9-23.
10. Cristofanilli M, Valero V, Buzdar AU, et al. Inflammatory breast cancer (IBC) and patterns of recurrence: understanding the biology of a unique disease. *Cancer*. 2007;110(7):1436-1444.
11. Gonzalez-Angulo AM, Hennessy BT, Broglio K, et al. Trends for inflammatory breast cancer: is survival improving? *Oncologist*. 2007;12(8):904-912.
12. Fouad TM, Kogawa T, Liu DD et al. Overall survival differences between patients with inflammatory and noninflammatory breast cancer presenting with distant metastasis at diagnosis. *Breast Cancer Res Treat*. 2015;152:407-416.
13. Schlichting JA, Soliman AS, Schairer C, Schottenfeld D, Merajver SD. Inflammatory and non-inflammatory breast cancer survival by socioeconomic position in the Surveillance, Epidemiology, and End Results database, 1990-2008. *Breast Cancer Res Treat-Breast Cancer Res Treat*. 2012;134(3):1257-1268.
14. Levine PH, Steinhorn SC, Ries LG, Aron JL. Inflammatory breast cancer: the experience of the surveillance, epidemiology, and end results (SEER) program. *J Natl Cancer Inst*. 1985;74(2):291-297.
15. Wingo PA, Jamison PM, Young JL, Gargiullo P. Population-based statistics for women diagnosed with inflammatory breast cancer (United States). *Cancer Causes Control*. 2004;15(3):321-328.
16. Schairer C, Li Y, Frawley P, et al. Risk factors for inflammatory breast cancer and other invasive breast cancers. *J Natl Cancer Inst*. 2013;105(18):1373-1384.
17. Chang S, Alderfer JR, Asmar L, Buzdar AU. Inflammatory breast cancer survival: the role of obesity and menopausal status at diagnosis. *Breast Cancer Res Treat*. 2000;64(2):157-163.
18. Dawood S, Broglio K, Gonzalez-Angulo AM, et al. Prognostic value of body mass index in locally advanced breast cancer. *Clin Cancer Res*. 2008;14(6):1718-1725.
19. Aziz SA, Pervez S, Khan S, Kayani N, Azam SI, Rahbar MH. Case control study of prognostic markers and disease outcome in inflammatory carcinoma breast: a unique clinical experience. *Breast J*. 2001;7(6):398-404.
20. Mourali N, Muenz LR, Tabbane F, Belhassen S, Bahi J, Levine PH. Epidemiologic features of rapidly progressing breast cancer in Tunisia. *Cancer*. 1980;46(12):2741-2746.
21. Bonnier P, Romain S, Dilhuydy JM, et al. Influence of pregnancy on the outcome of breast cancer: a case-control study. Societe Francaise de Senologie et de Pathologie Mammaire Study Group. *Int J Cancer*. 1997;72(5):720-727.
22. Ibrahim EM, Ezzat AA, Baloush A, Hussain ZH, Mohammed GH. Pregnancy-associated breast cancer: a case-control study in a young population with a high-fertility rate. *Medical Oncol*. 2000;17(4):293-300.
23. Chang S, Buzdar AU, Hursting SD. Inflammatory breast cancer and body mass index. *J Clin Oncol*. 1998;16(12):3731-3735.
24. Hachana M, Trimeche M, Ziadi S, et al. Prevalence and characteristics of the MMTV-like associated breast carcinomas in Tunisia. *Cancer Lett*. 2008;271(2):222-230.
25. Charafe-Jauffret E, Tarpin C, Viens P, Bertucci F. Defining the molecular biology of inflammatory breast cancer. *Semin Oncol*. 2008;35(1):41-50.
26. Van Laere SJ, Ueno NT, Finetti P, et al. Uncovering the molecular

secrets of inflammatory breast cancer biology: an integrated analysis of three distinct affymetrix gene expression datasets. *Clin Cancer Res*. 2013;19(17):4685-4696.

27. Bertucci F, Ueno NT, Finetti P, et al. Gene expression profiles of inflammatory breast cancer: correlation with response to neoadjuvant chemotherapy and metastasis-free survival. *Ann Oncol*. 2014;25(2):358-365.
28. Goldhirsch A, Wood WC, Coates AS, et al. Strategies for subtypes—dealing with the diversity of breast cancer: highlights of the St. Gallen International Expert Consensus on the Primary Therapy of Early Breast Cancer 2011. *Ann Oncol*. 2011;22(8):1736-1747.
29. Bertucci F, Finetti P, Rougemont J, et al. Gene expression profiling identifies molecular subtypes of inflammatory breast cancer. *Cancer Res*. 2005;65(6):2170-2178.
30. Masuda H, Baggerly KA, Wang Y, et al. Comparison of molecular subtype distribution in triple-negative inflammatory and non-inflammatory breast cancers. *Breast Cancer Res*. 2013;15(6):R112.
31. van Golen KL, Bao LW, Pan Q, Miller FR, Wu ZF, Merajver SD. Mitogen activated protein kinase pathway is involved in RhoC GTPase induced motility, invasion and angiogenesis in inflammatory breast cancer. *Clin Exp Metastasis*. 2002;19(4):301-311.
32. van Golen KL, Davies S, Wu ZF, et al. A novel putative low-affinity insulin-like growth factor-binding protein, LIBC (lost in inflammatory breast cancer), and RhoC GTPase correlate with the inflammatory breast cancer phenotype. *Clin Cancer Res*. 1999;5(9):2511-2519.
33. Kleer CG, Zhang Y, Pan Q, et al. WISP3 is a novel tumor suppressor gene of inflammatory breast cancer. *Oncogene*. 2002;21(20):3172-3180.
34. Colpaert CG, Vermeulen PB, Benoy I, et al. Inflammatory breast cancer shows angiogenesis with high endothelial proliferation rate and strong E-cadherin expression. *Br J Cancer*. 2003;88(5):718-725.
35. Kleer CG, van Golen KL, Braun T, Merajver SD. Persistent E-cadherin expression in inflammatory breast cancer. *Mod Pathol*. 2001;14(5):458-464.
36. Alpaugh ML, Tomlinson JS, Shao ZM, Barsky SH. A novel human xenograft model of inflammatory breast cancer. *Cancer Res*. 1999;59(20):5079-5084.
37. Alpaugh ML, Tomlinson JS, Kasraeian S, Barsky SH. Cooperative role of E-cadherin and sialyl-Lewis X/A-deficient MUC1 in the passive dissemination of tumor emboli in inflammatory breast carcinoma. *Oncogene*. 2002;21(22):3631-3643.
38. Pharoah PD, Day NE, Caldas C. Somatic mutations in the p53 gene and prognosis in breast cancer: a meta-analysis. *Br J Cancer*. 1999;80(12):1968-1973.
39. Gonzalez-Angulo AM, Sneige N, Buzdar AU, et al. p53 expression as a prognostic marker in inflammatory breast cancer. *Clin Cancer Res*. 2004;10(18 Pt 1):6215-6221.
40. Turpin E, Bieche I, Bertheau P, et al. Increased incidence of ERBB2 overexpression and TP53 mutation in inflammatory breast cancer. *Oncogene*. 2002;21(49):7593-7597.
41. Van der Auwera I, Van Laere SJ, Van den Eynden GG, et al. Increased angiogenesis and lymphangiogenesis in inflammatory versus noninflammatory breast cancer by real-time reverse transcriptase-PCR gene expression quantification. *Clin Cancer Res*. 2004;10(23):7965-7971.
42. McCarthy NJ, Yang X, Linnoila IR, et al. Microvessel density, expression of estrogen receptor alpha, MIB-1, p53, and c-erbB-2 in inflammatory breast cancer. *Clin Cancer Res*. 2002;8(12):3857-3862.
43. Shirakawa K, Kobayashi H, Heike Y, et al. Hemodynamics in vasculogenic mimicry and angiogenesis of inflammatory breast cancer xenograft. *Cancer Res*. 2002;62(2):560-566.
44. Fouad TM, Kogawa T, Reuben JM, Ueno NT. The role of inflammation in inflammatory breast cancer. *Adv Exp Med Biol*. 2014;816:53-73.
45. Van Laere S, Limame R, Van Marck EA, Vermeulen PB, Dirix LY. Is there a role for mammary stem cells in inflammatory breast carcinoma?: A review of evidence from cell line, animal model, and human tissue sample experiments. *Cancer*. 2010;116(11 Suppl):2794-2805.
46. Xiao Y, Ye Y, Yearsley K, Jones S, Barsky SH. The lymphovascular embolus of inflammatory breast cancer expresses a stem cell-like phenotype. *Am J Pathol*. 2008;173(2):561-574.
47. Charafe-Jauffret E, Ginestier C, Iovino F, et al. Aldehyde dehydrogenase 1-positive cancer stem cells mediate metastasis and poor clinical outcome in inflammatory breast cancer. *Clin Cancer Res*. 2010;16(1):45-55.
48. Van Laere S, Van der Auwera I, Van den Eynden GG, et al. Distinct molecular signature of inflammatory breast cancer by cDNA microarray analysis. *Breast Cancer Res Treat*. 2005;93(3):237-246.
49. Zhang D, LaFortune TA, Krishnamurthy S, et al. Epidermal growth factor receptor tyrosine kinase inhibitor reverses mesenchymal to epithelial phenotype and inhibits metastasis in inflammatory breast cancer. *Clin Cancer Res*. 2009;15(21):6639-6648.
50. Cabioglu N, Gong Y, Islam R, et al. Expression of growth factor and chemokine receptors: new insights in the biology of inflammatory breast cancer. *Ann Oncol*. 2007;18(6):1021-1029.
51. Lev DC, Kim LS, Melnikova V, Ruiz M, Ananthaswamy HN, Price JE. Dual blockade of EGFR and ERK1/2 phosphorylation potentiates growth inhibition of breast cancer cells. *Br J Cancer*. 2004;91(4):795-802.
52. Kleer CG, Zhang Y, Pan Q, Merajver SD. WISP3 (CCN6) is a secreted tumor-suppressor protein that modulates IGF signaling in inflammatory breast cancer. *Neoplasia*. 2004;6(2):179-185.
53. National Comprehensive Cancer Network. NCCN guidelines, version 3.2015, invasive breast cancer. 2015:IBC-1. http://www.nccn.org/professionals/physician_gls/pdf/breast.pdf. I don't believe it requires date of access as this is a versioned PDF document (date of access 11/09/2015).
54. Boutet G. Breast inflammation: clinical examination, aetiological pointers. *Diagn Interv Imaging*. 2012;93(2):78-84.
55. Haagensen CD. *Inflammatory Carcinoma*. 2nd ed. Philadelphia, PA: Saunders; 1971.
56. Hoffman HJ, Khan A, Ajmera KM, Zolfaghari L, Schenfeld JR, Levine PH. Initial response to chemotherapy, not delay in diagnosis, predicts overall survival in inflammatory breast cancer cases. *Am J Clin Oncol*. 2014;37(4):315-321.
57. Agrawal BL, Nath AR, Glynn TP Jr, Velazco D, Garnett RF Jr. Case 3. Simultaneous and synchronous bilateral inflammatory breast cancer. *J Clin Oncol*. 2003;21(11):2218-2220.
58. Dawood S, Merajver SD, Viens P, et al. International expert panel on inflammatory breast cancer: consensus statement for standardized diagnosis and treatment. *Ann Oncol*. 2011;22(3):515-523.
59. Robertson FM, Bondy M, Yang W, et al. Inflammatory breast cancer: the disease, the biology, the treatment. *CA Cancer J Clin*. 2010;60(6):351-375.
60. Hashmi S, Zolfaghari L, Levine PH. Does secondary inflammatory breast cancer represent post-surgical metastatic disease? *Cancers*. 2012;4(1):156-164.
61. Henderson MA, McBride CM. Secondary inflammatory breast cancer: treatment options. *South Med J*. 1988;81(12):1512-1517.
62. Schairer C, Brown LM, Mai PL. Inflammatory breast cancer: high risk of contralateral breast cancer compared to comparably staged non-inflammatory breast cancer. *Breast Cancer Res Treat*. 2011;129(1):117-124.

63. Wu M, Merajver SD. Molecular biology of inflammatory breast cancer: applications to diagnosis, prognosis, and therapy. *Breast Dis*. 2005;22:25-34.
64. Edge S, Byrd D, Compton C. *AJCC Cancer Staging Handbook*. 7th ed. New York, NY: American Joint Committee on Cancer, Springer; 2010.
65. Li J, Gonzalez-Angulo AM, Allen PK, et al. Triple-negative subtype predicts poor overall survival and high locoregional relapse in inflammatory breast cancer. *Oncologist*. 2011;16(12):1675-1683.
66. Zell JA, Tsang WY, Taylor TH, Mehta RS, Anton-Culver H. Prognostic impact of human epidermal growth factor-like receptor 2 and hormone receptor status in inflammatory breast cancer (IBC): analysis of 2,014 IBC patient cases from the California Cancer Registry. *Breast Cancer Res*. 2009;11(1):R9.
67. Chow CK. Imaging in inflammatory breast carcinoma. *Breast Dis*. 2005;22:45-54.
68. Yang WT, Le-Petross HT, Macapinlac H, et al. Inflammatory breast cancer: PET/CT, MRI, mammography, and sonography findings. *Breast Cancer Res Treat*. 2008;109(3):417-426.
69. Gunhan-Bilgen I, Ustun EE, Memis A. Inflammatory breast carcinoma: mammographic, ultrasonographic, clinical, and pathologic findings in 142 cases. *Radiology*. 2002;223(3):829-838.
70. Le-Petross CH, Bidaut L, Yang WT. Evolving role of imaging modalities in inflammatory breast cancer. *Semin Oncol*. 2008;35(1):51-63.
71. Lee KW, Chung SY, Yang I, et al. Inflammatory breast cancer: imaging findings. *Clin Imaging*. 2005;29(1):22-25.
72. Rieber A, Tomczak RJ, Mergo PJ, Wenzel V, Zeitler H, Brambs HJ. MRI of the breast in the differential diagnosis of mastitis versus inflammatory carcinoma and follow-up. *J Comput Assist Tomogr*. 1997;21(1):128-132.
73. Le-Petross HT, Cristofanilli M, Carkaci S, et al. MRI features of inflammatory breast cancer. *AJR Am J Roentgenol*. 2011;197(4):W769-W776.
74. Renz DM, Baltzer PA, Bottcher J, et al. Inflammatory breast carcinoma in magnetic resonance imaging: a comparison with locally advanced breast cancer. *Academic Radiol*. 2008;15(2):209-221.
75. Kuhl CK. High-risk screening: multi-modality surveillance of women at high risk for breast cancer (proven or suspected carriers of a breast cancer susceptibility gene). *J Exp Clin Cancer Res*. 2002;21(3 Suppl):103-106.
76. Rieber A, Brambs HJ, Gabelmann A, Heilmann V, Kreienberg R, Kuhn T. Breast MRI for monitoring response of primary breast cancer to neo-adjuvant chemotherapy. *Eur Radiol*. 2002;12(7):1711-1719.
77. Chen JH, Mehta RS, Nalcioglu O, Su MY. Inflammatory breast cancer after neoadjuvant chemotherapy: can magnetic resonance imaging precisely diagnose the final pathological response? *Ann Surg Oncol*. 2008;15(12):3609-3613.
78. Mogavero GT, Fishman EK, Kuhlman JE. Inflammatory breast cancer: CT evaluation. *Clin Imaging*. 1992;16(3):183-186.
79. Moyses B, Haegele P, Rodier JF, et al. Assessment of response by breast helical computed tomography to neoadjuvant chemotherapy in large inflammatory breast cancer. *Clin Breast Cancer*. 2002;2(4):304-310.
80. Akashi-Tanaka S, Fukutomi T, Watanabe T, et al. Accuracy of contrast-enhanced computed tomography in the prediction of residual breast cancer after neoadjuvant chemotherapy. *Int J Cancer*. 2001;96(1):66-73.
81. Carlson RW, McCormick B. Update: NCCN breast cancer Clinical Practice Guidelines. *J Natl Compr Canc Netw*. 2005;3(Suppl 1):S7-S11.
82. Niikura N, Liu J, Costelloe CM, et al. Initial staging impact of fluorodeoxyglucose positron emission tomography/computed tomography in locally advanced breast cancer. *Oncologist*. 2011;16(6):772-782.
83. Carkaci S, Sherman CT, Ozkan E, et al. (18)F-FDG PET/CT predicts survival in patients with inflammatory breast cancer undergoing neoadjuvant chemotherapy. *Eur J Nucl Med Mol Imaging*. 2013;40(12):1809-1816.
84. Kim T, Lau J, Erban J. Lack of uniform diagnostic criteria for inflammatory breast cancer limits interpretation of treatment outcomes: a systematic review. *Clin Breast Cancer*. 2006;7(5):386-395.
85. Kell MR, Morrow M. Surgical aspects of inflammatory breast cancer. *Breast Dis*. 2005;22:67-73.
86. Baldini E, Gardin G, Evagelista G, Prochilo T, Collecchi P, Lionetto R. Long-term results of combined-modality therapy for inflammatory breast carcinoma. *Clin Breast Cancer*. 2004;5(5):358-363.
87. Panades M, Olivotto IA, Speers CH, et al. Evolving treatment strategies for inflammatory breast cancer: a population-based survival analysis. *J Clin Oncol*. 2005;23(9):1941-1950.
88. Lyman GH, Giuliano AE, Somerfield MR, et al. American Society of Clinical Oncology guideline recommendations for sentinel lymph node biopsy in early-stage breast cancer. *J Clin Oncol*. 2005;23(30):7703-7720.
89. Stearns V, Ewing CA, Slack R, Penannen MF, Hayes DF, Tsangaris TN. Sentinel lymphadenectomy after neoadjuvant chemotherapy for breast cancer may reliably represent the axilla except for inflammatory breast cancer. *Ann Surg Oncol*. 2002;9(3):235-242.
90. Bristol IJ, Woodward WA, Strom EA, et al. Locoregional treatment outcomes after multimodality management of inflammatory breast cancer. *Int J Radiat Oncol Biol Phys*. 2008;72(2):474-484.
91. Hennessy BT, Gonzalez-Angulo AM, Hortobagyi GN, et al. Disease-free and overall survival after pathologic complete disease remission of cytologically proven inflammatory breast carcinoma axillary lymph node metastases after primary systemic chemotherapy. *Cancer*. 2006;106(5):1000-1006.
92. Hurley J, Doliny P, Reis I, et al. Docetaxel, cisplatin, and trastuzumab as primary systemic therapy for human epidermal growth factor receptor 2-positive locally advanced breast cancer. *J Clin Oncol*. 2006;24(12):1831-1838.
93. Liao Z, Strom EA, Buzdar AU, et al. Locoregional irradiation for inflammatory breast cancer: effectiveness of dose escalation in decreasing recurrence. *Int J Radiat Oncol Biol Phys*. 2000;47(5):1191-1200.
94. Barker JL, Nelson AJ, Montague ED. Inflammatory carcinoma of the breast. *Radiology*. 1976;121(1):173-176.
95. Krutchik AN, Buzdar AU, Blumenschein GR, et al. Combined chemoimmunotherapy and radiation therapy of inflammatory breast carcinoma. *J Surg Oncol*. 1979;11(4):325-332.
96. Ueno NT, Buzdar AU, Singletary SE, et al. Combined-modality treatment of inflammatory breast carcinoma: twenty years of experience at M. D. Anderson Cancer Center. *Cancer Chemother Pharmacol*. 1997;40(4):321-329.
97. Low JA, Berman AW, Steinberg SM, Danforth DN, Lippman ME, Swain SM. Long-term follow-up for locally advanced and inflammatory breast cancer patients treated with multimodality therapy. *J Clin Oncol*. 2004;22(20):4067-4074.
98. Cristofanilli M, Gonzalez-Angulo AM, Buzdar AU, Kau SW, Frye DK, Hortobagyi GN. Paclitaxel improves the prognosis in estrogen receptor negative inflammatory breast cancer: the M. D. Anderson Cancer Center experience. *Clin Breast Cancer*. 2004;4(6):415-419.
99. Costa SD, Loibl S, Kaufmann M, et al. Neoadjuvant chemotherapy shows similar response in patients with inflammatory or locally advanced breast cancer when compared with operable breast cancer: a secondary analysis of the GeparTrio trial data. *J Clin Oncol*. 2010;28(1):83-91.
100. Dawood S, Ueno NT, Valero V, et al. Differences in survival

among women with stage III inflammatory and noninflammatory locally advanced breast cancer appear early: a large population-based study. *Cancer*. 2011;117(9):1819-1826.
101. Rehman S, Reddy CA, Tendulkar RD. Modern outcomes of inflammatory breast cancer. *Int J Radiat Oncol Biol Phys*. 2012;84(3):619-624.
102. Tsai CJ, Li J, Gonzalez-Angulo AM, et al. Outcomes after multidisciplinary treatment of inflammatory breast cancer in the era of neoadjuvant HER2-directed therapy. *Am J Clin Oncol*. 2015;38(3):242-247.
103. Gianni L, Eiermann W, Semiglazov V, et al. Neoadjuvant chemotherapy with trastuzumab followed by adjuvant trastuzumab versus neoadjuvant chemotherapy alone, in patients with HER2-positive locally advanced breast cancer (the NOAH trial): a randomised controlled superiority trial with a parallel HER2-negative cohort. *Lancet*. 2010;375(9712):377-384.
104. Dawood S, Gong Y, Broglio K, et al. Trastuzumab in primary inflammatory breast cancer (IBC): high pathological response rates and improved outcome. *Breast J*. 2010 July 6. [Epub ahead of print]
105. Elias EG, Vachon DA, Didolkar MS, Aisner J. Long-term results of a combined modality approach in treating inflammatory carcinoma of the breast. *Am J Surg*. 1991;162(3):231-235.
106. Curcio LD, Rupp E, Williams WL, et al. Beyond palliative mastectomy in inflammatory breast cancer—a reassessment of margin status. *Ann Surg Oncol*. 1999;6(3):249-254.
107. Sutherland S, Ashley S, Walsh G, Smith IE, Johnston SR. Inflammatory breast cancer—The Royal Marsden Hospital experience: a review of 155 patients treated from 1990 to 2007. *Cancer*. 2010;116(11 Suppl):2815-2820.
108. Dawood S, Ueno NT, Valero V, et al. Identifying factors that impact survival among women with inflammatory breast cancer. *Ann Oncol*. 2012;23(4):870-875.
109. Dazzi C, Cariello A, Rosti G, et al. Neoadjuvant high dose chemotherapy plus peripheral blood progenitor cells in inflammatory breast cancer: a multicenter phase II pilot study. *Haematologica*. 2001;86(5):523-529.
110. Viens P, Tarpin C, Roche H, Bertucci F. Systemic therapy of inflammatory breast cancer from high-dose chemotherapy to targeted therapies: the French experience. *Cancer*. 2010;116(11 Suppl):2829-2836.
111. Boussen H, Cristofanilli M, Zaks T, DeSilvio M, Salazar V, Spector N. Phase II study to evaluate the efficacy and safety of neoadjuvant lapatinib plus paclitaxel in patients with inflammatory breast cancer. *J Clin Oncol*. 2010;28(20):3248-3255.
112. Wedam SB, Low JA, Yang SX, et al. Antiangiogenic and antitumor effects of bevacizumab in patients with inflammatory and locally advanced breast cancer. *J Clin Oncol*. 2006;24(5):769-777.
113. Overmoyer B, Fu P, Hoppel C, et al. Inflammatory breast cancer as a model disease to study tumor angiogenesis: results of a phase IB trial of combination SU5416 and doxorubicin. *Clin Cancer Res*. 2007;13(19):5862-5868.
114. Andreopoulou E, Vigoda IS, Valero V, et al. Phase I-II study of the farnesyl transferase inhibitor tipifarnib plus sequential weekly paclitaxel and doxorubicin-cyclophosphamide in HER2/neu-negative inflammatory carcinoma and non-inflammatory estrogen receptor-positive breast carcinoma. *Breast Cancer Res Treat*. 2013;141(3):429-435.

30 Special Situations in Breast Cancer

第三十章　乳腺癌中的特殊情况

Stacy Moulder-Thompson
Zahi Mitri

中文导读

本章介绍了乳腺癌中的一些特殊情况。①首先介绍了妊娠期乳腺癌。简单描述了其流行病学特征，并从活检和影像两个方面阐述妊娠期乳腺癌的诊断标准。随后简要概括妊娠期乳腺癌的病理特点和疾病分期。在妊娠期乳腺癌的治疗部分，从局部治疗和全身治疗两个方面着重阐述。此外，详细阐述了妊娠期乳腺癌的预后、疾病对哺乳的影响以及对后代的长远影响，概括了终止妊娠对妊娠期乳腺癌预后的可能影响。②其次介绍了乳腺癌患者确诊以后妊娠的流行病学情况，并介绍了化疗导致的闭经和患乳腺癌对妊娠的影响。③本章接下来介绍了男性乳腺癌这一情况，分别从流行病学概况、诊断和分期、病理特点以及治疗等方面逐一解析。关于治疗，分别从手术、放疗、辅助全身治疗和转移性疾病的治疗等方面阐述。④另外，本章介绍了激素替代治疗的风险和获益。⑤在导管内癌部分，简要阐述了流行病学的内容和病理特点，着重介绍了导管内癌的治疗，包括局部治疗和全身治疗。⑥本章简要介绍了高剂量化疗联合造血干细胞移植治疗乳腺癌。⑦本章最后介绍了乳腺癌中BRCA1和BRCA2基因突变携带者的风险降低策略，分别讲述了化学预防、预防性乳房切除、预防性双侧输卵管和卵巢切除的管理策略。

BREAST CANCER DURING PREGNANCY

Epidemiology

Pregnancy-associated breast cancer (PABC) or gestational breast cancer is defined as breast cancer that is diagnosed during pregnancy and the 12 months following delivery. Breast cancer is one of the most common cancers diagnosed during pregnancy. Given that many women are delaying childbearing ([1]), and age is a risk factor for breast cancer, the incidence of PABC appears to be on the rise. A study from the Swedish National Health Registry showed that the incidence of PABC increased from 16 to 37.4 per 100,000 deliveries between 1963 and 2002 ([2]). Factors associated with a diagnosis of breast cancer included age 35 years or older, women with private insurance, and women who delivered in an urban teaching hospital ([3]).

Diagnosis

The most common clinical presentation of PABC is a painless mass that is either self-detected or noted on clinical exam. The duration of symptoms was significantly longer in patients with PABC compared to their nonpregnant counterparts in a study from Japan. Physiologic changes in a pregnant woman's breast, especially in women younger than 30 years; physician familiarity with PABC; as well as socioeconomic and cultural factors may contribute to delays in diagnosis ([4]).

Biopsy

Although the majority of breast masses during pregnancy are benign, a breast mass that does not resolve within 2 weeks requires further investigation ([2]). Any clinically suspicious breast mass should be biopsied for a definitive diagnosis whether a patient is pregnant or not. Even though a number of small studies have shown the accuracy of fine-needle aspiration (FNA) in the diagnosis of PABC, a core or excisional biopsy of the breast lesion is necessary to make a diagnosis of invasion ([5]) (Fig. 30-1).

Two large surgical series of pregnant patients who had general anesthesia for a variety of underlying medical problems failed to demonstrate an increase in the risk of congenital malformations as compared with pregnant women who did not undergo surgery ([6, 7]). Ultimately, the least-invasive and most technically accurate method(s) available should be utilized to determine the nature of a breast mass in a pregnant woman.

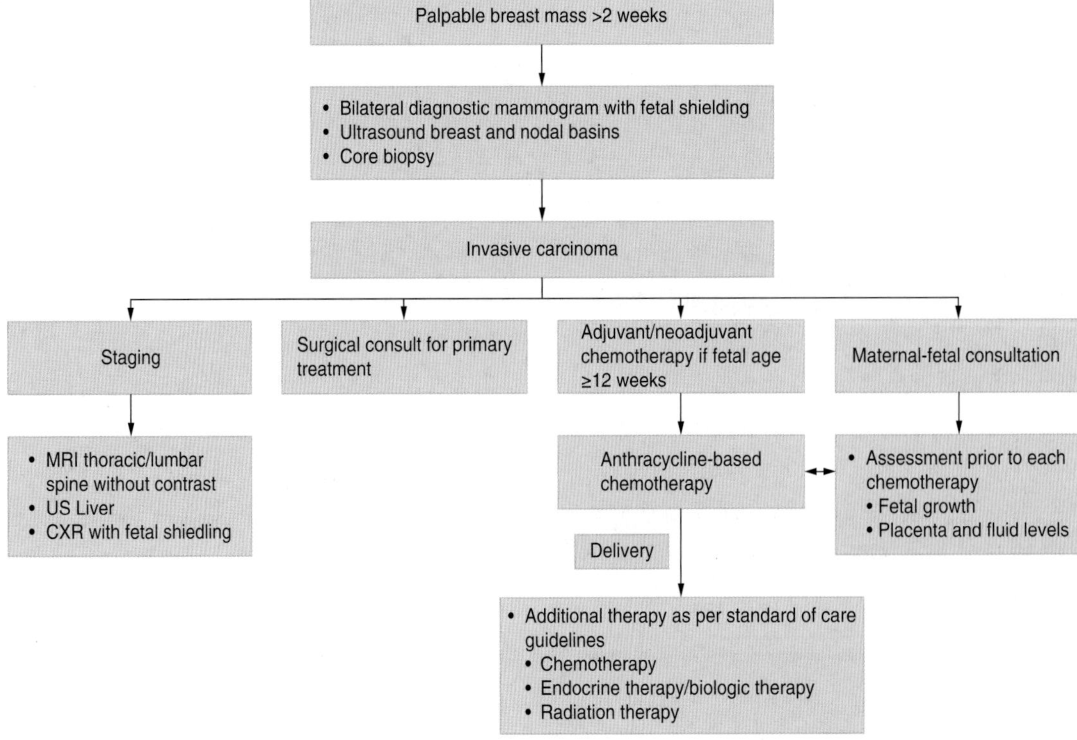

FIGURE 30-1 Algorithm for the evaluation and treatment of a suspicious breast mass during pregnancy. CXR, chest x-ray; US, ultrasound.

Diagnostic Imaging

Mammography and Ultrasound

Mammography can be safely ordered during pregnancy with abdominal shielding. The estimated fetal radiation exposure was 0.4 mrad, well below the 5-rad threshold for fetal malformations [2]. Ultrasound imaging is a preferred choice due to lack of radiation exposure and the better sensitivity for detecting breast masses in young patients. Ultrasound is also a valuable tool in evaluating nodal basins prior to treatment, as well as monitoring disease response in both in the breast and the nodal basins while on preoperative chemotherapy [8].

Magnetic Resonance Imaging

Magnetic resonance imaging (MRI) has not been studied for the diagnosis of breast masses in pregnant or lactating women. Gadolinium has been shown to cross the placenta and cause fetal abnormalities in animal studies. Given these safety concerns, Gadolinium is a Food and Drug Administration class C drug in pregnancy and should not be used routinely in the evaluation of breast masses in pregnancy [2].

Pathologic Features of Breast Cancer During Pregnancy

The most common pathology of PABC is invasive ductal carcinoma. In an MD Anderson Cancer Center (MDACC) case series of patients with breast cancer treated with chemotherapy during pregnancy, PABC was diagnosed at a more advanced stage, with lymph node involvement and poor histologic and prognostic features, including high Ki67 and estrogen receptor (ER) and progesterone receptor (PR) negativity. *HER2*–positive tumors comprised 28% of the specimens. The most common pathology was infiltrating ductal carcinoma. The authors concluded these features were similar to those reported in young nonpregnant women, and that age rather than pregnancy may be the determinant of tumor biology [9].

Staging

The American Joint Committee on Cancer (AJCC) tumor-node-metastasis (TNM) system is used for staging in pregnant patients with breast cancer. Given that stage of diagnosis may have significant psychosocial implications, accurate staging is important.

A complete history and physical examination and laboratory work, including complete blood cell counts and metabolic panel, should be done prior to initiation of treatment. Local imaging should include mammography and ultrasound of the breast and the draining lymphatics. Given that women with PABC often present with advanced-stage disease, the major sites of metastatic disease (lung, liver, and bone) should be evaluated in patients with stage II or higher cancers. Evaluation includes chest radiography with abdominal shielding, ultrasound of the liver, and MRI of the spine without contrast. A transthoracic echocardiogram prior to initiation of anthracycline chemotherapy is recommended [2].

Treatment of Breast Cancer During Pregnancy

The goal of treatment in both pregnant and nonpregnant patients is the same: the control of local and systemic disease. Although the treatment strategies for pregnant and nonpregnant patients are similar, the impact of the treatment on the fetus and the outcome of the pregnancy should be considered in the pregnant patient with breast cancer.

Local Therapy

Surgery and Radiation Therapy

As previously discussed, the use of anesthesia during pregnancy is not associated with an increased risk of fetal malformation [2]. Most patients and surgeons elect to wait until the end of the first trimester to operate to minimize the risk of spontaneous abortion. In most reports of pregnant patients with breast cancer, the majority of women underwent modified radical mastectomy with axillary lymph node dissection, possibly reflecting treatment practice during that time period, later stage of diagnosis, or concerns over the need for radiation if breast-conserving surgery is performed. In general, breast radiation is contraindicated during pregnancy because of the risk of radiation exposure to the fetus. With new practices recommending systemic therapy and surgery as initial treatment strategies, radiation therapy can usually be delayed until after delivery [2, 10].

In a recent series from MDACC, Dominici et al reported on 67 women diagnosed with PABC who received systemic chemotherapy during pregnancy and then proceeded to surgical management. Forty-seven patients underwent mastectomy, and 20 underwent breast-conserving surgery. There were a total of six postoperative complications, with all treated as outpatients; four complications were in the patients with mastectomy, and two were in the patients with breast-conserving surgery. The authors concluded breast-conserving surgery is feasible with no increase in the rate of complications [2].

Cardonick et al reported on 130 patients diagnosed with PABC from the Cancer and Pregnancy Registry. Ninety-five patients underwent surgery, 38 in the first, 48 in the second, and 9 in the third trimester. Fifty-four patients underwent mastectomy, 34 had a lumpectomy, and 15 had an excisional biopsy that did not require further surgery. There was no increase in the miscarriage rate in the first trimester ([2]).

There are limited data on the use of sentinel lymph node biopsy in pregnant patients with breast cancer. Isosulfane blue dye is not recommended due to reports of anaphylaxis in the patients as well as concerns for the safety of the fetus ([2]).

Systemic Therapy

The indications for systemic therapy in a pregnant patient with breast cancer patient are similar to those in the nonpregnant patient. Most of the chemotherapy agents used in pregnancy are rated category D. Limited data are available on pharmacokinetics of antineoplastic agents in the setting of physiologic changes of pregnancy. In a review of 289 pregnant cancer patients treated with chemotherapy for a variety of malignancies, the 14% to 19% incidence of fetal malformations with first-trimester exposure dropped to 1.3% with exposure in the second and third trimesters. Cardonick et al reported a rate of congenital malformations of 3.8% in their series of 104 women who received chemotherapy during pregnancy ([2]).

Chemotherapy

The only published prospective cohort of pregnant patients with breast cancer treated with systemic chemotherapy during the second and third trimesters of pregnancy did not report any congenital malformations, stillbirths, or spontaneous abortions ([11]). The 57 women in this prospective series were treated with chemotherapy with FAC (5-fluorouracil 500 mg/m^2 IV on days 1 and 4; doxorubicin 50 mg/m^2 IV continuous infusion over 72 hours; and cyclophosphamide 500 mg/m^2 IV on day 1; every 21 days if blood counts have recovered) for a median of four cycles while pregnant. Chemotherapy was held after 35 weeks to avoid maternal neutropenia at the time of delivery. All women had live births, one child had Down syndrome, and two children had congenital anomalies. One woman died of pulmonary embolism after a cesarean delivery. At MDACC, pregnant women with breast cancer continue to be treated with FAC chemotherapy during their second and third trimesters of pregnancy.

The European registry published a recent report detailing outcomes of 413 women who received systemic chemotherapy during pregnancy. Multiple regimens were used, including taxanes, Cyclophosphamide, Methotrexate, Fluorouracil (CMF), and anthracyclines. There was no difference in obstetric complications between women receiving chemotherapy during pregnancy and those who did not. Despite a similar rate of premature deliveries between the two groups, infants exposed to chemotherapy in utero had a lower birth weight as well as an increased risk of complications compared to infants with no exposure to chemotherapy in utero. The authors concluded that a full-term delivery seemed to be paramount to decrease the risk of infant complications ([12]).

A systematic review of the use of taxanes in pregnancy conducted by Zagouri et al looked at 50 women with breast cancer who received various taxane regimens after the first trimester. They reported that 76% of infants had a normal Apgar score, and at the 16-month follow-up, 90% of the children were completely healthy. One child had recurrent otitis media, one child had immunoglobulin (Ig) A deficiency and constipation, and one child had delayed speech ([13]). Given the scarcity of the evidence and the lack of long-term follow-up for the children, the routine use of taxanes in pregnant patients with breast cancer cannot be recommended. For our node-positive patients, taxanes are given after delivery.

Hormonal Therapy

The routine use of tamoxifen in pregnant patients with breast cancer is not recommended, given animal data suggesting that it could be teratogenic, as well as case reports in humans describing congenital malformations. These include Goldenhar syndrome, ambiguous genitalia, vaginal bleeding, and spontaneous abortions ([2]).

Biologic Agents

Trastuzumab use in pregnancy is currently not recommended given multiple reports of oligohydramnios and anhydramnios in the literature ([2]). Lapatinib exposure during pregnancy was described in one patient who received lapatinib until 11 weeks of gestation, then discontinued the drug. The pregnancy was uneventful, and there were no reported maternal or fetal outcomes ([2]). There are no current reports on the use of pertuzumab or ado-trastuzumab-emtansine during pregnancy.

Prognosis

There are mixed results in describing prognosis of PABC across the literature. In a series of 121 cases of breast cancer diagnosed during pregnancy, Ribeiro et al reported a 5-year survival rate of 39%. A case-control study from Saudi Arabia compared 28 patients with PABC to 84 women without PABCs and showed no difference in relapse-free or overall survival between the two groups. Beadle et al also showed no difference in locoregional recurrence, distant metastasis, and overall survival between the 104 women with PABC and their 564 non–pregnancy-associated counterparts treated at MDACC between 1973 and 2006 ([2]). Litton et al reported data on 75 patients treated for PABC on a protocol at MDACC with FAC chemotherapy during the second and third trimesters of pregnancy. In this controlled setting, with all patients receiving similar evaluation and treatment, PABC was associated with improved disease-free and overall survival compared to controls ([14]). These results show that by using a multidisciplinary approach to the management of PABC, we are able to provide patients with at least as favorable outcomes as their nonpregnant counterparts.

Monitoring the Pregnancy

The pregnant patient with breast cancer patient should be referred to a high-risk obstetrician skilled in maternal-fetal medicine, who will be charged with monitoring the health of the mother and the fetus while undergoing cancer therapy.

Prior to initiating treatment, ultrasound is used to determine fetal viability and gestational age and expected date of delivery because both will have a significant effect on treatment planning. In our practice, ultrasound is performed before every cycle of chemotherapy to assess fetal growth and development. Amniocentesis may be recommended by the maternal/fetal health team if the fetus is thought to be at higher-than-average risk for karyotype abnormalities or if there are abnormalities detected by ultrasound that should be investigated further. Although not part of the routine evaluation, amniocentesis may be necessary to assess fetal lung maturity, particularly if early induction of labor is being considered.

Timing of delivery should be optimized with relation to the systemic treatment of the breast cancer, occurring no less than 2 weeks after the last dose of anthracycline-based chemotherapy, to minimize the effects of cytopenias ([11]). Planned inductions of labor and cesarean deliveries are often done to minimize the risk of pregnancy-associated complications ([10]).

Breast Feeding

Given that many chemotherapeutic agents are excreted in breast milk, they can carry a risk of complications to the infant. Therefore, breast feeding should be avoided during the administration of chemotherapy, biologic agents, endocrine therapy, and radiation therapy.

Long-Term Implications for the Offspring

Of 57 children born to mothers who underwent chemotherapy for breast cancer in the second or third trimesters, MDACC has reported that the majority of children were healthy and had no developmental delays, with the exception of one child born with Down syndrome ([11]). A survey was sent to parents and guardians of children who were exposed to chemotherapy in utero to assess the child's health, development, and performance in school. Children's age ranged between 2 and 157 months, and only 2 of 40 evaluated by survey required special attention in school. One child had Down syndrome; the other had attention-deficit disorder. However, longer follow-up of these children will be needed to evaluate possible late side effects, such as impaired cardiac function and fertility. Another study by Aviles et al described similar outcomes for a cohort of 84 children born to mothers who received chemotherapy for hematologic malignancies while pregnant ([15]). They also evaluated 81 of these children for cardiac toxicity, using clinical evaluation and echocardiography, every 5 years after birth until 29 years of age. There was no evidence of cardiac dysfunction among the children, ranging in age from 9.3 to 29.5 years (mean 17.1 years) ([15]).

Pregnancy Termination

A number of case series do not appear to support the previously held belief that pregnancy termination improves the survival of pregnant patients with breast cancer. In contrast, there appears to be a trend toward shorter survival with termination of pregnancy ([2]). A pregnant woman with breast cancer must be fully aware of the evidence, or lack thereof, regarding pregnancy termination and survival. In situations of known or suspected fetal teratogenesis or if maternal health is in jeopardy, pregnancy termination may be an appropriate medical recommendation.

PREGNANCY AFTER A DIAGNOSIS OF BREAST CANCER

Epidemiology

Of the women diagnosed with breast cancer between 2007 and 2011 in the Surveillance Epidemiology and End Results (SEER) database, 1.8% were 20 to 34 years of age, and 9.3% were 35 to 44 years of age.

According to the National Center for Health Statistics, the average age of first-time mothers increased from 21.4 years in 1970 to 25 years in 2006 and to 25.8 years in 2012. From 1970 to 2006, the proportion of first births to women aged 35 years and older increased by almost eight times. In 2006, about 1 of 12 first births was to women aged 35 years and older compared with 1 of 100 in 1970. In the 2012 update, the birth rate for women in their early 20s declined to a record low, but continued to increase in women aged 30 to 44 years old.

Therefore, younger women diagnosed with breast cancer may not have had children at the time of their breast cancer diagnosis and may seek to do so after their breast cancer treatment is completed. Of course, patients with breast cancer who have had children before their diagnosis also may wish to have additional children after treatment.

Chemotherapy-Related Amenorrhea

Chemotherapy-related amenorrhea (CRA) is variably defined as cessation of menstruation for 3 to 12 months in women who have been exposed to chemotherapy ([16]). The incidence of CRA varies with age, cytotoxic agent used, and cumulative cytotoxic dose ([16]). A study by Goodwin et al looked at 183 women who underwent systemic therapy, including chemotherapy and tamoxifen for breast cancer. Multivariate analysis showed that age, chemotherapy, and tamoxifen were all predictors of menopause in patients with breast cancer receiving systemic therapy ([17]). Taxanes may result in a higher rate of CRA in the first year but have not been shown to cause a longer duration of CRA; this effect is primarily seen in older women, and when age is controlled for, adding a taxane appears to have little-to-no effect on subsequent risk of CRA ([18]). Lee et al reviewed the risk of permanent amenorrhea by chemotherapy regimen and patient age ([19]).

The current method recommended by the American Society of Clinical Oncology for fertility preservation is controlled ovarian stimulation followed by oocyte or embryo cryopreservation ([20, 21]). The efficacy of ovarian suppression by a gonadotropin-releasing hormone analogue (GNRHa) at reducing the risk of CRA has been evaluated in multiple studies. Gerber et al randomized 60 patients with hormone receptor–negative breast cancer to chemotherapy with or without goserelin. There was no difference in amenorrhea at 6 months between the two groups, and all but one patient had regular menses at 2 years ([22]). The PROMISE-GIM6 (Prevention of Menopause Induced by Chemotherapy: A Study in Early Breast Cancer Patients-Gruppo Italiano Mammella 6) trial randomized 281 patients with stage I to III breast cancer to chemotherapy with or without triptorelin. There was a significant decrease in the incidence of early menopause in the triptorelin group (26% vs 9%) ([23]). The POEMS/SWOG (Southwest Oncology Group) 0230 trial enrolled 257 hormone receptor–negative premenopausal patients with stage I to IIIA breast cancer randomized to receive cyclophosphamide-containing chemotherapy with or without goserelin. There was a decrease in the risk of premature ovarian failure (POF) at 2 years in the goserelin group (22% vs 8%), and more successful pregnancies were noted in the goserelin arm. A meta-analysis by Del Mastro et al revealed a significant decrease in the risk of POF, with an odds ratio of 0.43, in patients receiving GNRHa ([24]).

Impact of Pregnancy After Breast Cancer

A number of reviews have concluded that pregnancy after a diagnosis of breast cancer does not worsen survival ([25-27]). In a retrospective case-control study by Mueller et al, data from three SEER populations were linked to vital records data to identify women under the age of 45 at diagnosis who had live birth 10 months or longer after diagnosis. When these women were matched to nonpregnant women with a history of breast cancer, women who became pregnant after a diagnosis of breast cancer had a decreased risk of dying as compared with women who did not become pregnant ([28]). The improved survival noted in this and other studies may reflect a "healthy-mother effect," whereby women who become pregnant after a diagnosis of breast cancer may have already been at decreased risk of recurrence.

Women who are considering pregnancy after a diagnosis of breast cancer should understand that most data come from retrospective case-control studies in different populations and with different data collection techniques. Women with a history of breast cancer must be aware of their personal risk of recurrence and should weigh this against their desire to have a child. Although it has been suggested that women should wait 2 years after their breast cancer diagnosis before becoming pregnant, there are no data suggesting that a pregnancy in the first 2 years increases the risk of recurrence; rather, data indicate that this is the period of increased recurrence regardless of pregnancy ([29]).

MALE BREAST CANCER

Epidemiology

Male breast cancer is rare, accounting for less than 1% of male cancers. It was estimated that 2,360 new cases of breast cancer would be diagnosed in men in the United States in 2014 and that 430 men would die of the disease ([30]). A large population-based study done by Giordano et al suggested that the incidence of male breast carcinoma is increasing, from 0.86 to 1.08 per 100,000 population between 1973 and 1988, albeit at a slower rate than that of women ([31]). Men with *BRCA* mutations are at higher risk of male breast cancer compared to the general population, with a lifetime risk of 4% to 40% for *BRCA 2* mutation carriers and up to 4% for *BRCA 1* mutation carriers ([32]). Other risk factors for development of male breast cancer include testicular abnormalities, infertility, Klinefelter syndrome, positive family history, benign breast conditions, radiation exposure, increasing age, and Jewish ancestry. Other studies have also identified *PTEN* mutations, *CHEK 2* mutations, obesity, and gynecomastia as potential risk factors for male breast cancer. There is a 2.5-fold increase in risk in men who have female relatives with breast cancer ([32, 33]).

Diagnosis and Staging

The most common presenting symptom for men with breast cancer is a painless lump. Other symptoms include nipple retraction, local pain, nipple ulceration, nipple bleeding, and nipple discharge ([33]). The mean age of diagnosis is 67 years, compared to 62 years for women with breast cancer ([32]). Male breast cancer is more likely to have a delay in diagnosis when compared to women; this is thought to in part account for the later stage of disease and greater tumor size with lymph node involvement at diagnosis ([33]).

A biopsy should be performed of any suspicious mass. If breast cancer is diagnosed, the male patient with breast cancer should undergo staging evaluations appropriate for the given tumor stage, based on the AJCC TNM staging system.

Pathologic Features of Male Breast Cancer

As in women with breast cancer, increasing tumor size, lymph node involvement (including increasing numbers of positive lymph nodes), and higher histologic grade are poor prognostic features ([32, 33]). The majority of cases are infiltrating ductal carcinoma, with a high rate of hormone receptor–positive tumors (ER 80%-90%, PR 73%-81%). *HER2/neu*-positivity reports are inconsistent, initially reported as equivalent to female breast cancer, but more recently noted at 5% to 15% in different studies ([32, 33]).

Treatment of Male Breast Cancer

The overall prognosis for men with breast cancer is similar to that of women with similar stage disease, with studies showing an equivalent benefit of surgery, chemotherapy, and tamoxifen when compared to women with breast cancer ([34, 35]). The goals of treatment are the same: to control local and systemic disease (Fig. 30-2).

Surgery

There are no randomized trials that compare surgical interventions for localized male breast cancer. Clinical practice is based on retrospective data as well as extrapolation from female breast cancer. The current recommendation is a modified radical mastectomy,

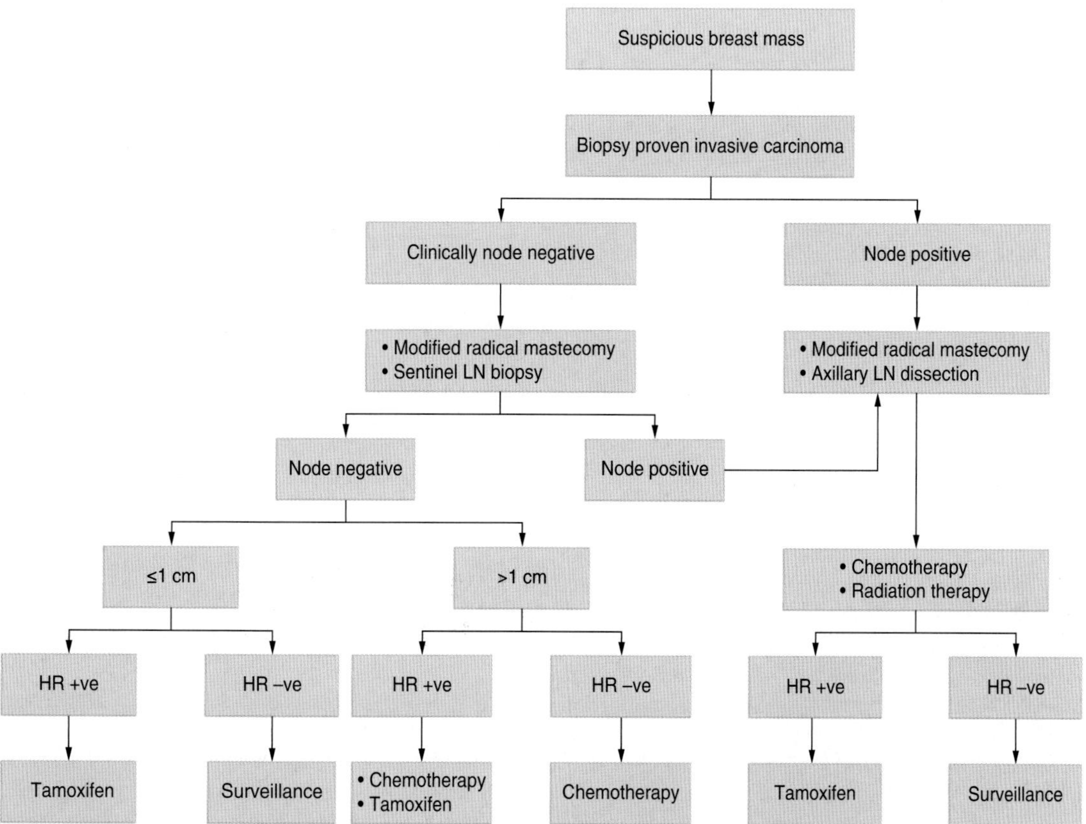

FIGURE 30-2 Algorithm for the treatment of male breast cancer. HR +ve, HR positive; HR -ve, HR negative; LN, lymph node.

which was found to be equivalent to a radical mastectomy ([33]). Given the scarce evidence available for breast-conserving surgery, and the potential lack of cosmetic benefit in men, modified radical mastectomy remains the standard of care for surgical management of male breast cancer.

As in women with breast cancer, evaluation of the axilla with a sentinel lymph node biopsy or axillary node dissection as indicated is considered part of standard of care ([33]).

Radiation Therapy

A study by Yu et al evaluated 81 male patients with breast cancer between 1977 and 2006 treated at London Regional Cancer Program in Ontario, Canada. The local therapy consisted of surgery alone for 26 patients and surgery with postmastectomy radiation therapy (PMRT) for 46 patients. There was no difference in overall survival between the two groups; however, there was a significant decrease in locoregional recurrence in the PMRT group ([36]). A study from MDACC looked at 142 male patients with breast cancer to determine factors associated with a benefit from adjuvant radiation therapy. In this cohort, 18% of patients had locoregional failure. Tumor size, margin status, and lymph node involvement were noted as predictors of locoregional recurrence ([37]).

Adjuvant Systemic Therapy

The MDACC experience was reported by Giordano et al. Between 1944 and 2001, there were 135 male patients with breast cancer evaluated and treated; 51 received adjuvant systemic therapy: 13 received chemotherapy alone, 19 received hormonal therapy alone, and 19 received both. There was a significant increase in time to recurrence (HR 0.49; 95% CI, 0.27-0.9) and survival (HR 0.45, 95% CI, 0.25-0.84) in patients receiving hormonal therapy. In patients with lymph node–positive disease, there was a nonsignificant trend toward improvement in time to recurrence and overall survival with the use of chemotherapy ([38]).

A review from MDACC on 64 men treated with tamoxifen revealed at a median follow-up of 3.9 years that 34/64 (53%) of patients experienced one or more toxicities while on tamoxifen therapy. The most common side effects were weight gain and sexual dysfunction; 13 patients discontinued tamoxifen due to side effects ([35]). A study by Xu et al revealed that adherence to tamoxifen decreased from 65% at year 1 to 18% at year 5 in a cohort of 116 hormone receptor–positive male patients with breast cancer. Five- and ten-year disease-free survivals, as well as overall survival, were significantly lower in the low-adherence group compared to the adherent group ([39]).

The role of aromatase inhibitors in the adjuvant setting of male breast cancer is currently limited. One study from the German Cancer Registry looked retrospectively at 257 male patients with breast cancer who were treated with either tamoxifen (n = 207) or an aromatase inhibitor (n = 50). The authors found that overall survival was significantly better following tamoxifen adjuvant therapy compared to aromatase inhibitors ([40]). Aromatase inhibitors are not currently recommended as adjuvant therapy for male patients with breast cancer.

Therapy for Metastatic Disease

Given the high proportion of hormone-sensitive tumors among men with breast cancer, a variety of hormonal therapies have been used for the treatment of metastatic disease ([41]). Tamoxifen has been established as first-line hormonal therapy because of its limited toxicity and established efficacy in men ([33]). The role of aromatase inhibitors in metastatic disease is not yet clear, although some case reports with disease response exist ([42, 43]). One study showed an overall response rate of 40% in 15 patients with metastatic breast cancer receiving an aromatase inhibitor ([44]). A phase II SWOG trial investigating anastrozole and goserelin for the treatment of male patients with hormone receptor–positive metastatic or recurrent breast cancer closed in 2007 because of lack of enrollment. Aromatase inhibitors may be used as a second-line option in metastatic male breast cancer following progression on tamoxifen, alone or in combination with a luteinizing hormone-releasing hormone analogue.

In men with hormone receptor–negative disease or who fail hormonal therapy, systemic chemotherapy may offer significant palliation for metastatic disease. Jaiyesimi et al reported an overall response rate of 40% for the use of chemotherapeutic agents or regimens such as FAC in men with metastatic breast cancer ([33]). The use of *HER2*-directed agents has not been formally studied in male breast cancer. Their use remains a consideration in *HER*-amplified male breast cancer, through extrapolation of the data from female breast cancer studies.

THE RISKS AND BENEFITS OF HORMONE REPLACEMENT THERAPY

A great debate occurred over several years regarding the value of hormone replacement therapy (HRT) in women as a cardiovascular protective agent when weighed against the risk of developing breast cancer. The combined estrogen and progesterone arm of the Women's Health Initiative (WHI), a large, randomized clinical trial designed to evaluate the role of HRT in the primary prevention of coronary artery disease, demonstrated an increased risk of breast cancer and ischemic stroke without any decrease in cardiovascular events ([45]). Combined HRT failed to improve cognitive function and health-related quality of life, although there was an improvement in vasomotor symptoms and sleep disturbances ([46, 47]). There was a nonsignificant increase in the incidence of ovarian cancer in the WHI study, with no difference in incidence of endometrial cancer ([48]). Combined HRT was effective at increasing bone mineral density and decreasing fractures in healthy postmenopausal women ([49]). Given the information obtained from the WHI, the decision to recommend combined HRT in a postmenopausal woman for either the vasomotor symptoms of menopause or bone health must be made carefully by weighing the risks and benefits for that individual.

The estrogen-only arm of the WHI closed for a lack of improvement in cardiovascular health among those treated with estrogen ([50]). Although there was a non–statistically significant decrease in breast cancer among those women randomized to the estrogen arm, the decision to recommend estrogen alone as HRT for a postmenopausal woman must be made carefully by weighing the risks and benefits for that individual.

A Cochrane review, last updated in 2012, evaluated the effect of long-term HRT by reviewing 19 trials involving 41,904 women ([51]). The results showed that continuous combined HRT significantly increased the risk of breast cancer, among other conditions. The continuous estrogen-only HRT did not significantly increase the risk of breast cancer. The HRT was only effective at decreasing the incidence of fractures. Given these findings, HRT is not indicated for the routine management of chronic disease at this time, and more evidence is needed regarding its safety.

Hormone Replacement Therapy in Breast Cancer Survivors

The first published, randomized trial evaluating the safety of HRT in breast cancer survivors was the HABITS (Hormone Replacement After Breast Cancer—Is It Safe?) trial ([52]). This study was a randomized, non–placebo-controlled, noninferiority trial that evaluated the risk of a new breast cancer in women with a history of breast cancer if they subsequently received HRT. Of the planned recruitment of 1,300, there 447 women randomized; 221 women received HRT, and 221 women acted as controls. This study was terminated early after the results of the WHI trials became available. With a median of 4 years of follow-up, the hazard ratio (HR) for the development of a new breast cancer in women receiving HRT in the HABITS trial was 2.4 (95% CI, 1.3-4.2). The cumulative incidence of breast cancer at 5 years was significantly increased in the HRT group at 22.2% compared to 8% in the control arm.

Given the results of the HABITS trial and the WHI data, one must carefully consider the use of HRT for postmenopausal breast cancer survivors. Among postmenopausal women without a history of breast cancer in the WHI cohort, combination HRT increased the risk of breast cancer and was most beneficial for the treatment of vasomotor symptoms and the prevention of bone loss and fracture. In women with a history of breast cancer, it may be best to pursue other pharmacologic therapies for bone health or vasomotor symptoms before prescribing HRT.

DUCTAL CARCINOMA IN SITU

Epidemiology

Ductal carcinoma in situ (DCIS), also called intraductal carcinoma, is a noninvasive breast cancer whose age-adjusted incidence rose from 5.8 per 100,000 to 32.5 per 100,000 women between 1975 and 2004 ([53, 54]). The increase in incidence is likely secondary to screening mammography and better detection of lower-grade lesions. The rates of noncomedo DCIS has increased across all age groups, whereas the rates of comedo DCIS have overall remained stable ([55]). The most common presentation of DCIS is an abnormal mammogram demonstrating clustered microcalcifications ([56]).

Pathologic Features

Traditionally, DCIS has been classified primarily on the basis of architectural pattern (solid, papillary, micropapillary, or cribriform), as well as the presence or absence of comedo necrosis. The comedo subtype is characterized by extensive central zonal necrosis ([56]). Bellamy et al reported that this classification correlates with the extent of disease. Micropapillary DCIS involved more than one quadrant in 71% of cases, compared to 18%, 17%, and 25% in comedo, solid, and cribriform subtypes, respectively. The solid DCIS subtype was the most likely to be excised fully at surgery ([57]). Nuclear grade (low, intermediate, or high) and the presence or absence of comedonecrosis has also been used to classify DCIS ([58]). High-grade DCIS is more frequently ER and PR negative, has a higher proliferation rate and higher expression of *HER2* when compared to low-grade DCIS. Intermediate grade is more heterogeneous and shows variability in its immunoprofile ([56]).

Ductal carcinoma in situ is classified as having microinvasion if the invasive component is 0.1 cm or less in greatest dimension ([59]). If there are multiple foci of microinvasion, the size of the largest area is used to classify the microinvasion.

Although an axillary or sentinel lymph node biopsy is not the standard of care for all women presenting with DCIS, a small proportion have axillary lymph node involvement. A National Cancer Data Base review of almost 11,000 women with DCIS who had a lymph node dissection between 1985 and 1991 found that 3.6% had axillary metastases ([60]). Silverstein et al evaluated 100 patients with DCIS treated with either mastectomy or radiation therapy who underwent axillary lymph node dissection. No patients were found to have positive axillary lymph nodes ([61]). Two studies looking at pure DCIS without evidence of microinvasion reported 1/102 (0.98%) sentinel lymph node positivity in one study ([62]) and 5/87 (6%) sentinel lymph node positivity in the other ([63]).

A study looking at high-risk DCIS and DCIS with microinvasion revealed that 9/76 (12%) of patients with high-risk DCIS had positive sentinel lymph nodes (7/9 were micrometastasis), and 3/31 (10%) of patients with DCIS with microinvasion had positive sentinel lymph nodes ([64]).

Currently, routine lymph node evaluation is not recommended for all patients with DCIS. However, nodal evaluation may be considered in patients with high risk of invasive carcinoma, that is, large (> 3 cm) tumors, which frequently have a high nuclear grade and are of the comedo subtype ([65, 66]). In addition, sentinel lymph node biopsy may be discussed as an option for those undergoing a simple mastectomy for DCIS as the opportunity for a sentinel lymph node biopsy is lost if invasive or microinvasive disease is subsequently found as the tumor bed is no longer in place.

Treatment

Local Therapy

The options for the surgical management of DCIS range from excision alone to mastectomy. Retrospective series of mastectomy for DCIS have shown 10-year breast cancer–specific survival rates in excess of 98% ([56]). The risk of local and distant recurrence following mastectomy is low, and recurrences usually present as invasive breast carcinomas ([67]). Mastectomy is a highly effective method for the treatment of DCIS; however, it is a radical procedure for a disease that carries a low probability of malignant transformation.

Multiple studies have evaluated the benefit of adjuvant radiation therapy at decreasing risk of recurrence in patients who undergo breast-conserving surgery for DCIS. A retrospective study by Vargas et al reviewed 405 patients treated at a single institution with lumpectomy alone (n = 54), lumpectomy and radiation therapy (n = 313), or mastectomy (n = 43). At a median follow-up of 7 years, the rates of ipsilateral breast tumor recurrence were 9.3% after lumpectomy alone, 8% after lumpectomy and radiation, and 4.7% after mastectomy. Of the 32 local failures, 20 involved invasive cancers. In this study, there was no difference in the rates of local control, cause-specific survival, and overall survival between the lumpectomy and mastectomy groups. Risk factors associated with local failure included young age (<45 years), close or positive margins (<2 mm), no breast radiation, and lower electron boost energies ([68]).

The National Surgical Adjuvant Breast and Bowel Project (NSABP) B-17 study compared lumpectomy to lumpectomy with radiation for women with primarily small-volume DCIS (≤2 cm) and negative resection margins. Through 8 years of follow-up, the use of radiation therapy significantly reduced the incidence of noninvasive breast cancer recurrence from 13.4% to 8.2% and that of invasive disease from 13.4% to 3.9% ([69]). Moderate-to-marked and absent-to-slight comedo necrosis was found to be an independent high- and low-risk predictor for ipsilateral breast tumor recurrence, respectively ([70]).

In a European trial, women with DCIS up to 5 cm in size at the time of excision were randomly assigned to no further treatment or radiation therapy ([71]). With a median follow-up of 10.5 years, the 10-year local recurrence-free rate was 74% in the group treated with excision alone compared with 85% in the women treated by excision and radiation ($P < .0001$; HR 0.53; 95% CI, 0.4-0.7). The HRs for DCIS and invasive local recurrence were 0.52 (95% CI, 0.34-0.77) and 0.58 (95% CI, 0.39-0.86), respectively. In multivariate analysis, factors significantly associated with an increased local recurrence risk in this study were young age, symptomatic detection of DCIS, intermediate or poorly differentiated DCIS, cribriform or solid growth pattern, involved or close margins, and treatment by local excision alone. The effect of radiation therapy was homogeneous across all assessed risk factors.

The need for radiation therapy in women with low-volume, good-prognosis DCIS was planned in a randomized trial conducted by the Radiation Therapy Oncology Group. Unfortunately, this study, which randomized women with good-prognosis DCIS to radiation with or without tamoxifen or to tamoxifen with or without observation, was closed due to slow accrual. A recent Cochrane review confirmed the benefit of adding radiation therapy to breast-conserving surgery in the treatment of all patients with DCIS ([72]).

Multiple randomized trials have confirmed the benefit of the addition of radiation therapy to lumpectomy in reducing the risk of ipsilateral breast cancer recurrence. It must be noted that DCIS overall has excellent prognosis, with a breast cancer–specific survival in excess of 95% across all trials in all treatment groups: mastectomy, lumpectomy, and lumpectomy plus radiation ([56]).

Systemic Therapy

The only approved therapy in the United States for the systemic treatment of DCIS is tamoxifen. In the NSABP B-24 study, 1,804 women with small-volume DCIS (most ≤2 cm), including some with positive margins, who had undergone a lumpectomy and radiation therapy were randomly assigned to either placebo or tamoxifen 20 mg by mouth daily for 5 years ([73]). There was a statistically significant absolute risk reduction of 5.2% in all breast cancer events (invasive and noninvasive combined) in women who received tamoxifen. This risk reduction was mainly the result of a decrease in ipsilateral invasive disease and contralateral noninvasive disease. The risk of the development of breast cancer at regional or distant sites was not significantly reduced among tamoxifen users. The most serious but rare side effects of tamoxifen were deep venous thrombosis (1%), nonfatal pulmonary embolism (0.2%), and uterine cancer (approximately 0.1%).

Subsequent analysis of available tumor tissue from women who participated in NSABP B-24 was performed to determine if response to tamoxifen was influenced by ER status ([74]). Although tamoxifen was beneficial among women with ER-positive DCIS, the number of women with ER-negative DCIS was small in this subanalysis, so the investigators concluded that the benefit of tamoxifen was unclear in this group of women. At MDACC, tamoxifen is recommended for women with ER-positive DCIS but not those with ER-negative DCIS. The benefit of tamoxifen in women with ER-negative but PR-positive DCIS is unclear.

Anastrozole is an aromatase inhibitor currently approved for the treatment of adjuvant and metastatic hormone receptor–positive breast cancer. The IBIS II trial assessed the efficacy and safety of anastrozole in the prevention of breast cancer in high-risk postmenopausal women. At 5-year follow-up, there was a significant benefit of anastrozole at reducing the risk of breast cancer (HR 0.47; 95% CI, 0.32-0.68). In this study, 366 patients had ER-positive DCIS, which was treated by mastectomy within 6 months of enrollment. The authors reported that the benefit of anastrozole was seen across all groups, including the DCIS subgroup, with an HR of 0.44 (95% CI, 0.11-1.15) ([75]). These results should be interpreted with caution as antiestrogen therapy is usually prescribed in patients following lumpectomy aiming at reducing the risk of ipsilateral invasive cancers, whereas all patients with DCIS in IBIS II underwent mastectomy. The NSABP B-24 data do not show any benefit of tamoxifen at reducing the incidence of contralateral invasive disease, and tamoxifen is not routinely prescribed in patients undergoing mastectomy for DCIS ([73]). Given these findings, the role of aromatase inhibitors in DCIS treatment remains to be elucidated. The NSABP-35 is a trial currently comparing anastrozole to tamoxifen in postmenopausal women with hormone-sensitive DCIS who have undergone lumpectomy and radiation therapy.

The role of trastuzumab for *HER2*-positive DCIS is currently being investigated in the NSABP B-43 trial. Trastuzumab is currently not recommended in the treatment of DCIS.

HIGH-DOSE CHEMOTHERAPY WITH TRANSPLANTATION

In an attempt at reducing the risk of death for women with early-stage, poor-prognosis, or metastatic breast cancer, the effectiveness of more aggressive chemotherapeutic regimens, including high-dose chemotherapy (HDC) with either bone marrow or stem cell support, has been investigated. Despite initial encouraging results, two meta-analyses failed to show a survival benefit in poor-prognosis, early-stage breast cancer or in metastatic breast cancer ([76, 77]). Given the results of these trials, HDC with stem cell support is not used in the management of breast cancer at MDACC.

RISK REDUCTION STRATEGIES FOR *BRCA 1* AND *BRCA 2* CARRIERS

Although a family history of breast cancer, especially in a first-degree relative, has been identified as a risk factor for the development of breast cancer, most women with breast cancer do not have a significant family history ([78-80]). It is believed that approximately 5% to 10% of breast cancer cases are due to the inheritance of rare, highly penetrant germline mutations, particularly in the *BRCA 1* and *BRCA 2* genes ([81]). Women with mutations in one of these two genes have a cumulative lifetime risk of invasive breast cancer (up to age 70 years) of 57% and 49%, invasive epithelial ovarian cancer of 40% and 18% for *BRCA 1* and *BRCA 2* mutations, respectively ([82]).

Chemoprevention

The benefit of tamoxifen for risk reduction among women with mutations in either the *BRCA 1* or *BRCA 2* gene is unclear. A subgroup analysis of the 288 patients in the P1 breast cancer prevention trial who developed breast cancer examined the protective effect of tamoxifen in the development of breast cancer among *BRCA 1* or *BRCA 2* mutation carriers. Of the 288 patients, 19 (6.6%) tested positive for deleterious *BRCA 1* or *BRCA 2* mutations. Within the *BRCA 1* mutation carriers (n = 8), 5 patients received tamoxifen and 3 received placebo (risk ratio 1.67; 95% CI, 0.32-10.7). Within the *BRCA 2* mutation carriers (n = 11), 3 received tamoxifen and 8 received placebo (risk ratio 0.38; 95% CI, 0.06-1.56). In this small subset of patients, tamoxifen did not reduce breast cancer incidence in *BRCA 1* mutation carriers; however, it was effective at reducing breast cancer incidence by 62% in *BRCA 2* carriers, a figure similar to the risk reduction among all women involved in the P1 trial. Of note, 83% of *BRCA 1* carriers had ER-negative tumors, compared to 76% of *BRCA 2* carriers who were ER positive ([83]). The Hereditary Breast Cancer Clinical Study group reported that tamoxifen protected against the development of contralateral breast cancer in *BRCA 1/BRCA 2* mutation carriers, with an odds ratio of 0.50 for *BRCA 1* carriers and 0.42 for *BRCA 2* carriers. In the small subgroup of patients who had undergone an oophorectomy, no benefit was noted from tamoxifen use. No information on hormone receptor status of the tumors was available in this study ([84]). Gronwald et al recently published a matched case-control study in 1,504 women (411 with bilateral breast cancer and 1,093 with unilateral breast cancer) with known *BRCA 1* or *BRCA 2* mutations, looking at the effect of tamoxifen in reducing incidence of contralateral breast cancer. Three hundred and thirty-one women (22%) used tamoxifen during the follow-up period. The use of tamoxifen was associated with a decrease in contralateral breast cancer in both *BRCA 1* (OR 0.58; 95% CI, 0.39–0.85) and *BRCA 2* (OR 0.39; 95% CI, 0.19–0.83) groups. The authors also found there was no additional protective effect with longer durations of tamoxifen use. The strongest protective effect was for women with 1 year or less of tamoxifen use (OR 0.37; 95% CI, 0.20-0.69; P = 0.001), followed by women with 1 to 4 years of tamoxifen use (OR 0.53; 95% CI, 0.32-0.87; P = 0.01), and nonsignificant in women with 4 or more years of tamoxifen (OR 0.83; 95% CI, 0.44-1.55; P = 0.55). The authors concluded that a short-term course of tamoxifen for chemoprevention may be as effective as a conventional 5-year treatment course in *BRCA 1/BRCA 2* carriers ([85]).

Given these results, the most effective chemoprevention strategy for women with known *BRCA 1* or *BRCA 2* mutations, the optimal duration of its use, and the age at which to begin have not yet been demonstrated ([86]). Patients with a known mutation in the *BRCA 1* or *BRCA 2* gene should be encouraged to participate in clinical trials evaluating the efficacy of chemoprevention agents for breast cancer.

Prophylactic Mastectomies

A woman with a mutation in either *BRCA 1* or *BRCA 2* gene should be counseled regarding the potential role of prophylactic mastectomy in reducing her future risk of developing breast cancer.

Both types of prophylactic mastectomies, subcutaneous or total, are likely to leave behind a small amount of residual breast tissue, making this a risk reduction strategy that is not 100% effective in preventing subsequent breast cancer.

Hartmann et al examined the effectiveness of prophylactic mastectomies among women at increased risk of breast cancer. In the moderate-risk group, 4 breast cancers were diagnosed, compared with 37.4 predicted by the Gail model, an 89.5% risk reduction. In the high-risk group, 214 women who underwent bilateral prophylactic mastectomies were compared to their sisters who did not undergo prophylactic mastectomies. At a median follow-up of 14 years, the incidence of breast cancer in the women who underwent prophylactic mastectomies as compared to their sisters who had not was 1.4% and 38.7%, respectively ([87]). As a follow-up to this study, the investigators then genotyped 176 of the women who had prophylactic mastectomies. Of these, 26 were found to carry germline mutations in *BRCA 1* or *BRCA 2*. None of these 26 women developed breast cancer over a median follow-up of 13 years ([88]).

Meijers-Heijboer et al prospectively followed 139 women with germline *BRCA 1* or *BRCA 2* gene mutations. After a mean follow-up of 2.9 years, no breast cancers were observed in the 76 women who underwent prophylactic mastectomy, compared to 8 breast cancers in the 63 women who did not undergo prophylactic mastectomies. The authors concluded that prophylactic bilateral total mastectomy was effective at reducing breast cancer incidence in *BRCA 1* or *BRCA 2* mutation carriers ([89]).

In the PROSE study group, Rebbeck et al prospectively followed 483 women with *BRCA 1* or *BRCA 2* gene mutations. Of those, 105 women underwent bilateral prophylactic mastectomy and 378 did not, serving as matched controls. With a mean follow-up of 6.1 years, 2/105 (1.9%) women in the surgery group were diagnosed with breast cancer, compared to 184/378 (48.7%) in the control group, a greater than 90% risk reduction ([90]).

Domcheck et al reported a prospective multicenter cohort study to evaluate the relationship between risk-reducing surgeries and cancer outcomes in *BRCA 1/BRCA 2* mutation carriers. Among 247 women who underwent prophylactic mastectomies, no breast cancers were diagnosed, compared to 98 breast cancers in 1,372 women who did not have risk-reducing mastectomy ([91]).

At MDACC, women with a known deleterious mutation in either the *BRCA 1* or *BRCA 2* gene are evaluated and counseled by our genetic counselors and breast surgeons regarding the potential breast cancer risk reduction of bilateral prophylactic mastectomies or bilateral mastectomies in patients who already carry a diagnosis of breast cancer.

Prophylactic Bilateral Salpingo-Oophorectomies

In addition to decreasing the risk of gynecologic cancer among women with a known mutation in either the *BRCA 1* or *BRCA 2* gene, prophylactic bilateral salpingo-oophorectomy (BSO) may decrease the risk of developing breast cancer ([92, 93]). A prospective study by Kauff et al followed 170 women 35 years of age or older with either a *BRCA 1* or *BRCA 2* mutation, of which 98 chose to undergo risk reduction BSO and 72 opted to undergo surveillance. With a median follow-up of 24.2 months, breast cancer and peritoneal cancer were diagnosed in 3 and 1, respectively, of the 98 women who chose prophylactic BSO. Of the 72 women who chose surveillance, breast cancer was diagnosed in 8 women, ovarian cancer in 4, and peritoneal cancer in 1. There was also a significant increase in the time to diagnosis of breast cancer of *BRCA*-related gynecologic malignancy in the BSO group (HR 0.25; 95% CI, 0.08-0.74). The authors concluded that prophylactic BSO was effective at decreasing the risk of breast and *BRCA*-associated gynecologic malignancies; there was still a residual risk of peritoneal cancer ([93]).

In a large, multicenter prospective study, 1,079 women 30 years of age and older with ovaries in situ and a deleterious *BRCA 1* or *BRCA 2* mutation were enrolled at 1 of 11 centers from November 1, 1994, to December 1, 2004 ([92]). Women self-selected prophylactic BSO or surveillance. Of 792 patients assessable for gynecologic cancers, 12/283 women in the surveillance group were diagnosed with gynecologic cancers (10 in *BRCA 1* carriers, 2 in *BRCA 2* carriers) compared to 3/509 diagnosed with peritoneal cancer in the BSO group (all in *BRCA 1* carriers). Of 597 patients assessable for breast cancer, 28/294 (19 in *BRCA 1* carriers, 9 in *BRCA 2* carriers) were diagnosed with breast cancer in the surveillance group, compared to 19/303 (15 in *BRCA 1* carriers, 4 in *BRCA 2* carriers) in the BSO group. The BSO was protective against ER-positive breast cancer but not against ER-negative breast cancer. The authors concluded that BSO was most effective at reducing the risk of *BRCA 1*–associated gynecologic malignancies (HR 0.15; 95% CI, 0.04-0.56) and at reducing the risk of *BRCA 2*–associated breast cancer (HR 0.28; 95% CI, 0.08-0.92).

Domchek et al reported a significantly lower incidence of ovarian cancer in patients undergoing BSO. These results were conserved in patients with or without a prior history of breast cancer. Patients undergoing BSO had a lower risk of first diagnosis of breast cancer in *BRCA 1* and *BRCA 2* mutation carriers. The authors also noted that BSO was associated with a significant reduction in all-cause mortality, breast cancer–specific mortality, as well as ovarian cancer–specific mortality ([91]).

Results from a meta-analysis of 10 studies in *BRCA 1*/*BRCA 2* carriers showed that prophylactic BSO was associated with a significant reduction in the risk of *BRCA*-associated gynecologic cancers (HR 0.21; 95% CI, 0.12-0.39). The same meta-analysis reported a statistically significant decrease in the risk of breast cancer in *BRCA 1*/*BRCA 2* mutation carriers (HR 0.49; 95% CI, 0.37-0.65). Similar risk reduction for breast cancer was observed in the *BRCA 1* and *BRCA 2* subgroups. Data were insufficient to stratify gynecologic cancer risk reduction by *BRCA 1* and *BRCA 2* mutations ([94]).

Our patients with germline mutations in either *BRCA 1* or *BRCA 2* are counseled by qualified professionals on the possible reduction in ovarian cancer as well as breast cancer risk through the use of prophylactic BSO. However, fertility is clearly impaired by this risk reduction strategy. Also, the premenopausal patient with a known mutation in *BRCA 1* or *BRCA 2* who is considering a prophylactic BSO should be counseled regarding the physiologic changes that may be associated with premature menopause, including bone loss and psychosocial changes, such as changes in mood and sexual function.

CHAPTER 30

REFERENCES

1. Hamilton BE, et al. Annual summary of vital statistics: 2010-2011. *Pediatrics*. 2013;131(3):548-558.
2. Litton JK, Theriault RL. Breast cancer and pregnancy: current concepts in diagnosis and treatment. *Oncologist*. 2010;15(12):1238-1247.
3. Abenhaim HA, et al. Incidence, risk factors, and obstetrical outcomes of women with breast cancer in pregnancy. *Breast J*. 2012;18(6):564-568.
4. Gwyn K, Theriault R. Breast cancer during pregnancy. *Oncology (Williston Park)*. 2001;15(1):39-46; discussion 46, 49-51.
5. Gupta, R.K., et al. The diagnostic impact of needle aspiration cytology of the breast on clinical decision making with an emphasis on the aspiration cytodiagnosis of male breast masses. *Diagn Cytopathol*. 1991;7(6):637-639.
6. Duncan PG, et al. Fetal risk of anesthesia and surgery during pregnancy. *Anesthesiology*. 1986;64(6):790-794.
7. Mazze RI, Kallen B. Reproductive outcome after anesthesia and operation during pregnancy: a registry study of 5405 cases. *Am J Obstet Gynecol*. 1989;161(5):1178-1185.
8. Yang WT, et al. Imaging of breast cancer diagnosed and treated with chemotherapy during pregnancy. *Radiology*. 2006;239(1):52-60.
9. Middleton LP, et al. Breast carcinoma in pregnant women: assessment of clinicopathologic and immunohistochemical features. *Cancer*. 2003;98(5):1055-1060.
10. Loibl S, et al. Breast carcinoma during pregnancy.

International recommendations from an expert meeting. *Cancer*. 2006;106(2):237-246.
11. Hahn KM, et al. Treatment of pregnant breast cancer patients and outcomes of children exposed to chemotherapy in utero. *Cancer*. 2006;107(6):1219-1226.
12. Loibl S, et al. Treatment of breast cancer during pregnancy: an observational study. *Lancet Oncol*. 2012;13(9):887-896.
13. Zagouri F, et al. Taxanes for breast cancer during pregnancy: a systematic review. *Clin Breast Cancer*. 2013;13(1):16-23.
14. Litton JK, et al. Case control study of women treated with chemotherapy for breast cancer during pregnancy as compared with nonpregnant patients with breast cancer. *Oncologist*. 2013;18(4):369-376.
15. Aviles A, Neri N. Hematological malignancies and pregnancy: a final report of 84 children who received chemotherapy in utero. *Clin Lymphoma*. 2001;2(3):173-177.
16. Bines J, Oleske DM, Cobleigh MA. Ovarian function in premenopausal women treated with adjuvant chemotherapy for breast cancer. *J Clin Oncol*. 1996;14(5):1718-1729.
17. Goodwin PJ, et al. Risk of menopause during the first year after breast cancer diagnosis. *J Clin Oncol*. 1999;17(8):2365-2370.
18. Han HS, et al. Analysis of chemotherapy-induced amenorrhea rates by three different anthracycline and taxane containing regimens for early breast cancer. *Breast Cancer Res Treat*. 2009;115(2):335-342.
19. Lee SJ, et al. American Society of Clinical Oncology recommendations on fertility preservation in cancer patients. *J Clin Oncol*. 2006;24(18):2917-2931.
20. Hachem HE, Atallah D, Grynberg M. Fertility preservation in breast cancer patients. *Future Oncol*. 2014;10(10):1767-1777.
21. Loren AW, et al. Fertility preservation for patients with cancer: American Society of Clinical Oncology clinical practice guideline update. *J Clin Oncol*. 2013;31(19):2500-2510.
22. Gerber B, et al. Effect of luteinizing hormone-releasing hormone agonist on ovarian function after modern adjuvant breast cancer chemotherapy: the GBG 37 ZORO study. *J Clin Oncol*. 2011;29(17):2334-2341.
23. Del Mastro L, et al. Effect of the gonadotropin-releasing hormone analogue triptorelin on the occurrence of chemotherapy-induced early menopause in premenopausal women with breast cancer: a randomized trial. *JAMA*. 2011;306(3):269-276.
24. Del Mastro L, et al. Gonadotropin-releasing hormone analogues for the prevention of chemotherapy-induced premature ovarian failure in cancer women: systematic review and meta-analysis of randomized trials. *Cancer Treat Rev*. 2014;40(5):675-683.
25. Surbone A, Petrek JA. Childbearing issues in breast carcinoma survivors. *Cancer*. 1997;79(7):1271-1278.
26. Upponi SS, et al. Pregnancy after breast cancer. *Eur J Cancer*. 2003;39(6):736-741.
27. Morrow PK, Theriault RL. Pregnancy after the diagnosis of breast cancer. *Clin Breast Cancer*. 2006;7(2):173-175.
28. Mueller BA, et al. Childbearing and survival after breast carcinoma in young women. *Cancer*. 2003;98(6):1131-1140.
29. Early Breast Cancer Trialists' Collaborative Group. Effects of chemotherapy and hormonal therapy for early breast cancer on recurrence and 15-year survival: an overview of the randomised trials. *Lancet*. 2005;365(9472):1687-1717.
30. Siegel R, et al. Cancer statistics, 2014. *CA Cancer J Clin*. 2014;64(1):9-29.
31. Giordano SH, et al. Breast carcinoma in men: a population-based study. *Cancer*. 2004;101(1):51-57.
32. Ottini L, et al. Male breast cancer. *Crit Rev Oncol Hematol*. 2010;73(2):141-155.
33. Fentiman IS, Fourquet A, Hortobagyi GN. Male breast cancer. *Lancet*. 2006;367(9510):595-604.
34. Fogh S, et al. Use of tamoxifen with postsurgical irradiation may improve survival in estrogen and progesterone receptor-positive male breast cancer. *Clin Breast Cancer*. 2011;11(1):39-45.
35. Pemmaraju N, et al. Retrospective review of male breast cancer patients: analysis of tamoxifen-related side-effects. *Ann Oncol*. 2012;23(6):1471-1474.
36. Yu E, et al. The impact of post-mastectomy radiation therapy on male breast cancer patients—a case series. *Int J Radiat Oncol Biol Phys*. 2012;82(2):696-700.
37. Perkins GH, et al. Male breast carcinoma: outcomes and predictors of local-regional failure in patients treated without radiation therapy. *Breast Cancer Res Treat*. 2002;76:S121-S121.
38. Giordano SH. A review of the diagnosis and management of male breast cancer. *Oncologist*. 2005;10(7):471-9.
39. Xu S, et al. Tamoxifen adherence and its relationship to mortality in 116 men with breast cancer. *Breast Cancer Res Treat*. 2012;136(2):495-502.
40. Eggemann H, et al. Adjuvant therapy with tamoxifen compared to aromatase inhibitors for 257 male breast cancer patients. *Breast Cancer Res Treat*. 2013;137(2):465-470.
41. Jepson AS, Fentiman IS. Male breast cancer. *Int J Clin Pract*. 1998;52(8):571-576.
42. Giordano SH, Hortobagyi GN. Leuprolide acetate plus aromatase inhibition for male breast cancer. *J Clin Oncol*. 2006;24(21):e42-e43.
43. Giordano SH, et al. Efficacy of anastrozole in male breast cancer. *Am J Clin Oncol*. 2002;25(3):235-237.
44. Doyen J, et al. Aromatase inhibition in male breast cancer patients: biological and clinical implications. *Ann Oncol*. 2010;21(6):1243-1245.
45. Rossouw JE, et al. Risks and benefits of estrogen plus progestin in healthy postmenopausal women: principal results from the Women's Health Initiative randomized controlled trial. *JAMA*. 2002;288(3):321-333.
46. Hays J, et al. Effects of estrogen plus progestin on health-related quality of life. *N Engl J Med*. 2003;348(19):1839-1854.
47. Rapp SR, et al. The effect of estrogen plus progestin on global cognitive function in postmenopausal women: results from the Women's Health Initiative Memory Study. *Menopause*. 2003;10(6):567.
48. Anderson GL, et al. Effects of estrogen plus progestin on gynecologic cancers and associated diagnostic procedures: the Women's Health Initiative randomized trial. *JAMA*. 2003;290(13):1739-1748.
49. Cauley JA, et al. Effects of estrogen plus progestin on risk of fracture and bone mineral density: the Women's Health Initiative randomized trial. *JAMA*. 2003;290(13):1729-1738.
50. Anderson GL, et al. Effects of conjugated equine estrogen in postmenopausal women with hysterectomy: the Women's Health Initiative randomized controlled trial. *JAMA*. 2004;291(14):1701-1712.
51. Marjoribanks J, et al. Long term hormone therapy for perimenopausal and postmenopausal women. *Cochrane Database Syst Rev*. 2012;7:CD004143.
52. Holmberg L, et al. Increased risk of recurrence after hormone replacement therapy in breast cancer survivors. *J Natl Cancer Inst*. 2008;100(7):475-482.
53. Brinton LA, et al. Recent trends in breast cancer among younger women in the United States. *J Natl Cancer Inst*. 2008;100(22):1643-1648.
54. Virnig BA, et al. Ductal carcinoma in situ of the breast: a systematic review of incidence, treatment, and outcomes. *J Natl Cancer Inst*. 2010;102(3):170-178.
55. Li CI, Daling JR, Malone KE. Age-specific incidence rates of in situ breast carcinomas by histologic type, 1980 to 2001. *Cancer Epidemiol Biomarkers Prev*. 2005;14(4):1008-1011.
56. Harris JR,. Lippman ME, Morrow M, Osborne CK, Diseases of the breast. 2014.

57. Bellamy CO, et al. Noninvasive ductal carcinoma of the breast: the relevance of histologic categorization. *Hum Pathol.* 1993;24(1):16-23.
58. Burstein HJ, et al. Ductal carcinoma in situ of the breast. *N Engl J Med.* 2004;350(14):1430-1441.
59. Greene FL, Page DL, Fleming ID, et al, eds. *AJCC Cancer Staging Manual.* 6th ed. Chicago, IL: American Joint Committee on Cancer; 2002.
60. Winchester DP, et al. Treatment trends for ductal carcinoma in situ of the breast. *Ann Surg Oncol.* 1995;2(3):207-213.
61. Silverstein MJ, et al. Axillary lymph node dissection for intraductal breast carcinoma—is it indicated? *Cancer.* 1987;59(10):1819-1824.
62. Zavagno G, et al. Role of axillary sentinel lymph node biopsy in patients with pure ductal carcinoma in situ of the breast. *BMC Cancer.* 2005;5:28.
63. Pendas S, et al. Sentinel node biopsy in ductal carcinoma in situ patients. *Ann Surg Oncol.* 2000;7(1):15-20.
64. Klauber-DeMore N, et al. Sentinel lymph node biopsy: is it indicated in patients with high-risk ductal carcinoma-in-situ and ductal carcinoma-in-situ with microinvasion? *Ann Surg Oncol.* 2000;7(9):636-642.
65. Sakorafas GH, Farley DR. Optimal management of ductal carcinoma in situ of the breast. *Surg Oncol.* 2003;12(4):221-240.
66. Cox CE, et al. Importance of lymphatic mapping in ductal carcinoma in situ (DCIS): why map DCIS? *Am Surg.* 2001;67(6):513-519; discussion 519-521.
67. Owen D, et al. Outcomes in patients treated with mastectomy for ductal carcinoma in situ. *Int J Radiat Oncol Biol Phys.* 2013;85(3):e129-e134.
68. Vargas C, et al. Factors associated with local recurrence and cause-specific survival in patients with ductal carcinoma in situ of the breast treated with breast-conserving therapy or mastectomy. *Int J Radiat Oncol Biol Phys.* 2005;63(5):1514-1521.
69. Fisher B, et al. Lumpectomy and radiation therapy for the treatment of intraductal breast cancer: findings from National Surgical Adjuvant Breast and Bowel Project B-17. *J Clin Oncol.* 1998;16(2):441-452.
70. Fisher ER, et al. Pathologic findings from the National Surgical Adjuvant Breast Project (NSABP) eight-year update of Protocol B-17: intraductal carcinoma. *Cancer.* 1999;86(3):429-438.
71. EORTC Breast Cancer Cooperative Group, EORTC Radiotherapy Group, Bijker N, et al. Breast-conserving treatment with or without radiotherapy in ductal carcinoma-in-situ: ten-year results of European Organisation for Research and Treatment of Cancer randomized phase III trial 10853—a study by the EORTC Breast Cancer Cooperative Group and EORTC Radiotherapy Group. *J Clin Oncol.* 2006;24(21):3381-3387.
72. Goodwin A, et al. Post-operative radiotherapy for ductal carcinoma in situ of the breast. *Cochrane Database Syst Rev.* 2009(4):CD000563.
73. Fisher B, et al. Tamoxifen in treatment of intraductal breast cancer: National Surgical Adjuvant Breast and Bowel Project B-24 randomised controlled trial. *Lancet.* 1999;353(9169):1993-2000.
74. Allred DC, et al. Estrogen receptor expression as a predictive marker of the effectiveness of tamoxifen in the treatment of DCIS: findings from NSABP Protocol B-24. *Breast Cancer Res Treat.* 2002;76:S36.
75. Cuzick J, et al. Anastrozole for prevention of breast cancer in high-risk postmenopausal women (IBIS-II): an international, double-blind, randomised placebo-controlled trial. *Lancet.* 2014;383(9922):1041-1048.
76. Berry DA, et al. High-dose chemotherapy with autologous stem-cell support as adjuvant therapy in breast cancer: overview of 15 randomized trials. *J Clin Oncol.* 2011;29(24):3214-3223.
77. Berry DA, et al. High-dose chemotherapy with autologous hematopoietic stem-cell transplantation in metastatic breast cancer: overview of six randomized trials. *J Clin Oncol.* 2011;29(24):3224-3231.
78. Adami HO, et al. Characteristics of familial breast cancer in Sweden: absence of relation to age and unilateral versus bilateral disease. *Cancer.* 1981;48(7):1688-1695.
79. Bain C, et al. Family history of breast cancer as a risk indicator for the disease. *Am J Epidemiol.* 1980;111(3):301-308.
80. Lubin JH, et al. Risk factors for breast cancer in women in northern Alberta, Canada, as related to age at diagnosis. *J Natl Cancer Inst.* 1982;68(2):211-217.
81. Easton DF, et al. Genetic linkage analysis in familial breast and ovarian cancer: results from 214 families. The Breast Cancer Linkage Consortium. *Am J Hum Genet.* 1993;52(4):678-701.
82. Chen S, Parmigiani G. Meta-analysis of BRCA1 and BRCA2 penetrance. *J Clin Oncol.* 2007;25(11):1329-1333.
83. Narod SA, et al. Tamoxifen and risk of contralateral breast cancer in BRCA1 and BRCA2 mutation carriers: a case-control study. Hereditary Breast Cancer Clinical Study Group. *Lancet.* 2000;356(9245):1876-1881.
84. Gronwald J, et al. Tamoxifen and contralateral breast cancer in BRCA1 and BRCA2 carriers: an update. *Int J Cancer.* 2006;118(9):2281-2284.
85. Gronwald J, et al. Duration of tamoxifen use and the risk of contralateral breast cancer in BRCA1 and BRCA2 mutation carriers. *Breast Cancer Res Treat.* 2014;146(2):421-427.
86. Pichert G, et al. Evidence-based management options for women at increased breast/ovarian cancer risk. *Ann Oncol.* 2003;14(1):9-19.
87. Hartmann LC, et al. Efficacy of bilateral prophylactic mastectomy in women with a family history of breast cancer. *N Engl J Med.* 1999;340(2):77-84.
88. Hartmann LC, et al. Efficacy of bilateral prophylactic mastectomy in BRCA1 and BRCA2 gene mutation carriers. *J Natl Cancer Inst.* 2001;93(21):1633-1637.
89. Meijers-Heijboer H, et al. Breast cancer after prophylactic bilateral mastectomy in women with a BRCA1 or BRCA2 mutation. *N Engl J Med.* 2001;345(3):159-164.
90. Rebbeck TR, et al. Bilateral prophylactic mastectomy reduces breast cancer risk in BRCA1 and BRCA2 mutation carriers: the PROSE Study Group. *J Clin Oncol.* 2004;22(6):1055-1062.
91. Domchek SM, et al. Association of risk-reducing surgery in BRCA1 or BRCA2 mutation carriers with cancer risk and mortality. *JAMA.* 2010;304(9):967-975.
92. Kauff ND, et al. Risk-reducing salpingo-oophorectomy for the prevention of BRCA1- and BRCA2-associated breast and gynecologic cancer: a multicenter, prospective study. *J Clin Oncol.* 2008;26(8):1331-1337.
93. Kauff ND, et al. Risk-reducing salpingo-oophorectomy in women with a BRCA1 or BRCA2 mutation. *N Engl J Med.* 2002;346(21):1609-1615.
94. Rebbeck TR, Kauff ND, Domchek SM. Meta-analysis of risk reduction estimates associated with risk-reducing salpingo-oophorectomy in BRCA1 or BRCA2 mutation carriers. *J Natl Cancer Inst.* 2009;101(2):80-87.

Section VIII

Gynecologic Malignancies

Section Editor: Karen H. Lu

第八篇 妇科恶性肿瘤

31

Ovarian Cancer

第三十一章　卵巢癌

Kari L. Ring
Jubilee Brown
Amir A. Jazaeri

中文导读

本章从卵巢上皮性肿瘤、恶性生殖细胞肿瘤、性索间质肿瘤3部分详细介绍了卵巢癌。在卵巢上皮癌部分，分别讲述了卵巢癌的流行病学、死亡率、病因学、危险因素、筛查手段、分子生物学、预后因素、组织学亚型（包括浆液性癌、黏液性癌、子宫内膜样腺癌、透明细胞癌、移行细胞癌及未分化癌）、分级、疾病分期、诊断方法和治疗。治疗主要分为手术治疗（初次减瘤手术及复发后的二次减瘤手术）、辅助治疗、随访及复发后的治疗，治疗部分又讲述了根据晚期患者对于铂类药物敏感或耐药的不同化疗方案的选择策略。另外本章对低级别浆液性卵巢癌做了简单介绍。在恶性生殖细胞肿瘤部分，本章阐述了病因学、诊断和治疗，随后对患者如何进行长期随访及放疗、化疗对患者生殖的影响进行了介绍。在性索间质肿瘤部分，本章介绍了该病的病因、诊断和治疗，治疗手段主要包括了手术、术后辅助化疗及内分泌治疗。

EPITHELIAL OVARIAN CANCER

Epidemiology

Ovarian cancer is the second most common cancer of the female genital tract, with approximately 21,290 cases expected in the United States in 2015 ([1]). Epithelial tumors comprise 90% of ovarian cancers, and the most common histologic subtype is high-grade serous carcinoma, followed by endometrioid, clear cell, and mucinous tumors. Ovarian cancer remains the number one cause of death due to gynecologic cancers in the United States, accounting for 14,180 deaths this year. Among women, ovarian cancer is the fifth most common cancer-related cause of death in the United States ([1]). The lifetime risk of a woman in the United States developing ovarian cancer is approximately 1 in 70 (1.37%). Ovarian cancer is also more common among white women compared to African American or Asian American women in the United States, although the differences are narrowing. In most parts of Europe and North America, the incidence of ovarian cancer was constant during the decades prior to the 1990s. However, among white women, ovarian cancer incidence rates are reported to have declined from 2001 to 2010 by 2.2% per year ([2]).

This cancer is predominantly a cancer of the perimenopausal and the postmenopausal period, with 80% to 90% of cases occurring after the age of 40. The incidence is higher in older women, and the median age at diagnosis is 63 years.

Mortality

Ovarian cancer accounts for 5.5% of the deaths from cancer that occur in women between 60 and 79 years of age ([1]). Prognosis among women with ovarian cancer is dependent on the stage of disease at the time of diagnosis. Five-year survival rates among women with localized, regional, and distant disease at the time of diagnosis are 92%, 72%, and 27%, respectively ([1]). Relative survival rates for ovarian cancer have improved substantially over the last decade by an average of 2% per year, and modern 5-year survival estimates are between 45% and 50% ([3]). Survival among white women with ovarian cancer in the United States is reportedly better than survival among black women, and the improvement noted was not observed in black women ([1, 4]).

Etiology

The etiology and the tissue of origin of ovarian cancer are not fully understood. Over the past decade, there has been an increased appreciation that epithelial ovarian cancers (EOCs) represent a heterogeneous group of malignancies. Some of this heterogeneity is related to distinct pathophysiology associated with the development of different histologic subtypes. For example, the majority of high-grade serous ovarian cancers are now believed to arise from fallopian tube fimbria rather than ovarian surface epithelium. This fallopian tube hypothesis originated from observations in women undergoing risk-reducing (prophylactic) salpingo-oophorectomy due to hereditary breast-ovarian cancer syndromes. Approximately 5% to 10% of these women are diagnosed with an occult ovarian cancer ([5-7]). The majority of these early cancers are either located in the fimbrial portion of the fallopian tube or, on close histologic examination, have a coexisting carcinoma in situ component in the fallopian tube fimbria. Subsequent investigations revealed that careful sectioning of fallopian tubes from high-risk women frequently revealed areas of marked cytologic atypia and disorganized growth within the fimbria. These areas have been called serous tubal intraepithelial carcinoma (STIC) or tubal dysplasia and are characterized by cytologic atypia, positive p53 immunostaining (which correlates with mutations in the *TP53* gene), abnormal proliferation (as evident by Ki67 staining), and DNA damage (Fig. 31-1) ([8-10]).

Based on their distinct molecular features and clinicopathologic characteristics, other carcinogenesis models have been proposed for endometrioid, clear cell, mucinous, and low-grade serous ovarian cancers. Endometrioid and clear cell tumors have a strong epidemiologic link with endometriosis, and there is accumulating

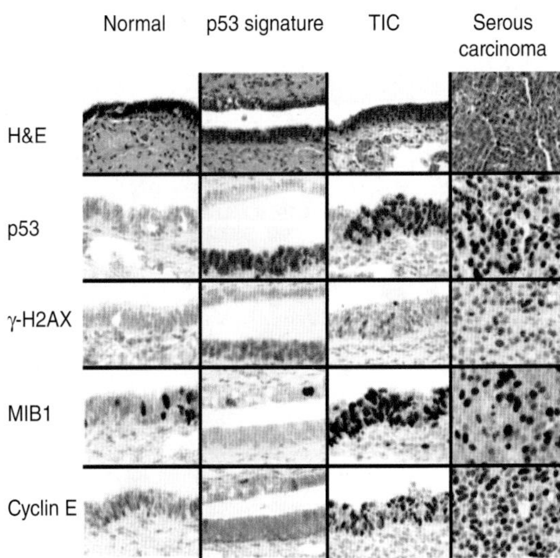

FIGURE 31-1 Overview of co-localization of p53, γ-H2AX, MIB1, and cyclin E in normal mucosa, p53 signature, tubal intraepithelial carcinoma, and serous carcinoma. H&E, hematoxylin and eosin. (Reproduced with permission from Lee Y, Miron A, Drapkin R, et al. A candidate precursor to serous carcinoma that originates in the distal fallopian tube. *J Pathol.* 2007;211:26-35.)

evidence that they may arise from endometriotic cysts or areas of atypical endometriosis. Low-grade serous carcinomas are thought to arise from borderline neoplasms. However, this remains a controversial area, and much research is focused on better understanding the pathophysiology of different subtypes of EOC.

Risk Factors

Numerous studies have attempted to demonstrate possible links between environmental, dietary, reproductive, endocrine, viral, and hereditary factors and the risk of developing ovarian cancer. These factors are summarized in Table 31-1.

The strongest risk factor for ovarian cancer is a genetic predisposition. Women with *BRCA1* and *BRCA2* mutations have a 39% to 46% and 10% to 27% lifetime risk of developing ovarian cancer, respectively, which is 18 to 36 times higher than that of the background risk. A smaller proportion of cases of familial ovarian cancer are associated with mutations in mismatch repair genes (*MLH1*, *MSH2*, *MHS6*, *PMS2*) related to Lynch syndrome, with a lifetime risk of ovarian cancer ranging from 0% to 24%. Patients with germline mutations in *MLH1* and *MSH2* seem to be at the highest risk for ovarian cancer compared to patients with *MSH6* and *PMS2* mutations. Most recently, germline mutations in *BRIP1*, *RAD51D*, and *RAD51C* have been associated with an increased lifetime risk of ovarian cancer, ranging from 10% to 15%.

Other factors associated with an increased risk of ovarian cancer include age, early menarche, late menopause, and obesity ([11-13]).

Protective factors that have been shown to reduce the risk of ovarian cancer include the use of oral contraceptives, multiparity, breast feeding, hysterectomy, and tubal ligation ([14]). Other factors, including exercise, perineal talc exposure, infertility treatment, and use of postmenopausal hormone replacement therapy, have not been definitively shown to alter a woman's risk of developing ovarian cancer.

Screening

Stage I ovarian cancer is associated with excellent survival; however, more than two-thirds of patients are diagnosed with stage III or IV disease. These observations have provided a compelling rationale in support of screening for early-stage disease. The most commonly used screening strategies include a combination of serum cancer antigen 125 (CA125) levels and pelvic sonography. While several large trials have demonstrated that screening can detect cancer in asymptomatic women, there are concerns regarding the poor positive predictive value for these strategies and lack of proven survival benefit. The findings of four key trials are summarized in Table 31-2 ([15-19]). Currently, the US Preventive Services Task Force recommends against screening for ovarian cancer in asymptomatic women of average risk. However, the United Kingdom Collaborative Trial of Ovarian Cancer Screening (UKCTOCS) is using the Risk of Ovarian Cancer (ROC) time series algorithm to interpret CA125, which has shown an encouraging sensitivity and specificity, and the mortality data are anticipated in 2015.

Table 31-1 Risk Factors for Developing Ovarian Cancer

Increased	Decreased	Indeterminate
Hereditary Family history of ovarian cancer Personal history of breast cancer *BRCA1* or *BRCA2* mutation Lynch syndrome	*Reproductive* Multiparity Breastfeeding	Fertility drugs Exercise Cigarette smoking Perineal talc exposure
Reproductive Advanced age Nulligravity Infertility	*Hormonal* Oral contraceptives Progestins	
Hormonal Early menarche Late age at natural menopause Hormone replacement therapy Estrogen Androgens	*Surgery* Hysterectomy Tubal ligation	
Inflammatory Endometriosis Pelvic inflammatory disease		
Lifestyle Obesity		
Geography Extremes in latitude		

Adapted with permission from Hunn J, Rodriguez GC. Ovarian cancer: etiology, risk factors, and epidemiology. *Clin Obstet Gynecol*. 2012;55(1):3-23.

CHAPTER 31

Table 31-2 Summary of Major Trials in Ovarian Cancer Screening

	Ovarian Cancer Screening Trials in the General Population			
	University of Kentucky Study ([19])	Japanese Shizuoka Cohort Study of Ovarian Cancer Screening ([8])	Prostate, Lung, Colorectal and Ovarian (PLCO) Cancer Screening Trial ([17])	United Kingdom Collaborative Trial of Ovarian Cancer Screening (UKCTOCS) ([15,16])
Study design	Single-arm prospective study	RCT with 1 screening strategy in study group	RCT with 1 screening strategy in study group	RCT with 2 screening strategies in the study group
Cohort	25,327	41,688	30,630	98,305
Screening strategy	Ultrasound	Physical exam, ultrasound and CA125	Ultrasound and CA125	Two screening arms (ultrasound, USS) and CA125 followed by ultrasound (multimodal, MMS)
Interpretation of CA125	35-kU/L cutoff	CA125 using a 35-kU/L cutoff	CA125 using a 35-kU/L cutoff	CA125 interpreted using the Risk of Ovarian Cancer (ROC) algorithm
Key screening findings	Encouraging sensitivity (81%) for primary OC/FT cancer; 76.3% for primary invasive OC/FT cancer	Encouraging sensitivity (77.1%) for primary OC/FT cancer	Lower sensitivity (69.5%) for primary OC/FT cancer; 68.2% for primary invasive OC/FT cancer when compared to the other trials (only 28% were stage I/II)	Encouraging sensitivity (89.4% MMS/84.9% USS) for primary OC/FT cancer; 84.9% MMS/75.0% USS for primary invasive OC/FT cancer (47% MMS/50% USS were stage I/II). Superior sensitivity (88.6% vs 65.8%) and PPV (21.7% vs 5.8%) of MMS compared to the USS arm for detection of primary invasive epithelial OC/FT cancers during incidence screening, with 40.3% in the MMS and 51.5% in the USS arm detected at early stage
Key mortality/ surrogates of mortality findings	Longer 5-year survival in the screened arm (74.8%) compared to unscreened women from the same institution treated by the same surgical and chemotherapeutic protocols (53.7%) ($P < 0.001$)	Stage shift: more stage I ovarian cancers in the screened group (63%) compared to the control (38%)	No mortality benefit: 118 ovarian cancer deaths in the screened arm, 100 in the control arm	Mortality data awaited in 2014/2015
Current status	Completed	Mortality data to be reported	Completed	Mortality data to be reported in 2015

Reproduced with permission from Menon U, Griffin M, Gentry-Maharaj A. Ovarian cancer screening—current status, future directions. *Gynecol Oncol.* 2014;132(2):490-495.
RCT, randomized controlled trial.

The Molecular Landscape of Epithelial Ovarian Cancer

Molecular Biology

Although the different subtypes of EOC possess unique molecular aberrations (Table 31-3) and transcriptional signatures, their morphologic features resemble the specialized epithelia of the reproductive tract that derive from the Müllerian ducts.

As noted, accumulating evidence points to the distal fallopian tube epithelium as the tissue of origin for most high-grade serous carcinomas. The most common molecular alterations in serous carcinomas are mutations in *TP53*, which are nearly ubiquitous. The Cancer Genome Atlas (TCGA) project has also significantly advanced our understanding of other molecular and genetic alterations in high-grade serous carcinoma. In addition to the expected *TP53* mutations in 96% of tumors, low prevalence recurrent somatic mutations in *NF1*, *BRCA1*, *BRCA2*, *RB1*, and *CDK12* were also observed. Serous carcinomas are also characterized by a high degree of chromosomal instability (gene copy number amplifications and deletions), and both total and regional instability are associated with tumor grade and altered patient outcomes ([20]). Somatic copy number analysis performed as part of TCGA also confirmed 8 and 22 chromosomal regions of recurrent gain and loss, respectively. Five of the gains and 18 of the losses occurred in more than half of the tumors. Although such aberrant areas of DNA frequently carry multiple genes, it is presently thought that only a limited number of genes are "key drivers" of the process. These key drivers are thought to be the most critical markers and potential treatment targets. Candidate drivers at areas of copy number gain and loss are frequently proposed. For example, it has been suggested that 45% of high serous cancers harbor altered phosphatidylinositol 3-kinase (PI3K)/RAS signaling mediated by multiple copy number alterations, including *PTEN* deletion and *PIK3CA*, *KRAS*, *AKT1*, and *AKT2* amplification. Low-grade serous carcinomas have been found to have alterations in the mitogen-activated protein kinase (MAPK) pathway. Approximately 20% to 40% of tumors have a *KRAS* mutation, while a smaller proportion of tumors demonstrate mutations in *BRAF*, accounting for 5% of low-grade serous carcinomas ([21]).

Clear cell and endometrioid cancers are epidemiologically and molecularly linked to endometriosis. Frequent somatic mutations of *PIK3CA* and ARID1A (AT-rich interactive domain-containing protein 1A) have been documented in tumors associated with endometriosis ([22, 23]). Common genetic abnormalities identified in endometrioid ovarian carcinomas include somatic mutations of *CTNNB1* and *PTEN* ([24]).

Cytokines and Growth Factors

Several cytokines and growth factors have been studied in ovarian carcinogenesis. For instance, levels of interleukin 10 (IL-10) and interleukin 6 (IL-6) are particularly elevated in ovarian cancer ascites. Endogenously produced IL-6 can protect tumor cells from natural killer cell–mediated killing, and IL-6 expression by immunohistochemistry was associated with poor prognosis ([25]). Furthermore, IL-6 has been identified as an etiologic paracrine factor in paraneoplastic

Table 31-3 Current Concepts Regarding the Origins and Molecular Pathology of Epithelial Ovarian Cancer

Histology	Precursor	Molecular Features
Low-grade serous carcinoma	Cystadenoma–borderline tumor–carcinoma sequence	Mutations in *K-RAS* and/or *b-RAF*
High-grade serous carcinoma	"De novo" in epithelial inclusion cysts	*p53* mutation and *BRCA1* dysfunction (usually promoter methylation) *PIK3CA*[b] amplification (25%-40%)
Low-grade endometrioid carcinoma	Endometriosis and endometrial-like hyperplasia[a]	Mutations in *CTNNB1* (B-catenin gene) and *PTEN* with microsatellite instability
High-grade endometrioid carcinoma	Epithelial inclusion glands/cysts	*p53* mutation and *BRCA1* dysfunction (usually promoter methylation) *PIK3CA* mutation
Mucinous carcinoma	Cystadenoma–borderline tumor–carcinoma sequence	Mutations in *K-RAS*; *p53* mutation associated with transition from borderline tumor to carcinoma.
Clear cell carcinoma	Endometriosis	*PTEN* mutation/loss of heterozygosity *PIK3CA* mutation

[a]Endometriosis and adjacent low-grade endometrioid carcinoma share common genetic events, such as loss of heterozygosity at the same loci involving the same allele (eg, PTEN). In contrast, high-grade and poorly differentiated endometrioid carcinomas are similar to high-grade serous carcinomas.
[b]*PIK3CA* is the gene at chromosome 3q26 that specifically encodes the p110α subunit of the phosphatidylinositol-3-kinase (PI3K) protein.

thrombocytosis and associated poor prognosis in ovarian cancer ([26]). When compared to high-grade serous tumors, ovarian clear cell carcinomas are associated with higher circulating levels of IL-6 ([27]).

A detailed review of growth factor pathways targeted in ovarian cancer is beyond the scope of this chapter. Instead, we briefly highlight the vascular endothelial growth factor (VEGF) pathway, which has proven to be the most clinically useful target to date. The VEGF signaling cascade is mediate through a partially redundant set of ligands and receptors, which have emerged as promising targets for antiangiogenic cancer therapy. The VEGF ligand family consists of seven ligands: VEGF A-E, placenta growth factor 1 (PlGF1), and PlGF2. The receptor tyrosine kinases involved in this signaling cascade include VEGF receptor type 1 (VEGFR1), VEGFR2, and VEGFR3. Vascular endothelial growth factor ligands are overexpressed in EOC cells, while the receptors are present mainly on the tumor endothelial cells ([28]). Vascular endothelial growth factor is a key mediator of angiogenesis, which is stimulated by hypoxia. Bevacizumab, a monoclonal anti-VEGF-A antibody, is the prototypical member of this class, and as a single agent has been the most promising biological compound for the treatment of recurrent ovarian cancer.

Prognostic Factors

Prognostic factors are tumor-related characteristics that determine the biologic behavior and risk of death from the disease; their predictive value may change during the course of treatment and thereafter.

Factors associated with poor prognosis in advanced ovarian cancer (stage III or IV) fall into two subgroups (as determined by multivariate analysis in clinical trials):

1. *Variables prior to systemic treatment predictive of survival:* age, stage at diagnosis, performance status, residual tumor volume, and tumor histology
2. *Variables at the time of relapse predictive of time to progression:* less than 6 months from last chemotherapy (platinum-resistant disease), poorer performance status, mucinous histology, larger number of sites of disease, best previous response to chemotherapy versus progression, serum CA 125 levels

Stage

Stage is a dominant prognostic factor in ovarian cancer. The main prognostic factors in early-stage ovarian cancer (stages I-IIA) are International Federation of Gynecology and Obstetrics (FIGO) stage, histologic grade, histologic type, and patient's age. Early-stage ovarian cancer is discovered early in fewer than 30% of patients; in such cases, the 5-year survival is good, ranging from 51% to 98% ([1]).

Cancer Antigen 125

Cancer antigen 125 is a high molecular weight glycoprotein that is elevated in 80% of EOCs ([29]). There is no definitive evidence that pretherapeutic CA125 levels correlate with survival in EOC ([30]). The most aggressive tumors are not necessarily those with the highest CA125 levels. However, there has been evidence that the kinetics of an individual's CA125 level during treatment may be related to best response to treatment as well as survival ([31]).

Residual Disease

It is logical to assume that the extent of postoperative residual tumor volume is affected by both the biology and the history of the disease, as well as the radicality, emphasis, and effort involved in the tumor reductive surgery. What remains controversial is the relative contribution of these factors to the prognostic significance of residual disease. On one hand, the tumors that are more aggressive and disseminated are more difficult to resect and therefore associated with larger residual disease. Therefore, how advanced the tumor was before debulking may be more important than how much disease was left behind. Other features—such as the type of chemotherapy, the intrinsic chemosensitivity of the tumor, and the presence of other biological variables—may be as important as or even more important than the extent of the surgery. Proponents of the importance of maximal surgical effort point to a wealth of retrospective data and the evolution of "optimal cytoreductive surgery" from less than 2 cm to R0 (no visible residual disease) as evidence for the importance of the surgical result ([32]). The only prospective randomized trial of the neoadjuvant approach versus up-front tumor reductive surgery in patients with advanced-stage EOC was carried out by the European Organization for Research and Treatment of Cancer (EORTC)–Gynaecological Cancer Group. In this trial, optimal resection (as defined by residual tumor of 1 cm or less) was noted in 41.6% of patients who underwent primary debulking compared to 80.6% of patients who underwent neoadjuvant chemotherapy interval debulking ([33]).

Histologic Subtypes

Serous Carcinoma

Serous carcinoma is the most common histologic subtype of EOC, and this subtype can further be divided into high-grade and low-grade serous carcinomas ([34]). Recently, MD Anderson developed a two-tier grading system in serous carcinomas based on nuclear atypia and mitotic rate to distinguish high-grade from low-grade tumors (Fig. 31-2). This has been adopted by the

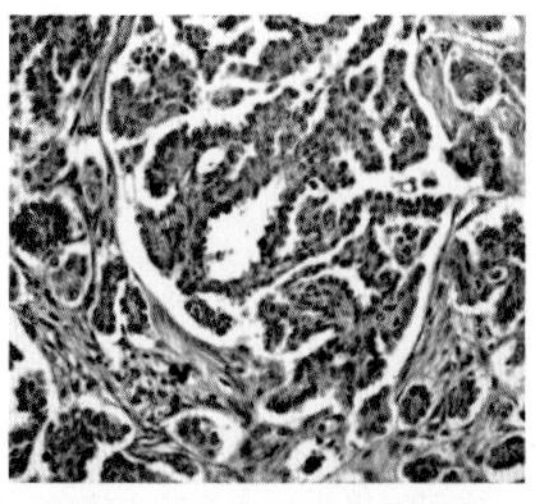

Low-grade serous carcinoma of the ovary is characterized by relative uniformity of the cells and up to 12 mitoses per 10 high-power fields. Courtesy of Anais Malpica, MD.

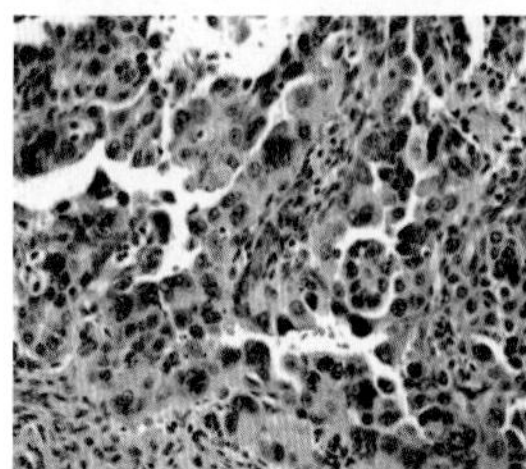

High-grade serous carcinoma of the ovary is characterized by pleomorphism; there is marked nuclear atypia and >12 mitoses per 10 high-power fields. Courtesy of Anais Malpica, MD.

FIGURE 31-2 Low-grade and high-grade serous carcinoma. (Used with permission from Anais Malpica, MD.)

gynecologic oncology community to further define these two diseases.

High-Grade Serous Carcinoma

High-grade serous carcinomas account for 70% to 80% of all ovarian cancers and are the most common type of EOC. High-grade serous carcinomas may present with varying architectural patterns, but the defining characteristic of these tumors is high mitotic activity (>12 mitoses per 10 high-power fields [HPFs]) and the presence of multinucleated cells ([34]).

Low-Grade Serous Carcinoma

Low-grade serous carcinoma accounts for 6% to 10% of serous ovarian cancers and 5% to 8% of all ovarian cancers. These tumors are now thought to arise from borderline tumors have distinct molecular aberrations and clinical behavior when compared to their high-grade counterpart. Low-grade serous tumors have low mitotic activity (<12 mitoses per 10 HPFs) and are distinguished from borderline tumors based on destructive invasion of more than 5 mm ([35]).

Mucinous Carcinoma

In older references, the proportion of mucinous ovarian cancers is as high as 30%. However, there is now increased recognition that many such tumors, on careful evaluation, are thought to represent metastases from the gastrointestinal tract. Contemporary estimates of the prevalence of primary ovarian mucinous carcinoma is approximately 3%. Primary ovarian origin is favored by unilaterality, large size greater than 12 cm, smooth external surface, and association with other ovarian pathology. Conversely, metastases tend to be bilateral, be less than 10 cm in size, exhibit surface involvement, and have colloid and signet ring morphology. True mucinous ovarian tumors are low-grade malignancies that have a low propensity for metastatic spread and are usually diagnosed as unilateral stage IA tumors even though they may reach enormous size (Fig. 31-3) ([36]). Newer studies have also dispelled the notion that pseudomyxoma peritonei is commonly secondary to an ovarian mucinous carcinoma. It is now recognized that pseudomyxoma peritonei is almost always associated with an appendiceal mucinous lesion ([37]).

Endometrioid Adenocarcinoma

Overall, 10% of epithelial ovarian tumors are of endometrioid histology and resemble endometrial adenocarcinoma, and both types occur simultaneously as synchronous primary tumors in as many as 25% of cases

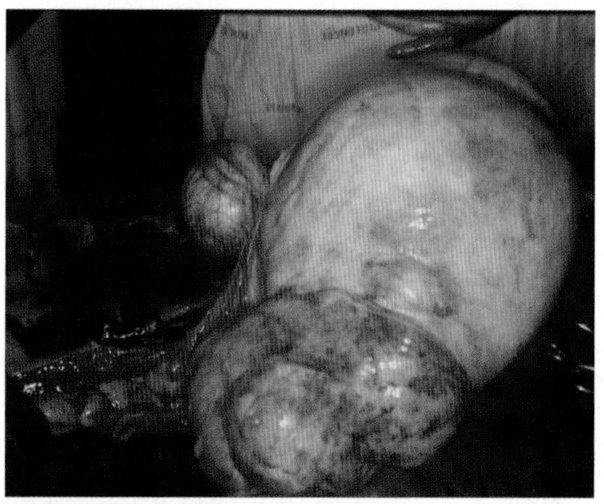

FIGURE 31-3 Operative removal of mucinous ovarian tumor.

in patients younger than 45 years of age ([38]). Identification of multifocal disease is important because patients with disease metastatic from the uterus to the ovaries have a 5-year survival rate of 30% to 40%. Those with synchronous multifocal disease have a 5-year survival rate of 70% to 80%. Concurrent endometriosis is present in 10% of cases. The malignant potential of endometriosis is very low, although a transition from benign to malignant epithelium may be seen.

Clear Cell Carcinoma

Clear cell carcinomas comprise 5% to 10% of ovarian cancers and, like endometrioid tumors, may be associated with endometriosis or endometrial cancer. Some studies indicated that clear cell carcinoma may be resistant to standard carboplatin-paclitaxel–based chemotherapy regimens. However, other investigators have shown that when the pathology was carefully reviewed by a gynecologic pathologist, only suboptimal cytoreduction and spread of disease were associated with a significantly increased risk of platinum resistance ([39]).

Transitional Cell Carcinoma

Transitional cell carcinomas were previously thought to represent malignant Brenner tumors; however, recent studies have shown that they are molecularly similar to high-grade serous carcinomas. These tumors are now classified as a subtype of high-grade serous carcinomas ([40]).

Undifferentiated Carcinoma

Undifferentiated carcinomas are thought to represent the most poorly differentiated high-grade serous carcinomas rather than a separate entity ([41]).

Histologic Grading

Previously, a three-tier grading system was used in the diagnosis of EOC; however, there was no consensus on the definition of this system. More recently, two-tier grading systems (high grade vs low grade) have been shown to have better prognostic and interobserver variability ([34, 42]). Consistent with their distinct pathophysiology and tumor biology, low-grade serous carcinomas are more resistant to chemotherapy and are associated with significantly higher rates of platinum-resistant disease ([43]).

Staging

Accurate staging is critical to the success of surgery and adjuvant therapy. The staging of ovarian cancer is based on the gross and pathologic findings of the initial surgical evaluation. The FIGO classification uses the sites and extent of the disease, including capsule rupture and ascites, to categorize ovarian cancer into four stages. This is summarized in Table 31-4.

Diagnosis

Symptoms of ovarian cancer are nonspecific and include early satiety, bloating, constipation, and weight loss. It is not uncommon for patients to have been referred for a gastrointestinal evaluation before the correct diagnosis is reached. Objective signs of ovarian carcinoma are also nonspecific and include a pelvic mass, ascites, carcinomatosis, possible pleural effusion(s), and occasionally supraclavicular lymphadenopathy.

Management

In general, the initial management and staging of EOC is surgical. In early-stage ovarian cancer, comprehensive staging allows for proper triage to adjuvant therapy. When comprehensive staging is performed, a substantial number of patients initially believed to have disease confined to the pelvis will be staged upward ([44]).

In advanced EOC, surgery and chemotherapy are both utilized in initial management. However, there remains debate regarding the sequence of these interventions in the treatment of advanced ovarian cancer. Patients have historically been candidates for neoadjuvant chemotherapy if they have multiple medical comorbidities, poor performance status, or extensive disease on imaging that is not felt to be amenable to up-front surgery. Despite this, there is no current consensus regarding which patients should have up-front cytoreduction or neoadjuvant chemotherapy. The current approach at MD Anderson is for all patients with suspected advanced ovarian cancer (based on computed tomographic [CT] imaging) to undergo a preoperative laparoscopic assessment (Fig. 31-4).

This laparoscopic evaluation provides the following: surgicopathologic diagnosis, assessment of metastatic disease burden and likelihood of complete resection (modified Fagotti score) ([45]), and research tissue acquisition. Our laparoscopic triage is accomplished by scoring made by two independent and blinded surgeons. Those patients scored less than 8 undergo primary cytoreduction (with up to a 2-week interval). Those with scores of 8 or more undergo neoadjuvant chemotherapy (consisting of three cycles of carboplatin and paclitaxel), followed by consideration of interval cytoreductive surgery and three additional cycles of chemotherapy (± maintenance therapy) ([46]). An outline of our treatment algorithm is shown in Fig. 31-5.

Table 31-4 FIGO Staging for Ovarian Cancer

FIGO		TNM
0	Primary tumor cannot be assessed	TX
	No evidence of primary tumor	T0
I	Tumor confined to ovaries	T1
IA	Tumor limited to one ovary, capsule intact	T1a
	No tumor on ovarian surface	
	No malignant cells in the ascites or peritoneal washings	
IB	Tumor limited to both ovaries, capsules intact	T1b
	No tumor on ovarian surface	
	No malignant cells in the ascites or peritoneal washings	
IC	Tumor limited to one or both ovaries	T1c
IC1	Surgical spill	
IC2	Rupture prior to surgery, tumor on ovarian surface, positive malignant cells in the ascites, or	
IC3	positive peritoneal washings	
II	Tumor involves one or both ovaries with pelvic extension	T2
IIA	Extension and/or implants in uterus and/or tubes	T2a
IIB	Extension to other pelvic organ	T2b
III	Tumor involves peritoneal metastasis outside the pelvis and/or regional lymph node metastasis	T3
IIIA1(i)	Positive retroperitoneal nodes only ≤10 mm	T1, T2,
IIIA1(ii)	Positive retroperotineal nodes only >10 mm	T3aN1
IIIA2	Microscopic, extrapelvic (above the brim) peritoneal involvement ± positive retroperitoneal lymph nodes	T3a/T3aN1
IIIB	Macroscopic, extrapelvic, peritoneal metastasis ≤2 cm ± positive retroperitoneal lymph nodes; includes extension to capsule of liver/spleen	T3b/T3bN1
IIIC	Macroscopic, extrapelvic, peritoneal metastasis >2 cm ± positive retroperitoneal lymph nodes; includes extension to capsule of liver/spleen	T3c/T3cN1
IVA	Pleural effusion with positive cytology	M1
IVB	Hepatic and/or splenic parenchymal metastasis, metastasis to extra-abdominal organs (including inguinal lymph nodes and lymph nodes outside the abdominal cavity)	

Other major recommendations are as follows:

- Histologic type including grading should be designated at staging.
- Primary site (ovary, fallopian tube or peritoneum) should be designated where possible.
- Tumors that may otherwise qualify for stage I but involved with dense adhesions justify upgrading to stage II if tumor cells are histologically proven to be present in the adhesions.

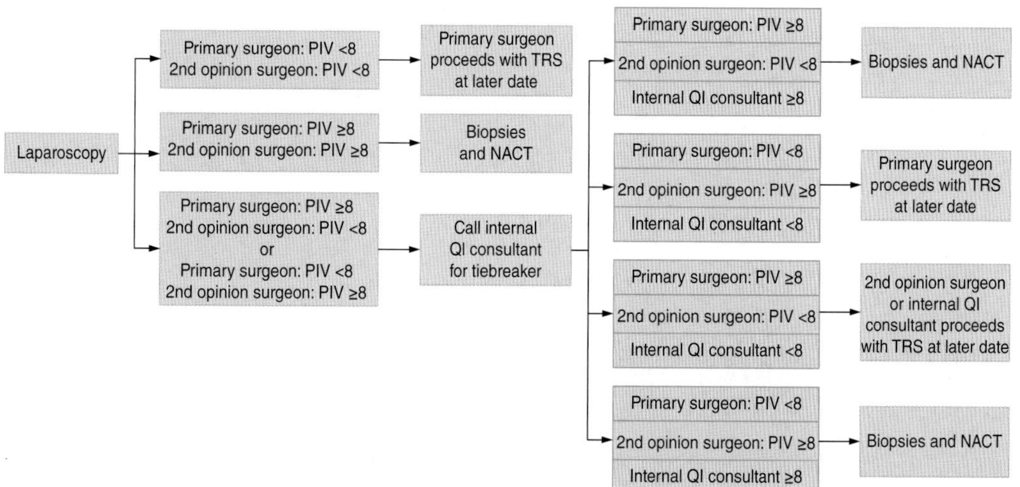

FIGURE 31-4 Laparoscopic scoring system utilized at MD Anderson to determine resectability of disease. PIV, predictive index value; QI, quality improvement; TRS, tumor reductive surgery; NACT, neoadjuvant chemotherapy. (Reproduced with permission from Nick AM, Coleman RL, Ramirez PT, et al: A framework for a personalized surgical approach to ovarian cancer. *Nat Rev Clin Oncol.* 2015;12(4):239-245.)

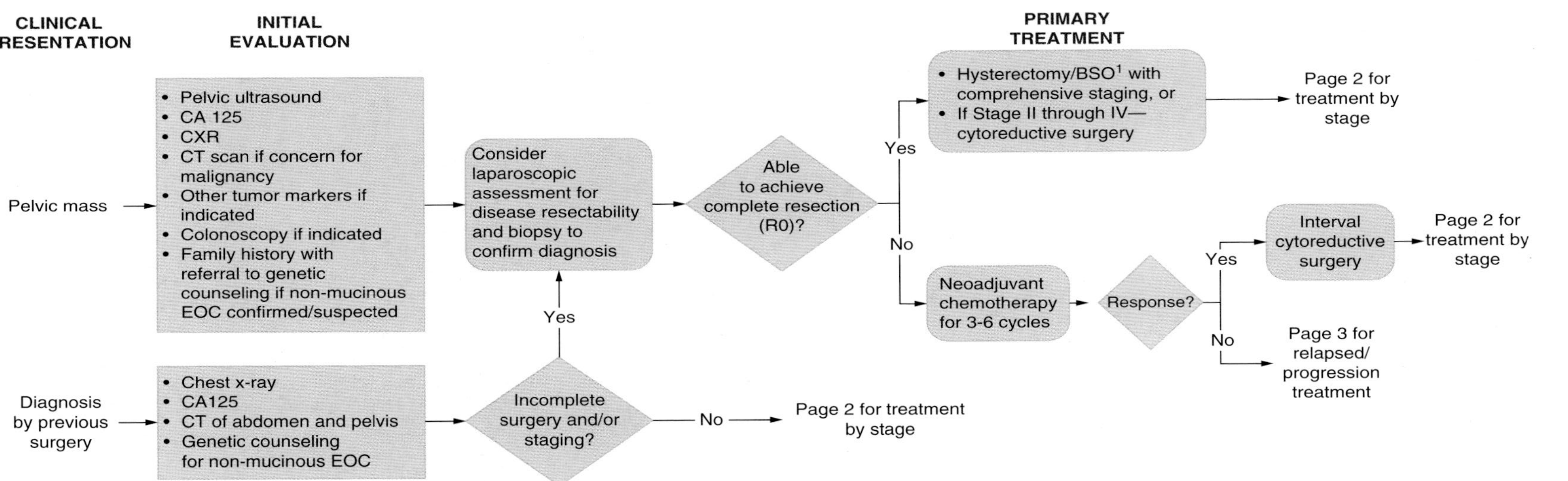

EOC = Epithelial Ovarian Cancer

[1]If Stage I and patient desires fertility preservation – consider USO and staging

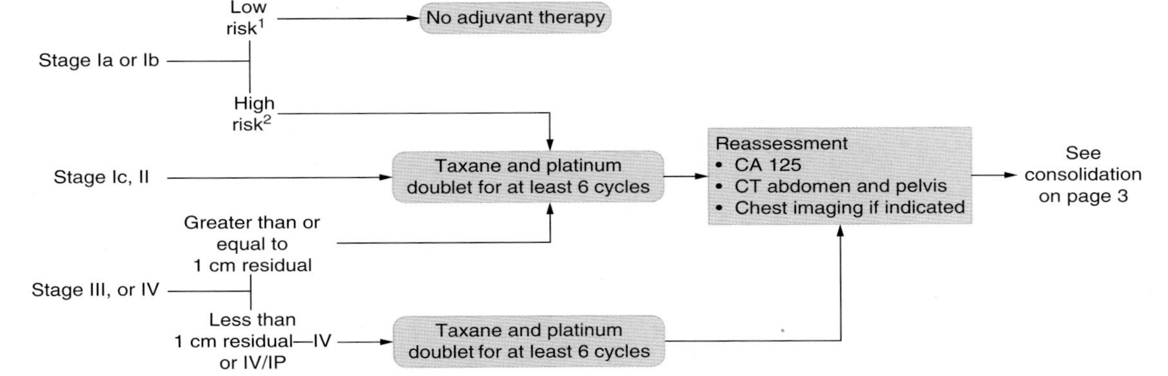

[1]Low risk—Grade 1 endometrioid; or low grade serous histology

[2]High risk—Grade 3 endometrioid; high grade serous, or clear cell histology

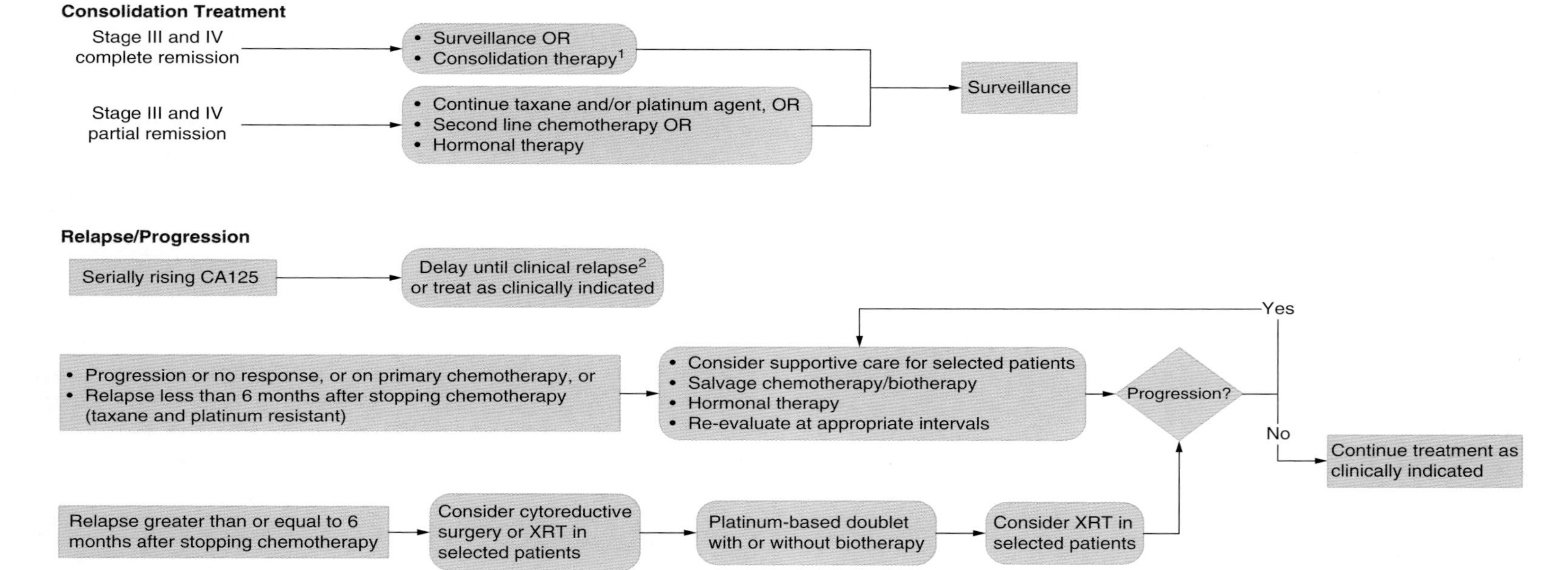

[1]Paclitaxel, hormonal therapy, or biologic therapy
[2]Symptomatic or radiologic

FIGURE 31-5 **Outline of treatment algorithms utilized at MD Anderson for the treatment of epithelial ovarian cancer. CXR, chest x-ray; BSO, bilateral salpingo-oophorectomy.**

In addition to a preoperative evaluation with lab testing, imaging, and office examination, the National Comprehensive Cancer Network (NCCN) now recommends genetic testing for all newly diagnosed high-grade serous ovarian cancers.

Primary Cytoreductive Surgery

A staging laparotomy involves the following steps:

1. Midline vertical incision
2. Evacuation and cytologic analysis of ascites
3. Inspection and palpation of all peritoneal (intraperitoneal and retroperitoneal) surfaces, including the subdiaphragmatic areas
4. Total abdominal hysterectomy and bilateral salpingo-oophorectomy
5. Omentectomy with debulking to no gross residual disease
6. If disease limited to ovaries, bilateral pelvic and para-aortic lymph node sampling; multiple biopsies, including the paracolonic gutters, cul-de-sac, lateral pelvic walls, vesicouterine reflection, subdiaphragmatic sites, and intra-abdominal areas
7. Appendectomy if a mucinous tumor is found

The goal of an initial cytoreductive surgery is to remove all visible tumor because the amount of residual disease left behind is inversely correlated with patient survival. Currently, an optimal tumor-reductive surgery is defined as no residual nodules greater than 1 cm in size. More recent studies have tried to refine the definition of *optimal* cytoreductive surgery by dividing patients into those with no visible residual disease and others as these patients have improved overall survival (OS), even compared to patients with less than 1 cm of residual disease ([32]).

The only prospective randomized trial of the neoadjuvant approach versus up-front tumor-reductive surgery in patients with advanced-stage EOC carried out by the EORTC demonstrated the noninferiority of the neoadjuvant approach with respect to progression-free survival (PFS) and OS ([33]). However, this study has been criticized by the lower rate (41.6%) of optimal cytoreductive surgery in the primary debulking group (which was defined as largest single tumor nodule <1cm in this study) compared to reports from institutions in the United States and elsewhere. Hence, this remains a controversial area in the management of ovarian cancer.

CHAPTER 31

Secondary Cytoreduction for Recurrent Disease

The benefits of secondary cytoreduction for recurrent disease are also unclear, although accumulating data suggest that, in certain circumstances, secondary cytoreduction may lead to a survival benefit. Eisenkop et al published a large series of patients with recurrent ovarian cancer undergoing cytoreduction for recurrent disease ([47]). There were 106 patients who had a complete clinical response to initial therapy. These patients had a disease-free interval of at least 6 months prior to recurrence. Sixty percent underwent reexploration and debulking, and 82% were rendered disease free at that time. The authors evaluated factors that might be predictive of surgical outcome (optimal debulking) as well as those that might be indicative of survival. Predictors of complete cytoreduction included the following:

1. Size of recurrent tumor less than 10 cm
2. The use of chemotherapy before cytoreduction
3. Good Karnofsky performance status

A study from MD Anderson Cancer Center (MDACC) looked at a similar group of patients who also had a disease-free interval of at least 6 months, with similar results. These investigators noted that there was significantly improved survival in women who underwent optimal cytoreduction of tumor to less than 2 cm (19.5 vs 8.3 months). Others have published similar findings, all noting that the duration of prior clinical response is important in terms of survival and chances of optimal cytoreduction.

Adjuvant Therapy

Chemotherapy

Early-Stage Disease

Previous studies have defined a subset of patients with early-stage disease who are at increased risk of relapse. These high-risk features include:

1. Stage IC disease
2. Clear cell histology
3. High-grade tumor

Patients with these features should be considered for adjuvant therapy. Two large meta-analyses have shown that adjuvant chemotherapy improved both recurrence-free survival (RFS) and OS in patients with early-stage disease; however, women who had no gross residual disease following surgery did not benefit from adjuvant treatment ([48]). Subgroup analysis showed that women with high-risk features who received chemotherapy did have improved OS compared to women who received no adjuvant therapy ([48]). Most recently, the ACTION trial randomized patients with early-stage disease to platinum-based chemotherapy or observation. Overall, adjuvant chemotherapy improved RFS (70% vs 62%); however, there was no improvement in patients who had complete surgical staging (RFS 78% vs 72%) ([49]). This trial supports the need for complete surgical staging in early-stage ovarian cancer to appropriately triage patients for adjuvant chemotherapy as well as prognostic counseling for the patient.

There is no consensus on the number of cycles of adjuvant chemotherapy to give in early disease. The main clinical trial targeting early stage ovarian cancer in the platinum and taxane era was conducted by the Gynecologic Oncology Group (GOG). The goal was to determine whether six cycles of carboplatin and paclitaxel would significantly lower the rate of cancer recurrence, compared to three cycles of the same agents following surgical staging operations on patients with stage IA grade 3, stage IB grade 3, stage IC, and completely resected stage II ovarian epithelial cancer. A secondary objective was to compare the toxicities of the two treatments. Following surgical staging, 321 patients were randomized to either three or six cycles of paclitaxel 175 mg/m^2 infused over 3 hours followed by carboplatin 7.5 AUC (area under the curve) infused over 30 minutes. Cycles were repeated every 21 days. A total of 70% of these patients had stage I disease. In the standard three-cycle arm, the estimated probability of cancer recurring within 5 years was 27%, compared to 19% in the six-cycle arm. The recurrence rate for six cycles was 24% lower (hazard ratio [HR] 0.761; 95% CI, 0.51–1.13; P = .18). It was concluded that the addition of three cycles of carboplatin and paclitaxel over the standard three cycles did not significantly alter the rate of cancer recurrence in patients with early-stage ovarian epithelial carcinoma. In addition, six cycles caused significantly more toxicity than three cycles ([50]). However, potential weaknesses of this study include the fact that it was likely underpowered to result in statistically significant differences, and that toxicity outcomes lacked external validity given that the high dose of carboplatin (AUC = 7.5) used in this trial is rarely used in clinical practice. At MD Anderson, we currently administer six cycles of neoadjuvant chemotherapy if utilized in the adjuvant setting for early-stage disease.

Advanced-Stage Disease

Carboplatin and paclitaxel remain the gold standard drugs in primary adjuvant treatment of EOC. The effect of incorporating additional cytotoxic agents (gemcitabine, liposomal doxorubicin, topotecan) in combination with carboplatin and paclitaxel was evaluated in GOG182. This randomized four-arm trial showed equivalent PFS and OS in all the arms and a better toxicity profile in the control carboplatin and paclitaxel alone arm ([51]). Addition of bevacizumab to carboplatin and paclitaxel in the frontline setting was tested in GOG218 and ICON7 ([52, 53]). Both studies showed that the addition of bevacizumab resulted in a modest improvement in PFS, but without an improvement in OS. Furthermore, the 4-month improvement in PFS observed in GOG218 was only associated with the arm receiving prolonged administration. There was no difference in the PFS of the control and carboplatin paclitaxel plus bevacizumab arms. Incidences of serious bowel toxicity (perforation or fistulas) and hypertension were about 2% and 23%, respectively ([52]). Given the significant costs of bevacizumab and the lack of OS improvement, cost-effective analysis has shown that the use of bevacizumab as part of frontline therapy in ovarian cancer is not cost-effective ([54]).

Intraperitoneal Chemotherapy

The frequent metastasis of EOC within the peritoneal cavity and the ability to achieve a much higher concentration of platinum and taxane drugs following intraperitoneal administration are the principal rationale for the use of intraperitoneal chemotherapy for the treatment of patients with advanced-stage EOC who have undergone optimal resection (largest residual tumor nodule less than 1 cm). Three randomized trials have revealed improved PFS and OS in patients receiving intraperitoneal chemotherapy ([55-57]). While all three trials have been criticized, the publication of GOG172 results, which revealed a 17-month OS benefit in the intraperitoneal arm, led the National Cancer Institute (NCI) to issue a Clinical Announcement recommending that women with stage III ovarian cancer who undergo optimal surgical cytoreduction be considered for intraperitoneal chemotherapy.

However, the better outcomes associated with intraperitoneal chemotherapy are associated with higher toxicity, illustrated by the fact that fewer than half of women randomized to the intraperitoneal arm were able to complete the six prescribed cycles ([55]). Furthermore, the regimen used in GOG172 included an inpatient administration of day 1 and 2 (for 24-hour paclitaxel and intraperitoneal cisplatin). While most centers have substituted a better-tolerated and outpatient regimen from the original GOG172, legitimate concerns regarding the equal efficacy of such regimens remain. In hopes of arriving at a better-tolerated and more efficacious intraperitoneal regimen, GOG252 was conducted to compare the GOG172-derived outpatient regimen to intraperitoneal carboplatin and weekly dose-dense paclitaxel and standard intravenous regimen (with bevacizumab included in all three arms). The results of this trial are anticipated in 2015.

Carboplatin and Dose-Dense (Weekly) Paclitaxel

The Japanese GOG protocol 3016 (JGOG3016) compared the administration of carboplatin (AUC = 6) with paclitaxel (180 mg/m^2) every 3 weeks or weekly paclitaxel

(80 mg/m^2 on days 1, 8, and 15 of a 21-day cycle). This study showed a significantly better median PFS and OS in the weekly dose regimen (PFS: 18.2 vs 17.5 months; OS: 100.5 vs 62.2 months) ([58, 59]). However, a peculiarity of this trial was that even the 62.2-month median OS survival in the control arm was much longer than in any of the platinum era GOG or European trials, especially given that the JGOG trial included patients with suboptimal cytoreductive surgery.

Additional questions about the external validity of the JGOG3016 trial were raised when the results of the MITO7 became available. This trial compared weekly carboplatin and paclitaxel (AUC = 2 and 60 mg/m^2, respectively) to conventional therapy (carboplatin AUC = 6; paclitaxel 175 mg/m^2) every 3 weeks. There was no significant difference in the median PFS between the two arms (median PFS 17.3 months in the every 3 weeks group vs 18.3 months in the weekly arm) ([60]). In addition, preliminary results from GOG262 showed no difference in PFS in patients with stage I to IV ovarian cancer. This study included both optimally and suboptimally debulked patients, but both arms also allowed bevacizumab administration. Interestingly, patients not treated with bevacizumab had a 4-month improvement in PFS if they received the dose-dense regimen, while there was no difference in PFS in patients who received bevacizumab in addition to the assigned treatment regimen ([61]).

Alternative Chemotherapeutic Agents

Docetaxel (Taxotere) is a semisynthetic compound structurally related to paclitaxel. The toxicity of docetaxel is similar to that of paclitaxel. However, docetaxel is associated with less neuropathy and more myelosuppression compared to paclitaxel. In addition, prolonged treatment with docetaxel increases skin and nail toxicity and can produce fluid retention and significant edema. Another important distinguishing feature is that docetaxel does not share the cremophor EL diluent used in the preparation of paclitaxel, which is the etiologic component responsible for many cases of paclitaxel hypersensitivity. A trial conducted by the Scottish Gynaecological Cancer Trials Group included 1,077 patients with FIGO stage IC to IV EOC who were randomized to receive carboplatin in combination with either paclitaxel or docetaxel. The median PFS for both arms was approximately 15 months ([62]). The authors concluded that the docetaxel combination appears to be a viable alternative to the paclitaxel combination as first-line chemotherapy in EOC because of an improved therapeutic index while maintaining similar efficacy.

Maintenance Therapy

The high risk of recurrent disease after treatment of advanced-stage EOC has prompted an intensive search for therapeutic strategies that can be given after standard-of-care therapy to improve patient outcomes. More than 12 phase III trials have been undertaken in this setting, including extension of frontline agents, administration of short-duration non–cross-resistant chemotherapy, high-dose chemotherapy, whole-abdominal or intraperitoneal radiotherapy, immunotherapy, vaccine therapy, biologic therapy, and single-agent paclitaxel; however, none has shown a survival advantage against various controls (usually no treatment) ([63]). The S9701/GOG178 phase III trial that administered paclitaxel intravenously for 12 months (vs 3 months) after an initial response to first-line chemotherapy showed improved PFS. However, the design of the trial (with PFS as the primary end point) led to early closure and lack of data on the effect of this consolidation strategy on OS. This improvement in PFS was associated with significant neurotoxicity, and overall this strategy has not been widely adopted in routine clinical practice ([64]). The chemotherapy regimens utilized at MD Anderson are outlined in Fig. 31-6.

Follow-up and Treatment of Recurrent Disease

Despite multimodality therapy, 75% to 80% of women with advanced-stage epithelial cancer will have a recurrence. Regular follow-up with tumor marker can detect disease recurrence ([65, 66]). In women with previously treated ovarian cancer that is in clinical remission, the NCCN has recommended assessment of serum CA125 concentration at every follow-up visit if this concentration was raised at initial diagnosis. After documentation of CA125 increase in such women, the median time to a clinical relapse of ovarian cancer is 2 to 6 months. There is, however, controversy over the benefit of early treatment versus treatment later. The results of a large study showed no survival benefit from early treatment on the basis of a raised serum CA125 concentration alone and therefore questioned the value of routine measurement of CA125 in the follow-up of patients with EOC ([66]). Some authors also suggested that smaller tumors are more often responsive to treatment, but this does not eliminate the lead-time bias. It is also argued that larger tumors have an inferior primary response and grow rapidly. Recurrent ovarian cancer is a mortal disease, but—in the absence of data showing that treatment improves quality of life—this does not justify haste in treating patients. At MD Anderson, we follow patients with CA125 levels in surveillance but in general do not treat patients based solely on a rising value (see Fig. 31-5).

One of the problems with recurrent ovarian cancer is the lack of a truly effective salvage therapy. The other problem is the inability to identify a predictive marker

Adjuvant Therapy	• Paclitaxel 135 mg/m² IV continuous infusion over 24 hours day 1; CISplatin 75-100 mg/m² IP day 2; Paclitaxel 60 mg/m² IP day 8. Every 3 weeks for 6 cycles. • Paclitaxel 175 mg/m² IV over 3 hours with Carboplatin AUC 5-6 IV over 1 hour every 3 weeks for 6 cycles. • Docetaxel 75 mg/m² IV over 1 hour with Carboplatin AUC 5 IV over 1 hours every 3 weeks for 6 cycles. • Paclitaxel 80 mg/m² IV over 1 hour on days 1, 8 and 15 with Carboplatin AUC 5-6 IV over 1 hour on day 1. Repeat every 3 weeks for 6 cycles. • Paclitaxel 175 mg/m² IV over 3 hours with Carboplatin AUC 5-6 IV over 1 hour every 3 weeks for 6 cycles. Starting day 1 of cycle 2 give Bevacizumab 15 mg/kg IV over 30 minutes ever 3 weeks.	
Neoadjuvant Therapy	• Paclitaxel 175 mg/m² IV over 3 hours with Carboplatin AUC 5-6 IV over 1 hour every 3 weeks for 3-6 cycles. • Docetaxel 75 mg/m² IV over 1 hour with Carboplatin AUC 5 IV over 1 hours every 3 weeks for 3-6 cycles. • Paclitaxel 80 mg/m² IV over 1 hour on days 1, 8 and 15 with Carboplatin AUC 5-6 IV over 1 hour on day 1. Repeat every 3 weeks for 3-6 cycles. • Paclitaxel 175 mg/m² IV over 3 hours with Carboplatin AUC 5-6 IV over 1 hour and Bevacizumab 15 mg/kg IV over 30 minutes every 3 weeks for 3-6 cycles. Bevacizumab should not be given in the cycle prior to surgery.	
	Platinum Sensitive	**Platinum Resistant**
Recurrence Therapy	• Paclitaxel and Carboplatin • Carboplatin and weekly Paclitaxel • Carboplatin and Docetaxel • Carboplatin and Gemcitabine • Carboplatin, Gemcitabine, and Bevacizumab • Carboplatin and Liposomal Doxorubicin • Carboplatin single agent	• Docetaxel • Oral Etoposide • Gemcitabine • Liposomal Doxorubicin • Weekly Paclitaxel • Cisplatin and Gemcitabine • Bevacizumab and oral Cyclophasphamide • Bevacizumab • Topotecan • Vinorelbine • Hormonal therapy

FIGURE 31-6 Chemotherapy regimens utilized at MD Anderson for the treatment of epithithelial ovarian cancer. AUC, area under the curve.

for recurrence. The treatment of recurrent ovarian cancer is stratified by the amount of time from completion of primary platinum-based chemotherapy. Patients who have a recurrence with a PFS of 6 months or longer are defined as having platinum-sensitive disease. Patients who have a recurrence less than 6 months from primary chemotherapy are classified as having platinum-resistant disease. Patients whose disease progresses on primary chemotherapy have tumors classified as platinum refractory and have a poor prognosis ([67]). A list of treatment regimens utilized at MD Anderson in platinum-sensitive and platinum-resistant disease can be found in Fig. 31-6.

Treatment of Platinum-Sensitive Disease

As mentioned, patients who have a treatment-free interval of 6 months or greater prior to recurrence are more likely to respond to repeat platinum treatment. As noted, depending on the pattern and extent of recurrence, some of these patients may also be good candidates for secondary cytoreductive surgery. While there are several options for second-line chemotherapy in platinum-sensitive disease, all regimens have a platinum backbone. Combination therapy has been shown to have an improved OS compared to single-agent therapy in this patient population and should be considered in patients with an acceptable performance status. As long as patients continue to respond to platinum and have more than a 6-month interval between each treatment, it seems reasonable to continue treatment with platinum, either as a single agent or in a combination regimen (see Fig. 31-5).

Carboplatin and Paclitaxel

Two phase III trials have shown the benefit of carboplatin and paclitaxel in the setting of platinum-sensitive recurrence, and the results were published together. The ICON4 and AGO-OVAR-2.2 studies randomized patients to receive conventional platinum-based chemotherapy or platinum plus paclitaxel or platinum plus a nontaxane ([68]). Results from this study showed an OS benefit (HR 0.82, $P = .02$), which led to a 7% absolute survival difference (57% vs 50%) and a 5-month improvement in median survival (29 vs 24 months) in favor of platinum plus paclitaxel. There were higher rates of neuropathy and alopecia in the platinum-plus-paclitaxel treatment group but a lower rate of myelosuppression ([68]). One critique of this study is that a large proportion of patients (30%) were not previously treated with taxane therapy, which may have led to an improved response in this patient population. Other options that may be utilized in the setting of platinum-sensitive ovarian cancer include docetaxel as well as the use of weekly paclitaxel, both in combination with carboplatin ([69, 70]).

Carboplatin and Liposomal Doxorubicin

A phase III study (CALYPSO) showed that a pegylated liposomal doxorubicin and carboplatin combination was better than paclitaxel with carboplatin in terms of PFS in relapsed platinum-sensitive cancer (11.3 vs 9.4 months); however, there was no difference in OS (30.7 vs 33 months). The combination of carboplatin plus liposomal doxorubicin led to fewer cases of severe neutropenia, fewer episodes of mild myalgias/arthalgias, and less neuropathy but did lead to more cases of severe thrombocytopenia, nausea/vomiting, hand-foot syndrome, and mucositis. Interestingly, the study combination also led to fewer episodes of carboplatin hypersensitivity reactions ([71]).

Carboplatin and Gemcitabine

A phase III trial was performed by the Gynecologic Cancer InterGroup (GCIG) to evaluate carboplatin alone versus carboplatin plus gemcitabine in patients with platinum-sensitive disease. Treatment with the combination regimen showed an improved PFS (8.6 vs 5.8 months), but no improvement in OS. Not surprisingly, there more toxicities seen in the combination arm, with increased neutropenia and thrombocytopenia. A second trial, OCEANS, was a randomized phase III trial that evaluated carboplatin plus gemcitabine with or without the addition of bevacizumab. Patients received the assigned treatment for 6 to 10 cycles and were then continued on bevacizumab or placebo maintenance until progression. The addition of bevacizumab led to an improved PFS (12.4 vs 8.4 months) with an improved objective response rate (78.5% vs 57.4%; $P < .001$). As seen with other antiangiogenesis studies, the addition of bevacizumab led to higher rates of hypertension and proteinuria ([72]).

Poly-ADP Ribose Inhibitors

The role for maintenance therapy with poly-ADP ribose (PARP) inhibitors has been evaluated in platinum-sensitive disease. In a randomized trial (Study 19), maintenance therapy with olaparib was given to patients who achieved a complete response to second-line therapy ([73]). Patients with germline *BRCA* mutations were found to have improved PFS (11 vs 4 months) with few adverse events ([74]). While there was no difference in OS, there was a 22.6% crossover rate in this study, which may prevent a true difference from being seen in this study population. While this did have significant results, olaparib is currently only approved by the Food and Drug Administration (FDA) for the treatment of advanced ovarian cancer in patients with germline *BRCA* mutation who have failed three or more prior lines of chemotherapy in the United States.

Treatment of Platinum-Resistant Disease

There are several treatment options for the treatment of platinum-resistant recurrent EOC. In general, single-agent treatment regimens are utilized in this patient population to minimize adverse effects, given incurable disease. While there are several options, no one therapy has been shown superior to others as first-line treatment for platinum-resistant disease. A Cochrane review of three of the most commonly used agents (paclitaxel, pegylated liposomal doxorubicin, and topotecan) showed similar efficacy. Thus, choice of first-line therapy is driven by side effect profiles of each of the therapies.

Liposomal Doxorubicin

A pegylated liposomal formulation of doxorubicin was first tested in patients with platinum-refractory disease; the resulting response rate was approximately 26%. Compared to topotecan in a phase III setting, liposomal doxorubicin was associated with lower toxicities, including lower rates of grade 3/4 neutropenia and thrombocytopenia, but with equivalent efficacy, with similar response rate (20% vs 17%) and time to progression (22 vs 20 weeks) ([75]). Based on the data from Gordon et al, the drug was FDA approved for use in ovarian cancer.

Gemcitabine

In a phase III study comparing gemcitabine and liposomal doxorubicin, both drugs had similar overall response rates (6.1% vs 8.3%), PFS (3.6 vs 3.1 months), and OS (12.7 vs 13.5 months) ([76]). Gemcitabine has been frequently studied in combination with cisplatin. The response rates ranged from 40% to 70%. However, the small number of patients treated as well as their heterogeneity disallows any further conclusion. Furthermore, it is difficult to justify the use of combination chemotherapy in patients without evidence that responses correlated with improvements in quality of life.

Weekly Paclitaxel

Paclitaxel is part of the backbone of treatment for advanced ovarian cancer. Several studies have shown activity of paclitaxel in platinum-resistant patients; however, a proportion of these studies were performed prior to the incorporation of paclitaxel in primary adjuvant therapy. Most recently, weekly paclitaxel produced a 21% response rate in patients with platinum-resistant disease. Not surprisingly, the main toxicity associated with this regimen is peripheral neuropathy ([77]).

Topotecan

Compared to paclitaxel in patients with refractory ovarian cancer, topotecan was found to produce a response rate of 20%, compared to the 13% in patients who received paclitaxel. This resulted in its approval for use by the FDA. In patients with relapsed platinum-resistant ovarian cancer, the overall response rates on treatment with topotecan ranged from 5% to 18%. The proportion of these patients who achieved stable disease was 17%. In phase III studies, topotecan was shown to have an efficacy equal to both paclitaxel and liposomal doxorubicin as second-line therapy in patients with relapsed ovarian cancer ([75]).

Etoposide

Etoposide, a topoisomerase II inhibitor, has the advantage of being administered as an oral agent. In patients with platinum-refractory disease who were given 100-mg doses of etoposide orally for 14 days every 21 days, the response rate was about 26%. Lower doses of etoposide, at 50 mg/d, produced similar response rates, ranging from 10% to 27%. The combination of cyclophosphamide and bevacizumab has also been shown to be active in this patient population. A phase II trial showed partial response in 24% of patients, with 56% of patients predicted to be alive and progression free at 6 months ([78]).

Bevacizumab

The phase III AURELIA study evaluated bevacizumab in addition to single-agent chemotherapy in platinum-resistant ovarian cancer. Patients with disease that progressed less than 6 months after completing adjuvant therapy were eligible, but platinum-refractory patients were excluded. The patients received the treating physician's choice of liposomal doxorubicin, weekly paclitaxel, or topotecan and were then randomized to chemotherapy alone or chemotherapy plus bevacizumab. Patients who received bevacizumab had an improved response rate (31% vs 13%) and a reduction in risk of disease progression (6.7 vs 3.4 months). There was no difference in OS; however, patients were allowed to cross over to receive bevacizumab following progression on chemotherapy alone, which may mask the survival advantage ([79]). Based on the results of this trial, bevacizumab is now FDA approved for use in combination with chemotherapy for the treatment of platinum-resistant recurrent EOC.

Low-Grade Serous Ovarian Carcinoma

The primary management of low-grade serous ovarian carcinoma, like its high-grade counterpart, is surgical with comprehensive surgical staging. However, low-grade serous carcinoma is relatively chemoresistant when compared to high-grade serous carcinoma ([43, 80]). Despite this, carboplatin and paclitaxel remain first-line adjuvant therapy in advanced disease as there is currently no better alternative. Recurrent disease can be treated with surgery, chemotherapy, hormone therapy, and targeted therapies, including MEK inhibitors. In a retrospective review of recurrent low-grade serous carcinoma, 78% of patients who had secondary cytoreduction had no gross residual disease at the conclusion of surgery, which translated into an improved PFS compared to patients who were left with gross residual disease ([81]). Similar to the adjuvant setting, low-grade serous carcinoma is also chemoresistant in the recurrent setting, with a response rate of less than 4%; however, 60% of patients did have stable disease ([82]). Numerous hormonal agents have been utilized in the treatment of recurrent low-grade serous carcinoma, with response rates that are only slightly improved compared to chemotherapy. Retrospective series have shown an overall response rate of 9%; however, similar to chemotherapy, 62% of patients achieved stable disease ([82]). Given the frequency of *KRAS* and *BRAF* mutations in this histologic subtype, a single-arm phase II trial of selumetinib, a MEK 1/2 inhibitor, was performed in recurrent low-grade serous carcinoma. The objective response rate was 15%, and 65% of patients had stable disease. Interestingly, there was no correlation between *KRAS* and *BRAF* mutational status and response to the study drug. Current trials are ongoing to evaluate therapy with MEK inhibitors in comparison to chemotherapy and hormonal therapy in the recurrent setting.

MALIGNANT GERM CELL TUMORS

Malignant ovarian germ cell tumors (MOGCTs) recapitulate normal embryonic and extraembryonic cells and structures and are derived from the primitive germ cells of the embryonic gonad. The MOGCTs comprise 2% to 3% of all ovarian malignancies, and they usually develop in girls, adolescents, and women of reproductive age. Advances in chemotherapy have yielded cure in the vast majority of patients with these tumors, and modifications in surgical technique have allowed fertility preservation in most patients ([83]). These tumors should always be considered in the differential diagnosis in a young woman with a solid ovarian mass, as the median age of diagnosis is 16 to 20 years (range 6-60 years), and the highest incidence occurs in 15- to 19-year-old girls.

The current classification of ovarian germ cell tumors includes both benign and malignant neoplasms. Most benign ovarian germ cell tumors are mature teratomas. The MOGCTs include primitive germ cell tumors, biphasic or triphasic teratomas, and monodermal teratomas (Table 31-5). Immature teratomas should be extensively sampled to determine the amount of immature neural, nonneural, and yolk sac elements and thereby malignant potential. While we continue to report grading criteria for immature teratomas using a three-tier system, we agree that a biphasic system may allow for greater consistency.

Etiology

The etiology of MOGCT is related to gonadal dysgenesis in a minority of patients. Patients with a mosaic variant of Turner syndrome including a Y chromosome

Table 31-5 World Health Organization Classification of Ovarian Germ Cell Tumors

Primitive Germ Cell Tumors	Biphasic or Triphasic Teratoma	Monodermal Teratoma and Somatic-Type Tumors
Dysgerminoma Endodermal sinus tumor (yolk sac tumor) Embryonal carcinoma Polyembryona Nongestational choriocarcinoma Mixed germ cell tumor	Immature teratoma (grades 1-3) Mature teratoma (solid, cystic, or fetiform teratoma)	Thyroid (struma ovarii) Carcinoid Neuroectodermal Carcinoma Melanocytic Sarcp, a Sebaceous Pituitary type Other

Adapted with permission from Tavassoli FA, Deville P, eds. In: *World Health Organization Classification of Tumors. Pathology and Genetics of Tumors of the Breast and Female Genital Organs*. Lyon, France: International Agency for Research on Cancer Press; 2003.

may develop gonadoblastoma ([84]). Patients with complete gonadal dysgenesis who have a 46, XY genotype and a female phenotype (Swyer syndrome) have up to a 30% risk of developing MOGCT, especially dysgerminomas, and prophylactic removal of both gonads is indicated if the diagnosis is made ([85]).

Diagnosis

The diagnosis of MOGCT may be suspected based on the young age of the patient with a solid, palpable ovarian mass, but histologic confirmation is required for the diagnosis. Eighty-five percent of patients present with abdominopelvic pain associated with a palpable mass. Other presenting symptoms and signs include abdominal distention, fever, ascites, and vaginal bleeding. Ten percent of patients present with acute abdominal pain associated with rupture, hemorrhage, or torsion of the mass. Isosexual pseudoprecocity may be caused by chorionic gonadotrophin (β-hCG) production by the tumor ([86]). Evaluation of the pelvic mass in the young patient may be aided by transvaginal ultrasound and magnetic resonance imaging (MRI). Supradiaphragmatic disease or pure choriocarcinoma is an indication for MRI of the brain ([83]).

Tumor markers may be especially helpful in MOGCT to suggest individual tumor histology, provide prognostic information, and provide a basis to follow the response of the disease to therapy (Table 31-6). Therefore, when MOGCT is suspected, these markers should be measured preoperatively. A karyotype should be performed if gonadal dysgenesis is suspected, as bilateral oophorectomy is indicated if the diagnosis is confirmed. The appropriate minimum diagnostic evaluation for the young woman with a suspicious adnexal mass should include routine blood studies, serum tumor marker analysis, chest radiography, and imaging of the abdomen and pelvis ([83]).

Management

Surgery is the mainstay of diagnosis and initial treatment of MOGCT. Laparotomy has been the standard of care, but minimally invasive surgery appears to be feasible when the tumor can be removed intact and complete staging can be performed ([87]). Patients who have completed childbearing should undergo total hysterectomy and bilateral salpingo-oophorectomy. However, most patients with MOGCT are of reproductive age, and since outcomes with conservative surgery are comparable to hysterectomy with bilateral salpingo-oophorectomy, fertility-sparing surgery should be considered in every patient of reproductive age. Whenever possible, the normal-appearing contralateral adnexa and uterus should be conserved. If both ovaries are

Table 31-6 Tumors Markers Helpful in MOGCT

Tumor	AFP	β-HCG	Lactic Dehydrogenase
Pure dysgerminoma	Normal	May be elevated	Elevated
Endodermal sinus tumor	Elevated	Normal	May be elevated
Embryonal carcinoma	Elevated	Elevated	Elevated
Choriocarcinoma	Normal	Elevated	Normal
Immature teratoma	May be elevated	Normal	Normal

grossly involved, bilateral salpingo-oophorectomy may be warranted, but this is the exception rather than the rule. Some discussion has centered on ovarian preservation with postoperative chemotherapy to treat this chemosensitive residual disease, thus allowing fertility preservation even with advanced disease or bilateral ovarian involvement. Even if both ovaries are removed, the uterus may be preserved to allow assisted reproduction with a donor egg.

Several treatment conundrums are encountered not infrequently. If a MOGCT is diagnosed postoperatively following an ovarian cystectomy for disease thought to be benign, subsequent removal of the remaining ovarian tissue may be avoided. Excellent survival has been reported in this setting, although most patients did receive adjuvant chemotherapy [88]. In addition, the occasional patient presents with widespread bulky abdominopelvic disease, and aggressive debulking surgery is followed by rapid tumor regrowth. While not yet considered standard, neoadjuvant chemotherapy after percutaneous biopsy has been increasingly utilized to allow for less-morbid, more effective, fertility-sparing interval cytoreductive surgery [89].

Staging for MOGCT follows FIGO staging for EOC (see Table 31-4). However, the extent of comprehensive surgical staging is controversial. Comprehensive surgical staging has traditionally been performed in adult patients, including peritoneal cytology, biopsies, omentectomy, bilateral pelvic and para-aortic lymphadenectomy, and removal of any suspicious tissue. In the pediatric setting, staging is typically limited to pelvic washing, tumor removal, and biopsy of suspicious implants. While proponents of limited staging cite the exquisite sensitivity of MOGCT to chemotherapy in the event of recurrence in untreated patients, we have performed comprehensive staging to administer chemotherapy up front in patients with nodal involvement and avoid chemotherapy in fully staged patients without metastatic disease. Regardless, patients with nondysgerminomatous MOGCT should receive chemotherapy unless their disease is stage IA with comprehensive surgical staging. Surveillance in low-risk patients has been proposed, and studies are ongoing.

Adjuvant Therapy

While patients with stage I dysgerminoma and stage IA grade 1 immature teratoma may be safely observed after surgery without chemotherapy, combination chemotherapy with three to four courses of bleomycin, etoposide, and cisplatin (BEP) results in the cure of most other patients with MOGCT (Table 31-7). Patients with completely resected disease usually receive three cycles of BEP, while patients with macroscopic residual disease receive four cycles, sometimes omitting bleomycin from cycle 4. Care should be taken to evaluate for

Table 31-7 Regimen for Administration of Bleomycin, Etoposide, and Cisplatin (BEP)

Following prehydration and premedications:
Cisplatin: 20 mg/m^2 per day in 1L normal saline with 50 g mannitol IV over 4 hours on days 1-5
Etoposide: 100 mg/m^2 per day in 1L 5% dextrose in normal saline IV over 2 hours on days 1-5
Bleomycin: 20 U/m^2 in 250 mL normal saline over 24 hours on day 1
OR
Bleomycin: 10 U/d on days 1-3
OR
Bleomycin: 10 U/d on days 1, 8, and 15 (United States)
OR
Bleomycin: 30,000 IU weekly for 12 weeks, with the fourth course consisting of EP alone (Europe/United Kingdom)[a]

[a]Maximum total bleomycin dose not to exceed 270 mg. Regimen repeated every 21 days.

bleomycin-related pulmonary toxicity, with periodic lung auscultation, chest radiography, and pulmonary function testing if the patient experiences symptoms. Rales, pulmonary consolidation, or a 30% decrease in the diffusion capacity of carbon monoxide prompts deletion of bleomycin from the regimen [83]. Radiation therapy is effective in the treatment of dysgerminoma but is rarely used due to the impact on ovarian function and subsequent fertility.

While most patients are cured, worse outcomes are related to advanced stage, yolk sac (endodermal sinus) tumor histology, incomplete surgical resection, and advanced age [90]. Patients with higher risk or who do not respond to BEP rapidly may be considered for alternate therapies, including paclitaxel combined with BEP (T-BEP) or dose-dense BEP [83].

Follow-up

Following treatment, patients receive imaging of the chest, abdomen, and pelvis and evaluation of tumor markers. Subsequently, they are monitored every 3 months for the first year, every 4 months for the second year, and every 6 months for years 3 to 5. We do not obtain routine imaging, although in high-risk patients transvaginal ultrasounds may be followed and initial abdominopelvic imaging may be obtained.

Treatment of Recurrent Disease

In the small percentage of patients who are thought to have a recurrence, evaluation must include repeat imaging of the chest, abdomen, and pelvis and evaluation of tumor markers, and a biopsy must confirm the diagnosis of recurrent disease since immature teratomas can recur with only mature benign elements (growing teratoma syndrome) or with benign gliosis. Both of these entities are benign and do not automatically require chemotherapy or surgical resection. In the event of true recurrence, surgical resection should be considered and appropriate salvage chemotherapy should be considered. Over half of patients who have a recurrence after 6 weeks following initial therapy (platinum sensitive) can achieve cure with VeIP (vinblastine, ifosfamide, and cisplatin) or TIP (paclitaxel, ifosfamide, and cisplatin); high-dose chemotherapy may also be administered [83]. Patients who progress during treatment or have a recurrence within 4 to 6 weeks (platinum resistant) are not curable; standard-dose VeIP may be administered, and in the event of response, high-dose etoposide and carboplatin with stem cell rescue may be given [83]. Other agents with activity include ifosfamide, taxanes, and gemcitabine.

Reproductive Outcomes

Reproductive outcomes following surgical or chemotherapeutic treatment for MOGCT are excellent, with little effect on menstrual cycling, reproductive function, conception, or childbirth. Chemotherapy-induced infertility appears to occur in 18% or less of patients treated with BEP and is unrelated to cisplatin dose. Eighty percent of women resume normal menstrual function. Long-term quality of life and psychosocial outcomes of survivors of MOGCT are also excellent.

SEX CORD STROMAL TUMORS

Sex cord stromal tumors (SCST) of the ovary comprise 7% of all ovarian malignancies and have an annual adjusted incidence rate of 2.1 per 1 million women [91]. These tumors can occur in females of all ages, but most occur in peri- and postmenopausal women. Some histologic subtypes, such as juvenile granulosa cell tumors (GCTs) and Sertoli-Leydig cell tumors (SLCTs) have a propensity to develop in adolescents; all histologic subtypes may develop in women of reproductive age. Overall, many of these tumors tend to be indolent, progressing slowly over decades.

Sex cord stromal tumors are a heterogeneous group of tumors classified in Table 31-8 [92]. The GCTs are the most common and consist of adult and juvenile forms, which differ in their histologic appearance, age of onset, and natural history. Juvenile GCTs usually affect adolescent females, may present with precocious puberty, may be associated with breast cancer, and have high mitotic activity. Adult GCTs represent 95% of GCTs, tend to occur in older women, produce estrogen, may be associated with endometrial hyperplasia or cancer, and are often quite indolent [92]. Sertoli-Leydig cell tumors arise from mesenchyme and sex cords, which recapitulate testicular development and may include various proportions of Sertoli and Leydig elements. Pure Sertoli cell tumors and pure Leydig cell tumors are benign, while tumors with Sertoli and Leydig cell components demonstrate degrees of malignant behavior and are classified based on differentiation. The benign differentiated form typically produces androgens; intermediate differentiated forms have immature Sertoli cells; and poorly differentiated forms with sarcomatoid or retiform patterns tend to be more aggressive. Gynandroblastomas are rare, tend to be virilizing, and are usually benign, but large tumors occurring in women aged 30 to 50 years may exhibit malignant behavior [92]. A sex cord tumor with annular tubules (SCTAT) may be associated with Peutz-Jeghers syndrome (PJS).

Table 31-8 Classification of Ovarian Sex Cord Stromal Tumors

Ovarian stromal tumors with sex cord elements
Adult granulosa cell tumor
Juvenile granulosa cell tumor
Sertoli-Leydig cell tumor
Gynandroblastoma
Sex cord tumor with annular tubules
Pure stromal tumors
Fibroma and thecomas: typical, cellular, mitotically active
Malignant tumors (fibrosarcoma)
Other ovarian stromal tumors
Ovarian stromal tumor with minor sex cord elements
Sclerosing stromal tumor
Signet ring stromal tumor
Microcystic stromal tumor
Ovarian myxoma
Stromal-Leydig cell tumor
Steroid cell tumors
Stromal luteoma
Leydig cell tumor
Steroid cell tumor, not otherwise specified

Etiology

The etiology for all SCSTs is unknown. However, a cytosine-to-guanine point mutation in the *FOXL2 403* gene has been identified as pathognomonic for adult granulosa cell tumor formation [93]. In addition, mutations in *DICER1* appear to be present in some patients with Sertoli-Leydig cell tumors (SLCT) and in patients with pleuropulmonary blastoma (PPB); children with SLCTs may be screened for *DICER1* mutations and thereby undergo early treatment for PPB, a potentially lifesaving intervention [94]. The SCTATs may be

CHAPTER 31

associated with PJS and potentially linked to *STK11* mutations in these patients.

Diagnosis

Most patients with SCSTs present with pelvic pain, pelvic pressure, and menstrual irregularities, including precocious puberty, menometrorrhagia, or postmenopausal bleeding ([92]). While these tumors cannot be diagnosed without histologic confirmation of surgical findings, preoperative studies such as pelvic ultrasound and analysis of certain tumor markers may suggest the diagnosis of SCST. When suspected, preoperative CT of the abdomen and pelvis is warranted. Preoperative laboratory testing should include analysis for serum hCG and routine laboratory testing.

Serum markers may be useful in the preoperative diagnosis of SCST when suspected or in establishing a baseline level with which to follow the tumor status of the patient during treatment and surveillance. Inhibin A, inhibin B, and antimüllerian hormone (AMH) are useful markers, and AMH may be highly specific for GCT in postmenopausal women or women whose ovaries have been removed. A karyotype should be obtained in cases of gonadoblastoma due to the risk of dysgenetic gonads, which should be removed based on the risk of subsequent neoplasia.

Management

Surgery remains the cornerstone of diagnosis and treatment for patients with SCSTs. While surgery has historically been performed via laparotomy, minimally invasive surgery appears to be safe and feasible for initial limited surgery and staging as well as restaging in many patients with SCSTs, as long as the tumor can be removed intact without contamination of the peritoneal cavity, using a specimen bag for removal ([92]). Staging procedures include examination of the entire abdominopelvic cavity, peritoneal washings, infracolic omentectomy, biopsy of any suspicious lesions and the diaphragmatic peritoneum, paracolic gutters, and pelvic peritoneum, but lymphadenectomy is omitted in the absence of suspicious lymph nodes due to absence of lymphatic metastasis ([92, 95]). While postmenopausal women and women who have completed childbearing should undergo total hysterectomy and bilateral salpingo-oophorectomy, young women and women of reproductive age who have not completed childbearing may undergo conservative surgery. This refers to removal of the entire involved adnexa and surgical staging. There is no role for ovarian cystectomy in definitive surgical treatment ([96]). Evaluation of the endometrium should be a part of any surgery for SCSTs as 55% of patients with GCTs have endometrial hyperplasia and 4% to 20% have endometrial adenocarcinoma ([97]). The FIGO staging for SCST is the same as that for EOCs (see Table 31-4) ([92]).

Adjuvant Therapy

Patients with stage IA and IB SCSTs do not require adjuvant therapy after surgery. Therapy for patients with stage IC disease is controversial and may include chemotherapy or hormonal therapy for patients with a high mitotic index. Patients with stage I SLCTs who have poorly differentiated tumors or heterologous elements should be treated with adjuvant chemotherapy. Any patient with advanced-stage (II or above) SCSTs should receive treatment with chemotherapy ([92]). The type of chemotherapy administered has historically been three to four cycles of BEP, but retrospective reports suggest that taxanes, especially when administered with platinum-based chemotherapy, have efficacy and less toxicity than BEP ([96, 98]). The GOG is currently comparing these two regimens in advanced-stage up front and recurrent chemonaive SCST patients.

Follow-up

Most patients with SCST are cured, but 20% have a recurrence; these patients may succumb to their disease ([92]). Tumor stage, tumor rupture, age over 50 years, and tumor size are reported prognostic factors ([99]). The SCSTs tend to have an indolent nature with a propensity for late recurrence. Therefore, patients require long-term surveillance. Our strategy is to follow patients every 3 months for the first year, every 4 months for the second year, every 6 months for years 3 to 5, then annually. At each visit, history, physical examination including pelvic examination, and tumor marker values (inhibin A, inhibin B, AMH, and sometimes CA125) are obtained; imaging is reserved for patients with new symptoms, signs, or elevated marker values.

Treatment of Recurrent Disease

Patients who have a recurrence require a biopsy to prove the initial recurrence. These patients may benefit from surgical resection in the event of limited resectable recurrent disease. Radiotherapy may also be an option. Treatment with hormonal agents may induce response or long-term stable disease. Chemotherapy utilizing BEP or taxane-platinum combinations may be useful. Most recently, bevacizumab has been shown to be an active agent in the recurrent setting ([100]).

REFERENCES

1. Siegel RL, Miller KD, Jemal A: Cancer statistics, 2015. *CA Cancer J Clin*. 2015;65:5-29.

2. Edwards BK, Noone A-M, Mariotto AB, et al. Annual report to the Nation on the status of cancer, 1975-2010, featuring prevalence of comorbidity and impact on survival among persons with lung, colorectal, breast, or prostate cancer. *Cancer.* 2014;120:1290-1314.
3. Surveillance End Results Program (SEER). *SEER Stat Fact Sheets: Ovary Cancer.* Bethesda, MD: SEER; 2014.
4. Edwards BK, Brown ML, Wingo PA, et al. Annual report to the nation on the status of cancer, 1975–2002, featuring population-based trends in cancer treatment. *J Natl Cancer Inst.* 2005;97:1407-1427.
5. Hirst JE, Gard GB, McIllroy K, et al. High rates of occult fallopian tube cancer diagnosed at prophylactic bilateral salpingo-oophorectomy. *Int J Gynecol Cancer.* 19:826-829.
6. Domchek S, Friebel T, Garber J, et al. Occult ovarian cancers identified at risk-reducing salpingo-oophorectomy in a prospective cohort of BRCA1/2 mutation carriers. *Breast Cancer Res Treat.* 2010;124:195-203.
7. Yates MS, Meyer LA, Deavers MT, et al. Microscopic and early-stage ovarian cancers in BRCA1/2 mutation carriers: building a model for early BRCA-associated tumorigenesis. *Cancer Prev Res.* 4:463-470.
8. Jarboe E, Folkins A, Nucci MR, et al. Serous carcinogenesis in the fallopian tube: a descriptive classification. *Int J Gynecol Pathol.* 2008;27:1-9.
9. Carlson JW, Jarboe EA, Kindelberger D, et al. Serous tubal intraepithelial carcinoma: diagnostic reproducibility and its implications. *Int J Gynecol Pathol.* 2010;29:310-314.
10. Lee Y, Miron A, Drapkin R, et al. A candidate precursor to serous carcinoma that originates in the distal fallopian tube. *J Pathol.* 2007;211:26-35.
11. Gates MA, Rosner BA, Hecht JL, et al. Risk factors for epithelial ovarian cancer by histologic subtype. *Am J Epidemiol.* 2010;171:45-53.
12. Tsilidis KK, Allen NE, Key TJ, et al. Oral contraceptive use and reproductive factors and risk of ovarian cancer in the European Prospective Investigation into Cancer and Nutrition. *Br J Cancer.* 2011;105:1436-1442.
13. Olsen CM, Green AC, Whiteman DC, et al. Obesity and the risk of epithelial ovarian cancer: a systematic review and meta-analysis. *Eur J Cancer.* 2007;43:690-709.
14. Collaborative Group on Epidemiological Studies of Ovarian C. Ovarian cancer and oral contraceptives: collaborative reanalysis of data from 45 epidemiological studies including 23,257 women with ovarian cancer and 87,303 controls. *Lancet.* 2008;371:303-314.
15. Menon U, Griffin M, Gentry-Maharaj A: Ovarian cancer screening—current status, future directions. *Gynecol Oncol.* 2014;132:490-495.
16. Skates SJ, Xu FJ, Yu YH, et al. Toward an optimal algorithm for ovarian cancer screening with longitudinal tumor markers. *Cancer.* 76:2004-2010.
17. Buys SS, Partridge E, Black A, et al. Effect of screening on ovarian cancer mortality: the prostate, lung, colorectal and ovarian (plco) cancer screening randomized controlled trial. *JAMA.* 2011;305:2295-2303.
18. Kobayashi H, Yamada Y, Sado T, et al. A randomized study of screening for ovarian cancer: a multicenter study in Japan. *Int J Gynecol Cancer.* 2008;18:414-420.
19. Van Nagell JR Jr, Miller RW, Desimone CP, et al. Long-term survival of women with epithelial ovarian cancer detected by ultrasonographic screening. *Obstet Gynecol.* 2011;118:1212-1221.
20. Cope L, Wu R-C, Shih I-M, et al. High level of chromosomal aberration in ovarian cancer genome correlates with poor clinical outcome. *Gynecol Oncol.* 2013;128:500-505.
21. Wong K-K, Tsang YTM, Deavers MT, et al. BRAF mutation is rare in advanced-stage low-grade ovarian serous carcinomas. *Am J Pathol.* 2010;177:1611-1617.
22. Kuo K-T, Mao T-L, Jones S, et al. Frequent activating mutations of PIK3CA in ovarian clear cell carcinoma. *Am J Pathol.* 2009;174:1597-1601.
23. Jones S, Wang T-L, Shih I-M, et al. Frequent mutations of chromatin remodeling gene ARID1A in ovarian clear cell carcinoma. *Science.* 2010;330:228-231.
24. Catasús L, Bussaglia E, Rodríguez I, et al. Molecular genetic alterations in endometrioid carcinomas of the ovary: similar frequency of beta-catenin abnormalities but lower rate of microsatellite instability and PTEN alterations than in uterine endometrioid carcinomas. *Hum Pathol.* 35:1360-1368.
25. Coward J, Kulbe H, Chakravarty P, et al. Interleukin-6 as a therapeutic target in human ovarian cancer. *Clin Cancer Res.* 2011;17:6083-6096.
26. Stone RL, Nick AM, McNeish IA, et al. Paraneoplastic thrombocytosis in ovarian cancer. *N Engl J Med.* 2012;366:610-618.
27. Anglesio MS, George J, Kulbe H, et al. IL6-STAT3-HIF signaling and therapeutic response to the angiogenesis inhibitor sunitinib in ovarian clear cell cancer. *Clin Cancer Res.* 2011;17:2538-2548.
28. Smith NR, Baker D, James NH, et al. Vascular endothelial growth factor receptors VEGFR-2 and VEGFR-3 are localized primarily to the vasculature in human primary solid cancers. *Clin Cancer Res.* 2010;16:3548-3561.
29. Bast RCJ, Badgwell D, Lu Z, et al. New tumor markers: CA125 and beyond. *Int J Gynecol Cancer.* 2005;15:274-281.
30. Steffensen KD, Waldstrøm M, Brandslund I, et al. Prognostic impact of prechemotherapy serum levels of HER2, CA125, and HE4 in ovarian cancer patients. *Int J Gynecol Cancer.* 2011;21:1040-1047.
31. Gadducci A, Cosio S, Tana R, et al. Serum and tissue biomarkers as predictive and prognostic variables in epithelial ovarian cancer. *Crit Rev Oncol Hematol.* 200969:12-27.
32. Chang S-J, Bristow RE. Evolution of surgical treatment paradigms for advanced-stage ovarian cancer: redefining "optimal" residual disease. *Gynecol Oncol.* 2012;125:483-492.
33. Vergote I, Tropé CG, Amant F, et al. Neoadjuvant chemotherapy or primary surgery in stage IIIC or IV ovarian cancer. *N Engl J Med.* 2010;363:943-953.
34. Bodurka DC, Deavers MT, Tian C, et al. Reclassification of serous ovarian carcinoma by a 2-tier system. *Cancer.* 2012;118:3087-3094.
35. Gourley C, Farley J, Provencher DM, et al. Gynecologic Cancer InterGroup (GCIG) consensus review for ovarian and primary peritoneal low-grade serous carcinomas. *Int J Gynecol Cancer.* 2014;24:S9-S13.
36. Leen SLS, Singh N. Pathology of primary and metastatic mucinous ovarian neoplasms. *J Clin Pathol.* 201265:591-595.
37. Rouzbahman M, Chetty R. Mucinous tumours of appendix and ovary: an overview and evaluation of current practice. *J Clin Pathol.* 2014;67:193-197.
38. Soliman PT, Slomovitz BM, Broaddus RR, et al. Synchronous primary cancers of the endometrium and ovary: a single institution review of 84 cases. *Gynecol Oncol.* 2004;94:456-462.
39. Rauh-Hain JA, Winograd D, Growdon WB, et al. Prognostic determinants in patients with uterine and ovarian clear carcinoma. *Gynecol Oncol.* 2012;125:376-380.
40. Ali RH SJ, Luck M, Kalloger S, Gilks CB. Transitional cell carcinoma of the ovary is related to high-grade serous carcinoma and is distinct from malignant brenner tumor. *Int J Gynecol Pathol.* 2012;31:499-506.
41. Shih I-M, Kurman RJ. Ovarian tumorigenesis: a proposed model based on morphological and molecular genetic analysis. *Am J Pathol.* 2004;164:1511-1518.
42. Malpica A, Deavers MT, Tornos C, et al. Interobserver and intraobserver variability of a two-tier system for grading ovarian serous carcinoma. *Am J Surg Pathol.* 2007;31:1168-1174.
43. Gershenson DM, Sun CC, Lu KH, et al. Clinical behavior of

stage II-IV low-grade serous carcinoma of the ovary. *Obstet Gynecol.* 2006;108:361-8.
44. Young RC, Decker DG, Wharton J, et al. Staging laparotomy in early ovarian cancer. *JAMA.* 1983;250:3072-3076.
45. Fagotti A, Ferrandina G, Fanfani F, et al. A laparoscopy-based score to predict surgical outcome in patients with advanced ovarian carcinoma: a pilot study. *Ann Surg Oncol.* 2006;13:1156-1161.
46. Nick AM, Coleman RL, Ramirez PT, et al. A framework for a personalized surgical approach to ovarian cancer. *Nat Rev Clin Oncol.* 2015;12(4):239-245.
47. Eisenkop SM FR, Spirtos NM. The role of secondary cytoreductive surgery in the treatment of patients with recurrent epithelial ovarian carcinoma. *Cancer.* 2000;188:144-53.
48. Winter-Roach BA, Kitchener H, Lawrie TA. Adjuvant (post-surgery) chemotherapy for early stage epithelial ovarian cancer. *Cochrane Database Syst Rev.* 2012:CD004706.
49. Trimbos B, Timmers P, Pecorelli S, et al. Surgical staging and treatment of early ovarian cancer: long-term analysis from a randomized trial. *J Natl Cancer Inst.* 2010;102:982-987.
50. Bell J, Brady MF, Young RC, et al. Randomized phase III trial of three versus six cycles of adjuvant carboplatin and paclitaxel in early stage epithelial ovarian carcinoma: a Gynecologic Oncology Group study. *Gynecol Oncol.* 2006;102:432-439.
51. Bookman MA, Brady MF, McGuire WP, et al. Evaluation of new platinum-based treatment regimens in advanced-stage ovarian cancer: a phase III trial of the Gynecologic Cancer InterGroup. *J Clin Oncol.* 2009;27:1419-1425.
52. Burger RA, Brady MF, Bookman MA, et al. Incorporation of bevacizumab in the primary treatment of ovarian cancer. *N Engl J Med.* 2011;365:2473-2483.
53. Perren TJ, Swart AM, Pfisterer J, et al. A phase 3 trial of bevacizumab in ovarian cancer. *N Engl J Med.* 2011;365:2484-2496.
54. Cohn DE, Kim KH, Resnick KE, et al. At what cost does a potential survival advantage of bevacizumab make sense for the primary treatment of ovarian cancer? A cost-effectiveness analysis. *J Clin Oncol.* 2011;29:1247-1251.
55. Armstrong DK, Bundy B, Wenzel L, et al. Intraperitoneal cisplatin and paclitaxel in ovarian cancer. *N Engl J Med.* 2006;354:34-43.
56. Alberts DS, Liu PY, Hannigan EV, et al. Intraperitoneal cisplatin plus intravenous cyclophosphamide versus intravenous cisplatin plus intravenous cyclophosphamide for stage III ovarian cancer. *N Engl J Med.* 1996;335:1950-1955.
57. Markman M, Bundy BN, Alberts DS, et al. Phase III trial of standard-dose intravenous cisplatin plus paclitaxel versus moderately high-dose carboplatin followed by intravenous paclitaxel and intraperitoneal cisplatin in small-volume stage III ovarian carcinoma: an intergroup study of the Gynecologic Oncology Group, Southwestern Oncology Group, and Eastern Cooperative Oncology Group. *J Clin Oncol.* 2001;19:1001-1007.
58. Katsumata N, Yasuda M, Takahashi F, et al. Dose-dense paclitaxel once a week in combination with carboplatin every 3 weeks for advanced ovarian cancer: a phase 3, open-label, randomised controlled trial. *Lancet.* 2009;374:1331-1338.
59. Katsumata N, Yasuda M, Isonishi S, et al. Long-term results of dose-dense paclitaxel and carboplatin versus conventional paclitaxel and carboplatin for treatment of advanced epithelial ovarian, fallopian tube, or primary peritoneal cancer (JGOG 3016): a randomised, controlled, open-label trial. *Lancet Oncol.* 2013;14:1020-1026.
60. Pignata S, Scambia G, Katsaros D, et al. Carboplatin plus paclitaxel once a week versus every 3 weeks in patients with advanced ovarian cancer (MITO-7): a randomised, multicentre, open-label, phase 3 trial. *Lancet Oncol.* 2014;15:396-405.
61. Chan J, Brady M, Penson R, et al. Phase III trial of every-3-weeks paclitaxel versus dose dense weekly paclitaxel wth carboplatin +/– bevacizumab in epithelial ovarian, peritoneal, fallopian tube cancer. Paper presented at GOG 262, European Society of Gynecologic Oncology Annual Meeting; 2013; Liverpool, UK. October 19-22, 2013.
62. Vasey PA, Jayson GC, Gordon A, et al. Phase III randomized trial of docetaxel–carboplatin versus paclitaxel–carboplatin as first-line chemotherapy for ovarian carcinoma. *J Natl Cancer Inst.* 2004;96:1682-1691.
63. Markman M. Maintenance chemotherapy in the management of epithelial ovarian cancer. *Cancer Metastasis Rev.* 2015;34:11-17.
64. Markman M, Liu PY, Moon J, et al. Impact on survival of 12 versus 3 monthly cycles of paclitaxel (175 mg/m2) administered to patients with advanced ovarian cancer who attained a complete response to primary platinum-paclitaxel: follow-up of a Southwest Oncology Group and Gynecologic Oncology Group phase 3 trial. *Gynecol Oncol.* 2009;114:195-198.
65. van der Burg MEL, Lammes FB, Verweij J. The role of CA 125 in the early diagnosis of progressive disease in ovarian cancer. *Ann Oncol.* 1990;1:301-302.
66. Rustin GJS, van der Burg MEL, Griffin CL, et al. Early versus delayed treatment of relapsed ovarian cancer (MRC OV05/EORTC 55955): a randomised trial. *Lancet.* 2010;376:1155-1163.
67. Friedlander M, Trimble E, Tinker A, et al. Clinical trials in recurrent ovarian cancer. *Int J Gynecol Cancer.* 2011;21:771-775.
68. Paclitaxel plus platinum-based chemotherapy versus conventional platinum-based chemotherapy in women with relapsed ovarian cancer: the ICON4/AGO-OVAR-2.2 trial. *Lancet.* 2003;361:2099-2106.
69. Strauss HG, Henze A, Teichmann A, et al. Phase II trial of docetaxel and carboplatin in recurrent platinum-sensitive ovarian, peritoneal and tubal cancer. *Gynecol Oncol.* 2007;104:612-616.
70. Rose PG, Smrekar M, Fusco N. A phase II trial of weekly paclitaxel and every 3 weeks of carboplatin in potentially platinum-sensitive ovarian and peritoneal carcinoma. *Gynecol Oncol.* 2005;96:296-300.
71. Wagner U, Marth C, Largillier R, et al. Final overall survival results of phase III GCIG CALYPSO trial of pegylated liposomal doxorubicin and carboplatin vs paclitaxel and carboplatin in platinum-sensitive ovarian cancer patients. *Br J Cancer.* 2012;107:588-591.
72. Aghajanian C, Blank SV, Goff BA, et al. OCEANS: a randomized, double-blind, placebo-controlled phase III trial of chemotherapy with or without bevacizumab in patients with platinum-sensitive recurrent epithelial ovarian, primary peritoneal, or fallopian tube cancer. *J Clin Oncol.* 2012;30:2039-2045.
73. Ledermann J, Harter P, Gourley C, et al. Olaparib maintenance therapy in platinum-sensitive relapsed ovarian cancer. *N Engl J Med.* 2012;366:1382-1392.
74. Ledermann J, Harter P, Gourley C, et al. Olaparib maintenance therapy in patients with platinum-sensitive relapsed serous ovarian cancer: a preplanned retrospective analysis of outcomes by BRCA status in a randomised phase 2 trial. *Lancet Oncol.* 2014;15:852-861.
75. Gordon AN, Fleagle JT, Guthrie D, et al. Recurrent epithelial ovarian carcinoma: a randomized phase III study of pegylated liposomal doxorubicin versus topotecan. *J Clin Oncol.* 2001;19:3312-3322.
76. Mutch DG, Orlando M, Goss T, et al. Randomized phase III trial of gemcitabine compared with pegylated liposomal doxorubicin in patients with platinum-resistant ovarian cancer. *J Clin Oncol.* 2007;25:2811-2818.
77. Markman M, Blessing J, Rubin SC, et al. Phase II trial of weekly paclitaxel (80 mg/m2) in platinum and paclitaxel-resistant ovarian and primary peritoneal cancers: a *Gynecol Oncol.* Group study. *Gynecol Oncol.* 2006;101:436-440.
78. Garcia AA, Hirte H, Fleming G, et al. Phase II clinical trial of bevacizumab and low-dose metronomic oral cyclophosphamide

in recurrent ovarian cancer: a trial of the California, Chicago, and Princess Margaret Hospital Phase II Consortia. *J Clin Oncol.* 2008;26:76-82.

79. Pujade-Lauraine E, Hilpert F, Weber B, et al. Bevacizumab combined with chemotherapy for platinum-resistant recurrent ovarian cancer: the AURELIA open-label randomized phase III trial. *J Clin Oncol.* 2014;32:1302-1308.
80. Schmeler KM, Sun CC, Bodurka DC, et al. Neoadjuvant chemotherapy for low-grade serous carcinoma of the ovary or peritoneum. *Gynecol Oncol.* 2008;108:510-514.
81. Crane EK, Sun CC, Ramirez PT, et al. The role of secondary cytoreduction in low-grade serous ovarian cancer or peritoneal cancer. *Gynecol Oncol.* 2015;136:25-29.
82. Gershenson DM, Sun CC, Bodurka D, et al. Recurrent low-grade serous ovarian carcinoma is relatively chemoresistant. *Gynecol Oncol.* 2009;114:48-52.
83. Brown J, Friedlander M, Backes FJ, et al. Gynecologic Cancer Intergroup (GCIG) consensus review for ovarian germ cell tumors. *Int J Gynecol Cancer.* 2014;24:S48-S54.
84. Brant WO, Rajimwale A, Lovell MA, et al. Gonadoblastoma and Turner syndrome. *J Urol.* 2006;175:1858-1860.
85. Jonson AL, Geller MA, Dickson EL. Gonadal dysgenesis and gynecologic cancer. *Obstet Gynecol.* 2010;116:550-552.
86. Gershenson DM. Management of ovarian germ cell tumors. *J Clin Oncol.* 2007;25:2938-2943.
87. Shim S-H, Kim D-Y, Lee S-W, et al. Laparoscopic management of early-stage malignant nonepithelial ovarian tumors: surgical and survival outcomes. *Int J Gynecol Cancer.* 2013;23:249-255.
88. Beiner ME, Gotlieb WH, Korach Y, et al. Cystectomy for immature teratoma of the ovary. *Gynecol Oncol.* 2004;93:381-384.
89. Nakamura H, Makino K, Kochi M, et al. Evaluation of neoadjuvant therapy in patients with nongerminomatous malignant germ cell tumors. *J Neurosurg Pediatr.* 2011;7:431-438.
90. Solheim O, Kærn J, Tropé CG, et al. Malignant ovarian germ cell tumors: Presentation, survival and second cancer in a population based Norwegian cohort (1953–2009). *Gynecol Oncol.* 2013;131:330-335.
91. Gatta G, van der Zwan JM, Casali PG, et al. Rare cancers are not so rare: the rare cancer burden in Europe. *Eur J Cancer.* 2011;47:2493-2511.
92. Ray-Coquard I, Brown J, Harter P, et al. Gynecologic Cancer InterGroup (GCIG) consensus review for ovarian sex cord stromal tumors. *Int J Gynecol Cancer.* 2014;24:S42-S47.
93. Shah SP, Köbel M, Senz J, et al. Mutation of FOXL2 in granulosa-cell tumors of the ovary. *N Engl J Med.* 2009;360:2719-2729.
94. Schultz KAP, Pacheco MC, Yang J, et al. Ovarian sex cord-stromal tumors, pleuropulmonary blastoma and DICER1 mutations: a report from the International Pleuropulmonary Blastoma Registry. *Gynecol Oncol.* 2011;122:246-250.
95. Brown J, Sood AK, Deavers MT, et al. Patterns of metastasis in sex cord-stromal tumors of the ovary: can routine staging lymphadenectomy be omitted? *Gynecol Oncol.* 2009;113:86-90.
96. Gershenson DM. Current advances in the management of malignant germ cell and sex cord-stromal tumors of the ovary. *Gynecol Oncol.* 2012;125:515-517.
97. Evans AT 3rd GT, Malkasian GD Jr, Annegers JF. Clinicopathologic review of 118 granulosa and 82 theca cell tumors. *Obstet Gynecol.* 1980;55:231-8.
98. Brown J, Shvartsman HS, Deavers MT, et al. The activity of taxanes in the treatment of sex cord-stromal ovarian tumors. *J Clin Oncol.* 2004;22:3517-3523.
99. Zhang M, Cheung MK, Shin JY, et al. Prognostic factors responsible for survival in sex cord stromal tumors of the ovary—an analysis of 376 women. *Gynecol Oncol.* 2007;104:396-400.
100. Brown J, Brady WE, Schink J, et al. Efficacy and safety of bevacizumab in recurrent sex cord-stromal ovarian tumors: results of a phase 2 trial of the Gynecologic Oncology Group. *Cancer.* 2014;120:344-351.

32

Tumors of the Uterine Corpus

第三十二章　子宫体恶性肿瘤

Michaela A. Onstad
Janelle B. Pakish
Karen H. Lu

中文导读

本章分为子宫上皮肿瘤、子宫非上皮源性肿瘤两部分介绍了子宫体恶性肿瘤。子宫上皮肿瘤部分重点讲述了子宫内膜癌的流行病学、危险因素、诊断、筛查、组织病理学，其中组织病理学部分详述了子宫内膜增生症、子宫内膜癌、乳头状浆液性癌、透明细胞癌、混合细胞瘤、癌肉瘤的内容；而后阐述了疾病分期、临床预后因素、病理预后因素、手术治疗、术后辅助治疗、内分泌治疗、复发后的治疗，其中术后辅助治疗根据患者疾病的特点和预后危险因素进行了危险分层，本章讲述了不同危险组患者的治疗决策；最后本章简单介绍了对癌肉瘤的定义、外科手术治疗、术后辅助治疗原则。在子宫非上皮源性肿瘤部分，本章对子宫平滑肌肉瘤、子宫内膜间质肉瘤、未分化的子宫内膜肉瘤、子宫腺肉瘤4个组织类型的肿瘤分别讲述了组织学、临床表现、诊断和治疗等内容。

EPITHELIAL UTERINE TUMORS

Epidemiology

Endometrial cancer is the most common gynecologic malignancy in the United States. In 2015, the American Cancer Society estimated there were 54,870 new cases and over 10,170 endometrial cancer–related deaths ([1]). Approximately 75% of women diagnosed with endometrial cancer are diagnosed at an early stage and have a 5-year overall survival of 74% to 91% ([2]). For women with stage III or IV disease, reported 5-year overall survival rates are 57% to 66% and 20% to 26%, respectively ([2]). This disease primarily affects women in their postmenopausal and perimenopausal years, and the average age at diagnosis is 61 years ([2]).

Risk Factors

The main risk factors for endometrial cancer are age, obesity, diabetes, and exposure to excess estrogen without adequate opposition by progesterone. This includes the historical use of exogenous unopposed estrogen therapy, the use of estrogen agonists (such as tamoxifen), and physiological states that lead to excess endogenous estrogen. Excess endogenous estrogen can be found in women with obesity, chronic anovulation, early age at menarche, nulliparity, late age of menopause, and in the setting of rare estrogen-secreting tumors.

Tamoxifen is a selective estrogen receptor modulator that is used for chemoprevention of breast cancer and as a part of adjuvant therapy for estrogen-receptor–positive breast cancer; it may also be used to treat metastatic breast cancer. It acts as an antagonist on estrogen receptors in the breast but also has a weak agonist effect on the estrogen receptors in the endometrium. These estrogenic effects on the endometrium lead to a significant increase in the risk of developing endometrial cancer, with a relative risk of 2.13 and an absolute annual risk of about 2 per 1,000 patients taking tamoxifen ([3]). In a study by the National Surgical Adjuvant Breast and Bowel Project (NSABP), women taking tamoxifen (20 mg/d) developed endometrial cancer at a rate of 1.6 per 1,000 patient years, compared to 0.2 per 1,000 patient years among women taking a placebo. At the same time, the 5-year survival rate from breast cancer was 38% higher among women taking tamoxifen compared to women in the placebo group. This suggested that the relatively small risk of developing endometrial cancer was outweighed by the greater survival benefit for women with breast cancer ([4]).

Obesity is a well-established risk factor for the development of endometrial cancer. A meta-analysis of 19 prospective studies showed that for every 5 kg/m^2 increase in body mass index (BMI), a women's risk of developing endometrial cancer significantly increases ([5]). One explanation for these findings is that women who are obese have higher levels of endogenous estrogen because of the conversion of androstenedione into estrone and the aromatization of androgens to estradiol, which occurs in the peripheral adipose tissue. There are additional proposed mechanisms for this association, including alterations in insulin signaling and insulin resistance, alterations in expression of circulating adipokines, as well as alterations in pathways involving inflammation ([6-8]). Obesity increases the risk of endometrial cancer in both post- and premenopausal women. In fact, the majority of young, premenopausal women diagnosed with endometrial cancer have a BMI greater than 30 ([9]).

Lynch syndrome is an autosomal dominant hereditary cancer syndrome characterized by an increased risk in endometrial cancer, colon cancer, and several other malignancies. It is associated with a germline defect in a DNA mismatch repair gene (MutL homolog 1 [*MLH1*], MutS homolog 2 [*MSH2*], MutS homolog 6 [*MSH6*], postmeiotic segregation 2 [*PMS2*]). Women who have Lynch syndrome have a 15% to 66% lifetime risk of developing endometrial cancer, a 15% to 68% lifetime risk of developing colon cancer, and a 1% to 20% lifetime risk of developing ovarian cancer, depending on the specific mutation involved ([10, 11]).

Diagnosis and Screening

Screening

Except for patients who have been diagnosed with Lynch syndrome, there is insufficient evidence to support screening for endometrial cancer in asymptomatic women in the general population, even those with risk factors such as tamoxifen use, history of unopposed estrogen, obesity, or diabetes. The American Cancer Society currently recommends that all women be informed about the risks and symptoms of endometrial cancer at menopause. Women should alert their physicians of any unexpected bleeding or spotting in the postmenopausal years and abnormal uterine bleeding in the pre- or perimenopausal years.

The American Cancer Society recommends yearly screening with endometrial biopsy beginning at age 35 for women who are known to carry Lynch syndrome–associated mutations, those who have a family member known to carry this mutation, or women from families with an autosomal dominant predisposition to colon cancer in the absence of genetic testing for Lynch syndrome ([12]). Prophylactic hysterectomy and salpingo-oophorectomy have been shown to be effective in decreasing the risk of endometrial and ovarian cancer and should be offered to women with Lynch syndrome after child-bearing is complete ([13]).

Diagnosis

The primary symptom of endometrial cancer is post-menopausal bleeding or abnormal uterine bleeding in pre- or perimenopausal women. A histologic diagnosis is most commonly obtained by office endometrial sampling or dilation and curettage.

Histopathology

Endometrial Hyperplasia

Women with histologic diagnoses of endometrial hyperplasia often present with postmenopausal bleeding or menometrorrhagia. The risk factors associated with the development of endometrial hyperplasia, including obesity and unopposed estrogen, are similar to those associated with endometrial cancer ([14]). The World Health Organization defined endometrial hyperplasia based on two characteristics: (1) simple or complex glandular/stromal architectural pattern and (2) the presence or absence of nuclear atypia. The presence of nuclear atypia correlates highest with the risk of developing malignancy. In this spectrum, those with simple hyperplasia without atypia are least likely to develop endometrial carcinoma, while women with complex hyperplasia with atypia are most likely to develop carcinoma. In a long-term follow-up study conducted by Kurman et al, endometrial carcinoma occurred in simple, complex, simple atypical, and complex atypical hyperplasia in 1%, 3%, 8%, and 29% of cases, respectively ([15]). A report from one meta-analysis showing a wider range of risk of cancer progression based on four prospective follow-up studies is summarized in Table 32-1 ([16]).

Endometrioid Carcinoma

Endometrioid adenocarcinoma is the most common subtype of endometrial cancer, accounting for 75% to 80% of endometrial cancer. Endometrioid adenocarcinomas are graded 1 to 3, based on degree of differentiation. Grade 1 tumors are well differentiated, composed of glands resembling normal endometrial tissue (Fig. 32-1A). In less-differentiated tumors, glandular formations are less evident or are replaced with solid areas (Fig. 32-1B). The percentage of tumor consisting of these nonsquamous or nonmorular solid areas is the criterion for grading, with grade 1 having a 5% or less solid component, grade 2 having more than 5% but less than or equal to 50%, and grade 3 having greater than 50%. Notably, the presence of nuclear atypia that does not correlate with the architectural features should lead to a one-step upgrade of the tumor.

Papillary Serous Carcinoma

Papillary serous carcinomas are highly aggressive tumors that should be distinguished from other types of uterine carcinoma. Papillary serous carcinomas tend to occur in older women, are usually present in advanced stages, and represent 1% to 5% of cases. Deep myometrial invasion, extensive lymphovascular space invasion (LVSI), and extrauterine spread are common. Intraperitoneal involvement is often observed even when the primary lesion is localized. The histologic features of papillary serous carcinoma resemble those of ovarian or tubal carcinoma. Cytologic atypia is so prominent that papillary serous carcinomas should always be graded as poorly differentiated tumors.

Clear Cell Carcinoma

Another aggressive form of uterine carcinoma, clear cell carcinoma, represents 5% to 10% of endometrial cancer cases and should also be considered a high-grade tumor. Clear cell carcinoma tends to occur in older women. Morphologically, it resembles clear cell carcinoma arising from other sites (eg, vagina, cervix, ovary), but clear cell carcinoma of the uterine corpus, unlike that of the vagina or cervix, is not associated with intrauterine exposure to diethylstilbestrol. The microscopic appearance varies and can include solid clear cell features, prominent glycogen content, and a glandular, tubulocystic, or papillary pattern. The cells have abundant clear or eosinophilic cytoplasm, sometimes containing periodic acid–Schiff-positive hyaline globules (Fig. 32-2). The

Table 32-1 Risk of Progression From Endometrial Hyperplasia to Endometrial Cancer

Hyperplastic Type	No. of Cases	Risk of Progression (%)	Mean Risk (%)
Simple hyperplasia	164	0-10	4.3
Complex hyperplasia	193	3-22	16.1[a]
Simple hyperplasia with atypia	27	7.8	7.4[a]
Complex hyperplasia with atypia	151	29-100	47.0

[a]Complex hyperplasia architecture carries a higher risk of progressing to carcinoma than does atypical simple hyperplasia.

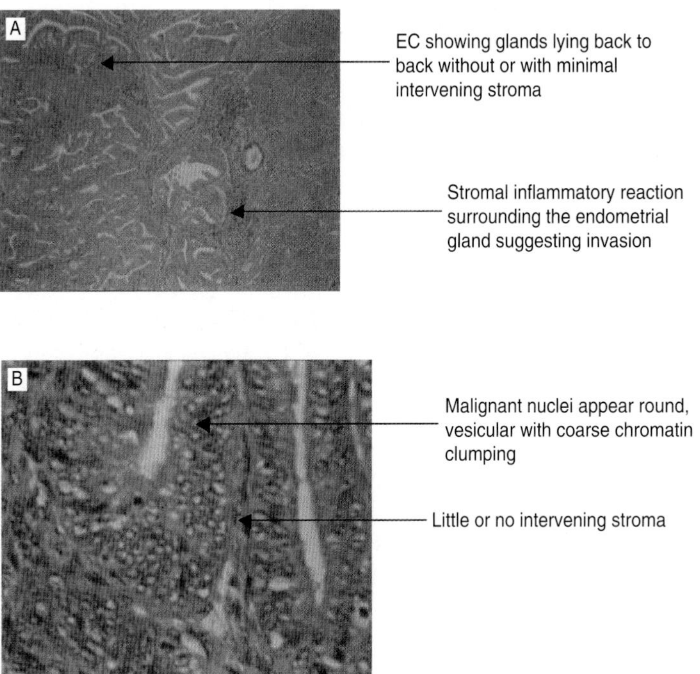

FIGURE 32-1 Endometrioid adenocarcinoma: A. Endometrial cancer with superficial myometrial invasion. The stromal inflammatory reaction surrounding the endometrial gland can aid in the diagnosis in some equivocal cases. B. High-power magnification shows malignant nuclei in the endometrial glands.

nuclei show marked atypia with frequent mitotic figures. The characteristic "hobnail" appearance is seen as cells with scanty cytoplasm and nuclei protruding into the lumen of the gland. At least half of the clear cell carcinomas are admixed with uterine papillary serous carcinoma (UPSC); this has contributed to ideas that the poor prognosis associated with clear cell carcinoma is due to the presence of UPSC.

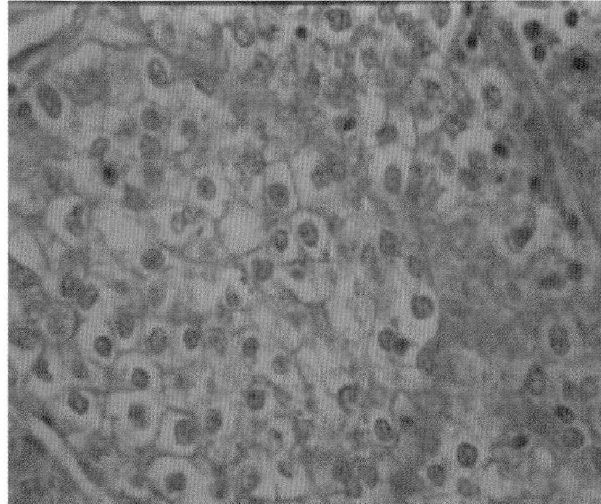

FIGURE 32-2 Clear cell carcinoma: A more aggressive type of endometrial cancer than the usual endometrioid carcinoma. The clear cytoplasmic content is glycogen rather than mucin.

Mixed Cell Type

As the name implies, mixed-cell endometrial cancers contain more than one type of tumor. The proportion of the minor component should exceed 10% for a tumor to be designated a mixed cell type.

Carcinosarcomas

Carcinosarcomas (also called mixed müllerian malignant tumors, MMMTs), consist of two components: malignant epithelial and mesenchymal tissue. In homologous MMMT, the sarcomatous component can be tissue that is normally found in the uterus; endometrial stromal sarcoma (ESS) or leiomyosarcoma are common. The so-called heterologous type of MMMT consists of tissue that does not normally appear in the uterus; rhabdomyosarcoma and chondrosarcoma are two common types ([17-19]). The MMMTs are believed to be aggressive carcinomas, rather than true sarcomas.

Staging

In 1988, the International Federation of Gynecology and Obstetrics (FIGO) committee established a surgical staging system for endometrial cancer (FIGO1988) (Table 32-2). In 2009, this staging system was updated to better stratify patients based on clinically relevant prognostic factors (FIGO 2009, Table 32-3).

Table 32-2 The 1988 FIGO Staging System

Stages	Characteristics
I	Tumor limited to uterus
IA	Confined to endometrium
IB	Invades ≤1/2 the myometrial depth[a]
IC	Invades >1/2 the myometrial depth[a]
II	Cervical extension
IIA	Involves endocervical gland only
IIB	Invades cervical stroma
III	Pelvic structures or intra-abdominal lymph node involvement
IIIA	Invades serosa or adnexa or is peritoneal cytology positive
IIIB	Vaginal metastasis
IIIC	Pelvic or para-aortic lymph node metastasis
IV	Other organ involvement
IVA	Invades bladder or rectal mucosa
IVB	Distant metastasis, including inguinal lymph node involvement

[a]Ideally, width (depth) of myometrial invasion should be measured and recorded with the depth (thickness) of the entire myometrium.

Prognostic Factors

There are clinical and pathologic factors that can be used to predict the behavior of endometrial cancer. Clinical factors include age, ethnicity, and stage of disease. Pathologic factors include histologic type, grade, depth of myometrial invasion, LVSI, and spread of tumor outside the uterine cavity, including the retroperitoneal lymph nodes.

Clinical Factors

Studies have shown that outcomes for women with endometrial cancer are more favorable among younger patients. A retrospective study showed that patients less than 45 years old were statistically more likely to have endometrioid histology, grade I tumors, and stage IA disease, while women over age 65 were significantly more likely to have papillary serous histology and grade 3 tumors. A subset analysis of patients greater than 75 years of age showed an increase in the percentage of patients with aggressive papillary serous histology, higher-grade (grade 3) disease, and advanced-stage disease compared to those less than 45 years old. Evaluation of patients with endometrioid tumors revealed a similar pattern of deeper myometrial invasion and higher tumor grade as age increased ([20]). Other studies have shown that the risks of locoregional relapse and death among patients older than 60 years were twice as high as the risks among those aged 60 years or younger ([21]).

Studies in the United States have demonstrated that white women are more likely to be diagnosed with endometrial cancer than black women. Interestingly, however, black women diagnosed with endometrial cancer are more likely to die of their disease. They

Table 32-3 The 2009 FIGO Surgical Staging for Endometrial Carcinoma

Stages	Characteristics
I[a]	Tumor confined to the corpus uteri
IA[a]	No or less than half myometrial invasion
IB[a]	Invasion equal to or more than one-half the myometrium
II[a]	Tumor invades cervical stroma but does not extend beyond the uterus[b]
III[a]	Local and/or parametrial involvement[c]
IIIA[a]	Tumor invades serosa and/or adnexae[c]
IIIB[a]	Vaginal and/or parametrial involvement[c]
IIIC[a]	Metastases to pelvic and/or para-aortic lymph nodes[c]
IIIC1[a]	Positive pelvic nodes
IIIC2	Positive para-aortic lymph nodes with or without positive pelvic lymph nodes
IV[a]	Tumor invasion of bladder and/or bowel mucosa and/or distant metastases
IVA[a]	Tumor invasion of bladder and/or bowel mucosa
IVB[a]	Distant metastases, including intra-abdominal metastases and/or inguinal lymph nodes

FIGO, International Federation of Gynecology and Obstetrics.
[a]Either G1, G2, or G3.
[b]Endocervical glandular involvement only should be considered as stage I and no longer as stage II.
[c]Positive cytology has to be reported separately without changing stage.
Reproduced with permission from Pecorelli S: Revised FIGO staging for carcinoma of the vulva, cervix, and endometrium, *Int J Gynaecol Obstet.* 2009 May;105(2):103-104.

tend to be diagnosed at a later stage, with higher-grade tumors, and are more likely to have papillary serous histology. However, after controlling for these factors as well as other comorbid factors, a higher disease-specific mortality rate among black women still exists ([22]).

Pathologic Factors

With regard to histologic subtype, papillary serous carcinoma and clear cell carcinoma are associated with worse prognosis than endometrioid carcinoma. Increasing tumor grade is associated with increased myometrial invasion, pelvic and para-aortic node involvement, recurrence, and a poorer overall survival ([23]) (Table 32-4, Fig. 32-3).

Lymphovascular space invasion, an independent risk factor for recurrence, is present in about 15% of endometrial cancer cases. Multivariate analyses have shown angioinvasion to be associated with survival in endometrial cancer regardless of disease stage. Independent of tumor grade or depth of myometrial invasion, LVSI is also associated with risk of pelvic and para-aortic node involvement and thus should lead to surgical nodal assessment or empiric radiation in patients with unstaged disease ([23]).

The depth of myometrial invasion is associated with degree of tumor differentiation, LVSI, lymph node involvement, extrauterine spread, recurrence, and overall survival (Fig. 32-4, Table 32-5). Adnexal metastasis correlates strongly with metastatic involvement of pelvic and para-aortic nodes; in one study, 32% of patients with adnexal involvement had positive pelvic nodes, as compared with 8% of those without adnexal disease ([23]). However, the alternative possibility of simultaneous ovarian and endometrial primaries must be ruled out as the surgical management and prognosis are vastly different. Up to 11% of patients with clinical stage I or II disease have lymph node involvement ([23]). The risk of para-aortic node involvement increases if the pelvic nodes are positive for tumor.

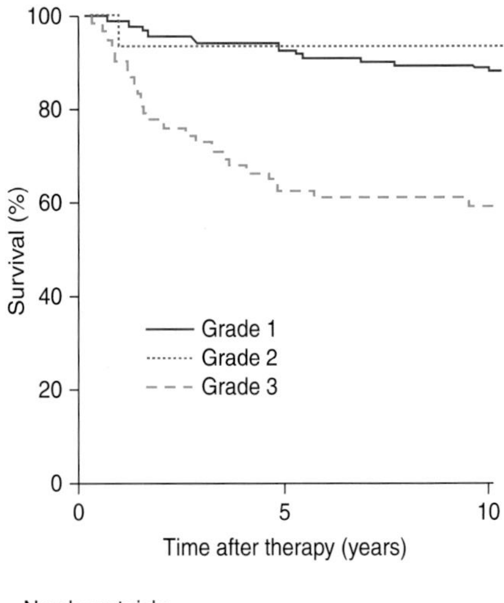

FIGURE 32-3 Tumor grade and survival in endometrial cancer. Use of the two-tier grading system is favored because of less interobserver variability and similar outcome for patients with grade 1 or 2 tumors (n = 243). (Reproduced with permission from Scholten AN, Creutzberg CL, Noordijk EM, Smit VT. Longterm outcome in endometrial carcinoma favors a two-instead of a three-tiered grading system. *Int J Radiat Oncol Biol Phys*, 2002;52:1067-1074.)

The current FIGO staging system does not incorporate peritoneal washings as the evidence for their prognostic value is weak. Positive findings on peritoneal cytology are often associated with other unfavorable prognostic factors, such as deep myometrial invasion, cervical extension, and extrauterine spread. In particular, UPSC demonstrates a high rate of positive washings. Even in clinical stage I disease that is confined to the uterus, cytologic findings have been positive in as many as 16% to 17% of cases ([24]). However, in at least two studies, the 5-year survival rates for patients with cytologically positive disease

Table 32-4 Pathologic Features of Endometrial Carcinoma Grades and Their Association With Depth of Myometrial Invasion

		Percentage of Patients With Each Depth of Myometrium Invasion			
Grade	Pathologic Features	Endometrial Only	Superficial	Middle	Deep
1	5% or less of nonsquamous solid area	24	53	12	10
2	6%-50% of nonsquamous solid area	11	45	24	20
3	>50% of nonsquamous solid area	7	35	16	42

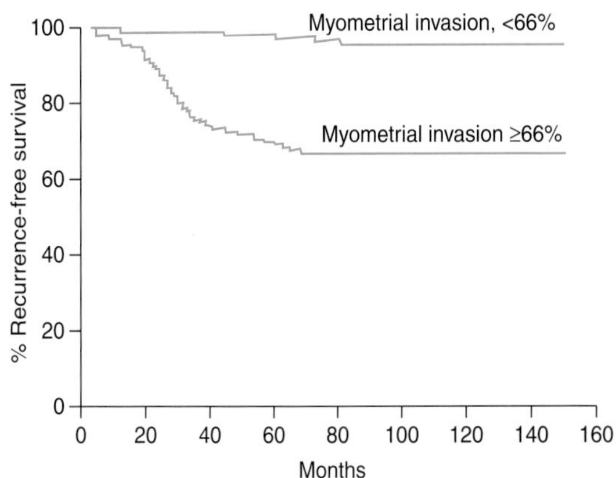

FIGURE 32-4 Recurrence-free survival rates for 282 patients with stage I endometrial cancer were significantly reduced when the depth of myometrial invasion exceeded two-thirds of the total thickness of the myometrium ($P < .001$). (Reproduced with permission from Mariani A, Webb MJ, Keeney GL, et al. Surgical stage I endometrial cancer: predictors of distant failure and death. *Gynecol Oncol.* 2002;87:274-280.)

but no other risk factors have been higher than 90% ([24]) (Fig. 32-5).

In conclusion, these prognostic factors correlate with clinical course of disease, recurrence, and risk of death. However, the relative importance of each factor is not always clear because of interrelations and interdependence among them. Results of a multivariate analysis by Zaino and colleagues of factors affecting survival in stages I and II endometrial cancer are summarized in Table 32-6 ([25]).

Evaluation

When evaluating a patient diagnosed with endometrial cancer, in addition to a history and physical examination, a chest x-ray should be performed, and imaging of the abdomen and pelvis should be considered. The measurement of cancer antigen 125 (CA125) may occasionally be useful (Fig. 32-6).

At MD Anderson, for patients with disease confined to the uterus, we recommend primary surgery with total hysterectomy and bilateral salpingo-oophorectomy, except in cases with significant medical comorbidities (see Fig. 32-6). Lymph node evaluation is based on intraoperative evaluation of grade and depth of invasion. Patients with gross cervical involvement may either undergo radical hysterectomy, bilateral salpingo-oophorectomy, with full staging, including pelvic and para-aortic lymph node sampling, or they may undergo primary radiation therapy (see Fig. 32-6). For disease that is not confined to the uterus, surgical debulking is considered (see Fig. 32-6).

Table 32-5 Association of Lymph Node Metastasis With Other Prognostic Factors in Endometrial Carcinoma

Risk Factors	Percentage of Patients With Positive Pelvic Nodes	Percentage of Patients With Positive Para-aortic Nodes
Histology		
Endometrioid carcinoma	9	5
Others	9	18
Tumor grade		
Grade 1	3	2
Grade 2	9	5
Grade 3	18	11
Depth of myometrial invasion		
None	1	1
Superficial	5	3
Middle	6	1
Deep	25	17
Tumor site		
Fundus	8	4
Isthmus or cervix	16	14
Lymphovascular space invasion		
Absent	7	9
Present	27	19
Peritoneal cytologic findings		
Negative	7	4
Positive	25	19
Extrauterine metastasis		
Absent	7	4
Present	51	23

Surgery

The standard staging procedure for endometrial cancer includes total hysterectomy, bilateral salpingo-oophorectomy, and pelvic and para-aortic lymphadenectomy. However, the indications for performing a pelvic and para-aortic lymphadenectomy for staging remain controversial among gynecologic oncologists. Some surgeons practice routine pelvic or pelvic and para-aortic lymphadenectomy for all patients with endometrial cancer, whereas others perform these procedures only for those patients with an increased risk of lymph node metastases based on preoperative and intraoperative assessments. The decision to selectively perform lymph node staging is based on multiple concerns. First, many believe there has been insufficient or unconvincing evidence in the literature that routinely

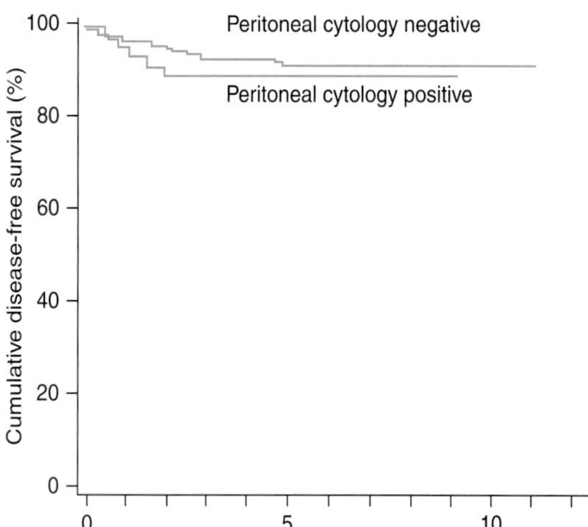

FIGURE 32-5 Five-year survival rates for patients with endometrial cancer confined to the uterus with positive findings on peritoneal cytology (91%) were not different from those with cytonegative findings (95%) (n = 280). (Reproduced with permission from Kasamatsu T, Onda T, Katsumata N, et al. Prognostic significance of positive peritoneal cytology in endometrial carcinoma confined to the uterus. *Br J Cancer*. 2003;88:245-250.)

performing lymphadenectomy for all patients results in improved overall survival. Second, performing a lymphadenectomy is associated with additional risks for the patient, including the risk of additional surgical complications and the long-term development of lower extremity lymphedema. Finally, there is a very low rate of lymph node metastases in patients with early disease, specifically those with low-grade endometrioid adenocarcinoma with less than 50% invasion of the myometrium. The absence of LVSI and a tumor size of 2 cm or less in diameter also add reassurance that the lymph nodes are not involved ([26])

Because of this, intraoperative gross inspection and frozen section of the uterus are commonly performed to evaluate the extent of uterine disease (see Fig. 32-6). This information may be used to further guide whether a lymph node dissection will be performed. The preoperative histologic findings and intraoperative pathologic findings that correlate with an increased risk of nodal involvement include grade 3 endometrioid histology; other aggressive histologies, including clear cell, serous, or squamous carcinoma; tumor invasion of

Table 32-6 Associations Between Pathologic Prognostic Factors and Relative Risk and Survival Rates

		Relative Risk of Surgical Stage I–II Tumors[a]		
Prognostic Factors	5-Year Survival Rate (%)	Grade 1	Grade 2	Grade 3
Histologic cell type				
Clear cell	67.7	5.1	3.5	2.5
Mucinous	100	—	—	—
Serous	55	2.2	3.1	4.4
Endometrioid	82.1	1.0	1.3	1.8
Endometrioid with squamous differentiation	89.4	1.2	1.0	0.8
Villoglandular	91.2	0.01	0.5[b]	41.9[b]
Myometrial invasion				
Endometrial only	92.9		1	
Superficial	87.6		0.5	
Middle	84.5		3.3	
Deep	62.6		4.6	
Lymphovascular space				
Invasion				
No	85.8		—	
Yes	60.9		1.4	
Grade				
1	91.1		—	
2	82		—	
3	66.4		—	
Peritoneal washings				
Negative	85.3		—	
Positive	56		—	

[a]Typical endometrioid grade 1 as the reference for all cell types.
[b]$P < .05$.

CHAPTER 32

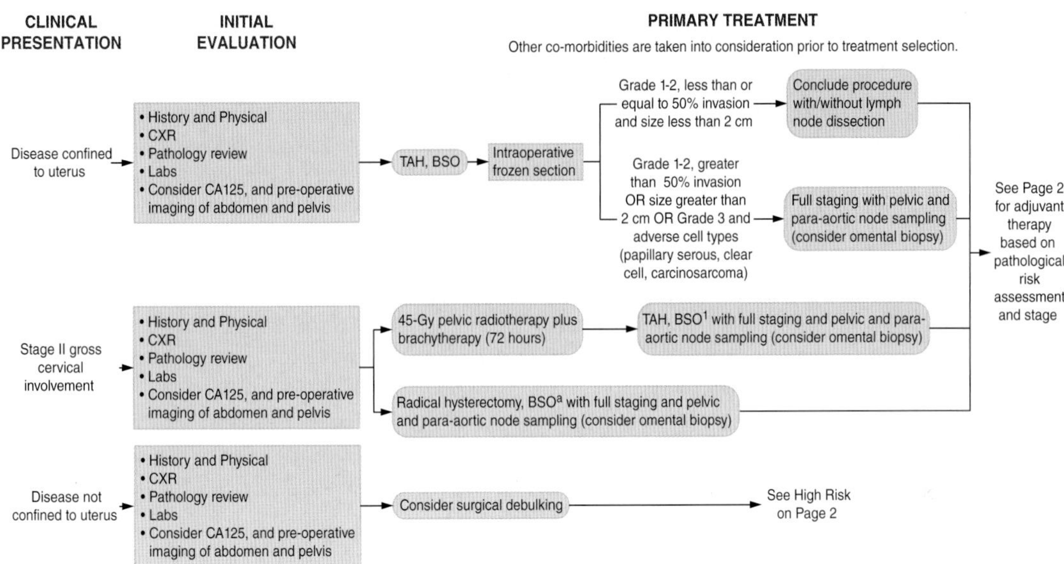

FIGURE 32-6 MD Anderson schema for initial evaluation and treatment of patients with endometrial cancer. TAH, Total Abdominal Hysterectomy; BSO, Bilateral Salpingo-Oophorectomy.

more than half of the myometrium; tumor size greater than 2 cm; and the presence of extrauterine disease ([23]). In the presence of these variables, there is a benefit for surgical resection of the pelvic and para-aortic lymph nodes (see Fig. 32-6).

In the process of lymph node evaluation, mere palpation of the fatty tissue of node-bearing areas is inadequate for the evaluation of nodal status because only about half of metastatic nodes are enlarged, and fewer than 30% can be identified as abnormal on palpation ([23]). A representative lymph node sampling or lymph node dissection should be performed to adequately evaluate the nodal basins.

The use of sentinel lymph node biopsy to identify patients with lymph node metastases without performing a complete lymph node dissection is currently under study. Theoretically, this could be performed even in patients at low risk for metastases, thereby avoiding the additional risks associated with performing a lymphadenectomy while accurately identifying those in need of additional adjuvant therapy.

Minimally Invasive Approaches

In two reports by the Gynecologic Oncology Group (GOG), laparoscopic surgical methods were compared to conventional laparotomy. The GOG LAP-2 study is the largest randomized trial ever performed in endometrial cancer. In this phase III prospective, multi-institutional, randomized study, 2,616 patients with stage I to IIA uterine cancer were assigned to laparoscopy (n = 1,696) or laparotomy (n = 920). Study end points were morbidity and mortality at 6 weeks, length of hospitalization, failure to complete laparoscopy, site of recurrence, and recurrence-free survival. Consistent with previous studies, laparoscopy required longer operative time but led to fewer postoperative adverse events and shorter hospitalization. The rate of intraoperative complications was similar. One unexpected outcome was that as many as 26% of patients in the laparoscopy arm were converted to laparotomy. Laparoscopic failure was associated with increasing age and body mass index ([27]).

In a companion report, patients undergoing surgical staging via laparoscopy versus laparotomy were assessed with quality-of-life (QOL) measures. The study's objective was to compare the QOL of patients with endometrial cancer undergoing surgical staging via laparoscopy versus laparotomy. Although patients in the laparoscopy arm had overall better QOL measures at 6 weeks postsurgery, except for better body image in the laparoscopy arm, no difference was detected between the two arms at 6 months ([28]).

Robot-assisted surgery is a newer minimally invasive technique commonly offered to women with endometrial cancer. A recent systematic review included eight studies, with a total of 589 patients undergoing surgery for endometrial cancer. When robot-assisted surgery was compared to laparotomy, it was found to be associated with lower estimated blood loss at time of surgery, lower rates of wound complications, and lower rates of other postoperative complications (including stroke, ileus, nerve palsy, lymphedema). The duration of surgery was significantly longer in robot-assisted surgery compared to laparotomy ([29]).

The decision to perform open or minimally invasive surgery depends on patient preference, the skill and experience of the surgeon, the availability of the equipment, the size of the uterus, the parity of the patient, and the patient's medical condition. At MD Anderson, minimally invasive approaches, both laparoscopic and robotic, are becoming the standard of care for the majority of women with endometrial cancer.

Adjuvant Therapy

At MD Anderson, we stratify patients according to features of the disease and various prognostic factors (Fig. 32-7). The risk group helps guide the choice of adjuvant treatment. Women with grade 1 or 2 endometrioid tumors with no myometrial invasion or LVSI are considered to have *low-risk* disease. Low-risk disease is associated with an excellent prognosis, with 5-year survival approaching 90% and a low risk for recurrence after surgery. Therefore, in general, we do not recommend adjuvant therapy for this group of patients (see Fig. 32-7). Women with stage III disease, regardless of histology or grade, and women with serous carcinoma or clear cell carcinoma at any stage are considered to have *high-risk* disease and typically undergo adjuvant therapy. *Intermediate-risk* disease, therefore, includes women with endometrial cancer confined to the uterus that invades the myometrium or the cervix. The intermediate-risk group can be further stratified based on the presence of specific prognostic factors, including outer one-third myometrial invasion, grade 2 or 3 disease, and the presence of LVSI. Women are considered to have *high-intermediate-risk* disease if they are (1) any age with all three factors, (2) age 50 to 69 with two factors, and (3) age greater than or equal to 70 years old with one factor. For patients with intermediate-risk disease, there are ongoing controversies regarding the benefit of adjuvant therapy.

Low-Risk Disease

As mentioned, most patients with low-risk disease are unlikely to benefit from adjuvant therapy. Therefore, it is not generally recommended for this group (see Fig. 32-7).

Intermediate-Risk Disease

A number of trials have addressed the question of adjuvant therapy in intermediate-risk endometrial cancers. *At this time, there is no evidence that adjuvant therapy improves overall survival for women with intermediate risk*

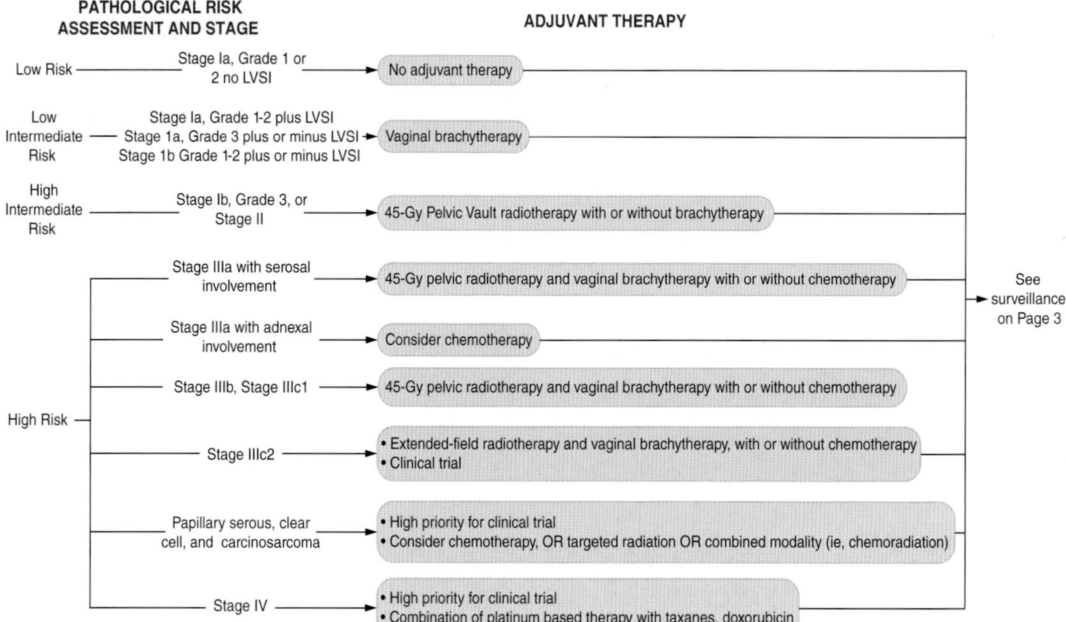

FIGURE 32-7 MD Anderson algorithm for adjuvant therapy in endometrial cancer based on postoperative pathological risk assessment and stage. LVSI, Lymphovascular space invasion.

CHAPTER 32

disease. For intermediate-risk patients, adjuvant radiation therapy reduces the incidence of pelvic recurrence without prolonging overall survival (Fig. 32-8) ([30]). Vaginal irradiation alone is adequate for preventing pelvic recurrence in patients who are at risk of only isolated vaginal recurrence. At MD Anderson, vaginal irradiation alone is offered to patients with low-intermediate risk (see Fig. 32-7). Vaginal irradiation has a higher therapeutic ratio than whole-pelvis radiation because it produces fewer long-term sequelae. The rate of recurrence after vaginal irradiation is low in women with negative or unknown lymph node status ([31, 32]). Patients with high-intermediate-risk disease at MD Anderson are offered adjuvant external pelvic radiation with or without brachytherapy (see Fig. 32-7).

Two large, randomized controlled trials compared external beam radiotherapy following surgery to no adjuvant therapy in intermediate-risk endometrial cancer. For GOG-99, 392 surgically staged patients were randomized to external beam radiation (50.4 Gy) or no treatment (control) ([31]). The study included patients with any degree of myometrial invasion, adenocarcinoma of any grade, with FIGO 1988 stages IB, IC, and occult stage II disease. The 2-year pelvic recurrence rate was 3% in the radiation arm versus 12% in the control arm (relative hazard 0.42; $P = .007$). In subgroup analysis, the treatment difference was particularly evident among the high-intermediate-risk subgroup (2-year cumulative incidence rate 6% vs 26% in radiation vs no radiation arms; relative hazard ratio [HR] 0.42). In fact, it was this study that defined the high-intermediate-risk subgroup described previously. In this study, the high-intermediate-risk subgroup was defined as those with: (1) moderate to poorly differentiated tumor, presence of lymphovascular invasion, and outer third myometrial invasion; (2) age 50 or greater with any two risk factors listed; or (3) age of at least 70 with any risk factor listed. However, the estimated 4-year survival was 92% in the radiation arm versus 92% for the control arm, which was not significantly different (HR 0.86; $P = .557$). The authors concluded that adjunctive radiation in early-stage intermediate-risk endometrial carcinoma decreases the risk of recurrence but should be limited to patients whose risk factors fit a high-intermediate-risk definition.

The PORTEC-1 (Post-Operative Radiation Therapy in Endometrial Carcinoma) study randomized 714 women with intermediate-risk endometrial cancer following surgical staging to either external beam radiotherapy (46 Gy) or no adjuvant treatment ([30]). At 5 years, local recurrence was significantly lower for patients in the experimental arm (4%) versus the control arm (14%) ([30]). At 10-year follow-up, the local recurrence rates were similar: 5% in the radiotherapy arm versus 14% in the control arm ([33]). There was no significant difference in distant recurrence rates at

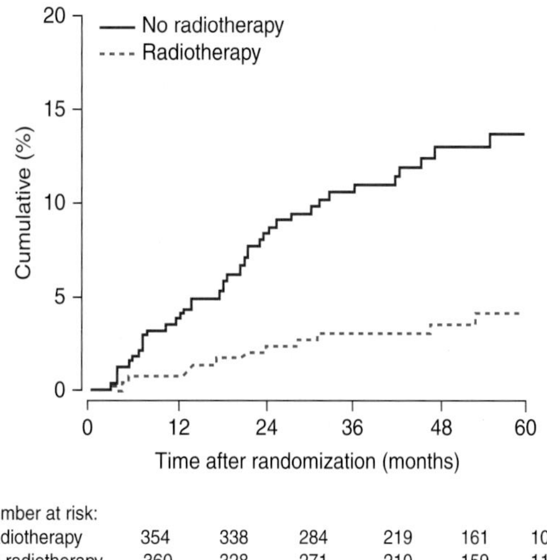

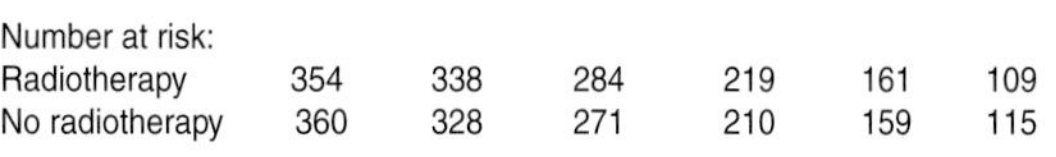

Number at risk:

Radiotherapy	354	338	284	219	161	109
No radiotherapy	360	328	271	210	159	115

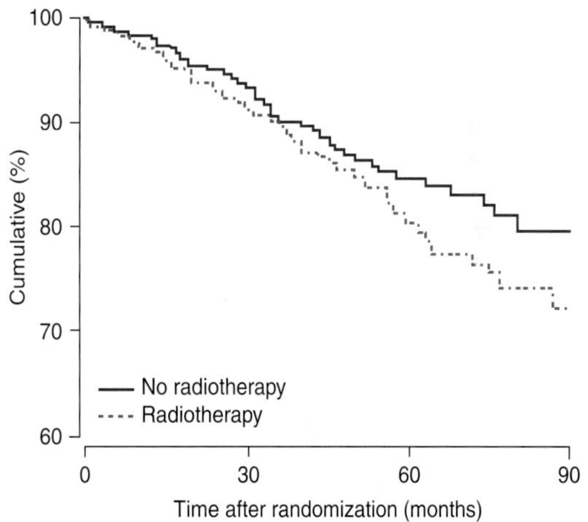

Number at risk:

Radiotherapy	354	260	111	24
No radiotherapy	360	257	125	23

FIGURE 32-8 Pelvic radiotherapy in stage I endometrial cancer. The PORTEC Study Group multicenter randomized trial of 715 patients with stage I endometrial cancer of any type (excluding grade 3 tumors or those with >50% myometrial invasion) showed that pelvic radiotherapy reduced locoregional relapse rates (4% vs 14%, *top panel*) but did not affect 5-year overall survival rates (81% radiotherapy vs 85% observation, *bottom panel*). (Reproduced with permission from Creutzberg CL, van Putten WL, Koper PC, et al. Surgery and postoperative radiotherapy versus surgery alone for patients with stage-1 endometrial carcinoma: multicentre randomized trial. *PORTEC Study Group. Post Operative Radiation Therapy in Endometrial Carcinoma. Lancet.* 2000;355:1404-1411.)

either 5 or 10 years and no overall survival benefit seen at either time point.

In both GOG-99 and PORTEC-1, patients with initial uterine-confined disease had local recurrences in the vagina, prompting evaluation of vaginal brachytherapy as a possible adjuvant therapy. Previously, Piver et al conducted a randomized controlled trial comparing (1) hysterectomy alone, (2) preoperative uterine radium followed by hysterectomy, and (3) hysterectomy and postoperative vaginal radium. This study reported no difference in local control rates, disease-free survival, or overall survival at a follow-up of 10 years ([34]).

More recently, PORTEC-2 randomized 427 women with high-intermediate-risk disease to vaginal brachytherapy or pelvic radiation. At 45 months, there were no statistically significant differences between the two treatment modalities in terms of locoregional recurrence, distant metastases, or 5-year disease-free survival. Vaginal brachytherapy was associated with a significantly lower rate of side effects, including treatment-related diarrhea and other bowel symptoms ([35, 36]).

At this time, the use of adjuvant chemotherapy to treat intermediate-risk disease is not supported by clinical evidence. Interestingly, however, it has been proposed that chemotherapy with or without vaginal cuff radiation may provide superior results to pelvic radiation in intermediate-risk patients. There are ongoing randomized clinical trials, including GOG 249 and PORTEC-3, attempting to evaluate this combined modality therapy in the high-intermediate-risk patient population.

High-Risk Disease

Women with high-risk disease have either serous or clear cell adenocarcinoma (any stage) or have pathologic stage III disease with extrauterine involvement. There are fewer high-quality studies to guide adjuvant therapy in this group. Treatment may involve radiation, chemotherapy, or a combination of the two modalities, based on histology, stage, and other factors (see Fig. 32-7). For patients with nodal disease, at MD Anderson Cancer Center (MDACC), we typically treat with chemoradiation followed by chemotherapy with four cycles of carboplatin and paclitaxel. A recent meta-analysis evaluated the use of chemotherapy alone versus radiation alone versus chemoradiation in women with stage III or IV endometrial cancer. Compared with radiation, the use of a combination platinum-based chemotherapy regimen resulted in a statistically significant improvement of overall survival (HR 0.75; 95% CI, 0.57-0.99) and progression-free survival (HR = 0.74; 95% CI, 0.59-0.92) ([37]). The MD Anderson algorithm further delineates our practice pattern for these patients (see Fig. 32-7).

Recurrent or Metastatic Disease

Women with disease outside the pelvis, either at their initial diagnosis or at the time of recurrence, are considered to have metastatic endometrial cancer. In general, these patients carry a poor prognosis and may benefit from systemic chemotherapy.

The GOG 209 study compared carboplatin plus paclitaxel to the combination of paclitaxel, doxorubicin, and cisplatin (TAP) in 1,300 women with chemotherapy naïve stage III, IV or recurrent metastatic endometrial cancer. Both regimens were administered every 3 weeks for a total of seven cycles. The data are not yet mature; however, initial findings were presented at the 2012 Society of Gynecologic Oncology Annual Meeting. Compared to TAP, carboplatin plus paclitaxel had a similar overall response rate (51% in each arm), similar progression-free survival (median of 13 months in each arm), and similar overall survival (37 months for carboplatin and paclitaxel vs 40 months for TAP). Importantly, the toxicity in the carboplatin-and-paclitaxel arm was significantly lower than the TAP arm. Peripheral neurotoxicity was 19% in the carboplatin/paclitaxel arm compared to 26% in patients assigned to receive TAP. Based on this study, carboplatin plus paclitaxel may often be preferred.

There is ongoing research about the use of biologic therapies in this setting. Single-agent bevacizumab demonstrated clinical activity and was well tolerated in GOG 229E ([38]). It is currently being studied in combination with cytotoxic chemotherapeutic regimens in GOG 86P, a recently closed randomized trial. The use of mTOR inhibitors has also been under investigation. A recent phase II trial of the mTOR (mechanistic target of rapamycin) inhibitor everolimus plus letrozole demonstrated a high clinical benefit rate and response rate ([39]). Additional research with these agents is also under way.

Endocrine Therapy

Progestins have been used to treat advanced endometrial cancer for over 50 years. These medications tend to be well tolerated with relatively minor side effects, including weight gain, thrombophlebitis, headache, and occasional hypertension. Response rates tend to be modest, ranging from 11% to 24% ([40, 41]). In GOG 121, women with no previous chemotherapy or hormonal treatment were given megesterol acetate (800 mg/d). The overall response rate was 24%, with progression-free survival of 2.5 months and overall survival of 7.6 months ([40]). Unlike in breast cancer, there does not appear to be a dose-response effect for progestins in endometrial cancer. In a randomized trial of oral medroxyprogesterone acetate (GOG 81), women who received a low-dose regimen (200 mg/d) actually had a higher response rate compared to women who received the high-dose regimen (1,000 mg/d) ([41]).

Certain characteristics improve the likelihood that a patient will have a favorable response to hormone therapy. These include having a low tumor grade (1 or 2), endometrioid histology, the presence of estrogen and progesterone receptors, having a longer disease-free interval, and being asymptomatic or minimally symptomatic.

Tamoxifen has been shown to have some efficacy in this population, with improved rates among women with hormone receptor–positive disease. Interestingly, it has been shown that short-term use of tamoxifen may lead to an increase in progesterone receptors. In GOG 153, women were given a regimen of tamoxifen for 3 weeks, alternating with megestrol acetate for 3 weeks. The overall response rate was 27%, with a median progression-free survival of 2.7 months and overall survival of 14 months ([42]). Letrozole and anastrazole are both aromatase inhibitors that have been evaluated in advanced or recurrent endometrial cancer in phase II trials. Both agents have shown a response rate of less than 10% ([43, 44]).

Surgery for Relapsed Disease

At MD Anderson, we evaluate all patients who have experienced an isolated central pelvic recurrence after radiotherapy for radical pelvic surgery or pelvic exenteration; these procedures remain the only potentially curative options that offer the possibility of long-term survival. However, given the high incidence of major postoperative complications, such as urinary/intestinal tract fistulas, pelvic abscesses, septicemia, pulmonary emboli, and cerebrovascular accidents, we consider only selected patients with isolated central recurrences for this treatment.

Postoperative Surveillance

There are no prospective studies to guide frequency of postoperative follow-up. At MD Anderson, for patients with low-risk disease, we schedule office visits every 6 months for the first year and annually during years 2 to 5. For patients with intermediate- and high-risk disease, we schedule office visits every 3 months for year 1, every 4 months for year 2, and every 6 months for years 3 to 5 (Fig. 32-9). At each visit, patients undergo a physical and pelvic examination. Performing routine vaginal cytology in endometrial cancer survivors is not recommended by the SGO. This is because multiple studies have suggested that Papanicolaou tests are not as effective in detecting endometrial cancer recurrences compared to physical examination alone ([45, 46]) and are costly and inefficient ([47]). In one of these studies, abnormal vaginal cytology had a sensitivity of 40% and specificity of 88% for detecting a vaginal recurrence. The positive predictive value was 7.3%, and negative predictive value was 98.4% ([46]).

Serum CA125 level measurements may be helpful for certain patients. In patients with elevated serum CA125 levels at diagnosis, they can be used as a marker for recurrent disease. In one study, among patients with advanced endometrial cancer who initially had high CA125 levels, 26% to 58% showed elevated CA125 levels at recurrence ([48]). The use of serial CA125 assays is most beneficial in diagnosing recurrence in a high-risk population, although there have been no studies to show that their use improves survival. False elevations may occur following radiation therapy.

Hormone Replacement Therapy Following Treatment

The use of estrogen replacement therapy in women who have been treated for endometrial cancer is controversial. Most of the evidence regarding the effects of hormone replacement therapy in women with previously treated endometrial cancer comes from retrospective studies. In one study, Chapman et al found no significant difference in disease-free survival rates between women who used estrogen replacement therapy and those who did not ([49]). However, in this study, the group that used estrogen had earlier-stage disease with less depth of invasion compared to the control group. A subsequent cohort study by Suriano et al, who matched cases for tumor status and treatment, also found lower recurrence rates and longer disease-free survival among women who used estrogen ([50]). Notably, 49% of patients in the estrogen replacement group in that study were also given progestin, which might have influenced the apparent improvement in outcome.

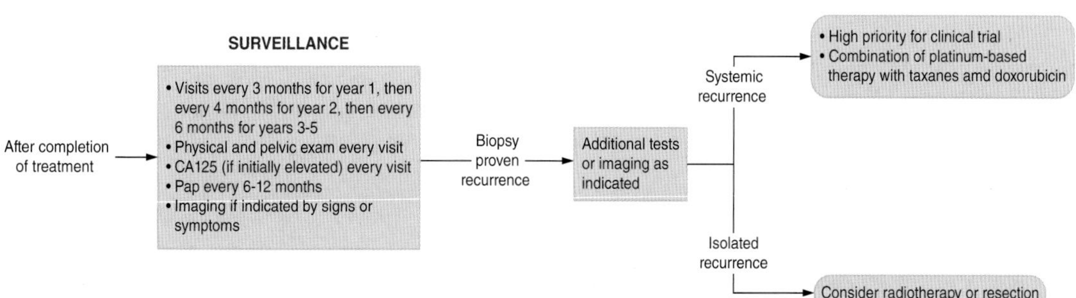

FIGURE 32-9 Sample surveillance protocol for patients with intermediate- and high-risk disease.

In a study reported in 2006, the GOG conducted a double-blind, randomized, phase III trial to evaluate the safety of estrogen replacement therapy following treatment for endometrial cancer (GOG 137) ([51]). Within 20 weeks following surgery, 1,236 women with a history of stage I or occult stage II endometrial cancer were enrolled. All enrolled patients had an indication for treatment with estrogen replacement therapy, including hot flashes, vaginal atrophy, increased risk of cardiovascular disease, or an increased risk of osteoporosis, and were randomized to receive estrogen replacement or placebo for 3 years following surgery. This study closed early when the results of the Women's Health Initiative (WHI) study showed increased overall risks in the estrogen and progestin arm ([52]). Based on the results of the WHI study, GOG 137 closed prematurely, and the study was left with insufficient power to detect a difference in patients with intermediate- or high-risk early endometrial cancers. The results of this study are inconclusive. However, the authors noted that in the low-risk population, the absolute recurrence rate (2.1%) was low. The relative risk of recurrence/death in the estrogen replacement therapy group was 1.27 compared with the placebo group (80% CI, 0.916-1.77).

At MD Anderson, we approach the use of estrogen replacement therapy on an individual basis. Overall risk of disease recurrence in low-risk patients is low, even in the setting of exogenous estrogen replacement. Therefore, estrogen replacement therapy may be considered for this population. If adjuvant therapy is given following surgery, we recommend a 6- to 12-month waiting period prior to initiation of hormone replacement therapy.

Carcinosarcomas

Carcinosarcomas, or MMMTs, account for less than 5% of malignant neoplasms of the uterus ([53-57]). The gross appearance of a polypoid carcinosarcoma mass protruding into the endometrial cavity is shown in Fig. 32-10. Although not pathognomonic of carcinosarcoma, this feature in a postmenopausal woman should alert the clinician to the possibility of carcinosarcoma.

Carcinosarcomas, although historically classified as a sarcoma, are now thought to represent a dedifferentiated variety of endometrial carcinoma ([58]). Epidemiologically, carcinosarcomas usually appear in older women aged 60 or above ([53, 54, 59]).

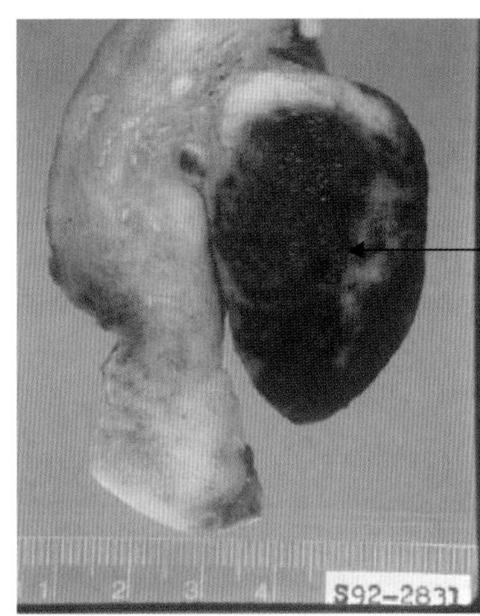

FIGURE 32-10 Gross appearance of a fleshy hemorrhagic polypoid MMMT protruding into the endometrial cavity in a hemiuterus specimen. Such tumors, which typically present with vaginal bleeding, must be distinguished from submucous myoma. Several endometrial tissue biopsies are sometimes needed for diagnosis because of the necrotic and hemorrhagic nature of this tumor.

Treatment

Surgery

Carcinosarcoma is an aggressive type of endometrial carcinoma, and surgical management of carcinosarcoma includes total abdominal hysterectomy with bilateral salpingo-oophorectomy and pelvic and aortic lymph node dissection ([60-63]). Peritoneal cytology, omentectomy, and peritoneal biopsies are also recommended ([60, 64-67]). Approximately 20% to 60% of patients will have more advanced disease during surgical staging ([55, 68, 69]). A recent study reported that in patients with stages I to III uterine carcinosarcomas, 5-year overall survival, disease-free survival, and median survival were significantly improved for patients receiving lymph node dissection compared to those who did not ([70]). In regard to the role of cytoreductive surgery in carcinosarcoma, a recent series of 44 patients demonstrated increased overall survival in those patients who had a complete cytoreductive surgery versus those that had residual disease (52.3 vs 8.6 months, respectively) ([71]). Complete cytoreductive surgery should be attempted, when possible, in patients with carcinosarcoma.

Adjuvant Therapy

Adjuvant therapy for stage IA tumors is left to the discretion of the provider as studies have been inconclusive, and the benefit of adjuvant therapy in these patients is unclear ([72, 73]). A phase III study by the European Organization for Research and Treatment of Cancer of radiotherapy versus observation in early-stage uterine sarcomas showed a trend toward improved local control but higher rates of distant recurrence in carcinosarcomas ([73]). There was also no significant difference seen in overall survival ([73]). Another study of adjuvant therapy in early-stage carcinosarcomas showed treatment with chemotherapy to significantly increase progression-free survival; however, overall survival was not significantly increased ([72]).

For stage IB and greater carcinosarcomas, adjuvant chemotherapy is generally recommended. A meta-analysis showed improved overall survival (HR 0.75; 95% CI 0.60-0.94) and reduced disease progression (HR 0.72; 95% CI, 0.58-0.90) with combination chemotherapy versus single-agent ifosfamide ([74-76]). Combination regimens included ifosfamide plus paclitaxel or cisplatin ([76]). A phase II study of combination carboplatin and paclitaxel also showed an overall response rate of 54% and median progression-free survival of 7.6 months ([77]). A phase III study, GOG 261, is currently being conducted to further evaluate combination chemotherapy. This study compares combination ifosfamide and paclitaxel to carboplatin and paclitaxel in patients with stage I through IV previously untreated carcinosarcomas (NCT00954174). Examples of these combination chemotherapy regimens are shown in Table 32-7.

NONEPITHELIAL UTERINE TUMORS

Uterine sarcoma is uncommon, accounting for only 3% to 9% of all tumors arising from the uterine corpus ([55, 58, 68]). Most uterine sarcomas originate from mesodermal tissue, although some are derived from specialized müllerian mesenchyme, such as endometrial stroma, and a few originate from nonspecific or nonmüllerian mesenchyme (eg, smooth or skeletal muscle, vessels, or lymphoid tissue). The three most common types of uterine sarcoma are leiomyosarcoma, endometrial stromal sarcoma (ESS), and adenosarcomas. Overall, uterine sarcomas are aggressive tumors with a 5-year overall survival rate of 17.5% to 54.7% ([78]).

The 2009 FIGO staging system includes three classifications for staging uterine sarcomas (Table 32-8) ([79]).

EPIDEMIOLOGY

Leiomyosarcoma and ESS usually affect women in their early 50s. Adenosarcomas have been reported in women 14 to 84 years old; the median age at appearance is in the late 50s ([80-82]).

Although uterine sarcoma differs somewhat from endometrial cancer in its clinical and pathologic characteristics, some risk factors—such as hypertension, diabetes mellitus, and obesity—are common to both. Previous history of pelvic irradiation has been associated with carcinosarcomas and undifferentiated sarcomas, occurring in 2% to 29% of patients so exposed at an interval ranging from 1 to almost 40 years ([83, 84]). Prior exposure to pelvic radiation, however, is not felt to be associated with leiomyosarcomas ([84]). Although the link between estrogen and endometrial cancer is well established, no such clear relationship is evident for estrogen and uterine sarcoma. An association between tamoxifen use and uterine sarcoma was confirmed in a study by Bergman et al, showing increased numbers of uterine sarcomas among women taking tamoxifen and sarcomas constituting about 10% of total malignancies in these cases ([85]).

Leiomyosarcoma

Histology

Leiomyosarcomas represent only 1% to 2% of uterine malignancies; however, they are the most frequent of the uterine sarcomas ([55-58, 86, 87]). Gross features of leiomyosarcoma (Fig. 32-11) are typified by variegation at the cut surface (unlike the whorllike surface typical of a benign leiomyoma).

Cells are spindle shaped and arranged in fascicles with eosinophilic cytoplasm. The nuclei are usually elongated with rounded ends, appearing hyperchromatic with coarse chromatin and prominent

Table 32-7 Drug Combinations Used to Treat Uterine Carcinosarcomas

Type of Tumor	Drug Regimen	First Author and Year of Study (Reference)	No. of Patients	Intent	Results
Carcinosarcoma	Ifosfamide vs ifosfamide + cisplatin	Sutton, 2000 (154)	194	Pall	36% vs 54%, median PFS 4 vs 6 months ($P < .05$)
	Ifosfamide vs ifosfamide + paclitaxel	Homesley, 2007 (155)	88	Pall	OR 29% vs 45%
	Paclitaxel + carboplatin	Powell, 2010 (157)	46	Pall	OR 54%

OR, overall response rate; Pall, palliative; PFS, progression-free survival.

Table 32-8 FIGO Staging for Uterine Sarcomas

Leiomyosarcomas and Endometrial Stromal Sarcomas[a]	
Stage	**Definition**
I	Tumor limited to uterus
IA	≤5 cm
IB	≥5 cm
II	Tumor extends beyond the uterus, within the pelvis
IIA	Adnexal involvement
IIB	Involvement of other pelvic tissues
III	Tumor invades abdominal tissues (not just protruding into the abdomen)
IIIA	One site
IIIB	More than one site
IIIC	Metastasis to pelvic and/or para-aortic lymph nodes
IV	
IVA	Tumor invades bladder and/or rectum
IVB	Distant metastasis
Adenosarcomas	
Stage	**Definition**
I	Tumor limited to uterus
IA	Tumor limited to endometrium/endocervix with no myometrial invasion
IB	Less than or equal to half myometrial invasion
IC	More than half myometrial invasion
II	Tumor extends beyond the uterus, within the pelvis
IIA	Adnexal involvement
IIB	Involvement of other pelvic tissues
III	Tumor invades abdominal tissues (not just protruding into the abdomen)
IIIA	One site
IIIB	More than one site
IIIC	Metastasis to pelvic and/or para-aortic lymph nodes
IV	
IVA	Tumor invades bladder and/or rectum
IVB	Distant metastasis
Carcinosarcomas	
Carcinosarcomas should be staged as carcinomas of the endometrium.	

[a]*Note*: Simultaneous endometrial stromal sarcomas of the uterine corpus and ovary/pelvis in association with ovarian/pelvic endometriosis should be classified as independent primary tumors.
FIGO, International Federation of Gynecology and Obstetrics.
Reproduced with permission from Prat J: FIGO staging for uterine sarcomas, *Int J Gynaecol Obstet* 2009 Sep;106(3):277.

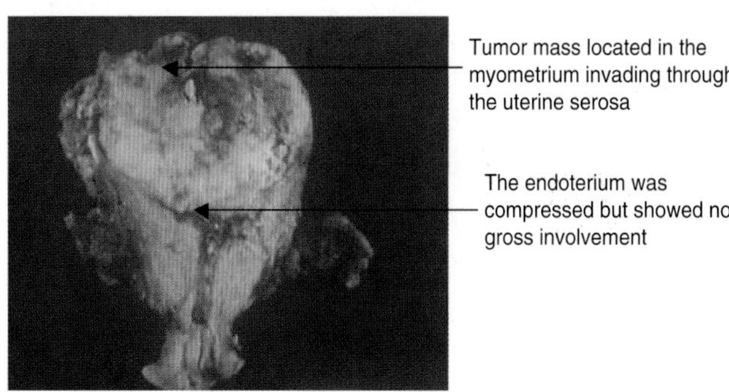

FIGURE 32-11 Gross appearance of a leiomyosarcoma in the upper uterus. The cut surface shows a grayish-tan tumor with hemorrhage and necrosis, without the whorllike appearance typical of benign leiomyoma. The mass clearly involves most of the myometrium but not the endometrium.

nucleoli. The most important criterion for the diagnosis of leiomyosarcoma is a high mitotic rate, generally exceeding 15 mitotic figures per 10 high-power fields. Other features, such as extrauterine extension, large size, and infiltrating border, necrosis, and atypical mitotic figures can also aid in the diagnosis ([58]).

Other variants of leiomyosarcoma include myxoid and epithelioid leiomyosarcoma. In myxoid leiomyosarcoma, tumor cellularity is low, cells are separated by myxoid material, and the tumor cells are still characterized by nuclei atypia and high mitotic index ([58, 88, 89]). The tumor cells in epithelioid leiomyosarcoma, in contrast, exhibit epithelioid features distinct from the usual characteristics of leiomyosarcoma ([90]).

Smooth Muscle Tumor of Uncertain Malignant Potential

Uterine smooth muscle tumors with histologic features of necrosis, nuclear atypia, or mitoses that do not meet all diagnostic criteria for leiomyosarcoma fall into the category of smooth muscle tumor of uncertain malignant potential (STUMP) ([91]). The STUMPs are a group of smooth muscle tumors for which a diagnosis of sarcoma cannot be made because of their uncertain malignant characteristics. Most of these tumors are associated with favorable prognosis, and only follow-up of the patients is recommended ([92]). In a study conducted at MD Anderson of 41 cases of STUMP, the recurrence rate was 7%. One of the three recurrences was a leiomyosarcoma; the others were STUMPs ([93]).

Clinical Presentation

Vaginal bleeding is the most common presenting symptom of uterine sarcomas. Other symptoms, such as back pain, urinary retention or hematuria, gastrointestinal symptoms, or weight loss may indicate an invading or metastasizing tumor ([94-96]).

Diagnosis

Definitive diagnosis of uterine sarcomas is usually made following hysterectomy, with the diagnosis based on histologic examination. Methods utilizing pulsed Doppler ultrasonography to preoperatively distinguish between a benign leiomyoma and uterine sarcoma are reported, but not clinically useful ([97]). Although useful for detecting extrauterine disease, imaging studies such as computed tomography and magnetic resonance imaging are not specific for diagnosing sarcomas ([98]).

Prognosis and Clinical Course

Many prognostic factors affect outcome in uterine sarcoma, but the most important is the clinical stage at presentation ([56, 87, 99-102]). Disease stage directly affects disease-free and overall survival rates ([56, 102, 103]).

Leiomyosarcomas are aggressive tumors with a recurrence rate of 50% to 70% even at early stages ([68]). The overall 5-year survival rate ranges from 15% to 25%, and the 5-year survival rate for patients with stages I and II is 40% to 70% ([104, 105]). There has been no consensus on prognostic indicators for leiomyosarcoma. Previous studies have reported mitotic index, cellular atypia, vascular invasion, and tumor size to correlate with survival.

Treatment

Surgery

Surgery remains the mainstay of treatment for uterine sarcoma, regardless of histologic type. However, there is some controversy regarding the need for oophorectomy or lymph node dissection for each subtype of uterine sarcoma. In general, hysterectomy, including oophorectomy with or without lymph node dissection, is the treatment of choice. In addition, morcellation should not be utilized in women undergoing surgery for uterine sarcoma or suspected uterine sarcoma.

Oophorectomy for early-stage leiomyosarcomas, particularly in premenopausal women, is controversial, as the incidence of adnexal metastases is low ([68]). In one study, multivariate analysis showed that oophorectomy for leiomyosarcoma was associated with significantly worse disease-specific survival. Furthermore, case-control investigations implied that ovarian preservation does not adversely affect survival ([106]). In another study, ovarian metastases were found in about 10% of all cases, despite most having been detected at an early stage ([107]). Hence, the choice of oophorectomy for the treatment of early-stage leiomyosarcoma should be judged on an individual basis.

The need for lymph node dissection is also controversial. Leiomyosarcoma has substantially lower risk of nodal involvement than clinical stage I or stage II endometrial cancer with other risk factors. A GOG study of early-stage sarcoma found that nodal metastases were present in only 3.5% of leiomyosarcoma cases, and the pelvic nodes were twice as likely to be involved as the para-aortic nodes ([94]). However, the patients in this series underwent lymph node sampling rather than intended dissection, so the reported incidence may be falsely low. Goff et al found lymph node involvement in about 27% of leiomyosarcoma cases, but only in those cases that involved recurrent or disseminated intraperitoneal disease ([94]). Two more recent studies identified lymph node metastases in 7% to 11% of patients who underwent lymph node dissection ([106, 107]). In the series by Kapp et al, the 5-year disease-specific survival rate was 26% in patients who had positive lymph nodes compared with 64% in those who had negative nodes ([107]).

Adjuvant Therapy

For early-stage leiomyosarcomas, there has been no clear benefit shown for adjuvant chemotherapy ([108-110]). In these patients, surveillance versus referral to a clinical trial are reasonable treatment options. Currently, the GOG is conducting a study of stage I completely resected leiomyosarcomas comparing adjuvant chemotherapy to observation (GOG 277). The chemotherapy arm consists of gemcitabine on days 1 and 8 and docetaxel on day 8 repeated every 21 days for up to four cycles (NCT01533207).

Advanced-stage leiomyosarcomas, on the other hand, have a high risk of recurrence, and individuals so affected are typically offered adjuvant therapy. We work closely with our sarcoma medical oncology colleagues for treatment recommendations. Combination chemotherapy, specifically, for leiomyosarcoma improves response rates. Various combinations have been investigated, with response rates ranging from 18% to 53% ([109, 111-114]). The two most common combination regimens used at MD Anderson are doxorubicin plus ifosfamide or gemcitabine plus paclitaxel. Examples of these combination chemotherapies are shown in Table 32-9.

ENDOMETRIAL STROMAL SARCOMA

Histology

Endometrial stromal sarcoma accounts for about 23% of all uterine sarcomas ([53-57]). The ESSs originate from endometrial stromal cells that invade the myometrium. Low- and high-grade variants differ in their clinical behavior. Gross features of a low-grade ESS presenting as multiple, small, lobulated tumor masses in the myometrium are shown in Fig. 32-12A.

In fresh specimens, tumor invading the lymphovascular spaces can sometimes be compressed out of the vascular lumen, giving a vermiform appearance. Tumor cells resemble endometrial stromal cells during the proliferative phase of the menstrual cycle and are monotonous and of uniform shape and size ([93]). The presence of spiral arteriole-like vessels is a characteristic finding of ESS, as is the propensity of the tumor cells to invade the lymphovascular spaces (Fig. 32-12B).

Endometrial stromal sarcoma tumors contain both estrogen and progesterone receptors ([58]). In addition, these tumors are generally positive for CD10 and frequently have a t(1;17) chromosomal translocation that expresses a fusion protein composed of JAZF1 and JJAZ1 ([58]).

Clinical Presentation

Like leiomyosarcomas, vaginal bleeding is the most common presenting symptom. Another common presenting symptom in ESS and adenosarcoma is the appearance of a prolapsed polypoid mass through the cervical os ([94-96]).

Prognosis and Clinical Course

Low-grade ESSs are indolent tumors ([115]). Generally, patients with ESS have favorable prognoses; however, recurrence can appear late after primary diagnosis and treatment, even in stage I disease ([116, 117]). The FIGO stage, depth of myometrial invasion, tumor grade, positive margins, and patient characteristics such as age, race, and menopausal status have been reported to be prognostic factors ([53, 118-120]). Mitotic activity and cytologic atypia were found to be important by some ([53, 104, 121]) but not by others ([122, 123]). Extrauterine and nodal disease is prevalent in ESS.

Treatment

Surgery

Initial treatment for ESS is largely surgical, and hysterectomy with bilateral salpingo-oophorectomy is

Table 32-9 Drug Combinations Used to Treat Leiomyosarcomas

Type of Tumor	Drug Regimen	First Author and Year of Study (Reference)	No. of Patients	Intent	Results
Leiomyosarcoma	Dox vs dox + dacarbazine	Omura, 1983 (111)	48	Pall	OR 25% vs 30%
	Dox + ifosfamide	Sutton, 1996 (113)	33	Pall	OR 30.3%
	Eto + hydroxyurea + dacarbazine	Currie, 1996 (112)	39	Pall	OR 18.4%
	Mitomycin C + dox + cisplatin	Edmonson, 2002 (114)	23	Pall	OR 23%
	Gemcitabine + docetaxel	Hensley, 2009 (109)	25	Adj	2-year PFS 45%

Adj, adjuvant; dox, doxorubicin; eto, etoposide; OR, overall response rate; Pall, palliative; PFS, progression-free survival.

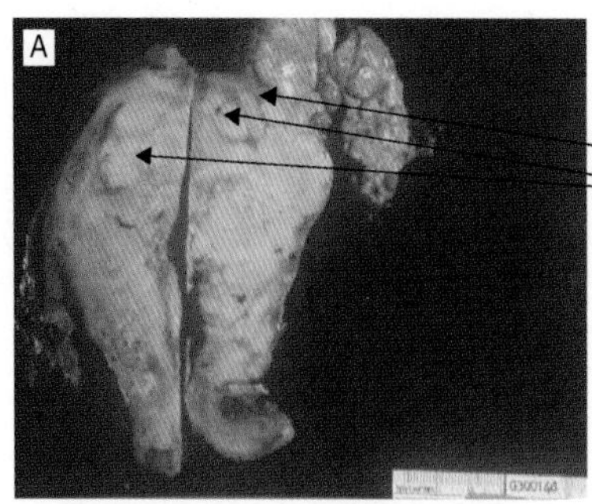

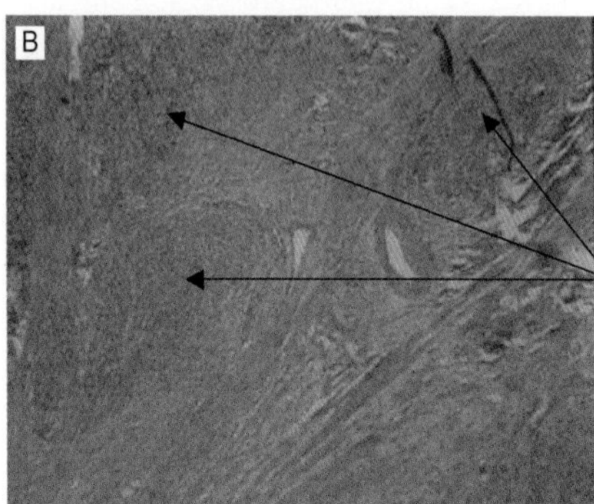

FIGURE 32-12 A. Gross appearance of an endometrial stromal sarcoma infiltrating most of the myometrium. The lobulated appearance corresponds with the presence of tumor in the lymphovascular spaces, as verified on microscopy in panel B. B. Endometrial stromal sarcoma cells with invasion of the intralymphatic spaces.

recommended. Endometrial stromal sarcoma is often sensitive to hormones, and patients with intact ovaries may be at a higher risk for recurrence ([124-127]). However, there is no consensus on the absolute need for oophorectomy in early-stage ESS. In a study by Li et al, bilateral salpingo-oophorectomy did not appear to affect time to recurrence or overall survival in patients with stage I ESS ([125]). In a recent report of 384 women with low-grade ESS, lymph node metastasis and ovarian preservation were not significant prognostic factors for survival in this study. Lymph node metastasis was found in 7% of patients ([126]). In two smaller series, only two of the nine patients with ESS who had undergone lymph node sampling were found to have lymph node metastases ([94, 121]). The choice of lymph node dissection for ESS should be individualized.

Adjuvant Therapy

Observation is generally recommended for stage I ESS. More advanced stages are typically offered additional therapy after surgical resection, although the data are limited given this rare tumor type. As these tumors typically express estrogen and progesterone receptors, hormonal therapy is considered first-line treatment. Limited retrospective data have reported response of metastatic and recurrent ESS to hormonal agents such as medroxyprogesterone acetate or letrazole ([124, 128]). Tamoxifen is contraindicated in the treatment of ESS due to its stimulatory effect on the endometrial stromal cells ([128]).

Because of its rarity and because low-grade ESS usually responds well to hormonal therapy, ESS has not been well studied in chemotherapeutic trials. A cisplatin-based chemotherapy regimen was tested in a study of uterine sarcoma in which about 10% of the cases were ESS ([129]). Despite a relatively high response rate of 54%, the regimen was too toxic to be clinically useful. Radiotherapy may help to improve local control, but its role as adjuvant therapy in ESS is unclear ([130]).

Undifferentiated Endometrial Sarcoma

Histology

In undifferentiated endometrial sarcomas, previously considered high-grade ESS, the tumor cells tend to be larger, with more vesicular nuclei, coarse clumps of chromatin, and more prominent nucleoli ([131]). Mitotic counts are usually low in low-grade ESS, and this is the principal criterion for distinguishing between the low- and high-grade forms ([131]). However, numerous mitotic figures can be present in otherwise-typical low-grade tumors, and high-grade tumors can have only a few mitotic figures ([123, 132]). Flow cytometry with DNA ploidy seems to be associated more with the behavior of the tumor than with mitotic count ([133]). In the 2002 classification of ESS by the World Health Organization, high-grade tumors were considered as pleomorphic or undifferentiated sarcoma rather than as a type of ESS because of their distinctive and aggressive clinical behavior. Undifferentiated sarcomas generally stain for Ki67, p16, and p53 and not for estrogen and progesterone receptors. These tumors also do not have any known chromosomal abnormalities ([58]).

Prognosis and Clinical Course

In contrast to low-grade ESS, individuals with undifferentiated sarcomas have poor overall survival regardless of stage. The median progression-free survival, in one series, was 7.3 months, and overall survival was only 11.8 months ([134]). Patients are also likely to progress quickly despite an initial response to treatment ([134]).

Treatment

Surgery

Undifferentiated endometrial sarcomas are treated with up-front surgical management, including hysterectomy and oophorectomy with or without lymphadenectomy. Due to the aggressive nature of this disease, these patients require adjuvant therapy.

Adjuvant Therapy

Unlike ESS, undifferentiated endometrial sarcomas are not responsive to hormone therapy. Adjuvant chemotherapy is similar to that for leiomyosarcoma, as discussed previously.

Adenosarcoma

Histology

Adenosarcomas have two tissue components: The mesenchymal tissue is malignant, and the epithelial part is benign. The epithelial component commonly resembles a proliferative or inactive endometrial gland, often appearing as cleftlike spaces dispersed throughout the proliferative stroma in a phyllode pattern. Slight atypia may be present ([81]). The mesenchymal stromal component is usually homologous tissue, such as stromal sarcoma, fibrosarcoma, or leiomyosarcoma ([81, 135]). The pattern of stromal cell hypercellularity surrounding the glands is characteristic, and the stromal cells show variable atypia and mitosis ([80]). Adenosarcomas with extensive stromal sarcoma proliferation are called *adenosarcoma with sarcoma overgrowth* if the sarcomatous component constitutes more than 25% of the tumor ([80, 81]). This subtype should be recognized because its prognosis is worse than that of a typical adenosarcoma and more similar to that of carcinosarcoma ([136]).

Prognosis and Clinical Course

Adenosarcoma is considered a low-grade malignant tumor with an excellent prognosis ([80-82]). Most cases are confined to the uterus at time of diagnosis and require no adjuvant therapy. Distant metastases have been reported in 5% of cases, and the recurrence rate is approximately 23%, with about one-third of recurrences occurring more than 5 years after initial treatment ([80, 81, 137]). Extrauterine spread at diagnosis, deep infiltrating tumors, sarcomatous overgrowth, and tumor cell necrosis have all been associated with increased risk of recurrence, but again are rare ([80, 104, 120, 138]).

Treatment

Surgery

Management of adenosarcomas consists of hysterectomy and, as discussed previously, additional therapy is generally not required given the excellent prognosis.

Adjuvant Therapy

Only a few reports have described cases in which adenosarcoma was successfully treated with chemotherapeutic drugs such as liposomal doxorubicin ([82]). Krivak and colleagues reported adjuvant chemotherapeutic treatment of nine patients with residual or recurrent adenosarcoma with sarcomatous overgrowth. The drugs used were cisplatin and ifosfamide; doxorubicin; and cisplatin and doxorubicin. The progression-free interval for four patients ranged from 7 to 22 months; all patients had died of recurrent or progressive disease by 39 months ([136]).

REFERENCES

1. Siegel R, Miller K, Jemal A. Cancer statistics, 2015. *CA Cancer J Clin.* 2015;65:5-29
2. Creasman WT, Odicino F, Maisonneuve P, et al. Carcinoma of the corpus uteri. *J Epidemiol Biostat/* 2001;6:47-86.
3. Nelson HD, Fu R, Griffin JC, Nygren P, Smith ME, Humphrey L. Systematic review: effectiveness of medications to reduce risk for primary breast cancer. *Ann Intern Med.* 2009;151(10):703-715.
4. Fisher B, Costantino JP, Redmond CK, et al. Endometrial cancer in tamoxifen-treated breast cancer patients: findings from the National Surgical Adjuvant Breast and Bowel Project (NSABP) B-14. *J Natl Cancer Inst.* 1994;86:527-537.
5. Renehan AG, Tyson M, Egger M, Heller RF, Zwahlen M. Body-mass index and incidence of cancer: a systematic review and

meta-analysis of prospective observational studies. *Lancet.* 2008;371(9612):569.
6. Mu N, Zhu Y, Wang Y, Zhang H, Xue F. Insulin resistance: a significant risk factor of endometrial cancer. *Gynecol Oncol.* 2012;125(3):751-757.
7. Wang T, Rohan TE, Gunter MJ, et al. A prospective study of inflammation markers and endometrial cancer risk in postmenopausal hormone nonusers. *Cancer Epidemiol Biomarkers Prev.* 2011;20(5):971-977.
8. Luhn P, Dallal CM, Weiss JM, et al. Circulating adipokine levels and endometrial cancer risk in the prostate, lung, colorectal, and ovarian cancer screening trial. *Cancer Epidemiol Biomarkers Prev.* 2013;22(7):1304-1312.
9. Soliman PT, Oh JC, Schmeler KM, et al. Risk factors for young premenopausal women with endometrial cancer. *Obstet Gynecol.* 2005;105:575-580.
10. Hampel H, Stephens J, Pukkala E, et al. Cancer risk in hereditary nonpolyposis colorectal cancer syndrome: later age of onset. *Gastroenterology.* 2005;129:415.
11. Watson P, Vasen HFA, Mecklin JP, et al. The risk of extra-colonic, extra-endometrial cancer in the Lynch syndrome. *Int J Cancer.* 2008;123:444.
12. Smith RA, Cokkinides V, Brawley OW. Cancer screening in the United States, 2009: a review of current American Cancer Society guidelines and issues in cancer screening. *CA Cancer J Clin.* 2009;59:27-41.
13. Schmeler KM, Lynch HT, Chen LM, et al. Prophylactic surgery to reduce the risk of gynecologic cancers in the Lynch syndrome. *N Engl J Med.* 2006;354(3):261-269.
14. Epplein M, Reed SD, Voigt LF, et al. Risk of complex and atypical endometrial hyperplasia in relation to anthropometric measures and reproductive history. *Am J Epidemiol.* 2008;168:563-570; discussion 71-76.
15. Kurman RJ, Kaminski PF, Norris HJ. The behavior of endometrial hyperplasia. A long-term study of "untreated" hyperplasia in 170 patients. *Cancer.* 1985;56:403-412.
16. Silverberg SG. Problems in the differential diagnosis of endometrial hyperplasia and carcinoma. *Mod Pathol.* 2000;13:309-327.
17. Larson B, Silfverswärd C, Nilsson B, et al. Prognostic factors in uterine leiomyosarcoma. A clinical and histopathological study of 143 cases. The Radiumhemmet series 1936-1981. *Acta Oncol.* 1990;29:185-191.
18. Nielsen SN, Podratz KC, Scheithauer BW, et al. Clinicopathologic analysis of uterine malignant mixed mullerian tumors. *Gynecol Oncol.* 1989;34:372-378.
19. Silverberg SG, Major FJ, Blessing JA, et al. Carcinosarcoma (malignant mixed mesodermal tumor) of the uterus. A Gynecologic Oncology Group pathologic study of 203 cases. *Int J Gynecol Pathol.* 1990;9:1-19.
20. Lachance JA, Everett EN, Greer B, et al. The effect of age on clinical/pathologic features, surgical morbidity, and outcome in patients with endometrial cancer. *Gynecol Oncol.* 2006;101:470-475
21. Alektiar KM, Venkatraman E, Abu-Rustum N, et al. Is endometrial carcinoma intrinsically more aggressive in elderly patients? *Cancer.* 2003;98:2368-2377.
22. Ruterbusch JJ, Ali-Fehmi R, Olson SH, et al. The influence of comorbid conditions on racial disparities in endometrial cancer survival. *Am J Obstet Gynecol.* 2014;211(6):612.
23. Creasman WT, Morrow CP, Bundy BN, et al. Surgical pathologic spread patterns of endometrial cancer. A Gynecologic Oncology Group study. *Cancer.* 1987;60:2035-2041.
24. Kasamatsu T, Onda T, Katsumata N, et al. Prognostic significance of positive peritoneal cytology in endometrial carcinoma confined to the uterus. *Br J Cancer.* 2003;88:245-250.
25. Zaino RJ, Kurman RJ, Diana KL, et al. Pathologic models to predict outcome for women with endometrial adenocarcinoma: the importance of the distinction between surgical stage and clinical stage—a Gynecologic Oncology Group study. *Cancer.* 1996;77:1115-1121.
26. Morrow CP. *Gynecologic Cancer Surgery.* 2nd ed. Encinitas, CA: South Coast Medical; 2013.
27. Walker JL, Piedmonte MR, Spirtos NM, et al. Laparoscopy compared with laparotomy for comprehensive surgical staging of uterine cancer: Gynecologic Oncology Group study LAP2. *J Clin Oncol.* 2009;27:5331-5336.
28. Kornblith AB, Huang HQ, Walker JL, et al. Quality of life of patients with endometrial cancer undergoing laparoscopic International Federation of Gynecology and Obstetrics staging compared with laparotomy: a Gynecologic Oncology Group study. *J Clin Oncol.* 2009;27:5337-5342.
29. Gaia G, Holloway RW, Santoro L, Ahmad S, Di Silverio E, Spinillo A. Robotic-assisted hysterectomy for endometrial cancer compared with traditional laparoscopic and laparotomy approaches: a systematic review. *Obstet Gynecol.* 2010;116(6):1422.
30. Creutzberg CL, van Putten WL, Koper PC, et al. Surgery and postoperative radiotherapy versus surgery alone for patients with stage-1 endometrial carcinoma: multicentre randomised trial. PORTEC Study Group. Post operative radiation therapy in endometrial carcinoma. *Lancet.* 2000;355:1404-1411.
31. Keys HM, Roberts JA, Brunetto VL, et al. A phase III trial of surgery with or without adjunctive external pelvic radiation therapy in intermediate risk endometrial adenocarcinoma: a Gynecologic Oncology Group study. *Gynecol Oncol.* 2004;92:744-751.
32. Aalders J, Abeler V, Kolstad P, et al. Postoperative external irradiation and prognostic parameters in stage I endometrial carcinoma: clinical and histopathologic study of 540 patients. *Obstet Gynecol.* 1980;56:419-427.
33. Scholten AN, van Putten WL, Beerman H, et al. Postoperative radiotherapy for stage 1 endometrial carcinoma: Long-term outcome of the randomized PORTEC trial with central pathology review. *Int J Radiat Oncol Biol Phys.* 2005;63:834-838.
34. Piver MS, Yazigi R, Blumenson L, et al. A prospective trail comparing hysterectomy, hysterectomy plus vaginal radium, and uterine radium plus hysterectomy in stage I endometrial carcinoma. *Obstet Gynecol.* 1979;54:85-89.
35. Nout RA, Smit VT, Putter H, et al. Vaginal brachytherapy versus pelvic external beam radiotherapy for patients with endometrial cancer of high-intermediate risk (PORTEC-2): an open-label, non-inferiority, randomized trial. *Lancet.* 2010:375(9717):816.
36. Nout RA, Putter, H., Jürgenliemk-Schulz IM, et al. Vaginal brachytherapy versus external beam pelvic radiotherapy for high-intermediate risk endometrial cancer: results of the randomized PORTEC-2 trial [abstract]. *J Clin Oncol.* 2008;26:LBA5503.
37. Galaal K, Al Moundhri M, Bryant A, Lopes AD, Lawrie TA. Adjuvant chemotherapy for advanced endometrial cancer. *Cochrane Database Syst Rev.* 2014;5:CD010681.
38. Agahajanian C, Sill MW, Darcy KM,. Phase II trial of bevacizumab in recurrent or persistent endometrial cancer: a Gynecologic Oncology Group study. *J Clin Oncol.* 2011;29(16):2259-2265.
39. Slomovitz BM, Jiang Y, Yates MS, et al. Phase II study of everolimus and letrozole in patients with recurrent endometrial carcinoma. *J Clin Oncol.* 2015;33(8):930-936.
40. Podratz KC, O'Brien PC, Malkasian GD Jr, Decker DG, Jeffries JA, Edmonson JH. Effects of progestational agents in treatment of endometrial carcinoma. *Obstet Gynecol.* 1985,66(1):106.
41. Lentz SS, Brady MF, Major FJ, Reid GC, Soper JT. High-dose megestrol acetate in advanced or recurrent endometrial carcinoma:

a Gynecologic Oncology Group Study. *J Clin Oncol.* 1996;14(2):357.
42. Fiorica JV, Brunetto VL, Hanjani P, et al. Phase II trial of alternating courses of megestrol acetate and tamoxifen in advanced endometrial carcinoma: a Gynecologic Oncology Group study. *Gynecol Oncol.* 2004;92(1):10.
43. Ma BB, Oza A, Eisenhauer E, Stanimir G, et al. The activity of letrozole in patients with advanced or recurrent endometrial cancer and correlation with biological markers—a study of the National Cancer Institute of Canada Clinical Trials Group. *Int J Gynecol Cancer.* 2004;14(4):650.
44. Rose PG, Brunetto VL, VanLe L, Bell J, Walker JL, Lee RB. A phase II trial of anastrozole in advanced recurrent or persistent endometrial carcinoma: a Gynecologic Oncology Group study. *Gynecol Oncol.* 2000;78(2):212.
45. Salani R, Backes FJ, Fung MF, et al. Posttreatment surveillance and diagnosis of recurrence in women with gynecologic malignancies: Society of Gynecologic Oncologists recommendations. *Am J Obstet Gynecol.* 2011;204(6):466.
46. Novetsky AP, Kuroki LM, Massad LS, et al. The utility and management of vaginal cytology after treatment for endometrial cancer. *Obstet Gynecol.* 2013;121(1):129-135.
47. Bristow RE, Purinton SC, Santillan A, Diaz-Montes TP, Gardner GJ, Guintoli RL 2nd. Cost-effectiveness of routine vaginal cytology for endometrial cancer surveillance. *Gynecol Oncol.* 2006;103(2):709.
48. Rose PG, Sommers RM, Reale FR, et al. Serial serum CA 125 measurements for evaluation of recurrence in patients with endometrial carcinoma. *Obstet Gynecol.* 1994;84:12-16.
49. Chapman JA, DiSaia PJ, Osann K, et al. Estrogen replacement in surgical stage I and II endometrial cancer survivors. *Am J Obstet Gynecol.* 1996;175:1195-1200.
50. Suriano KA, McHale M, McLaren CE, et al. Estrogen replacement therapy in endometrial cancer patients: a matched control study. *Obstet Gynecol.* 2001;97:555-560.
51. Barakat RR, Bundy BN, Spirtos NM, et al. Randomized double-blind trial of estrogen replacement therapy versus placebo in stage I or II endometrial cancer: a Gynecologic Oncology Group study. *J Clin Oncol.* 2006;24:587-592.
52. Rossouw JE, Anderson GL, Prentice RL, et al. Risks and benefits of estrogen plus progestin in healthy postmenopausal women: principal results from the Women's Health Initiative randomized controlled trial. *JAMA.* 2002;288:321-333.
53. Trope CG, Abeler VM, Kristensen GB. Diagnosis and treatment of sarcoma of the uterus. A review. *Acta Oncol.* 2012;51:694-705.
54. Piura B, Rabinovich A, Yanai-Inbar I, et al. Uterine sarcoma in the south of Israel: study of 36 cases. *J Surg Oncol.* 1997;64:55-62.
55. Amant F, Dreyer L, Makin J, et al. Uterine sarcomas in South African black women: A clinicopathologic study with ethnic considerations. *Eur J Gynaecol Oncol.* 2001;22:194-200.
56. Jereczek B, Jassem J, Kobierska A. Sarcoma of the uterus. A clinical study of 42 patients. *Arch Gynecol Obstet.* 1996;258:171-180.
57. Tinkler SD, Cowie VJ. Uterine sarcomas: a review of the Edinburgh experience from 1974 to 1992. *Br J Radiol.* 1993;66:998-1001.
58. D'Angelo E, Prat J. Uterine sarcoma. A review. *Gynecol Oncol.* 2010;116:131-139.
59. Olah KS, Dunn JA, Gee H. Leiomyosarcomas have a poorer prognosis than mixed mesodermal tumours when adjusting for known prognostic factors: the result of a retrospective study of 423 cases of uterine sarcoma. *Br J Obstet Gynaecol.* 1992;99:590-594.
60. Gadducci A, Cosio S, Romanini A, et al. The management of patients with uterine sarcoma: a debated clinical challenge. *Crit Rev Oncol Hematol.* 2008;65:129-142.
61. Callister M, Ramondetta LM, Jhingran A, et al. Malignant mixed Mullerian tumors of the uterus: analysis of patterns of failure, prognostic factors, and treatment outcome. *Int J Radiat Oncol Biol Phys.* 2004;58:786-796.
62. Livi L, Paiar F, Shah N, et al. Uterine sarcoma: twenty-seven years of experience. *Int J Radiat Oncol Biol Phys.* 2003;57:1366-1373.
63. Villena-Heinsen C, Diesing D, Fischer D, et al. Carcinosarcomas–a retrospective analysis of 21 patients. *Anticancer Res.* 2006;26:4817-4823.
64. Ali S, Wells M. Mixed Mullerian tumors of the uterine corpus: a review. *Int J Gynecol Cancer.* 1993;3:1-11.
65. Morice P, Rodriguez A, Rey A, et al. Prognostic value of initial surgical procedure for patients with uterine sarcoma: analysis of 123 patients. *Eur J Gynaecol Oncol.* 2003;24:237-240.
66. Sartori E, Bazzurini L, Gadducci A, et al. Carcinosarcoma of the uterus: a clinicopathological multicenter CTF study. *Gynecol Oncol.* 1997;67:70-75.
67. Vaccarello L, Curtin JP. Presentation and management of carcinosarcoma of the uterus. *Oncology (Williston Park).* 1992;6:45-49; discussion 53-54, 59.
68. Nordal RR, Thoresen SO. Uterine sarcomas in Norway 1956-1992: incidence, survival and mortality. *Eur J Cancer.* 1997;33:907-911.
69. Yamada SD, Burger RA, Brewster WR, et al. Pathologic variables and adjuvant therapy as predictors of recurrence and survival for patients with surgically evaluated carcinosarcoma of the uterus. *Cancer.* 2000;88:2782-2786.
70. Nemani D, Mitra N, Guo M, et al. Assessing the effects of lymphadenectomy and radiation therapy in patients with uterine carcinosarcoma: a SEER analysis. *Gynecol Oncol.* 2008; 111:82-88.
71. Tanner EJ, Leitao MM Jr, Garg K, et al. The role of cytoreductive surgery for newly diagnosed advanced-stage uterine carcinosarcoma. *Gynecol Oncol.* 2011;123:548-552.
72. Cantrell LA, Havrilesky L, Moore DT, et al. A multi-institutional cohort study of adjuvant therapy in stage I-II uterine carcinosarcoma. *Gynecol. Oncol.* 2012;127:22-26.
73. Reed NS, Mangioni C, Malstrom H, et al. Phase III randomized study to evaluate the role of adjuvant pelvic radiotherapy in the treatment of uterine sarcomas stages I and II: an European Organisation for Research and Treatment of Cancer Gynaecological Cancer Group Study (protocol 55874). *Eur J Cancer.* 2008;44:808-818.
74. Sutton G, Brunetto VL, Kilgore L, et al. A phase III trial of ifosfamide with or without cisplatin in carcinosarcoma of the uterus: a Gynecologic Oncology Group study. *Gynecol Oncol.* 2000;79:147-153.
75. Homesley HD, Filiaci V, Markman M, et al. Phase III trial of ifosfamide with or without paclitaxel in advanced uterine carcinosarcoma: a Gynecologic Oncology Group study. *J Clin Oncol.* 2007;25:526-531.
76. Galaal K, van der Heijden E, Godfrey K, et al. Adjuvant radiotherapy and/or chemotherapy after surgery for uterine carcinosarcoma. *Cochran Database Syst Rev.* 2013;2:CD006812.
77. Powel MA, Filiaci VL, Rose PG, et al. Phase II evaluation of paclitaxel and carboplatin in the treatment of carcinosarcoma of the uterus: a Gynecologic Oncology Group Study. *J Clin Oncol.* 2010;28:2727-2731.
78. Koivisto-Korander R, Butzow R, Koivisto AM, et al. Clinical outcome and prognostic factors in 100 cases of uterine sarcoma: experience in Helsinki University Central Hospital 1990-2001. *Gynecol Oncol.* 2008;111:74-81.
79. Prat J. FIGO staging for uterine sarcomas. *Int J Gynaecol Obstet.* 2009;104:177-178.
80. Kaku T, Silverberg SG, Major FJ, et al. Adenosarcoma of the uterus: a Gynecologic Oncology Group clinicopathologic study of 31 cases. *Int J Gynecol Pathol.* 1992;11:75-88.
81. Clement PB, Scully RE. Mullerian adenosarcoma of the uterus: A clinicopathologic analysis of 100 cases with a review of the literature. *Hum Pathol.* 1990;21:363-381.
82. Verschraegen CF, Vasuratna A, Edwards C, et al. Clinicopatho-

logic analysis of mullerian adenosarcoma: the M.D. Anderson Cancer Center experience. *Oncol Rep*. 1998;5:939-944.
83. Meredith RF, Eisert DR, Kaka Z, et al. An excess of uterine sarcomas after pelvic irradiation. *Cancer*. 1986;58:2003-2007.
84. Leitao MM, Tornos C, Wolfson AH, et al. Corpus: mesenchymal tumors. In: Barakat RR, Berchuck A, Randall ME, (eds). *Principles and Practice of Gynecologic Oncology*, 6th ed. Baltimore, MD: Lippincott Williams & Wilkins; 2013:715-749.
85. Bergman L, Beelen ML, Gallee MP, et al. Risk and prognosis of endometrial cancer after tamoxifen for breast cancer. Comprehensive Cancer Centres' ALERT Group. Assessment of Liver and Endometrial cancer Risk following Tamoxifen. *Lancet*. 2000;356:881-887.
86. Gonzalez-Bosquet E, Martinez-Palones JM, Gonzalez-Bosquet J, et al. Uterine sarcoma: a clinicopathological study of 93 cases. *Eur J Gynaecol Oncol*. 1997;18:192-195.
87. El Husseiny G, Al Bareedy N, Mourad WA, et al. Prognostic factors and treatment modalities in uterine sarcoma. *Am J Clin Oncol*. 2002;25:256-260.
88. Kunzel KE, Mills NZ, Muderspach LI, et al. Myxoid leiomyosarcoma of the uterus. *Gynecol Oncol*. 1993;48:277-280.
89. Schneider D, Halperin R, Segal M, et al. Myxoid leiomyosarcoma of the uterus with unusual malignant histologic pattern—a case report. *Gynecol Oncol*. 1995;59:156-158.
90. Clement PB. The pathology of uterine smooth muscle tumors and mixed endometrial stromal-smooth muscle tumors: a selective review with emphasis on recent advances. *Int J Gynecol Pathol*. 2000;19:39-55.
91. Bell SW, Kempson RL, Hendrickson MR. Problematic uterine smooth muscle neoplasms. A clinicopathologic study of 213 cases. *Am J Surg Pathol*. 1994;18:535-558.
92. Ip PP, Cheung AN, Clement PB. Uterine smooth muscle tumors of uncertain malignant potential (STUMP): a clinicopathologic analysis of 16 cases. *Am J Surg Pathol*. 2009;33:992-1005.
93. Guntupalli SR, Ramirez PT, Anderson ML, et al. Uterine smooth muscle tumor of uncertain malignant potential: a retrospective analysis. *Gynecol Oncol*. 2009;113:324-326.
94. Goff BA, Rice LW, Fleischhacker D, et al. Uterine leiomyosarcoma and endometrial stromal sarcoma: lymph node metastases and sites of recurrence. *Gynecol Oncol*. 1993;50:105-109.
95. Iwasa Y, Haga H, Konishi I, et al. Prognostic factors in uterine carcinosarcoma: a clinicopathologic study of 25 patients. *Cancer*. 1998;82:512-519.
96. Larson B, Silfversward C, Nilsson B, et al. Endometrial stromal sarcoma of the uterus. A clinical and histopathological study. The Radiumhemmet series 1936-1981. *Eur J Obstet Gynecol Reprod Biol*. 1990;35:239-249.
97. Hata K, Hata T, Maruyama R, et al. Uterine sarcoma: can it be differentiated from uterine leiomyoma with Doppler ultrasonography? A preliminary report. *Ultrasound Obstet Gynecol*. 1997;9:101-104.
98. Rha SE, Byun JY, Jung SE, et al. CT and MRI of uterine sarcomas and their mimickers. *AJR Am J Roentgenol*. 2003;181:1369-1374.
99. Kahanpaa KV, Wahlstrom T, Grohn P, et al. Sarcomas of the uterus: a clinicopathologic study of 119 patients. *Obstet Gynecol*. 1986;67:417-424.
100. Peters WA 3rd, Kumar NB, Fleming WP, et al. Prognostic features of sarcomas and mixed tumors of the endometrium. *Obstet Gynecol*. 1984;63:550-556.
101. Wolfson AH, Wolfson DJ, Sittler SY, et al. A multivariate analysis of clinicopathologic factors for predicting outcome in uterine sarcomas. *Gynecol Oncol*. 1994;52:56-62.
102. Soumarova R, Horova H, Seneklova Z, et al. Treatment of uterine sarcoma. A survey of 49 patients. *Arch Gynecol Obstet*. 2002;266:92-95.
103. Knocke TH, Kucera H, Dorfler D, et al. Results of postoperative radiotherapy in the treatment of sarcoma of the corpus uteri. *Cancer*. 1998;83:1972-1979.
104. Abeler VM, Royne O, Thoresen S, et al. Uterine sarcomas in Norway. A histopathological and prognostic survey of a total population from 1970 to 2000 including 419 patients. *Histopathology*. 2009;54:355-364.
105. D'Angelo E, Spagnoli LG, Prat J. Comparative clinicopathologic and immunohistochemical analysis of uterine sarcomas diagnosed using the World Health Organization classification system. *Hum Pathol*. 2009;40:1571-1585.
106. Giuntoli RL 2nd, Metzinger DS, DiMarco CS, et al. Retrospective review of 208 patients with leiomyosarcoma of the uterus: prognostic indicators, surgical management, and adjuvant therapy. *Gynecol Oncol*. 2003;89:460-469.
107. Kapp DS, Shin JY, Chan JK. Prognostic factors and survival in 1396 patients with uterine leiomyosarcomas: emphasis on impact of lymphadenectomy and oophorectomy. *Cancer*. 2008;112:820-830.
108. Omura GA, Blessing JA, Major F, et al. A randomized clinical trial of adjuvant adriamycin in uterine sarcomas: a Gynecologic Oncology Group study. *J Clin Oncol*. 1985;3:1240-1245.
109. Hensley ML, Ishil N, Soslow R, et al. Adjuvant gemcitabine plus docetaxel for completely resected stage I-IV high grade uterine leiomyosarcoma: results of a prospective study. *Gynecol Oncol*. 2009;112:563-567.
110. Hensley ML, Wathen JK, Maki RG, et al. Adjuvant therapy for high-grade, uterus-limited leiomyosarcoma: results of a phase 2 trial (SARC 005). *Cancer*. 2013;119:1555-1561.
111. Omura GA, Major FJ, Blessing JA, et al. A randomized study of adriamycin with and without dimethyl triazenoimidazole carboxamide in advanced uterine sarcomas. *Cancer*. 1983;52:626-632.
112. Currie J, Blessing JA, Muss HB, et al. Combination chemotherapy with hydroxyurea, dacarbazine (DTIC), and etoposide in the treatment of uterine leiomyosarcoma: a Gynecologic Oncology Group study. *Gynecol Oncol*. 1996;61:27-30.
113. Sutton G, Blessing JA, Malfetano JH. Ifosfamide and doxorubicin in the treatment of advanced leiomyosarcomas of the uterus: a Gynecologic Oncology Group study. *Gynecol Oncol*. 1996;62:226-229.
114. Edmonson JH, Blessing JA, Cosin JA, et al. Phase II study of mitomycin, doxorubicin, and cisplatin in the treatment of advanced uterine leiomyosarcoma: a Gynecologic Oncology Group study. *Gynecol Oncol*. 2002;85:507-510.
115. Dionigi A, Oliva E, Clement PB, et al. Endometrial stromal nodules and endometrial stromal tumors with limited infiltration: a clinicopathologic study of 50 cases. *Am J Surg Pathol*. 2002;26:567-581.
116. Chang KL, Crabtree GS, Lim-Tan SK, et al. Primary uterine endometrial stromal neoplasms. A clinicopathologic study of 117 cases. *Am J Surg Pathol*. 1990;14:415-438.
117. Thomas MB, Keeney GL, Podratz KC, et al. Endometrial stromal sarcoma: treatment and patterns of recurrence. *Int J Gynecol Cancer*. 2009;19:253-256.
118. Chan JK, Kawar NM, Shin JY, et al. Endometrial stromal sarcoma: a population-based analysis. *Br J Cancer*. 2008;99:1210-1215.
119. Haberal A, Kayikcioglu F, Boran N, et al. Endometrial stromal sarcoma of the uterus: analysis of 25 patients. *Eur J Obstet Gynecol Reprod Biol*. 2003;109:209-213.
120. Nordal RR, Kristensen GB, Kaern J, et al. The prognostic significance of surgery, tumor size, malignancy grade, menopausal status, and DNA ploidy in endometrial stromal sarcoma. *Gynecol Oncol*. 1996;62:254-259.
121. Gadducci A, Sartori E, Landoni F, et al. Endometrial stromal sarcoma: analysis of treatment failures and survival. *Gynecol Oncol*. 1996;63:247-253.
122. Evans HL. Endometrial stromal sarcoma and poorly differentiated endometrial sarcoma. *Cancer*. 1982;50:2170-2182.

123. Chang KL, Crabtree GS, Lim-Tan SK, et al. Primary uterine endometrial stromal neoplasms. A clinicopathologic study of 117 cases. *Am J Surg Pathol.* 1990;14:415-438.
124. Chu MC, Mor G, Lim C, et al. Low-grade endometrial stromal sarcoma: hormonal aspects. *Gynecol Oncol.* 2003;90:170-176.
125. Li AJ, Giuntoli RL 2nd, Drake R, et al. Ovarian preservation in stage I low-grade endometrial stromal sarcomas. *Obstet Gynecol.* 2005;106:1304-1308.
126. Shah JP, Bryant CS, Kumar S, et al. Lymphadenectomy and ovarian preservation in low-grade endometrial stromal sarcoma. *Obstet Gynecol.* 2008;112:1102-1108.
127. Spano JP, Soria JC, Kambouchner M, et al. Long-term survival of patients given hormonal therapy for metastatic endometrial stromal sarcoma. *Med Oncol.* 2003;20:87-93.
128. Pink D, Lindner T, Mrozek A, et al. Harm or benefit of hormonal treatment in metastatic low-grade endometrial stromal sarcoma: single center experience with 10 cases and review of the literature. *Gynecol Oncol.* 2006;101:464-469.
129. Pautier P, Genestie C, Fizazi K, et al. Cisplatin-based chemotherapy regimen (DECAV) for uterine sarcomas. *Int J Gynecol Cancer.* 2002;12:749-754.
130. Li N, Wu LY, Zhang HT, et al. Treatment options in stage I endometrial stromal sarcoma: a retrospective analysis of 53 cases. *Gynecol Oncol.* 2008;108:306-311.
131. Zaloudek C, Hendrickson MR. *Mesenchymal Tumor of the Uterus,* 5th ed. New York, NY: Springer-Verlag; 2002.
132. Berchuck A, Rubin SC, Hoskins WJ, et al. Treatment of endometrial stromal tumors. *Gynecol Oncol.* 1990;36:60-65.
133. August CZ, Bauer KD, Lurain J, et al. Neoplasms of endometrial stroma: histopathologic and flow cytometric analysis with clinical correlation. *Hum Pathol.* 1989;20:232-237.
134. Tanner EJ, Garg K, Leitao MM Jr, et al. High grade undifferentiated uterine sarcoma: surgery, treatment, and survival outcomes. *Gynecol Oncol.* 2012;127:27-31.
135. Fehmian C, Jones J, Kress Y, et al. Adenosarcoma of the uterus with extensive smooth muscle differentiation: Ultrastructural study and review of the literature. *Ultrastruct Pathol.* 1997;21:73-79.
136. Krivak TC, Seidman JD, McBroom JW, et al. Uterine adenosarcoma with sarcomatous overgrowth versus uterine carcinosarcoma: comparison of treatment and survival. *Gynecol Oncol.* 2001;83:89-94.
137. Moinfar F, Azodi M, Tavassoli FA. Uterine sarcomas. *Pathology.* 2007;39:55-71.
138. Seidman JD, Wasserman CS, Aye LM, et al. Cluster of uterine mullerian adenosarcoma in the Washington, DC metropolitan area with high incidence of sarcomatous overgrowth. *Am J Surg Pathol.* 1999;23:809-814.

33

Tumors of the Uterine Cervix

第三十三章　子宫颈恶性肿瘤

Maria D. Iniesta
Kathleen M. Schmeler
Pedro T. Ramirez

中文导读

本章首先讲述了宫颈癌患者的流行病学，紧接着讲述了病因和危险因素，主要包括：人乳头状瘤病毒、人类免疫缺陷病毒、多位性伴侣、过早开始性生活、避孕、吸烟。组织病理学部分包括了宫颈鳞癌、宫颈腺癌及其癌前病变的内容。在筛查部分重点介绍了宫颈巴氏涂片和贝塞斯达系统的应用。随后阐述了疾病临床表现、FIGO分期、诊断方法、预后因素及相关肿瘤标志物，其中预后因素包括了疾病分期、肿瘤体积、浸润深度、组织学类型和组织学分级。治疗部分首先阐述了不同分级宫颈上皮内瘤变的治疗选择策略；而后重点讲述了宫颈癌的治疗手段，主要包括宫颈癌手术、根治性放疗及化疗。治疗方法的选择主要取决于患者的一般情况和疾病分期。治疗后的监测是指根据患者危险分级定期进行体检，内容主要包括体格检查和细胞学涂片检查。本章最后简述了宫颈癌复发后的治疗原则，而此主要取决于患者初始治疗时所采用的治疗方案。

EPIDEMIOLOGY

Demographics

Cancer of the cervix is the third most common gynecologic malignancy in the United States. In 2015, a total of 12,900 new cases of cervical cancer and 4,100 deaths are estimated ([1]). The incidence of this disease has decreased steadily over the past several decades. However, cervical cancer remains one of the most common cancers in women worldwide with approximately 527,600 new cases diagnosed each year and 265,700 related deaths ([2]).

Squamous cell carcinoma (SCC) of the cervix may occur at any age from the second decade of life onward. The mean age at diagnosis is approximately 51.4 years, with the number of cases evenly divided between patients at 30 to 39 and 60 to 69 years of age ([3]). Adenocarcinoma makes up to 15% to 25% of all invasive cervical cancers.

Etiology and Risk Factors

Risk factors for cervical cancer are listed in Table 33-1.

Human Papillomavirus

To understand the current methods for cervical screening, a basic understanding of the nature of cervical abnormalities is essential. Human papillomavirus (HPV) is the critical factor for the development of preinvasive and invasive cervical lesions. More than 14 million incident cases are reported annually, the majority of which occur in persons age 15 to 24 years ([4-6]). HPV is a small, nonenveloped, double-stranded DNA virus predominantly transmitted through sexual intercourse. The most consistent risk factors for acquiring HPV are number of sexual partners, age of first sexual intercourse, and a partner infected with HPV.

More than 40 genotypes of HPV infect the epithelial lining of the anogenital tract and other mucosal areas of the body ([7]). These subtypes are further classified into high-risk HPV (HR-HPV) and low-risk HPV (LR-HPV) depending on their oncogenic potential for cervical cancer and its precursors. Low-risk HPV genotypes include HPV-6 and -11 and typically cause benign anogenital warts, although they may occasionally be associated with neoplastic cervical changes ([8]). Invasive lesions, on the other hand, are much more commonly caused by HR-HPV including, in order of frequency, types 16, 18, 31, 45, 52, and 33 ([9]). Although the majority of premalignant and invasive disease can be directly attributed to types 16 or 18, HPV DNA from any genotype is detectable in greater than 99% of all cervical cancer specimens ([8]).

Table 33-1 Risk Factors for Cervical Cancer

Gynecologic Factor	Male Factor	Others
Human papillomavirus	History of penile cancer	Immunodeficiency
Number of sexual partners	Cervical cancer in ex-wife	Smoking
Age at first intercourse	Multiple sexual partners	Genetic predisposition
Multiparity		Nutrient deficiency
Sexually transmitted disease		
Oral contraception		

Immunodeficiency Status

Many studies have reported an increased risk of HPV infection and preinvasive and invasive cervical cancer in women who have low immunity, such as those with human immunodeficiency virus (HIV) infection ([10]). It was found that rare HR-HPV types are more common in cervical dysplasia of HIV-infected women. It is possible that these other HPV types (35, 45, 52, and 59) are not able to evade the immune system as efficiently as HPV types 16 and 18, except in HIV-infected individuals who are immunocompromised ([11]).

Number of Sexual Partners

The number of sexual partners is an important risk factor for both preinvasive and invasive cervical cancer. Many studies have found an increased relative risk of cervical cancer in women who have had more than six sexual partners ([12]). This is related to a higher risk of acquiring HPV infection.

Age at First Intercourse

Women who have intercourse early in life (<16 years of age) are more prone to develop cervical cancer ([13]). This increase in risk has been proposed because the process of transformation of columnar epithelium to squamous epithelium is active and is vulnerable to carcinogenic agents during early adolescence. However, these women frequently have other associated risk factors, such as multiple sexual partners and HPV infection.

Contraception

Many studies have produced controversial results on the effect of oral contraception on cervical cancer risk.

The relative risk of cervical cancer is increased in current users of oral contraceptives and declines after use ceases ([14]).

Smoking

Tobacco use is a well-established risk factor for cancer of the cervix. Cigarette smoking confers a 1.5- to 2.5-fold increase in cancers of the cervix. Overall, tobacco smoking is estimated to account for 21% of cancer deaths worldwide, of which 2% (2% in high-income countries and 11% in low- and middle-income countries) are due to cervical cancer. Therefore, it is the most preventable risk factor for smoking-related cancer deaths ([15]).

Male Factors

Women with cervical cancer frequently report a history of having a male partner who has multiple other female partners, a history of condyloma infection, a history of intercourse with prostitutes, or an ex-wife or former partner with cervical cancer ([12]).

HISTOPATHOLOGY

Squamous Cell Tumors and Precursors

Squamous Intraepithelial Lesions

Cervical SCCs are believed to develop from precursor or preinvasive lesions, which have been classified in a variety of ways but are generally based on the degree of disruption of epithelial differentiation. The oldest such system is the dysplasia–carcinoma in situ (CIS) system, with mild dysplasia at one end and severe dysplasia/CIS at the other. Another is the cervical intraepithelial neoplasia (CIN) classification, with mild dysplasia termed CIN1 and CIS termed CIN3. The Bethesda System for reporting cervical/vaginal cytologic abnormalities categorizes squamous abnormalities as follows: low-grade squamous intraepithelial lesion (LSIL), encompassing HPV infection and CIN1; high-grade squamous intraepithelial lesion HSIL, encompassing CIN2 and CIN3; and SCC. These systems are compared in Table 33-2 ([16]).

Microinvasive Carcinoma

Microinvasion has been defined variably depending on the recommendations of the International Federation of Gynecology and Obstetrics (FIGO) ("preclinical invasive carcinoma diagnosed microscopically only"; depth of lesion, ≤5 mm; width, ≤7 mm) or Society of Gynecologic Oncology (depth of invasion, ≤3 mm with no lymphovascular space invasion [LVSI] or confluent pattern) ([17]). The depth of stromal invasion is measured from the base of the epithelium, either squamous or glandular, to the deepest point of invasion. Microinvasion can be diagnosed only with a conization specimen containing the entire lesion, having uninvolved margins, and having a sufficient number of sections examined by the pathologist.

The histology of invasive foci is usually better differentiated than that of the nearby squamous intraepithelial lesion (Figs. 33-1 and 33-2).

Invasive Squamous Cell Carcinoma

The histopathology of SCC is shown in Figs. 33-3 and 33-4.

Table 33-2 Classification of HPV-Associated Intraepithelial Lesions of the Cervix and Cytologic Classification

Comparison of Classification Systems			
HPV Risk Category	Dysplasia/CIN	Pap System	Bethesda System
—	Normal	Class I	Normal
Low risk	Inflammation	Class II	LSIL
Low risk	Inflammation	Class II	LSIL
Low and high risk	Inflammation	Class II	LSIL
Low and high risk	Mild dysplasia/CIN1	Class III	LSIL
High risk	Moderate dysplasia/CIN2	Class III	HSIL
High risk	Severe dysplasia/CIS/CIN3	Class IV	HSIL
	Cancer	Class V	

CIN, cervical intraepithelial neoplasia; CIS, carcinoma in situ; HPV, human papillomavirus; HSIL, high-grade squamous intraepithelial lesion; LSIL, low-grade squamous intraepithelial lesion.

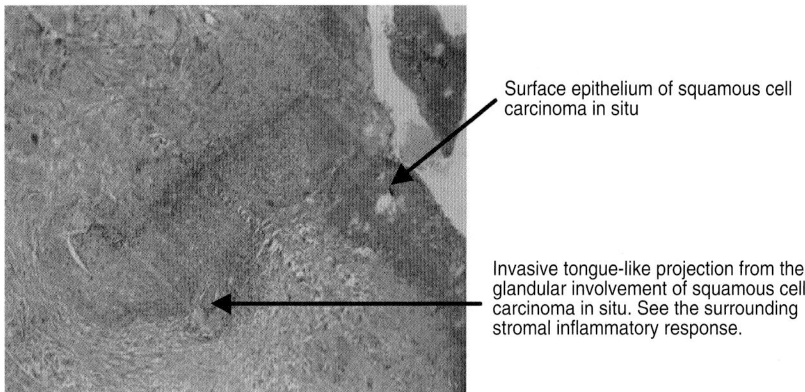

FIGURE 33-1 Microinvasive squamous cell carcinoma (hematoxylin and eosin stain, ×100).

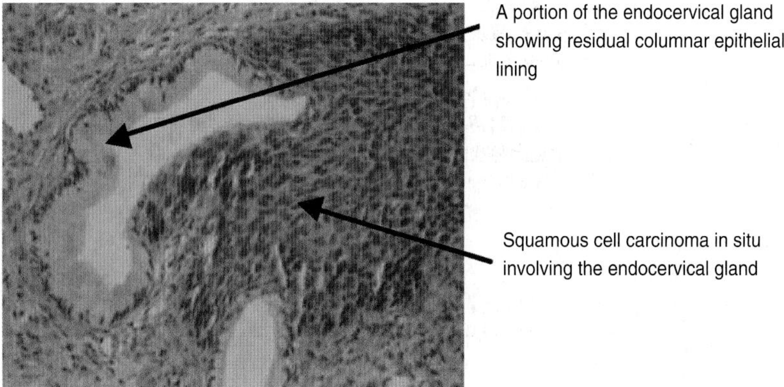

FIGURE 33-2 Squamous cell carcinoma in situ with glandular involvement (hematoxylin and eosin stain, ×400). This should not be interpreted as invasive carcinoma.

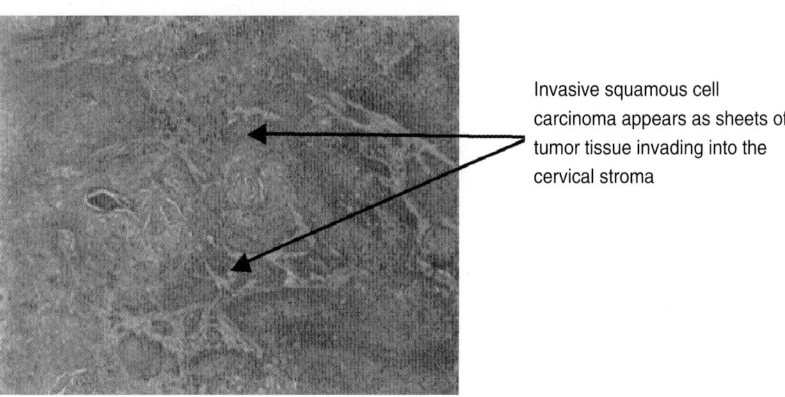

FIGURE 33-3 Invasive squamous cell carcinoma (hematoxylin and eosin stain, ×10).

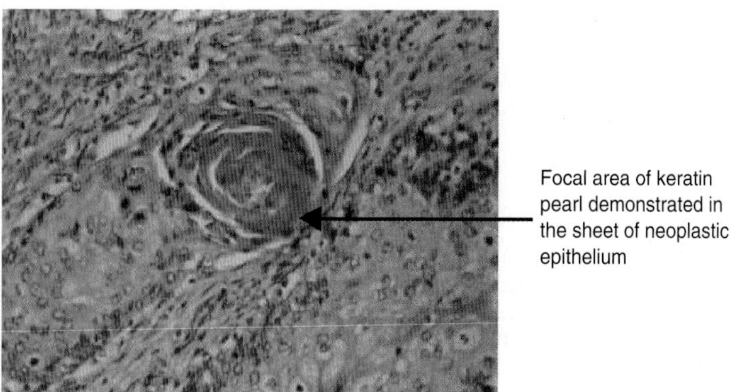

FIGURE 33-4 High-power magnification (×40) of epithelial sheets of squamous cell carcinoma.

Glandular Tumors and Precursors

The World Health Organization (WHO) has classified cervical adenocarcinoma into eight categories: (1) adenocarcinoma in situ, (2) early invasive adenocarcinoma, (3) adenocarcinoma not otherwise specified, (4) mucinous adenocarcinoma (including endocervical, intestinal, minimal deviation adenocarcinoma or adenoma malignum, signet ring cell, and villoglandular adenocarcinoma), (5) endometrioid adenocarcinoma, (6) clear cell adenocarcinoma, (7) serous adenocarcinoma, and (8) mesonephric adenocarcinoma.

Adenocarcinoma in Situ

Adenocarcinoma in situ (AIS) is an intraepithelial glandular neoplasm that occurs in women at a younger age than invasive adenocarcinoma ([18]). Adenocarcinoma in situ is typically located at the transformation zone, although it may be present high up in the endocervical canal (between 20 and 30 mm, measured from the maximum convexity of the portio vaginalis). The principal morphologic features are cytologic malignant glandular epithelium with stratification, atypia, mitotic activity, and frequent apoptosis without stromal invasion. The cellular changes may be found focally in the glands and may have features of endocervical, endometrial, intestinal, or mixed cell types. The distinction between AIS and nonneoplastic glandular epithelium may at times be difficult; some authors have coined terms such as *glandular dysplasia* and *glandular atypia* for these lesser changes.

Early Invasive or Microinvasive Adenocarcinoma

Although the concept of microinvasive adenocarcinoma has not been universally accepted, published literature suggests that patients with LVSI-negative cervical adenocarcinoma with depth of stromal invasion of <5 mm and a tumor volume of <500 μL can be treated with nonradical management (extrafascial hysterectomy with excision of the anterior leaf of the vesicouterine ligament, without lymph node dissection and oophorectomy) ([19]).

Adenocarcinoma

Various subtypes of adenocarcinoma have been noted due to their differentiation, as their respective names imply, such as mucinous adenocarcinoma, which can have endocervical or intestinal goblet cell features and the appearance of endometrioid, clear cell, serous, or mesonephric types. Adenoma malignum is usually an extremely benign-appearing cancer that is often diagnosed late and thus has a clinically poor prognosis. Clear cell adenocarcinomas may or may not be associated with diethylstilbestrol exposure in utero, but they have no known association with HPV ([20]). Serous adenocarcinoma is rare, with histology identical to its ovarian counterpart, and it carries a similarly bad prognosis. Mesonephric carcinomas are rare and are found in embryonal remnants of wolffian ducts, such as the uterine cervix, broad ligament, mesosalpinx, and exceptionally in the uterine corpus. The primary histologic pattern is tubular glands that vary in size and are lined by one to several layers of columnar cells ([21]) (Fig. 33-5).

SCREENING

Pap Smear and Bethesda System

Pap Smear

Guidelines for screening have been put forth by American College of Obstetricians and Gynecologists ([22]) and are summarized below:

- Cervical cancer screening should begin at age 21 years. Women younger than age 21 years should not be screened regardless of the age of sexual initiation or the presence of other behavior-related risk factors.

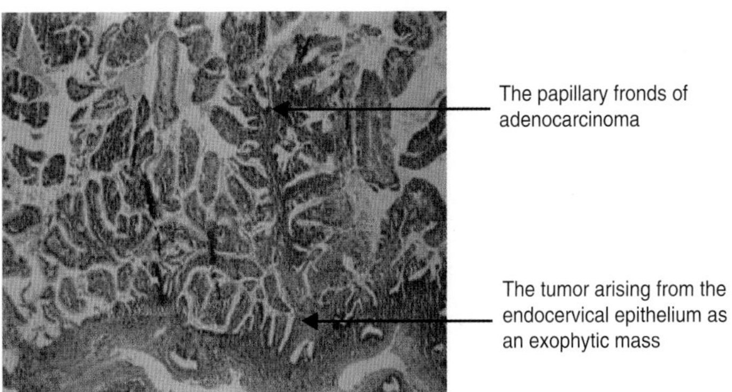

FIGURE 33-5 Endocervical papillary adenocarcinoma (hematoxylin and eosin stain, ×10).

- Women age 21 to 29 years should be tested with cervical cytology alone, and screening should be performed every 3 years. Human papillomavirus testing should not be performed in women younger than 30 years.
- For women age 30 to 65 years, co-testing with cytology and HPV testing every 5 years is preferred.
- In women age 30 to 65 years, screening with cytology alone every 3 years is acceptable. Annual screening should not be performed.
- Women who have a history of cervical cancer, have HIV infection, are immunocompromised, or were exposed to diethylstilbestrol in utero should not follow routine screening guidelines.
- Both liquid-based and conventional methods of cervical cytology collection are acceptable for screening.
- In women who have had a hysterectomy with removal of the cervix (total hysterectomy) and have never had CIN2 or higher, routine cytology screening and HPV testing should be discontinued and not restarted for any reason.
- Screening by any modality should be discontinued after age 65 years in women with evidence of adequate negative prior screening results and no history of CIN2 or higher. Adequate negative prior screening results are defined as three consecutive negative cytology results or two consecutive negative co-test results within the previous 10 years, with the most recent test performed within the past 5 years.

Since the Pap smear was initially developed, there have been several changes in nomenclature and interpretation to make the results more clinically relevant. At present, the Bethesda System is being used worldwide for cytologic diagnosis (see Table 33-2).

Bethesda System

The Bethesda System is another procedure used for the cytologic diagnosis of cervical cancer. It was developed in 1988 and last updated in 2001 and is now used widely ([23]). The Bethesda System report is divided into three sections:

1. *Specimen adequacy*
   Satisfactory for evaluation
   Unsatisfactory for evaluation
2. *General categorization (optional)*
   Negative for intraepithelial lesion or malignancy
   Epithelial cell abnormality
   Other
3. *Interpretation/result*
   Negative for intraepithelial lesion or malignancy
     Organism
     Other nonneoplastic findings (optional to report; list not comprehensive)
       Reactive cellular changes associated with (descriptive findings)
       Glandular cells status post hysterectomy
       Atrophy
   Epithelial cell abnormalities
   Squamous cell
     Atypical squamous cells (ASCs); ASC of undetermined significance (ASC-US) and ASC cannot exclude HSIL (ASC-H)
      LSIL
      HSIL
     Glandular cell (specify endocervical, endometrial, or not otherwise specified)
       Atypical glandular cells (AGCs)
       AGCs, favor neoplastic
       Endocervical AIS
     Adenocarcinoma
       Other (list not comprehensive)
       Endometrial cells in a woman ≥40 years of age
       Automated review and ancillary testing (include as appropriate)
   Educational notes and suggestions (optional)

Note the following:

1. ASC: Some cells were seen that cannot be called normal but do not meet the requirements to call them precancerous. The abnormal cells may be caused by an infection, irritation, or intercourse or may be precancerous.

   a. ASC-US
   b. ASC-H
2. Squamous intraepithelial lesion: Changes were seen in the cells that may show precancerous signs. Squamous intraepithelial lesion can be low or high grade.
   a. LSIL: Early, mild changes in the size or shape of cells were seen.
   b. HSIL: Moderate or severe cell changes are seen; HSIL changes on a Pap smear suggest an increased risk of "precancer" when compared with LSIL changes.
3. AGC: Cell changes were seen that represent an abnormality that must be evaluated more closely. The type of evaluation depends on patient age and other factors.

Example of cytologic features of HPV and CIN are shown in Fig. 33-6.

NATURAL HISTORY

The natural history of growth of a cervical lesion is believed to progress through a state of microscopic invasion into the stroma and radial growth on the surface. Ultimately, a mass is formed, which, in general, grows locally to invade first the deeper stroma and later the paracervical and parametrial tissues. If left untreated, the disease will expand through these tissues to involve the lateral pelvic side wall and nearby viscera, such as the urinary bladder and rectum. Cancer arising from the cervix has been reported to involve the uterine corpus in 10% to 30% of cases. The incidence of ovarian metastasis in patients with cervical cancer is estimated at 0.22% for stage IB, 0.75% for stage IIA, and 2.2% for stage IIB with SCC, and 3.7%, 5.3%, and 9.9%, respectively, in adenocarcinoma ([24]).

A retrospective review of 360 patients with carcinoma of the cervix with clinical stage IB and IIA who had undergone radical hysterectomy and pelvic node dissection showed that lymph node metastasis was present in 21.9% of patients. In patients with and without lymph node metastasis, lymphovascular space invasion positivity, full-thickness stromal invasion, involvement of the uterine isthmus, positive parametrium, positive vaginal margins, and involvement of uterine corpus were seen in 25.3% and 9.2% ($P < .001$), 63% and 32% ($P < .001$), 32.9% and 13.8% ($P < .001$), 15.2% and 5% ($P < .004$), 24% and 14.2% ($P < .005$), and 17.7% and 13.8% ($P = .11$) of patients, respectively. In patients with lymph node metastases, 79.7% had grade 3 tumor compared with 69.5% of patients without lymph node metastases ($P = .19$). Multiple logistic regression indicated that only LVSI and full-thickness stromal invasion were statistically significant ($P < .001$ and $P < .002$, respectively) for lymph node metastasis ([25]). Distant metastasis to bones, lungs, breast, brain, and abdominal viscera often has a late presentation. Variant cell types, such as neuroendocrine and glassy cell carcinoma, may be associated with distant disease in the absence of local involvement.

CLINICAL PRESENTATION

Symptoms

The clinical signs and symptoms of patients with cervical cancer vary depending on the stage and characteristic

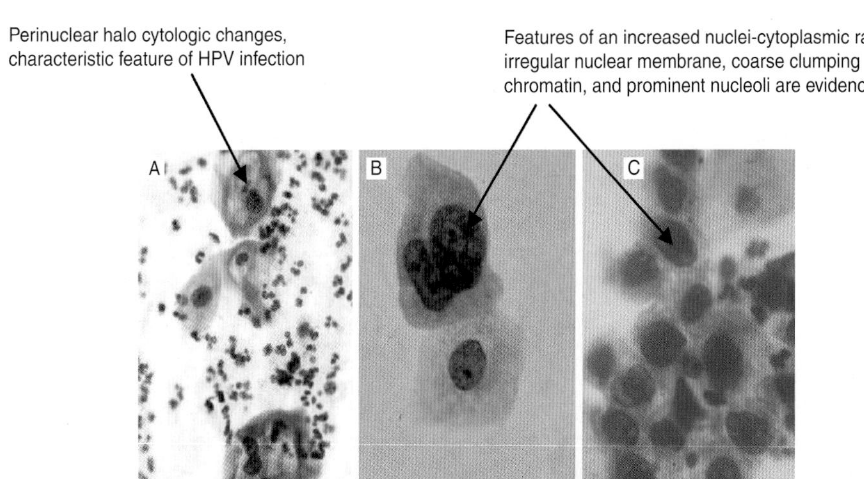

FIGURE 33-6 Cytologic changes associated with cervical intraepithelial neoplasia (CIN), including A. CIN1 with koilocytotic feature of human papillomavirus (HPV) infection (×600 magnification), B. CIN2 (×1,000 magnification), and C. CIN3 (×1,000 magnification).

features of their lesions. Patients with early-stage disease may not have any abnormal symptoms; rather, their lesions may be discovered incidentally on a Pap smear. In patients with gross lesions, the most common presenting symptom is vaginal bleeding, which may have a characteristic pattern of mucous bloody discharge, postcoital bleeding, and/or intermenstrual, intermittent, or continuous vaginal bloody discharge. Vaginal bleeding is often found with exophytic cervical lesions. Tumor necrosis with superimposed infection may cause a mucopurulent bloody discharge with a foul smell due to anaerobic organisms. The symptoms in patients with more advanced disease include leg swelling due to compression of the venous or lymphatic system, pain due to nerve or bone involvement, and other urinary or bowel symptoms due to cancer invasion, such as hematuria or hematochezia.

INTERNATIONAL FEDERATION OF GYNECOLOGY AND OBSTETRICS STAGING

Cervical cancer is currently staged clinically using the FIGO system ([17]). Routine evaluation includes physical examination, pelvic and rectal examination, and pathologic review of cervical or cone biopsy specimens. Basic imaging studies such as chest x-ray, intravenous pyelography, cystoscopy, and proctoscopy are allowed in order to classify the disease into four stages, as shown in Table 33-3.

DIAGNOSTIC IMAGING

Imaging plays an important role in the pretreatment evaluation of patients with common gynecologic

Table 33-3 FIGO Staging of Cervical Carcinoma

Stage	Description
Stage I	The carcinoma is strictly confined to the cervix (extension to the uterine corpus should be disregarded).
Stage IA	Invasive cancer identified only microscopically. (All gross lesions even with superficial invasion are Stage IB cancers.) Invasion is limited to measured stromal invasion with a maximum depth of 5 mm[a] and no wider than 7 mm.
Stage IA1	Measured invasion of stroma ≤3 mm in depth and ≤7 mm in width.
Stage IA2	Measured invasion of stroma >3 mm and <5 mm in depth and ≤7 mm in width.
Stage IB	Clinical lesions confined to the cervix, or preclinical lesions greater than stage IA.
Stage IB1	Clinical lesions no greater than 4 cm in size.
Stage IB2	Clinical lesions >4 cm in size.
Stage II	The carcinoma extends beyond the uterus, but has not extended onto the pelvic wall or to the lower third of vagina.
Stage IIA	Involvement of up to the upper 2/3 of the vagina. No obvious parametrial involvement.
Stage IIA1	Clinically visible lesion ≤4 cm
Stage IIA2	Clinically visible lesion >4 cm
Stage IIB	Obvious parametrial involvement but not onto the pelvic sidewall.
Stage III	The carcinoma has extended onto the pelvic sidewall. On rectal examination, there is no cancer-free space between the tumor and pelvic sidewall. The tumor involves the lower third of the vagina. All cases of hydronephrosis or nonfunctioning kidney should be included unless they are known to be due to other causes.
Stage IIIA	Involvement of the lower vagina but no extension onto pelvic sidewall.
Stage IIIB	Extension onto the pelvic sidewall, or hydronephrosis/nonfunctioning kidney.
Stage IV	The carcinoma has extended beyond the true pelvis or has clinically involved the mucosa of the bladder and/or rectum.
Stage IVA	Spread to adjacent pelvic organs.
Stage IVB	Spread to distant organs.

[a]The depth of invasion should not be more than 5 mm taken from the base of the epithelium, either surface of glandular, from which it originates. Vascular space invasion should not alter the staging.

malignancies. Magnetic resonance imaging (MRI) is the best imaging technique for evaluation of extent of disease in patients with cervical cancer. Magnetic resonance imaging is also useful in the pretreatment evaluation of young women with small-volume disease who wish to preserve fertility. Computed tomography (CT) is able to identify extra-uterine spread of disease, including enlarged pelvic and/or retroperitoneal lymph nodes, extension to the pelvic sidewalls and hydronephrosis, fistulation into bladder or into rectum, and the presence of distant parenchymal metastases. Positron emission tomography (PET)/CT is useful in the detection of lymph node metastases, with sensitivities of 75% to 100% and specificities of 87% to 100%, demonstrating abnormal tracer uptake even in normal-size nodes ([26]).

PROGNOSTIC FACTORS

Stage IA

The depth of stromal invasion correlates with the risk of pelvic lymph node metastases and progression-free interval. In tumors with a depth of invasion <1, 1 to 3, and <3 mm, the risk of lymph node involvement (LNI) was 0% to 1.6%, 0% to 5.3%, and 1.3% to 13.8%, respectively; the risk of parametrial invasion was 0%, 0% to 2.3%, and 0% to 3.3%, respectively ([27]). Positive LVSI status has significant adverse prognostic effects on relapse-free survival and overall survival in tumors with increasing depth of invasion (P < .001) ([28]). In a study by Milam et al ([29]), the authors aimed to determine the association between findings on review of preoperative biopsy specimens and the risk of LNI at radical hysterectomy in patients with early-stage (stage IA-IB1) cervical cancer. In that study, the authors found that 12 patients (14.8%) had LNI at radical hysterectomy. Stage, grade, and histologic subtype were not associated with LNI. Lymphovascular space invasion and depth of invasion >4 mm were both significantly associated with LNI (25.6% vs 4.8%, P = .01; and 25.0% vs 4.5%, P = .01, respectively). Patients with LVSI with >4 mm invasion were 6.6 times more likely to have LNI at the time of radical hysterectomy (relative risk, 6.6; 95% confidence interval [CI], 2.1-21.9). The authors concluded that patients with preoperative LVSI are at higher risk for LNI at radical hysterectomy and should be counseled regarding potential implications for management.

Stage IB-IIA

The incidence of lymph node metastasis in patients with stage IB1 and IB2 cervical cancer has been reported to be as high as 15% to 20% and 30% to 50%, respectively. Parametrial invasion is related to the grade of the tumor, depth of stromal invasion, and presence of LVSI. A study by Frumovitz et al ([30]) evaluated the incidence of parametrial involvement and the factors associated with parametrial spread in women with early-stage cervical cancer. In that study, the authors sought to also identify a cohort of patients at low risk for parametrial spread who may benefit from less radical surgery. Three hundred fifty patients met the inclusion criteria. Overall, 27 women (7.7%) had parametrial involvement. The majority of specimens with parametrial involvement (52%) had tumor spread through direct microscopic extension. Patients with parametrial involvement were more likely to have a primary tumor size larger than 2 cm (>2 cm, 14%; <2 cm, 4%; P = .001), higher histologic grade (grade 3, 12%; grades 1 and 2, 3%; P = .01), LVSI (positive, 12%; negative, 3%; P = .002), and metastasis to the pelvic lymph nodes (positive, 31%; negative, 4%; $P \leq .001$). One hundred twenty-five women (36%) had squamous, adenocarcinoma, or adenosquamous lesions, all grades, with primary tumor size ≤2 cm and no LVSI. In this group of patients, there was no pathologic evidence of parametrial involvement. Significant prognostic factors include tumor diameter, positive lymphangiography, and adenocarcinoma histology.

VACCINATIONS

Preventive Setting

Koutsky et al ([31]) conducted a double-blinded randomized study in 2,392 women at risk for infection who received three doses of a placebo or HPV-16–like particle vaccine (40 mg/dose). After a median follow-up duration of 17.4 months from administration of the last dose, the incidence of HPV-16 infection was significantly lower in the study group (3.8% in the placebo group, 0.0% in the vaccinated group; P < .001).

The first HPV vaccine was licensed for use in the United States in June 2006. At present, there are two HPV vaccines available in the United States. Human papillomavirus quadrivalent, or HPV4 (types 6, 11, 16, 18), vaccine, recombinant (Gardasil) and HPV bivalent, or HPV2 (types 16 and 18), vaccine, recombinant (Cervarix). Both vaccines have greater than 95% efficacy in preventing HPV-16– and HPV-18–related cervical precancer lesions ([32]).

The WHO has changed its previous recommendation of a three-dose schedule to a two-dose schedule, with increased flexibility in the interval between doses, which may facilitate vaccine uptake. For both the bivalent and quadrivalent HPV vaccines, a two-dose schedule with a 6-month interval between doses is recommended for females younger than 15 years.

Those who are >15 years old at the time of the second dose are also adequately covered by two doses. There is no maximum recommended interval between doses. However, an interval no greater than 12 to 15 months is suggested in order to complete the schedule promptly and before becoming sexually active. If the interval between doses is shorter than 5 months, a third dose should be given at least 6 months after the first dose. A three-dose schedule (at 0, 1-2, and 6 months) is recommended for females age 15 years and older and for those known to be immunocompromised and/or infected with HIV (regardless of whether they are receiving antiretroviral therapy) ([33]).

The data from the National Health and Nutrition Examination Surveys (NHANES) continue to show good efficacy for the HPV vaccines. Data comparing 2003 to 2006 with 2007 to 2010, the first 4 years of the HPV vaccination program in the United States, have shown that there was a 56% reduction in prevalence of HPV types 6, 11, 16, and 18 in girls age 14 to 19 years and 36% reduction in genital warts in US girls age 15 to 19 years from 2006 to 2010 ([32]).

Apter et al ([34]) conducted the double-blinded randomized PATRICIA trial on the immunogenicity and efficacy of the HPV-16/18 AS04-adjuvantedvaccine in young women age 15 to 25 years. The total vaccinated cohort (TVC) included all randomized participants who received at least one vaccine dose (vaccine, n = 9,319; control, n = 9,325) at months 0, 1, and/or 6. The TVC-naïve group (vaccine, n = 5,822; control, n = 5,819) had no evidence of high-risk HPV infection at baseline, approximating adolescent girls targeted by most HPV vaccination programs. It was concluded that vaccinating adolescents before sexual debut has a substantial impact on the overall incidence of high-grade cervical abnormalities, and catch-up vaccination up to 18 years of age is most likely effective.

TUMOR MARKERS

Squamous Cell Carcinoma Antigen

A study was conducted to identify patient-, disease-, and treatment-related factors associated with unusual levels of SCC antigen (SCC-Ag) and to determine whether SCC-Ag is a useful tumor marker in patients. Among 129 patients with recurrence, 14 who showed a normal SCC-Ag level at diagnosis but an elevated level at recurrence were classified as group I; 22 patients with an elevated SCC-Ag level at diagnosis but not at recurrence were classified as group II; and 76 patients with an elevated SCC-Ag level at both diagnosis and recurrence were classified as group III. In univariate analysis, unusual SCC-Ag showed statistically significant relationships with pathology and biochemical response to treatment. However, in the multivariate analysis, none of the clinicopathologic factors showed a statistical relationship with unusual levels of SCC-Ag. The 5-year disease-free survival rates for groups I, II, and III were 7.1%, 9.1%, and 0% (P = .418), and the 5-year overall survival rates were 34.3%, 58.4%, and 33.3%, respectively (P = .142). It was found that patients with a high initial SCC-Ag and elevated SCC-Ag at relapse have poor prognosis due to high SCC-Ag level ([35]).

TREATMENTS

Management of Abnormal Pap Smears

The current consensus guidelines from the American Society for Colposcopy and Cervical Pathology (ASCCP) for the management of abnormal Pap tests and treatment of cervical dysplasia are summarized below ([36]).

Atypical Squamous Cells

Treatment of ASC depends on the subcategory based on the Pap smear: undetermined significance (ASC-US) or cannot exclude HSIL (ASC-H).

1. ASC-US: Atypical squamous cells of undetermined significance is the most common cytologic abnormality, but it carries the lowest risk of CIN3+, partly because one- to two-thirds of cases are not HPV associated. For women >25 years old with ASC-US cytology, HPV testing is recommended. If HPV-negative ASC-US is present, repeat co-testing (Pap and HPV testing) at 3 years is recommended. If HPV-positive ASC-US is present, colposcopy is recommended. For women age 21 to 24 years with ASC-US, repeat cytology in 12 months is recommended. Immediate colposcopy or repeat HPV testing is not recommended. Management of pregnant women with ASC-US is identical to that described for nonpregnant women, with the exception that deferring colposcopy until 6 weeks postpartum is acceptable. Endocervical curettage in pregnant women should not be performed.
2. ASC-H: For women with ASC-H cytology, colposcopy is recommended regardless of HPV result.

Low-Grade Squamous Intraepithelial Lesion

For women with LSIL who are 21 to 24 years old, follow-up with cytology at 12-month intervals is recommended. For women >25 years old, colposcopy is recommended. For pregnant women with LSIL, colposcopy is preferred and can be performed immediately or deferred until 6 weeks postpartum.

High-Grade Squamous Intraepithelial Lesion

For women >25 years old with HSIL cytology, colposcopy or immediate treatment with loop electrosurgical excision or colposcopy is recommended. For women age 21 to 24 years with HSIL, colposcopy is recommended. When CIN2+ is not identified histologically, observation for up to 24 months using both colposcopy and cytology at 6-month intervals is recommended, provided the colposcopic examination is adequate and endocervical assessment is negative or CIN1.

Atypical Glandular Cells, Adenocarcinoma In Situ, and Benign Glandular Changes

For women with AGC or AIS on Pap test, colposcopy with endocervical sampling is recommended regardless of HPV result. Endometrial sampling is recommended in conjunction with colposcopy and endocervical sampling in women 35 years of age and older with all subcategories of AGC and AIS. Endometrial sampling is also recommended for women younger than 35 years with risk factors for endometrial cancer (obesity, chronic anovulation, Lynch syndrome, or family history of endometrial and/or colorectal cancer). For women with atypical endometrial cells, initial evaluation limited to endometrial and endocervical sampling is preferred, with colposcopy acceptable either at the initial evaluation or deferred until the results of endometrial and endocervical sampling are known; if colposcopy is deferred and no endometrial pathology is identified, colposcopy is then recommended.

For women with AGC not otherwise specified cytology in whom CIN2+ is not identified, co-testing at 12 months and 24 months is recommended. If both co-tests are negative, return for repeat co-testing in 3 years is recommended.

For women with AGC "favor neoplasia" or AIS cytology, if invasive disease is not identified during the initial colposcopic workup, a diagnostic excisional procedure is recommended. It is recommended that the type of diagnostic excisional procedure used in this setting provide an intact specimen with interpretable margins. Endocervical sampling above the cone bed is recommended. The initial evaluation of AGC in pregnant women should be identical to that of nonpregnant women, except that endocervical curettage and endometrial biopsy are not performed.

For asymptomatic premenopausal women with Pap showing benign endometrial cells, endometrial stromal cells, or histiocytes, no further evaluation is recommended. For postmenopausal women with benign endometrial cells, endometrial biopsy is recommended.

TREATMENT OF CERVICAL INTRAEPITHELIAL NEOPLASIA

Cervical Intraepithelial Neoplasia Grade 1

The recommended management of women with a histologic diagnosis of CIN1 preceded by an ASC-US, ASC-H, or LSIL cytology is follow-up with either HPV DNA testing every 12 months or repeat cervical cytology every 6 to 12 months. If the HPV DNA test is positive or if repeat cytology shows ASC-US or greater, colposcopy is recommended. If the HPV test is negative or two consecutive repeat cytology tests are negative, return to routine cytologic screening is recommended. If CIN1 persists for at least 2 years, either continued follow-up or treatment with excision or ablation can be performed. Hysterectomy as the primary and principal treatment for histologically diagnosed CIN1 is not recommended. For CIN1 preceded by HSIL or AGC not otherwise specified cytology, either a diagnostic excisional procedure or observation with colposcopy and cytology at 6-month intervals for 1 year is acceptable. If observation with cytology and colposcopy is elected, a diagnostic excisional procedure is recommended for women with repeat HSIL or AGC not otherwise specified cytologic results at either the 6- or 12-month visit. The recommended management of pregnant women with a histologic diagnosis of CIN1 is follow-up without treatment.

Cervical Intraepithelial Neoplasia Grades 2 and 3

Both excision and ablation are acceptable treatment modalities for women with a histologic diagnosis of CIN2/3 and satisfactory colposcopy. If the colposcopy is unsatisfactory or the lesion is large, excision should be performed with ablation not recommended.

For women <25 years of age with a histologic diagnosis of CIN2, either treatment or observation for up to 24 months using both colposcopy and cytology at 6-month intervals is acceptable, provided colposcopy is satisfactory. Treatment is recommended if CIN3 is subsequently identified or if CIN2/3 persists for 24 months.

In the absence of invasive disease, additional colposcopic and cytologic examinations are acceptable in pregnant women with a histologic diagnosis of CIN2/3 at intervals no more frequent than every 12 weeks. Repeat biopsy is recommended only if the appearance of the lesion worsens or if cytology suggests invasive cancer. Reevaluation with cytology and colposcopy is recommended 6 weeks postpartum.

Treatment of Adenocarcinoma In Situ

Hysterectomy is preferred for women who have completed childbearing and have a histologic diagnosis of AIS. Conservative management with cervical conization is acceptable if future fertility is desired. If the margins of the specimen are involved or endocervical sampling obtained above the cone bed contains CIN or AIS, reexcision to increase the likelihood of complete excision is recommended. Long-term follow-up is recommended for women who do not undergo hysterectomy.

Treatment of Invasive Cervical Carcinoma

Type of Treatment

Treatment of invasive cervical cancer depends on many factors, including disease stage, patient age, performance status, fertility of the patient, and skill and resources of the care providers. The treatment of cervical cancer is described by stage of disease in the following sections.

Hysterectomy Classification According to Piver et al ([37])

In 1974, Piver et al ([37]) categorized hysterectomy into five classes according to the extent of tissue resection.

Class I

Simple hysterectomy is removal of the uterus along with the cervix in an extrafascial manner without incision into the cervical or uterine tissue.

Class II

Modified radical hysterectomy is removal of the uterus with part of the paracervical and parametrial tissue in the lateral aspect of the cervix after dissecting the ureters away. Half of the cardinal ligament (lateral aspect), the uterosacral ligament (posterior aspect), and one-third of the upper vagina are all removed. This is usually performed in cases of stage IA2 or persistent or local recurrent cervical cancer after radiation therapy.

Class III

Radical hysterectomy is removal of the uterus in a manner similar to that of class II hysterectomy, but the tissue structure is removed to a greater extent, generally close to the pelvic side wall laterally and sacrum posteriorly; the upper half of the vagina is also removed. Conventionally, this class of hysterectomy is done for cases of stage IB to IIA disease. However, it can be performed for persistent or recurrent cervical cancer after primary radiation therapy as an alternative procedure to exenteration in highly selected patients. These include patients with stage IB to IIA disease at primary diagnosis, no clinical parametrial involvement, and a tumor diameter of ≤4 cm at the time of recurrence.

Class IV

Extended radical hysterectomy is complete removal of the cervix, uterus, parametrial tissue, cardinal, and uterosacral ligaments. In addition, the ureter is completely dissected from the vesicouterine ligament, and the superior vesical artery is sacrificed. This is a possible procedure for central locoregional recurrence.

Class V

Partial exenteration is partial excision of the involved organs. In addition to the above procedures, this encompasses the removal of the distal ureter and urinary bladder. This procedure is performed in cases of central recurrence.

Hysterectomy Classification According to Cibula et al ([38])

A more recent classification has been introduced by Cibula et al ([38]).

Type A: Minimum Resection of Paracervix

This resection is an extrafascial hysterectomy, in which the position of the ureters is determined by palpation or direct vision (after opening of the ureteral tunnels) without freeing the ureters from their beds. The paracervix is transected medial to the ureter but lateral to the cervix. The uterosacral and vesicouterine ligaments are not transected at a distance from the uterus. Vaginal resection is generally at a minimum, routinely less than 10 mm, without removal of the vaginal part of the paracervix (paracolpos).

Type B: Transection of Paracervix at the Ureter

Partial resection of the uterosacral and vesicouterine ligaments is a standard part of this category. The ureter is unroofed and rolled laterally, permitting transection of the paracervix at the level of the ureteral tunnel. The caudal (posterior, deep) neural component of the paracervix caudal to the deep uterine vein is not resected. At least 10 mm of the vagina from the cervix or tumor is resected.

Type C: Transection of Paracervix at Junction With Internal Iliac Vascular System

The Q–M classification system distinguishes between a type C1 procedure, which corresponds to the nerve-sparing modification, and the type C2 procedure, which aims for a complete parametrial resection. Type C1 requires separation of two parts of the dorsal parametria; the medial part, which entails rectouterine and rectovaginal ligaments, and the lateral laminar structure, also called mesoureter, which contains the hypogastric plexus. Furthermore, type C1 requires only a partial dissection of the ureter from the ventral parametria, which is usually asymmetric towards more extensive resection of the medial leaf of the cranial (above the ureter) part of the ventral parametria. In the C2 type, the ureter is completely dissected from the ventral parametria up to the urinary bladder wall. Defining the resection limits on the longitudinal (deep parametrial or vertical) plane is crucial for distinguishing between types C1 and C2.

Type D: Laterally Extended Resection

This type differs from type C2 only in the lateral extent of the lateral parametria resection. Ureteral dissection and resection of both dorsal and ventral parametria is identical to the type C2. Laterally, however, it requires ligation and removal of the internal iliac artery and vein, together with their branches, including the gluteal, internal pudendal, and obturator vessels.

Treatment by Stage of Disease

Stage IA1

Stage IA1 cervical cancer should be diagnosed using a conization specimen, because small tissue biopsy study may not be accurate enough to rule out other areas of a more extensive lesion. The treatment depends on the need for fertility preservation.

Conization

In a recent study, He et al ([39]) evaluated the value of cold knife conization (CKC) as a conservative management in patients with microinvasive cervical SCC. A total of 108 patients with stage IA1 were enrolled. Eighty-three patients (76.9%) underwent further hysterectomy, out of which 48 (57.8%) underwent extrafascial hysterectomy, 30 (36.1%) underwent extensive hysterectomy, and 5 (6.1%) underwent radical hysterectomy. All patients were followed up for 1 year. The 18 patients with positive resection margins had greater likelihood of cervical residual lesions (CIN1-3) than the 65 patients with clear resection margins, but there were no significant differences (P = .917). Twenty-five patients who underwent CKC as final therapy were followed up for 1 year. Two patients with positive resection margins had a second CKC surgery; one patient was diagnosed with CIN1, and the other was diagnosed with cervicitis by pathology. Twenty-three patients had clear resection margins; two patients underwent a second CKC 3 months after the first CKC because of the abnormal ThinPrep Cytologic Test (TCT) result, and they were both diagnosed with microinvasive cervical SCC (stage IA1) by pathology with clear resection margins. No one enrolled in this study presented with metastasis or progression within 1 year of follow-up. This provided the clinical evidence for the possibility of fertility-sparing treatments, especially CKC, as conservative treatment for microinvasive cervical SCC.

Simple Hysterectomy

Simple hysterectomy may be performed in women with stage IA1 cervical cancer in whom preservation of fertility function is not required. However, in patients with LVSI, a modified radical hysterectomy may be the procedure of choice.

Stage IA2

The incidence of LNI in patients with this stage of cervical cancer is as high as 7% with a recurrence rate of 3% to 5%, and these patients should be treated with a radical hysterectomy with pelvic lymph node dissection. In women who want to conserve fertility, another approach that has been reported to have a successful outcome is radical trachelectomy with laparoscopic pelvic lymphadenectomy, in which the body of uterus is preserved for fertility function ([40]). Individualization of therapy based on findings from extensive pathologic review of an adequate cone biopsy specimen is important for treatment planning.

Stage IB1

The standard surgical treatment for FIGO stage IB1 cervical cancer consists of a radical hysterectomy or trachelectomy and systematic pelvic lymphadenectomy.

Radical Hysterectomy

Traditionally, surgery for stage IB disease consists of radical hysterectomy performed in conjunction with pelvic lymphadenectomy. Lately, some have recommended class II hysterectomy rather than conventional class III hysterectomy in stages IB and IIA disease with a tumor size <2 cm due to fewer complications from the former and no difference in the 5-year survival ([41]) (Figs. 33-7 and 33-8).

Sentinel Lymph Node Mapping

The concept of the sentinel node (SN) was first clinically developed by Cabanas in association with penile carcinoma ([42]). It is based on the principle that if the SN or the first node receiving drainage from tumor is negative, more extensive lymphadenectomy may be exempted to avoid the morbidity of the procedure.

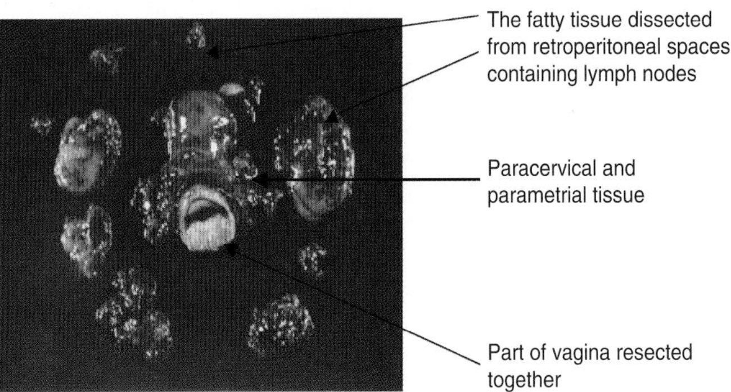

FIGURE 33-7 Gross specimen from a radical hysterectomy with lymph nodes dissected.

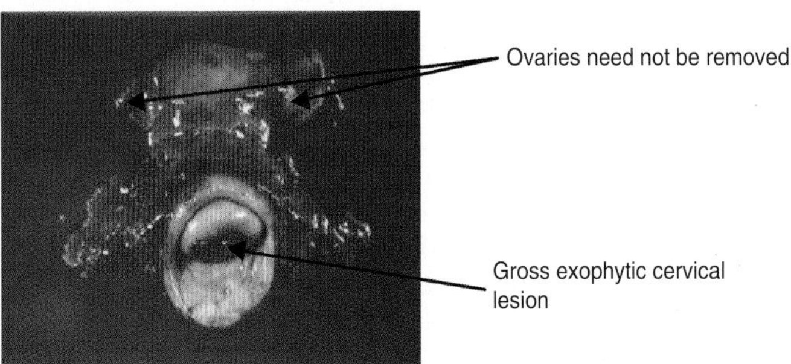

FIGURE 33-8 A radical hysterectomy specimen with a portion of upper vagina. Note that the ovaries need not be removed unless indicated by the associated pathology.

Generally, the techniques used to map SNs involve identification of the lymphatic duct by injecting isosulfan blue dye or lymphoscintigraphy, using gamma probe detection of technetium 99m–labeled colloid, which is injected into the cervix. This can be done either before or during the operation. A number of studies of SN mapping for cervical cancer have been published; in these instances, the investigators used either blue dye, lymphoscintigraphy, or both with varying degrees of success. The introduction of indocyanine green (ICG) as another tool for SN mapping may be revolutionizing the field because it is now being used in patients undergoing minimally invasive surgery, both by the laparoscopic and robotics approach. Indocyanine green is a dye that fluoresces in the near-infrared (NIR) spectrum when illuminated with 806-nm light. When a laser emitted from the NIR imager excites ICG, it produces a wavelength that is converted to a fluorescent image. The emitted fluorescence is captured with a video camera device that allows for the ICG to be displayed in the visible light spectrum ([43]).

Jewell et al ([44]) assessed the detection rate of SNs using ICG in patients with uterine and cervical cancer. A total of 227 cases were performed. The median SN count was 3 (range, 1-23). An SN was identified in 216 cases (95%), with bilateral pelvic mapping in 179 cases (79%). The authors found that there was no difference in the detection rate when ICG alone was used versus the combination of both dyes (ICG and isosulfan blue). The authors concluded that combined use of ICG and blue dye appears unnecessary.

In the SENTICOL study by Lécuru et al ([45]), the authors aimed to determine if bilateral negative SNs accurately predict absence of lymph node metastasis in early cervical cancer patients with stage IA1 disease with LVSI to stage IB1. One hundred forty-five patients were enrolled, and 139 were included in a modified intent-to-diagnose analysis. Intraoperative radioisotope-blue dye mapping detected at least one SN in 136 patients (97.8%; 95% CI, 93.8%-99.6%), 23 of whom had true-positive results and two of whom had false-negative results, yielding 92.0% sensitivity (23 of 25 patients; 95% CI, 74.0%-99.0%) and 98.2% negative predictive value (111 of 113 patients; 95% CI, 74.0%-99.0%) for node metastasis detection. No false-negative results were observed in the 104 patients (76.5%) in whom SNs were identified bilaterally. Therefore, the authors concluded that SN biopsy was fully reliable only when SNs were detected bilaterally.

Radical Trachelectomy

Radical trachelectomy (RT) is resection of the cervix together with paracervical and parametrial tissue, with retention of the corpus uteri. The procedure is indicated in reproductive-age women with disease stage IA1 (with LVSI), IA2, or IB1 (<2 cm) disease who wish to preserve fertility ([46]).

Abu-Rustum and Sonoda ([40]) analyzed a prospectively maintained database of all patients with FIGO stage IA1 to IB1 cervical cancer admitted to the operating room for planned fertility-sparing abdominal RT. Sentinel node mapping was performed through cervical injection. Between November 2001 and May 2010, 98 consecutive patients with FIGO stage IA1 to IB1 cervical cancer and a median age of 32 years (range, 6-45 years) underwent a fertility-sparing RT. The most common histology was adenocarcinoma in 54 patients (55%) and squamous carcinoma in 42 patients (43%). Lymphovascular invasion was seen in 38 patients (39%). The FIGO stages included IA1 (with lymphovascular invasion) in 10 patients (10%), IA2 in 9 patients (9%), and IB1 in 79 patients (81%). Only 15 patients (15%) needed immediate completion radical hysterectomy because of intraoperative findings. Median number of nodes evaluated was 22 (range, 3-54), and 16 patients (16%) had positive pelvic nodes on final pathology. Final trachelectomy pathology showed no residual disease in 44 patients (45%), dysplasia in 5 patients (5%), and AIS in 3 patients (3%). Overall, 27 patients (27%) needed hysterectomy or adjuvant pelvic radiation postoperatively. One documented recurrence (1%) was fatal at the time of this report. It was thus concluded that cervical adenocarcinoma and lymphovascular invasion are common features of patients selected for RT, and most patients can undergo the operation successfully, with approximately 65% having no residual invasive disease; however, nearly 27% of all selected cases will require hysterectomy or postoperative chemoradiation for oncologic reasons.

Diaz et al ([47]) compared the oncologic outcomes of women who underwent a fertility-sparing RT to those who underwent a radical hysterectomy for stage IB1 cervical carcinoma. Forty stage IB1 patients underwent an RT, and 110 patients underwent a radical hysterectomy. There were no statistical differences between the two groups for the following prognostic variables: histology, median number of lymph nodes removed, node-positive rate, LVSI, or deep stromal invasion. The median follow-up time for the entire group was 44 months. The 5-year recurrence-free survival rate was 96% for the RT group compared with 86% for the radical hysterectomy group (*P* value not significant). On multivariate analysis in this group of stage IB1 lesions, tumor size <2 cm was not an independent predictor of outcome, but both LVSI and deep stromal invasion retained independent predictive value ($P = .033$ and $P = .005$, respectively). The authors concluded that for selected patients with stage IB1 cervical cancer, fertility-sparing RT appears to have a similar oncologic outcome to radical hysterectomy. Lymphovascular space invasion and deep stromal invasion appear to be more valuable predictors of outcome than tumor diameter in this subgroup of patients.

In 2013, Pareja et al ([48]) published a systematic literature review of patients with early-stage cervical cancer who underwent abdominal RT. A total of 485 patients age 6 to 44 years were identified. The most common stage was IB1 (71%), and the most common histologic subtype was SCC (70%). Operative times ranged from 110 to 586 minutes. Blood loss ranged from 50 to 5568 mL. Forty-seven patients (10%) had conversion to radical hysterectomy. One hundred fifty-five patients (35%) had a postoperative complication. The most frequent postoperative complication was cervical stenosis (n = 42; 9.5%). The median follow-up time was 31.6 months (range, 1-124 months). Sixteen patients (3.8%) had disease recurrence. Two patients (0.4%) died of disease. A total of 413 patients (85%) were able to maintain their fertility. A total of 113 patients (38%) attempted to get pregnant, and 67 of these patients (59.3%) were able to conceive. Therefore, the authors concluded that abdominal RT is a safe treatment option in patients with early-stage cervical cancer interested in preserving fertility.

Conservative Treatment

The possibility of less radical surgery may be appropriate not only for patients desiring to preserve fertility but also for all patients with low-risk early-stage cervical cancer. Recently, a number of studies have explored less radical surgical options for early-stage cervical cancer, including simple hysterectomy, simple trachelectomy, and cervical conization with or without SN biopsy and pelvic lymph node dissection. Criteria that define this low-risk group include squamous carcinoma, adenocarcinoma, or adenosquamous carcinoma, tumor size <2 cm, stromal invasion <10 mm, and no LVSI ([49]).

The ConCerv study is one of the several prospective studies evaluating the role of conservative surgery in women with newly diagnosed, early-stage cervical cancer.

Retrospective data have shown that low-risk cervical cancer may not require radical hysterectomy because the risk for parametrial involvement is less than 1% in these patients. In this study, eligible women undergo CKC or simple hysterectomy and pelvic lymphadenectomy with SN based on their desire for future fertility. The primary outcome of this study is the safety and feasibility of a conservative approach ([49]).

More recently, a Gynecologic Cancer Intergroup (GCIG) trial was led by the National Cancer Institute of Canada Clinical Trials Group, called the SHAPE trial. In this trial, patients with stage IA2 to IB1 cervical cancer with low-risk qualities (early-stage cervical cancer [IA2, IB1 <2 cm], limited stromal invasion <10 mm on loop electrosurgical excision procedure/cone biopsy, <50% stromal invasion on pelvic MRI) are randomized to either simple or radical hysterectomy. The study is currently ongoing and is aiming to accrue a total of 700 patients ([50]).

Stage IB2-IVA

Concurrent Chemoradiation

In 1999, the US National Cancer Institute announced its support of concurrent cisplatin-based chemotherapy and radiation therapy in women who require radiation therapy for the management of cervical cancer. This was based on data from five randomized controlled trials that showed a significant benefit of concurrent chemoradiation either as postoperative adjuvant therapy in patients with high-risk factors or primary therapy in patients with locally advanced cervical cancer. All five trials sed concurrent cisplatin either alone or in combination with 5-fluorouracil (5-FU) or 5-FU and hydroxyurea. Peters et al ([51]) applied concurrent chemoradiation as postoperative adjuvant therapy in patients with risk factors found from radical hysterectomy in stage IA2 to IIA disease and indicated that it was superior to radiation therapy alone. Keys et al ([52]) compared chemoradiation and radiation with adjuvant hysterectomy as the definitive treatment in patients with stage IB2 disease. Significant improvement of 3-year survival was found in the chemoradiation group (83% vs 74%). Pathologic examination of the hysterectomy specimens demonstrated a significant decrease in persistent disease with chemoradiation.

Three other studies comprised patients with more advanced disease ([53-55]). The Radiation Therapy Oncology Group trial (RTOG) 9001 by Morris et al randomized stage IB-IVA patients to concurrent chemoradiation with cisplatin and 5-FU versus extended-field radiation ([53]). Chemoradiation was superior, with an increase in overall survival of 73%, compared with 58% for radiation alone. Acute toxicity was more common with chemoradiation, but the rates of late complications (>60 days after treatment) were similar. A trial by Rose et al ([54]) studied the optimal chemoradiation regimen by randomizing patients with stage IIB-IVA disease to receive radiation therapy concurrent with one of the following chemotherapy regimens: cisplatin alone; cisplatin, 5-FU, and hydroxyurea; or hydroxyurea alone. With a median follow-up time of 35 months, the results demonstrated superior survival rates for both concurrent cisplatin regimens (66% and 64%, respectively) compared with concurrent hydroxyurea alone (39%). The toxicity of treatment was least with the single-agent cisplatin regimen. Another Gynecologic Oncology Group trial in stage IIB to IVA cervical cancer by Whitney et al ([55]) compared the efficacy of a chemotherapy regimen in the concurrent chemoradiation setting. The results showed superiority of cisplatin and 5-FU over hydroxyurea; survival rates at a median follow-up of 8.7 years were 55% and 43%, respectively. Leukopenia occurred less often in the group receiving cisplatin and 5-FU than in those receiving hydroxyurea.

A summary of these five trials is presented in Table 33-4.

Neoadjuvant Chemotherapy

A review by the Neoadjuvant Chemotherapy for Locally Advanced Cervical Cancer Meta-Analysis Collaboration group discovered seven randomized controlled trials available for analysis, comprising 872 patients ([56]). The overall analysis and analysis of each individual trial showed significant improvement of all outcomes with neoadjuvant chemotherapy: hazard ratio of 0.65 for survival, with 14% absolute improvement in 5-year survival rate (50% to 64%); hazard ratio of 0.68 for disease-free survival, with 13% absolute improvement of disease-free survival (45% to 58%); and hazard ratio of 0.63 for metastasis-free survival, with 15% absolute improvement in metastasis-free survival (45% to 60%). However, many confounding factors were inherent and unavoidable in this systematic analysis: these factors were that a number of patients, ranging from 28% to 90% in each trial, also received postoperative adjuvant radiation therapy or triple-modality treatment compared with radiation therapy, the route of cisplatin administration differed (intra-arterial in one trial), and patients recruited to each trial had different stages of disease.

Eddy et al ([57]) published a phase III trial from the Gynecologic Oncology Group to determine whether neoadjuvant chemotherapy (NACT) prior to radical hysterectomy and pelvic/para-aortic lymphadenectomy (RHPPL) could improve progression-free survival and overall survival, as well as operability, with acceptable levels of toxicity. Two hundred eighty-eight eligible patients with bulky FIGO stage IB cervical cancer, tumor diameter ≥4 cm, adequate bone marrow, renal, and hepatic function, and performance status ≤2 were randomly allocated to RHPPL (n = 143) or NACT + RHPPL (n = 145). The NACT + RHPPL group had a similar recurrence rate (relative risk, 0.998) and death rate (relative risk, 1.008) compared with the RHPPL group. Seventy-nine percent of patients had surgery in the RHPPL group compared to 78% in the NACT + RHPPL group. Fifty-two percent of patients received postoperative RT in the RHPPL group compared to 45% in the NACT + RHPPL group (not statistically significant). The authors concluded that NACT offered no additional objective benefit to patients undergoing RHPPL for stage IB cervical cancer.

Another phase III trial was conducted by Katsumata et al ([58]) to determine whether NACT before radical surgery improved overall survival. A total of 134 patients with stage IB2, IIA2, or IIB SCC of the uterine

Table 33-4 Five Randomized Control Trials of Concurrent Chemoradiation for Cervical Cancer

Study (Protocol)	Setting	No. of Patients	Treatment	Outcome[a]	Remarks
Keys et al ([52]), 1999 (GOG 123)	IB2	369	1. RT + weekly C 2. RT (followed by TAH in both groups)	RR of progression and death, 0.51 and 0.54 in CRT arm	Higher severe hematologic and GIT toxicity in CRT arm (21% vs 4% and 14% vs 5%)
Peters et al ([51]), 2000 (SWOG 8797/GOG 109)	PO IA2-IIA with risk factors	243	1. RT + CF 2. RT alone	4-year PFS and SVR, 80% and 81% in group 1 4-year PFS and SVR, 63% and 71% in group 2	ACA had similar outcomes as SCC in CRT arm; ACA did worse in RT arm
Whitney et al ([55]), 1999 (GOG 85)	IIB-IVA	368	1. RT + CF 2. RT + HU	RR of progression and death, 0.79 and 0.74 of group 1 compared to group 2 (21% and 26% decreased risk of progression and death)	Severe leukopenia more common in HU arm (24% vs 4%)
Morris et al ([53]), 1999 (RTOG 9001)	IB-IVA	388	1. RT + CF 2. RT + extended-field radiation	5-year OS and DFS, 73% and 67% 5-year OS and DFS, 58% and 40%	Higher reversible hematologic side effects in CRT arm
Rose et al ([54]), 1999 (GOG 120)	IIB-IVA	526	1. RT + weekly C 2. RT + CF + HU 3. RT + HU	2-year PFS, 67% and 64% in groups 1 and 2 and 47% in group 3 RR of death, 0.61 and 0.58 in groups 1 and 2 compared with group 3	Group 1 least toxic

[a]There was a significant difference in all outcomes between the study and control groups.
ACA, adenocarcinoma; C, cisplatin; CF, cisplatin plus 5-fluorouracil; CRT, concurrent chemoradiation; DFS, disease-free survival; GIT, gastrointestinal tract; GOG, Gynecologic Oncology Group; HU, hydroxyurea; OS, overall survival; PFS, progression-free survival; PO, postoperative; RR, relative risk; RT, radiation therapy; RTOG, Radiation Therapy Oncology Group; SCC, squamous cell carcinoma; SVR, survival rate; SWOG, Southwest Oncology Group; TAH, total abdominal hysterectomy.

cervix were randomly assigned to receive either BOMP (bleomycin, vincristine, mitomycin, cisplatin) plus radical surgery (NACT group) or radical surgery alone (radical surgery group). Patients with pathologic high-risk factors received postoperative radiotherapy. This study was prematurely terminated at the first planned interim analysis because overall survival in the NACT group was inferior to that in the radical surgery group. The 5-year overall survival was 70.0% in the NACT group and 74.4% in the radical surgery group ($P = .85$). Hence, it was concluded that NACT with BOMP regimen before radical surgery did not improve overall survival but reduced the number of patients who received postoperative radiotherapy.

Stage IVB

In patients with stage IVB cervical cancer, which implies systemic disease, treatment is palliative rather than curative. Radiation therapy has a role for local primary disease to alleviate symptoms such as bleeding and pain. In patients who have distant metastasis, symptoms such as bone pain can be relieved with high-dose radiation. Chemotherapy is also an option for patients with stage IVB disease, but the response is modest because of factors like poor vascular supply and bone marrow reserve.

POSTTREATMENT SURVEILLANCE

The recommended surveillance is based on patients' risk for recurrence and personal preferences. History and physical examination are recommended every 3 to 6 months for 2 years, every 6 to 12 months for another 3 to 5 years, and then annually. Patients with high-risk disease can be assessed more frequently (eg, every 3 months for the first 2 years). Annual cervical/vaginal cytology tests can be considered as indicated for detection of lower genital tract dysplasia. Patient education regarding symptoms suggestive of recurrence is recommended (eg, vaginal discharge; weight loss; anorexia; pain in the pelvis, hips, back, or legs; persistent coughing). Patients who have received RT for cervical cancer may experience vaginal stenosis and dryness and should receive education on important issues regarding sexual health and vaginal health. Cervical cancer survivors are at risk for second cancers; therefore, careful surveillance is appropriate for these patients ([59]).

RECURRENT CERVICAL CANCER

It is generally accepted that any lesions detected within 6 months after treatment should be considered persistent. The diagnosis of recurrence is usually made after 6 months. If a lesion is noted within 3 months after radiation therapy, no treatment is recommended due to the ongoing effects of irradiation at this time period.

Choosing the type of therapy for recurrent cervical cancer depends on many factors, including site of recurrence, previous therapy, and performance status of the patients.

Locoregional

Concurrent platinum-based chemotherapy reduces the risk of pelvic recurrence by approximately 50% and extends overall survival by an absolute 5% to 20% compared to radiation therapy alone; this includes tumor-directed radiation therapy and platinum-based chemotherapy with (or without) brachytherapy; surgical resection can be considered if feasible. Typically, the chemoradiation for recurrence uses cisplatin as a single agent or cisplatin plus 5-FU. Patients with central pelvic recurrent disease after radiotherapy should be evaluated for pelvic exenteration, with (or without) intraoperative radiotherapy. Surgical mortality is generally 5% or less, with survival rates approaching 50% in carefully selected patients. Although exenteration is the common surgical approach in postradiation patients with isolated central pelvic relapse, radical hysterectomy or brachytherapy may be an option in patients with small central lesions (<2 cm) ([59]).

Westin et al ([60]) conducted a study to determine the impact of clinical and pathologic factors on 5-year survival after pelvic exenteration for gynecologic malignancies. A total of 160 women who underwent pelvic exenteration were evaluated. Five-year recurrence-free survival was 33% (95% CI, 0.25-0.40). Factors that negatively impacted recurrence-free survival included shorter treatment-free interval ($P = .050$), vulvar primary ($P = .032$), positive margins ($P < .001$), LVSI ($P < .001$), positive lymph nodes ($P < .001$), and perineural invasion ($P = .030$). Factors that negatively impacted overall survival included vulvar primary ($P =.04$), positive margins ($P < .001$), LVSI ($P < .001$), positive lymph nodes ($P < .001$), and perineural invasion ($P = .008$). Hence, it was concluded that the 5-year overall survival after pelvic exenteration was 40%.

Distant

Distant recurrence with or without associated locoregional lesions denotes systemic disease and carries a poor prognosis and minimal chance of a cure. Monk et al ([61]) published the phase III trial from the Gynecologic Oncology Group evaluating the toxicity and efficacy of cisplatin doublet combinations in advanced and recurrent cervical carcinoma. Patients were randomly assigned to paclitaxel 135 mg/m^2 over 24 hours plus cisplatin 50 mg/m^2 on day 2 every 3 weeks (PC, reference arm); vinorelbine 30 mg/m^2 on days 1 and 8 plus cisplatin 50 mg/m^2 on day 1 every 3 weeks (VC); gemcitabine 1,000 mg/m^2 on days 1 and 8 plus cisplatin 50 mg/m^2 on day 1 every 3 weeks (GC); or topotecan 0.75 mg/m^2 on days 1, 2, and 3 plus cisplatin 50 mg/m^2 on day 1 every 3 weeks (TC). Survival was the primary end point, with a 33% improvement relative to PC considered important (85% power, $\alpha = 5\%$). Quality-of-life data were prospectively collected. A total of 513 patients were enrolled when a planned interim analysis recommended early closure for futility. The experimental-to-PC hazard ratios of death were 1.15 (95% CI, 0.79-1.67) for VC, 1.32 (95% CI, 0.91-1.92) for GC, and 1.26 (95% CI, 0.86-1.82) for TC. The hazard ratios for progression-free survival were 1.36 (95% CI, 0.97-1.90) for VC, 1.39 (95% CI, 0.99-1.96) for GC, and 1.27 (95% CI, 0.90-1.78) for TC. Response rates for PC, VC, GC, and TC were 29.1%, 25.9%, 22.3%, and 23.4%, respectively. The arms were comparable with respect to toxicity except for leukopenia, neutropenia, infection, and alopecia. The authors concluded that none of the regimens studied was superior to PC in terms of overall survival. However, the trends in response rate, progression-free survival, and overall survival favored PC.

Until recently, no chemotherapy combination or single agent had shown a survival advantage in phase III trials. Tewari et al ([62]) evaluated the effectiveness of bevacizumab and nonplatinum combination chemotherapy in patients with recurrent, persistent, or metastatic cervical cancer. A total of 452 patients were randomly assigned to chemotherapy with or without bevacizumab at a dose of 15 mg/kg of body weight. Groups were well balanced with respect to age, histologic findings, performance status, previous use or nonuse of a radiosensitizing platinum agent, and disease status. The addition of bevacizumab to chemotherapy was associated with increased overall survival (17.0 vs 13.3 months; hazard ratio for death, 0.71; 98% CI, 0.54-0.95; $P = .004$ in a one-sided test) and higher response rates (48% vs 36%, $P = .008$). Bevacizumab, as compared with chemotherapy alone, was associated with an increased incidence of hypertension of grade 2 or higher (25% vs 2%), thromboembolic events of grade 3 or higher (8% vs 1%), and gastrointestinal fistulas of grade 3 or higher (3% vs 0%). Therefore, it was concluded that the addition of bevacizumab to combination chemotherapy in patients with recurrent, persistent, or metastatic cervical cancer was associated with an improvement of 3.7 months in median overall survival.

REFERENCES

1. Siegel RL, Miller KD, Jemal A. Cancer statistics, 2015. *CA Cancer J Clin.* 2015;65:5-29.
2. Torre LA, Bray F, Siegel RL, Ferlay J, Lortet-Tieulent J, Jemal A. Global cancer statistics, 2012. *CA Cancer J Clin.* 2015;65(2):87-108.
3. Hacker NF. Cervical cancer. In: Berek JS, Hacker NF, eds. *Gynecologic Oncology.* 5th ed. Philadelphia, PA: Lippincott Williams & Wilkins; 2010:341-394.
4. Kjaer SK, Chackerian B, van den Brule AJ, et al. High-risk human papillomavirus is sexually transmitted: evidence from a follow-up study of virgins starting sexual activity (intercourse). *Cancer Epidemiol Biomarkers Prev.* 2001;10:101-106.
5. Schiffman M, Castle PE. Human papillomavirus: epidemiology and public health. *Arch Pathol Lab Med.* 2003;127:930-934.
6. Satterwhite CL, Torrone E, Meites E, et al. Sexually transmitted infections among U.S. women and men: prevalence and incidence estimates, 2008. *Sex Transm Dis.* 2013;40:187-193.
7. Trottier H, Franco EL. The epidemiology of genital human papillomavirus infection. *Vaccine.* 2006;24:S1-S15.
8. Castellsague X, Diaz M, de Sanjose S, et al. Worldwide human papillomavirus etiology of cervical adenocarcinoma and its cofactors: implications for screening and prevention. *J Natl Cancer Inst.* 2006;98:303-315.
9. Joste NE, Ronnett BM, Hunt WC, et al. Human papillomavirus genotype-specific prevalence across the continuum of cervical neoplasia and cancer. *Cancer Epidemiol Biomarkers Prev.* 2015;24:230-240.
10. Ferenczy A, Coutlee F, Franco E, Hankins C. Human papillomavirus and HIV coinfection and the risk of neoplasias of the lower genital tract: a review of recent developments. *CMAJ.* 2003;169:431-434.
11. McKenzie ND, Kobetz EN, Ganjei-Azar P, et al. HPV in HIV-infected women: implications for primary prevention. *Front Oncol.* 2014;4:179.
12. Juneja A, Sehgal A, Mitra AB, Pandey A. A survey on risk factors associated with cervical cancer. *Indian J Cancer.* 2003;40:15-22.
13. Louie KS, de Sanjose S, Diaz M, et al. Early age at first sexual intercourse and early pregnancy are risk factors for cervical cancer in developing countries. *Br J Cancer.* 2009;100:1191-1197.
14. International Collaboration of Epidemiological Studies of Cervical Cancer, Appleby P, Beral V, et al. Cervical cancer and hormonal contraceptives: collaborative reanalysis of individual data for 16,573 women with cervical cancer and 35,509 women without cervical cancer from 24 epidemiological studies. *Lancet.* 2007;370:1609-1621.
15. Lee YC, Hashibe M. Tobacco, alcohol, and cancer in low and high income countries. *Ann Glob Health.* 2014;80:378-383.
16. International Agency for Research on Cancer. Tumours of the uterine cervix. In: Tavassoli FA, Devilee P, eds. *Pathology and Genetics of Tumours of the Breast and Female Genital Organs. World Health Organization Classification of Tumours.* Lyon, France: International Agency for Research on Cancer; 2003:259-290.
17. International Federation of Gynecology and Obstetrics Committee on Gynecologic Oncology. FIGO staging for carcinoma of the vulva, cervix, and corpus uteri. *Int J Gynecol Obstet.* 2014;125:97-98.
18. Lee KR, Flynn CE. Early invasive adenocarcinoma of the cervix. *Cancer.* 2000;89:1048-1055.
19. Murakami I, Fujii T, Kameyama K, et al. Tumor volume and lymphovascular space invasion as a prognostic factor in early invasive adenocarcinoma of the cervix. *J Gynecol Oncol.* 2012;23:153-158.
20. Pirog EC, Kleter B, Olgac S, et al. Prevalence of human papillomavirus DNA in different histological subtypes of cervical adenocarcinoma. *Am J Pathol.* 2000;157:1055-1062.
21. Wu H, Zhang L, Cao W, Hu Y, Liu Y. Mesonephric adenocarcinoma of the uterine corpus. *Int J Clin Exp Pathol.* 2014;7:7012-7019.
22. ACOG Practice Bulletin Number 131: Screening for cervical cancer. *Obstet Gynecol.* 2012;120:1222-1238.
23. Solomon D, Davey D, Kurman R, et al. Forum Group Members; Bethesda 2001 Workshop. The 2001 Bethesda System: terminology for reporting results of cervical cytology. *JAMA.* 2002;287:2114-2119.
24. Shimada M, Kigawa J, Nishimura R, et al. Ovarian metastasis in carcinoma of uterine cervix. *Gynecol Oncol.* 2006; 101:234-237.
25. Pallavi VR, Devi KU, Mukherjee G, Ramesh C, Bafna UD. Relationship between lymph node metastases and histopathological parameters in carcinoma cervix: a multivariate analysis. *J Obstet Gynaecol.* 2012;32:78-80.
26. Loft A, Berthelsen AK, Roed H, et al. The diagnostic value of PET/CT scanning in patients with cervical cancer: a prospective study. *Gynecol Oncol.* 2007;106:29-34.
27. Raspagliesi F, Ditto A, Solima E, et al. Microinvasive squamous cell cervical carcinoma. *Crit Rev Oncol Hematol.* 2003;48:251-61.
28. Singh P, Tripcony L, Nicklin J. Analysis of prognostic variables, development of predictive models, and stratification of risk groups in surgically treated FIGO early-stage (IA-IIA) carcinoma cervix. *Int J Gynecol Cancer.* 2012;22:115-122.
29. Milam MR, Frumovitz M, dos Reis R, Broaddus RR, Bassett RL Jr, Ramirez PT. Preoperative lymph-vascular space invasion is associated with nodal metastases in women with early-stage cervical cancer. *Gynecol Oncol.* 2007;106:12-15.
30. Frumovitz M, Sun CC, Schmeler KM, et al. Parametrial involvement in radical hysterectomy specimens for women with early-stage cervical cancer. *Obstet Gynecol.* 2009;114:93-99.
31. Koutsky LA, Ault KA, Wheeler CM, et al. Proof of Principle Study Investigators. A controlled trial of a human papillomavirus type 16 vaccine. *N Engl J Med.* 2002;347:1645-1651.
32. Gilmer LS. Human papillomavirus vaccine update. *Prim Care.* 2015;42:17-32.
33. Human papillomavirus vaccines: WHO position paper, October 2014–Recommendations. *Vaccine.* 2015;33(36):4383-4384.
34. Apter D, Wheeler CM, Paavonen J, et al. Efficacy of HPV-16/18 AS04-adjuvanted vaccine against cervical infection and precancer in young women: final event-driven analysis of the randomised, double-blind PATRICIA trial. *Clin Vaccine Immunol.* 2015;22:361-373.
35. Jeong BK, Huh SJ, Choi DH, Park W, Bae DS, Kim BG. Prognostic value of different patterns of squamous cell carcinoma antigen level for the recurrent cervical cancer. *Cancer Res Treat.* 2013;45:48-54.
36. Massad LS, Einstein MH, Huh WK, et al. 2012 ASCCP Consensus Guidelines Conference. 2012 updated consensus guidelines for the management of abnormal cervical cancer screening tests and cancer precursors. *Obstet Gynecol.* 2013;121:829-846.
37. Piver MS, Rutledge F, Smith JP. Five classes of extended hysterectomy for women with cervical cancer. *Obstet Gynecol.* 1974;44:265-272.
38. Cibula D, Abu-Rustum NR, Benedetti-Panici P, et al. New classification system of radical hysterectomy: emphasis on a

three-dimensional anatomic template for parametrial resection. *Gynecol Oncol.* 2011;122:264-268.
39. He Y, Wu YM, Zhao Q, et al. Clinical value of cold knife conization as conservative management in patients with microinvasive cervical squamous cell cancer (stage IA1). *Int J Gynecol Cancer.* 2014;24:1306-1311.
40. Abu-Rustum NR, Sonoda Y. Fertility-sparing surgery in early-stage cervical cancer: indications and applications. *J Natl Compr Canc Netw.* 2010;8:1435-1438.
41. Landoni F, Maneo A, Cormio G, et al. Class II versus class III radical hysterectomy in stage IB-IIA cervical cancer: a prospective randomized study. *Gynecol Oncol.* 2001;80:3-12.
42. Cabanas R. An approach for the treatment of penile carcinoma. *Cancer.* 1977;39:456-466.
43. Ramirez PT, Frumovitz M. Optimizing sentinel node identification: a step toward novel tools and improved strategies-exciting times are here! *J Minim Invasive Gynecol.* 2015;22:153-154.
44. Jewell EL, Huang JJ, Abu-Rustum NR, et al. Detection of sentinel lymph nodes in minimally invasive surgery using indocyanine green and near-infrared fluorescence imaging for uterine and cervical malignancies. *Gynecol Oncol.* 2014;133:274-277.
45. Lécuru F, Mathevet P, Querleu D, et al. Bilateral negative sentinel nodes accurately predict absence of lymph node metastasis in early cervical cancer: results of the SENTICOL study. *J Clin Oncol.* 2011;29:1686-1691.
46. Roy M, Plante M. Radical vaginal trachelectomy for invasive cervical cancer. *J Gynecol Obstet Biol Reprod.* 2000;29:279-281.
47. Diaz JP, Sonoda Y, Leitao MM, et al. Oncologic outcome of fertility-sparing radical trachelectomy versus radical hysterectomy for stage IB1 cervical carcinoma. *Gynecol Oncol.* 2008; 111:255-260.
48. Pareja R, Rendón GJ, Sanz-Lomana CM, Monzón O, Ramirez PT. Surgical, oncological, and obstetrical outcomes after abdominal radical trachelectomy: a systematic literature review. *Gynecol Oncol.* 2013;131:77-82.
49. Ramirez PT, Pareja R, Rendón GJ, Millan C, Frumovitz M, Schmeler KM. Management of low-risk early-stage cervical cancer: should conization, simple trachelectomy, or simple hysterectomy replace radical surgery as the new standard of care? *Gynecol Oncol.* 2014;132:254-259.
50. ClinicalTrials.gov. Radical versus simple hysterectomy and pelvic node dissection in patients with early stage cervical cancer. https://clinicaltrials.gov/show/NCT01658930. Accessed May 9, 2014.
51. Peters WA 3rd, Liu PY, Barrett RJ 2nd, et al. Cisplatin and 5-fluorouracil plus radiation therapy are superior to radiation therapy as adjunctive in high-risk early stage carcinoma of the cervix after radical hysterectomy and pelvic lymphadenectomy: report of a phase III intergroup study. *J Clin Oncol.* 2000;18:1606-1613.
52. Keys HM, Bundy BN, Stehman FB, et al. Cisplatin, radiation, and adjuvant hysterectomy compared with radiation and adjuvant hysterectomy for bulky stage IB cervical carcinoma. *N Engl J Med.* 1999;340:1154-1161.
53. Morris M, Eifel PJ, Lu J, et al. Pelvic radiation with concurrent chemotherapy versus pelvic and para-aortic radiation for high-risk cervical cancer: a randomized Radiation Therapy Oncology Group clinical trial. *N Engl J Med.* 1999;340:1137-1143.
54. Rose PG, Bundy BN, Watkins EB, et al. Concurrent cisplatin-based chemoradiation improves progression free and overall survival in advanced cervical cancer: results of a randomized Gynecologic Oncology Group study. *N Engl J Med.* 1999;340:1144-1153.
55. Whitney CW, Sause W, Bundy BN, et al. A randomized comparison of fluorouracil plus cisplatin versus hydroxyurea as an adjunct to radiation therapy in stages IIB-IVA carcinoma of the cervix with negative para-aortic lymph nodes. A Gynecologic Oncology Group and Southwest Oncology Group study. *J Clin Oncol.* 1999;17:1339-1348.
56. Neoadjuvant Chemotherapy for Locally Advanced Cervical Cancer Meta-Analysis Collaboration. Neoadjuvant chemotherapy for locally advanced cervical cancer: a systematic review and meta-analysis of individual patient data from 21 randomised trials. *Eur J Cancer.* 2003;39:2470-2486.
57. Eddy GL, Bundy BN, Creasman WT, et al. Treatment of ("bulky") stage IB cervical cancer with or without neoadjuvant vincristine and cisplatin prior to radical hysterectomy and pelvic/para-aortic lymphadenectomy: a phase III trial of the Gynecologic Oncology Group. *Gynecol Oncol.* 2007;106:362-369.
58. Katsumata N, Yoshikawa H, Kobayashi H, et al. Phase III randomised controlled trial of neoadjuvant chemotherapy plus radical surgery vs radical surgery alone for stages IB2, IIA2, and IIB cervical cancer: a Japan Clinical Oncology Group trial (JCOG 0102). *Br J Cancer.* 2013;108:1957-1963.
59. National Comprehensive Cancer Network. Guidelines Version 2. 2015. Cervical cancer. www.NCCN.org.
60. Westin SN, Rallapalli V, Fellman B, et al. Overall survival after pelvic exenteration for gynecologic malignancy. *Gynecol Oncol.* 2014;134:546-551.
61. Monk BJ, Sill MW, McMeekin DS, et al. Phase III trial of four cisplatin-containing doublet combinations in stage IVB, recurrent, or persistent cervical carcinoma: a Gynecologic Oncology Group study. *J Clin Oncol.* 2009;27:4649-4655.
62. Tewari KS, Sill MW, Long HJ 3rd, et al. Improved survival with bevacizumab in advanced cervical cancer. *N Engl J Med.* 2014;370:734-743.

34

Gestational Trophoblastic Disease

第三十四章　妊娠滋养细胞疾病

Jubilee Brown

中文导读

妊娠滋养细胞疾病泛指胎盘滋养细胞组织来源的肿瘤疾病。本章首先介绍妊娠滋养细胞疾病的流行病学，之后重点讲述了疾病的组织学分型，根据组织学类型将其分为葡萄胎、绒毛膜癌、侵蚀性葡萄胎、胎盘部位滋养细胞肿瘤、上皮样滋养细胞肿瘤。在发病机制部分包括了细胞生物学、生长因子和癌基因的内容。临床表现部分分别对完全性葡萄胎、部分性葡萄胎、恶性妊娠滋养细胞疾病3种类型进行了阐述。诊断部分重点讲述了超声影像检查及实验室检查，并对错觉绒毛膜癌综合征做了简单介绍。在分期和预后部分，简述了妊娠滋养细胞疾病的分期标准及预后影响因素。在治疗部分，分别讲述了葡萄胎、恶性妊娠滋养细胞疾病的治疗方案，其中恶性妊娠滋养细胞的疾病又根据预后危险因素进行了危险分层，并阐述了不同危险组患者的治疗策略。本章最后对双胎妊娠、患者未来的生育和生存状况进行了简单的介绍。

Gestational trophoblastic disease (GTD) comprises a wide spectrum of neoplastic disorders that arise from placental trophoblastic tissue after abnormal fertilization (Fig. 34-1). The spectrum includes benign disease (complete and partial hydatidiform moles) and malignant gestational trophoblastic neoplasia (GTN), which includes choriocarcinoma, placental site trophoblastic tumor (PSTT), and epithelioid trophoblastic tumor (ETT) ([1]). Invasive moles may also occur and are best categorized as malignant, since they can metastasize. Gestational trophoblastic neoplasia is also described as gestational trophoblastic tumor (GTT) and is further designated as nonmetastatic or metastatic ([2]).

The hydatidiform mole is the most common type of GTD. It is essentially a benign condition with variable potential for malignant transformation. Most molar pregnancies resolve spontaneously after uterine evacuation, with no further events or adverse outcomes. At any time during or after gestation, approximately 20% undergo malignant transformation to invasive nonmetastatic or metastatic GTN and require further treatment ([3]). Nearly two-thirds of these lesions develop into persistent nonmetastatic GTN; the remaining one-third develop distant metastases ([2, 4]).

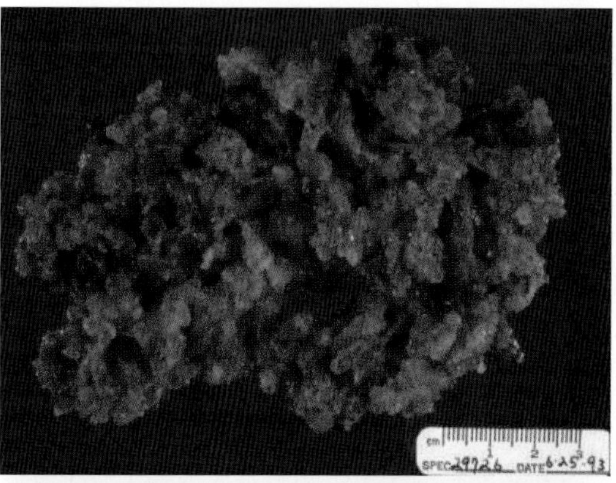

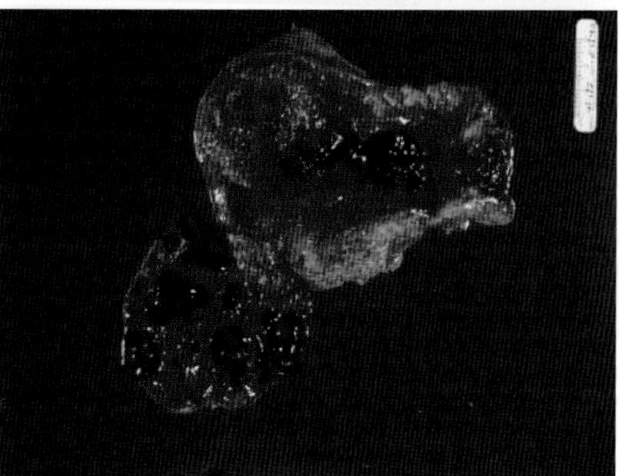

FIGURE 34-1 Gross specimen of two complete molar pregnancies. Note the absence of fetal tissue, which is replaced by abundant trophoblastic tissue.

These tumors were first described around 400 B.C. by Hippocrates and subsequently termed "dropsy" of the uterus. During the 1950s, the 5-year survival of patients with choriocarcinoma was less than 5%. The treatment of these tumors has been revolutionized with effective chemotherapy, leading to a cure rate approaching 100% and fertility preservation in most patients ([1, 5, 6]). Successful outcomes rely on individualized management based on careful staging and treatment planning by a multidisciplinary team.

EPIDEMIOLOGY

The prevalence of GTD depends on geography, maternal age, previous GTD history, socioeconomic factors, dietary factors, and blood grouping. True estimates of the incidence of molar pregnancy are difficult to obtain because of the vast variation in presentation and management of normal and abnormal pregnancies around the world. In North America and in Europe, GTD develops in approximately 1 in 100 to 2,000 pregnancies ([1, 7, 8]). A higher rate of 1.5 to 6 per 1,000 pregnancies has been reported in South America. Early observations comparing East and Southeast Asian countries with the United States suggest a 5- to 15-fold higher incidence, as high as 1 in 120 pregnancies in East Asia ([1, 8, 9]). Native Alaskans have an incidence three- to fourfold that of white women. Native Americans had a higher incidence than other ethnic groups in New Mexico ([10]). Not all data confirm the importance of ethnic background. Recent analyses suggest that the incidence in Southeast Asia is similar to that in Europe, which may reflect modifications in diet, improved diagnosis, and improved capture of population statistics ([1, 2, 8]).

Extremes of age at conception appear to influence the rate of GTD ([1, 2, 11]). Women older than 40 years have a fivefold greater risk of molar pregnancy ([11]); those younger than 20 years have a 1.5- to 2-fold relative risk ([11]). Women with a history of hydatidiform mole have a 10-fold greater risk for a second molar pregnancy and a more than 1,000-fold greater risk of choriocarcinoma than women with normal pregnancies ([11]). The New England Trophoblastic Disease Center demonstrated the increased risk of subsequent molar pregnancy to be 1% ([12]).

Women of lower socioeconomic status have a 10-fold greater rate of molar pregnancy than more affluent counterparts. This trend has been reported in East Asia, the Middle East, the United States, and Brazil ([2, 13]). This relationship between GTD incidence and geographic region, culture, and socioeconomic status suggests that diet and nutrition may contribute to the etiology. Low β-carotene and high animal fat consumption are associated with GTD. There is strong association between cigarette smoking and GTD.

Historically 80% of GTDs are hydatidiform moles, 15% are invasive moles, and 5% are choriocarcinomas. Placental site trophoblastic tumor occurs in 0.2% to 2% of all GTD but is responsible for the highest mortality rate of all GTD histologies ([14, 15]). Choriocarcinoma is associated with an antecedent complete hydatidiform mole in 50% of the cases, a history of abortion in 25%, term delivery in 20%, and ectopic pregnancy in 5%. Occurrence after partial mole is rare ([1, 2]). The precise rate of choriocarcinoma may be underreported because tissue is not recommended for the diagnosis based on the risk of hemorrhage with biopsy ([1, 2]).

In the United States, molar pregnancies are reported in approximately 3,000 patients per year, and malignant transformation occurs in 2% to 19% of these cases ([1, 2, 4]). Complete molar pregnancies occur 1 in 15,000 abortions and 1 in 150,000 normal pregnancies. The estimated incidence of twin pregnancy consisting of a molar pregnancy and a normal fetus is 1 per 22,000 to 100,000 pregnancies.

PATHOLOGY

A hydatidiform mole is confined to the uterine cavity. When a hydatidiform mole persists, it is termed malignant and may be designated GTT or GTN and may be metastatic or nonmetastatic. Most malignant GTDs occur after evacuation of a mole and exhibit the histologic features of either hydatidiform moles or choriocarcinomas. Choriocarcinomas are highly malignant and tend to metastasize extensively. Conversely, persistent GTD after a nonmolar pregnancy almost always has the histologic pattern of choriocarcinoma. Invasive moles and placental site tumors are locally invasive but rarely metastatic. Both tumors are rare, but they can be distinguished histologically ([2]). Specific pathologic criteria exist for each of these histologic subtypes.

Complete Mole (See Fig. 34-1)

Based on morphologic and cytogenetic features, hydatidiform moles are divided into two unique syndromes: complete (classic) and partial (Table 34-1). Complete hydatidiform mole is characterized by the lack of a fetus and a characteristic abnormal budding edematous villous structure with nonpatchy trophoblastic hyperplasia, stromal karyorrhectic debris, and collapsed, abnormal villous blood vessels ([2]). A complete mole is usually detected during the second trimester and is identified by total hydatidiform enlargement of the villi, which are enveloped by hyperplastic and atypical trophoblasts. There is a notable absence of any embryonic or amniotic remnant. In questionable cases, p57 immunohistochemistry can be useful in confirming the diagnosis ([16]). Approximately 20% of complete moles give rise to persistent trophoblastic disease.

Table 34-1 Features of Complete and Partial Hydatidiform Moles

	Complete	Partial
Fetal or embryonic tissue	Absent	Present
Hydatidiform swelling of chorionic villi	Diffuse	Focal
Trophoblastic hyperplasia	Diffuse	Focal
Trophoblastic stromal inclusions	Absent	Present
Genetic parentage	Paternal	Biparental
Karyotype	46XX; 46XY	69XXY; 69XYY
Persistent β-hCG elevation	20%	0.5%

Partial Mole (Fig. 34-2)

Partial moles, in contrast to complete moles, are typically accompanied by an identifiable embryo or amniotic membranes. These moles are described as partial because the hydatidiform changes in the villi tend to be focal. They demonstrate patchy villous hydrops with scattered abnormally shaped and scalloped irregular villi with trophoblastic pseudo inclusions and patchy trophoblastic hyperplasia ([2]). The villous capillaries appear to be functional because they possess the same proportion of nucleated fetal erythrocytes as the embryo. In partial moles, hydatidiform change occurs at a slower rate, and the proportion of relatively normal villi appears to correlate with fetal survival rate.

Diagnosis of molar pregnancies based on histology alone can be problematic. Negative immunostaining for *P57KIP2*, an imprinted gene expressed by the maternal allele, is diagnostic of a complete mole, as the placenta of all other gestations demonstrates nuclear staining of cytotrophoblast and villous mesenchyme ([2, 6]). Ploidy analysis can help differentiate partial (triploid) from complete (diploid) mole, but cannot distinguish between this and other etiologies of triploidy. Selective molecular genotyping allows for definitive diagnosis when histologic review is equivocal, but the cost of such testing may prohibit widespread adoption of this technique.

Maturation of mesenchymal elements is only minimally delayed in partial moles, and there is a paucity of fibroblast karyorrhexis. Approximately 2% to 6% of partial moles undergo malignant degeneration ([3]).

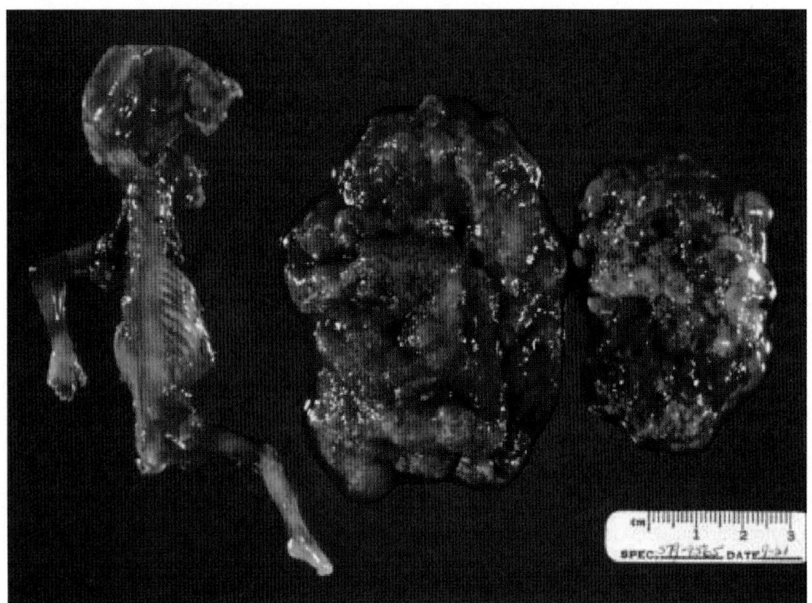

FIGURE 34-2 Partial molar pregnancy removed along with partially formed fetal tissue.

Because of this sporadic malignant potential, follow-up and treatment of patients with partial moles are the same as for patients with complete moles.

Invasive Mole

Locally invasive moles have the same histologic features as complete mole. In addition, they are characterized by myometrial invasion without involvement of intervening endometrial stroma. Invasive moles are typically diagnosed clinically approximately 6 months after molar evacuation when human chorionic gonadotropin (hCG) remains elevated. They tend to invade locally, causing hemorrhage and necrosis. Rarely, uterine perforation results. Hematogenous metastasis may occur, often to the lungs. Occasionally, metastatic deposits display hydropic villi rather than the sheets of anaplastic cells that typify metastatic choriocarcinoma. Invasive moles are scored using the World Health Organization (WHO) scoring system, and treatment is predicated based on the score. If childbearing is complete, hysterectomy is recommended, but if fertility preservation is desired, the appropriate form of chemotherapy based on the WHO score is administered.

Choriocarcinoma

Choriocarcinoma is a malignant tumor with a unique histology distinct from that of moles ([2]). The tumor is grossly red and granular and exhibits extensive necrosis and hemorrhage. On microscopic examination, the neoplasm is composed of a disordered array of syncytiotrophoblastic and cytotrophoblastic elements, absence of chorionic villi, frequent mitoses, and multinucleated giant cells. Direct myometrial and vascular invasion occur early, with resultant metastases to the lungs, vagina, brain, kidneys, liver, pelvis, spleen, and gastrointestinal tract ([1,2,6]).

Placental Site Trophoblastic Tumor

Placental site tumors are rare and most often develop after nonmolar gestations but can occur after evacuation of a complete hydatidiform mole ([14]). These tumors occur at the placental implantation site and consist of numerous nodules in the endometrium or myometrium. Histologically, these consist of a homogeneous population of mononuclear intermediate trophoblast cells of the placenta infiltrating in sheets or cords between myometrial fibers, sometimes with a few syncytial elements ([17]). The intermediate trophoblastic cells have oval nuclei with abundant eosinophilic cytoplasm, and no chorionic villi are seen. Syncytiotrophoblastic and cytotrophoblastic populations are absent, and less vascular invasion, necrosis, and hemorrhage are seen than in choriocarcinoma ([17]). Lymphatic metastasis is common. Placental site trophoblastic tumor secretes placental lactogen and small amounts of β-hCG and is usually diploid ([1,2]).

Epithelioid Trophoblastic Tumor

Epithelioid trophoblastic tumor is a rare variant of PSTT that mimics carcinoma but histologically is composed of chorionic-type intermediate trophoblast.

PATHOGENESIS

Pathologic characteristics alone generally do not allow adequate discrimination of molar pregnancies. With the advent of cytogenetic techniques, such as chromosomal banding and restriction fragment length polymorphism analysis of DNA, unique chromosomal patterns of molar pregnancies were discovered ([18]), allowing complete and partial moles to be distinguished from one another ([19]).

Cell Biology (Fig. 34-3)

Normal fertilization results from the union of a single sperm and an egg, followed by rapid cellular division and the creation of a diploid embryo. Early embryonic differentiation gives rise to trophoblasts, specialized epithelial cells responsible for developing the placenta and the villi. Gestational trophoblastic tumors arise from abnormal unions of sperm with the ovum, resulting in distinct pathologic characteristics involving activated transcription factors, cytokines, hormone secretion, cell adhesion molecules, and immunologic activity ([20]).

A complete mole contains nuclear chromosomes of paternal origin and mitochondrial DNA of maternal origin ([2, 21]). Chromosomal banding studies reveal that complete moles contain only paternal chromosomes. This finding has been confirmed by showing that when paternal heterozygotes for the human leukocyte antigen (HLA) locus give rise to a mole, the HLA expression of the molar tissue is homozygous ([22]). Approximately 80% to 92% of complete moles have a 46,XX karyotype derived from fertilization of an empty egg, the chromosomes of which were lost during meiosis, by a haploid sperm (23X) that then undergoes duplication to create a diploid set of identical chromosomes (46,XX) ([23]). Complete moles can also result from postzygotic diploidization of a triploid conception. Approximately 4% to 20% of complete moles result from dispermy, in which two spermatozoa (each of which may be 23X or 23Y) fertilize an empty ovum, resulting in a 46,XX or 46,XY karyotype containing all paternal nuclear chromosomes ([2, 24]). Most are 46,XY, but approximately 5% of all complete moles are heterozygous 46,XX resulting from such dispermy. A 46,YY mole has not been reported, suggesting that the X chromosome is required for survival. There is no strong evidence that dispermic or Y chromosome–containing moles have greater malignant potential than the monospermic 46,XX karyotype ([21]).

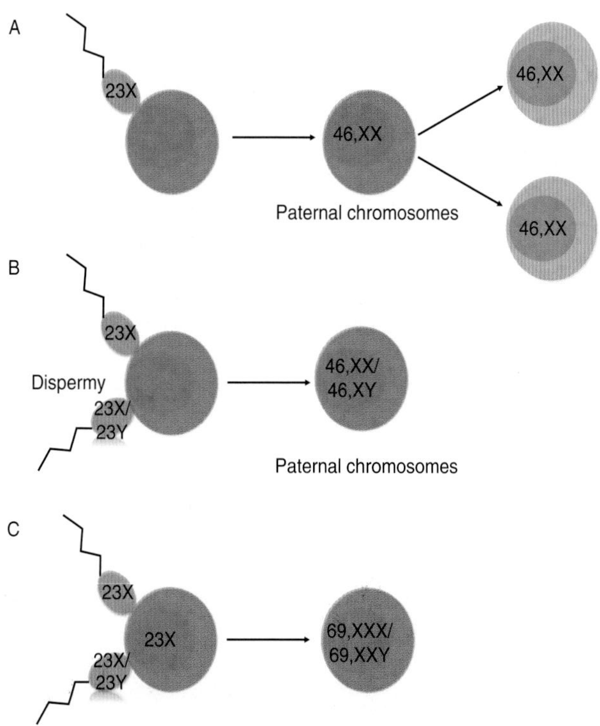

FIGURE 34-3 Schematic diagram of the pathogenesis of molar pregnancies. (A) Complete mole. Most common pathogenesis, in which a haploid sperm (23X) fertilizes an empty egg which then undergoes duplication (46,XX). (B) Complete mole. Dispermy, in which two spermatozoa (23X or 23Y) fertilize an empty egg yielding a complete mole (46,XX or 46,XY). (C) Partial mole. Two spermatozoa (23X or 23Y) fertilize an ovum (23X) yielding a triploid mole (69,XXY or 69,XXX).

A partial mole results from the abnormal union of two spermatozoa with one ovum with intact chromosomes, resulting in a triploid karyotype. Occasionally, a normal ovum can be fertilized by an abnormal diploid sperm ([2]). Therefore, the classic partial mole has a triploid karyotype (69 chromosomes), and both paternal and maternal chromosomes are present. The most common sex chromosome arrangement is XXY, but XXX and XYY do exist ([2]). Of note, in triploid pregnancies, a partial mole results when the extra haploid chromosome is of paternal origin, and a fetus develops when the extra haploid chromosome is of maternal origin. In the event that a partial mole is reported as diploid, the diagnosis is usually a misdiagnosed complete mole, hydropic abortion, or twin pregnancy ([2]).

Rarely, familial recurrent hydatidiform mole syndrome may be present, leading to recurrent molar pregnancies. This is an autosomal recessive disorder with mutations in *NLRP7* (70% of cases) or *KHDC3L* (5% of cases) resulting in diploid complete moles of biparental origin, as opposed to exclusively paternal origin. Live birth in these patients is rare, but egg donation from unaffected women may result in successful live birth ([25]).

Growth Factors and Oncogenes

Our improved understanding of the activities of protooncogenes, tumor suppressor genes, cytokines, and growth factors is contributing to our understanding of GTN and tumor progression ([22]).

The excess of paternal chromosomes in moles probably contributes to the induction of trophoblastic hyperplasia. The genomic imbalance may cause changes in expression of growth factor genes located on the paternal allele. Both normal placentas and molar pregnancies contain paternal antigens. Upon implantation, an immunologic response is initiated, with infiltration of lymphocytes and macrophages and secretion of cytokines.

The growth of choriocarcinomas may be related to the abundant expression of epidermal growth factor (EGF) receptor. Macrophage-derived cytokines—interleukin-1 (IL-1-α, IL-1-β) and tumor necrosis factor—can suppress cell growth and increase the expression of EGF receptor in choriocarcinoma cell lines, thus acting as paracrine mediators of cell growth ([26]).

The contribution of several oncogenes to the malignant transformation of GTD has also been examined. Growth regulation in the trophoblast is associated with expression of the transcription factor Mash-2 ([27]). Complete moles demonstrate increased expression of c-fms RNA compared with that in normal placentas ([28]). In choriocarcinoma, increased expression of oncogenes has been observed, and progression of some tumors has been associated with inactivation of tumor suppressor genes ([29]). The significance of these findings is uncertain. Because trophoblasts are by nature rapidly dividing and invasive, increased expression of these oncogenes may be essential for normal cell function. Table 34-2 lists other genes whose overexpression has been implicated in GTD ([30-32]). Human placental growth hormone has recently been detected in all variants of GTD and may serve as a novel biomarker for diagnosis ([33]).

CLINICAL PRESENTATION

Complete Moles

The most common presenting symptom of the complete mole is vaginal bleeding in the first or early second trimester of pregnancy, although the classic signs of a molar pregnancy include vaginal bleeding as well as absence of fetal heart sounds and physical evidence of a uterus that is larger than expected for the gestational age ([2]).

A constellation of symptoms and signs has historically been associated with molar pregnancy, but such events are becoming less common due to routine ultrasonography in early pregnancy and the resulting early diagnosis of molar pregnancy ([34]). In the event that molar pregnancy is detected later in the first or early second trimester, patients may present with abdominal pain due to the enlarged uterus, which may be larger than expected for gestational age. Intrauterine blood clots may liquefy and produce the pathognomonic prune juice–like vaginal discharge. Because of recurrent bleeding, patients may also present with iron deficiency beyond that expected for a normal pregnancy. Symptoms of anemia have been noted in approximately 50% of patients at diagnosis ([35]). Theca lutein cysts, caused by β-hCG–induced hyperstimulation of both ovaries in about 50% of patients, may result in a sensation of pelvic pressure or fullness. Usually, these cysts regress spontaneously after

Table 34-2 Genes That Have Been Implicated in Gestational Trophoblastic Disease

p53
p21$^{WAF1/CIP1}$
Mdm2
Rb (retinoblastoma)
C-myc7q21–q31
C-erbB2
C-fms
bcl-2
Telomerase

uterine evacuation, although their rupture or tension can cause acute abdominal symptoms occasionally requiring surgery ([35]).

In the past, 20% to 30% of patients have presented with early pre-eclampsia, thought to be precipitated by the release of large amounts of vasoactive substances from necrotic trophoblastic tissue, but seizures are rare ([12]). Ten percent of patients have presented with hyperemesis gravidarum, and 7% have presented with hyperthyroidism, presumably due to the structural similarities of β-hCG to thyroid-stimulating hormone ([36, 37]). Thyroid storm has been reported. Other rare presentations include respiratory distress, disseminated intravascular coagulation, and microangiopathic hemolytic anemia ([35]).

Partial Moles

Unlike complete moles, fewer than 10% of patients with partial moles present with an enlarged uterus. An intact fetus can coexist with a partial mole, though this occurs in fewer than 1 in 100,000 pregnancies. Patients with partial moles typically do not have the hormonal symptoms experienced by patients with complete moles, and pre-eclampsia is rare. Among 81 patients with partial moles, none had prominent theca lutein cysts, hyperthyroidism, or respiratory insufficiency and only one had toxemia ([37]). Patients with partial moles present with signs and symptoms of a missed or incomplete abortion, and the diagnosis of a partial mole is made only after histologic review of curettage specimens.

Malignant Gestational Trophoblastic Disease

Although spontaneous remission occurs in approximately 80% of patients with GTD after evacuation, malignant GTD is most commonly diagnosed after evacuation of a molar pregnancy when serum β-hCG titers plateau or rise ([2, 15]). Patients treated surgically for molar pregnancy should be monitored closely for malignant transformation with symptoms, signs, and serum evaluation. Previously referred to as persistent trophoblastic disease, a plateaued or rising β-hCG level (three consecutive measurements) indicates malignant change and the development of GTN.

Fifty percent of all malignant GTNs follow molar pregnancy, 25% follow normal pregnancy, and the remaining 25% follow ectopic pregnancy or abortion. Persistent invasive nonmetastatic GTN usually presents with recurrence of symptoms or signs such as irregular vaginal bleeding, theca lutein cysts, asymmetric uterine enlargement, or persistently elevated serum β-hCG levels. The tumor may even perforate the myometrium causing intraperitoneal bleeding, or the tumor may invade into uterine vessels causing vaginal hemorrhage. Irregular vaginal bleeding may be due to a vascular uterine mass or a vaginal metastasis. Patients can also present with sepsis and abdominal pain, as the uterine tumor presents a nidus for infection ([2]). Placental site trophoblastic tumor and ETT present in the same manner as invasive moles and nearly always present with abnormal vaginal bleeding, because the disease remains localized to the uterus prior to metastasis ([14]). Only small amounts of β-hCG are produced relative for their size, and in some cases, the β-hCG is normal ([2]).

Metastatic GTN occurs in about 20% of patients who have undergone molar evacuation ([35]). Metastatic GTN most often arises from choriocarcinoma. Molar pregnancy is the most common antecedent of choriocarcinoma, but this tumor may also occur after normal pregnancy, ectopic pregnancy, or abortion. These highly vascular tumors tend to metastasize extensively and may cause spontaneous hemorrhage at the metastatic foci, causing symptoms. The metastases are sometimes histologically identical to molar disease, but the vast majority are choriocarcinomas. Metastatic spread is hematogenous. Because of its extensive vascular network, metastatic GTN often produces local spontaneous bleeding. Common metastatic sites of GTN as reported by the New England Trophoblastic Disease Center are summarized in Table 34-3 ([38]).

Pulmonary metastases are common, occurring in 80% of patients with metastatic disease ([38]), and result when trophoblastic tissue enters the circulation via uterine venous sinuses. Most often, this happens spontaneously, but it may also occur after molar evacuation. Because choriocarcinoma is a vascular tumor, hemoptysis is frequent with lung involvement. Other symptoms include chest pain, dyspnea, and cough.

Pulmonary hypertension and pleural effusions may develop. An asymptomatic lesion on a chest x-ray or

Table 34-3 Common Metastatic Sites in Order of Frequency

Lungs	80%
Vagina	30%
Pelvis	20%
Brain	10%
Liver	10%
Bowel, kidney, spleen	<5%
Other	<5%
Serum[a]	<5%

[a]Persistent hCG after hysterectomy.
Data from Berkowitz RS, Goldstein DP. Pathogenesis of gestational trophoblastic neoplasms. *Pathol Annu.* 1981;11:391–411.

computed tomography (CT) scan may be the only sign of pulmonary involvement. Radiologic features may be subtle and include alveolar, nodular, and miliary patterns ([39]). Pulmonary metastases (Fig. 34-4) can be extensive and can cause respiratory failure and death.

Patients may experience right-upper-quadrant pain when hepatic metastases stretch the Glisson capsule. Gastrointestinal lesions can result in severe hemorrhage or perforation with peritonitis, either of which requires emergency intervention. Vaginal examination may reveal bluish metastatic deposits. Biopsy of these and other metastatic sites is contraindicated because severe uncontrolled bleeding may occur ([35]).

Central nervous system (CNS) involvement from metastatic GTN suggests widespread disease. Central nervous system metastases occur in 7% to 28% of patients with metastatic choriocarcinoma ([38, 39]). The presenting neurologic symptoms include headache, hemiparesis, vomiting, dizziness, coma, grand mal seizure, visual disturbances, aphasia, and slurred speech. Weight loss and anorexia may also occur. In one-third of cases with cerebral metastases, there is no vaginal bleeding ([2]). Cerebral metastases tend to respond favorably to both radiotherapy and chemotherapy (Fig. 34-5).

DIAGNOSIS

The diagnosis of molar pregnancy is usually made by the histologic examination of curettage specimens. The diagnosis of persistent GTN or malignant GTN is most often indicated by plateauing or rising hCG titers after evacuation during surveillance. Histologic diagnosis of invasive mole, choriocarcinoma, or metastatic deposits should never be attempted because a biopsy of these neoplasms can cause massive, life-threatening hemorrhage. The hCG level in this setting is sensitive enough to make the diagnosis of malignant GTN without histologic confirmation. Beause PSTT and ETT do not typically arise after molar pregnancy, their diagnosis is usually made upon examination of the curettage, biopsy, or hysterectomy specimens ([2]). Presenting symptoms of PSTT are most commonly irregular vaginal bleeding, amenorrhea, and a pelvic mass ([17]).

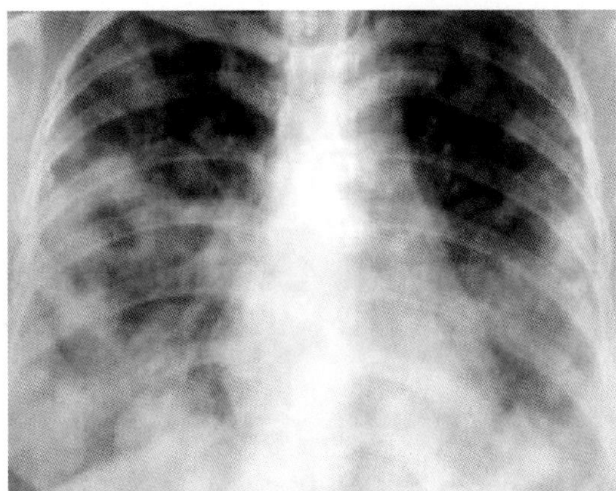

FIGURE 34-4 Chest radiograph of a patient with metastatic choriocarcinoma. This patient had refused treatment and died of the disease.

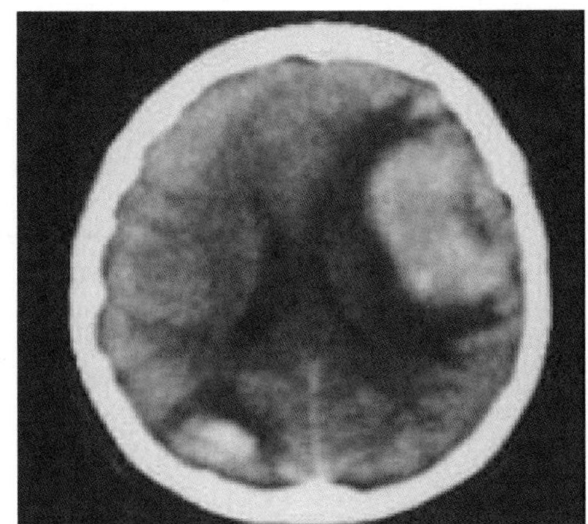

FIGURE 34-5 Magnetic resonance imaging scan of patient with metastatic choriocarcinoma

Radiologic Imaging

Ultrasonography is useful for the confirmation of molar pregnancy but is not diagnostic, because diagnosis depends on histologic examination of evacuated material. Ultrasonography is the first modality of radiographic imaging used when GTD is considered and may reveal the classic "snowstorm" appearance, which is due to the numerous chorionic villi exhibiting diffuse hydatidiform swelling ([40]) (see Fig. 34-5; Figs. 34-6 and 34-7). Such a classic appearance is less common now, because the diagnosis is often made in the first trimester prior to the development of significant hydropic change. More common is a mixed echogenic vascular mass. In the setting of partial mole, fetal parts may also be detected ([1]).

A chest x-ray should be performed in all patients because 70% to 80% of patients with metastatic GTN have lung involvement ([35]) (see Fig. 34-4). Brain imaging is not routinely warranted in the absence of symptoms or pulmonary abnormalities, because 97% to 100% of patients with CNS disease from choriocarcinoma have concomitant pulmonary metastases ([41]).

An abnormal chest x-ray associated with a β-hCG level that plateaus or rises during treatment is an indication for a more extensive evaluation for metastatic disease. Computed tomography scans of the brain, abdomen, and pelvis should be performed to evaluate other likely sites of metastatic spread.

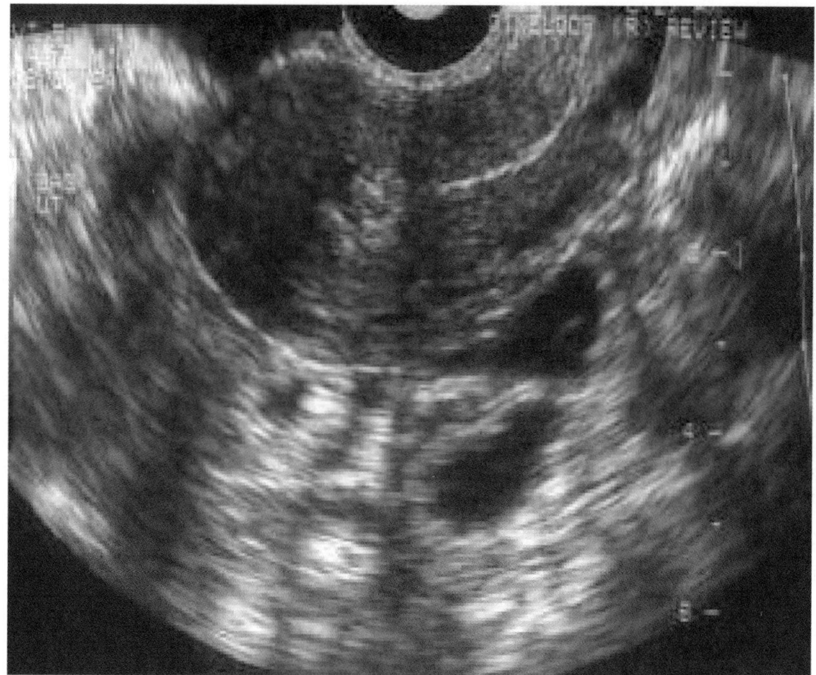

FIGURE 34-6 Ultrasound of a gestational trophoblastic tumor

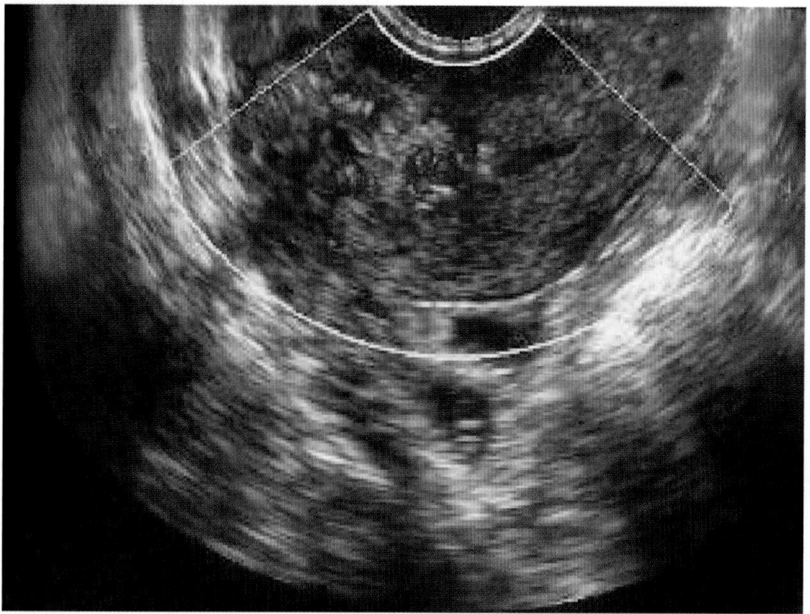

FIGURE 34-7 Doppler ultrasound of a gestational trophoblastic tumor

Magnetic resonance imaging (MRI) is the preferred modality for localized disease to delineate invasiveness and tumor vascularity (Fig. 34-8) ([42]).

Laboratory Tests

Chorionic gonadotropin is a glycoprotein hormone secreted by the syncytiotrophoblast: it is essential for the maintenance of normal function of the corpus luteum during pregnancy. This hormone has an α subunit identical to the α subunit of the pituitary hormones and a β subunit (β-hCG) unique to trophoblastic tissue that confers its specific biologic activity. The hormone becomes detectable 8 days after ovulation, and its level doubles every 2 to 4 days, reaching its peak at 10 to 12 weeks of gestation. After that, the

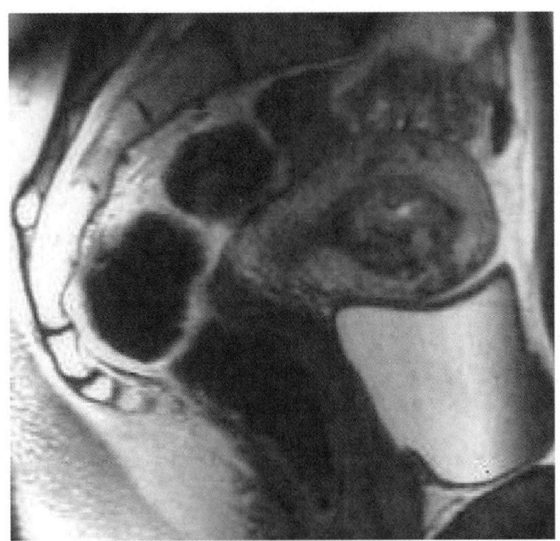

FIGURE 34-8 Magnetic resonance imaging scan of a gestational trophoblastic tumor.

β-hCG level declines steadily. Because all trophoblastic tumors secrete β-hCG, its level serves as an excellent marker for tumor activity in the nonpregnant patient ([2, 43]).

In normal pregnancy, hCG exists intact with both subunits and is hyperglycosylated in the first trimester. In GTD, hCG can exist as a free β subunit, nicked free β subunit, c-terminal peptide, β-core, or hyperglycosylated forms ([44]). The assay used to detect or follow hCG in the setting of GTD must recognize all of these forms; for this reason, home pregnancy tests should be avoided in favor of commercial assays ([1, 2]). Even some commercial assays only work well for pregnancy-related hCG. These assays may be unreliable for detecting hCG isoforms, occasionally leading to false-negative readings, or may cross-react with heterophile antibodies leading to false-positive results ([1, 2]). Because the heterophile antibodies are large, they are filtered in the renal glomerulus and do not pass through into the urine. Therefore, urine pregnancy tests may be useful to exclude a false-positive result (serum positive, urine negative) but are not sufficient for making the diagnosis of GTD, only for excluding a false-positive result.

Monitoring of the serial β-hCG levels is mandatory during therapy for GTD to ensure adequate treatment. The level of β-hCG can be considered approximately proportional to the tumor burden and inversely proportional to therapeutic outcome. The 10% to 20% of patients with hydatidiform mole who are not cured by local therapy or do not achieve a spontaneous remission can be identified by a rising or plateaued β-hCG titer on serial determinations after evacuation of a mole. These patients may have persistent trophoblastic disease and require additional therapy, as outlined later. A new pregnancy should be excluded by correlating the hCG level with the ultrasound findings prior to assuming malignant GTD; that is, once the hCG level rises to a level where a fetal pole should be identified, an ultrasound should exclude conception.

At one time, the ratio of β-hCG in serum to that in cerebrospinal fluid (CSF) was used to detect brain metastases in GTD. A serum:CSF β-hCG ratio of less than 60:1 was considered a positive predictor for brain metastases ([41]). With the availability of MRI, this test is rarely used. CA-125 may also have a role as a marker for GTD. In at least one study of patients with hydatidiform mole, the CA-125 level was elevated; more significant was the association of the degree of CA-125 elevation with the development of persistent GTD ([45]).

The complete blood count usually reveals anemia and thrombocytopenia. Clotting times may be prolonged, and consumption of coagulation factors may be unusually high in patients with disseminated intravascular coagulation. Hepatic or renal impairments are rare. Thyroid function studies are mandated in patients with a clinical history or physical examination findings suggestive of hyperthyroidism.

PHANTOM HUMAN CHORIONIC GONADOTROPIN SYNDROME

Phantom hCG or phantom choriocarcinoma syndrome is also called pseudohypergonadotropinemia. It refers to persistent mild elevation of hCG when no true hCG or trophoblastic tissue is present. This may result in the patient being treated further by her physician during the follow-up period either after primary surgery for molar pregnancy or chemotherapy for metastatic disease. It is mentioned here because clinicians may encounter this problem during the follow-up period and should rule out this syndrome before deciding to label a patient as having persistent disease.

Human chorionic gonadotropin is a glycoprotein whose two subunits, α and β, are held together by charge and hydrophobic interactions. Over 40 different professional laboratory tests are available for assaying the level of serum hCG. Most of these work through the multiantibody "sandwich assay," using the labeled-enzyme or chemoimmunoassay (radioimmunoassay) method developed in the 1950s. The mechanism by which heterophilic antibodies cause false-positive results relates to the nature of this immunometric assay. One antibody, commonly a mouse monoclonal immunoglobulin (IgG), immobilizes hCG by binding one site on the molecule. A second antibody, commonly a polyclonal antibody labeled with an enzyme or chemiluminescent agent, marks the first antibody. Heterophilic antibodies usually bind the assay of IgG at sites common to humans and other species. They are bivalent and therefore link the capture and tracer antibodies, mimicking hCG immunoactivity. Binding of human antibodies to mouse IgG is the most common form of interference. The positivity of this test in the serum, however, is not correlated with positivity in the urine. These large heterophile antibodies are filtered out at the level of the glomerulus, and the urine hCG test is therefore negative in the setting of heterophile antibodies. Therefore, a simple urine hCG test can support or refute a "phantom hCG" test result. If both the urine test and the serum test results are positive, this likely represents true malignant GTD, and searching for occult disease is prudent. If the urine test is negative, assuming that no clear radiologic sites of disease are identified, different assay systems can then be used to confirm the first serum result, which may indicate heterophile antibodies and exclude true malignant GTD ([46]). It is recommended that the serum be tested by a reference laboratory in these cases.

Phantom hCG emphasizes the clinical dilemma that arises when patient care is based primarily on laboratory data. It is the clinician's responsibility to interpret test results with caution. The prevalence of false-positive hCG results is not well recognized. It has been found to be 3.4% of healthy individuals.

STAGING AND PROGNOSIS

There are many staging and prognostic systems in GTD. Each of these systems attempts to define prognostic groups in order to identify patients most likely to become resistant to single-agent methotrexate or dactinomycin and direct a rational therapeutic strategy, thereby optimizing treatment and achieving the highest possible cure rate ([2]). Patients are classified into different prognostic groups based on factors such as tumor histologic subtype, extent of disease, human gonadotropin titer, duration of disease, nature of the antecedent pregnancy, and extent of prior treatment. The staging system of the International Federation of Gynecology and Obstetrics (FIGO 2000) is the most commonly used system (Table 34-4). This staging system was developed from the WHO scoring system, shown in Table 34-5 ([47, 48]). Patients with a score of 0 to 6 have a low risk of developing resistance to single-agent therapy and may be appropriately treated with dactinomycin or methotrexate. Patients scoring greater than 6 have a higher risk of developing disease resistant to treatment with a single chemotherapy agent and are best treated with combination chemotherapy ([2, 48, 49]).

The FIGO 2000 system is not universally predictive of individual patient outcome. Patients with a score of 0 to 3 will almost all be cured with single-agent chemotherapy, but 70% of patients who score 5 to 6 will fail single-agent treatment and require combination chemotherapy. Because almost all failures can be cured by transitioning to combination chemotherapy, single-agent therapy is still used initially for patients who score 5 to 6 to spare the 30% of responders the more toxic effects of combination chemotherapy ([6]).

Table 34-4 Figo Staging of Gestational Trophoblastic Tumors

Stage I: GTT confined to the uterus	
Stage IA	Disease confined to the uterus with no risk factors
Stage IB	Disease confined to the uterus with one risk factor
Stage IC	Disease confined to the uterus with two risk factors
Stage II: GTT extends outside the uterus but is limited to the genital structures (ovary, tube, vagina, broad ligament)	
Stage IIA	Disease involving genital structures without risk factors
Stage IIB	Disease extends outside the uterus but is limited to the genital structures with one risk factor
Stage IIC	Disease extents outside of the uterus but is limited to the genital structures with two risk factors
Stage III: GTT extends to the lungs with or without known genital tract involvement	
Stage IIIA	Disease extends to the lungs with or without known genital tract involvement and no risk factors
Stage IIIB	Disease extends to the lungs with or without known genital tract involvement with one risk factor
Stage IIIC	Disease extends to the lungs with or without known genital tract involvement with two risk factors
Stage IV: All other metastatic sites	
Stage IVA	All other metastatic sites without risk factors
Stage IVB	All other metastatic sites with one risk factor
Stage IVC	All other metastatic sites with two risk factors

Table 34-5 FIGO 2000 Prognostic Scoring for Gestational Trophoblastic Disease

FIGO (WHO) Risk Factor Scoring With FIGO Staging	0	1	2	4
Age (year)	<40	>40		
Antecedent pregnancy	Hydatidiform mole	Abortion	Term	
Interval months from index pregnancy	<4	4-6	7-12	>12
Pretreatment in hCG mIU/ml	$<10^3$	10^3-10^4	10^4-10^5	$>10^5$
Largest tumor size including uterus	3-4 cm	≥5 cm		
Site of metastases including uterus		Spleen, kidney	Gastrointestinal tract	Brain, liver
Number of metastases identified	0	1-4	5-8	>8
Previous failed chemotherapy			Single drug	Two or more drugs

Low risk ≤6, High risk ≥7.
This combination of the modified WHO risk factor scoring system with the FIGO Cancer Staging and Nomenclature Committee in September 2000 and ratified in June 2002 with the FIGO announcement.
Modified with permission from Kohorn EI: The new FIGO 2000 staging and risk factor scoring system for gestational trophoblastic disease: description and critical assessment, *Int J Gynecol Cancer* 2001 Jan-Feb;11(1):73-77.

Certain other factors can be used to predict and identify early development of resistance to therapy. Pulsatility index, measured with Doppler ultrasonography, can measure uterine vascularity and predict methotrexate-resistant disease ([6]). Additionally, hCG regression nomograms and kinetics may predict early onset of resistant disease during treatment with a single agent, although this is not yet in common practice ([50]). Patients infected with human immunodeficiency virus who have CD4 counts less than 200 cells/µL do not tolerate chemotherapy and have poor outcomes with higher mortality ([51]).

Although outcomes for patients treated with GTD are favorable, the mortality rate for patients primarily treated at a trophoblast center is lower than that in patients referred after failure of primary treatment, prompting the recommendation for early referral to a trophoblast center when possible ([3, 52]).

MANAGEMENT

Using the FIGO 2000 scoring system, each patient is considered individually and treated by a multidisciplinary team. Figure 34-9 outlines the general diagnostic and therapeutic approaches used at the University of Texas MD Anderson Cancer Center.

Molar Pregnancy

Primary Treatment

Hydatidiform mole is curable. The treatment is mainly surgical ([53]), but optimal management is dependent on the desire to preserve reproductive capability. All patients are evaluated for any medical condition secondary to the mole and treated appropriately before surgery. Most patients are of reproductive age, wish to maintain fertility, and are treated with suction dilation and curettage, often with ultrasound guidance to remove all molar tissue and avoid uterine perforation ([1, 53]). The procedure has less than a 1% incidence of mortality ([15]). If the uterus is greater than 16 weeks in size, there is a risk of pulmonary embolization of molar tissue, and care in a referral center is warranted ([2]). Depending on the trophoblastic elements, the amount of bleeding can vary. Oxytocin is often infused immediately prior to surgery to limit the volume of blood lost, although caution is necessary in patients with medical complications due to the risk of hyponatremia and fluid overload ([54]). Specimens from surgery are sent for pathologic evaluation. Labor induction and hysterectomy are not recommended due to the increased incidence of post-molar GTN requiring chemotherapy ([38]). Patients maintaining fertility should be counseled with regard to the possibility of another molar pregnancy and of malignant transformation. Patients with partial moles should be given anti-D immunoglobulin prophylaxis.

In the rare patient who has completed childbearing and no longer desires fertility, hysterectomy to remove the uterus with the mole intact is reasonable. The ovaries may be preserved, even in the setting of theca lutein cysts. After hysterectomy, patients must be followed with hCG levels.

Postsurgical Care and Indications for Chemotherapy

After primary surgical treatment, all patients undergo weekly serum β-hCG tests until the level returns to

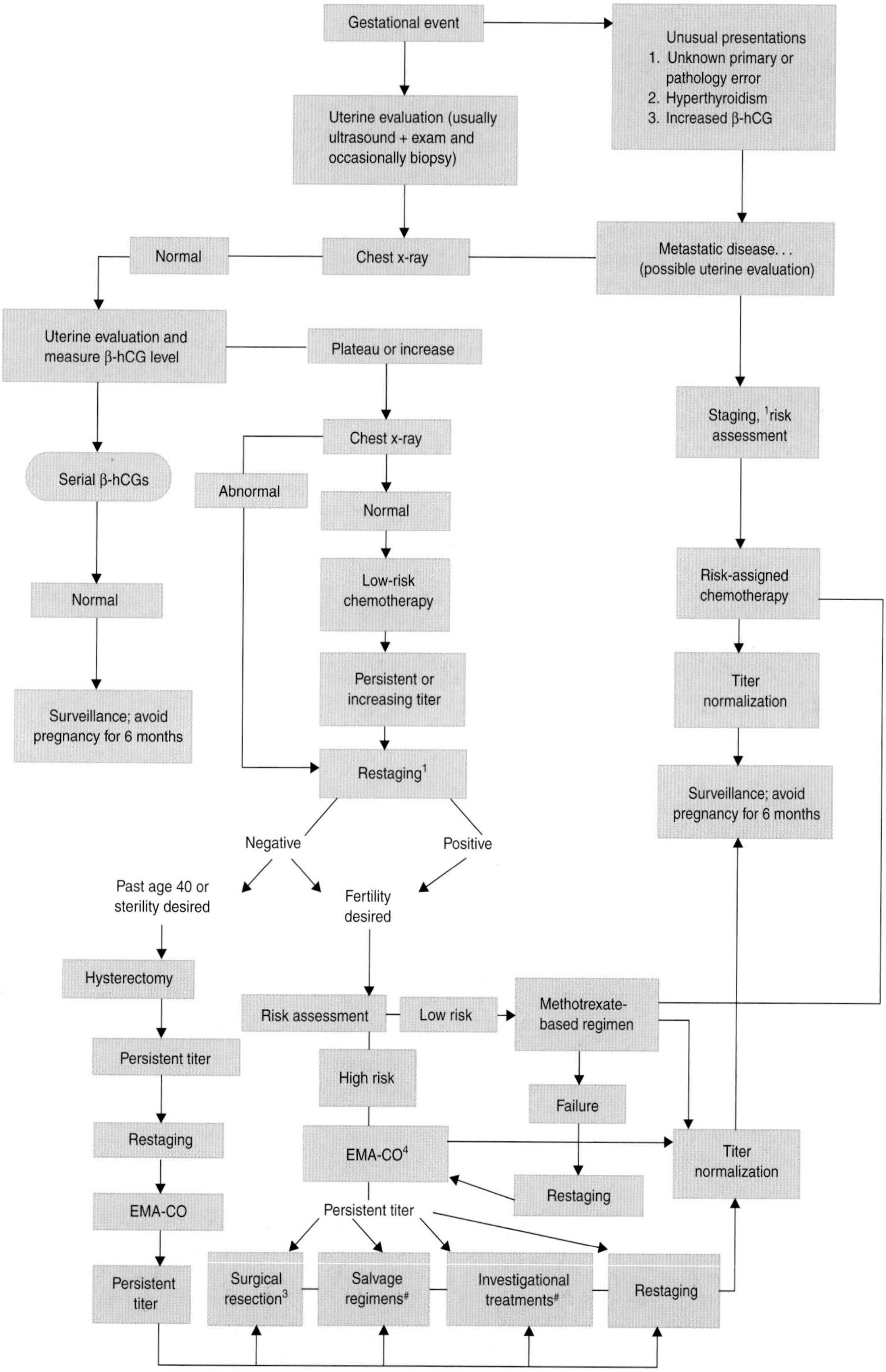

Gestational event

Unusual presentations
1. Unknown primary or pathology error
2. Hyperthyroidism
3. Increased β-hCG

Uterine evaluation (usually ultrasound + exam and occasionally biopsy)

Normal

Chest x-ray

Metastatic disease. . . (possible uterine evaluation)

Uterine evaluation and measure β-hCG level

Plateau or increase

Staging, [1]risk assessment

Chest x-ray

Serial β-hCGs

Abnormal

Normal

Normal

Low-risk chemotherapy

Risk-assigned chemotherapy

Persistent or increasing titer

Titer normalization

Surveillance; avoid pregnancy for 6 months

Restaging[1]

Surveillance; avoid pregnancy for 6 months

Negative

Positive

Past age 40 or sterility desired

Fertility desired

Hysterectomy

Risk assessment

Low risk

Methotrexate-based regimen

Persistent titer

High risk

Failure

Restaging

EMA-CO[4]

Titer normalization

Restaging

EMA-CO

Persistent titer

Persistent titer

Surgical resection[3]

Salvage regimens#

Investigational treatments#

Restaging

FIGURE 34-9 **Management algorithm for gestational trophoblastic disease. β-hCG, β-human chorionic gonadotropin; EMA-CO, etoposide/methotrexate/Adriamycin (dactinomycin)/cyclophosphamide/vincristine. [1]Includes radiologic evaluation of brain, liver, kidney, and lungs (magnetic resonance imaging of brain preferred). [2]β-hCG titers every month for 1 year, then every 4 months for 1 year, and then every 12 months for 2 years. [3]Of prior or suspected disease sites, including uterus. #No other active sites on radiologic restaging. [4]No prior EMA-CO.**

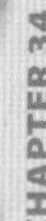

normal on three consecutive assays (ie, 3 consecutive weeks). Three consecutive normal β-hCG levels define complete remission.

Urine pregnancy tests alone are considered inadequate for monitoring. The level of β-hCG typically normalizes within 8 weeks, but this may take up to 14 to 16 weeks in 20% of patients. In patients with complete moles, the β-hCG should be checked monthly for 6 months. Patients with partial moles have less than 1 in 3,000 risk of subsequent GTD, but rates in the literature range up to 6% ([2, 3]). Although international guidelines do not require follow-up serum hCG testing, this is still performed at our institution ([2, 6]).

Contraception should be used for 6 months, but no increased risk of recurrent molar pregnancy has been demonstrated in the 6-month period ([2]). Because luteinizing hormone (LH) interferes with the detection of β-hCG at low levels, the use of oral contraceptives may be useful, because they suppress endogenous LH. Historically, oral contraceptive use prior to normalization of hCG was linked to GTD, but modern oral contraceptives do not appear to pose this risk ([2, 6]).

Eighty percent of patients need no further treatment ([4, 55]). The other 20% who develop malignant sequelae are treated as appropriate for their status, as either low- or high-risk patients as defined by the FIGO 2000 criteria (see Table 34-5) ([15]). These patients are considered to have malignant GTN rather than molar pregnancies. The initial pathologic results of the previous gestation were complete mole in 78%, partial mole in 9%, and choriocarcinoma in 8% ([15]). Of these patients, 81% had low-risk disease, 18% had high-risk disease, and 1% had PSTT. Risk factors include a pre-evacuation hCG level >100,000 IU/L, excessive uterine growth, theca lutein cysts over 6 cm in diameter, and age over 40 years ([56, 57]). These patients are identified through the following events ([2, 3, 49]):

- Rising or plateaued β-hCG level for 2 weeks measured over three separate intervals
- Tissue diagnosis of choriocarcinoma
- Evidence of metastatic disease
- Elevation of β-hCG level after a normal result
- Postevacuation bleeding not due to retained tissues

An elevated but falling hCG 6 months after molar evacuation does not mandate chemotherapy because hCG levels eventually normalize in patients ([58]). However, a serum hCG level greater than 20,000 IU/L more than 4 weeks after evacuation prompts chemotherapy because of the risk of uterine perforation and hemorrhage ([1, 2]). Patients who receive treatment for molar pregnancy are encouraged to use effective contraception with hormonal or barrier methods during the 6-month interval of β-hCG follow-up. Intrauterine devices are not used because of the potential for uterine perforation. It is essential to exclude a new pregnancy in a patient under surveillance, rather than assume GTD. This is done by correlating the rise in β-hCG levels and ultrasonic findings based on the hCG level.

Prophylactic Chemotherapy

Prophylactic adjuvant chemotherapy after molar evacuation is controversial and usually not advised. The postevacuation risk of developing GTN is 15% to 20% after complete mole and 0.5% to 1% after partial mole. In one study, administering dactinomycin intravenously for 5 days starting 3 days after molar evacuation reduced the risk of GTN to 3% to 8% ([59]). However, such prophylaxis exposes approximately 80% of women to unnecessary chemotherapy and its attendant side effects, as the hCG levels would have been expected to decline without chemotherapy. Additionally, surveillance is still required after chemotherapy, and unnecessary chemotherapy may induce drug resistance ([60]). Because the vast majority of patients with GTN are detected and cured with hCG surveillance and directed chemotherapy without prophylaxis, prophylactic chemotherapy has not improved survival. Thus, the benefit of prophylaxis is outweighed by the risk, except in unique circumstances where compliant patient follow-up is not possible ([2, 61]).

A minority of patients who have undergone removal of a complete hydatidiform mole may develop the unusual complication of intermediate trophoblastic disease ([19]). They usually present with vaginal bleeding and a slightly elevated β-hCG titer. Examination of the uterus may reveal multiple nodules involving the endometrium and myometrium. Surgical intervention is warranted because progressive disease tends to develop, and the disease does not readily respond to chemotherapy.

Malignant Gestational Trophoblastic Disease

For malignant GTD, the treatment depends on the cell type, stage, level of serum β-hCG, duration of the disease, specific sites of metastases, and extent of prior treatment. Patients should be stratified for risk prior to initiating a treatment plan. The FIGO 2000 system incorporating the modified WHO scoring system is the most commonly used risk stratification system (see Table 34-4) ([47-49]). A score of 0 to 6 indicates a low risk of developing resistance to single-agent chemotherapy; a score over 6 indicates a high risk of resistance to single-agent chemotherapy and mandates combination chemotherapy.

To assign a risk category and stage, patients must undergo history, physical, and directed imaging. Patients who are detected early by hCG monitoring are evaluated by history, examination, serum hCG, pelvic ultrasound (excludes pregnancy, measures uterine size, and excludes pelvic extension), and chest x-ray. If the chest x-ray suggests lung metastasis, a chest CT may be ordered, but only lesions visible on chest x-ray should be scored ([2, 49]). If a patient is found to have lung metastasis, an MRI of the brain is obtained to exclude brain metastasis ([6]). If a patient has choriocarcinoma or suspected GTN following a nonmolar pregnancy, imaging should include a CT of the chest and abdomen, MRI of the brain and pelvis, and a pelvic ultrasound to evaluate for metastases to the lung, liver, pelvis, and brain ([2]). Positron emission tomography (PET)/CT may be useful in imaging patients with recurrent disease prior to consideration of surgical resection ([6]). Lumbar puncture to measure the CSF:serum hCG ratio is of historical interest but is not routinely used since the advent of MRI.

Low-Risk Disease, Nonmetastatic

Hysterectomy is the treatment of choice for patients who do not wish to maintain fertility. Posthysterectomy chemotherapy may be considered but is not routine. The rationale behind chemotherapy is to reduce the likelihood of disseminating viable tumor cells at surgery and during the immediate postoperative period as well as to eliminate any occult metastases. Outcomes data are not convincing. Patients who wish to retain fertility should receive chemotherapy as primary treatment for low-risk disease. Each patient must be stratified for risk prior to initiating chemotherapy.

Acceptable chemotherapy regimens are listed in Table 34-6. Either methotrexate, with or without folinic acid rescue, or dactinomycin is acceptable with the schedules as outlined. The differences in inclusion criteria in studies comparing these regimens make determining superiority of one regimen over another difficult, although dactinomycin may result in superior outcomes. The only published randomized trial compared low-dose methotrexate (30 mg/m^2) with dactinomycin and found dactinomycin to be superior ([62]). Advocates of methotrexate cite less toxicity, no hair loss, less nausea, less vomiting, and less myelosuppression. Advocates of dactinomycin cite the above trial and less frequent infusion schedule ([2]). An ongoing trial conducted by the Gynecologic Oncology Group compares pulsed dactinomycin with intravenous methotrexate. Regardless, patient outcome for low-risk nonmetastatic GTN is cure.

Response to treatment is determined by monitoring serum β-hCG levels every 1 to 2 weeks during treatment ([2]). Persistent elevation over three consecutive samples or an increase in titer of β-hCG over two consecutive samples over more than 2 weeks indicates disease resistant to first-line therapy and requires restaging ([2]). Phantom hCG syndrome must be excluded in the setting of low-level persistent positive results. Assuming this represents a true result, if the tumor is still limited to the uterus and the patient is older than 40 years and/or has no wish to retain fertility, hysterectomy is offered. If the patient prefers to retain fertility and belongs to the low-risk category, she can be treated with other chemotherapy. Patients who are initially treated with methotrexate but fail with hCG levels less than 300 IU/L can often be cured with dactinomycin administered as a single agent. Patients with higher levels of hCG should be treated with combination EMA-CO chemotherapy (etoposide, methotrexate, dactinomycin, cyclophosphamide, and vincristine) ([2, 6]). Despite a high rate of resistance to first-line chemotherapy, a cure rate of almost 100% is achieved with combination chemotherapy. In the rare instances of tumor resistance to combination chemotherapy in a patient who wishes to retain fertility, localized resection should be offered after careful evaluation by perioperative MRI, ultrasonography, and/or arteriography.

Once the serum hCG has normalized, three additional treatments of chemotherapy past normal are administered to minimize the chance of recurrence ([2]). A comparison of two versus three cycles of methotrexate past normalization of hCG level showed a doubling in recurrence rates in patients receiving only two consolidation courses, so it is important to administer three cycles past titer normalization ([63]).

Low-Risk Disease, Metastatic

More than 50 years ago, metastatic GTD was not curable. Since then, treatments have improved such that

Table 34-6 Chemotherapy Regimes for Low-Risk[a] Gestational Trophoblastic Disease

Drug	Administration	Cycle[b]
Methotrexate and folinic acid	1 mg/kg (up to 70 mg) IM or IV days 1, 3, 5, 7 0.1 mg/kg IM or IV days 2, 4, 6, 8	14 days
Methotrexate	0.4 mg/kg IM or IV daily for 5 days	14 days
Methotrexate	30 to 50 mg/m^2 IM	7 days
Dactinomycin	10 μg/kg (max 0.5 mg) IV daily for 5 days	14 days
Dactinomycin	1.25 mg/m^2	14 days

[a]Therapy based on WHO risk criteria.
[b]Withhold treatment for marrow recovery if necessary

the cure rate now exceeds 90% ([5]). This success is the result of a combination of factors:

- The discovery that these tumors are chemosensitive
- The ability to diagnose and monitor therapy by using β-hCG levels
- Identification of prognostic factors
- Use of combination therapy
- Referral of patients to specialized centers for treatment

Patients with metastatic low-risk disease as determined by the WHO prognostic scoring system have a high potential for cure with chemotherapy alone ([1, 2]). Single-agent chemotherapy with methotrexate or dactinomycin is indicated as in low risk nonmetastatic disease (see Table 34-6). Complete response occurs in 90% of patients with low-risk disease, with little short- or long-term toxicity ([64]). In patients who fail single-agent therapy with methotrexate and have hCG levels less than 300 IU/L, dactinomycin can still result in cure ([6]). Patients who fail single-agent chemotherapy are still cured with combination regimens ([64]).

Patients in whom treatment does not produce a complete response may have undetected metastatic disease. Mutch et al reported that at least 40% of patients with a negative chest radiograph result will have a positive chest CT scan and may be at higher risk of resistance to single-agent therapy ([65]). The cure rate for patients with low-risk disease is essentially 100% ([2, 6]).

High-Risk Disease

High-risk disease is not likely to be cured by single-agent chemotherapy, and patients with high-risk disease are at the highest risk of treatment failure. These patients should be treated with combination chemotherapy, most commonly EMA-CO (Table 34-7) ([1, 2, 5]). The ACE regimen (dactinomycin, cisplatin, and etoposide) has recently been reported to have outstanding efficacy but is not yet regarded as standard of care for upfront high-risk disease ([66]).

Historically, a combination of MAC (methotrexate, dactinomycin, and cyclophosphamide) was used, producing cure rates of 63% to 80% ([67]). In intermediate- or high-risk GTT, MAC is most effective when used as initial chemotherapy (65% survival) rather than second-line treatment (39% survival) following failed single-agent therapy ([67]).

An older regimen, CHAMOCA (cyclophosphamide, hydroxyurea, dactinomycin, methotrexate with leucovorin rescue, vincristine, cyclophosphamide, and doxorubicin), resulted in a remission rate of 82%, but this regimen was inferior to MAC in terms of toxicity and efficacy and is not used in current practice ([68]).

Because etoposide was identified to have activity against trophoblastic disease, Bagshawe developed the EMA-CO regimen and reported a survival rate of 83% in patients with high-risk choriocarcinoma ([69]). The efficacy of this combination has been confirmed and this remains the preferred regimen for high-risk GTT ([70-72]). It is generally well tolerated. Toxicity includes alopecia, mild anemia, neutropenia, and stomatitis. Reproductive function is preserved in 75% of patients. In patients with significant tumor volume, rapid tumor necrosis may result in hemorrhage, and consideration may be given to lower dose induction therapy. After normalization of hCG, three additional consolidation cycles (6 weeks) of EMA-CO are administered ([2]).

Table 34-7 Chemotherapy Regimes for Intermediate- and High-Risk[a] Gestational Trophoblastic Disease

Drug Regimen		Administration
EMA-CO[b] (preferred regimen)		
Course I (EMA)		
Day 1	Etoposide	100 mg/m² IV over 30 min
	Methotrexate	100 mg/m² IV bolus
	Methotrexate[c]	200 mg/m² IV as 12-h continuous infusion
	Dactinomycin	0.5 mg IV bolus
Day 2	Etoposide	100 mg/m² IV over 30 min
	Folinic acid	15 mg IV/IM/PO every 6 h for four doses, beginning 24 h after start of methotrexate
	Dactinomycin	0.5 mg IV bolus
Course II (CO)		
Day 8	Cyclophosphamide	600 mg/m² IV over 30 min
	Vincristine	1 mg/m² (up to 2 mg) IV bolus

[a]Therapy based on the WHO risk criteria.
[b]Repeat each regimen in sequence every 14 days as toxicity permits.
[c]In case of CNS metastases, the dose of infused methotrexate is increased to 1000 mg/m² IV over 12 h after alkalinization of the urine. Increase the number of folinic acid doses to eight given every 6 h. This regimen is called "high-dose methotrexate EMA-CO."

Metastases Requiring Special Care

In the setting of high-risk disease and bulky tumor in areas susceptible to massive hemorrhage or worsening

CHAPTER 34

organ failure, consideration may be given to induction chemotherapy followed by full-dose combination chemotherapy. Patients with massive pulmonary or liver metastases or brain metastases may benefit from a 25% dose reduction for the first two cycles, with monitoring in an intensive care unit setting until the disease shrinks enough to allow full-dose chemotherapy with less significant risk of hemorrhage. An alternative strategy is to use low-dose etoposide 100 mg/m^2 and cisplatin 20 mg/m^2 on days 1 and 2 every week up to three times prior to initiating standard EMA-CO. Additionally, consideration can be given to using EMA-EP (EMA with etoposide and cisplatin) rather than EMA-CO in patients with the worst prognosis, namely with liver and brain metastases.

Significant vaginal hemorrhage should prompt resuscitative transfusion but is expected to resolve within 3 to 4 days. Additional strategies for management may include embolization, hysterectomy, and arterial ligation. Nearly all patients experiencing hemorrhage can be expected to survive with appropriate resuscitation and management ([73]). Twenty-five percent of patients with high-risk disease do not attain complete remission, in which case salvage chemotherapy is administered.

Pulmonary Metastases

Pulmonary metastases can be extensive and may cause respiratory failure and death ([74]). Some factors that predict a worse outcome or early death from respiratory compromise include cyanosis, pulmonary hypertension, dyspnea, anemia, tachycardia, extensive (>50%) lung opacification, mediastinal involvement, bilateral pleural effusion, and a high WHO prognostic score ([75, 76]). In patients with extensive pulmonary metastases, reduced doses of initial chemotherapy have been suggested to abate the risk of respiratory failure, although this strategy does not protect completely against pulmonary failure and death ([75, 76]).

Central Nervous System Metastases

Like pulmonary metastases, CNS metastases pose a significant threat. Although clinically apparent in only 7% to 28% of patients with choriocarcinoma, CNS involvement is found in as many as 40% of patients on postmortem examination. Multimodality therapy seems to be optimal, yielding a remission rate of 50% (7 of 14 patients) with disease-free intervals of 12 to 120 months.

Athanassiou et al reported that 8.8% of 782 patients had CNS metastases ([41]). The overall survival rate of patients who had CNS metastases at diagnosis was 80%. The overall survival of patients who developed CNS metastases after initial diagnosis and treatment was only 25%. Two other studies found similar outcomes and concluded that CNS prophylaxis may improve prognosis ([77, 78]). However, Gillespie et al showed no benefit of CNS prophylaxis in 69 patients with lung metastases ([79]). We do not advocate CNS prophylaxis in the absence of definite CNS disease.

Patients with known CNS disease benefit from chemotherapy and whole-brain irradiation. In a retrospective analysis of 70 patients, half died before therapy was initiated. Of the remaining patients, 24% of those given chemotherapy alone survived, but 50% of patients given concurrent chemotherapy plus whole-brain irradiation achieved long-term remission and none died of CNS disease ([80]).

When patients present with CNS metastases, primary treatment of the brain with surgical resection or radiotherapy prior to EMA-CO chemotherapy is indicated to decrease the risk of hemorrhage. Surgical resection is appropriate only for patients with solitary metastasis. Surgical decompression should be considered for patients who have symptoms of raised intracranial pressure ([81]).

The optimal dose of radiation appears to be 30 Gy. Patients with less than 25 Gy had a lower cure rate ([80]). The local control rate was 91% if >22 Gy was administered but 24% if <22 Gy was administered ([82]). For CNS disease, it is prudent to administer 30 Gy over 10 fractions initiated simultaneously with the start of chemotherapy. Stereotactic radiotherapy or gamma-knife treatment has been advocated at the end of chemotherapy to treat any residual unresectable lesions as an alternative to whole-brain radiation, due to the toxicity and limited evidence of improvement with whole-brain irradiation ([6]).

The EMA-CO chemotherapy regimen should be administered following surgery or radiation ([83]). The dose of methotrexate is escalated to 1,000 mg/m^2. Intrathecal methotrexate 12.5 mg may be given with the CO component of EMA-CO or with whole-brain radiotherapy (20-30 Gy in two daily fractions) concurrent with chemotherapy ([6, 84]). Extracranial sites of metastases at the time of CNS metastasis are common. Overall survival in patients with CNS metastases is 67% ([83]).

Patients in First Remission

Patients in first remission thought to have a high risk of recurrence are observed closely with serum β-hCG levels and posttherapy baseline radiologic imaging. For patients who had lung metastases, a repeat high-resolution CT scan at the end of chemotherapy serves as a baseline for follow-up. Many patients who have had lung metastases have residual nodules in the lung field on CT scans or chest x-ray, signifying fibrous scar tissue. For patients who had brain metastases, an MRI of the head would be obtained. Likewise, for patients who had liver metastases, a CT scan of the liver would be obtained. If the uterus is in place and was a site of previous disease, consideration is also given to baseline MRI of the uterus. The rationale is that modest increases in the β-hCG level, signifying relapse, may be accompanied by subtle changes in "sterile" lesions noted on earlier images. This finding raises the issue of surgical resection of a chemotherapy-resistant site. If the imaging obtained after chemotherapy reveals suspicious nodules or masses and the β-hCG level is normal, a baseline PET-CT scan is sometimes obtained to serve as a baseline. If the β-hCG level rises during follow-up, a PET-CT scan would help identify active disease.

Salvage Therapy

One-quarter of patients with high-risk metastatic disease do not achieve complete remission with EMA-CO or experience relapse later. These patients require identification of chemotherapy-resistant sites for possible surgical resection and salvage therapy with alternative platinum-based regimens. These regimens may include EMA-EP (omitting day 2 etoposide and dactinomycin and alternating weekly with etoposide and cisplatin); TE/TP (paclitaxel and etoposide alternating weekly with paclitaxel and cisplatin); ACE (dactinomycin, cisplatin, and etoposide); VIP (etoposide, ifosfamide, and cisplatin); BEP (bleomycin, etoposide, and cisplatin); cisplatin, vincristine, and methotrexate; PVB (cisplatin, vinblastine, and bleomycin); PEBA (cisplatin, etoposide, bleomycin, and doxorubicin); and ICE (high-dose ifosfamide, carboplatin, and etoposide) ([2, 5, 66, 85-95]). Response rates range from 20% to 75%. The most commonly used regimens are EMA-EP, which is toxic but results in a cure rate greater than 75%, and TE/TP, which may be equally efficacious and less toxic ([2]).

Cure can also be achieved with surgery in a subset of chemoresistant patients who have one to three disease sites after combination chemotherapy. In this setting, PET-CT may be useful to detect metastatic sites ([6, 96]). Total or radical hysterectomy to remove the disease, with or without adnexectomy and lymphadenectomy, can be curative in 90% of patients with primary drug-resistant and relapsed GTN ([97, 98]).

Patients who fail these approaches may be candidates for high-dose chemotherapy. Limited outcomes data exist, but reports suggest that high-dose chemotherapy alone combined with surgical resection may lead to salvage in one-third of patients. The most common regimen is CarbopEC-T (carboplatin, etoposide, cyclophosphamide, and paclitaxel) ([2, 6]).

Placental Site Trophoblastic Tumor

Originally known as trophoblastic pseudotumor, these tumors have been designated as PSTT to better reflect their malignant potential. The median age at diagnosis is 33 years (range, 18-47 years). The most common presenting symptoms are irregular vaginal bleeding, amenorrhea, and a pelvic mass ([17]). The median interval from antecedent pregnancy is 3.4 years. These tumors present with lung metastases in 10% to 20% of cases, and 10% of patients develop metastases during the follow-up interval ([17]).

The FIGO scoring is not used to determine the treatment of PSTT ([2]). Hysterectomy is the preferred treatment for nonmetastatic disease, which is highly curable. Postoperative chemotherapy is indicated for patients with certain risk factors, including metastatic disease, mitotic index, hCG level, and time from antecedent pregnancy. The latter is the most prognostic factor ([2]). The long-term survival rate of patients presenting with PSTT within 4 years of antecedent pregnancy was 98%, compared with 100% mortality for patients presenting with PSTT more than 4 years after antecedent pregnancy, but these findings have been inconsistent ([14, 17]).

The general strategy is to perform hysterectomy for patients with nonmetastatic disease who present less than 4 years after antecedent pregnancy. Premenopausal patients with limited disease may preserve their ovaries, and lymphadenectomy is of limited utility ([17]). Patients with metastatic disease at presentation receive EMA-EP ([2, 14, 94, 99, 100]) and, upon response, undergo resection of residual disease sites and hysterectomy. Recurrent disease not amenable to surgical resection may require radiation or combination chemotherapy with EMA-CO ([94, 99]). Patients who present more than 4 years after antecedent pregnancy have poor survival and should be considered for clinical trials or high-dose chemotherapy, even when the disease appears to be localized ([1, 2, 7]). Patients with limited disease who desire fertility may be considered for focal uterine resection with or without chemotherapy, but this is investigational ([1, 2]).

Placental site trophoblastic tumor produces β-hCG inconsistently, so the serum β-hCG level is not uniformly helpful in diagnosis, treatment, or follow-up ([17, 64]). Placental site trophoblastic tumor is less responsive to chemotherapy than choriocarcinoma, but chemotherapy remains effective in many patients, and the prognosis depends on the extent of disease at presentation ([2, 17]). The overall mortality rate of PSTT is 16% to 21% ([3]). The median overall survival is 86 months; 88% of patients with early-stage disease and 11% of patients with advanced-stage disease were without evidence of disease 28 months after diagnosis ([17]).

Epithelioid Trophoblastic Tumor

This rare disease entity appears to be distinct from PSTT but is treated in a similar fashion. The

International Society for the Study of Trophoblastic Disease database is collecting information on both of these tumor entities and will inform future treatment decisions ([2]).

CO-TWIN PREGNANCY

The estimated incidence of twin pregnancy consisting of a molar pregnancy and a normal fetus is 1 per 22,000 to 100,000 pregnancies. This has been described in both spontaneous and in vitro fertilization (IVF) gestations, although the incidence may be greater in women undergoing assisted reproduction. Gestational trophoblastic tumors in such cases have been either molar pregnancies or malignant neoplasms.

A patient with this rare condition poses a therapeutic dilemma. Although some have suggested termination for these pregnancies due to a low successful birth rate and an increased risk of GTN, recent studies have reported that 38% to 57% of women deliver a healthy baby, with a slight increase in maternal complications but no increase in malignant transformation of molar pregnancy ([101]). The decision on any therapy is made after consultation with the patient, a perinatologist, and a gynecologic oncologist, with careful assessment of the risk to the mother and the fetus.

FUTURE CHILDBEARING AND SURVIVORSHIP

Women who have undergone effective treatment for molar pregnancy have a risk of future molar pregnancy of 1% to 2% ([102]). Strict contraception is required during the surveillance period because pregnancy would obviate the usefulness of β-hCG as a tumor marker. Patients are advised to use effective hormonal or barrier contraception. Intrauterine devices are not employed as contraception for patients with intact uteri because of concerns of uterine perforation. In general, once a 6-month surveillance establishes disease-free status, conception is acceptable, although these women are always at higher risk for future molar disease and will require close observation during future pregnancies ([103]). Previous studies suggested a 12-month conception-free period, but 6 months confers the same protection and allows the patient to pursue fertility earlier without an increased risk of GTD relapse. The recommendation to avoid pregnancy relates to the importance of hCG surveillance and does not relate to the risk of recurrence, as GTN-related outcomes, miscarriage, and the incidence of birth defects appear to be unrelated to conception ([6, 56]).

Standard chemotherapy has minimal impact on subsequent ability to reproduce ([104, 105]). In one study, 83% of women who received prior chemotherapy subsequently conceived ([6]). In general, no increase in adverse events such as first- or second-trimester abortions or stillbirths, prematurity, or need for cesarean section has been noted, except for one report documenting a slight increase in stillbirth in subsequent pregnancies after chemotherapy ([102]). Similarly, their offspring have no increased risk of anomalies ([56]). Patients are monitored closely throughout any subsequent pregnancy, especially in the first trimester, to confirm that gestation is normal ([79]). Patients who have difficulty with conception are considered for fertility treatment but are at increased risk of repeat molar pregnancy.

Combination chemotherapy with EMA-CO induces menopause an average of 3 to 5 years earlier than otherwise anticipated ([6, 105]). The previously identified increased risk of second primary cancers (eg, acute myelogenous leukemia and thyroid cancer) after chemotherapy for choriocarcinoma was not observed in recent studies ([106]). Issues of survivorship concern sexual dysfunction and reproductive quality of life and appear to be greater in socially disadvantaged patients ([2, 107]).

CONCLUSION

Gestational trophoblastic disease represents a wide spectrum of neoplastic disorders that arise from placental trophoblastic tissue after abnormal fertilization. Patients are classified into different prognostic groups based on factors such as tumor histologic subtype, extent of disease, human gonadotropin titer, duration of disease, nature of the antecedent pregnancy, and extent of prior treatment. Each patient should receive individualized management after careful prognostication under the care of a multidisciplinary team. Surgery and chemotherapy each play an important role in effective management. Patients with GTD are followed long term with regular laboratory tests of complete blood count and β-hCG. Survivors of GTD are also followed for management of psychosocial problems that may be associated with GTD and their treatment.

REFERENCES

1. Seckl MJ, Sebire NJ, Berkowitz RS. Gestational trophoblastic disease. *Lancet*. 2010;376(9742):717-729.
2. Mangili G, Lorusso D, Brown J, et al. Trophoblastic disease review for diagnosis and management: a joint report from the International Society for the Study of Trophoblastic Disease, European Organisation for the Treatment of Trophoblastic Disease, and the Gynecologic Cancer InterGroup. *Int J Gynecol Cancer*. 2014;24(9 Suppl 3):S109-S116.

3. Kohorn EI. Worldwide survey of the results of treating gestational trophoblastic disease. *J Reprod Med*. 2014;59(3-4):145-153.
4. Lurain JR, Brewer JI, Torok EE, et al. Natural history of hydatidiform mole after primary evacuation. *Am J Obstet Gynecol*. 1983;145:591-595.
5. Lurain JR. Advances in management of high-risk gestational trophoblastic tumors. *J Reprod Med*. 2002;47(6):451-459.
6. Seckl MJ, Sebire NJ, Fisher RA, et al. Gestational trophoblastic disease: ESMO Clinical Practice Guidelines for diagnosis, treatment and follow-up. *Ann Oncol*. 2013;24(Suppl 6):vi39-50.
7. Hayashi K, Bracken MB, Freeman DH, et al. Hydatidiform mole in the United States (1970-1977): a statistical and theoretical analysis. *Am J Epidemiol*. 1982;115:67-77.
8. Berkowitz RS, Goldstein DP. Clinical practice. Molar pregnancy. *N Engl J Med*. 2009;360(16):1639-1645.
9. Wei PY, Ouyang PC. Trophoblastic diseases in Taiwan. *Am J Obstet Gynecol*. 1963;85:844-849.
10. Smith HO, Hilgers RD, Bedrick EJ, et al. Ethnic differences at risk for gestational trophoblastic disease in New Mexico: a 25-year population based study. *Am J Obstet Gynecol*. 2003;188(2):357-366.
11. Savage P, Williams J, Wong SL, et al. The demographics of molar pregnancies in England and Wales from 2000-2009. *J Reprod Med*. 2010;55(7-8):341-345.
12. Berkowitz RS, Bernstein MR, Laborde O, et al. Subsequent pregnancy experience in patients with gestational trophoblastic disease. New England Trophoblastic Disease Center, 1965-1992. *J Reprod Med*. 1994;39(3):228-232.
13. Soares PD, Maestesresedpregnanc et al. Geographical distribution and demographic characteristics of gestational trophoblastic disease. *J Reprod Med*. 2010;55(7-8):305-310.
14. Schmid P, Nagai Y, Agarwal R, et al. Prognostic markers and long-term outcome of placental-site trophoblastic tumours: a retrospective observational study. *Lancet*. 2009;374(9683):48-55.
15. Braga A, Uberti EM, Fajardo Mdo C, et al. Epidemiological report on the treatment of patients with gestational trophoblastic disease in 10 Brazilian referral centers: results after 12 years since International FIGO 2000 Consensus. *J Reprod Med*. 2014;59(5-6):241-247.
16. Buza N, Hui P. Immunohistochemistry and other ancillary techniques in the diagnosis of gestational trophoblastic diseases. *Semin Diagn Pathol*. 2014;31(3):223-232.
17. Hyman DM, Bakios L, Gualtiere G, et al. Placental site trophoblastic tumor: analysis of presentation, treatment, and outcome. *Gynecol Oncol*. 2013;129(1):58-62.
18. Lawler S, Fisher RA, Dent J. A prospective genetic study of complete and partial hydatidiform moles. *Am J Obstet Gynecol*. 1991;164:1270-1277.
19. Jacobs PA, Wilson CM, Sprenkle JA, et al. Mechanisms of origin of complete hydatidiform moles. *Nature*. 1980;286:714-716.
20. Cross JC, Werb Z, Fisher SJ. Implantation and the placenta: key pieces of the development puzzle. *Science*. 1994;266:1508-1518.
21. Wallace DC, Surti U, Adams CW, et al. Complete moles have paternal chromosomes but maternal mitochondrial DNA. *Hum Genet*. 1982;61:145-147.
22. Yamashita K, Wake N, Araki T, et al. Human lymphocyte antigen expression in hydatidiform mole: androgenesis following fertilization by a haploid sperm. *Am J Obstet Gynecol*. 1979;135:597-600.
23. Hoffner L, Surti U. The genetics of gestational trophoblastic disease: a rare complication of pregnancy. *Cancer Genet*. 2012;205(3):63-77.
24. Ohama K, Kajii T, Okamoto E, et al. Dispermic origin of XY hydatidiform moles. *Nature*. 1981;292:551-552.
25. Fisher RA, Lavery SA, Carby A, et al. What a difference an egg makes. *Lancet*. 2011;378(9807):1974.
26. Steller MA, Mok SC, Yeh J. Effects of cytokines on epidermal growth factor receptor expression by malignant trophoblast cells in vitro. *J Reprod Med*. 1994;39:209-216.
27. Guillemot F, Nagy A, Auerbach A, et al. Essential role of Mash2 in extraembryonic development. *Nature*. 1994;371:333-336.
28. Cheung AN, Srivastava G, Pittaluga S, et al. Expression of c-myc and c-fins oncogenes in hydatidiform mole and normal human placenta. *J Clin Pathol*. 1993;46:204-207.
29. Sarkar S, Kacinski BM, Kohorn EI, et al. Demonstration of myc and ras oncogene expression by hybridization in situ in hydatidiform mole and in the BeWo choriocarcinoma cell line. *Am J Obstet Gynecol*. 1986;154:390-393.
30. Cheung AN, Shen DH, Khoo US, et al. p21WAF1/CIP1 expression in gestational trophoblastic disease: correlation with clinicopathological parameters, and Ki67 and p53 gene expression. *J Clin Pathol*. 1998;51(2):159-162.
31. Fulop V, Mok SC, Genest DR, et al. p53, p21, Rb and mdm2 oncoproteins: expression in normal placenta, partial and complete mole, and choriocarcinoma. *J Reprod Med*. 1998;43:119-127.
32. Li HW, Tsao SW, Cheung AN. Current understandings of the molecular genetics of gestational trophoblastic diseases. *Placenta*. 2002;23(1):20-31.
33. Hubener C, Bidlingmaier M, Wu Z, et al. Human placental growth hormone: a potential new biomarker in gestational trophoblastic disease. *Gynecol Oncol*. 2015;136(2):264-268.
34. Mangili G, Garavaglia E, Cavoretto P, et al. Clinical presentation of hydatidiform mole in northern Italy: has it changed in the last 20 years? *Am J Obstet Gynecol*. 2008;198(3):302 e1-4.
35. Page RD, Freedman RS, Gestational trophoblastic tumors, in Pazdur R (ed): Medical Oncology: A Comprehensive Review, Huntington, NY: PRR Inc; 1993.
36. Amir SM, Osathanondh R, Berkowitz RS, et al. Human chorionic gonadotropin and thyroid function in patients with hydatidiform mole. *Am J Obstet Gynecol*. 1984;150:723-728.
37. Goldstein DP, Berkowitz RS. Current management of complete and partial molar pregnancy. *J Reprod Med*. 1994;39:139-146.
38. Berkowitz RS, Goldstein DP. Current management of gestational trophoblastic diseases. *Gynecol Oncol*. 2009;112(3):654-662.
39. Kumar J, Ilancheran A, Ratnam SS. Pulmonary metastases in gestational trophoblastic disease: a review of 97 cases. *Br J Obstet Gynaecol*. 1988;95(1):70-74.
40. Bakri Y, Berkowitz RS, Goldstein DP, et al. Brain metastases of gestational trophoblastic tumor. *J Reprod Med*. 1994;39:179-183.
41. Benson CB, Genest DR, Bernstein MR, et al. Sonographic appearance of first trimester complete hydatidiform moles. *Ultrasound Obstet Gynecol*. 2000;16(2):188-191.
42. Athanassiou A, Begent RHL, Newlands ES, et al. Central nervous system metastases of choriocarcinoma: Twenty-three years' experience at Charing Cross Hospital. *Cancer*. 1983;52:1728-1735.
43. Ha HK, Jung JK, Jee MK, et al. Gestational trophoblastic tumors of the uterus: MR imaging—pathologic correlation. *Gynecol Oncol*. 1995;57(3):340-350.
44. Pastorfide GB, Goldstein DP, Kosasa TS. The use of a radioimmunoassay specific for human chorionic gonadotropin in patients with molar pregnancy and gestational trophoblastic disease. *Am J Obstet Gynecol*. 1974;120:1025-1028.
45. Cole LA. hCG, its free subunits and its metabolites. Roles in pregnancy and trophoblastic disease. *J Reprod Med*. 1998;43(1):3-10.
46. Koonings PP, Schalerth JB. CA-125: a marker for persistent gestational trophoblastic disease? *Gynecol Oncol*. 1993;49(2):240-242.
47. Rotmensch S, Cole LA. False diagnosis and needless therapy of presumed malignant disease in women with false-positive human chorionic gonadotropin concentrations. *Lancet*. 2000;355(9205):712-715.
48. Kohorn EI, Goldstein DP, Hancock BW, et al. Combining the

staging system of the International Federation of Gynecology and Obstetrics with the scoring system of the World Health Organization for trophoblastic neoplasia. Report of the Working Committee of the International Society for the Study of Trophoblastic Disease and the International Gynecologic Cancer Society. *Int J Gynecol Cancer.* 2000;10:84-88.
49. Kohorn EI. The new FIGO 2000 staging and risk factor scoring system for gestational trophoblastic disease: description and critical assessment. *Int J Gynecol Cancer.* 2001;11(1):73-77.
50. Ngan HY, Bender H, Benedet JL, et al. Gestational trophoblastic neoplasia, FIGO 2000 staging and classification. *Int J Gynaecol Obstet.* 2003;83(Suppl 1):175-177.
51. You B, Harvey R, Henin E, et al. Early prediction of treatment resistance in low-risk gestational trophoblastic neoplasia using population kinetic modelling of hCG measurements. *Br J Cancer.* 2013;108(9):1810-1816.
52. Moodley M, Budhram S, Connolly C. Profile of mortality among women with gestational trophoblastic disease infected with the human immunodeficiency virus (HIV): argument for a new poor prognostic factor. *Int J Gynecol Cancer.* 2009;19(2):289-293.
53. Dantas PR, Maestastascol Cancearry R, et al. Influence of hydatidiform mole follow-up setting on postmolar gestational trophoblastic neoplasia outcomes: a cohort study. *J Reprod Med.* 2012;57(7-8):305-309.
54. Hancock BW, Tidy JA. Current management of molar pregnancy. *J Reprod Med.* 2002;47(5):347-354.
55. Soper JT. Surgical therapy for gestational trophoblastic disease. *J Reprod Med.* 1994;39(3):168-174.
56. Miller JM Jr, Surwit EA, Hammond CB. Choriocarcinoma following term pregnancy. *Obstet Gynecol.* 1979;53(2):207-212.
57. Berkowitz RS, Tuncer ZS, Bernstein MR, Goldstein DP. Management of gestational trophoblastic diseases: subsequent pregnancy experience. *Semin Oncol.* 2000;27(6):678-685.
58. Savage P, Seckl M, Short D. Practical issues in the management of low-risk gestational trophoblast tumors. *J Reprod Med.* 2008;53(10):774-780.
59. Agarwal R, Teoh S, Short D, et al. Chemotherapy and human chorionic gonadotropin concentrations 6 months after uterine evacuation of molar pregnancy: a retrospective cohort study. *Lancet.* 2012;379(9811):130-135.
60. Goldstein DP. Prevention of gestational trophoblastic disease by use of actinomycin D in molar pregnancies. *Obstet Gynecol.* 1974;43(4):475-479.
61. Kim DS, Hyung M, Kyung TK, et al. Effects of prophylactic chemotherapy for persistent trophoblastic disease in patients with complete hydatidiform mole. *Obstet Gynecol.* 1986;67:690-694.
62. Fu J, Fang F, Xie L, et al. Prophylactic chemotherapy for hydatidiform mole to prevent gestational trophoblastic neoplasia. *Cochrane Database Syst Rev.* 2012;10:CD007289.
63. Osborne RJ, Filiaci V, Schink JC, et al. Phase III trial of weekly methotrexate or pulsed dactinomycin for low-risk gestational trophoblastic neoplasia: a Gynecologic Oncology Group study. *J Clin Oncol.* 2011;29(7):825-831.
64. Lybol C, Sweep FC, Harvey R, et al. Relapse rates after two versus three consolidation courses of methotrexate in the treatment of low-risk gestational trophoblastic neoplasia. *Gynecol Oncol.* 2012;125(3):576-579.
65. Berkowitz RS, Goldstein DP, Bernstein MR. Ten years' experience with methotrexate and folinic acid as primary therapy for gestational trophoblastic disease. *Gynecol Oncol.* 1986;23(1):111-118.
66. Mutch DG, Soper JT, Baker ME, et al. Role of computed axial tomography of the chest in staging patients with nonmetastatic gestational trophoblastic disease. *Obstet Gynecol.* 1986;68(3):348-352.
67. Even C, Pautier P, Duvillard P, et al. Actinomycin D, cisplatin, and etoposide regimen is associated with almost universal cure in patients with high-risk gestational trophoblastic neoplasia. *Eur J Cancer.* 2014;50(12):2082-2089.
68. Lurain JR, Brewer JI. Treatment of high-risk gestational trophoblastic disease with methotrexate, actinomycin D, and cyclophosphamide chemotherapy. *Obstet Gynecol.* 1985;65(6):830-836.
69. Curry SL, Blessing JA, Disaia PJ, et al. A prospective randomized comparison of methotrexate, actinomycin D, and chlorambucil (MAC) versus modified Bagshawe regimen in "poor-prognosis" gestational trophoblastic disease. *Obstet Gynecol.* 1989;73:357-362.
70. Bagshawe KD. Treatment of high-risk choriocarcinoma. *J Reprod Med.* 1984;29:813-820.
71. Quinn M, Murray J, Friedlander M, et al. EMACO in high risk gestational trophoblast disease—The Australian experience. Gestational Trophoblast Subcommittee, Clinical Oncological Society of Australia. *Aust N Z J Obstet Gynaecol.* 1994;34(1):90-92.
72. Soper JT, Evans AC, Clarke-Pearson DL, et al. Alternating weekly chemotherapy with etoposide-methotrexate-dactinomycin/cyclophosphamide-vincristine for high-risk gestational trophoblastic disease. *Obstet Gynecol.* 1994;83(1):113-117.
73. Bower M, Newlands ES, Holden L, et al. EMA/CO for high-risk gestational trophoblastic tumors: results from a cohort of 272 patients. *J Clin Oncol.* 1997;15(7):2636-2643.
74. Tse KY, Chan KK, Tam KF, Ngan HY. 20-year experience of managing profuse bleeding in gestational trophoblastic disease. *J Reprod Med.* 2007;52(5):397-401.
75. DuBeshter B, Berkowitz RS, Goldstein DP, et al. Analysis of treatment failure in high-risk metastatic gestational trophoblastic disease. *Gynecol Oncol.* 1988;29(2):199-207.
76. Dobkin GR, Berkowitz RS, Goldstein DP, et al. Duplex ultrasonography for persistent gestational trophoblastic tumor. *J Reprod Med.* 1991;36(1):14-16.
77. Bakri YN, Berkowitz RS, Khan J, et al. Pulmonary metastases of gestational trophoblastic tumor: Risk factors for early respiratory failure. *J Reprod Med.* 1994;38:175-178.
78. Evans AC Jr, Soper JT, Clarke-Pearson DL, et al. Gestational trophoblastic disease metastatic to the central nervous system. *Gynecol Oncol.* 1995;59(2):226-230.
79. Ayhan A, Tuncer ZS, Tanir M, et al. Central nervous system involvement in gestational trophoblastic neoplasia. *Acta Obstet Gynecol Scand.* 1996;75(6):548-550.
80. Gillespie AM, Siddiqui N, Coleman RE, et al. Gestational trophoblastic disease: Does central nervous system chemoprophylaxis have a role? *Br J Cancer.* 1999;79(7-8):1270-1272.
81. Yordan EL Jr, Schlaerth JB, Gaddis O, et al. Radiation therapy in the management of gestational choriocarcinoma metastatic to the central nervous system. *Obstet Gynecol.* 1987;69:627-630.
82. Kobayashi T, Kida Y, Yoshida J, et al. Brain metastasis of choriocarcinoma. *Surg Neurol.* 1982;17(6):395-403.
83. Schechter NR, Mychalczak B, Jones W, et al. Prognosis of patients treated with whole-brain radiation therapy for metastatic gestational trophoblastic disease. *Gynecol Oncol.* 1998;68(2):183-192.
84. Altintas A, Vardar MA. Central nervous system involvement in gestational trophoblastic neoplasia. *Eur J Gynaecol Oncol.* 2001;22(2):154-156.
85. Neubauer NL, Latif N, Kalakota K, et al. Brain metastasis in gestational trophoblastic neoplasia: an update. *J Reprod Med.* 2012;57(7-8):288-292.
86. Gordon AN, Kavanagh JJ, Gershenson DM, et al. Cisplatin, vincristine, and bleomycin combination therapy in resistant gestational trophoblastic disease. *Cancer.* 1986;58:1407-1410.
87. Surwit EA, Childers JM. High-risk metastatic gestational

trophoblastic disease: a new dose-intensive, multiagent chemotherapeutic regimen. *J Reprod Med.* 1991;36:45-48.
88. Sutton GP, Soper JT, Blessing JA, et al. Ifosfamide alone and in combination in the treatment of refractory malignant gestational trophoblastic disease. *Am J Obstet Gynecol.* 1992;167:489-495.
89. Chen LP, Cai SM, Fan JX, Li ZT. PEBA regimen (cisplatin, etoposide, bleomycin, and adriamycin) in the treatment of drug-resistant choriocarcinoma. *Gynecol Oncol.* 1995;56(2):231-234.
90. Garris PD, Gallup DG, Melton K. Long-term remission of previously resistant choriocarcinoma with a combination of etoposide, ifosfamide, and cisplatin. *Gynecol Oncol.* 1995;57(2):254-256.
91. Hartenbach EM, Saltzman AK, Carter JR, Twiggs LB. A novel strategy using G-CSF to support EMA/CO for high-risk gestational trophoblastic disease. *Gynecol Oncol.* 1995;56(1):105-108.
92. Lotz JP, Andre T, Donsimoni R, et al. High dose chemotherapy with ifosfamide, carboplatin, and etoposide combined with autologous bone marrow transplantation for the treatment of poor-prognosis germ cell tumors and metastatic trophoblastic disease in adults. *Cancer.* 1995;75:874-885.
93. Soper JT, Evans AC, Rodriguez G, et al. Etoposide-platin combination therapy for chemorefractory gestational trophoblastic disease. *Gynecol Oncol.* 1995;56(3):421-424.
94. Piamsomboon S, Kudelka AP, Termrungruanglert W. Remission of refractory gestational trophoblastic disease in the brain with ifosfamide, carboplatin, and etoposide (ICE): first report and review of literature. *Eur J Gynaecol Oncol.* 1997;18(6):453-456.
95. Newlands ES, Mulholland PJ, Holden L, et al. Etoposide and cisplatin/etoposide, methotrexate, and actinomycin D (EMA) chemotherapy for patients with high-risk gestational trophoblastic tumors refractory to EMA/cyclophosphamide and vincristine chemotherapy and patients presenting with metastatic placental site trophoblastic tumors. *J Clin Oncol.* 2000;18(4):854-859.
96. Lurain JR, Schink JC. Importance of salvage therapy in the management of high-risk gestational trophoblastic neoplasia. *J Reprod Med.* 2012;57(5-6):219-224.
97. Mapelli P, Mangili G, Picchio M, et al. Role of 18F-FDG PET in the management of gestational trophoblastic neoplasia. *Eur J Nucl Med Mol Imaging.* 2013;40(4):505-513.
98. Doumplis D, Al-Khatib K, Sieunarine K, et al. A review of the management by hysterectomy of 25 cases of gestational trophoblastic tumours from March 1993 to January 2006. *BJOG.* 2007;114(9):1168-1171.
99. Alazzam M, Hancock BW, Tidy J. Role of hysterectomy in managing persistent gestational trophoblastic disease. *J Reprod Med.* 2008;53(7):519-524.
100. Newlands ES, Bower M, Fisher RA, et al. Management of placental site trophoblastic tumors. *J Reprod Med.* 1998;43(1):53-59.
101. Feltmate CM, Genest DR, Wise L, et al. Placental site trophoblastic tumor: a 17-year experience at the New England Trophoblastic Disease Center. *Gynecol Oncol.* 2001;82(3):415-419.
102. Vargas R, Barroilhet LM, Esselen K, et al. Subsequent pregnancy outcomes after complete and partial molar pregnancy, recurrent molar pregnancy, and gestational trophoblastic neoplasia: an update from the New England Trophoblastic Disease Center. *J Reprod Med.* 2014;59(5-6):188-194.
103. Sebire NJ, Foskett M, Paradinas FJ, et al. Outcome of twin pregnancies with complete hydatidiform mole and healthy co-twin. *Lancet.* 2002;359(9324):2165-2166.
104. Walden PA, Bagshawe KD. Pregnancies after chemotherapy for gestational trophoblastic tumours. *Lancet.* 1979;2(8154):1241.
105. Garner EI, Lipson E, Bernstein MR, et al. Subsequent pregnancy experience in patients with molar pregnancy and gestational trophoblastic tumor. *J Reprod Med.* 2002;47(5):380-386.
106. Wong JM, Liu D, Lurain JR. Reproductive outcomes after multiagent chemotherapy for high-risk gestational trophoblastic neoplasia. *J Reprod Med.* 2014;59(5-6):204-208.
107. Sisti G, Kanninen TT, Asciutti S, et al. Rate of second primary tumors following diagnosed choriocarcinoma: a SEER analysis (1973-2010). *Gynecol Oncol.* 2014;134(1):90-95.
108. Stafford L, McNally OM, Gibson P, Judd F. Long-term psychological morbidity, sexual functioning, and relationship outcomes in women with gestational trophoblastic disease. *Int J Gynecol Cancer.* 2011;21(7):1256-1263.

Section IX

Genitourinary Malignancies

Section Editor: Nizar M. Tannir

第九篇　泌尿生殖系统恶性肿瘤

35

Renal Cell Carcinoma

第三十五章　肾细胞癌

Matthew T. Campbell
Eric Jonasch
Christopher G. Wood
Nizar M. Tannir

中文导读

本章节首先介绍了肾细胞癌的流行病学，指出自2000年以来，肾细胞癌的死亡率呈下降趋势。肾细胞癌是肾脏肿瘤中最常见的类型，而肾透明细胞癌是其中最常见的组织学亚型。本章后续介绍了肾细胞癌的分期、危险因素，以及影响预后的临床病理及生物标志物。随后分别讲述了非转移性肾细胞癌和转移性肾细胞癌的处理原则。对于转移性肾细胞癌，主要介绍了肾透明细胞癌的治疗原则，包括原发灶切除的价值、全身治疗药物的种类、如何合理选择药物以及相关副作用的综合管理等，并对近年来新型治疗手段如疫苗、免疫检查点抑制剂的研究现状做了阐述。针对肾非透明细胞癌，由于多数临床研究均排除了肾非透明细胞癌，可供参考的数据较少，因此主要推荐此类患者参加临床研究。文章列举了几种肾非透明细胞癌亚型的治疗原则，包括肉瘤样肾细胞癌、集合管癌，以及Xp11.2 转位型肿瘤。本章最后总结性描绘了肾脏肿瘤的全程管理模式以供临床医生在实践中遵循和参考。

INCIDENCE AND DIAGNOSIS

The American Cancer Society predicts that in 2015 there will be over 64,000 new cases of renal neoplasms in the United States and that 14,000 patients will die as a consequence of disease progression ([1]). Renal cell carcinoma (RCC) is the most common histology found in kidney tumors, with clear cell RCC (ccRCC) being the most common histologic subtype (Fig. 35-1). Non–clear cell RCC (nccRCC) subtypes include chromophobe, papillary, oncocytoma, collecting duct carcinoma (CDC), renal medullary, translocation, and unclassified RCC.

Work by Chow et al ([1]) found the worldwide incidence of RCC appearing to plateau after a steady increase over several decades. To examine the incidence in the United States, the group used the database of the National Cancer Institute's Surveillance, Epidemiology, and End Results (SEER) Program to track patients with a diagnosis of kidney cancer from 1977 to 2006. The rate of localized cancer detection has continued to increase, whereas the rates of regional, metastatic, and unstaged RCC have declined. In this work, the mortality rate associated with RCC appears to begin declining in the early 2000s across both gender and racial lines. Although the direct causal relationship for the decline in RCC mortality in this study is unclear, early detection in the era of computed tomography (CT) imaging may be contributing to this finding.

STAGING, EPIDEMIOLOGY, AND RISK FACTORS

The American Joint Commission on Cancer staging schema for RCC was updated in 2010. Major staging

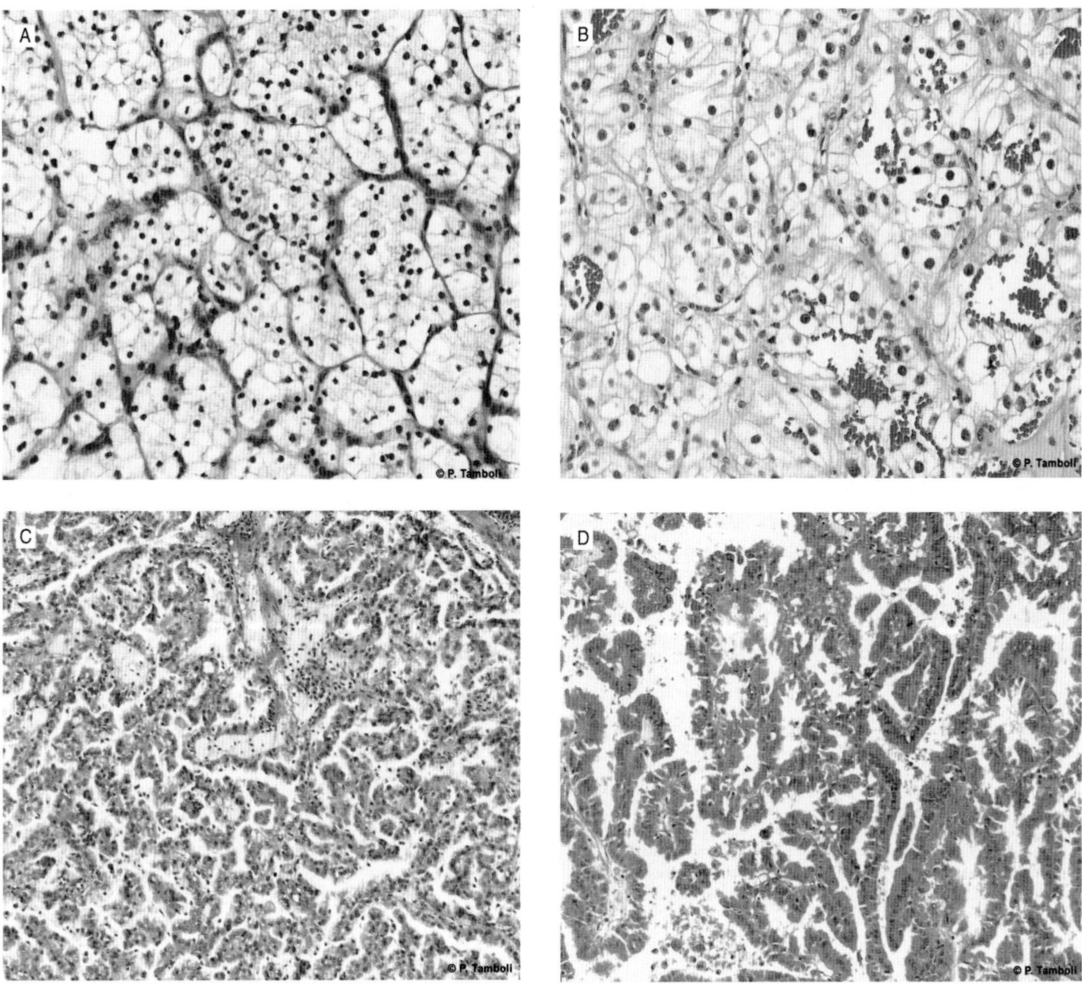

FIGURE 35-1 Photomicrographs of clear cell (conventional) renal cell carcinoma (RCC) with low-grade (A) and high-grade (B) nuclear features. Photomicrographs of a type 1 papillary RCC (C) showing papillae lined by short cuboidal cells and a type 2 papillary RCC (D) showing papillae lined by tall columnar cells, with eosinophilic cytoplasm and high-grade nuclear features. (Used with permission from Pheroze Tamboli, MD.)

categories are as follows: stage 1: T1 tumors that are 7 cm in maximum diameter or less and are confined to the kidney; stage 2: T2 tumors that exceed 7 cm in diameter but are confined to the kidney; stage 3: T3 tumors that demonstrate extracapsular invasion into the perinephric adipose tissue or renal sinus or extend into the renal vein or inferior vena cava (stage 3 also includes tumors with regional lymph node metastasis); and stage 4: extension of the primary tumor into the ipsilateral adrenal gland or beyond Gerota's fascia or distant metastases ([2]).

The link between germline genetic mutations and the development of RCC is well established and applies to a small but biologically important subset of RCC cases ([3]). Although these genetic alterations certainly play an important role in the biology of RCC in both familial and sporadic cases, there are also some environmental factors that contribute to the risk of developing a renal neoplasm. Smoking has long been linked to an increase in the risk of developing RCC, in addition to its association with multiple other malignancies ([4]). As is the case with other malignancies, cessation of smoking can be associated with a diminution in the risk of developing RCC ([5]). Interestingly, this diminution in risk appears to be slower and requires a significantly longer time to reach baseline than that seen with other malignancies, such as lung cancer.

Obesity or increased body mass index (BMI) has also been linked to increased risk of developing RCC. Several studies have demonstrated a higher incidence of obesity or increased BMI in patients with RCC, suggesting an epidemiologic linkage ([6]). As is the case in most retrospective epidemiologic studies, these observations are confounded by other associated variables, including diet, occupational history, and smoking. In a report by Kamat et al., overweight and obese patients had a more favorable prognosis following surgery than did patients with a lower BMI ([7]). Additional possible risk factors identified retrospectively in epidemiologic studies include diabetes, hypertension, and treatment with diuretics; in addition, certain diets have been linked to higher or lower risk than the general population.

PROGNOSTIC FACTORS, PATHOLOGY, AND MOLECULAR MARKERS

The natural history is variable, depending on tumor genetic factors, the general medical condition of the patient, and factors such as angiogenesis and immune response. Patients who undergo nephrectomy for localized disease remain at risk of recurrence for many years and require appropriate counseling and surveillance.

The traditional measures of performance status, tumor stage, and tumor grade each demonstrate good correlation with clinical outcome ([8]). Integration of these parameters and other clinical prognostic variables allows the classification of patients into groups with statistically significant differences in survival. There are a variety of clinical, pathologic, and molecular features that have been proposed and studied as prognostic factors (Table 35-1) ([9, 10]). As the genomic landscape continues to be more clearly defined in ccRCC and the genetic drivers of metastasis are identified, more

Table 35-1 Prognostic Factors in Advanced Renal Cell Carcinoma

Patient- or Treatment-Related Factors	Laboratory Studies	Tumor-Related Factors	Molecular Markers
Performance status	Lactate dehydrogenase	Site and/or number of metastatic sites	*VHL* mutation or hypermethylation
Age, gender, race	Alkaline phosphatase	Disease-free interval	Carbonic anhydrase IX expression
Symptoms: weight loss, fatigue, pain, loss of appetite, fever	Calcium	Metastasis-free interval	Phospho-extracellular signal regulated kinase (pERK)
Overweight	Albumin	Tumor burden	Cytoplasmic mTOR staining
Prior nephrectomy	Liver dysfunction	Histologic type	*PTEN* deletion
Prior therapy	Anemia Neutrophilia	Sarcomatoid dedifferentiation	p53 overexpression
	Thrombocytosis	Ploidy	MMP-2 and MMP-9 overexpression *BAP1* and *PBRM1* mutation

refined putative biomarkers are needed to more effectively treat this heterogeneous disease ([11, 12]).

Clinical Prognostic Variables

In 1999, Motzer et al identified five risk factors (elevated serum corrected calcium level, anemia, lactate dehydrogenase >1.5× the upper limit of normal [ULN], Karnofsky performance score [KPS] <80, and primary tumor in place) that segregated patients into three risk groups (good, zero factors; intermediate, one to two factors; and poor, three or more factors) ([13]). In 2002, an updated version, now referred to as the Memorial Sloan-Kettering Cancer Center (MSKCC) risk criteria (also referred to as the "Motzer criteria"), was published with the original four risk factors, with the fifth being treatment of interferon within 1 year of diagnosis ([14]). For clinical trial purposes, the fifth factor is often considered time to initiation of systemic therapy within 1 year from initial diagnosis of RCC. With the introduction of targeted therapy, the International Metastatic Renal Cell Carcinoma Database Consortium (IMDC) was formed, and a modified prognostic scoring system was put forth in 2009 and externally validated in 2013 ([15, 16]). The IMDC prognostic scoring system (also referred to as the "Heng score") has six risk factors (elevated serum corrected calcium level, anemia, KPS <80, systemic treatment for metastatic disease within 1 year, absolute neutrophil count >ULN, and platelet count >ULN). Similar to the MSKCC scoring system, good risk is defined as zero risk factors, intermediate risk as one to two risk factors, and poor risk as three or more risk factors. Although other systems have been proposed, the MSKCC and IMDC remain the most widely used (Table 35-2).

Non–clear cell histology has been associated with lower response to systemic therapy ([17]). In an attempt to improve on the MSKCC clinical prognostic model, we investigated the role of cytokines and angiogenic factors (CAFs) in serum of patients treated with interferon-α (IFN-α) and found elevated baseline levels of interleukin (IL)-5, IL-6, IL-12p40, and vascular endothelial growth factor A (VEGFA) to be independent risk factors associated with inferior survival. Incorporating the CAF model with the MSKCC clinical model improved the concordance index for predicting overall survival (OS). Patients with three or more of the four CAFs or with MSKCC poor-risk status had a median OS of 9 months, compared with a median OS of 32 months for patients with two or fewer CAFs ([18]). Similar efforts have been undertaken to develop serum and plasma-based prognostic and predictive biomarkers in individuals who received antiangiogenic therapy ([19, 20]).

Pathology and Molecular Markers

There are several major histologic subtypes in RCC, including clear cell, papillary, and chromophobe RCC (see Fig. 35-1). Historically, patients with nccRCC variants except chromophobe do poorly once they develop metastatic disease, mainly due to the dearth of effective systemic therapy.

The *VHL* gene product regulates the hypoxia-induced pathway and is commonly mutated in ccRCC ([11]). The hypoxia-induced pathway leads to the activation of survival genes that mediate glucose transport, proliferation, angiogenesis, and pH regulation and is also implicated in the other tumor types. In a study of 187 patients undergoing nephrectomy for ccRCC in Japan, mutation or hypermethylation of the *VHL* gene was found

Table 35-2 The Memorial Sloan-Kettering Cancer Center (MSKCC) Modified Risk Score for Metastatic Renal Cell Carcinoma and the International Metastatic Renal Cell Database Consortium (IMDC) Risk Score With Survival by Risk Stratification

MSKCC 2002 Factors (1 point each)	Risk Group (points)	Overall Survival (months)	IMDC or Heng Score (1 point each)	Risk Group (points)	Overall Survival (months)
Anemia	Good (0)	30	Anemia	Good (0)	43
Elevated calcium			Elevated calcium		
KPS <80	Intermediate (1-2)	14	KPS <80	Intermediate (1-2)	22.5
Metastatic Tx within 1 year of Dx			Metastatic Tx within 1 year		
LDH >1.5× ULN	Poor (3-5)	5	Platelet count >ULN	Poor (3-6)	7.8
			Neutrophil count >ULN		

Dx, diagnosis; KPS, Karnofsky performance score; LDH, lactate dehydrogenase; Tx, treatment; ULN, upper limit of normal.

in 58% of tumors, and was associated with significantly improved disease-free and cancer-specific survival in patients with organ-confined tumors (n = 134), but not in those with stage IV disease at the time of nephrectomy (n = 53) ([21]). *VHL* loss occurs early in the development of clear cell carcinoma ([12]), potentially identifying a subset of patients who do well after surgery.

In ccRCC, loss of the short arm of chromosome 3 was the most common genetic alteration identified in The Cancer Genome Atlas (TCGA) analysis. The most common genetic mutations related to this loss include *VHL*, *SETD2* (a histone methyltransferase), *BAP1* (histone deubiquitinase), and *PBRM1* (part of chromatin remodeling complex), and all lie on chromosome 3p ([11]). The University of Texas Southwestern group identified *BAP1* mutations to be associated with poor survival, with a median OS of 4.6 years from nephrectomy in patients who present with nonmetastatic disease compared with a median OS of 10.6 years in patients whose tumors harbor *PBRM1* mutations. The investigators validated these findings from tumor specimens included in the TCGA analysis ([22]).

MANAGEMENT OF NONMETASTATIC RENAL CELL CARCINOMA

With the introduction of improved cross-sectional imaging including CT and magnetic resonance imaging (MRI), the detection of renal masses has increased substantially. The ability to characterize renal masses as benign or malignant appearing has also evolved with improved technology and the use of specific contrast-enhancing sequences. The management of small renal masses (<4 cm) will not be extensively covered in this chapter but includes options such as active surveillance, partial nephrectomy (PN), radical nephrectomy (RN), or thermal ablation depending on factors including patient comorbidities and surgical expertise ([23]). Current surgical approaches to both PN and RN include open, laparoscopic, and robotic-assisted techniques ([24, 25]). Loss of nephrons associated with RN compared to PN increases patient risk for development of chronic kidney disease (CKD)([26]). In the general population, CKD is associated with increased risk of mortality and cardiovascular disease. Retrospectively, patients treated with RN were found to have higher all-cause mortality and an increased incidence of cardiovascular events ([27]).

With the introduction of robotic partial nephrectomy, the warm ischemia and suturing times are reduced compared to laparoscopic PN even among experienced laparoscopic surgeons ([28]). The management algorithm of potential tumors amenable to PN continues to evolve and should take into account the health of the contralateral kidney, familial cancer syndromes leading to multiple renal masses, proximity to the hilum and vascular structures, baseline kidney function, and surgeon experience and volume.

With larger, more locally advanced tumors requiring nephrectomy, the decision to perform a lymph node dissection remains an area of debate. In the European Organization for Research and Treatment of Cancer (EORTC) 30881 trial, 772 patients were randomized between lymph node resection or no resection during nephrectomy procedure. The majority of patients had ≤T2 disease ([29]). The study found no difference in recurrence-free survival or OS. However, other series have found the presence of lymph node positivity to be directly correlated with increasing T stage. As a result, at the University of Texas MD Anderson Cancer Center (MDACC) when patients have radiographic evidence of lymph node involvement or T stage ≥T3a, a therapeutic or staging lymph node dissection is typically undertaken.

The decision to perform ipsilateral adrenalectomy as part of the standard RN procedure has evolved. In a retrospective review of the literature, O'Malley et al estimated a negative predictive value of 96% when cross-sectional imaging of the ipsilateral adrenal gland was compared to surgical pathology ([30]). Unless there is evidence of involvement either by direct extension, radiographic evidence of metastatic spread of disease, or concern for involvement during gross inspection during surgery, the ipsilateral adrenal gland is typically spared.

Locally advanced tumors staged as T3b or higher require considerable institutional and surgeon experience in the management of these patients and will not be covered here in detail.

METASTATIC DISEASE WITH CLEAR CELL HISTOLOGY

Role of Cytoreductive Nephrectomy in Metastatic Disease

Renal cell carcinoma remains a relatively rare malignancy where addressing the primary tumor in selected patients with metastatic disease leads to an improvement in OS ([31, 32]). In a pooled analysis of the results of the Southwest Oncology Group (SWOG) 8949 and EORTC 30947 studies, improvement in OS favored the nephrectomy arm, with a median survival of 13.6 months versus 7.8 months for those randomized to the surgical arm ([33]). Because the initial studies compared patients treated with IFN-α with or without cytoreductive nephrectomy, the question of benefit of cytoreductive nephrectomy in the era of targeted therapy has reemerged. In a retrospective analysis, the IMDC found that patients treated in the targeted era appear to benefit from cytoreductive nephrectomy if they have three or fewer prognostic risk factors as outlined in Table 35-2, whereas those with four or more factors do not appear to benefit ([34]). Two ongoing prospective trials, SURTIME (NCT01099423) and CARMENA (NCT0093033), are attempting to address two questions regarding targeted therapy and cytoreductive nephrectomy. The SURTIME trial is investigating whether cytoreductive surgery is better performed before or after first-line sunitinib. The CARMENA trial is an EORTC effort investigating whether cytoreductive nephrectomy is beneficial in patients treated with sunitinib. Based on the available data and our institutional experience, patients at MDACC with synchronous metastatic disease who have a good performance status, a good or intermediate prognosis based on MSKCC or IMDC score, ccRCC, and a sizable renal primary compared to metastatic disease burden are generally offered upfront cytoreductive nephrectomy.

Patients who present with metastatic disease and primary tumor in situ offer an ideal presurgical setting for clinical and translational research studies ([35]). Retrospectively, patients at MDACC treated with targeted agents prior to cytoreductive nephrectomy compared to upfront cytoreductive nephrectomy experienced similar rates of serious adverse events ([36]). With the ability to analyze treated tissue paired with time blood samples and clinical and radiographic parameters at defined intervals, presurgical clinical trials offer an opportunity to enhance our understanding of metastatic RCC and determinants of response and resistance to targeted and immunotherapeutic agents.

Role of Metastasectomy

In carefully selected patients, metastasectomy plays an important role in the multidisciplinary treatment of patients with metastatic RCC (mRCC). Retrospective series have found survival benefit in resecting oligometastatic disease from multiple sites. Interpretation of these results is always limited due to the highly selected and retrospective nature of these studies. However, appropriate patient selection, complete resection of disease, and metachronous single site or oligometastatic disease positively impact patient outcomes. In a pooled retrospective analysis from three centers including patients from MDACC, 22 patients who had received targeted therapy underwent consolidative metastasectomy with an acceptable postoperative complication rate. After 108 weeks of follow-up, 11 patients remained disease free, and the median time to resumption of targeted therapy was 55 weeks ([37]). An ongoing randomized phase II study (NCT01575548) is addressing the role of pazopanib versus placebo in patients with no evidence of disease after metastasectomy. Further treatment decisions are based on the timing of recurrence, sites of recurrence, and individual patient characteristics. At MDACC, we strongly believe a multidisciplinary approach at high-volume centers is required to optimally manage these patients.

An algorithm to select candidates for metastasectomy and for the approach to postmetastasectomy systemic treatment is shown in Fig. 35-2.

SYSTEMIC THERAPY

Cytokine Therapy

Until the introduction of targeted therapy (discussed in more detail in the later section on targeted therapy), metastatic resection and cytokine therapy remained the only viable treatment options in mRCC. Interferon-α and IL-2 have been extensively evaluated over the past three decades. In a randomized phase II study from MDACC, treatment with low-dose IFN-α-2b compared to intermediate-dose IFN-α-2b resulted in no significant differences in progression-free survival (PFS) or OS, but patients had an improved quality of life while on low-dose therapy ([38]). Sustained complete remissions with IFN-α are rare (1%-2%), and with the relatively low response rate of approximately 7%, IFN-α monotherapy never received US Food and Drug Administration (FDA) approval for treatment of mRCC and is no longer considered as a single agent for mRCC at MDACC.

High-dose IL-2 (HD IL-2) received FDA approval in the treatment of mRCC in 1992 based on the results of several phase II trials that found an overall response rate of 15% to 20% and a durable response in the majority of patients who achieved a complete response. A phase III trial comparing HD IL-2 with an outpatient low-dose IL-2 plus IFN-α regimen yielded a higher response rate to HD IL-2 of 23% versus 10% but no statistically significant differences in PFS and OS. However, durable responses of greater than 3 years were seen in 7% of those treated with HD IL-2 versus 0% of patients in the other arm, supporting HD IL-2 as a viable standard-of-care option for patients who are candidates for this therapy ([39]). Although the management of toxicity related to the delivery of HD IL-2 is challenging, high-volume centers have published a toxic death rate of less than 1%, with response rates of roughly 15% to 20% and durable remissions in the range of 5% to 7% ([40, 41]). Given the ability to produce a sustained remission with likely cure in a small subset of patients, at MDACC, we offer frontline HD IL-2 therapy to patients with excellent performance status, previous nephrectomy, limited or no comorbidities,

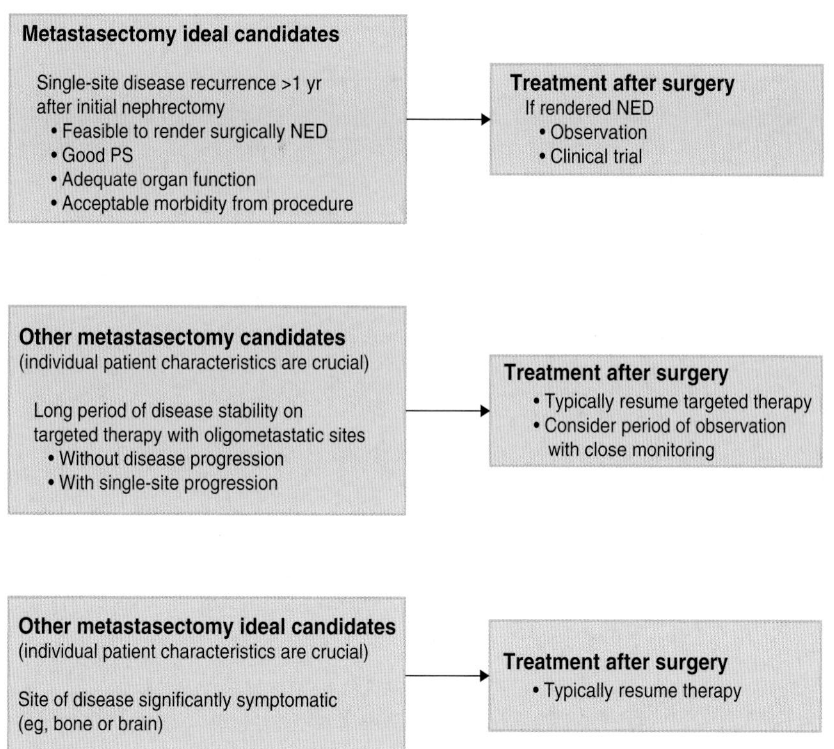

FIGURE 35-2 Metastasectomy candidates and treatment after procedure. NED, no evidence of disease; PS, performance status.

and low-volume metastatic disease burden, especially lung-only disease.

Targeted Therapy

Over the last decade, seven agents have been FDA approved for the treatment of mRCC. Of these agents, five are vascular endothelial growth factor (VEGF) pathway–blocking agents, with four being within the small-molecule tyrosine kinase inhibitor family and one, bevacizumab, being a monoclonal antibody directed against VEGF on the cell surface. The remaining two agents are mammalian target of rapamycin (mTOR) inhibitors. These agents target both the tumor cells and the tumor microenvironment.

Vascular Endothelial Growth Factor, or Vascular Endothelial Growth Factor Receptor–Targeted Agents

The presence of a *VHL* mutation in up to 80% of patients with ccRCC and the resultant increased production of angiogenic factors has made this axis the most exploited treatment target. A number of agents that target either VEGF or its receptors (VEGFR) were FDA approved in the past 10 years (Table 35-3).

Bevacizumab is a humanized recombinant anti-VEGF antibody. Two large randomized phase III studies demonstrated an improved PFS in patients who received a combination of bevacizumab plus IFN-α, when compared to IFN-α alone in patients with mRCC who had not received prior systemic therapy ([42, 43]). The AVOREN study compared patients treated with the combination of bevacizumab plus IFN versus placebo plus IFN and found that the bevacizumab combination resulted in a superior median PFS of 10.2 months compared to 5.4 months. The Cancer and Leukemia Group B (CALGB) 90206 study yielded a median PFS of 8.5 months for the combination arm versus 5.2 months for IFN monotherapy, a difference that was statistically significant. Of note, the OS for both studies was numerically superior in the bevacizumab-containing arm but did not reach statistical significance. Bevacizumab plus IFN was FDA approved for advanced RCC in 2009.

Sorafenib is an orally bioavailable small-molecule inhibitor of VEGFR, platelet-derived growth factor receptor (PDGFR), and Raf and was FDA approved in 2005 for the treatment of advanced RCC. In a randomized phase III trial, sorafenib yielded a significant improvement in PFS compared to placebo (median, 5.5 vs 2.8 months) in patients who had failed one prior

Table 35-3 Phase III Studies Leading to Approval of Molecularly Targeted Agents in Renal Cell Carcinoma

Agent	Year FDA Approved	Trial Design	Setting	No. of Patients	MSKCC Risk (%)	Median PFS (months)	Median OS (months)
Sorafenib	2005	Sorafenib vs placebo	Cytokine failures ccRCC	903	Good: 50 Int: 49 Missing: 1	5.5 vs 2.8	19.3 vs 15.9 (NS)
Sunitinib	2006	Sunitinib vs IFN	Frontline ccRCC	750	Good: 34 Int: 59 Poor: 7	11.0 vs 5.0	26.4 vs 21.8 (P = .051)
Temsirolimus	2007	Temsirolimus vs temsirolimus plus IFN vs IFN	Frontline Any histology	626	Good: 0 Int: 26 Poor: 74	5.5 vs 4.7 vs 3.1	10.9 vs 8.4 vs 7.3
Everolimus	2009	Everolimus vs placebo	Sorafenib or sunitinib failures ccRCC	416	Good: 28.5 Int: 56.5 Poor: 15	4.9 vs 1.9	14.8 vs 14.4
Bevacizumab plus IFN-α	2009	Bevacizumab plus IFN vs IFN plus placebo	Frontline ccRCC	649	Good: 28 Int: 56 Poor: 9 Unknown: 8	10.2 vs 5.4	23.3 vs 21.8
		Bevacizumab plus IFN vs IFN	Frontline ccRCC	732	Good: 26 Int: 64 Poor: 10	8.5 vs 5.2	18.3 vs 17.4
Pazopanib	2009	Pazopanib vs placebo	Frontline and cytokine failures ccRCC	435	Good: 39 Int: 54 Poor: 3	11.1 vs 2.8	22.9 vs 20.5
Axitinib	2012	Axitinib vs sorafenib	Second line ccRCC	723	Good: 28 Int: 37 Poor: 33	6.7 vs 4.7	20.1 vs 19.2

ccRCC, clear cell renal cell carcinoma; FDA, US Food and Drug Administration; IFN, interferon; Int, intermediate; MSKCC, Memorial Sloan-Kettering Cancer Center; NS, not significant; OS, overall survival; PFS, progression-free survival.

therapy, with the majority having received prior cytokines ([44]). A phase II study compared sorafenib monotherapy to sorafenib plus IFN-α and found similar overall response rates, toxicity, and median PFS, leading further exploration of this combination to be abandoned ([45]).

Sunitinib is an oral inhibitor of VEGFR and PDGFR. When it was first tested in the cytokine-refractory population, a time to progression of 8.7 months was achieved ([46]), earning it provisional FDA approval in early 2006. A follow-up first-line phase III trial randomizing patients between sunitinib and IFN showed a median PFS of 11.0 months for sunitinib versus 5.0 months for IFN ([47]). Median OS of sunitinib-treated patients was 26.4 months versus 21.8 months for the IFN-treated group (P = .051), which although not statistically significant was likely due to crossover from IFN to sunitinib and salvage therapy after protocol ([48]). When a subgroup analysis of the individuals who did not receive any subsequent therapy was performed, it was found that those who received sunitinib had a median OS of 28 months versus 14 months for the IFN group.

Pazopanib is an oral small molecule with a lower half-maximal inhibitory concentration (IC_{50}) for VEGFR when compared to sorafenib and sunitinib ([49]). A randomized, phase III trial compared pazopanib to placebo in patients treated with a cytokine and previously untreated patients and demonstrated an overall PFS of 9.2 versus 4.2 months (hazard ratio, 0.46; 95% confidence interval, 0.34-0.62; P < .0000001 ([50]). Pazopanib was FDA approved in 2009 for the first-line treatment of advanced RCC. Pazopanib has not been evaluated prospectively after first-line targeted therapy. At MDACC, we retrospectively studied 93 patients who received targeted therapy preceding pazopanib and observed an overall response rate of 15%, a median PFS of 6.5 months, and a median OS of 18.1 months ([51]). Adverse events were similar to those described in the large prospective trials with the agent.

Axitinib is a selective small-molecular inhibitor of the VEGFR-1, VEGFR-2, and VEGFR-3 signaling pathways ([52]). In a randomized phase III trial, axitinib was compared to sorafenib as second-line therapy after sunitinib, cytokines, bevacizumab plus IFN, or temsirolimus. The overall median PFS time was 6.7 versus 4.7 months in favor of axitinib ([53]). Median OS was not statistically different between the two groups (20.1 months for axitinib and 19.2 months for sorafenib) ([54]). The largest difference between the two arms was in patients previously treated with cytokines. Patients who developed hypertension with a diastolic blood pressure of greater than 90 mm Hg on trial had a significantly improved survival in both treatment arms as compared to patients who remained normotensive. When axitinib was compared with sorafenib in the first-line setting, the median PFS was 10.1 months with axitinib and 6.5 months with sorafenib with overlapping confidence intervals. Despite the numerically longer PFS with axitinib, the difference did not reach the trial's prespecified threshold of statistical significance ([55]).

Mammalian Target of Rapamycin Inhibitors

Temsirolimus is an intravenous sirolimus ester that was tested in intermediate- and poor-risk patients after phase II data had suggested that this was the subgroup of patients most likely to benefit from temsirolimus ([56]). This first-line phase III trial randomized patients to temsirolimus, temsirolimus plus IFN, or IFN monotherapy. The median OS in the temsirolimus arm was 10.9 months versus 8.4 months for the combination arm and 7.3 months for IFN monotherapy ([57]). An elevated pretreatment serum lactate dehydrogenase was found to be both a predictive and prognostic biomarker in patients treated with temsirolimus compared to IFN (OS, 6.9 vs 4.2 months, $P < .002$) ([58]).

Everolimus is an orally bioavailable sirolimus ester that was evaluated in patients who had progressed on sorafenib, sunitinib, or both. This phase III trial (RECORD-1) randomized patients between everolimus 10 mg by mouth daily versus placebo in a 2:1 fashion. Median PFS was 4.0 months with everolimus versus 1.9 months with placebo ([59]).

Because everolimus and temsirolimus are mTORC1 inhibitors, agents capable of blocking both the mTORC1 and mTORC2 pathways have been developed. In a recent study comparing everolimus with GDC-0980, a pan PI3K and TORC1/2 inhibitor, the median PFS was 6.1 months with everolimus versus 3.7 months with the investigational agent, with a higher rate of adverse events in the investigational arm ([60]).

The reasons for this surprising result are unclear at this time.

Side Effect Profiles

The major side effects of the targeted agents are summarized in Table 35-4.

Blockade of VEGFRs or depletion of the VEGF ligand causes class effects, which include hypertension, fatigue, proteinuria, and a slightly increased risk of bleeding and thromboembolic events. All of the anti-VEGF agents will cause these side effects to varying degrees. Sorafenib, sunitinib, and pazopanib are also inhibitors of PDGF, Flt3, and a number of other receptor tyrosine kinases and thus will induce hand-foot syndrome, diarrhea, and dysgeusia. Sunitinib appears to be particularly prone to inducing hypothyroidism ([61, 62]) and, in some cases, cardiomyopathy with decreased ejection fraction ([63]). The frequency of cardiac toxicity may be underappreciated. A single-institution experience from Stanford found that 33% of patients had evidence of cardiac toxicity even when excluding hypertension ([64]). The rate of heart failure induced by sunitinib at MDACC in the treatment of a variety of tumor types including mRCC was 2.7% ([65]). Emerging data suggest that scrupulous control of blood pressure in patients on sunitinib will decrease cardiac stress and resultant cardiac failure.

Other side effects include wound dehiscence and increased thromboembolic events. Our group reported perioperative complications in patients with mRCC and primary in situ who received antiangiogenic agents in the presurgical setting prior to cytoreductive nephrectomy. In a single-arm phase II trial ([35]), perioperative wound healing complications in patients who received 8 weeks of bevacizumab therapy were increased when compared to a set of matched controls. The retrospective study, which looked at 44 individuals who received sorafenib, sunitinib, or bevacizumab preoperatively, did not detect a significant elevation of any perioperative events ([66]).

The mTOR inhibitors demonstrate several unique side effects, including hyperglycemia, hypertriglyceridemia, and noninfectious pneumonitis. However, these agents are not as likely to induce hypertension or hand-foot skin reaction.

Agent Selection and Side Effect Management

A number of different factors are important when choosing the best initial agent for patients with metastatic ccRCC. Clearly, evidence-based criteria for selection are vital, but as seen in Fig. 35-3, there are several agents available for a particular treatment stage.

Table 35-4 Summary of Side Effects of Targeted Agents Approved in Renal Cell Carcinoma

Agent	Sorafenib	Sunitinib	Bevacizumab	Pazopanib	Temsirolimus	Everolimus	Axitinib
Hypertension	X/X	XX/–	XX/X	XX/X			XX/X
Fatigue	XX/X	XXX/X	XX/X	X/X	XX/X	X/X	XX/X
Hand-foot skin reaction	XX/X	XX/X		XX/X			XX/X
Diarrhea	XX/X	XX		XXX/X	XX/X	X/X	XXX/X
Dysgeusia	X /–	XX/X		X/			
Stomatitis	X/X	X/X			X/X	XX/X	X/X
Cardiac toxicity	X/X	X/X	X/X	X/X			
Nausea	X/X	XX/X				X/0	XX/X
Asthenia	XX/X	X/X	XX/XX		XX/X	X/X	X/X
Pulmonary toxicity	X/X				X/X	X/X	
Hepatotoxicity		XX/X		XXX/XX		XX/X	
Hypertriglyceridemia					XX/X	XXX/X	
Rash	XX/X	X/X			XX/X	XX/X	X/X
Hyperglycemia				XX/X	XX/X	XX/X	
Hypothyroidism	X/–	X/0	?	X/–			X/X
Proteinuria	X/X	X/X	X/X	X/X			
Cytopenias	X/X	XXX/X	X/X	XX/X	XX/X	XXX/X	XX/X
Increased creatinine	X/X	XXX/X	X/X	XX/X	X/X	X/X	X/0

X, XX, and XXX: Low (0%-25%), intermediate (25%-50%), and high incidence (>50%), all grades/grade 3 or higher.

For example, if we are dealing with a patient who has undergone nephrectomy, has good-risk characteristics, and is younger than age 70 years, HD IL-2, sunitinib, bevacizumab plus IFN, and pazopanib are all reasonable options. In the COMPARZ trial, a noninferiority phase III trial with PFS as the primary end point, sunitinib and pazopanib were directly compared ([67]). The trial showed noninferiority of pazopanib. Importantly, the side effect profile and quality-of-life assessment favored pazopanib. Consequently, we prefer pazopanib over the standard dosing schedule of sunitinib and over bevacizumab plus IFN given the relative ease of patient administration. Although HD IL-2 is often offered, many patients are not interested to receive it because of the low likelihood of success and the formidable toxicity.

Table 35-4 provides a summary of some of the most common side effects seen with these agents. A review of these side effects may aid in treatment selection for specific patients. Some may have occupational considerations that make hand-foot skin reaction a particular problem. Others may have cardiac comorbidities that make an agent like sunitinib, with a known effect on cardiac output in a subset of patients, less favorable. Table 35-5 summarizes the standard dose-reduction algorithms used in clinical trials of these agents.

In addition to dose interruptions and dose reductions, a change in schedule may be beneficial for some patients. Our group and others have retrospectively compared cohorts of patients treated on the standard sunitinib schedule of 4 weeks on, 2 weeks off with a schedule of 2 weeks on and 1 week off ([68]). The 2-week-on, 1-week-off schedule has a better toxicity profile and retrospectively has similar treatment efficacy compared with the standard approach ([69]). However, prospective comparison of the two treatment schedules has not been reported.

Symptom control is essential for patients receiving molecularly targeted agents. Table 35-6 outlines supportive care measures that can mitigate or prevent specific side effects. It is essential that the patient and health-care team maintain an ongoing dialogue during each cycle of therapy to ensure that patients proactively and appropriately manage these adverse events. Successful adverse event management will translate into higher drug compliance and a greater probability of achieving a successful outcome.

A retrospective review of patients treated with temsirolimus or everolimus at MDACC found a rate of noninfectious pneumonitis (NIP) of 6% with temsirolimus and 23% with everolimus ([70]). We observed that patients who developed NIP had longer treatment

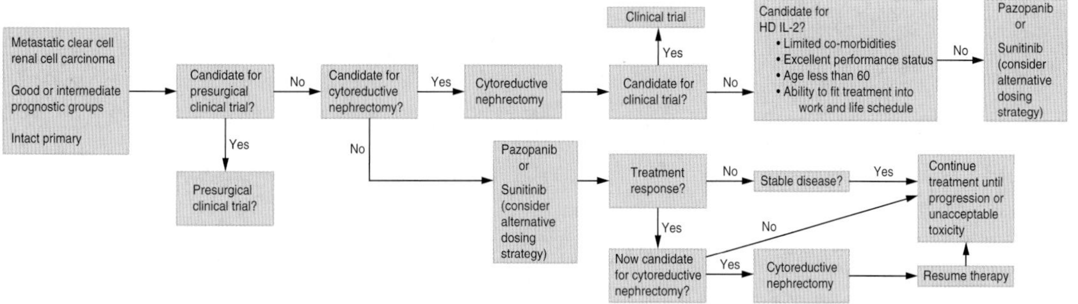

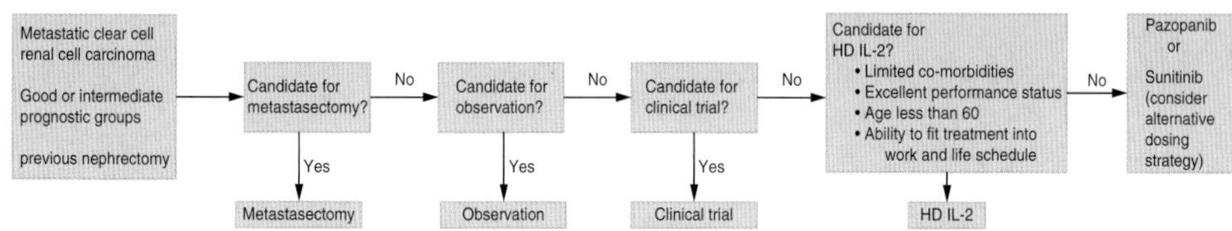

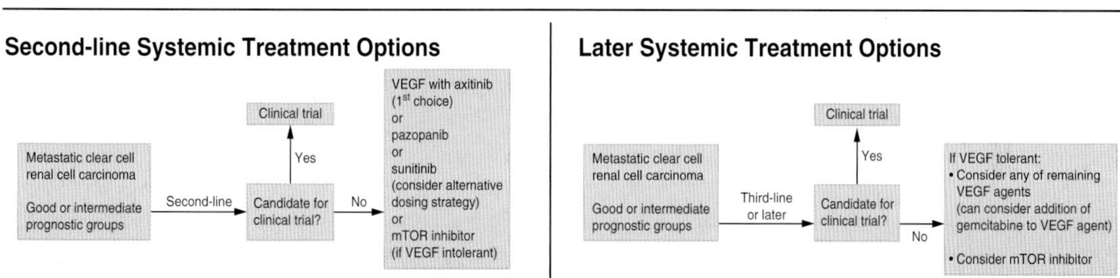

FIGURE 35-3 The University of Texas MD Anderson Cancer Center approach to initial systemic treatment lines for patients with metastatic clear cell renal cell carcinoma. HD IL-2, high-dose interleukin-2; mTOR, mammalian target of rapamycin VEGF, vascular endothelial growth factor.

duration and longer OS. Recent guidelines have been established to diagnose and treat NIP with the important caveats that patients with radiographic findings but lacking symptoms can continue therapy and patients with radiographic findings with mild to moderate cough can continue therapy with close monitoring ([71]). More severe symptoms require corticosteroids with a consideration of break or permanent discontinuation of mTOR inhibitor therapy depending on the severity of the event.

The decision for second-line and later therapy has become increasingly complex. Sequencing of VEGF-VEGF–directed therapy or VEGF-mTOR–directed therapy has been compared prospectively. In a randomized phase III trial of second-line therapy in patients who received first-line sunitinib, temsirolimus was compared to sorafenib. The trial's primary end point of detecting a superior PFS with temsirolimus was not met, with a median PFS of 4.1 months with temsirolimus and 3.7 months with sorafenib. Interestingly, the secondary end point of median OS favored the sorafenib arm (16.6 vs 12.3 months, $P = .01$). Although median OS was not the primary end point of the trial, the authors hypothesized that VEGF-VEGF sequencing may be more beneficial compared with the so-called "sandwich approach" of VEGF-mTOR-VEGF sequence ([72]). In the community, VEGF-mTOR-VEGF sequencing is the most common current treatment approach ([73]). In the AXIS trial, axitinib was compared to sorafenib in the second-line setting (although first-line treatment could be cytokine-based treatment) and led to an improved PFS ([53]). A phase II, single-arm, single-institution study found that after failure of frontline sunitinib or bevacizumab, pazopanib had activity, with a median PFS of 7.5 months ([74]). As such, a reasonable treatment approach for patients with good- or intermediate-risk disease by Heng criteria who are deemed good candidates for targeted therapy

Table 35-5 Dose Reduction Algorithm Used in Pivotal Trials of Approved Targeted Agents[a]

Agent	Standard Dose	Dose Reduction Schema
Sorafenib	400 mg PO bid	Dose level 1: 400 mg PO daily
		Dose level 2: 400 mg PO every other day
		Alternate[b]: Dose reduction to 600 mg PO daily
Sunitinib	50 mg PO daily 4 weeks on, followed by 2 weeks off	Dose level 1: 37.5 mg PO daily, 4 weeks on, 2 weeks off
		Dose level 2: 25 mg PO daily, 4 weeks on, 2 weeks off
		Alternate[b]: Schedule change to 50 mg PO 14 days on and 7 days off
Temsirolimus	25 mg IV weekly	Dose level 1: 20 mg IV weekly
		Dose level 2: 15 mg IV weekly
Everolimus	10 mg PO daily	Dose level 1: 5 mg PO daily Dose level 2: 5 mg PO every other day
Bevacizumab plus IFN	Bevacizumab 10 mg/kg IV every 14 days; IFN 9 MU SC TIW	IFN: Dose level 1: 6 MU SC TIW Dose level 2: 3 MU SC TIW
		Bevacizumab: for proteinuria: If greater than 2 g/dL hold until below 500 mg/dL
Pazopanib	800 mg PO daily	600 mg/d (dose level 1); 400 mg/d (dose level 2)
Axitinib	5 mg PO bid	3 mg PO bid (dose level 1); 2 mg PO bid (dose level 2)

bid, twice a day; IFN, interferon; IV, intravenous; MU, million units; PO, oral; SC, subcutaneous; TIW, three times a week.

[a]Once patients are on therapy, there are several ways to mitigate side effects. The package inserts of each agent outline the standard algorithm for dose reduction. This table summarizes the standard dose reduction algorithms used in clinical trials of these agents.

[b]Not prospectively validated but used empirically with good effect.

and do not elect to pursue HD IL-2 therapy can receive pazopanib as first-line therapy and receive axitinib or everolimus as second-line therapy. Depending on performance status and comorbidities, the decision can be made to continue with an alternative VEGF-directed therapy with sorafenib or sunitinib or change to an mTOR-directed therapy at progression. Certainly, consideration of a clinical trial should be entertained in the frontline and later line settings.

Patients who fall into the poor prognostic group remain a considerable unmet need in the care of patients with mRCC. At this time, temsirolimus remains the only agent with category 1 evidence to support its use. Ongoing trials in this setting include the FLIPPER trial (NCT01521715), which is a phase IV trial evaluating pazopanib in poor-risk mRCC, and a randomized phase II trial at MDACC comparing temsirolimus to pazopanib in the frontline setting (NCT01392183).

Combinations of Targeted Therapy

In an attempt to improve on the success of single-agent targeted therapy, combinations of VEGF and mTOR pathway blockade have been pursued. To date, combinations are associated with significant toxicity without a positive impact on response rate, PFS, or OS, as compared with sequential single-agent targeted therapy. A phase III trial compared the standard of bevacizumab plus IFN-α versus bevacizumab plus temsirolimus ([75]). The response rate, median PFS, and median OS were not found to be statistically different between the two treatment arms. As a result of early phase and later phase clinical trials to date, combinations of VEGF and mTOR inhibitors are unlikely to yield significant clinical benefit.

EMERGING THERAPIES

Vaccine Strategies

Given the rare durable responses to cytokine therapy, investigators have searched for vaccine-based strategies. At this time, no vaccine has proven successful in rigorous phase III testing. Currently, two phase III trials are ongoing. The first trial compares a multipeptide vaccine, IMA-901, paired with sunitinib versus sunitinib alone (NCT01265901). The second trial, the ADAPT phase III trial, involves a dendritic cell–based RNA vaccine, AGS-003, plus standard therapy versus standard therapy alone (NCT01582672).

Immune Checkpoint Inhibitors

A class of agents known as the immune checkpoint inhibitors has been developed allowing the targeting of molecules on both T cells and tumor cells important in downregulating the immune system, allowing for

Table 35-6 Management Recommendations for Commonly Experienced Toxicities

Side Effect	Preventative Measures	Supportive Care Measures		
Diarrhea	In patients with prior history of diarrhea on agent, consider loperamide once daily in morning	Loperamide 1-2 tabs after diarrhea	Diphenoxylate plus atropine	1 scoop psyllium with 1 oz water daily
Hand-foot syndrome	Heavy emollients applied to hands and feet bid and prn	As in preventive measures, plus urea-based callus creams		
Fatigue	Regular physical activity	Consider modafenil or methylphenidate	Check thyroid function	Short naps Regular exercise Regularized diet
Hypertension		Maintain BP below 140/90 using: 1. Calcium channel blockers (amlodipine okay but not diltiazem) 2. Angiotensin-converting enzyme inhibitors 3. β-Blockers		
Hypothyroidism		Levothyroxine		
Dysgeusia	Salt and soda mouthwash 4 times a day	Avoidance of hot and spicy foods Salt and soda mouthwash	Carafate	
Mouth sores	Salt and soda mouthwash 4 times a day	Xylocaine-based mouthwash		
Hyperglycemia	Scrupulous glycemic control	Scrupulous glycemic control		
Rash (sorafenib)		Dose adjustment Aveeno baths		
Rash (temsirolimus and everolimus)		Topical steroids		
Noninfectious pneumonitis (temsirolimus and everolimus)		Corticosteroids		

bid, twice a day; BP, blood pressure; prn, as needed.

a sustained antitumor response. Agents including the cytotoxic T lymphocyte-associated antigen 4 antibody (anti-CTLA-4; ipilimumab) ([76]) and the programmed death receptor-1 antibody (anti-PD-1; nivolumab and MK-3475) ([77]) and its ligand antibody (anti-PDL-1; MPDL3280A) ([78]) have shown significant, sustained antitumor responses in mRCC ([79]).

Table 35-7 shows the available clinical results for these agents. The VEGF pathway has been found preclinically to play an important role in tumor microenvironment immunosuppression ([80]). At this time, 10 ongoing studies are evaluating a variety of immune checkpoint inhibitors alone, in combination with other checkpoint inhibitors, or in combination with anti-VEGF therapy. Table 35-8 outlines the registered trials with these agents as of December 2014.

NON–CLEAR CELL RENAL CELL CARCINOMA

The large majority of studies performed to date excluded nccRCC. The exception was the phase III temsirolimus study, where 20% of the 626 patients

CHAPTER 35

Table 35-7 Results of Clinical Trials of Immune Checkpoint Inhibitors in Patients With Metastatic Clear Cell Renal Cell Carcinoma

Check Point Inhibitor	Phase of Trial, Malignancy	Dosing	Response Rate in mRCC	Toxicity: Grade 3 or Higher
Ipilimumab ([77])	Phase II, mccRCC, any number of previous treatments allowed All risk groups	Arm A: 3 mg/kg × 1 then 1 mg/kg Arm B: 3 mg/kg	1/29 (3.4%) 5/40 (12.5%)	14% 43%, 2 deaths
Nivolumab (anti-PD-1) ([78]) Abstract only	Phase II, mccRCC, one prior VEGF, ≤3 prior therapies All risk groups	Arm A: 0.3 mg/kg Arm B: 2 mg/kg Arm C: 10 mg/kg	20% 22% 20%	5% 17% 13%
Nivolumab (Nivo) plus ipilimumab (Ipi) ([79]) Abstract only	Phase I, mccRCC No or any prior treatments allowed Good-/intermediate-risk groups only	Arm A: Nivo 3 mg/Ipi 1 mg Arm B:Nivo 1 mg/Ipi 3 mg Arm C: Nivo 3 mg/Ipi 3 mg	6/21 (29%) 9/23 (39%) Not available	24% 61% Not available
MPDL3280A (anti-PD-L1) [(80)] Abstract only	Phase I, mRCC expansion cohort 83% prior treatment ccRCC and nccRCC	Dosing arms 3 mg/kg 10 mg/kg 15 mg/kg 20 mg/kg	Overall RR, 13% PFS, 50% at 24 wk	43% (13% attributed to study drug)

ccRCC, clear cell renal cell carcinoma; mccRCC, metastatic clear cell renal cell carcinoma; mRCC, metastatic renal cell carcinoma; nccRCC, non–clear cell renal cell carcinoma; PFS, progression-free survival; RR, response rate; VEGF, vascular endothelial growth factor.

Table 35-8 Registered Clinical Trials With Immune Checkpoint Inhibitors in Metastatic Renal Cell Carcinoma

Trial Name ± Sponsor	Drugs	Phase and setting	Identifying Number
CheckMate 025 Bristol-Meyer Squibb (BMS)	Nivolumab (anti-PD-1) vs everolimus	Phase III, mccRCC pretreated with anti-VEGF	NCT01668784, accrual complete
CheckMate 214 BMS	Nivolumab + ipilimumab (anti-CTLA-4) vs sunitinib	Phase III, mccRCC, untreated	NCT02231749
MD Anderson with BMS	Nivolumab vs nivolumab + bevacizumab vs nivolumab + ipilimumab	Phase I, presurgical, eligible for cytoreductive nephrectomy	NCT02210117
GlaxoSmithKline (GSK)	Pazopanib vs MK3475 (anti-PD-1) vs pazopanib + MK3475	Phase I/II, mccRCC, untreated	NCT02014636
Beth-Israel Deaconess	CT-011 (anti-PD-1) ± vaccine	Phase II, mRCC (any histology), any prior number of therapies	NCT02014636
Hoffman-La-Roche	MPDL3280A (anti-PDL-1) ± bevacizumab	Phase II, untreated mccRCC	NCT01984242
BMS	Anti-LAG-3 ± anti-PD-1	Phase I, solid tumors	NCT01968109
Pfizer and Merck, Sharp & Dohme	MK3475 + axitinib	Phase I, mccRCC	NCT02133742
Keynote-029 Merck, Sharp & Dohme Corp.	MK3475 + pegylated IFN-2α MK3475 + ipilimumab	Phase I/II, mRCC eligible only for phase I portion, melanoma eligible for all portions	NCT02089685
Merck, Sharp & Dohme Corp.	MK3475	Phase I, presurgical	NCT02212730

IFN, interferon; mccRCC, metastatic clear cell renal cell carcinoma; mRCC, metastatic renal cell carcinoma; VEGF, vascular endothelial growth factor;

had non–clear cell histology. A post hoc analysis of papillary RCC showed outcomes similar to ccRCC after treatment with temsirolimus ([81]). At MDACC, we conducted a phase II single-arm study of sunitinib in advanced nccRCC histologies including patients who had up to two previous lines of treatment and reported a median PFS of 2.7 months and an overall response rate of 5% ([82]). Our group recently presented the findings of the ESPN randomized phase II clinical trial comparing everolimus to sunitinib for frontline systemic therapy in patients with metastatic non–clear cell histologies ([83]). The primary end point was PFS after first-line treatment. The trial was stopped early due to futility of satisfying the primary end point, with a median PFS of 4.1 months with everolimus compared to 6.1 months with sunitinib. Foretinib, a c-MET, RET, and VEGFR-2 inhibitor, was tested with two different dosing schedules in a phase II trial enrolling patients with papillary RCC ([84]). The study found an overall response rate of 13.5% and a median PFS of 9.5 months, and foretinib is no longer being developed in this setting. Of note, a subset of 10 patients with a germline *c-MET* mutation had a 50% response rate, and alternative c-MET inhibitors should be explored in this setting. An actuarial 45-patient trial evaluating erlotinib in papillary RCC showed a response rate of 11%, and an OS of 27 months ([85]). Unfortunately, choosing the right agent for this relatively heterogeneous group of patients is hampered by a lack of studies and relatively small patient numbers. With the paucity of available data for clinical treatment decisions, we recommend enrolling patients with non–clear cell histologies on clinical trials when available.

Sarcomatoid Renal Cell Carcinoma

Approximately 5% of all patients with RCC will demonstrate sarcomatoid dedifferentiation in their tumors ([86]). Varying percentages of sarcomatoid involvement can be seen, and in cases where there is a predominance of sarcomatoid cells, it is difficult to determine the underlying histologic background. In these extreme cases, epithelial tumor markers are still present on the tumor cells, distinguishing these tumors from sarcomas.

Presence of sarcomatoid features in the tumor portends a poor prognosis ([87]). The results of chemotherapy and immunotherapy have been largely disappointing in patients with metastatic disease. Therapy targeting VEGF has been retrospectively reviewed, and in a series of 43 patients from several institutions, this approach had limited utility, with a median PFS of 5.3 months and median OS of 11.7 months ([88]). At MDACC, we retrospectively reviewed 28 patients with mRCC who received the combination of gemcitabine, capecitabine, and bevacizumab, including 8 patients with sarcomatoid features, and reported a median PFS of 5.9 months and a median OS of 10.4 months. These observations formed the basis of a prospective study at MDACC using this three-drug combination in patients with sarcomatoid histology. Preliminary findings from this study in the the first 18 patients treated (out of a planned 40 patients) revealed time to treatment failure of 5.5 months and median OS of 12 months.

Collecting Duct Carcinoma

Tumors arising from the collecting duct epithelium are located in the medulla or center portion of the kidney, in contrast to RCC tumors, which arise from tubules in the cortex ([89]). The diagnosis of CDC is based on both clinical and histologic features. Sarcomatoid dedifferentiation is not uncommon, and patterns of metastasis are similar to those of a high-grade, rapidly progressive RCC. There is no established effective systemic therapy for metastatic CDC, although marginal benefit is occasionally seen with chemotherapy regimens developed for transitional cell carcinoma ([90, 91]).

Medullary Carcinoma

Renal medullary carcinoma is a rare and virulent malignancy, afflicting patients with sickle cell hemoglobinopathies, usually sickle cell trait ([92]). It arises from the caliceal epithelium and can be morphologically distinguished from RCC and CDC. Some investigators have suggested that it is a dedifferentiated form of transitional cell carcinoma. Other kidney disorders associated with sickle cell hemoglobinopathies include unilateral hematuria, papillary necrosis, nephrotic syndrome, renal infarction, inability to concentrate urine, and pyelonephritis. These associated conditions may contribute to the development of renal medullary carcinoma. The majority of cases reported have a highly aggressive clinical course, presenting with metastatic disease and with a survival historically of about 4 months. It is refractory to most forms of systemic therapy ([93]), with some responses to cytotoxic chemotherapy.

Outcomes of patients with renal medullary carcinoma treated at four institutions found the median OS for all patients to be approximately 1 year from diagnosis ([94]). Of 16 patients who received targeted therapy, one response was noted. An updated effort from seven institutions that evaluated clinical outcomes for 39 patients with renal medullary carcinoma was presented in abstract form at the 2015 Genitourinary Cancer Symposium ([95]). Again, the median OS was 1 year, with the majority of patients presenting with advanced disease. Of seven patients who received presurgical treatment, one patient had a complete response, three had a partial response, and three had stable disease. The patient with the complete response had a near-complete pathologic response at the time of nephrectomy and remains without evidence of disease 27 months after diagnosis. Continued efforts to gain insight into the biology of this devastating entity are ongoing. In our experience, initial systemic therapy with chemotherapy with or without the addition of bevacizumab is a reasonable initial approach.

Xp11.2 Translocation Carcinoma

Xp11.2 translocation carcinoma is a rare disease entity that is proportionally more common in children but can also occur in young adults ([96]). A strong female predominance is observed. The *TFE3* gene located at Xp11.2 has a number of potential translocation partners leading to fusion of a novel gene. A recent analysis of 16 patients with translocation RCC found significant genomic heterogeneity, with 17q gain, 9p loss, 3p loss, and 17p loss being the most common findings ([97]). Histologically, these tumors may resemble ccRCC or show mixed clear and papillary features. These histologic findings in a young adult should prompt further histologic and molecular characterization of the tumor. Staining for *TFE3* permits relatively specific identification of this disease entity, but if it is highly suspected, a break apart fluorescent in situ hybridization assay should be used to increase sensitivity ([98, 99]). Response to standard immunotherapy or chemotherapy is poor, and patients have a relatively short OS. A retrospective review of 15 adult patients (12 females; median age, 40 years) with translocation carcinoma who were treated with targeted therapy at four centers in the United States showed an overall response rate of 20%, with a median PFS of 7.1 months and median OS of 14.3 months ([100]). A French study reported on 21 patients with adult translocation carcinoma treated with anti-VEGF agents or mTOR inhibitors. The authors reported objective responses, PFS, and OS results in the range of those previously reported for ccRCC ([101]).

CONCLUSION

Figure 35-4 succinctly outlines the current approach at MDACC for diagnosing and treating patients with a renal mass. With rapidly improving understanding of

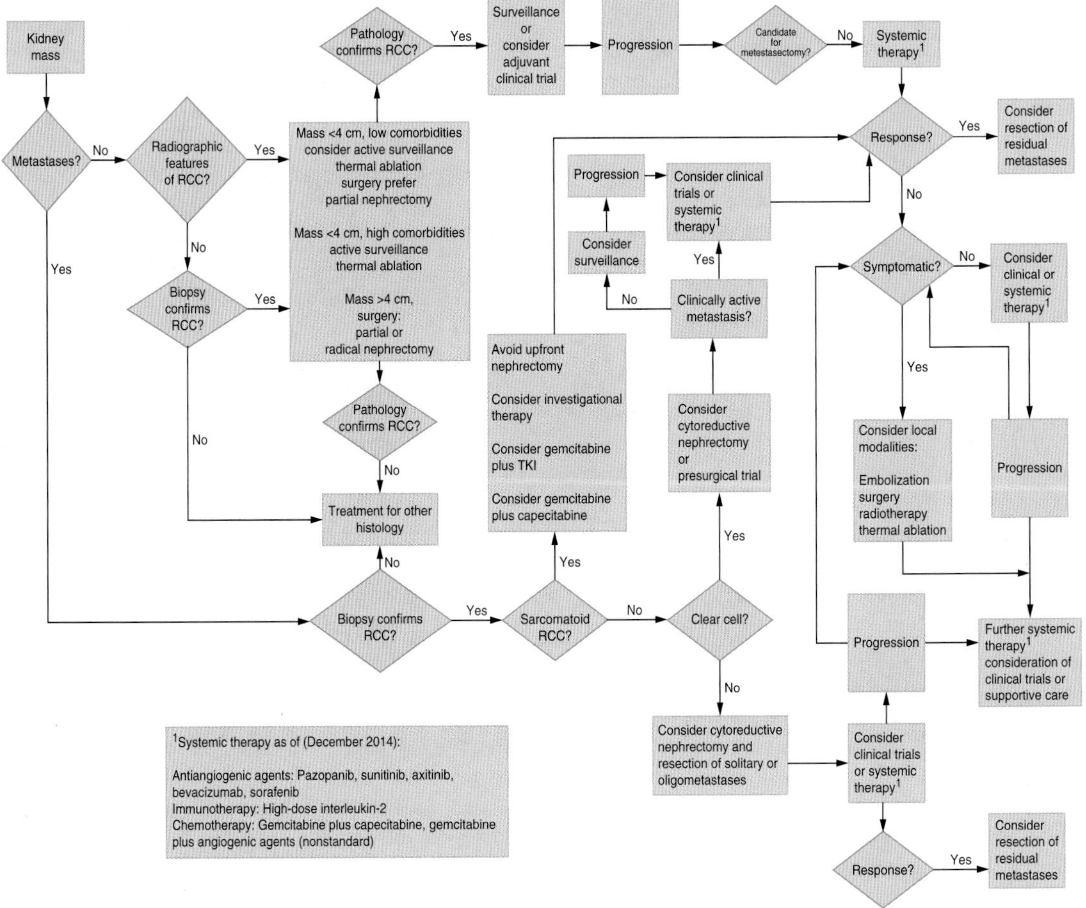

FIGURE 35-4 Management algorithm for patients diagnosed with a renal mass. RCC, renal cell carcinoma; TKI, tyrosine kinase inhibitor.

the biology of RCC, better patient selection and surgical techniques, an enriched arsenal of targeted agents, and the promise of new immunotherapy agents in late-phase clinical testing, the future of treatment for patients with RCC appears bright. We need to continue to focus on patients in the poor-risk clinical prognostic categories with metastatic clear cell carcinoma and patients with non–clear cell histologies because these represent major areas of unmet clinical need.

REFERENCES

1. Chow WH, Dong LM, Devesa SS. Epidemiology and risk factors for kidney cancer. *Nat Rev Urol.* 2010;7:245-257.
2. Edge SB, Byrd DR, Compton CC, Fritz AG, Greene FL, Trotti A (eds). *American Joint Committee on Cancer (AJCC). Cancer Staging Manual* (7th ed). New York: Springer; 2009.
3. Linehan WM, Walther MM, Zbar B. The genetic basis of cancer of the kidney. *J Urol.* 2003;170:2163-2172.
4. Hunt JD, van der Hel OL, McMillan GP, Boffetta P, Brennan P. Renal cell carcinoma in relation to cigarette smoking: meta-analysis of 24 studies. *Int J Cancer.* 2005;114:101-108.
5. Parker PS, Cerhan JR, Janney CA, Lynch CF, Cantor KP. Smoking cessation and renal cell carcinoma. *Ann Epidemiol.* 2003;13:245-251.
6. Chow WH, Gridley G, Fraumeni JF Jr, Jarvholm B. Obesity, hypertension, and the risk of kidney cancer in men. *N Engl J Med.* 2000;343:1305-1311.
7. Kamat AM, Shock RP, Naya Y, Rosser CJ, Slaton JW, Pisters LL. Prognostic value of body mass index in patients undergoing nephrectomy for localized renal tumors. *Urology.* 2004;63:46-50.
8. Zisman A, Pantuck AJ, Dorey F, et al. Improved prognostication of renal cell carcinoma using an integrated staging system. *J Clin Oncol.* 2001;19:1649-1657.
9. Eichelberg C, Junker K, Ljungberg B, Moch H. Diagnostic and prognostic molecular markers for renal cell carcinoma: a critical appraisal of the current state of research and clinical applicability. *Eur Urol.* 2009;55:851-863.
10. Maroto P, Rini B. Molecular biomarkers in advanced renal cell carcinoma. *Clin Cancer Res.* 2014;20:2060-2071.
11. The Cancer Genome Atlas Research Network. Comprehensive molecular characterization of clear cell renal cell carcinoma. *Nature.* 2013;499:43-49.
12. Gerlinger M, Rowan AJ, Horswell S, et al. Intratumor heterogeneity and branched evolution revealed by muliregion sequencing. *N Engl J Med.* 2012;366:883-892.
13. Motzer RJ, Mazumdar M, Bacik J, Berg W, Amsterdam A, Ferrara J. Survival and prognostic stratification of 670 patients with advanced renal cell carcinoma. *J Clin Oncol.* 1999;17:2530-2540.
14. Motzer RJ, Bacik J, Murphy BA, Russo P, Mazumdar M. Interferon-alfa as a comparative treatment for clinical trials of new therapies against advanced renal cell carcinoma. *J Clin Oncol.* 2002;20:289-296.
15. Heng D, Wanling X, Meredith M, et al. Prognostic factors for overall survival in patients with metastatic renal cell carcinoma treated with vascular endothelial growth factor-targeted agents: results from a large multicenter study. *J Clin Oncol.* 2009;27:5794-5799.
16. Heng DYC, Xie W, Regan MM, et al. External validation and comparison with other models of the International Metastatic Renal-Cell Carcinoma Database Consortium prognostic model: a population-based study. *Lancet Oncol.* 2013;14:141-148.
17. Motzer RJ, Bacik J, Mariani T, Russo P, Mazumdar M, Reuter V. Treatment outcome and survival associated with metastatic renal cell carcinoma of non-clear cell histology. *J Clin Oncol.* 2002;20:2376-2381.
18. Montero AJ, Diaz-Montero CM, Millikan RE, et al. Cytokines and angiogenic factors in patients with metastatic renal cell carcinoma treated with interferon-alpha: association of pretreatment serum levels with survival. *Ann Oncol.* 2009;20:1682-1687.
19. Zurita AJ, Jonasch E, Wu HK, Tran HT, Heymach JV. Circulating biomarkers for vascular endothelial growth factor inhibitors in renal cell carcinoma. *Cancer.* 2009;115:2346-2354.
20. Tran HT, Liu Y, Zurita AJ, et al. Prognostic or predictive plasma cytokines and angiogenic factors for patients treated with pazopanib for metastatic renal cell cancer: a retrospective analysis of phase 2 and phase 3 trials. *Lancet Oncol.* 2012;13:827-837.
21. Yao M, Yoshida M, Kishida T, et al. VHL tumor suppressor gene alterations associated with good prognosis in sporadic clear-cell renal carcinoma. *J Natl Cancer Inst.* 2002;94:1569-1575.
22. Kapur P, Pena-Llopis S, Christie A, et al. Effects on survival of BAP1 and PBRM1 mutations in sporadic clear-cell renal-cell carcinoma: a retrospective analysis with independent validation. *Lancet Oncol.* 2013;14:159-167.
23. Campbell SC, Novick AC, Belldegrun A, et al. Guideline for management of the clinical T1 renal mass. *J Urol.* 2009; 182:1271-1279.
24. Permpongkosol S, Bagga HS, Romero FR, Sroka M, Jarrett TW, Kavoussi LR. Laparoscopic versus open partial nephrectomy for the treatment of pathological T1N0M0 renal cell carcinoma: a 5-year survival rate. *J Urol.* 2006;176:1984-1988.
25. Kyllo RL, Tanagho YS, Kaouk JH, et al. Prospective multi-center study of oncologic outcomes of robot-assisted partial nephrectomy for pT1 renal cell carcinoma. *BMC Urol.* 2012;12:11.
26. Huang WC, Levey AS, Serio AM, et al. Chronic kidney disease after nephrectomy in patients with renal cortical tumours: a retrospective cohort study. *Lancet Oncol.* 2006;7:735-740.
27. Huang WC, Elkin EB, Levey AS, Jang TL, Russo P. Partial nephrectomy versus radical nephrectomy in patients with small renal tumors: is there a difference in mortality and cardiovascular outcomes? *J Urol.* 2009;181:55-62.
28. Benway BM, Bhayani SB, Rogers CG, et al. Robot assisted partial nephrectomy versus laparoscopic partial nephrectomy for renal tumors: a multi-institutional analysis of perioperative outcomes. *J Urol.* 2009;182:866-872.
29. Blom ML, van Poppel H, Marechal JM, et al. Radical nephrectomy with and without lymph-node dissection: final results of European Organization for Research and Treatment of Cancer (EORTC) randomized phase 3 trial 30881. *Eur Urol.* 2009;55:28-34.
30. O'Malley RL, Godoy G, Kanofsky JA, Taneja SS. The necessity of adrenalectomy at the time of radical nephrectomy: a systemic review. *J Urol.* 2009;181:2009-2017.
31. Mickisch GH, Garin A, van Poppel H, de Prijick L, Sylvester R. Radical nephrectomy plus interferon-alfa-based immunotherapy compared with interferon alfa alone in metastatic renal-cell carcinoma: a randomised trial. *Lancet.* 2001;358:966-970.
32. Flanigan RC, Salmon SE, Blumenstein BA, et al. Nephrectomy followed by interferon alfa-2b compared with interferon alfa-2b alone for metastatic renal-cell cancer. *N Engl J Med.* 2001;345:1655-1659.
33. Flanigan RC, Mickisch G, Sylvester R, Tangen C, Van Poppel H, Crawford ED. Cytoreductive nephrectomy in patients with metastatic renal cancer: a combined analysis. *J Urol.* 2004;171:1071-1076.
34. Heng DYC, Wells JC, Rini BI, et al. Cytoreductive nephrectomy in patients with synchronous metastases from renal cell carcinoma: results from the international metastatic renal cell carcinoma database consortium. *Eur Urol.* 2014;66:704-710.
35. Jonasch E, Wood CG, Matin SF, et al. Phase II presurgical

CHAPTER 35

feasibility study of bevacizumab in untreated patients with metastatic renal cell carcinoma. *J Clin Oncol*. 2009;27:4076-4081.
36. Chapin BF, Delacroix Jr SE, Culp SH, et al. Safety of presurgical targeted therapy in the setting of metastatic renal cell carcinoma. *Eur Urol*. 2011;60:964-971.
37. Karam JA, Rini BI, Varella L, et al. Metastasectomy after targeted therapy in patients with advanced renal cell carcinoma. *J Urol*. 2011;185:439-444.
38. Tannir NM, Cohen L, Wang X, et al. Improved tolerability and quality of life with maintained efficacy using twice-daily low-dose interferon-alpha-2b. *Cancer*. 2006;107:2254-2261.
39. McDermott DF, Regan MM, Clark JI, et al. Randomized phase III trial of high-dose interleukin-2 versus subcutaneous interleukin-2 and interferon in patients with metastatic renal cell carcinoma. *J Clin Oncol*. 2005;23:133-141.
40. Belldegrun AS, Klatte T, Shuch B, et al. Cancer-specific survival outcomes among patients treated during the cytoking era of kidney cancer (1989-2005). *Cancer*. 2008;113:2457-2463.
41. Klapper JA, Downey SG, Smith FO, et al. High-dose interleukin-2 for the treatment of metastatic renal cell carcinoma: a retrospective analysis of response and survival in patients treated in the surgery branch at the National Cancer Institute between 1986 and 2006. *Cancer*. 2008;113:293-301.
42. Escudier B, Pluzanska A, Koralewski P, et al. Bevacizumab plus interferon alfa-2a for treatment of metastatic renal cell carcinoma: a randomised, double-blind phase III trial. *Lancet*. 2007;370:2103-2111.
43. Rini BI, Halabi S, Rosenberg JE, et al. Bevacizumab plus interferon alfa compared with interferon alfa monotherapy in patients with metastatic renal cell carcinoma: CALGB 90206. *J Clin Oncol*. 2008;26:5422-5428.
44. Escudier B, Eisen T, Stadler WM, et al. Sorafenib in advanced clear-cell renal-cell carcinoma. *N Engl J Med*. 2007;356: 125-134.
45. Jonasch E, Corn P, Pagliaro LC, et al. Upfront, randomized, phase 2 trial of sorafenib versus sorafenib and low-dose interferon alfa in patients with advanced renal cell carcinoma: clinical and biomarker analysis. *Cancer*. 2010;116:57-65.
46. Motzer RJ, Michaelson MD, Redman BG, et al. Activity of SU11248, a multitargeted inhibitor of vascular endothelial growth factor receptor and platelet-derived growth factor receptor, in patients with metastatic renal cell carcinoma. *J Clin Oncol*. 2006;24:16-24.
47. Motzer RJ, Hutson TE, Tomczak P, et al. Sunitinib versus interferon alfa in metastatic renal cell carcinoma. *N Engl J Med*. 2007;356:115-124.
48. Motzer RJ, Hutson TE, Tomczak P, et al. Overall survival and updated results for sunitinib compared with inferferon alfa in patients with metastatic renal cell carcinoma. *J Clin Oncol*. 2009;27:3584-3590/
49. Harris PA, Boloor A, Cheung M, et al. Discovery of 5-[[4-[(2,3-dimethyl-2H-indazol-6-yl)methylamino]-2-pyrimidinyl]amino]-2-methyl-benzenesulfonamide(Pazopanib), a novel and potent vascular endothelial growth factor receptor inhibitor. *J Med Chem*. 2008;51:4632-4640.
50. Sternberg CN, Davis ID, Mardiak J, et al. Pazopanib in locally advanced or metastatic renal cell carcinoma: results of a randomized phase III trial. *J Clin Oncol*. 2010;28:1061-1068.
51. Matrana MR, Duran C, Shetty A, et al. Outcomes of patients with metastatic clear-cell renal cell carcinoma treated with pazopanib after disease progression with other targeted therapies. *Eur J Cancer*. 2013;49:169-175.
52. Hu-Lowe DD, Zou HY, Grazzini ML, et al. Nonclinical antiangiogenesis and antitumor activities of axitinib (AG-013736), an oral, potent, and selective inhibitor of vascular endothelial growth factor receptor tyrosine kinases 1,2,3. *Clin Cancer Res*. 2008;14:7272-7283.
53. Rini BI, Escudier B, Tomczak P, et al: Comparative effectiveness of axitinib versus sorafenib in advanced renal cell carcinoma (AXIS): a randomised phase 3 trial. *Lancet*. 2011;378:1931-1939.
54. Motzer RJ, Escudier B, Tomczak P, et al. Axitinib versus sorafenib as second-line treatment for advanced renal cell carcinoma: overall survival analysis and updated results from a randomised phase 3 trial. *Lancet Oncol*. 2013;14:552-562.
55. Hutson TE, Lesovoy V, Al-Shukri S, et al. Axitinib versus sorafenib as first-line therapy in patients with metastatic renal-cell carcinoma: a randomised open-label phase 3 trial. *Lancet Oncol*. 2013;14:1287-1294.
56. Atkins MB, Hidalgo M, Stadler WM, et al. Randomized phase II study of multiple dose levels of CCI-779, a novel mammalian target of rapamycin kinase inhibitor, in patients with advanced refractory renal cell carcinoma. *J Clin Oncol*. 2004;22:909-918.
57. Hudes G, Carducci M, Tomczak P, et al. Temsirolimus, interferon alfa, or both for advanced renal-cell carcinoma. *N Engl J Med*. 2007;356:2271-2281.
58. Armstrong AJ, George DJ, Halabi S. Serum lactate dehydrogenase predicts for overall survival benefit in patients with metastatic renal cell carcinoma treated with inhibition of mammalian target of rapamycin. *J Clin Oncol*. 2012;30:3402-3407.
59. Motzer RJ, Escudier B, Oudard S, et al. Efficacy of everolimus in advanced renal cell carcinoma: a double-blind, randomised, placebo-controlled phase III trial. *Lancet*. 2008;327:449-456.
60. Powles T, Oudard S, Ecudier BJ, et al. A randomized phase II study of GDC-0980 versus everolimus in metastatic renal cell carcinoma (mRCC) patients (pts) after VEGF-targeted therapy (VEGF-TT) [abstract]. *J Clin Oncol*. 2014;32:4525.
61. Brown RL. Tyrosine kinase inhibitor-induced hypothyroidism: incidence, etiology, and management. *Target Oncol*. 2011;6:217-226.
62. Rini BI, Tamaskar I, Shaheen P, et al. Hypothyroidism in patients with metastatic renal cell carcinoma treated with sunitinib. *J Natl Cancer Inst*. 2007;99:81-83.
63. Schmidinger M, Zielinski CC, Vogl UM, et al. Cardiac toxicity of sunitinib and sorafenib in patients with metastatic renal cell carcinoma. *J Clin Oncol*. 2008;26:5204-5212.
64. Hall PS, Harshman LC, Srinivas S, Witteles RM. The frequency and severity of cardiovascular toxicity from targeted therapy in advanced renal cell carcinoma patients. *J Am Coll Cardiol*. 2013;1:72-78.
65. Khakoo AY, Kassiotis CM, Tannir N, et al. Heart failure associated with sunitinib malate a multitargeted receptor tyrosine kinase inhibitor. *Cancer*. 2008;112:2500-2508.
66. Margulis V, Matin SF, Tannir N, et al. Surgical morbidity associated with administration of targeted molecular therapies before cytoreductive nephrectomy or resection of locally recurrent renal cell carcinoma. *J Urol*. 2008;180:94-98.
67. Motzer RJ, Hutson TE, Cella D, et al. Pazopanib versus sunitinib in metastatic renal-cell carcinoma. *N Engl J Med*. 2013;369:722-731.
68. Atkinson BJ, Kalra S, Wang X, et al. Clinical outcomes for patients with metastatic renal cell carcinoma treated with alternative sunitinib schedules. *J Urol*. 2014;191:611-618.
69. Naijar YG, Mittal K, Wood L, Garcia JA, Dreicer R, Rini BI. A 2 weeks on and 1 week off schedule of sunitinib is associated with decreased toxicity in metastatic renal cell carcinoma. *Eur J Cancer*. 2014;50:1084-1089.
70. Atkinson BJ, Cauley DH, Ng C, et al. Mammalian target of rapamycin (mTOR) inhibitor-associated non-infectious pneumonitis in patients with renal cell cancer: predictors, management, and outcomes. *BJU Int*. 2014;113:376-382.
71. Porta C, Osanto S, Ravaud A, et al. Management of adverse events associated with the use of everolimus in patients with advanced renal cell carcinoma. *Eur J Cancer*. 2011;47:1287-1298.
72. Hutson TE, Escudier B, Esteban E, et al. Randomized phase III

trial of temsirolimus versus sorafenib as second-line therapy after sunitinib in patients with metastatic renal cell carcinoma. *J Clin Oncol.* 2014;32:760-767.

73. Jonasch E, Signorovitch JE, Lin PL, et al. Treatment patterns in metastatic renal cell carcinoma: a retrospective review of medical records from US community oncology practices. *Curr Med Res Opin.* 2014;30:2041-2050.
74. Hainsworth JD, Rubin MS, Arrowsmith ER, Khatcheressian J, Crane EJ, Franco LA. Pazopanib as second-line treatment after sunitinib or bevacizumab in patients with advanced renal cell carcinoma: a Sarah Cannon Oncology Research Consortium Phase II trial. *Clin Genitourin Cancer.* 2013;11:270-275.
75. Rini BI, Bellmunt J, Clancy J, et al. Randomized phase III trial of temsirolimus and bevacizumab versus interferon alfa and bevacizumab in metastatic renal cell carcinoma: INTORACT Trial. *J Clin Oncol.* 2014;32:752-759.
76. Yang Y, Hughes M, Kammula U, et al. Ipilimumab (Anti-CTLA-4 Antibody) causes regression of metastatic renal cell cancer associated with enteritis and hypophysitis. *J Immunother.* 2007;30:825-830.
77. Motzer RJ, Rini BI, McDermott DF, et al. Nivolumab for metastatic renal cell carcinoma (mRCC): Results of a randomized, dose-ranging phase II trial [abstract]. *J Clin Oncol.* 2014;32:5009.
78. Cho D, Sosman JA, Sznol M, et al. Clinical activity, safety, and biomarkers of MPDL3280A, an engineered PD-L1 antibody in patients with metastatic renal cell carcinoma (mRCC) [abstract]. *J Clin Oncol.* 2013;31:4505.
79. Hammers HJ, Plimack ER, Infante JR, et al. Phase I study of nivolumab in combination with ipilimumab in metastatic renal cell carcinoma (mRCC) [abstract]. *J Clin Oncol.* 2014;32:4504.
80. Johnson BF, Clay TM, Hobeika AC, Lyerly HK, Morse MA. Vascular endothelial growth factor and immunosuppression in cancer: current knowledge and potential for new therapy. *Exp Opin Biol Ther.* 2007;7:449-460.
81. Dutcher JP, de Souza P, McDermott D, et al. Effect of temsirolimus versus interferon-alpha on outcome of patients with advanced renal cell carcinoma of different tumor histologies. *Med Oncol.* 2009;26:202-209.
82. Tannir NM, Plimack E, Ng C, et al. A phase 2 trial of sunitinib in patients with advanced non-clear cell renal cell carcinoma. *Eur Urol.* 2012;62:1013-1019.
83. Tannir NM, Jonasch E, Altinmakas E, et al. Everolimus versus sunitinib prospective evaluation in metastatic non-clear cell renal cell carcinoma (The ESPN Trial): a multicenter randomized phase 2 trial [abstract]. *J Clin Oncol.* 2014;32:4505.
84. Choueiri TK, Vaishampayan U, Rosenberg JE, et al. Phase II and biomarker study of the dual MET/VEGFR2 inhibitor foretinib in patients with papillary renal cell carcinoma. *J Clin Oncol.* 2013;31:181-186.
85. Gordon MS, Hussey M, Nagle RB, et al. Phase II study of erlotinib in patients with locally advanced or metastatic papillary histology renal cell cancer: SWOG S0317. *J Clin Oncol.* 2009;27:5788-5793.
86. Cheville JC, Lohse CM, Zincke H, et al. Sarcomatoid renal cell carcinoma: an examination of underlying histologic subtype and an analysis of associations with patient outcome. *Am J Surg Pathol.* 2004;28:435-441.
87. Mian BM, Bhadkamkar N, Slaton JW, et al. Prognostic factors and survival of patients with sarcomatoid renal cell carcinoma. *J Urol.* 2002;167:65-70.
88. Golshayan AR, George S, Heng DY, et al. Metastatic sarcomatoid renal cell carcinoma treated with vascular endothelial growth factor-targeted therapy. *J Clin Oncol.* 2009;27:235-241.
89. Peyromaure M, Thiounn N, Scotte F, Vieillefond A, Debre B, Oudard S. Collecting duct carcinoma of the kidney: a clinicopathological study of 9 cases. *J Urol.* 2003;170:1138-1140.
90. Cheville JC, Lohse CM, Zincke H, Weaver AL, Blute ML. Comparisons of outcome and prognostic features among histologic subtypes of renal cell carcinoma. *Am J Surg Pathol.* 2003;27:612-624.
91. Gollob A, Upton MP, DeWolf WC, Atkins MB. Long-term remission in a patient with metastatic collecting duct carcinoma treated with taxol/carboplatin and surgery. *Urology.* 2001;58:1058.
92. Davis CJ Jr, Mostofi FK, Sesterhenn IA. Renal medullary carcinoma. The seventh sickle cell nephropathy. *Am J Surg Pathol.* 1995;19:1-11.
93. Avery RA, Harris JE, Davis CJ Jr, Borgaonkar DS, Byrd JC, Weiss RB. Renal medullary carcinoma: clinical and therapeutic aspects of a newly described tumor. *Cancer.* 1996;78:128-132.
94. Tannir NM, Dbuauskas Z, Bekele BN, et al. Outcome of patients (pts) with renal medullary carcinoma (RMC) treated in the era of targeted therapies (TT): a multicenter experience [abstract]. *J Clin Oncol.* 2011;29:386.
95. Shah AY, Karam JA, Rao P, et al. Management and outcomes of patients with renal medullary carcinoma (RMC): a multicenter retrospective study of 39 patients [abstract]. *J Clin Oncol.* 2015;33:438.
96. Argani P, Olgac S, Tickoo SK, et al. Xp11 translocation renal cell carcinoma in adults: exanded clinical, pathologic, and genetic spectrum. *Am J Surg Pathol.* 2007;31:1149-1160.
97. Malouf GG, Monzon FA, Couturier J, et al. Genomic heterogeneity of translocation renal cell carcinoma. *Clin Cancer Res.* 2013;19:4673-4684.
98. Rao Q, Williamson SR, Zhang S, et al. TFE3 break-apart FISH has a higher sensitivity for XP11.2 translocation-associated renal cell carcinoma compared with TFE3 or cathepsin K immunohistochemical staining alone: expanding the morphologic spectrum. *Am J Surg Pathol.* 2013;37:804-815.
99. Argani P, Lal P, Hutchinson B, Lui MY, Reuter VE, Ladanyi M. Aberrant nuclear immunoreactivity for TFE3 in neoplasms with TFE3 gene fusions: a sensitive and specific immunohistochemical assay. *Am J Surg Pathol.* 2003;27:750-761.
100. Choueiri TK, Dubauskas Z, Hirsch MS, et al. Vascular endothelial growth factor-targeted therapy for the treatment of adult metastatic Xp11.2 translocation renal cell carcinoma. *Cancer.* 2010;116:5219-5225.
101. Malouf GC, Camparo P, Oudard S, et al. Targeted agents in metastatic Xp11 translocation/TFE3 gene fusion renal cell carcinoma (RCC): a report from the Juvenile RCC Network. *Ann Oncol.* 2010;21:1834-1838.

CHAPTER 35

36 Bladder Cancer

第三十六章　膀胱癌

Arlene O. Siefker-Radtke
Bogdan A. Czerniak
Colin P.N. Dinney
Commentary: David J. McConkey

中文导读

自20世纪80年代以来，尿路上皮癌的药物治疗一直处于平台期，局限于以顺铂为基础的化疗。直至近些年，一些新兴药物，如免疫检查点抑制剂、成纤维生长因子受体抑制剂、血管内皮生长因子抑制剂等的相继出现，使得人们对尿路上皮癌的生物学行为有了全新的认识。本章首先介绍了膀胱癌的流行病学，并从分子层面阐述了发病机制。接着介绍了肿瘤生物学行为，包括尿路上皮癌的发生发展、新兴药物如免疫检查点抑制剂和成纤维细胞生长因子受体（FGFR）抑制剂等的研发现状以及组织学类型。随后本章从临床角度阐述了膀胱癌的诊断及分期要点、影响预后的危险因素分层。本章重点介绍了膀胱癌的临床处理原则，针对不同分期的肿瘤，包括表浅型、微浸润型、局部进展型（可切除及不可切除）以及伴有远处转移的膀胱癌，采取不同的治疗措施。本章最后介绍了尿路上皮癌的系统性药物治疗，阐述了从传统的化疗向新兴的分子靶向和免疫治疗的变更过程。在展望中，指出目前有更多的药物用于尿路上皮癌的临床研究，期待尿路上皮癌的治疗真正进入个体化治疗的时代。

Expectant optimism is now pervading the field of urothelial cancer as we anticipate that we will soon be soaring above the plateaus established with cisplatin-based chemotherapy in the 1980s and finally have new agents approved for the treatment of urothelial carcinoma. Immune checkpoint inhibitors, which are transforming the field of oncology, are showing evidence of clinical activity in early clinical trials in this disease ([1]). In addition, there are several ongoing trials of targeted agents including fibroblast growth factor (FGF) receptor inhibitors and vascular endothelial growth factor (VEGF) inhibitors currently in clinical trials with the goal of obtaining US Food and Drug Administration (FDA) approval. Our fundamental understanding of the biology of urothelial cancer is changing as well, with molecular characterization suggesting that urothelial cancer is no longer only one disease ([2]). These nascent technologies suggest we will soon be able to personalize therapy for urothelial cancer and reliably predict which patients will benefit from specific chemotherapy and/or other targeted agents, transforming our current treatment of urothelial cancer.

OVERVIEW

The urinary tract conveys urine from the confluence of urinary tubules in the renal papillae to the outside world. This entire path is lined by a specialized epithelial surface known as the urothelium, which is composed primarily of transitional cells, and extends from the renal pelvis through the ureters, bladder, and urethra. In males, it also lines the terminal prostatic ducts and prostatic urethra. Although tumors arising from the urothelium can involve any organ along this path, about 90% of these cancers arise in the urinary bladder.

EPIDEMIOLOGY

Urothelial cancer is the fifth most common cancer diagnosis in the United States and is strikingly related to cigarette smoking. In 2015, about 80,000 new cases were expected, with about 74,000 arising in the bladder. Altogether, these cases account for just over 18,000 deaths ([3]). These incidence figures are somewhat misleading, however, because it is a historical anomaly that only in the bladder are histologically bland hyperplastic lesions counted as cancers. In other sites, such lesions would be counted as benign or at most premalignant, and thus the incidence figures include many patients with lesions that do not meet the conventional definition of malignancy. Imagine what the incidence figures for colon cancer would be if every patient with a polyp was counted as a case of colon cancer! Many such lesions recur; however, few progress to true malignancy. Thus, it is critically important to separate risk models that are designed to predict recurrence from those that predict progression, which is far more biologically significant. Because of this anomaly of classification, the literature on "risk of bladder cancer," both for incidence and recurrence, must be interpreted very carefully.

In contrast to most other carcinomas, the majority of patients with urothelial cancer (even after excluding the low-grade papillary "cancers") have early-stage, potentially curable disease at presentation. Only about 20% of patients present with disease that invades into the muscle wall. Fewer than 5% of patients present with locally advanced (ie, clinically extravesical) disease, and another 5% or so present with clinically apparent metastatic disease. Once clinically metastatic, urothelial cancer is remarkably aggressive, exhibiting a natural history reminiscent of small cell carcinoma of the lungs: untreated, the survival is measured in weeks; it is markedly chemotherapy sensitive; responses are typically short lived; the brain is a typical "sanctuary" site of relapse after response to initial therapy; and cure of patients with distant metastases, although well documented, remains anecdotal.

The ready accessibility of urine and the fact that the urothelium itself can be accessed via minimally invasive cystoscopy makes urothelial cancer an important context for understanding the processes of carcinogenesis and clonal evolution and an important platform for the development of human gene therapy.

The current state of the art is rather sobering:

- Careful patient selection has made it possible for some patients to have organ preservation, but this strategy clearly results in some patients dying unnecessarily.
- Although the combination of chemotherapy and surgery does improve the cure fraction for patients with locally advanced disease, a disturbing fraction (30%-40% even at referral centers) of patients with invasive disease but no detectable involvement beyond the bladder at the time of diagnosis still succumb to the disease.
- There have been no substantive advances in systemic treatment since the introduction of methotrexate, vinblastine, doxorubicin, and cisplatin (M-VAC) in the early 1980s, and indeed, reported outcomes for patients with metastatic urothelial cancer are getting worse as marginally effective systemic therapies (such as gemcitabine and carboplatin) are now widely used.

However, there is optimism for the following reasons:

- Recent developments in immunology with checkpoint inhibitors suggest their utility in urothelial cancer.
- The molecular characterization of urothelial cancer may help us choose which patients are most likely to benefit from a specific therapy, leading to a personalized approach to care.

CLASSICAL EPIDEMIOLOGY

Malignant transformation of the urothelium parallels observations with other epithelial tumors ([4]), in that it is distinctly uncommon before age 40 and has a peak incidence in the seventh decade. The male-to-female ratio is about 3:1, reflecting, in part, differences in exposure to smoking and industrial toxins. Malignant transformation is the result of a multistep process in which multiple genes are implicated. The appearance of clinical cancer typically follows carcinogenic exposure by decades. Fluid intake is inversely associated with risk ([5]), supporting the concept that contact time of excreted carcinogens with the urothelial surface contributes to carcinogenesis.

There is a striking correlation of urothelial cancer incidence with exposure to certain environmental toxins. About half of all cases are related to smoking. Industrial exposures, especially to petrochemicals, account for another 10% to 15%. Many occupations with "chemical" exposures have been linked to an excess risk of urothelial cancer. An association with aniline dye exposure was noted more than a century ago, and many aromatic amines (prototypically β-naphthyl amine) have now been shown to be potent urothelial carcinogens. Cigarette smoke is rich in both aromatic amines and the highly reactive bladder toxin acrolein. Another source of acrolein, which is strongly linked to urothelial carcinogenesis, is the metabolism of cyclophosphamide and ifosfamide. In one report, prolonged exposure to oral cyclophosphamide (as was a common intervention for some forms of cancer and for autoimmune disease in the 1970s) increased the risk of bladder cancer by a factor of nine ([6]). Also noteworthy are exposures to the analgesic phenacetin and to the plant toxin–related "Balkan nephropathy" in which the risk of upper tract tumors is increased ([7, 8]).

As is generally true for epithelial carcinogenesis, chronic irritation and inflammation have also been associated with malignant transformation. This is seen prototypically in settings such as staghorn calculus and other cases of chronic urolithiasis, chronic bladder catheterization (a particularly distressing complication of spinal cord injury ([9]) or congenital malformations), and classically, chronic schistosomiasis in the Middle East. Urothelial cancers that arise in the context of chronic irritation typically show squamous differentiation.

Molecular Epidemiology

Assessment of genomic variations, as well as functional assessment of certain metabolic pathways, is now routinely integrated with classical aspects of cancer risk assessment. As might have been anticipated from the classical epidemiologic studies of environmental exposures, it has now been confirmed that polymorphisms of various genes involved in xenobiotic metabolism are correlated with the risk of developing bladder cancer. However, these pathways are complex, and the impact of genetic changes is of course context dependent. A classic example of this is provided by *N*-acetyltransferase 2 (NAT-2)–mediated *N*-acetylation, which constitutes a detoxification step for some carcinogens but can be an activation step for others ([10, 11]). A meta-analysis suggests a possible role for some of these variants in risk of bladder cancer and clearly demonstrates an interaction with smoking status ([12]), as would be expected on the hypothesis that these genes are important for the response to smoking-induced DNA damage ([13]).

Telomere length, which also contributes to the maintenance of genetic integrity, may also be relevant to urothelial carcinogenesis because patients with bladder cancer have been found to have shortened telomeres or telomerase abnormalities ([14, 15]).

TUMOR BIOLOGY

Carcinogenesis

A dual track concept has been proposed in urothelial cancer carcinogenesis (Fig. 36-1) ([16]). The majority of urothelial cancers, approximately 80% to 85%, arise from a hyperplastic epithelium and most commonly present as low-grade papillary tumors. Although these tumors tend to recur, they are much less likely to evolve into a more aggressive form of urothelial cancer. Earlier studies suggested that preservation of E-cadherin expression is classic in these tumors and associated with a low risk of recurrence ([17]), with additional studies suggesting that ratios of E-cadherin to matrix metalloproteinase-9, which is a surrogate for epithelial to mesenchymal transformation (EMT), are inversely correlated with outcome ([18, 19]). Additional proliferative drivers including FGF receptor (FGFR)-3 have been observed in a much higher frequency in these superficial papillary urothelial cancers of low malignant potential ([20]).

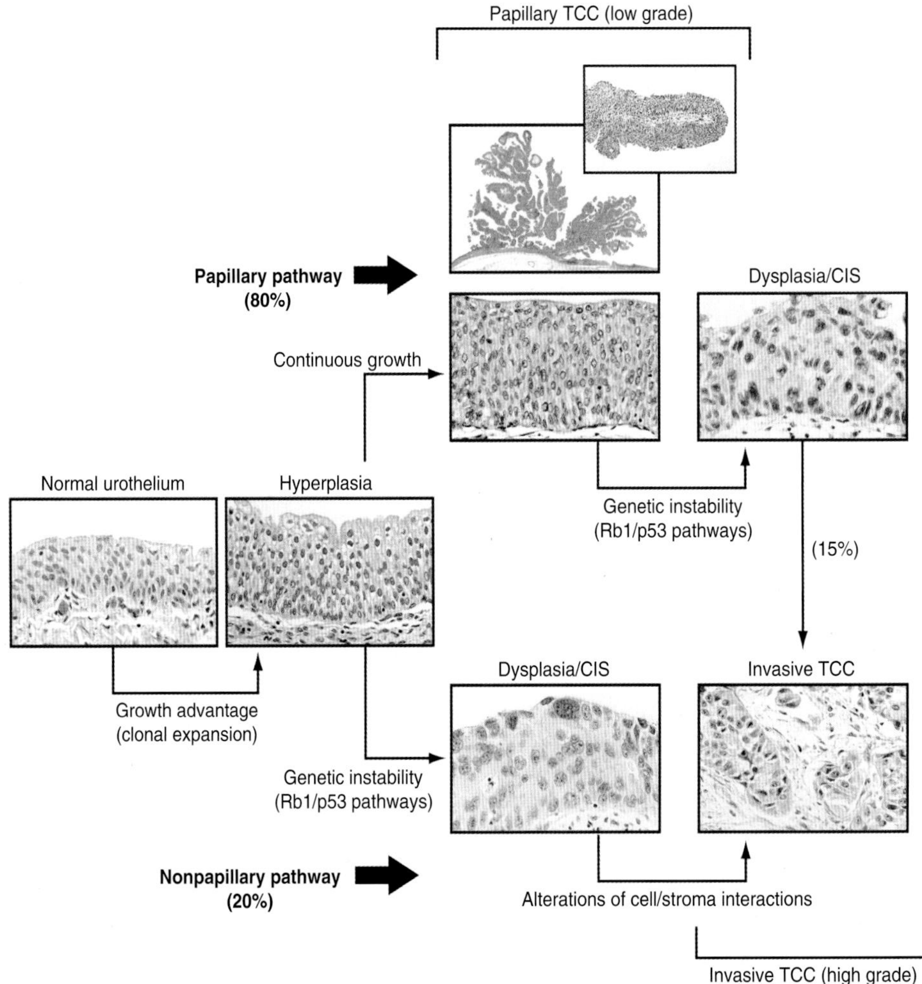

FIGURE 36-1 Dual track pathway of urothelial cancer. CIS, carcinoma in situ; TCC, transitional cell carcinoma. (Reproduced with permission from Dinney CP, McConkey DJ, Millikan RE, et al: Focus on bladder cancer, *Cancer Cell* 2004 Aug;6(2):111-116.)

Because the bladder is readily accessible, with most patients presenting before life-threatening progression is apparent, bladder cancer is well suited for studying the details of the molecular pathogenesis of transformation, invasion, and metastasis. Molecular genetics investigations have revealed that numerous loci are lost and have confirmed that clonal expansion is an early event; that is, morphologically normal urothelium in bladders harboring urothelial tumors is genetically altered, and multifocal disease generally represents multifocal expansion of a preexisting clonal lesion ([21]). Thus, the classical notion of "field carcinogenesis" is amply confirmed by these molecular genetic studies. These studies demonstrate that early carcinogenesis involves relatively few key loci that provide the fertile context for more generalized chromosomal instability that is apparent in grossly established invasive tumors.

Following along the dual track concept of bladder carcinogenesis, the nonpapillary pathway is associated with early genetic instability (see Fig. 36-1). These flat, infiltrative tumors typically behave more aggressively and invade the muscularis propria with a much higher probability of impacting survival. Loss of the retinoblastoma gene (*RB*) or any inactivation of *RB* function is clearly associated with an adverse prognosis in these tumors ([22]). The *p53* gene is also frequently mutated in these tumors ([23]) and appears to interact with *RB* ([24]). Abnormal p53 immunohistochemical staining is highly correlated with a nonfunctional mutation associated adverse prognosis ([25]).

Tumors from the nonpapillary pathway typically have mesenchymal features associated with their invasive nature. However, recent studies suggest that the EMT concept is indeed more complex as some epithelial markers, including TP63 expression, have been associated with adverse outcome in the setting of invasive disease ([26, 27]). TP63 expression has been noted to be at high levels within the basal layer of the urothelium, which typically contains the stem cell compartments. In addition, most p63 isoforms are felt to act as dominant negatives, potentially suppressing p53-dependent transactivation ([28]). Recent studies using gene expression profiling continue to suggest a strong role for p63 controlling basal gene expression in these lethal basal tumors ([2]).

Recently, three distinct subtypes of urothelial cancer have been identified using gene expression profiling (GEP) (Fig. 36-2) ([2, 29]). Basal urothelial carcinomas, which have immunohistochemical markers associated with the basal layer, are often characterized by TP63 activation and rapid proliferation with more aggressive disease and may be prognostic for poor outcomes. The angiogenic signature is expressed in the basal subtype. Luminal urothelial carcinomas, which share immunohistochemical markers associated with the umbrella cell layer, show evidence of PPARγ activation. Enrichment of *FGFR3* mutations has been noted in this group of tumors. A third group of p53-like urothelial cancers show a high degree of resistance to typical chemotherapy agents and are associated with a stromal infiltrate. A recent series of patient treated on clinical trial suggests a high incidence of bone metastasis in this subtype (in press, Evr. Urol.). Furthermore, data from this clinical trial suggest that clinical outcomes are improved when the basal subtype tumors are treated with neoadjuvant chemotherapy, suggesting this is a potential predictive marker for clinical outcomes. Therefore, subtyping strategies may aid in the development of personalized treatment for urothelial cancer and appropriate selection of patients for systemic chemotherapy and specific targeting agents.

Novel Therapeutic Targets

The use of immune checkpoint inhibitors appears to be transforming the world of cancer, including the field of urothelial cancer. Early results from clinical trials suggest that response rates with programmed cell death (PD)-1 inhibitors maybe as high as 20% to 40% ([1]). Combined checkpoint inhibition using PD1 inhibitors in combination with cytotoxic T lymphocyte-associated antigen 4 (CTLA4) antibodies potentially may yield improved responses, although trials are still accruing in this group of patients. Expression of PD ligand 1 (PDL1) either on the tumor cell or on the lymphocyte infiltrate has been proposed as one method of determining which patients are most likely respond to checkpoint inhibition. Because the response rates in PDL1 negative disease maybe anywhere from 15% to 20% and PDL1 expression is dynamic and may be influenced by chemotherapy and intravesical agents including bacillus Calmette-Guérin (BCG), the clinical utility of this biomarker remains problematic. Approval of a checkpoint inhibitor in the treatment of urothelial cancer is an event that is highly anticipated and will likely be the first novel agent approved for urothelial cancer in more than 20 years.

The FGFR inhibitors are also showing promise, with early phase I studies suggesting response rates as high as 40% to 50% in patients with *FGFR3* mutations or translocations. Although FGFR mutations and translocations are predicted to occur in less than 20% of muscle-invasive bladder cancers, approvals of such agents may also play a role in earlier stage disease where the presence of these mutations maybe as high as 50%. Trials are currently accruing in the second-line setting in hopes of obtaining FDA approval.

Angiogenesis inhibitors still remain of interest in the treatment of urothelial cancer. Early studies suggested that overexpression of VEGF was associated with adverse outcomes and poor prognosis in patients treated with neoadjuvant chemotherapy ([18]). One mouse model suggested that these effects could be enhanced when angiogenesis inhibitors are combined with taxanes ([30]). Preliminary results of a randomized phase II trial of docetaxel plus or minus the VEGF inhibitor ramucirumab suggested an improvement in progression-free survival for the combination as a second-line therapy for metastatic urothelial carcinoma ([31]). A frontline trial of gemcitabine with cisplatin plus or minus bevacizumab is still completing accrual. Phase II results were promising, with an objective response rate of 72% and a median overall survival (OS) of 19.1 months ([32]). In the neoadjuvant setting, a trial of dose-dense M-VAC) with bevacizumab showed pT0N0 rates of 39%, with 5-year OS and disease-specific survival rates of 63% and 64%, respectively ([33]). Using GEP to molecularly characterize the tumors from this trial. we found that the 5-year survival for the basal subtype was 91% (in press, Evr. Urol.). Because the angiogenic signature is enriched in the basal subtype, one would hypothesize that to promote personalized medicine in urothelial cancer, future studies should focus on enrichment of basal tumors on clinical trials of antiangiogenic therapies.

Histology

In the United States, approximately 90% of all urothelial malignancies are within the histologic spectrum of transitional cell carcinoma (TCC), which, in our view, merges without obvious demarcation with the sarcomatoid and small cell variants at the extreme of dedifferentiation. Most of the remainder exhibit squamous histology (especially prominent in the more distal urethra) or glandular differentiation (ie, adenocarcinoma). The finding of adenocarcinoma apart from the context of bladder exstrophy or a urachal tumor (see below) should prompt consideration of metastatic disease from some other primary site because bona fide

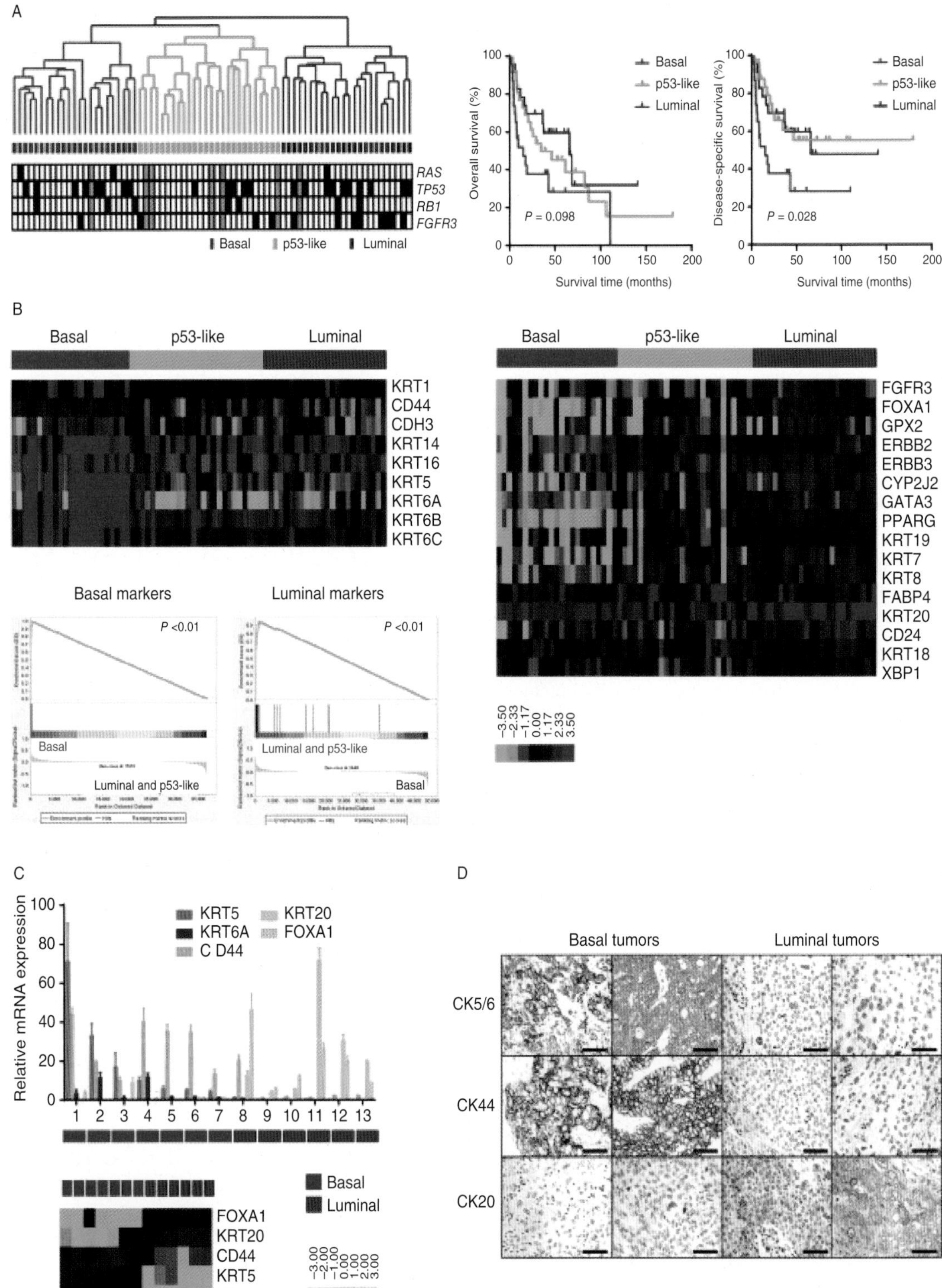

FIGURE 36-2 Molecular characterization of bladder cancer suggesting three intrinsic subtypes: basal, luminal, and p53-like. (Reproduced with permission from Choi W, Porten S, Kim S, et al: Identification of distinct basal and luminal subtypes of muscle-invasive bladder cancer with different sensitivities to frontline chemotherapy, *Cancer Cell* 2014 Feb 10;25(2):152-165.)

primary adenocarcinomas originating from the urothelium are distinctly uncommon.

As noted earlier, primarily hyperplastic lesions, biologically akin to polyps in the gastrointestinal tract, account for a large portion of incident cases. In 1999, the World Health Organization (WHO) put forward a new classification of noninvasive papillary urothelial tumors in recognition of the fact that the malignant potential of these lesions varies widely ([34]). The WHO terminology for these lesions, which together account for more than half of all new cases of urothelial neoplasia, is as follows:

Papillary urothelial neoplasm of low malignant potential. This lesion is characterized by orderly progression of morphology within the urothelium and no cellular atypia. Recurrence is seen in about 25% of cases, but progression is rare.

Noninvasive papillary urothelial carcinoma, low grade. This lesion shows some architectural variation and mild atypia. Such lesions commonly recur (in 50% or more of cases), but progression is seen in only 5% to 10%. It is classified by the WHO as a borderline tumor.

Noninvasive papillary urothelial carcinoma, high grade. This lesion shows predominantly disorganized architecture and moderate to marked cytologic atypia. Such lesions do not invade below the basement membrane, but they have substantial biologic potential, with progression to invasive, potentially life-threatening disease in up to 65% of cases. These are classified by the WHO as malignant. Note that in the WHO system, grades are collapsed to a two-tier system of low grade and high grade. In general, this would map to the older three-tier system as follows: grade 1 = low grade and grades 2 and 3 = high grade.

In contrast to these papillary cancers, some urothelial cancers exhibit dysplasia and chromosomal instability early on and constitute a "second pathway" of carcinogenesis ([16, 35, 36]), and most of the cases with lethal potential are in this class (see Fig. 36-1). In contrast to the classic "mulberry" appearance, the nonpapillary lesions have a grossly flat or infiltrative appearance at cystoscopy. In older literature, such cancers have been known as *flat, sessile, solid,* or *tentacular.* Currently, the preferred nomenclature is simply *nonpapillary,* although *flat* persists in the American Joint Committee on Cancer (AJCC) *Cancer Staging Manual* (seventh edition). These morphologic differences were noted long before an understanding of the genetic changes associated with cancer was appreciated. As expected for such distinct phenotypes, the characteristic genetic lesions have been found to be distinct.

In addition to papillary and nonpapillary variants, a *micropapillary* pattern is increasingly recognized ([37-40]). The term *micropapillary* originally came from the recognition of morphologic resemblance to an aggressive variant of ovarian cancer. Indeed, this general histologic pattern has been reported in many epithelial malignancies and invariably identifies a more aggressive subset, as was first reported for bladder cancer in 1994. Thus, the biologic potential of urothelial neoplasia extends from relatively nonthreatening in papillary lesions, to potentially life-threatening in nonpapillary lesions, to remarkably aggressive micropapillary lesions, all of which are recognizable as TCC.

Depending on the series, about 30% (or more) of muscle-invasive urothelial cancers are found to have focal areas of squamous or glandular morphology when examined in detail. It is not clear that such "mixed" tumors have a different prognosis than "pure" TCC, and we do not consider this a meaningful subset at University of Texas MD Anderson Cancer Center (MDACC). Certainly, tumors with only focal areas of squamous or glandular differentiation do not exhibit the distinctive natural history of pure squamous cancers or pure adenocarcinomas. Primary nonepithelial cancers (eg, sarcomas, lymphomas, melanomas) are exceedingly uncommon in the bladder. When they do occur, they do not appear to have a distinctive natural history or clinical management from what would be expected of similar tumors arising in more typical sites.

Urothelial cancers can dedifferentiate to include spindled ("sarcomatoid"), small cell, and plasmacytoid variants. In these cases, the clinical expression of the overall disease process is dominated by the aggressive component, even if most of the primary cancer is well within the typical morphologic spectrum of TCC.

Small cell carcinoma of the urothelium is a remarkably aggressive malignancy and exhibits a similar propensity for spread to the brain as small cell carcinoma arising in other sites. Even in the setting of clinically localized disease, the prognosis with local therapy alone remains poor, reflecting the early development of micrometastases. We strongly favor management of patients with cT2 or lower disease that is based on neoadjuvant chemotherapy, followed by surgical consolidation ([41, 42]). In our hands, this provides about 70% cure ([42, 43]). Patients with locally advanced disease have a high incidence (8 of 16 patients in our series) of relapse in the brain ([43]), and thus, we feel these patients are candidates for prophylactic cranial irradiation. Patients with metastatic disease at presentation continue to have nearly a 100% response rate, with a 100% relapse rate and a median survival of only 11 months ([43]).

Plasmacytoid urothelial cancer is a rare histology with limited series reported to date ([44]). These tumors typically appear mesenchymal with downregulation of E-cadherin ([45, 46]) and consist of poorly cohesive tumor cells with perinuclear clearing reminiscent of plasma cells ([46, 47]). They also tend to be highly proliferative with abundant mitosis and staining for Ki-67. These tumors tend to have a unique spread pattern, often appearing as a linitis plastica with diffuse thickening of the bladder and rectum. Although plasmacytoid tumors appear to be sensitive to chemotherapy, even in the neoadjuvant setting with adequate downstaging to pathologic T0 disease, there are few long-term survivors ([44]). These tumors have also been shown to have a high incidence of recurrence in the peritoneum (>50% of patients) ([44]).

Cancers arising in a urachal remnant, although not strictly "bladder cancers" in the sense of this chapter, merit a comment. These cancers typically involve the dome of the bladder and histologically are enteric-type adenocarcinomas. They are thought to reflect malignant transformation of an enteric epithelial rest within the urachal remnant, producing a cancer readily recognized as a mucinous adenocarcinoma ([48]). An early MDACC series suggested that the risk of relapse was increased when an en bloc resection was not performed and in the setting of positive margins, lymph node involvement, and tumor involving the peritoneal surface ([49]). The Memorial Sloan-Kettering Cancer Center experience in 50 patients demonstrated long-term survival in 26 (93%) of 28 patients with pathologically localized disease, in 9 (69%) of 13 patients with extension through the bladder or urachal cavity, and in none of 9 patients with peritoneal involvement initially ([50]). Similarly, the Mayo Clinic experience ([51]) in 49 patients demonstrated apparent cure in the majority of patients with confined disease and relapse in the majority of patients with nonconfined disease, with the latter group having a median survival of only 16 months ([52]). All investigators have emphasized the importance of an attempt at margin-negative, en bloc resection if at all possible.

Urachal cancers have a tendency to recur locally, often with peritoneal carcinomatosis, and the typical metastatic sites are (about equally) the lungs and liver. Although dramatic responses are infrequent, the use of modern combination regimens with activity in enteric adenocarcinoma is associated with about a 40% objective response rate. Thus, in essentially every clinical respect, urachal cancer behaves like colon cancer and, based on the available data, should be treated accordingly. Median survival from the recognition of metastases was 24 months in our retrospective series of 26 patients with metastatic disease, although some patients with grossly metastatic disease have been long-term survivors ([49]).

DIAGNOSIS, STAGING, AND PROGNOSIS

Presentation

About 80% of patients present with hematuria, usually painless. The "typical" patient is a smoker in his late 60s. Such patients frequently suffer from pulmonary disease and cardiovascular disease, magnifying the morbidity of both chemotherapy and surgery. They are also at high risk for other smoking-related malignancies. A high percentage of patients have diminished renal function as a result of hypertension and obstructive nephropathy. Thus, the use of nephrotoxic chemotherapy is especially challenging in this population. Hospitalization and meticulous attention to detail are typically required to safely deliver multiple cycles of cisplatin- or ifosfamide-based therapy.

Irritative voiding symptoms, including frequency, dysuria, and dribbling, are important points in the medical history because the presence of irritative symptoms raises the possibility of extensive carcinoma in situ (CIS) or large, infiltrative tumors that may be far more extensive than is revealed by the initial cystoscopy. Obstructive symptoms (nocturia, double voiding, overflow incontinence, low anterior abdominal pain) are often encountered from tumors of the bladder neck or prostatic urethra. Tumors in these locations are far less likely to be anatomically confined (ie, curable with surgery) than are similarly muscle-invasive bladder cancers that are well away from these areas where the detrusor muscle is discontinuous.

In evaluating patients presenting with hematuria, it is mandatory to evaluate the upper urinary tracts. Even if a bladder tumor is confirmed on initial cystoscopy, excretory urography is still appropriate because synchronous or metachronous tumors of the upper tracts typically are not associated with specific symptoms.

Recently, several urine tests for cancer-associated antigens have been promulgated for diagnosis. None of these tests is yet sensitive and specific enough to replace cystoscopy and biopsy. The role of these tests for widespread screening is also not defined. Likewise, the role of urine cytology in initial diagnosis is unsettled. The yield is highly dependent on sample collection technique and the skill of the cytopathologist. As with many epithelial cancers, it is likely that DNA-based tests will eventually be widely used to find pathognomonic genetic alterations in urine and thus revolutionize the detection and clinical follow-up of bladder cancer. The role of some form of surveillance in high-risk populations (such as petrochemical workers) remains controversial. The relatively low positive and negative predictive value of cytology, even when applied to a high-risk group, makes such screening difficult to justify.

Stage and Prognostic Classification

Excepting the extremes of histology (eg, small cell), the dominant prognostic clinical variable is anatomic stage at diagnosis. Classically, this is defined by depth of invasion. The currently used staging system is summarized in Fig. 36-3. This system is, of course, historically rooted in pathologic findings related to cystectomy specimens. As a result, it is not well suited for *clinical* staging. For example, the distinction between deep muscle invasion (T2b) and more superficial muscle invasion (T2a) cannot be reliably made by cystoscopic biopsy, and indeed the differentiation of muscle fibers in the lamina propria from muscularis propria (ie, the distinction between deep cT1 and cT2) is often problematic. As with most solid tumors, one must be extraordinarily careful regarding staging information, especially when comparing surgical and radiotherapy series, which necessarily rely on different primary information.

Unfortunately the AJCC staging system does not account for available information about tumor biology. Although "staging" has come to be understood as "prognostic assessment" for most cancers, urologic oncology lags behind in laying aside the historical notion of stage as essentially an anatomic concept. As noted earlier, the biology of papillary cancers is fundamentally different from that of nonpapillary cancers. Other biologic characteristics such as location of tumor within the bladder, the presence or absence of lymphovascular invasion, and the presence or absence of specific markers are known to influence prognosis, and thus, there is a significant need to fully evaluate and standardize how such features are reported.

A suggested refinement to the currently dominant AJCC system relates to the subdivision of cT1. Several ways of doing this have been suggested, including measuring the depth of invasion (with a break point at 1.5 mm) or determining whether muscle fibers consistent with muscularis mucosa are invaded (T1b) or not (T1a). Although many subspecialty pathologists have found such a subdivision to be strongly prognostic ([53]), it is not yet widely reported, and there are questions about both intra- and interobserver variability ([54, 55]). We tend to think of the commonly reported "extensive involvement" of lamina propria as a useful way of identifying higher risk cT1 disease. What is clear is that there is significant variability of prognosis among patients with cT1 disease, and better ways of refining this group remain a worthy goal for clinical investigators.

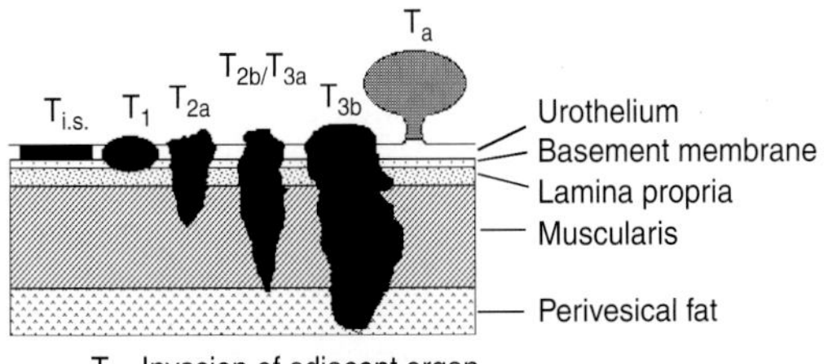

FIGURE 36-3 Current scheme for tumor (T) staging of urothelial cancer. EUA, examination under anesthesia.

Although there is no official system for *clinical* staging, there are several important factors that largely define prognosis that can be reasonably well assessed by clinical evaluation:

- The presence or absence of muscle invasion (ie, T1 vs ≥T2). This is fairly reliably established by transurethral resection (TUR), especially if the surgeon provides deep enough samples that contain muscularis propria.
- The presence or absence of a definable mass (ie, assessable in three dimensions) by examination under anesthesia (EUA) following a complete TUR. This is the clinical definition of cT3b disease and is of critical prognostic importance. The role of cross-sectional imaging criteria for cT3b disease is controversial. We do not believe that routinely available studies can make this distinction reliably at the present time. The EUA is an essential component of the evaluation of a patient with muscle-invasive bladder cancer ([56]) and is most informative when it is done following drainage of the bladder once the TUR has been completed. A proper EUA provides important staging information complementing data obtained by imaging modalities such as computed tomography (CT) scan or magnetic resonance imaging (MRI). The presence of induration indicates deep muscle invasion, whereas the palpation of a discreet, mobile, three-dimensional mass implies gross invasion into extravesical tissue and carries a significant risk (30%-40%) of occult lymph node metastasis. At EUA, it is possible to identify masses extending directly into the prostate in men or into the vagina in women. These findings are also associated with a high risk of occult lymph node metastasis. The finding of a mass by EUA that extends and is fixed to the pelvic sidewall (ie, cT4b) indicates an unresectable cancer. These patients have a similar prognosis to those with overt distant metastases.
- The presence or absence of nodal disease, as assessed clinically by CT or MRI imaging of the pelvis. Patients with radiographically detectable adenopathy should have a biopsy prior to surgery. If positive, primary chemotherapy is appropriate, because distant recurrence dominates the clinical course in these patients. That being said, we certainly advocate surgical consolidation with cystectomy and pelvic node dissection in patients with no clinical evidence of disease after chemotherapy.

- The presence or absence of lymphovascular invasion (LVI) on the TUR biopsy specimen is also a powerful prognostic feature. Although it must be admitted that TUR samples are often difficult to assess secondary to crush and cautery artifact, the unequivocal finding of tumor cells in vascular spaces identifies a group of patients with a high risk of occult nodal involvement. In fact, LVI is associated with a risk of pN+ status of about 35%, comparable to the risk associated with a large cT3b tumor. (It should be noted that tumors in the dome are both difficult to completely resect by TUR and more difficult to evaluate by EUA, and thus, clinical staging is even less reliable in this subset.)

Other clinical factors that routinely "stay in the model" when investigators construct Cox proportional hazard models for the prognosis of urothelial cancer patients treated with cystectomy are age, gender (females consistently do worse), and time from diagnosis to definitive therapy.

From a medical oncology perspective, the most important issue is how to recognize which patients will benefit from the addition of systemic chemotherapy to definitive surgery. The current management guidelines for bladder cancer as promulgated by the National Comprehensive Cancer Network (NCCN) ([54]) suggest the use of neoadjuvant chemotherapy for patients with cT2 disease. In our view, this is a wonderful example of how evidence-based medicine can pave the way for uncritical and even irrational management guidelines.

In evaluating this recommendation, it should first be noted that cT2 cancers could easily be pT0 (ie, no residual disease in cystectomy specimen after initial TUR), pTis, pTa, pT1, pT2a, pT2b, or pT3a without constituting a clinical staging error. However, it is abundantly clear that the burden of residual disease (ie, the burden of disease found at cystectomy) after TUR is strongly related to the risk of disease relapse and death. In a series of 208 patients, Isbarn et al recently demonstrated that those with residual invasive disease (ie, pT1 and pT2) were cured about 70% of the time, whereas all 55 patients with no residual invasive disease (pTa, pTis, or pT0) were cured ([57]).

To further highlight the enormous heterogeneity of patients with cT2 cancers, consider that we know of many features that have a dramatic influence on prognosis:

1. Cancers arising at the bladder neck are notoriously difficult to adequately stage and monitor and have a higher rate of occult nodal involvement.
2. Cancers presenting with hydronephrosis from tumors in the region of the ureterovesical junctions have a very high rate of pT3b extension, occult nodal involvement, and inferior outcome. This was first reported in the 1980s and has been amply confirmed. In a recent study of 241 patients with cT2 disease treated by cystectomy ([58]), the 5-year cause-specific survival (a good surrogate for cure) was 63% for those without this feature versus 12% for those with hydronephrosis. This remained prognostically significant after accounting for pathologic stage. Similar results were obtained by Bartsch et al ([59]), who observed survival rates of 68% versus 30%, again remaining significant after accounting for pathologic stage.
3. As noted earlier, cancers exhibiting micropapillary, sarcomatoid, plasmacytoid, and small cell histology have a much more aggressive biology and inferior stage-for-stage outcome with cystectomy.
4. Large nonpapillary tumors (cut points range from 3-5 cm) that are muscle invasive over a broad front are much worse (ie, much more likely to be upstaged at cystectomy) than those with focal muscle invasion.
5. Cancers showing LVI, especially when appreciated in the TUR specimen, are associated with about a 30% rate of occult nodal involvement ([60]).
6. Cancers with an abnormal immunophenotype for *p53* and *RB* gene products have a decreased probability of cure with cystectomy, and the prognosis is especially unfavorable when both are altered. In a large study of patients with cT2 disease, the cure rate for patients with both genes showing wild-type expression was 80%, whereas only 20% of patients with both genes altered were cured ([22]).
7. Cancers with prominent neovascularity in the tumor (ie, microvessel density as revealed by CD34 staining or other methods) or strong expression of VEGF are consistently associated with a higher risk of recurrent disease after cystectomy ([18, 61]).
8. Cancers with an invasive or mesenchymal phenotype characterized, for example, by high expression of matrix metalloprotease-9 and/or low expression of E-cadherin are consistently associated with an increased risk of recurrent and metastatic disease ([62]).
9. In addition to these tumor characteristics, it is now well established that circulating levels of tumor markers are independent predictors of outcome. This has been demonstrated for human chorionic gonadotropin (hCG), CA19-9, and CA-125 ([63-65]).

It is apparent that based on information that can be gathered preoperatively, it is possible to substantially refine the clinical risk of a patient with cT2 bladder cancer. Vickers et al ([66]) have provided a compelling numerical analysis of just how powerful the application of a multivariate model to decision making can be and how this consistently outperforms the simple-minded notion that all patients with cT2 cancer should get chemotherapy.

In addition to these clinical features that can be ascertained preoperatively, there are surgical factors that impact outcome. For example, we know that outcome is dependent on the experience of both the surgeon and the center where surgery is performed ([67, 68]) and that cure is consistently related to extent of pelvic node dissection ([69]), and of course, patients with involved surgical margins nearly always relapse.

CLINICAL MANAGEMENT

Management of Superficial Disease (cTa, cTis)

The management of low-grade papillary disease is by TUR, and because these lesions recur but rarely progress, there is generally no thought of cystectomy except in the rare case that the bladder surface is a carpet of lesions. In such a case, just as with overwhelming colon polyposis, radical surgery prior to progression to more threatening disease is appropriate.

High-grade noninvasive cancers present a difficult dilemma for the urologist, who must balance the risk of recurrent, invasive disease (which occurs despite therapy and surveillance in at least 20% of patients) with the risk of overtreating patients not destined to have a threatening cancer. As noted earlier, there is currently much interest in finding markers that will stratify the risk of progression and allow optimized management. The presence of CIS increases the probability of both recurrence and progression. Typically, patients with either high-grade Ta disease or CIS (or both) are now treated with both TUR and BCG.

Intravesical BCG was introduced in 1976, and since the first controlled trial establishing the efficacy of BCG was reported by Lamm et al in 1980 ([70]), it has had a remarkable impact on the clinical management of bladder cancer. Although standard criteria for therapy are still evolving, BCG has been shown in randomized trials to be superior to intravesical chemotherapy and TUR alone and will delay recurrence and progression, decreasing the need for immediate cystectomy. It is important to note that complete responses to BCG are required for significant alteration of the natural history of the disease ([71]). Partial responses should prompt referral for experimental therapy or consideration of early cystectomy. Especially in the context of any invasive component, BCG therapy will be associated with progression to potentially life-threatening disease in a substantial fraction, and thus, persistent treatment with BCG in the context of less than complete response is a major cause of potentially avoidable mortality from bladder cancer. In our experience, urologists are likely to emphasize the advantages of avoiding cystectomy but place less emphasis on the dangers of progression to the point that a cystectomy will no longer be curative. The decision to delay cystectomy in the face of less than an initial complete response to BCG is responsible for many deaths from disease that was not caught early enough, despite close surveillance ([72]).

The other feature of BCG therapy of particular interest from a medical oncology perspective (because it relates to assessment of the need for perioperative systemic therapy) is the increasing incidence of cancers in the distal ureter and prostatic urethra. In each case, these lesions are a challenge for cystoscopic surveillance. Particularly for ureteral lesions, minimal progression can be associated with a sharply increasing risk of life-threatening disease. Therapy with BCG can clear the bladder proper, while urothelial carcinogenesis and progression continue just millimeters away. Patients treated with BCG (especially those with CIS) who have negative cystoscopy but positive cytology are at substantial risk of having such disease, and it is often fatal if definitive management is delayed ([73]).

Management of Minimally Invasive Disease (cT1)

Patients with cancers that are invasive into the lamina propria (cT1) are at high risk of developing muscle-invasive disease. In general, patients with an invasive or high-grade component recognized on the initial TUR should have a re-excision approximately 4 weeks later ([74]). A second TUR provides another opportunity to sample muscle and thus more definitively establish the status of muscle invasion, which is a key prognostic feature. In addition, the re-resection establishes which patients have or do not have persistent disease. Those with persistent disease have a prognosis similar to cT2 patients and should be informed of the risk associated with bladder-preserving therapy. Conversely, a complete TUR, as demonstrated by a negative re-resection, may be adequate therapy for many patients with cT1 disease, especially if there is no CIS present and noninvolved muscle has been sampled. In this context, it is especially important to have a highly sensitive test for CIS. Although not yet standard, there is substantial interest in looking at tissue fluorescence to enhance conventional cystoscopy ([75]). In the United States, most patients with cT1 disease receive BCG, and the caveats about BCG use as noted earlier apply even more strongly to this group. It is also important to recognize that tumors that overlie the ureteral orifices or involve the bladder neck are sometimes difficult to confirm as only T1 lesions and require a lower threshold for definitive surgery.

Men with a positive cytology and no obvious tumor within the bladder should undergo transurethral biopsy of the prostate at 5 and 7 o'clock at the verumontanum in addition to random bladder biopsies. Prostate recurrence is detected in approximately 10% to 15% of patients within 5 years of treatment of their bladder tumor and in 20% to 40% by 10 years.

At MDACC, patients with persistent T1 disease despite resection and intravesical therapy are generally cautioned against second-line therapy and guided toward radical cystectomy. Esrig et al have provided a useful perspective on this situation ([76]).

Management of Clinically Localized, Muscle-Invasive Disease (cT2)

In the United States, cystectomy is the standard therapy for muscle-invasive bladder cancer. In older surgical series, cystectomy was curative in about half of these patients. More contemporary series typically report cure in the range of 80%, but this is based on *pathologic stage*. Thus, although it is true that in experienced centers 80% to 85% of patients undergoing cystectomy for cancers that are found to be pathologically confined to the muscular wall of the bladder (ie, pT2b or less, N0) will be cured, it is not absolutely clear that the old figure of about 50% cure for *clinical stage* T2 patients is now obsolete, although modern series do seem better ([77]). At the very least, the finding of muscle invasion signals a potentially life-threatening problem; in fact, this seems to constitute an oncologic urgency. In a study of 214 patients treated with cystectomy at the University of Michigan ([78]), a cut point of 93 days from recognition of muscle invasion to surgery was associated with statistically inferior cause-specific survival and OS. Specifically, about 60% of patients with timely surgery were long-term survivors versus about 40% of those with delay, even though there was no clinical or pathologic stage migration.

In view of available knowledge of prognostic features reviewed earlier, it is clearly inappropriate in the current era to speak of muscle-invasive bladder cancer as though it were a single disease state with a well-defined prognosis and a single best management. We know that there are many patients with cT2 bladder cancer with such a favorable prognosis that no available systemic therapy would be expected to improve outcome over that achieved with radical cystectomy and template pelvic node dissection ([79]). Likewise, we know that some patients at high risk will benefit from currently available chemotherapy in addition to surgery. The challenge for clinicians, and especially for clinical investigators, is to better define those at each end of this spectrum and then continue to work on subdivision of the remaining patients where we currently do not know how to define the role of systemic chemotherapy. This issue of identifying the appropriate patients for systemic chemotherapy is the single most important question related to bladder cancer from a medical oncology perspective. There is no longer any question that perioperative chemotherapy can improve outcome for some patients; likewise, it is all too obvious that it can do much harm. Thus, as always, the central question for the medical oncologist is: How are we to balance risk and benefit for each patient?

Based on our understanding of the impact of currently available therapy, it is our sense that patients with a ≥70% chance of cure should not be offered chemotherapy as it currently exists. Conversely, when the probability of surgical cure falls to about ≤40%, then it seems clear that chemotherapy should be offered. In between these extremes, the decision is a highly personal issue of risk abatement versus burden of therapy. As a practical implementation of this intuitive sense that 40% cure probability is about the right threshold for chemotherapy plus surgery, we offer chemotherapy to patients with any of the following: direct invasion of the prostate or vagina (ie, cT4a disease), a three-dimensional mass on EUA (ie, cT3b disease), LVI on TUR material, bladder neck involvement, and hydronephrosis or an excessive delay (ie, >4 months) between the finding of muscle-invasive disease and definitive management. We look forward to implementing more refined prognostic tools in our own practice.

Primary Radiotherapy

In our view, radiotherapy is inferior to surgery as a local modality for bladder cancer. Available data clearly demonstrate that long-term control can be achieved in about 40% of patients with small primary tumors amenable to complete resection, not associated with CIS, not arising at the bladder neck or ureterovesical junction, and without hydronephrosis ([80]). This is precisely the subset that has about an 80% cure with surgery, and to claim that the available results are comparable to surgical series is not justified ([81]). Clearly some patients could decide that the risks are acceptable and rationally choose radiotherapy, but this must not be presented as an option associated with a comparable outcome to surgery. When chosen as an option, we would recommend the use of concomitant radiosensitizing chemotherapy ([82]).

Management of Locally Advanced, Resectable Disease (High-Risk cT2, cT3, cT4A)

Since the publication of the Southwest Oncology Group (SWOG) intergroup trial of neoadjuvant chemotherapy ([83]), many guidelines, including the NCCN guidelines, advocate for neoadjuvant chemotherapy as the standard of care for patients with muscle-invasive urothelial carcinoma. Because, in our experience, the cure fraction for patients with muscle-invasive disease only with surgery is approximately 85% and the use of systemic chemotherapy can be toxic in this often frail and elderly patient population, we have advocated for a more refined approach relying on the probability of recurrence as a guide for the use of neoadjuvant treatment. Tumors that are clinically beyond the bladder wall (ie, those with a three-dimensional mass at exam under anesthesia) after thorough TUR of intravesical tumor carry a worse prognosis with a surgical cure rate of about 35%. Many patients with cT2 disease and high-risk features have a similar chance for surgical cure. The presence of LVI is associated with a high risk of nodal involvement, even in the setting of clinically negative lymph nodes on CT scan.

Patients with prostatic stromal involvement (from the bladder, *not* from TCC of prostatic ducts) or extension into the vaginal wall (ie, anatomic clinical stage cT4a) have a surgical cure rate in the range of 5% to 20%. A recent retrospective multicenter study of 583 patients with pT4 disease (all obviously deemed resectable on clinical grounds) found a cause-specific survival rate of about 30% ([84]). Univariate analysis confirmed female gender, LVI, nodal involvement, positive surgical margins, and pT4b substage to be associated with inferior outcome. None of these patients received neoadjuvant therapy. Collectively, these groups have what we term *locally advanced but resectable* disease, and at MDACC, they are treated primarily with chemotherapy, followed by surgical consolidation as appropriate. Although this is a patient cohort with truly threatening disease, it is also true that this is the population for whom combined application of best systemic therapy and best surgical therapy has the greatest patient benefit. In the MDACC experience ([85, 86]), the benchmark outcome in this cohort is cure in about 60% of patients (by intent to treat), with about 40% having no residual invasive cancer in the resected specimen following chemotherapy (so-called "p-zero" status), which we and others ([83]) have noted to be a reliable indicator of long-term disease-free survival.

Recently, several centers have reported on the use of dose-dense M-VAC in the neoadjuvant setting for urothelial carcinoma ([87-89]). The use of the dose-dense strategy has had multiple benefits including a faster time to surgery, with chemotherapy given on a 2-week schedule, and an improved tolerance for chemotherapy. In one study, 93% of patients completed at least three cycles of neoadjuvant chemotherapy ([87]). Pathologic T0 rates have been quite promising, on the order of 39% ([87-89]), with long-term survival at one center suggesting a cure fraction of approximately 63% ([87]). Molecular characterization of urothelial tumors from the MDACC trial suggests that the basal subtype may be predictive for benefit from neoadjuvant chemotherapy ([90]). Further efforts in subtyping bladder cancer may yield a prognostic test available for community use that would allow us to discriminate which patients are most likely to benefit from a neoadjuvant approach.

Management of Locally Advanced, Unresectable Disease (cT4B, cN+)

This group of patients has a dismal prognosis. In our experience, patients presenting with large tumors that are clinically fixed to the rectum, pelvic sidewall, or pubic symphysis actually have a worse prognosis than patients with extrapelvic nodes or lung-only metastases. These patients are considered unresectable and are treated with chemotherapy initially, and then reassessed for the possibility of surgical consolidation in light of the quality of response and their fitness for surgery after chemotherapy ([91]).

Investigators from Memorial Sloan-Kettering Cancer Center ([92]) and MDACC ([93]) have published their experience with this strategy. These data suggest that response to systemic therapy is the dominant prognostic feature and that surgical consolidation is both feasible and associated with long-term survival. This experience also confirmed that patients with significant residual disease after chemotherapy did not benefit from surgery and that, overall, the prognosis is still poor. Still, a 22% to 40% survival rate among initially unresectable bladder cancer patients is much better than what could be expected of any single modality.

Radiotherapy has not been useful as a single modality with these large cancers. As with surgery, there probably is a role for radiotherapy in the consolidation of patients who show an excellent response to primary chemotherapy. It is worth emphasizing that sensitivity to chemotherapy and radiotherapy does tend to be parallel in the context of urothelial cancer. We have never seen a chemotherapy-refractory cancer respond to radiation, and we have seen some excellent long-term results from use of radiotherapy to consolidate an initially unresectable mass after an excellent response to combination chemotherapy.

Management of Distant Metastatic Disease

Bladder cancer typically spreads first to regional nodes and then disseminates with about equal frequency to the lungs, liver, and bone. Late in the course, subcutaneous and brain metastases are common. Brain involvement is especially likely in patients who have elevated serum levels of β-hCG or variant histology, including small cell.

Even with strictly palliative goals in mind, most patients with metastatic bladder cancer should be treated with multicomponent chemotherapy, pitched at their level of physiologic tolerance. Metastatic urothelial cancer remains a clinical situation in which toxic side effects are typically encountered if chemotherapy is given in a way that has any chance of substantially altering the natural history of the disease. Unfortunately, "kinder, gentler" therapy is likely to be of little benefit. Metastatic urothelial cancer is an aggressive malignancy, with an untreated natural history from the time it causes symptoms to death of approximately 3 to 4 months. Quality of life is essentially completely dependent on the efficacy of therapy. Even extraordinarily toxic regimens can be truly palliative in light of how rapidly (and morbidly) the disease progresses.

Since the mid-1980s, the use of cisplatin-based combination chemotherapy has been standard. In the modern era with a bit of lead time bias compared to practice in the early 1980s, such treatment results in median survival of about 16 months, with few survivors beyond 3 years. This is the benchmark where therapy has plateaued for more than a decade.

Of course, some patients with distant metastatic disease still have disease restricted to one (or a few) anatomic areas, and one might imagine that local therapy would have a role in such a setting. However, in contrast to the situation with renal cell carcinoma for example, surgery is almost never an appropriate initial intervention for metastatic urothelial cancer. Almost always, the disease is not really localized, and one finds rapid progression in the postoperative setting. Thus, even in cases of anatomically threatening lesions such as threatened cord compression, we generally advocate primary chemotherapy to get the disease under some control that will then permit safe surgical intervention. Nonetheless, it is only natural to ask if there is a role for surgical consolidation after a good response to chemotherapy for (highly) selected patients with metastatic urothelial cancer. The MDACC experience with this strategy has been published in the setting of retroperitoneal lymph node metastases ([91]) and in a very small, select subset of patients with visceral metastases ([94]). Selection criteria for this approach have not yet matured. In the absence of more data, we have adopted the following guidelines. For patients with pelvic or retroperitoneal nodal involvement (below the renal vessels), we typically offer an extended node dissection to patients with a complete radiographic response to initial chemotherapy. Because judging the completeness of response in a lymph node is problematic, we include in our working definition a negative biopsy for any node that is large enough for CT-guided biopsy. For patients with visceral involvement, we typically treat to maximum response and observe. Only when patients progress in the initially involved area (with no progression elsewhere) and then go on to have a significant response to a second course of chemotherapy do we consider surgical removal of residual metastatic disease. Just as with patients with germ cell cancers, failure of markers to normalize is nearly an absolute contraindication to surgical consolidation.

The exception to this is the rare patient with a long interval from initial management to the onset of resectable, oligometastatic visceral disease. In this setting, we typically give systemic therapy and then excise the lesions. Note that in our view surgery without some chemotherapy is essentially never appropriate because these cancers have a high propensity of seeding surgical wounds. Even in the face of cord compression, chemotherapy followed by surgery is usually the preferred management.

Patients relapsing after cystectomy essentially always have systemic disease, but a substantial fraction have clinically detectable involvement confined to local and/or regional nodes. We know that some of these patients will have an excellent response to chemotherapy and, with surgical consolidation, will be long-term survivors. Thus, although it has not been rigorously shown to produce a better overall outcome, surveillance by periodic CT is usually performed. Relapse is stereotypically circumscribed between 9 and 18 months, by which time about 85% of those destined to relapse will have done so, and this is when we advocate surveillance.

In our experience, CIS of the distal ureter is the pathologic feature most closely associated with upper tract recurrence ([95]). In fact, 15% of those with post-cystectomy tumor within the distal intramural ureter developed an upper tract recurrence. Intraoperative ureteral margin status by itself was of little consequence. Patients with TCC involving the prostatic urethra also had a higher incidence of upper tract recurrence following cystectomy, in keeping with the field-change hypothesis of urothelial carcinogenesis. Upper tract surveillance of these patients can be accomplished with urine cytology and upper tract imaging. Traditionally, the intravenous pyelogram was the primary imaging tool for surveillance of the upper tract because it provides visualization of filling defects and can detect obstruction. More recently, CT urography has been found to be a more sensitive surveillance tool following cystectomy because it can identify not only local and distant recurrences but also early upper tract recurrences.

SYSTEMIC THERAPY FOR UROTHELIAL CANCER

Currently, *combination therapy is standard* in the treatment of metastatic TCC. The development of M-VAC at Memorial Sloan-Kettering Cancer Center ([96]) was an important achievement. Subsequent landmark trials have confirmed that M-VAC is superior to single-agent cisplatin ([97]); the combination of cyclophosphamide, doxorubicin, and cisplatin ([98]); the combination of 5-fluorouracil, interferon-α, and cisplatin ([93]); and the combination of docetaxel and cisplatin ([99]). In fact, there are at least nine randomized trials involving M-VAC, and to date, the only challenger to even suggest improved clinical outcome was a trial of a dose-dense variant of M-VAC given with granulocyte colony-stimulating factor support versus classic M-VAC ([100]). The dose-dense version was associated with markedly less mucositis, and the cycles are only 14 days (compared to 28 in the classic schedule), and thus, dose-dense M-VAC has supplanted classic M-VAC. With overall response rates in the 50% to 60% range and up to a 30% clinical complete response rate, there is no doubt that dose-dense M-VAC provides meaningful palliation for most patients and can significantly change the natural history of the disease for a few.

Nonetheless, for most oncologists, M-VAC has overstayed its welcome. Despite having been the standard of care for 20 years, it is nearly completely abandoned because of significant toxicity and the availability of regimens of similar efficacy that are slightly less toxic. Although we freely acknowledge the considerable shortcomings of M-VAC, it is distressing to us to see phase II studies of newer doublets consistently show survival results inferior to the well-established benchmark established by M-VAC and to see widespread use of these regimens. Although one might argue that this is acceptable in the metastatic setting, where a shorter OS might be associated with "more good days" if one uses a less toxic treatment, we see no rationale for the widespread use of inferior regimens in the setting of perioperative therapy for locally advanced disease. In that context, improvement of cure fraction has been demonstrated for M-VAC, but not established for other regimens. Thus, in the absence of a clinical trial, the dose-dense version of M-VAC is the standard frontline therapy at MDACC when chemotherapy is given with curative intent.

In the setting of metastatic disease, for which the goals are clearly palliative, the doublet of gemcitabine and cisplatin has become a standard option. Gemcitabine-cisplatin was compared to M-VAC in a large international phase III trial ([101]). The doublet was shown to be similar with respect to median survival and was associated with significantly less mucositis and neutropenic fever. Gemcitabine-cisplatin did cause more thrombocytopenia, however. As expected for two regimens with comparable efficacy, quality-of-life measures were not different between the two treatments, despite the favorable treatment-related side effect profile of gemcitabine-cisplatin. In our view, this is not a surprising finding, but rather reinforces the notion that the burden of morbidity in patients with metastatic bladder cancer is far more likely to be due to the disease, rather than secondary to the treatment.

Gemcitabine, the taxanes ([102, 103]), and ifosfamide ([86, 104, 105]) all have activity in urothelial cancer, and there have been many new doublets and triplets investigated over the past 10 years. From this experience, it is clear that all regimens substituting carboplatin for cisplatin show inferior results, or even increased toxicity, as was seen with the triplet combination of gemcitabine, paclitaxel, and carboplatin ([106]).

Urothelial cancer is a disease of the elderly. The lifetime accumulation of risk factors predisposing patients to bladder cancer often leads to other comorbid conditions such as coronary artery disease and chronic obstructive pulmonary disease. These diseases, in addition to other conditions found in an aging population, such as diabetes and hypertension, often contribute to poor renal function or a performance status unable to tolerate aggressive cisplatin- or ifosfamide-based therapy.

Ureteral obstruction is also a frequent factor contributing to diminished renal function, and nephrostomy tubes are an indispensable tool in the treatment of advanced bladder cancer. Nephrostomy tubes are much preferred over ureteral stents in patients undergoing chemotherapy for locally advanced bladder cancer. This is because chemotherapy often engenders periods of neutropenia that can lead to chronic infection associated with foreign bodies. Nephrostomies are much more easily changed out than stents. Furthermore, stents are far more irritating and likely to bleed during periods of thrombocytopenia. It is not uncommon to have stents clog from bleeding, and this is much less problematic with nephrostomies. Finally, nephrostomies will reliably decompress the kidneys, even if the cancer grows, whereas stents can be collapsed by tumor and even by desmoplastic reaction to therapy.

Relatively effective chemotherapy for patients with impaired renal function is now fairly easy to come by. Vinblastine, gemcitabine, taxanes, and doxorubicin can all be given safely in the context of renal insufficiency. At the present time, we favor a triplet of gemcitabine (900 mg/m^2 given over 90 minutes), paclitaxel (100 mg/m^2), and doxorubicin (30 mg/m^2) repeated every 14 days for patients with poor renal function. This regimen is reliably deliverable and has useful clinical activity ([107]).

FUTURE PROSPECTS

The ready availability of the bladder surface makes bladder cancer an ideal clinical model for the development of gene therapy. Investigators at MDACC have reported that adenoviral-mediated gene expression (in this case of interferon-α-2b) within the bladder can be achieved using the detergent Syn3 ([108]). A phase I trial has been completed, and further work with this and other intravesical gene transfer therapies is ongoing.

The efficacy of BCG strongly suggests that immune recognition and reaction to bladder cancer antigens is a clinical strategy that could be further developed. Moreover, tumor-infiltrating CD8-expressing T cells are predictive of survival in patients with urothelial carcinoma ([109]). Clinical trials are currently in the planning stages to evaluate the impact of the immune checkpoint inhibitors in patients with superficial disease who have failed BCG.

Further building upon the immunologic platform are studies of immune checkpoint inhibitors in patients with metastatic disease. The PD1 and PDL1 inhibitors are currently in late-phase clinical trials. With early reported response rates of 20% to 40% ([1]), their approval as the first targeted agents in metastatic urothelial cancer is eagerly anticipated. Future trials combining these agents with other therapies targeting the immune system, including CTLA4 antibodies, are currently ongoing.

Current optimism is high that we are now entering the era of personalized medicine for urothelial cancer. In addition to agents targeting mutations, including *FGFR3*, we are gaining an understanding of the underlying biology of urothelial cancer. The molecular characterization of urothelial cancer is expected to provide the framework of underlying biology and help us predict which patients are candidates for chemotherapy. One might predict that the basal subtype, which is sensitive to chemotherapy, may also benefit from angiogenesis inhibition. The luminal subtype, which is enriched for *FGFR3* mutations and downstream markers of FGFR activation, may be more susceptible to FGFR inhibition. Recently, ERBB2 expression, which appears associated with subtype, may predict which of the luminal tumors are more likely to respond to systemic chemotherapy. Finally, further study of the p53-like subtype will help us in finding agents in chemotherapy-resistant disease. The presence of stroma in these tumors may correlate with the higher incidence of bone metastases and guide us toward therapies that impact the stromal environment.

Thus, urothelial cancer is no longer just one disease. Novel agents and selection strategies have now come to this disease, with an energy and optimism that we are moving from cytotoxic strategies to immunologic and targeted interventions that will be embraced by physicians and enhance the lives of our patients. The era of personalized medicine is indeed upon us.

Commentary: Molecular Markers for Risk Stratification and Personalized Therapy in Urothelial Tumors

As the authors of this chapter appropriately emphasize, the clinical management of bladder cancer appears to be on the verge of a remarkable transformation. Several large-scale cancer genomics projects (including the first phase of The Cancer Genome Atlas's bladder cancer project) have provided the first detailed molecular "parts lists" of the disease, and the information suggests clear implications for prognostication and precision therapy. Converging with these basic biological breakthroughs are the exciting, game-changing results of ongoing clinical trials with immune checkpoint inhibitors, which provide the first examples of targeted therapies that are active against tumors that are resistant to the current frontline therapies. This chapter provides an excellent and comprehensive description of the current state of the science with insightful predictions regarding where the field is heading in the near future.

David J. McConkey

REFERENCES

1. Powles T, Eder JP, Fine G, Braiteh F, et al. MPDL3280A (anti-PD-L1) treatment leads to clinical activity in metastatic bladder cancer. *Nature*. 2014;515:558-562.
2. Choi W, Porten S, Kim S, et al. Identification of distinct basal and luminal subtypes of muscle-invasive bladder cancer with different sensitivities to frontline chemotherapy. *Cancer Cell*. 2014;25:152-165.
3. Siegel RL, Miller KD, Jemal A. Cancer statistics, 2015. *CA Cancer J Clin*. 2015;65:5-29.
4. Wu X, Ros MM, Gu J, et al. Epidemiology and genetic susceptibility to bladder cancer. *BJU Int*. 2008;102:1207-1215.
5. Michaud DS, Spiegelman D, Clinton SK, et al. Fluid intake and the risk of bladder cancer in men [see comment]. *N Engl J Med*. 1999;340:1390-1397.
6. Levine LA, Richie JP. Urological complications of cyclophosphamide. *J Urol*. 1989;141:1063-1069.
7. Ross RK, Paganini-Hill A, Landolph J, et al. Analgesics, cigarette smoking, and other risk factors for cancer of the renal pelvis and ureter. *Cancer Res*. 1989;49:1045-1048.
8. Jelakovic B, Karanovic S, Vukovic-Lela I, et al. Aristolactam-DNA adducts are a biomarker of environmental exposure to aristolochic acid. *Kidney Int*. 2012;81:559-567.
9. Groah SL, Weitzenkamp DA, Lammertse DP, et al. Excess risk of bladder cancer in spinal cord injury: evidence for an association between indwelling catheter use and bladder cancer. *Arch Phys Med Rehabil*. 2002;83:346-351.
10. Taylor JA, Umbach DM, Stephens E, et al. The role of N-acetylation polymorphisms in smoking-associated bladder cancer: evidence of a gene-gene-exposure three-way interaction. *Cancer Res*. 1998;58:3603-3610.
11. Reszka E, Wasowicz W. Genetic polymorphism of N-acetyltransferase and glutathione S-transferase related to neoplasm of genitourinary system. Minireview. *Neoplasma*.

2002;49:209-216.
12. Wang M, Gu D, Zhang Z, et al. XPD polymorphisms, cigarette smoking, and bladder cancer risk: a meta-analysis. *J Toxicol Environ Health A*. 2009;72:698-705.
13. Stern MC, Lin J, Figueroa JD, et al. Polymorphisms in DNA repair genes, smoking, and bladder cancer risk: findings from the international consortium of bladder cancer. *Cancer Res*. 2009;69:6857-6864.
14. Wu X, Amos CI, Zhu Y, et al. Telomere dysfunction: a potential cancer predisposition factor. *J Natl Cancer Inst*. 2003;95:1211-1218.
15. McGrath M, Wong JY, Michaud D, et al. Telomere length, cigarette smoking, and bladder cancer risk in men and women. *Cancer Epidemiol Biomarkers Prev*. 2007;16:815-819.
16. Dinney CPN, McConkey DJ, Millikan RE, et al. Focus on bladder cancer. *Cancer Cell*. 2004;6:111-116.
17. Mhawech-Fauceglia P, Fischer G, Beck A, et al. Raf1, Aurora-A/STK15 and E-cadherin biomarkers expression in patients with pTa/pT1 urothelial bladder carcinoma; a retrospective TMA study of 246 patients with long-term follow-up. *Eur J Surg Oncol*. 2006;32:439-444.
18. Inoue K, Slaton JW, Karashima T, et al. The prognostic value of angiogenesis factor expression for predicting recurrence and metastasis of bladder cancer after neoadjuvant chemotherapy and radical cystectomy. *Clin Cancer Res*. 2000;6:4866-4873.
19. Imao T, Koshida K, Endo Y, et al. Dominant role of E-cadherin in the progression of bladder cancer. *J Urol*. 1999;161:692-698.
20. Barbisan F, Santinelli A, Mazzucchelli R, et al. Strong immunohistochemical expression of fibroblast growth factor receptor 3, superficial staining pattern of cytokeratin 20, and low proliferative activity define those papillary urothelial neoplasms of low malignant potential that do not recur. *Cancer*. 2008;112:636-644.
21. Majewski T, Lee S, Jeong J, et al. Understanding the development of human bladder cancer by using a whole-organ genomic mapping strategy. *Lab Invest*. 2008;88:694-721.
22. Cote RJ, Dunn MD, Chatterjee SJ, et al. Elevated and absent pRb expression is associated with bladder cancer progression and has cooperative effects with p53. *Cancer Res*. 1998;58:1090-1094.
23. Esrig D, Elmajian D, Groshen S, et al. Accumulation of nuclear p53 and tumor progression in bladder cancer. *N Engl J Med*. 1994;331:1259-1264.
24. Sarkar S, Julicher KP, Burger MS, et al. Different combinations of genetic/epigenetic alterations inactivate the p53 and pRb pathways in invasive human bladder cancers. *Cancer Res*. 2000;60:3862-3871.
25. Shariat SF, Lotan Y, Karakiewicz PI, et al. p53 predictive value for pT1-2 N0 disease at radical cystectomy. *J Urol*. 2009;182:907-913.
26. Choi W, Shah JB, Tran M, et al. p63 expression defines a lethal subset of muscle-invasive bladder cancers. *PloS One*. 2012;7:e30206.
27. Karni-Schmidt O, Castillo-Martin M, HuaiShen T, et al. Distinct expression profiles of p63 variants during uothelial development and bladder cancer progression. *Am J Pathol*. 2011;178:1350-1360.
28. Yang A, Kaghad M, Wang Y, et al. p63, a p53 homolog at 3q27-29, encodes multiple products with transactivating, death-inducing, and dominant-negative activities. *Mol Cell*. 1998;2:305-316.
29. The Cancer Genome Atlas: Comprehensive molecular characterization of urothelial bladder carcinoma. *Nature*. 2014;507:315-322.
30. Inoue K, Slaton JW, Davis DW, et al. Treatment of human metastatic transitional cell carcinoma of the bladder in a murine model with the anti-vascular endothelial growth factor receptor monoclonal antibody DC101 and paclitaxel. *Clin Cancer Res*. 2000;6:2635-2643.
31. Petrylak D, Tagawa, S, Kohli, M, et al. Interim results of a randomized phase 2 study of docetaxel with ramucirumab versus docetaxel in second-line advanced or metastatic urothelial carcinoma [abstract]. *J Clin Oncol*. 2015;33:295.
32. Hahn NM, Stadler WM, Zon RT, et al. Phase II trial of cisplatin, gemcitabine, and bevacizumab as first-line therapy for metastatic urothelial carcinoma: Hoosier Oncology Group GU 04-75. *J Clin Oncol*. 2011;29:1525-1530.
33. Siefker-Radtke AO, Kamat AM, Corn PG, et al. Neoadjuvant chemotherapy with DD-MVAC and bevacizumab in high-risk urothelial cancer: results from a phase II trial at the University of Texas M. D. Anderson Cancer Center [abstract]. *J Clin Oncol*. 2012;30:4523.
34. Epstein JI, Amin MB, Reuter VR, et al. The World Health Organization/International Society of Urological Pathology consensus classification of urothelial (transitional cell) neoplasms of the urinary bladder. Bladder Consensus Conference Committee. *Am J Surg Pathol*. 1998;22:1435-1448.
35. Mitra AP, Datar RH, Cote RJ. Molecular pathways in invasive bladder cancer: new insights into mechanisms, progression, and target identification. *J Clin Oncol*. 2006;24:5552-5564.
36. Spiess PE, Czerniak B. Dual-track pathway of bladder carcinogenesis: practical implications. *Arch Pathol Lab Med*. 2006;130:844-852.
37. Amin MB, Ro JY, el-Sharkawy T, et al. Micropapillary variant of transitional cell carcinoma of the urinary bladder. Histologic pattern resembling ovarian papillary serous carcinoma. *Am J Surg Pathol*. 1994;18:1224-1232.
38. Kamat AM, Dinney CPN, Gee JR, et al. Micropapillary bladder cancer: a review of the University of Texas M. D. Anderson Cancer Center experience with 100 consecutive patients. *Cancer*. 2007;110:62-67.
39. Ohtsuki Y, Kuroda N, Umeoka T, et al. KL-6 is another useful marker in assessing a micropapillary pattern in carcinomas of the breast and urinary bladder, but not the colon. *Med Mol Morphol*. 2009;42:123-127.
40. Sangoi AR, Higgins JP, Rouse RV, et al. Immunohistochemical comparison of MUC1, CA125, and Her2Neu in invasive micropapillary carcinoma of the urinary tract and typical invasive urothelial carcinoma with retraction artifact. *Mod Pathol*. 2009;22:660-667.
41. Siefker-Radtke AO, Dinney C, Abrahams N, et al. Is there a role for pre-operative chemotherapy in small cell carcinoma? The M.D. Anderson Experience. *J Urol*. 2003;169:335.
42. Lynch S, Shen Y, Kamat A, et al. Neoadjuvant chemotherapy in small cell urothelial cancer improves pathologic down-staging and long-term outcomes: results from a retrospective study at the M. D. Anderson Cancer Center. *Eur Urol*. 2013;64:307-313.
43. Siefker-Radtke AO, Kamat AM, Grossman HB, et al. Phase II clinical trial of neoadjuvant alternating doublet chemotherapy with ifosfamide/doxorubicin and etoposide/cisplatin in small-cell urothelial cancer. *J Clin Oncol*. 2009;27:2592-2597.
44. Dayyani F, Czerniak BA, Sircar K, et al. Plasmacytoid urothelial carcinoma, a chemosensitive cancer with poor prognosis, and peritoneal carcinomatosis. *J Urol*. 2013;189:1656-1661.
45. Keck B, Wach S, Stoehr R, et al. Plasmacytoid variant of bladder cancer defines patients with poor prognosis if treated with cystectomy and adjuvant cisplatin-based chemotherapy. *BMC Cancer*. 2013;13:71.
46. Lopez-Beltran A, Requena MJ, Montironi R, et al. Plasmacytoid urothelial carcinoma of the bladder. *Hum Pathol*. 2009;40:1023-1028.
47. Ro JY, Shen SS, Lee HI, et al. Plasmacytoid transitional cell carcinoma of urinary bladder: a clinicopathologic study of 9 cases.

Am J Surg Pathol. 2008;32:752-757.

48. Siefker-Radtke A. Urachal adenocarcinoma: a clinician's guide for treatment. *Semin Oncol*. 2012;39:619-624.
49. Siefker-Radtke AO, Gee J, Shen Y, et al. Multimodality management of urachal carcinoma: the M. D. Anderson Cancer Center experience. *J Urol*. 2003;169:1295-1298.
50. Herr HW, Bochner BH, Sharp D, et al. Urachal carcinoma: contemporary surgical outcomes. *J Urol*. 2007;178:74-78.
51. Molina JR, Quevedo JF, Furth AF, et al. Predictors of survival from urachal cancer: a Mayo Clinic study of 49 cases. *Cancer*. 2007;110:2434-2440.
52. Ashley RA, Inman BA, Sebo TJ, et al. Urachal carcinoma: clinicopathologic features and long-term outcomes of an aggressive malignancy. *Cancer*. 2006;107:712-720.
53. Mhawech-Fauceglia P, Fischer G, Alvarez V Jr, et al. Predicting outcome in minimally invasive (T1a and T1b) urothelial bladder carcinoma using a panel of biomarkers: a high throughput tissue microarray analysis. *BJU Int*. 2007;100:1182-1187.
54. Platz CE, Cohen MB, Jones MP, et al. Is microstaging of early invasive cancer of the urinary bladder possible or useful? *Mod Pathol*. 1996;9:1035-1039.
55. Engel P, Anagnostaki L, Braendstrup O. The muscularis mucosae of the human urinary bladder. Implications for tumor staging on biopsies. *Scand J Urol Nephrol*. 1992;26:249-252.
56. Wijkstrom H, Norming U, Lagerkvist M, et al. Evaluation of clinical staging before cystectomy in transitional cell bladder carcinoma: a long-term follow-up of 276 consecutive patients. *Br J Urol*. 1998;81:686-691.
57. Isbarn H, Karakiewicz PI, Shariat SF, et al. Residual pathological stage at radical cystectomy significantly impacts outcomes for initial T2N0 bladder cancer. *J Urol*. 2009;182:459-465.
58. Resorlu B, Baltaci S, Resorlu M, et al. Prognostic significance of hydronephrosis in bladder cancer treated by radical cystectomy. *Urol Int*. 2009;83:285-288.
59. Bartsch GC, Kuefer R, Gschwend JE, et al. Hydronephrosis as a prognostic marker in bladder cancer in a cystectomy-only series. *Eur Urol*. 2007;51:690-697; discussion 697-698.
60. Quek ML, Stein JP, Nichols PW, et al. Prognostic significance of lymphovascular invasion of bladder cancer treated with radical cystectomy. *J Urol*. 2005;174:103-106.
61. Goddard JC, Sutton CD, Furness PN, et al. Microvessel density at presentation predicts subsequent muscle invasion in superficial bladder cancer. *Clin Cancer Res*. 2003;9:2583-2586.
62. Slaton JW, Millikan R, Inoue K, et al. Correlation of metastasis related gene expression and relapse-free survival in patients with locally advanced bladder cancer treated with cystectomy and chemotherapy. *J Urol*. 2004;171:570-574.
63. Margel D, Tal R, Baniel J. Serum tumor markers may predict overall and disease specific survival in patients with clinically organ confined invasive bladder cancer. *J Urol*. 2007;178:2297-2300; discussion 2300-2301.
64. Margel D, Tal R, Neuman A, et al. Prediction of extravesical disease by preoperative serum markers in patients with clinically organ confined invasive bladder cancer. *J Urol*. 2006;175:1253-1257; discussion 1257.
65. Pectasides D, Bafaloucos D, Antoniou F, et al. TPA, TATI, CEA, AFP, beta-HCG, PSA, SCC, and CA 19-9 for monitoring transitional cell carcinoma of the bladder. *Am J Clin Oncol*. 1996;19:271-277.
66. Vickers AJ, Cronin AM, Kattan MW, et al. Clinical benefits of a multivariate prediction model for bladder cancer: a decision analytic approach. *Cancer*. 2009;115:5460-5469.
67. Herr HW. Extent of surgery and pathology evaluation has an impact on bladder cancer outcomes after radical cystectomy. *Urology*. 2003;61:105-108.
68. Elting LS, Pettaway C, Bekele BN, et al. Correlation between annual volume of cystectomy, professional staffing, and outcomes: a statewide, population-based study. *Cancer*. 2005;104:975-984.
69. Herr HW, Faulkner JR, Grossman HB, et al. Pathologic evaluation of radical cystectomy specimens: a cooperative group report. *Cancer*. 2004;100:2470-2475.
70. Lamm DL, Thor DE, Harris SC, et al. Bacillus Calmette-Guerin immunotherapy of superficial bladder cancer. *J Urol*. 1980;124:38-40.
71. Lerner SP, Tangen CM, Sucharew H, et al. Failure to achieve a complete response to induction BCG therapy is associated with increased risk of disease worsening and death in patients with high risk non-muscle invasive bladder cancer. *Urol Oncol*. 2009;27:155-159.
72. Herr HW, Sogani PC. Does early cystectomy improve the survival of patients with high risk superficial bladder tumors? *J Urol*. 2001;166:1296-1299.
73. Cookson MS, Herr HW, Zhang ZF, et al. The treated natural history of high risk superficial bladder cancer: 15-year outcome. *J Urol*. 1997;158:62-67.
74. Herr HW. The value of a second transurethral resection in evaluating patients with bladder tumors. *J Urol*. 1999;162:74-76.
75. Fradet Y, Grossman HB, Gomella L, et al. A comparison of hexaminolevulinate fluorescence cystoscopy and white light cystoscopy for the detection of carcinoma in situ in patients with bladder cancer: a phase III, multicenter study. *J Urol*. 2007;178:68-73; discussion 73.
76. Esrig D, Freeman JA, Stein JP, et al. Early cystectomy for clinical stage T1 transitional cell carcinoma of the bladder. *Semin Urol Oncol*. 1997;15:154-160.
77. Madersbacher S, Hochreiter W, Burkhard F, et al. Radical cystectomy for bladder cancer today—a homogeneous series without neoadjuvant therapy. *J Clin Oncol*. 2003;21:690-696.
78. Lee CT, Madii R, Daignault S, et al. Cystectomy delay more than 3 months from initial bladder cancer diagnosis results in decreased disease specific and overall survival. *J Urol*. 2006;175:1262-1267; discussion 1267.
79. Herr HW. Extent of pelvic lymph node dissection during radical cystectomy: where and why! *Eur Urol*. 2010;57:212-213.
80. Shipley WU, Zietman AL, Kaufman DS, et al. Selective bladder preservation by trimodality therapy for patients with muscularis propria-invasive bladder cancer and who are cystectomy candidates—the Massachusetts General Hospital and Radiation Therapy Oncology Group experiences. *Semin Radiat Oncol*. 2005;15:36-41.
81. Logothetis CJ. Organ preservation in bladder carcinoma: a matter of selection. *J Clin Oncol*. 1991;9:1525-1526.
82. James ND, Hussain SA, Hall E, et al. Radiotherapy with or without chemotherapy in muscle-invasive bladder cancer. *N Engl J Med*. 2012;366:1477-1488.
83. Grossman HB, Natale RB, Tangen CM, et al. Neoadjuvant chemotherapy plus cystectomy compared with cystectomy alone for locally advanced bladder cancer [see comment] [erratum appears in *N Engl J Med*. 2003 Nov 6;349(19):1880]. *N Engl J Med*. 2003;349:859-866.
84. Tilki D, Svatek RS, Karakiewicz PI, et al. Characteristics and outcomes of patients with pT4 urothelial carcinoma at radical cystectomy: a retrospective international study of 583 patients. *J Urol*. 2010;183:87-93.
85. Millikan R, Dinney C, Swanson D, et al. Integrated therapy for locally advanced bladder cancer: final report of a randomized trial of cystectomy plus adjuvant M-VAC versus cystectomy with both preoperative and postoperative M-VAC. *J Clin Oncol*. 2001;19:4005-4013.
86. Siefker-Radtke AO, Dinney CP, Shen Y, et al. A phase 2 clinical trial of sequential neoadjuvant chemotherapy with ifosfamide, doxorubicin, and gemcitabine followed by cisplatin, gemcitabine, and ifosfamide in locally advanced urothelial cancer:

final results. *Cancer.* 2013;119:540-547.

87. Siefker-Radtke A, Kamat A, Corn P, et al. Neoadjuvant chemotherapy with DDMVAC and bevacizumab in high-risk urothelial cancer: results from a phase II trial at the M. D. Anderson Cancer Center [abstracr]. *J Clin Oncol.* 2012;30:261.
88. Plimack ER, Hoffman-Censits JH, Viterbo R, et al. Accelerated methotrexate, vinblastine, doxorubicin, and cisplatin is safe, effective, and efficient neoadjuvant treatment for muscle-invasive bladder cancer: results of a multicenter phase II study with molecular correlates of response and toxicity. *J Clin Oncol.* 2014;32:1895-1901.
89. Choueiri TK, Jacobus S, Bellmunt J, et al. Neoadjuvant dose-dense methotrexate, vinblastine, doxorubicin, and cisplatin with pegfilgrastim support in muscle-invasive urothelial cancer: pathologic, radiologic, and biomarker correlates. *J Clin Oncol.* 2014;32:1889-1894.
90. Siefker-Radtke AO, Choi W, Melquist J, et al. Gene expression profiling in the context of neoadjuvant chemotherapy with DDMVAC+B (dose-dense methotrexate, vinblastine, doxorubicin, cisplatin, and bevacizumab) can predict clinical outcomes and tumor biology [abstract]. *Cancer Res.* 2014;74:241.
91. Sweeney P, Millikan R, Donat M, et al. Is there a therapeutic role for post-chemotherapy retroperitoneal lymph node dissection in metastatic transitional cell carcinoma of the bladder? *J Urol.* 2003;169:2113-2117.
92. Donat SM, Herr H, Bajorin DF, et al. Methotrexate, vinblastine, doxorubicin and cisplatin chemotherapry and cystectomy for unresectable bladder cancer. *J Urol.* 1996;156:368-371.
93. Siefker-Radtke AO, Millikan RE, Tu SM, et al. Phase III trial of fluorouracil, interferon alpha-2b, and cisplatin versus methotrexate, vinblastine, doxorubicin, and cisplatin in metastatic or unresectable urothelial cancer. *J Clin Oncol.* 2002;20:1361-1367.
94. Siefker-Radtke AO, Walsh GL, Pisters LL, et al. Is there a role for surgery in the management of metastatic urothelial cancer? The M. D. Anderson experience. *J Urol.* 2004;171:145-148.
95. Kenworthy P, Tanguay S, Dinney CP. The risk of upper tract recurrence following cystectomy in patients with transitional cell carcinoma involving the distal ureter [see comment]. *J Urol.* 1996;155:501-503.
96. Sternberg CN, Yagoda A, Scher HI, et al. Preliminary results of M-VAC (methotrexate, vinblastine, doxorubicin and cisplatin) for transitional cell carcinoma of the urothelium. *J Urol.* 1985;133:403-407.
97. Loehrer PJ Sr, Einhorn LH, Elson PJ, et al. A randomized comparison of cisplatin alone or in combination with methotrexate, vinblastine, and doxorubicin in patients with metastatic urothelial carcinoma: a cooperative group study. *J Clin Oncol.* 1992;10:1066-1073.
98. Logothetis CJ, Dexeus FH, Finn L, et al. A prospective randomized trial comparing MVAC and CISCA chemotherapy for patients with metastatic urothelial tumors. *J Clin Oncol.* 1990;8:1050-1055.
99. Bamias A, Aravantinos G, Deliveliotis C, et al. Docetaxel and cisplatin with granulocyte colony-stimulating factor (G-CSF) versus MVAC with G-CSF in advanced urothelial carcinoma: a multicenter, randomized, phase III study from the Hellenic Cooperative Oncology Group. *J Clin Oncol.* 2004;22:220-228.
100. Sternberg CN, de Mulder PH, Schornagel JH, et al. Randomized phase III trial of high-dose-intensity methotrexate, vinblastine, doxorubicin, and cisplatin (MVAC) chemotherapy and recombinant human granulocyte colony-stimulating factor versus classic MVAC in advanced urothelial tract tumors: European Organization for Research and Treatment of Cancer Protocol no. 30924. *J Clin Oncol.* 2001;19:2638-2646.
101. von der Maase H, Hansen SW, Roberts JT, et al. Gemcitabine and cisplatin versus methotrexate, vinblastine, doxorubicin, and cisplatin in advanced or metastatic bladder cancer: results of a large, randomized, multinational, multicenter, phase III study. *J Clin Oncol.* 2000;18:3068-3077.
102. Tu SM, Hossan E, Amato R, et al. Paclitaxel, cisplatin and methotrexate combination chemotherapy is active in the treatment of refractory urothelial malignancies. *J Urol.* 1995;154:1719-1722.
103. Bellmunt J, Guillem V, Paz-Ares L, et al. Phase I-II study of paclitaxel, cisplatin, and gemcitabine in advanced transitional-cell carcinoma of the urothelium. Spanish Oncology Genitourinary Group. *J Clin Oncol.* 2000;18:3247-3255.
104. Milowsky MI, Nanus DM, Maluf FC, et al. Final results of sequential doxorubicin plus gemcitabine and ifosfamide, paclitaxel, and cisplatin chemotherapy in patients with metastatic or locally advanced transitional cell carcinoma of the urothelium. *J Clin Oncol.* 2009;27:4062-4067.
105. Pagliaro LC, Millikan RE, Tu SM, et al. Cisplatin, gemcitabine, and ifosfamide as weekly therapy: a feasibility and phase II study of salvage treatment for advanced transitional-cell carcinoma. *J Clin Oncol.* 2002;20:2965-2970.
106. Smith DC, Mackler NJ, Dunn RL, et al. Phase II trial of paclitaxel, carboplatin and gemcitabine in patients with locally advanced carcinoma of the bladder. *J Urol.* 2008;180:2384-2388; discussion 2388.
107. Pagliaro L, Munsell M, Harris D, Carolla R, Siefker-Radtke A. Gemcitabine, paclitaxel, and doxorubisin for patients with urothelial carcinoma and renal insufficiency: preliminary results of a multlicenter phase II study [abstract]. *J Clin Oncol.* 2011;29:246.
108. Nagabhushan TL, Maneval DC, Benedict WF, et al. Enhancement of intravesical delivery with Syn3 potentiates interferon-alpha2b gene therapy for superficial bladder cancer. *Cytokine Growth Factor Rev.* 2007;18:389-394.
109. Sharma P, Shen Y, Wen S, et al. CD8 tumor-infiltrating lymphocytes are predictive of survival in muscle-invasive urothelial carcinoma. *Proc Natl Acad Sci USA.* 2007;104:3967-3972.

37

Prostate Cancer

第三十七章　前列腺癌

Mehmet A. Bilen
Christopher J. Logothetis
Paul G. Corn

中文导读

前列腺癌的治疗近年来得到了很大的进步和提高。本章首先介绍了前列腺癌的流行病学及临床特征，特别是与种族的关系以及遗传易感性。接着介绍了前列腺癌的组织形态学相关内容，包括Gleason分级系统、前列腺活检标本及手术切除标本的评估、分子遗传学特征、组织变异（特殊的形态学亚型）、可能的癌前病变、分期、早期筛查及化学预防等。随后根据疾病的风险分层状态和分期介绍了临床处理原则。针对局限期疾病，强调在风险分层的前提下采取不同强度的治疗手段：如对于低风险的局限期疾病，可采取主动监测或适当的局部治疗；而对于高风险或局部晚期前列腺癌，更强调全身和局部治疗联合的综合治疗。针对转移性前列腺癌，雄激素阻断为主的全身治疗仍是标准策略。对于雄激素依赖性疾病，列举了雄激素阻断治疗的临床应用原则，包括用药时机、药物类型和选择以及药物不良反应的处理；对于雄激素剥夺治疗耐药的肿瘤，介绍了二线内分泌治疗药物选择、不同的化疗方案以及新兴的针对肿瘤基质或免疫系统的靶向治疗等。

Over the past decade, insight into the biological basis of prostate cancer development and progression has influenced our approach to treating patients with the disease. While research efforts have historically focused on the prostate cancer epithelial cell, there is growing evidence that interactions between the host tissue microenvironment and the cancer epithelial cell are critical for tumorigenesis. Understanding the bidirectional cancer cell–host interaction now dominates prostate cancer research.

Prostate cancers have recognizable clinical features that allow anticipation of their clinical behavior. Fortunately, the progression from localized, androgen-dependent disease to castration-resistant disease with bone-forming metastases occurs in only a minority of patients. To conceptualize the clinical heterogeneity displayed along this continuum, patients have historically been assigned to different "clinical states" (eg, metastatic castrate vs noncastrate) to help structure treatment recommendations and therapy development ([1, 2]). However, this approach has been limited by the fact that patients within each state display wide biological heterogeneity and response to therapy. To address this, improved classification of the disease based on the underlying molecular mechanisms of progression is necessary. This effort will create a "marker-driven" strategy to more reliably predict prostate cancer progression, permit optimal selection of specific therapies for individual patients, and apply therapy to only those patients who need it. This strategy will favorably improve the outcome of selected patients threatened by their disease while avoiding unnecessary morbidity to the majority who are not.

EPIDEMIOLOGY AND CLINICAL FEATURES

Prostate cancer is a major health-care challenge in the United States ([3]). It is the second most common cancer in men (behind skin cancer) and the second leading cause of cancer death (behind lung cancer). There are a number of unique clinical features of prostate cancer that distinguish it from other solid tumor types:

1. Despite the high prevalence of prostate cancer, the majority of patients diagnosed with the disease eventually die from other causes. This is in striking contrast to lung cancer, where the majority of patients diagnosed with the disease die from it.
2. Cancer of the prostate often has a prolonged natural history. This is evidenced by a high incidence of occult malignancy in autopsy series of men who die from nonprostate cancer causes and in clinically normal prostates of men undergoing cystoprostatectomy for bladder cancer. Therefore, over the course of a normal lifetime, most men will develop "clinically occult" prostate cancer that will never produce symptoms, require treatment, or cause death.
3. The incidence of detected carcinoma increases with age.
4. Androgens are a major driving force in normal prostate development and are implicated in tumorigenesis.
5. Prostate cancer is typically multifocal, commonly presenting as synchronous carcinomas arising in multiple locations, and the malignant potential is determined by the sum of the primary and secondary grades (Gleason score). Thus, biologic heterogeneity is an inherent property of each tumor.
6. Clinical prostate cancer is more prevalent in Western than Eastern societies, although incidence rates increase for men from China and Japan who immigrate to the United States. This observation implicates environmental factors (diet, lifestyle, etc) in prostate cancer development.
7. Prostate cancers have a predictable rate and pattern of progression, with bone-forming metastases dominating the clinical progression in the majority of patients with advanced disease. This observation supports the view that the bone-epithelial interaction is central to the progression of prostate cancer.

Aging

It has long been recognized that prostate cancer is a disease of the elderly, and epidemiologic data demonstrate that rates of prostate cancer incidence and mortality increase with age ([4]). While prostate-specific antigen (PSA) screening has led to an earlier average age at diagnosis, mortality is still largely seen in patients 70 years of age or older. As the longevity of populations increases worldwide, the burden of prostate cancer creates a significant health-care challenge. This has generated a sense of urgency among physicians to refine our ability to predict cancer virulence and apply therapy to those patients who need it.

Endocrine

Androgens are central to the normal growth, differentiation, and function of the prostate gland, although the role of androgen receptor (AR) signaling in prostate carcinogenesis and progression has not been fully elucidated. Even in the clinically castrate state (serum testosterone <50 ng/mL), there is growing evidence that prostate cancer cells continue to rely on AR signaling for proliferation ([5]). One of the principal mechanisms for this involves a gradual shift from endocrine sources of androgens (ie, from the testes and adrenal glands) to paracrine/autocrine/intracrine (ie, intratumoral) sources during prostate cancer progression (Fig. 37-1). This occurs through the peripheral conversion of adrenal steroid precursors (eg, dehydroepiandrosterone and androstenedione) in prostate and bone tissues expressing CYP17 enzymes ([6]). Other mechanisms accounting for castrate resistance include intratumoral amplification of AR, mutations of AR, changes in levels of AR cofactors, and ligand-independent activation of AR (Fig. 37-1).

Diet and Obesity

Several lines of clinical and experimental evidence support a central role for diet, caloric intake, and obesity in the development of prostate cancer with lethal potential. Obesity, defined as body mass index (BMI) above 30, is manifested by overgrowth of white adipose tissue (WAT). Obesity has been associated with incidence, progression, and mortality of prostate cancer ([7, 8]). The mechanism for the association between obesity and prostate cancer progression is poorly understood. Current models suggest that predetermined genetic traits associated with both obesity and cancers are influenced by lifestyle components such as diet and physical activity. However, epidemiological studies show that cancer can be accelerated in obese patients irrespective of their lifestyle. Thus, it has been proposed that WAT itself may have a direct effect on cancer progression.

Mechanisms linking obesity and aggressive prostate cancer include signaling through insulin-like growth factor 1 (IGF-1) and adipokines ([9]). The insulin/IGF-1 axis has been widely implicated in obesity-induced tumorigenesis, including prostate cancer ([10]). Primary human prostate cancer commonly expresses the insulin receptor, suggesting insulin may stimulate tumor growth ([11]). Both excess body weight and a high plasma concentration of C-peptide are associated with increased prostate cancer–specific mortality ([12]). In addition, the antidiabetic agent metformin has been shown to reduce all-cause and prostate cancer–specific mortality among diabetic men ([13]).

Beyond changes in insulin, obesity alters levels of adipokines (such as leptin, adiponectin) due to chronic subclinical inflammation. Leptin is associated with in vitro protumor effect in human prostate cancer cell lines ([14]), but epidemiologic studies have failed to consistently establish an association with prostate cancer risk and mortality ([15]). In contrast to leptin, adiponectin serum levels are reduced in obesity and have largely antitumor effects ([16]).

Race and Ethnicity

African Americans have a higher frequency of death from prostate cancer compared to Caucasian and Hispanic Americans. This has variably been attributed to differences in steroid metabolism, genetics, environmental effects, or social factors ([17, 18]). There is a reduced incidence of prostate cancer among Chinese and Japanese Americans, but their incidence is higher than that reported in native Chinese or Japanese persons. Of interest is the fact that northern European men have a higher frequency of prostate cancer than men from southern Europe. A similar finding has been reported in the United States, suggesting that the incidence of prostate cancer is inversely related to sun exposure. These findings have epidemiologically linked prostate cancer to vitamin D metabolism.

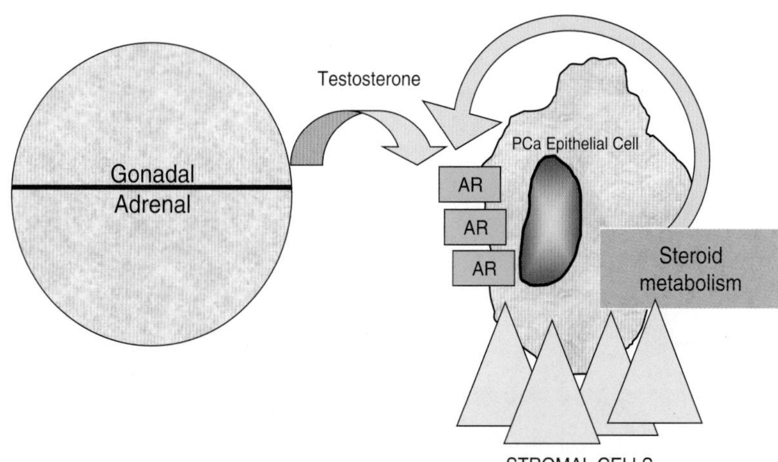

FIGURE 37-1 Androgen sources switch from endocrine to paracrine/autocrine during disease progression. PCa, prostate cancer.

Genetic Predisposition

As with breast and colon cancer, familial clustering of prostate cancer has been reported. Unlike with breast and colon cancer, however, specific genetic lesions have not been identified to merit the routine use of genetic screening for prostate cancer. The search for "prostate cancer genes" has identified candidate genetic events implicated in tumorigenesis, but these findings have been more useful in understanding the underlying etiology of prostate cancer than in screening. For example, a major hereditary prostate cancer susceptibility locus resides at 1q24, although the responsible gene(s) remains under investigation ([19, 20]). More recently, men carrying *BRCA1/BRCA2* (breast cancer 1 and 2) mutations have been shown to be at increased risk of developing prostate cancer ([21, 22]). In addition, it has been suggested that BRCA-associated prostate cancer cases may be more virulent than nonfamilial cases ([23, 24]). However, it remains unclear how this information will influence management decisions for individual patients.

RELEVANT HISTOMORPHOLOGY OF PROSTATE CANCER

Most epithelial cancers arise from the prostatic acinus, with fewer than 10% having a pure ductal origin (this is the opposite of the pattern seen in cancers of the pancreas and breast, where ductal cancers are far more common than those arising in the acinar portion of the secretory unit). The majority show glandular differentiation (ie, adenocarcinoma) (Fig. 37-2A). Importantly, mucin is essentially never seen in prostate cancer. Historically, numerous grading systems have been devised, using all of the typical morphologic criteria by which pathologists can sometimes infer biologic potential. While more than 20 systems have been put forward, prostate cancers are now almost universally graded according to the system of Gleason.

Gleason Grading System

The Gleason system is unique among pathologic grading systems because it is a composite classification based on a combination of architectural and cellular features often considered in the grading of other epithelial cancers. As originally described, the Gleason system includes two components:

1. There are five patterns, or grades, ranging from normal architecture to arrays of cells without any glandular organization at all. At our institution, because unequivocal criteria for malignancy already correspond to Gleason grade 2 and the Gleason grade 1 category is rarely reported, prostate cancers are assigned Gleason grades ranging from 3 through 5.
2. The Gleason score is obtained by assigning one Gleason grade to the most dominant (ie, "primary") pattern and another to the next most common (ie, "secondary") pattern. By convention, such data are expressed as a sum, with the primary pattern listed first. Thus, the Gleason score can range from 2 (ie, 1 + 1) to 10 (5 + 5). At MD Anderson, these scores range from 6 to 10, reflecting our decision not to assign a Gleason grade of 1.

A major advantage of the Gleason grading system is its reproducibility and ability to distinguish different cancer phenotypes that influence clinical management. The system is most useful for tumors falling at one the extremes (eg, Gleason 6 or less versus Gleason 8 to 10). However, a major disadvantage of the system is that it does not provide a refined view of Gleason 7 tumors, the most commonly reported type. Gleason 7 cancers (ie, 3 + 4 or 4 + 3) represent a clinically heterogeneous

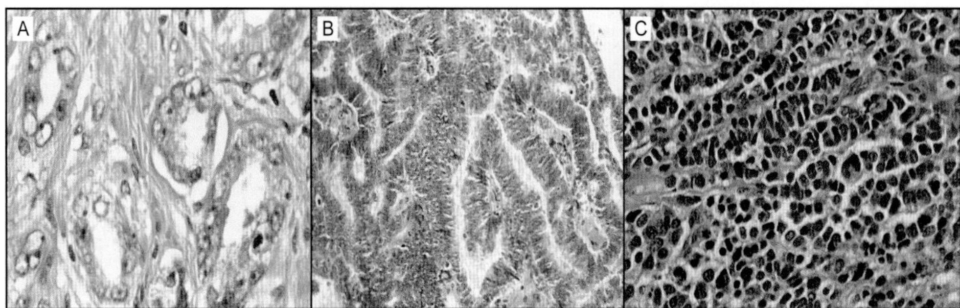

FIGURE 37-2 A. Architecture of prostate adenocarcinoma. B. Architecture of prostate ductal carcinoma. C. Architecture of prostate small cell carcinoma.

group with variable biologic potential and clinical outcome ([25]). Despite efforts to improve stratification of Gleason 7 tumors, it is clear the Gleason system is inherently limited by light microscopic methodology to evaluate morphology. Thus, most investigators are now looking to incorporate molecular characterization of tumors into the current grading system.

Assessment of Prostate Biopsies and Prostatectomy Specimens

Gleason grading is a validated system to prognosticate untreated prostate cancers sampled at initial diagnosis. However, the common practice of applying Gleason grading to treated cancers may be misleading. At MD Anderson, for example, pathology reports of specimens obtained after hormone ablation typically indicate "hormonal treatment effect" rather than a Gleason grade per se. Thus, Gleason scores from serial biopsies obtained pre- and posttherapy from the same patient should be interpreted with careful regard to treatment effects. To address this problem, our group has proposed a novel "posttherapy" histologic classification to introduce uniformity in analysis of treated tissue specimens ([26]). If prospectively validated, this system should prove useful in prognosticating preoperatively treated prostate cancers.

An additional confounding variable is tissue sampling. We recognize that there is intratumoral heterogeneity of grade within individual prostate cancers. Thus, it logically follows that the extent and areas of sampling will affect the accuracy of grading and staging. The development of techniques to obtain prostate tissue samples with ultrasound guidance and limited patient morbidity has had a major effect on stage and grade assignment. We increasingly find that the completeness of tissue sampling as measured by the number and distribution of transrectal biopsies greatly influences the adequacy of tumor staging and grading. Biopsy algorithms have been developed to ensure adequate number and distribution of the biopsies ([27]).

Many of the challenges attributed to the sampling errors that occur with needle biopsies can be overcome with proper handling of the prostate following surgery. Assigning a primary and secondary Gleason score is straightforward in a properly processed specimen. This requires great attention to detail in assessing whether the cancer has invaded beyond the prostate capsule (extracapsular) or beyond the margin of resection (margin positive). Effective communication between the surgeon and pathologist is essential to properly identify the extent and site of surgical margin involvement. As the therapeutic benefit of postoperative radiation therapy is better appreciated, the importance of these aspects has proportionally increased.

Molecular Genetics of Prostate Cancer

In prostate cancer, gene fusions between *TMPRSS2* (21q22.3), an androgen-regulated gene, and *ERG*, from the ETS family of transcription factors (21q22.2), are common ([28]). However, the functional and prognostic significance of *TMRPSS2-ERG* remain poorly understood. Currently, detection and measurement of *TMPRSS2-ERG* are not performed in standard clinical practice.

Additional studies have sought to refine the diagnostic classification of prostate cancer through molecular methods. Unfortunately, no consensus yet exists about the usefulness of molecular phenotypic (or genotypic) characterization in prostate cancer. Using immunohistochemistry, we do know that expression of specific proteins in human specimens has been linked to the clinical course of the disease. For example, loss of functional PTEN, mutations in p53, and increased expression of Bcl-2 are some of the widely reported gain- and loss-of-function changes that have been correlated with prostate cancer progression and mechanistically linked to castration-resistant growth ([29, 30]). Despite this link to biology and correlation with clinical outcome, the methods provide insufficient additional clinical information to justify their routine use.

Prostate Cancer Variants

The two most prominent morphologic subtypes are ductal and small cell/anaplastic variants.

Ductal Cancers

The ductal variant of prostate cancer in its pure form is unusual. More often, ductal and acinar components are mixed, and the relative contribution of the ductal variant to the clinical phenotype of the cancer is unclear. Our impression of the behavior of ductal cancers of the prostate is based on those tumors that are either dominant or pure ductal in origin (Fig. 37-2B). The clinical features that lead us to suspect its presence include the lack of proportional rises in serum PSA concentrations with invasion of the base of the bladder (occasionally mistaken for urothelial cancer), soft tissue distribution of metastases, or lytic bone metastases. For localized disease, patients with pure ductal adenocarcinoma have a better clinical outcome after radical prostatectomy than patients with mixed ductal adenocarcinoma ([31]). However, metastatic cancers as more aggressive and demonstrate a higher probability of developing visceral metastases than pure acinar adenocarcinomas.

Small Cell/Anaplastic Cancers

Small cell carcinoma of the prostate is clinically distinguishable from prostate adenocarcinoma in predictable ways. It is castration resistant, is highly metastatic, produces little or no PSA, and causes lytic rather than blastic bone metastases. In addition, in comparison to adenocarcinoma, small cell prostate cancer more frequently metastasizes to lymph nodes and visceral organs (eg, liver or lung). It can arise de novo or more commonly as a delayed manifestation of progression in patients with a history of high-grade adenocarcinomas following therapy (hormone ablation, radiation therapy, or chemotherapy). The classic clinical presentation is a patient with a precipitously enlarging prostate associated with obstructive symptoms and very little (to no) PSA production. Interestingly, the evolution to a neuroendocrine phenotype is often associated with expression of carcinoembryonic antigen (CEA). For many patients, the CEA will be a much more useful monitoring tool than PSA.

In our experience, small cell carcinomas are also frequently detected in metastatic sites. Our approach is to biopsy sites with unusual features (lytic as opposed to blastic metastases or soft tissue metastases), particularly in those patients whose PSA concentration is judged to be lower than would be expected for the volume of cancer. Requests are made to pathology to analyze the tissue for neuroendocrine markers (chromogranin, synaptophysin, etc). Although standard criteria for establishing a diagnosis have not emerged, most of these cancers will show "salt-and-pepper" chromatin, express synaptophysin and chromogranin, and display a high nuclear/cytoplasm ratio (Fig. 37-2C), However, the diagnosis of small cell carcinoma does not require proof of neuroendocrine differentiation.

For this reason, we have added the term *anaplastic* to our nomenclature to describe aggressive tumors presenting clinically as "neuroendocrine-like" but lacking neuroendocrine markers. Until more precise genotype-phenotype associations are elucidated, we recognize that tumors displaying the clinical phenotype described may display heterogeneity with respect to neuroendocrine differentiation. Small cell/anaplastic carcinomas are highly responsive to etoposide and cisplatin-based chemotherapy but are generally incurable [32-34].

Candidate Premalignant Lesions

Prostatic Intraepithelial Neoplasia

The search for premalignant lesions of the prostate has resulted in the identification of two candidate morphologic lesions [35]. The first and most promising premalignant lesion is prostatic intraepithelial neoplasia (PIN). Grades I and II PIN are observed but have not been reliably associated with cancer or linked with confidence to prostate cancer development or progression. Thus, the reporting of grades I and II PIN has fallen into disfavor at MD Anderson and at most leading institutions. Grade III PIN has been linked to the presence of cancer in many studies, but it does not justify a therapeutic intervention (eg, prostatectomy). Rather, its presence leads to the recommendation of a more thorough biopsy to search for coexistent cancer or a repeat biopsy within 6 to 12 months. Grade III PIN is frequently linked to the presence of established cancer in other regions of the prostate, and as a consequence it rarely serves as a useful early predictive marker. Therein lies the difficulty of performing prevention studies targeting PIN. Most MD Anderson clinicians share the view that a report of multifocal PIN III is nearly identical to a report of low-grade prostate cancer, but with the important caveat that there is insufficient evidence to justify routine intervention (surgery or radiation).

The second potential premalignant lesion is proliferative inflammatory atrophy (PIA) [36]. Histologically, these lesions are characterized by inflammatory infiltrates associated with atrophic epithelium. Compared with normal epithelium, there is an increased fraction of proliferating epithelial cells within PIAs. These lesions are thought to provide a mechanistic link between chronic infection or inflammation and the predisposition to develop prostate cancer. However, in contrast to PINs, adenocarcinomas rarely arise from PIAs, and PIAs are often observed in prostate biopsies that have no evidence of cancer. Thus, it remains unclear if PIAs are truly precursor lesions for prostate cancer. Ongoing studies seek to address this.

Staging

It is difficult to precisely assess the extent of prostate cancer on clinical criteria alone. The major benchmark of local extent that influences treatment—organ confined versus non–organ confined—is essentially impossible to distinguish by rectal examination and is not easily appreciated by any imaging modality. Furthermore, PSA levels do not accurately inform about extraprostatic extension of disease. Thus, it is common to employ an array of modalities, including transrectal ultrasound, computed tomography, conventional magnetic resonance imaging (MRI), MRI with an endorectal receiver coil, complex biopsy strategies designed to sample the seminal vesicles and extraprostatic space, and even pelvic lymph node sampling, to determine disease extent. Clearly, each of these modalities offers a different level of sensitivity for detecting lesions and can vary markedly in efficacy. In the final analysis, the concept of clinical stage is meaningless without proper context. One must ask, What is the clinical stage by a particular set of diagnostic tests?

The Case for Prostate Cancer Screening

With the advent of PSA screening, there has been a dramatic increase in the number of younger men detected with localized disease. Along with improved outcomes for local therapy (surgery or radiation), it logically follows that PSA screening has contributed to the improved survival rates for men diagnosed with localized prostate cancer. However, the benefits of PSA screening remain controversial for clinicians and a source of confusion for patients. For clinicians, there has been a lack of level 1 evidence supporting the use of PSA screening. The two large randomized screening trials (with greater than 250,000 patients) has not helped clarify the issue because one trial did not show a survival benefit (the PLCO Cancer Screening Trial in the United States), while the other one did (the ERSPC trial in Europe) ([37, 38]). While confounding factors to each study limit a definitive conclusion about PSA screening, the enormous expense and time required may discourage future PSA screening trials. Available evidence favors clinician discussion of the pros and cons of PSA screening with average-risk men aged 55 to 69 years. Other strategies to mitigate the potential harms of screening include considering biennial screening, a higher PSA threshold for biopsy, and conservative therapy for men receiving a new diagnosis of prostate cancer.

Although the US Preventive Services Task Force no longer recommends routine screening ([39]), in our practice, we recommend annual PSA and digital rectal examination (DRE) for all healthy men starting at age 50 or age 40 for those at high risk (eg, those men with a family history or African Americans). Early inclusion of the patient in the decision-making process is essential to optimize patient care given the ambiguities regarding the cost effectiveness and clinical value of widespread screening for prostate cancer. The rationale for routine screening that justifies routine application is outlined in Table 37-1.

The Case for Chemoprevention

Given the high prevalence of prostate cancer and the significant burden of therapy for patients, there is great interest in preventing the disease altogether or preventing lethal progression of the disease. Inhibitors of 5α-reductase enzymes (types 1 and 2 enzymes convert testosterone to dihydrotestosterone, the predominant and more potent agonist of AR signaling in prostate tissues) have demonstrated potential in this regard. Two randomized, placebo-controlled clinical trials utilizing finasteride (a type II inhibitor) and dutasteride (a type I/II inhibitor) have demonstrated a reduction in prostate cancer in healthy men who had no evidence for prostate cancer at enrollment but did have risk for developing disease (based on age and PSA) ([40, 41]). A third clinical trial evaluated the ability of dutasteride to prevent prostate cancer progression in patients with low-grade, low-risk, localized prostate cancer at study entry (REDEEM), and dutasteride could provide a favorable addition to active surveillance for men with low-risk prostate cancer ([42]). While we have not adapted chemoprevention as standard of care, we are encouraging patients with low-risk prostate cancer to participate in preoperative trials that offer short-duration 5α-reductase inhibition prior to radical prostatectomy. Our goal is to elucidate molecular signatures that (1) predict response (or resistance) to 5α-reductase inhibition, (2) characterize therapy-specific effects on epithelial-stromal compartments, and (3) refine existing risk stratification schemas.

Table 37-1 Rationale for Prostate Cancer Screening

• Reduction in prostate cancer mortality coincides with the introduction of routine PSA screening.
• Patients whose cancers are detected with PSA screening have early-stage disease.
• Long-term disease-free survival is linked to treatment of early-stage disease.
• Randomized trials demonstrate a survival advantage for early surgical intervention for early-stage disease.

PATIENT MANAGEMENT BY DISEASE STATE

Clinically Localized Disease at Presentation

As a result of widespread screening of men by PSA and DRE, the majority of patients are seen with clinically localized disease at diagnosis. Unfortunately, it is not always obvious how to match the individual patient with the most appropriate management. In an abstract sense, patients with clinically localized prostate cancer fall into one of four theoretical categories:

- *Those not destined to have any clinical manifestations of their disease.* These patients are actually harmed by any intervention, including further surveillance.
- *Those destined to have a clinical manifestation of cancer but will not to die of it.* These patients might benefit from definitive therapy (such as prostatectomy or radiation) but would likely benefit equally from less-morbid intervention (eg, minimally invasive surgery).
- *Those destined to have life-threatening disease for whom definitive therapy will be curative.* Patients who can be cured, or for whom there will be a substantial alteration of the natural history of their disease, constitute the group that will unequivocally benefit from definitive local therapy.
- *Those destined to have life-threatening disease for whom the opportunity to cure by means of local therapy either*

never existed or passed. For these patients, however, control of the primary could still be an important component of an overall treatment strategy that considers the probability of local versus distant progression, comorbidity, and other factors.

The common practice of urologists and radiation therapists is to assume that nearly every patient falls into the third category, and thus they recommend definitive therapy for the vast majority of newly diagnosed cases of localized prostate cancer. Unfortunately, available evidence suggests that less than half of patients are in category 3, so it is not surprising that understanding the role of definitive therapy in eliminating prostate cancer morbidity and mortality has been both difficult and controversial. In fact, these issues underscore the fact that overtreatment of "clinically insignificant" prostate cancers certainly occurs. The significant cost and morbidity associated with local treatment also adds to the difficulty of managing these patients (whether the patient ultimately benefited from the therapy or not).

In patients with newly diagnosed localized disease, current prognostic and predictive models rely on data derived from large prostatectomy series conducted at major academic centers. For example, investigators at Johns Hopkins initially published a predictive model relating the rate of finding disease that is not confined to the prostate (by assessing the surgical specimen) as a function of three readily available preoperative clinical parameters: PSA, Gleason score from the core biopsy, and the clinical stage based on DRE ([43, 44]). The correlation of these features with pathologically organ-confined disease, summarized in the famous "Partin tables," provided sobering evidence that commonly encountered subsets of patients had a surprisingly high risk of disease that was not confined to the prostate. Of course, not all patients with pathologically organ-confined disease relapse, and not all patients with pathologically organ-confined cancers are cured. Thus, the importance of this particular surrogate outcome was and remains uncertain. Nevertheless, the effect of the Partin tables on clinical practice has been profound. They have driven the application of prostatectomy to patients with smaller and smaller volumes of cancer. It is clear that although more patients are remaining free of disease after prostatectomy, this comes paradoxically at the cost of operating on many patients who may not have needed surgery or not operating on many patients who would have benefited from good local control even if the surgery were not curative.

Additional models have been developed to predict outcomes following radical prostatectomy or radiation therapy. Based on the work of D'Amico, a combination of pretherapy PSA, Gleason score, and clinical stage can be used to stratify patients into low (T1-T2a and Gleason score 2-6 and PSA <10 ng/mL); intermediate (T2b-T2c or Gleason score 7 or PSA 10-20 ng/mL); high (T3a or Gleason score 8-10 or PSA >20 ng/mL); and locally advanced (T3b-T4) groups that predict risk for both biochemical recurrence and survival following definitive local therapy (radical prostatectomy or radiation) ([45]). Similarly, Kattan et al developed postoperative nomograms for predicting prostate cancer recurrence after radical prostatectomy ([46]). These tools not only help guide recommendations for individual patients, but also help stratify patients for clinical trials. For example, low-risk patients can be directed toward "active surveillance" trials, while high-risk patients can be direct toward adjuvant/neoadjuvant trials. The rationale for the use of predictive nomograms is outlined in Table 37-2.

Despite the efforts detailed previously, tumors with identical morphology and clinicopathologic characteristics often display biologic heterogeneity (ie, some "low-risk" tumors rapidly progress, while some "high-risk" tumors are relatively indolent). Thus, more refined models are needed. Recent efforts have sought to incorporate genetic tests to enhance current clinicopathologic risk stratification for patients newly diagnosed with localized prostate cancer. For example, PROLARIS (Myriad Genetics, Inc.) directly measures expression of 46 different genes in formalin-fixed paraffin-embedded tissue obtained by biopsy or prostatectomy ([47-49]), including 31 cell cycle progression (CCP) genes and 15 housekeeper genes that correlate with proliferation of prostate cancer. Low expression is associated with a low risk of disease progression, whereas high expression is more indicative of higher risk of disease progression, suggesting either close monitoring or additional therapy for the latter group of patients.

Other investigational approaches to improve risk stratification include assessing suspicious nodes or small-volume extracapsular extension by MRI or positron emission tomography, staging biopsies of seminal vesicles and extraprostatic tissue, and incorporation of molecular signatures. Within our group, a significant effort is under way to relate the expression of genes that may affect apoptotic threshold, invasion, angiogenesis, and AR signaling to biologic potential and

Table 37-2 Rationale for Use of Predictive Nomograms

- Gleason grade, clinical stage, and initial PSA are predictive of surgical stage, risk of subsequent relapse, and risk of cancer-specific mortality.
- Improving the ability to predict outcome will inform both physicians and patients about the risk/benefits of local therapy.
- Fewer patients will undergo unnecessary or futile surgery.

ultimately clinical outcome of localized tumors. These data suggest that both loss of tumor suppressor pathways (eg, p53) and gain of oncogene/antiapoptotic pathways (eg, Bcl-2) contributes to prostate cancer progression. In addition to these and other "epithelial" events, the importance of the host-epithelial interaction in prostate cancer progression has been supported by evidence that pathways involved in paracrine regulation of normal stromal-epithelial interactions have also been implicated in prostate cancer progression ([50-52]).

Therapy

Localized Low-Stage Prostate Cancer

In patients with localized low-stage disease (generally including low- and intermediate-risk groups based on the D'Amico risk stratification groups), the options offered include active surveillance, surgery, radiation, or presurgical clinical trials. Educating the patient about his treatment options is critical to make the best decision for each individual. Patients who are undecided or request more information about treatments and side effects are seen in our multidisciplinary clinic.

Critical evaluation of the relative merits of different therapies for localized low-stage prostate cancer is difficult. This is because patients in this category have a greater than 80% chance of 10-year progression-free survival following local therapy ([53-55]). Prostate cancer has a long natural history, and 10-year data for patients with low-risk prostate cancer remain immature with respect to cause-specific and disease-free survival. The contribution of delayed hormonal therapy and the appreciation that not all patients with a delayed PSA recurrence after local therapy are threatened by their disease have made comparisons between different treatment modalities difficult. As a consequence, the modification of older therapies or the application of new ones (such as brachytherapy, cryoablation, or proton beam therapy) is often judged by their complication profile and the rate of PSA-free survival with a relatively short follow-up. While seemingly logical, interpreting potential benefit from "new and improved" therapies is challenged by the impact of "stage migration" on outcomes. Stage migration refers to the fact that, as a consequence of awareness and PSA screening, younger patients with lower-stage cancer are diagnosed with increasing frequency. This trend of earlier therapy in younger patients with earlier-stage disease likely has an effect on the analysis of therapy efficacy and morbidity for low-stage cancer. Therefore, the practice of deriving conclusions from the comparison of nonrandomized study groups in low-stage prostate cancer is a dubious exercise.

In fact, in localized, low-stage prostate cancer, the principal therapeutic dilemma is whether to intervene at all. Increasingly, many investigators are recognizing that not all patients diagnosed with prostate cancer by histologic criteria have a disease that has lethal potential ([56]). Hence, many clinicians have explored a strategy of observation followed by delayed therapy if required. This strategy has historically been called "watchful waiting," but in recent years we have adopted the term *active surveillance*. This is because the definition of watchful waiting is ambiguous and includes the practice of not following or evaluating patients after diagnosis until they present with a prostate cancer–associated symptom(s). In contrast, active surveillance implies regular follow-ups with PSA evaluation, DRE, and repeat biopsies as indicated to inform the need for local therapy. Active surveillance acknowledges the reality that many patients with prostate cancer survive despite diagnosis and therapy, as opposed to benefiting directly from the intervention. At MD Anderson, the rationale for offering active surveillance is the idea that carefully monitored patients will require therapy with curative intent only if accompanied by objective evidence that their cancer has become life threatening. In this way, patients with truly indolent disease can be spared the morbidities of local therapy, while patients who show progression over time to potentially lethal disease will preserve the opportunity for curative therapy.

Active Surveillance With Deferred Treatment

Two categories of patients with low-stage disease are generally considered for active surveillance: (1) men who have a higher probability of dying from a comorbid illness (such as coronary artery disease) than from prostate cancer and (2) men whose cancer poses some risk for lethality but choose active surveillance because of concerns about consequences of therapy (eg, impotence or incontinence). The rationale for active surveillance is outlined in Table 37-3.

There are two central challenges of the active surveillance strategy. The first is that we do not yet have a validated method to anticipate progression of the disease to avoid "closing the window" on curative therapy. The second is that we lack methods to ensure reliable selection of all patients in whom the disease will be unlikely to spread while excluding all patients

Table 37-3 Rationale for Active Surveillance

• A significant portion of newly diagnosed patients will not develop clinical progression.
• Complications of local therapy exceed benefits in some patients.
• Close monitoring of selected patients with serial PSA measurements may avoid or delay initiation of potentially morbid or unnecessary therapy.

who will have lethal progression of the disease despite its initial morphologic appearance as low stage. Thus, this strategy, while supported by compelling logic, must be regarded as unproven. This is particularly true for those patients with a life expectancy of 15 years or more. As a patient's life span shortens due to comorbid conditions, the unproven nature of this strategy has less predicted impact on outcome. Thus, outside a clinical trial, active surveillance in our practice is routinely reserved for patients with low-stage disease and an expected survival of less than 10 years due to comorbidities.

Active surveillance for category 1 patients is not codified, and follow-up strategies (such as annual PSA checks) are designed by mutual agreement between the physician and patient. Select elderly patients whose cancer diagnosis was precipitated by an ill-advised PSA screening test may choose no further follow-up. In contrast, active surveillance for category 2 patients involves close observation with quarterly PSA checks and annual prostate biopsies. Often, these patients elect to undergo local therapy as the physical and emotional burden of close observation becomes more obvious. Despite the intensity of follow-up, the ability to anticipate progression of disease based on true biologic evidence as opposed to apparent progression caused by the randomness of the biopsies remains a major problem. These problems will be clarified with prospective studies accruing at several institutions.

Treatment of Low-Stage Disease With Available Therapy

Although there is much debate about the relative merits of radiation therapy and surgery for patients with localized low-stage prostate cancer, the inescapable conclusion is that both treatment groups have excellent survival, and the principal issues influencing choice are related to therapy-associated morbidity. Interestingly, competition between radiation therapy and surgery has resulted in the reduction of morbidity to both therapies. The morbidity of radiation therapy—while retaining its effectiveness—has been greatly reduced, as has morbidity related to improvements in surgical techniques. Thus, for low-stage prostate cancer, the principal therapeutic recommendation is to treat those patients who have a greater than 15-year expected life expectancy. The primary recommendation is surgery or radiation therapy, with a bias toward surgery for those patients with an expected longevity of more than 20 years and a bias toward radiation therapy for those patients with an expected longevity of 15 years or less (Table 37-4).

Presurgical Trials for Low-Stage Disease

Presurgical trials facilitate the development of novel therapies and treatment strategies in prostate cancer by providing proof of "target engagement" by the drug(s) and modulation of the tumor phenotype in a therapeutically favorable manner ([57]). The principal goal of a *preoperative* clinical trial is to identify short-term molecular and pathologic tissue surrogates that establish target engagement and modulation of key signaling pathways by the drug(s). Because surgery is performed before cytoreduction or significant changes in the tumor phenotype are expected (as opposed to *neoadjuvant* trials), preoperative trials provide only limited inferences about the therapeutic potential of the drug(s) being tested. However, data from preoperative trials help identify the most promising therapeutic candidates worthy of further study. Preoperative studies of low-stage prostate cancer seek to identify molecular markers that characterize response to therapy and predict tumor biology.

Table 37-4 Rationale for Selection of Local Treatment Modality

- There are no clinical trials showing a therapeutic advantage of surgery over radiation therapy for localized disease.
- Either approach is associated with some risk of significant morbidity (initial impotence rates are higher with surgery).
- There is a reduction in impotence rates over time with radiation.
- Surgery provides better assessment of risk for future relapse by allowing molecular-pathologic analysis of the radical prostatectomy specimen.
- Radiation is ideally suited for patients who are physically unfit for surgery or those who have disease extending beyond the bounds of traditional surgical fields.
- Surgery improves symptom-free and overall survival in patients with localized disease.

High-Risk and Locally Advanced Prostate Cancer

As a general principle of oncology, high-risk and locally advanced tumors (based on the D'Amico risk stratification groups) are best treated with a combination of systemic therapy and aggressive local therapy. This strategy addresses occult disseminated disease while preventing local complications of the primary tumor. Despite the widely recognized poor outcomes for patients with seminal vesicle or regional node involvement, the application of optimum local control with systemic therapy has only recently become accepted ([58]).

Current multimodal therapies include radiation plus hormones and neoadjuvant therapy plus surgery. It is now well established that the addition of hormones to radiation therapy is superior to radiation therapy or hormones alone for patients with high-risk and locally advanced tumors ([59]). The duration and sequence of the combination are important in maximizing therapy benefit from the combination. Several lines of evidence suggest that initiating the androgen ablation 2 months prior to the radiation therapy is more effective than combined therapy from the outset or sequential therapy with radiation followed by androgen ablation. The available data demonstrate an increase in survival with a 3-year period of androgen ablation. However, the optimal duration of androgen ablation in the context of locally advanced prostate cancer treated with radiation remains an area of investigation.

It also appears that improved local control represents another strategy to improve overall survival (OS) in patients with T3N0M0 (TNM, tumor-node-metastasis) tumors. Randomized controlled trials have demonstrated that adjuvant radiation therapy following radical prostatectomy for T3N0M0 tumors significantly reduces the risk of metastases and improves OS ([60]). These data support the hypothesis that untreated residual disease at the primary site can act as a source for metastatic progression.

Neoadjuvant Trials in High-Risk and Locally Advanced Prostate Cancer

At MD Anderson, we recognize two different categories of patients with high-risk or locally advanced disease: (1) those we believe can be effectively treated with hormones and radiation therapy and (2) those we believe will not be effectively treated with this approach because of the extent of their disease, adverse histologic features of the tumor, or the relative youth and expected long survival of the patient. Patients in the second category are candidates for a novel preoperative therapy given prior to prostatectomy. The rationale for neoadjuvant therapy in this setting is based on progress made in other cancer types and is described as follows: (1) In high-risk and locally advanced disease, the posttherapy pathology specimen will inform both prognosis and future treatment decisions, and (2) controlling the primary tumor is an essential part of an integrated strategy for patients with high-risk and locally advanced disease (although this strategy is not always curative) ([61]). We are using neoadjuvant trial designs with increasing frequency to develop novel agents (eg, angiogenesis inhibitors) in prostate cancer. Analysis of the prostatectomy specimen permits detailed analysis of molecular (eg, apoptosis) and pathologic surrogates for therapy benefit (eg, achievement of Pathologic 0 stage-P0). We believe the preoperative model will significantly enhance our ability to identify the most promising agents worthy of development in a time-efficient manner.

A promising combined modality approach has recently been reported utilizing maximal androgen blockade of both endocrine (using luteinizing hormone-releasing hormone agonists) and paracrine/autocrine/intracrine (using abiraterone, a CYP17 inhibitor) testosterone sources. Two recent phase 2 studies demonstrated that combination leuprolide/abiraterone was clinically superior to leuprolide alone with respect to PSA responses and cytoreduction ([62, 63]). A subset of patients in both trials achieved P0 (or near P0) in the surgical specimen, a relatively common phenomenon in neoadjuvant trials of other epithelial cancers (eg, breast and bladder) but essentially unprecedented in prostate cancer.

Castration-Resistant Locally Advanced Prostate Cancer

Castration-resistant prostate cancer (CRPC) is an "umbrella" term that encompasses a spectrum of disease states ranging from rising PSA alone to rising PSA associated with osseous or soft tissue metastases ([1]). Furthermore, patients receiving combined androgen blockade are typically screened for an antiandrogen withdrawal response before being considered castration resistant. Patients with CRPC and PSA-only recurrence are discussed in the next section.

For patients with castration-resistant locally advanced prostate cancer, clinical progression presents significant clinical symptoms (pain, hematuria, bladder outlet and bowel obstruction), but optimal management remains a difficult therapeutic problem. The critical decision is whether to offer consolidative therapy. For patients without metastatic disease, we offer neoadjuvant chemotherapy followed by surgery for consolidation. If not used as primary therapy, salvage radiation therapy is another rational strategy, particularly for patients who are not candidates for salvage surgery.

For patients with both castration-resistant locally advanced and metastatic disease, these approaches are more controversial. Nonetheless, we recognize that these patients experience significant morbidity from local tumor progression that is comparable to patients without metastases. Thus, for select candidates, we still offer consolidative therapy. As an example, consider the case of a patient who presented with metastatic prostate cancer at diagnosis and was successfully treated with androgen ablation for 10 years. He then developed castration-resistant progression and presented with invasion of his primary tumor into the bladder (Fig. 37-3). To relieve painful voiding symptoms attributed to the bladder invasion, induction chemotherapy followed by salvage cystoprostatectomy was performed. At 3 years follow-up, the patient continued to have evidence of active metastases but was free of cancer-associated local symptoms. While this patient benefited longer than most, striking relief of intractable symptoms is common using this approach. The clinical rationale to apply chemotherapy followed by salvage surgery is summarized in Table 37-5.

Rising Prostate-Specific Antigen After Definitive Local Therapy

The utility of PSA measurements is greatest in monitoring cancer progression and effects of therapy in patients with radiographic evidence of disease. In contrast, the significance of PSA in patients without detectable disease is less clear. Although available evidence suggests that patients with a measurable PSA following prostatectomy will eventually develop a recurrence given sufficient time, these recurrences are not uniformly fatal. Furthermore, in patients treated with radiation therapy, interpretation of PSA post-therapy is very different compared to patients treated with surgery.

Significance of Prostate-Specific Antigen Following Prostatectomy

The serum PSA concentration should be undetectable using standard commercial assays within 6 weeks of prostatectomy. Persistent PSA following surgery usually indicates persistent cancer secondary to inadequate surgery, persistent cancer despite adequate surgery, or the presence of occult metastases. The experience from Johns Hopkins suggests that, given sufficient time, patients with early PSA recurrence (≤2 years) or short PSA doubling time (<10 months) will develop metastatic disease within 15 years of surgery ([64-66]). In contrast, patients with late PSA recurrence or a longer PSA doubling time are more likely to have a recurrence confined to the prostatic fossa. Patients who have a striking discordance between the predicted behavior of the cancer (eg, low stage) and early elevations of postoperative serum PSA may have had inadequate surgery and are considered for adjuvant radiation therapy. In patients who undergo nerve-sparing prostatectomy, consideration must also be given to the possibility that normal prostate gland left behind at surgery is producing PSA.

Table 37-5 Rationale for Salvage Surgery

• Patients can avoid significant morbidity associated with local progression.
• Improved local control may contribute to longer overall survival.
• Patients who develop a delayed local relapse after treatment with primary radiation therapy may still have surgically curable disease.

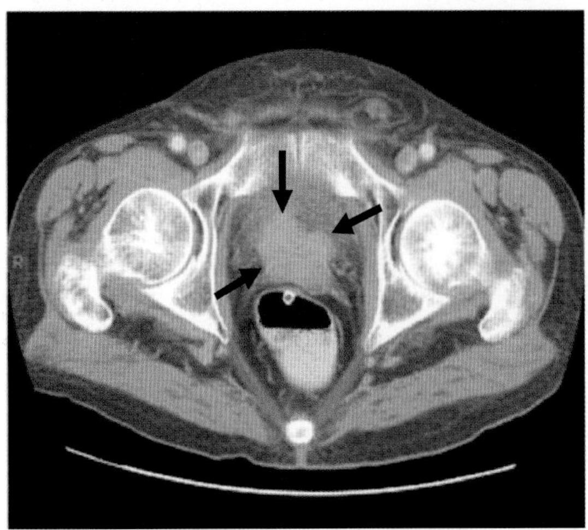

FIGURE 37-3 Recurrent prostate cancer invading the base of the bladder.

Significance of Prostate-Specific Antigen Following Radiation Therapy

In contrast to surgery, serum PSA concentrations are not expected to become undetectable following curative therapy. In addition, the phenomenon of a PSA "bounce" is well described following radiation of the primary tumor ([67]). The PSA bounce is a modest, self-limited rise in PSA concentration without evidence of cancer progression. It typically occurs within the first 18 months following completion of radiation and can last for as long as 3 months before reaching a plateau and then declining. The central clinical dilemma with PSA bounces is that their presence can only be determined with confidence in retrospect. Thus, clinicians need to be aware of this phenomenon and show restraint in introducing therapy to patients displaying delayed PSA elevation after radiation without evidence for metastases.

Management of the Patient With Prostate-Specific Antigen–Only Recurrence

The scenario of the patient with prostate-specific antigen–only recurrence poses a therapeutic dilemma for physicians and considerable anxiety for patients. As experience with this disease state matures, it is becoming clear that PSA-only recurrences do not uniformly portend morbidity/mortality from the disease. Our general approach is to offer hormone ablative therapy (commonly using an intermittent strategy) during the androgen-dependent phase of the disease ([68]). Notably, we never use chemotherapy for PSA-only recurrences that occur in the setting of CRPC. Instead, we advocate placing these patients on clinical trials testing novel compounds.

Currently, we are conducting a clinical trial at our institution (NCT01786265) that is testing whether more potent inhibition of androgen synthesis will help. The goal of this clinical research study is to determine whether inhibition of paracrine/autocrine/intracrine androgens (using abiraterone) in addition to endocrine androgens (using leuprolide) will improve efficacy in this patient group. A key data point will be *PSA-free survival*, defined as duration of time "off" therapy with an undetectable PSA and return of testosterone levels.

Metastatic Cancer

Metastatic Androgen-Dependent Disease

For patients with visible disease in the bone or lymph nodes, the standard approach is continuous androgen ablation. The clinical rationale for the use of androgen ablation is summarized in Table 37-6. For patients with de novo metastatic disease and primary tumors

Table 37-6 Clinical Rationale for Androgen Ablation

1. Androgen ablation enhances local therapy: • Concurrent androgen ablation and radiation therapy increase survival in selected patients. • Early use of androgen ablation in patients noted to be node positive following radical prostatectomy increases overall survival.
2. Timing of androgen ablation: • The decision to introduce androgen ablation among patients with a rising PSA following local therapy should be based on assessment of risk for recurrence and cancer-associated mortality. • Androgen ablation therapy reduces the duration of time patients experience symptomatic progression. • Symptoms are reliably relieved and should be initiated in the presence of symptomatic progression.
3. Types of androgen ablation: • Surgical castration and LHRH agonists or antagonists are considered to be equally effective. • Combined androgen ablation is not convincingly superior to serial use of an LHRH agonist followed by an antiandrogen on progression. However, antiandrogen therapy should precede the use of an LHRH agonist in the setting of threatening disease to avoid a "surge."
4. Secondary hormonal therapy: • Experimental and clinical data demonstrate that some prostate cancers growing in a castrate environment still rely on androgen signaling for continued growth.
5. Management of complications associated with androgen ablation: • Patients on sustained androgen ablation should be monitored for bone complications and considered for bisphosphonate therapy to reduce the risk of osteopenia. • Supplementation with calcium (500 mg) and vitamin D (400 IU) is recommended. • Antidepressants should be considered for androgen ablation–associated depression.

in place, we are currently conducting a clinical trial (NCT01751438) to test best systemic therapy versus best systemic therapy plus definitive treatment (radiation or surgery) of the prostate. The goal of this clinical research study is to learn if control of the primary tumor improves the clinical outcome in patients with metastatic disease. The safety of this combined modality treatment combination will also be studied.

The role of cytotoxic chemotherapy in patients with androgen-dependent disease remains controversial. Most recently, data from the CHAARTED trial comparing "up-front" chemotherapy plus androgen deprivation therapy (ADT) to ADT alone in men with metastatic prostate cancer was reported. The results showed that, in men with high-volume disease (defined as visceral metastasis and/or ≥4 bone metastases), median OS was 49.2 months with docetaxel plus ADT compared with 32.2 months with ADT, a difference of 17 months ([69]). Although the final manuscript is pending publication at this point, this study suggests that patients with high-volume, androgen-dependent disease may benefit from up-front docetaxel.

However, in contrast to those data, other large phase 3 studies of similar design have been negative ([70, 71]). The GETUG-AFU 15 trial recently reported no differences in OS between patients with noncastrate metastatic disease receiving ADT plus docetaxel versus ADT alone (median OS was 58.9 months in the group given ADT plus docetaxel and 54.2 months in the group given ADT) ([71]). It is likely that differences in patient populations (eg, volume of disease at baseline) and treatments postprogression explain the disparate results between these trials. At our institution, while our clinical experience strongly supports the notion that some patients with metastatic disease will benefit from early application of cytotoxic chemotherapy (eg, patients with small cell/anaplastic features), we offer it on a case-by-case basis rather than routinely.

Castration-Resistant Progression

Second-Line Hormonal Therapies

During castrate-resistant progression, there is a gradual "switch" in sources of androgens that sustain tumor growth from endocrine to intratumoral (paracrine/autocrine/intracrine). Second-line hormonal therapies that block these alternative sources have long been of interest as cancer therapeutics. For example, considerable advances have been made in developing small molecule inhibitors that block CYP17, a key enzyme involved in androgen biosynthesis expressed in testes, adrenal glands, and tumor tissues ([72]). Ketoconazole is an antifungal agent with weak and nonspecific CYP17 inhibitory properties that has been available for decades. While ketoconazole is active in prostate cancer, its application has been limited due to extremely poor tolerance. In contrast, several new agents, including abiraterone, have proven more successful. Abiraterone is a potent irreversible inhibitor of CYP17, and two large randomized phase 3 studies have demonstrated clinical benefit in both chemotherapy-naïve and docetaxel-treated patients with metastatic castration-resistant prostate cancer (mCRPC) ([73,74]).

Enzalutamide (Xtandi; Medivation/Astellas) is a small molecule that directly binds the AR to competitively inhibit endogenous androgen binding and antagonize AR function. It has a higher affinity for the AR than first-generation nonsteroidal antiandrogens (eg, bicalutamide). Randomized phase 3 studies have demonstrated that enzalutamide is clinically beneficial in both chemotherapy-naïve and docetaxel-treated patients with mCRPC ([75]). Because enzaluatmide can potentially address molecular resistance mechanisms to abiraterone monotherapy and vice versa, studies of combination abiraterone and enzalutmide are also under way. More specifically, resistance to abiraterone is associated with increased nuclear AR copy number (theoretically blocked with enzalutamide), and resistance to enzalutamide is associated with increased microenvironment testosterone levels (theoretically blocked with abiraterone) ([76,77]). Preliminary analysis suggested that a higher percentage of patients experience favorable PSA response profiles than seen with either agent alone, and the combination appears to be well tolerated ([78]).

Although abiraterone and enzalutamide represent breakthroughs in the treatment of mCRPC, approximately 20% to 40% of patients have no response to these agents (primary refractory). Furthermore, among patients who initially have a response to enzalutamide or abiraterone, virtually all eventually acquire secondary resistance. For example, the emergence of mutations (such as a single F876L amino acid substitution) in the AR can confer resistance to enzalutamide. Recently, Antonarakis et al reported detection of AR-V7 in circulating tumor cells from patients with CRPC may be associated with resistance to enzalutamide and abiraterone ([79]).

Chemotherapy

Prostate cancer has now entered the realm of the other adult common solid tumors in that chemotherapy is routinely applied to patients with castration-resistant locally advanced or metastatic disease. For more than a decade, patients have been treated with docetaxel-based regimens. However, while these therapies improve quality of life, prolongation in survival is modest. Faced with these challenges, the approach at MD Anderson has been to delay cytotoxic therapy until second-line hormonal (or experimental options) have been explored. Of course, patients with rapidly progressive disease causing (or expecting to cause) symptoms are offered chemotherapy sooner rather than later, particularly when additional hormonal manipulations are predicted to fail (eg, in patients with small cell/anaplastic tumors). The rationale for the use of chemotherapy is outlined in Table 37-7.

Given the limitations of docetaxel-based chemotherapy, there has been a global research initiative to improve on it, principally by combining docetaxel with other agents. However, these efforts have met with little success. For example, antiangiogenic drugs such as sunitinib and avastin did not improve OS compared with placebo in docetaxel-refractory mCRPC ([80, 81]). Similarly, bone microenviroment targeting agents such as zibotentan, atrasentan, and dasatinib were each tested in phase III trials and all failed to improve on standard docetaxel ([82-84]). Interestingly, each of these agents showed promise in phase II studies, and some (eg, avastin and sunitinib) did result in improvements in median progression-free survival. These results suggest that a subset of patients did benefit and that moving forward, clinical trial designs that incorporate predictive biomarkers to enrich for patients most likely to respond will be necessary to develop novel treatment strategies.

Optimizing Therapy Benefit Using Different Cytotoxic Agents in Metastatic Castration-Resistant Prostate Cancer

The concept that patients can respond to another taxane after progressing on docetaxel is important. The recent approval of cabazitaxel by the Food and Drug Administration (FDA), based on the results of the phase III TROPIC study, provided further validation of this concept ([85]). Cabazitaxel is a novel semisynthetic taxane developed specifically to overcome docetaxel resistance, and it is typically offered as second-line therapy for patients with mCRPC previously treated with docetaxel. This promising advance suggests that further study of cabazitaxel is warranted to explore its potential to overcome taxane resistance.

Beyond docetaxel and cabazitaxel, multiple chemotherapy regimens with modest activity are routinely applied in a sequential manner to patients in the salvage

Table 37-7 Rationale for the Use of Chemotherapy

- Chemotherapy palliates or prevents symptoms associated with progression of disease.
- Docetaxel-based regimens result in modest improvements in survival in patients with metastatic castration-resistant cancer.
- Other active agents in prostate cancer (eg, mitoxantrone and prednisone) can be used as second-line therapy.

setting. Examples include CVD (cyclophosphamide, vincristine, and dexamethasone); KAVE (ketoconazole plus doxorubicin alternating with vinblastine plus estramustine); TEC (paclitaxel, estramustine, and carboplatin); and TEE (paclitaxel, estramustine, and etoposide). However, there is no standard chemotherapy in the salvage setting, and we do not have randomized comparisons testing whether the sequential application of therapy prolongs survival.

More recent studies have demonstrated clinical responses to platinum-based therapy in combination with taxanes ([86-88]). Ross et al tested the activity of docetaxel/carboplatin in patients that had progressed during or within 45 days after the completion of docetaxel ([89]). PSA declines of 50% or greater were noted in 18% of patients, and measurable responses occurred in 14% of patients. As patients in this study would not be anticipated to respond to "rechallenge" with docetaxel alone, these results support the hypothesis that carboplatin has the potential to overcome docetaxel resistance mechanisms.

We are presently conducting a randomized phase I/II study of cabazitaxel with or without carboplatin in patients with mCRPC (NCT01505868). Patients are stratified by prior docetaxel exposure, performance status, and presence of anaplastic features. Preliminary results suggest excellent safety and efficacy of the two-drug combination.

Stromal-Targeting Therapies

Bone-targeting radiopharmaceuticals are examples of stromal-targeting agents in prostate cancer. The merits of targeting the bone microenvironment have been established by the use of strontium 89 (pure β-emitter radiopharmaceutical) as a single agent or in combination with cytotoxic therapy ([90]) (Table 37-8). Emerging data support the view that targeting bone will prolong overall patient survival, even in those with advanced-stage disease. Samarium-153 conjugated to ethylenediamine-tetra-methylenephosphonic acid is a β- and γ-emitter radiopharmaceutical. It was approved by the FDA in 1997 after the landmark study that showed palliation of pain associated with metastatic bone cancer using samarium-153 lexidronam ([91]). However,

Table 37-8 Rationale for Bone-Targeted Therapy

• Osseous metastases are the preferred site of castration-resistant progression.
• Osseous metastases significantly contribute to the morbidity and mortality of prostate cancer.
• Bone-targeting radiopharmaceuticals prolong symptom-free survival in patients with castration-resistant progression and skeletal metastases.

marrow toxicity remains the principal side effect. The radioactive calcium mimetic radium-223 dichloride (Xofigo; Bayer), which specifically targets bone metastases (present in 80%–90% of patients with metastatic CRPC), is the newest treatment for mCRPC. A phase III, randomized, double-blind, placebo-controlled study (ALSYMPCA) investigated the use of radium-223 in men with CRPC and bone metastases; radium-223 showed improved OS in this patient population ([92]). This study led to its FDA approval for CRPC with bone metastases in 2013.

Bisphosphonates were the first class of agents investigated for prevention of skeletal-related events (SREs) in patients with mCRPC. A randomized, placebo-controlled trial of zoledronic acid in patients with hormone-refractory metastatic prostate carcinoma showed zoledronic acid reduced SREs in patients with prostate cancer with bone metastases ([93]). Currently, zoledronic acid is the only bisphosphonate approved to prevent SREs in patients with mCRPC.

Denosumab is a fully humanized monoclonal antibody that binds to the RANK-L, which results in inhibition of RANK-L–mediated bone resorption. In a phase III study, men with CRPC with bone metastases and no previous exposure to intravenous bisphosphonate compared denosumab with zoledronic acid for prevention of SREs ([94]). Denosumab was superior to zoledronic acid in delaying or preventing SREs, but there was no significant difference between treatments in survival or disease progression ([94]). It was approved by the FDA in 2010 for prevention of SREs in patients with bone metastases.

Immune-Based Therapies

Historically, there has been long-standing interest in stimulating a patient's immune system as a therapy strategy for prostate cancer. Despite enthusiasm for this paradigm, studies have consistently demonstrated no clinical benefit. Recently, several new strategies have emerged that reveal the potential of immunotherapy in treating prostate cancer. Randomized, placebo-controlled phase III trials demonstrated an OS benefit for men with CRPC treated with sipuleucel-T ([95]). GVAX, a cellular vaccine product that uses exogenous tumor cells that secrete granulocyte-macrophage colony-stimulating factor, has shown promising activity in phase II studies ([96]), although it failed to meet its primary end point of OS when compared with docetaxel in a phase III study ([97, 98]). Ipilimumab is a humanized anti-CTLA-4 antibody; recent data from a phase III trial of a single dose of radiation treatment followed by ipilimumab or placebo in previously treated patients showed the primary end point (ie, OS) was not met (ipilimumab vs placebo, 11.2 vs 10.0 months, respectively; however, there was an improvement in progression-free survival and PSA responses) ([99]). Another phase III trial has completed enrolling patients with less-advanced, chemotherapy-naïve mCRPC. Further development of these agents (and others) could dramatically change the way we treat prostate cancer in the coming decade.

FUTURE DIRECTIONS

The majority of patients with advanced prostate cancer demonstrate a predictable clinical pattern of progression. As elucidation of the biologic events responsible for prostate cancer progression evolves, better classification of the disease based on the underlying molecular mechanisms of progression will facilitate the implementation of current and emerging therapies. To reflect this, we have recently proposed a "spiral" model for prostate cancer progression that describes underlying biology to predict response to therapy ([100]) (Fig. 37-4). The model proposes three main phases in prostate cancer progression: (1) DHT-dependent phase, (2) microenvironment-dependent phase, and (3) cell-autonomous phase.

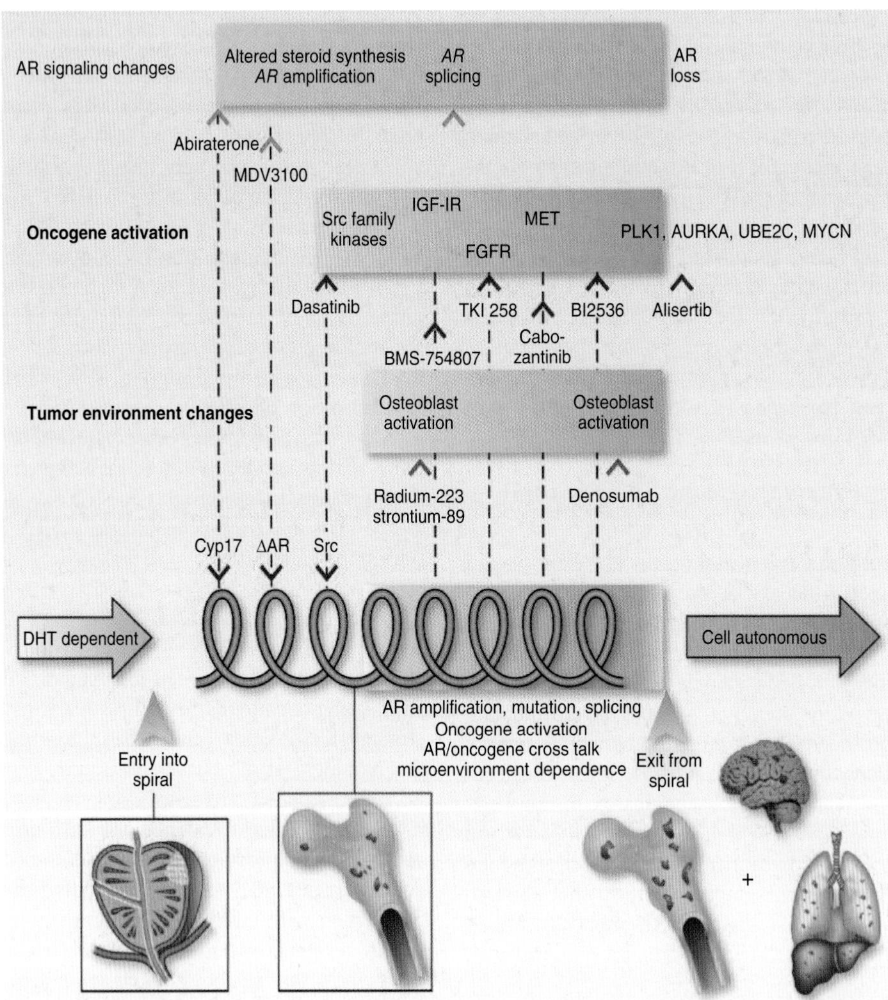

FIGURE 37-4 Spiral model for prostate cancer progression. The first phase is the *DHT-dependent phase*. The second phase is the *microenvironment-dependent phase*. The third phase is the *cell-autonomous phase*. Each "turn" is defined by a predictive marker(s) that can be targeted. The pitch in each spiral reflects the duration that the tumors remain responsive to a specific therapy. The adaptive changes in tumors in response to therapy account for resistance, leading the tumor to progress to the next turn of the progression spiral, which signals additional alterations in the tumor and its microenvironment. Tumors in this new "turn" will require different therapeutics that specifically target the altered properties that define the turn. Markers that reflect the biology that drives each turn can be used to guide timely therapy application in anticipation of progression. DHT, dihydrotesterone; AR, Androgen Receptor; IGF, Insulin Like Growth Factor; FGF, Fibroblast Growth Factor. (Reproduced with permission from Logothetis CJ, Gallick GE, Maity SN, et al. Molecular classification of prostate cancer progression: foundation for marker-driven treatment of prostate cancer, *Cancer Disco*. 2013 Aug;3(8):849-861.)

The first phase is the *DHT-dependent phase*, during which the tumor is responsive to 5-α-reductase inhibitor treatments. In the PSA era, this phase typically occurs when patients are initially diagnosed with early-stage, localized prostate cancer. Tumors in this phase would be predicted to respond optimally to chemoprevention strategies.

The second phase is the *microenvironment-dependent phase*, when the tumor enters a progression spiral where multiple factors, including AR signaling changes, oncogene activation, tumor suppressor gene loss, and microenvironment changes, affect tumor progression. Tumors in this phase would be predicted to respond optimally to inhibitors of intratumoral androgen signaling (eg, with abiraterone and enzalutamide). Over time, however, adaptive changes in response to therapy promote resistance, leading the tumor to progress to the next turn of the progression spiral, which signals additional molecular alterations in the tumor and its microenvironment. Tumors in a new turn of the spiral will require different therapeutics that specifically target the altered molecular events that drive each turn (eg, inhibitors of Src, FGF, c-Met). Predictive biomarkers corresponding to each turn can be used to guide timely therapy application.

The third phase is the *cell-autonomous phase*, whereby cancers exit the spiral when a series of mutations arise, including the loss of AR, RB, or p53; upregulation of polo-like kinase 1 (PLK1), Aurora kinase A (AURKA); and amplification of *MYCN*. At this stage, the prostate cancer cells are no longer regulated by the microenvironment and become tumor cell autonomous. Cancers in this phase would be predicted to respond optimally to chemotherapy.

Along with the integration of improved predictive and prognostic markers, we believe it is realistic to expect individualized treatment algorithms for prostate cancer patients as details of the spiral evolve. The application of biologically based, rational therapy is the foundation of our mission at MD Anderson to cure prostate cancer. Recent progress has created a strong sense of hope that we are well on our way to achieving this goal.

REFERENCES

1. Scher HI, Heller G. Clinical states in prostate cancer: toward a dynamic model of disease progression. *Urology*. 2000;55(3):323-327.
2. Chang AJ, Autio KA, Roach M 3rd, Scher HI. High-risk prostate cancer-classification and therapy. *Nat Rev Clin Oncol*. 2014;11(6):308-323.
3. Siegel R, Ma J, Zou Z, Jemal A. Cancer statistics, 2014. *CA Cancer J Clin*. 2014;64(1):9-29.
4. Patel AR, Klein EA. Risk factors for prostate cancer. *Nat Clin Pract Urol*. 2009;6(2):87-95.
5. Scher HI, Sawyers CL. Biology of progressive, castration-resistant prostate cancer: directed therapies targeting the androgen-receptor signaling axis. *J Clin Oncol*. 2005;23(32):8253-8261.
6. Ebos JM, Lee CR, Bogdanovic E, Alami J, Van Slyke P, Francia G, et al. Vascular endothelial growth factor-mediated decrease in plasma soluble vascular endothelial growth factor receptor-2 levels as a surrogate biomarker for tumor growth. *Cancer Res*. 2008;68(2):521-529.
7. Renehan AG, Tyson M, Egger M, Heller RF, Zwahlen M. Body-mass index and incidence of cancer: a systematic review and meta-analysis of prospective observational studies. *Lancet*. 2008;371(9612):569-578.
8. Golabek T, Bukowczan J, Chlosta P, Powroznik J, Dobruch J, Borowka A. Obesity and prostate cancer incidence and mortality: a systematic review of prospective cohort studies. *Urol Int*. 2014;92(1):7-14.
9. Roberts DL, Dive C, Renehan AG. Biological mechanisms linking obesity and cancer risk: new perspectives. *Annu Rev Med*. 2010;61:301-316.
10. Rowlands MA, Gunnell D, Harris R, Vatten LJ, Holly JM, Martin RM. Circulating insulin-like growth factor peptides and prostate cancer risk: a systematic review and meta-analysis. *Int J Cancer*. 2009;124(10):2416-2429.
11. Cox ME, Gleave ME, Zakikhani M, et al. Insulin receptor expression by human prostate cancers. *Prostate*. 2009;69(1):33-40.
12. Ma J, Li H, Giovannucci E, et al. Prediagnostic body-mass index, plasma C-peptide concentration, and prostate cancer-specific mortality in men with prostate cancer: a long-term survival analysis. *Lancet Oncol*. 2008;9(11):1039-1047.
13. Margel D, Urbach DR, Lipscombe LL, et al. Metformin use and all-cause and prostate cancer-specific mortality among men with diabetes. *J Clin Oncol*. 2013;31(25):3069-3075.
14. Huang CY, Yu HS, Lai TY, et al. Leptin increases motility and integrin up-regulation in human prostate cancer cells. *J Cell Physiol*. 2011;226(5):1274-1282.
15. Baillargeon J, Platz EA, Rose DP, et al. Obesity, adipokines, and prostate cancer in a prospective population-based study. *Cancer Epidemiol Biomarkers Prev*. 2006;15(7):1331-1335.
16. Goktas S, Yilmaz MI, Caglar K, Sonmez A, Kilic S, Bedir S. Prostate cancer and adiponectin. *Urology*. 2005;65(6):1168-1172.
17. Martin DN, Starks AM, Ambs S. Biological determinants of health disparities in prostate cancer. *Curr Opin Oncol*. 2013;25(3):235-241.
18. Taksler GB, Keating NL, Cutler DM. Explaining racial differences in prostate cancer mortality. *Cancer*. 2012;118(17):4280-4289.
19. Smith JR, Freije D, Carpten JD, et al. Major susceptibility locus for prostate cancer on chromosome 1 suggested by a genome-wide search. *Science*. 1996;274(5291):1371-1374.
20. Xu J, Gillanders EM, Isaacs SD, et al. Genome-wide scan for prostate cancer susceptibility genes in the Johns Hopkins hereditary prostate cancer families. *Prostate*. 2003;57(4):320-325.
21. Ford D, Easton DF, Bishop DT, Narod SA, Goldgar DE. Risks of cancer in BRCA1-mutation carriers. Breast Cancer Linkage Consortium. *Lancet*. 1994;343(8899):692-695.
22. Gayther SA, de Foy KA, Harrington P, et al. The frequency of germ-line mutations in the breast cancer predisposition genes BRCA1 and BRCA2 in familial prostate cancer. The Cancer Research Campaign/British Prostate Group United Kingdom Familial Prostate Cancer Study Collaborators. *Cancer Res*. 2000;60(16):4513-4518.
23. Castro E, Goh C, Olmos D, et al. Germline BRCA mutations are associated with higher risk of nodal involvement, distant metastasis, and poor survival outcomes in prostate cancer. *J Clin Oncol*. 2013;31(14):1748-1757.
24. Castro E, Goh C, Leongamornlert D, et al. Effect of BRCA

mutations on metastatic relapse and cause-specific survival after radical treatment for localised prostate cancer. *Eur Urol.* 2015;68(2):186-193.
25. Stark JR, Perner S, Stampfer MJ, et al. Gleason score and lethal prostate cancer: does 3 + 4 = 4 + 3? *J Clin Oncol.* 2009;27(21):3459-3464.
26. Efstathiou E, Abrahams NA, Tibbs RF, et al. Morphologic characterization of preoperatively treated prostate cancer: toward a post-therapy histologic classification. *Eur Urol.* 2010;57(6):1030-1038.
27. Srigley JR, Humphrey PA, Amin MB, et al. Protocol for the examination of specimens from patients with carcinoma of the prostate gland. *Arch Pathol Lab Med.* 2009;133(10):1568-1576.
28. Petrovics G, Liu A, Shaheduzzaman S, et al. Frequent overexpression of ETS-related gene-1 (ERG1) in prostate cancer transcriptome. *Oncogene.* 2005;24(23):3847-3852.
29. McDonnell TJ, Navone NM, Troncoso P, et al. Expression of bcl-2 oncoprotein and p53 protein accumulation in bone marrow metastases of androgen independent prostate cancer. *J Urol.* 1997;157(2):569-574.
30. Assikis VJ, Do KA, Wen S, et al. Clinical and biomarker correlates of androgen-independent, locally aggressive prostate cancer with limited metastatic potential. *Clin Cancer Res.* 2004;10(20):6770-6778.
31. Tu SM, Lopez A, Leibovici D, et al. Ductal adenocarcinoma of the prostate: clinical features and implications after local therapy. *Cancer.* 2009;115(13):2872-2880.
32. Papandreou CN, Daliani DD, Thall PF, et al. Results of a phase II study with doxorubicin, etoposide, and cisplatin in patients with fully characterized small-cell carcinoma of the prostate. *J Clin Oncol.* 2002;20(14):3072-3080.
33. Beltran H, Rickman DS, Park K, et al. Molecular characterization of neuroendocrine prostate cancer and identification of new drug targets. *Cancer Discov.* 2011;1(6):487-495.
34. Aparicio AM, Harzstark AL, Corn PG, et al. Platinum-based chemotherapy for variant castrate-resistant prostate cancer. *Clin Cancer Res.* 2013;19(13):3621-3630.
35. Epstein JI. Precursor lesions to prostatic adenocarcinoma. *Virchows Arch.* 2009;454(1):1-16.
36. De Marzo AM, Platz EA, Sutcliffe S, et al. Inflammation in prostate carcinogenesis. *Nat Rev Cancer.* 2007;7(4):256-2569.
37. Andriole GL, Crawford ED, Grubb RL 3rd, et al. Mortality results from a randomized prostate-cancer screening trial. *N Engl J Med.* 2009;360(13):1310-1319.
38. Schroder FH, Hugosson J, Roobol MJ, et al. Screening and prostate-cancer mortality in a randomized European study. *N Engl J Med.* 2009;360(13):1320-1328.
39. US Preventive Services Task Force. Prostate cancer: screening. 2012, May. http://www.uspreventiveservicestaskforce.org/Page/Topic/recommendation-summary/prostate-cancer-screening.
40. Thompson IM, Goodman PJ, Tangen CM, et al. The influence of finasteride on the development of prostate cancer. *N Engl J Med.* 2003;349(3):215-224.
41. Andriole GL, Bostwick DG, Brawley OW, et al. Effect of dutasteride on the risk of prostate cancer. *N Engl J Med.* 2010;362(13):1192-1202.
42. Fleshner NE, Lucia MS, Egerdie B, et al. Dutasteride in localised prostate cancer management: the REDEEM randomised, double-blind, placebo-controlled trial. *Lancet.* 2012;379(9821):1103-1111.
43. Partin AW, Kattan MW, Subong EN, et al. Combination of prostate-specific antigen, clinical stage, and Gleason score to predict pathological stage of localized prostate cancer. A multi-institutional update. *JAMA.* 1997;277(18):1445-1451.
44. Makarov DV, Trock BJ, Humphreys EB, et al. Updated nomogram to predict pathologic stage of prostate cancer given prostate-specific antigen level, clinical stage, and biopsy Gleason score (Partin tables) based on cases from 2000 to 2005. *Urology.* 2007;69(6):1095-1101.
45. Hernandez DJ, Nielsen ME, Han M, Partin AW. Contemporary evaluation of the D'amico risk classification of prostate cancer. *Urology.* 2007;70(5):931-935.
46. Kattan MW, Wheeler TM, Scardino PT. Postoperative nomogram for disease recurrence after radical prostatectomy for prostate cancer. *J Clin Oncol.* 1999;17(5):1499-1507.
47. Cuzick J, Berney DM, Fisher G, et al. Prognostic value of a cell cycle progression signature for prostate cancer death in a conservatively managed needle biopsy cohort. *Br J Cancer.* 2012;106(6):1095-1099.
48. Cooperberg MR, Simko JP, Cowan JE, et al. Validation of a cell-cycle progression gene panel to improve risk stratification in a contemporary prostatectomy cohort. *J Clin Oncol.* 2013;31(11):1428-1434.
49. Cuzick J, Swanson GP, Fisher G, et al. Prognostic value of an RNA expression signature derived from cell cycle proliferation genes in patients with prostate cancer: a retrospective study. *Lancet Oncol.* 2011;12(3):245-255.
50. Sanchez P, Hernandez AM, Stecca B, et al. Inhibition of prostate cancer proliferation by interference with SONIC HEDGEHOG-GLI1 signaling. *Proc Natl Acad Sci U S A.* 2004;101(34):12561-12566.
51. Zunich SM, Douglas T, Valdovinos M, et al. Paracrine sonic hedgehog signalling by prostate cancer cells induces osteoblast differentiation. *Mol Cancer.* 2009;8:12.
52. Park SI, Zhang J, Phillips KA, et al. Targeting SRC family kinases inhibits growth and lymph node metastases of prostate cancer in an orthotopic nude mouse model. *Cancer Res.* 2008;68(9):3323-3333.
53. Holmberg L, Bill-Axelson A, Helgesen F, et al. A randomized trial comparing radical prostatectomy with watchful waiting in early prostate cancer. *N Engl J Med.* 2002;347(11):781-789.
54. Bill-Axelson A, Holmberg L, Ruutu M, et al. Radical prostatectomy versus watchful waiting in early prostate cancer. *N Engl J Med.* 2005;352(19):1977-1984.
55. D'Amico AV, Moul J, Carroll PR, Sun L, Lubeck D, Chen MH. Cancer-specific mortality after surgery or radiation for patients with clinically localized prostate cancer managed during the prostate-specific antigen era. *J Clin Oncol.* 2003;21(11):2163-2172.
56. Johansson JE, Holmberg L, Johansson S, Bergstrom R, Adami HO. Fifteen-year survival in prostate cancer. A prospective, population-based study in Sweden. *JAMA.* 1997;277(6):467-471.
57. Efstathiou E, Kim J, Logothetis CJ. Informative clinical investigation: a demanding taskmaster. *J Clin Oncol.* 2009;27(30):4937-498.
58. Messing EM, Manola J, Sarosdy M, Wilding G, Crawford ED, Trump D. Immediate hormonal therapy compared with observation after radical prostatectomy and pelvic lymphadenectomy in men with node-positive prostate cancer. *N Engl J Med.* 1999;341(24):1781-1788.
59. Bolla M, Collette L. pT3N0M0 prostate cancer: a plea for adjuvant radiation. *Nat Rev Urol.* 2009;6(8):410-412.
60. Thompson IM, Tangen CM, Paradelo J, et al. Adjuvant radiotherapy for pathological T3N0M0 prostate cancer significantly reduces risk of metastases and improves survival: long-term followup of a randomized clinical trial. *J Urol.* 2009;181(3):956-962.
61. Pettaway CA, Pisters LL, Troncoso P, et al. Neoadjuvant chemotherapy and hormonal therapy followed by radical prostatectomy: feasibility and preliminary results. *J Clin Oncol.* 2000;18(5):1050-1057.
62. Taplin ME, Montgomery B, Logothetis CJ, et al. Intense androgen-deprivation therapy with abiraterone acetate plus leuprolide

acetate in patients with localized high-risk prostate cancer: results of a randomized phase II neoadjuvant study. *J Clin Oncol*. 2014;32(33):3705-3715.
63. Efstathiou E, Davis J, Troncoso P, et al. Cytoreduction and androgen signaling modulation by abiraterone acetate (AA) plus leuprolide acetate (LHRHa) versus LHRHa in localized high-risk prostate cancer (PCa): Preliminary results of a randomized preoperative study [Abstract 4556]. *J Clin Oncol*. 2012;30(Suppl).
64. Pound CR, Partin AW, Eisenberger MA, Chan DW, Pearson JD, Walsh PC. Natural history of progression after PSA elevation following radical prostatectomy. *JAMA*. 1999;281(17):1591-1597.
65. Han M, Partin AW, Pound CR, Epstein JI, Walsh PC. Long-term biochemical disease-free and cancer-specific survival following anatomic radical retropubic prostatectomy. The 15-year Johns Hopkins experience. *Urol Clin North Am*. 2001;28(3):555-565.
66. Cannon GM J., Walsh PC, Partin AW, Pound CR. Prostate-specific antigen doubling time in the identification of patients at risk for progression after treatment and biochemical recurrence for prostate cancer. *Urology*. 2003;62(Suppl 1):2-8.
67. Rosser CJ, Kuban DA, Levy LB, et al. Prostate specific antigen bounce phenomenon after external beam radiation for clinically localized prostate cancer. *J Urol*. 2002;168(5):2001-2005.
68. Bhandari MS, Crook J, Hussain M. Should intermittent androgen deprivation be used in routine clinical practice? *J Clin Oncol*. 2005;23(32):8212-8218.
69. Sweeney C, Chyen Y-H, Carducci MA, et al. Impact on overall survival (OS) with chemohormonal therapy versus hormonal therapy for hormone-sensitive newly metastatic prostate cancer (mPrCa): an ECOG-led phase III randomized trial [Abstract LBA2]. *J Clin Oncol*. 2014;32(Suppl):5s.
70. Millikan RE, Wen S, Pagliaro LC, et al. Phase III trial of androgen ablation with or without three cycles of systemic chemotherapy for advanced prostate cancer. *J Clin Oncol*. 2008;26(36):5936-5942.
71. Gravis G, Fizazi K, Joly F, et al. Androgen-deprivation therapy alone or with docetaxel in non-castrate metastatic prostate cancer (GETUG-AFU 15): a randomised, open-label, phase 3 trial. *Lancet Oncol*. 2013;14(2):149-158.
72. Reid AH, Attard G, Barrie E, de Bono JS. CYP17 inhibition as a hormonal strategy for prostate cancer. *Nat Clin Pract Urol*. 2008;5(11):610-620.
73. de Bono JS, Logothetis CJ, Molina A, et al. Abiraterone and increased survival in metastatic prostate cancer. *N Engl J Med*. 2011;364(21):1995-2005.
74. Ryan CJ, Smith MR, de Bono JS, et al. Abiraterone in metastatic prostate cancer without previous chemotherapy. *N Engl J Med*. 2013;368(2):138-148.
75. Beer TM, Armstrong AJ, Rathkopf DE, et al. Enzalutamide in metastatic prostate cancer before chemotherapy. *N Engl J Med*. 2014;371(5):424-433.
76. Efstathiou E, Titus M, Tsavachidou D, et al. Effects of abiraterone acetate on androgen signaling in castrate-resistant prostate cancer in bone. *J Clin Oncol*. 2012;30(6):637-643.
77. Efstathiou E, Titus M, Wen S, et al. Molecular characterization of enzalutamide-treated bone metastatic castration-resistant prostate cancer. *Eur Urology*. 2015;67(1):53-60.
78. Efstathiou E TM, Wen S, SanMiguel A, Hoang A, De Haas-Amatsaleh A, Perabo F, Phung D, Troncoso P, Ouatas T, Logothetis C. Enzalutamide (ENZA) in combination with abiraterone acetate (AA) in bone metastatic castration resistant prostate cancer (mCRPC) [Abstract 5000]. *J Clin Oncol*. 2014;32(Suppl):5s.
79. Antonarakis ES, Lu C, Wang H, et al. AR-V7 and resistance to enzalutamide and abiraterone in prostate cancer. *N Engl J Med*. 2014;371(11):1028-1038.
80. Michaelson MD, Oudard S, Ou YC, et al. Randomized, placebo-controlled, phase III trial of sunitinib plus prednisone versus prednisone alone in progressive, metastatic, castration-resistant prostate cancer. *J Clin Oncol*. 2014;32(2):76-82.
81. Kelly WK, Halabi S, Carducci M, et al. Randomized, double-blind, placebo-controlled phase III trial comparing docetaxel and prednisone with or without bevacizumab in men with metastatic castration-resistant prostate cancer: CALGB 90401. *J Clin Oncol*. 2012;30(13):1534-1540.
82. Fizazi K, Higano CS, Nelson JB, et al. Phase III, randomized, placebo-controlled study of docetaxel in combination with zibotentan in patients with metastatic castration-resistant prostate cancer. *J Clin Oncol*. 2013;31(14):1740-1747.
83. Quinn DI, Tangen CM, Hussain M, et al. Docetaxel and atrasentan versus docetaxel and placebo for men with advanced castration-resistant prostate cancer (SWOG S0421): a randomised phase 3 trial. *Lancet Oncol*. 2013;14(9):893-900.
84. Araujo JC, Trudel GC, Saad F, et al. Docetaxel and dasatinib or placebo in men with metastatic castration-resistant prostate cancer (READY): a randomised, double-blind phase 3 trial. *Lancet Oncol*. 2013;14(13):1307-1316.
85. de Bono JS, Oudard S, Ozguroglu M et al. Prednisone plus cabazitaxel or mitoxantrone for metastatic castration-resistant prostate cancer progressing after docetaxel treatment: a randomised open-label trial. *Lancet*. 2010;376(9747):1147-1154.
86. Kelly WK, Curley T, Slovin S, et al. Paclitaxel, estramustine phosphate, and carboplatin in patients with advanced prostate cancer. *J Clin Oncol*. 2001;19(1):44-53.
87. Oh WK, Halabi S, Kelly WK, et al. A phase II study of estramustine, docetaxel, and carboplatin with granulocyte-colony-stimulating factor support in patients with hormone-refractory prostate carcinoma: Cancer and Leukemia Group B 99813. *Cancer*. 2003;98(12):2592-2598.
88. Regan MM, O'Donnell EK, Kelly WK, et al. Efficacy of carboplatin-taxane combinations in the management of castration-resistant prostate cancer: a pooled analysis of seven prospective clinical trials. *Ann Oncol*. 2010;21(2):312-318.
89. Ross RW, Beer TM, Jacobus S, et al. A phase 2 study of carboplatin plus docetaxel in men with metastatic hormone-refractory prostate cancer who are refractory to docetaxel. *Cancer*. 2008;112(3):521-526.
90. Tu SM, Lin SH. Current trials using bone-targeting agents in prostate cancer. *Cancer J*. 2008;14(1):35-39.
91. Serafini AN, Houston SJ, Resche I, et al. Palliation of pain associated with metastatic bone cancer using samarium-153 lexidronam: a double-blind placebo-controlled clinical trial. *J Clin Oncol*. 1998;16(4):1574-1581.
92. Parker C, Nilsson S, Heinrich D, et al. Alpha emitter radium-223 and survival in metastatic prostate cancer. *N Engl J Med*. 2013;369(3):213-223.
93. Saad F, Gleason DM, Murray R, et al. A randomized, placebo-controlled trial of zoledronic acid in patients with hormone-refractory metastatic prostate carcinoma. *J Natl Cancer Inst*. 2002;94(19):1458-1468.
94. Fizazi K, Carducci M, Smith M, et al. Denosumab versus zoledronic acid for treatment of bone metastases in men with castration-resistant prostate cancer: a randomised, double-blind study. *Lancet*. 2011;377(9768):813-822.
95. Kantoff PW, Higano CS, Shore ND, et al. Sipuleucel-T immunotherapy for castration-resistant prostate cancer. *N Engl J Med*. 2010;363(5):411-422.
96. Higano CS, Corman JM, Smith DC, et al. Phase 1/2 dose-escalation study of a GM-CSF-secreting, allogeneic, cellular immunotherapy for metastatic hormone-refractory prostate cancer. *Cancer*. 2008;113(5):975-984.
97. Higano C, Saad, F, Somer SB, et al. A phase III trial of GVAX immunotherapy for prostate cancer vs docetaxel plus

prednisone in asymptomatic, castration-resistant prostate cancer (CRPC). Genitourinary Cancer Symposium [Abstract LBA150]. *Proc Am Soc Clin Oncol.* 2009.
98. Small E, Demkow T, Gerritsen W, et al. A phase III trial of GVAX immunotherapy for prostate cancer in combination with docetaxel vs docetaxel plus prednisone in symptomatic, castration-resistant prostate cancer (CRPC). Genitourinary Cancer Symposium [Abstract 7]. *Proc Am Soc Clin Oncol.* 2009.
99. Kwon ED, Drake CG, Scher HI, et al. Ipilimumab versus placebo after radiotherapy in patients with metastatic castration-resistant prostate cancer that had progressed after docetaxel chemotherapy (CA184-043): a multicentre, randomised, double-blind, phase 3 trial. *Lancet Oncol.* 2014;15(7):700-712.
100. Logothetis CJ, Gallick GE, Maity SN, et al. Molecular classification of prostate cancer progression: foundation for marker-driven treatment of prostate cancer. *Cancer Discov.* 2013;3(8):849-861.

38 Penile Cancer

第三十八章　阴茎癌

Lance C. Pagliaro

中文导读

本章首先介绍了阴茎癌的发病率及流行病学，阴茎癌在美国多见于50～70岁男性，年轻人少见。阴茎癌危险因素包括未进行环切手术、HPV感染、HIV感染等。阴茎癌具有独特的分子特征，包括过表达不同的HPV亚型、与RB及TP53通路相关、基质金属蛋白酶的参与以及表皮生长因子受体过表达等。就转移模式而言，阴茎癌更容易发生淋巴道转移，但也可发生远处转移，并且多数于2年内死亡。本章接着详细阐述了对患者的评估，包括分期系统评估、TNM系统的局限性、淋巴结的评估、CT及PET的影像学评估等方法及要点。针对阴茎癌的治疗，分别从局部控制、淋巴结清扫、ⅢB/Ⅳ期阴茎癌的化疗以及多学科综合治疗等角度阐述，并强调了新辅助化疗及辅助化疗在综合治疗中的作用，以及放疗联合手术或放疗、化疗联合的综合治疗模式。本章最后总结了阴茎癌的全程管理模式。

INCIDENCE AND ETIOLOGY

Incidence in United States

Penile cancer most commonly affects men between 50 and 70 years of age. The tumor is not unusual in younger men; in one large series, 22% of patients were younger than 40 years, and 7% were younger than 30 years ([1]). In 2015, there were an estimated 1,820 new cases in the United States ([2]).

Epidemiology

Penile carcinoma accounts for less than 1% of all malignant neoplasms among men in the United States and Europe, but it may represent up to 20% of malignant neoplasms in men in some Asian, African, and South American countries ([1]). These differences are thought to be related to the prevalence of neonatal circumcision, human papillomavirus (HPV) infection, and hygienic practices. Rates of HPV vaccination will likely become a factor in the future ([3]).

Incidence and Significance Worldwide

Among uncircumcised tribes of Africa and within uncircumcised Asian cultures, penile cancer may amount to 10% to 20% of all malignant neoplasms in men ([1]). Carcinoma of the penis is particularly rare among the Jewish population, for whom neonatal circumcision is a universal practice ([4]). The annual number of new cases in total per year worldwide has been estimated at approximately 26,000 ([5]). Squamous cell carcinoma is the most common histologic subtype, accounting for over 95% of cases (Table 38-1) ([6]).

RISK FACTORS

Lack of Circumcision

The risk of penile cancer varies according to circumcision practice, hygienic standard, phimosis, number of sexual partners, HPV infection, exposure to tobacco products, and other factors ([1,5]). Neonatal circumcision has been well established as a prophylactic measure that removes most of the risk of penile carcinoma because it eliminates the closed preputial environment where penile carcinoma most commonly develops. Phimosis is found in 25% to 75% of patients with penile carcinoma described in most large series. Reddy et al ([7]) studied the foreskins of 26 men undergoing circumcision because of phimosis and found epithelial atypia in one-third of the specimens. Data from most large series show that neonatal circumcision is protective, whereas circumcision delayed until after puberty is not ([8]).

Table 38-1 Histopathology Subtypes of Penile Cancer

Squamous cell carcinoma
Adenocarcinoma
Lymphoma
Melanoma
Kaposi sarcoma
Leiomyosarcoma

Human Papillomavirus

Although HPV is not a reportable sexually transmitted disease, the number of new genital HPV infections has been estimated at 500,000 to 1 million annually in the United States ([9]). The terms *genital condyloma, venereal warts, genital warts,* and *genital HPV infection* all refer to a sexually transmitted disease caused by HPV. Factors associated with higher rates of infection with HPV include presence of foreskin, increasing numbers of sexual partners, lack of condom use, and smoking ([10]). The overall prevalence of HPV in females was found to be 26.8% among US females aged 14 to 59 years and was highest among women aged 20 to 24 years (44.8%) ([11]). Human papillomavirus is recognized as the principal etiologic agent in cervical dysplasia and cervical cancer ([12]).

On histologic examination, the koilocyte—a cell characterized by an empty cavity surrounding an atypical nucleus—is pathognomonic for HPV infection (Fig. 38-1) ([13]). DNA hybridization techniques have been used to identify and classify HPV infections, and some 60 genotypes of HPV virus have been identified that involve the genital tract ([14]). Virus types 6, 11, and 42 to 44 are associated with gross condylomata and low-grade dysplasia, whereas types 16, 18, 31, 33, 35, and 39 have a higher association with malignant disease ([15]).

In men, a personal history of genital condylomata has been associated with squamous cell carcinoma of the penis ([10]). Malignant transformation of condylomata to squamous cell carcinoma has been reported ([16]). Condylomata acuminata located in the perianal, scrotal, and oral areas have also demonstrated malignant degeneration. An increased incidence of penile intraepithelial neoplasia has been found in the male partners of women with cervical intraepithelial neoplasia ([3]).

More than 25 types of HPV infect genital sites. It appears that HPV-16 is the most frequently detected type in primary carcinomas and has also been detected in metastatic lesions ([17]). Thus, preventive strategies are relevant, and prophylactic HPV vaccines are available

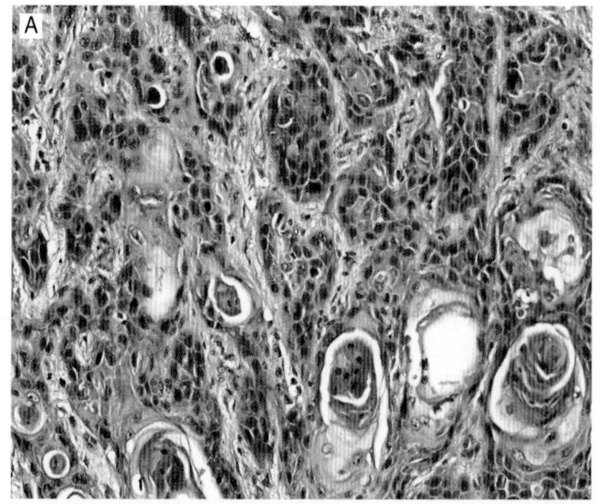

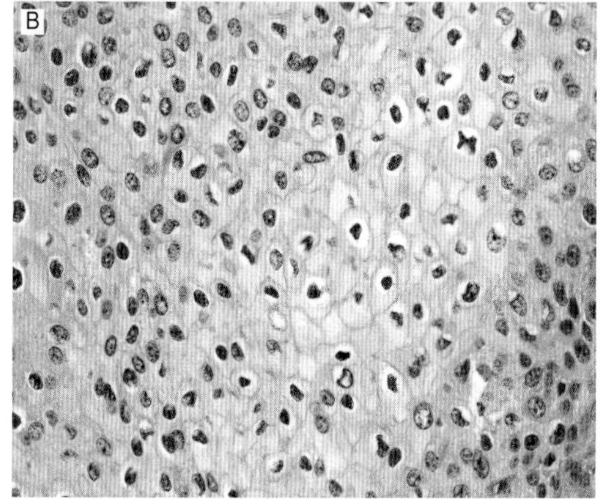

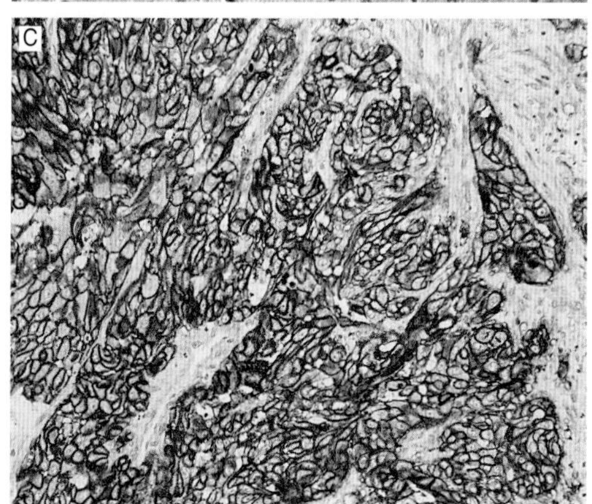

FIGURE 38-1 A. Moderately differentiated keratinizing squamous cell carcinoma. B. Human papilloma virus–related changes, including koilocytosis. C. Immunohistochemical stain for epidermal growth factor receptor. (Used with permission from Pheroze Tamboli, MD.)

for both men and women ([3]). The prevalence of HPV vaccination in the United States, however, remains disappointingly low.

Although HPV infection is probably an important factor in the development of penile cancer, with evidence that 31% to 63% of tumors are HPV related, its presence is not invariable ([18]). Other factors must be involved in the development of the disease or its subtypes. Human papillomavirus is most associated with the basaloid and warty tumor subtypes, which were found to contain HPV DNA in 80% to 100% of cases.

Patients with HPV-related penile cancer appear to have a better prognosis than those with HPV-unrelated tumors. A population-based study found that the detection of HPV DNA in penectomy specimens was associated with a significant advantage in disease-specific survival (96% vs 82%) ([19]). Immunohistochemical detection of p16, which is a marker for HPV infection, was also associated with improved outcome ([20]). Whether HPV is predictive of response to treatment (eg, chemotherapy) is unknown.

Human Immunodeficiency Virus

Human immunodeficiency virus (HIV) infection may predispose affected patients to rapid development of squamous carcinoma from preexisting condyloma infection ([21]). Poblet et al ([22]) reported on two cases of coexisting HIV-1 and HPV infection and postulated that HIV-1 could synergize with HPV to increase the progression of HPV penile lesions into penile carcinoma. Whereas there is evidence supporting this effect in cervical and anal neoplasia ([23]), definitive proof for penile cancer awaits further study.

MOLECULAR FEATURES

Overview of Molecular Features

The viral genes *E6* and *E7* are overexpressed in HPV-transformed cells, and they are known to interact with the *RB1* and *TP53* tumor suppressor pathways. These molecular events are known to play a critical role in the development of cervical cancer ([12]), and a similar mechanism probably exists in HPV-related cases of penile cancer ([3, 18]).

The tumor suppressor gene *TP53* is commonly mutated in human solid tumors, where the abnormal protein accumulates and can be detected by positive immunostaining. In penile cancer, positive p53 immunostain is an independent predictor of lymph node metastasis ([24]). In a study by Lopes et al ([25]), the p53-positive cases had a lower overall survival and higher incidence of lymph node metastasis. Martins et al ([24]) studied 50 patients, of which 14 had clinically positive lymph nodes. After penectomy, tumors were stained for p53 and proliferating cell nuclear antigen (PCNA), and these results were compared with stage, grade, nodal status, and cause of death. Overexpression of p53 was associated with pT classification, grade, nodal metastasis, and cause-specific survival. Also, PCNA was associated with nodal metastasis but not survival. Of note, *TP53* mutations would not be expected to occur in HPV-related tumors because p53 is inactivated by HPV viral proteins.

Matrix metalloproteinases (MMPs) and cellular adhesion molecules have been studied in penile cancer. Campos et al ([26]) measured MMP-2 and MMP-9 expression and found that MMP-9 was an independent risk factor for disease recurrence. In the same study, low E-cadherin was associated with a greater risk of lymph node metastasis. A Chinese study ([27]) found that 45% of tumors had low E-cadherin, and that it was associated with shorter cause-specific survival. These alterations have been found in both HPV-related and unrelated penile tumors ([5]).

Epidermal Growth Factor Receptor

Multiple studies have shown that the epidermal growth factor receptor (*EGFR*) is overexpressed in the majority of penile cancer cases ([28, 29]). Activating mutations of *EGFR* or *KRAS*, on the other hand are uncommon. Several published case reports and one case series suggested that *EGFR* is a useful target for therapy in metastatic penile cancer ([30-32]).

PATTERN OF METASTASIS

Anatomy of Lymphatic Drainage

Penile cancers have a predictable pattern of local, regional, and systemic spread. The earliest route of dissemination from the penis is metastasis to the regional femoral and iliac nodes. The lymphatics of the prepuce form a connecting network that joins with the lymphatics from the skin of the shaft. These tributaries drain into the superficial inguinal nodes. The lymphatics of the glans join the lymphatics draining the corporal bodies, and they form a collar of connecting channels at the base of the penis that also drain by way of the inguinal lymph nodes. From there, drainage is to the pelvic nodes (external iliac, internal iliac, and obturator). Multiple cross connections exist at all levels of drainage, so that penile lymphatic drainage is bilateral to both inguinal areas ([33]).

Frequency of Metastases: Prognostic Factors

Tumor grade, lymphovascular invasion, and perineural invasion appear to be the most important pathologic prognostic factors for nodal spread and mortality ([34]). Other frequently cited risk factors are pT classification, tumor thickness, anatomical site (proximal vs distal), pathologic subtype, urethral invasion, and positive margins of resection.

Lymphovascular invasion in the primary tumor has significant prognostic importance. Studies have assessed its presence or absence and found that it was an important predictor of nodal metastasis ([35]). The pathologist should specifically comment on the presence or absence of vascular invasion in the surgical specimen. Perineural invasion was found to be present in 36% of cases analyzed in a multi-institutional data set of 134 patients and was also a strong predictor of lymph node metastasis ([36]).

Distant Metastasis and Mortality

Metastatic penile cancer is characterized by a relentlessly progressive course, causing death for the majority of untreated patients within 2 years ([37]). Metastatic enlargement of the regional nodes eventually leads to skin necrosis, chronic infection, and death from sepsis, hemorrhage secondary to erosion into the femoral vessels, and failure to thrive.

Clinically detectable distant metastatic lesions to the lung, liver, bone, or brain are uncommon at initial presentation. Such metastases usually occur late in the course of the disease after the local lesion has been treated. Distant metastases in the absence of regional node metastases are unusual.

EVALUATION OF THE PATIENT

Staging System

The American Joint Committee on Cancer (AJCC) seventh edition TNM staging system for penile cancer (Table 38-2) differs from the sixth edition in that pT1 tumors are stratified regarding whether there is high-grade histology or lymphovascular invasion (pT1b) ([38]). Considering pathologic nodal factors further, the seventh edition distinguishes patients with a single positive node (N1) from those with multiple or bilateral nodes (N2) and further recognizes the ominous prognosis (5%-18% 5-year survival) associated with extranodal extension of cancer.

Limitations of the Staging System

A study from the Netherlands Cancer Institute evaluated the practical and prognostic value of the sixth edition TNM classification for penile carcinoma (Table 38-3) ([39]). The current T2 category combines tumors that invade either the corpus spongiosum or the corpora cavernosa ([38]). The 5-year disease-specific survival for tumors invading the corpus spongiosum

Table 38-2 Definitions of TNM

Primary Tumor (T)	
TX	Primary tumor cannot be assessed
T0	No evidence of primary tumor
Tis	Carcinoma in situ
Ta	Noninvasive verrucous carcinoma
T1a	Tumor invades subepithelial connective tissue without lymph vascular invasion and is not poorly differentiated (ie, grades 3-4)
T1b	Tumor invades subepithelial connective tissue and exhibits lymph vascular invasion or is poorly differentiated
T2	Tumor invades corpus spongiosum or cavernosum
T3	Tumor invades urethra
T4	Tumor invades other adjacent structures
Regional Lymph Nodes (N)	
Clinical Stage Definition	
CNX	Regional lymph nodes cannot be assessed
cN0	No palpable or visibly enlarged inguinal lymph nodes
cN1	Palpable mobile unilateral inguinal lymph node
cN2	Palpable mobile multiple or bilateral inguinal lymph nodes
cN3	Palpable fixed inguinal nodal mass or pelvic lymphadenopathy unilateral or bilateral
Pathologic Stage Definition	
PNX	Regional lymph nodes cannot be assessed
pN0	No regional lymph node metastasis
pN1	Metastasis in a single inguinal lymph node
pN2	Metastasis in multiple or bilateral inguinal lymph nodes
pN3	Extranodal extension of lymph node metastasis or pelvic lymph nodes(s) unilateral or bilateral
Distant Metastasis (M)	
M0	No distant metastasis
M1	Distant metastasis[a]

[a]Lymph node metastasis outside the true pelvis in addition to visceral or bone sites.
Reproduced with permission from Edge SB, Byrd DR, Compton CC (eds): *AJCC Cancer Staging Manuarl*, 7th ed. New York, NY: Springer; 2010.

in the Dutch series was 77.7% and for tumors invading the corpora cavernosa was 52.6%, suggesting that the capacity of a tumor to penetrate the tunica albuginea covering the corpora cavernosa is a more invasive characteristic. The Dutch investigators also suggested that the T3 category appears to be obsolete because a distally located tumor that invades the urethra can still be treated with good prognosis; they proposed that invasion of the corpora cavernosa should be designated T3 ([40]).

The Dutch study did not find a significant difference in 5-year disease-specific survival between the N1 and N2 category (70.2% and 58.3%, respectively; $P = .18$), and the authors proposed designating all unilateral inguinal (mobile) lymph node metastases as N1, bilateral inguinal (mobile) lymph nodes as N2, and any fixed groin mass as N3 ([39]). They also noted the difficulty of distinguishing superficial from deep inguinal lymph nodes, which is not always possible to do either clinically or on histopathologic analysis of a surgical specimen. The seventh edition TNM does not distinguish superficial from deep inguinal lymph nodes and does recognize the prognostic significance of a fixed groin mass as N3. The N2 category, however, still includes two or more unilateral, mobile lymph nodes, where the prognosis with two to three nodes is probably better than with more than three nodes involved ([38, 40]).

Thus, the 2010 TNM classification, while an improvement over previous versions, still necessitates caution with respect to prognosis in the assessment of deep inguinal lymph nodes (regarding whether they are truly inguinal or pelvic lymph nodes) and in considering laterality as well as the number of inguinal lymph

Table 38-3 Stage Grouping for Penile Cancer

Stage 0	Tis	N0	M0
	Ta	N0	M0
Stage I	T1a	N0	M0
Stage II	T1b	N0	M0
	T2	N0	M0
	T3	N0	M0
Stage IIIa	T1-T3	N1	M0
Stage IIIb	T1-T3	N2	M0
Stage IV	T4	Any N	M0
	Any T	N3	M0
	Any T	Any N	M1

Reproduced with permission from Edge SB, Byrd DR, Compton CC (eds): *AJCC Cancer Staging Manuarl*, 7th ed. New York, NY: Springer; 2010.

nodes involved. Also, bulky inguinal lymph nodes that are mobile and suspected of having extranodal extension based on imaging are still classified as N1 or N2; such cases would likely be pN3 on histopathologic confirmation of extranodal involvement ([41]). Patients with clinical N1 or N2 and computed tomographic (CT) scan appearance suggestive of extranodal extension should be regarded as being at higher risk.

Evaluation of Palpable Lymph Nodes

Palpable inguinal lymph nodes are found at presentation in 28% to 64% of patients with penile cancer, but not all of these represent metastatic tumor. Lymphadenopathy is caused by metastasis in 47% to 85% of cases, whereas the rest are secondary to inflammation ([35]). Approximately 25% of patients with palpable lymph nodes will have bilateral metastases. Careful note should be made of the uni- or bilateral location of palpable adenopathy, diameter, number in each inguinal area, whether mobile or fixed, relationship to other structures (eg, skin) with respect to infiltration or perforation, and presence of leg or scrotal edema. The National Comprehensive Cancer Network and European Association of Urology guidelines for penile cancer recommend fine-needle aspiration (FNA) of palpable inguinal lymph nodes ([42, 43]).

Staging Groin Dissection

While treatment of the primary tumor and a period of antibiotics may be useful to help sterilize the inguinal region, this practice is no longer advocated as a tool to select patients who either should or should not undergo lymphadenectomy. One alternative to immediate lymphadenectomy for all patients has been to observe patients with normal findings on inguinal examination. Lymphadenectomy is subsequently reserved for those patients who develop palpable lymph nodes. The reluctance to advocate automatic ilioinguinal lymphadenectomy in all patients with penile cancer stems from the substantial morbidity the procedure can produce. Early complications of phlebitis, pulmonary embolism, wound infection, flap necrosis, and permanent and disabling lymphedema of the scrotum and lower limbs were frequent after both inguinal and ilioinguinal node dissections ([35]). Postoperative complications have been reduced by improved preoperative and postoperative care and advances in surgical technique. The mortality of complete inguinal lymph node dissection by an experienced surgeon is about 3% ([44]).

Several studies have analyzed the survival of men undergoing early versus delayed lymphadenectomy according to pathologic evaluation of nodal status. McDougal et al ([45]) reported a series of 23 patients with invasive primary lesions and nonpalpable nodes; 9 patients were treated with immediate adjunctive lymph node dissection (6 were positive), and 14 were treated with surveillance and delayed lymph node dissection. The 5-year survival in the node-positive immediate adjunctive lymphadenectomy group was 83% (5 of 6 patients), whereas in the surveillance group, the 5-year survival was 36% (5 of 14 patients). A third subset in this series had palpable nodes at presentation and had immediate therapeutic lymph node dissection, with 10 of 15 patients (66%) surviving 5 years. The best results were from immediate adjunctive lymph node dissection (83%), with the next best from immediate therapeutic lymphadenectomy (66%). The worst results were from the surveillance and delayed lymphadenectomy group (36%), in whom dissection was delayed until palpable nodes developed. The interval of opportunity for cure in this third group appears to have been lost.

Similarly, Fraley et al ([46]) reported that immediate adjunctive lymphadenectomy resulted in a 5-year disease-free survival in 6 of 8 node-positive patients (75%) compared with 1 of 12 patients (8%) who had been followed up and then treated by delayed lymphadenectomy when nodal enlargement occurred. Six other patients in that series also presented with unresectable adenopathy after initial surveillance, and all died of disease. Although only two of six immediate lymphadenectomy patients had more than two positive nodes, all the patients treated by delayed lymph node dissection had three or more positive nodes.

A series from MD Anderson Cancer Center ([47]) compared 5-year disease-free survival of 14 patients undergoing early lymphadenectomy for clinically suspicious and histologically node-positive disease with that of 8 patients who were followed up and later underwent lymphadenectomy when clinical nodal enlargement was undisputed. The primary tumors were of similar stage. The 5-year disease-free survival was 57% for early lymphadenectomy compared with 13% for delayed node dissection. Of note, the number of involved nodes in the immediate lymphadenectomy group (median 2) was half that of the delayed lymphadenectomy group (median 4), and no patient with more than two positive nodes survived more than 5 years.

Data from these and other studies suggest that a policy of immediate adjunctive or early lymphadenectomy gives greater assurance that surgical intervention will occur when tumor volume is small. For patients at highest risk of lymph node metastases based on features in the primary tumor, surgical staging can be performed by complete bilateral inguinal lymph node dissection, which may also be curative in cases of small-volume metastases. Moreover, experience has suggested that lymphadenectomy in the setting of microscopic disease may be less likely to produce complications than node dissection in the presence of bulky nodal metastases. This is presumably due to the reduced amount of lymphatic tissue removed, preservation of venous drainage, and blood supply compromised, which affect the viability of skin flaps and lymphatic flow.

In patients with nonpalpable inguinal lymph nodes, if ultrasound-guided FNA of any questionable lymph node is tumor negative, dynamic sentinel lymph node biopsy (DSNB) can be performed if the equipment and expertise are available ([35, 48]). In patients at intermediate risk of inguinal lymph node metastases, sentinel lymph node biopsy or modified (superficial) inguinal lymph node dissection may be performed if DSNB is not feasible.

Computed Tomographic Imaging

Patients with clinically palpable lymph nodes should undergo imaging to define the full extent of disease. Both CT and magnetic resonance imaging (MRI) scanning techniques depend primarily on lymph node enlargement for detection of metastases but are unable to define the internal architecture of normal-size nodes ([48]). Because CT and MRI have similar accuracy in detecting lymphadenopathy in other cancers, CT has often been the imaging modality chosen in penile cancer to examine the inguinal and pelvic areas as well as to rule out more distant metastases (Fig. 38-2).

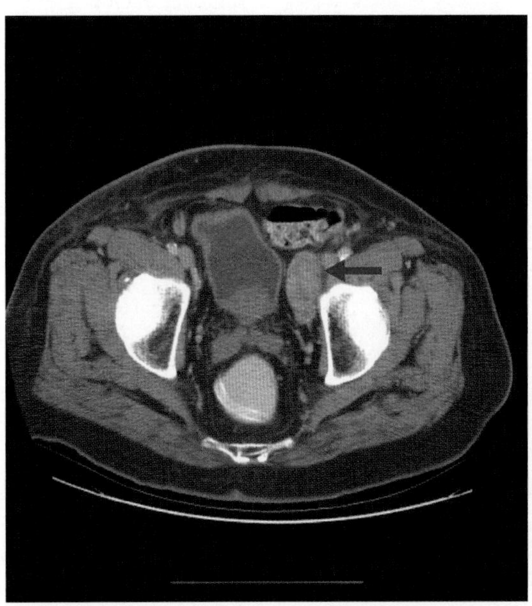

FIGURE 38-2 A CT scan showing bulky metastasis in left external iliac lymph node.

Computed tomographic scanning facilitates the examination of the inguinal region in obese patients or in those who have had prior inguinal surgery, for whom the physical examination may be unreliable. In addition, in patients with known inguinal metastases, CT-guided biopsy of enlarged pelvic nodes may provide important information for consideration of neoadjuvant chemotherapy. Otherwise, the addition of CT imaging does not appear to improve the sensitivity or specificity of lymph node detection when compared to physical examination in patients with a normal inguinal examination.

Positron Emission Tomographic Imaging

Scher et al ([49]) evaluated positron emission tomography (PET)/CT among 13 patients with penile cancer. Five of thirteen patients had metastatic disease, and PET/CT detected four of five patients (80% sensitivity). There may be a role for PET/CT in the detection of lymph node disease in penile cancer; however, the sensitivity of PET/CT is limited for smaller size lymph nodes (Fig. 38-3).

TREATMENT

Local Control

Surgical amputation of the primary tumor remains the oncologic gold standard for rapid definitive treatment of the penile primary tumor; local recurrence rates range from 0% to 8% ([45]). Amputation is often necessary for bulky stage T2-T4 tumors, but it has been shown to decrease sexual quality of life ([50]). It is generally accepted that patients with penile primary tumors exhibiting favorable histologic features (stages Tis, Ta, T1; grades 1 and 2 tumors) are at a lower risk for metastases. These patients are also best suited for organ-sparing or glans-sparing procedures, with the goal of preserving glans sensation where possible or at least to maximize penile shaft length. Such approaches include topical treatments (fluorouracil or imiquimod cream for Tis only), radiotherapy, Mohs surgery, limited excision strategies (eg, circumcision), and laser ablation ([51-55]).

Partial or total penectomy should be considered in patients exhibiting adverse features that defy adequate control by organ preservation strategies. These include tumors of size 4 cm or more, grade 3 lesions, and those invading deeply into the glans, urethra, or corpora cavernosa.

Therapeutic Lymph Node Dissection

The biology of penile cancer is such that it exhibits a prolonged locoregional phase before distant dissemination. Lymphadenectomy alone can be curative and should be incorporated into the treatment planning for most patients. However, due to the morbidity of traditional lymphadenectomy, especially among those patients with clinically negative groins, contemporary controversial issues include the following: (1) the selection of patients for lymphadenectomy versus careful observation; (2) the types of procedures to correctly stage the inguinal region with low morbidity; and (3) multimodality strategies (eg, neoadjuvant chemotherapy, see further in the chapter) to improve survival among patients with bulky inguinal metastases.

The presence and the extent of metastasis to the inguinal region are the most important prognostic factors for survival in patients with squamous cell carcinoma of the penis. The survival rates for

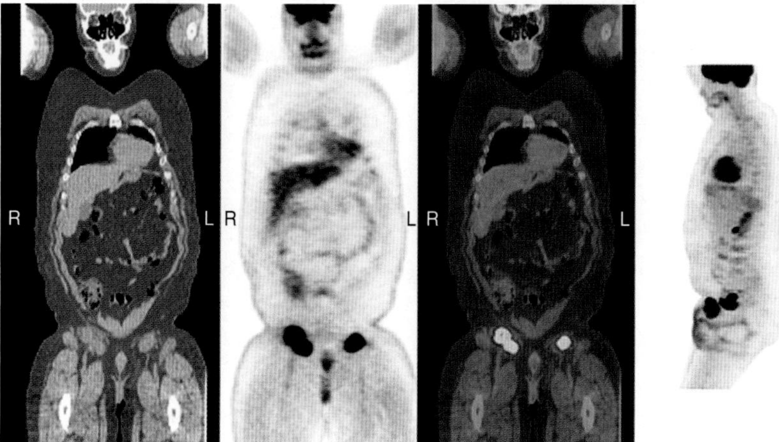

FIGURE 38-3 Computed tomographic and PET images of bilateral inguinal and left external iliac lymph node metastases.

therapeutic lymph node dissection in patients with established regional lymph node metastases are variable, averaging about 60% (range, 0%-86%) ([35, 46, 48]). This variability in survival rates is directly attributable to the extent of nodal metastasis. Patients with pN1 or pN2 with a minimal number of lymph nodes involved have an average 5-year survival of 77%, compared with only 25% when a greater degree of nodal involvement is present. In one study ([56]), the 5-year survival of patients with extranodal involvement was only 6% (1 of 17 patients). The combined results of several small series suggest an average 5-year survival of 15% when pelvic lymph nodes are present.

Taken together, these data suggest that the pathologic criteria that predict long-term survival (ie, 80% 5-year survival rate) after attempted curative surgical resection of inguinal metastases are (1) minimal nodal disease (up to two involved nodes in most series); (2) unilateral involvement; (3) no evidence of extranodal extension of cancer; and (4) absence of pelvic nodal metastases.

Chemotherapy for Stage IIIB/IV Penile Carcinoma

The first candidate drugs for the chemotherapeutic treatment of stage IIIB/IV penile carcinoma included cisplatin, vincristine, methotrexate, fluorouracil, mitomycin, and bleomycin ([37, 57]). In a multicenter study conducted by the Southwest Oncology Group (SWOG) ([58]), 26 patients with metastatic penile cancer received single-agent cisplatin at a dosage of 50 mg/m^2 on days 1 and 8 of each 28-day cycle. Only four patients (15%) experienced responses that persisted for 1 to 3 months.

The combination of bleomycin, methotrexate, and cisplatin (BMP) was studied in phase II clinical trials. In a single-institution study conducted at MD Anderson Cancer Center ([59]), 30 patients with squamous cell carcinoma of the urinary tract, including 21 men with metastatic penile carcinoma, received bleomycin at a dosage of 50 mg/m^2 on days 2 to 6, cisplatin at 20 mg/m^2 on days 2 to 6, and methotrexate at 200 mg/m^2 with leucovorin rescue on days 1, 15, and 22 of each 28-day cycle. There were 12 responses (55%) in the group with penile carcinoma, and the median duration of response was 4.7 months for the entire study. A second phase II study was conducted by the SWOG ([60]), in which patients received bleomycin at a dosage of 10 U/m^2 on days 1 and 8, methotrexate at 25 mg/m^2 on days 1 and 8, and cisplatin 75 mg/m^2 on day 1 of each 21-day cycle. Among 40 evaluable patients, there were 5 complete and 8 partial responses for an overall response rate of 32.5%, which narrowly exceeded the predetermined target rate of 30%. The median response duration was 16 weeks, and the estimated median survival time was 28 weeks. The toxicity of the regimen was considerable, however, with five treatment-related deaths due to bleomycin lung toxicity, other pulmonary causes, and infection. The BMP regimen and bleomycin in particular are no longer recommended for the treatment of penile cancer because of the unacceptable toxicity.

Other cisplatin-based drug combinations demonstrated response rates of 8% to 50% (Table 38-4) ([61-65]). A regimen would be of interest if it has an overall response

Table 38-4 Cisplatin-Based Chemotherapy Regimens Without Bleomycin

Reference	Regimen	Overall Response Rate (PR + CR)	Median Overall Survival (Months)
Theodore et al (2008)	Irinotecan Cisplatin	31%	Not reported
Pagliaro et al (2010)	Paclitaxel Ifosfamide Cisplatin	50%[a]	17.1[a]
Di Lorenzo et al (2012)	5-Fluorouracil Cisplatin	32%	8
Nicholson et al (2013)	Docetaxel Cisplatin 5-Fluorouracil	38.5%	13.9
Houede et al (2015)	Gemcitabine Cisplatin	8%	15

[a]Patients in this study had metastases confined to inguinal or pelvic lymph nodes (Tx N2-N3 M0) and underwent surgical consolidation when possible.

rate greater than 30% with acceptable toxicity. The study of irinotecan/cisplatin conducted by the European Organization for Research and Treatment of Cancer ([61]) was a prospective study with 26 evaluable patients, but was interpreted as having a negative result by the authors because the response rate had an 80% confidence interval of 18.8% to 45.1%, extending well below 30%. In another study, paclitaxel, ifosfamide, and cisplatin was given to patients with metastases limited to the inguinal and pelvic lymph nodes ([62]). In this neoadjuvant study, patients with response or stable disease after four courses underwent surgery with curative intent. The response rate was 50%, and the safety profile of this regimen was an improvement over BMP, with no treatment-related deaths. In another study of taxane drugs for the treatment of metastatic penile cancer, docetaxel, 5-fluorouracil, and cisplatin resulted in a response rate of 38.5% ([63]). The response rate was not high enough to recommend this regimen in preference to 5-fluorouracil and cisplatin, and grade 3 and 4 toxicities were frequent.

5-Fluorouracil and cisplatin were studied in a retrospective series of patients with metastatic penile cancer ([64]). Partial responses had been seen in 8 of 25 evaluable patients (32%). While there have been no randomized controlled trials to establish a single standard of chemotherapy treatment for metastatic penile cancer, either 5-fluorouracil plus cisplatin or paclitaxel, ifosfamide, and cisplatin have been endorsed by contemporary guidelines ([42, 43]).

Multimodality Therapy

Neoadjuvant Chemotherapy

As discussed in the section on therapeutic lymph node dissection, the 5-year overall and disease-free survival rates with surgery alone are as high as 80% for unilateral, superficial inguinal lymph node involvement with no more than two nodes (stage N1 or limited N2), only 10% to 20% for stages N2 and N3 (multiple, bilateral, or pelvic lymph nodes involved), and less than 10% in the presence of extranodal extension ([66]). Nearly all recurrences are detected within 2 years of surgery, and an aggressive, multimodality approach to the treatment of high-risk patients could result in better overall survival ([37, 57, 67]).

In 1988, a team of Italian investigators reported their experience with adjuvant or preoperative (neoadjuvant) bleomycin, vincristine, and methotrexate for patients with penile carcinoma and metastases confined to the inguinal lymph nodes ([68]). In the neoadjuvant group, five patients with fixed inguinal nodes received weekly bleomycin (30 mg intramuscularly), vincristine (1 mg intravenously), and methotrexate (30 mg orally). Three of those five patients had a sufficient tumor response that they could undergo surgical consolidation, and they were reported to be alive and disease free at 20, 27, and 72 months after surgery. The other two patients experienced less-than-partial responses, did not undergo surgery, and survived less than 12 months. This study, although small, demonstrated that perioperative chemotherapy for locally advanced penile carcinoma was feasible.

A group from the Netherlands reported on their retrospective analysis of 20 patients who had received preoperative chemotherapy to downstage unresectable disease ([69]). Seventeen patients had had bulky lymph node metastases (Tx, N3), and the other three had had advanced primary tumors (T3-T4, N0-N1). The most commonly used regimens in the Dutch series, which spanned a 34-year period, had been BMP (n = 10); bleomycin, vincristine, and methotrexate (n = 5); and single-agent bleomycin (n = 3). Severe toxicity had occurred in four patients, including three treatment-related deaths. Twelve patients had experienced an objective tumor response; nine of the twelve had undergone surgery, and eight had achieved long-term disease-free survival. Two patients had no residual tumor in the surgical specimen. The finding of pathologic complete responses suggested that this finding could be used as a screen for efficacy.

A retrospective study from MD Anderson Cancer Center reported a series of 10 patients who had received neoadjuvant chemotherapy ([70]). The reported experience spanned a 15-year period at one institution and was limited to patients who had undergone aggressive lymph node dissections after having experienced a response or stable disease after chemotherapy. The regimens given preoperatively had been BMP (n = 3); paclitaxel and carboplatin (n = 2); and paclitaxel, ifosfamide, and cisplatin (n = 5). Four patients had complete responses, and one had a partial response. Three patients had a pathologic complete response in the lymph nodes; all of these patients had received paclitaxel, ifosfamide, and cisplatin, and all had biopsy-confirmed metastases prior to chemotherapy. Four patients had experienced long-term disease-free survival.

Neoadjuvant chemotherapy was next studied prospectively in a phase II clinical trial conducted at MD Anderson Cancer Center ([62]). Thirty patients with clinical TX N2-N3, M0 penile cancer received four courses of paclitaxel, ifosfamide, and cisplatin prior to a planned complete bilateral inguinal lymph node dissection and uni- or bilateral pelvic lymph node dissection. Fifteen patients (50%) experienced a partial or complete response to chemotherapy. Twenty-two patients (73%) were able to complete the neoadjuvant chemotherapy and surgery, of whom there were three patients (14%) with a pathologic complete response in the lymph nodes (see Fig. 38-4). Objective response to chemotherapy, absence of bilateral residual tumor, and absence of extranodal extension

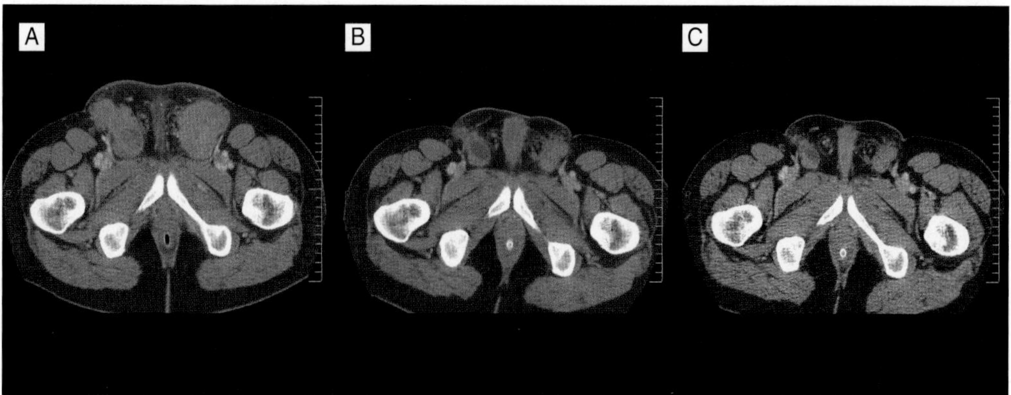

FIGURE 38-4 **A patient with bilateral bulky superficial and deep inguinal lymph node metastases, shown (A) at baseline, (B) after two courses, and (C) after four courses of paclitaxel, ifosfamide, and cisplatin chemotherapy. Bilateral inguinal and pelvic lymph node dissections revealed no viable tumor (ie, a pathologic complete response).**

in residual tumor were associated with a higher rate of overall and progression-free survival in a univariable analysis (Fig. 38-5).

The overall and progression-free survival rates in N2-N3 disease achieved with neoadjuvant paclitaxel, ifosfamide, and cisplatin are an improvement over the expected survival with surgery alone. Despite the absence of a randomized controlled trial, contemporary guidelines have recommend neoadjuvant paclitaxel, ifosfamide, and cisplatin for patients presenting with bulky/high-risk regional lymph node metastases ([42]).

Adjuvant Chemotherapy

Adjuvant chemotherapy has the advantage of allowing patient selection based on accurate pathologic staging. Unfortunately, a randomized controlled trial of adjuvant chemotherapy would not be feasible due to the low incidence of penile carcinoma and the large number of patients necessary to power such a trial. The development of neoadjuvant chemotherapy as standard treatment appears to be more achievable and has advantages of downstaging to facilitate surgery, better tolerance of chemotherapy in the preoperative setting, and earlier exposure of micrometastases to the chemotherapy agents. Tumor response can be detected in the neoadjuvant setting, but not in the adjuvant setting, and the histopathologic findings of postchemotherapy surgery provide an early indicator of the treatment effect and prognosis (Fig. 38-6) ([71]).

In cases where patients have undergone surgery without neoadjuvant chemotherapy and are found to have multiple inguinal or any pelvic lymph nodes involved or extranodal extension, then a regimen such as paclitaxel, ifosfamide, and cisplatin can be administered as adjuvant therapy on the basis of extrapolation from the neoadjuvant data.

Radiotherapy Combined With Surgery or Chemotherapy

Studies of radiotherapy in penile carcinoma have included penis-sparing treatment for small (T1-T2, <4 cm) primary tumors, treatment of lymph node metastases, postoperative radiotherapy, and chemoradiotherapy ([54, 57]). There are no published randomized trials of multimodality treatment with radiotherapy in penile cancer, as there are in squamous cell carcinomas from other sites. For example, radiotherapy with surgical lymphadenectomy has been studied in women with cancer of the vulva, a disease site that has natural history and nodal drainage similar to those of the penis. On the basis of these studies, the standard of care for metastatic vulvar cancer is radiotherapy to the pelvis rather than pelvic lymph node dissection ([72]). Pelvic lymph node dissection remains the standard of care for penile cancer patients following definitive treatment of inguinal lymph node metastases ([42]). Thus, a randomized trial in penile cancer would be informative concerning the optimal method for consolidation of pelvic lymph nodes.

International Randomized Trial

It has not been possible to conduct randomized controlled trials in penile cancer to answer basic questions. One of the studies currently being developed and discussed by the International Rare Tumors Initiative (IRCI) is a 400-patient trial to be conducted in the United Kingdom, United States, and Canada ([73]). The International Penile Advanced Cancer Trial (InPACT) uses a Bayesian design for randomized treatment of patients with inguinal lymph node metastases from penile cancer. The trial has two independent randomizations, addressing key questions in the clinical pathway: first, the role of neoadjuvant therapy prior to standard surgery, by randomizing to chemotherapy, chemoradiotherapy, or no

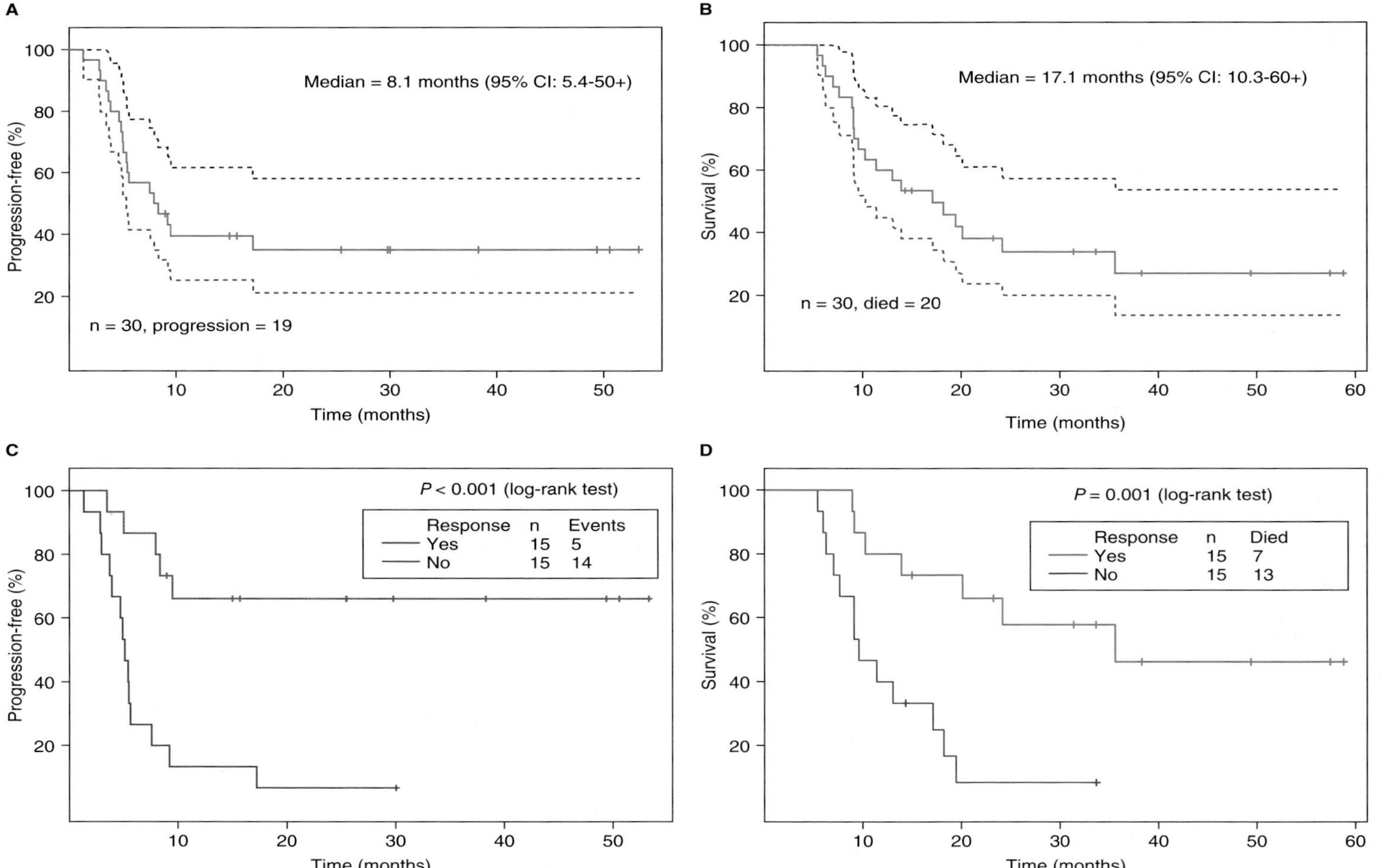

FIGURE 38-5 Kaplan-Meier plots (with 95% CIs as dotted lines) of (A) time to progression of disease, (B) overall survival; patients are grouped by response for (C) time to progression and (D) overall survival. Treatment consisted of neoadjuvant paclitaxel, ifosfamide, and cisplatin. (Reproduced with permission from Pagliaro LC, Williams DL, Daliani D, et al: Neoadjuvant paclitaxel, ifosfamide, and cisplatin chemotherapy for metastatic penile cancer: a phase II study, *J Clin Oncol*. 2010 Aug 20;28(24):3851-3857.)

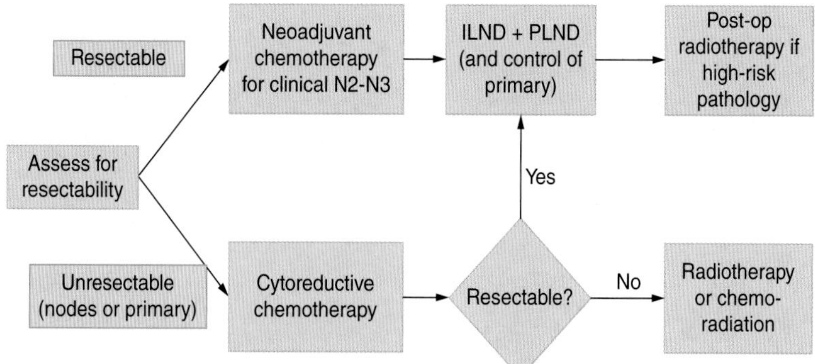

FIGURE 38-6 Treatment algorithm for penile cancer with or without bulky/unresectable regional lymph node metastases.

neoadjuvant therapy; and second, the role of prophylactic pelvic lymph node dissection following the standard surgery with therapeutic inguinal lymph node dissection. The primary outcome measure of the InPACT study is overall survival.

CONCLUSION

The treatment of men with squamous cell carcinoma of the penis has evolved considerably in recent years, along with our understanding of its molecular biology. Penis-sparing strategies for early-stage disease allow for better outcomes in terms of comfort, dignity, and quality of life. Neoadjuvant chemotherapy is now standard of care for patients presenting with bulky regional lymph nodes. An ambitious international randomized trial proposes to compare neoadjuvant and adjuvant as well as surgical and radiotherapeutic strategies in this clinical setting. Meanwhile, vaccination of both men and women against HPV offers to reduce the risk of cancer, particularly for uncircumcised men who are already at increased risk. Viral antigens are a promising target for the immunotherapeutic treatment of penile cancer and suggest a possible role in this disease for drugs that exert immune checkpoint blockade. On the basis of these considerations, one could conclude that we are entering a period of rapid development in the treatment of patients with penile cancer.

REFERENCES

1. Nardi AC, et al. Epidemiology and natural history of penile cancer. In: Pompeo ACL, Heyns CF, Abrams P, eds. *Penile Cancer*. Montreal: Societe Internationale d'Urologie; 2009.
2. Siegel RL, Miller KD, Jemal A. Cancer statistics, 2015. *CA Cancer J Clin*. 2015;65(1):5-29.
3. Flaherty A, et al. Implications for human papillomavirus in penile cancer. *Urol Oncol*. 2014;32(1):53e1-8.
4. Licklider S. Jewish penile carcinoma. *J Urol*. 1961;86:98.
5. Bleeker MC, et al. Penile cancer: epidemiology, pathogenesis and prevention. *World J Urol*. 2009;27(2):141-150.
6. Muneer A, et al. Molecular prognostic factors in penile cancer. *World J Urol*. 2009;27(2):161-167.
7. Reddy CR, Devendranath V, Pratap S. Carcinoma of penis—role of phimosis. *Urology*. 1984;24(1):85-88.
8. Minhas S, et al. Penile cancer—prevention and premalignant conditions. In Pompeo ACL, Heyns CF, Abrams P, eds, *Penile Cancer*. Montreal: Societe Internationale d'Urologie; 2009.
9. Stone KM. Epidemiologic aspects of genital HPV infection. *Clin Obstet Gynecol*. 1989;32(1):112-116.
10. Giuliano AR, et al. Circumcision and sexual behavior: factors independently associated with human papillomavirus detection among men in the HIM study. *Int J Cancer*. 2009;124(6):1251-1257.
11. Dunne EF, et al. Prevalence of HPV infection among females in the United States. *JAMA*. 2007;297(8):813-819.
12. Schiffman M, Wentzensen N. Human papillomavirus infection and the multistage carcinogenesis of cervical cancer. *Cancer Epidemiol Biomarkers Prev*. 2013;22(4):553-560.
13. Schneider V. Microscopic diagnosis of HPV infection. *Clin Obstet Gynecol*. 1989;32(1):148-156.
14. Schneider A, Grubert T. Diagnosis of HPV infection by recombinant DNA technology. *Clin Obstet Gynecol*. 1989;32(1):127-140.
15. Smotkin D. Virology of human papillomavirus. *Clin Obstet Gynecol*. 1989;32(1):117-126.
16. Malek RS, et al. Human papillomavirus infection and intraepithelial, in situ, and invasive carcinoma of penis. *Urology*. 1993;42(2):159-170.
17. Heideman DA, et al. Human papillomavirus-16 is the predominant type etiologically involved in penile squamous cell carcinoma. *J Clin Oncol*. 2007;25(29):4550-4556.
18. Chaux A, Cubilla AL. The role of human papillomavirus infection in the pathogenesis of penile squamous cell carcinomas. *Semin Diagn Pathol*. 2012;29(2):67-71.
19. Djajadiningrat RS, et al. Human papillomavirus prevalence in invasive penile cancer and association with clinical outcome. *J Urol*. 2015;193(2):526-531.
20. Gunia S, et al. p16(INK4a) is a marker of good prognosis for primary invasive penile squamous cell carcinoma: a multi-institutional study. *J Urol*. 2012;187(3):899-907.
21. Sanders CJ. Condylomata acuminata of the penis progressing rapidly to invasive squamous cell carcinoma. *Genitourin Med*. 1997;73(5):402-403.
22. Poblet E, et al. Human papillomavirus-associated penile squamous cell carcinoma in HIV-positive patients. *Am J Surg Pathol*. 1999;23(9):1119-1123.
23. Northfelt DW. Cervical and anal neoplasia and HPV infection in persons with HIV infection. *Oncology (Williston Park)*. 1994;8(1):33-37; discussion 38-40.
24. Martins AC, et al. Immunoexpression of p53 protein and proliferating cell nuclear antigen in penile carcinoma. *J Urol*.

2002;167(1):89-92; discussion 92-93.
25. Lopes A, et al. p53 as a new prognostic factor for lymph node metastasis in penile carcinoma: analysis of 82 patients treated with amputation and bilateral lymphadenectomy. *J Urol.* 2002;168(1):81-86.
26. Campos RS, et al. E-cadherin, MMP-2, and MMP-9 as prognostic markers in penile cancer: analysis of 125 patients. *Urology.* 2006;67(4):797-802.
27. Zhu Y, et al. The prognostic significance of p53, Ki-67, epithelial cadherin and matrix metalloproteinase-9 in penile squamous cell carcinoma treated with surgery. *BJU Int.* 2007;100(1):204-208.
28. Chaux A, et al. The epidermal growth factor receptor is frequently overexpressed in penile squamous cell carcinomas: a tissue microarray and digital image analysis study of 112 cases. *Hum Pathol.* 2013;44(12):2690-2695.
29. Spiess PE, et al. Current concepts in penile cancer. *J Natl Compr Canc Netw.* 2013;11(5):617-624.
30. Necchi A, et al. Proof of activity of anti-epidermal growth factor receptor-targeted therapy for relapsed squamous cell carcinoma of the penis. *J Clin Oncol.* 2011;29(22):e650-e652.
31. Brown A, et al. Epidermal growth factor receptor-targeted therapy in squamous cell carcinoma of the penis: a report of 3 cases. *Urology.* 2014;83(1):159-165.
32. Carthon BC, et al. Epidermal growth factor receptor-targeted therapy in locally advanced or metastatic squamous cell carcinoma of the penis. *BJU Int.* 2014;113(6):871-877.
33. Cabanas RM. Anatomy and biopsy of sentinel lymph nodes. *Urol Clin North Am.* 1992;19(2):267-276.
34. Cubilla AL. The role of pathologic prognostic factors in squamous cell carcinoma of the penis. *World J Urol.* 2009;27(2):169-177.
35. Heyns CF. Management of the lymph nodes in penile cancer. In Pompeo ACL, Heyns CF, Abrams P, eds, *Penile Cancer.* Montreal: Societe Internationale d'Urologie; 2009.
36. Velazquez EF, et al. Histologic grade and perineural invasion are more important than tumor thickness as predictor of nodal metastasis in penile squamous cell carcinoma invading 5 to 10 mm. *Am J Surg Pathol.* 2008;32(7):974-979.
37. Pagliaro LC. Role of chemotherapy in treatment of squamous cell carcinoma of the penis. *Curr Probl Cancer.* 2015;39(3):166-172.
38. Edge S, Byrd DR, Compton CC. Penis. In Edge S, Byrd DR, Compton CC, Fritz AG, Greene FL, Trotti A, eds. *AJCC Cancer Staging Manual.* 7th ed. New York: Springer; 2010.
39. Leijte JA, et al. Evaluation of current TNM classification of penile carcinoma. *J Urol.* 2008;180(3):933-938; discussion 938.
40. Leijte JA, Horenblas S. Shortcomings of the current TNM classification for penile carcinoma: time for a change? *World J Urol.* 2009;27(2):151-154.
41. Graafland NM, et al. Identification of high risk pathological node positive penile carcinoma: value of preoperative computerized tomography imaging. *J Urol.* 2011;185(3):881-887.
42. Clark PE, et al. Penile cancer: clinical practice guidelines in oncology. *J Natl Compr Canc Netw.* 2013;11(5):594-615.
43. Hakenberg OW, et al. EAU guidelines on penile cancer: 2014 update. *Eur Urol.* 2015;67(1):142-150.
44. Bevan-Thomas R, Slaton JW, Pettaway CA. Contemporary morbidity from lymphadenectomy for penile squamous cell carcinoma: the M.D. Anderson Cancer Center Experience. *J Urol.* 2002;167(4):1638-1642.
45. McDougal WS, et al. Treatment of carcinoma of the penis: the case for primary lymphadenectomy. *J Urol.* 1986;136(1):38-41.
46. Fraley EE, et al. The role of ilioinguinal lymphadenectomy and significance of histological differentiation in treatment of carcinoma of the penis. *J Urol.* 1989;142(6):1478-1482.
47. Johnson DE, Lo RK. Management of regional lymph nodes in penile carcinoma. Five-year results following therapeutic groin dissections. *Urology.* 1984;24(4):308-311.
48. Inman BA, Stewart SB, Kattan MW. Staging and risk stratification in penile cancer. In: Spiess PE, ed. *Penile Cancer: Diagnosis and Treatment.* New York: Springer, 2013.
49. Scher, B, et al. 18F-FDG PET/CT for staging of penile cancer. *J Nucl Med.* 2005;46(9):1460-1465.
50. Opjordsmoen S, Fossa SD. Quality of life in patients treated for penile cancer. A follow-up study. *Br J Urol.* 1994;74(5):652-657.
51. Mohs FE, Snow, Larson PO. Mohs micrographic surgery for penile tumors. *Urol Clin North Am.* 1992;19(2):291-304.
52. Windahl T, et al. Sexual function and satisfaction in men after laser treatment for penile carcinoma. *J Urol.* 2004;172(2):648-651.
53. Minhas S, et al. What surgical resection margins are required to achieve oncological control in men with primary penile cancer? *BJU Int.* 2005;96(7):1040-1043.
54. Crook J, Ma C, Grimard L. Radiation therapy in the management of the primary penile tumor: an update. *World J Urol.* 2009;27(2):189-196.
55. Alnajjar HM, Shabbir M, Watkin NA. Penile-sparing approaches to primary penile tumours. In: Spiess PE, ed. *Penile Cancer: Diagnosis and Treatment.* New York: Springer, 2013.
56. Ravi R. Correlation between the extent of nodal involvement and survival following groin dissection for carcinoma of the penis. *Br J Urol.* 1993;72(5 Pt 2):817-819.
57. Pagliaro LC, Crook J. Multimodality therapy in penile cancer: when and which treatments? *World J Urol.* 2009;27(2):221-225.
58. Gagliano RG, et al. *cis*-Diamminedichloroplatinum in the treatment of advanced epidermoid carcinoma of the penis: a Southwest Oncology Group Study. *J Urol.* 1989;141(1):66-67.
59. Corral DA, et al. Combination chemotherapy for metastatic or locally advanced genitourinary squamous cell carcinoma: a phase II study of methotrexate, cisplatin and bleomycin. *J Urol.* 1998;160(5):1770-1774.
60. Haas GP, et al. Cisplatin, methotrexate and bleomycin for the treatment of carcinoma of the penis: a Southwest Oncology Group study. *J Urol.* 1999;161(6):1823-1825.
61. Theodore C, et al. A phase II multicentre study of irinotecan (CPT 11) in combination with cisplatin (CDDP) in metastatic or locally advanced penile carcinoma (EORTC PROTOCOL 30992). *Ann Oncol.* 2008;19(7):1304-1307.
62. Pagliaro LC, et al. Neoadjuvant paclitaxel, ifosfamide, and cisplatin chemotherapy for metastatic penile cancer: a phase II study. *J Clin Oncol.* 2010;28(24):3851-3857.
63. Nicholson S, et al. Phase II trial of docetaxel, cisplatin and 5FU chemotherapy in locally advanced and metastatic penis cancer (CRUK/09/001). *Br J Cancer.* 2013;109(10):2554-2559.
64. Di Lorenzo G, et al. Cisplatin and 5-fluorouracil in inoperable, stage IV squamous cell carcinoma of the penis. *BJU Int.* 2012;110(11 Pt B):E661-E666.
65. Houédé N, Dupuy L, Fléchon A, et al. Intermediate analysis of a phase II trial assessing gemcitabine and cisplatin in locoregional or metastatic penile squamous cell carcinoma. *BJU Int.* 2015 Jan 20. doi:10.1111/bju.13054.
66. Zhu, Y, et al. New N staging system of penile cancer provides a better reflection of prognosis. *J Urol.* 2011;186(2):518-523.
67. Pettaway CA, et al. Treatment of visceral, unresectable, or bulky/unresectable regional metastases of penile cancer. *Urology.* 2010;76(2 Suppl 1):S58-S65.
68. Pizzocaro G, Piva L. Adjuvant and neoadjuvant vincristine, bleomycin, and methotrexate for inguinal metastases from squamous cell carcinoma of the penis. *Acta Oncol.* 1988;27(6b):823-824.
69. Leijte JA, et al. Neoadjuvant chemotherapy in advanced penile carcinoma. *Eur Urol.* 2007;52(2):488-494.
70. Bermejo C, et al. Neoadjuvant chemotherapy followed by aggressive surgical consolidation for metastatic penile squamous cell carcinoma. *J Urol.* 2007;177(4):1335-1338.
71. Dickstein RJ, Munsell MF, Pagliaro LC, Pettaway CA. Prognostic factors influencing survival from regionally advanced squamous

cell carcinoma of the penis after preoperative chemotherapy. *BJU Int*. Jan 2016;117(1):118-125.
72. Kunos C, et al. Radiation therapy compared with pelvic node resection for node-positive vulvar cancer: a randomized controlled trial. *Obstet Gynecol*. 2009;114(3):537-546.
73. Bogaerts, J, et al. Clinical trial designs for rare diseases: studies developed and discussed by the International Rare Cancers Initiative. *Eur J Cancer*. 2015;51(3):271-281.

39 Testicular Cancer

第三十九章　睾丸癌

Maryam N. Shafaee
Nizar M. Tannir
Lance C. Pagliaro

中文导读

睾丸生殖细胞肿瘤占睾丸癌的绝大多数，具有高度治愈性。本章重点讨论来源于睾丸的生殖细胞肿瘤，包括精原细胞瘤和非精原细胞瘤两种类型，来源于其他部位如纵隔、腹膜后等的生殖细胞肿瘤则较为少见。针对精原细胞肿瘤，分别介绍了流行病学、危险因素、肿瘤生物学、组织学类型、临床表现、诊断、血清肿瘤标志物、转移途径等。随后介绍了疾病分期及保留生育能力的考虑。针对睾丸来源的精原细胞瘤，介绍了组织学特点、临床特征、预后以及针对不同分期及风险分层的治疗原则。接着针对非精原生殖细胞肿瘤，介绍了组织学类型、临床表现、预后以及不同分期肿瘤的处理原则。最后，本章介绍了发生于性腺外部位的生殖细胞肿瘤的诊疗原则。

INTRODUCTION

Testicular germ cell tumors (GCTs) account for the majority of testicular cancers and are highly curable. This chapter primarily discusses GCTs arising in the testicle, dividing this category into seminoma versus nonseminoma germ cell tumors (NSGCTs). Then, the rare entity of extragonadal GCTs, which can arise in the mediastinum, retroperitoneum, or pineal body, is described.

OVERVIEW OF GERM CELL TUMORS

Epidemiology

The GCTs are the most common new cancer diagnosis in young men. Roughly an estimated 8,430 new cases were expected to be diagnosed in 2015 ([1]). Highlighting the high curability of this cancer, GCTs only claimed approximately 380 lives in 2015 ([1]) and carry a 5-year overall survival (OS) rate of approximately 95% ([2, 3]). The GCTs have a bimodal age distribution, with most men diagnosed between ages 15 and 25. There is a second peak of diagnosis around age 60, which largely represents seminoma histology and a lower mortality risk. Lifetime risk for the development of GCTs is approximately 0.5% or 1 in 200 ([4]).

Worldwide, GCTs are six times more common in developed countries, with the largest incidence reported in Denmark and Switzerland and the lowest in Japan, Finland, and Israel ([4]). In the United States, the overall incidence of GCTs appears to be gradually increasing. The incidence has specifically increased among African Americans, with the greatest increase in seminoma histology. This does not appear to be related to screening or earlier diagnosis ([5]). Caucasian men, although still representing the group most likely to be diagnosed, are more likely to be identified at an earlier stage than in the past ([6]).

Risk Factors

Cryptorchidism is one of the few identifiable risk factors for the development of GCTs, although representing at most about 10% of cases. When present, cryptorchidism imparts a relative risk between 2.5 and 17.1 ([7, 8]). This increased risk includes the contralateral testicle, even if descended normally or via orchiopexy. It is unclear if orchiopexy reduces the lifetime risk of GCTs, although data showing increased incidence even in the contralateral testicle support the theory that the etiology of GCTs lies in abnormal gonadal development rather than anatomic malposition ([9, 10]). Men with a prior history of GCTs also have an increased risk of GCTs in the contralateral testicle, suggesting a genetic predisposition, although men with a family history of GCTs account for only 1.5% of patients with new diagnosis ([11]). A personal history of GCT carries an increased lifetime risk of secondary cancers, irrespective of histologic type ([12]).

Tumor Biology

The most common genetic abnormality found in GCTs is an isochromosome of the short arm of chromosome 12, which has been identified in approximately 80% of GCTs ([13]). This abnormality can be found in all histologic subtypes except spermatocytic seminoma ([14, 15]). Overexpression of *c-kit* is seen in seminoma ([16]). Of note, p53 is rarely altered in GCTs, and single-gene mutations in general are uncommon ([17]).

Carcinoma in situ (CIS), or intratubular germ cell neoplasia (ITGCN), has been identified as the precursor lesion in most GCTs. It is histologically described as atypical germ cells in the seminiferous tubules. Such changes are found adjacent to most invasive GCTs, with the notable exception of spermatocytic seminoma. The ITGCN cells express numerous proto-oncogenic proteins that play a role in tumorigenesis, including the receptor tyrosine kinase CD-117 or *c-kit*, a protein normally involved in germ cell migration and early differentiation ([18, 19]).

Histologic Classification

The main histologies encountered in GCTs are seminoma, embryonal carcinoma, endodermal sinus tumor (EST, also known as yolk sac tumor), choriocarcinoma, and teratoma. The last can be further classified as mature, immature, or teratoma with malignant transformation. It is common to see more than one histologic subtype within a tumor. Importantly, the clinical course can be largely inferred from the histology. The GCTs that show exclusively the seminoma histology constitute pure seminomas, while those containing any other histologic pattern are classified as NSGCTs, even if the dominant histologic pattern is seminoma. Thus, the term *seminoma* is used in two very different ways: as a histologic pattern and as a main subdivision of GCTs. The biology and clinical expression are dominated by the nonseminoma component, and thus the presence of any histologic component other than seminoma places the tumor in the category of NSGCT.

Clinical Presentation

Most patients with GCTs present with painless testicular swelling or a nodule. In some cases, testicular swelling can be accompanied by pain secondary to bleeding or infarction within the tumor. In the presence of pain or a history of injury, an appropriate differential diagnosis would include testicular torsion, epididymitis, orchitis, hydrocele, spermatocele, and hematoma. *It is extremely important that regardless of pain or other associated symptoms, all scrotal masses should be approached as if they were malignant.* In patients who present with gynecomastia, especially bilateral, GCTs should be considered [20]. Other symptoms can include fever, weight loss, back pain, and hemoptysis (most often seen in patients presenting with high-volume disease).

Diagnosis

The importance of prompt diagnosis and treatment cannot be stressed enough because the extent of disease at presentation predicts overall prognosis. Awareness of GCT prevalence among young men is important for both general practitioners and the general public. Radiographic evaluation of a suspected primary should include high-resolution, trans-scrotal ultrasonography with color Doppler of both testicles, and any suspicious lesion should be definitively evaluated with radical orchiectomy.

Trans-scrotal biopsy is contraindicated in the diagnostic workup of a suspected testicular neoplasm, as this procedure can disrupt regional lymphatics, potentially altering the otherwise-predictable nodal spread. Because the diagnosis of GCTs is rarely in question, the preferred diagnostic and therapeutic procedure for a testicular mass is radical inguinal orchiectomy. If a tissue diagnosis is felt to be necessary prior to orchiectomy, an open biopsy should be performed via an inguinal incision to allow for proper examination and tissue sampling with minimal risk of inguinal or scrotal contamination.

Serum Tumor Markers

Serum markers, specifically human chorionic gonadotropin (hCG), α-fetoprotein (AFP) and lactate dehydrogenase (LDH), have unique diagnostic and prognostic significance in GCTs. These markers enable the clinician to infer clinical behavior, monitor therapy, decide when to apply surgical consolidation, and detect residual or recurrent disease.

Elevated in pregnancy, hCG is not normally detectable in males except in the setting of GCTs. With a half-life of 18 to 36 hours, hCG can also be markedly elevated in gestational trophoblastic disease and occasionally in epithelial cancers [21]. It is composed of two subunits, α and β, which exist in multiple isoforms. The α subunit has sequence similarity to the α subunit of thyroid-stimulating hormone (TSH), follicle-stimulating hormone (FSH), and luteinizing hormone (LH), which leads to "cross-talk" between these hormones and hCG. For this reason, hCG assays measure the β subunit. This "cross talk" can be clinically significant in high-volume disease accompanied by high levels of hCG, where hCG causes hyperthyroidism by binding to the TSH receptor. *Extreme elevation of hCG in males should be considered pathognomonic for GCTs and, in selected cases of threatening disease, justifies initiation of therapy even before tissue confirmation.*

Normally produced by the fetal yolk sac, AFP also exists in multiple isoforms. It is elevated in GCT cells derived from the embryological yolk sac, including endodermal sinus tumor and embryonal carcinoma. It has also been found to be elevated in other neoplasms, such as hepatocellular carcinoma and pancreatic, gastric, and lung cancer, and has a serum half-life of approximately 5 days [22]. Seminoma does not produce AFP, and in the setting of GCT, an elevated AFP implies a nonseminomatous histology [23].

Lactate dehydrogenase is neither cancer specific nor germ cell specific. Of the LDH isoforms, LDH-1 is most specific for GCTs; however, there is no established routine use for the fractionation of LDH and precise measurement of LDH-1. Total LDH can be used to estimate the prognosis in advanced NSGCT at the time of diagnosis or to detect recurrent disease [24].

Anatomic Progression

The GCTs follow a distinct pattern of spread and metastasis. The lymphatic drainage from the testicle reflects embryologic origin, and thus the right testicle drains to the interaortocaval lymph nodes, and the left testicle drains to the left para-aortic lymph nodes. These initial nodes of spread are termed the "landing zone." Epididymal lymphatics drain via the external iliac chain and scrotal lymphatics via the pelvic chain; therefore, locally advanced disease (involving the epididymis and scrotum) can present with involvement of these nodal basins. Distant metastasis involves the lungs principally, followed by the liver, brain, and bones.

STAGING

Table 39-1 shows the American Joint Commission on Cancer (AJCC) TNM staging of testicular cancer [25]. This system is based on the anatomic characteristics of the tumor, the presence of elevated tumor markers, and the presence of distant disease. These well-defined risk factors are used to group patients into stages I-III. In general, stage I disease is confined to the testis, stage II disease has nodal metastases confined to the retroperitoneum with markers in the good prognosis range (S1), and stage III disease includes nodes

Table 39-1 Germ Cell Tumor: The New AJCC TNM Staging of Testicular Cancer

Primary Tumor (T)	
The extent of primary tumor is usually classified after radical orchiectomy, and for this reason a pathologic stage is assigned.	
PTX	Primary tumor cannot be assessed
pT0	No evidence of primary tumor (eg, histologic scar in testis)
PTis	Intratubular germ cell neoplasia (carcinoma in situ)
pT1	Tumor limited to the testis and epididymis without vascular/lymphatic invasion; tumor may invade into the tunica albuginea but not the tunica vaginalis
pT2	Tumor limited to the testis and epididymis with vascular/lymphatic invasion, or tumor extending through the tunica albuginea with involvement of the tunica vaginalis
pT3	Tumor invades the spermatic cord with or without vascular/lymphatic invasion
pT4	Tumor invades the scrotum with or without vascular/lymphatic invasion
Regional Lymph Nodes (N) Clinical	
NX	Regional lymph nodes cannot be assessed
N0	No regional lymph node metastasis
N1	Metastasis with a lymph node mass ≤2 cm in greatest dimension or multiple lymph nodes, none >2 cm in greatest dimension
N2	Metastasis with a lymph node mass >2 cm but not >5 cm in greatest dimension; or multiple lymph nodes, any one mass >2 cm but not >5 cm in greatest dimension
N3	Metastasis with a lymph node mass >5 cm in greatest dimension
Pathologic (PN)	
PNX	Regional lymph nodes cannot be assessed
pN0	No regional lymph node metastasis
pN1	Metastasis with a lymph node mass ≤2 cm in greatest dimension and ≤5 nodes positive, none >2 cm in greatest dimension
pN2	Metastasis with a lymph node mass >2 cm but not >5 cm in greatest dimension; or >5 nodes positive, none >5 cm; or evidence of extranodal extension of tumor
pN3	Metastasis with a lymph node mass >5 cm in greatest dimension
Distant Metastasis (M)	
M0	No distant metastasis
M1	Distant metastasis
M1a	Nonregional nodal or pulmonary metastasis
M1b	Distant metastasis other than to nonregional lymph nodes and lungs
Serum Tumor Markers (S)	
SX	Marker studies not available or not performed
S0	Marker study levels within normal limits
S1	LDH <1.5 × N AND
	hCG (mIU/mL) <5,000 AND
	AFP (ng/mL) <1,000
S2	LDH >1.5-10 × N OR
	hCG (mIU/mL) 5,000-50,000 OR
	AFP (ng/mL) 1,000-10,000
S3	LDH >10 × N OR
	hCG (mIU/mL) >50,000 OR
	AFP (ng/mL >10,000
N indicates the upper limit of normal for the LDH assay.	

(Continued)

Table 39-1 Germ Cell Tumor: The New AJCC TNM Staging of Testicular Cancer (*Continued*)

Stage Grouping				
Stage 0	pTis	N0	M0	S0
Stage I	pT1-pT4	N0	M0	SX
Stage IA	pT1	N0	M0	S0
Stage IB	pT2	N0	M0	S0
	pT3	N0	M0	S0
	pT4	N0	M0	S0
Stage IS	Any pT/Tx	N0	M0	S1-S3
Stage II	Any pT/Tx	N1-N3	M0	SX
Stage IIA	Any pT/Tx	N1	M0	S0
	Any pT/Tx	N1	M0	S1
Stage IIB	Any pT/Tx	N2	M0	S0
	Any pT/Tx	N2	M0	S1
Stage IIC	Any pT/Tx	N3	M0	S0
	Any pT/Tx	N3	M0	S1
Stage III	Any pT/Tx	Any N	M1	SX
Stage IIIA	Any pT/Tx	Any N	M1a	S0
	Any pT/Tx	Any N	M1a	S1
Stage IIIB	Any pT/Tx	N1-N3	M0	S2
	Any pT/Tx	Any N	M1a	S2
Stage IIIC	Any pT/Tx	N1-N3	M0	S3
	Any pT/Tx	Any N	M1a	S3
	Any pT/Tx	Any N	M1b	Any S

Reproduced with permission from Edge SB, Byrd DR, Compton CC (eds): *AJCC Cancer Staging Manuarl*, 7th ed. New York, NY: Springer; 2010.

that extend beyond the retroperitoneum, extranodal metastases, or elevation of tumor markers to the intermediate- or poor-prognosis range (S2-S3).

Fertility Considerations

Of particular importance to men with GCTs is the preservation of fertility. Both the diagnosis and treatment of GCTs are associated with impaired fertility. It is recommended that, if clinically feasible, the patient be counseled about and offered the opportunity to pursue sperm banking prior to starting chemotherapy. It is not recommended to delay chemotherapy in symptomatic poor-risk patients, as poor physical condition often makes sperm donation difficult or even impossible ([26]).

TESTICULAR SEMINOMA

Histology

Under microscopic visualization, classic seminoma has a "fried-egg" appearance, defined as a monotonous proliferation of large, rounded cells arranged in sheets or cords with large centralized nuclei and nucleoli. These tumors can be difficult to distinguish from lymphoma if there is a background of lymphocytic infiltration. Further confirmation (ie, negativity for lymphocyte markers such as common leukocyte antigen) is often required. Although not specific, seminomas stain positive for placental alkaline phosphatase (PLAP) and are routinely negative for AFP and hCG. Figure 39-1 shows the histological appearance of classic seminoma.

On pathologic examination of the testis, seminoma tends to be a semisolid tumor that readily oozes onto the gross examination table. This makes the presence of malignant cells on the surface of the spermatic cord and at the margins of resection a ubiquitous finding. Thus, the clinician must be careful not to be unduly influenced by reports of "margin positivity" and "involvement of the spermatic cord" in the pathology report ([27]). Figure 39-2 shows the typical gross appearance of seminoma.

Even in the presence of significant metastatic disease, it is not uncommon to find only a scar in the testicle. This phenomenon is known as "burned-out"

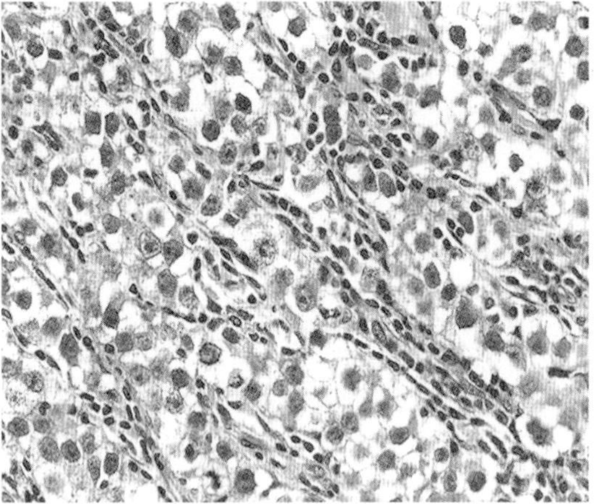

FIGURE 39-1 Histological appearance of classic seminoma.

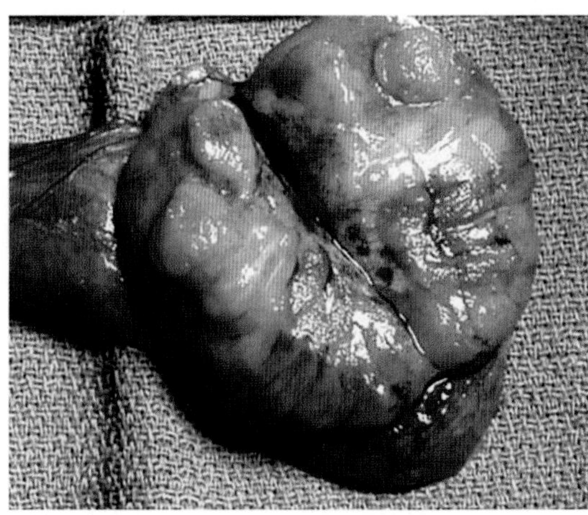

FIGURE 39-2 Gross appearance of seminoma.

seminoma and can also occur in NSGCT. The biological basis for this spontaneous regression of the primary is not known. Seminomas are typically associated with significant inflammatory infiltration, and metastatic deposits characteristically leave a dense desmoplastic residual mass after treatment, often making them difficult to resect.

Clinical Features

Pure seminoma is the most common GCT of the testicle, accounting for approximately 50% of GCTs. By definition, seminomas have no evidence of a nonseminoma component and do not produce AFP but may have modest elevation of β-hCG. Spermatocytic seminomas, a rare variant comprising only 10% of seminomas, are not associated with ITGCN. These tumors typically occur in men over 50 years old, in stage I disease, and have a low metastatic rate. This subtype portends an excellent prognosis with resection alone (with or without radiotherapy) ([28]). Seminomas tend to spread via lymphatics initially, with late hematogenous spread, and are more likely to spread locally, as evidenced by positive margins and involvement of the spermatic cord on histology. The most common hematogenous spread is to the lungs, and metastatic seminomas rarely metastasize to the brain. Remarkably, bulky tumors rapidly respond, with dramatic loss of tumor bulk, but tumor lysis syndrome is never encountered.

Prognosis

The International Germ Cell Cancer Collaborative Group (IGCCCG) established a standard risk classification for both seminomas and NSGCTs (Table 39-2). Patients with metastatic seminoma are divided into either good- or intermediate-risk categories, with no definable "poor-risk" seminoma. The one characteristic that predicted worse outcome for seminoma was the presence of nonpulmonary visceral metastases (intermediate prognosis). The prechemotherapy tumor markers do not predict prognosis (unlike in NSGCTs, discussed further in the chapter). Ninety percent of patients with seminoma fall into the good-prognosis category, with a 5-year OS of 86%. Patients with seminoma in the intermediate-prognosis category have a 5-year OS of 72% ([2]).

Management of Clinical Stage I Seminoma

Patients with clinical stage I seminoma, representing 70% of patients at diagnosis, have disease confined to the testicle with no evidence of nodal or distant metastasis. Most patients will be cured by radical orchiectomy alone, but approximately 20% recur without adjuvant intervention. The disease-specific survival is nearly 100% with or without adjuvant treatment because patients who recur on surveillance are readily salvaged with standard treatment.

Active Surveillance

The benefits of surveillance include avoidance of unnecessary treatment in patients who are likely to be already cured by orchiectomy. Warde et al reported data on 638 patients with clinical stage I seminoma managed with surveillance with a median follow-up of 7 years. Patients with a primary tumor less than 4 cm maximum dimension and without invasion of rete testis had 5-year risk of relapse of only 12%. Patients with both risk factors had a risk of recurrence of 32%, while one of the two risk factors portends a 16% risk of relapse ([29]). Because of excellent outcomes of patients later treated for recurrent disease, active surveillance is considered a reasonable option for most patients, including those with both risk factors.

Radiotherapy

The recurrence rate after prophylactic radiotherapy for clinical stage I seminoma is about 4%, and most of those patients who recur after radiation survive with additional treatment (chemotherapy). Treatment of para-aortic lymph nodes to a dose of 20 Gy was associated with excellent local control approaching 100%. A randomized trial of 20 Gy versus 30 Gy showed no difference in rate of recurrence. Omission of ipsilateral iliac lymph nodes from the treatment field resulted in less toxicity (infertility, gastrointestinal effects) and minimal loss of efficacy. Radiotherapy is contraindicated for patients with horseshoe kidney or inflammatory bowel disease.

Radiotherapy was once viewed favorably because it reduced the number of computed tomographic (CT) scans that were necessary for follow-up, with a net reduction in the cost of treatment. There is, however, a risk of second malignant neoplasms related to treatment. Studies of testicular cancer survivors 25 or more years after treatment have revealed an increase in midline cancers, such as gastrointestinal and genitourinary malignancies. This added risk has brought about a reassessment of whether radiotherapy is warranted, especially considering that 80% of patients with clinical stage I seminoma will be treated unnecessarily, and that there is no survival benefit. At MD Anderson Cancer Center (MDACC), we no longer offer prophylactic radiation to men with stage I testicular seminoma.

Table 39-2 IGCCCG Classification Prognostic Risk Stratification

Seminoma	Nonseminoma
Good Risk	
Any primary site	Testis/retroperitoneal primary
and	and
No nonpulmonary visceral metastases	No nonpulmonary visceral metastases
and	and
Normal AFP, any hCG, any LDH	AFP <1000 ng/mL
	hCG <5000 mIU/mL
	LDH <1.5 × ULN
82% 5-year PFS; 86% 5-year OS	86% 5-year PFS; 90% 5-year OS
Intermediate Risk	
Any primary site	Testis/retroperitoneal primary
and	and
Nonpulmonary visceral metastases	No nonpulmonary visceral metastases
and	and
Normal AFP, any hCG, any LDH	AFP 1,000-10,000 ng/mL
	hCG 5,000-50,000 mIU/mL
	LDH 1.5-10 × ULN
67% 5-year PFS; 72% 5-year OS	75% 5-year PFS; 80% 5-year OS
Poor Risk	
—	Mediastinal primary
	or
—	Nonpulmonary visceral metastases
	or
	AFP >10,000 ng/mL
—	hCG >50,000 mIU/mL
	LDH >10 × ULN
—	41% 5-year PFS; 48% 5-year OS

Chemotherapy

A randomized controlled trial was conducted to compare a single infusion of carboplatin, with dose based on area under the curve (AUC) of 7, versus radiotherapy for the adjuvant treatment of clinical stage I seminoma ([30]). Median follow-up was 4 years, and the relapse-free survival was similar in both treatment arms, 96.7% and 97.7%, respectively, showing noninferiority of the one-cycle, single-agent carboplatin. There are limited data comparing the long-term safety of carboplatin to that of radiotherapy, leading many practitioners to adopt surveillance as the preferred option. Figure 39-3 outlines an approach to therapy for stage I seminoma.

Management of Nonbulky, Good-Risk Seminoma (Stages IIA/IIB)

Patients with stage II seminoma are often divided into nonbulky versus bulky disease for treatment discussion. In general, nonbulky disease is defined as nodes less than 5 cm in cross-sectional dimension on CT or magnetic resonance imaging (MRI) at MDACC. The primary mode of therapy for patients in this category is radiotherapy unless the patient has a contraindication or is unable to tolerate radiation treatment.

Radiotherapy

It is no longer recommended that patients with stages IIA and IIB seminoma receive high-dose radiation (30-35 Gy), mediastinal radiation, or left supraclavicular radiation. At MDACC, our current approach is to give 20 Gy to the para-aortic and ipsilateral iliac nodal fields with a 6-Gy

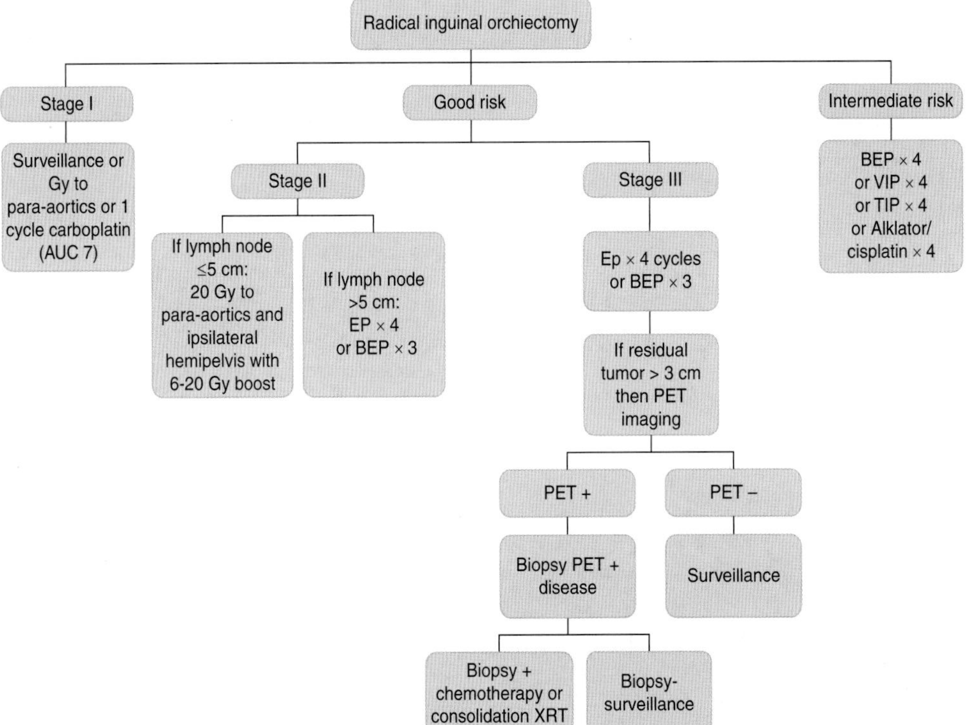

FIGURE 39-3 Management of testicular cancer (seminoma). BEP, bleomycin, etoposide, and cisplatin; EP, etoposide and cisplatin; TIP, paclitaxel, ifosfamide, cisplatin; VIP, etoposide, ifosfamide, cisplatin.

boost to the para-aortic lymph nodes ([31]). Occasionally, radiographic evidence for residual disease is present post-radiotherapy, but if the abnormality is less than 3 cm, observation is recommended.

Alternatives to Radiotherapy

A subset of patients exists who will not be able to receive radiation therapy for various reasons. These reasons may include patient refusal, inflammatory bowel disease, horseshoe or pelvic kidney, and history of abdominal surgery. In this setting, systemic chemotherapy could be offered. In a series published by Xiao et al ([32]), patients with good-prognosis seminoma were included in the analysis and were treated with four cycles of etoposide and cisplatin (EP). Although this does not represent the standard of care for stages IIA and IIB seminoma, it is a reasonable alternative for patients who absolutely cannot receive radiation therapy.

Management of Advanced, Good-Risk Seminoma (Stages IIC/III)

This treatment group includes patients with stage II with bulky lymphadenopathy (≥5 cm) and patients with stage III with good-risk disease. In this group of patients, the risk of recurrence remains high despite local therapy; therefore, the primary treatment recommendation is systemic chemotherapy. It is also in this category of patients that the role of positron emission tomographic (PET) scan may be introduced in its limited role for GCTs.

Chemotherapy

The recommended systemic chemotherapy regimen for patients with good-risk advanced seminoma (stage IIC or IIIA) is three cycles of bleomycin, etoposide, and cisplatin (BEP) or its equivalent. The evidence for use of three cycles of BEP versus four cycles was presented by de Wit et al ([33]). These investigators showed that three cycles of BEP are equivalent to four cycles, with 2-year progression-free survival (PFS) of 90.4% and 89.4%, respectively ([33]). Alternatively, patients who are unable or refuse to receive bleomycin or are older than 50 years can be successfully treated with four cycles of EP.

Residual Disease After Chemotherapy and the Role of Positron Emission Tomography

After completion of chemotherapy, restaging CT scans are performed. If a patient is found to have residual mass measuring 3 cm or less in size with normal tumor markers, active surveillance should be pursued. After chemotherapy, residual disease measuring greater than 3 cm can be further evaluated by PET imaging. Evidence for the role of PET imaging in the setting of residual disease greater than 3 cm was presented by De Santis et al ([34]). In this evaluation of 33 patients with follow-up time of 23 months, the positive predictive value of fluorodeoxyglucose (FDG) PET was 100%, with specificity and sensitivity of 100% and 89%, respectively, for the identification of residual disease in lesions larger than 3 cm. Although encouraging, the role of PET imaging in this setting is being reexamined because several false-positive cases from our institution have been recently identified ([35]).

Positron Emission Tomography–Negative Disease Postchemotherapy

If there is no evidence of avid uptake on PET after chemotherapy, the patient enters the active surveillance strategy. If the patient is unable to have PET imaging, surgical biopsy can be considered for those patients with residual disease measuring greater than 3 cm.

Positron Emission Tomography–Positive Disease Postchemotherapy

At MD Anderson, a positive PET scan requires a confirmatory biopsy. If residual disease is confirmed, several options can be considered. First, salvage radiation therapy to the residual mass can be offered, but this does not provide long-term control. Second, the patient can be offered salvage chemotherapy. Finally, the patient may undergo high-dose chemotherapy with autologous stem cell transplantation. See Fig. 39-3 for the algorithm of our management strategy.

Management of Advanced, Intermediate-Risk Seminoma

Patients with advanced, intermediate-risk seminoma have nonpulmonary visceral metastasis. The most common sites of disease are the liver and bone. These rare patients are offered systemic chemotherapy on presentation (see Fig. 39-3). The chemotherapy regimens commonly used are four cycles of BEP, four cycles of etoposide, ifosfamide, cisplatin (VIP), or four cycles of paclitaxel, ifosfamide, cisplatin (TIP) ([36]).

Salvage Therapy for Refractory/Recurrent Seminoma

The primary treatment for recurrence after radiotherapy is salvage chemotherapy. For patients with lung metastasis (good-risk category), the standard of care is administration of either three cycles of BEP or four cycles of EP. In patients with bone or liver metastasis (intermediate-risk category), salvage chemotherapy is pursued with four cycles of BEP, TIP, or VIP. Bleomycin should be avoided in men older than 50 years.

Clinical signs of chemotherapy-refractory disease should be approached with an aggressive change of strategy, including the option of high-dose chemotherapy and stem cell transplantation. Usually reserved for BEP failures, the role of stem cell transplantation in refractory/recurrent advanced seminoma was addressed by Einhorn et al ([37]). Nineteen percent of a series of 184 patients were patients with metastatic testicular seminoma. At a median follow-up of 48 months, 26 of 35 patients with seminoma treated were in complete remission. Patients in this category should be considered for referral to transplant centers if possible.

NONSEMINOMATOUS GERM CELL TUMORS

Histology

Embryonal Carcinoma

Embryonal carcinoma is the second most common pure presentation of GCT. It is rarely seen at the extremes of age, most commonly presenting in the 20- to 30-year age group, and presents with metastasis in one-third of cases. Microscopically, embryonal carcinoma cells

Case 39-1: Seminoma Presenting With Renal Insufficiency

A 37-year-old man had a left inguinal orchiectomy for classic seminoma. Laboratory data at presentation to MDACC revealed serum creatinine of 1.8 mg/dL, calcium 12.7 mg/dL, hemoglobin 10.5 g/dL, hCG 113 mIU/mL, alkaline phosphatase 194 IU/L, and LDH 1,773 IU/L (ULN 618). A CT scan of abdomen and pelvis revealed a large retroperitoneal mass with marked left hydronephrosis (Fig. 39-4A). The patient initially received one cycle of cyclophosphamide and carboplatin. Repeat laboratory data revealed serum creatinine of 1.1 mg/dL, calcium 8.2 mg/dL, LDH 483 IU/L, and undetectable hCG. He subsequently received three full cycles of EP with excellent response. Repeat imaging shown in Fig. 39-4B revealed marked improvement in the size of the mass (from 14 to 7 cm). Postchemotherapy PET imaging showed the residual mass to be metabolically inactive.

Comment: A patient with advanced seminoma presenting with hydronephrosis and renal insufficiency may receive induction chemotherapy with cyclophosphamide and carboplatin rather than placing nephrostomy tubes to allow administration of BEP or EP in the first cycle. The patient can subsequently receive standard therapy after normalization of renal function.

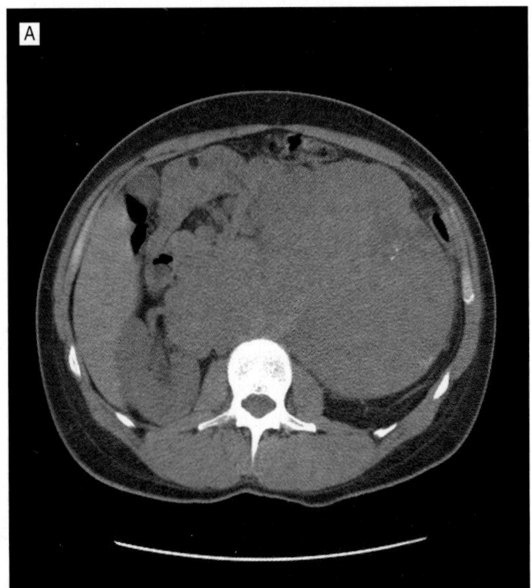

FIGURE 39-4A Baseline imaging from Case 39-1 showing a large left retroperitoneal mass with left hydronephosis.

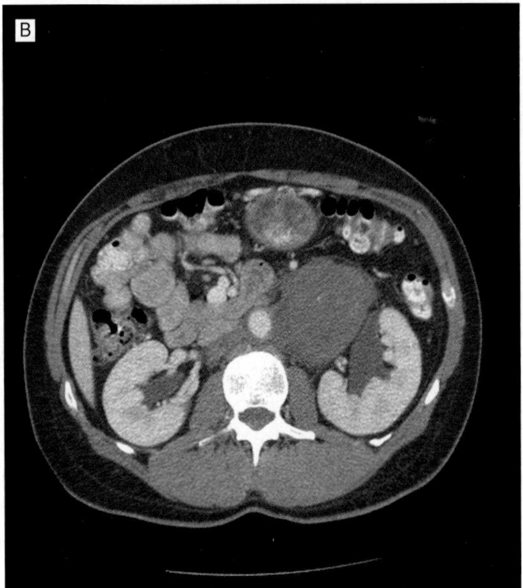

FIGURE 39-4B Repeat imaging from patient in Case 39-1 showing marked improvement in mass after three cycles of chemotherapy.

are the most undifferentiated of the GCT types and are characterized by microscopically varied cells with indistinct borders and scant cytoplasm, giving the appearance of overlapping nuclei. Tumor cells can be seen in sheets or arranged as papillary or tubular structures with a high mitotic rate. There is a propensity for vascular invasion. Phenotypic characterization can reveal positivity for cytokeratin, CD30, PLAP, AFP, and hCG. Modest elevations of both AFP and hCG are typical, but importantly, pure embryonal cancers can be marker negative in the serum. Figure 39-5 shows the typical histologic appearance of embryonal carcinoma.

Endodermal Sinus Tumors (or Yolk Sac Tumors)

Pure yolk sac tumors are extremely rare in the adult patient but account for the majority of childhood GCTs. In adults, EST or yolk sac elements are commonly seen as a component of mixed NSGCTs. Microscopically, EST can manifest as macrocystic, papillary, solid, or a glandular/alveolar pattern with perivascular arrangements of epithelial cells known as glomeruloid or Schiller-Duval bodies. Very high serum AFP levels generally reflect the presence of an EST component, and serum levels of AFP immediately prior to the start of chemotherapy are important prognostically in the classification of good- (AFP <5,000 ng/mL), intermediate- (5,000-10,000 ng/mL), and poor-risk (>10,000 ng/mL) metastatic NSGCTs. Figure 39-6 shows the typical histological appearance of an EST carcinoma.

Choriocarcinoma

Also rare in the pure form in the adult population, choriocarcinoma frequently presents as a component of mixed NSGCTs. Choriocarcinomas comprise both syncytiotrophoblasts and cytotrophoblasts, typically arranged in sheets or nests. Choriocarcinomas generally make copious amounts of hCG, and the level of this marker is also an indication of prognosis in metastatic NSGCTs. Levels of hCG greater than 50,000 mIU/mL are a marker of poor-prognosis NSGCT and are typical of metastatic choriocarcinoma. Half of choriocarcinomas are PLAP positive. Choriocarcinoma elements tend to dominate the clinical course and frequently metastasize to the brain. Symptoms of hyperthyroidism are common, owing to stimulation of the TSH receptor by hCG, and treatment such as a β-blocker is indicated while chemotherapy is initiated. Figure 39-7 shows the typical histological appearance of choriocarcinoma.

Teratoma

Teratomas possess somatic cells from at least two germ cell layers (ectoderm, endoderm, and mesoderm). Variable degrees of differentiation allow for the subclassification of mature and immature forms. A mature teratoma consists of terminally differentiated tissues and can form cystic structures. Although histologically bland, this low-grade malignancy can grow to a threatening dimension and become unresectable. Only about 2% to 3% of all GCTs show mature teratoma as the only histologic component, but teratoma is commonly present as an element of a mixed GCT. An adult

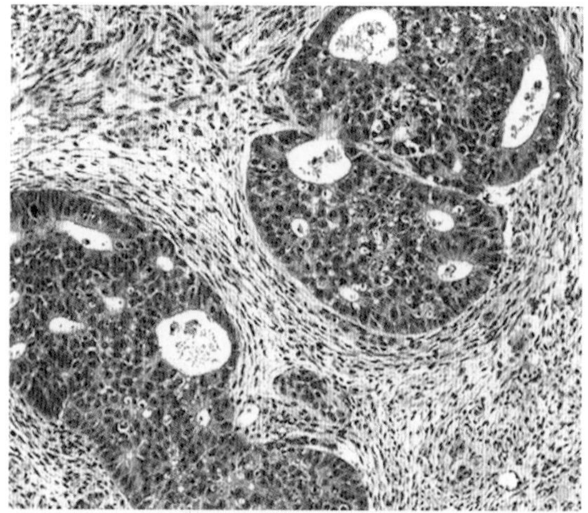

FIGURE 39-5 Histological appearance of embryonal carcinoma.

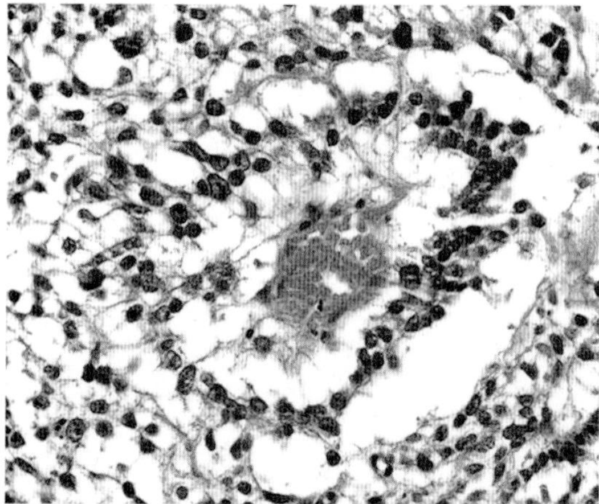

FIGURE 39-6 Histological appearance of EST carcinoma.

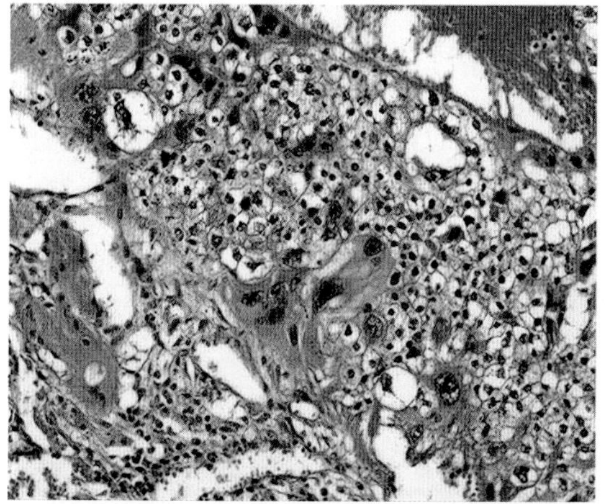

FIGURE 39-7 Histological appearance of choriocarcinoma.

man presenting with teratoma as the only histologic pattern should be presumed to have a mixed GCT and be treated as such. An immature teratoma is less differentiated, although this distinction has no known clinical significance.

One of the unfortunate manifestations is the development of somatic (non-GCT) malignancy within a teratoma. Sometimes known as "teratoma with malignant transformation," this entity typically displays the biology of whatever histology develops and can range from leukemias to sarcomas to carcinomas. In general, transformation to somatic malignancy carries a poor prognosis, and the best prevention is to surgically remove all residual teratoma whenever possible ([38]). Figures 39-8 and 39-9 represent the typical histological and gross appearance of teratoma, respectively.

Clinical Features

As described previously, approximately half of testicular GCTs show histologic elements other than seminoma or produce serum elevation of AFP indicating nonseminoma. These cancers are collectively known as mixed GCTs or NSGCTs, and they form a group of histologically and clinically diverse cancers ([39]). The NSGCTs are more likely to spread hematogenously with increased risk of distant metastasis when compared to seminomas. Because of the unique and heterogeneous nature of NSGCTs, there are several clinical presentations that warrant further discussion because of their significance to patient care and prognosis.

Growing Teratoma Syndrome

Residual teratoma is a low-grade, slow-growing malignancy that can be fatal by inexorable growth. This can take 10 or even 20 years to become threatening and thus can be missed without dedicated lifelong follow-up of patients with NSGCTs. One of the most remarkable and clinically important features of teratomas is that they are often "pushing" and rarely invasive. Thus, at surgery, even very large masses are sometimes removed far more easily than would be expected on the basis of the preoperative imaging. It is important to consult a center where sufficient surgical experience is available before concluding that a residual teratoma is "unresectable" ([40]).

Choriocarcinoma Syndrome

As the name implies, choriocarcinoma syndrome is seen in the setting of high-volume NSGCT that shows predominantly choriocarcinoma histology and is associated with very high (in some cases over 1 million mIU/mL) levels of β-hCG. This syndrome is characterized by prominent constitutional symptoms that represent the effects of both a bulky cancer and secondary

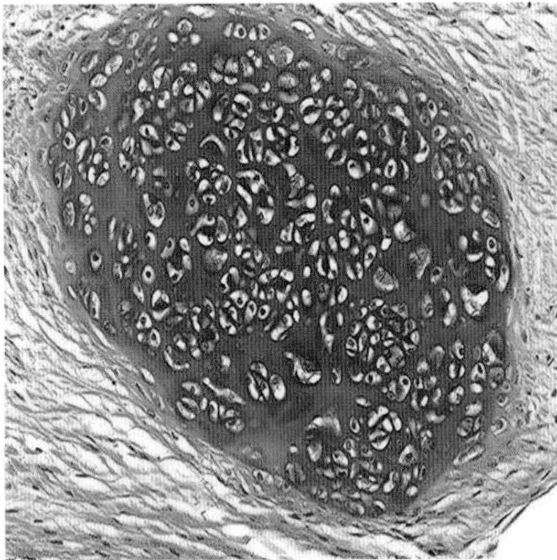

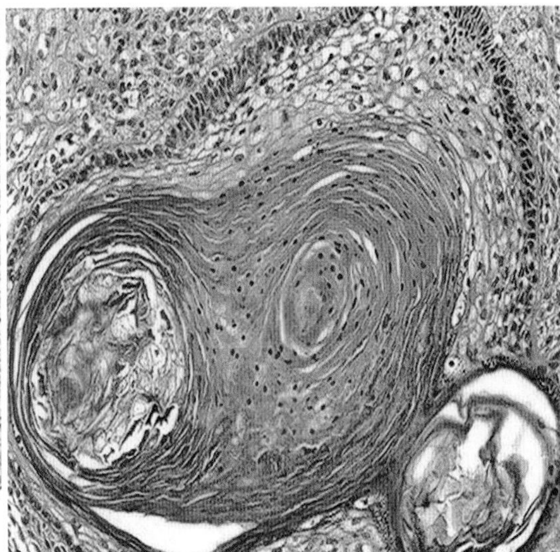

FIGURE 39-8 Histological appearance of teratoma.

hyperthyroidism caused by cross-reaction of hCG with TSH receptors. Typically, patients are rapidly losing weight, tachycardic, anxious, and diaphoretic and have tender gynecomastia from secondary hyperprolactinemia. In addition, most patients have high-volume lung metastases with impending respiratory compromise from the burden of pulmonary metastasis. This is a medical emergency, and treatment should not be delayed for histologic confirmation because this is a pathognomonic constellation in a young man. Metastatic choriocarcinoma has a propensity for brain metastasis, although this is not always apparent on baseline imaging.

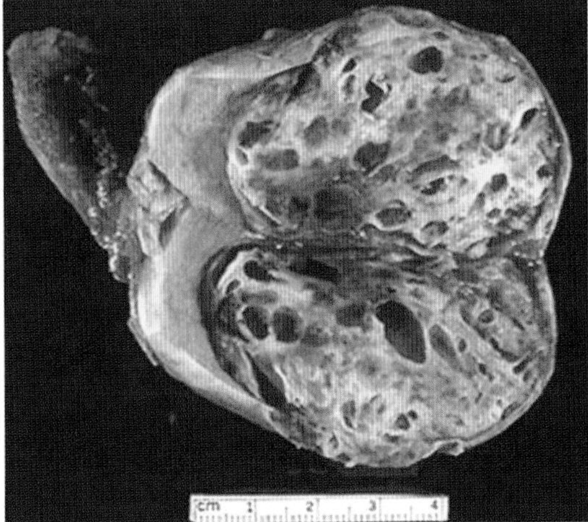

FIGURE 39-9 Gross appearance of teratoma.

Prognosis

As described for seminoma, the IGCCCG developed a prognostic staging system for NSGCTs, with extrapulmonary visceral metastasis found as a major factor in prognosis. Unlike seminoma, prechemotherapy tumor markers were identified as significant in the prognosis of these patients. The prognostic categories are outlined in Table 39-2. In general, patients with mediastinal primary, nonpulmonary visceral metastasis and "poor-risk markers" as defined in the table are considered to have a poor prognosis and have a 5-year OS of 48% with standard treatment. Patients with testis or retroperitoneal primary and no extrapulmonary visceral metastasis are placed in the good-prognosis category based on tumor marker levels as described in the table. Patients with a good prognosis have a 5-year OS of 92%. All others are placed in the intermediate-risk group and have a 5-year OS of 80% ([2]). Van Dijk et al ([3]) updated the 5-year OS data for NSGCTs in a pooled meta-analysis. The authors reported a 5-year OS of 94% for good prognosis, 83% for intermediate prognosis, and 71% for poor prognosis. This illustrates the improving survival rates in the high-risk group.

Management of Clinical Stage I Nonseminoma Germ Cell Tumors

In general, individuals with clinical stage I NSGCT include patients with normal markers postorchiectomy and no evidence of disease outside the resected testis, epididymis, or cord. As with seminoma, radical inguinal orchiectomy is the initial therapy for early-stage NSGCT. Appropriate surgery will cure approximately 70% of patients in clinical stage I. The two identified risk factors in these patients include percentage of embryonal histology and presence of lymphovascular invasion (LVI), with LVI the most predictive ([41]). Patients are considered low risk for recurrence postorchiectomy if there is less than 50% embryonal component in the tumor and no evidence of LVI. The role of percentage of embryonal component is debatable, as it is often seen together with LVI. In fact, European guidelines utilize only absence of LVI for determination of "low risk" for recommendation of observation ([42]).

Observation

Observation is a reasonable strategy for the reliable low-risk patient, which in practice can be those with absence of LVI. The active surveillance schedule as outlined by the National Comprehensive Cancer Network (NCCN) Clinical Practice Guidelines in Oncology recommends that patients should have a physical examination and tumor marker measurements every 2 months during the first year, every 3 months during the second year, and every 4 to 6 months during the third year. Chest x-ray is recommended at 4 and 12 months, then annually. Abdominal and pelvic CT is recommended approximately every 4 months during the first year and annually for years 2 and 3 ([43]).

Observation is also acceptable for high-risk patients. The NCCN guidelines recommend more frequent imaging, with chest x-ray every 2 months in the first year, every 3 months in the second year, and every 4 to 6 months in the third year. Also recommended are abdominal and pelvic CT every 4 months in the first year, every 4 to 6 months in the second year, and every 6 months in the third year.

Retroperitoneal Lymph Node Dissection

Retroperitoneal lymph node dissection (RPLND) is a surgical removal of the "landing zone" lymph nodes and is an accurate staging strategy. However, its role in primary prevention of recurrence in patients with stage I NSGCT is controversial. Morbidity of RPLND includes sympathetic nerve damage that may lead to failure of ejaculation and infertility; however, use of a modified surgical template is a nerve-sparing approach that can preserve the sympathetic nerves and may facilitate anterograde ejaculation in 90% or more patients. Stephenson et al ([44]) reported that RPLND in patients with clinical stage I yielded a 4-year progression-free probability of 96% and is an option for therapy in this patient population. Higher failure rates have been reported for patients with high-risk clinical stage I NSGCT. Patients who do not undergo prophylactic RPLND must undergo periodic CT scanning of the abdomen to rule out growing teratoma in the retroperitoneum. At MDACC, we have abandoned prophylactic RPLND for stage I NSGCT in favor of active surveillance.

Chemotherapy

Adjuvant chemotherapy for clinical stage I NSGCT consists of one or two cycles of BEP. In a randomized controlled trial, Albers et al ([45]) compared RPLND to one cycle of BEP in 382 patients with a median follow-up of 4.7 years. The 2-year recurrence-free survival was 99.46% in the chemotherapy group and 91.87% in the RPLND group, suggesting an advantage of one cycle of BEP chemotherapy. Tandstad et al ([46]), in the Swedish and Norwegian Testicular Cancer Project (SWENOTECA) study, reported that one cycle of BEP reduced the risk of recurrence by 90% in patients with or without LVI. In practice, adjuvant chemotherapy should only be offered to patients with either LVI, embryonal carcinoma-predominant tumor, or both. Our algorithm for management of nonseminoma testicular cancer is shown in Fig. 39-10.

Management of Good-Risk Clinical Stages IIA and IIB Nonseminoma Germ Cell Tumors

Patients with tumor marker—negative stages IIA or IIB NSGCTs—present a unique clinical situation. At our institution, these patients are divided into groups by CT evidence of disease greater than or less than 3 cm. If patients have negative tumor markers with a retroperitoneal mass less than 3 cm after orchiectomy, the options are close follow-up or primary RPLND. Patients with elevated serum tumor markers or retroperitonal mass larger than 3 cm are treated with primary chemotherapy with three cycles BEP or four cycles EP. If residual mass greater than 1cm is detected on follow-up staging, surgical resection is recommended.

Management of Good-Risk Stages IIC and III Nonseminoma Germ Cell Tumors

Patients with bulky retroperitoneal disease of greater than 5 cm or pulmonary metastasis with relatively low serum markers constitute those with advanced disease, but still with favorable prognosis. These patients may be either stage IIC or IIIA according to the AJCC criteria and are considered together in this discussion. The primary mode of treatment in this patient population is systemic chemotherapy. This may be administered before or after radical orchiectomy as long as surgical resection of the primary is performed after completion of therapy. Once again, three cycles of BEP chemotherapy are considered standard of care, and four cycles of EP are considered a reasonable alternative for patients with a contraindication to receive

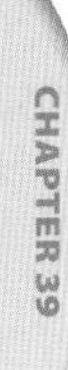

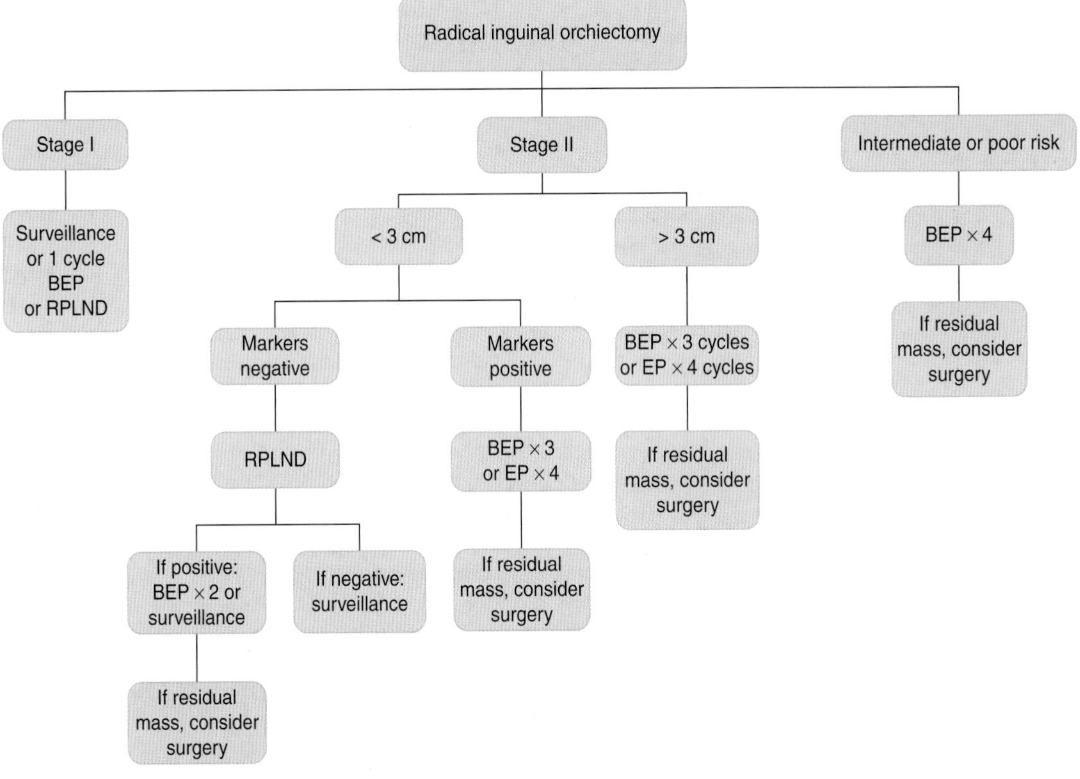

FIGURE 39-10 Management of testicular cancer (nonseminoma).

bleomycin. Resection of residual disease present on restaging should be performed.

Pathology of the resected tumor after salvage chemotherapy is different from after primary chemotherapy. Following primary chemotherapy, viable GCT, fibrosis, and teratoma are found in approximately 20%, 40%, and 40% of pathological specimens, respectively, compared to 50%, 10%, and 40% following salvage chemotherapy, respectively. Patients with greater than 10% viable GCT in the residual pathology specimen after primary chemotherapy should receive an additional two cycles of platinum-based chemotherapy (see Fig. 39-10).

Management of Intermediate- and Poor-Risk Advanced-Stage IIIB and IIIC Nonseminoma Germ Cell Tumors

Patients with advanced NSGCTs who present with intermediate- or poor-risk features are managed with systemic chemotherapy consisting of four cycles of BEP or its equivalent (VIP or TIP). In selected cases, the treatment may be started based on clinical diagnosis prior to radical orchiectomy. Patients with persistent elevation of tumor markers after four courses of first-line chemotherapy in most cases should go on to receive salvage chemotherapy or high-dose chemotherapy with autologous stem cell transplantation.

Personalized Strategy Based on Tumor Marker Decline

Failure of either AFP or hCG to normalize is a well-recognized feature of chemotherapy resistance ([47]). The rate of tumor marker decline has also been studied as a predictor of poor outcome. For patients presenting with stage IIIC NSGCT, it is possible to identify a subgroup of about 25% who, based on favorable marker decline, will do comparatively well and a larger group of about 75% whose outcome with standard therapy is poor ([48]). This observation led to a phase III clinical trial in which patients with stage IIIC NSGCT received BEP in the first cycle, and at completion of the first cycle, those with normalization or favorable decline in both tumor markers remained on BEP (four courses total) and the rest were randomized (1:1) to BEP or an intensified regimen. Final results of this study confirmed superior PFS and OS in the group with favorable decline compared to unfavorable decline (treated with BEP) and demonstrated a statistically significant improvement in 3-year PFS for patients randomized to intensified treatment versus BEP ([49]).

Management of Recurrent and Refractory Nonseminoma Germ Cell Tumors

Several chemotherapy regimens with clinical activity in the salvage setting have been reported, and these include VIP, TIP, VeIP (vinblastine, ifosfamide, cisplatin), or gemcitabine/oxaliplatin. In general, many patients respond and some are even cured with salvage chemotherapy and surgical consolidation, especially those with a small or moderate volume of disease.

High-Dose Chemotherapy

High-dose induction chemotherapy with autologous peripheral blood stem cell transplantation has been studied in first recurrence and later recurrence of GCT. Einhorn et al ([37]) retrospectively reviewed 184 patients (149 patients with advanced NSGCT) with a median follow-up of 48 months. Ninety of the 149 patients (60%) with NSGCT treated with high-dose chemotherapy and subsequent autologous stem cell transplantation were disease free at follow-up. The authors advocated the use of this aggressive treatment as second-line therapy, suggesting that it is more advantageous than when it is used in the third-line setting. Based on this study and despite the absence of a randomized trial, patients with recurrent or refractory advanced-stage NSGCT may be considered for this aggressive, yet effective, treatment strategy.

Special Considerations

Pitfalls in Tumor Marker Elevation

Mild elevation of β-hCG (usually <20 mIU/mL) may occur secondary to hypogonadism or marijuana use and therefore should not always be attributed to residual or recurrent tumor. Modest elevation of AFP may be present with residual teratoma and will normalize following surgical resection, but it may also be constitutionally elevated or indicate the presence of liver disease. In addition, elevated tumor markers may indicate unidentified central nervous system disease or residual primary testicular tumor.

Role of Desperation Surgery

There are patients with NSGCTs who have rising tumor markers despite optimal systemic therapy. In these instances, "desperation surgery" to resect all visible disease may be the only option. It is estimated that up to 20% of patients who fit these criteria can be cured with surgical resection. Patients with isolated retroperitoneal lymph node disease, those with AFP-only elevation, and those who undergo a complete resection of residual disease have the most favorable outcome. Referral to a center with high surgical expertise in this setting is recommended, as potentially large

Case 39-2: BEP/TIP Failure

A 24-year-old man presented with lower back pain, anorexia, night sweats, and weight loss. Imaging studies revealed extensive retroperitoneal lymphadenopathy, a right testicular mass, and bilateral lung nodules. Tumor markers were hCG 33,261, AFP 4.1, and LDH 1,847. A fine-needle aspiration of the retroperitoneal mass revealed embryonal carcinoma. Chemotherapy with BEP was initiated. The kinetics of decline of serum hCG levels were as shown next for the first three of four planned cycles:

- s/p cycle 1: 1,507
- s/p cycle 2: 279
- s/p cycle 3: 323

Salvage chemotherapy commenced after the third cycle of BEP. The patient received four cycles of TIP, with decrease in adenopathy and decline of serum hCG to an undetectable level. The patient was then referred for RPLND and right radical orchiectomy. Pathology revealed no viable tumor. Two months postoperatively, serum hCG rose to 161. He received one cycle of irinotecan, paclitaxel, and oxaliplatin with tumor marker normalization. He then underwent tandem peripheral blood stem cell transplantation with high-dose Ifosfamide, Carboplatin and Etoposide (ICE). He remains disease free 3.5 years later.

Comments: For symptomatic patients with intermediate- or poor-risk GCTs, chemotherapy can be initiated before orchiectomy. Rising tumor markers during BEP chemotherapy signal BEP failure and dictate a change of therapy. The best results are achieved with high-dose chemotherapy and stem cell transplantation.

Case 39-3: The Challenge of Managing Intercurrent Illness

A 35-year-old man who was a heavy smoker and marijuana user underwent a left orchiectomy for a 3.5-cm mixed NSGCT and presented 2 months later to MDACC with left groin pain and left thigh numbness. Tumor markers were AFP 6,575, hCG 1,059, and LDH 2,441. Computed tomographic scans revealed bilateral lung nodules, a large (14.7-cm) retroperitoneal mass, left hydronephrosis, and multiple other enlarged abdominal and pelvic lymph nodes. During the first BEP chemotherapy cycle, he suffered an inferior myocardial infarction (MI) secondary to an occluding atherosclerotic plaque in the right coronary artery. After coronary stenting and optimal medical therapy, the patient was able to complete four cycles of BEP on schedule and at full dose, without delay or significant complications, except for moderate peripheral neuropathy. His tumor markers declined as follows:

- s/p cycle 1 AFP = 3,853, hCG = 34.7
- s/p cycle 2 AFP = 542, hCG = 5.2
- s/p cycle 3 AFP = 88.1, hCG = 4.6
- s/p cycle 4 AFP = 42, hCG = 4.7

The patient received intramuscular testosterone injection for a low serum testosterone level, and 3 weeks later serum hCG was <1.0. Six months after his MI, the patient had resection of the large left retroperitoneal mass, the left kidney, and left adrenal gland; RPLND; and segmental resection of the left psoas muscle. Pathology of the specimen revealed 98% necrosis and only two microscopic foci of residual viable EST in transition to adenocarcinoma. The patient has been recurrence free for 3 years.

Comments: This case illustrates three points. The first is the importance of pursuing chemotherapy while managing an intercurrent illness. The second point is to remember that there are causes of elevated tumor markers other than tumor. The third point is that we do not treat foci of Malignant transformation of Teratoma (MTT).

en bloc resections may be required to achieve the desired outcome of complete resection.

Treatment of Late Relapse

Late relapse is defined as disease recurrence after 24 months from chemotherapy treatment. Teratoma and EST are the most common histologies in this setting, with pure teratoma conferring a better prognosis. Surgery is the preferred initial treatment in these cases if the tumor is anatomically resectable.

Late Complications of Therapy

Although rare, there are specific complications associated with treatment of GCTs that are especially important in this patient population because curability may lead to a normal life expectancy. Secondary leukemias occur in fewer than 0.5% of patients and are associated with use of etoposide. Bleomycin toxicity can appear early and is most associated with dose greater than 200 IU. Patients may also have increased risk of vascular side effects, including Raynaud's syndrome and hypertension. Up to 25% of patients may develop the metabolic syndrome. Additional complications include renal insufficiency, chemotherapy-induced peripheral neurotoxicity, sensorineural hearing loss, chronic electrolyte abnormalities, and neuropsychiatric abnormalities.

EXTRAGONADAL GERM CELL TUMORS

Patients with pure seminoma arising in the mediastinum have similar prognosis as patients with testicular seminomas and are treated with four cycles of EP at our institution, provided they do not have extrapulmonary visceral metastasis. Nonseminomatous extragonadal GCTs represent a distinct subset of GCTs and carry a poor prognosis. The most common origin is the mediastinum, but they can also arise in the retroperitoneum or pineal region. Rare cases involve the vagina, prostate, liver, and orbit.

Mediastinal extra-gonadal germ cell tumors (EGCT) appear as large anterior masses on radiographs. This subset is characterized by prominence of EST and teratoma histology compared to primary testicular GCTs ([50]). Initial diagnosis may be aided by elevations of AFP or hCG. Klinefelter syndrome is associated with increased risk of primary mediastinal NSGCTs ([51]). Additional associations include acute megakaryoblastic leukemia, acute myeloid leukemia, myelodysplastic syndrome, and malignant

Case 39-4: Desperation Surgery

A 46-year-old man presented with back pain and was found to have an 11-cm retroperitoneal mass, biopsy of which revealed high-grade GCT (Fig. 39-11**A**). He underwent a left radical orchiectomy for a 2.8-cm mixed GCT (99% seminoma, 1% teratoma). Postoperatively, serum AFP was greater than 10,000. He received six cycles of EP, followed by one cycle of VeIP but never achieved tumor marker normalization (Fig. 39-11B). At presentation to MDACC, his serum AFP was 604. The patient received multiple additional cycles of rotating salvage chemotherapy, including actinomycin-D, cyclophosphamide, and etoposide (ACE); TIP, cisplatin, vincristine, methotrexate, and bleomycin (POMB); doxorubicin, paclitaxel, and gemcitabine (ATG); and cisplatin, cyclophosphamide, and doxorubicin (CisCA) (Fig. 39-11C). The patient developed renal insufficiency, recalcitrant anemia, and grade 3 peripheral neuropathy and had transient normalization of serum tumor markers while awaiting surgical resection. At the time of surgery, serum AFP was 46.9. The patient underwent RPLND with excision of retroperitoneal masses, left radical nephrectomy, and excision of retrocrural lymph node masses. Pathology demonstrated metastatic mixed GCT, including areas of EST, mature teratoma, and focal areas suspicious for embryonal carcinoma and choriocarcinoma. He remains disease free past 5 years from the time of his salvage surgery.

Comments: Four cycles of BEP and not EP is the standard for patients with intermediate- and poor-risk NSGCT. In rare cases, where the tumor markers do not normalize, even after exhausting all chemotherapeutic options, patients may be salvaged surgically. Patients who have primarily AFP elevation and EST or teratoma benefit the most from such an approach.

histiocytosis. Some of these cases represent malignant transformation of immature teratoma elements.

Mediastinal NSGCTs are classified as poor-prognosis GCTs ([2]), and data suggest that long-term survival is approximately 50% ([52-54]). The aggressive nature of this entity is coupled with the surgical difficulty of resection of residual disease after therapy. Early diagnosis and aggressive resection of mediastinal NSGCTs may improve the outcome. At our institution, the treatment strategy for this rare entity includes presurgical chemotherapy to optimum response and then consolidation surgery.

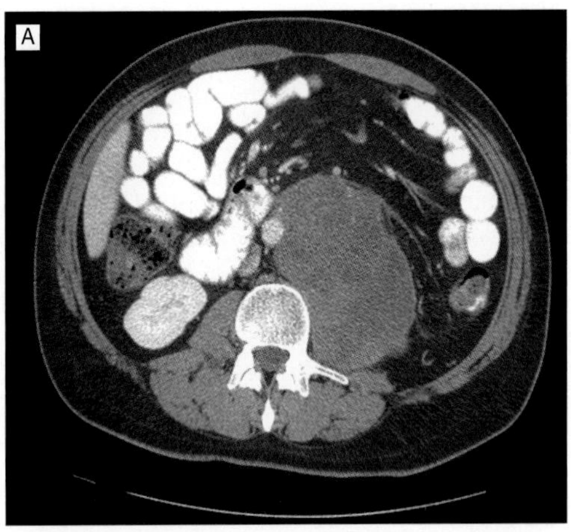

FIGURE 39-11A Baseline imaging of patient described in Case 39-4 with large retroperitoneal mass.

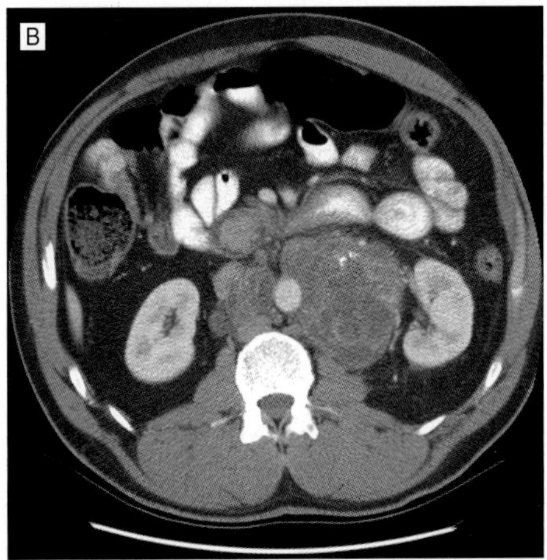

FIGURE 39-11B Repeat imaging of patient in Case 39-4 after six cycles of EP.

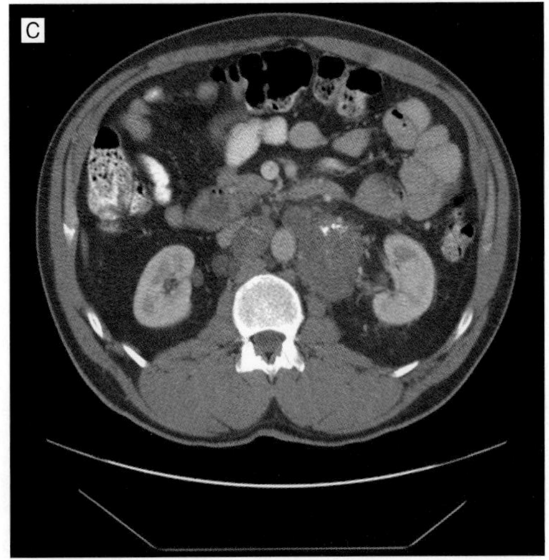

FIGURE 39-11C Imaging of patient from Case 39-4 showing residual disease despite multiple lines of salvage chemotherapy prior to desperation surgery.

CHAPTER 39

Case 39-5: Germ Cell Tumors With Occult Primary

A 29-year-old man presented with weight loss and left supraclavicular lymphadenopathy (Fig. 39-12A) but had a negative testicular examination and ultrasound. Imaging studies confirmed a 5-cm left supraclavicular lymph node and showed a small left pleural effusion. A biopsy of the supraclavicular lymph node demonstrated poorly differentiated adenocarcinoma. Embryonal carcinoma could not be excluded. Immunostains for PLAP and Ki-1 were positive but were negative for AFP and inconclusive for hCG. Laboratory evaluation revealed azoospermia but normal serum chemistries and tumor markers. The patient was treated with three cycles of BEP and achieved a complete remission; he is now disease free for 5 years without surgical consolidation (Fig. 39-12B).

Comments: The case of unknown primary carcinoma in a young man, even if tumor markers are negative, should raise the diagnosis of GCT and should be treated as such. Surgical consolidation is not always necessary when a clinical complete response is achieved with chemotherapy.

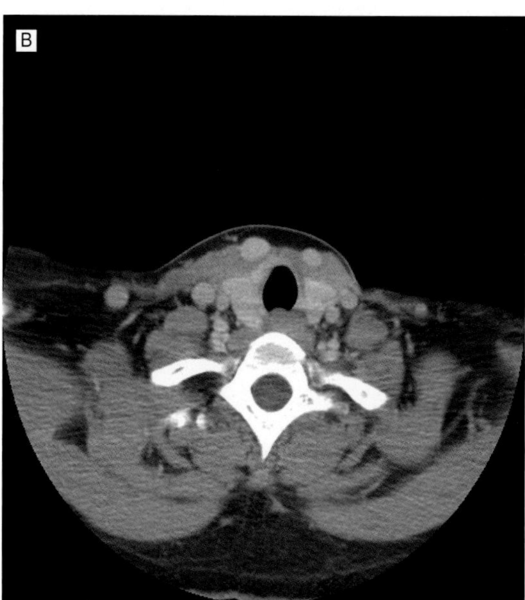

FIGURE 39-12B Imaging after three cycles of chemotherapy.

CONCLUSION

The GCTs represent the paradigm of curable solid tumors. Optimal management of patients with GCTs requires a multidisciplinary approach, integrating chemotherapy and surgery, to achieve the highest cure rates. Patients who pose a unique diagnostic or therapeutic challenge should be considered for early referral to a large tertiary care center.

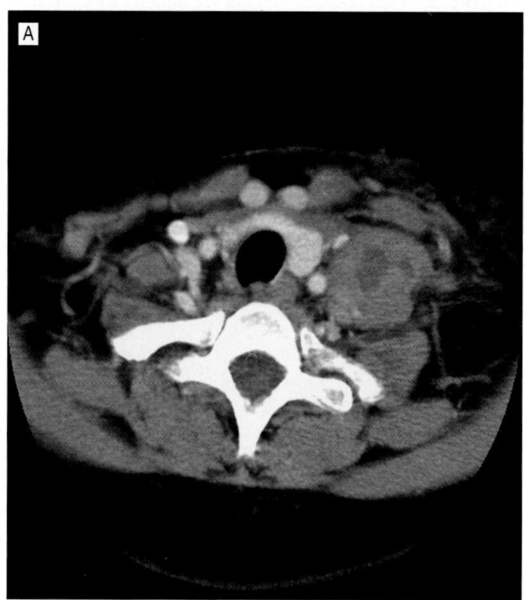

FIGURE 39-12A Baseline imaging of patient described in Case 39-5 showing bulky left supraclavicular adenopathy.

REFERENCES

1. Siegel RL, Miller KD, Jemal A. Cancer statistics, 2015. *CA Cancer J Clin*. 2015;65(1):5-29.
2. International Germ Cell Consensus Classification: a prognostic factor-based staging system for metastatic germ cell cancers. International Germ Cell Cancer Collaborative Group. *J Clin Oncol*. 1997;15(2):594-603.
3. van Dijk MR, Steyerberg EW, Habbema JD. Survival of non-seminomatous germ cell cancer patients according to the IGCC classification: an update based on meta-analysis. *Eur J Cancer*. 2006;42(7):820-826.
4. Bray F, Ferlay J, Devesa SS, McGlynn KA, Møller H. Interpreting the international trends in testicular seminoma and nonseminoma incidence. *Nat Clin Pract Urol*. 2006;3(10):532-543.
5. McGlynn KA, et al. Increasing incidence of testicular germ cell tumors among black men in the United States. *J Clin Oncol*. 2005;23(24):5757-5761.
6. McGlynn KA, et al. Trends in the incidence of testicular germ cell tumors in the United States. *Cancer*. 2003;97(1):63-70.
7. Dieckmann KP, Pichlmeier U. Clinical epidemiology of testicular germ cell tumors. *World J Urol*. 2004;22(1):2-14.
8. Hanna N, Timmerman R, Foster RS, Roth BJ, Einhorn LH, Nichols CR. Testis cancer. In: Kufe DW, Pollock RE, Weichselbaum RR, et al, eds. *Cancer Medicine*. Hamilton, ON, Canada: Decker; 1747-1768.
9. Moller H, et al. Risk of testicular cancer with cryptorchidism and with testicular biopsy: cohort study. *BMJ*. 1998;317(7160):729.
10. Giwercman A, et al. Prevalence of carcinoma in situ and other histopathological abnormalities in testes of men with a history

of cryptorchidism. *J Urol.* 1989;142(4):998-1001; discussion 1001-1002.
11. Dieckmann KP, Pichlmeier U. The prevalence of familial testicular cancer: an analysis of two patient populations and a review of the literature. *Cancer.* 1997;80(10):1954-1960.
12. Travis LB, et al. Risk of second malignant neoplasms among long-term survivors of testicular cancer. *J Natl Cancer Inst.* 1997;89(19):1429-1439.
13. Bosl GJ, et al. Clinical relevance of the i(12p) marker chromosome in germ cell tumors. *J Natl Cancer Inst.* 1994;86(5):349-355.
14. Atkin NB, Baker MC. Specific chromosome change, i(12p), in testicular tumours? *Lancet.* 1982;2(8311):1349.
15. Rodriguez E, et al. Cytogenetic analysis of 124 prospectively ascertained male germ cell tumors. *Cancer Res.* 1992;52(8):2285-2291.
16. Summersgill B, et al. Molecular cytogenetic analysis of adult testicular germ cell tumours and identification of regions of consensus copy number change. *Br J Cancer.* 1998;77(2):305-313.
17. Kersemaekers AM, et al. Role of P53 and MDM2 in treatment response of human germ cell tumors. *J Clin Oncol.* 2002;20(6):1551-1561.
18. Horie K, et al. The expression of c-kit protein in human adult and fetal tissues. *Hum Reprod.* 1993;8(11):1955-1962.
19. Hoei-Hansen CE, et al. Carcinoma in situ testis, the progenitor of testicular germ cell tumours: a clinical review. *Ann Oncol.* 2005;16(6):863-868.
20. Braunstein GD. Clinical practice. Gynecomastia. *N Engl J Med.* 2007;357(12):1229-1237.
21. Wehmann RE, Nisula BC. Metabolic and renal clearance rates of purified human chorionic gonadotropin. *J Clin Invest.* 1981;68(1):184-194.
22. Light PA. Tumour markers in testicular cancer. *J R Soc Med.* 1985;78(Suppl 6):19-24.
23. Yuasa T, et al. Detection of alpha-fetoprotein mRNA in seminoma. *J Androl.* 1999;20(3):336-340.
24. Mencel PJ, et al. Advanced seminoma: treatment results, survival, and prognostic factors in 142 patients. *J Clin Oncol.* 1994;12(1):120-126.
25. Edge S, Byrd DR, Compton CC. Penis. In Edge S, Byrd DR, Compton CC, Fritz AG, Greene FL, Trotti A, eds. *AJCC Cancer Staging Manual.* 7th ed. New York: Springer; 2010.
26. Jeruss JS, Woodruff TK. Preservation of fertility in patients with cancer. *N Engl J Med.* 2009;360(9):902-911.
27. Nazeer T, et al. Spermatic cord contamination in testicular cancer. *Mod Pathol.* 1996;9(7):762-766.
28. Chung PW, et al. Spermatocytic seminoma: a review. *Eur Urol.* 2004;45(4):495-498.
29. Warde P, et al. Prognostic factors for relapse in stage I seminoma managed by surveillance: a pooled analysis. *J Clin Oncol.* 2002;20(22):4448-4452.
30. Oliver RT, et al. Radiotherapy versus single-dose carboplatin in adjuvant treatment of stage I seminoma: a randomised trial. *Lancet.* 2005;366(9482):293-300.
31. Classen J, et al. Radiotherapy for stages IIA/B testicular seminoma: final report of a prospective multicenter clinical trial. *J Clin Oncol.* 2003;21(6):1101-1106.
32. Xiao H, et al. Long-term follow-up of patients with good-risk germ cell tumors treated with etoposide and cisplatin. *J Clin Oncol.* 1997;15(7):2553-2558.
33. de Wit R, et al. Equivalence of three or four cycles of bleomycin, etoposide, and cisplatin chemotherapy and of a 3- or 5-day schedule in good-prognosis germ cell cancer: a randomized study of the European Organization for Research and Treatment of Cancer Genitourinary Tract Cancer Cooperative Group and the Medical Research Council. *J Clin Oncol.* 2001;19(6):1629-1640.
34. De Santis M, et al. Predictive impact of 2-18fluoro-2-deoxy-D-glucose positron emission tomography for residual postchemotherapy masses in patients with bulky seminoma. *J Clin Oncol.* 2001;19(17):3740-3744.
35. Bilen MA, et al. Positive FDG-PET/CT scans of a residual seminoma after chemotherapy and radiotherapy: case report and review of the literature. *Clin Genitourin Cancer.* 2014;12(4):e147-e150.
36. Vuky J, et al. Salvage chemotherapy for patients with advanced pure seminoma. *J Clin Oncol.* 2002;20(1):297-301.
37. Einhorn LH, et al. High-dose chemotherapy and stem-cell rescue for metastatic germ-cell tumors. *N Engl J Med.* 2007;357(4):340-348.
38. Spiess P.E, et al. Malignant transformation of testicular teratoma: a chemoresistant phenotype. *Urol Oncol.* 2008;26(6):595-599.
39. Bosl GJ, et al. Interrelationships of histopathology and other clinical variables in patients with germ cell tumors of the testis. *Cancer.* 1983;51(11):2121-2125.
40. Logothetis CJ, et al. The growing teratoma syndrome. *Cancer.* 1982;50(8):1629-1635.
41. Albers P, et al. Risk factors for relapse in clinical stage I nonseminomatous testicular germ cell tumors: results of the German Testicular Cancer Study Group Trial. *J Clin Oncol.* 2003;21(8):1505-1512.
42. Krege S, et al. European consensus conference on diagnosis and treatment of germ cell cancer: a report of the second meeting of the European Germ Cell Cancer Consensus group (EGCCCG): part I. *Eur Urol.* 2008;53(3):478-496.
43. Motzer RJ, et al. Testicular cancer. Clinical practice guidelines in oncology. *J Natl Compr Canc Netw.* 2006;4(10):1038-1058.
44. Stephenson AJ, et al. Retroperitoneal lymph node dissection in patients with low stage testicular cancer with embryonal carcinoma predominance and/or lymphovascular invasion. *J Urol.* 2005;174(2):557-560; discussion 560.
45. Albers P, et al. Randomized phase III trial comparing retroperitoneal lymph node dissection with one course of bleomycin and etoposide plus cisplatin chemotherapy in the adjuvant treatment of clinical stage I Nonseminomatous testicular germ cell tumors: AUO trial AH 01/94 by the German Testicular Cancer Study Group. *J Clin Oncol.* 2008;26(18):2966-2972.
46. Tandstad T, et al. Risk-adapted treatment in clinical stage I nonseminomatous germ cell testicular cancer: the SWENOTECA management program. *J Clin Oncol.* 2009;27(13):2122-2128.
47. Murphy BA, et al. Serum tumor marker decline is an early predictor of treatment outcome in germ cell tumor patients treated with cisplatin and ifosfamide salvage chemotherapy. *Cancer.* 1994;73(10):2520-2526.
48. Pagliaro LC, Logothetis CJ. Cancer of the testis. In: DeVita VT, Lawrence, TS, Rosenberg SA, eds. *DeVita, Hellman, and Rosenberg's Cancer: Principles and Practice of Oncology.* Philadelphia: Lippincott Williams & Wilkins; 2015:988-1004.
49. Fizazi K, et al. Personalised chemotherapy based on tumour marker decline in poor prognosis germ-cell tumours (GETUG 13): a phase 3, multicentre, randomised trial. *Lancet Oncol.* 2014;15(13):1442-1450.
50. Moran CA, Suster S. Primary germ cell tumors of the mediastinum: I. Analysis of 322 cases with special emphasis on teratomatous lesions and a proposal for histopathologic classification and clinical staging. *Cancer.* 1997;80(4):681-690.
51. Nichols CR, et al. Klinefelter's syndrome associated with mediastinal germ cell neoplasms. *J Clin Oncol.* 1987;5(8):1290-1294.
52. Logothetis CJ, et al. Chemotherapy of extragonadal germ cell tumors. *J Clin Oncol.* 1985;3(3):316-325.
53. Toner GC, et al. Extragonadal and poor risk nonseminomatous germ cell tumors. Survival and prognostic features. *Cancer.* 1991;67(8):2049-2057.
54. Moran CA, Suster S, Koss MN. Primary germ cell tumors of the mediastinum: III. Yolk sac tumor, embryonal carcinoma, choriocarcinoma, and combined nonteratomatous germ cell tumors of the mediastinum—a clinicopathologic and immunohistochemical study of 64 cases. *Cancer.* 1997;80(4):699-707.

Section X Neurologic Tumors

Section Editors: John de Groot and Michael Fisch

第十篇 神经系统肿瘤

40 Tumors of the Central Nervous System

第四十章　中枢神经系统肿瘤

Shiao-Pei Weathers
Barbara O'Brien
John de Groot
Commentary: Anita Mahajan
Commentary: Sujit S. Prabhu

中文导读

本章首先回顾了中枢神经系统肿瘤目前的治疗现状，由于异质性和脑部原发肿瘤的耐药性，中枢神经系统肿瘤患者的处理十分复杂，生存期很短，应鼓励患者积极参加临床实验。本章分别从中枢神经系统肿瘤的WHO分型和发生率、流行病学（包括脑部转移性肿瘤和原发性脑部肿瘤）、生物学和分子基因组学、临床表现、诊断、病理、治疗和预后详细进行了阐述。生物学和分子基因组学部分包括：① 神经胶质肿瘤的信号通路改变，肿瘤发生相关基因，以及预测和预后因素；② 脑膜瘤；③ 脑部转移性肿瘤。在治疗和预后部分，着重讲述了低级别胶质瘤的临床处理策略。本章对Ⅲ～Ⅳ级恶性胶质瘤进行了详尽的阐述，内容包括间变性少突胶质瘤，间变性星型细胞瘤，成胶质细胞瘤，癫痫的控制，脑膜瘤，原发性中枢神经系统淋巴瘤，脑部转移性肿瘤，脑部转移性肿瘤的化疗。最后，本章针对放疗对脑部肿瘤的作用和原发性脑部肿瘤的手术处理进行了简要的评述。

OVERVIEW

Brain tumors are a heterogeneous group of lesions that range from benign, slow-growing tumors found only incidentally on autopsy, to malignant, rapidly growing tumors that cause death within months. The most common intracranial tumors are brain metastases from systemic cancer, estimated at 200,000 new cases per year in the United States, based on a 10% to 15% incidence ([1]). In comparison, the incidence of primary brain and spinal cord tumors for 2014 was estimated at 23,380 new cases (American Cancer Society 2014 Facts and Figures [http://www.cancer.org/acs/groups/content/@research/documents/webcontent/acspc-042151.pdf (or, cancer.org]).

Because of the heterogeneous histology and often-refractory nature of primary brain tumors, their management is complex, ideally requiring a multidisciplinary team and individualized treatment. The diagnosis is made on the basis of histology, so an accurate characterization of the lesion pathology is crucial, often necessitating confirmation at a specialized cancer center. Optimal outcomes involve the coordination of neurosurgery, radiation oncology, and neuro-oncology specialists. Despite advances in neurosurgical techniques, radiation therapy, and chemotherapy, the prognosis for patients with high-grade gliomas such as glioblastoma (GBM), the most common form of glioma, remains dismal. Recent large clinical trials have reported a median survival of only 14 to 16 months with a 26% to 33% 2-year survival rate ([2, 3]). A review of eight consecutive phase II chemotherapy trials for recurrent GBM demonstrated only a 6% response rate (complete response [CR] and partial response [PR]), with a 6-month progression-free survival (PFS) of 15% and a 1-year survival of 21% ([4]). It is therefore important to consider patients with high-grade gliomas for entry into clinical trials at all stages of disease because new therapies target patients from initial diagnosis, with presurgical protocols, to salvage therapy at relapse. This chapter provides basic principles that can be used for diagnosing and treating patients with brain tumors along with an introduction to the molecular mechanisms underlying gliomagenesis.

CLASSIFICATION AND INCIDENCE

Brain tumors are either primary tumors that arise de novo or secondary metastases, the latter being far more common. Most commonly, brain metastases result from lung cancer, followed by breast, melanoma, renal, and colorectal cancers. Most patients with brain metastases die from progression of their systemic cancer, although, because of improvements in systemic therapy, brain metastases are now seen more frequently and with increasing morbidity and mortality. On a more hopeful note, advances in treating brain metastasis with surgery and radiotherapy (RT) have improved overall survival when systemic disease is controlled.

Primary brain tumors are classified by the World Health Organization (WHO) grading system (Table 40-1), which is based on the histologic pattern of cell differentiation in the tumor, in addition to histologic features associated with biological aggressiveness (ie, mitotic figures, necrosis, vascular proliferation). Tumor grade is inversely correlated with prognosis. The most common primary brain tumors are gliomas (all glial tumors), followed by meningiomas, nerve sheath tumors, and pituitary tumors ([5]).

EPIDEMIOLOGY

Brain Metastases

Brain metastases occur far more commonly than primary brain tumors. Nearly any type of primary cancer can metastasize to the brain, including hematologic malignancies. Most commonly, brain metastases

Table 40-1 World Health Organization (WHO) Classification of Tumors of the Central Nervous System

WHO grade I	
Pilocytic astrocytoma	Meningioma
Myxopapillary ependymoma	Craniopharyngioma
Subependymoma	
WHO grade II	
Diffuse astrocytoma	Ependymoma
Pleomorphic xanthoastrocytoma	Pineocytoma
Oligodendroglioma	Atypical meningioma
Oligoastrocytoma	
WHO grade III	
Anaplastic astrocytoma	Anaplastic oligoastrocytoma
Anaplastic oligodendroglioma	Anaplastic ependymoma
Anaplastic (malignant) meningioma	
WHO grade IV	
Glioblastoma	Pineoblastoma
Gliosarcoma	Medulloblastoma

originate from lung cancer, which represents the second most common systemic cancer in men and women ([6]). The next most common pathology to metastasize to the brain is breast cancer, followed by melanoma, renal cancer, and colorectal cancer ([7]). Among solid tumors, melanoma has the highest propensity to metastasize to the brain. Based on autopsy findings, 40% to 60% of patients with melanoma develop brain metastases ([8]). Most brain metastases, particularly melanoma, present with multiple lesions, although when renal cancer metastasizes to the brain, it often results in a single lesion. Approximately 10% of metastatic lesions will present as an intraparenchymal hemorrhage. Hemorrhagic metastases are most commonly seen in patients with melanoma, renal cell carcinoma, thyroid carcinoma, and choriocarcinoma. The pattern of distribution of metastases in the brain varies depending on the primary cancer.

The incidence of brain metastases appears to be rising, which may be a consequence of increasingly sensitive imaging modalities such as magnetic resonance imaging (MRI), greater use of imaging, and the increasingly prolonged survival of patients with metastatic disease. The development of brain metastases usually occurs in the context of systemic relapse, although relapses can be isolated to the central nervous system (CNS). The impermeability of the blood–brain barrier (BBB), which often limits chemotherapy penetration into the CNS, may be the culprit in circumstances of isolated brain relapse.

Primary Brain Tumors

Gliomas are the most frequently occurring primary brain tumors and include astrocytomas, oligodendrogliomas (ODs), and ependymomas. Combined, these histologies account for approximately 40% of all primary brain tumors and over 80% of all malignant CNS tumors ([9]). The next most common tumor is meningioma (32%), followed by nerve sheath tumor (9%) and pituitary tumor (8%) ([9]). The most recent data from the Central Brain Tumor Registry of the United States reported an incidence of all primary benign and malignant CNS tumors of 21.03 cases per 100,000 for a total count of 326,711 incident tumors ([10]).

The incidence of primary brain tumors differs by age. Glioblastomas, which account for more than half of all gliomas, typically peak in incidence between ages 65 and 74, anaplastic gliomas peak between ages 45 and 54, and low-grade gliomas are most typically seen between ages 20 and 34 ([5]). In addition to the disparities of age, gender differences are seen in the incidence of primary brain tumors. The incidence of malignant brain tumors per 100,000 person-years in males is 7.7, compared with 5.4 for females ([10]) (Fig. 40-1).

Primary CNS lymphoma (PCNSL), concordant with AIDS, has decreased since its peak in the early 1990s, when it reached 10.2 per 1 million person-years. By 1998, the incidence decreased to 5.1 per

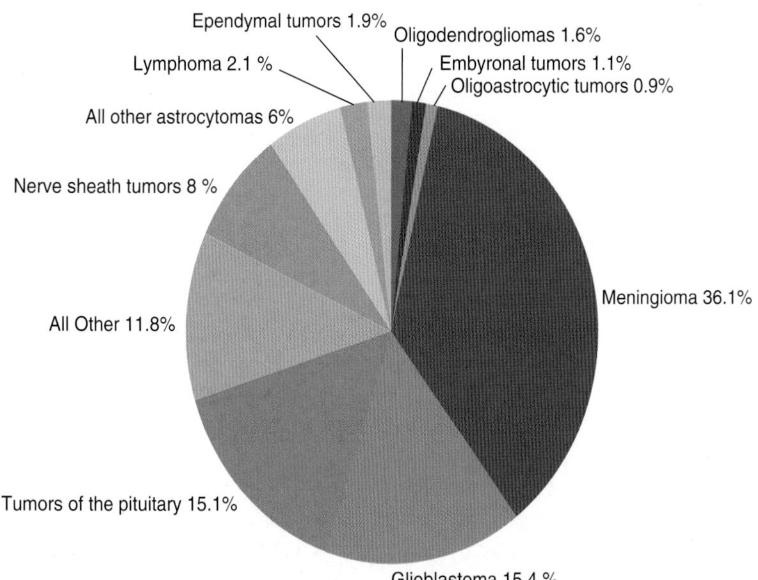

FIGURE 40-1 Distribution of all primary brain and central nervous system tumors by histology, Central Brain Tumor Registry of the United States (CBTRUS) 2007-2011 (n = 343,175). (Reproduced with permission from Ostrom QT, Gittleman H, Liao P, et al: CBTRUS statistical report: primary brain and central nervous system tumors diagnosed in the United States in 2007-2011, Neuro Oncol 2014 Oct;16 Suppl 4:iv1-63).

CHAPTER 40

1 million person-years, which was attributed to the treatment of human immunodeficiency virus (HIV) with highly active antiretroviral therapy (HAART) in males under the age of 60 ([11]). An increased incidence in PCNSL is seen not only in HIV/AIDS but also in iatrogenic immunosuppression, such as organ transplant, autoimmune disease, and cancer. The rate for persons over 60 years of age, however, has remained stable since 1994, at approximately 16 per 1 million person-years ([11]).

Although many factors have been considered as putatively involved in gliomagenesis, therapeutic ionizing radiation is the strongest established causative agent underlying the development of brain tumors. Children with acute lymphoblastic leukemia (ALL), following prophylactic cranial irradiation, have an increased risk for both gliomas and meningiomas ([12]). Increased risk of brain tumors has been seen following therapeutic irradiation for pituitary tumors. Even low doses of radiation previously used to treat scalp ringworm increased the risk of developing nerve sheath tumors, meningiomas, and gliomas ([13]). Fortunately, diagnostic radiation does not appear to be strongly associated with the development of gliomas ([14]).

While a link between brain tumors and chemical exposure has been suggested, no specific agent has been identified with a link to brain tumors that can be validated with an exposure-disease correlation. No consistent link has been proven for the occurrence of cancer in agricultural workers. Positive correlations, but not causation, have been drawn between the occurrence of brain tumors and occupations involving exposure to synthetic rubber, vinyl chloride, and petroleum refining ([15]). Whereas smoking is implicated in an increased risk for many cancers, it is not associated with an increased risk of brain tumors. Exposure to cured foods has been linked to meningiomas, and nitrosamines have been associated with gliomas with a relative risk of 1.48 in adults with a high intake of cured meat ([16]). No correlation between alcohol intake or cosmetic use and brain tumors has been found ([17]).

There has been concern, particularly in the popular press, about the relationship between exposure to cell phones and the risk for brain tumors. Thus far, several case-control studies and a cohort study have failed to establish such a link.

Other than the increased incidence of PCNSL in patients with HIV infection, associations between viral exposures and brain tumors have not been consistent. Human cytomegalovirus (CMV) has recently garnered increasing attention in regard to its role in gliomagenesis. There is sufficient evidence that CMV sequences and viral gene expression exist in most gliomas and that CMV could modulate the malignant phenotype in GBM, but a specific role of CMV in glioma development has yet to be defined ([18]).

A protective effect of allergies (asthma, eczema, and hay fever) was noted in a meta-analysis of over 3,000 patients, with a relative risk of glioma incidence of 0.61 ([19]), supporting a role for immune modulation in brain tumor genesis. A retrospective case-control series demonstrated a decreased incidence of glioma in patients who reported histories of chickenpox, shingles, herpes simplex virus and Epstein-Barr virus ([20]), and as a surrogate for exposure to infections in early life, birth order was correlated with increased risk for the development of glioma in adulthood ([21]).

Relatively few brain tumors are attributable to heredity; studies have cited from 1% to 5% ([22]). Brain tumors can arise as a component of familial tumor syndromes, such as neurofibromatosis type 1 (NF1). Patients with NF1 are at increased risk for the development of gliomas originating predominantly in the optic pathway and brainstem. These neoplasms are typically pilocytic astrocytomas with a tendency toward a more indolent course in comparison to their sporadic counterparts. Neurofibromatosis type 1 is caused by a mutation of the *NF-1* gene and is also associated with leukemia and pheochromocytoma. Neurofibromatosis type II is marked by a mutation of the *NF-2* gene and is associated with bilateral vestibular schwannomas, meningiomas, and gliomas, including an increased risk for ependymomas. The Li-Fraumeni syndrome results from an autosomal dominant mutation of the *p53* tumor suppressor gene, located on chromosome 17p. This *p53* mutation results in many types of malignancies, including glioma and medulloblastoma, as well as sarcoma, breast cancer, leukemia, and adrenocortical cancer. Turcot syndrome is an autosomal dominant disease characterized by multiple polyps of the gastrointestinal tract as well as brain tumors. Two separate mutations have been identified in Turcot syndrome. One involves the *APC* (adenomatous polyposis coli) gene, which is associated with medulloblastoma. A mutation of the *hMLH1* DNA mismatch repair gene is associated with GBM.

BIOLOGY AND MOLECULAR GENETICS

The understanding of cancer relies on uncovering the underlying molecular biologic mechanisms and signaling pathways that drive tumorigenesis. Delineating such mechanisms is complicated by the tremendous degree of intertumoral and intratumoral heterogeneity. Newer drugs target specific extracellular receptors or block intracellular signal transduction systems.

Glial Tumors

Pathway Alterations

Malignant glial tumors often exhibit significant histologic heterogeneity, which is reflected at the molecular level. Large-scale profiling efforts have accelerated our understanding of gliomas. The landscape of somatic genomic alterations has been comprehensively characterized by The Cancer Genome Atlas (TCGA). In the most recent publication by TCGA in 2013, alterations in three core overlapping pathways were described: receptor tyrosine kinase/RAS/phosphatidylinositol 3 kinase (RTK/RAS/PI3K) signaling (altered in 90% of GBMs), p53 signaling (altered in 86% of GBMs), and RB signaling (altered in 79% of GBMs). The alterations affecting the p53 pathway (*MDM2, MDM4,* and *TP53*); the Rb pathway (*CDK4, CKD6, CCND2, CDKN2A/B,* and *RB1*); and the PI3K pathway (*PIK3CA, PIK3R1, PTEN, EGFR, PDGFRA,* and *NF1*) were found to be mutually exclusive ([23]). Of the 251 GBMs analyzed, at least one RTK was found altered: *EGFR* (57.4%), *PDGFRA* (13.1%), *MET* (1.6%), and *FGFR2/3* (3.2%). Mutations of PI3Kinase were found in 25.1% of GBMs and were found to be mutually exclusive for *PTEN* mutations/deletions. The p53 pathway was found to be altered in 85.3% of tumors through mutations/deletion of *TP53* (27.9%), amplification of *MDM1/2/4* (15.1%), or deletion of *CDKN2A* (57.8%) ([23]). The most recent TCGA analysis also identified mutations in genes for which targeted therapies have been developed, including *BRAF* ([24]) and *FGFR1/FGFR2/FGFR3* ([25]).

The epidermal growth factor (EGF) pathway was found to be altered in 57.4% of GBMs in the most recent TCGA data. An alternate mutation in the external domain generates a truncated receptor, the EGFRvIII mutant, which is constitutively activated in gliomas ([26]). Growth factors such as EGF and platelet-derived growth factor (PDGF) activate multiple signal transduction pathways that lead to cell survival and proliferation. The *EGFR* can activate the PI3Kinase pathway, which is also frequently mutated in glioma. When the PI3Kinase pathway is activated, the activation of *AKT* (protein kinase B) is triggered, in turn activating multiple prosurvival pathways, such as nuclear factor kappa B (NFκB), forkhead, and glycolysis. The activation of the PI3Kinase pathway has been associated with the reduced survival of patients with glioma ([27]). Growth factors can also stimulate the *ras* pathway, which initiates a signal cascade through *Raf/MEK/Erk* and also promotes cell survival and tumorigenesis ([28]). PTEN has phosphatase activity that inhibits the PI3Kinase pathway. The deletion of *MMAC/PTEN* leads to *AKT* pathway activation. The activation of *p53* can result in either apoptosis or cell cycle arrest and initiation of DNA repair mechanisms. The abrogation of *p53* activity would be expected to increase proliferation and mutations, leading to genetic instability, the prodrome of tumorigenesis.

Cell cycle regulation is a key target of carcinogenesis. Cell cycle checkpoints are affected by multiple proteins, acting either as accelerators or inhibitors of cell regulation. Important molecules in this process include *p53, p21,* and *MDM*. Another cell cycle regulation pathway important for glial tumors involves the retinoblastoma (*RB*) gene. When the *RB* gene is phosphorylated, the E2F transcription factor is released and activates cellular proliferation. The regulation of *RB* activity is complex and involves multiple cyclins (cyclin D), cyclin-dependent kinases (CDK4/6), and CDK inhibitors (p16), whose activities are under investigation ([29]).

Gliomagenesis

The majority of GBMs (~90%) are primary, characterized by rapid development in the absence of any clinical or histologic evidence of a lower-grade lesion, in contrast to secondary GBMs, which progress from a low-grade astrocytoma or anaplastic astrocytoma (AA). Primary and secondary GBMs arise from distinctly different genetic pathways. Primary GBMs are postulated to develop quickly from glial progenitor cells over a period of a few months, potentially acquiring mutations in *EGFR, TP53,* or *PTEN*. In contrast, secondary GBMs are believed to arise from a stepwise accumulation of mutations.

Isocitrate dehydrogenase (*IDH*) mutations are believed to be a very early event in gliomagenesis that persist during progression to secondary GBM. The *IDH1/2* mutations likely occur prior to the acquisition of a *TP53* mutation, a driving force toward astrocytic differentiation, and prior to the acquisition of 1p/19q loss, believed to be the driving force toward oligodendroglial differentiation. Codeletion of 1p/19q has been classified as the genetic signature of ODs. Recent exomic sequencing has revealed that mutations in the *CIC* gene at 19q13.2 and *FUBP1* gene at 1p are also frequently observed in ODs. In addition to the acquisition of *TP53* mutations, *ATRX* mutations are often noted in WHO grade II and III astrocytomas and secondary GBMs ([30]).

Predictive and Prognostic Factors

In anaplastic oligodendrogliomas (AODs), allelic losses of chromosomes 1p and 19q (1p19q LOH) have emerged as markers of chemotherapeutic response and longer survival ([31]), qualifying 1p19q loss as a prognostic factor. Recent studies have confirmed that 1p/19q

LOH is also predictive of response to chemotherapy. In independent seminal studies by the European Organization for Research and Treatment of Cancer (EORTC) and Radiation Therapy Oncology Group (RTOG), patients with AODs harboring 1p/19q LOH did significantly better when treated with a combination of radiation and chemotherapy compared to treatment with radiation alone. Tumors without 1p/19q LOH did not incur a survival benefit [32-34].

O6-Methylguanine-DNA methyltransferase (MGMT) is a DNA repair protein that reverses DNA damage induced by alkylating agents such as temozolomide and has been implicated as a major mechanism of resistance to alkylating agents. Hypermethylation of the promoter region of the *MGMT* gene, which inactivates *MGMT* gene transcription, has been associated with response to alkylating agents and increased survival in glioma patients [35].

Isocitrate dehydrogenase mutations were first reported in 2008 [36] and quickly became a seminal discovery. The *IDH* mutations now definitively distinguish primary from secondary GBM and have been established as a positive prognostic factor with an increase in overall survival noted in patients harboring an *IDH* mutation over those with wild-type *IDH* [37]. In low-grade glioma, anaplastic glioma, and GBM, *IDH* mutation status appears to be the most important prognostic factor [36, 38]. In a study of 382 patients with high-grade gliomas, *IDH1* mutation was found to be of greater prognostic relevance than histological diagnosis according to the current WHO classification system. The sequence of more favorable to poorer outcome was (1) AA with *IDH1* mutation, (2) GBM with *IDH1* mutation, (3) AA without *IDH1* mutation, and (4) GBM without *IDH1* mutation [38].

Meningiomas

A mutation in the tumor suppressor *NF2* gene on chromosome 22q12, has been closely associated with meningiomas and is disrupted in approximately half of meningiomas [39]. Germline mutations of this gene result in neurofibromatosis type 2, an autosomal dominant disorder that can manifest as multiple meningiomas, bilateral schwannomas, gliomas, and intracranial calcifications [40]. Merlin, the product of the *NF2* gene, functions as a tumor suppressor gene and is a member of a family of cytoskeleton-associated proteins linked to RTK activity and ECM interactions [41].

In a recent study, whole-genome or whole-exome sequencing was performed on 17 sporadic meningiomas. The majority of meningiomas harbored simple genomes, with fewer mutations, rearrangements, and copy number alterations than observed in other adult tumors. Focal *NF2* inactivation was confirmed in 43% of tumors. A subset of meningiomas lacking *NF2* alterations exhibited recurrent oncogenic mutations in *AKT1* and *SMO* with immunohistochemical (IHC) evidence of activation of their pathways. Mutations involving *SMO* were observed in 3/17 tumors, and *AKT*1 mutations were noted in 5/17 samples. Interestingly, these mutations were seen in the more therapeutically challenging tumors involving the skull base and were of higher grade [42]. Hyperactive Hedgehog (Hh) signaling has been linked to many other cancers and is under active investigation in meningiomas highlighting SMO as a potential therapeutic target [43]. Inhibitors of PI3K/AKT/mTOR are also under active investigation for meningiomas harboring *AKT1* mutations.

Brain Metastases

The development of brain metastases is an intricate sequential process. In addition to proliferating, tumor cells must migrate and enter the systemic circulation, survive, travel/transport through the blood to the brain, adhere to and extravasate through the endothelium, invade the brain parenchyma, and proliferate, which requires the recruitment of a secondary blood supply. Failure at any of these steps will halt the metastatic process. Each of these steps requires complex interactions between the tumor cell and its changing microenvironment.

An understanding of the biological processes of brain metastases and the role of the BBB provides potential targets for intervention to improve treatment. There are multiple complex regulators of cell adhesion, including molecules such as integrins, cadherins, selectins, and heparin sulfate proteoglycans [44]. In addition, integrins can recruit intracellular signaling molecules such as focal adhesion kinase and src, which can lead to a cascade of cellular signaling that affects cell cycle control and proliferation. Integrins also play a part in regulating angiogenesis and tumor invasion. Other molecules that mediate invasion include the MMP family, serine proteases, and heparinase [45].

Tumor cells must generate their own blood supply if they are to grow successfully and remain viable. Important activators of angiogenesis include vascular endothelial growth factor (VEGF), angiopoietin, hypoxia-inducible transcription factor (HIF), cyclooxygenase 2 (COX-2), PDGF, integrins, MMPs, and others. Important inhibitors of angiogenesis include angiostatin, endostatin, tissue inhibitors of matrix metalloproteinases (TIMPs), interferons, and platelet factor 4 [46]. Upregulation of activators or downregulation of inhibitors favors angiogenesis. As tumors grow, they begin to produce increasing numbers of angiogenic molecules that can participate in metastasis [46]. Because a multitude of pathways are involved in tumor growth and invasion, it is likely that if one pathway is inhibited, cells may escape through alternate pathways.

Effective drug delivery through the BBB to tumor cells is a significant obstacle to chemotherapy, both for brain metastases and primary brain tumors. The P-glycoprotein family of transporters actively exports drugs such as anthracyclines, Vinca alkaloids, taxanes, and etoposide [47]. The BBB can be breached by circulating cancer cells, which migrate across the BBB without degrading its permeability and proliferate. Once the tumor reaches a size that requires recruitment of new vessels, the BBB is disrupted, which allows imaging of brain tumors with contrast agents. In experimental models, brain metastases smaller than 0.25 mm in diameter are associated with an intact BBB, whereas larger tumors demonstrate BBB permeability [48]. Despite the presence of the BBB, studies of drug levels in brain tumors from systemic delivery have demonstrated pharmacologically relevant concentrations of drugs such as etoposide, cisplatin, cytarabine, and methotrexate. Measurements of drug levels in cerebrospinal fluid are not accurate indicators of tissue drug levels and also vary widely depending on the agent [49].

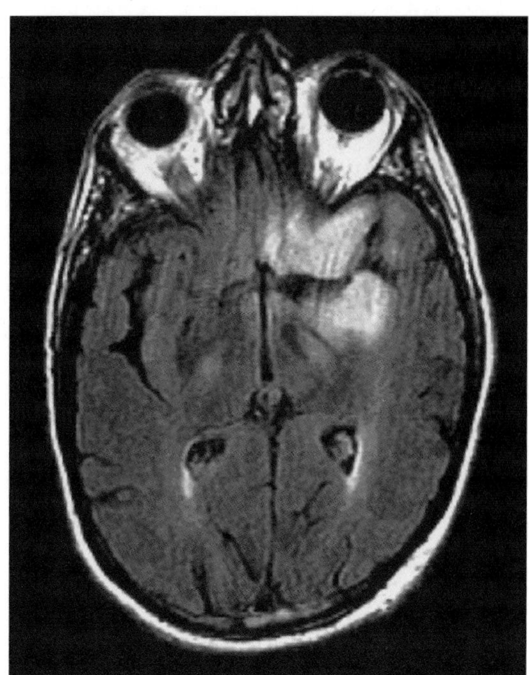

FIGURE 40-2 Low-grade glioma.

CLINICAL PRESENTATION, DIAGNOSIS, AND PATHOLOGY

Clinical Presentation

Brain tumors are usually diagnosed following presentation with symptoms such as seizure, headache, or focal neurologic deficits. We commonly see high-grade, malignant tumors presenting with headache, which reflects elevated intracranial pressure, and focal neurologic signs, such as weakness or aphasia. Low-grade glial tumors often come to attention with seizure, while other slow-growing tumors, such as meningioma, may be clinically silent and incidentally detected during imaging for an unrelated problem. We use contrast-enhanced MRI, the diagnostic standard, for brain tumor imaging. In addition to its superior sensitivity compared with computed tomography (CT), MRI provides more detailed anatomic as well as physiologic information that can contribute to a differential diagnosis. While contrast-enhanced CT can detect high-grade lesions that cause BBB breakdown, low-grade lesions may be detectable only on MRI, using sequences sensitive for edema and tissue changes. However, even in the case of known systemic primary cancer, contrast-enhanced CT may miss small foci of metastatic disease that are visible on MRI (Figs. 40-2 to 40-9).

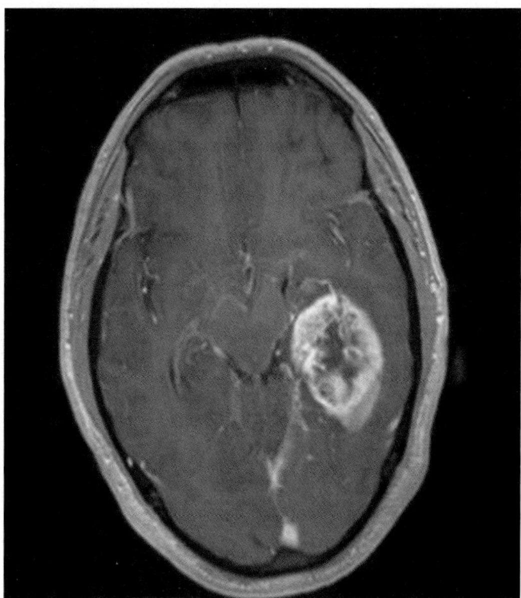

FIGURE 40-3 Glioblastoma.

The brain tumor imaging characteristics seen on MRI are helpful in making a diagnosis. However, confirmation of the diagnosis with pathology is necessary in nearly all cases. Noncancerous brain lesions that may be mistaken for malignancy include infection, demyelinating disease, vascular malformations, and stroke. A particular variant of demyelinating disease (tumefactive multiple sclerosis) with large focal tumor-like lesions, is known to resemble a malignant brain tumor. Unfortunately, some of these lesions have been irradiated, under the presumptive diagnosis of GBM, which only increases the severity of the demyelination.

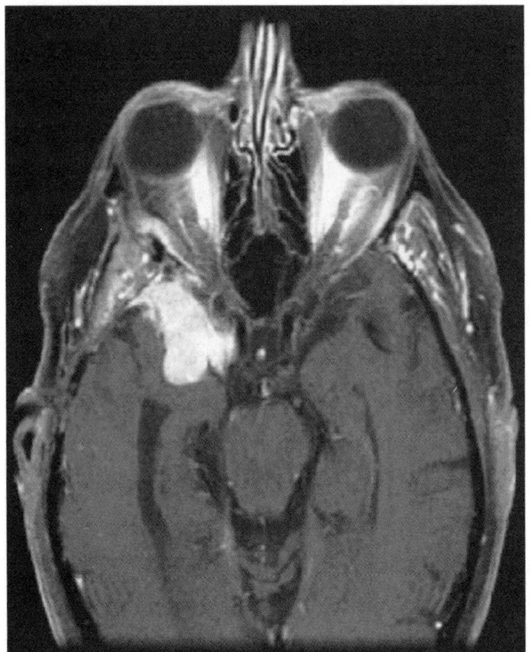

FIGURE 40-4 Meningioma.

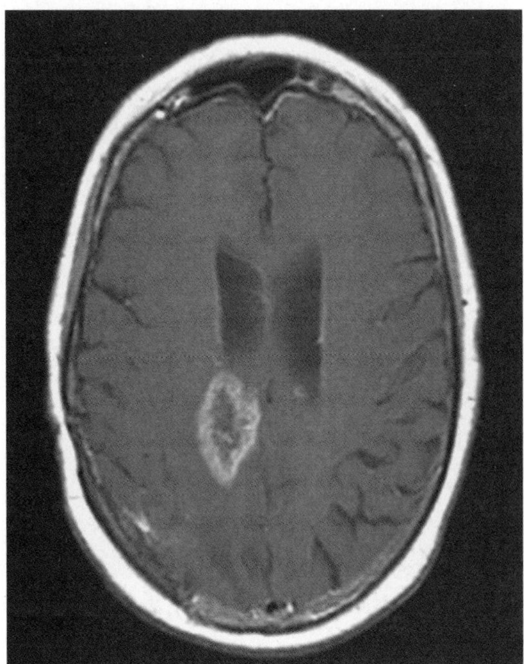

FIGURE 40-5 Radiation necrosis.

Conversely, patients with primary brain tumors are sometimes initially diagnosed with stroke or demyelinating disease. Further complicating the picture are patients who have brain tumors in addition to stroke, which is far more prevalent with increasing age. Patients with systemic cancer, often in remission, or in stable condition, can present with brain lesions that are suspected to be brain metastases but turn out to be a primary brain tumor. These types of cases often benefit from an interpretation by a specialized neuroradiologist who has been provided with a relevant

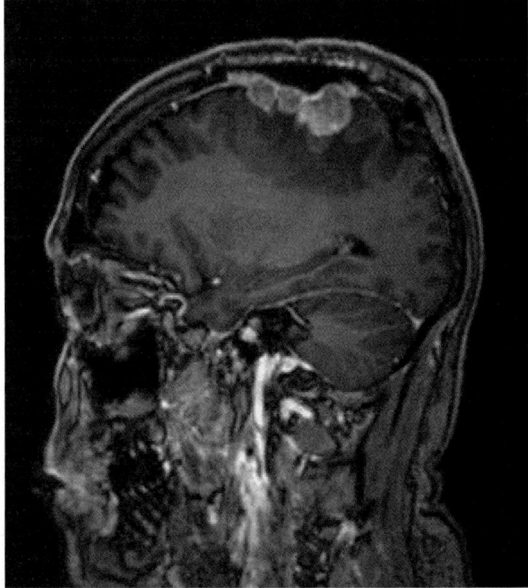

FIGURE 40-6 Anaplastic meningioma.

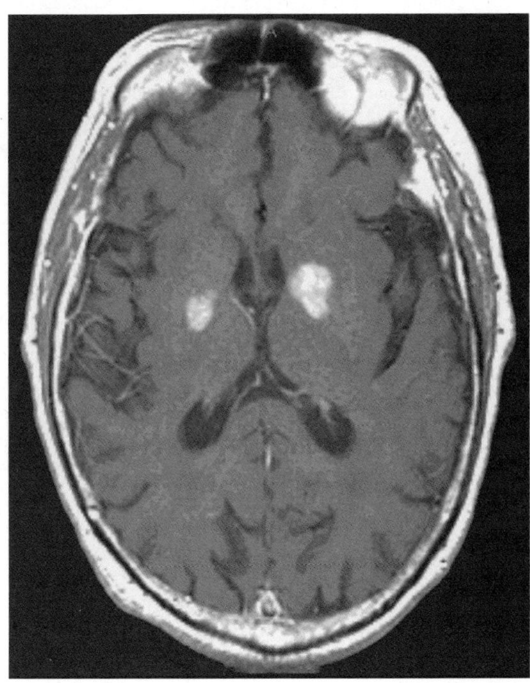

FIGURE 40-7 Central nervous system lymphoma.

patient history. A history of immunosuppression and multiple subcortical enhancing lesions may prompt the suspicion of a PCNSL or infection with toxoplasmosis. Further testing with brain thallium single-photon emission computed tomography (SPECT) scanning or fluorodeoxyglucose positron emission tomography (FDG-PET) imaging may serve to distinguish between the two possibilities.

Several classic radiographic appearances of brain tumors suggest malignancy. An irregular enhancing lesion with extensive edema following white matter pathways suggests a malignant glioma. Non–contrast-enhancing lesions with increased diffuse signals on FLAIR (fluid-attenuated inversion recovery) imaging suggest a low-grade astrocytoma. As a general rule for glial tumors, the presence of contrast enhancement suggests a high-grade malignancy. The WHO grade IV tumors nearly always enhance, as opposed to grade II tumors, which are typically nonenhancing. Two notable exceptions include pilocytic astrocytoma (WHO grade I) and pleomorphic xanthoastrocytoma (WHO grade II), which typically have an enhancing nodule and associated cyst. Meningiomas are typically homogeneously enhancing dural-based lesions associated with calcification. The appearance of multiple enhancing subcortical lesions with homogeneous enhancement suggests PCNSL. However, the same lesions, if associated with a known primary malignancy, may indicate brain metastases.

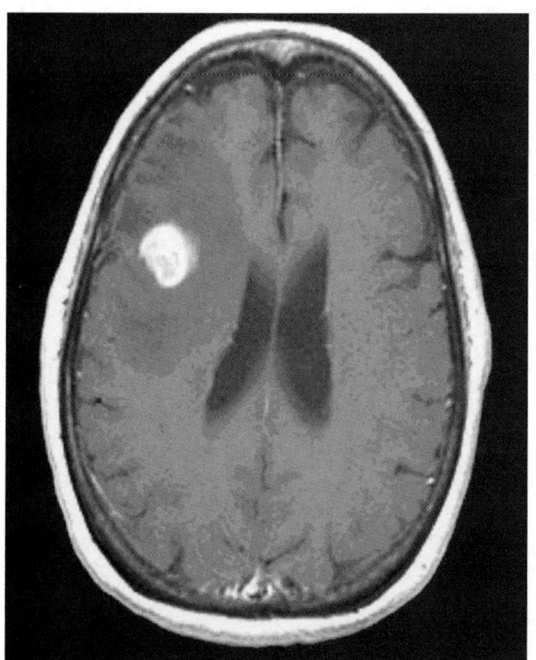

FIGURE 40-8 Single brain metastasis, lung adenocarcinoma.

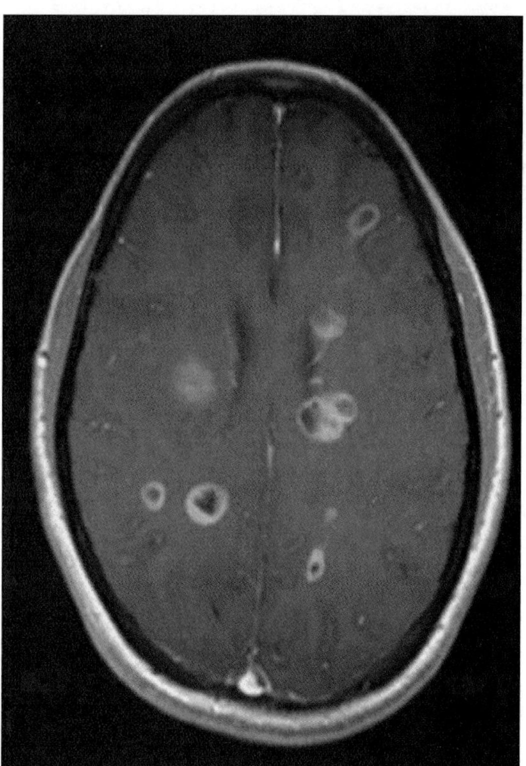

FIGURE 40-9 Multiple brain metastases, breast.

Diagnosis

The discovery of a brain lesion should prompt referral to a neurosurgeon for consideration of biopsy or resection. The management of brain tumors is critically dependent on a definitive pathology for diagnosis. A referral to a specialized neuropathologist may be necessary for diagnosis of uncommon or rare tumors and also in cases where there is only limited biopsy tissue available. Biopsies must be of adequate quality and be representative of the overall tumor to allow accurate diagnosis. Our institution insists on reviewing patient diagnostic slides prior to rendering a treatment recommendation, and it is not uncommon for our neuropathologists to disagree with the diagnosis provided by the referring physician. Primary brain glial tumors are graded according to the most malignant portion of the tumor. A brain lesion that is predominantly grade III astrocytoma but has a few regions that meet the criteria for grade IV astrocytoma (GBM) should be graded as a GBM. The tumor grade may be underestimated if the most malignant portion of the tumor is not sampled. Typically, the most malignant region corresponds to an area of contrast enhancement. If a patient is suspected of having PCNSL, the use of corticosteroids should be avoided. Primary CNS lymphoma can be sensitive to steroids which are lymphocytolytic during initial presentation, and the preoperative use of even small doses of corticosteroids can lead to a nondiagnostic biopsy. These patients usually require repeat biopsy after steroid discontinuation. Patients may present with deep central lesions involving the brainstem or thalamus. These cases may require referral to a specialized neurosurgical center to evaluate whether open biopsy, resection, or stereotactic-guided biopsy is appropriate. In these cases, close coordination with a department of neuropathology will be critical in obtaining adequate tissue for diagnosis.

Pathology

Diffuse astrocytomas are characterized by well-differentiated astrocytes—either fibrillary, gemistocytic, or rarely protoplasmic—with mildly increased cellularity. The cellular morphology of the tumor cells may differ within the same tumor sample and show great variability between tumors. Necrosis and microvascular proliferation are absent. Rare mitotic figures may occur, and nuclear atypia may be present, but not sufficiently to characterize the tumor as AA. The typical MIB-1 labeling index is less than 4% (Figs. 40-10 and 40-11).

Oligodendrogliomas are characterized by moderately cellular tumor cells with rounded, homogeneous nuclei, giving a "fried egg" artifactual appearance that is referred to as "classical OD." A recent RTOG trial found that 80% of tumors with classical oligodendroglial morphology were associated with 1p/19q deletion, compared with only 13% of 1p and 19q deletions seen in nonclassical ODs ([50]). Microcalcifications, microcyst formation, extracellular mucin deposition, and a dense network of branching capillaries are other oligodendrogliomal features. Nuclear

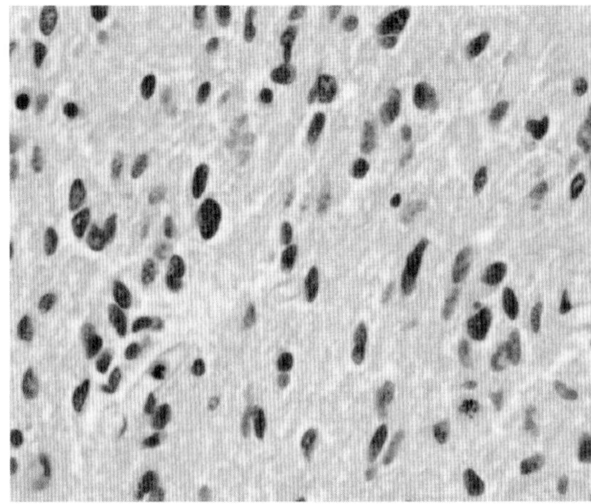

FIGURE 40-11 Low-grade astrocytoma, WHO grade II (×400). (Used with permission from Dr. Gregory N. Fuller.)

atypia may be seen, but significant mitotic activity or microvascular proliferation is suggestive of an anaplastic tumor. The MIB-1 index is typically less than 5% (Figs. 40-12 and 40-13).

Anaplastic ODs are characterized by oligodendroglial cells, with signs of increased cellularity, nuclear atypia, and mitotic activity. Cellular pleomorphism may be present, with formation of multinucleated giant cells or spindle cells. Gliofibrillary oligodendrocytes and minigemistocytes are common. Although microvascular proliferation and necrosis may be present, their presence does not change the diagnosis to GBM. There is currently no designation for a WHO grade IV OD. The MIB-1 ratio is usually greater than 5% (Figs. 40-14 to 40-16.)

Anaplastic astrocytoma is characterized by diffusely infiltrating astrocytes with increased cellularity, nuclear atypia, and mitotic activity. They are more cellular than low-grade astrocytomas, and the nuclear

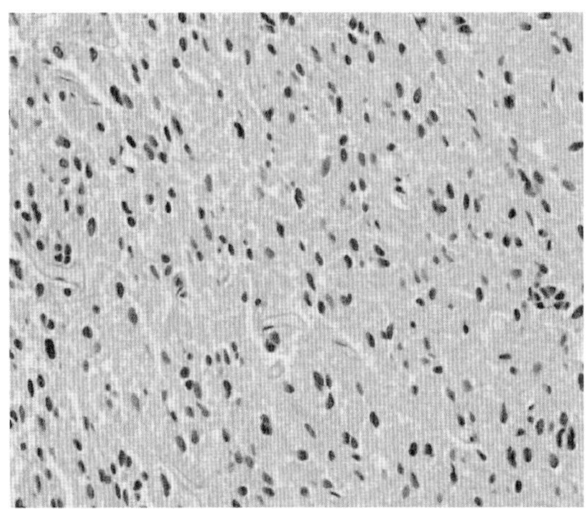

FIGURE 40-10 Low-grade astrocytoma, WHO grade II (×200). (Used with permission from Dr. Gregory N. Fuller.)

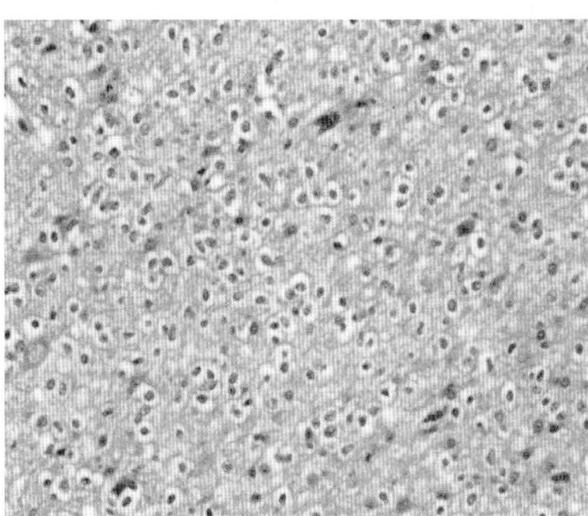

FIGURE 40-12 Oligodendroglioma, WHO grade II (×200).

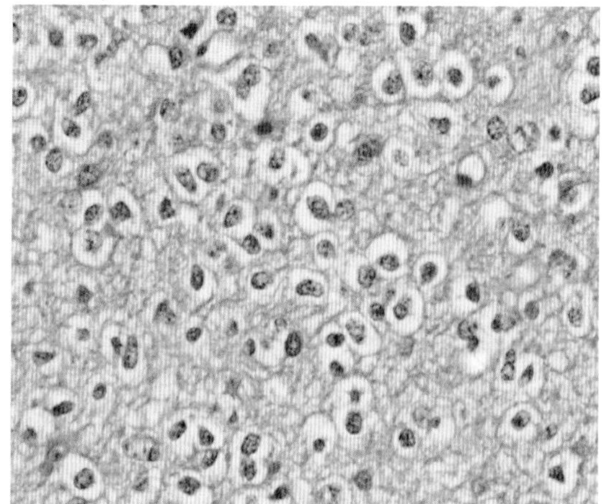

FIGURE 40-13 Oligodendroglioma, WHO grade II (×400).

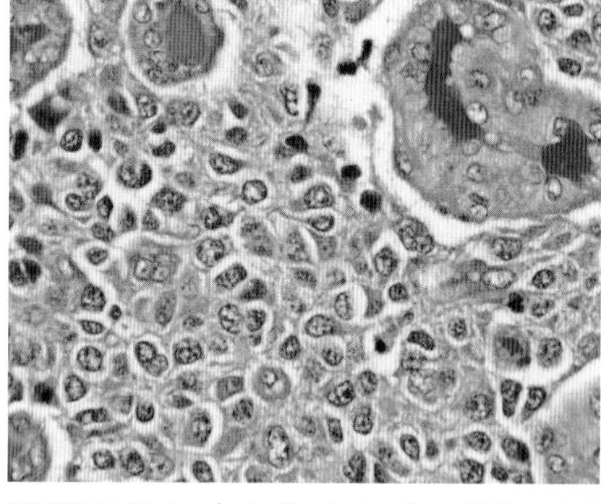

FIGURE 40-16 Anaplastic oligodendroglioma, WHO grade III (×400).

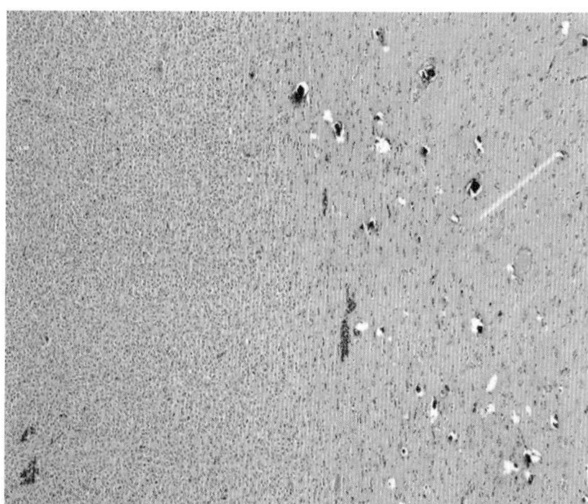

FIGURE 40-14 Anaplastic oligodendroglioma, WHO grade III (×40).

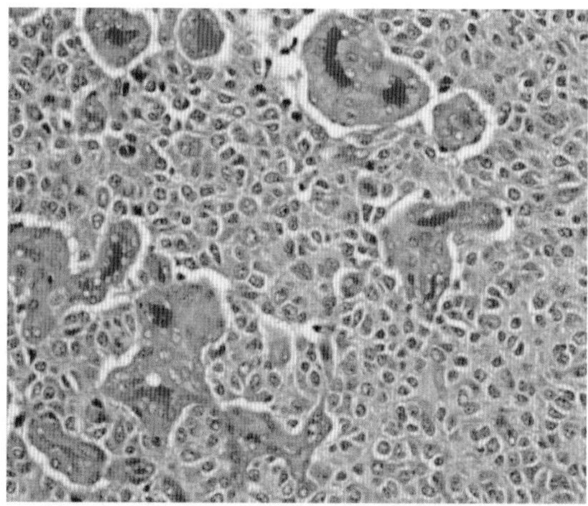

FIGURE 40-15 Anaplastic oligodendroglioma, WHO grade III (×200).

atypia include formation of nuclear inclusions, multinucleated cells, and abnormal mitoses. Microvascular proliferation is absent; if present, it would upgrade the tumor to GBM. The typical MIB-1 labeling index ranges from 5% to 10% and can occasionally overlap with index values for low-grade astrocytoma and GBM (Figs. 40-17 and 40-18).

Glioblastoma and glioblastoma multiforme are synonymous; "multiforme" was dropped from the name in the 2007 WHO classification book, although glioblastoma is still commonly referred to as GBM. Glioblastoma is an anaplastic cellular tumor with marked nuclear atypia and mitotic activity, often with marked regional heterogeneity and cellular polymorphism. The presence of either microvascular proliferation or necrosis differentiate this lesion from AA. Other features associated with GBM include formation of epithelial "adenoid" structures, multinucleated giant cells, granular cells, lipidized cells,

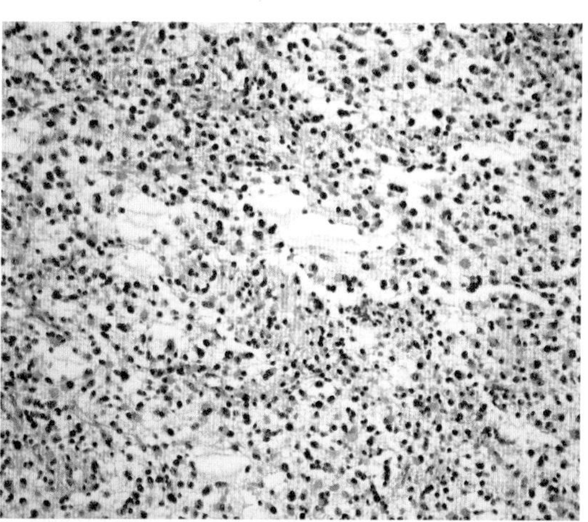

FIGURE 40-17 Anaplastic astrocytoma, WHO grade III (×100).

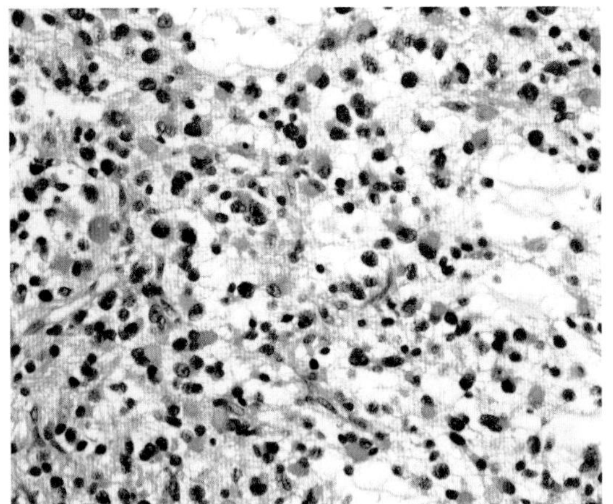

FIGURE 40-18 Anaplastic astrocytoma, WHO grade III (×200).

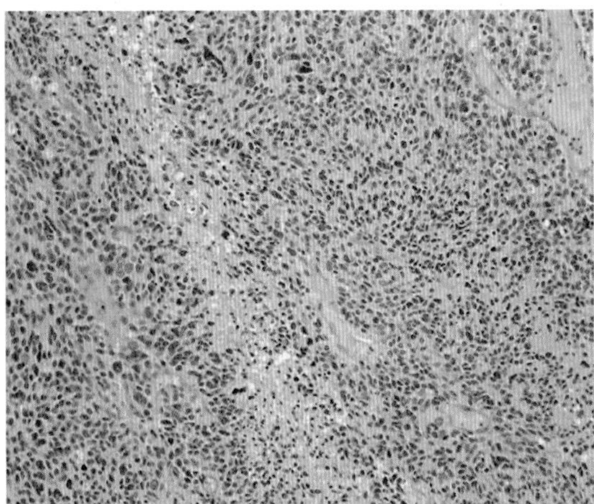

FIGURE 40-19 Glioblastoma, WHO grade IV (×100).

perivascular lymphocytes, and metaplasia. Glioblastoma is associated with a high proliferative rate, and MIB-1 labeling typically ranges from 15% to 20% (Figs. 40-19 to 40-21).

The accumulating evidence regarding the prognostic significance of *IDH* mutation status and gene expression profiling has highlighted the limitations of the current WHO criteria for the classification of diffuse gliomas. Molecular profiling is becoming an increasingly important tool in the separation of prognostic groups in diffuse gliomas. At our institution, molecular classification of diffuse gliomas has become standard. IDH and 1p/19q status are now routinely reported as part of an integrated diagnosis in addition to other pathologic features, including morphologic characteristics such as oligodendroglial or astrocytic phenotype, the results of other relevant IHC stains or diagnostic molecular tests (eg, p53, *EGFR* amplification, proliferation indices), and the method of molecular feature determination (eg, fluorescence in situ hybridization, IHC, comparative genomic hybridization) ([51]). This comprehensive format helps inform clinical decision making and patient counseling.

Meningiomas can have a wide range of appearances and are subtyped according to their appearance. Most meningiomas are grade I. The transitional variant has numerous concentric "onion bulb" structures. The psammomatous variant has calcified psammoma bodies. Pleomorphic nuclei and occasional mitoses are allowed, although four or more mitoses per 10 high-power fields would qualify in diagnosing atypical meningioma, grade II. Increased cellularity, high nuclear-to-cytoplasmic ratio, prominent nucleoli and foci of necrosis will also upgrade these to a grade II. Anaplastic meningiomas, grade III, have more than 20 mitoses per 10 high-power fields or obviously malignant cytology resembling

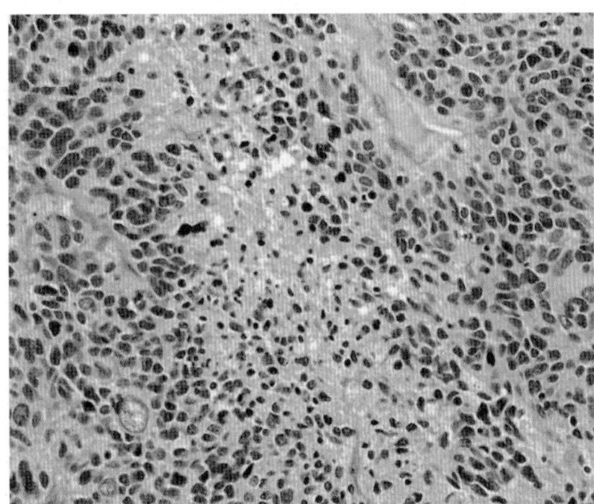

FIGURE 40-20 Glioblastoma, WHO grade IV (×200).

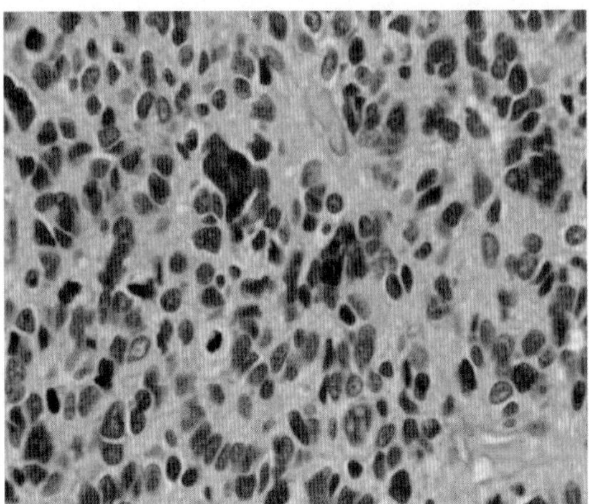

FIGURE 40-21 Glioblastoma, WHO grade IV (×400).

carcinoma, melanoma, or high-grade sarcoma ([52]) (Figs. 40-22 and 40-23).

TREATMENT AND PROGNOSIS

Low-Grade Glioma

Diffuse astrocytomas are infiltrative low-grade brain tumors. Patients commonly present with new-onset seizures. Their peak incidence is in the third decade, followed by the second decade. Overall, these low-grade tumors represent 4% of glial tumors ([9]). The median survival time of patients with diffuse astrocytoma is between 5 and 8 years ([53]). Variation in length of survival depends on patient age, performance status at diagnosis, and total versus partial tumor (as visualized on MRI) resection ([53, 54]).

The OD is a diffusely infiltrative, well-differentiated tumor composed of oligodendrocytes. These tumors comprise 3% to 4% of all primary brain tumors and approximately 7% of glial tumors, with an incidence of 0.3 per 100,000 per year. The peak incidence is from the ages of 30 to 50. Tumors with pure OD differentiation behave more indolently than astrocytomas. The ODs appear to be more sensitive to both chemotherapy and radiation therapy than astrocytomas, and the benefit from these therapies is more pronounced and durable. Median survival ranges from 4 to 12 years, and both OD and oligoastrocytoma (OA) have been included in the reported data ([53]).

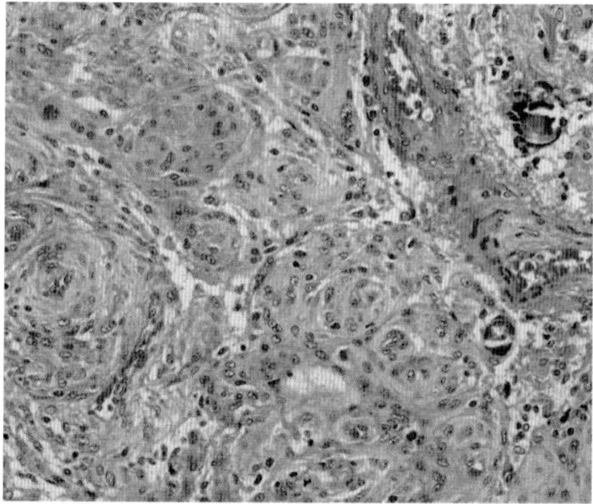

FIGURE 40-22 Meningioma (×100).

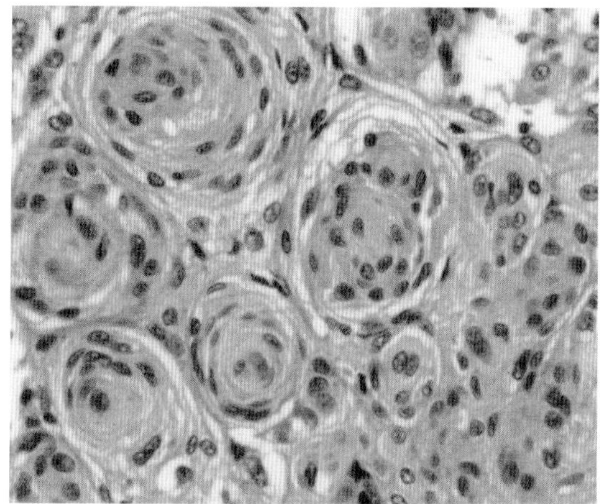

FIGURE 40-23 Meningioma (×200).

The OA is a mixed tumor composed of cells that resemble both OD and diffuse astrocytoma. Based on only a few cytogenetic studies, these tumors are thought to be of monoclonal origin. Clinically, these tumors present in a similar fashion to other low-grade glial tumors, which are best imaged with MRI and have imaging characteristics that indicate a diffuse, nonenhancing tumor. There has been no demonstration of a better prognosis with an increased proportion of the OD component. We treat these similarly to other low-grade glial tumors. Median survival ranges from 3 to 6 years. In general, these mixed tumors behave more aggressively than pure ODs but are possibly less malignant than pure astrocytomas ([55]).

Clinical Management

Once a diagnosis of low-grade glioma is suspected, we recommend proceeding with a biopsy or resection to differentiate between a low-grade glioma and a nonenhancing anaplastic glioma (Tables 40-2 and 40-3).

If gross total resection or a major resection is possible without significant morbidity, neuro-oncologists generally recommend a complete resection, which may obviate the need for irradiation and decrease the risk of malignant transformation from residual tumor cells. In multiple retrospective series, total resection of nonenhancing tumor improves survival ([53]). A volumetric analysis of the preoperative tumor, in addition to analysis of postoperative residual tumor, showed a correlation with time to recurrence and the likelihood of malignant transformation ([56]). There are several low-grade tumors—such as pilocytic astrocytoma,

Table 40-2 Initial Brain Tumor Workup

Contrast-enhanced MRI
Magnetic resonance spectroscopy may help diagnose nonenhancing tumors
Referral to neurosurgery for resection versus biopsy for tissue diagnosis
Confirmation of pathologic diagnosis
Postoperative MRI obtained within 3 days of surgery

MRI, magnetic resonance imaging.

Table 40-3 Evaluation by Tumor Type

Astrocytoma, oligodendroglioma, anaplastic astrocytoma, anaplastic oligodendroglioma, glioblastoma
MRI brain (with and without contrast)
MRI spine (with and without contrast), only if patient is symptomatic
Primary CNS lymphoma
MRI brain and spine (with and without contrast)
Lumbar puncture
Ophthalmology evaluation including slit-lamp examination
CT chest/abdomen/pelvis
Consider bone marrow biopsy

CNS, central nervous system; CT, computed tomography; MRI, magnetic resonance imaging.

Table 40-4 Management of Low-Grade Gliomas

Confirmation of diagnosis with biopsy/resection is preferred, although observation is acceptable with close follow-up.
Maximal safe resection should be considered.
Observation for low-risk patients is reasonable.
For high-risk patients (age >40 or subtotal resection), consider radiation therapy followed by chemotherapy.
Radiation therapy is the current standard of treatment (focal brain irradiation to 54 Gy).
Formal serial neuropsychologic testing is helpful in assessing cognitive function.
Consider use of psychostimulants to improve cognitive function and quality of life.
Consider biopsy/resection of progressive tumor to confirm diagnosis and consider same salvage regimens as for malignant glioma.

ependymoma and subependymoma, pleomorphic xanthoastrocytoma, ganglioglioma, and dysembryoplastic neuroepithelial tumor—that may be definitively treated by complete surgical resection alone. These patients may benefit from treatment at a specialized neurosurgical center that treats a large volume of patients with brain tumors (Table 40-4 and Fig. 40-24).

If a complete resection is not recommended, therapeutic options range from observation to treatment with focal brain irradiation or chemotherapy. Older studies of low-grade astrocytomas suggested that radiation improved survival. The 5-year survival rates ranged from 49% to 68% for irradiated tumors compared with 32% for nonirradiated tumors ([57]). The EORTC 22845 trial randomized patients to either up-front RT (54 Gy in 6 weeks) or delayed radiation therapy at progression. The PFS was 5.3 years in the early radiation group and 3.4 years in the control group. Overall survival, however, was 7.4 years in the up-front radiation group versus 7.2 years in the control group ([2]). No data were collected on quality of life. These data suggest that it is acceptable to delay radiation therapy until there are signs of tumor progression, especially for asymptomatic patients or patients who have had a complete tumor resection.

Patients with low-grade glioma should be carefully assessed to determine whether their symptoms are caused by the tumor. Formal neuropsychological testing may reveal cognitive deficits that are not apparent in the simple mental status screening used for dementia. In addition, these tests can be repeated to detect subtle cognitive decline, which may lead to a decision to alter a prescribed therapy. Patients who are symptomatic from their tumor from seizures, who have altered mental status due to tumor bulk or location, or who have other focal neurologic signs would be expected to improve with treatment of the tumor.

The etiology of cognitive decline in patients with a primary brain tumor is multifactorial. The causes include direct tumor effects from invasion and destruction as well as side effects from radiation therapy, chemotherapy, and anticonvulsants ([58]). We have found the use of psychostimulants such as methylphenidate to be helpful in improving cognitive function, mood, and fatigue ([59]).

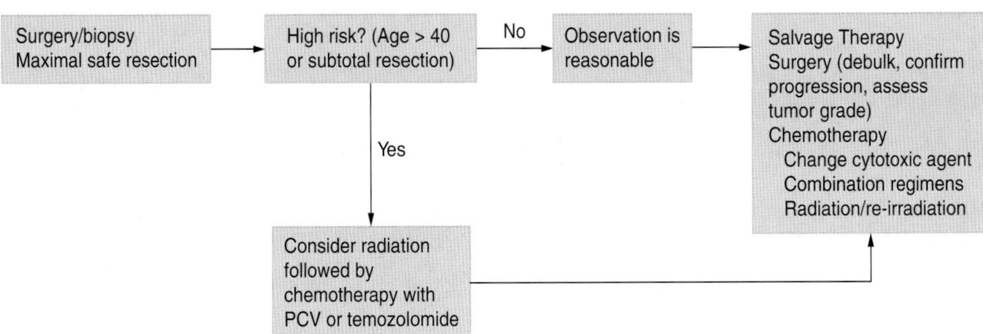

FIGURE 40-24 Treatment algorithm for low-grade glioma.

Although there are concerns about the long-term effects of brain irradiation, radiation therapy is the current treatment standard ([58]). The dose of RT currently used by the RTOG for low-grade glioma is 54 Gy to localized treatment fields as defined by the tumor appearance on T2-weighted MRI and including a 2-cm margin. A European trial involving 379 patients with low-grade glioma did not demonstrate a benefit for higher radiation dose when comparing 45 Gy with 59.4 Gy ([60]). A second prospective study that randomized 203 patients with low-grade glioma to radiation therapy with either 50.4 or 64.8 Gy found a slightly lower survival (64% vs 72% at 5 years) and higher incidence of radiation necrosis in the group receiving the higher dose of 64.8 Gy ([61]).

Much less is known about the usefulness of chemotherapy for low-grade tumors. A small study of patients with incompletely resected tumors randomized to RT alone or RT with CCNU (lomustine) demonstrated a median survival time of 4.5 years with no difference between the two treatment arms ([62]). An RTOG trial (RTOG 98-02) randomized patients with low-grade glioma and a high risk of recurrence (age ≥40 or subtotal resection/biopsy) to either radiation therapy alone or radiation therapy followed by six cycles of procarbazine, CCNU, and vincristine (PCV). The early results of this trial were presented at the American Society of Clinical Oncology (ASCO) meeting in 2014. The combination of PCV and radiation therapy prolonged both overall survival and PFS compared with radiation therapy alone in patients with high-risk grade 2 glioma, defined as patients with less than a subtotal resection and age over 40 years (ASCO abstract, *J Clin Oncol.* 2014;32:5s) ([62a]).

The usefulness of chemotherapy as an initial treatment for patients with low-grade gliomas without high-risk features is unproven. The rationale for using chemotherapy as an alternative to radiation therapy for these patients is that although radiation therapy has a proven record of treatment response, it does not improve survival and may be associated with the significant long-term side effect of cognitive decline. It is hoped that chemotherapy will delay the need for radiation therapy without reducing treatment efficacy or survival ([63]). Several limited studies have demonstrated an encouraging radiographic response by low-grade gliomas (primarily ODs but also astrocytomas) after treatment with temozolomide or PCV ([34, 64, 65]). Patients who have residual tumor and would be at a high risk of cognitive side effects from radiation therapy may benefit from this strategy. However, there are no results from prospective randomized studies to recommend this approach. Patients with OD or OA may be more attractive candidates for applying this strategy, as they tend to have higher response rates to chemotherapy than patients with astrocytoma. The cytogenetic analysis of the tumor sample for LOH at 1p and 19q may predict patients who might benefit from this strategy.

MALIGNANT GLIOMAS—GRADES III AND IV

Anaplastic Oligodendroglioma

The AODs comprise between 20% and 50% of all oligodendroglial tumors and approximately 5% of anaplastic tumors. The peak incidence is between ages 40 and 50. The clinical presentation of these tumors is similar to that of other anaplastic tumors, with focal neurologic signs, seizures, or symptoms of increased intracranial pressure. These lesions, which are usually contrast enhancing, can show calcification on CT scans as well as cystic structures, necrosis, and hemorrhage.

The initial standard therapy for an AOD is surgery, with the goal of gross total resection. In RTOG 9402, random assignment of 291 eligible patients with AO/AOA was made for the patients to receive PCV plus RT versus RT alone. There was no difference in median survival by treatment between the 148 patients randomized to PCV plus RT and the 143 patients randomized to RT ([66]). However, the significance of codeletion of 1p/19q was supported by the results of EORTC 26951 with increased survival of both AOD and AOA with 1p/19q codeletion noted regardless of the treatment given: radiation alone versus radiation with chemotherapy ([67]). The prognostic significance of 1p/19q was validated in the long-term results of RTOG 9402. Patients with co-deleted tumors lived longer than those with non–co-deleted tumors with the median survival of those patients with co-deleted tumors treated with PCV plus RT being twice that of patients who received RT alone. Neither timing (before, during, or following radiation treatment) nor dose intensity of PCV was found to be significant. No difference in median survival by treatment arm was appreciated in patients with non–co-deleted tumors ([66]). A phase III study (CATNON) is under way to examine the appropriate treatment of anaplastic gliomas without 1p/19q codeletion.

Although PCV is the most studied regimen, in clinical practice temozolomide is typically favored for its more tolerable toxicity profile. Further study is ongoing from the RTOG/NCCTG/EORTC trial to determine if chemotherapy (PCV or temozolomide) can replace radiation and maintain the survival benefit. Despite initially high response rates, these tumors usually recur. Median survival for AOD treated with surgery, irradiation, and chemotherapy ranges from 3 to 5 years, although some patients survive past 10 years ([55]). Recurrent disease is often treated with salvage regimens similar to those used for AA and GBM (Tables 40-5 and 40-6).

Anaplastic Astrocytoma

Anaplastic astrocytomas are diffusely infiltrating with nuclear atypia and anaplasia as well as marked proliferation, features that distinguish them from low-grade astrocytomas. A lack of vascular proliferation or necrosis distinguishes these tumors histologically from GBM. The highest incidence of AA is in the fourth decade, followed by the third decade, with nearly equal incidence rates in the second, fifth, and sixth decades. These tumors account for 7.5% of all glial tumors ([9]). Some patients may have a history of prior low-grade astrocytoma. Brain imaging shows diffuse hypointense tumor on CT scans and T1-weighted MRI. There is usually more mass effect and edema compared with low-grade astrocytomas, and contrast enhancement is typical. Because these tumors can occasionally be nonenhancing, neuroimaging alone is not sufficient to distinguish these lesions from low-grade astrocytomas. The median survival for patients with AA ranges from 5 to 7 years.

Optimal initial management begins with surgery with the goal of maximal, safe resection, both to provide adequate tissue for accurate analysis of pathology and to improve survival. Following surgery, limited-field radiation therapy to a target dose of 60 Gy is commonly recommended. The target radiation field typically includes the contrast-enhancing region of the tumor as well as the surrounding edema or nonenhancing tumor plus a 2-cm margin. The size of this field is often reduced after a 46-Gy dose has been applied to the contrast-enhancing lesion alone plus a 2-cm margin. Clinical trials using alternate radiation schemes of hyperfractionation or accelerated fractionation have not demonstrated an increased survival benefit over conventional fractionated conformal radiation therapy ([68]). Adjuvant chemotherapy following radiation therapy increases time to progression and survival. Standard agents include combination therapy composed of PCV or (see Table 40-6) temozolomide ([69]).

Patients with recurrent AA should be considered for clinical trials. Surgical resection should also be considered to provide a palliative benefit, relieve mass effect, allow dose reduction of steroids, and confirm histology. The recurrent tumor may actually have progressed to GBM from AA, and such patients are often eligible for a wider array of clinical trials than are available for recurrent AA. Trials have used temolozomide in combination with agents such as interferon alfa (IFN-α), *cis*-retinoic acid, metalloproteinase inhibitors, carmustine, irinotecan, and thalidomide ([70-72]). Other agents that have been used for recurrent AA include tamoxifen, carboplatin, etoposide, irinotecan, and combination chemotherapy. To date, no single trial has proven to be superior (Fig. 40-25). Reirradiation can be considered for patients who are over 2 years beyond their original radiation treatment and for patients whose site of recurrent disease lies outside the initial radiation treatment field.

Table 40-5 Management of High-Grade Gliomas

Consider clinical trials at all stages: up front, adjuvant, and at relapse (especially at first or second recurrence).
Multidisciplinary approach is necessary for optimal outcome:
Neurosurgery
Neuro-oncology
Radiation therapy
Psychiatry
Neuropsychology
Rehabilitation
Social work
Maximal, safe resection
Concurrent chemoradiotherapy with temozolomide for glioblastoma.
Adjuvant chemotherapy for glioblastoma (temozolomide).
For 1p/19q co-deleted anaplastic oligodendroglioma, PCV or temozolomide following radiation therapy or vice versa.
For 1p/19q intact anaplastic glioma, the role of adjuvant chemotherapy is under investigation.
Avoid use of anticonvulsants that induce cytochrome P-450 3A4 metabolism when possible (Table 40-7).
Progressive disease
Consider clinical trials.
Consider surgical resection at relapse (especially to rule out radiation necrosis).
Salvage chemotherapy agents include single-agent and combination regimens incorporating temozolomide, nitrosoureas, irinotecan, and platinum agents.
Consider re-irradiation.

PCV, procarbazine, CCNU, and vincristine.

Table 40-6 Chemotherapy Regimens for Gliomas

Newly diagnosed gliomas:
Temozolomide *Newly diagnosed glioblastoma:* 75 mg/m²/d by mouth days 1-42 during radiotherapy followed by 150-200 mg/m²/d[a] by mouth days 1-5 of a 28-day cycle
PCV[b] *Newly diagnosed oligodendroglioma and anaplastic oligodendroglioma:* Procarbazine 60-75 mg/m²/d by mouth days 8-21 of a 42-day cycle and Lomustine 110-130 mg/m²/d by mouth day 1 of a 42-day cycle and Vincristine 1.4 mg/m²/d IV days 8 and 29 (maximum dose = 2 mg) of a 42-day cycle
Recurrent gliomas:
Temozolomide 150-200 mg/m²/d[a] by mouth days 1-5 of a 28-day cycle
Lomustine monotherapy 90-110 mg/m² by mouth day 1 of a 42-day cycle
Carboplatin monotherapy AUC 4-5 IV day 1 of a 28-day cycle
Bevacizumab monotherapy or in combination with chemotherapy 10 mg/kg/dose IV days 1 and 15 of a 28-day cycle *or* days 1, 15, and 29 of a 42-day cycle
Bevacizumab and lomustine Bevacizumab 10 mg/kg/dose IV days 1, 15, and 29 of a 42-day cycle and Lomustine 90 mg/m² by mouth day 1 of a 42-day cycle
Bevacizumab and carboplatin Bevacizumab 10 mg/kg/dose IV days 1 and 15 of a 28-day cycle and Carboplatin AUC 4-5 IV on day 1 of a 28-day cycle

[a]Begin at 150 mg/m²/d for cycle 1; increase to 200 mg/m²/d for cycle 2 if no myelosuppression.
[b]Dose adjusted based on timing of radiotherapy.

Glioblastoma

Glioblastoma is the most common and most malignant glial tumor of the brain. It comprises 50% of all glial tumors, with an incidence of approximately two to three per 100,000 per year ([9]). Glioblastomas are characterized by poorly differentiated astrocytes with cellular polymorphism, nuclear atypia, microvascular proliferation, and necrosis. The peak incidence is in the fifth decade, followed by the sixth and fourth decades. Glioblastoma is rare in children and young adults ([9]). Clinically, these tumors often present with signs of increased intracranial pressure, such as headache. They can also present with seizures or focal neurologic symptoms such as hemiparesis and aphasia, often with a short history of symptoms.

Imaging with CT or MRI usually reveals a contrast-enhancing lesion with irregular borders, frequently with a necrotic center. Vasogenic edema and nonenhancing tumor often surround the area of contrast enhancement and are best seen on T2-weighted or FLAIR imaging on MRI. Glioblastomas commonly spread through white matter tracts across the corpus callosum, internal capsule, and optic radiations. Multifocal lesions are seen. If these multiple lesions truly arise independently as opposed to spreading diffusely through tracts that are not visualized by imaging or pathology, they may have a polyclonal origin.

Glioblastomas are highly lethal. Despite extensive clinical research, survival has not changed greatly during the last 20 years. Prognostic factors include age and Karnofsky performance status (KPS). Surgical resection has shown some benefit, especially gross total resection, described when 90% or more of the enhancing tumor is removed ([73]) (Fig. 40-26).

The addition of chemotherapy to radiation emerged as the standard of care for GBM based on the seminal large prospective, randomized, phase III trial from the EORTC. This trial randomized 573 patients to receive either standard RT (60 Gy in 30 daily fractions) or concurrent temozolomide (75 mg/m²/d) with RT followed by adjuvant temozolomide for 6 months (150 to 200 mg/m²/d for 5 days every 28 days). The group receiving concurrent and adjuvant temozolomide had a significant improvement in PFS (median 7.2 vs 5.0 months), survival (median 14.6 vs 12 months), and 2-year survival rate (median 26% vs 8%). Both groups had similar age, KPS, and surgical resection rates.

Our center strongly recommends patient participation in clinical trials, which enroll patients from initial resection to radiation therapy and salvage therapy at relapse. Patients are eligible for entry into a clinical protocol for recurrent disease if it has been greater than 12 weeks since completion of concurrent chemoradiation to avoid enrolling patients with pseudoprogression (radiographic change that can mimic tumor progression but is actually due to radiation-induced changes). If a patient is not enrolled in an "up-front" trial, we recommend evaluation by our neurosurgery service to explore the prospect of gross total resection. It is not unusual for our patients to have repeat resection of tumor following biopsy or subtotal resection at an outside institution. Following resection, we treat

CHAPTER 40

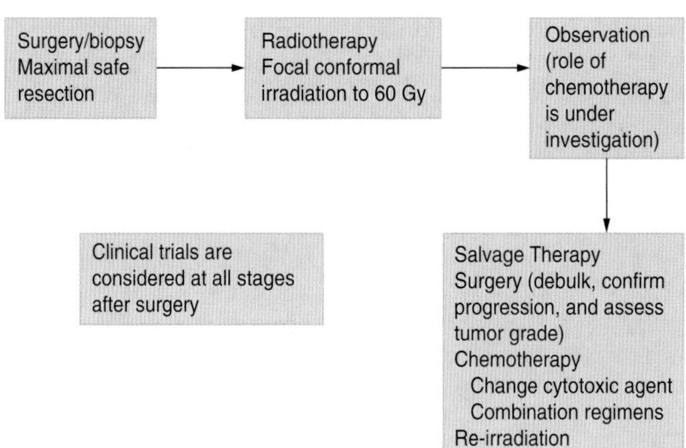

FIGURE 40-25 Treatment algorithm for anaplastic astrocytoma.

patients with concurrent temozolomide (75 mg/m^2/d throughout radiation therapy) and standard conformal radiation therapy (59.4 Gy in 1.8-Gy fractions). Following radiation therapy, we use adjuvant temozolomide or temozolomide combination therapy. Although the EORTC study only used adjuvant temozolomide for 6 months, we typically continue treatment for at least 1 year, given the lethal natural history of GBM.

Dose-dense scheduling of temozolomide was evaluated in a large randomized, phase III trial based on the premise that prolonged exposure to temozolomide would result in prolonged depletion of MGMT, possibly translating into an improved survival in patients with newly diagnosed GBM. Standard adjuvant temozolomide (days 1-5 every 28 days) was compared to a dose-dense schedule (days 1-21 every 28 days). No statistically significant difference in either median OS or median PFS was observed between the two treatment arms. Treatment toxicity was higher with the dose-dense schedule ([3]).

Patients with GBM and progressive disease are offered salvage therapy if their KPS is adequate. We consider options including resection of tumor, chemotherapy, and stereotactic radiation therapy. Some novel neurosurgical clinical trials have offered local therapy with gene therapy using *p53*, although this was limited by lack of dispersion of the therapy into surrounding tissues ([74]). An interleukin 13–conjugated *Pseudomonas*

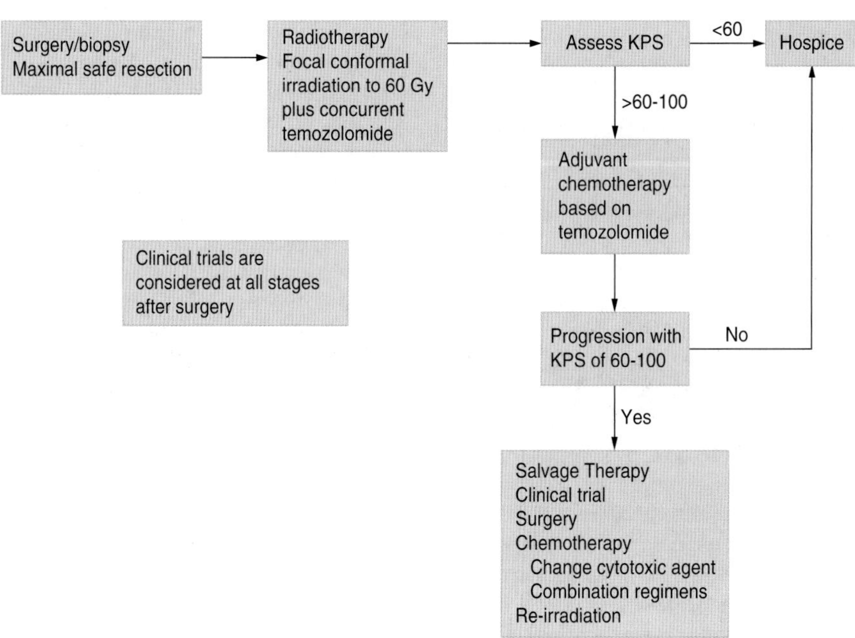

FIGURE 40-26 Treatment algorithm for glioblastoma.

exotoxin has been studied using convection-enhanced delivery to lead to higher tissue concentration with larger volumes of distribution in phase I ([75, 76]). Another ongoing trial uses a conditionally replication-competent adenovirus (Delta-24-RGD) injected into the resection cavity for recurrent malignant gliomas.

One advantage of re-resection of progressive disease is to confirm pathology and specifically to determine whether the progressive enhancement on MRI represents tumor or radiation necrosis. Magnetic resonance imaging dynamic contrast and MR spectroscopy imaging, FDG-PET scanning, and brain SPECT thallium imaging sometimes help to distinguish between these two possibilities. However, all of these modalities have limited sensitivity and specificity, and sometimes the pathology reveals both treatment-related necrosis and foci of active tumor. Patients with pathology-confirmed radiation necrosis are often treated with steroids. More recently, bevacizumab, a monoclonal antibody targeted against the VEGF, has been utilized to treat radiation necrosis ([77]).

Chemotherapy for recurrent disease typically produces response rates less than 10% and a 6-month PFS of 15% ([4]). Response rates that include stable disease and complete or PRs are 40% at best, but as the 6-month PFS value indicates, these responses are not durable. It is hypothesized that the multiple mutations and alterations in GBM and the heterogeneity of the tumor cell population may partially explain the striking resistance of these tumors to therapy. Younger patients respond best to chemotherapy, although responses to alkylating agents can be seen in patients older than 60 years of age. Long-term survivors of GBM (over 5 years) have typically had gross total resection, radiation therapy to a dose of 60 Gy, and chemotherapy, generally with temozolomide or a nitrosourea or other alkylating agent.

Salvage agents used for malignant glioma are identical to those used for recurrent AA (see Table 40-6). Rechallenging with continuous dose-intense temozlomide 50 mg/m^2/d is a valuable therapeutic option as evidenced by the RESCUE study. The overall 6-month PFS for recurrent progressive GBM was 23.9% ([78]) in contrast to 15% based on a pooled analysis of eight consecutive phase II trials of cytostatic and cytotoxic agents. In this study, the greatest therapeutic benefit was observed in patients with progressive disease during the first six cycles of conventional adjuvant temozolomide therapy (150-200 mg/m^2 × 5 days every 28 days) or after a treatment-free interval ([4]).

Bevacizumab has been approved by the Food and Drug Administration (FDA) for progressive disease following prior therapy, based on two trials. One study showed a 6-month PFS of 42% and overall survival of 8.7 months in patients receiving bevacizumab alone ([79]). Another study showed a response rate of 19.6% with median duration of 3.9 months. The 6-month PFS was 29%, and 6-month survival was 57%. In addition, 50% of patients experienced decreased cerebral edema, 58% were able to decrease corticosteroid dependency, and 52% had improvement in neurologic symptoms ([80]).

Bevacizumab was subsequently evaluated in phase III clinical trials for newly diagnosed GBM. Unfortunately, no effect was seen on overall patient survival. Two recent large randomized, phase III trials, AVAglio and RTOG 0825, demonstrated that the addition of bevacizumab to up-front treatment with radiation and temozolomide conferred no benefit in terms of overall survival. Progression-free survival was prolonged in both studies by approximately 3 to 4 months, reaching statistical significance in the AVAglio study but not in the RTOG 0825 study based on predefined criteria ([81, 82]).

Other active agents include irinotecan and carboplatin, which have been investigated as single agents in the salvage setting and in combination with bevacizumab in bevacizumab-naïve recurrent GBM ([83]). The optimal schedule and combination of bevacizumab with alternative drugs has not been identified. Agents targeting angiogenesis have also been studied, although the use of interferon, thalidomide, EGF-RTK antagonists, and integrin receptor antagonists is not standard. Many of these targeted therapies demonstrated only limited activity as single agents, and efforts are under way to combine them with cytotoxic therapy ([84]). Other cellular pathways being investigated with small-molecule inhibitors include the *ras* pathway with farnesyl-transferase inhibitors and the PI3Kinase pathway with *mTOR* inhibitors. Other novel approaches to malignant brain tumor therapy include use of oncolytic adenovirus, vaccine and dendritic cell immunotherapy, and histone deacetylase inhibitors. An important reaction has been discovered from the interaction between anticonvulsants that induce the hepatic cytochrome P-450 3A4 enzyme and other chemotherapy agents also metabolized by this same enzyme. Pharmacokinetic studies of patients with malignant glioma on single-agent irinotecan and sirolimus found significantly lower levels of active drug in patients on enzyme-inducing anticonvulsant drugs ([85]). We recommend that patients on chemotherapy avoid the use of anticonvulsants that induce the expression of the P-450 3A4 enzyme whenever possible (Table 40-7).

Seizure Control

The management of seizures in patients with brain tumor is important to improve patient functioning and quality of life. A decline in seizure control may indicate tumor progression or worsening edema. It may also indicate a systemic infection or a drug interaction leading to decreased anticonvulsant drug effectiveness. In the case of tumor progression, a reduction in

Table 40-7 Cytochrome P-450 3a4-Inducing Agents (Anticonvulsants in bold)

Carbamazepine	Phenytoin
Dexamethasone	Primidone
Ethosuximide	**Progesterone**
Glucocorticoids	**Rifabutin**
Griseofulvin	**Rifampin**
Nafcillin	**Rofecoxib (mild)**
Nelfinavir	**St. John's wort**
Nevirapine	**Sulfadimidine**
Oxcarbazepine	**Sulfinpyrazone**
Phenobarbital	**Troglitazone**
Phenylbutazone	

the amount of brain edema with high-potency corticosteroids (dexamethasone) may be sufficient to prevent further seizures. A second anticonvulsant is often necessary. Dexamethasone is a hepatic cytochrome P-450 3A4–inducing agent and often causes a reduction in serum levels of antiepileptic medications such as phenytoin and carbamazepine (also enzyme inducers) when the dose is increased. Similarly, patients can become symptomatic with toxic levels of anticonvulsants in the midst of a dexamethasone taper. It is important to follow serum anticonvulsant levels when using agents metabolized by the cytochrome P-450 system. Anticonvulsants that are highly protein bound can demonstrate significant changes in levels of circulating free drug without significantly changing the total serum level. It is useful to check serum-free phenytoin or valproic acid levels when patients taking these agents have seizures or show signs of toxicity.

Despite the numerous choices of anticonvulsants, it can be difficult to control seizures. Of the newer generation of anticonvulsants, we have had success using levetiracetam and lacosamide, which are easily titrated without significant drug interactions. Phenobarbital and clonazepam can be useful in resistant cases of seizures. Short-term use of lorazepam can help bridge changes in anticonvulsant regimens.

Quality-of-Life Considerations

It is critical to provide effective supportive care to patients with brain tumors to improve their functional status and quality of life for themselves and their caregivers. This care is typically labor intensive and often beyond the means of patients and their families to provide. We involve social work and case management early in the treatment of patients. They can provide interventions that may prevent a later breakdown in care.

The incidence of depression is high among this population and should be treated early. The causes of depression are typically multifactorial and may include direct effects of the tumor, side effects of chemotherapy and radiation therapy, and side effects of steroids in addition to issues associated with a loss of independence and a diagnosis of cancer. We suggest referral to psychiatry to optimally address these issues. A related concern is the impact of fatigue and somnolence, common side effects of brain radiation. We advocate the use of psychostimulants such as methylphenidate to treat both fatigue and cognitive side effects ([59]). Although there are theoretical concerns that the use of stimulants may exacerbate seizures, we have not observed this in practice.

Patients often require high doses of steroids to manage edema and experience both acute and chronic toxicities from their administration. Acutely, the steroids may induce hyperglycemia requiring an insulin sliding scale. Patients often become agitated and irritable, suffer extreme mood swings, and even become psychotic when taking steroids. Low-dose neuroleptics can be effective in treating these side effects. Clinicians should aim to taper steroid use to the lowest doses necessary. Patients typically tolerate initial steroid weaning but often experience fatigue or worsening of neurologic function as dexamethasone doses are reduced to below 4 mg daily. This can be ameliorated with an extremely slow steroid taper and only lowering doses every 1 to 2 weeks by decrements of 1 mg or even 0.5 mg. Psychostimulants can help treat the inevitable fatigue experienced with the steroid taper. There is no effective treatment for steroid myopathy other than tapering off steroids and initiating physical therapy and rehabilitation as early as possible.

Meningioma

Meningiomas comprise 32% of primary brain tumors, with a rate of 5.35 per 100,000 person-years. The incidence of meningioma increases with age; the median age at diagnosis is 64 years ([9]). The tumor is often discovered incidentally without any symptoms. Clinically, these tumors typically present with headache, cognitive or personality changes, persistent focal neurologic deficits, and sometimes seizure. The main treatment is surgical resection, with the goal of complete resection when possible, accounting for relative risks and benefits depending on the patient's age and condition ([86]).

Options for residual tumor include observation and radiation therapy, which can incorporate stereotactic delivery to minimize effects to local tissue ([87]).

Chemotherapy for meningioma has been used for patients who have progressive disease after resection and RT; it is sometimes used adjuvantly following RT when pathology indicates malignant meningioma. Response rates have been disappointing in small case series. Agents that have been used include hydroxyurea ([88]), IFN-α ([89]), and liposomal doxorubicin ([90]). Results using temozolomide have been discouraging, with no responders ([91]). As there are no established treatments after surgery and radiation have been exhausted and response to chemotherapy has been disappointing, the use of molecularly targeted therapy is being explored in aggressive meningioma. Frequently, EGF, PDGF, and VEGF receptors are overexpressed in meningiomas. Clinical trials using small-molecule signal transduction inhibitors such as erlotinib, gefitinib, and imatinib are being explored but have not yet shown significant efficacy ([92, 93]). In a recent phase II trial, sunitinib, a small-molecule tyrosine kinase inhibitor that targets VEGF and PDGF receptors, was found to have activity in patients with recurrent atypical/malignant meningiomas and warrants investigation in a randomized trial ([94]). A novel genomic-driven clinical trial currently in development will examine the efficacy of SMO and AKT inhibitors in patients with surgery-confirmed mutations in these oncogenes.

Primary Central Nervous System Lymphoma

In contrast to most other brain tumors, chemotherapy is the initial treatment of choice for CNS lymphoma. Efforts at surgical resection have largely been discouraged as PCNSL has a tendency to involve deep brain structures and a multifocal pattern of growth. The traditional view has been that gross total resection conferred no survival benefit over biopsy, but this view has been challenged recently. In a phase III trial of 526 patients, PFS was found to be significantly shorter in patients who were biopsied compared to patients who had undergone subtotal or gross total resections, with no difference in outcome attributable to KPS or age, suggesting that surgical resection could be considered for patients with single lesions for which resection is deemed safe ([95]).

Methotrexate-based, multiagent chemotherapy has been viewed as the treatment of choice in PCNSL. The incorporation of high-dose methotrexate (greater than 1 g/m^2) has resulted in a significantly greater response and improved survival compared with previous regimens using a CHOP regimen prior to whole-brain radiation therapy (WBRT). A report by DeAngelis, incorporating methotrexate (1 g/m^2), followed by whole-brain irradiation and two cycles of high-dose cytarabine (ara-C) (3 g/m^2), demonstrated a median survival of 42.5 months ([96]). This strategy is the basis for current CNS lymphoma protocols that have increased the dose of methotrexate and incorporated agents that more easily cross the BBB, such as procarbazine. A follow-up clinical trial incorporating methotrexate at 3.5 g/m^2 with procarbazine and vincristine, followed by whole-brain irradiation and cytarabine demonstrated a median survival of 60 months ([97]). The improvement in patient survival has also brought to attention significant rates of cognitive decline and radiation-induced dementia, especially in patients older than 60 years ([98]).

Current approaches to therapy of CNS lymphoma are investigating whether radiation therapy can be avoided or delayed to reduce cognitive decline and dementia without adversely affecting survival. Preliminary results from a trial using single-agent methotrexate at 8 g/m^2 every 2 weeks demonstrated a PFS of 12.8 months. Median survival had not been reached at more than 22.8 months ([99]). Many clinicians at our center are cautiously delaying radiation therapy until relapse and continuing to use high-dose–based methotrexate regimens. In hoping to improve the results of single-agent methotrexate ([99]), some regimens continue to incorporate procarbazine. Other agents that may be active in this setting include temozolomide and rituximab.

Patients with recurrent disease may respond again to methotrexate. Other regimens used include PCV ([100]), high-dose cytarabine ([101]), temozolomide ([102]), rituximab ([103]), and the combination of temozolomide and rituximab ([104]). High-dose chemotherapy with autologous stem cell rescue may also be effective ([105]).

Brain Metastasis

The treatment of brain metastasis involves optimal interactions between oncology, neurosurgery, and radiation therapy. Depending on the setting of relapse, patient survival may depend more on local tumor control in the brain or on systemic control for progressive metastasis. Advances in local brain tumor control with surgery and radiosurgery will not improve patient survival if the patient ultimately succumbs to progressive systemic disease or continues to develop new brain metastases. The median survival of patients with brain metastases is 3 to 6 months ([106]).

The options for therapy include surgical resection, WBRT, stereotactic radiosurgery (SRS), and systemic chemotherapy. Surgical resection is the treatment option considered primarily in patients with single large tumors. Resection of brain metastases has emerged as a standard treatment option for patients with surgically accessible single lesions, good performance status, and controlled or absent extracranial disease. The advantages of surgical resection is that the mass effect can be immediately ameliorated and removal of the tumor decreases edema. Surgical resection also provides pathologic confirmation of the diagnosis. Stereotactic radiosurgery utilizes multiple convergent beams to deliver a single high dose of radiation to a discrete target volume and is usually reserved for lesions whose maximum diameter is 3 cm or less. The ability to treat locations that were otherwise considered surgically inaccessible is a distinct advantage of SRS. Whole-brain radiation therapy via 30 to 40 Gy (in daily fractions of 2 to 3 Gy) is the standard therapy for brain metastasis, with an established body of literature supporting its use for multiple metastases. This therapy has the ability to eradicate micrometastatic disease to delay recurrence ([106, 107]) and is often used in conjunction with surgical resection or radiosurgery. It is well tolerated and can be effective for radiosensitive tumors such as metastases from small cell lung cancer or germ cell tumors. The greatest concern about WBRT has been the risk of neurocognitive effects, which can range from mild impairment to dementia. Hippocampal-sparing WBRT has been under active investigation in a large multicenter clinical trial (clinicaltrials.gov, identifier NCT01227954) as a technique to reduce neurotoxicity. Overall, the neurocognitive impact of WBRT in patients with brain metastases has not been well studied, and future research efforts will focus on the identification of risk factors predicting vulnerability. Neurocognitive end points should also be integrated into clinical trial designs.

We frequently treat patients at our institution with surgery if the lesions are greater than 3 cm and the patients are symptomatic. If the patient's medical condition makes a surgical procedure risky, the patient may receive WBRT. Patients who have lesions smaller than 3 cm can receive radiosurgery if they are asymptomatic or if the lesion is in a deep region not amenable to resection. However, patients with symptoms resulting from the lesions more frequently receive surgery to remove mass effect as long as their medical condition permits. There is also debate over the role of whole-brain irradiation following surgery or radiosurgery to single lesions.

Chemotherapy for Brain Metastasis

Several small clinical trials and case reports support the concept that systemic chemotherapy demonstrates activity in treating brain metastases. Chemosensitive tumor types include breast cancer, small cell lung cancer, and germ cell tumors. The primary consideration in choosing a given regimen of chemotherapy is to use agents with known activity in a given tumor type. In many trials, response rates of brain metastases have been comparable to response rates of systemic disease. Patients who have had prior chemotherapy usually respond at lower rates.

Most clinical trials of investigational agents for solid tumors explicitly exclude patients with brain metastases. Compounding this omission is their common inclusion in studies of a heterogeneous group of patients with mixed tumor types and differing prior exposures to chemotherapy. Patients might also be expected to be more resistant to treatment with chemotherapeutic agents if they had failed RT. If chemotherapy is given during and after RT, it may be difficult to separate the efficacy due to RT versus chemotherapy. These factors make it difficult to compare treatment regimens and interpret studies ([108]).

Newer drugs targeting specific extracellular receptors or blocking intracellular signal transduction systems are under investigation. Owing to their specificity, they often lack the side effects commonly associated with standard cytotoxic chemotherapy. If the therapeutic target is crucial for the cancer cell's continued viability, the drug can be especially effective. The identification of *BRAF* mutations in 50% to 60% of advanced melanomas resulted in the development of potent and selective inhibitors. Vemurafenib and dabrafenib are FDA approved for the treatment of advanced melanoma and have transformed melanoma therapy, with high response rates seen in patients even with advanced, symptomatic, metastatic disease ([109]).

Immune checkpoint blockade is emerging as a highly effective immunotherapeutic strategy in metastatic melanoma and other solid tumors. Ipilimumab, a human immunoglobulin (Ig) G1 monoclonal antibody to cytotoxic T-lymphocyte antigen 4 (CTLA-4), has been demonstrated to result in a durable response and improved overall survival when compared to non–ipilimumab-containing treatment arms in randomized trials ([110]). Ipilimumab has also been shown to be efficacious in the treatment of patients with melanoma with brain metastases, as evidenced by the measurable tumor reduction seen with ipilimumab used as monotherapy ([111]).

The use of chemotherapy for brain metastases is faced with great challenges. The most important imperative is to discover new agents that can overcome tumor resistance to standard chemotherapy, whether through selection by prior pretreatment or inherent chemoresistance of tumor cell clones that metastasize from a primary site. Because most patients with brain metastases succumb to progressive systemic disease, improvement of local brain control will likely have a limited effect on survival. Conversely, the development of agents that are effective in establishing durable tumor control, both systemically and in the brain, will improve survival, as in the unique case of germ cell tumors.

Clinical variables associated with survival in the setting of brain metastases have been studied. The most well-known prognostic scoring system is the recursive partitioning analysis classification developed from 1,200 patients who received WBRT in the RTOG database. Patients were categorized into one of three classes based on age, KPS, status of primary tumor, and extent of extracranial disease ([106]). Recently, the Graded Prognostic Assessment scale was developed based on the analysis of 1,960 patients in the RTOG database; it also incorporates the number of metastatic lesions in the scoring system ([112]) These prognostic scoring systems may help identify patients who might benefit from chemotherapy and help design clinical trials that account for specific tumor histology and prior exposure to chemotherapy. Improvement in patient survival will result from improved local control of CNS disease if the primary disease site remains dormant, illustrating the need for a multimodality approach to the treatment of the patient with brain metastases.

Commentary: The Role of Radiation Therapy for Brain Tumors

Radiation therapy is used to enhance local control and overall survival as a sole modality or in combination with surgery or chemotherapy for many benign and malignant CNS tumors.

Radiotherapy is prescribed in the unit of Gray, which measures the energy absorbed in a material (J/kg). Typically, radiation treatments are fractionated as 1.8 to 2 Gy per day. The prescribed dose of radiation depends on the inherent radiosensitivity of the lesion and the risk to the normal tissues that are in or close to the RT volumes. For example, CNS leukemia is treated with 18 to 24 Gy in 10 to 12 fractions, whereas, GBM requires 60 Gy delivered in 30 fractions. The risk of cataract formation increases after a total dose of only 2 Gy, but brain necrosis typically will not occur below a dose of 60 Gy.

A variety of different RT techniques and modalities are available for the treatment of CNS tumors. All current treatment techniques—three-dimensional conformal radiotherapy (3DCRT), intensity-modulated radiotherapy (IMRT), SRS, proton therapy, and intensity-modulated proton therapy (IMPT)—use three-dimensional algorithms that calculate dose distributions in all planes and display dose in the axial, coronal, and sagittal views. The tumor and normal tissues are delineated using the planning CT scan and other imaging modalities, such as MRI or PET, that may facilitate this process. The tumor delineation involves determination of the gross tumor volume (GTV), which represents the macroscopic visible tumor; the clinical target volume, which is GTV with a margin that incorporates areas of possible microscopic extension; and planning target volume, which gives an additional margin for day-to-day setup differences.

The basic form of three-dimensional planning is 3DCRT. These plans use conformal fields from different angles optimized to the individual patient's needs. Any RT modality, that is, photons, electrons, or protons, can be used for 3DCRT.

Stereotactic radiosurgery and fractionated stereotactic radiotherapy (FSRT) are techniques that use stereotactic positioning by using an external fiducial system to immobilize and position patients allowing submillimeter precision for RT treatments. A large single fraction of radiation is given with SRS, whereas FSRT uses multiple fractions of repeated doses of radiation with a noninvasive stereotactic frame. Stereotactic radiosurgery is typically used for noninfiltrating tumors that are less than 3 cm and away from critical structures such as the optic chiasm. Fractionated stereotactic radiotherapy may be used for a tumor that is close to a critical structure where the highest precision for delivery is required.

Intensity-modulated radiotherapy is typically used with photon beams with a few centers now using it with proton beams (IMPT). Intensity modulation can also be implemented with the stereotactic approach, which may allow an increase in precision of delivery and conformality. The IMRT plans use multiple beams optimized for the tumor location and patient. For each beam, the multileaf collimation varies during the dose delivery to modulate the dose from that beam to "paint" a dose to allow improved conformality and reduction in normal tissue doses.

Proton RT is a modality that is becoming more available worldwide and allows treatment of larger, deeper tumors without an exit dose, thereby reducing the volume of normal tissue receiving low-to-moderate doses, which could result in a reduction in acute and late toxicities. Proton RT may be a useful technology in young patients with curable tumors.

The results of RT vary according to the type of tumor being treated. Benign tumors such as meningiomas or acoustic schwannomas have control rates as high as 90%; malignant tumors such as GBM have lower durable control rates.

Anita Mahajan

Commentary: Surgical Management of Primary Brain Tumors

The primary goal in the surgical management of primary brain tumors, like gliomas, is maximum safe resection. The decision to resect or not to resect should be made after close collaboration between the neurosurgeons, neuro-oncologists, and radiation oncologists. The surgeon must consider a number of critical factors prior to making the decision to operate: age, neurologic status, location and size of the tumor, number and extent of recurrences, and whether the patient would be suitable for adjuvant treatments, including radiation and chemotherapy. In both low-grade gliomas and high-grade gliomas, compared with patients having lesser degrees of resection, those undergoing gross total resections have a better neurologic outcome on long-term follow-up without added perioperative morbidity or mortality. Recent surgical series in low-grade gliomas have shown maximum safe resection if the tumor is an independent predictor of both PFS and OS. Lacroix et al described 416 consecutive patients with GBM and demonstrated that radical resection of the main tumor mass (≥98% by volumetric analysis) was an independent variable that significantly prolonged survival ([73]). The median survival for these patients was 13.4 months compared with 8.8 months for patients who had lesser resections ($P < .0001$). The study relied on a prospective computerized measurement of the volume of tumors, with the extent of resection expressed as a percentage of the preoperative volume. A 90% resection did not result in a statistically significant survival prolongation; the greatest benefit was noted when the extent of resection was 98% or greater. These data are particularly important because of their precision of volumetric assessments and their avoidance of subjective terms such as "gross total" or "subtotal" to describe the degree of resection.

Beyond extending survival, several other benefits can result from more radical resections of gliomas in our experience. These include: (1) a diagnostic advantage in terms of better sampling of tumors and better tissue quality acquired for IHC and molecular diagnosis; (2) a symptomatic advantage through relief of mass effect, leading to improved performance status and enhanced tolerance to RT; (3) an oncologic advantage by reducing the number of neoplastic cells by almost two logs; and (4) a research advantage by harvesting ample tissue material for molecular analysis and fingerprinting, with the eventual identification of novel and specific molecular targets that will form the basis of future therapies.

Several technological adjuncts to surgery are available to aid in localizing the brain mass, in identifying zones of brain function, and in aiding the surgeon to maintain proper orientation in reference to the mass and to its surrounding anatomic structures. Of these, intraoperative ultrasound is an inexpensive, readily accessible surgical tool that allows localization of the mass in real time and aids in the assessment of the completeness of tumor resection. Most gliomas and metastases are hyperechoic with respect to normal brain and thus can be localized easily with the ultrasound probe. It is almost inconceivable to perform such procedures without intraoperative ultrasound.

Frameless stereotactic systems have provided significant assistance on many levels, including adequate placement and sizing of the bone flap, identification of the surface margins, and localization of the mass and the navigational direction for the dissection around or into the mass. The obvious drawback of these systems is their inability to provide a true assessment of residual tumor because of brain shifts that occur necessarily during surgery. Experience with these systems and correlation of the image-derived data with the ultrasound data and with what is visible in the operative field are necessary for the safe use of these techniques in obtaining maximum tumor resection. Recently, intraoperative MRI has been introduced in a few centers, including ours. This technique identifies residual tumor more accurately than other methods. Its main drawback is that it is expensive to install and can prolong operation times. Early systems had low field magnetic strength and as such were less sensitive and provided more indistinct images than the current generation of high-field (1.5-T and higher) magnets.

Neurophysiologic techniques are employed primarily when the tumor is in or adjacent to eloquent brain (those parts of the brain that control language, motor, or sensory function). The most commonly used techniques for cortical mapping include somatosensory evoked potentials, continuous motor evoked potentials, and direct cortical and subcortical stimulation. For motor and sensory localization, the patient is usually (although not invariably) under general anesthesia; for speech localization, however, an awake craniotomy is necessary. The introduction of these techniques has made it possible to perform larger resections with an increased margin of safety in both high- and low-grade gliomas.

Existing data concerning the benefits of surgical resection suggest a survival advantage in patients with gliomas who undergo complete tumor mass resection. Careful preoperative planning should allow for the gross total resection of most gliomas. Until convincing data to the contrary, the goal of a neuro-oncologic operation should be a complete resection of the tumor mass.

Sujit S. Prabhu

REFERENCES

1. Schouten LJ, Rutten J, Huveneers HA, Twijnstra A. Incidence of brain metastases in a cohort of patients with carcinoma of the breast, colon, kidney, and lung and melanoma. *Cancer.* 2002;94:2698-2705.
2. Stupp R, Mason WP, van den Bent MJ, et al. Radiotherapy plus concomitant and adjuvant temozolomide for glioblastoma. *N Engl J Med.* 2005;352:987-996.
3. Gilbert MR, Wang M, Aldape KD, et al. Dose-dense temozolomide for newly diagnosed glioblastoma: a randomized phase III clinical trial. *J Clin Oncol.* 2013;31:4085-4091.
4. Wong ET, Hess KR, Gleason MJ, et al. Outcomes and prognostic factors in recurrent glioma patients enrolled onto phase II clinical trials. *J Clin Oncol.* 1999;17:2572-2578.
5. Dolecek TA, Propp JM, Stroup NE, Kruchko C. CBTRUS statistical report: primary brain and central nervous system tumors diagnosed in the United States in 2005-2009. *Neuro Oncol.* 2012;14(Suppl 5):v1-v49.
6. Fan YS, Lui PC, Tam FK, et al. A 33-year-old Chinese woman with a left frontal tumor. *Brain Pathol.* 2009;19:337-340.
7. Sawaya R, Bindal, RK, Lang FF. Metastatic brain tumors. *Brain Tumors.* 2001;999-1026.
8. Skibber JM, Soong SJ, Austin L, et al. Cranial irradiation after surgical excision of brain metastases in melanoma patients. *Ann Surg Oncol.* 1996;3:118-123.
9. CBTRUS. *Statistical Report: Primary Brain Tumors in the United States 2000-2004.* Central Brain Tumor Registry of the United States; 2008. http://www.cbtrus.org
10. Ostrom QT, Gittleman H, Farah P, et al. CBTRUS statistical report: Primary brain and central nervous system tumors diagnosed in the United States in 2006-2010. *Neuro Oncol.* 2013;15(Suppl 2):ii1-56.
11. Kadan-Lottick NS, Skluzacek MC, Gurney JG. Decreasing incidence rates of primary central nervous system lymphoma. *Cancer.* 2002;95:193-202.
12. Neglia JP, Robison LL, Stovall M, et al. New primary neoplasms of the central nervous system in survivors of childhood cancer: a report from the Childhood Cancer Survivor Study. *J Natl Cancer Inst.* 2006;98:1528-1537.
13. Sadetzki S, Flint-Richter P, Ben-Tal T, Nass D. Radiation-induced meningioma: a descriptive study of 253 cases. *J Neurosurg.* 2002;97:1078-1082.
14. Sodickson A, Baeyens PF, Andriole KP, et al. Recurrent CT, cumulative radiation exposure, and associated radiation-induced cancer risks from CT of adults. *Radiology.* 2009;251:175-184.
15. Wrensch M, Minn Y, Chew T, et al. Epidemiology of primary brain tumors: current concepts and review of the literature. *Neuro Oncol.* 2002;4:278-299.
16. Huncharek M, Kupelnick B, Wheeler L. Dietary cured meat and the risk of adult glioma: a meta-analysis of nine observational studies. *J Environ Pathol Toxicol Oncol.* 2003;22:129-137.
17. Hurley SF, McNeil JJ, Donnan GA, et al. Tobacco smoking and alcohol consumption as risk factors for glioma: a case-control study in Melbourne, Australia. *J Epidemiol Community Health.* 1996;50:442-446.
18. Dziurzynski K, Chang SM, Heimberger AB, et al. Consensus on the role of human cytomegalovirus in glioblastoma. *Neuro Oncol.* 2012;14:246-255.
19. Linos E, Raine T, Alonso A, Michaud D. Atopy and risk of brain tumors: a meta-analysis. *J Natl Cancer Inst.* 2007;99:1544-1550.
20. Scheurer ME, El-Zein R, Thompson PA, et al. Long-term anti-inflammatory and antihistamine medication use and adult glioma risk. *Cancer Epidemiol Biomarkers Prev.* 2008;17:1277-1281.
21. Amirian E, Scheurer ME, Bondy ML. The association between birth order, sibship size, and glioma development in adulthood. *Int J Cancer.* 2009;126(11):2752-2756.
22. Preston-Martin S. Epidemiology of primary CNS neoplasms. *Neurol Clin.* 1996;14:273-290.
23. Brennan CW, Verhaak RG, McKenna A, et al. The somatic genomic landscape of glioblastoma. *Cell.* 2013;155:462-477.
24. Chapman PB, Hauschild A, Robert C, et al. Improved survival with vemurafenib in melanoma with BRAF V600E mutation. *N Engl J Med.* 2011;364:2507-2516.
25. Singh D, Chan JM, Zoppoli P, et al. Transforming fusions of FGFR and TACC genes in human glioblastoma. *Science.* 2012;337:1231-1235.
26. Wong AJ, Ruppert JM, Bigner SH, et al. Structural alterations of the epidermal growth factor receptor gene in human gliomas. *Proc Natl Acad Sci U S A.* 1992;89:2965-2969.
27. Chakravarti A, Zhai G, Suzuki Y, et al. The prognostic significance of phosphatidylinositol 3-kinase pathway activation in human gliomas. *J Clin Oncol.* 2004;22:1926-1933.
28. Guha A, Feldkamp MM, Lau N, et al. Proliferation of human malignant astrocytomas is dependent on Ras activation. *Oncogene.* 1997;15:2755-2765.
29. Maher EA, Furnari FB, Bachoo RM, et al. Malignant glioma: genetics and biology of a grave matter. *Genes Dev.* 2001;15:1311-1333.
30. Ohgaki H, Kleihues P. The definition of primary and secondary glioblastoma. *Clin Cancer Res.* 2013;19:764-772.
31. Ino Y, Betensky RA, Zlatescu MC, et al. Molecular subtypes of anaplastic oligodendroglioma: implications for patient management at diagnosis. *Clin Cancer Res.* 2001;7:839-845.
32. Cairncross JG, Ueki K, Zlatescu MC, et al. Specific genetic predictors of chemotherapeutic response and survival in patients with anaplastic oligodendrogliomas. *J Natl Cancer Inst.* 1998;90:1473-1479.
33. Ino Y, Betensky RA, Zlatescu MC, et al. Molecular subtypes of anaplastic oligodendroglioma: implications for patient management at diagnosis. *Clin Cancer Res.* 2001;7:839-845.
34. Hoang-Xuan K, Capelle L, Kujas M, et al. Temozolomide as initial treatment for adults with low-grade oligodendrogliomas or oligoastrocytomas and correlation with chromosome 1p deletions. *J Clin Oncol.* 2004;22:3133-3138.
35. Hegi ME, Diserens AC, Gorlia T, et al. MGMT gene silencing and benefit from temozolomide in glioblastoma. *N Engl J Med.* 2005;352:997-1003.
36. Parsons DW, Jones S, Zhang X, et al. An integrated genomic analysis of human glioblastoma multiforme. *Science.* 2008;321:1807-1812.
37. Yan H, Parsons DW, Jin G, et al. IDH1 and IDH2 mutations in gliomas. *N Engl J Med.* 2009;360:765-773.
38. Hartmann C, Hentschel B, Wick W, et al. Patients with IDH1 wild type anaplastic astrocytomas exhibit worse prognosis than IDH1-mutated glioblastomas, and IDH1 mutation status accounts for the unfavorable prognostic effect of higher age: implications for classification of gliomas. *Acta Neuropathol.* 2010;120:707-718.
39. Choy W, Kim W, Nagasawa D, et al. The molecular genetics and tumor pathogenesis of meningiomas and the future directions of meningioma treatments. *Neurosurg Focus.* 2011;30:E6.
40. Louis D, Stemmer-Rachamimov AO, Wiestler OD. Neurofibromatosis type 2. In: Kleihues P, Cavenee K, eds. *Pathology and Genetics of Tumors of the Nervous System.* Lyons, France: IARC Press; 2000:219-222.
41. Xiao GH, Chernoff J, Testa JR. NF2: the wizardry of merlin. *Genes Chromosomes Cancer.* 2003;38:389-399.
42. Brastianos PK, Horowitz PM, Santagata S, et al. Genomic sequencing of meningiomas identifies oncogenic SMO and AKT1 mutations. *Nat Genet.* 2013;45:285-289.

43. Ruat M, Hoch L, Faure H, Rognan D. Targeting of Smoothened for therapeutic gain. *Trends Pharmacol Sci*. 2014;35:237-246.
44. Puduvalli VK. Brain metastases: biology and the role of the brain microenvironment. *Curr Oncol Rep*. 2001;3:467-475.
45. Marchetti D, Nicolson GL. Human heparanase: a molecular determinant of brain metastasis. *Adv Enzyme Regul*. 2001;41:343-359.
46. Carmeliet P, Jain RK. Angiogenesis in cancer and other diseases. *Nature*. 2000;407:249-257.
47. Gottesman MM, Fojo T, Bates SE. Multidrug resistance in cancer: role of ATP-dependent transporters. *Nat Rev Cancer*. 2002;2:48-58.
48. Fidler IJ, Yano S, Zhang RD, et al. The seed and soil hypothesis: vascularisation and brain metastases. *Lancet Oncol*. 2002;3:53-57.
49. Muldoon LL, Soussain C, Jahnke K, et al. Chemotherapy delivery issues in central nervous system malignancy: a reality check. *J Clin Oncol*. 2007;25:2295-2305.
50. Giannini C, Burger PC, Berkey BA, et al. Anaplastic oligodendroglial tumors: refining the correlation among histopathology, 1p 19q deletion and clinical outcome in Intergroup Radiation Therapy Oncology Group Trial 9402. *Brain Pathol*. 2008;18:360-369.
51. Theeler BJ, Yung WK, Fuller GN, De Groot JF. Moving toward molecular classification of diffuse gliomas in adults. *Neurology*. 2012;79:1917-1926.
52. World Health Organization. *WHO Classification of Tumours of the Central Nervous System*. Lyon, France: International Agency for Research on Cancer; 2007.
53. Shaw E. Management of low-grade gliomas in adults. *Brain Cancer*. 2002;279-302.
54. Bauman G, Lote K, Larson D, et al. Pretreatment factors predict overall survival for patients with low-grade glioma: a recursive partitioning analysis. *Int J Radiat Oncol Biol Phys*. 1999;45:923-929.
55. Berger M, Leibel S, Bruner J, et al. Primary cerebral tumors. In: Levin V, ed. *Cancer in the Nervous System*. New York: Oxford University Press; 2002:75-157.
56. Berger MS, Deliganis AV, Dobbins J, Keles GE. The effect of extent of resection on recurrence in patients with low grade cerebral hemisphere gliomas. *Cancer*. 1994;74:1784-1791.
57. Shaw EG, Daumas-Duport C, Scheithauer BW, et al. Radiation therapy in the management of low-grade supratentorial astrocytomas. *J Neurosurg*. 1989;70:853-861.
58. Taphoorn MJ. Neurocognitive sequelae in the treatment of low-grade gliomas. *Semin Oncol*. 2003;30:45-48.
59. Meyers CA, Weitzner MA, Valentine AD, Levin VA. Methylphenidate therapy improves cognition, mood, and function of brain tumor patients. *J Clin Oncol*. 1998;16:2522-2527.
60. Karim AB, Maat B, Hatlevoll R, et al. A randomized trial on dose-response in radiation therapy of low-grade cerebral glioma: European Organization for Research and Treatment of Cancer (EORTC) Study 22844. *Int J Radiat Oncol Biol Phys*. 1996;36:549-556.
61. Shaw E, Arusell R, Scheithauer B, et al. Prospective randomized trial of low- versus high-dose radiation therapy in adults with supratentorial low-grade glioma: initial report of a North Central Cancer Treatment Group/Radiation Therapy Oncology Group/Eastern Cooperative Oncology Group study. *J Clin Oncol*. 2002;20:2267-2276.
62. Eyre HJ, Crowley JJ, Townsend JJ, et al. A randomized trial of radiotherapy versus radiotherapy plus CCNU for incompletely resected low-grade gliomas: a Southwest Oncology Group study. *J Neurosurg*. 1993;78:909-914.
62a. Buckner, Jan C., et al. "Phase III study of radiation therapy (RT) with or without procarbazine, CCNU, and vincristine (PCV) in low-grade glioma: RTOG 9802 with Alliance, ECOG, and SWOG." ASCO Annual Meeting Proceedings. Vol. 32. No. 15_suppl. 2014.
63. van den Bent M. Can chemotherapy replace radiotherapy in low-grade gliomas? Time for randomized studies. *Semin Oncol*. 2003;30:39-44.
64. Buckner JC, Gesme D Jr, O'Fallon JR, et al. Phase II trial of procarbazine, lomustine, and vincristine as initial therapy for patients with low-grade oligodendroglioma or oligoastrocytoma: efficacy and associations with chromosomal abnormalities. *J Clin Oncol*. 2003;21:251-255.
65. Sanson M, Cartalat-Carel S, Taillibert S, et al. Initial chemotherapy in gliomatosis cerebri. *Neurology*. 2004;63:270-275.
66. Cairncross G, Wang M, Shaw E, et al. Phase III trial of chemoradiotherapy for anaplastic oligodendroglioma: long-term results of RTOG 9402. *J Clin Oncol*. 2013;31:337-343.
67. van den Bent MJ, Carpentier AF, Brandes AA, et al. Adjuvant procarbazine, lomustine, and vincristine improves progression-free survival but not overall survival in newly diagnosed anaplastic oligodendrogliomas and oligoastrocytomas: a randomized European Organisation for Research and Treatment of Cancer phase III trial. *J Clin Oncol*. 2006;24:2715-2722.
68. Levin VA, Yung WK, Bruner J, et al. Phase II study of accelerated fractionation radiation therapy with carboplatin followed by PCV chemotherapy for the treatment of anaplastic gliomas. *Int J Radiat Oncol Biol Phys*. 2002;53:58-66.
69. Yung WK, Albright RE, Olson J, et al. A phase II study of temozolomide vs. procarbazine in patients with glioblastoma multiforme at first relapse. *Br J Cancer*. 2000;83:588-593.
70. Jaeckle KA, Hess KR, Yung WK, et al. Phase II evaluation of temozolomide and 13-cis-retinoic acid for the treatment of recurrent and progressive malignant glioma: a North American Brain Tumor Consortium study. *J Clin Oncol*. 2003;21:2305-2311.
71. Groves MD, Puduvalli VK, Hess KR, et al. Phase II trial of temozolomide plus the matrix metalloproteinase inhibitor, marimastat, in recurrent and progressive glioblastoma multiforme. *J Clin Oncol*. 2002;20:1383-1388.
72. Gilbert M. Phase I/II study of combination temozolomide (TMZ) and irinotecan (CPT-11) for recurrent malignant gliomas: a North American Brain Tumor Consortium (NABTC) study [Abstract 410]. *Proc Am Soc Clin Oncol*. 2003;22.
73. Lacroix M, Abi-Said D, Fourney DR, et al. A multivariate analysis of 416 patients with glioblastoma multiforme: prognosis, extent of resection, and survival. *J Neurosurg*. 2001;95:190-198.
74. Lang FF, Bruner JM, Fuller GN, et al. Phase I trial of adenovirus-mediated p53 gene therapy for recurrent glioma: biological and clinical results. *J Clin Oncol*. 2003;21:2508-2518.
75. Kunwar S. Convection enhanced delivery of IL13-PE38QQR for treatment of recurrent malignant glioma: presentation of interim findings from ongoing phase 1 studies. *Acta Neurochir Suppl*. 2003;88:105-111.
76. Kunwar S, Prados MD, Chang SM, et al. Direct intracerebral delivery of cintredekin besudotox (IL13-PE38QQR) in recurrent malignant glioma: a report by the Cintredekin Besudotox Intraparenchymal Study Group. *J Clin Oncol*. 2007;25:837-844.
77. Torcuator R, Zuniga R, Mohan YS, et al. Initial experience with bevacizumab treatment for biopsy confirmed cerebral radiation necrosis. *J Neurooncol*. 2009;94:63-68.
78. Perry JR, Belanger K, Mason WP, et al. Phase II trial of continuous dose-intense temozolomide in recurrent malignant glioma: RESCUE study. *J Clin Oncol*. 2010;28:2051-2057.
79. Vredenburgh JJ, Desjardins A, Herndon JE, 2nd, et al. Phase II trial of bevacizumab and irinotecan in recurrent malignant glioma. *Clin Cancer Res*. 2007;13:1253-1259.
80. Kreisl TN, Kim L, Moore K, et al. Phase II trial of single-agent bevacizumab followed by bevacizumab plus irinotecan at

tumor progression in recurrent glioblastoma. *J Clin Oncol.* 2009;27:740-745.

81. Gilbert MR, Dignam JJ, Armstrong TS, et al. A randomized trial of bevacizumab for newly diagnosed glioblastoma. *N Engl J Med.* 2014;370:699-708.
82. Chinot OL, Wick W, Mason W, et al. Bevacizumab plus radiotherapy-temozolomide for newly diagnosed glioblastoma. *N Engl J Med.* 2014;370:709-722.
83. Reardon DA, Desjardins A, Peters KB, et al. Phase II study of carboplatin, irinotecan, and bevacizumab for bevacizumab naive, recurrent glioblastoma. *J Neurooncol.* 2012;107:155-164.
84. Reardon DA. A phase I/II trial of PTK787/ZK 222584 (PTK/ZK): a novel oral angiogenesis inhibitor in combination with either temozolomide or lomustine for patients with recurrent glioblastoma multiforme (GBM). ASCO Annual Meeting Proceedings. *J Clin Oncol.* 2004;22(suppl 14S):1513.
85. Prados MD, Yung WK, Jaeckle KA, et al. Phase 1 trial of irinotecan (CPT-11) in patients with recurrent malignant glioma: a North American Brain Tumor Consortium study. *Neuro Oncol.* 2004;6:44-54.
86. Mcdermott M, Quinones-Hinosa A, Bollen AW. Meningiomas. *Brain Cancer.* 2002;333-364.
87. Ojemann SG, Sneed PK, Larson DA, et al. Radiosurgery for malignant meningioma: results in 22 patients. *J Neurosurg.* 2000;93(Suppl 3):62-67.
88. Mason WP, Gentili F, Macdonald DR, et al. Stabilization of disease progression by hydroxyurea in patients with recurrent or unresectable meningioma. *J Neurosurg.* 2002;97:341-346.
89. Kaba SE, DeMonte F, Bruner JM, et al. The treatment of recurrent unresectable and malignant meningiomas with interferon alpha-2B. *Neurosurgery.* 1997;40:271-275.
90. Travitzky M, Libson E, Nemirovsky I, et al. Doxil-induced regression of pleuro-pulmonary metastases in a patient with malignant meningioma. *Anticancer Drugs.* 2003;14:247-250.
91. Chamberlain MC, Tsao-Wei DD, Groshen S. Temozolomide for treatment-resistant recurrent meningioma. *Neurology.* 2004;62:1210-1212.
92. Gupta V, Samuleson CG, Su S, Chen TC. Nelfinavir potentiation of imatinib cytotoxicity in meningioma cells via survivin inhibition. *Neurosurg Focus.* 2007;23:E9.
93. Norden AD, Raizer JJ, Abrey LE, et al. Phase II trials of erlotinib or gefitinib in patients with recurrent meningioma. *J Neurooncol.* 2010;96:211-217.
94. Kaley TJ, Wen P, Schiff D, et al. Phase II trial of sunitinib for recurrent and progressive atypical and anaplastic meningioma. *Neuro Oncol.* 2015;17:116-121.
95. Weller M, Martus P, Roth P, et al. Surgery for primary CNS lymphoma? Challenging a paradigm. *Neuro Oncol.* 2012;14:1481-1484.
96. DeAngelis LM, Yahalom J, Thaler HT, Kher U. Combined modality therapy for primary CNS lymphoma. *J Clin Oncol.* 1992;10:635-643.
97. Abrey LE, Yahalom J, DeAngelis LM. Treatment for primary CNS lymphoma: the next step. *J Clin Oncol.* 2000;18:3144-3150.
98. Harder H, Holtel H, Bromberg JE, et al. Cognitive status and quality of life after treatment for primary CNS lymphoma. *Neurology.* 2004;62:544-547.
99. Batchelor T, Carson K, O'Neill A, et al. Treatment of primary CNS lymphoma with methotrexate and deferred radiotherapy: a report of NABTT 96-07. *J Clin Oncol.* 2003;21:1044-1049.
100. Herrlinger U, Brugger W, Bamberg M, et al. PCV salvage chemotherapy for recurrent primary CNS lymphoma. *Neurology.* 2000;54:1707-1708.
101. Abrey LE, DeAngelis LM, Yahalom J. Long-term survival in primary CNS lymphoma. *J Clin Oncol.* 1998;16:859-863.
102. Lerro KA, Lacy J. Case report: a patient with primary CNS lymphoma treated with temozolomide to complete response. *J Neurooncol.* 2002;59:165-168.
103. Pels H, Schulz H, Schlegel U, Engert A. Treatment of CNS lymphoma with the anti-CD20 antibody rituximab: experience with two cases and review of the literature. *Onkologie.* 2003;26:351-354.
104. Enting RH, Demopoulos A, DeAngelis LM, Abrey LE. Salvage therapy for primary CNS lymphoma with a combination of rituximab and temozolomide. *Neurology.* 2004;63:901-903.
105. Soussain C, Suzan F, Hoang-Xuan K, et al. Results of intensive chemotherapy followed by hematopoietic stem-cell rescue in 22 patients with refractory or recurrent primary CNS lymphoma or intraocular lymphoma. *J Clin Oncol.* 2001;19:742-749.
106. Gaspar L, Scott C, Rotman M, et al. Recursive partitioning analysis (RPA) of prognostic factors in three Radiation Therapy Oncology Group (RTOG) brain metastases trials. *Int J Radiat Oncol Biol Phys.* 1997;37:745-751.
107. Gaspar LE, Scott C, Murray K, Curran W. Validation of the RTOG recursive partitioning analysis (RPA) classification for brain metastases. *Int J Radiat Oncol Biol Phys.* 2000;47:1001-1006.
108. Gilbert M. Brain metastases: still an "orphan" disease? *Curr Oncol Rep.* 2001;3:463-466.
109. Ribas A, Flaherty KT. BRAF targeted therapy changes the treatment paradigm in melanoma. *Nat Rev Clin Oncol.* 2011;8:426-433.
110. Hodi FS, O'Day SJ, McDermott DF, et al. Improved survival with ipilimumab in patients with metastatic melanoma. *N Engl J Med.* 2010;363:711-723.
111. Schartz NE, Farges C, Madelaine I, et al. Complete regression of a previously untreated melanoma brain metastasis with ipilimumab. *Melanoma Res.* 2010;20:247-250.
112. Sperduto PW, Berkey B, Gaspar LE, et al. A new prognostic index and comparison to three other indices for patients with brain metastases: an analysis of 1,960 patients in the RTOG database. *Int J Radiat Oncol Biol Phys.* 2008;70:510-514.
113. Ostrom QT, Gittleman H, Liao P, et al. CBTRUS statistical report: primary brain and central nervous system tumors diagnosed in the United States in 2007-2011. *Neuro Oncol.* 2014;16(Suppl 4):iv1-63.

SECTION XI

Melanoma and Sarcomas

Section Editors: Michael A. Davies and Sapna P. Patel

第十一篇 黑色素瘤和肉瘤

41

Melanoma

第四十一章　黑色素瘤

Dae Won Kim
Jeffrey E. Gershenwald
Sapna P. Patel
Michael A. Davies

中文导读

黑色素瘤是高度侵袭性的皮肤肿瘤，占所有皮肤相关肿瘤死亡的75%。本章首先介绍了黑色素瘤的流行病学史和相关危险因素；接着介绍了黑色素瘤的分类，其按原发部位可分为皮肤型、葡萄膜型、黏膜型、增生性和原发中枢神经系统的黑色素瘤，按分子特点可分为BRAF突变、NRAS突变、KIT突变和CNAQ/GNA11基因改变几种类型。随之阐述了该病的分子生物学，皮肤型黑色素瘤有较高的体细胞突变，主要包括：RAS-RAF-MEK-ERK通路、PI3K-Akt等通路的激活；而其他非皮肤型黑色素瘤的分子特点主要是KIT和CNAQ/GNA11的突变。然后介绍了黑色素瘤的分期，主要依据第7版AJCC分期。最后本章重点介绍了针对不同分期黑色素瘤的治疗手段。无淋巴结转移的早期黑色素瘤以手术治疗为主，主要包括原发病灶的广泛切除和区域淋巴结评估；对于存在区域转移的黑色素瘤，治疗主要包括辅助放疗、干扰素治疗、辅助生物治疗联合化疗等；转移性黑色素瘤的治疗手段主要包括化疗、靶向治疗（BRAF抑制剂、MEK抑制剂、KIT抑制剂）、免疫治疗（白介素-2、抗CTLA-4单抗治疗、抗PD-1单抗治疗、肿瘤浸润淋巴细胞的治疗和生化治疗）等。

INTRODUCTION

Melanoma is the most aggressive form of skin cancer. Although its incidence pales in comparison to basal cell carcinoma and squamous cell carcinoma (SCC), melanoma is the cause of approximately 75% of all skin cancer–related deaths. The majority of patients who are diagnosed with early-stage melanoma have very good outcomes with appropriate surgical management. In contrast, patients with regional and distant metastases have historically had poorer outcomes, because agents that have proven efficacious in other malignancies (eg, chemotherapy) generally have had limited activity in this disease. However, the management of melanoma is evolving rapidly due to parallel breakthroughs in the understanding and targeting of the molecular drivers of this disease and the regulators of the antitumor immune response. These advances are rapidly translating into improved outcomes in patients with advanced melanoma and the consideration of new diagnostic and therapeutic approaches across the full continuum of this disease.

EPIDEMIOLOGY AND RISK FACTORS

Melanoma is the fifth most common cancer in men and the sixth most common cancer in women in the United States ([1]). The age-adjusted incidence for cutaneous melanoma from 2007 to 2011 was 21.3 per 100,000 per year in the United States ([2]). In contrast to the favorable trends that have been observed with almost all other major cancers, the annual incidence of melanoma continues to rise by approximately 2% to 3% per year and has increased overall more than 500-fold since the 1950s ([3]).

A number of factors have been identified that correlate with an increased risk of being diagnosed with melanoma (Table 41-1). Many of these factors reflect the strong association between melanoma and ultraviolet radiation (UVR) exposure, which is supported by epidemiologic studies ([4]). More recently, whole-exome sequencing studies have demonstrated that melanomas are characterized by a higher rate of somatic mutations than almost all other solid tumors and that the majority of mutations that are identified bear the molecular signature of UVR-related DNA damage ([5]). Several risk assessment aids have been developed to identify high-risk individuals, including the Melanoma Risk Assessment Tool (MRAT), which is available online (http://www.cancer.gov/melanomarisktool/). Individuals at increased risk of developing melanoma should have awareness of the signs of melanoma and regular screening examinations.

Patients with dysplastic (atypical) nevi with irregular borders, multiple colors, and >5 mm diameter have a 3- to 20-fold higher risk of developing melanomas than the general population ([6]). Although the majority of melanomas are sporadic, these nevi can be inherited in a familial pattern. The familial atypical multiple mole and melanoma (FAMMM) syndrome is an autosomal dominant disorder characterized by the occurrence of melanoma in one or more first- or second-degree relatives and the presence of a high number of acquired nevi or atypical nevi. This syndrome is associated with germline mutations of the *CDKN2A* gene and is also associated with an increased risk of other cancers, especially pancreatic cancer ([7]). Congenital nevi can also be a precursor of melanoma, and individuals with large congenital nevi (>20 cm) have been shown to be at increased risk of developing melanoma ([8]).

CLASSIFICATION

Cutaneous melanomas, which are the most common manifestation of this disease, arise from melanocytes in the skin. The four major types of cutaneous melanoma are superficial spreading, nodular, lentigo maligna, and acral lentiginous melanoma. Melanomas can also arise from melanocytes in other areas, including the uveal tract of the eye (uveal melanomas) and mucosal surfaces throughout the body (mucosal melanoma). Desmoplastic melanomas represent a distinct subtype that arise from melanocytes in the skin, generally in areas with chronic sun exposure, that are characterized by highly invasive local growth that often tracks along nerves. Very rare subtypes include primary central nervous system (CNS) melanomas, which arise from melanocytes in the leptomeninges, and melanomas of soft parts (also known as clear cell sarcoma), which arise in soft tissues and dermis. Although the melanoma subtypes are not independent prognostic factors, they can be associated with distinct clinical (Table 41-2) and molecular (Table 41-3) features ([9]).

MOLECULAR BIOLOGY

Cutaneous melanomas are characterized by an extremely high rate of somatic mutations. The first cutaneous melanoma analyzed by whole-genome sequencing identified more than 33,000 somatic changes in the tumor ([10]). The majority of the somatic changes detected in cutaneous melanomas are typical of DNA damage induced by UVR. Despite the challenges presented by this overall high background mutation rate, confirmed driver mutations are detectable in the majority of cutaneous melanomas. A number of important molecular events have also been identified in other melanoma subtypes.

Table 41-1 Factors Associated With Increased Risk of Melanoma

Risk Factor	Features
Personal history of melanoma	9× increased risk of developing a second melanoma (vs general population)
Family history of melanoma	First-degree relatives have a higher risk, and 10% of all melanomas are familial (FAMMM syndrome and dysplastic nevus syndrome)
Total number of nevi	Relative risk of 5 to 17 with presence of >50 nevi
Congenital nevi	6% lifetime risk with large (>20 cm) congenital nevi
Dysplastic nevi	3- to 20-fold higher risk of developing melanoma than general population
Immunosuppression	Chronic immune suppressant use, HIV infection, and organ transplantation
MC1R variants	Associated with fair skin, red hair, and freckles
Exposure to ultraviolet light	Tanning bed use, sunburn

FAMMM, familial atypical multiple mole and melanoma.

RAS-RAF-MEK-ERK Pathway

The RAS-RAF-MEK-ERK pathway promotes cellular proliferation and survival, and activation of this pathway has been implicated in multiple tumor types. Genetic events that activate this pathway are detected in almost all cutaneous melanomas [11]. The most common alterations detected are point mutations in the *BRAF* gene. *BRAF* encodes a serine-threonine kinase in the RAS-RAF-MEK-ERK cascade. Point mutations in *BRAF* are detected in approximately 45% of cutaneous melanomas, and approximately 95% of these mutations result in substitutions for valine at position 600 in the BRAF protein [12]. The most common mutations result in the substitution of a glutamic acid (*BRAF*^{V600E}, 70%) or lysine (*BRAF*^{V600K}, 20%) residue. These and other substitutions at codon 600 increase the kinase activity of the BRAF protein ≥200-fold and result in

Table 41-2 Melanoma Subtypes

Type	Frequency	Sites	Features
Cutaneous			
Superficial Spreading	70%	Any site (more common on the upper back in both sexes and the lower extremities in women)	Most common subtype of cutaneous melanomas
Nodular	15%-30%	Any site (common on the trunk or legs)	Presents with vertical growth phase without radial growth phase
Lentigo maligna	4%-15%	Sun-exposed area (the head and neck and arms)	
Acral lentiginous	2%-8%	The palms, soles, and beneath the nail plate	More common in African Americans and Asians
Uveal	Rare	Uveal tract of the eye (iris, ciliary body, and the choroid)	Frequent, and often exclusive, metastatic involvement of the liver
Mucosal	Rare	Mucosal surfaces (head and neck, respiratory, gastrointestinal, and genitourinary tracts)	Poor prognosis, potentially due to delayed diagnosis and the rich lymphovascular supply of the mucosa
Desmoplastic	Rare	Areas with chronic sun exposure, especially head and neck	High risk for local recurrence and growth along nerves
Primary CNS	Rare	Leptomeninges	
Melanoma of soft parts (clear cell sarcoma)	Rare	Soft tissues, dermis	Associated with fusions involving the *EWSR1* gene

CNS, central nervous system.

Table 41-3 Classification of Melanoma by Oncogenic Mutations

Melanoma Subtype	Mutations			
	BRAF	*NRAS*	*KIT*	*GNAQ/GNA11*
Cutaneous without CSD	50%	15%-20%	1%-2%	—
Cutaneous with CSD	5%-30%	10%-15%	2%-17%	—
Acral lentiginous	10%-15%	10%-15%	15%-20%	—
Mucosal	5%	5%-10%	15%-20%	—
Uveal	—	—	—	85%

CSD, chronic sun damage.

constitutive activation of downstream components of the RAS-RAF-MEK-ERK pathway. The *BRAF*^{V600E} mutation is also frequently detected in benign nevi, supporting that this molecular event occurs very early in melanoma development ([13]). Consistent with this theory, *BRAF* mutation status is highly concordant between primary melanomas and their metastases. Mutations at other sites in *BRAF* (*BRAF*$^{Non-V600}$) are detected in approximately 5% of cutaneous melanomas. These mutations have variable effects on BRAF's catalytic activity, but preclinical data supports that they still activate the RAS-RAF-MEK-ERK pathway ([14]). Recently, translocations involving the *BRAF* locus have also been identified as rare events in melanoma ([15]). These translocations generate fusion proteins that again appear to activate the RAS-RAF-MEK-ERK pathway.

Mutations in *NRAS* are detected in 20% of cutaneous melanomas ([11]). These mutations overwhelmingly occur in hotspot regions that result in substitutions at amino acid residues Q61 (approximately 80%) or G12/G13 (approximately 20%). Similar to *BRAF*^{V600E}, the mutant NRAS proteins potently activate the RAS-RAF-MEK-ERK pathway, and they are also commonly detected in benign nevi. Notably, hotspot mutations in *NRAS* are essentially mutually exclusive (<1% co-occurrence) with *BRAF*^{V600E} mutations, but they co-occur relatively frequently with *BRAF*$^{Non-V600}$ mutations ([16]). Mutations in *KRAS* and *HRAS*, which are members of the RAS family of GTPases, are also detected as rare events (<2%) in melanoma. Loss-of-function mutations of *NF1*, a negative regulator of RAS, are detected in approximately 15% of cutaneous melanomas, predominantly in melanomas without *NRAS* or *BRAF*^{V600} mutations.

Additional Pathways Implicated in Cutaneous Melanomas

The PI3K-AKT pathway is a key regulator of many cellular processes, including proliferation, survival, motility, and metabolism. As studies in multiple cancer types have shown that oncogenic *RAS* mutations use this pathway in addition to RAS-RAF-MEK-ERK to transform cells, the identification of *NRAS* mutations was the first evidence supporting a role for PI3K-AKT activation in melanoma. This pathway may also be activated by loss of function of *PTEN*, which is a lipid phosphatase that normally inhibits the activation of the PI3K-AKT pathway. Loss-of-function mutations and deletions involving *PTEN* are detected in up to 30% of cutaneous melanomas ([11]). Loss of *PTEN* appears to be largely mutually exclusive in melanomas with *NRAS* mutations, but it occurs frequently in tumors with concurrent *BRAF*^{V600} mutations. Experiments in preclinical models have shown that loss of *PTEN* cooperates with *BRAF*^{V600} mutations to promote transformation, invasiveness, and metastasis of melanocytes, providing functional support for this clinical association ([17]). Rare (<2% each) activating mutations in *AKT1*, *AKT3*, and *PIK3CA* have also been detected in cutaneous melanomas, again generally in tumors with *BRAF*^{V600} mutations.

Alterations in key cell cycle regulators are also pervasive in cutaneous melanomas. Germline loss-of-function mutations in the *CDKN2A* gene are the most common events detected in familial melanoma. The *CDKN2A* gene encodes two different proteins, P14^{ARF} and P16^{INK4A}. P16^{INK4A} regulates cell cycle progression by binding to cyclin-dependent kinase 4 (CDK4). Point mutations in the gene that encodes CDK4 are the most common germline event detected in familial melanoma cases without *CDKN2A* mutations. The mutations alter the site in CDK4 that P16^{INK4A} normally binds to, thereby promoting cell cycle progression ([18]). Somatic mutations and copy number changes in both *CDKN2A* and *CDK4* are detected commonly in cutaneous melanomas. Cyclin D1, which forms a protein complex with CDK4 or CDK6 to promote cell cycle progression, can also be amplified in this disease ([19]). Loss of function of P14^{ARF} inhibits the function of *TP53* via increased MDM2 activity. In addition, mutations in *TP53* are present in approximately 20% of cutaneous melanomas ([11]).

Molecular Features of Noncutaneous Melanomas

Activating mutations in *BRAF* are relatively rare events in acral lentiginous (approximately 15%) and mucosal (approximately 5%) melanomas, and they are not detected at all in uveal melanomas ([9]). However, several other prevalent oncogenic events have been identified in these melanoma subtypes.

KIT is a type III transmembrane receptor tyrosine kinase that activates several pro-survival signaling pathways following binding of its ligand, stem cell factor (SCF). *KIT* amplifications and mutations are frequently (20%-30%) detected in acral, mucosal, and cutaneous melanoma with chronic sun-induced damage, whereas few are detected in cutaneous melanoma without chronic sun-induced damage (<5%) ([20]). The two most common *KIT* mutations in melanoma are *L576P* (34% of *KIT* mutations) and *K642E* (15%) in exons 11 and 13, respectively, and overall, 70% of *KIT* mutations occur in exon 11, which encodes the juxtamembrane domain ([21]). *KIT* mutations in exon 11 prevent the juxtamembrane domain's inhibitory function and induce the constitutive activation of KIT and its associated pathways.

GNAQ and *GNA11* encode regulatory subunits of G-protein-coupled receptors that are frequently mutated in uveal melanomas. Hotspot mutations affecting residues Q209 (exon 5) and R183 (exon 4) in these genes are mutually exclusive events. Combined, mutations in either *GNAQ* or *GNA11* are present in 85% of uveal melanomas ([22]). The mutant GNAQ/11 proteins hyperactivate a number of cellular signaling pathways, including RAS-RAF-MEK-ERK and PI3K-AKT. *GNAQ* and *GNA11* mutations appear to be extremely rare (≤1%) in cutaneous melanomas, but they have been detected in both blue nevi and primary CNS melanoma.

STAGING

Once patients are diagnosed with melanoma, staging of melanoma is important for prognosis and treatment. The seventh edition of the American Joint Committee on Cancer (AJCC) staging system for cutaneous melanoma based on the primary tumor (T), regional lymph node (N), and distant metastasis (M) was published in 2009 and took effect in 2010 (Tables 41-4 and 41-5) ([23]). Prognostic factors for primary tumor staging are Breslow thickness, ulceration, and (for melanomas with Breslow thickness <1 mm) mitoses ([24]). For regional lymph nodal staging, the number of involved lymph nodes is the strongest predictor of outcome, but tumor burden (microscopic vs macroscopic) and pattern of involvement (lymph nodes, in-transit disease) are also prognostic ([24]). In patients with distant metastasis, staging is organized into three subgroups (M1a, M1b, and M1c) reflecting the site(s) of metastasis and serum lactate dehydrogenase (LDH) levels.

SURGICAL MANAGEMENT OF EARLY-STAGE MELANOMA

For patients with primary cutaneous melanoma and clinically negative regional lymph nodes, surgery represents the mainstay of initial clinical management. It is useful to consider this approach in the context of two themes: (1) wide excision and (2) approach to the regional nodal basin. Prior to definitive surgery, it is important to identify other lesions suspicious for a second primary melanoma; evidence, if any, of regional metastasis; and signs/symptoms that may raise suspicion for distant metastatic disease. Such findings may alter treatment plans.

Recommended wide excision margins are based on primary tumor thickness (Breslow thickness), and they are measured from the melanoma biopsy site edges or residual intact disease ([25]). Wide excision includes subcutaneous tissue down to the level of, but generally not including, underlying muscular fascia. Recommended margins of excision are summarized in Table 41-6.

The surgical approach to the regional nodal basin is guided by Breslow thickness and other tumor and host factors. The technique of lymphatic mapping and sentinel node biopsy (SNB) is based on the observation that finite regions of skin drain via afferent lymphatics to regional lymph nodes, termed sentinel nodes, and that these represent the most likely nodes to contain occult metastatic disease, if any are involved ([26]). Overall, for patients with clinically negative regional nodes, the risk of regional lymph node metastasis ranges from <1% for patients with very thin primary tumors to approximately 50% for patients with thick, ulcerated primary tumors. Sentinel node biopsy has been widely recommended for patients with primary cutaneous melanomas ≥1 mm in tumor thickness ([27]). In contrast, a selective approach to SNB is entertained for patients with thin (T1) melanomas due to the overall low risk of microscopic regional metastasis. Although indications for SNB among patients with thin melanoma continue to evolve, SNB should be considered for a patient whose primary tumor is ≥0.75 mm and/or has other high-risk features ([28]). Preoperative

Table 41-4 American Joint Committee on Cancer Staging System for Melanoma (Seventh Edition)

T Classification	Primary Tumor (Breslow) Thickness (mm)	Ulceration Status/Mitoses
Tis	NA	melanoma in situ
T1	≤1.00	a: without ulceration and mitosis <1/mm^2 b: with ulceration and/or mitoses ≥1/mm^2
T2	1.01-2.00	a: without ulceration b: with ulceration
T3	2.01-4.00	a: without ulceration b: with ulceration
T4	>4.00	a: without ulceration b: with ulceration
N Classification	**No. of Metastatic Nodes**	**Nodal Metastatic Burden**
N1	1	a: micrometastasis[a] b: macrometastasis[b]
N2	2-3	a: micrometastasis[a] b: macrometastasis[b] c: in-transit met(s)/satellite(s) without metastatic lymph nodes
N3	4+ metastatic nodes, or matted lymph nodes, or in-transit met(s)/satellite(s) with metastatic node(s)	
M Classification	**Distant Metastatic Site(s)**	**Serum Lactate Dehydrogenase (LDH) Level**
M1a	Distant skin, subcutaneous, or nodal met(s)	Normal
M1b	Lung met(s)	Normal
M1c	All other visceral met(s) Any distant met(s)	Normal Elevated

LDH, lactate dehydrogenase; mets, metastases; NA, not applicable.
[a]Micrometastases are diagnosed after sentinel lymph node biopsy.
[b]Macrometastases are defined as clinically detectable lymph node metastases confirmed pathologically (or by finding of gross [not microscopic] extracapsular extension).
Reproduced, with permission, from Balch CM, Gershenwald JE, Soong SJ, et al. Final version of 2009 AJCC melanoma staging and classification. *J Clin Oncol.* 2009;27(36):6199-6206.

lymphoscintigraphy is generally recommended to identify regional nodal basins at risk and to localize the sentinel nodes; a dual-modality approach (ie, in the United States, isosulfan blue dye and technetium-99 sulfur colloid) along with a hand-held gamma probe is used intraoperatively ([26, 29]). Following surgery, enhanced histologic analysis is performed, generally as a combination of step sectioning and immunohistochemical analysis. In contrast to many other solid tumors, intraoperative frozen section assessment is rarely employed.

Sentinel node pathologic status is an important independent predictor of survival ([30, 31]). Although complete lymph node dissection (CLND; also known as completion lymphadenectomy or early therapeutic lymph node dissection) has been a standard of care for patients with a positive sentinel node for over two decades, its role continues to evolve. The recently completed Multicenter Selective Lymphadenectomy Trial-I (MSLT-I) prospective, randomized, clinical trial compared wide excision and SNB (with CLND for patients with a positive SNB) to wide excision and nodal observation (followed by lymphadenectomy for patients who developed nodal recurrence). This trial confirmed the strong prognostic significance of SNB in patients with early-stage melanoma, but it did not demonstrate an overall survival (OS) benefit for the procedure. However, subset analysis among all node-positive patients did show a survival advantage to SNB-positive patients who had CLND compared to patients who had nodal observation and subsequently recurred in regional nodes ([31]). The role of CLND for patients with at least one positive sentinel node is currently being investigated in the randomized international MSLT-II trial and the European Organization for Research and Treatment of Cancer (EORTC) registry-based MINITUB clinical trial.

Table 41-5 American Joint Committee on Cancer Stage Groupings for Cutaneous Melanoma (Seventh Edition)

Clinical Staging[a]				Pathologic Staging[b]			
	T	N	M		T	N	M
0	Tis	N0	M0	0	Tis	N0	M0
IA	T1a	N0	M0	IA	T1a	N0	M0
IB	T1b	N0	M0	IB	T1b	N0	M0
	T2a	N0	M0		T2a	N0	M0
IIA	T2b	N0	M0	IIA	T2b	N0	M0
	T3a	N0	M0		T3a	N0	M0
IIB	T3b	N0	M0	IIB	T3b	N0	M0
	T4a	N0	M0		T4a	N0	M0
IIC	T4b	N0	M0	IIC	T4b	N0	M0
III	Any T	N > N0	M0	IIIA	T1-4a	N1a	M0
					T1-4a	N2a	M0
				IIIB	T1-4b	N1a	M0
					T1-4b	N2a	M0
					T1-4a	N1b	M0
					T1-4a	N2b	M0
					T1-4a	N2c	M0
				IIIC	T1-4b	N1b	M0
					T1-4b	N2b	M0
					T1-4b	N2c	M0
					Any T	N3	M0
IV	Any T	Any N	M1	IV	Any T	Any N	M1

[a]Clinical staging includes microstaging of the primary melanoma and clinical/radiologic evaluation for metastases. By convention, it should be used after complete excision of the primary melanoma with clinical assessment for regional and distant metastases.
[b]Pathologic staging includes microstaging of the primary melanoma and pathologic information about the regional lymph nodes after partial (ie, sentinel node biopsy) or complete lymphadenectomy. Pathologic stage 0 or stage IA patients are the exception; they do not require pathologic evaluation of their lymph nodes.
Reproduced, with permission, from Balch CM, Gershenwald JE, Soong SJ, et al. Final version of 2009 AJCC melanoma staging and classification. *J Clin Oncol.* 2009;27(36):6199-6206.

MANAGEMENT OF REGIONAL DISEASE

Adjuvant Radiation

Recurrences at the primary tumor site after surgery are rare and occur in <5% of cutaneous melanomas ([32]). However, in some cases, the risk of regional recurrence may be increased and the use of adjuvant radiation may improve local disease control. Inadequate margins due to anatomic restrictions, satellitosis in the surgical specimen, or recurrence at the primary site are relative indications for adjuvant radiation at the primary tumor site. Thick (>4 mm) tumors, especially those that originate in the head and neck region, are also sometimes considered for adjuvant radiation. In particular, desmoplastic melanomas, which overall are rare but frequently (>60%) occur in the head and neck region ([33]) and tend toward neurotropic spread rather than classical lymphatic spread, have a high local failure rate (20%-50%). Retrospective reports of postoperative adjuvant radiation in desmoplastic melanoma patients have demonstrated a significant decrease in recurrence rate with

Table 41-6 Recommended Wide Local Excision Surgical Margins

Primary Tumor Thickness (mm)	Excision Margin (cm)
In situ	0.5–1
0–1	1
1–2	1 or 2[a]
2–4	2
>4	2

[a]A 1 cm margin is appropriate in anatomically restricted areas; otherwise a 2 cm margin is preferred.

postoperative adjuvant radiation versus observation alone (local recurrence, 24% vs 7%; $P = .009$) ([33]).

Retrospective analyses have also established risk factors that correlate with increased risk of nodal basin recurrence, including involvement of more than three nodes, nodal size >3 cm, presence of extracapsular extension in the lymph node(s), and recurrent disease in the nodal basin ([34]). The Trans-Tasman Radiation Oncology Group (TROG) and Australia and New Zealand Melanoma Trials Group (ANZMTG) completed a prospective, randomized trial of patients with high risk of nodal basin relapse ([35]). Two-hundred fifty patients were randomized to receive observation or adjuvant radiation consisting of 48 Gy in 20 fractions. Adjuvant radiation treatment significantly reduced the risk of lymph node recurrence (hazard ratio [HR], 0.56; $P = .041$). However, this did not translate into an OS benefit (HR, 1.37; $P = .12$). Adjuvant radiation is not without complications. In the head and neck region there is a 10% rate of associated hearing loss, ear pain, wound dehiscence, and bone exposure ([36]). Outside of this area, chronic lymphedema remains an impediment with significant morbidity to afflicted patients. Patients with a body mass index defined as obese and those undergoing groin radiation are at increased risk for complications from therapy ([37]).

Adjuvant Interferon

Early reports of activity of interferon α-2b (IFN) in metastatic melanoma led to it being studied in the adjuvant setting following definitive surgery. The Eastern Cooperative Oncology Group (ECOG) 1684 trial randomized 287 patients to receive 1 year of treatment with IFN, a regimen known as high-dose IFN (HDI), or observation ([38]). Eligible patients included those with melanomas greater than 4 mm in depth without lymph node involvement (T4N0M0), melanomas of any thickness with lymph node involvement (TxN1-3M0), or regional lymph node recurrence after definitive therapy for primary melanoma. Patients in the HDI arm received induction intravenous IFN 20 million units (MU)/m^2/d for 5 days per week for 4 weeks followed by maintenance subcutaneous IFN 10 MU/m^2/d three times a week for 48 weeks. Treatment with HDI resulted in a statistically significant improvement in relapse-free survival (RFS) compared to observation (1.72 vs 0.98 years, $P = .0023$) as well as an improvement in median OS (3.82 vs 2.78 years, $P = .0237$). High-dose IFN is associated with significant toxicities including flu-like symptoms of fever, myalgia, and malaise; biochemical abnormalities including transaminitis, leukopenia, and thrombocytopenia; and psychological symptoms such as depression with suicidal ideation. On the basis of ECOG 1684, the US Food and Drug Administration (FDA) approved HDI as adjuvant therapy for patients with high-risk melanoma (Table 41-7). Long-term follow-up studies of the patients included in this trial confirmed the significant improvement in RFS. However, the difference in OS initially observed between the two groups was not significant with additional follow-up ($P = .18$) ([39]). The unclear impact of HDI on OS led to several follow-up studies investigating intermediate-dose IFN, duration

Table 41-7 Approved Systemic Therapies for Melanoma

Agent	Year of FDA Approval	Indication
Dacarbazine	1974	Unresectable or metastatic disease
Interferon	1995	Stage IIB/IIC/III (adjuvant)
Interleukin-2	1998	Unresectable or metastatic disease
Pegylated interferon	2011	Stage III (adjuvant)
Ipilimumab	2011	Unresectable or metastatic disease
Vemurafenib	2011	Unresectable or metastatic disease with *BRAF*^{V600} mutation
Dabrafenib	2013	Unresectable or metastatic disease with *BRAF*^{V600} mutation
Trametinib	2013	Unresectable or metastatic disease with *BRAF*^{V600} mutation
Dabrafenib + trametinib	2014	Unresectable or metastatic disease with *BRAF*^{V600} mutation
Pembrolizumab	2014	Unresectable or metastatic disease after ipilimumab (and after BRAF inhibitor if *BRAF*^{V600} mutation present)[a]
Nivolumab	2014	Unresectable or metastatic disease after ipilimumab (and after BRAF inhibitor if *BRAF*^{V600} mutation present)[a]
Ipilimumab + nivolumab	2015	*BRAF*^{V600} wild-type, unresectable or metastatic disease
Vemurafenib + cobimetinib	2015	Unresectable or metastatic disease with *BRAF*^{V600} mutation

[a]Additional indications in stage IV patients under consideration.

CHAPTER 41

of IFN treatment, and induction IFN alone. None of these studies demonstrated a significant OS benefit.

Pegylation of IFN increases the half-life of the drug in the body, diminishing the need for frequent injections compared with standard IFN. The EORTC 18991 trial was a phase III randomized controlled trial comparing pegylated IFN (PEG-IFN) for 5 years versus observation ([40]). In this trial, 1,256 patients with node-positive stage III melanoma were randomized with a primary end point of recurrence-free survival, a composite end point defined as the length of time from randomization to the first of local or regional or distant recurrence or death from any cause. Pegylated IFN did significantly improve recurrence-free survival (34.8 vs 25.6 months, $P = .01$), but it did not significantly impact time to distant relapse or OS. These results were maintained with additional follow-up ([41]). Subset analysis found that patients with an ulcerated primary tumor and microscopic nodal involvement appear to have the greatest benefit from PEG-IFN treatment, as they were characterized by statistically significant improvements in recurrence-free survival, distant metastasis–free survival, and OS. These findings support previous evidence that ulceration and lower nodal burden are predictive factors associated with response to IFN-based adjuvant treatments ([42]). An important feature of EORTC 18991 was the ability to dose reduce PEG-IFN early during treatment to keep patients on study. Prolonged therapy even with dose reduction had already been shown to delay relapse (EORTC 18952), and EORTC 18991 continued this modification to maintain patients at an ECOG performance status of 0 to 1 ([43]). After year 1, only 12% of patients discontinued due to toxicity. Adjuvant PEG-IFN was approved by the FDA in 2011 (Table 41-7).

Adjuvant Biochemotherapy

Biochemotherapy consists of cisplatin, vinblastine, and dacarbazine chemotherapy combined with interleukin-2 and IFN biotherapy. In the metastatic setting, response rates up to 30% to 60% have been seen in treatment-naïve patients using this regimen ([44, 45]). The S0008 trial was a cooperative intergroup randomized phase III trial comparing the efficacy of three cycles of biochemotherapy, with cycles given every 3 weeks, versus 1 year of HDI in improving RFS and OS in patients with resected stage III melanoma ([46]). With a median follow-up of 7.2 years, biochemotherapy treatment resulted in a significantly prolonged RFS (median, 4.0 vs 1.9 years; $P = .029$) but not OS (median, 9.9 vs 6.7 years; $P = .55$). Biochemotherapy was associated with more grade 4 toxicity, but it was of shorter duration than that seen with HDI. The grade 3 and 4 toxicity combined rates were similar between biochemotherapy and HDI (76% vs 64%, respectively), as were discontinuation rates (15% vs 19%, respectively). Biochemotherapy may be considered based on S0008 for select patients who can tolerate higher grade toxicities for a shorter duration, at centers with experience in managing the toxicities of biochemotherapy, and in patients for whom HDI or 1 year's worth of adjuvant therapy is not appropriate.

Adjuvant Therapy for Mucosal Melanoma

Mucosal melanoma is the only subtype of melanoma with OS data supporting the use of adjuvant systemic therapy. A randomized three-arm phase II trial assigned 189 patients with surgically resected mucosal melanoma to observation versus HDI versus cisplatin 25 mg/m^2 on days 1 to 3 and temozolomide 200 mg/m^2 on days 1 to 5 every 3 weeks for six cycles ([47]). Chemotherapy with cisplatin and temozolomide showed statistically significant improvements in both RFS and OS compared to both HDI and observation. High-dose IFN resulted in improved RFS and OS versus observation as well. Fever and fatigue were more common in the HDI arm, whereas anorexia and nausea/vomiting were more common in the chemotherapy arm. Both HDI and chemotherapy are safe and effective therapies for patients with resected mucosal melanoma.

MANAGEMENT OF METASTATIC DISEASE

Chemotherapy

Dacarbazine is the only chemotherapy agent approved for the treatment of metastatic melanoma (see Table 41-7). Approved in 1975, dacarbazine achieves clinical responses in 5% to 10% of patients. The overwhelming majority of these responses are short-lived, and dacarbazine has never been proven to be superior to another agent in a phase III trial. Temozolomide is an orally available prodrug that is metabolized to the same active intermediate as dacarbazine. Temozolomide was shown to be noninferior to dacarbazine in a phase III trial ([48]). Temozolomide is able to cross the intact blood-brain barrier. However, in a large phase II trial, temozolomide achieved clinical responses in only 7% of patients with previously untreated melanoma brain metastases and in 3% of patients with previous brain-directed treatments ([49]). Fotemustine was shown to achieve a higher response rate than dacarbazine (15.2% vs 6.8%, $P = .04$), and there was a trend for improved OS (median, 7.3 vs 5.6 months; $P = .067$) in a randomized phase III trial. However, its use remains limited ([50]).

In addition to these single agents, a variety of combination chemotherapy regimens have been evaluated in melanoma ([51]). Although these regimens achieve clinical responses in up to 20% to 25% of patients, none have been shown to significantly improve OS versus single-agent chemotherapy, and all are associated with increased toxicity.

Targeted Therapy

Targeted therapies are agents that inhibit the proteins and/or pathways that are activated in tumors by oncogenic events. Targeted therapies demonstrated efficacy in a number of cancers in which critical oncogenes have been identified, including chronic myelogenous leukemia (*BCR-ABL*), breast cancer (*HER2/neu*), and gastrointestinal stromal tumors (*KIT*), among others. The extremely high rate of somatic mutations suggested that such strategies might be effective in melanoma as well.

BRAF Inhibitors

As noted previously, point mutations that cause substitutions at the V600 residue of the BRAF protein (*BRAF*^{V600}) are the most common oncogenic event in cutaneous melanoma. Shortly after the identification of these mutations, several clinical trials of sorafenib were initiated in metastatic melanoma patients. Sorafenib is a small-molecule inhibitor of many kinases, including BRAF. However, sorafenib achieved clinical responses in <5% of metastatic melanoma patients as a single agent, and it failed to improve outcomes when it was combined with paclitaxel and carboplatin in a randomized phase III study ([52, 53]). Analyses of smaller trials support that sorafenib failed to achieve significant inhibition of the RAS-RAF-MEK-ERK signaling pathway at clinically tolerated doses, likely explaining its lack of activity ([54]).

Although the results of sorafenib were disappointing, much more impressive activity has been observed with second-generation BRAF inhibitors. These agents are highly selective for inhibition of BRAF over other kinases, and they have greater affinity for the *BRAF*^{V600} mutant proteins than the wild-type *BRAF* protein. The first such agent to enter into clinical trials was vemurafenib (also known as PLX4032 or RO5185426). After promising early-phase trials, the BRIM-3 trial, a phase III randomized clinical trial, compared vemurafenib versus dacarbazine chemotherapy ([55]). A total of 675 metastatic patients were randomized, and all patients had a *BRAF*^{V600} mutation. This trial was halted at its first interim analysis because vemurafenib resulted in significant improvements in progression-free survival (median, 5.3 vs 1.6 months; HR, 0.26; $P < .001$) and OS (HR, 0.37; $P < .001$). The overall response rates were 48% for vemurafenib and 5% for dacarbazine; the disease control rate for vemurafenib was approximately 90%. Vemurafenib was approved for the treatment of metastatic melanoma patients with a *BRAF*^{V600} mutation in 2011 (Table 41-7).

Dabrafenib was the second mutant-selective BRAF inhibitor to enter into clinical testing. The clinical efficacy of dabrafenib appears to be similar to vemurafenib. In the BREAK-3 phase III trial, 250 metastatic melanoma patients with *BRAF*^{V600} mutations were randomized to treatment with dabrafenib or dacarbazine ([56]). The overall response rate was 50% for dabrafenib and 6% for dacarbazine, and dabrafenib treatment significantly improved progression-free survival (median, 5.1 vs 2.7 months; HR, 0.30; $P < .0001$). In this trial, dabrafenib did not achieve a statistically significant improvement in OS (HR, 0.61). However, in this trial, patients randomized to chemotherapy were allowed to cross over at the time of disease progression to treatment with dabrafenib, whereas the BRIM-3 study did not allow cross-over. Dabrafenib was approved for the treatment of metastatic melanoma patients with a *BRAF*^{V600} mutation in 2013 (Table 41-7).

Both vemurafenib and dabrafenib are well tolerated by most patients. The most common side effects of the mutant BRAF inhibitors are rash, fever, fatigue, and arthralgias ([55, 56]). Up to 25% of patients treated in early-phase clinical trials with vemurafenib, and a slightly lower percentage of patients treated with dabrafenib, developed cutaneous SCCs or keratoacanthomas, which are hyperproliferative skin lesions. Such lesions are generally removed surgically, and the BRAF inhibitors may be resumed safely without dose adjustment after appropriate treatment. Fevers, which occur in up to 30% of patients treated with dabrafenib, are generally controlled with dose interruptions and antipyretics, with treatment resumed safely after fevers resolve. For patients who develop frequent and severe fevers, dose reductions may provide relief, or the fevers can usually be controlled by concurrent treatment with steroids.

A key limitation to the use of vemurafenib and dabrafenib is their restriction to patients with a *BRAF*^{V600} mutation. A total of 10 metastatic melanoma patients without a *BRAF*^{V600} mutation were included in the phase I studies of these agents ([57, 58]). None of those patients responded, and eight patients had disease progression at their initial restaging. Although it is possible that this could be simply due to the aggressive nature of this disease, preclinical testing has demonstrated that the mutant-selective BRAF inhibitors can increase the growth of cancer cells that do not have a *BRAF*^{V600} mutation ([59]). This is due to an unexpected effect of the inhibitors, known as paradoxical activation, which produces increased signaling through the RAS-RAF-MEK-ERK signaling pathway when there is no *BRAF*^{V600} mutation present. As a result, molecular testing for the *BRAF*^{V600} mutation is an absolute prerequisite for any patient in whom vemurafenib or dabrafenib is considered.

MEK Inhibitors

Although almost all metastatic melanoma patients with a *BRAF*^{V600} mutation derive some clinical benefit with BRAF inhibitor treatment, nearly all patients develop resistance. The median progression-free survival of both vemurafenib and dabrafenib is approximately 6 months, and 90% of patients develop resistance within 1 year. Analyses of both patient samples and cell lines with acquired resistance to the BRAF inhibitors have identified a number of resistance mechanisms ([60]). To date, all resistant tumors have retained the *BRAF*^{V600} mutation, and no new mutations in the coding region of the *BRAF* gene have been identified. However, both amplifications and splice variants of the *BRAF*^{V600} mutation have been identified in resistant tumors, as have concurrent activating mutations in *NRAS* and *MEK1/2*. Each of these events reactivates signaling by MEK and downstream components of the RAS-RAF-MEK-ERK signaling pathway. These findings supported the rationale for determining the safety and efficacy of MEK inhibitors in *BRAF*^{V600} mutant melanomas.

Trametinib is a selective and potent inhibitor of MEK1 and MEK2. The safety and efficacy of trametinib were compared to chemotherapy (dacarbazine or paclitaxel) in 322 metastatic melanoma patients with *BRAF*^{V600} mutations in a phase III trial ([61]). Trametinib resulted in improved overall response rate (22% vs 8%), progression-free survival (median, 4.8 vs 1.5 months; HR, 0.45; $P < .001$), and OS (HR, 0.54; $P = .01$). Trametinib is well tolerated, with side effects including rash, diarrhea, edema, and fatigue. Ocular events are a relatively rare but clinically important side effect of trametinib, including blurred vision, retinal pigment epithelium detachment, and retinal vein occlusion. Trametinib can also cause reversible cardiomyopathy. Single-agent trametinib was approved for the treatment of metastatic melanoma patients with a *BRAF*^{V600} mutation in 2013 (Table 41-7). Notably, trametinib was approved for patients who had not previously been treated with a selective BRAF inhibitor, because it fails to achieve clinical benefit in pretreated patients ([62]). Although no head-to-head clinical trials have compared single-agent trametinib to single-agent BRAF inhibitor therapy, it appears that the BRAF inhibitors have higher response rates and longer progression-free survival ([55, 61]). Trametinib is an option for patients who cannot tolerate BRAF inhibitors.

Much more compelling data supports the use of MEK inhibitors in combination with BRAF inhibitors in *BRAF*^{V600} mutant melanoma patients. Phase I testing of dabrafenib and trametinib demonstrated that they could be combined safely at the maximally tolerated dose of each single agent ([63]). In fact, the combination had a much lower rate of cutaneous SCCs (7% vs 19%) and hyperkeratosis (9% vs 30%) than was observed with single-agent dabrafenib. This protective effect appears to be due to MEK inhibitor–induced blockade of dabrafenib's paradoxical activation of the RAS-RAF-MEK-ERK pathway in keratinocytes ([64]). The combination does have a higher rate of pyrexia (71%) than is observed with dabrafenib alone (26%). In a randomized phase II trial of 162 metastatic melanoma patients with *BRAF*^{V600} mutations who were treated with dabrafenib alone or in combination with trametinib, the combination achieved a significant improvement in progression-free survival (median, 9.4 vs 5.8 months; HR, 0.39; $P < .001$), and none of the patients treated with the combination of dabrafenib and trametinib had disease progression as their best response (76% overall response rate). Combined treatment with dabrafenib and trametinib was approved for metastatic melanoma patients with a *BRAF*^{V600} mutation in 2014 (Table 41-7). Subsequent to this approval, phase III trials demonstrated that dabrafenib and trametinib produce significant improvements in progression-free survival versus single-agent dabrafenib and versus single-agent vemurafenib ([65, 66]). Combined treatment with vemurafenib and cobimetinib, another MEK1/2 inhibitor, has also demonstrated superiority to single-agent vemurafenib treatment in a phase III trial (see Table 41-7) ([67]). Although the clinical results with combined BRAF and MEK inhibition are impressive in patients who are BRAF inhibitor naïve, these combination regimens achieve clinical responses in only approximately 15% of patients who have already developed resistance to single-agent BRAF inhibitors ([68, 69]).

MEK inhibitors have also been tested in selected melanoma patients without *BRAF*^{V600} mutations. Treatment with MEK162, also known as binimetinib, achieved clinical responses in 20% of metastatic melanoma patients with activating *NRAS* mutations in a phase II trial, and randomized clinical trials versus chemotherapy in this patient population are under way ([70]). Preclinical studies have also identified candidate combinatorial strategies with MEK inhibitors to achieve increased efficacy in *NRAS*-mutant melanomas, a number of which are in early-phase clinical trials ([71]). Both preclinical studies and the clinical outcomes of a small number of patients enrolled in early-phase clinical trials also support that MEK inhibitors may be effective for patients with *BRAF* mutations that affect sites other than V600 ([72]). Prospective clinical trials with MEK inhibitors in this population are ongoing.

KIT Inhibitors

Three different phase II clinical trials of the KIT inhibitor imatinib, which is approved for the treatment of gastrointestinal stromal tumor (GIST), in metastatic melanoma patients reported a combined clinical response rate of approximately 1% ([21]). However, these trials were performed without any molecular selection criteria, because they predated the discovery of frequent *KIT* mutations in mucosal, acral, and sun-damaged cutaneous melanomas ([20]). Phase II studies of imatinib in metastatic melanoma patients with *KIT* mutations or amplifications have demonstrated much more promising results than were observed in unselected patients ([73-75]). The response rates reported in these trials range from 15% to 30%, with subgroup analyses demonstrating response rates of up to 50% in patients with the most common recurrent mutations detected in melanomas. Although these results are a marked improvement compared to those observed in unselected patients, the response rates are not as high as those in GIST patients with *KIT* mutations treated with the same inhibitors. Studies are ongoing to identify the *KIT*-mutant melanoma patients who are most likely to benefit from KIT inhibitors and combinatorial strategies that are more effective.

Immunotherapy

Melanoma is a highly immunogenic tumor. In the last 20 years, immunotherapeutic approaches such as cytokine therapy, cancer vaccines, immune checkpoint inhibition, and adoptive T-cell transfer have been extensively studied in metastatic melanoma. In contrast to direct cytotoxic chemotherapy, immunotherapy aims to control cancer by stimulating the patient's own immune systems to attack it. Over time, it has been demonstrated that effective immunotherapies can achieve remarkably durable disease control and survival in melanoma, even in patients with very advanced disease. Such results appear to be achievable in an increasing number of patients as the key regulators of the antitumor immune response are identified, understood, and targeted.

Interleukin-2

Interleukin-2 (IL-2) is a growth factor normally secreted by CD4 helper cells that can activate effector CD8 T cells and natural killer (NK) cells. In nonrandomized studies, high-dose IL-2 (HD IL-2) therapy (600,000-720,000 IU/kg intravenously every 8 hours for up to a maximum of 14 doses per cycle for two cycles) achieved clinical responses in 16% of patients, including approximately 6% of patients who had complete responses ([76]). Long-term follow-up showed that the majority of complete responders remained disease free for more than 10 years. Although it was never proven superior to another therapy in a randomized trial, HD IL-2 therapy was approved for the treatment of metastatic melanoma patients in 1998 based on this potential for durable disease control (see Table 41-7) ([77]). Retrospective analyses demonstrated that higher response rates may be observed in patients with only cutaneous and/or subcutaneous metastases, whereas patients with brain metastases have very poor outcomes with this treatment ([78]). High-dose IL-2 therapy is complicated by capillary leak syndrome that can cause hypotension, pulmonary edema, and renal failure; hepatic, gastrointestinal, endocrine, and cutaneous toxicities; arrhythmias; and psychiatric disturbances. Although these toxicities generally resolve quickly (within days) after stopping HD IL-2 therapy, the treatment-related mortality for HD IL-2 is 1% to 2%. Thus, safe administration requires adequate prescreening of patients to ensure adequate cardiac and pulmonary function, as well as significant training and experience of the health care team.

Combinations of IL-2 with other therapeutic agents have been investigated. A randomized multicenter phase III trial of HD IL-2 with or without gp100 cancer vaccine in 185 metastatic melanoma patients demonstrated that the addition of gp100 significantly improved overall response rate (16% vs 6%) and progression-free survival (median, 2.2 vs 1.6 months, $P = .008$) ([79]). Patient treated with combination therapy also had a trend for improved OS, but this did not reach statistical significance (17.8 vs 11.1 months, $P = .06$).

Ipilimumab (Anti–Cytotoxic T Lymphocyte-Associated Antigen 4 Antibody)

Cytotoxic T lymphocyte-associated antigen 4 (CTLA4) is an inhibitory immune checkpoint molecule that is expressed on the surface of activated T cells and regulatory T cells. Ipilimumab is a fully human immunoglobulin (Ig) G1 anti-CTLA4 monoclonal antibody that binds to the T cells and enhances antitumor immunity. Two randomized phase III studies have demonstrated that ipilimumab improves OS in metastatic melanoma patients. In the first phase III study, previously treated patients with advanced melanoma were randomized to receive gp100 vaccine, ipilimumab, or ipilimumab with gp100 vaccine ([80]). Ipilimumab was given at 3 mg/kg every 3 weeks for a total of four treatments. The response rate was only 10.9% for ipilimumab and only 5.7% for ipilimumab with gp100. However, both regimens resulted in improved progression-free survival and OS compared to gp100 vaccine alone. Patient had a median survival of 10.0 months with single-agent ipilimumab (HR, 0.68; $P < .001$ vs gp100) and 10.1 months with ipilimumab plus gp100 (HR, 0.66; $P = .003$), in comparison to 6.4 months with gp100. Because treatment with ipilimumab alone demonstrated greater progression-free survival (HR, 0.64 vs gp100) than treatment with ipilimumab with gp100 (HR, 0.81), there was concern that gp100 could be having a detrimental effect on patient outcomes, as had been observed previously in other vaccine trials in melanoma ([51]). A subsequent phase III trial randomized 502 treatment-naïve metastatic melanoma patients to treatment with dacarbazine alone or in combination with ipilimumab ([81]). Ipilimumab was dosed at 10 mg/kg for four doses followed by maintenance therapy every 12 weeks. Both OS (median, 11.2 vs 9.1 months; HR, 0.72; $P < .001$) and progression-free survival (HR, 0.76; $P = .006$) were significantly improved in the patients who received ipilimumab. The overall response rate was 15.2% with ipilimumab plus dacarbazine and 10.3% with dacarbazine alone. Ipilimumab (3 mg/kg every 3 weeks for four doses) was subsequently approved for the treatment of metastatic melanoma patients in 2011 (see Table 41-7). Recently, long-term follow-up of almost 5,000 patients treated on clinical trials with ipilimumab demonstrated that the 3-year OS rate was 22% for all patients in the cohort (26% for treatment-naïve patients and 20% for previously treated patients), with Kaplan-Meier analysis suggesting that very few patients died from melanoma after this time point ([82]).

As noted earlier, the clinical response rate of ipilimumab is modest. In addition, the clinical responses seen with ipilimumab are often significantly delayed and can even develop after an initial increase in tumor size. In recognition of this potential for delayed but significant clinical benefit, immune-related response criteria (irRC) were developed to assess clinical responses in patients treated with immunotherapy ([83]). In irRC, new lesions do not necessarily define progression, and progressive disease must be confirmed in two consecutive observations at least 4 weeks apart. In addition to the potential for delayed responses, it also appears that re-initiation of ipilimumab can benefit some patients who experience disease progression after this therapy. In a study of 31 patients with initial clinical response or stable disease for at least 3 months with initial ipilimumab treatment that subsequently progressed, investigators demonstrated that re-induction of ipilimumab (3 mg/kg for four doses) led to clinical responses in up to 38% of patients and disease control in up to 75% ([84]). Thus, re-induction of ipilimumab is a reasonable therapeutic option for patients with disease progression who had disease control lasting at least 3 months from previous ipilimumab treatment. Ipilimumab can also provide clinical benefit in appropriately selected patients with brain metastases. A phase II trial in 72 patients with active brain metastases demonstrated that ipilimumab achieved disease control in up to 24% of patients with small, asymptomatic brain tumors that did not require steroids ([85]). However, disease control was only achieved in 5% of patients with tumors that required steroids to controls symptoms and/or cerebral edema.

Immune-related adverse effects (irAEs) are frequently seen with ipilimumab. These effects include hypophysitis, rash, colitis, and hepatitis. Approximately 60% of patients treated with ipilimumab have irAEs, including up to 20% with grade 3 or 4 toxicities. Because high-grade irAEs can be life threatening, particularly autoimmune colitis leading to bowel perforation, early recognition of irAEs is critical to the safe administration of ipilimumab. Treatment of irAEs includes symptomatic and supportive care, as well as high-dose systemic steroids (1-2 mg/kg/d of prednisone or equivalent) depending on the severity of irAEs. Ipilimumab retreatment can be considered in patients with grade 1 or 2 irAEs once symptoms resolve. However, any grade 3 or 4 irAEs other than grade 3 skin toxicity are contraindications to further ipilimumab treatment. Interestingly, systemic steroid use to control severe irAEs does not appear to affect tumor response to ipilimumab ([86]).

Anti–Programmed Death 1 Protein Antibodies

The programmed death 1 protein (PD-1) is another important immune checkpoint receptor expressed on the surface of activated T cells. PD-1 has two known ligands, PD-L1 (B7-H1) and PD-L2 (B7-DC); PD-L1 is broadly expressed on immune and nonhematopoietic cells including tumor cells, and the expression on tumor cells can be upregulated by IFN, which is predominantly produced by T cells. The ligation of PD-1 and PD-L1 inhibits T-cell proliferation and activation and induces apoptosis of antigen-specific T cells to prevent collateral tissue damage and autoimmune disease. The PD-1/PD-L1 pathway is hijacked by tumor cells to suppress antitumor immunity. Therefore, blocking the interaction of PD-1 and PD-L1 has been studied as a therapeutic approach for cancers.

Pembrolizumab

Pembrolizumab, a humanized anti–PD-1 IgG4 monoclonal antibody, was approved by the FDA in 2014 for metastatic melanoma patients with disease progression following ipilimumab (and BRAF inhibitor therapy if *BRAF*^{V600} mutation positive) (see Table 41-7). In a phase I study, 135 patients with advanced melanoma received pembrolizumab at a dose of 10 mg/kg every 2 or 3 weeks or 2 mg/kg every 3 weeks ([87]). The objective response rate was 38% across all dose cohorts, with the highest confirmed response of 52% in in the 10 mg/kg every 2 weeks cohort, regardless of previous ipilimumab treatment. In patients with ipilimumab-refractory advanced melanoma, pembrolizumab has demonstrated a 26% clinical response rate ([88]). Notably, most clinical responses to pembrolizumab were ongoing at the time of those reports, and the median OS had yet to be reached. More recently, a randomized clinical phase III clinical trial demonstrated that pembrolizumab (2 mg/kg dosed either every 2 or 3 weeks for up to 2 years) achieved significant improvements in response rate (33% for both dosing regimens vs 12%, $P < .001$), progression-free survival (HR, 0.58; $P < .001$ for both dosing regimens), and OS (HR, 0.63; $P < .0005$ for every-2-week dosing; HR, 0.69; $P = .0036$) versus treatment with ipilimumab (3 mg/kg every 3 weeks for four cycles) ([89]).

In contrast to ipilimumab, less than 5% of patients treated with pembrolizumab experienced grade 3 or 4 irAEs, and only approximately 10% experience grade 3 or 4 toxicity of any kind ([89]). Fatigue (~20%), rash (~15%), pruritus (~15%), diarrhea (~15%), and hypothyroidism (~10%) are the most frequent toxicities observed, and they are generally not severe. While rare with ipilimumab, treatment-related pneumonitis has been reported in 1% to 4% of the patients treated with pembrolizumab, usually grade 1 or 2.

Nivolumab

Nivolumab is another human anti–PD-1 IgG4 monoclonal antibody. In a phase I study, 296 previously treated patients with advanced solid cancers received nivolumab at a dose of 0.1 to 10 mg/kg every 2 weeks for up to 2 years ([90]). Objective responses were observed in 28% of 96 evaluable melanoma patients, and the responses were durable, lasting at least 1 year in 13 of 18 patients treated for 1 year or more. The most common adverse events were fatigue, decreased appetite, diarrhea, nausea, rash, and pruritus. Grade 3 or 4 drug-related adverse events occurred in 14% of patients. Pneumonitis developed in nine patients (3%) and was the cause of drug-related death in three patients (1%). Nivolumab was approved in 2014 for the treatment of metastatic melanoma patients previously treated with ipilimumab (and a BRAF inhibitor for patients with a *BRAF*^{V600} mutation) (see Table 41-7). Nivolumab has also been shown to be more effective than chemotherapy in treatment-naïve patients. In a randomized phase III study of 418 previously untreated metastatic melanoma patients, the 1-year OS rate was 72.9% with nivolumab and 42.1% with dacarbazine (HR, 0.42; $P < .001$) ([91]). The response rates with nivolumab and dacarbazine were 40% and 14%, respectively, and the median progression-free survival times were 5.1 and 2.2 months, respectively (HR, 0.43; $P < .001$). Grade 3 or 4 treatment-related adverse events were also less common with nivolumab (11.7%) than with dacarbazine (17.6%).

Preclinical studies demonstrated that combined blockade of both CTLA4 and PD-1 was more effective than either alone ([92]). This strategy is now being evaluated in patients. A phase I study of concurrent ipilimumab and nivolumab found that the maximum-tolerated dose of the concurrent administration of both agents was 3 mg/kg of ipilimumab and 1 mg/kg of nivolumab ([93]). In the phase I trial, the overall response rate was 40%. Impressively, most of the responding patients experienced >80% tumor regression, and the median OS in the trial was 39.7 months. Although the regimen was very active, 53% of patients developed grade 3 or 4 adverse events, and 21% of patients discontinued therapy due to treatment-related toxicities. A subsequent phase III clinical trial comparing outcomes with ipilimumab (3 mg/kg every 3 weeks for four doses) with or without nivolumab (1 mg/kg every 3 weeks for four doses, then 3 mg/kg every 2 weeks for up to 2 years) showed that the combination resulted in higher response rates (61% vs 11%, $P < .001$), with 22% of patients achieving complete responses, and improved progression-free survival (HR, 0.40; $P < .001$) ([94]). The combination was more toxic, with 54% of patients experiencing grade 3 or 4 toxicities (24% with single-agent ipilimumab). A randomized, three-arm, phase III study comparing single-agent nivolumab, single-agent ipilimumab, and concurrent nivolumab with ipilimumab showed similar outcomes with the combination therapy, with statistically superior outcomes to treatment with ipilimumab. Concurrent treatment with ipilimumab and nivolumab for *BRAF*^{V600} wild-type, unresectable or metastatic melanoma was approved by the FDA in 2015 ([94a]).

Tumor-Infiltrating Lymphocytes

Adoptive cell transfer with autologous ex vivo–expanded tumor-infiltrating lymphocytes (TILs) is a promising therapy that builds on the initial development of HD IL-2. Tumor-infiltrating lymphocytes, which are isolated from a surgically resected tumor, are expanded with IL-2 ex vivo. If a sufficient number of TILs are generated in this process, then the patient is eligible to be infused with these TIL cells as therapy. Prior to this infusion, patients undergo lymphodepletion, and then after the TIL infusion, patients receive HD IL-2. There are a number of potential benefits of the lymphodepletion, including the reduction or elimination of immune suppressive lymphocytes (ie, regulatory T cells), increased availability of homeostatic cytokines such as IL-7 and IL-15 that promote the expansion and activation of TILs ([95, 96]), and stimulation of toll-like receptor signaling ([97]). In addition, the cytoreductive nature of lymphodepletion also results in the TILs having no competition for the IL-2 that is administered. In sum, these features promote the likelihood that the IL-2 treatment will support the growth and activity of T cells that can recognize and attack melanoma metastases. Preclinical and clinical studies support that more aggressive lymphodepletion regimens may result in improved outcomes with TIL treatment ([96, 98]).

For example, a retrospective analysis of TIL trials reported that patients who received 12 Gy or 2 Gy of total-body irradiation with lymphodepleting chemotherapy prior to TIL infusion had higher clinical response rates than patients who received lymphodepleting chemotherapy alone (72% vs 52% vs 49%) ([99]). However, to date, no randomized trial has compared the safety and benefits of different conditioning regimens.

Overall, the clinical response rate of adoptive cell transfer with lymphodepletion and IL-2 is 40% to 50%. Many of these responses are durable, and 5-year OS rates are approximately 30% ([99]). However, adoptive cell transfer is only available for patients who are capable of tolerating the significant toxicities caused by lymphodepletion and HD IL-2. In addition, a significant proportion of patients (30% to 40%) fail to have sufficient TIL expansion from their tumor harvests to allow treatment, and it is currently unknown if successful TIL growth portends a better disease biology and/or improved outcomes with other therapies as well. In addition to planning randomized trials, multiple efforts are under way using genetically modified TILs, including with recombinant T-cell receptors that recognize tumor antigens or expressing chimeric antigen receptors fused to costimulatory molecules. Trials are also under way and planned to test the safety and efficacy of combining TIL with checkpoint inhibitors.

Biochemotherapy

Biochemotherapy refers to regimens that combine cytotoxic chemotherapy with immunotherapy. Although a variety of regimens exist, the chemotherapy background generally consists of cisplatin, vinblastine, and dacarbazine, wherea the immunotherapy component includes IFN α-2b and IL-2 (given as an infusion instead of boluses). Results of both randomized and nonrandomized clinical trials have demonstrated that biochemotherapy regimens can achieve response rates in 30% to 50% of patients, but at the cost of significantly increased toxicity versus either chemotherapy or immunotherapy alone. Retrospective analyses support that a subset of patients treated with biochemotherapy achieve long-term survival (ie, 15% to 17% OS at 5 and 10 years) ([100]). However, multiple prospective randomized clinical trials failed to demonstrate significant improvements in survival compared to chemotherapy alone ([51]). Due to its high response rate and potential for long-term survival, biochemotherapy can be considered for selected patients, particularly patients without *BRAF*^{V600} mutations with rapidly progressive or symptomatic disease after progression on other effective therapies. Similar to HD IL-2 therapy, careful patient selection and an experienced health care team are necessary for safe administration of biochemotherapy.

REFERENCES

1. Siegel R, Ma J, Zou Z, Jemal A. Cancer statistics, 2014. *CA Cancer J Clin*. 2014;64(1):9-29.
2. SEER Cancer Statistics Review, 1975-2011. Bethesda, MD: National Cancer Institute, 2014. Available at: http://seer.cancer.gov/csr/1975_2011/. Accessed October 22, 2015.
3. Jemal A, Saraiya M, Patel P, et al. Recent trends in cutaneous melanoma incidence and death rates in the United States, 1992-2006. *J Am Acad Dermatol*. 2011;65(5, Suppl 1):S17-S25.e13.
4. Kanavy HE, Gerstenblith MR. Ultraviolet radiation and melanoma. *Semin Cutan Med Surg*. 2011;30(4):222-228.
5. Berger MF, Hodis E, Heffernan TP, et al. Melanoma genome sequencing reveals frequent PREX2 mutations. *Nature*. 2012;485(7399):502-506.
6. Olsen CM, Carroll HJ, Whiteman DC. Estimating the attributable fraction for melanoma: a meta-analysis of pigmentary characteristics and freckling. *Int J Cancer*. 2010;127(10):2430-2445.
7. Lynch HT, Fusaro RM, Lynch JF, Brand R. Pancreatic cancer and the FAMMM syndrome. *Fam Cancer*. 2008;7(1):103-112.
8. Vourc'h-Jourdain M, Martin L, Barbarot S, aRED. Large congenital melanocytic nevi: therapeutic management and melanoma risk: a systematic review. *J Am Acad Dermatol*. 2013;68(3):493-498 e491-414.
9. Curtin JA, Fridlyand J, Kageshita T, et al. Distinct sets of genetic alterations in melanoma. *N Engl J Med*. 2005;353(20):2135-2147.
10. Pleasance ED, Cheetham RK, Stephens PJ, et al. A comprehensive catalogue of somatic mutations from a human cancer genome. *Nature*. 2010;463(7278):191-196.
11. Hodis E, Watson Ian R, Kryukov Gregory V, et al. A landscape of driver mutations in melanoma. *Cell*. 2012;150(2):251-263.
12. Davies H, Bignell GR, Cox C, et al. Mutations of the BRAF gene in human cancer. *Nature*. 2002;417(6892):949-954.
13. Pollock PM, Harper UL, Hansen KS, et al. High frequency of BRAF mutations in nevi. *Nat Genet*. 2003;33(1):19-20.
14. Wan PTC, Garnett MJ, Roe SM, et al. Mechanism of activation of the RAF-ERK signaling pathway by oncogenic mutations of B-RAF. *Cell*. 2004;116(6):855-867.
15. Botton T, Yeh I, Nelson T, et al. Recurrent BRAF kinase fusions in melanocytic tumors offer an opportunity for targeted therapy. *Pigment Cell Melanoma Res*. 2013;26(6):845-851.
16. Siroy AE, Boland GM, Milton DR, et al. Beyond BRAFV600: clinical mutation panel testing by next-generation sequencing in advanced melanoma. *J Invest Dermatol*. 2015;135(2):508-515.
17. Dankort D, Curley DP, Cartlidge RA, et al. Braf(V600E) cooperates with Pten loss to induce metastatic melanoma. *Nat Genet*. 2009;41(5):544-552.
18. Wolfel T, Hauer M, Schneider J, et al. A p16INK4a-insensitive CDK4 mutant targeted by cytolytic T lymphocytes in a human melanoma. *Science*. 1995;269(5228):1281-1284.
19. Sauter ER, Yeo U-C, von Stemm A, et al. Cyclin D1 is a candidate oncogene in cutaneous melanoma. *Cancer Res*. 2002;62(11):3200-3206.
20. Curtin JA, Busam K, Pinkel D, Bastian BC. Somatic activation of KIT in distinct subtypes of melanoma. *J Clin Oncol*. 2006;24(26):4340-4346.
21. Woodman SE, Davies MA. Targeting KIT in melanoma: a paradigm of molecular medicine and targeted therapeutics. *Biochem Pharmacol*. 2010;80(5):568-574.
22. Van Raamsdonk CD, Griewank KG, Crosby MB, et al. Mutations in GNA11 in uveal melanoma. *N Engl J Med*. 2010;363(23):2191-2199.
23. Edge SB, Byrd DR, Compton CC. *Melanoma of the Skin*. In American Joint Committee on Cancer Staging Manual (Seventh edition). New York: Springer; 2009.
24. Balch CM, Gershenwald JE, Soong SJ, et al. Final version of 2009 AJCC melanoma staging and classification. *J Clin Oncol*.

CHAPTER 41

2009;27(36):6199-6206.
25. Thomas JM, Newton-Bishop J, A'Hern R, et al. Excision margins in high-risk malignant melanoma. *N Engl J Med.* 2004;350(8):757-766.
26. Gershenwald JE, Ross MI. Sentinel-lymph-node biopsy for cutaneous melanoma. *N Engl J Med.* 2011;364(18):1738-1745.
27. Wong SL, Balch CM, Hurley P, et al. Sentinel lymph node biopsy for melanoma: American Society of Clinical Oncology and Society of Surgical Oncology joint clinical practice guideline. *J Clin Oncol.* 2012;30(23):2912-2918.
28. Gershenwald JE, Coit DG, Sondak VK, Thompson JF. The challenge of defining guidelines for sentinel lymph node biopsy in patients with thin primary cutaneous melanomas. *Ann Surg Oncol.* 2012;19(11):3301-3303.
29. Morton DL, Wen D-R, Wong JH, et al. Technical details of intraoperative lymphatic mapping for early stage melanoma. *Arch Surg.* 1992;127(4):392-399.
30. Gershenwald JE, Thompson W, Mansfield PF, et al. Multi-institutional melanoma lymphatic mapping experience: the prognostic value of sentinel lymph node status in 612 stage I or II melanoma patients. *J Clin Oncol.* 1999;17(3):976-983.
31. Morton DL, Thompson JF, Cochran AJ, et al. Final trial report of sentinel-node biopsy versus nodal observation in melanoma. *N Engl J Med.* 2014;370(7):599-609.
32. Ballo MT, Ang KK. Radiotherapy for cutaneous malignant melanoma: rationale and indications. *Oncology (Williston Park).* 2004;18(1):99-107; discussion 107-110, 113-104.
33. Guadagnolo BA, Prieto V, Weber R, Ross MI, Zagars GK. The role of adjuvant radiotherapy in the local management of desmoplastic melanoma. *Cancer.* 2014;120(9):1361-1368.
34. Agrawal S, Kane JM, Guadagnolo BA, Kraybill WG, Ballo MT. The benefits of adjuvant radiation therapy after therapeutic lymphadenectomy for clinically advanced, high-risk, lymph node-metastatic melanoma. *Cancer.* 2009;115(24):5836-5844.
35. Burmeister BH, Henderson MA, Ainslie J, et al. Adjuvant radiotherapy versus observation alone for patients at risk of lymph-node field relapse after therapeutic lymphadenectomy for melanoma: a randomised trial. *Lancet Oncol.* 2012;13(6):589-597.
36. Guadagnolo BA, Zagars GK. Adjuvant radiation therapy for high-risk nodal metastases from cutaneous melanoma. *Lancet Oncol.* 2009;10(4):409-416.
37. Kingham TP, Panageas KS, Ariyan CE, Busam KJ, Brady MS, Coit DG. Outcome of patients with a positive sentinel lymph node who do not undergo completion lymphadenectomy. *Ann Surg Oncol.* 2010;17(2):514-520.
38. Kirkwood J, Strawderman M, Ernstoff M, Smith T, Borden E, Blum R. Interferon alfa-2b adjuvant therapy of high-risk resected cutaneous melanoma: the Eastern Cooperative Oncology Group Trial EST 1684. *J Clin Oncol.* 1996;14(1):7-17.
39. Kirkwood JM, Manola J, Ibrahim J, Sondak V, Ernstoff MS, Rao U. A pooled analysis of Eastern Cooperative Oncology Group and Intergroup Trials of adjuvant high-dose interferon for melanoma. *Clin Cancer Res.* 2004;10(5):1670-1677.
40. Eggermont AM, Suciu S, Santinami M, et al. Adjuvant therapy with pegylated interferon alfa-2b versus observation alone in resected stage III melanoma: final results of EORTC 18991, a randomised phase III trial. *Lancet.* 2008;372(9633):117-126.
41. Eggermont AM, Suciu S, Testori A, et al. Long-term results of the randomized phase III trial EORTC 18991 of adjuvant therapy with pegylated interferon alfa-2b versus observation in resected stage III melanoma. *J Clin Oncol.* 2012;30(31):3810-3818.
42. Eggermont AM, Suciu S, Testori A, et al. Ulceration and stage are predictive of interferon efficacy in melanoma: results of the phase III adjuvant trials EORTC 18952 and EORTC 18991. *Eur J Cancer.* 2012;48(2):218-225.
43. Eggermont AM, Suciu S, MacKie R, et al. Post-surgery adjuvant therapy with intermediate doses of interferon alfa 2b versus observation in patients with stage IIb/III melanoma (EORTC 18952): randomised controlled trial. *Lancet.* 2005;366(9492):1189-1196.
44. Legha SS, Ring S, Eton O, et al. Development of a biochemotherapy regimen with concurrent administration of cisplatin, vinblastine, dacarbazine, interferon alfa, and interleukin-2 for patients with metastatic melanoma. *J Clin Oncol.* 1998;16(5):1752-1759.
45. Kim KB, Eton O, East MJ, et al. Pilot study of high-dose, concurrent biochemotherapy for advanced melanoma. *Cancer.* 2004;101(3):596-603.
46. Flaherty LE, Othus M, Atkins MB, et al. Southwest Oncology Group S0008: a phase III trial of high-dose interferon alfa-2b versus cisplatin, vinblastine, and dacarbazine, plus interleukin-2 and interferon in patients with high-risk melanoma—an intergroup study of Cancer and Leukemia Group B, Children's Oncology Group, Eastern Cooperative Oncology Group, and Southwest Oncology Group. *J Clin Oncol.* 2014;32(33):3771-3778.
47. Lian B, Si L, Cui C, et al. Phase II randomized trial comparing high-dose IFN-alpha2b with temozolomide plus cisplatin as systemic adjuvant therapy for resected mucosal melanoma. *Clin Cancer Res.* 2013;19(16):4488-4498.
48. Middleton MR, Grob JJ, Aaronson N, et al. Randomized phase III study of temozolomide versus dacarbazine in the treatment of patients with advanced metastatic malignant melanoma. *J Clin Oncol.* 2000;18(1):158-166.
49. Agarwala SS, Kirkwood JM, Gore M, et al. Temozolomide for the treatment of brain metastases associated with metastatic melanoma: a phase II study. *J Clin Oncol.* 2004;22(11):2101-2107.
50. Avril MF, Aamdal S, Grob JJ, et al. Fotemustine compared with dacarbazine in patients with disseminated malignant melanoma: a phase III study. *J Clin Oncol.* 2004;22(6):1118-1125.
51. Garbe C, Eigentler TK, Keilholz U, Hauschild A, Kirkwood JM. Systematic review of medical treatment in melanoma: current status and future prospects. *Oncologist.* 2011;16(1):5-24.
52. Eisen T, Ahmad T, Flaherty KT, et al. Sorafenib in advanced melanoma: a phase II randomised discontinuation trial analysis. *Br J Cancer.* 2006;95(5):581-586.
53. Flaherty KT, Lee SJ, Zhao F, et al. Phase III trial of carboplatin and paclitaxel with or without sorafenib in metastatic melanoma. *J Clin Oncol.* 2013;31(3):373-379.
54. Davies MA, Fox PS, Papadopoulos NE, et al. Phase I study of the combination of sorafenib and temsirolimus in patients with metastatic melanoma. *Clin Cancer Res.* 2012;18(4):1120-1128.
55. Chapman PB, Hauschild A, Robert C, et al. Improved survival with vemurafenib in melanoma with BRAF V600E mutation. *N Engl J Med.* 2011;364(26):2507-2516.
56. Hauschild A, Grob JJ, Demidov LV, et al. Dabrafenib in BRAF-mutated metastatic melanoma: a multicentre, open-label, phase 3 randomised controlled trial. *Lancet.* 2012;380(9839):358-365.
57. Flaherty KT, Puzanov I, Kim KB, et al. Inhibition of mutated, activated BRAF in metastatic melanoma. *N Engl J Med.* 2010;363(9):809-819.
58. Kefford RF, Arkenau H, Brown MP, et al. Phase I/II study of GSK2118436, a selective inhibitor of oncogenic mutant BRAF kinase, in patients with metastatic melanoma and other solid tumors. *J Clin Oncol.* 2010;28(15s):8503.
59. Hatzivassiliou G, Song K, Yen I, et al. RAF inhibitors prime wild-type RAF to activate the MAPK pathway and enhance growth. *Nature.* 2010;464(7287):431-435.
60. Bucheit AD, Davies MA. Emerging insights into resistance to BRAF inhibitors in melanoma. *Biochem Pharmacol.* 2014;87(3):381-389.
61. Flaherty KT, Robert C, Hersey P, et al. Improved survival with MEK inhibition in BRAF-mutated melanoma. *N Engl J Med.* 2012;367(2):107-114.
62. Kim KB, Kefford R, Pavlick AC, et al. Phase II study of the MEK1/MEK2 inhibitor trametinib in patients with metastatic

BRAF-mutant cutaneous melanoma previously treated with or without a BRAF inhibitor. *J Clin Oncol.* 2013;31(4):482-489.

63. Flaherty KT, Infante JR, Daud A, et al. Combined BRAF and MEK inhibition in melanoma with BRAF V600 mutations. *N Engl J Med.* 2012;367(18):1694-1703.
64. Su F, Viros A, Milagre C, et al. RAS mutations in cutaneous squamous-cell carcinomas in patients treated with BRAF inhibitors. *N Engl J Med.* 2012;366(3):207-215.
65. Long GV, Stroyakovskiy D, Gogas H, et al. Combined BRAF and MEK inhibition versus BRAF inhibition alone in melanoma. *N Engl J Med.* 2014;371(20):1877-1888.
66. Robert C, Karaszewska B, Schachter J, et al. Improved overall survival in melanoma with combined dabrafenib and trametinib. *N Engl J Med.* 2015;372(1):30-39.
67. Larkin J, Ascierto PA, Dréno B, et al. Combined vemurafenib and cobimetinib in BRAF-mutated melanoma. *N Engl J Med.* 2014;371(20):1867-1876.
68. Ribas A, Gonzalez R, Pavlick A, et al. Combination of vemurafenib and cobimetinib in patients with advanced BRAF(V600)-mutated melanoma: a phase 1b study. *Lancet Oncol.* 2014;15(9):954-965.
69. Johnson DB, Flaherty KT, Weber JS, et al. Combined BRAF (dabrafenib) and MEK inhibition (trametinib) in patients with BRAFV600-mutant melanoma experiencing progression with single-agent BRAF inhibitor. *J Clin Oncol.* 2014;32(33):3697-3704.
70. Ascierto PA, Schadendorf D, Berking C, et al. MEK162 for patients with advanced melanoma harbouring NRAS or Val600 BRAF mutations: a non-randomised, open-label phase 2 study. *Lancet Oncol.* 2013;14(3):249-256.
71. Kwong LN, Davies MA. Targeted therapy for melanoma: rational combinatorial approaches. *Oncogene.* 2014;33(1):1-9.
72. Dahlman KB, Xia J, Hutchinson K, et al. BRAF(L597) mutations in melanoma are associated with sensitivity to MEK inhibitors. *Cancer Discov.* 2012;2(9):791-797.
73. Carvajal RD, Antonescu CR, Wolchok JD, et al. KIT as a therapeutic target in metastatic melanoma. *JAMA.* 2011;305(22):2327-2334.
74. Guo J, Si L, Kong Y, et al. Phase II, open-label, single-arm trial of imatinib mesylate in patients with metastatic melanoma harboring c-Kit mutation or amplification. *J Clin Oncol.* 2011;29(21):2904-2909.
75. Hodi FS, Corless CL, Giobbie-Hurder A, et al. Imatinib for melanomas harboring mutationally activated or amplified KIT arising on mucosal, acral, and chronically sun-damaged skin. *J Clin Oncol.* 2013;31(26):3182-3190.
76. Atkins MB, Lotze MT, Dutcher JP, et al. High-dose recombinant interleukin 2 therapy for patients with metastatic melanoma: analysis of 270 patients treated between 1985 and 1993. *J Clin Oncol.* 1999;17(7):2105-2116.
77. Rosenberg SA. IL-2: the first effective immunotherapy for human cancer. *J Immunol.* 2014;192(12):5451-5458.
78. Phan GQ, Attia P, Steinberg SM, White DE, Rosenberg SA. Factors associated with response to high-dose interleukin-2 in patients with metastatic melanoma. *J Clin Oncol.* 2001;19(15):3477-3482.
79. Schwartzentruber DJ, Lawson DH, Richards JM, et al. gp100 peptide vaccine and interleukin-2 in patients with advanced melanoma. *N Engl J Med.* 2011;364(22):2119-2127.
80. Hodi FS, O'Day SJ, McDermott DF, et al. Improved survival with ipilimumab in patients with metastatic melanoma. *N Engl J Med.* 2010;363(8):711-723.
81. Robert C, Thomas L, Bondarenko I, et al. Ipilimumab plus dacarbazine for previously untreated metastatic melanoma. *N Engl J Med.* 2011;364(26):2517-2526.
82. Schadendorf D, Hodi FS, Robert C, et al. Pooled analysis of long-term survival data from phase II and phase III trials of ipilimumab in unresectable or metastatic melanoma. *J Clin Oncol.* 2015;33(17):1889-1894.
83. Wolchok JD, Hoos A, O'Day S, et al. Guidelines for the evaluation of immune therapy activity in solid tumors: immune-related response criteria. *Clin Cancer Res.* 2009;15(23):7412-7420.
84. Robert C, Schadendorf D, Messina M, Hodi FS, O'Day S, Investigators MDX. Efficacy and safety of retreatment with ipilimumab in patients with pretreated advanced melanoma who progressed after initially achieving disease control. *Clin Cancer Res.* 2013;19(8):2232-2239.
85. Margolin K, Ernstoff MS, Hamid O, et al. Ipilimumab in patients with melanoma and brain metastases: an open-label, phase 2 trial. *Lancet Oncol.* 2012;13(5):459-465.
86. Amin A, De Pril V, Hamid O, et al. Evaluation of the effect of systemic corticosteroids for the treatment of immune-related adverse events (irAEs) on the development or maintenance of ipilimumab clinical activity [abstract]. *J Clin Oncol.* 2009;27:9037.
87. Hamid O, Robert C, Daud A, et al. Safety and tumor responses with lambrolizumab (anti-PD-1) in melanoma. *N Engl J Med.* 2013;369(2):134-144.
88. Robert C, Ribas A, Wolchok JD, et al. Anti-programmed-death-receptor-1 treatment with pembrolizumab in ipilimumab-refractory advanced melanoma: a randomised dose-comparison cohort of a phase 1 trial. *Lancet.* 2014;384(9948):1109-1117.
89. Robert C, Schachter J, Long GV, et al. Pembrolizumab versus ipilimumab in advanced melanoma. *N Engl J Med.* 2015;372(26):2521-2532.
90. Topalian SL, Hodi FS, Brahmer JR, et al. Safety, activity, and immune correlates of anti–PD-1 antibody in cancer. *N Engl J Med.* 2012;366(26):2443-2454.
91. Robert C, Long GV, Brady B, et al. Nivolumab in previously untreated melanoma without BRAF mutation. *N Engl J Med.* 2015;372(4):320-330.
92. Curran MA, Montalvo W, Yagita H, Allison JP. PD-1 and CTLA-4 combination blockade expands infiltrating T cells and reduces regulatory T and myeloid cells within B16 melanoma tumors. *Proc Natl Acad Sci.* 2010;107(9):4275-4280.
93. Wolchok JD, Kluger H, Callahan MK, et al. Nivolumab plus ipilimumab in advanced melanoma. *N Engl J Med.* 2013;369(2):122-133.
94. Postow MA, Chesney J, Pavlick AC, et al. Nivolumab and ipilimumab versus ipilimumab in untreated melanoma. *N Engl J Med.* 2015;372(21):2006-2017.

94a. Larkin, J., Chiarion-Sileni, V., Gonzalez, R. et al. Combined nivolumab and ipilimumab or monotherapy in untreated melanoma. New England J Med. 2015; 373 (1): 23-34.

95. Dudley ME, Yang JC, Sherry R, et al. Adoptive cell therapy for patients with metastatic melanoma: evaluation of intensive myeloablative chemoradiation preparative regimens. *J Clin Oncol.* 2008;26(32):5233-5239.
96. Gattinoni L, Finkelstein SE, Klebanoff CA, et al. Removal of homeostatic cytokine sinks by lymphodepletion enhances the efficacy of adoptively transferred tumor-specific CD8+ T cells. *J Exp Med.* 2005;202(7):907-912.
97. Paulos CM, Wrzesinski C, Kaiser A, et al. Microbial translocation augments the function of adoptively transferred self/tumor-specific CD8+ T cells via TLR4 signaling. *J Clin Invest.* 2007;117(8):2197-2204.
98. Rosenberg SA. Cell transfer immunotherapy for metastatic solid cancer: what clinicians need to know. *Nat Rev Clin Oncol.* 2011;8(10):577-585.
99. Rosenberg SA, Yang JC, Sherry RM, et al. Durable complete responses in heavily pretreated patients with metastatic melanoma using T-cell transfer immunotherapy. *Clin Cancer Res.* 2011;17(13):4550-4557.
100. Bedikian AY, Johnson MM, Warneke CL, et al. Systemic therapy for unresectable metastatic melanoma: impact of biochemotherapy on long-term survival. *J Immunotoxicol.* 2008;5(2):201-207.

42

Soft Tissue and Bone Sarcomas

第四十二章　软组织和骨肉瘤

J. Andrew Livingston
Anthony Conley
Vinod Ravi
Shreyaskumar Patel

中文导读

肉瘤是一类起源于间充质组织的罕见的异质性肿瘤。本章首先介绍了肉瘤的流行病学和发病机制。虽然病因和发病机制尚不清楚，但某些散在和遗传的基因突变以及一些遗传性家族癌症综合征与软组织和骨肉瘤的发生有关，如李法美尼综合征、遗传性视网膜母细胞瘤、1型神经纤维瘤变、基底细胞痣综合征、沃纳综合征、家族性腺瘤性息肉病、Gardner综合征等。骨和软组织肉瘤根据基因特征分成3类：① 具有复杂核型的遗传不稳定的肉瘤；② 具有特定的，复发遗传改变（如易位、缺失、拷贝数异常）的肿瘤；③ 具有分子畸变（如扩增、突变或杂合性丧失）的肿瘤。文中列出了不同类型肉瘤的基因改变，并推荐将分子病理学应用于肉瘤的诊断，建议对肉瘤进行分子检测，识别特定亚型的基因异常。这些改变在肉瘤的诊断和预后中起重要作用，并可作为潜在的治疗靶点，如针对KIT突变的伊马替尼用于治疗胃肠间质细胞瘤取得了巨大的成功。随后两部分，本章从临床表现、影像评估、病理诊断、分期与预后、治疗、随访等多方面分别对软组织肉瘤和骨肉瘤进行了详细的阐述。在软组织肉瘤部分，本章分别介绍了血管肉瘤、平滑肌肉瘤、脂肪肉瘤、肺泡性软组织肉瘤及胃肠间质细胞瘤。在骨肿瘤的治疗部分，则单独介绍了软骨肉瘤、骨尤文肉瘤和骨巨细胞瘤。

INCIDENCE

Sarcomas are a rare and heterogeneous group of tumors that arise from mesenchymal tissues. According to the estimates of the American Cancer Society, approximately 1.6 million people were estimated to be diagnosed with cancer in the United States in the year 2013, with only 14,420, or just less than 1% of cases, representing sarcomas ([1]); 11,410 of these cases represent new soft tissue sarcomas and 3,010 represent bone sarcomas, with 4,390 and 1,440 deaths, respectively, resulting from these tumors ([1]).

EPIDEMIOLOGY AND PATHOGENESIS

The etiology and pathogenesis of sarcomas is not well understood. Multiple environmental factors including radiation and chemical exposures, trauma, and infection have been associated with the development of soft tissue and bone sarcomas. Both sporadic and inherited molecular and genetic aberrations have been identified in specific subsets of sarcoma and have been implicated in sarcomagenesis.

Several inherited familial cancer syndromes have been associated with a predisposition to development of soft tissue and bone sarcomas. The Li-Fraumeni syndrome resulting from a germline mutation of the *p53* tumor suppressor gene is associated with increased risk of soft tissue sarcomas and osteosarcoma among several other cancers in children and young adults ([2]). Inherited retinoblastoma is also associated with the development of sarcomas, both osteosarcoma and soft tissue sarcoma ([2]). Neurofibromatosis type 1 is associated with an increased risk of development of sarcoma in a preexisting neurofibroma, resulting in a malignant peripheral nerve sheath tumor ([3]). Sarcomas have been associated with other cancer family syndromes including basal cell nevus syndrome, Werner syndrome, familial adenomatous polyposis, and Gardner syndrome, among others ([2]).

Recurrent cytogenetic abnormalities have been identified in many sarcomas and are thought to contribute to sarcomagenesis. Genetic profiling of bone and soft tissue sarcomas has expanded the characterization of mesenchymal tumors beyond translocation-positive/translocation-negative categorizations to identify three distinct groups: (1) genetically unstable sarcomas with complex karyotypes; (2) tumors with specific, recurrent genetic alterations such as translocations, deletions, or copy number variations; or (3) tumors with molecular aberrations such as amplifications, mutations, or loss of heterozygosity (Table 42-1). These alterations serve an important role in diagnosis as well as prognosis and have potential implications for therapy.

Molecular testing has become more widely used for diagnosis in soft tissue sarcoma, identifying specific abnormalities in certain histologic subtypes ([4]). For example the t(x;18) translocation is a specific marker for synovial sarcomas. The transcript formed from this translocation (*SYT-SSX*) can be detected using polymerase chain reaction (PCR) testing. In one study, the *SYT-SSX* transcript was positive in 84.5% of tumors where the diagnosis of synovial sarcoma was certain based on histology and 24.3% of tumors in which synovial sarcoma was considered but not first in the differential diagnosis ([5]). Another example is the *FUS-DDIT3* translocation in myxoid liposarcoma where the presence of *DDIT3* rearrangement confirms the diagnosis ([6]). These data suggest that molecular pathology may also be a useful adjunct in the diagnosis of some sarcomas.

Specific translocations have also been investigated as prognostic biomarkers and potential therapeutic targets. For example, the *EWS-FLI1* transcript in Ewing sarcoma was previously identified as an independent prognostic factor ([7]), but more recent studies have not found an association potentially due to improved therapeutic regimens ([8]). Alternatively, in alveolar rhabdomyosarcoma, translocation-negative tumors have better outcomes than translocation-positive tumors despite histologic appearance ([9]). Although genomic profiling has increased our understanding of sarcomageneis, to date no routine therapies have been identified to target specific translocations in sarcoma. However, the success of the targeted therapy imatinib in the treatment of gastrointestinal stromal tumors, directed at an oncogenic mutation in *KIT*, suggests a role for subtype-specific molecular therapies.

SOFT TISSUE SARCOMA

Soft tissues include fibrous, adipose, and vascular structures as well as muscles and tendons and are mesenchymal in origin. Soft tissue sarcomas are a heterogeneous group encompassing approximately 60 different subtypes, based on their resemblance to normal tissues rather than the tissue of origin.

Clinical Presentation

Soft tissue sarcomas can occur in any anatomic region. The majority of soft tissue sarcomas arise from the extremities (60%), followed by the trunk (30%) and the head and neck region (10%). The most common presenting symptom is a soft tissue mass or swelling. Pain is reported by only about one-third of patients at presentation. Therefore, because of the lack of symptoms,

Table 42-1 Genetic Alterations in Soft Tissue Sarcomas

Tumor	Cytogenetic Abnormality	Gene Product
Alveolar rhabdomyosarcoma	t(2;13)(q35;q14) t(1;13)(p36;q14) t(X;2)(q13;q35)	*PAX3-FOXO1A* *PAX7-FOXO1A* *PAX3-AFX*
Alveolar soft tissue sarcoma	t(X;17)(p11.2;q25)	*ASPL-TFE3*
Clear cell sarcoma	t(12;22)(q13;q12) t(2;22)(q32;q12)	*EWSR1-ATF1* *EWSR1-CREB1*
Congenital fibrosarcoma	t(12;15)(p13;q25)	*ETV6-NTRK3*
Dermatofibrosarcoma protuberans	t(17;22)(q22;q13)	*COL1A1-PDGFB*
Desmoplastic small round cell tumor Epithelioid hemangioendothelioma	t(11;22)(p13;q12) t(1;3)(p36;q25)	*EWSR1-WT1* *WWTR1-CAMTA1*
Endometrial stromal sarcoma	t(7;17)(p15;q11)	*JAZF1-SUZ12*
Gastrointestinal stromal tumor	Activating mutations Overexpression Loss of 14q LOH of 22q Loss of 1p	*KIT, PDGFR, BRAF* *ETV1*
Inflammatory myofibroblastic tumor	t(1;2)(q22-23;p23) t(2;19)(p23;p13.1)	*TPM3-ALK* *TPM4-ALK*
Low-grade fibromyxoid sarcoma Lipoma	t(7;16)(q32–34;p11) t(11;16)(p11;p11) t(3;12)(q27-28, q14-15)	*FUS-CREB3L2* *FUS-CREB3L1* *HMGA2-LPP*
Malignant peripheral nerve sheath tumor	Inactivating	Deletion of *NF1*
Myxoid chondrosarcoma	t(9;22)(q22-31;q11-12) t(9;17)(q22;q11) t(9;15)(q22;q21)	*EWSR1-NR4A3* *TAF15-NR4A3* *TCF12-NR4A3*
Myxoid liposarcoma	t(12;16)(q13;p11)	*FUS-DDIT3*
	t(12;22)(q13;q12)	*EWSR1-DDIT3* *PIK3CA* mutation
Synovial sarcoma	t(X;18)(p11;q11)	*SS18-SSX1* *SS18-SSX2* *SS18-SSX4*
WDLPS/ALT and DDLPS	12q14-15 (supernumerary ring chromosomes; giant marker chromosomes)	Amplification of *MDM2, CDK4, HMGA2, SAS, GLI,* and *JUN*
Uterine leiomyosarcoma	t(12;14)(q7-)	

DDLPS, dedifferentiated liposarcoma; LOH, loss of heterozygosity; WDLPS/ALT, well-differentiated liposarcoma/atypical lipomatous tumor.

there is often a delay in the diagnosis. Patients with a soft tissue mass that is increasing in size, a mass >5 cm, or a mass that is deep to deep fascia, regardless of pain, should be referred for evaluation of a suspected soft tissue sarcoma ([10]).

Evaluation

Evaluation of a suspected soft tissue sarcoma begins with a comprehensive history and physical examination. Imaging evaluation is dependent on the site of disease. For soft tissue tumors of the extremities, head and neck, and pelvis, magnetic resonance imaging (MRI) is preferred. Soft tissue sarcomas found in the retroperitoneum and abdomen are generally best evaluated by computed tomography (CT). Positron emission tomography (PET) imaging can distinguish histologic grade to a degree based on tumor standardized uptake values (SUV) ([11]). For both soft tissue sarcomas and bone sarcomas, PET imaging has a predictive role in determining response to chemotherapy and targeted agents such as imatinib, but it has also been shown to predict survival after initial cycle of therapy among patients receiving neoadjuvant chemotherapy for high-grade soft tissue sarcoma ([12, 13]).

A biopsy is essential to diagnosis, and the method of biopsy chosen should be the least invasive technique available to make a definitive diagnosis. A core-needle biopsy is sufficient; however, multiple cores should be obtained to improve diagnostic yield. If an open biopsy is performed, it should be planned such that the biopsy tract can be removed at the time of definitive surgical resection to reduce the risk of seeding and recurrence ([14]). An excisional biopsy may be used for small or superficial lesions; however, careful examination of margins and planning of the orientation of the resection should always be performed. Fine-needle aspiration (FNA) is not recommended but can be useful in confirming recurrence, assuming that an experienced sarcoma cytopathologist is available ([15]).

Pathology

Sarcomas are classified primarily according to their tissue appearance, histologic grade, and sometimes the cell of origin. This can be difficult, as approximately 60 different histologic types of soft tissue sarcoma are recognized (Table 42-2). Histologic diagnosis is classified by the updated 2013 World Health Organization criteria ([16]).

Pathologists often separate sarcomas into three histologic grades using the Federation Nationale des Centres de Lutte Contre le Cancer (FNCLCC) grading system. Biological aggressiveness can be predicted based on histologic grade, and this spectrum varies among the histologic subtypes of sarcoma ([17]). Immunohistochemistry, cytogenetics, and molecular pathology can aid in making a diagnosis; however, some poorly differentiated spindle cell neoplasms cannot be categorized further.

Staging and Prognosis

The American Joint Committee on Cancer (AJCC) staging system may be used for soft tissue sarcomas (Table 42-3) ([18]). All soft tissue sarcoma subtypes are included except Kaposi sarcoma, dermatofibrosarcoma protuberans, infantile fibrosarcoma, and angiosarcoma. This system is designed to classify tumors of the extremities, trunk, head and neck, and retroperitoneum, but it was not designed for evaluation of sarcomas of the gastrointestinal (GI) tract. This system has its limitations because anatomic site and certain histologic subtypes (eg, small cell histologies) that are known to influence outcome are not taken into account ([19]).

Several clinicopathologic factors are important for treatment planning and prognosis assessment. These form the basis for the AJCC classification system and include tumor grade, size of the primary tumor, depth

Table 42-2 Soft Tissue Sarcoma: Histologic Diagnosis

Sarcomas of adipose tissue
Liposarcoma
Atypical lipomatous tumor
Myxoid liposarcoma
Cellular myxoid liposarcoma
Round cell liposarcoma
Dedifferentiated liposarcoma
Pleomorphic liposarcoma
Sarcomas of peripheral nervous tissue
Malignant peripheral nerve sheath tumor
(Malignant schwannoma, neurofibrosarcoma, neurogenic sarcoma)
Sarcomas of smooth muscle
Leiomyosarcoma
Sarcomas of fibrous tissue
Desmoid fibromatosis
Dermatofibrosarcoma protuberans
Low-grade fibromyxoid sarcoma
Fibrosarcoma
Malignant fibrous histiocytoma (MFH)
Sarcomas of blood vessels and lymphatics
Epithelioid hemangioendothelioma
Hemangiopericytoma
Angiosarcoma/lymphangiosarcoma
Sarcomas of skeletal muscle
Embryonal rhabdomyosarcoma
Alveolar rhabdomyosarcoma
Pleomorphic rhabdomyosarcoma
Sarcomas of unknown origin
Synovial sarcoma
Monophasic
Biphasic
Alveolar soft tissue sarcoma
Epithelioid sarcoma
Unclassified sarcoma
Extraskeletal osteosarcoma
Extraskeletal chondrosarcoma
Extraskeletal Ewing sarcoma (PNET)
Soft tissue tumors of melanocytic tissue
Melanoma of soft tissue or clear cell sarcoma

PNET, primitive neuroectodermal tumor.

Table 42-3 Staging From the American Joint Committee on Cancer

Primary tumor (T)						
TX	Primary tumor cannot be assessed					
T0	No evidence of primary tumor					
T1	Tumor 5 cm or less in greatest dimension					
	T1a superficial tumor[a]					
	T1b deep tumor[a]					
T2	Tumor more than 5 cm in greatest dimension					
	T2a superficial tumor					
	T2b deep tumor					
Regional lymph nodes (N)						
NX	Regional lymph nodes cannot be assessed					
N0	No regional lymph node metastasis					
N1	Regional lymph node metastasis					
Distant metastasis (M)						
MX	Distant metastasis cannot be assessed					
M0	No distant metastasis					
M1	Distant metastasis					
Histologic grade (G)						
GX	Grade cannot be assessed					
G1	Well differentiated					
G2	Moderately differentiated					
G3	Poorly differentiated					
G4	Poorly differentiated or undifferentiated (four-tiered systems only)					
Stage grouping						
Stage I	T1a, 1b, 2a, 2b	N0	M0	G1-2	G1	Low
Stage II	T1a, 1b, 2a	N0	M0	G3-4	G2-3	High
Stage III	T2b	N0	M0	G3-4	G2-3	High
Stage IV	Any T	N1	M0	Any G	Any G	High or low

[a]Superficial tumors are located exclusively above the superficial fascia without invasion of the fascia; deep tumors are located either exclusively beneath the superficial fascia, superficial to the fascia with invasion of or through the fascia, or both superficial yet beneath the fascia. Retroperitoneal, mediastinal, and pelvic sarcomas are classified as deep tumors.

Reproduced with permission from Edge SB, Byrd DR, Compton CC (eds): *AJCC Cancer Staging Manuarl*, 7th ed. New York, NY: Springer; 2010 ([18]).

of invasion, and extent of disease ([17]). High-risk features for local recurrence or distant metastases are high-grade lesions, primary tumor >5 cm, and deep tumor location. Approximately 50% of patients with intermediate- and high-grade soft tissue sarcoma will develop metastatic disease requiring systemic therapy ([20]). The 5-year overall survival for soft tissue sarcoma is around 50%, with local control and distant disease being the key determinants ([21]).

Treatment

Treatment of sarcoma requires a multidisciplinary approach with experienced medical, surgical, and radiation oncologists, pathologists, and radiologists. An improved understanding of soft tissue sarcoma subtypes in regard to natural history, response to chemotherapy, and potential for targeted therapies has led to more subtype-specific treatment according to individual histology.

Treatment of Local Disease

Surgery

For local disease, surgical resection is the mainstay of treatment. Sarcomas tend to expand and compress tissue planes, which produce a pseudo-capsule comprising normal tissue interlaced with tumor tissue. Wide local excision with a margin of normal tissue surrounding the tumor is associated with lower local recurrence rates of approximately 10% to 30% ([17]). The ideal surgical margins should be 2 to 3 cm without tumor involvement. If positive margins are confirmed by pathology, re-excision to obtain negative margins is important when feasible to improve local control and relapse-free survival. For patients with borderline resectable tumors, consideration should be given to neoadjuvant therapy depending on the tumor histology and patient's performance status.

Adult sarcomas have a less than 4% prevalence of lymph node metastases ([22]). For this reason, routine regional lymph node dissection is often not required. However, patients with synovial sarcoma, clear cell sarcoma, rhabdomyosarcoma, angiosarcoma, and epithelioid sarcomas have a higher incidence of lymph node metastases and should be evaluated closely for lymphadenopathy.

Improved surgical techniques and multimodality treatment have resulted in a decrease in radical resection of extremity tumors with a corresponding rise in limb-sparing procedures combining wide local resection with preoperative or postoperative chemotherapy and radiotherapy. Approximately 90% of patients with localized sarcomas of the extremities can safely undergo limb-sparing procedures to preserve limb function and adequately maintain local control ([23]). A study conducted at the National Cancer Institute (NCI) showed no survival advantage to amputation over limb-sparing surgery with postoperative radiation ([24]).

Radiation

Although radiation is not effective for the treatment of gross disease, it has been a useful adjunct to surgery in the treatment of microscopic local disease and for palliation of symptoms. Radiation therapy is commonly used in the preoperative or postoperative adjuvant setting. Because there are pros and cons as to the timing of radiation therapy, this topic remains controversial; appropriate discussion between radiation oncologists, medical oncologists, and surgeons is required in planning the treatment of each patient.

Preoperative radiation has several advantages over postoperative radiation, including smaller radiation portals, conversion to a limb-sparing procedure, reduction of the extent of the surgical procedure, and lower radiation doses, which can be used because there are theoretically fewer radio-resistant hypoxic cells within the tumor and surgical removal can supplement the boost ([25]). However, preoperative radiotherapy may lead to difficulty in assessing pathologic responses to preoperative chemotherapy and may also contribute to delayed wound healing. Several studies have shown improved local control rates with preoperative radiation, especially with larger tumors that were initially considered unresectable ([26]). The modality of choice is external beam radiotherapy (EBRT), and a dose of 50 Gy or more is often required to obtain local control. At these dose levels, the entire circumference of the extremity must not be irradiated in order to avoid lymphedema. A period of 4 to 6 weeks is needed following preoperative radiation to prevent wound complications. Following the surgical resection, close or positive margins could be treated with a radiation boost if feasible. Brachytherapy, EBRT, or intraoperative radiotherapy can be used by experienced clinicians in appropriate situations ([27]).

Postoperative radiation therapy should be considered in patients with high-grade soft tissue sarcomas of the extremities with positive microscopic margins (<1 mm from the inked margin). In this setting, adjuvant radiation improved the 5-year local control rate compared to the no RT group (74% vs 56%; $P = .01$) ([28]). More recently, adjuvant intensity-modulated radiation therapy has been shown to reduce local recurrence as compared to conventional EBRT for primary soft tissue sarcoma of the extremity (hazard ratio [HR], 0.46; $P = .02$) ([29]). The interval of time between surgery and initiation of radiation therapy is a controversial but legitimate concern. The most recent soft tissue sarcoma guidelines issued by the National Comprehensive Cancer Network (NCCN) suggest the interval should be no greater than 6 weeks ([30]).

Radiation therapy is occasionally used as the sole treatment modality for palliation for some patients with soft tissue sarcomas. These patients are often those who have unresectable disease or who are not appropriate candidates for surgery and/or chemotherapy. There have been reports of 5-year survival rates ranging from 25% to 40% with radiation therapy alone and of local control rates of approximately 30%, depending on the primary tumor's size and biology ([31]).

Chemotherapy

Systemic therapy for soft tissue sarcomas is primarily used in the metastatic/advanced disease setting, whereas the role of chemotherapy in the neoadjuvant and adjuvant setting is less well established. Treatment relies primarily upon conventional chemotherapy agents, which are largely unchanged over the past two decades. In general, tumors with a higher grade are more likely to responds to chemotherapy; however, chemosensitivity varies based on histologic subtype (Table 42-4) ([32]). An understanding of chemosensitivity and molecular aberrations based on subtype has led to histology-driven treatment algorithms for specific soft tissue sarcomas such as leiomyosarcoma, myxoid liposarcoma, and angiosarcomas (Fig. 42-1). This approach is particularly important in considering targeted therapies for specific subtypes that are considered chemoresistant such as alveolar soft parts sarcoma.

Table 42-4 Relative Chemosensitivity of Soft Tissue Sarcomas

Relative Chemosensitivity	Example
Highly sensitive (chemotherapy standard of care in management)	Ewing sarcoma family of tumors/PNET Embryonal and alveolar rhabdomyosarcoma
Sensitive to chemotherapy	Synovial sarcoma Small cell sarcoma Myxoid/round cell liposarcoma Uterine leiomyosarcoma
Moderate sensitivity to chemotherapy	Pleomorphic liposarcoma Myxofibrosarcoma Epithelioid sarcoma Pleomorphic rhabdomyosarcoma Leiomyosarcoma Malignant peripheral nerve sheath tumor (MPNST) Angiosarcoma Desmoplastic small round cell tumor (DSRCT)
Insensitive to chemotherapy	Dedifferentiated liposarcoma Clear cell sarcoma Endometrial stromal sarcoma
Chemoresistant (chemotherapy risk clearly outweighs benefit)	Gastrointestinal stromal tumor (GIST) Alveolar soft parts sarcoma (ASPS) Extraskeletal myxoid chondrosarcoma

PNET, primitive neuroectodermal tumor.

The two most active agents in the treatment of soft tissue sarcoma are doxorubicin and ifosfamide. Doxorubicin is most active at doses of ≥75 mg/m^2, with single-agent response rates of approximately 20% to 35% ([33]). Ifosfamide has been shown to produce single-agent response rates similar to those of single-agent doxorubicin when used at doses of 10 g/m^2 or higher ([34]). Ifosfamide has also been shown to have greater efficacy when administered as a 2- to 3-hour infusion as opposed to a 24-hour infusion ([34, 35]). Studies have shown that both doxorubicin and ifosfamide also exhibit a positive dose-response curve ([33, 34]). The response rate in soft tissue sarcoma patients whose disease failed doxorubicin-based therapy and who then received high-dose ifosfamide as a single agent was 29% ([34]). Therefore, high-dose ifosfamide as a single agent at doses of 14 g/m^2 is sometimes used as a salvage regimen at the University of Texas MD Anderson Cancer Center (MDACC) for selected histologies.

Combination therapy with dose-intense doxorubicin and ifosfamide has been shown to improve response rates and progression-free survival (PFS) and possibly overall survival ([36]). The combination of doxorubicin (75 or 90 mg/m^2) and ifosfamide (at 10 g/m^2) was evaluated at MDACC in patients with soft tissue sarcomas and demonstrated a 75% response rate (95% confidence interval [CI], 59%-71%; complete response [CR], 12%) in patients with primary tumors of the extremities and a 68% response rate (95% CI, 56%-80%; CR, 12%) in patients with primary disease at any site ([37]). The response rates according to histology were as follows: malignant fibrous histiocytoma, 69%; synovial sarcoma, 88%; unclassified sarcomas, 60%; non-GI leiomyosarcomas, 50%; liposarcomas, 56%; angiosarcomas, 83%; and neurogenic sarcomas, 40%; other miscellaneous histologies demonstrated objective response rates of 45% ([37]). In the large randomized phase III European Organization for Research and Treatment of Cancer (EORTC) 62012 trial comparing single-agent doxorubicin with doxorubicin in combination with ifosfamide, the combination group had a significantly higher response rate (26% vs 14%) and increased median PFS (7.4 vs 4.6 months) but also had an increase it grade 3 and 4 toxicities. Although overall survival at 1 year was increased in the combination group (60% vs 51%, $P = .076$), this failed to meet statistical significance ([38]). At our center, we continue to use combination dose-intense doxorubicin and ifosfamide in appropriately selected patients and preferentially in the neoadjuvant setting for large (≥5 cm), high-grade, resectable soft tissue sarcomas.

Dacarbazine has activity as a single agent, with response rates of 10% to 15%. The three-drug regimen MAID (mesna, doxorubicin [Adriamycin], ifosfamide, dacarbazine) has been studied and has shown response rates varying from 25% to 47% ([39]). When the MAID regimen was studied at MDACC, significant toxicities related to the addition of dacarbazine were seen ([40]). The combination of doxorubicin and dacarbazine (ADIC) is often used in extrauterine leiomyosarcoma or as a second-line regimen in other soft tissue sarcomas. In patients with advanced/metastatic leiomyosarcoma or liposarcoma treated with ADIC as first-line therapy, Response Evaluation Criteria in Solid Tumors (RECIST) response rates of 57% and 40% were observed, respectively ([41]).

Gemcitabine alone or in combination with docetaxel is frequently used for the treatment of advanced, recurrent, or metastatic disease once patients fail doxorubicin- and ifosfamide-based therapy or in patients who may not tolerate intensive chemotherapy. An initial phase II study using gemcitabine as a single agent demonstrated a response rate of 18% (95% CI, 7%-29%), including many pretreated patients ([42]). The synergistic effect of docetaxel when added to gemcitabine was evaluated in

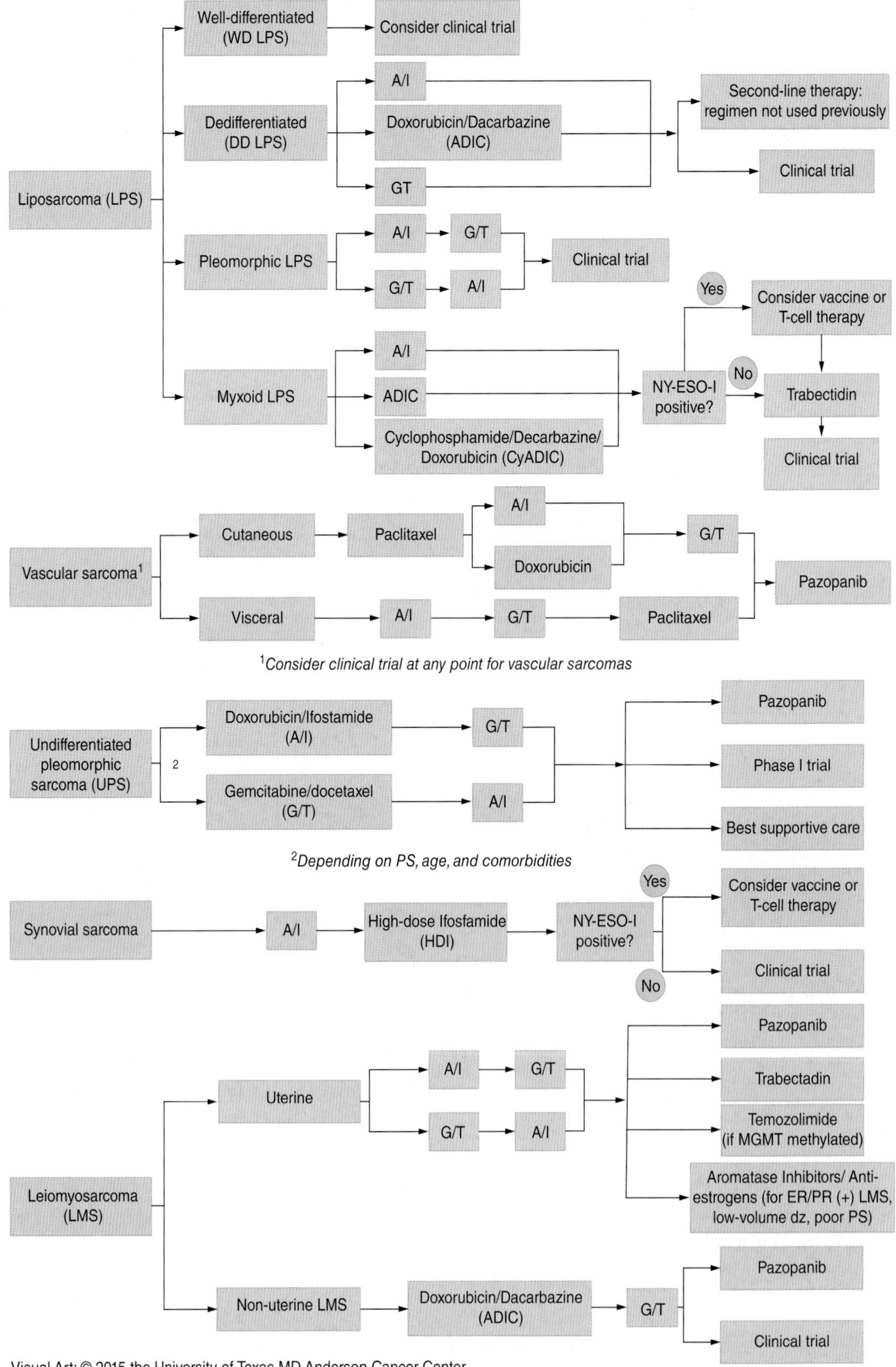

FIGURE 42-1 Approach to systemic therapies for advanced soft tissue sarcomas. A/I doxorubicin/ifosfamide; ADIC doxorubicin, dacarbazine; CyADIC, cyclophosphamide, doxorubicin, dacarbazine; ER, estrogen receptor; G/T gemcitabine/docetaxel; MGMT, O6-methylguanine-DNA methyltransferase; PR, progesterone receptor; PS, performance status.

CHAPTER 42

a randomized phase II study, SARC002 ([43]). By RECIST, response rates for the gemcitabine-docetaxel arm and gemcitabine arm was 16% and 8%, respectively. Furthermore, an improvement in median PFS (6.2 vs 3.0 months) and overall survival (17.9 vs 11.5 months) was noted in the gemcitabine-docetaxel arm compared to the gemcitabine arm. The two histologies most responsive to the gemcitabine-docetaxel arm were leiomyosarcoma and high-grade undifferentiated pleomorphic sarcoma.

Trabectedin, a novel antitumor compound initially isolated from extracts of sea squirt *Ecteinascidia turbinata* through the NCI drug screening program in the 1960s, has shown activity in the second-line treatment of soft tissue sarcomas. The mechanism of action of trabectedin is complex but is thought to involve displacement of transcription factors from their promoter ([44]). Additionally, sensitivity of myxoid liposarcoma, a translocation-related soft tissue sarcoma, has been shown to correlate with expression of the *FUS-DDIT3* fusion gene ([45]). Taken together, these factors suggest a role for trabectedin in translocation-related sarcomas and pose a potential mechanism of action. In a single-arm phase II trial of trabectedin as second- or third-line therapy in advanced soft tissue sarcoma, the overall response rate was 8% ([46]). However, many patients demonstrated prolonged disease stabilization, with 26% with stable disease >6 months with minimal toxicities. This benefit was greatest in leiomyosarcomas and translocation-related sarcomas. A retrospective review of eight phase II trials of trabectedin in translocation-related soft tissue sarcomas demonstrated encouraging results in regard to disease control, with greatest activity in myxoid liposarcoma ([47]). This has led to a current phase III trial of first-line therapy with trabectedin versus doxorubicin-based chemotherapy in translocation-related sarcomas. Currently, trabectedin is approved in Europe for second-line treatment of soft tissue sarcoma and has been granted orphan drug status by the US Food and Drug Administration.

Adjuvant/Neoadjuvant Chemotherapy

The goals of chemotherapy in the treatment of high-risk local disease are to eradicate micrometastasis, decrease risk of local recurrence, and downsize tumors to facilitate either limb-sparing procedures for extremity tumors or resection for tumors initially deemed unresectable (Fig. 40-2). At MDACC, preoperative chemotherapy is preferred in patients with high-risk (>5 cm or high-grade) tumors and in patients who are considered borderline resectable with chemosensitive soft tissue sarcoma subtypes.

Postoperative chemotherapy and its benefits continue to be controverted as trials of adjuvant therapy have yielded conflicting results. In the most recent update to the Sarcoma Meta-Analysis Collaboration (SMAC) conducted in 2008, the benefit of adjuvant chemotherapy was analyzed among 1,953 patients with soft tissue sarcoma across 18 trials ([48]). This update incorporated five trials evaluating doxorubicin and ifosfamide in combination, a regimen not previously represented in the initial SMAC analysis. This updated meta-analysis detected favorable odds ratios (ORs) of local recurrence and distant recurrence for chemotherapy. Although the absolute risk reduction (ARR) in distant recurrence with adjuvant doxorubicin-based chemotherapy for all studies was 9% (95% CI, 5%-14%; $P = .000$), the ARR with adjuvant doxorubicin-ifosfamide chemotherapy was 10% (95% CI, 1%-19%; $P = .03$) ([48]). By pooling the data, the number needed to treat (NNT) to prevent distant recurrence was 12. Although a survival benefit was not noted with single-agent doxorubicin, a statistically significant survival advantage was observed with the doxorubicin-ifosfamide combination. The OR for overall survival in the doxorubicin-ifosfamide cohort was 0.56 (95% CI, 0.36-0.85; $P = .01$). Combining all trials in the meta-analysis, the NNT to prevent one death was 17. A recent randomized controlled trial of adjuvant therapy with doxorubicin 75 mg/m^2 and ifosfamide 5 g/m^2 in patients with intermediate- or high-grade STS failed to demonstrate a benefit in overall survival (HR, 0.94; $P = .72$) or relapse-free survival (HR, 0.91; $P = .51$) ([49]). Although the data regarding adjuvant therapy are conflicting, within our institution, we continue to offer adjuvant therapy with doxorubicin in combination with ifosfamide to healthy patients with intact organ function who have high-risk disease (tumor size >5 cm, high-grade histology, and deep soft tissue involvement).

Targeted Therapy

As in other tumor types, increased knowledge of cancer genomics and identification of oncogenic driver mutations in soft tissue sarcomas have led to much enthusiasm and investigation of molecular-based targeted therapies. A comprehensive review of targeted therapies under development for soft tissue sarcoma is beyond the scope of this chapter, and therefore, the focus will be on currently approved therapies. Targeting cKIT with the tyrosine kinase inhibitor (TKI) imatinib in gastrointestinal stromal tumors (GISTs) is perhaps the best-known and most successful example in sarcoma. Although targeted agents have shown promise in specific histologies, the multitargeted TKI pazopanib has shown activity across multiple subtypes of soft tissue sarcomas. Pazopanib is a small-molecule inhibitor with activity against VEGF1-3, PDGFRA, PDGFRB, and KIT. A phase II trial of pazopanib in advanced soft tissue sarcoma evaluating 12-week PFS as the primary end point showed benefit in leiomyosarcoma (44%), synovial sarcoma (49%), and other nonlipomatous soft tissue sarcoma (39%) ([50]). Subsequently, a placebo-controlled

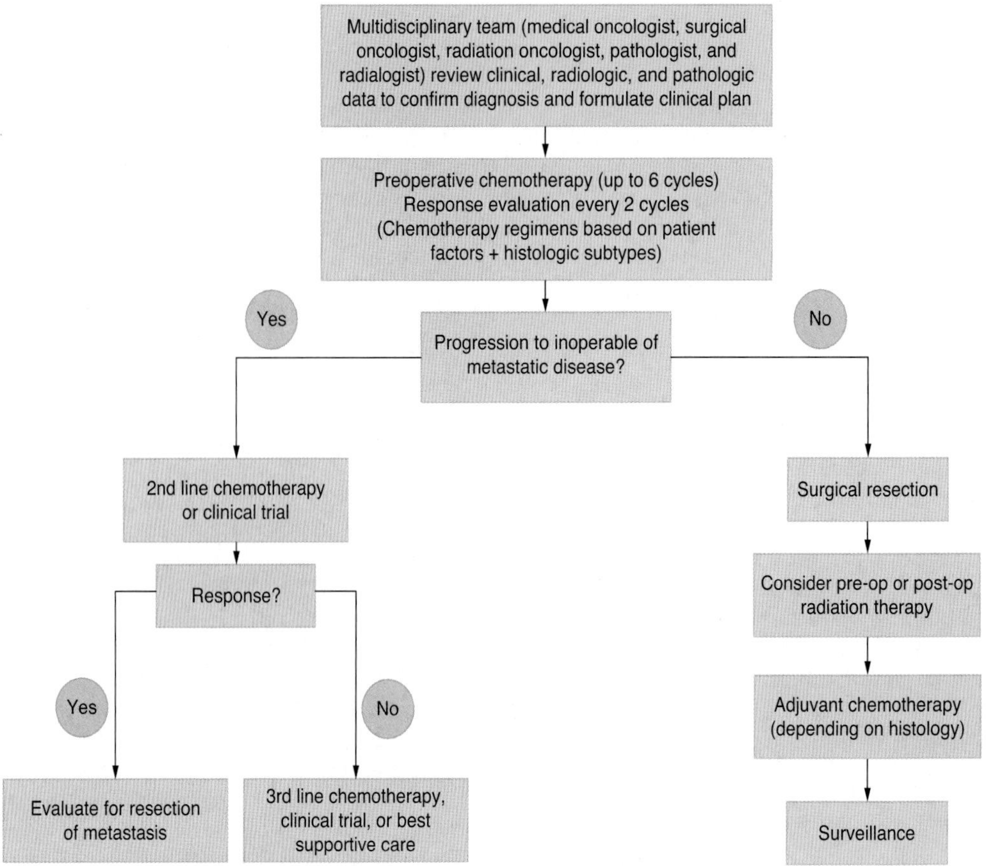

FIGURE 42-2 Treatment approach for patients with stage III soft tissue sarcomas.

phase III trial of pazopanib in metastatic soft tissue sarcoma demonstrated a low response rate (partial response [PR], 6%) but significant improvement in PFS (4.6 months vs 1.6 months with placebo; HR, 0.31; $P < .0001$) ([51]). In a multivariate Cox model, favorable prognostic factors in patients treated with pazopanib were good performance status and low or intermediate tumor grade. Additional targeted therapies in soft tissue sarcoma are primarily being developed and studied in specific soft tissue sarcoma subtypes.

Metastatic Disease and Metastasectomy

Patients with metastatic disease involving multiple organs are generally incurable and considered appropriate for palliative systemic therapy as described earlier. The subset of patients with lung-only metastatic disease, especially with a greater than 12-month disease-free interval, have a favorable biology and prognosis and therefore should be considered for resection if feasible. This approach results in 3- to 5-year survival of up to 20%. Chemotherapy is the mainstay of therapy for patients with metastatic disease, although surgical resection of residual disease to render patients free of gross disease is often pursued. The sequencing of chemotherapy is similar to that of isolated local disease. In a study conducted at MDACC, patients with metastatic disease showed a 57% response rate to doxorubicin (75-90 mg/m^2) and ifosfamide (10 g/m^2) ([37]). If patients fail this regimen, the choice of treatment depends on the histology of the tumor and the performance status of the patient.

Specific Soft Tissue Sarcomas

Vascular Sarcomas

Vascular sarcomas are tumors that originate from or differentiate toward the endothelium with varying malignant potential. Although epithelioid hemangioendotheliomas have an intermediate malignant potential and indolent clinical course, angiosarcomas, at the other end of the spectrum, have a highly malignant biologic behavior with early propensity for distant metastasis and dismal outcomes. These tumors also differ in their response to chemotherapy and targeted therapy and, therefore, are discussed separately below.

Epithelioid hemangioendotheliomas (EHE) are considered to be of intermediate malignant potential with development of metastasis and recurrence. They typically are associated with a blood vessel, usually a medium sized or large vein. Epithelioid hemangioendothelioma most commonly occurs in the soft tissues, but liver, lung, and bone may be sites of primary involvement. In over 42% of patients with hepatic EHE, symptoms are often absent and the lesions are discovered incidentally. Some patients experience constitutional symptoms such as fatigue, anorexia, nauseam and poor exercise tolerance. Most cases of EHE affecting soft tissues are localized, whereas multifocality is more common with EHE involving liver or lung, and these patients develop metastatic disease during the course of their illness. Multifocal or metastatic disease does not equate to mortality, and many patients can survive long term with metastatic disease. Sixty-three percent of patients with liver EHE and less than half of patients with metastatic EHE of soft tissues die from their disease.

Localized EHE of soft tissue should be treated with surgical resection with adequate margins. Following resection, these tumors can recur locally in about 12% of patients ([52]). Preoperative radiation therapy should be considered in patients where good margins are unlikely, and postoperative radiation therapy should be considered in cases where the margins are positive and no preoperative radiation was administered. Localized EHE does not require the use of chemotherapy or targeted therapies.

Metastatic EHE of soft tissue may be followed without therapy until there is evidence of progressive disease on serial imaging over a 3-month period. When systemic therapy is needed, conventional chemotherapy and antiangiogenic therapy may be considered. Systemic therapy options include gemcitabine, taxanes, and doxorubicin. Targeted therapy with bevacizumab (PR, 29%; stable disease, 57%; and progressive disease, 14%) ([53]), sorafenib (30.7% without progression at 9 months) ([54]), and interferon α-2b ([55]) has been reported to have utility in patients with metastatic EHE.

Angiosarcomas are highly malignant tumors with endothelial differentiation with a propensity for recurrence and distant metastasis. These tumors are extremely rare, representing <2% of all sarcomas, and can develop de novo or in the setting of prior radiation therapy or chronic lymphedema. Due to their endothelial location, these tumors are particularly well poised for early dissemination and development of metastasis. Angiosarcoma has a propensity for cutaneous involvement, and 60% of cases have skin or soft tissue involvement. Other sites of visceral involvement include spleen, liver, lung, pleura, heart, and GI tract. Clinical behavior and response to therapy can vary from one site to another, with cardiac angiosarcomas carrying the worst prognosis.

Even when these tumors are nonmetastatic, multifocality is often present locally, resulting in high recurrence rates. Therefore, it is critical to approach localized disease with a multidisciplinary approach that combines chemotherapy, radiation, and surgery to produce better outcomes ([56]). At our institution, we prefer to treat these patients with neoadjuvant chemotherapy followed by surgery and radiation. Chemotherapy can utilize either doxorubicin-based or taxane-based approaches, both of which have excellent outcomes, and the choice of the regimen depends on the primary location of disease, histologic subtype, performance status of the patient, and potential for toxicity. For cutaneous angiosarcoma, taxanes are as good as doxorubicin-based approaches, but for visceral angiosarcoma, doxorubicin-based approaches may have better activity.

Patients with metastatic disease can be treated with single-agent or multiagent chemotherapy. Monotherapy with doxorubicin (response rate, 29%-33%; PFS, 3-5 months) and paclitaxel (response rate, 18%-89%; PFS, 4-5 months) appears to have significant activity in patients with angiosarcomas ([57-61]). Based on a retrospective study of 117 patients with metastatic angiosarcoma, weekly paclitaxel (response rate, 53%) may have comparable efficacy to doxorubicin as a single agent in patients with cutaneous angiosarcoma ([57]). Doxorubicin may have advantages over paclitaxel in visceral angiosarcomas. Gemcitabine also appears to have single-agent activity (response rate, 64%; PFS, 7 months) ([62]), but this drug is more commonly used in combination with taxanes.

The most commonly used combination therapies in angiosarcoma are doxorubicin-ifosfamide and gemcitabine-docetaxel. The doxorubicin-ifosfamide combination is preferred for visceral angiosarcomas and has better durability than any other treatment for angiosarcoma, with a median PFS of 5.4 months ([59]). The gemcitabine-docetaxel combination appears to have good activity both in the visceral and cutaneous angiosarcomas.

Antiangiogenic therapies with activity in angiosarcomas include bevacizumab (PR, 9%; stable disease, 48%; median PFS, 12 weeks) ([53]), sunitinib ([63]), and sorafenib (CR, 3%; PR, 11%; stable disease, 57%; median PFS, 3.2 months) ([64]). Although responses with targeted therapies appear to be low compared to conventional chemotherapy, this may be a result of using an unselected study population for treatment.

Leiomyosarcoma

Leiomyosarcoma (LMS) is a common soft tissue sarcoma subtype and can arise anywhere in the body. The site of origin and grade are important prognostic factors and also guide treatment. Patients with vascular origin LMS have a worse prognosis compared with nonvascular LMS patients. Additionally, patients with uterine LMS tend to fare better compared with extrauterine LMS patients, although this may be in part due to a higher rate of complete resection in uterine LMS ([65]). Leiomyosarcoma is responsive to multiple chemotherapeutic agents used in soft tissue sarcoma but has been shown to be less responsive to ifosfamide-containing regimens than single-agent doxorubicin ([66]). Gemcitabine is active in LMS. A subtype-specific phase II trial of gemcitabine versus gemcitabine in combination with docetaxel in metastatic or relapsed LMS ([67]) showed significant response rates with both single-agent gemcitabine and the combination (19% vs 24%, respectively) in patients with uterine LMS. In the non–uterine LMS subgroup, combination therapy resulted in higher objective response rates (14% vs 5%) and prolonged PFS (6.3 vs 3.8 months). Hormonal treatment may be considered for patients with uterine LMS. In the largest retrospective study of aromatase inhibitors in uterine LMS, response rates included PR in 9% and stable disease in 32%. Patients with hormone receptor–positive disease demonstrated better PFS ([68]). The treatment algorithm for advanced LMS should take into account the site of origin (uterine vs extrauterine), hormone expression in uterine LMS, and O^6-methylguanine-DNA methyltransferase (MGMT) methylation status (see Fig. 42-1).

CHAPTER 42

Liposarcoma

Liposarcomas represent the second most common soft tissue sarcoma. There are several histologic subtypes of liposarcoma with unique clinical and biological features. Myxoid liposarcoma represents the most common variant of liposarcoma. Other subsets include well-differentiated, dedifferentiated, and pleomorphic subtypes. Myxoid liposarcomas often occur in the third through fifth decades of life and generally develop in the extremities. Although regarded a low-grade tumor, local recurrence and distant metastasis occur in about 30% of patients. Sites of metastasis include lungs and soft tissue regions such as the axilla, retroperitoneum, the pleural lining, and even the pericardium. A rare variant of myxoid liposarcoma, round cell liposarcoma, is considered to be a more malignant variant of a spectrum of this disease. An increase in round cell percentage correlates to metastasis and poor survival in myxoid liposarcomas ([69]). The balanced translocation t(12;16)(q13;p11) results in the oncoprotein FUS-DDIT3, which is pathognomonic for myxoid liposarcoma ([70, 71]). The product of this arrangement is thought to contribute to the oncogenesis through transcription of angiogenic, inflammatory, and adipocytic maturation factors resulting in myxoid liposarcoma ([72]). Treatment options for myxoid liposarcoma depend on the location and size of the lesion. Whereas surgery and radiation are more feasible for extremity locations, retroperitoneal involvement is less amenable to surgery for curative intent. Importantly, myxoid liposarcoma is considered a chemosensitive disease. Reports from MDACC using doxorubicin-based chemotherapy yield response rates of 44%. Trabectedin has been shown to be active in myxoid liposarcoma across multiple trials ([45, 73]). Aside from binding to the minor groove of DNA and forming covalent adducts and displacement of transcription factors, this agent is thought to promote differentiation of myxoid liposarcoma lipoblasts. Surgery is the mainstay of treatment for well-differentiated/dedifferentiated liposarcoma; however, recurrence rates are high, especially in the retroperitoneum. Benefit from chemotherapy has been reported to be minimal, with objective response rates of approximately 12% ([74]). In a recent review of 89 patients with dedifferentiated liposarcoma of the retroperitoneum treated at MDACC, response rates were higher (23% by RECIST) with a clinical benefit rate (PR + stable disease >6 months) of 37%, suggesting a potential role for chemotherapy in select patients with unresectable or borderline resectable disease.

Alveolar Soft Parts Sarcoma

Alveolar soft parts sarcoma (ASPS) is a rare soft tissue sarcoma subtype predominantly affecting adolescents and young adults and accounting for <1% of all soft tissue sarcomas. Although the disease course is indolent with a prolonged natural history, ASPSs have a high rate of metastasis and a median overall survival of approximately 90 months. Although lung metastases are most common, ASPS can also metastasize to the brain, an otherwise uncommon site for sarcoma. In a review of our institutional experience with ASPS, 65% of patients presented with stage IV disease. Among those with localized disease at presentation, 5-year overall survival was 88%, whereas those who presented with metastatic disease had a median overall survival of 40 months and 5-year overall survival of 20% ([75]). Despite its propensity for metastasis, ASPS is resistant to conventional chemotherapy. Highly vascular, these tumors are characterized by an unbalanced translocation t(X;17)(p11:q25) resulting in the ASPL-TFE3 fusion protein and overexpression of *MET*, leading to angiogenesis. Cediranib, a highly potent vascular endothelial growth factor (VEGF) inhibitor, has recently shown promise in the treatment of ASPS. In a single-arm phase II study of 43 patients, cediranib demonstrated an overall response rate of 35% and a disease control rate of 84% at 6 months [76]. Sunitinib, a multitargeted small-molecule inhibitor including VEGF, has also been shown to be active in ASPS [77].

Follow-Up Management

The major goals of follow-up surveillance and management should be early identification of potentially curable recurrences, identification of treatment-related complications, and patient reassurance. Surveillance of patients treated for soft tissue sarcomas is based on known prognostic factors, outcomes in individual subsets of patients, and patterns of tumor recurrence.

For patients with low-risk T1 primaries who have undergone treatment with curative intent and are free of any gross evidence of disease, follow-up should include a history and physical, cross-sectional imaging of the tumor bed to evaluate for local recurrence, and routine chest x-rays for surveillance of metastatic disease [78]. For tumors of the head and neck and extremities, MRI is appropriate; for tumors of the chest cavity, abdomen, and retroperitoneum, CT scans are appropriate [78]. The routine use of chest CT for evaluation of metastatic disease in soft tissue sarcomas has been studied and found not to be cost effective. The NCCN guidelines recommend follow-up with annual scanning of the primary site for at least 5 years; however, often these patients are seen every 3 to 4 months in the immediate postoperative period for the first 2 years, then every 4 to 6 months for the next 2 years, and yearly thereafter.

Patients with high-risk T2 (>5 cm) soft tissue sarcomas are at a greater risk for distant lung metastases. In patients with high-risk tumors who have undergone treatment with curative intent and are free of any gross evidence of disease, follow-up should include a history and physical, cross-sectional imaging of the tumor bed, and routine chest x-rays for surveillance of metastatic disease [78]. These patients are followed in the same manner as low-risk patients, with follow-up visits with the above studies every 3 months for the first 1 to 2 years, then visits every 4 months for the next 1 to 2 years, followed by visits every 6 months for 1 to 2 years, and yearly visits thereafter [78]. As for local recurrence surveillance, the cross-sectional imaging is omitted after 5 years, because most local recurrences appear within 5 years of initial treatment [78].

Gastrointestinal Stromal Tumors

Gastrointestinal stromal tumors are the most common mesenchymal tumors of the GI tract [79]. Previously, they were often designated smooth muscle tumors of the GI tract—specifically, GI LMS, leiomyoblastoma, LMS, and leiomyomas. Investigators discovered that GISTs express the KIT (CD-117) receptor tyrosine kinase and possibly originate from the interstitial cell of Cajal, the intestinal pacemaker cell responsible for peristalsis [80]. These tumors most commonly arise in the stomach (60%-70%), small intestine (20%-30%), colon and rectum (5%), and esophagus (<5%), although they can arise anywhere in the GI tract or omentum/peritoneum. The liver, peritoneum, and abdominal wall are the most common sites of metastatic disease; however, there are reports of associated central nervous system (CNS), lymph node, lung, and bone metastasis [81]. The incidence of GIST is equal in men and women; it generally peaks between the fourth and sixth decades of life, and patients are more commonly Caucasian. Presenting symptoms often represent the site of tumor origin but may be vague, including abdominal pain, anorexia, weight loss, and dyspepsia.

Historically, the mainstay of treatment for GIST was surgical resection. Conventional chemotherapy or radiotherapy has not been effective in the treatment of GIST. The identification of specific oncogenic driver mutations involving the c-KIT protein has led to the development and approval of multiple TKIs that have greatly improved the prognosis of patients with metastatic GIST. Previously, median overall survival was approximately 18 months. In the era of imatinib, this has improved to around 5 years [82].

Molecular profiling of patients with GIST has now become standard of care, as the mutational status has important implications in regard to diagnosis, prognosis, and guiding treatment decisions. Approximately 70% to 80% of GISTs harbor a *KIT* gene mutation, with another 5% to 8% with *PDGFRA* mutations, and the remaining 12% to 15% deemed wild-type GIST [83]. Wild-type GIST constitutes a heterogeneous grouping, with additional mutations identified in succinate dehydrogenase (*SDH*) and *BRAF* V600E, among others. Deletions in exon 11 are the most common *KIT* mutation and portend a more aggressive disease course with shorter overall survival and higher risk of recurrence. Internal tandem repeats involving exon 11, however, are associated with gastric GIST and tend to be more indolent. Exon 9 mutations have been associated with GIST of the small intestine and a clinically aggressive course. *PDGFRA* mutations can occur in multiple exons (12, 14, and 18) and are observed primarily in gastric GIST.

Imatinib mesylate, an oral TKI that selectively inhibits BCR-ABL, KIT, and PDGFR, is approved for adjuvant therapy and for unresectable/metastatic GIST. Early trials with imatinib showed objective response rates of 53% to 69% and significant improvement in 5-year overall survival of about 50% [82, 84]. These trial results led to two phase III trials (EORTC 62005 and Southwest Oncology Group [SWOG] S0033) that were designed to compare imatinib at two dose levels (400 mg/d vs 800 mg/d) ([85, 86]). In both studies, the higher dose arm failed to show a statistically significant difference in response or overall survival as compared to the once-daily dosing schedule. Gastrointestinal stromal tumors with exon 11 mutations are the most responsive to imatinib therapy, whereas those with exon 9 mutations tend to be more resistant. Patients with exon 9 mutations demonstrated shorter PFS and overall survival as compared to those with exon 11 mutations when treated with imatinib ([87]). Patients with exon 9 mutations may benefit from an increased dose of imatinib (800 mg daily). Patients with non-KIT non-PDGFRA mutated or wild-type GIST rarely show significant or sustained response to treatment. The optimal duration of imatinib therapy is not known. In one study, investigators randomized patients who had control of disease at 3 years with imatinib to either continue or discontinue treatment ([88]). The 2-year PFS was 80% in the continuous treatment cohort compared with 16% in the treatment interruption group. Relapse in the continuous treatment group was thus attributed to resistance.

Imatinib has also shown efficacy in the adjuvant setting ([89]). As in the metastatic setting, the optimal duration of adjuvant imatinib therapy has not been well established. A randomized trial comparing 1 year versus 3 years of adjuvant imatinib therapy for *KIT*-positive resected GIST showed benefit to longer duration of adjuvant therapy ([90]). Patients receiving 36 months of adjuvant imatinib had longer recurrence-free survival (5-year recurrence-free survival, 65.6% vs 47.9%; HR, 0.46; $P < .001$) and improved 5-year overall survival (92% vs 81.7%; HR, 0.45; $P = .02$). The benefit of extending therapy beyond 3 years is not known.

Approximately 10% of GIST patients have primary resistance to imatinib, with higher rates seen in exon 9 mutated and wild-type GIST. Secondary resistance is often due to new mutations in the *KIT* gene involving exon 13 or exon 17 ([91]). Sunitinib, a multikinase inhibitor that targets VEGF, appears to have activity in patients with primary resistance and secondary *KIT* mutations ([92, 93]). The overall objective response rate, however, was less than 10%. Several additional targeted therapies targeting the KIT and PDGFRA pathways have also been evaluated. Nilotinib, a second-generation TKI, was evaluated as third-line therapy following imatinib and sunitinib and showed a low response rate of 3% ([94]). Regorafenib, a multitargeted TKI, has shown better efficacy in patients after failure of both imatinib and sunitinib. In a phase II trial, an objective response rate of 12% and clinical benefit rate (PR or stable disease >16 weeks) of 79% were observed in patients, leading to a current phase III trial ([95]).

Response evaluation in GIST uses the Choi criteria rather than the standard RECIST measures used in most other solid tumors. Positron emission tomography imaging may also be used and was initially noted to show treatment response at an earlier time point compared to standard CT imaging ([12]). Certain molecular events, such as apoptosis, occur early on and may partially explain the rationale behind early PET response related to imatinib ([96]). Our institution also demonstrated that RECIST criteria may underestimate early tumor response seen in GIST. Patients who respond to imatinib clinically may show a decrease in tumor size and/or a decrease in tumor radiodensity by CT radiography (Fig. 42-3). Further analysis of patients treated with imatinib at MDACC revealed that, when tumor density is taken into account, sensitivity of CT imaging is comparable to PET response ([97, 98]). This data culminated in the development of the Choi criteria of response assessment (Table 42-5). These criteria have been prospectively validated and are considered in response assessment in current trials of GIST. It is our experience that decisions to discontinue therapy should not be based solely on CT radiography or PET imaging but instead should also take into consideration the patient's overall clinical condition.

In summary, the front-line therapy for patients with newly diagnosed, metastatic GIST is imatinib at 400 mg daily. Patients with exon 9 mutations should initiate therapy with imatinib at 800 mg daily. Imatinib should be continued indefinitely or until progression, as defined by Choi criteria. Computed tomography imaging is used to assess response initially at 2 months and then at 3-month intervals for at least the first 2 years. At the time of progression, we check the plasma imatinib level, and if tolerable, we increase the dose of imatinib to a total of 800 mg daily. If or when this strategy fails, we proceed to second-line therapy sunitinib and subsequent third-line therapy with regorafenib. For patients with isolated or resectable metastatic disease, surgery and/or

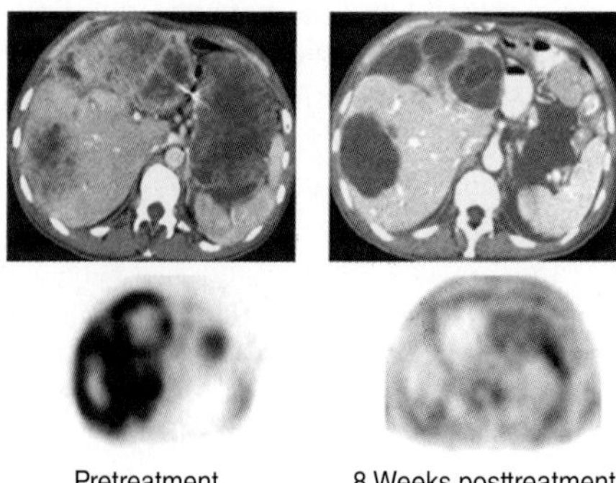

FIGURE 42-3 Gastrointestinal stromal tumor response to imatinib therapy on computed tomography and positron emission tomography imaging. (Used with permission from Dr. Haesun Choi, Department of Diagnostic Radiology, The University of Texas MD Anderson Cancer Center.)

Table 42-5 Choi Response Criteria

Response	Response Definition
Complete response (CR)	Disappearance of all disease No new lesions
Partial response (PR)	A decrease in size of >10% OR a decrease in CT density (HU) >15% No new lesions No obvious progression of nonmeasurable disease
Stable disease (SD)	Does not meet the criteria for CR, PR, or PD No symptomatic deterioration attributed to tumor progression
Progression of disease (PD)	An increase in unidimensional tumor size of >10% AND did not meet criteria for PR by CT density Any new lesions, including new tumor nodules in a previous cystic tumor

CT, computed tomography; HU, Hounsfield unit.

hepatic artery embolization or radiofrequency ablation is offered if feasible. For resectable GIST patients with high-risk features, such as a high mitotic count and/or large tumor size, adjuvant imatinib for at least 3 years should be administered to increase recurrence-free survival. The optimal duration of imatinib use in the adjuvant setting beyond 3 years remains unknown.

BONE SARCOMA

Bone sarcomas are rare tumors, making up less than 0.2% of all cancers. In 2013, an estimated 3,010 new cases of bone sarcomas were diagnosed in the United States, and 1,440 deaths were attributed to this group of diseases ([1]). The most common malignant tumor of bone is osteosarcoma followed by chondrosarcoma and then the Ewing sarcoma/primitive neuroectodermal tumor (PNET) family of tumors. Malignant fibrous histiocytoma, fibrosarcoma, chordoma, and giant cell tumor of bone are rare bone tumors and account for <5% of all primary malignant bone tumors. The Ewing sarcoma/PNET family of tumors tend to occur more frequently in children and adolescents, whereas osteosarcoma has a biphasic pattern of incidence that peaks in adolescents, with the growth of long bones, and in the elderly, with tumors arising in association with Paget disease or previously radiated tissues. Chondrosarcomas are usually seen in patients after the fifth decade of life, but they can also occur in younger patients, where the tumors tend to be of a higher grade malignancy. Features of common bone tumors are listed in Table 42-6.

Clinical Presentation

The clinical presentation of any bone tumor depends on its location. Most osteosarcomas arise in the metaphyseal region of long bones, specifically the distal femur, proximal tibia, and proximal humerus. Approximately 55% of osteosarcomas occur around the knee joint. Chondrosarcomas can also arise in any bone of the body; however, they generally occur in the pelvis and other flat bones. Ewing sarcoma/PNET tumors tend to occur in the diaphyseal portion of the long bones and in flat bones of the body (eg, the pelvis and scapula).

The most common presenting symptom is pain and swelling or a mass. Patients who have pelvic tumors may have neurologic impairment and severe pain, typically because these tumors are often not recognized until late in the disease course. In the case of Ewing

Table 42-6 Features of Common Bone Tumors

Type	Frequency	Age Distribution	Gender	Common Sites	Radiologic Features	Pathologic Features
Osteosarcoma	45%	10-20 years	M > F	Metaphysis	Sunburst calcifications	Spindle cells, osteoid matrix
MFH	8%	20-80 years	M > F	Long bones	Radiolucent with ill-defined margins	Pleomorphic spindle cells, NO osteoid
Chondrosarcoma	22%	20-80 years	M > F	Pelvis/shoulder girdles	Lobulated appearance	Lobules, chondroid matrix
Ewing/PNET	15%	10-20 years	F > M	Diaphyses	Lytic with soft tissue component	Small round blue cells

F, female; M, male; MFH, malignant fibrous histiocytoma; PNET, primitive neuroectodermal tumor.

CHAPTER 42

sarcoma, patients often present with constitutional symptoms of night sweats and fevers.

Evaluation

Evaluation of suspected bone sarcoma should begin with a careful history, physical examination, and routine laboratory tests, followed by imaging directed to the given complaint. The imaging of any bone tumor should begin with a plain film of the involved area. X-ray images are often helpful in the diagnosis of bone sarcomas; for example, osteosarcoma often has a "sunburst" appearance of calcification on x-ray imaging, which is virtually diagnostic (Fig. 42-4). The amount of calcification associated with osteosarcoma depends on the histologic subtype (eg, osteoblastic osteosarcoma usually has very dense calcification, whereas telangiectatic osteosarcoma is primarily lytic). Chondrosarcoma also has a distinct appearance on x-ray imaging, with destruction of the bone and endosteal scalloping of the bony cortex and a chondroid matrix, which appears lobulated (See Fig. 42-4). Ewing sarcoma has a typical "onion-skin" appearance on x-ray imaging (See Fig. 42-4). Additional initial imaging should include a CT scan and/or MRI of the primary lesion to further evaluate involvement of the neurovascular structures, surrounding soft tissues, and adjacent joints and to better evaluate any associated soft tissue mass.

Biopsy of bone sarcomas is critical to the diagnosis, and careful planning is essential. When patients are diagnosed with bone sarcoma or the diagnosis is suspected, it is important to have a multidisciplinary team approach with physicians who are experienced in the treatment of bone sarcomas. Core-needle biopsy has been shown to be accurate in making a diagnosis in up to 91% of cases ([99]). An open biopsy should be performed only when core-needle biopsy is nondiagnostic. Current guidelines recommend either a core or open biopsy to confirm the diagnosis prior to any surgical procedure. When surgery is ultimately performed, care should be taken to assure that the biopsy tract is completely resected.

Complete staging should include chest x-ray, CT scan of the chest, and bone scan to evaluate for metastatic disease. Chest imaging is warranted in all patients, because the most common site of metastasis from bone sarcoma is the lungs. A bone scan should be included in the workup for metastatic disease in patients with bone sarcoma to evaluate for distant bone metastases or skip metastases. For patients with Ewing sarcoma, an MRI of the spine should be performed, because there is a risk of bone marrow metastases. We do not routinely obtain bone marrow biopsy in the staging evaluation of Ewing sarcoma. Marrow involvement has been shown to highly correlate with bone metastasis ([100]).

Positron emission tomography/CT is being used more frequently in the initial diagnostic evaluation,

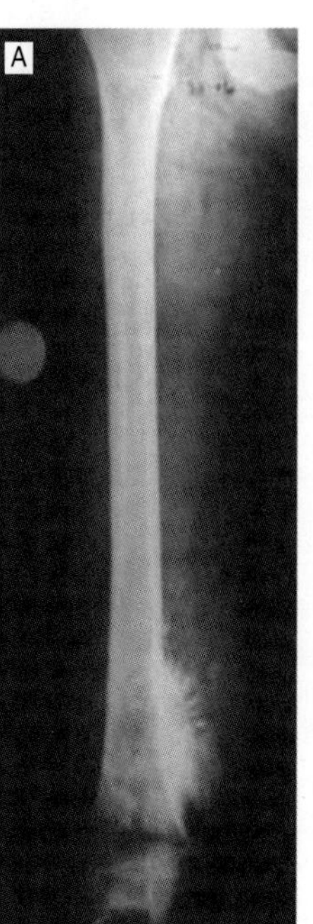

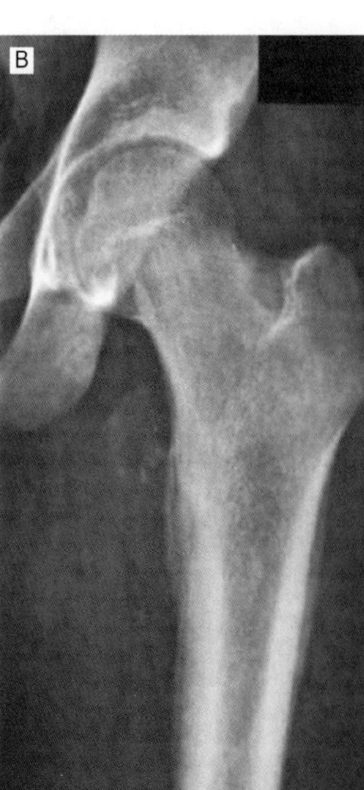

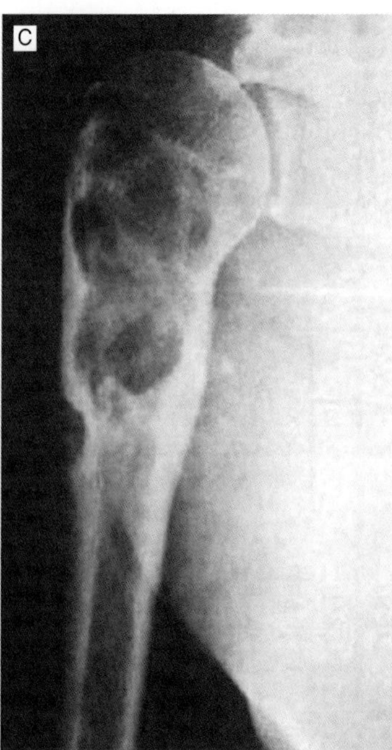

FIGURE 42-4 X-ray imaging of osteosarcoma, Ewing sarcoma, and chondrosarcoma. **A.** The typical "sunburst" appearance of osteosarcoma. **B.** The "onion-skin" appearance often seen in Ewing sarcoma. **C.** The lobulated appearance of chondrosarcoma.

staging, and response assessment for bone sarcomas. However, fluorodeoxyglucose (FDG) uptake alone is not adequate for characterization of primary bone tumors; morphologic evaluation is key ([101]). Positron emission tomography/CT imaging can also play an important role in response assessment because bone sarcomas do not demonstrate typical RECIST responses to chemotherapy (Fig. 42-5). Multiple studies have reported the utility of PET/CT in evaluating chemotherapy response in osteosarcoma and Ewing family tumors ([102, 103]). In one study of osteosarcoma, a 25% to 50% reduction of SUV following 1 week of neoadjuvant chemotherapy has been shown to correlate with >90% tumor necrosis on pathologic evaluation ([104]). At our center, we routinely use PET/CT in the evaluation and response assessment for osteosarcoma and Ewing family tumors.

Pathology

There are multiple histologic subtypes of bone sarcoma, with the most common cytogenetic and molecular aberrations summarized in Table 42-7. Osteosarcoma can be broken down into two major categories: conventional osteosarcoma and variant osteosarcoma (Fig. 42-6). Conventional osteosarcoma comprises approximately 60% to 75% of all osteosarcomas, whereas the 11 variants comprise the other 35% to 40% ([105]). Conventional osteosarcoma includes osteoblastic osteosarcoma, chondroblastic osteosarcoma, and fibroblastic osteosarcoma. These classifications are made based on the histologic features of the tumor, such as the amount of matrix present within the tumor and whether bone or cartilage is predominant. The classification of the osteosarcoma variants relies more on the clinical correlation, such as the site of disease (ie, jaw, skull, or pelvis), the setting in which the disease presents (ie, postradiation, Paget disease, multifocal, and retinoblastoma), and the morphology, such as telangiectatic, small cell, malignant fibrous histiocytoma (MFH) of bone, dedifferentiated chondrosarcoma, and surface lesions such as parosteal, periosteal, and high-grade surface osteosarcoma. High-grade osteosarcomas demonstrate significant genomic instability and therefore possess complex and heterogeneous chromosomal alterations. Copy number loss or gain in multiple chromosomes as well as amplifications in the *MDM2* gene, *CDK4*, *MYC*, and *VEGF* have been described. To date, sequencing of osteosarcomas has yet to identify effective molecular targets ([106]).

Malignant fibrous histiocytoma of bone is similar to MFH of soft tissue histologically and often appears to constitute the high-grade component of dedifferentiated chondrosarcoma. Malignant fibrous histiocytoma is thought to be part of a spectrum of osteosarcoma where the spindle cells do not produce osteoid visible by light microscopy; however, it may become possible to visualize these at some time in the future, especially following chemotherapy in responding tumors.

Chondrosarcomas are malignant tumors of bone characterized by cartilaginous proliferation. These tumors produce chondroid matrix and can arise from benign processes such as enchondroma. Chondrosarcoma is characterized by the permeation of cartilage into the bone marrow. This process is virtually pathognomonic for chondrosarcoma. Dedifferentiated chondrosarcoma is a unique subset of chondrosarcomas typified by a low-grade conventional chondrosarcoma juxtaposed with a high-grade soft tissue component. Several less common variants exist including mesenchymal chondrosarcoma and clear cell chondrosarcoma. Next-generation sequencing has identified somatic mutations in isocitrate dehydrogenase 1 and 2 (*IDH1/2*) in central conventional chondrosarcomas and dedifferentiated chondrosarcomas ([107]). This finding may aid in distinguishing chondrosarcoma from chondroblastic osteosarcoma and could serve as a unique therapeutic target ([108]).

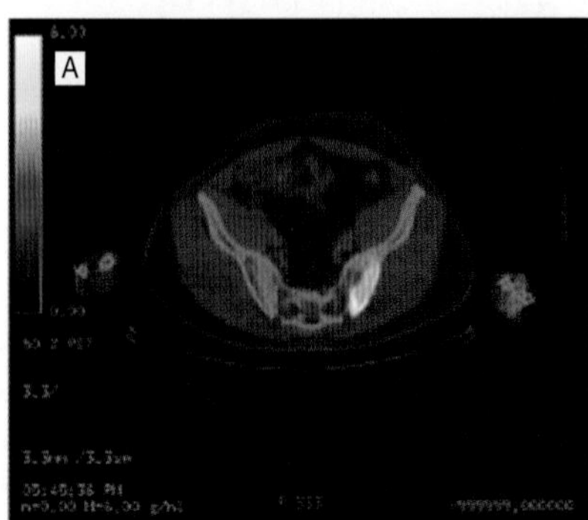

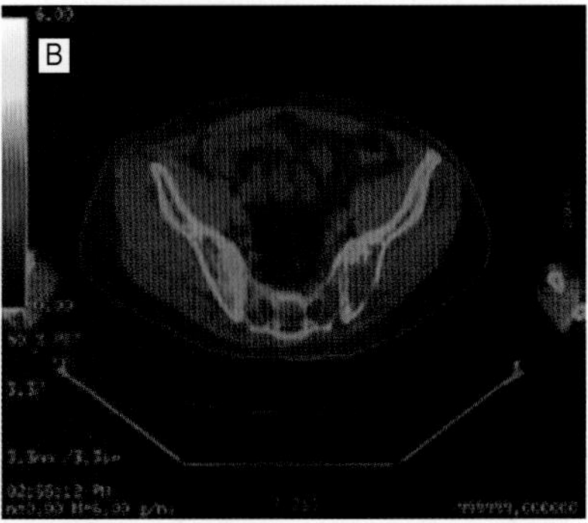

FIGURE 42-5 Osteosarcoma response assessment by positron emission tomography/computed tomography. Left ilium osteosarcoma (A) at baseline and (B) after treatment with extensive therapeutic effect and 99% tumor necrosis at resection. (Used with permission from Dr. Robert Benjamin, Department of Sarcoma Medical Oncology, The University of Texas MD Anderson Cancer Center.)

Table 42-7 Genetic Alterations in Bone Tissue Sarcomas

Tumor	Cytogenetic Abnormality	Gene Product
Aneurysmal bone cyst	t(16;17)(q22;p13) t(1;17)(p34.3;p13) t(3;17)(q21;p13) t(9;17)(q22;p13) t(17;17)(q21;p13)	*CDH11-USP6* *THRAP3-USP6* *CNBP-USP6* *OMD-USP6* *COL1A1-USP6*
Chondrosarcoma or chondroma		*IDH1* or *IDH2* Point mutation
Ewing sarcoma/PNET family	t(11;22)(q24;q12) t(21;22)(q22;q12) t(7;22)(p22;q12) t(2;22)(q33;q12) t(17;22)(q12;q12) inv(22)(q12;q12) t(16;21)(p11;q22)	*EWS1-FLI1* *EWS1-ERG* *EWSR1-ETV1* *EWSR1-FEV* *EWSR1-E1AF* *EWSR1-ZSG* *FUS-ERG*
Fibrous dysplasia	Activating oncogenic mutations	*GNAS1*
Mesenchymal chondrosarcoma	t(8;8)(q13;q21)	*HEY1-NCOA2*
Osteosarcoma, low-grade (parosteal and intramedullary)	12q14-15 (ring chromosomes, giant marker chromosomes)	Amplification of *CDK4, MDM2, HMGA2, GLI*, and *SAS*
Osteosarcoma		Multiple genetic aberrations

PNET, primitive neuroectodermal tumor.

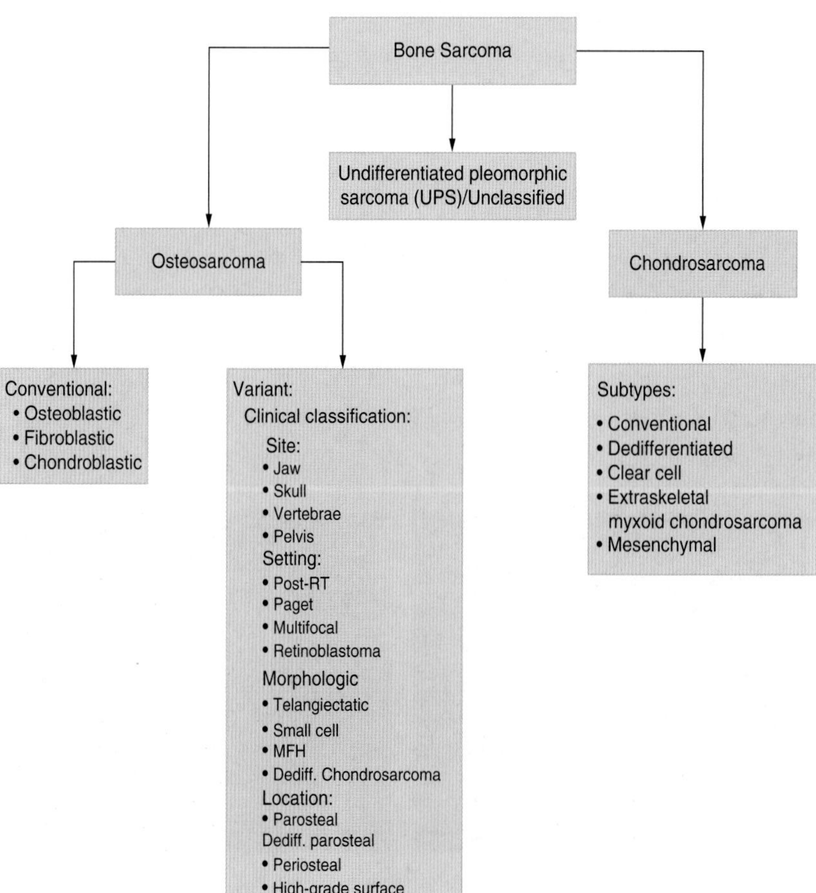

FIGURE 42-6 Pathologic classification of bone sarcomas. Dediff, dedifferentiated; MFH, malignant fibrous histiocytoma; RT, radiotherapy. (Visual Art: © 2015 the University of Texas MD Anderson Cancer Center).

Ewing sarcoma family of tumors (ESFT) represent a completely separate histology and are grouped with the PNETs due to their similarities in histology, immunohistochemical staining, and molecular genetics. This family of tumors includes Ewing tumors of bone, extraosseous Ewing tumors, PNETs, and Askin tumors (PNET of the chest wall). These tumors are often referred to as "small round blue cell tumors" because, under the microscope, the cells contain scanty cytoplasm and round to oval nuclei with fine chromatin that are tightly packed together. The ESFTs possess recurrent translocations involving the *EWS* gene, with identification of an *EWS* translocation considered pathognomonic in the diagnosis of ESFT. The translocation t(11;22)(q24;q12) *EWS-FLI-1* fusion was the first described and most common translocation. Several additional translocations have also been identified (see Table 42-7).

Bone sarcomas are classified as either high- or low-grade lesions, similar to the three-tier grading system of soft tissue sarcomas. Grading is an important factor that helps to determine the overall stage and prognosis. Finally, the pathologist should be provided with the diagnostic imaging and x-ray findings because these provide important information to assist in making a final diagnosis in bone sarcomas.

Staging and Prognosis

There are two widely accepted staging systems, that of the AJCC and that of the Musculoskeletal Tumor Society ([109, 110]). In a comparison of these systems, there was no significant difference between them, and neither had any notable advantage ([111]). At MDACC, instead of routinely using a staging system, we prefer to emphasize prognostic factors (eg, size of the primary, location and extent of bone involvement, soft tissue involvement, histologic grade, and presence or absence of distant metastases). The prognosis of patients with bone sarcomas largely depends on the specific histology, grade, location, and presence of metastatic disease. The most important and well-established prognostic factor for patients with bone sarcoma is the percentage of tumor necrosis achieved with preoperative chemotherapy.

Treatment

The treatment of bone sarcomas is best accomplished by a multidisciplinary team comprising medical oncologists, surgical oncologists, pathologists, and radiation oncologists working together to provide comprehensive care. The treatment required depends on the tumor type, location, and extent of disease. Treatment algorithms for high-grade bone sarcomas and Ewing sarcoma are show in Figs. 42-7 and 42-8.

Osteosarcoma

Osteosarcoma is the prototype of most other bone sarcomas. Chemotherapy is the mainstay of treatment for osteosarcoma, which is considered a systemic disease, because most patients have micrometastatic disease at presentation. This is evidenced by the historic long-term survival rate of <20% in patients treated with surgery alone as compared to the nearly 70% cure rate among patients with localized osteosarcoma of an extremity treated with aggressive combination chemotherapy followed by adjuvant surgery ([112]).

At MDACC, adolescent and adult patients with conventional high-grade osteosarcoma of an extremity receive treatment consisting of preoperative chemotherapy followed by limb-sparing surgery, followed by postoperative chemotherapy (see Fig. 42-7). The postoperative therapy is tailored based on the knowledge of the percent necrosis found in the pathologic specimen after surgery. This approach is based on a series of patients treated within our center in which tailored postoperative therapy demonstrated improved survival and differs from the current standard treatment of pediatric osteosarcoma ([113]).

The most active agents for the treatment of osteosarcoma are cisplatin, doxorubicin, ifosfamide, and high-dose methotrexate ([34]). Intra-arterial administration of cisplatin (120 mg/m^2) in combination with doxorubicin (90 mg/m^2 continuous infusion over 96 hours) given preoperatively has been studied by investigators at MDACC ([112]). Imaging of osteosarcoma has limited utility in response assessment; the percentage of tumor necrosis is the single most important predictor of long-term disease-free and overall survival ([114]). Generally, patients with ≥90% tumor necrosis after preoperative chemotherapy have a 5-year continuous disease-free survival of approximately 80% ([112]). The 5-year continuous disease-free survival of patients with <90% tumor necrosis after preoperative chemotherapy is significantly worse, ranging from 13% up to 67% depending on the postoperative chemotherapy regimen ([112]). To address this, we analyzed a consecutive series of 123 patients with osteosarcoma of the extremity treated within our center who were divided into three cohorts based on the time period in which they were treated and the postoperative chemotherapy given. All patients received preoperative doxorubicin and cisplatin induction. Patients received the sequential addition of high-dose methotrexate (8 g/m^2) and then methotrexate plus ifosfamide postoperatively in the second and third groups depending on the time period in which they were treated. Among patients with ≥90% tumor necrosis, relapse-free survival was

CHAPTER 42

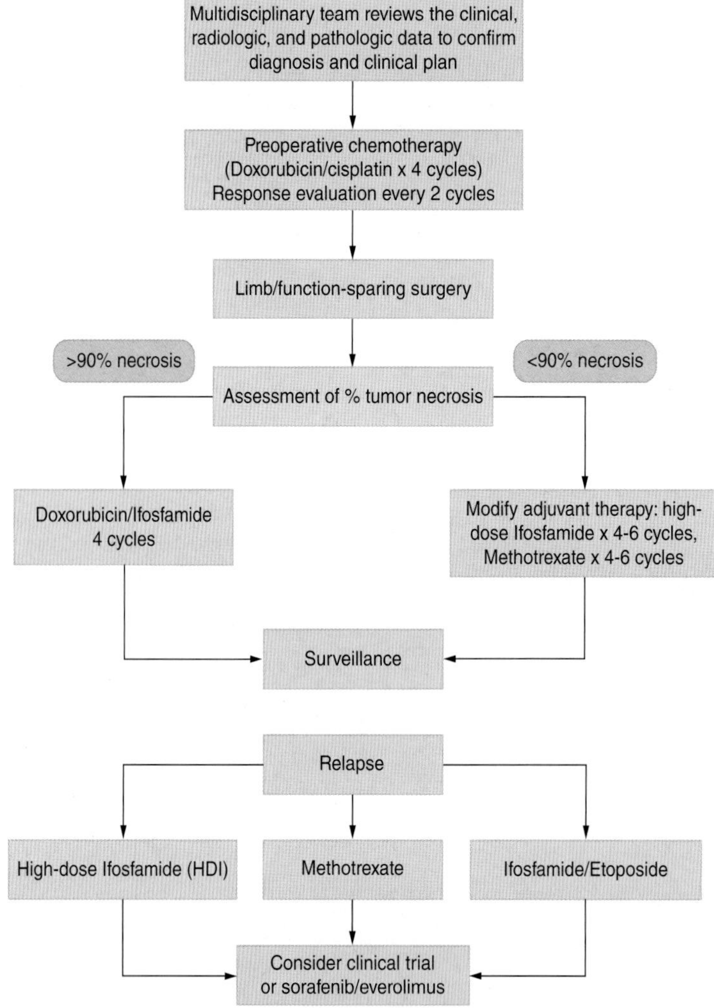

FIGURE 42-7 Treatment approach for high-grade primary bone sarcomas. (Visual Art: © 2015 the University of Texas MD Anderson Cancer Center).

not significantly different among the three groups. In patients with poor response, with <90% tumor necrosis, the addition of methotrexate and then methotrexate plus ifosfamide improved the 5-year relapse-free survival from 13% to 34% and 67%, respectively ([113]).

The role of postoperative switch therapy or intensified therapy among patients guided by histologic response to preoperative chemotherapy remains controversial. In the EURAMOS-1 study, 618 patients with high-grade osteosarcoma who received preoperative methotrexate, doxorubicin, and cisplatin (MAP) with ≥10% viable tumor at surgery were randomized 1:1 after surgery to receive either continuation of MAP or intensification with the addition of ifosfamide and etoposide to the same MAP backbone (MAPIE) ([115]). Intensification with MAPIE failed to show an advantage in terms of event-free survival (HR, 1.01) and overall survival (HR, 0.99) and was associated with additional toxicity at a median follow up of 4.5 years.

For patients who achieve ≥90% tumor necrosis with four cycles of doxorubicin and cisplatin preoperatively, we recommend four additional cycles of doxorubicin (75 mg/m^2) combined with ifosfamide (10 g/m^2). For those with <90% tumor necrosis after preoperative doxorubicin and cisplatin, we favor six cycles of high-dose ifosfamide and six cycles of high-dose methotrexate given sequentially.

Patients with high-grade osteosarcomas of other sites are treated in a similar fashion; however, their overall outcome appears to be worse than that of patients with extremity tumors. This may be due in part to poor sensitivity to the chemotherapy agents and also to difficulties in achieving a negative surgical margin of resection owing to anatomic constraints. Patients

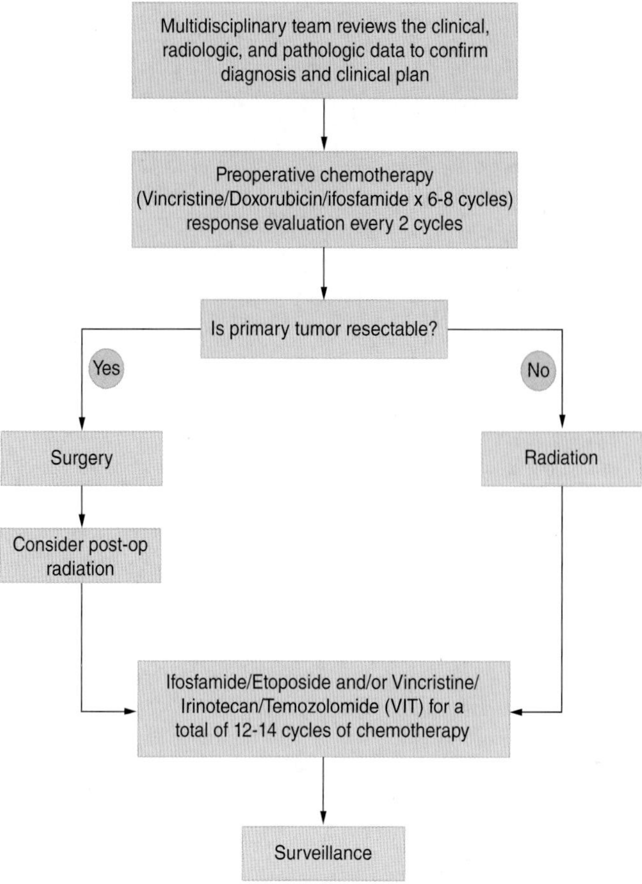

FIGURE 42-8 Treatment approach for patients with Ewing sarcoma/primitive neuroectodermal tumor and mesenchymal chondrosarcoma. (Visual Art: © 2015 the University of Texas MD Anderson Cancer Center).

with low-grade and variant osteosarcomas—such as well-differentiated intramedullary osteosarcoma or parosteal osteosarcoma and jaw osteosarcoma, typically arising in the mandible, which have a lower tendency to produce distant metastases—are treated with surgical resection with negative margins alone without routine use of adjuvant chemotherapy. If surgical resection with negative margins cannot be achieved in osteosarcoma of the jaw, preoperative chemotherapy should be considered. Patients with intermediate-grade periosteal osteosarcoma should also receive preoperative chemotherapy.

Malignant fibrous histiocytoma of bone is treated according to the same basic principles as conventional osteosarcoma. Studies performed at MDACC showed that with preoperative doxorubicin and cisplatin, approximately 50% of the patients with localized MFH of bone had percent tumor necrosis of ≥90% ([116]). The median survival was 23 months for all patients who received this preoperative regimen, with the patients who achieved ≥90% having a median survival of 66 months and patients with <90% necrosis having a median survival of 20 months. The European Osteosarcoma Intergroup had similar results in studies using doxorubicin and cisplatin preoperatively and postoperatively, with 5-year PFS and overall survival rates of 56% and 59%, respectively ([117]).

Extraskeletal osteosarcomas, chondrosarcomas, and Ewing sarcomas are treated in a similar fashion as soft tissue sarcomas. In our experience at the MDACC, extraskeletal osteosarcomas are not as responsive to chemotherapy as osseous osteosarcomas and do not respond to cisplatin or high-dose methotrexate, unlike their skeletal counterparts ([118]).

Metastatic and Recurrent Disease

Approximately 10% to 20% of patients with osteosarcoma present with metastatic disease. Lung is the most common site of metastasis in osteosarcoma; however, osteosarcoma can also metastasize to almost any bone in the body. Lymph node metastases are rare. Patients who have resectable pulmonary metastases are treated with curative intent with primary chemotherapy, as described earlier, followed by surgical resection of all lesions either at the same time or in staged operations. With this approach, patients have a 15% to 30% chance of long-term disease-free survival and potential cure. Patients with bone metastasis have a poorer prognosis, with therapy usually directed at palliation.

Relapse is seen in about 30% of patients presenting with localized disease and up to 80% of patients who present with primary metastatic disease. Patients with relapsed or recurrent disease are approached similarly to patients with primary metastatic disease with chemotherapy and/or resection when possible. Several agents have demonstrated some activity in relapsed or refractory osteosarcoma including gemcitabine alone or in combination with docetaxel; ifosfamide or cyclophosphamide in combination with etoposide; as well as others. Targeted therapies are under investigation in osteosarcoma. The multikinase inhibitor sorafenib demonstrated benefit in a phase II trial of relapsed osteosarcoma, with a PFS of 46% at 4 months and clinical benefit rate of 29% ([119]). Subsequently, a phase II trial of sorafenib and everolimus demonstrated 45% PFS at 6 months, but failed to meet its prespecified end point of 50% PFS at 6 months ([120]).

Chondrosarcoma

Chondrosarcomas are resistant to most chemotherapeutic agents used for the treatment of bone sarcomas. Surgical resection is the primary treatment modality, regardless of the grade of the tumor. Conventional chondrosarcoma patients with unresectable/metastatic disease should be enrolled onto clinical trials, and genomic profiling should be considered for potential target identification. Unlike other chondrosarcoma subtypes, mesenchymal chondrosarcoma and dedifferentiated chondrosarcoma should be treated with multimodality therapy.

Dedifferentiated chondrosarcoma is associated with low-grade chondrosarcoma, and foci of high-grade soft tissue sarcoma may resemble osteosarcoma of MFH of bone and are often thought of as variants of osteosarcoma ([121]). These tumors can respond to doxorubicin/cisplatin-based chemotherapy and are treated in the same manner as conventional osteosarcomas ([122]), although tumor necrosis at resection is less than optimal compared to conventional chondrosarcomas. Patients with refractory/recurrent disease should be considered for clinical trials and molecular testing. Approximately 60% of dedifferentiated chondrosarcomas harbor mutations in the *IDH1* gene, which makes IDH oncometabolite inhibitors an attractive option to consider ([123]). Mesenchymal chondrosarcomas are a rare variant that present in the jaw, spinal column, and ribs with lytic lesions on x-ray. The histology consists of a bimorphic appearance of benign to low-grade cartilaginous components with poorly differentiated small cell components ([124]). The majority of these tumors harbor a unique *HEY1-NCOA2* fusion, which is thought to affect Notch signaling ([125]). Mesenchymal chondrosarcomas do respond to chemotherapy; a recent series of 54 patients with localized disease treated with combination chemotherapy demonstrated a reduced risk of fracture (HR, 0.482; 95% CI, 0.213-0.996; $P = .046$) and death (HR, 0.445; 95% CI, 0.256-0.774; $P = .004$) ([126]). This disease is treated in a similar fashion as Ewing sarcoma, discussed in the next section. In our experience, responsive tumors typically exhibit more calcification with an associated decrease in FDG avidity (when PET/CT is used for response assessment), and they are less apt to show decreases in tumor size, as opposed to Ewing sarcomas, which typically exhibit dramatic tumor size reduction. This makes RECIST a less reliable tool for adequate response assessment of mesenchymal chondrosarcoma.

Ewing Sarcoma

Like osteosarcoma, Ewing sarcoma and the PNET family of tumors are treated primarily with chemotherapy prior to surgery, because patients with localized disease most likely have occult metastasis at the time of diagnosis. These tumors are extremely responsive to the following chemotherapeutic agents: doxorubicin, dactinomycin, ifosfamide, cyclophosphamide, vincristine, and etoposide. The most commonly used combinations are vincristine, doxorubicin, and cyclophosphamide (VAC); ifosfamide and etoposide (IE); and vincristine, doxorubicin, and ifosfamide (VAI). Multiple trials have shown that with these combinations of chemotherapy, survival rates greater than 50% can be achieved ([127, 128]). At MDACC, we usually give vincristine (up to 2 mg) with doxorubicin (75-90 mg/m^2) and ifosfamide (10 g/m^2) as our preoperative chemotherapy regimen. This is followed by surgical resection, if possible, or radiation therapy. Ewing sarcoma is very radiosensitive; often, when surgical resection is not an option or positive margins remain, consolidative radiation therapy is used. Studies show good survival results in patients who have consolidative radiation therapy when needed ([129]). After definitive resection, tumor necrosis is assessed and postoperative therapy modified as needed (see Fig. 42-8). A recent retrospective review of 66 patients from our institution treated with chemotherapy and R0 resection identified histologic response (necrosis ≤95%), radiographic response by RECIST, and metastasis to be independent predictors of outcome ([130]). Based on these data, additional study is needed to determine the role of adjuvant radiation in patients with poor histologic response after preoperative chemotherapy and R0 resection.

Metastatic/Recurrent Disease

Metastatic or recurrent Ewing sarcoma is treated in a similar manner as metastatic or recurrent disease in osteosarcoma. Patients who have metastatic disease in their lungs at the time of presentation are treated as outlined earlier, with curative intent. Patients with recurrent or metastatic disease after primary therapy are treated on the basis of their disease-free interval. If there is a long interval (>12 months), a retrial of previous chemotherapeutic regimens, preferably at higher dose intensity (eg, high-dose ifosfamide), is reasonable. For patients with a shorter interval between therapy and recurrence or metastasis, investigational therapies are appropriate.

Targeted therapy for metastatic ESFT has recently focused on inhibition of the insulin-like growth factor 1 receptor (IGF1R). This tyrosine kinase receptor is expressed on the cell surface of Ewing sarcoma cells and is thought to play a key role in the pathogenesis of Ewing sarcoma ([131]). Single-agent studies with IGF1R antibodies have only shown modest activity, with objective response rates ranging from 6% to 14% ([132, 133]). To date, efforts focused on targeting the *ETS* tumor-specific gene fusions have been unsuccessful.

Giant Cell Tumor of Bone

Giant cell tumor of bone is another rare primary tumor of bone. Although considered benign, these tumors have a propensity for local recurrence to metastasize to lung. Tumors most commonly involve the epiphyses of long bones and usually result in pain, swelling, and decreased range of motion. Giant cell tumors appear as lytic, eccentrically located lesions in the epiphyses of a long bone on x-ray imaging. The primary treatment of giant cell tumors of bone consists of surgical intervention, either wide excision or intralesional curettage and cementation. Radiation therapy can be used as primary treatment or following surgery and has been shown to improve local control and disease-free survival, but has also been associated with an increased risk of malignant transformation ([134]). When the primary location precludes surgical resection due to morbidity or patients develop distant metastatic disease, consideration is given to systemic therapy ([135]). At MDACC, we have previously treated patients with interferon α-2b therapy with either 3 million units subcutaneously every day for 6 to 12 months or 10 million units subcutaneously every Monday, Wednesday, and Friday for 6 to 12 months ([136]). Clinicians should be aware, however, that these tumors respond gradually and can even grow initially on treatment and that often responses are not fully appreciated until after interferon therapy has been completed. More recently, denosumab, an antibody to the RANK ligand, which inhibits osteoclastic function and increases calcification, has been shown to improve pain in patients with recurrent or metastatic giant cell tumor. In a phase II study of denosumab in unresectable or recurrent giant cell tumor, treatment with denosumab resulted in tumor response in 86% of evaluable patients (defined as elimination of >90% of giant cells or no radiographic progression of target lesion for up to 25 weeks) ([135]). For patients with unresectable disease, we currently employ a combination of embolization, interferon, and denosumab on a case-by-case basis.

Follow-Up Management

Regular and long-term follow-up is essential. Patients are followed at MDACC with x-rays and physical examination every 3 months for the first 2 years, every 4 months for the next 2 years, every 6 months for the next 2 years, and then yearly thereafter. Surveillance includes high-quality chest imaging with either chest x-ray or chest CT in high-risk patients, plain films of the primary tumor site to evaluate for recurrence and stability of any prosthesis, and routine laboratories. Bone scans and/or PET/CT scans are useful in patients with specific symptoms or history of bony metastasis. Monitoring should also include an assessment of the potential late effects of chemotherapy including anthracycline-induced cardiomyopathy, nephrotoxicity, neuropathy, and secondary malignancies.

REFERENCES

1. Siegel R, Naishadham D, Jemal A. Cancer statistics, 2013. *CA Cancer J Clin*. 2013;63(1):11-30.
2. Zahm SH, Fraumeni JF Jr. The epidemiology of soft tissue sarcoma. *Semin Oncol*. 1997;24(5):504-514.
3. Helman LJ, Meltzer P. Mechanisms of sarcoma development. *Nat Rev Cancer*. 2003;3(9):685-694.
4. Sandberg AA, Bridge JA. Updates on the cytogenetics and molecular genetics of bone and soft tissue tumors: osteosarcoma and related tumors. *Cancer Genet Cytogenet*. 2003;145(1):1-30.
5. Coindre JM, Pelmus M, Hostein I, Lussan C, Bui BN, Guillou L. Should molecular testing be required for diagnosing synovial sarcoma? A prospective study of 204 cases. *Cancer*. 2003;98(12):2700-2707.
6. Mertens F, Antonescu CR, Hohenberger P, et al. Translocation-related sarcomas. *Semin Oncol*. 2009;36(4):312-323.
7. de Alava E, Kawai A, Healey JH, et al. EWS-FLI1 fusion transcript structure is an independent determinant of prognosis in Ewing's sarcoma. *J Clin Oncol*. 1998;16(4):1248-1255.
8. van Doorninck JA, Ji L, Schaub B, et al. Current treatment protocols have eliminated the prognostic advantage of type 1 fusions in Ewing sarcoma: a report from the Children's Oncology Group. *J Clin Oncol*. 2010;28(12):1989-1994.
9. Stegmaier S, Poremba C, Schaefer KL, et al. Prognostic value

of PAX–FKHR fusion status in alveolar rhabdomyosarcoma: a report from the cooperative soft tissue sarcoma study group (CWS). *Pediatr Blood Cancer*. 2011;57(3):406-414.
10. Grimer R, Judson I, Peake D, Seddon B. Guidelines for the management of soft tissue sarcomas. *Sarcoma*. 2010;2010:506182.
11. Folpe AL, Lyles RH, Sprouse JT, Conrad EU 3rd, Eary JF. (F-18) fluorodeoxyglucose positron emission tomography as a predictor of pathologic grade and other prognostic variables in bone and soft tissue sarcoma. *Clin Cancer Res*. 2000;6(4):1279-1287.
12. Van den Abbeele AD, Badawi RD. Use of positron emission tomography in oncology and its potential role to assess response to imatinib mesylate therapy in gastrointestinal stromal tumors (GISTs). *Eur J Cancer*. 2002;38(Suppl 5):S60-S65.
13. Herrmann K, Benz MR, Czernin J, et al. 18F-FDG-PET/CT imaging as an early survival predictor in patients with primary high-grade soft tissue sarcomas undergoing neoadjuvant therapy. *Clin Cancer Res*. 2012;18(7):2024-2031.
14. Schwartz HS, Spengler DM. Needle tract recurrences after closed biopsy for sarcoma: three cases and review of the literature. *Ann Surg Oncol*. 1997;4(3):228-236.
15. Kilpatrick SE, Cappellari JO, Bos GD, Gold SH, Ward WG. Is fine-needle aspiration biopsy a practical alternative to open biopsy for the primary diagnosis of sarcoma? Experience with 140 patients. *Am J Clin Pathol*. 2001;115(1):59-68.
16. Doyle LA. Sarcoma classification: an update based on the 2013 World Health Organization Classification of tumors of soft tissue and bone. *Cancer*. 2014;120(12):1763-1774.
17. Pisters PW, Leung DH, Woodruff J, Shi W, Brennan MF. Analysis of prognostic factors in 1,041 patients with localized soft tissue sarcomas of the extremities. *J Clin Oncol*. 1996;14(5):1679-1689.
18. Green FL, Page DL, Fleming ID, et al. Soft tissue sarcoma. In: *AJCC Cancer Staging Handbook*. 6th ed. Philadelphia: Lippincott-Raven; 2002:221-228.
19. Kattan MW, Leung DH, Brennan MF. Postoperative nomogram for 12-year sarcoma-specific death. *J Clin Oncol*. 2002;20(3):791-796.
20. Coindre JM, Terrier P, Guillou L, et al. Predictive value of grade for metastasis development in the main histologic types of adult soft tissue sarcomas. *Cancer*. 2001;91(10):1914-1926.
21. Kotilingam D, Lev DC, Lazar AJ, Pollock RE. Staging soft tissue sarcoma: evolution and change. *CA Cancer J Clin*. 2006;56(5):282-291.
22. Behranwala KA, A'Hern R, Omar AM, Thomas JM. Prognosis of lymph node metastasis in soft tissue sarcoma. *Ann Surg Oncol*. 2004;11(7):714-719.
23. Williard WC, Collin C, Casper ES, Hajdu SI, Brennan MF. The changing role of amputation for soft tissue sarcoma of the extremity in adults. *Surg Gynecol Obstet*. 1992;175(5):389-396.
24. Rosenberg SA, Tepper J, Glatstein E, et al. The treatment of soft-tissue sarcomas of the extremities: prospective randomized evaluations of (1) limb-sparing surgery plus radiation therapy compared with amputation and (2) the role of adjuvant chemotherapy. *Ann Surg*. 1982;196(3):305-315.
25. Zagars GK, Ballo MT, Pisters PW, Pollock RE, Patel SR, Benjamin RS. Preoperative vs. postoperative radiation therapy for soft tissue sarcoma: a retrospective comparative evaluation of disease outcome. *Int J Radiat Oncol Biol Phys*. 2003;56(2):482-488.
26. Pollack A, Zagars GK, Goswitz MS, Pollock RA, Feig BW, Pisters PW. Preoperative vs. postoperative radiotherapy in the treatment of soft tissue sarcomas: a matter of presentation. *Int J Radiat Oncol Biol Phys*. 1998;42(3):563-572.
27. Sadoski C, Suit HD, Rosenberg A, Mankin H, Efird J. Preoperative radiation, surgical margins, and local control of extremity sarcomas of soft tissues. *J Surg Oncol*. 1993;52(4):223-230.
28. Alektiar KM, Velasco J, Zelefsky MJ, Woodruff JM, Lewis JJ, Brennan MF. Adjuvant radiotherapy for margin-positive high-grade soft tissue sarcoma of the extremity. *Int J Radiat Oncol Biol Phys*. 2000;48(4):1051-1058.
29. Folkert MR, Singer S, Brennan MF, et al. Comparison of local recurrence with conventional and intensity-modulated radiation therapy for primary soft-tissue sarcomas of the extremity. *J Clin Oncol*. 2014;32(29):3236-3241.
30. von Mehren M, Randall RL, Benjamin RS, et al. Soft Tissue Sarcoma, Version 2.2014. *J Natl Compr Canc Netw*. 2014;12(4):473-483.
31. Slater JD, McNeese MD, Peters LJ. Radiation therapy for unresectable soft tissue sarcomas. *Int J Radiat Oncol Biol Phys*. 1986;12(10):1729-1734.
32. Sleijfer S, Ouali M, van Glabbeke M, et al. Prognostic and predictive factors for outcome to first-line ifosfamide-containing chemotherapy for adult patients with advanced soft tissue sarcomas: an exploratory, retrospective analysis on large series from the European Organization for Research and Treatment of Cancer-Soft Tissue and Bone Sarcoma Group (EORTC-STBSG). *Eur J Cancer*. 2010;46(1):72-83.
33. O'Bryan RM, Baker LH, Gottlieb JE, et al. Dose response evaluation of adriamycin in human neoplasia. *Cancer*. 1977;39(5):1940-1948.
34. Patel SR, Vadhan-Raj S, Papadopolous N, et al. High-dose ifosfamide in bone and soft tissue sarcomas: results of phase II and pilot studies—dose-response and schedule dependence. *J Clin Oncol*. 1997;15(6):2378-2384.
35. Benjamin RS, Legha SS, Patel SR, Nicaise C. Single-agent ifosfamide studies in sarcomas of soft tissue and bone: the M.D. Anderson experience. *Cancer Chemother Pharmacol*. 1993;31(Suppl 2):S174-179.
36. Patel SR, Vadhan-Raj S, Burgess MA, et al. Results of two consecutive trials of dose-intensive chemotherapy with doxorubicin and ifosfamide in patients with sarcomas. *Am J Clin Oncol*. 1998;21(3):317-321.
37. Patel SR. *Dose Intensive Chemotherapy for Soft Tissue Sarcoma*. Alexandria, VA: Lippincott Williams & Wilkins; 2000.
38. Judson I, Verweij J, Gelderblom H, et al. Doxorubicin alone versus intensified doxorubicin plus ifosfamide for first-line treatment of advanced or metastatic soft-tissue sarcoma: a randomised controlled phase 3 trial. *Lancet Oncol*. 2014;15(4):415-423.
39. Elias A, Ryan L, Sulkes A, Collins J, Aisner J, Antman KH. Response to mesna, doxorubicin, ifosfamide, and dacarbazine in 108 patients with metastatic or unresectable sarcoma and no prior chemotherapy. *J Clin Oncol*. 1989;7(9):1208-1216.
40. Vadhan-Raj S, Patel S, Burgess MA, et al. Phase II trial of adriamycin (A), ifosfamide (I), mesna (M) uroprotection, dacarbazine (D)(MAID) with PIXY321 (GM-CSF/IL-3 fusion protein) of G-CSF in patients (PTS) with soft tissue sarcoma (STS) [abstract]. *Proc Am Soc Clin Oncol*. 1996:525.
41. Bitz U, Pink D, Busemann C, Reichardt P. Doxorubicin (Doxo) and dacarbacin (DTIC) as first-line therapy for patients (pts) with locally advanced or metastatic leiomyosarcoma (LMS) and liposarcoma (LPS) [abstract]. *J Clin Oncol*. 2011;29(15 suppl):10094.
42. Patel SR, Gandhi V, Jenkins J, et al. Phase II clinical investigation of gemcitabine in advanced soft tissue sarcomas and window evaluation of dose rate on gemcitabine triphosphate accumulation. *J Clin Oncol*. 2001;19(15):3483-3489.
43. Maki RG, Wathen JK, Patel SR, et al. Randomized phase II study of gemcitabine and docetaxel compared with gemcitabine alone in patients with metastatic soft tissue sarcomas: results of sarcoma alliance for research through collaboration study 002 [corrected]. *J Clin Oncol*. 2007;25(19):2755-2763.
44. Di Giandomenico S, Frapolli R, Bello E, et al. Mode of action of trabectedin in myxoid liposarcomas. *Oncogene*. 2014;33(44):5201-5210.

45. Grosso F, Jones RL, Demetri GD, et al. Efficacy of trabectedin (ecteinascidin-743) in advanced pretreated myxoid liposarcomas: a retrospective study. *Lancet Oncol.* 2007;8(7):595-602.
46. Le Cesne A, Blay J-Y, Judson I, et al. Phase II study of ET-743 in advanced soft tissue sarcomas: a European Organisation for the Research and Treatment of Cancer (EORTC) soft tissue and bone sarcoma group trial. *J Clin Oncol.* 2005;23(3):576-584.
47. Cesne AL, Cresta S, Maki RG, et al. A retrospective analysis of antitumour activity with trabectedin in translocation-related sarcomas. *Eur J Cancer.* 2012;48(16):3036-3044.
48. Pervaiz N, Colterjohn N, Farrokhyar F, Tozer R, Figueredo A, Ghert M. A systematic meta-analysis of randomized controlled trials of adjuvant chemotherapy for localized resectable soft-tissue sarcoma. *Cancer.* 2008;113(3):573-581.
49. Woll PJ, Reichardt P, Le Cesne A, et al. Adjuvant chemotherapy with doxorubicin, ifosfamide, and lenograstim for resected soft-tissue sarcoma (EORTC 62931): a multicentre randomised controlled trial. *Lancet Oncol.* 2012;13(10):1045-1054.
50. Sleijfer S, Ray-Coquard I, Papai Z, et al. Pazopanib, a multikinase angiogenesis inhibitor, in patients with relapsed or refractory advanced soft tissue sarcoma: a phase II study from the European Organisation for Research and Treatment of Cancer–Soft Tissue and Bone Sarcoma Group (EORTC study 62043). *J Clin Oncol.* 2009;27(19):3126-3132.
51. van der Graaf WT, Blay J-Y, Chawla SP, et al. Pazopanib for metastatic soft-tissue sarcoma (PALETTE): a randomised, double-blind, placebo-controlled phase 3 trial. *Lancet.* 2012;379(9829):1879-1886.
52. Mentzel T, Beham A, Calonje E, Katenkamp D, Fletcher CD. Epithelioid hemangioendothelioma of skin and soft tissues: clinicopathologic and immunohistochemical study of 30 cases. *Am J Surg Pathol.* 1997;21(4):363-374.
53. Agulnik M, Yarber JL, Okuno SH, et al. An open-label, multicenter, phase II study of bevacizumab for the treatment of angiosarcoma and epithelioid hemangioendotheliomas. *Ann Oncol.* 2013;24(1):257-263.
54. Ray-Coquard I, Italiano A, Bompas E, et al. Sorafenib for patients with advanced angiosarcoma: a phase II Trial from the French Sarcoma Group (GSF/GETO). *Oncologist.* 2012;17(2):260-266.
55. Kayler LK, Merion RM, Arenas JD, et al. Epithelioid hemangioendothelioma of the liver disseminated to the peritoneum treated with liver transplantation and interferon alpha-2B. *Transplantation.* 2002;74(1):128-130.
56. Torres KE, Ravi V, Kin K, et al. Long-term outcomes in patients with radiation-associated angiosarcomas of the breast following surgery and radiotherapy for breast cancer. *Ann Surg Oncol.* 2013;20(4):1267-1274.
57. Italiano A, Cioffi A, Penel N, et al. Comparison of doxorubicin and weekly paclitaxel efficacy in metastatic angiosarcomas. *Cancer.* 2012;118(13):3330-3336.
58. Skubitz KM, Haddad PA. Paclitaxel and pegylated-liposomal doxorubicin are both active in angiosarcoma. *Cancer.* 2005;104(2):361-366.
59. Fury MG, Antonescu CR, Van Zee KJ, Brennan MF, Maki RG. A 14-year retrospective review of angiosarcoma: clinical characteristics, prognostic factors, and treatment outcomes with surgery and chemotherapy. *Cancer J.* 2005;11(3):241-247.
60. Penel N, Bui BN, Bay JO, et al. Phase II trial of weekly paclitaxel for unresectable angiosarcoma: the ANGIOTAX Study. *J Clin Oncol.* 2008;26(32):5269-5274.
61. Fata F, O'Reilly E, Ilson D, et al. Paclitaxel in the treatment of patients with angiosarcoma of the scalp or face. *Cancer.* 1999;86(10):2034-2037.
62. Stacchiotti S, Palassini E, Sanfilippo R, et al. Gemcitabine in advanced angiosarcoma: a retrospective case series analysis from the Italian Rare Cancer Network. *Ann Oncol.* 2012;23(2):501-508.
63. Lu HJ, Chen PC, Yen CC, et al. Refractory cutaneous angiosarcoma successfully treated with sunitinib. *Br J Dermatol.* 2013;169(1):204-206.
64. Maki RG, D'Adamo DR, Keohan ML, et al. Phase II study of sorafenib in patients with metastatic or recurrent sarcomas. *J Clin Oncol.* 2009;27(19):3133-3140.
65. Farid M, Ong WS, Tan MH, et al. The influence of primary site on outcomes in leiomyosarcoma: a review of clinicopathologic differences between uterine and extrauterine disease. *Am J Clin Oncol.* 2013;36(4):368-374.
66. Sleijfer S, Ouali M, van Glabbeke M, et al. Prognostic and predictive factors for outcome to first-line ifosfamide-containing chemotherapy for adult patients with advanced soft tissue sarcomas: an exploratory, retrospective analysis on large series from the European Organization for Research and Treatment of Cancer-Soft Tissue and Bone Sarcoma Group (EORTC-STBSG). *Eur J Cancer.* 2010;46(1):72-83.
67. Pautier P, Floquet A, Penel N, et al. Randomized multicenter and stratified phase II study of gemcitabine alone versus gemcitabine and docetaxel in patients with metastatic or relapsed leiomyosarcomas: a Federation Nationale des Centres de Lutte Contre le Cancer (FNCLCC) French Sarcoma Group Study (TAXOGEM study). *Oncologist.* 2012;17(9):1213-1220.
68. O'Cearbhaill R, Zhou Q, Iasonos A, et al. Treatment of advanced uterine leiomyosarcoma with aromatase inhibitors. *Gynecol Oncol.* 2010;116(3):424-429.
69. Kilpatrick SE, Doyon J, Choong PF, Sim FH, Nascimento AG. The clinicopathologic spectrum of myxoid and round cell liposarcoma. A study of 95 cases. *Cancer.* 1996;77(8):1450-1458.
70. Forni C, Minuzzo M, Virdis E, et al. Trabectedin (ET-743) promotes differentiation in myxoid liposarcoma tumors. *Mol Cancer Ther.* 2009;8(2):449-457.
71. Perez-Losada J, Pintado B, Gutierrez-Adan A, et al. The chimeric FUS/TLS-CHOP fusion protein specifically induces liposarcomas in transgenic mice. *Oncogene.* 2000;19(20):2413-2422.
72. Riggi N, Cironi L, Provero P, et al. Expression of the FUS-CHOP fusion protein in primary mesenchymal progenitor cells gives rise to a model of myxoid liposarcoma. *Cancer Res.* 2006;66(14):7016-7023.
73. Le Cesne A, Blay JY, Judson I, et al. Phase II study of ET-743 in advanced soft tissue sarcomas: a European Organisation for the Research and Treatment of Cancer (EORTC) soft tissue and bone sarcoma group trial. *J Clin Oncol.* 2005;23(3):576-584.
74. Italiano A, Toulmonde M, Cioffi A, et al. Advanced well-differentiated/dedifferentiated liposarcomas: role of chemotherapy and survival. *Ann Oncol.* 2012;23(6):1601-1607.
75. Portera CA Jr, Ho V, Patel SR, et al. Alveolar soft part sarcoma. *Cancer.* 2001;91(3):585-591.
76. Kummar S, Allen D, Monks A, et al. Cediranib for metastatic alveolar soft part sarcoma. *J Clin Oncol.* 2013;31(18):2296-2302.
77. Stacchiotti S, Negri T, Zaffaroni N, et al. Sunitinib in advanced alveolar soft part sarcoma: evidence of a direct antitumor effect. *Ann Oncol.* 2011;22(7):1682-1690.
78. Patel SR, Zagars GK, Pisters PW. The follow-up of adult soft-tissue sarcomas. *Semin Oncol.* 2003;30(3):413-416.
79. Fletcher CD, Berman JJ, Corless C, et al. Diagnosis of gastrointestinal stromal tumors: a consensus approach. *Hum Pathol.* 2002;33(5):459-465.
80. Kindblom LG, Remotti HE, Aldenborg F, Meis-Kindblom JM. Gastrointestinal pacemaker cell tumor (GIPACT): gastrointestinal stromal tumors show phenotypic characteristics of the interstitial cells of Cajal. *Am J Pathol.* 1998;152(5):1259-1269.
81. DeMatteo RP, Lewis JJ, Leung D, Mudan SS, Woodruff JM, Brennan MF. Two hundred gastrointestinal stromal tumors: recurrence patterns and prognostic factors for survival. *Ann Surg.* 2000;231(1):51-58.

82. Blanke CD, Demetri GD, von Mehren M, et al. Long-term results from a randomized phase II trial of standard- versus higher-dose imatinib mesylate for patients with unresectable or metastatic gastrointestinal stromal tumors expressing KIT. *J Clin Oncol*. 2008;26(4):620-625.
83. Corless CL, Barnett CM, Heinrich MC. Gastrointestinal stromal tumours: origin and molecular oncology. *Nat Rev Cancer*. 2011;11(12):865-878.
84. Demetri GD, von Mehren M, Blanke CD, et al. Efficacy and safety of imatinib mesylate in advanced gastrointestinal stromal tumors. *N Engl J Med*. 2002;347(7):472-480.
85. Verweij J, Casali PG, Zalcberg J, et al. Progression-free survival in gastrointestinal stromal tumours with high-dose imatinib: randomised trial. *Lancet*. 2004;364(9440):1127-1134.
86. Blanke CD, Rankin C, Demetri GD, et al. Phase III randomized, intergroup trial assessing imatinib mesylate at two dose levels in patients with unresectable or metastatic gastrointestinal stromal tumors expressing the kit receptor tyrosine kinase: S0033. *J Clin Oncol*. 2008;26(4):626-632.
87. Heinrich MC, Owzar K, Corless CL, et al. Correlation of kinase genotype and clinical outcome in the North American Intergroup Phase III Trial of imatinib mesylate for treatment of advanced gastrointestinal stromal tumor: CALGB 150105 Study by Cancer and Leukemia Group B and Southwest Oncology Group. *J Clin Oncol*. 2008;26(33):5360-5367.
88. Le Cesne A, Ray-Coquard I, Bui BN, et al. Discontinuation of imatinib in patients with advanced gastrointestinal stromal tumours after 3 years of treatment: an open-label multicentre randomised phase 3 trial. *Lancet Oncol*. 2010;11(10):942-949.
89. Dematteo RP, Ballman KV, Antonescu CR, et al. Adjuvant imatinib mesylate after resection of localised, primary gastrointestinal stromal tumour: a randomised, double-blind, placebo-controlled trial. *Lancet*. 2009;373(9669):1097-1104.
90. Joensuu H, Eriksson M, Hall KS, et al. One vs three years of adjuvant imatinib for operable gastrointestinal stromal tumor: a randomized trial. *JAMA*. 2012;307(12):1265-1272.
91. Antonescu CR, Besmer P, Guo T, et al. Acquired resistance to imatinib in gastrointestinal stromal tumor occurs through secondary gene mutation. *Clin Cancer Res*. 2005;11(11):4182-4190.
92. Demetri GD, van Oosterom AT, Garrett CR, et al. Efficacy and safety of sunitinib in patients with advanced gastrointestinal stromal tumour after failure of imatinib: a randomised controlled trial. *Lancet*. 2006;368(9544):1329-1338.
93. Heinrich MC, Maki RG, Corless CL, et al. Primary and secondary kinase genotypes correlate with the biological and clinical activity of sunitinib in imatinib-resistant gastrointestinal stromal tumor. *J Clin Oncol*. 2008;26(33):5352-5359.
94. Sawaki A, Nishida T, Yamada Y, et al. Phase 2 study of nilotinib as third-line therapy for patients with gastrointestinal stromal tumor. *Cancer*. 2011;117(20):4633-4641.
95. George S, Wang Q, Heinrich MC, et al. Efficacy and safety of regorafenib in patients with metastatic and/or unresectable GI stromal tumor after failure of imatinib and sunitinib: a multicenter phase II trial. *J Clin Oncol*. 2012;30(19):2401-2407.
96. McAuliffe JC, Hunt KK, Lazar AJ, et al. A randomized, phase II study of preoperative plus postoperative imatinib in GIST: evidence of rapid radiographic response and temporal induction of tumor cell apoptosis. *Ann Surg Oncol*. 2009;16(4):910-919.
97. Choi H, Charnsangavej C, Faria SC, et al. Correlation of computed tomography and positron emission tomography in patients with metastatic gastrointestinal stromal tumor treated at a single institution with imatinib mesylate: proposal of new computed tomography response criteria. *J Clin Oncol*. 2007;25(13):1753-1759.
98. Benjamin RS, Choi H, Macapinlac HA, et al. We should desist using RECIST, at least in GIST. *J Clin Oncol*. 2007;25(13):1760-1764.
99. Adams SC, Potter BK, Pitcher DJ, Temple HT. Office-based core needle biopsy of bone and soft tissue malignancies: an accurate alternative to open biopsy with infrequent complications. *Clin Orthop Relat Res*. 2010;468(10):2774-2780.
100. Kopp LM, Hu C, Rozo B, et al. Utility of bone marrow aspiration and biopsy in initial staging of Ewing sarcoma. *Pediatr Blood Cancer*. 2015;62(1):12-15.
101. Costelloe CM, Chuang HH, Madewell JE. FDG PET/CT of primary bone tumors. *Am J Roentgenol*. 2014;202(6):W521-W531.
102. Hawkins DS, Conrad EU, Butrynski JE, Schuetze SM, Eary JF. [F18] fluorodeoxy-D-glucose–positron emission tomography response is associated with outcome for extremity osteosarcoma in children and young adults. *Cancer*. 2009;115(15):3519-3525.
103. Hawkins DS, Schuetze SM, Butrynski JE, et al. [18F] Fluorodeoxyglucose positron emission tomography predicts outcome for Ewing sarcoma family of tumors. *J Clin Oncol*. 2005;23(34):8828-8834.
104. Brenner W, Bohuslavizki KH, Eary JF. PET imaging of osteosarcoma. *J Nucl Med*. 2003;44(6):930-942.
105. National Comprehensive Cancer Network. Bone cancer. *NCCN Clinical Practice Guidelines in Oncology*. 2010. Available at: http://www.nccn.org/professionals/physician_gls/f_guidelines.asp. Accessed October 20, 2015.
106. Martin JW, Squire JA, Zielenska M. The genetics of osteosarcoma. *Sarcoma*. 2012;2012:627254.
107. Amary MF, Bacsi K, Maggiani F, et al. IDH1 and IDH2 mutations are frequent events in central chondrosarcoma and central and periosteal chondromas but not in other mesenchymal tumours. *J Pathol*. 2011;224(3):334-343.
108. Kerr DA, Lopez HU, Deshpande V, et al. Molecular distinction of chondrosarcoma from chondroblastic osteosarcoma through IDH1/2 mutations. *Am J Surg Pathol*. 2013;37(6):787-795.
109. Enneking WF, Spanier SS, Goodman MA. A system for the surgical staging of musculoskeletal sarcoma. *Clin Orthop Relat Res*. 1980;153:106-120.
110. Green FL, Page DL, Fleming ID, et al. Bone. In: *AJCC Cancer Staging Handbook*. 6th ed. New York: Springer-Verlag; 2002:213-319.
111. Heck RK Jr, Stacy GS, Flaherty MJ, Montag AG, Peabody TD, Simon MA. A comparison study of staging systems for bone sarcomas. *Clin Orthop Relat Res*. 2003;415:64-71.
112. Jaffe N, Patel SR, Benjamin RS. Chemotherapy in osteosarcoma. Basis for application and antagonism to implementation; early controversies surrounding its implementation. *Hematol Oncol Clin North Am*. 1995;9(4):825-840.
113. Benjamin RS, Patel SR. Pediatric and adult osteosarcoma: comparisons and contrasts in presentation and therapy. *Cancer Treat Res*. 2009;152:355-363.
114. Raymond AK, Chawla SP, Carrasco CH, et al. Osteosarcoma chemotherapy effect: a prognostic factor. *Semin Diagn Pathol*. 1987;4(3):212-236.
115. Marina N, Smeland S, Bielack S, et al. MAPIE vs MAP as postoperative chemotherapy in patients with a poor response to preoperative chemotherapy for newly-diagnosed osteosarcoma: results from EURAMOS-1 (Paper 032). 2014. Available at: http://discovery.ucl.ac.uk/1453874/.
116. Patel SR, Armen T, Carrasco CH, et al. Primary chemotherapy in malignant fibrous histiocytoma of bone. In: Banzet P, Holland J, Khayat D, eds. *U.T.M.D. Anderson Cancer Center Experience*. Houston, TX: MDACC; 1994:577-580.
117. Bramwell VH, Steward WP, Nooij M, et al. Neoadjuvant chemotherapy with doxorubicin and cisplatin in malignant fibrous histiocytoma of bone: a European Osteosarcoma Intergroup study. *J Clin Oncol*. 1999;17(10):3260-3269.
118. Ahmad SA, Patel SR, Ballo MT, et al. Extraosseous osteosarcoma: response to treatment and long-term outcome. *J Clin*

Oncol. 2002;20(2):521-527.
119. Grignani G, Palmerini E, Dileo P, et al. A phase II trial of sorafenib in relapsed and unresectable high-grade osteosarcoma after failure of standard multimodal therapy: an Italian Sarcoma Group study. *Ann Oncol.* 2012;23(2):508-516.
120. Grignani G, Palmerini E, Ferraresi V, et al. Sorafenib and everolimus for patients with unresectable high-grade osteosarcoma progressing after standard treatment: a non-randomised phase 2 clinical trial. *Lancet Oncol.* 2015;16(1):98-107.
121. Frassica FJ, Unni KK, Beabout JW, Sim FH. Dedifferentiated chondrosarcoma. A report of the clinicopathological features and treatment of seventy-eight cases. *J Bone Joint Surg Am.* 1986;68(8):1197-1205.
122. Benjamin RS, Chu P, Patel SR, et al. De-differentiated chondrosarcoma: a treatable disease [abstract]. *Proc Am Assoc Cancer Res.* 1995;36:243.
123. Schaap FG, French PJ, Bovée JV. Mutations in the isocitrate dehydrogenase genes IDH1 and IDH2 in tumors. *Adv Anat Pathol.* 2013;20(1):32-38.
124. Nakashima Y, Unni KK, Shives TC, Swee RG, Dahlin DC. Mesenchymal chondrosarcoma of bone and soft tissue. A review of 111 cases. *Cancer.* 1986;57(12):2444-2453.
125. Wang L, Motoi T, Khanin R, et al. Identification of a novel, recurrent HEY1-NCOA2 fusion in mesenchymal chondrosarcoma based on a genome-wide screen of exon-level expression data. *Genes Chromosomes Cancer.* 2012;51(2):127-139.
126. Frezza AM, Cesari M, Baumhoer D, et al. Mesenchymal chondrosarcoma: Prognostic factors and outcome in 113 patients. A European Musculoskeletal Oncology Society study. *Eur J Cancer.* 2015;51(3):374-381.
127. Paulussen M, Ahrens S, Dunst J, et al. Localized Ewing tumor of bone: final results of the cooperative Ewing's Sarcoma Study CESS 86. *J Clin Oncol.* 2001;19(6):1818-1829.
128. Rosito P, Mancini AF, Rondelli R, et al. Italian Cooperative Study for the treatment of children and young adults with localized Ewing sarcoma of bone: a preliminary report of 6 years of experience. *Cancer.* 1999;86(3):421-428.
129. Dunst J, Schuck A. Role of radiotherapy in Ewing tumors. *Pediatr Blood Cancer.* 2004;42(5):465-470.
130. Pan HY, Morani A, Wang W-L, et al. Prognostic factors and patterns of relapse in Ewing sarcoma patients treated with chemotherapy and R0 resection. *Int J Radiat Oncol Biol Phys.* 2015;92(2):349-357.
131. Ludwig JA. Ewing sarcoma: historical perspectives, current state-of-the-art, and opportunities for targeted therapy in the future. *Curr Opin Oncol.* 2008;20(4):412-418.
132. Pappo AS, Patel SR, Crowley J, et al. R1507, a monoclonal antibody to the insulin-like growth factor 1 receptor, in patients with recurrent or refractory Ewing sarcoma family of tumors: results of a phase II Sarcoma Alliance for Research through Collaboration study. *J Clin Oncol.* 2011;29(34):4541-4547.
133. Tap WD, Demetri G, Barnette P, et al. Phase II study of ganitumab, a fully human anti–type-1 insulin-like growth factor receptor antibody, in patients with metastatic Ewing family tumors or desmoplastic small round cell tumors. *J Clin Oncol.* 2012;30(15):1849-1856.
134. Bhatia S, Miszczyk L, Roelandts M, et al. Radiotherapy for marginally resected, unresectable or recurrent giant cell tumor of the bone: a rare cancer network study. *Rare Tumors.* 2011;3(4):e48.
135. Thomas D, Henshaw R, Skubitz K, et al. Denosumab in patients with giant-cell tumour of bone: an open-label, phase 2 study. *Lancet Oncol.* 2010;11(3):275-280.
136. Benjamin RS, Patel SR, Gutterman JU, et al. Interferon alpha-2b as anti-angiogenesis therapy of giant cell tumor of bone: implications for the study of newer angiogenesis-inhibitors [abstract]. *Proc Am Soc Clin Oncol.* 1999:548a1999.

SECTION XII

Other Tumors

Section Editors: Michael Fisch and John de Groot

第十二篇 其他肿瘤

43

Endocrine Malignancies

第四十三章　内分泌恶性肿瘤

Lily Kwatampora
Steven P. Weitzman
Mouhammed A. Habra
Naifa L. Busaidy

中文导读

本章重点介绍了包括甲状腺癌、甲状旁腺癌、嗜铬细胞瘤、副神经节瘤及肾上腺皮质癌在内的内分泌肿瘤。甲状腺癌是最常见的内分泌恶性肿瘤，在美国的发病率最高。首先介绍良恶性孤立甲状腺结节的诊断流程，并根据不同病理类型分节描述甲状腺癌。分化型甲状腺癌约占所有甲状腺癌的90%，除介绍疾病危险因素、发病机制、诊断分期外，着重阐述包括手术、放射性核素治疗、激素治疗、放疗等治疗策略，并对随访进行建议。在晚期分化型甲状腺癌中，强调综合治疗的重要性。并简单介绍了儿童分化型甲状腺癌。对于髓样癌，重点介绍诊治流程，治疗首选手术，高危患者可行放疗，晚期疾病以靶向治疗为主。未分化癌预后极差，主要行姑息治疗，推荐手术、放疗、化疗及靶向治疗，建议患者参加临床试验。甲状旁腺癌较罕见，临床常出现高钙血症，推荐进行多学科会诊。嗜铬细胞瘤和副神经节瘤是一类罕见疾病，主要来源于肾上腺髓质及交感或副交感神经节。临床症状以高血压常见，严重时可出现心血管休克，甚至死亡。确诊需要生化检测，并结合影像学检查。此类疾病常与多种家族综合征相关，因此建议行基因检测。在血压控制良好的情况下，手术为首选治疗。恶性嗜铬细胞瘤的治疗则包括手术、放疗、射频消融及化疗。肾上腺皮质癌同样罕见，多发生于白种人，预后较差。需行激素检测、影像学、病理学及基因检测进行诊断。治疗方式包括手术和化疗，放疗及射频消融的使用尚有争议。

THYROID CANCER

Introduction

Thyroid cancer is the most common endocrine malignancy. It has the highest incidence in the United States and is increasing worldwide. In 2014, approximately 63,000 new cases of thyroid carcinoma were diagnosed in the United States, accounting for 4% of all new malignant disease. Three of four all new thyroid cancer diagnoses are made in women, corresponding to the threefold higher rates seen in women between 2007 and 2011 ([1]). Thyroid cancer occurs less frequently in children compared to adults, with a peak incidence of around 50 years. Despite this, overall long-term survival remains favorable ([2]). Histologic types (Table 43-1) include those that derive from the follicular epithelial cells (papillary and follicular), which account for the majority of thyroid cancers, and from the parafollicular C cells (medullary) ([2]). Other thyroid tumors, including primary lymphomas of the thyroid, which are usually metastases from other primary sites, are also encountered, although rarely.

EVALUATION OF SOLITARY THYROID NODULES

Introduction

Thyroid cancer usually presents as a nodule identified on physical examination or discovered incidentally on imaging studies performed for unrelated reasons. However, most thyroid nodules are benign, with about 10% to 15% found to be malignant on biopsy ([3]). The main diagnostic challenge is accurately differentiating benign from malignant disease in order to ensure appropriate definitive therapy and avoid unnecessary treatments.

Diagnosis

Clinically palpable nodules are found in approximately 5% of the population ([4]). Benign and malignant nodules are almost always clinically indistinguishable. Features indicating increased likelihood of carcinoma are summarized in Table 43-2. Initial evaluation and management of patients presenting with thyroid nodules is detailed in Fig. 43-1.

Thyroid ultrasonography with fine-needle aspiration (FNA) and cytologic examination is the modality of choice for evaluating nodules with suspicious characteristics ([5]). Papillary, medullary, and anaplastic carcinomas can be readily diagnosed by FNA or biopsy, but distinguishing benign from malignant follicular lesions proves more difficult. Histologic examination showing capsular or vascular invasion is necessary to classify a lesion as malignant. Because follicular adenoma and carcinoma cannot be differentiated cytologically, they are grouped as "indeterminate or suspicious follicular neoplasms." The rate of carcinoma for suspicious follicular neoplasms is about 20%. The incidence of malignancy increases with larger nodule size, male sex, and increasing age. Testing for molecular markers should be considered for patients with indeterminate or suspicious follicular neoplasm on cytology. Fifteen to 25% of the time, the FNA will yield "inadequate diagnostic material," and this necessitates repeat aspiration. The majority (85%-95%) of thyroid nodules are benign. Radionuclide scans usually show malignant lesions as hypofunctioning or "cold," although 85% of "cold" nodules are still benign.

DIFFERENTIATED THYROID CANCER

Introduction

Differentiated thyroid cancer (DTC) includes papillary, follicular, and poorly differentiated histology types and composes about 90% of all thyroid cancers ([6]). The factors associated with increased risk of thyroid carcinoma are summarized in Table 43-3.

Traditionally, exposure to ionizing radiation, family history, and genetic syndromes have been the main risks associated with DTC ([7,8]). However, a recent meta-analysis of 21 observational studies suggests an association with obesity (adjusted relative risk [RR], 1.33; 95% confidence interval [CI], 1.24-1.42) ([9]). On average, thyroid tumors are recognized ten years following radiation exposure, but can be seen as long as 30 years. Malignancy occurs in up to 30% of cases with head or neck irradiation. Exposure to external sources of radiation after the Chernobyl nuclear accident led to a 3- to 75-fold increase in the incidence of papillary thyroid carcinoma (PTC) in fallout regions, especially in younger children ([7]). Familial PTC is reported in 5% of all patients with PTC and may portend a more aggressive disease course ([9a]). Additionally, DTC has also been associated with other tumors, particularly breast and renal cancer ([10]).

Pathogenesis

Understanding the follicular cell tumorigenesis pathways is central to the development of novel therapies to treat thyroid cancer. The MAPK pathway is the main oncogenic propagator of PTC. *BRAF* and *Ras* genes in this pathway normally code for growth and function in normal and tumor cells. Chromosomal rearrangements of the gene encoding the transmembrane tyrosine kinase receptors ret and trk have been implicated as an early step in the development of these

Table 43-1 Types of Thyroid Cancer

Type	Frequency	Prognosis (10-year overall survival)
Originating from follicular cells		
Papillary	80%	93%
Follicular	11%	85%
Hürthle cell	3%	76%
Anaplastic (undifferentiated)	2%	14%
Originating from C cells		
Medullary	4%	75%

Data from Hundahl SA, Fleming ID, Fremgen AM, Menck HR. A National Cancer Data Base report on 53,856 cases of thyroid carcinoma treated in the U.S., 1985-1995. *Cancer.* 1998;83(12):2638-2648.

Table 43-2 Clinical Features Associated With Increased Risk of Malignancy

Age <20 years
Presence of cervical lymphadenopathy
History of radiation to the head and neck during childhood
Family history of medullary thyroid cancer or MEN types 2A and 2B
Hard fixed nodule
Recent nodule growth
Hoarseness of voice (indicating invasion of recurrent laryngeal nerve)

MEN, multiple endocrine neoplasia.

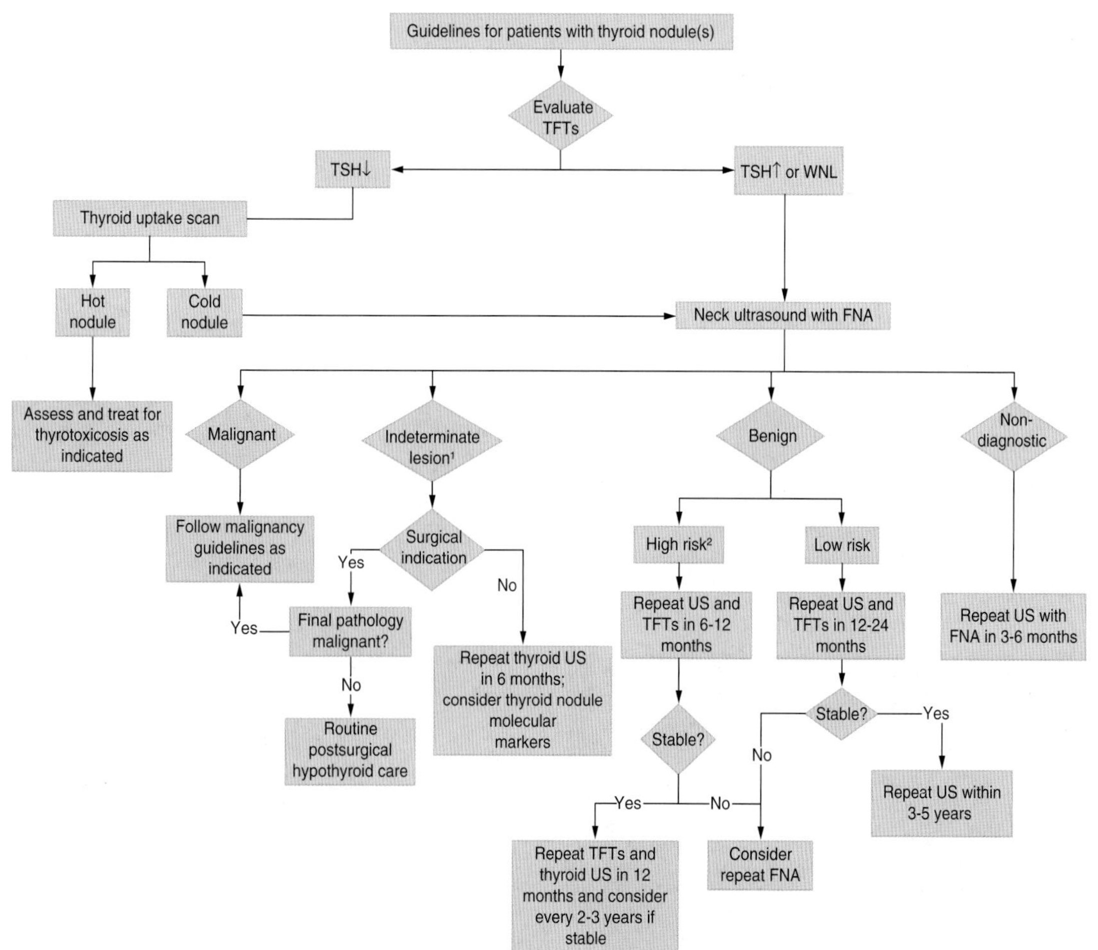

[1]Includes: suspicious for papillary, follicular neoplasm or lesion, Hürthle cell neoplasm, or lesion or atyptical cells of undetermined significance.
[2]History of radiation exposure to the head and neck or family history of thyroid cancer.

FIGURE 43-1 Evaluation of thyroid nodules. FNA, fine-needle aspiration; TFT, thyroid function test; TSH, thyroid-stimulating hormone; US, ultrasound; WNL, within normal limits.

Table 43-3 Risk Factors Associated With Differentiated Thyroid Carcinoma

Exposure to ionizing radiation, especially during childhood
Familial adenomatous polyposis (Gardner syndrome)
Carney complex
Werner syndrome
Cowden syndrome (phosphatase and tensin homolog [PTEN]-hamartoma tumor syndrome)
Pendred syndrome
Familial papillary thyroid cancer

Data from Nose V. Familial follicular cell tumors: classification and morphological characteristics. *Endocr Pathol.* 2010;21(4):219-226; and Ivanov VK, Kashcheev VV, Chekin SY, et al. Radiation-epidemiological studies of thyroid cancer incidence in Russia after the Chernobyl accident (estimation of radiation risks, 1991-2008 follow-up period). *Radiat Prot Dosimetry.* 2012;151(3):489-499.

tumors. Mutations in either *BRAF* (40%-60%) or *Ras* (10%-15%) or *RET/PTC* rearrangements (10%-15%) are present in most DTCs ([11, 12]) (Fig. 43-2)

Activating *ret* mutations may be the result of ionizing radiation and were the most common mutations found in the Chernobyl radiation-induced thyroid carcinomas ([13, 14]). *BRAF* mutation has been implicated in more aggressive disease and greater mortality from PTC ([15]). In addition, when present in combination with *BRAF*, a recent novel driver, telomerase reverse transcriptase (*TERT*) mutation, which is implicated in advanced thyroid cancer, results in the most aggressive PTC with the highest recurrence rate ([16, 17]). Of follicular thyroid cancers, 30% are driven by Pax8-peroxisome proliferator-activating receptor (*PPAR*)-γ rearrangements, and 10% to 15% are driven by *Ras* mutations ([12]).

Thyroid tumors are dependent upon angiogenesis, which is important for tumor cell growth, promotion and development of metastases ([18]). Vascular endothelial growth factor (VEGF), an important proangiogenic factor, binds to VEGF receptors. This then activates MAP-kinase signalling and promotes further tumor growth. Vascular endothelial growth factor receptors play a contributory role in the development and progression of thyroid cancer ([11]).

Diagnosis

Thyroid cancer is subdivided into well-differentiated neoplasms characterized by slow growth and high curability and a small group of poorly differentiated tumors with poor outcome. There are four major sub-types of thyroid cancer which are based on morphology and biological behavior. This classification is advantageous as it relates morphology to methods of treatment and prognosis.

Histologic characteristics of conventional PTCs include numerous papillae lined by cuboidal to low columnar follicular cells with enlarged irregular nuclei with longitudinal grooves, intranuclear cytoplasmic pseudoinclusions, and solitary or multiple marginally placed micronucleoli ([19]) (Fig. 43-3). Follicular variant of PTC and other PTC variants are also recognized. Follicular tumors, although frequently encapsulated, can exhibit vascular and capsular invasion microscopically; it is this invasion that, when identified histopathologically, distinguishes benign neoplasms from malignant follicular neoplasms (Fig. 43-4). Hürthle cell carcinomas are considered a type of follicular cancer. Tall cell variants, columnar cell variants, Hürthle cell variant, and insular type are histologic subtypes that may portend a worse prognosis.

Staging

The TNM (tumor, node, metastasis) method may be most useful for prediction of disease-free survival and is generally used in our institution. Tumor size and presence of extrathyroidal invasion carry prognostic

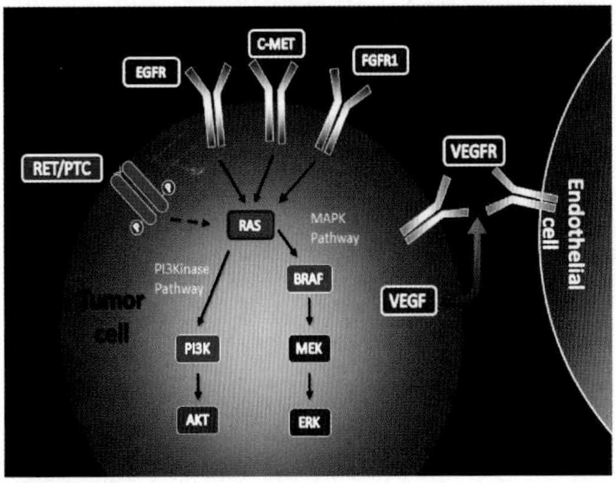

FIGURE 43-2 Tumorigenesis of thyroid cancer. Image courtesy of Dr. Steven I. Sherman.

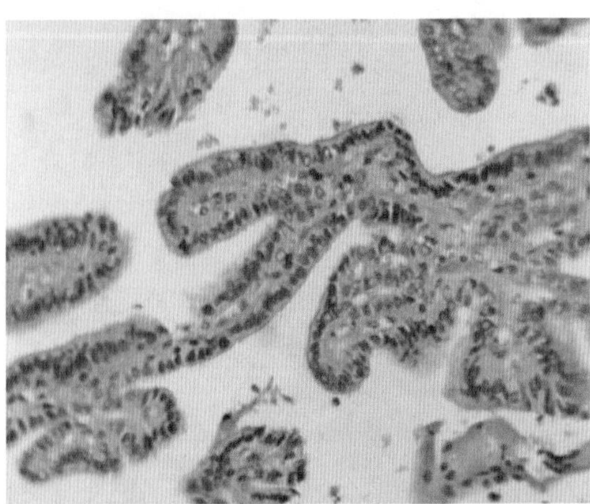

FIGURE 43-3 Classic histology for papillary thyroid carcinoma.

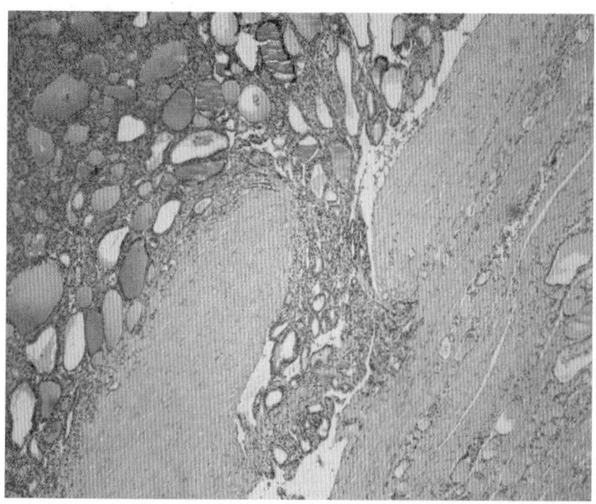

FIGURE 43-4 Follicular carcinoma with invasion of capsule. Capsular and vascular invasion distinguish benign neoplasms from carcinoma.

importance and thus should consistently be included in the pathologist's synoptic report. Anaplastic thyroid carcinoma by convention is always stage IV (Tables 43-4 and 43-5).

Management

Surgical Management

Preoperative ultrasound of the entire neck (not just of the thyroid) is indicated to help identify the presence of nodal metastases and help the surgeon to perform the appropriate surgery. Total thyroidectomy is the preferred initial surgical procedure for most patients with DTC at our institution (Fig. 43-5). Arguments for total thyroidectomy rather than lobectomy are that: (1) papillary foci are seen in bilateral lobes in 60% to 85% of patients ([20]) and (2) 5% to 10% of recurrences of PTC after a unilateral lobectomy arise in the contralateral lobe ([21]). A third reason that supports total thyroidectomy is that treatment with radioiodine and the specificity of serum thyroglobulin (Tg) concentrations as a tumor marker become most efficacious.

Consideration for lobectomy is reasonable in patients with no or low risk with localized small tumors ([5]). Neck dissection should be performed on patients with identifiable nodal disease, because their presence impacts recurrence. Calcium and parathyroid hormone levels should be monitored postoperatively due to the risk of hypoparathyroidism from either vascular damage intraoperatively or inadvertent removal.

Postoperative Iodine-131 Therapy (Radioactive Iodine Treatment)

Iodine-131 (^{131}I) is used as adjuvant therapy for thyroid carcinoma; iodine is preferentially taken up and trapped by the thyroid follicular cells and malignant counterparts. Iodine-131 destroys cells of follicular origin by first becoming concentrated in the cell where β rays are released, and the high-energy electrons spewed induce radiation cytotoxicity; simultaneously, γ rays are released that allow for detection of the emission by a camera. Therefore, postoperative examination with radioiodine scanning allows the identification of residual regional or distant foci of disease, and radioiodine can be used therapeutically to ablate such tumor deposits. The rationale for using ^{131}I as adjuvant therapy is as follows: (1) it destroys any residual microscopic foci of disease, (2) it increases specificity of subsequent ^{131}I scanning for detection of recurrent or metastatic disease by elimination of uptake by residual normal tissue, and (3) it improves the value of measurements of serum Tg as a serum marker; hence, any elevation in Tg would be representative of recurrent or metastatic disease and not residual normal thyroid tissue ([5, 6]). Combined retrospective data suggest that radioiodine ablation reduces long-term, disease-specific mortality in patients with primary tumors >4 cm in diameter or larger, those with multicentric disease, or those in whom there is evidence of soft tissue invasion at presentation ([22, 23]). Low-risk patients (Fig. 43-5) may not benefit from radioiodine, and selective use is advocated in these patients. The use of postoperative Tg measured 1 to 2 months after surgery is a useful tool to gauge residual or metastatic disease. Undetectable stimulated or unstimulated Tg indicates very low likelihood of residual disease. Nonstimulated Tg levels <5 ng/mL or stimulated Tg levels <10 ng/mL are also reassuring ([24]). However, the decision to give ^{131}I should not rely solely on the level of Tg.

Postoperatively, patients who require ^{131}I therapy should be started on liothyronine (synthetic T_3) at 25 mg twice daily and discontinued 2 weeks prior to the radioiodine scan. Lower doses are given to elderly patients and patients with coronary artery disease. During this time, patients should avoid foods rich in iodine. Urinary iodine concentrations can be checked to assess total-body iodine content prior to the radioiodine therapy. For maximum radioiodine uptake, the thyroid-stimulating hormone (TSH) should be allowed rise to >30 μIU/mL because this facilitates uptake of iodine by follicular cells. Increased iodide stores decrease radioiodine uptake. For patients in whom a preoperative contrast computed tomography (CT) was done, radioiodine therapy should be avoided for at least 3 months. A pretreatment scan using a 2- to 5-mCi ^{123}I or ^{131}I radioiodine scan for localization of uptake prior to ablation is recommended but not mandatory. Twenty-four to 96 hours after dosing, a whole-body scan showing <5% uptake is presumed to be normal residual tissue. An uptake of more than 5% indicates excessive thyroid tissue and warrants consideration

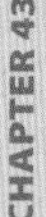

Table 43-4 Staging of Thyroid Carcinoma

Primary Tumor (T)	
Note: all categories may be subdivided into (a) solitary tumor and (b) multifocal tumor (the largest determines the classification).	
TX	Primary tumor cannot be assessed
T0	No evidence of primary tumor
T1	Tumor 2 cm or less in greatest dimension limited to the thyroid
T2	Tumor more than 2 cm but not more than 4 cm in greatest dimension limited to the thyroid
T3	Tumor more than 4 cm in greatest dimension limited to the thyroid or any tumor with minimal extrathyroid extension (eg, extension to sternothyroid muscle or perithyroid soft tissues)
T4a	Tumor of any size extending beyond the thyroid capsule to invade subcutaneous soft tissues, larynx, trachea, esophagus, or recurrent laryngeal nerve
T4b	Tumor invades prevertebral fascia or encases carotid artery or mediastinal vessels
	All anaplastic carcinomas are considered T4 tumors
T4a	Intrathyroidal anaplastic carcinoma—surgically resectable
T4b	Extrathyroidal anaplastic carcinoma—surgically unresectable
Regional Lymph Nodes (N)	
Regional lymph nodes are those of the central compartment as well as lateral cervical and upper mediastinal lymph nodes.	
NX	Regional lymph nodes cannot be assessed
N0	No regional lymph node metastasis
N1	Regional lymph node metastasis
N1a	Metastasis to level VI (pretracheal, paratracheal, and prelaryngeal/Delphian lymph nodes)
N1b	Metastasis to unilateral, bilateral, or contralateral cervical or superior mediastinal lymph nodes
Distant Metastasis (M)	
MX	Distant metastasis cannot be assessed
M0	No distant metastasis
M1	Distant metastasis

Reproduced with permission from Edge SB, Byrd DR, Compton CC (eds): *AJCC Cancer Staging Manuarl*, 7th ed. New York, NY: Springer; 2010.

for further surgical resection. The dose of radioactive iodine is determined by extent of residual disease: 30 to 100 mCi for adjuvant ablation, approximately 150 mCi for nodal disease, and 200 mCi or more for metastatic disease outside the lungs ([24]). A posttreatment scan is performed to assess for further uptake of radioactive iodine that was not previously seen on the pretreatment scan (ie, regional or distant metastases). The posttreatment scan is a more sensitive technique to detect metastatic disease, because the ability to demonstrate radioactive iodine–avid lesions is directly proportional to the amount of radioactive iodine given (Fig. 43-6).

Short-term complications, although rare, include radiation thyroiditis, neck edema, sialoadenitis, and tumor hemorrhage. These occur more often in the presence of bulky disease. Long-term complications, which increase with cumulative doses, include xerostomia, nasolacrimal duct obstruction ([25]), pulmonary fibrosis (if pulmonary metastasis is present and treated at high doses), and secondary malignancies such as acute myelogenous leukemia ([26]). There are no reports of congenital abnormalities in children conceived after radioactive iodine treatment; however, most physicians recommend waiting for 6 months before conceiving. Radioactive iodine should not be given to pregnant women due to the potential teratogenic effects for the fetus's growth and thyroid development; all women of childbearing age must have a negative pregnancy test prior to treatment.

Thyroid Hormone Therapy

Thyroid hormone replacement targeting TSH suppression has been shown to increase disease-free survival two- to threefold, especially in high-risk patients. It minimizes potential TSH-stimulated growth of thyroid cancer cells. Oversuppression of TSH to undetectable levels can present morbid consequences including

Table 43-5 Stage Grouping for Thyroid Carcinoma

Separate stage groupings are recommended for papillary or follicular, medullary, and anaplastic (undifferentiated) carcinomas.			
Papillary or Follicular (<45 Years)			
Stage I	Any T	Any N	M0
Stage II	Any T	Any N	M1
Papillary or Follicular (≥45 Years)			
Stage I	T1	N0	M0
Stage II	T2	N0	M0
Stage III	T3	N0	M0
	T1/T2/T3	N1a	M0
Stage IVA	T4a	N0/N1a	M0
	T1/T2/T3/T4a	N1b	M0
Stage IVB	T4b	Any N	M0
Stage IVC	Any T	Any M	M1
Medullary Carcinoma			
Stage I	T1	N0	M0
Stage II	T2	N0	M0
Stage III	T3	N0	M0
	T1/T2/T3	N1a	M0
Stage IVA	T4a	N0/N1a	M0
	T1/T2/T3/T4a	N1b	M0
Stage IVB	T4b	Any N	M0
Stage IVC	Any T	Any N	M1
Anaplastic Carcinoma			
All anaplastic carcinomas are stage IV.			
Stage IVA	T4a	Any N	M0
Stage IVB	T4b	Any N	M0
Stage IVC	Any T	Any N	M1

Reproduced with permission from Edge SB, Byrd DR, Compton CC (eds): *AJCC Cancer Staging Manuarl*, 7th ed. New York, NY: Springer; 2010.

osteopenia, atrial fibrillation, and possible cardiac hypertrophy. Moderate TSH suppression (subnormal but not undetectable) during follow-up was associated with better outcomes in all stages, including those with distant metastatic disease ([27]). For high risk patients, moderate TSH suppression continued for the first 3 years after initial diagnosis may be indicated.

External Beam Radiotherapy

External beam radiotherapy (EBRT) has a limited role in the treatment of PTC. Our institutional review of postoperative conformal EBRT in high-risk DTC patients showed durable locoregional control in those with residual microscopic disease after initial surgery. However, patients with gross residual disease had significantly worse outcomes, and EBRT in these instances should be avoided ([28]). Guidelines recommend consideration for EBRT in patients >45 years old with gross non–iodine-avid macroscopic disease in whom further surgery would not be beneficial ([5]).

Management After Initial Therapy

Imaging

Following initial therapy, patients with DTC need lifelong monitoring using both clinical and radiographic data. In high-risk patients, follow-up radioiodine scan 12 months after initial radioiodine ablation should be considered for reassessment of disease burden. The TSH should be allowed to increase to a value >30 μIU/mL by either withdrawal of thyroid hormone or using recombinant human

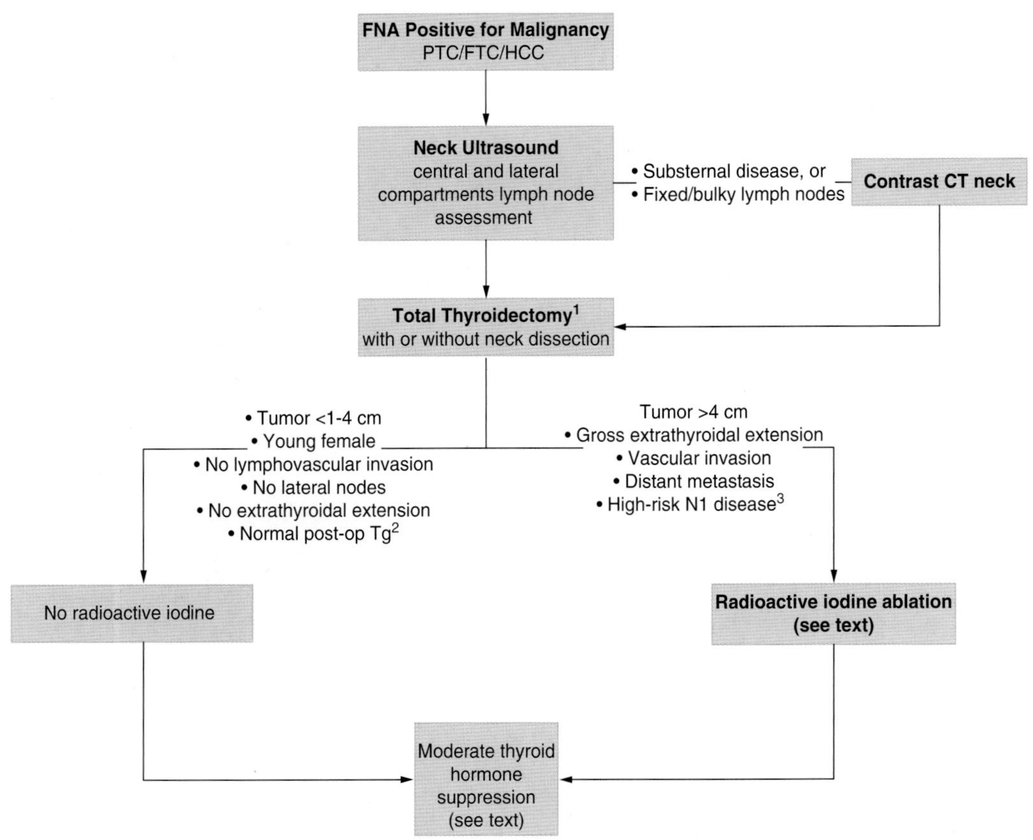

[1]Consider lobectomy for small tumors <4 cm; no history of radiation; no gross extrathyroidal extension; no cervical lymph node disease; age <4; no family history.
[2]Nonstimulated Tg <5 ng/mL or stimulated Tg <10 ng/mL and negative Tg antibodies.
[3]High-risk N1 disease: >10 involved nodes if all are less than 5 mm; >5 involved nodes if most are 5-15 mm; or any single lymph node more than 15 mm.

FIGURE 43-5 Initial approach to management of differentiated thyroid cancer. CT, computed tomography; FNA, fine-needle aspiration; FTC, follicular thyroid carcinoma; HCC, Hürthle cell carcinoma; PTC, papillary thyroid carcinoma; Tg, thyroglobulin. Data from Tuttle RM, Sabra MM. Selective use of RAI for ablation and adjuvant therapy after total thyroidectomy for differentiated thyroid cancer: a practical approach to clinical decision making. *Oral Oncol*. 2013;49(7):676-683.

TSH (rhTSH). Thyrotropin alfa, an rhTSH, administered as two injections on 2 consecutive days may be used in lieu of standard thyroid hormone withdrawal to increase thyrotropin concentrations and for adequate stimulation of both radioiodine uptake for scanning and serum Tg concentrations. The use of rhTSH is of particular benefit in the patient in whom endogenous TSH levels cannot rise due to hypopituitarism or in whom the clinician prefers to avoid prolonged hypothyroidism and its resultant complications due to concurrent medical problems. Radioiodine scanning beyond this first follow-up scan needs to be individualized and is no longer routine for all thyroid cancer patients including high-risk patients.

Ultrasonography of the neck (thyroid bed and cervical neck compartments) with FNA of suspicious accessible lesions is used 6 to 12 months postoperatively as part of routine follow-up.

Other non–radioiodine imaging techniques include CT of the neck and chest, chest radiographs, fluorodeoxyglucose (FDG) positron emission tomography (PET) or PET, and magnetic resonance imaging (MRI). Magnetic resonance imaging and CT of the neck play important roles in the detection of recurrent disease; they are not as sensitive as ultrasound but are much less operator dependent. Chest CT shows both micronodular and macronodular pulmonary metastases. Fluorodeoxyglucose-PET/CT imaging is useful in patients with a Tg >10 ng/mL who have negative radioiodine

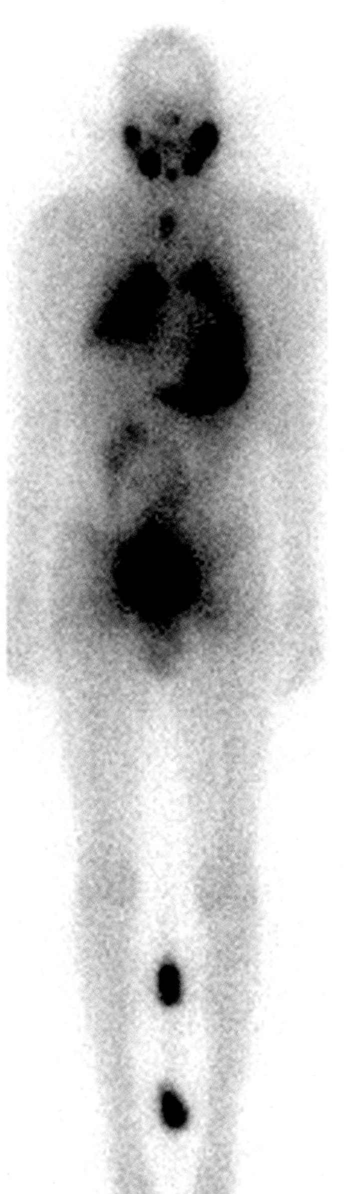

FIGURE 43-6 Whole-body scan with iodine-131 (^{131}I) showing multiple metastatic deposits in the neck and lungs, with physiologic uptake in the salivary gland, stomach, intestines, and bladder.

imaging but is not routinely used in follow-up of other thyroid cancer patients (5). Patients with DTC with little to no iodine activity generally have higher glucose metabolism and positivity on FDG-PET scans. Lack of iodine uptake denotes tumor dedifferentiation. Although PET is sensitive in detecting metastatic disease, it is not specific for thyroid cancer, and caution should be exercised when evaluating recurrent disease (Fig. 43-7). The use of CT imaging in conjunction with

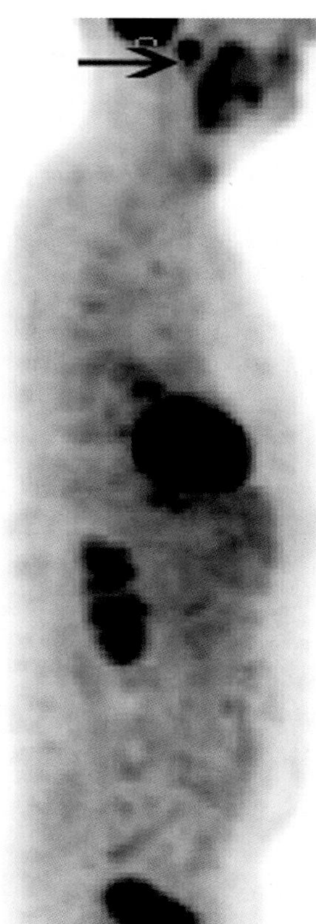

FIGURE 43-7 Positron emission tomography (PET) scan showing posterior pharyngeal metastatic papillary thyroid carcinoma. Thyroglobulin level was 35 ng/mL, and radioiodine whole-body scan was negative for disease.

FDG-PET improves the sensitivity for small subcentimeter metastatic disease seen with DTC.

Monitoring Serum Thyroglobulin

Thyroglobulin is a unique protein synthesized only by the thyroid follicular cells (both benign and differentiated malignant tissue) and, therefore, is a good biochemical test to assess for the presence of residual, recurrent, or metastatic disease. Dedifferentiated tumors lose the ability to secrete Tg, and it cannot be used as a tumor marker. Following total thyroidectomy with or without radioiodine ablation, the Tg falls to its nadir usually within 3 months, but may take as long as 2 years. Subsequent Tg measurements (stimulated or unstimulated) are used to monitor for disease recurrence and should be repeated in the same laboratory to avoid erroneous misinterpretations of interassay variability (29). Simultaneously Tg and Tg antibody (TgAb) should always be measured together because TgAb can falsely lower the Tg concentrations in immunometric assays. These antibodies, which are present in approximately 25%

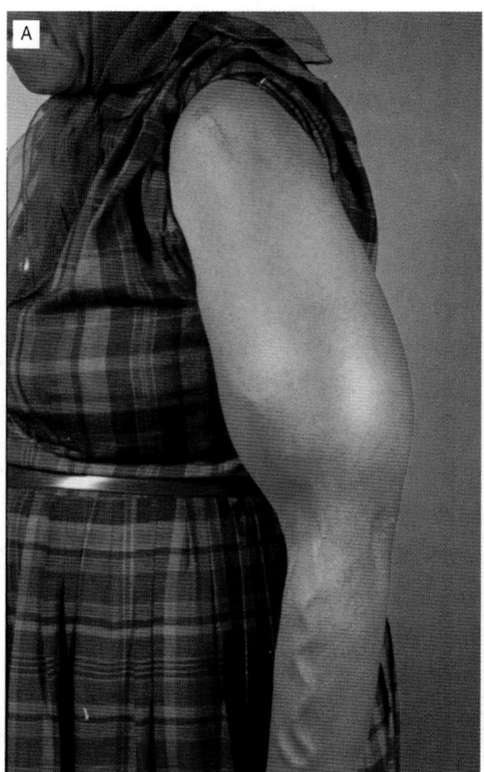

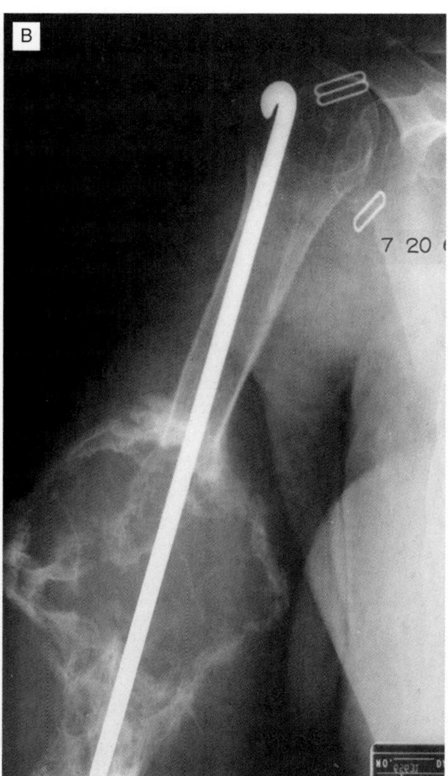

FIGURE 43-8 A. A woman with metastatic follicular thyroid carcinoma to left humerus. **B.** Radiograph of metastatic follicular thyroid carcinoma to left humerus in the same patient.

of patients, interfere with the assay's ability to bind to Tg. Thyroglobulin measurements by radioimmunoassay or liquid chromatography tandem mass spectrometry are more resistant to interference by TgAb and are used when antibody presence is detected. The median time to TgAb disappearance after total thyroidectomy and radioiodine ablation is about 3 years ([30]). Therefore, increases in TgAb after the nadir has been reached should alert the clinician to the possibility of recurrent disease. Although in general the diagnostic accuracy of serum Tg is higher after TSH stimulation than during thyroxine treatment, an unstimulated Tg measured by second-generation assays may be used to follow up patients with stimulated Tg of <2 ng/mL with no evidence of recurrent disease on imaging ([31]).

Metastatic Disease

Distant metastases are evident in about 15% of patients with DTC. Half of these patients have notable metastases at the time of initial presentation ([12]). The most common sites of metastasis, in decreasing order of frequency, are the lungs, bones, and other soft tissues (Figs. 43-8A, 43-8B, and 43-9). Older patients have a higher risk for distant metastases. For resectable locoregional and isolated metastasis, surgery is preferred.

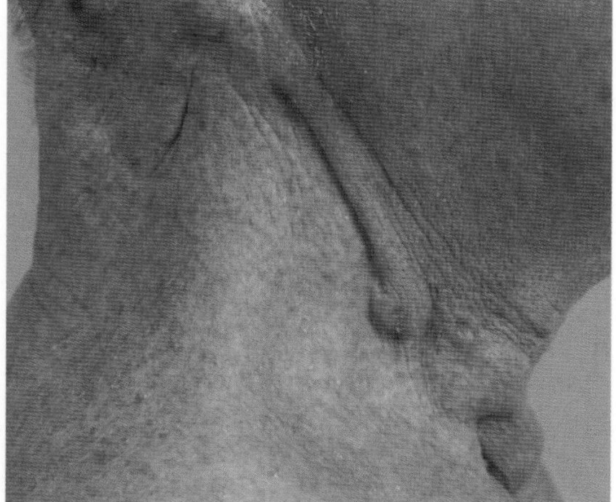

FIGURE 43-9 Patient with multiple metastatic deposits of papillary thyroid carcinoma to the skin.

In those with iodine-avid unresectable disease or distant metastasis, ^{131}I treatment should be recommended, and higher doses (150-200 mCi) are typically used. Although this treatment may be repeated 6 to 12 months later, caution and careful monitoring for side effects should be exercised. Moderate TSH suppression should also be continued in these patients. Metastases at different sites require management by multimodality approaches. Bone lesions may be surgically resected or treated with ^{131}I treatment or EBRT ([32]). In follicular thyroid carcinoma, where the lesions are highly vascular, arterial embolization has been used anecdotally with successful reduction in pain at our institution. In addition, intravenous bisphosphonates (pamidronate or zoledronic acid) and denosumab are prescribed for painful bony metastases with some success. Experience at our institution also showed improved median survival for patients with one or more brain metastases after surgical resection. Stereotactic radiosurgery is also an option. We suggest a multidisciplinary approach and discussion with the surgeon, radiation oncologist, and endocrinologist about the risks and benefits of each modality in the management of metastatic disease.

Systemic Therapy

In patients with progressive metastatic disease that does not respond to standard therapy, long-term overall survival is <10%. For this subset of patients, the understanding of the molecular model for thyroid cancer and the discovery of targeted therapies have led to a new era of treatment ([12]). Consequently, over the last 5 years, two tyrosine kinase inhibitors (TKIs), sorafenib (2013) and lenvatinib (2015), have been approved by the US Food and Drug Administration (FDA) for the treatment of locally recurrent or metastatic, progressive DTC refractory to radioactive iodine treatment. Previously recommended cytotoxic therapies with agents such as doxorubicin have had poor outcomes with significant toxicities ([12]). The TKIs target intercellular signaling pathways (MAPK pathway in the tumor cells) but also play a role in the surrounding tumor vasculature ([12]). Trials evaluating the efficacy of the approved drugs have shown better progression-free survival (PFS) than in the placebo groups (5 months with sorafenib and 14.7 months with lenvatinib) ([33, 34]). The recently approved TKI lenvatinib had an overall response rate of 64.8% versus 1.5% in the placebo group (odds ratio, 28.87; 95% CI, 12.46-66.86). However, it is important to note the deleterious effects of these drugs, most commonly hypertension, gastrointestinal effects such as diarrhea, altered taste and stomatitis, palmar-plantar erythrodysesthesia syndrome (hand and foot syndrome), and weight loss.

Indications for therapy include patients with progressive or symptomatic unresectable disease that is refractory to ^{131}I treatment. Patients with asymptomatic stable or very slowly progressive disease on thyroid hormone suppression may be closely monitored. Prior to initiation of therapy, a comprehensive evaluation to ascertain appropriate selection of patients should be conducted. This should include a candid discussion with the patient and family about the benefits and risks of these agents. Furthermore due to the life-threatening adverse effects of these drugs, only clinicians who are well versed with use of these agents should initiate and monitor these patients. We have previously published an adverse event monitoring tool used at our institution to guide clinicians initiating patients on these agents ([35]).

Differentiated Thyroid Carcinoma in Children

As in adults, PTC followed by follicular thyroid cancer occur most frequently in children. Exposure to radiation is the major risk factor. It is not unusual for children with PTC to present with multifocal disease with lymph node involvement, extrathyroidal extension, and pulmonary metastasis ([36]). Despite this, children overall have high cure rates, with 10-year survival of almost 100%. Those diagnosed before the age of 10 years, however, seem to have a higher risk of recurrence and death. The treatment of thyroid cancer in children mirrors that of adults. Total thyroidectomy (rarely lobectomy) with nodal dissection done at a high-volume center due to higher complication rates is recommended ([36]). Postoperative universal radioiodine therapy is no longer advocated, and careful selection based on risk of recurrence, residual or distant disease remaining after surgery, and Tg levels is used to determine the need for therapy ([36]). Moderate TSH suppression (0.1-0.5 μIU/mL) with relaxation when there is no evidence of recurrent disease is suggested. Lifelong surveillance is essential in monitoring children for recurrent disease because recurrence may occur 20 to 30 years later. For the few children with progressive radioiodine-refractory DTC, referral to a center with pediatric endocrine neoplasia expertise for consideration for systemic therapy is recommended.

MEDULLARY THYROID CARCINOMA

Introduction

Medullary thyroid carcinomas (MTCs) are derived from C cells (calcitonin-secreting cells) that are part of neural crest origin (see Table 43-1). The majority—80% of patients with MTC have sporadic disease. The other 20% have an inherited form that occurs as an autosomal dominant trait as part of the multiple endocrine neoplasia (MEN) clinical syndromes, MEN type 2A or type 2B or familial MTC ([37]). In MEN 2A, MTC occurs in association with pheochromocytoma and multigland parathyroid tumors; MTC is usually the first manifested disease of the three components of this syndrome. In MEN 2B, MTC occurs in association with pheochromocytoma and mucosal neuromas (Figs. 43-10A and 43-10B) or neurofibromas and marfanoid habitus. Familial MTC is a variant of MEN 2A where only MTC is clinically evident ([38]). Most patients with sporadic MTC present in the fifth or sixth decade of life with a male-to-female ratio of 1.4:1.

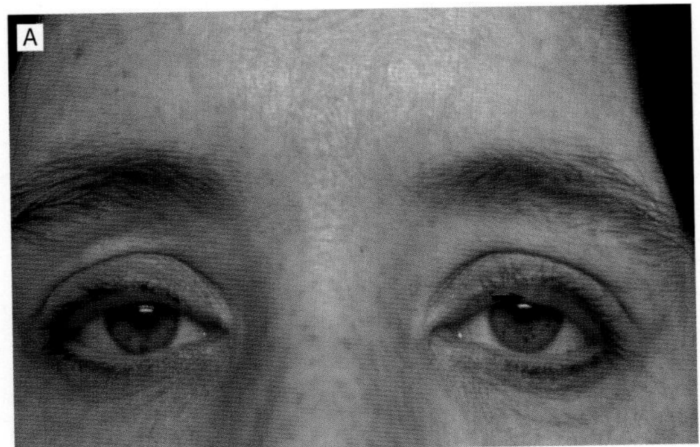

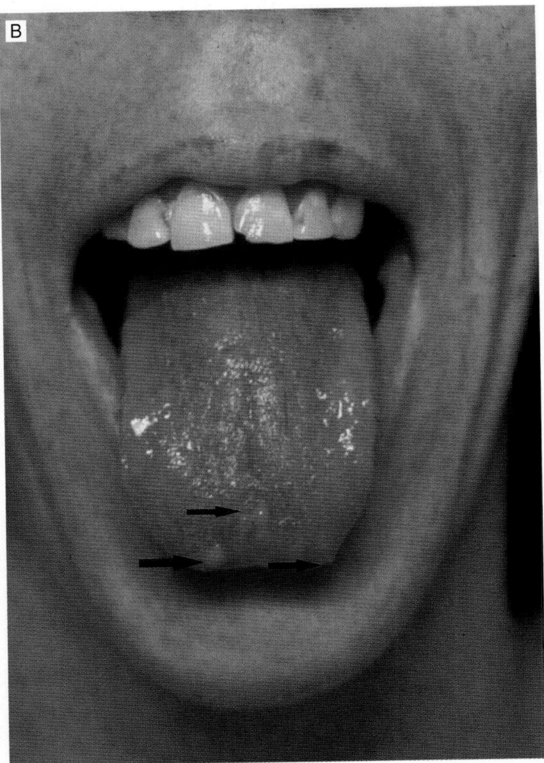

FIGURE 43-10 A. Patient with multiple endocrine neoplasia (MEN) type 2B, with typical thickening of the palpebrum. Note also the ganglioneuroma on the left superior eyelid. B. Multiple ganglioneuromas on the tongue of a patient with MEN type 2B.

Clinical Features and Diagnosis

The most common clinical presentation of sporadic MTC is a solitary thyroid mass found incidentally during routine examination. Other symptoms such as secretory diarrhea and facial flushing may also be seen with hormone overproduction. Fine-needle aspiration should be performed for suspicious nodules, and once MTC is suspected, calcium, calcitonin, and carcinoembryonic antigen (CEA) levels should be obtained, with screening for pheochromocytoma and a thorough history and physical examination also performed. Because about 6% of patients with sporadic MTC carry a germline *RET* mutation, genetic counseling and testing are offered to all patients with newly diagnosed apparent sporadic disease ([39]). If pheochromocytoma is confirmed, appropriate control of catecholamine hypersecretion and removal should precede thyroid surgery.

Medullary thyroid cancer occurs as a solid mass or cluster of C-cell hyperplasia interspersed between normal thyroid follicles and can be visualized with calcitonin immunostaining. (Fig. 43-11). It appears as variable amounts of fibrosis as well as deposits of amyloid in 60% to 80% of tumors. Notably, even the smallest visible tumors can be associated with metastases.

Metastases to cervical and mediastinal lymph nodes are found in about 50% of the patients at the time of initial presentation. Distant metastases to the lungs, liver, bones, and adrenal glands most commonly occur late in the course of the disease (Fig. 43-12).

Inherited Medullary Thyroid Cancer

Inherited syndromes of MTC are all transmitted in an autosomal dominant form. In kindreds with inherited MTC, prospective family screening is essential due to the 90% to 95% penetrance of the disease ([40]). In these cases, MTC is usually present by the third to fourth decade of life. The mutation is detected in *RET* and can be identified in 98% of affected family members with appropriate screening. Patients with MEN 2B tend to exhibit more locally aggressive MTC ([40]). Screening with *RET* testing is recommended at age <6 months for familial MTC, and MEN 2A screening is recommended by 5 years of age ([38]).

Analysis of the *RET* gene should include the most common sites of mutation, exons 10 and 11, and if no mutation is found, testing should proceed with exons

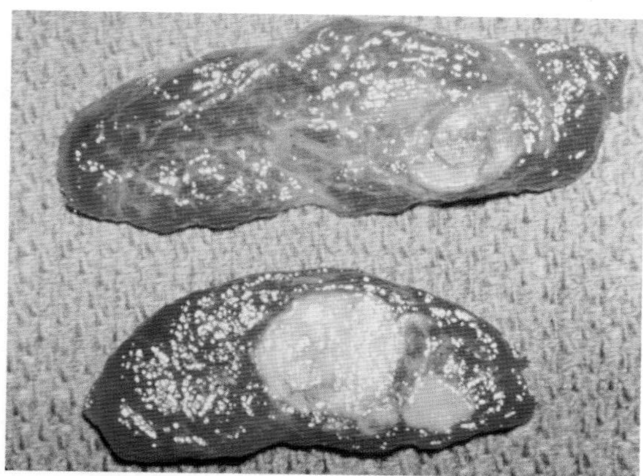

FIGURE 43-11 Gross specimen of thyroid gland containing medullary thyroid carcinoma.

13 to 16 ([38, 41]). Appropriate genetic counseling must be a part of the initial evaluation, including the possibilities of errors in testing, the potential for discrimination, and changes that may occur in quality of life.

Management

Surgery

In MTC, there is a high propensity for bilateral disease in both the sporadic and familial forms, and therefore, the usual treatment is total thyroidectomy with central neck compartment dissection in all patients. In unilateral sporadic disease, if the primary tumor is greater than 1 cm or central compartment disease is present, strong consideration should be given to ipsilateral modified radical neck or mediastinal dissections, or both ([41]). Bilateral neck dissections are usually performed in many institutions, including our own. Hypoparathyroidism and recurrent laryngeal nerve damage are the most frequently encountered complications in both children and adults. We recommend referral to centers with high volume and experienced surgeons to decrease these complications.

For carriers of a familial *RET* mutation, current guidelines recommend prophylactic total thyroidectomy by age 5 years or when the mutation is identified for adults, particularly for those with codon 609, 611, 618, 620, 630, or 634 *RET* mutations. For MEN 2B patients and patients with codon 883 *RET*, 918 *RET*, or compound heterozygous (V804M + E805K, V804M + Y806C, or V804M + S904C) *RET* mutations, prophylactic thyroidectomy is recommended in the first year of life or at diagnosis ([38, 41]). For patients with less lethal MTC codon 768, 790, 791, 804, and 891 *RET* mutations, surgery can be delayed if stringent criteria are met and good follow-up is adhered to ([5]).

There is no role for thyroid hormone suppression therapy; hence, the goal should be to maintain the TSH and free thyroxine (T_4) concentrations within normal levels. There is also no role of radioactive iodine therapy in the treatment of MTC, and therefore, thyroid hormone replacement may be started immediately after surgery.

External Beam Radiotherapy

External beam radiotherapy should be considered for patients who are at high risk for locoregional recurrence, due to improved relapse-free rate ([42]). In general, 20 fractions totaling 40 Gy are given to the cervical, supraclavicular, and upper mediastinal lymph nodes over 4 weeks; subsequent booster doses of 10 Gy are then given to the thyroid bed, especially if there was gross residual disease ([41]). External beam radiotherapy can also be given to treat painful skeletal metastases.

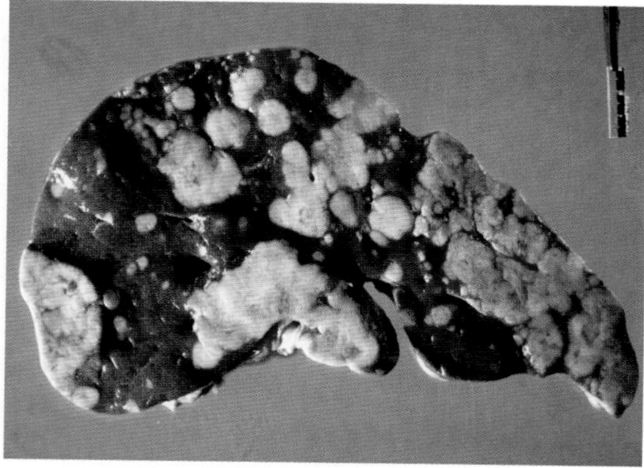

FIGURE 43-12 Gross specimen of liver containing metastatic lesions of medullary thyroid carcinoma.

Monitoring and Follow-Up

Biochemical testing with serum calcitonin and CEA is used in the routine follow-up of patients with MTC. About 3 months postoperatively, these markers should be within the normal ranges (a nadir of 6 months has been reported). Patients with palpable recurrent/residual disease, in general, will have stimulated calcitonin levels of at least 10 pg/mL except for tumors that are dedifferentiated and no longer secrete calcitonin (these tumors usually secrete CEA). Values of serum calcitonin >100 pg/mL are indicative of residual neck disease or distant metastases particularly in the liver, and these patients should be aggressively assessed clinically and radiographically ([41]). Because of MTC's propensity for neck, mediastinal, and liver metastasis, diagnostic imaging should include ultrasonography of the neck, CT of the chest, and MRI of the liver. Routine use of PET, metaiodobenzylguanidine (MIBG), and bone scans is not recommended.

Recurrent or Persistent Disease

Patients with stable and asymptomatic recurrent disease can be monitored closely without therapy. Once the disease is progressive, symptomatic treatment is recommended. For those with locoregional disease without metastases, surgery is preferred. Similar to metastatic DTC, treatment of individual metastatic sites causing symptoms or problems can be addressed individually (see earlier "Differentiated Thyroid Carcinoma" section). As with DTC, recently the FDA has approved two TKIs, vandetanib (2011) and cabozantinib (2012), for progressive metastatic MTC. Initiation of these therapies should be done by clinicians who are well versed with use of these agents and are able to monitor these patients closely.

ANAPLASTIC THYROID CARCINOMA

Introduction

Anaplastic thyroid carcinoma (ATC) is a locally and systemically aggressive undifferentiated tumor with a disease-specific mortality rate approaching 100%. More than 90% of patients are over the age of 50 years, and more females than males are affected.

Diagnosis

Anaplastic thyroid carcinoma most commonly presents as rapid growth of a thyroid mass. A history of long-standing thyroid enlargement is noted in about 80% of the patients. Fine-needle aspiration or surgical biopsy can usually establish the diagnosis. Preoperative imaging (CT of brain to pelvis including FDG-PET) to assess extent of disease and planning for surgery and/or radiation therapy is recommended but should not delay therapy. Vocal cord paralysis is common in patients with ATC and should be assessed. Anaplastic thyroid carcinoma frequently arises from preexisting well-differentiated thyroid carcinoma, which supports the opinion that some ATCs develop by dedifferentiation from well-differentiated DTC (Fig. 43-13). Immunohistochemical staining for Tg, TTF1, and paired box protein Pax 8 (PAX8) should be used to aid in identifying better-differentiated sections ([43]). However, because undifferentiated carcinoma cells lose their ability to synthesize Tg, Tg immunoreactivity in ATCs may be absent. Although various mutations are found in ATC including *TP53* and β-catenin (*CTNNB1*), *RAS*, *BRAF*, *PIK3CA*, and others, molecular testing is currently not required for diagnosis or management ([43, 44]).

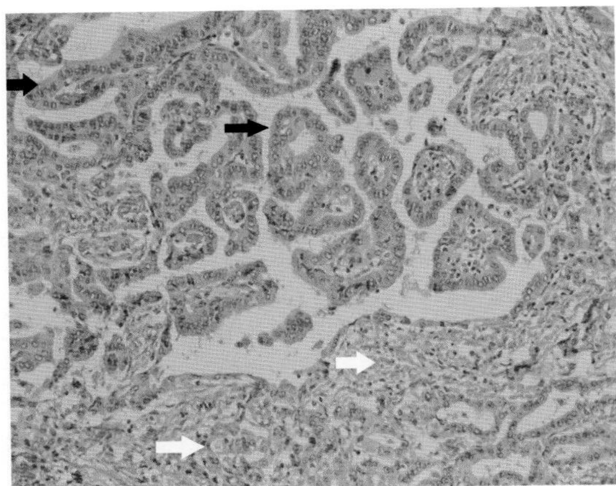

FIGURE 43-13 Hematoxylin and eosin staining of thyroid illustrating papillary thyroid carcinoma (*black arrows*) in transition to anaplastic thyroid carcinoma (*white arrows*).

Median survival is about 5 months, with 1-year survival of 20% ([44]). Better survival rates are seen only in patients with well-localized anaplastic tumors. Favorable prognostic features seem to be age <60 years, tumor size less than 5 cm, extent of surgery, radiotherapy, chemotherapy, coexisting DTC, and absence of distant metastases ([44]).

Therapy

Treatment is generally palliative in nature because ATC is rarely cured and almost always fatal. Death occurs from upper airway obstruction and suffocation in half of patients and complications of therapy or distant metastases in the others. A multidisciplinary thyroid cancer team approach is needed in the management of these patients. The potential risks and benefits of all treatment modalities including palliative care should be discussed with the patient and family.

For primary lesions with no distant metastases for which effective resection can be safely achieved, then surgery is recommended as first-line treatment followed by adjuvant conformal radiotherapy with or without chemotherapy. In the presence of distant metastases, primary tumor resection should be considered to avoid invasion of surrounding structures. For unresectable lesions, neoadjuvant conformal radiotherapy with or without chemotherapy should be considered first because this may render the tumor resectable ([43]). Patients with poor performance status should be offered palliative doses of radiotherapy if tolerable. The chemotherapeutic agents doxorubicin, paclitaxel or docetaxel, and cisplatin are the currently recommended agents ([45, 46]). Combretastatin, an antimicrotubule agent, and TKIs including sorafenib, gefitinib, and imatinib have also been used with varied responses ([43]). However, because no systemic therapies are known to improve survival or quality of life in advanced ATC, patients seeking an aggressive approach should be considered for participation in clinical trials.

PARATHYROID CARCINOMA

Introduction

Parathyroid carcinoma is a rare endocrine malignancy, with a prevalence of 0.005% of all cancers ([47]). The etiology of parathyroid carcinoma remains largely unknown. No well-recognized risk factors have been identified. Predisposing factors identified with some cases are outlined in Table 43-6. Parathyroid carcinoma also occurs sporadically or as part of a genetic syndrome. Patients with parathyroid carcinoma are about a decade younger than patients with benign hyperparathyroidism. The disease occurs with similar frequency in both sexes.

Clinical Features

Hypercalcemia is common and ranges from mild to severe and may manifest with peripheral target organ complications such as kidney stones and osteoporosis. Parathyroid hormone levels are generally greater than five times normal, and patients may present with a discrete neck mass. However, parathyroid cancer is an uncommon cause of primary hyperparathyroidism. The presence of severe hypercalcemia (>12 mg/dL), extremely elevated parathyroid hormone, and a palpable neck mass should raise the suspicion for parathyroid cancer ([48]).

Diagnosis

The presence of personal or family history of associated conditions and the constellation of clinical features described earlier significantly increase the likelihood of parathyroid cancer. Confirming the diagnosis prior to histologic confirmation remains challenging. Imaging modalities routinely used to aid diagnosis include parathyroid ultrasonography and technetium-99m sestamibi. Chest CT and bone scintigraphy may also be useful for initial staging ([49]). FNA is not routinely recommended due to the risk of seeding the tumor and lack of sufficient sample to definitely make a diagnosis. Screening for mutations in the *CDC73* gene, which encodes parafibromin, a protein that inhibits mitogenic function, is considered an integral part of the diagnostic workup of patients with sporadic or familial parathyroid cancer. Patients with familial hyperparathyroidism are also considered at high risk for *CDC73* mutation and should also be screened.

Table 43-6 Risk Factors and Syndromes Associated With Parathyroid Carcinoma

Predisposing factors
Prior diagnosis of thyroid cancer
Prior hyperfunctioning parathyroid gland
Secondary and tertiary hyperparathyroidism resulting from chronic renal failure and dialysis
Radiation exposure to the head and neck region
Genetic syndromes
Multiple endocrine neoplasia type 1
Familial isolated hyperparathyroidism
Hereditary hyperparathyroidism-jaw tumor syndrome

Pathology

Histopathologic diagnosis following the World Health Organization (WHO) criteria is defined by the presence of capsular invasion and soft tissue invasion or histologic evidence of vascular invasion with or without invasion of vital organs or presence of locoregional or distant metastasis ([50]). The classic histopathologic criteria initially described by Schantz and Castleman, including the presence of a trabecular or lobular pattern, mitotic figures, thick fibrous bands, and capsular or blood vessel invasion, are also still used today ([51]) (Fig. 43-14).

However, in some cases, the histopathologic diagnosis still remains quite challenging, and some highly differentiated tumors without distinct nuclear atypia or classic histopathologic criteria are initially considered to be adenomas but are later reclassified when recurrence or metastases appear. Immunohistochemical staining for parafibromin may increase the diagnostic accuracy, and although not widely used, we have used this at our institution for various cases. Mutations in the *CDC73* gene are seen not only in the majority of patients with hyperparathyroidism-jaw tumor syndrome but also in cases of sporadic and familial parathyroid cancer ([52, 53]). Fifteen percent of the parathyroid tumors associated with HPT-JT are carcinomas ([54]). On the contrary, mutations in *MEN1* seldom result in parathyroid carcinoma. To improve the accuracy of diagnosis of malignant parathyroid disease, pathologic specimens of suspected cases should be reviewed by experienced pathologists. We are currently exploring the role of molecular profiling of parathyroid cancer in prognostication and also to identify targetable mutations that could result in novel targeted therapies.

To date, there no currently agreed upon staging criteria for parathyroid carcinoma.

The 5-year survival rate has improved over the years to approximately 85%, and the 10-year survival rate is approximately 50% ([47]). Death usually results from hypercalcemia and its associated complications.

Management

Because of its rarity and unpredictable clinical course, a multidisciplinary approach to caring for the patient with parathyroid carcinoma that involves the endocrinologist, surgeon, oncologist, and radiotherapist offers the best chance for cure.

Preoperative suspicion and intraoperative identification of malignancy and appropriate initial surgery are critical in the therapy for parathyroid carcinoma. Comprehensive resection of the tumor along with the ipsilateral lobe of the thyroid and abnormal or involved adjacent tissues (the so-called "en bloc" resection) is indicated ([55]). Every effort should be made to maintain the integrity of the capsule to prevent seeding of tumor, because this will contribute to recurrence. Because this tumor does not typically metastasize to lymph nodes, routine lymph node dissection is not indicated unless involved by tumor. For recurrences, a wide excision of locally recurrent tumor and an aggressive surgical resection of metastases whenever possible are recommended. Although these repeat operations are not always curative, they usually offer palliation for the marked hypercalcemia (the cause of true morbidity in these patients) for a considerable although variable period. Nevertheless, surgical resection, where possible, remains the most effective treatment for both primary and recurrent disease.

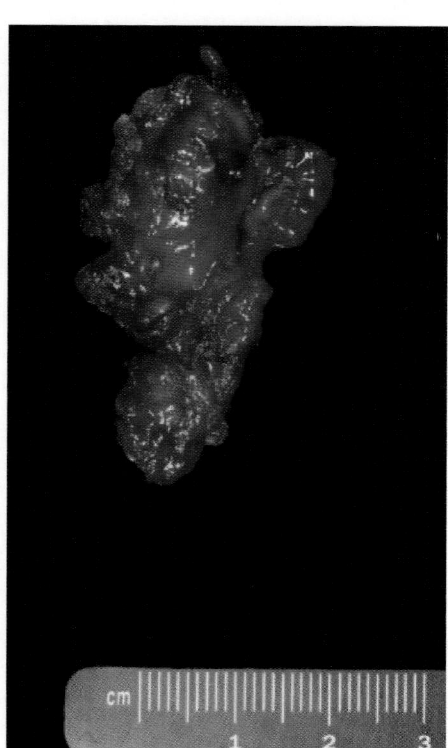

FIGURE 43-14 Parathyroid gland carcinoma.

Radiotherapy has not become the standard of care in patients with parathyroid carcinoma because it is difficult to prove its efficacy with such small numbers of patients being treated in reported series ([56]). It may be considered in select patients at high risk of local relapse (those with gross or local invasion or tumor spillage intraoperatively) or those left with gross disease.

Chemotherapeutic agents, as of yet, do not seem to be efficacious in this disease. We have had success with sorafenib in a patient with metastatic disease who has shown sustained improvements in hypercalcemia ([57]).

Morbidity and mortality are generally caused by the effects of unremitting hypercalcemia rather than tumor growth. Medical treatments, especially in patients with unresectable disease, such as bisphosphonates, denosumab, or calcimimetics, offer only temporary and palliative control of hypercalcemia. Lifetime surveillance of serum calcium and parathyroid hormone levels is essential because of the protracted and unpredictable course of malignant parathyroid disease.

PHEOCHROMOCYTOMA AND PARAGANGLIOMA

Introduction

The term pheochromocytoma refers to a neoplasm derived from chromaffin cells. Although the majority of these tumors occur in the adrenal medulla, about 15% to 20% of cases arises from sympathetic or parasympathetic ganglia and are known as paragangliomas. Pheochromocytomas and paragangliomas are rare, with an estimated incidence of 0.95 per 100,000 person-years ([58]), and they have a slight female predominance (54% female) ([59]). Although pheochromocytoma is a possible cause of secondary hypertension, it represents less than 1% of cases. Nonetheless, it is important to consider this diagnosis in the proper clinical setting because it is potentially curable. Furthermore, failure to treat or improper treatment can lead to serious complications or death (Fig. 43-15).

The rule of 10 is a classic teaching in regard to pheochromocytoma. This rule states that among pheochromocytomas, 10% are bilateral, 10% are extra-adrenal, 10% are familial, and 10% are malignant. However, this does not capture our current understanding. Data now suggest that nearly 25% of apparently sporadic pheochromocytomas are

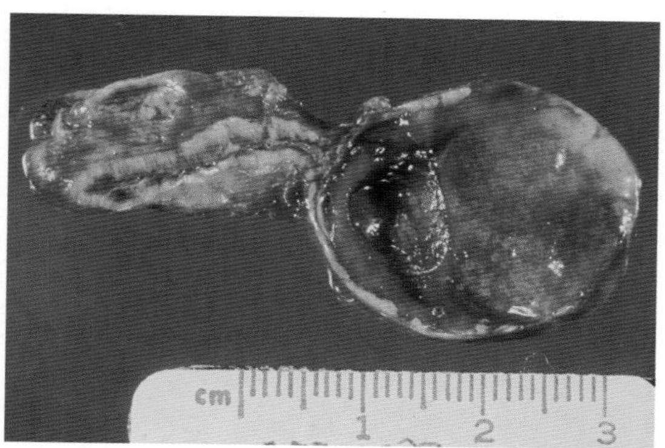

FIGURE 43-15 Adrenal gland with pheochromocytoma.

Table 43-7 Signs and Symptoms of Pheochromocytoma (list not all inclusive)

Hypertension	Anxiety
Headache	Constipation
Sweating	Nausea
Palpitations	Insulin resistance
Pallor	Orthostasis
Flushing	Weight loss

hereditary and associated with germline mutations such as *RET*, *VHL*, *SDHD*, and *SDHB* ([60]). These are patients who were thought to have sporadic disease but have a higher risk of bilateral disease, malignancy, or extra-adrenal disease on the basis of their germline mutation.

Clinical Features

The presentation of pheochromocytomas and paragangliomas ranges from incidental discovery to cardiovascular shock and death. A classic presentation is described as the five Ps. These five Ps are spells of pressure (hypertension), pain (headache), palpitations, perspiration, and pallor. Although none of these signs and symptoms is universally present, it is reasonable to screen patients with hypertension and symptomatology suggestive of hyperadrenergic episodes. The spells can last from minutes to hours and may be triggered by exercise, stress, micturition, Valsalva maneuver, or anesthesia induction (Table 43-7).

Additional findings include hyperglycemia (due to suppression of insulin release), orthostasis/volume depletion (due to vasoconstriction), and constipation/abdominal distention (due to inhibition of gut motility). Rarely, there is co-secretion of other hormones resulting in distinct endocrine syndromes. These include vasoactive intestinal peptide causing Verner Morrison syndrome, adrenocorticotropic hormone (ACTH) causing Cushing syndrome, growth hormone–releasing hormone causing acromegaly, and parathyroid hormone–related protein causing hypercalcemia ([61]) (Figs. 43-16 and 43-17).

Diagnosis

Laboratory

Biochemical testing is the cornerstone of diagnosis. At our institution, plasma-free metanephrines and

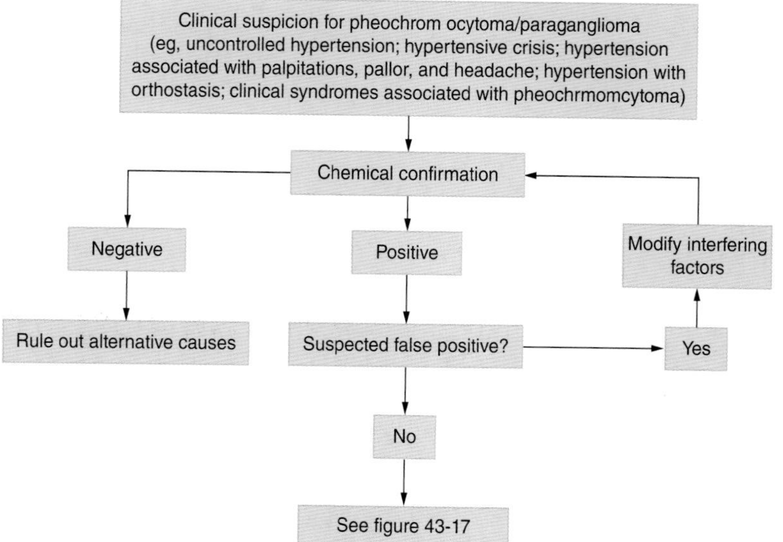

FIGURE 43-16 Biochemical confirmation of pheochromocytoma or paraganglioma.

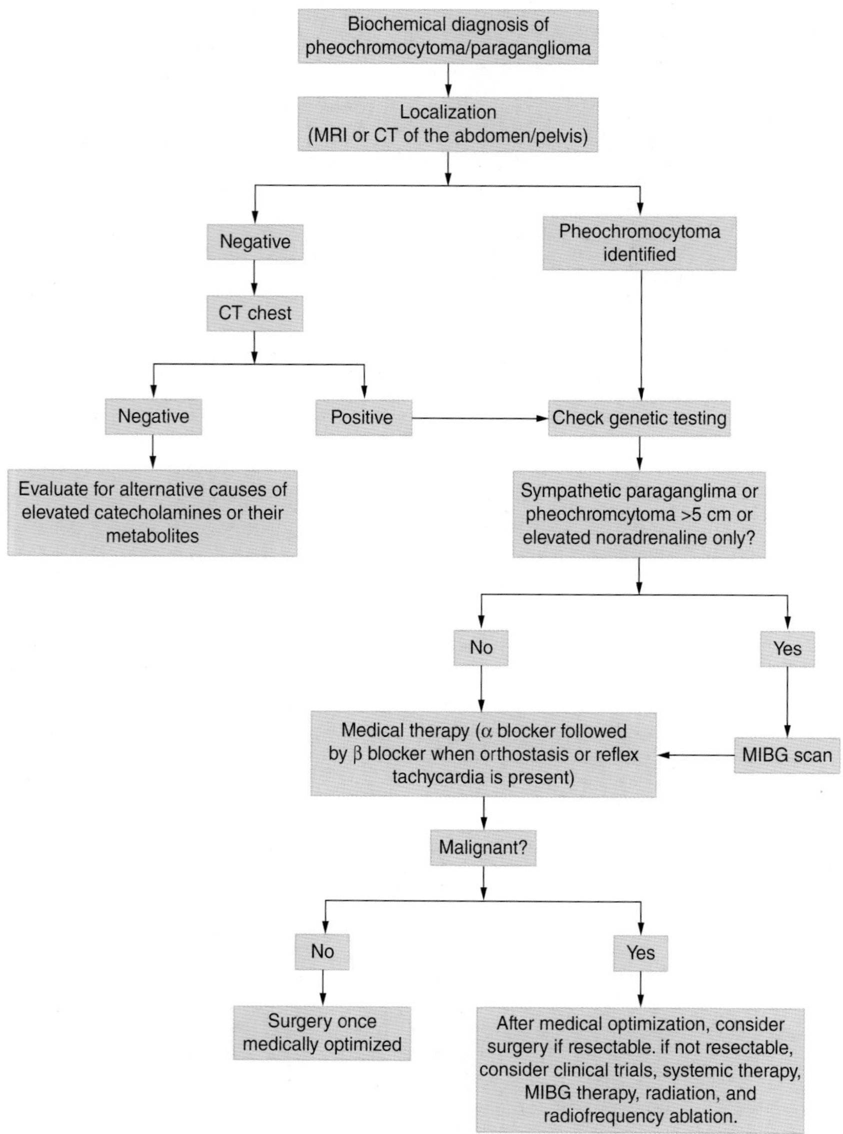

FIGURE 43-17 Algorithm for clinical approach to pheochromocytoma or paraganglioma following biochemical confirmation. CT, computed tomography; MIBG, metaiodobenzylguanidine; MRI, magnetic resonance imaging.

24-hour urine fractionated metanephrines are the two most commonly used laboratory tests to diagnose pheochromocytoma or paraganglioma. The high sensitivity and specificity of these tests are the main reasons they are preferred over alternatives such as plasma or urinary catecholamines, urinary total metanephrines, or urinary vanillylmandelic acid. For low-risk patients, however, the 24-hour urine fractionated metanephrines may be preferable in order to reduce the number of false-positive results. Of course, note should be taken of any drugs or other factors that may cause false-positive results ([62, 63]) (Table 43-8).

Even in patients without signs or symptoms of pheochromocytoma or paraganglioma, testing is suggested in the following situations: (1) features or family history suggestive of syndromes associated with pheochromocytoma listed in Table 43-9; (2) personal history of pheochromocytoma; or (3) adrenal incidentalomas.

Imaging

Imaging is not recommended for screening in the absence of biochemical evidence of pheochromocytoma or paraganglioma. However, once biochemical confirmation of the diagnosis is obtained, the next

Table 43-8 Potential Sources of False-Positive Laboratory Results for Pheochromocytoma

Related to time of collection
- Posture (fewer false positives if done supine after resting in a dark, quiet room for 30 minutes) - Nonfasting state - Exercise - Stress - Cold exposure - Hypoglycemia
Dietary or habits
- Caffeine - Nicotine - Alcohol - Ingestion of foods high in tyramine - Cocaine
Medications listed here are those most frequently encountered (many are test dependent)
- Tricyclic antidepressants (most other antidepressants can also interfere to a lesser degree) - Phenoxybenzamine - Labetalol - Acetaminophen - Amphetamines - Ephedrine - L-Dopa - Mesalamine - Sulfasalazine

Table 43-9 Syndromes Associated With Pheochromocytoma

Syndrome	Gene	Inheritance	Clinical Findings
MEN2a	*RET*	Autosomal dominant	Primary hyperparathyroidism, medullary thyroid carcinoma, Hirschsprung disease
MEN2b	*RET*	Autosomal dominant	Primary hyperparathyroidism, medullary thyroid carcinoma, mucosal ganglioneuromas, Marfanoid body habitus
Neurofibromatosis type 1	*NF1*	Autosomal dominant	Café-au-lait spots, axillary/inguinal freckling, neurofibromas, Lisch nodules, scoliosis, malignant nerve sheath tumors
von Hippel–Lindau syndrome	*VHL*	Autosomal dominant	Hemangiomas or the CNS, retinal angiomas, renal cell cancer, pancreatic neuroendocrine tumors, endolymphatic sac tumors
Carney triad	Unknown	Unknown	Gastrointestinal stromal tumors, pulmonary chondromas
Carney-Stratakis dyad	*SDHx*	Autosomal dominant	Gastrointestinal stromal tumors
Familial paraganglioma syndromes			
Paraganglioma syndrome 1	*SDHD*	Autosomal dominant	Head and neck parasympathetic paragangliomas (parent of origin effect—paternal)
Paraganglioma syndrome 2	*SDHAF2*	Autosomal dominant	Head and neck parasympathetic paragangliomas (parent of origin effect—paternal)
Paraganglioma syndrome 3	*SDHC*	Autosomal dominant	Head and neck parasympathetic paragangliomas
Paraganglioma syndrome 4	*SDHB*	Autosomal dominant	Renal cell cancer, papillary thyroid cancer, paragangliomas located in the chest/abdomen/pelvis

CNS, central nervous system; MEN, multiple endocrine neoplasia.
Data from Waguespack SG, Rich T, Grubbs E, et al. A current review of the etiology, diagnosis, and treatment of pediatric pheochromocytoma and paraganglioma. *J Clin Endocrinol Metab*. 2010;95(5):2023-2037; and Jimenez C, Cote G, Arnold A, Gagel RF. Review: should patients with apparently sporadic pheochromocytomas or paragangliomas be screened for hereditary syndromes? *J Clin Endocrinol Metab*. 2006;91(8):2851-2858.

step is localization with imaging studies. Because the majority of pheochromocytomas and paragangliomas are located in the adrenal gland or elsewhere in the abdomen, cross-sectional imaging (CT or MRI) of the abdomen with attention to the adrenal glands has the highest yield. If an adrenal mass is not seen, the paraspinous region and urinary bladder should be carefully examined. Less commonly, extra-adrenal tumors may be located in the head and neck region.

There are certain imaging characteristics considered typical of pheochromocytoma or paraganglioma. Although helpful when present, their absence cannot be used to exclude the possibility that a mass is a pheochromocytoma or paraganglioma. On CT scan, they are usually heterogeneous with a density of greater than 10 Hounsfield units (HU) and delayed washout of contrast. On MRI, they are also usually heterogeneous and hyperintense on T2-weighted images with no dropout of signal on opposed phase imaging ([64]). Functional imaging, such as MIBG scintigraphy or PET scan, may be useful when cross-sectional imaging is nonlocalizing despite a high clinical suspicion. Because these tests are more often used to complement cross-sectional imaging when there is suspicion of metastases, they will be discussed in the section on malignant pheochromocytomas and paraganglioma (Figs. 43-18 and 43-19).

Genetics

Because pheochromocytoma and paraganglioma are associated with multiple familial syndromes (the majority of which are inherited in an autosomal dominant fashion), it is important to consider genetic testing. Features associated with familial cases include young age at diagnosis, positive family history, bilateral or multiple adrenal pheochromocytomas, and any paraganglioma. The syndromes in which pheochromocytomas or paragangliomas are seen include MEN type 2, familial paraganglioma syndromes, neurofibromatosis type 1, von Hippel–Lindau syndrome, Carney triad, and Carney-Stratakis syndrome ([65]) (see Table 43-9).

Although some suggest genetic testing only in those with features suggesting a familial syndrome, others advocate more widespread testing due to a reported incidence of somatic mutations in more than 20% of patients with apparently sporadic disease. At our institution, genetic testing is performed on all patients with pheochromocytoma or paraganglioma. In any case, patients should always meet with a knowledgeable genetic counselor to discuss the risks and benefits prior to and after any familial testing. When a decision is made to test, it is recommended that genetic testing be performed taking into account the most likely diagnoses rather than checking all mutations at once ([60, 65, 66]).

Therapy

Medical

Although surgery is the treatment of choice for pheochromocytoma or paraganglioma, patients must be medically optimized prior to surgery to reduce the risk of perioperative mortality. Preparation for surgery includes management of hypertension along with volume expansion. The first step is initiating α blockade with either a nonspecific α-blocker (phenoxybenzamine) or a selective α-1 blocker (eg, doxazosin, prazosin, or terazosin) ([67]). The dose is titrated until adequate control of hypertension is achieved without inducing severe orthostatic hypotension. Once the patient starts

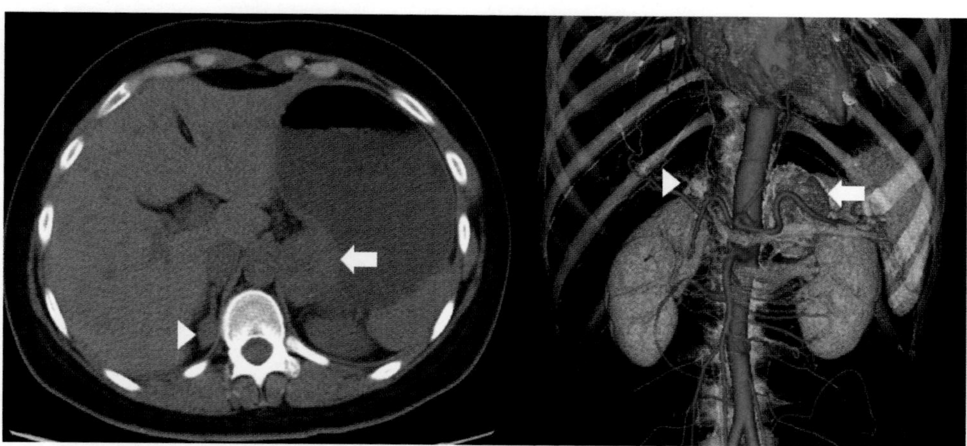

FIGURE 43-18 This is a patient with multiple endocrine neoplasia type 2A and bilateral adrenal pheochromocytomas. The computed tomography (CT) scan (*left*) and CT angiogram (*right*) show a 1.6-cm pheochromocytoma in the medial limb of the right adrenal gland (*white arrowheads*) and a 4.6-cm pheochromocytoma in the left adrenal gland (*white arrows*).

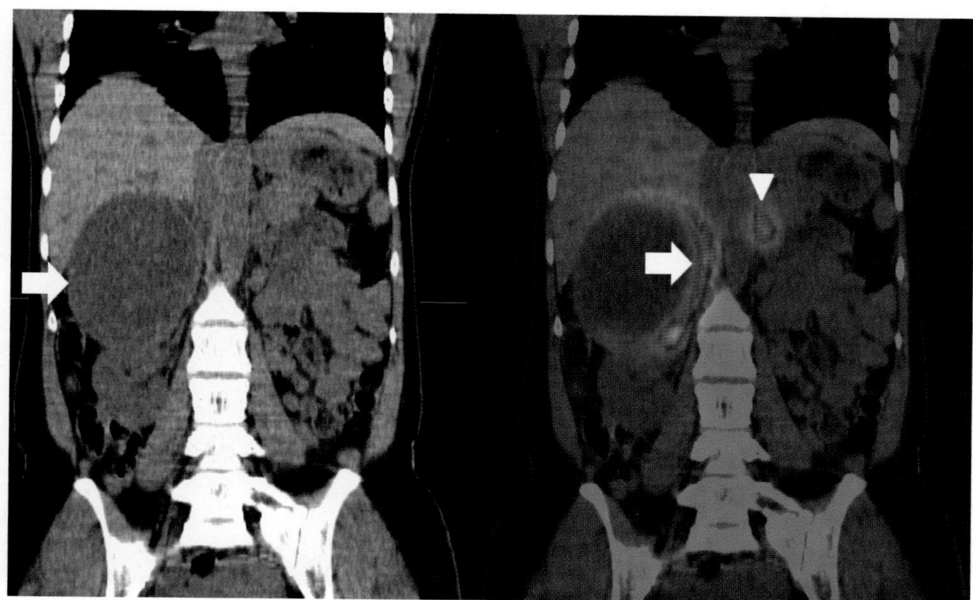

FIGURE 43-19 This is a patient with bilateral adrenal pheochromocytomas. These images are coronal views from a single photon emission computed tomography on the left and a metaiodobenzylguanidine scan on the right. They show increased uptake in the periphery of a cystic right-sided adrenal pheochromocytoma (*white arrows*) as well as a smaller left-sided adrenal pheochromocytoma (*white arrowhead*).

to develop orthostasis or reflex tachycardia, β blockade should be initiated. A high-sodium diet starting at the same time as α blockade is helpful for some patients to promote volume expansion. Medical optimization prior to surgery may be accomplished in 1 to 2 weeks. However, each patient is unique, and preparation may take longer for some patients.

Keep in mind that it is of utmost importance to avoid β-blockers before achieving adequate α blockade because lone β blockade leaves α receptors unopposed and open for activation by circulating catecholamines. This situation could potentially promote a hypertensive crisis. Although it is not currently the standard of care, calcium channel blockers have also been effective in the preoperative management of these patients ([67]).

Surgical

Surgical resection following appropriate medical therapy is the primary mode of treatment for benign pheochromocytoma or paraganglioma. For smaller tumors, minimally invasive surgeries can reduce blood loss and hospital length of stay. As a result, the preferred procedures are laparoscopic or posterior retroperitoneoscopic adrenalectomy ([68]). However, in some cases, a larger tumor or a lack of local surgical experience with these techniques may make an open procedure preferable.

Close hemodynamic monitoring with pre- and intraoperative volume repletion is important to avoid hypotension following tumor resection. Short-acting intravenous vasodilators (eg, nitroprusside, nitroglycerine, phentolamine) may be needed intraoperatively to decrease the risk of precipitating a hypertensive crisis during tumor manipulation. Intravenous fluids should contain dextrose because patients are prone to hypoglycemia as a result of rebound insulin secretion following the precipitous drop in catecholamine levels after successful tumor resection. In patients who have pheochromocytoma associated with a germline mutation or bilateral adrenal disease, cortical-sparing adrenalectomy is the procedure of choice to minimize the risk of lifelong adrenal insufficiency. However, these patients require long-term follow-up because recurrence may develop many years after their primary surgery, and some may develop adrenal insufficiency despite a cortical-sparing technique ([69, 70]).

MALIGNANT PHEOCHROMOCYTOMA

Introduction

Unfortunately, there are no reliable clinical or pathologic features of the primary tumor that have been shown to consistently identify malignant pheochromocytoma or paraganglioma. As a result, the diagnosis can only be made after the discovery of metastatic disease. The most common sites of metastasis are the axial skeleton, followed by the liver, lymph nodes, lungs, and peritoneum. Although a generally quoted statistic is that 10% of pheochromocytomas are malignant, this is not true for all patients. In hereditary forms, rates less than 10% have been seen in patients with germline *RET* and *VHL* mutations. In contrast, rates in excess of 80% have been reported in patients with a germline *SDHB* mutation ([71]).

In a large retrospective review, it was found that almost half of patients with malignant pheochromocytoma or paraganglioma are diagnosed with metachronous metastases (ie, they were thought to have benign disease until they were later found to have metastatic disease). This review identified tumor size (>5 cm) and site of primary tumor (infradiaphragmatic para-aortic paraganglia or the mediastinum) as being associated with a higher incidence of malignancy. However, there were no criteria that reliably excluded the possibility of malignancy ([72]), and newly noted metastatic disease can be found up to 20 years after resection of an apparently benign pheochromocytoma ([73, 74]). It is for these reasons that lifelong surveillance of patients with seemingly benign pheochromocytoma or paraganglioma is always recommended.

Diagnosis

Because the diagnosis is made based on identification of metastatic disease, a combination of laboratory testing, imaging, and pathologic confirmation is generally relied upon. Typical staging studies include cross-sectional imaging (ie, CT or MRI) of the chest, abdomen, and pelvis. In the setting of malignant pheochromocytoma or paraganglioma, functional studies may be used to complement cross-sectional imaging. For example, MIBG scintigraphy has been used since 1981 to localize pheochromocytoma ([75]). Its usefulness is based on the fact that MIBG structurally resembles norepinephrine and is stored in the catecholamine-storage vesicles. For patients in whom dedifferentiation has occurred as well as patients with an *SDHB* mutation, PET scans using FDG have been a useful adjunct to cross-sectional imaging. Furthermore, 6-[^{18}F]fluorodopamine PET scanning may have a role in the future but is not widely available ([75, 76]) (Fig. 43-20).

Given the rarity of this entity, precise data do not exist regarding prognosis. However, in a series of 10 patients with malignant pheochromocytomas, the 5-year survival was reported as 20%, and all patients died within 10 years ([77]).

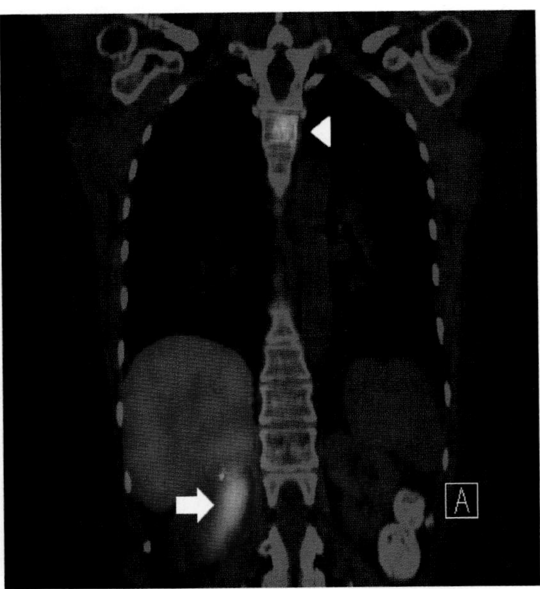

FIGURE 43-20 Metaiodobenzylguanidine scan showing uptake in recurrent malignant pheochromocytoma in the right adrenal bed (*white arrow*) as well as metastatic disease in the T2 vertebral body (*white arrowhead*).

Therapy

Medical/Surgical

Medical therapy is recommended following the same process as for benign tumors. For patients whose disease is potentially curable, surgery via an open approach is the preferred strategy. In patients for whom surgical cure is not feasible, palliative surgery may be recommended as needed for improved control of catecholamine secretion or for the prevention of complications related to the location of the disease. Because skeletal metastases are commonly seen, it is important to consider antiresorptive therapy to reduce the risk of skeletal-related events and associated morbidity ([78]).

Radiation and Radiofrequency Ablation

If there is evidence of MIBG avidity, it can be used as a carrier for ^{131}I delivery as targeted therapy. Although it is not widely available, it has shown efficacy in selected patients. Unfortunately, patients with MIBG-avid lesions will sometimes have additional nonavid lesions. Furthermore, the dose of radiation is limited by bone marrow toxicity. As a result, it is generally given with palliative intent ([79, 80]).

External beam radiation can also be used for symptomatic relief of metastases not amenable to surgical resection. Retrospective studies have demonstrated improvement in symptoms but no dramatic response of the tumor on imaging ([81]). Radiofrequency ablation (RFA) has also been attempted in a limited number of patients with metastatic pheochromocytoma and can be considered as part of the treatment armamentarium ([82]).

Chemotherapy

Traditional cytotoxic chemotherapy has been used with some success. Because these tumors are rare, there are no trials that definitively identify the most effective regimen. The regimens most often used are CVD (cyclophosphamide, vincristine, and dacarbazine) and CVAD (cyclophosphamide, vincristine, doxorubicin, and dacarbazine). In a retrospective review at a large cancer center, the response rate was 33%. Furthermore, the patients who responded to chemotherapy had a better overall survival compared with those who were nonresponders (6.4 vs 3.7 years) ([83]). Although initial reports using a multityrosine kinase inhibitor (sunitinib) suggested partial short-term responses in a very small number of patients, data regarding the long-term efficacy and validation of these findings are still lacking ([84, 85]).

ADRENOCORTICAL CARCINOMA

Introduction

Adrenocortical carcinoma (ACC) is a rare malignancy with significant morbidity and mortality. A review of the National Cancer Institute's Surveillance, Epidemiology, and End Results (SEER) database found the majority of patients (87%) were Caucasian and diagnosis occurred at an average age of 51 years. A bimodal distribution of incidence was seen in the first and fourth decades of life. The age-adjusted annual incidence was 0.72 per million in the United States, and there was a slight female predominance (54%) ([86]).

A review at our institution found that 42% of cases were hormonally productive, but there have been reports as high as two-thirds of cases. The majority of cases (55%) were associated with hypercortisolemia, and smaller numbers were associated with hyperaldosteronism or hyperandrogenism. Furthermore, the production of multiple hormones was present in almost 20% of these patients ([87]). The various syndromes seen with functioning adrenal cancers are presented in Table 43-10. Of course, ACC can also present as a nonfunctioning tumor with only nonspecific symptoms of abdominal discomfort or pain, indigestion, or site-specific symptoms based on the location of metastatic disease.

Diagnosis

Laboratory

The suggested hormonal evaluation includes morning serum cortisol, ACTH, plasma renin activity, plasma aldosterone concentration, plasma free metanephrines, and 24-hour urine free cortisol. Additionally, total testosterone, dehydroepiandrosterone sulfate (DHEAS), and estradiol may be obtained if there is clinical suspicion of increased sex hormone secretion (ie, virilizing or feminizing features) (Fig. 43-21).

Imaging

Computed tomography or MRI of the chest, abdomen, and pelvis is generally the first step in staging. On CT, ACC is usually a large, heterogeneous mass with attenuation values greater than 10 HU showing

Table 43-10 Clinical Syndromes Associated With Functional Adrenocortical Carcinoma (ACC)

Clinical Syndrome	Suggestive Clinical Features	Suggested Laboratory Workup
Cushing syndrome	Obesity, moon facies, purple striae, cervical fat pads, easy bruising, myopathy, hypertension, diabetes mellitus	Plasma electrolytes, plasma glucose, adrenocorticotropic hormone (ACTH), cortisol, 24-h urine free cortisol
Virilizing syndrome	Hirsutism, clitoromegaly, temporal balding, increased muscle mass, amenorrhea, male precocious puberty, advanced bone age in children	Dehydroepiandrosterone sulfate (DHEAS), testosterone, 17-OH progesterone
Feminizing syndrome	Gynecomastia, loss of libido	Estradiol, prolactin, testosterone
Hyperaldosteronism	Hypertension, hypokalemia	Plasma renin activity, plasma aldosterone concentration, plasma electrolytes, 18-OH corticosterone
Mixed syndromes	Combinations of features above	Testing as appropriate based on clinical features

Data from Ayala-Ramirez M, Jasim S, Feng L, et al. Adrenocortical carcinoma: clinical outcomes and prognosis of 330 patients at a tertiary care center. *Eur J Endocrinol.* 2013;169(6):891-899.

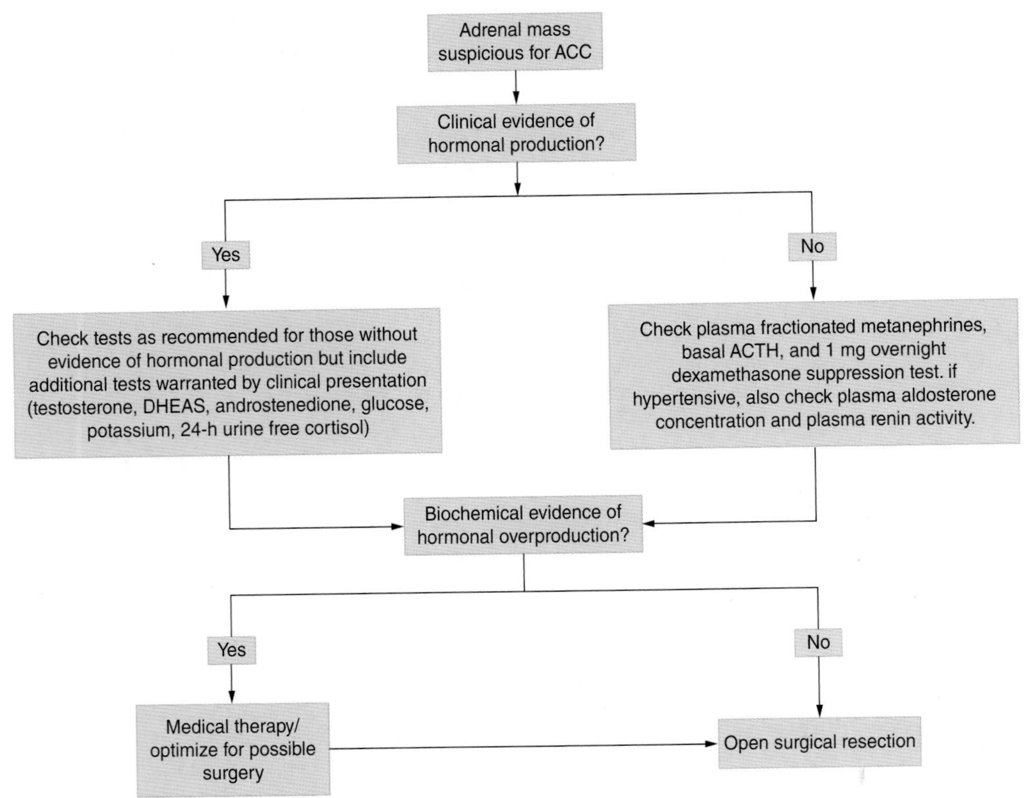

FIGURE 43-21 Hormonal testing for adrenocortical carcinoma (ACC). ACTH, adrenocorticotropic hormone; DHEAS, dehydroepiandrosterone sulfate.

heterogeneous contrast enhancement, poor contrast washout, and necrosis. Special attention should be devoted to assessment for metastatic disease in the lungs, liver, bones, and regional lymph nodes. The MRI appearance of ACC is also heterogeneous and hyperintense on T2-weighted images. As seen on CT, contrast enhancement on MRI is heterogeneous with poor washout. Of note, MRI is particularly useful in assessing for tumor invasion of the inferior vena cava. Although FDG-PET scan is a sensitive tool for detecting malignant tissue, its low specificity limits its usefulness. However, FDG-PET can play an important role in the identification of metastatic disease in the setting of known ACC ([88, 89]) (Figs. 43-22 and 43-23).

Pathology

Weiss proposed a scoring system consisting of nine criteria to aid in the diagnosis of adrenal cancer, and this has proved helpful in assessing malignant potential (Fig. 43-24). The criteria include: (1) mitotic rate greater than 5 mitoses per 50 high-power fields in the most active areas of the tumor, (2) atypical mitoses, (3) venous invasion, (4) clear cells comprising 25% or less of the tumor, (5) tumor necrosis, (6) nuclear grade 3 or 4 tumor (Fuhrman method), (7) diffuse (solid) architecture in more than one-third of the tumor, (8) invasion of sinusoidal structures, and (9) capsular invasion. The presence of three or more of these nine features is highly suggestive of ACC ([90]). Despite this system, there remain borderline cases in which a systematic approach is needed to make a definitive diagnosis. The staging of ACC is detailed in Table 43-11. We have also found the use of Ki-67 expression useful in assessing prognosis.

In general, FNA of suspected ACC is not recommended due to the risk of seeding the needle track with tumor. However, FNA may be considered after pheochromocytoma has been ruled out in the context of a known primary malignant tumor with possible metastasis to the adrenal gland (ie, small cell lung cancer, breast cancer, renal cell cancer, and gastric cancer). Nonetheless, FNA is only recommended if it will alter the treatment strategy.

Genetics

An association has been observed between ACC and Li-Fraumeni syndrome, Lynch syndrome, Beckwith-Wiedemann syndrome. Very rarely has ACC been seen in association with MEN1, familial adenomatous

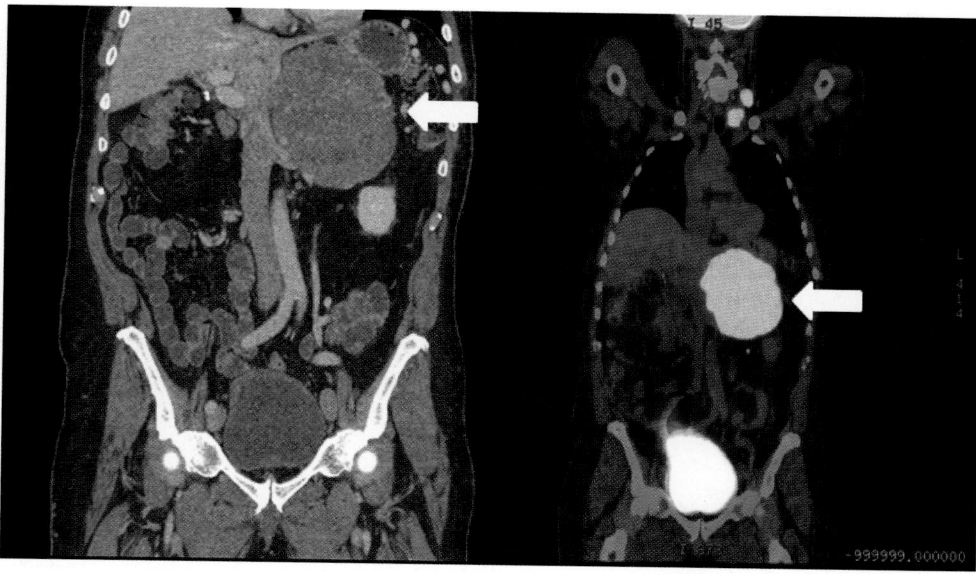
FIGURE 43-22 Coronal images from computed tomography (CT; *left*) and fluorodeoxyglucose–positron emission tomography/CT (*right*) showing left-sided adrenocortical carcinoma (*white arrows*).

polyposis, neurofibromatosis type 1, and Carney complex ([91]). As a result, it is important to keep this in mind when seeing patients with these syndromes as well as to keep these syndromes in mind when seeing patients with ACC (Table 43-12).

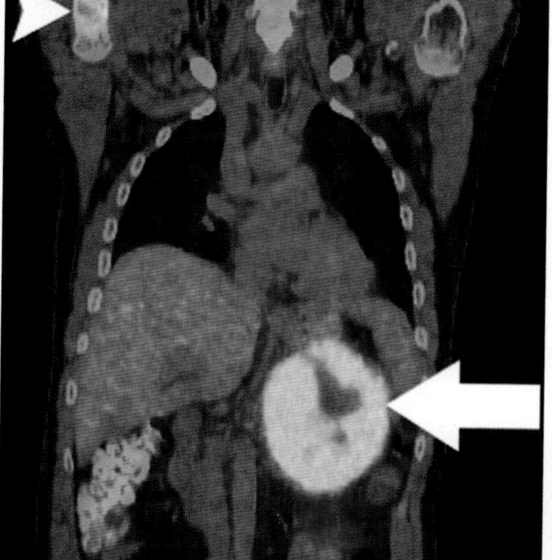
FIGURE 43-23 Fluorodeoxyglucose (FDG) positron emission tomography (PET) scan (coronal view) of a patient with adrenocortical carcinoma (ACC) showing FDG-avid left adrenal mass (*white arrow*) with bone metastases (*arrowhead*).

Prognosis

A diagnosis of ACC carries high mortality. A review of the National Cancer Institute's SEER database found a 1-year cause-specific mortality rate of 58% and a 5-year rate of 88% ([86]). However, long-term survival is possible in these patients if complete resection with tumor-free margins can be achieved. At our institution, the 5-year survival rate has been found to be 38%, with a median overall survival of 3.21 years for all patients. As is seen in many other cancers, survival is inversely correlated with disease stage at diagnosis. For example, those with stage I disease had a mean

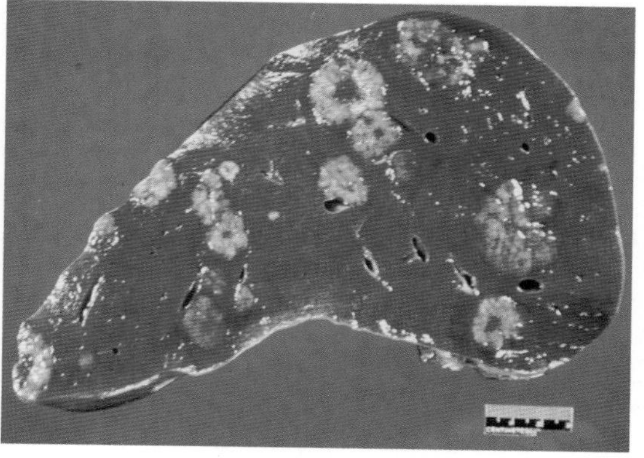
FIGURE 43-24 Liver metastases from adrenocortical carcinoma.

Table 43-11 Staging for Adrenocortical Carcinoma (ACC)

Stage	AJCC	ENSAT
I	Primary tumor ≤5 cm with no nodal or distant metastasis	Primary tumor ≤5 cm with no nodal or distant metastasis
II	Primary tumor >5 cm with no extra-adrenal spread	Primary tumor >5 cm with no extra-adrenal spread
III	Primary tumor not invasive but lymph node metastasis present *or* Primary tumor locally invasive without lymph node metastasis	Primary tumor not invasive but lymph node metastasis present *or* Primary tumor locally invasive or invading adjacent organs but without distant metastasis (lymph node metastasis may be present)
IV	Tumor locally invasive with lymph node metastasis *or* Tumor invading adjacent organs *or* Distant metastasis present	Distant metastasis present (no other requirements)

AJCC, American Joint Committee on Cancer; ENSAT, European Network for the Study of Adrenal Tumors.
Data from Lughezzani G, Sun M, Perrotte P, et al. The European Network for the Study of Adrenal Tumors staging system is prognostically superior to the international union against cancer-staging system: a North American validation. *Eur J Cancer*. 2010;46(4):713-719; and Asare EA, Wang TS, Winchester DP, Mallin K, Kebebew E, Sturgeon C. A novel staging system for adrenocortical carcinoma better predicts survival in patients with stage I/II disease. *Surgery*. 2014;156(6):1378-1386.

survival of 24.1 years as compared to 0.89 years for those with stage IV disease ([87]).

Therapy

Surgical

Complete surgical resection is the most important treatment for ACC and offers the best chance for prolonged disease-free survival. If ACC is suspected, laparoscopic adrenalectomy is not recommended because it can result in early locoregional recurrence and peritoneal carcinomatosis. Furthermore, it may decrease the ability to achieve tumor-free margins or adequate lymph node dissection ([92]). Tumor encasement of the celiac axis, aorta, or proximal superior mesenteric artery may make the tumor unresectable. In contrast, the presence of tumor thrombus in the inferior vena cava or renal vein, or tumor invasion of the pancreas, spleen, or kidney is not a

Table 43-12 Genetic Syndromes Associated With Adrenocortical Carcinoma

Syndrome	Gene(s)	Inheritance	Common Clinical Findings
Li-Fraumeni syndrome	*TP53*	Autosomal dominant	Sarcoma, breast cancer, leukemia, brain tumors, radiation-induced cancers
Beckwith-Wiedemann syndrome	Multiple	Majority of cases are sporadic	Macrosomia, macroglossia, cleft palate, omphalocele, advanced bone age, Wilms tumor, hepatoblastoma
MEN1	*MENIN*	Autosomal dominant	Parathyroid adenoma, pituitary adenoma, pancreatic islet cell tumors, carcinoid, angiofibromas, collagenomas
Familial adenomatous polyposis	*APC*	Autosomal dominant	Colon polyps/cancer, pancreatic cancer, thyroid cancer, medulloblastomas, osteomas
Lynch syndrome	*MLH1, MLH2, MSH6, PMS2*	Autosomal dominant	Colorectal cancer, endometrial cancer, ovarian cancer, glioma, gastric cancer
Carney complex	*PRKAR1A*	Autosomal dominant	Primary pigmented nodular adrenocortical disease, lentigines, testicular cancer (Sertoli cell), thyroid cancer, pancreatic cancer, atrial myxoma
Congenital adrenal hyperplasia	*CYP21A2*	Autosomal recessive	Ambiguous genitalia, precocious puberty, infertility, hirsutism, electrolyte abnormalities

Data from Else T, Kim AC, Sabolch A, et al. Adrenocortical carcinoma. *Endocr Rev*. 2014;35(2):282-326; Libe R, Arlt W, Louiset E, et al. A feminizing adrenocortical carcinoma in the context of a late onset 21-hydroxylase deficiency. *J Clin Endocrinol Metab*. 2014;99(6):1943-1944; and Varma T, Panchani R, Goyal A, Maskey R. A case of androgen-secreting adrenal carcinoma with non-classical congenital adrenal hyperplasia. *Indian J Endocrinol Metab*. 2013;17(Suppl 1):S243-S245.

contraindication for complete resection in selected patients. Although there is limited evidence of benefit from resection of the primary tumor in the presence of metastatic disease, there may still be a role for resection of the primary tumor and all visible metastases in an otherwise young, healthy patient, especially in cases of symptomatic hormonally active tumors.

In corticosteroid-producing ACC, there is speculation that preoperative blockade of steroid production using agents such as ketoconazole or metyrapone may reduce postoperative morbidity. In these cases, the contralateral adrenal gland is usually atrophic, and patients may require peri- and postoperative corticosteroid replacement. In fact, relative adrenal insufficiency may last for months following successful resection.

Chemotherapy

In 1949, it was found that oral administration of the insecticide dichlorodiphenyltrichloroethane (DDT) to dogs caused selective necrosis of zona fasciculata and zona reticularis of the adrenal cortex. Since 1960, a DDT analog known as mitotane has been used to treat ACC. Research has shown that maintaining mitotane levels of 14 to 20 mg/L improve recurrence-free survival but not necessarily overall survival ([93]). Mitotane is believed to be useful in the adjuvant setting and also for inoperable disease. Mitotane has even been used successfully in a small number of patients in the neoadjuvant setting, resulting in improved surgical outcomes ([94]). In addition to adrenal toxicity, mitotane also increases corticosteroid-binding globulin and enhances steroid clearance. As a result, there are increased glucocorticoid requirements during mitotane therapy, and failure to adequately replace glucocorticoids can result in adrenal crisis. Furthermore, lipid changes have been well described in patients taking mitotane ([95]) (Fig. 43-25).

In terms of other chemotherapeutic agents, an international phase III study (FIRM-ACT) was carried out to compare mitotane plus EDP (etoposide, doxorubicin, cisplatin) with mitotane plus streptozotocin. In this study, it was found that mitotane-EDP showed better tumor response (23% vs 9%) and PFS (5.3 vs 2.1 months). However, there was no significant improvement in overall survival ([96]). Our current practice in managing ACC is summarized in Figs. 43-26 and 43-27.

Targeted therapies are also a fertile area for clinical investigation. Potential candidates include insulin-like growth factor-1R inhibitors, epidermal growth factor receptor inhibitors, multitarget TKIs, mammalian target of rapamycin (mTOR) inhibitors, and agents targeting steroidogenic factor-1 ([97, 98]). Enrollment in clinical trials for use of investigational agents is favored to help answer important clinical questions regarding safety and efficacy.

Radiation and Radiofrequency Ablation

Adrenocortical carcinoma is generally considered a radioresistant tumor, and adjuvant radiation may not reduce the risk of recurrence or increase overall survival ([99]).

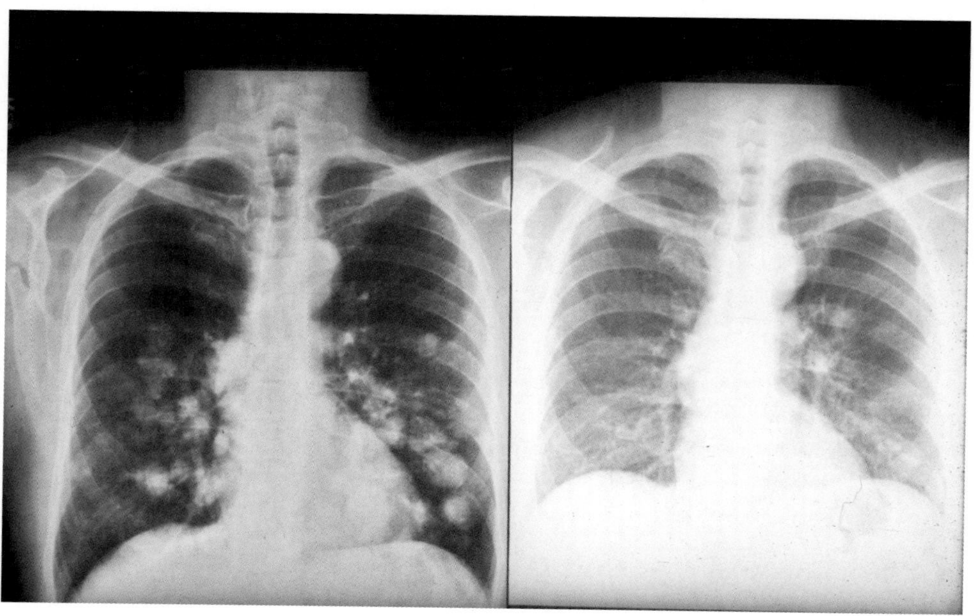

FIGURE 43-25 These are chest x-rays of a patient with metastatic adrenocortical carcinoma. These images demonstrates the extent of disease before mitotane (*left*) and after mitotane (*right*).

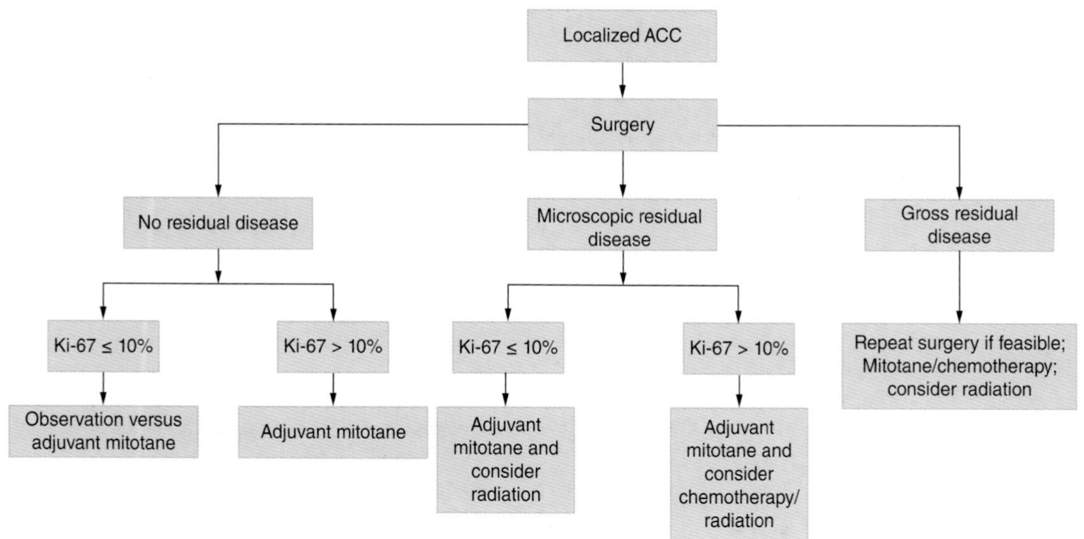

FIGURE 43-26 Management of localized adrenocortical carcinoma (ACC).

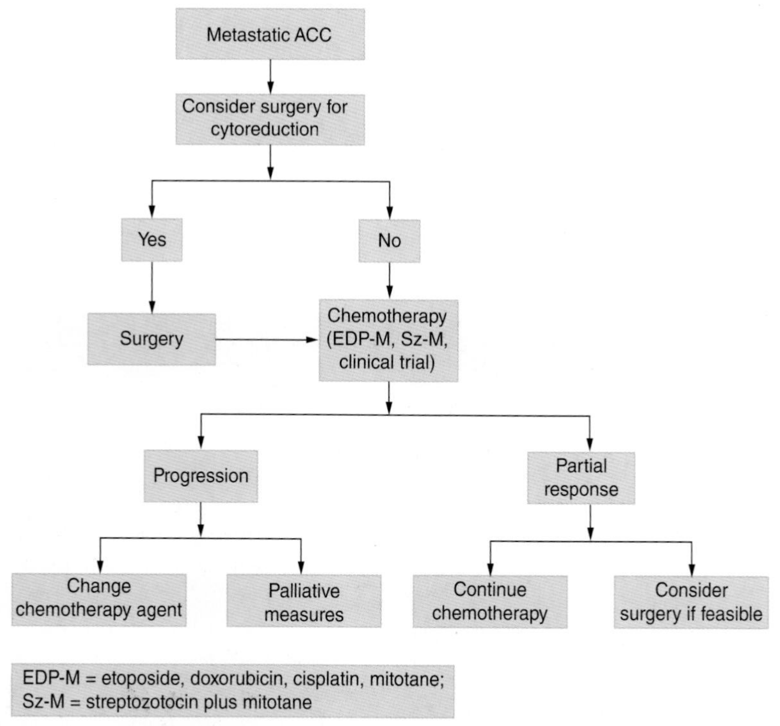

FIGURE 43-27 Management of metastatic adrenocortical carcinoma (ACC).

At the University of Texas MD Anderson Cancer Center, radiation treatment is used in selected patients with metastatic ACC for palliation ([100]). Percutaneous image-guided RFA has also been attempted in the setting of unresectable primary or metastatic ACC. This procedure may be useful for short-term, local control of small adrenal tumors, but further data are needed to elucidate the long-term efficacy and potential impact on survival.

REFERENCES

1. American Cancer Society. Cancer Facts and Figures. 2014. http://www.cancer.org/acs/groups/content/@research/documents/webcontent/acspc-042151.pdf. Accessed September 21, 2014.
2. Hundahl SA, Fleming ID, Fremgen AM, Menck HR. A National Cancer Data Base report on 53,856 cases of thyroid carcinoma treated in the U.S., 1985-1995. *Cancer.* 1998;83(12):2638-2648.
3. Yassa L, Cibas ES, Benson CB, et al. Long-term assessment of a multidisciplinary approach to thyroid nodule diagnostic evaluation. *Cancer.* 2007;111(6):508-516.
4. Mazzaferri EL. Management of a solitary thyroid nodule. *N Engl J Med.* 1993;328(8):553-559.
5. American Thyroid Association Guidelines Taskforce on Thyroid Nodules and Differentiated Thyroid Cancer, Cooper DS, Doherty GM, et al. Revised American Thyroid Association management guidelines for patients with thyroid nodules and differentiated thyroid cancer. *Thyroid.* 2009;19(11):1167-1214.
6. Sherman SI. Thyroid carcinoma. *Lancet.* 2003;361(9356):501-511.
7. Ivanov VK, Kashcheev VV, Chekin SY, et al. Radiation-epidemiological studies of thyroid cancer incidence in Russia after the Chernobyl accident (estimation of radiation risks, 1991-2008 follow-up period). *Radiat Prot Dosimetry.* 2012;151(3):489-499.
8. Nose V. Familial follicular cell tumors: classification and morphological characteristics. *Endocr Pathol.* 2010;21(4):219-226.
9. Ma J, Huang M, Wang L, Ye W, Tong Y, Wang H. Obesity and risk of thyroid cancer: evidence from a meta-analysis of 21 observational studies. *Med Sci Monit.* 2015;21:283-291.

9a. Mazeh H, Benavidez J, Poehls JL, Youngwirth L, Chen H, Sippel RS. In patients with thyroid cancer of follicular cell origin, a family history of nonmedullary thyroid cancer in one first-degree relative is associated with more aggressive disease. Thyroid 2012;22(1):3-8.

10. Carhill AA, Litofsky DR, Sherman SI. Unique characteristics and outcomes of patients diagnosed with both primary thyroid and primary renal cell carcinoma. *Endocr Pract.* 2014:1-19.
11. Fagin JA. How thyroid tumors start and why it matters: kinase mutants as targets for solid cancer pharmacotherapy. *J Endocrinol.* 2004;183(2):249-256.
12. Haugen BR, Sherman SI. Evolving approaches to patients with advanced differentiated thyroid cancer. *Endocr Rev.* 2013;34(3):439-455.
13. Bounacer A, Wicker R, Caillou B, et al. High prevalence of activating ret proto-oncogene rearrangements, in thyroid tumors from patients who had received external radiation. *Oncogene.* 1997;15(11):1263-1273.
14. Jhiang SM. The RET proto-oncogene in human cancers. *Oncogene.* 2000;19(49):5590-5597.
15. Xing M, Alzahrani AS, Carson KA, et al. Association between BRAF V600E mutation and recurrence of papillary thyroid cancer. *J Clin Oncol.* 2015;33(1):42-50.
16. Xing M, Liu R, Liu X, et al. BRAF V600E and TERT promoter mutations cooperatively identify the most aggressive papillary thyroid cancer with highest recurrence. *J Clin Oncol.* 2014;32(25):2718-2726.
17. Liu X, Bishop J, Shan Y, et al. Highly prevalent TERT promoter mutations in aggressive thyroid cancers. *Endocr Relat Cancer.* 2013;20(4):603-610.
18. Carmeliet P, Jain RK. Molecular mechanisms and clinical applications of angiogenesis. *Nature.* 2011;473(7347):298-307.
19. Auger M, Stelow E, Yang G, et al. Papillary thyroid carcinoma and variants. In: Cibas E, Ali SZ, eds. *The Bethesda System for Reporting Thyroid Cytopathology.* New York, NY: Springer; 2010:91-116.
20. Katoh R, Sasaki J, Kurihara H, Suzuki K, Iida Y, Kawaoi A. Multiple thyroid involvement (intraglandular metastasis) in papillary thyroid carcinoma. A clinicopathologic study of 105 consecutive patients. *Cancer.* 1992;70(6):1585-1590.
21. Silverberg SG, Hutter RV, Foote FW Jr. Fatal carcinoma of the thyroid: histology, metastases, and causes of death. *Cancer.* 1970;25(4):792-802.
22. Mazzaferri EL, Jhiang SM. Long-term impact of initial surgical and medical therapy on papillary and follicular thyroid cancer. *Am J Med.* 1994;97(5):418-428.
23. Taylor T, Specker B, Robbins J, et al. Outcome after treatment of high-risk papillary and non-Hurthle-cell follicular thyroid carcinoma. *Ann Intern Med.* 1998;129(8):622-627.
24. Tuttle RM, Sabra MM. Selective use of RAI for ablation and adjuvant therapy after total thyroidectomy for differentiated thyroid cancer: a practical approach to clinical decision making. *Oral Oncol.* 2013;49(7):676-683.
25. Shepler TR, Sherman SI, Faustina MM, Busaidy NL, Ahmadi MA, Esmaeli B. Nasolacrimal duct obstruction associated with radioactive iodine therapy for thyroid carcinoma. *Ophthal Plast Reconstr Surg.* 2003;19(6):479-481.
26. Sawka AM, Thabane L, Parlea L, et al. Second primary malignancy risk after radioactive iodine treatment for thyroid cancer: a systematic review and meta-analysis. *Thyroid.* 2009;19(5):451-457.
27. Carhill A, Ain K, Brierley J, et al. Long-term moderate thyroid hormone suppression therapy is associated with improved outcomes in differentiated thyroid carcinoma: National Thyroid Cancer Treatment Cooperative Study Group Registry analysis 1987–2012. Paper presented at the 84th Annual Meeting of the American Thyroid Association, San Diego, CA, October 29-November 2, 2014.
28. Schwartz DL, Lobo MJ, Ang KK, et al. Postoperative external beam radiotherapy for differentiated thyroid cancer: outcomes and morbidity with conformal treatment. *Int J Radiat Oncol Biol Phys.* 2009;74(4):1083-1091.
29. Spencer CA, Lopresti JS. Measuring thyroglobulin and thyroglobulin autoantibody in patients with differentiated thyroid cancer. *Nat Clin Pract Endocrinol Metab.* 2008;4(4):223-233.
30. Chiovato L, Latrofa F, Braverman LE, et al. Disappearance of humoral thyroid autoimmunity after complete removal of thyroid antigens. *Ann Intern Med.* 2003;139(5 Pt 1):346-351.
31. Spencer C, Fatemi S, Singer P, Nicoloff J, Lopresti J. Serum basal thyroglobulin measured by a second-generation assay correlates with the recombinant human thyrotropin-stimulated thyroglobulin response in patients treated for differentiated thyroid cancer. *Thyroid.* 2010;20(6):587-595.
32. Wexler JA. Approach to the thyroid cancer patient with bone metastases. *J Clin Endocrinol Metab.* 2011;96(8):2296-2307.
33. Brose MS, Nutting CM, Jarzab B, et al. Sorafenib in radioactive iodine-refractory, locally advanced or metastatic differentiated thyroid cancer: a randomised, double-blind, phase 3 trial. *Lancet.* 2014;384(9940):319-328.
34. Schlumberger M, Tahara M, Wirth LJ, et al. Lenvatinib versus placebo in radioiodine-refractory thyroid cancer. *N Engl J Med.* 2015;372(7):621-630.
35. Carhill AA, Cabanillas ME, Jimenez C, et al. The noninvestigational use of tyrosine kinase inhibitors in thyroid cancer: establishing a standard for patient safety and monitoring. *J Clin Endocrinol Metab.* 2013;98(1):31-42.
36. Waguespack SG, Francis G. Initial management and follow-up of differentiated thyroid cancer in children. *J Natl Compr Canc Netw.* 2010;8(11):1289-1300.
37. Pelizzo MR, Boschin IM, Bernante P, et al. Natural history, diagnosis, treatment and outcome of medullary thyroid cancer: 37 years experience on 157 patients. *Eur J Surg Oncol.* 2007;33(4):493-497.
38. American Thyroid Association Guidelines Task Force, Kloos

RT, Eng C, et al. Medullary thyroid cancer: management guidelines of the American Thyroid Association. *Thyroid*. 2009;19(6):565-612.
39. Wohllk N, Cote GJ, Bugalho MM, et al. Relevance of RET proto-oncogene mutations in sporadic medullary thyroid carcinoma. *J Clin Endocrinol Metab*. 1996;81(10):3740-3745.
40. Brandi ML, Gagel RF, Angeli A, et al. Guidelines for diagnosis and therapy of MEN type 1 and type 2. *J Clin Endocrinol Metab*. 2001;86(12):5658-5671.
41. Tuttle RM, Ball DW, Byrd D, et al. Medullary carcinoma. *J Natl Compr Canc Netw*. 2010;8(5):512-530.
42. Brierley J, Tsang R, Simpson WJ, Gospodarowicz M, Sutcliffe S, Panzarella T. Medullary thyroid cancer: analyses of survival and prognostic factors and the role of radiation therapy in local control. *Thyroid*. 1996;6(4):305-310.
43. Smallridge RC, Ain KB, Asa SL, et al. American Thyroid Association guidelines for management of patients with anaplastic thyroid cancer. *Thyroid*. 2012;22(11):1104-1139.
44. Smallridge RC, Copland JA. Anaplastic thyroid carcinoma: pathogenesis and emerging therapies. *Clini Oncol*. 2010;22(6):486-497.
45. Shimaoka K, Schoenfeld DA, DeWys WD, Creech RH, DeConti R. A randomized trial of doxorubicin versus doxorubicin plus cisplatin in patients with advanced thyroid carcinoma. *Cancer*. 1985;56(9):2155-2160.
46. Ain KB, Egorin MJ, DeSimone PA. Treatment of anaplastic thyroid carcinoma with paclitaxel: phase 2 trial using ninety-six-hour infusion. Collaborative Anaplastic Thyroid Cancer Health Intervention Trials (CATCHIT) Group. *Thyroid*. 2000;10(7):587-594.
47. Hundahl SA, Fleming ID, Fremgen AM, Menck HR. Two hundred eighty-six cases of parathyroid carcinoma treated in the U.S. between 1985-1995: a National Cancer Data Base Report. The American College of Surgeons Commission on Cancer and the American Cancer Society. *Cancer*. 1999;86(3):538-544.
48. Schulte KM, Talat N. Diagnosis and management of parathyroid cancer. *Nat Rev Endocrinol*. 2012;8(10):612-622.
49. Talat N, Schulte KM. Clinical presentation, staging and long-term evolution of parathyroid cancer. *Ann Surg Oncol*. 2010;17(8):2156-2174.
50. Bondeson L, DeLellis RA, Lloyd R, et al. Parathyroid carcinoma. In: DeLellis RA, Heitz PU, Eng C, eds. Vol 8. *World Health Organisation Classification of Tumours, Pathology and Genetics: Tumour of Endocrine Organs*. Lyon, France: International Agency for Research on Cancer Press; 2004:124-127.
51. Schantz A, Castleman B. Parathyroid carcinoma. A study of 70 cases. *Cancer*. 1973;31(3):600-605.
52. Newey PJ, Bowl MR, Cranston T, Thakker RV. Cell division cycle protein 73 homolog (CDC73) mutations in the hyperparathyroidism-jaw tumor syndrome (HPT-JT) and parathyroid tumors. *Hum Mutat*. 2010;31(3):295-307.
53. Cetani F, Pardi E, Borsari S, et al. Genetic analyses of the HRPT2 gene in primary hyperparathyroidism: germline and somatic mutations in familial and sporadic parathyroid tumors. *J Clin Endocrinol Metab*. 2004;89(11):5583-5591.
54. DeLellis RA. Parathyroid tumors and related disorders. *Mod Pathol*. 2011;24(Suppl 2):S78-S93.
55. Rodgers SE, Perrier ND. Parathyroid carcinoma. *Curr Opin Oncol*. 2006;18(1):16-22.
56. Busaidy NL, Jimenez C, Habra MA, et al. Parathyroid carcinoma: a 22-year experience. *Head Neck*. 2004;26(8):716-726.
57. Naifa L, Busaidy MEC, Dadu R, et al. Metastatic parathyroid carcinoma and hypercalcemia responds to treatment with sorafenib. Presented at the Endocrine Society's 96th Annual Meeting and Expo, Chicago, IL, June 21–24, 2014.
58. Beard CM, Sheps SG, Kurland LT, Carney JA, Lie JT. Occurrence of pheochromocytoma in Rochester, Minnesota, 1950 through 1979. *Mayo Clin Proc*. 1983;58(12):802-804.
59. Mannelli M, Ianni L, Cilotti A, Conti A. Pheochromocytoma in Italy: a multicentric retrospective study. *Eur J Endocrinol*. 1999;141(6):619-624.
60. Neumann HP, Bausch B, McWhinney SR, et al. Germ-line mutations in nonsyndromic pheochromocytoma. *N Engl J Med*. 2002;346(19):1459-1466.
61. Tsirlin A, Oo Y, Sharma R, Kansara A, Gliwa A, Banerji MA. Pheochromocytoma: a review. *Maturitas*. 2014;77(3):229-238.
62. Eisenhofer G, Peitzsch M. Laboratory evaluation of pheochromocytoma and paraganglioma. *Clin Chem*. 2014;60(12):1486-1499.
63. van Berkel A, Lenders JW, Timmers HJ. Diagnosis of endocrine disease: biochemical diagnosis of phaeochromocytoma and paraganglioma. *Eur J Endocrinol*. 2014;170(3):R109-R119.
64. Baez JC, Jagannathan JP, Krajewski K, et al. Pheochromocytoma and paraganglioma: imaging characteristics. *Cancer Imaging*. 2012;12:153-162.
65. Jimenez C, Cote G, Arnold A, Gagel RF. Review: should patients with apparently sporadic pheochromocytomas or paragangliomas be screened for hereditary syndromes? *J Clin Endocrinol Metab*. 2006;91(8):2851-2858.
66. Jafri M, Maher ER. The genetics of phaeochromocytoma: using clinical features to guide genetic testing. *Eur J Endocrinol*. 2012;166(2):151-158.
67. Brunaud L, Boutami M, Nguyen-Thi PL, et al. Both preoperative alpha and calcium channel blockade impact intraoperative hemodynamic stability similarly in the management of pheochromocytoma. *Surgery*. 2014;156(6):1410-1418.
68. Dickson PV, Alex GC, Grubbs EG, et al. Posterior retroperitoneoscopic adrenalectomy is a safe and effective alternative to transabdominal laparoscopic adrenalectomy for pheochromocytoma. *Surgery*. 2011;150(3):452-458.
69. Grubbs EG, Rich TA, Ng C, et al. Long-term outcomes of surgical treatment for hereditary pheochromocytoma. *J Am Coll Surg*. 2013;216(2):280-289.
70. Yip L, Lee JE, Shapiro SE, et al. Surgical management of hereditary pheochromocytoma. *J Am Coll Surg*. 2004;198(4):525-534; discussion 534-525.
71. Eisenhofer G, Bornstein SR, Brouwers FM, et al. Malignant pheochromocytoma: current status and initiatives for future progress. *Endocr Relat Cancer*. 2004;11(3):423-436.
72. Ayala-Ramirez M, Feng L, Johnson MM, et al. Clinical risk factors for malignancy and overall survival in patients with pheochromocytomas and sympathetic paragangliomas: primary tumor size and primary tumor location as prognostic indicators. *J Clin Endocrinol Metab*. 2011;96(3):717-725.
73. Tanaka S, Ito T, Tomoda J, Higashi T, Yamada G, Tsuji T. Malignant pheochromocytoma with hepatic metastasis diagnosed 20 years after resection of the primary adrenal lesion. *Intern Med (Tokyo, Japan)*. 1993;32(10):789-794.
74. Parida GK, Dhull VS, Sharma P, Bal C, Kumar R. Pheochromocytoma presenting with remote bony recurrence twenty years after initial surgery: detection with 68Ga-DOTANOC PET/CT. *Clin Nucl Med*. 2014;39(4):365-366.
75. Sisson JC, Frager MS, Valk TW, et al. Scintigraphic localization of pheochromocytoma. *N Engl J Med*. 1981;305(1):12-17.
76. Timmers HJ, Kozupa A, Chen CC, et al. Superiority of fluorodeoxyglucose positron emission tomography to other functional imaging techniques in the evaluation of metastatic SDHB-associated pheochromocytoma and paraganglioma. *J Clin Oncol*. 2007;25(16):2262-2269.
77. John H, Ziegler WH, Hauri D, Jaeger P. Pheochromocytomas: can malignant potential be predicted? *Urology*. 1999;53(4):679-683.
78. Ayala-Ramirez M, Palmer JL, Hofmann MC, et al. Bone metastases and skeletal-related events in patients with malignant pheochromocytoma and sympathetic paraganglioma. *J Clin Endocrinol Metab*. 2013;98(4):1492-1497.

79. Plouin PF, Fitzgerald P, Rich T, et al. Metastatic pheochromocytoma and paraganglioma: focus on therapeutics. *Horm Metab Res*. 2012;44(5):390-399.
80. Loh KC, Fitzgerald PA, Matthay KK, Yeo PP, Price DC. The treatment of malignant pheochromocytoma with iodine-131 metaiodobenzylguanidine (131I-MIBG): a comprehensive review of 116 reported patients. *J Endocrinol Investigation*. 1997;20(11):648-658.
81. Vogel J, Atanacio AS, Prodanov T, et al. External beam radiation therapy in treatment of malignant pheochromocytoma and paraganglioma. *Front Oncol*. 2014;4:166.
82. Venkatesan AM, Locklin J, Lai EW, et al. Radiofrequency ablation of metastatic pheochromocytoma. *J Vasc Interv Radiol*. 2009;20(11):1483-1490.
83. Ayala-Ramirez M, Feng L, Habra MA, et al. Clinical benefits of systemic chemotherapy for patients with metastatic pheochromocytomas or sympathetic extra-adrenal paragangliomas: insights from the largest single-institutional experience. *Cancer*. 2012;118(11):2804-2812.
84. Jimenez C, Cabanillas ME, Santarpia L, et al. Use of the tyrosine kinase inhibitor sunitinib in a patient with von Hippel-Lindau disease: targeting angiogenic factors in pheochromocytoma and other von Hippel-Lindau disease-related tumors. *J Clin Endocrinol Metab*. 2009;94(2):386-391.
85. Ayala-Ramirez M, Chougnet CN, Habra MA, et al. Treatment with sunitinib for patients with progressive metastatic pheochromocytomas and sympathetic paragangliomas. *J Clin Endocrinol Metab*. 2012;97(11):4040-4050.
86. Kebebew E, Reiff E, Duh QY, Clark OH, McMillan A. Extent of disease at presentation and outcome for adrenocortical carcinoma: have we made progress? *World J Surg*. 2006;30(5):872-878.
87. Ayala-Ramirez M, Jasim S, Feng L, et al. Adrenocortical carcinoma: clinical outcomes and prognosis of 330 patients at a tertiary care center. *Eur J Endocrinol*. 2013;169(6):891-899.
88. Bharwani N, Rockall AG, Sahdev A, et al. Adrenocortical carcinoma: the range of appearances on CT and MRI. *AJR Am J Roentgenol*. 2011;196(6):W706-714.
89. Takeuchi S, Balachandran A, Habra MA, et al. Impact of (1)(8)F-FDG PET/CT on the management of adrenocortical carcinoma: analysis of 106 patients. *Eur J Nucl Med Mol Imaging*. 2014;41(11):2066-2073.
90. Lau SK, Weiss LM. The Weiss system for evaluating adrenocortical neoplasms: 25 years later. *Hum Pathol*. 2009;40(6):757-768.
91. Else T, Kim AC, Sabolch A, et al. Adrenocortical carcinoma. *Endocr Rev*. 2014;35(2):282-326.
92. Cooper AB, Habra MA, Grubbs EG, et al. Does laparoscopic adrenalectomy jeopardize oncologic outcomes for patients with adrenocortical carcinoma? *Surg Endosc*. 2013;27(11):4026-4032.
93. Terzolo M, Baudin AE, Ardito A, et al. Mitotane levels predict the outcome of patients with adrenocortical carcinoma treated adjuvantly following radical resection. *Eur J Endocrinol*. 2013;169(3):263-270.
94. Bednarski BK, Habra MA, Phan A, et al. Borderline resectable adrenal cortical carcinoma: a potential role for preoperative chemotherapy. *World J Surg*. 2014;38(6):1318-1327.
95. Shawa H, Deniz F, Bazerbashi H, et al. Mitotane-induced hyperlipidemia: a retrospective cohort study. *Int J Endocrinol*. 2013;2013:624962.
96. Fassnacht M, Terzolo M, Allolio B, et al. Combination chemotherapy in advanced adrenocortical carcinoma. *N Engl J Med*. 2012;366(23):2189-2197.
97. Tacon LJ, Prichard RS, Soon PS, Robinson BG, Clifton-Bligh RJ, Sidhu SB. Current and emerging therapies for advanced adrenocortical carcinoma. *Oncologist*. 2011;16(1):36-48.
98. Fay AP, Elfiky A, Telo GH, et al. Adrenocortical carcinoma: the management of metastatic disease. *Crit Rev Oncol Hematol*. 2014;92(2):123-132.
99. Habra MA, Ejaz S, Feng L, et al. A retrospective cohort analysis of the efficacy of adjuvant radiotherapy after primary surgical resection in patients with adrenocortical carcinoma. *J Clin Endocrinol Metab*. 2013;98(1):192-197.
100. Ho J, Turkbey B, Edgerly M, et al. Role of radiotherapy in adrenocortical carcinoma. *Cancer J*. 2013;19(4):288-294.

The Acquired Immunodeficiency Syndrome–Related Cancers

第四十四章　获得性免疫缺陷综合征相关癌症

Adan Rios
Fredrick B. Hagemeister

中文导读

随着高效抗逆转录病毒疗法（HAART）的展开，获得性免疫缺陷综合征（即艾滋病）相关癌症的疾病谱也出现了明显变化。在广泛开展HAART后，艾滋病定义性恶性肿瘤的发病率出现了明显的下降，而其他某些肿瘤的发病率则有所增加。本章首先介绍了人类免疫缺陷病毒（HIV）及其对免疫系统的影响。接着，本章又进一步着重阐述艾滋病定义性恶性肿瘤，包括卡波氏肉瘤、艾滋病相关非霍奇金淋巴瘤（包括系统性淋巴瘤和原发性中枢神经系统淋巴瘤）和霍奇金淋巴瘤。在每一个瘤种部分，本章都详细讲述了流行病学、致病机制、HAART的影响、病理特征、临床表现、诊断方法以及治疗手段。尽管某些恶性肿瘤与HIV免疫的抑制并无直接联系，但鉴于其在HIV患者中的高发状态，本章也进行了简要介绍，如伯基特淋巴瘤和HPV相关癌症（宫颈肿瘤、直肠肛管癌）。最后，本章简要阐述了在艾滋病治疗中可出现的免疫重组炎性综合征和MD安德森癌症中心在艾滋病流行中所做的工作。

THE CHANGING INCIDENCE OF MALIGNANCIES IN PATIENTS WITH HUMAN IMMUNODEFICIENCY VIRUS DISEASE

The relationship between malignancies and acquired immunodeficiency syndrome (AIDS) changed in 1996 when highly active antiretroviral therapy (HAART) was introduced in industrial nations. Thanks to the United Nations and other philanthropy programs, HAART has also been successfully introduced into a number of developing nations ([1]). Africa, the pandemic epicenter, is the exception, due to the epidemic magnitude on that continent and its significant political and social turmoil. Prior to 1996, epidemiologists noted specific malignancies afflicting patients with AIDS, with a risk proportional to host immune status. Before HAART, AIDS patients could be separated into two groups: patients with an opportunistic infection as their first manifestation of AIDS (60%) and those with a malignancy as its mode of presentation (40%) ([2]).

Of those with an AIDS-related malignancy, up to 90% would have Kaposi sarcoma (KS) and the rest non-Hodgkin lymphomas (NHLs), including primary central nervous system lymphoma (PCNSL) and systemic diffuse large B-cell lymphoma (DLBCL). Despite an increase in human papilloma virus (HPV)-related invasive cervical cancers in women with high-grade uterine cervical dysplasia, recent findings of a lack of clear association between cervical cancer and human immunodeficiency virus (HIV)-related immunosuppression questions the validity of including cervical cancer among AIDS-defining or associated malignancies ([3]). After HAART, previously obvious relationships between AIDS and some malignancies have been challenged. An example is HIV-related Burkitt lymphoma, initially associated with AIDS-induced immunosuppression. Investigators have found that HAART improvement of immunity is associated with significant reductions in KS, PCNSL, and systemic DLBCL, but this is not the case with Burkitt lymphoma. Together with invasive cervical cancer, the incidence of Burkitt lymphoma has remained stable across the pre- and post-HAART eras, increasing its proportional frequency. Epithelial dysplasia and squamous cell carcinomas of the anal canal, rectum, and oral cavity are also observed in men infected by HIV. There has been a post-HAART era increase in Hodgkin lymphoma (Epstein-Barr virus related), lung cancer, and nonmelanoma skin cancer, with implications related to the complex relationship between immunity, aging, chronic antigenic stimulation, and viral oncogenesis. Overall, the excess risk of a malignancy in HIV disease is observed mostly in cancers with an established or suspected infectious cause ([4]).

In this chapter, we first discuss HIV and its effect on the immune system. We then concentrate on malignancies associated with AIDS immunosuppression. We include a discussion of malignancies (Burkitt lymphoma and HPV-related cancers) not directly associated with HIV immunosuppression occurring with a high enough incidence in HIV-infected patients to merit study.

HUMAN IMMUNODEFICIENCY VIRUS DISEASE

Historical Significance of the Virus

The AIDS pandemic came into the medical world in 1980 with the publication in the Center for Diseases Control and Prevention (CDC) journal *Morbidity and Mortality Weekly Report* of a series of patients afflicted by de novo opportunistic infections, mostly *Pneumocystis jiroveci* (formerly known as *Pneumocystis carinii*) pneumonia and cytomegalovirus (CMV) infections ([5]). At about that time, these conditions were known to occur in immunodeficient patients. It was followed by a report of KS in 26 homosexual men thought to be immunologically healthy. The number of similar cases increased exponentially throughout the United States and Europe, with reports from other parts of the world confirming a new pandemic with an epicenter in sub-Saharan Africa. The high number of cases with similar clinical presentations gave way to a new syndrome, the acquired immunodeficiency syndrome, or AIDS. Twenty-five years after, much is known and much is to be learned about the cause of the syndrome, HIV, and its complications, including opportunistic infections and malignancies ([6]).

Human immunodeficiency virus disease is caused by infection of a human subject with a retrovirus, HIV. Human immunodeficiency virus is only transmitted through blood or unprotected sexual contact, causing a progressive destruction of the immune system with occurrence of opportunistic infections and malignancies. When an opportunistic infection or a malignancy occurs, it signals a significant degree of immunodeficiency. The association of opportunistic infections and immune suppression is well established in the medical literature and clinical practice. The relationship between immune surveillance dysfunction and development of malignancies has also been described in the medical literature. In the early 1970s, kidney transplantation programs in Canada reported an increased incidence of malignancies in patients treated with the immunosuppressant azathioprine ([7]). Similar reports indicated that pharmacologically immune-suppressed patients had increases of several folds of magnitude of certain types of cancers and opportunistic infections. Typically, they had KS or lymphoproliferative malignancies, although other types of malignancies were also reported. In a sense, these patients had a chemically induced AIDS, whereas HIV patients have a biologically induced AIDS.

Origin of the Disease

Human immunodeficiency virus was discovered in 1983 ([8]), dispelling much of the mystery surrounding AIDS. Acquired immunodeficiency syndrome (AIDS) in humans is caused by a retrovirus, HIV, a lentivirus (Latin *lentus*, meaning "slow," + virus), endemic in African primates, which entered the human population as a result of a cross-species transmission or zoonosis. Two types of HIV have infected humans: HIV-1 and HIV-2. The HIV-1 virus originated from chimpanzees infected by a retrovirus, the SIVcpz (the chimpanzee simian immunodeficiency virus), and HIV-2 originated from sooty mangabeys monkeys, endemically infected by another retrovirus, SIVsm. SIVcpz is the product of recombination in chimpanzees of two monkeys' retroviruses preyed upon by chimpanzees: the SIVrcm and the SIVgsn (the red capped mangabeys, *Cerocebus torquatus*, and the great spot-nosed monkeys, *Ceropithecus nictitans*, respectively). These viruses do not cause disease in their natural hosts and were named simian immunodeficiency viruses, or SIV, after their genetic and structural similarities with HIV. Each HIV type (1 and 2) is phylogenetically classified in groups and clades; HIV-1 has three groups, M (major), N (non-M, non-O), and O (outlier), with the predominant group M comprising 11 clades A to K, and HIV-2 has six clades, A to F. The HIV-1 and HIV-2 clades can recombine giving origin to genetically complex viral quasispecies. Transmission from animals to humans occurs when infected animals enter in contact with humans as a result of hunting and butchering (SIVcpz from chimpanzees) or through contact with infected animals used as domestic pets (sooty mangabeys monkeys) ([9]).

The HIV-2 virus is endemic and contained in coastal West Africa. The HIV-1 virus is endemic in west equatorial Africa with several clades from the group M responsible for the majority of worldwide infections. In the Western world, HIV-1B is responsible for over 90% of infections, whereas in Africa, subtypes A, C, D, and G, and in Asia, subtype C and the circulating recombinant forms (CRFs) 01 and 02 can be found. The disease is diagnosed by detecting serum anti-HIV antibodies using an enzyme-linked immunoabsorbent assay (ELISA) test. The initial result can be corroborated by a repeated Elisa test (Explanation: saying "with another Elisa test" implies a different type of ELISA) or by a Western blot blood test. The amount of replicating virus can be measured by quantitative polymerase chain reaction (PCR) or via signal amplification such as branch-DNA HIV viral load test ([10]).

Status of the Pandemic and Its Effects on the Immune System

Human immunodeficiency virus disease and AIDS are responsible for a human tragedy of incalculable proportions. Since the pandemic's beginning, there have been over 25 million deaths and more than 50 million infected persons, including those who have died. The estimated rate of new infections is 7,500 new infections per day. Most of these new infections occur in developing nations, affecting many women and children. The most frequent modes of transmission are unprotected sex and intravenous (IV) drugs. The main epicenter of the pandemic continues to be sub-Saharan Africa, with new epicenters in the former Soviet Union, China, India, and Latin America. In the United States, minority groups such as Hispanics and African Americans as well as younger generations of gay men are disproportionately affected by HIV ([11]).

Human immunodeficiency virus is an enveloped diploid RNA virus (two RNA ribbons per particle), each with an armamentarium of enzymes essential for the virus life cycle. The viral particle membrane is composed of human leukocyte antigen (HLA) groups, other cell surface membrane proteins, and the viral protein gp120 in a trimer form. Among the enzymes within the viral particle are reverse transcriptase, integrase, and proteases. Eighty percent of transmitted mucosal HIV infections are established by a single Transmitted/Founder (T/F) variant, or Transmitted/Founder virus. The other 20% are transmitted by two to five variants (ie, IV drug users). These T/F viruses have specific phenotypic characteristics, including enhanced infectivity, higher envelope content, more efficient binding of dendritic cells, and relative resistance to interferon (IFN)-α ([12]). Once HIV enters a susceptible host, the viral envelope spikes (gp120 trimers) bind to receptors (CD4) and co-receptors (CCR-5) of cells of the immune system, entering through a membrane fusion. The particle content is released into the cytoplasm, and viral RNA is transcribed into DNA. This viral DNA is then randomly integrated into the genome of the infected cell. Through a complex process of transcription activators and as result of the frequent replication cycles of the immune system's cells, new viral particles are generated. These new particles are released through budding and lysis, continuing to infect new susceptible cells with this process, occurring at an unusually fast pace. Infection with HIV is characterized in simian models of AIDS and in man by a rapid destruction of memory cells of the gut-associated lymphoid tissue (GALT). This process occurs in days to few weeks in animal models and in weeks in man. GALT harbors the majority of body lymphocytes in comparison to the 2% to 5% of lymphocytes located in the peripheral circulation.

The result of GALT's destruction, together with the activation of B cells and inhibition of the immune system function by HIV viral gene products such as the vif protein, which inhibits the APOBEC3 gene family, implicated in the control of HIV infection including the production of neutralizing antibodies , inducing a severe immune dysfunction and depletion. (This is an important piece of information that address the mechanistic question of why we have such a difficult time developing neutralizing antibodies against HIV) ([13]). Once HIV is integrated into the genome of the susceptible cells, there is a gradual destruction of the immune system, leading to a progressive status of immunodeficiency, with development of opportunistic infections and tumors. This early senescence of the immune system is implicated in changes at a molecular level resulting in loss of control of oncogenic viruses and associated with the malignant transformations observed in AIDS.

ACQUIRED IMMUNODEFICIENCY SYNDROME–DEFINING MALIGNANCIES

Kaposi Sarcoma

Epidemiology

Kaposi sarcoma was described by Dr. Moritz Kaposi in 1872 as an indolent dermatologic disease characterized by the appearance of purplish nodules or plaques, particularly in the lower extremities of older men of Eastern European, Mediterranean, or Jewish descent (classical KS). Canadian investigators were one of the first ones to note in the 1970s that KS occurred in renal transplant patients exposed to immunosuppressant regimens (ie, azathioprine; transplant or iatrogenic KS). Their observations included reports of remissions when immunosuppressant regimens were temporarily discontinued, suggesting a relationship between immunodeficiency and the malignancies. They also noted a high incidence of NHL. In the 1960s, British investigators reported an aggressive lymphadenopathic form of KS confined to equatorial Africa (African KS). This form occurred in younger patients with aggressive involvement of lymph nodes and appearance of nodules and plaques of the lower extremities that rapidly became ulcerated. With the CDC *Morbidity and Mortality Weekly Report* of 26 gay men with KS, the disease became one of the hallmarks of the AIDS epidemic (epidemic or AIDS-related KS).

In contrast to the classical form, the AIDS-related KS lesions appear with an aggressive pattern of distribution that includes the trunk, arms, and face in addition to the lower extremities ([14]). Prior to antiretroviral therapies, patients died of a combination of tumor progression and opportunistic infections. Despite HAART, KS continues to be a prevalent cancer among HIV-infected patients, although HAART has significantly changed the incidence of the disease. From 1990 to 1995, the incidence of KS in the United States was 1,838.9 cases per 100,000 person-years in contrast to 334.6 cases per 100,000 person-years from 1996 to 2002. In the United States and Europe, AIDS-related KS has been almost exclusively diagnosed in homosexual men, suggesting that its prevalence may vary among different categories of AIDS patients. In Africa, where the human herpesvirus 8 (HHV-8), or KS herpesvirus (KSHV), is endemic, the male-to-female ratio of AIDS-related KS in some countries is 2:1, almost the same ratio observed in transplant- or iatrogenic-related KS. Thus, in the presence of profound immune suppression, factors that made the disease more prevalent in males than in females prior to the AIDS pandemic appear to be of little relevance. What is clear is that the incidence of AIDS-related KS is related to the degree of the immune suppression of the infected hosts, with most afflicted patients having $CD4^+$ cell counts of 200 $CD4^+$ cells/μL or less.

The Viral Etiology of Kaposi Sarcoma

The etiologic agent of all forms of KS is HHV-8, also called KSHV ([15]). Early in the pandemic, other viruses or agents were implicated as the cause of AIDS-related KS, including CMV. In 1994, sequences of a new herpes-like virus were isolated from the lesions of an AIDS-related KS patient. Using a subtractive PCR technique called representative differential analysis, investigators found sequences isolated from KS lesions homologous but not identical to other known herpesviruses, and thus it was named HHV-8, because it became the eighth known herpesvirus. Not all patients infected with HHV-8 develop KS; however, viral DNA and seroconversion can be detected in patients prior to the development of KS, confirming the role of HHV-8 as the cause of all forms of KS and the relationship of its pathogenesis to immunosuppression in addition to other cofactors.

Human herpes virus 8 belongs to the γ-herpesvirus subfamily and the subgroup γ-2 or rhadinovirus (from the Latin term *rhadino*, referring to the tendency of the viral genome to break apart when it is isolated) and is the first human virus of this subfamily identified. The detection of the infection relies on the presence of antibodies against viral antigens using immunofluorescence assays based on the use of B lymphocytes as the antigen source or ELISA with recombinant immunogenic proteins or peptides of HHV-8. The infection seroprevalence mirrors the geographic distribution of AIDS-related KS, with the highest infection rates in central African countries (80%), rates of 25% to 50% among homosexual men in the Western world, and an intermediate level in the Mediterranean regions. The adult general population of blood donors in North America and Europe has an HHV-8 seroprevalence ranging from 0% to 8%. In addition to being the etiologic agent of AIDS-related KS, HHV-8 has been associated with two other lymphoproliferative disorders: primary effusion lymphoma (PEL, a subset of body cavity–based lymphomas [Fig. 44-1], subsequently called PELs) and multicentric Castleman disease ([15]).

Pathogenesis of Kaposi Sarcoma

Human herpes virus 8 incorporates a significant number of host genes such as cyclin D and growth factor interleukin (IL)-6 ([16]). These genes participate in the replication, survival, and transformation of the infected tumor cells. The viral K1 gene kaposin and viral G protein–coupled receptor (vGPCR) have transformation potential. Others deregulate cell growth and lead to transformation including viral IL-6, viral IL-10, viral cc-class chemokines, and viral FLICE-inhibitory protein (vFLIP). The expression of the different key genes is related to the latency and lytic cycles of HHV-8. During the latency phase, genes such as *LANA-1* (latency-associated nuclear antigen 1), in addition to the maintenance of latency, inactivate p53, inhibiting apoptosis. In addition, a viral cyclin prevents cell cycle arrest by cyclin-dependent kinases, pRB and vFLIP, avoiding the activation of the Fas death receptor pathway. During the lytic phase, homologues of replication genes including the K1 kaposin gene, a Bcl-2 homologue, a viral G protein–coupled receptor gene (*vGPCRP*), a viral homologue of IL (IL-6), and viral macrophages and IFN regulatory factors become active. Some of these genes have immunosuppression functions, such as the inhibition by vFLIP including cytotoxicity of T cells against HHV-8–infected cells and the inhibition of HHV-8 class 2 major histocompatibility complex (MHC)-mediated T-cell activation by K1 ([17]). Finally, other viral proteins such as K3 and K5 downregulate the presentation of MHC class 1 molecules on the cell surface.

Pathology of Kaposi Sarcoma

The histology of KS is characterized by the abundance of spindle cells in a matrix of neovascular formation and a rich background of mononuclear inflammatory cells and collagen. Vascular spaces are dilated and contain extravasated erythrocytes. Involvement of the reticular dermis, reflected by patchy lesions and the involvement of all the layers of the skin, clinically presents as nodular or plaque lesions that can coalesce, interfering with the lymphatic circulation, and are histologically

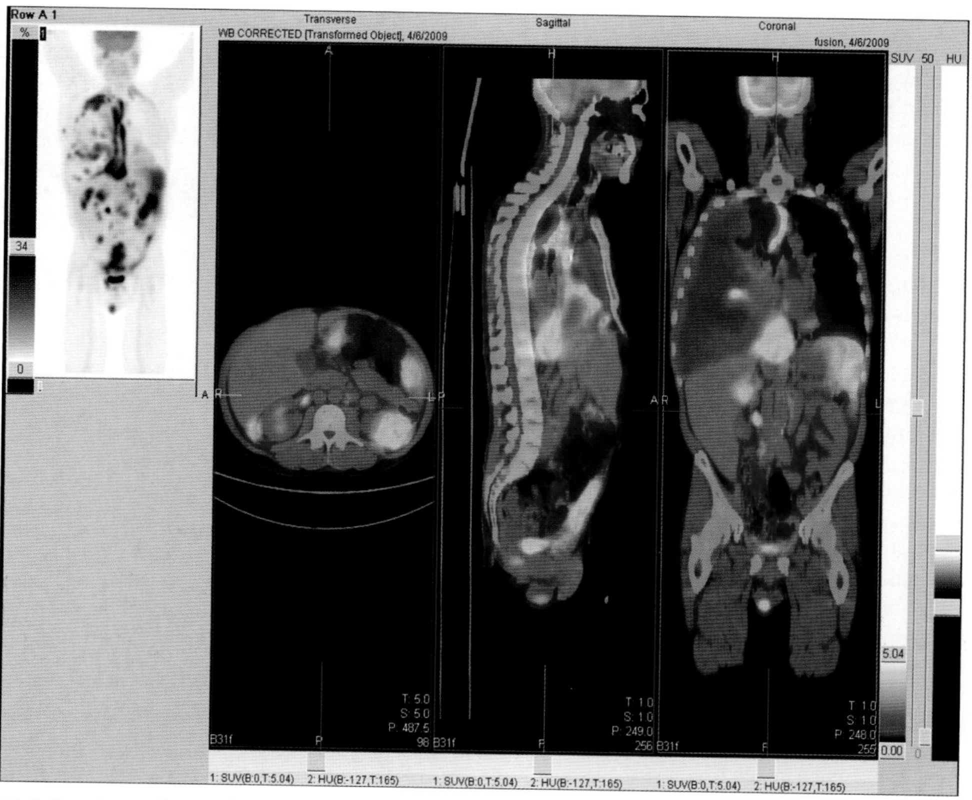

FIGURE 44-1 Scan in a patient with primary effusion lymphoma (PEL) showing multiple sites of increased fluorodeoxyglucose activity and a large right pleural effusion.

and clinically associated with surrounding hemorrhage and subcutaneous edema. The spindle KS cells are rich in endothelial factor VIII. Recent microarray studies have demonstrated that the origin of the KS cell is from a virally transformed lymphatic endothelial cell. Kaposi sarcoma spindle cells express angiogenic/inflammatory cytokines and growth factors, including vascular endothelial growth factor (VEGF), basic fibroblast growth factor (bFGF), IL-1, and IL-6, among others. Kaposi sarcoma cells also overexpress receptors for cytokines, suggesting growth through autocrine or paracrine mechanisms. They also proliferate in response to IL-1, IFN-γ, IL-6, and tumor necrosis factor (TNF), which are abundantly present in the serum of patients with poorly controlled HIV infection, and matrix metalloproteinases (MMPs), enzymes involved in the destruction of extracellular matrix proteins required for angiogenesis and metastasis. In AIDS-related KS, Tat (the trans-activator of transcription protein) stimulates KS spindle and endothelial cell replication, promoting an increase in the concentrations of bFGF. This, in turn, upregulates the integrins $\alpha_5\beta_1$ and $\alpha_v\beta_3$, receptors for fibronectin and vitronectin, which are highly expressed in AIDS-related KS.

Clinical Features of Kaposi Sarcoma

Most patients with AIDS-related KS have CD4+ cell counts of 200 CD4+ cells/μL of blood, with an increased number and aggressiveness of lesions in those who are more severely immunosuppressed. There are periods of exacerbation alternated with quiescence related to oscillations of the patient's immunity. Kaposi sarcoma rarely invades the central nervous system. This is of biological interest because many other human malignancies are characterized by the invasion of the central nervous system ([18]).

The distribution of skin lesions in patients with AIDS-related KS often follows the Langer's folds of the skin. The occurrence of lesions in acral regions of the body such as the tip of the nose is common. The evolution of the skin lesions correlates with the patient's immune system status. In the pre-HAART era, severe involvement of the skin of the face by raised purplish lesions was frequent. With KS progression, there is frequent involvement of the gastrointestinal tract. Lesions of the palate and gums are often the first ones to be noted, and diarrhea and occasional bleeding can suggest KS involvement of the gastrointestinal tract. In the case of involvement of the lower extremities, progressive edema with nodular and coalescing plaque lesions can cause significant discomfort and pain. Prior to HAART, this was a frequent and serious complication of KS, because "elephantiasis" secondary to the progression of KS was extremely difficult to treat. Advanced cases often involve ulceration of lesions, particularly when located in the lower extremities. Lymph node involvement is frequent, and when there is only generalized lymph node involvement, a biopsy is required for confirmation of diagnosis. In advanced cases, lung involvement is manifested by bilateral basilar infiltrates mixed with a nodular appearance; however, severe hemoptysis or gastrointestinal bleeding is infrequent. During the early years of the epidemic, a significant number of patients experienced involvement by large masses of KS in vital organs such as the liver and heart, and death was due to from progression of their KS tumors and associated opportunistic infections.

Staging and Prognostic Factors for Kaposi Sarcoma

The usual TNM system used in other solid tumors is not easily applicable to AIDS-related KS. A system based on the work of Chachoua and colleagues was proposed in 1989 by the AIDS Clinical Trial Group (ACTG) (Table 44-1). This staging system included the

Table 44-1 TIS Staging System for AIDS-Related Kaposi Sarcoma and Risk Status

	Good Risk (0)	Poor Risk (1)
Characteristics	All of the Following	Any of the Following
Tumor (T)	Tumor confined to skin and lymph nodes and/or minimal oral disease[a]	Tumor-associated edema or ulceration; extensive oral KS; gastrointestinal KS; KS in other nonnodal viscera
Immune system (I)	CD4 cells ≥150/mm³	CD4 cells <150/mm³
Systemic illness (S)	No history of opportunistic infection or thrush; no B symptoms[b]; performance status ≥70 (Karnofsky)	History of opportunistic infection and/ or thrush; B symptoms; performance status <70 (Karnofsky); other HIV-related illness (eg, neurologic disease, lymphoma)

AIDS, acquired immunodeficiency syndrome; HIV, human immunodeficiency virus; KS, Kaposi sarcoma.
[a]Minimal oral disease defined as nonnodular KS confined to the palate.
[b]B symptoms: fever, drenching night sweats, and/or >10% involuntary weight loss.
Reproduced, with permission, from Levine AM, Tulpule A. Clinical aspects and management of AIDS-related Kaposi's sarcoma. *Eur J Cancer*. 2001;37:1288-1295.

extent of tumor involvement, the immune status measured by the level of CD4+ cell count, and presence or absence of any systemic illness (B symptoms). In addition to a complete physical examination, it included a complete blood count, serum chemistries, HIV viral load, panendoscopy of the gastrointestinal tract, computed tomography (CT) of the abdomen and pelvis, and when indicated, the performance of bronchoscopy when pulmonary involvement by KS was suspected. Biopsies of skin or lymph nodes were also suggested when indicated to rule out entities that could be similar in presentation, such as bacillary angiomatosis or pyoderma gangrenosum. After HAART, the extent of disease and the presence of HIV systemic symptoms became the most important prognostic factors; however, pulmonary involvement by KS still carries a particularly poor prognosis. Correlations with the levels of HIV viral load and the status of HHV-8 infection are under study in relationship to their impact on survival ([19]).

Therapy of Kaposi Sarcoma

Highly Active Antiretroviral Therapy

Highly active antiretroviral therapy brought a dramatic decrease in the incidence of AIDS-related KS. Highly active antiretroviral therapy consists of the administration of a combination of agents with anti-HIV activity, including inhibitors of HIV reverse transcriptase and protease inhibitors. The consensus of experts in the field about frontline components of HAART is periodically published in *Guidelines for the Use of Antiretroviral Agents in HIV-1 Infected Adults and Adolescents* by the Department of Human and Health Services (DHHS; available online by visiting the DHHS website). For patients in whom KS is part of the initial diagnosis of AIDS, HAART therapy should be started irrespective of the extent of the disease. For patients with minimal tumor burden, HAART initiation constitutes frontline therapy of their AIDS-related KS. This approach can control these lesions for long periods of time, often more than 1 year, and in many instances results in complete disappearance of KS lesions ([20]). Patients with extensive disease or visceral involvement can receive systemic chemotherapy in addition to HAART.

Radiation Therapy for Kaposi Sarcoma

Radiotherapy can be useful for treatment of minimal local disease and when the use of systemic treatment other than HAART is not indicated. It can also be used as an adjunct treatment modality for patients in whom the administration of chemotherapy leads to incomplete results, enhancing the beneficial effects of the systemic treatment. Depending on the general condition of the patient and the size of the lesions to be treated, doses range from the administration of a single fraction to fractionated doses over periods of 2 to 4 weeks. For single lesions and frail patients, the administration of a single 800-cGy dose can be used. Radiotherapy can be used for cosmetic reasons, although this should be done carefully to avoid secondary side effects such as postradiation cataracts in the case of periorbital lesions. For larger lesions or when the therapeutic intent is cosmetic, fractionated doses between 200 and 4,000 cGy are effective and carry less risk. For patients receiving systemic therapy, radiotherapy can be an adjuvant for the treatment of complicated single lesions, particularly when they are bleeding, ulcerated, or painful, or when they affect the well-being of the patient. Such is the case of patients with disseminated disease receiving systemic treatment and in whom oral lesions may affect eating due to local pain or size.

Local Therapy Other Than Radiotherapy for Kaposi Sarcoma

In the modern era, the use of local therapies such as cryotherapy and laser therapy may have a role for patients with few and small lesions. The use of surgery may be appropriate in selected cases such as large skin lesions or when there are complications (bleeding of obstruction of a hollow viscus). Other treatments, such as intralesional injection of chemotherapeutic agents, particularly of the oral cavity, and application of alitretinoin gel, have been abandoned and replaced by a more sophisticated use of radiotherapy techniques, HAART, and systemic chemotherapy.

Immunomodulators in Therapy of Kaposi Sarcoma

After the demonstration of the activity of IFN-α in hairy cell leukemia and renal cell cancer in 1984 ([21]), there was an impetus to use the same doses of IFN in patients with AIDS-related KS. Low doses of IFN-α effective against hairy cell leukemia and renal cell carcinoma were ineffective against AIDS-related KS (Rios A, personal observation). A dose-response study unequivocally demonstrated the therapeutic effect of IFN-α in KS when used at doses of 20 to 30 MU/m^2 ([22, 23]). A different situation was observed with IFN-γ. Under the angiogenic stimuli of IFN-γ, KS has the capacity to replicate, resulting in a deleterious impact on patients treated with this agent in pilot studies. As a result of these trials, recombinant IFNs α-2a (Roferon-A) and α-2b (Intron-A) were approved for the systemic treatment of patients with AIDS-related KS. Expanded use of these agents has revealed their true activity to be in the range of 15% to 20%.

Interferon can block the synthesis of viral proteins and the budding of viral particles from infected cells in addition to other complex pleiotropic effects. Interferon actions are accompanied by significant systemic side effects including tiredness, fatigue, anorexia, hepatotoxicity, and severe myelosuppression. With the development of HAART and the use of more effective systemic chemotherapy regimens in the treatment of AIDS-related KS, the interest in the use of IFN-α in the treatment of AIDS-related KS has declined.

Chemotherapy for Kaposi Sarcoma

Indications for the use of systemic chemotherapy in AIDS-related KS includes extensive skin, mucocutaneous, and visceral involvement by tumor. In patients who require systemic chemotherapy, local radiotherapy is used to treat local complications in addition to systemic disease. The introduction of HAART has resulted in better and more durable responses with increased tolerability and durability than those observed prior to HAART.

Before the discovery of antiretrovirals, a variety of chemotherapeutic agents had modest to significant activity as monotherapy for KS. These agents included etoposide, vinblastine, vincristine, bleomycin, doxorubicin, vinorelbine, and epirubicin, which induced responses in 40% to 69% of patients. After HAART, ABV (doxorubicin 20 mg/m^2, bleomycin 10 U/m^2, and vincristine at maximum doses of 1 to 2 mg) became the first standard treatment of AIDS-related KS. It produced a response rate of 60%, with complications and tolerance depending on the performance status and general condition of the patient ([23]). Antiretroviral and other supportive therapies with growth factors (granulocyte-macrophage colony-stimulating factor [CSF] and granulocyte CSF [G-CSF]) paired with vigorous prophylaxis of opportunistic infections reduce the risks of treatment. Complications of ABV were the expected ones with systemic chemotherapy including the potential for cardiac toxicity induced by doxorubicin.

The ABV regimen was followed by the introduction of agents considered today the standard of care for AIDS-related KS, including liposomal encapsulated anthracyclines (doxorubicin and daunorubicin) and taxanes (paclitaxel). The last of these promotes apoptosis and downregulates Bcl-2 protein expression in KS cells in vitro and in KS-like lesions in mice. In addition, it has an important antimitotic effect associated with its capacity for the disruption of tubulin activity during mitosis.

The current treatment of AIDS-related KS is based on the combination of an anthracycline (liposomal doxorubicin 20 mg/m^2 or liposomal daunorubicin 40 mg/m^2 but *not both* together) with paclitaxel 25 mg/m^2 with or without bleomycin or vincristine. Escalation of the dose of liposomal doxorubicin is not recommended due to a syndrome of desquamation of the skin of the palms and soles of the feet, known as palmar-plantar erythrodysesthesia. In contrast, the dose of liposomal-encapsulated daunorubicin can be increased to up to 60 mg/m^2 or even higher for patients who tolerate lower doses. This is of particular relevance in patients with advanced disease or significant pulmonary involvement and for whom prompt control and achievement of a quick therapeutic response is of great importance (Fig. 44-2).

Future Therapies for Kaposi Sarcoma

Only patients with early disease and relatively good performance status consistently achieve durable remissions with current therapies for KS. For the rest of the patients, only palliation and stabilization of disease is achieved with current treatments. For these reasons, efforts are under way to develop new therapies based on the knowledge of the pathophysiology of the disease. For example, because angiogenesis is an important component of AIDS-related KS, agents such as thalidomide and anti-VEGF agents such as bevacizumab are of great interest in the therapy of this disease. Metalloprotease inhibitors are also of great interest, and active clinical trials are in progress. Viruses associated with the production of malignancies tend to constitutively activate the nuclear factor-κB (NF-κB) pathway, and agents that can inhibit this pathway such as bortezomib may be of some value. Inhibition of signaling cell receptors implicated in the stimulation of angiogenesis such as platelet-derived growth factor receptor (PDGFR) and C-kit receptor by agents such as imatinib, an orally administered tyrosine kinase inhibitor, approved by the US Food and Drug Administration (FDA) for treatment of chronic myeloid leukemia and gastrointestinal stromal tumor, is being investigated.

There is significant interest in the development of therapies against the latent phase of HHV-8, the most common form of HHV-8 in KS cells, which does not respond to standard antiherpetic drugs such as foscarnet and cidofovir. This area of research has led to potential development of a vaccine against HHV-8. Despite all these new potential therapeutic developments, the impact of HAART in the incidence of AIDS-related KS cannot be overemphasized. The development of more potent and less toxic HAART regimens and the acceptance of earlier therapeutic intervention against HIV seem to be the main paths to control the epidemic of AIDS-related KS.

Acquired Immunodeficiency Syndrome–Related Non-Hodgkin Lymphoma: Systemic Non-Hodgkin Lymphoma

Epidemiology

Non-Hodgkin lymphoma is the second most frequent AIDS-associated malignancy. Both KS and NHL were

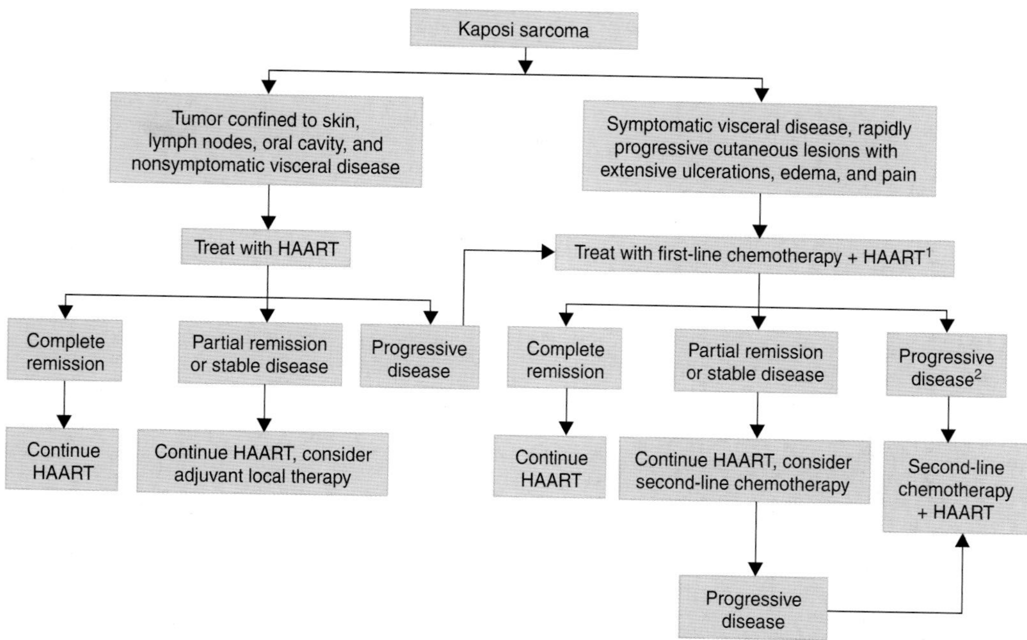

FIGURE 44-2 Algorithm for the management of acquired immunodeficiency syndrome (AIDS)-related Kaposi sarcoma. [1]Monthly evaluation of Kaposi sarcoma clinical response and estimation of $CD4^+$ cell count and HIV-RNA levels. [2]Highly active antiretroviral therapy (HAART) regimen should be changed in the case of immunovirologic failure. (Reproduced, with permission, from Catellan AM, Trevenzoli M, Aversa SM. Recent advances in the treatment of AIDS-related Kaposi sarcoma. *Am J Clin Dermatol*. 2002;3:451-462.)

occurring with an incidence almost linear in its relationship to the patient's immunodeficiency status ([24]). In 1985, high- or intermediate-grade B-cell NHLs were considered part of the spectrum of AIDS-related malignancies. Eighty percent of AIDS-related NHLs were systemic (peripheral) lymphomas, involving nodal or extranodal sites, with 15% to 20% originating in the primary central nervous system (PCNSL). A small proportion, less than 3%, of systemic AIDS-related NHL patients had PELs, known as body cavity lymphomas. In general, the risk of AIDS-related NHL in patients with HIV appears to be higher in those who have poor immune function with average $CD4^+$ cell counts of 150 $CD4^+$ cells/μL of blood.

A viral relationship is implicated in the development of AIDS-associated lymphomas. Epstein-Barr virus (EBV) contributes to the development of most of these tumors, although HHV-8 is associated with the development of PEL ([24]). There is no relationship between the risk of development of AIDS-related NHL and modes of HIV transmission. The incidence of pre-HAART AIDS-related NHL was 60 to 200 times higher than in a matched HIV-seronegative population; the relative risk was higher for PCNSL. Age, nadir of $CD4^+$ cell count, and absence of anti-HIV therapy were critical factors that predicted the development of AIDS-related NHL. In the pre-HAART era, 80% of these NHLs, including systemic and PCNSL cases, were immunoblastic variants associated with $CD4^+$ cell count depletion and EBV infection. In the post-HAART era, there has been a 30% reduction of peripheral cases and a 70% reduction in PCNSL, indicating the impact of immune reconstitution in the incidence of immunosuppression-related lymphomas. In contrast, the incidence of Burkitt lymphoma and of centroblastic DLBCL has remained stable without significant change from the pre- to the post-HAART eras ([25]). When comparing the AIDS-related lymphomas with non–AIDS-related NHL, the former tend to be of higher histologic grade, with increased frequency of B symptoms, extranodal presentations, and an increased incidence of leptomeningeal and primary CNS involvement ([26]). In the post-HAART era, the World Health Organization (WHO) has expanded the categories of lymphomas that can occur in HIV patients to include extranodal marginal zone B-cell lymphoma of mucosa-associated lymphoid tissue type (MALT lymphoma), peripheral T-cell lymphoma (PTCL), and classical Hodgkin lymphoma (HL), as well as lymphomas that more specifically occur in AIDS patients, including plasmablastic lymphomas of the oral cavity, polymorphic B-cell lymphomas (posttransplant lymphoproliferative disorder–like), and PEL ([27]). Finally, the demographics of AIDS-related NHL patients have changed in the last decade, reflecting changes in the demographics of the AIDS epidemic, with increasing incidence in Hispanic and African American patients and patients who have acquired HIV through heterosexual contact (Table 44-2).

Pathogenesis of Acquired Immunodeficiency Syndrome–Related Non-Hodgkin Lymphomas

The development of NHLs in HIV patients is similar to that of malignancies associated with other congenital or posttransplant immunodeficiency disorders ([28, 29]). In such conditions, most of the malignancies consist of NHL and KS. In the case of HIV, immunodeficiency and cofactors, including oncogenic viruses, chronic antigenic stimulation, and cytokine overproduction, are responsible for the development of AIDS-related NHL malignancies. In contrast to AIDS-associated KS, no one has yet found HIV sequences in tumor cells of AIDS-related NHLs ([30]), although PCR analysis has revealed the presence of HIV in infiltrating T cells. For patients with severe HIV immunodeficiency, the oncogenic nature of both EBV and HHV-8 is responsible for the development of the immunoblastic subtype of DLBCL, PCNSL, plasmablastic lymphoma of the oral cavity, and PEL. The last of these often results from coinfection with HHV-8 and EBV. These lymphomas are the result of active oncogenic viruses released from control by an effective immune surveillance.

Epstein-Barr virus is central to the pathogenesis of AIDS-related NHLs, including those that are related to immunodeficiency and those that occur with a

Table 44-2 Demographic Profile of 369 Patients With AIDS-Related Lymphoma Over Different Time Intervals

	1982-1986 (%)	1987-1990 (%)	1991-1994 (%)	1995-1998 (%)	Total (%)	*P* Value
No. of patients	44	88	132	105	369	
Median age (years)	40	36	38	39	38	.18
Sex						.25
Female	0 (0)	2 (2)	6 (5)	7 (7)	15 (4)	
Male	44 (100)	86 (98)	126 (95)	98 (93)	354 (96)	
Race						.001
Caucasian	33 (75)	50 (57)	64 (48)	42 (40)	189 (51)	a
Hispanic	7 (16)	26 (33)	51 (39)	58 (55)	145 (39)	b
Black	4 (9)	4 (5)	17 (13)	5 (5)	30 (8)	
Asian	0 (0)	5 (6)	0 (0)	0 (0)	5 (1)	
Risk						.039
MSM	37 (84)	67 (76)	105 (80)	69 (66)	278 (75)	c
IDU +/– MSM	3 (7)	7 (8)	4 (3)	3 (3)	17 (5)	
Hetero	2 (5)	4 (5)	13 (10)	19 (18)	38 (10)	d
Transfusion	0	3 (3)	1 (0.5)	4 (4)	8 (2)	
Unknown	2 (5)	7 (8)	9 (7)	10 (10)	28 (8)	
KPS						.0008
>80%	14 (32)	28 (32)	75 (57)	45 (43)	162 (44)	
<80%	30 (68)	60 (68)	57 (43)	60 (57)	207 (56)	
Prior OI[e]	14 (32)	40 (45)	58 (44)	53 (50)	165 (45)	.22
Prior KS[e]	2 (5)	13 (15)	11 (8)	14 (13)	40 (11)	.20
Median CD4[f]	177	113	54	53	66	.0006
Range	0-1703	2-1927	0-710	0-700	0-1927	

AIDS, acquired immunodeficiency syndrome; Hetero, heterosexual risk factor for HIV; HIV, human immunodeficiency virus; IDU, injection drug use; KPS, Karnofsky performance status; KS, Kaposi sarcoma; MSM, men who have sex with men; OI, opportunistic infection.

[a] $P = .0007$, comparing Caucasian versus all other races.

[b] $P = < .0001$, comparing Hispanics versus all other races.

[c] $P = .045$, comparing MSM with all other HIV-risk groups.

[d] $P = .011$, comparing heterosexual transmission with all other HIV-risk groups.

[e] Patients without a diagnosis of OI or KS prior to development of lymphoma presented with lymphoma as the first AIDS-defining condition.

[f] CD4 cell count at time of diagnosis of AIDS-related lymphoma.

Reproduced, with permission, from Levine AM, Seneviratne L, Espina BM, et al. Evolving characteristics of AIDS-related lymphoma. *Blood*. 2000;96(13):4084-4090.

reconstituted immune system, such as centroblastic DLBCL and Burkitt lymphoma. The EBV genome presence is very high in immunodeficiency-associated AIDS-related NHLs (100%) ([31]), although it can only be detected in approximately 60% of centroblastic DLBCLs and 30% of Burkitt lymphomas. This suggests that other factors, including other common latent or chronic viral infections, may be involved in the development of these tumors.

In EBV-infected cells, the EBV virus is, for the most part, in a state of latency with brief periods of lytic activity. The malignant transformation of B cells occurs in the latent phase, requiring multiple molecular events ([32]). Epstein-Barr virus contributes to the cellular transformation process through expression of genes with oncogenic activity such as *LMP-1*, *LMP-2*, *EBNA-1*, and *EBNA-2*. There is also expression of small EBV-encoded, nonpolyadenylated nuclear RNAs (EBERs), all of which participate in the oncogenic transformation phenomenon. These proteins can rescue cells from apoptosis by mimicking cell receptors such as CD40 and B-cell receptor. For example, LMP-1 (latent membrane protein-1) is capable of replacing the function of CD40 in germinal B cells which otherwise would follow an apoptotic fate.

The Impact of Highly Active Antiretroviral Therapy on Distribution of Acquired Immunodeficiency Syndrome–Related Non-Hodgkin Lymphoma

In the post-HAART era there has been a decline in the incidence of NHLs associated with immunodeficiency due to AIDS. In contrast, the incidence of centroblastic DLBCL and Burkitt lymphoma appears to be similar before and after introduction of HAART. Factors influencing the pathogenesis of these diseases include an increase in regulatory cells of the immune system, associated with recovery of the immune status of the host, and effects of chronic antigenic stimulation by HIV with a resultant overproduction of cytokines. The existence of more than one pathogenic mechanism for the occurrence of AIDS-related NHLs can be inferred from the variety of genetic abnormalities displayed by the malignant cells ([33]). The number and type of these genetic abnormalities vary according to the anatomic site and tumor histology. They include *c-myc* rearrangement, *bcl-6* gene rearrangement, *ras* gene mutations, and *p53* mutations/deletions ([34]).

Pathology of Systemic Non-Hodgkin Lymphomas

The hallmark of AIDS-related NHL is a high-grade histology, regardless of the histologic subtype, including diffuse large cell, immunoblastic, and small noncleaved cell lymphomas and Burkitt and Burkitt-like lymphomas. The cells of PEL express CD45, activation-associated antigens such as HLA-DR, CD30, CD38, CD71, epithelial membrane antigen, and CD 138/syndecan-1. Primary effusion lymphoma cells often lack B-cell antigens and *c-myc* gene rearrangements and mutations and uniformly contain HHV-8 and frequently also contain EBV ([33, 34]). Other hematologic neoplasms, including low-grade B-cell lymphomas and lymphocytic leukemia, multiple myeloma/plasmacytomas, T-cell neoplasms, and various acute myeloid leukemias and myeloproliferative disorders, have been reported in patients with HIV infection. However, there is no evidence that the incidence of these neoplasms has increased in parallel with the AIDS epidemic ([35-39]).

Clinical Features of Systemic Non-Hodgkin Lymphomas

Patients with AIDS-related NHLs usually present with advanced stages of the disease and B symptoms, including fever, loss of weight, night sweats, and enlarged lymph nodes or masses. Over 60% of the patients will present with stage III or IV disease. Frequent extranodal sites of involvement are bone marrow, CNS parenchyma and meninges, lungs, and spleen. Patients with PEL present with ascites or a pleural effusion and less frequently with a pericardial effusion. Masses are typically absent in the presentation of PEL, although occasionally a mass may accompany the development of the effusion ([40]) (see Fig. 44-1).

The staging of patients with AIDS-related NHL is similar to non-HIV patients with NHL and should be reported according to the Ann Arbor system (Table 44-3). The International Prognostic Index has been validated in pre-HAART studies, and significant changes in treatment outcomes have occurred since the initiation of HAART ([41]). Complete blood count, β_2-microglobulin, lactic dehydrogenase, and complete blood chemistries should be performed, and a radiologic staging should include magnetic resonance imaging (MRI) of the brain and positron emission tomography (PET)/CT scan. Patients in remission after two courses of treatment will tend to remain in remission for the duration of induction therapy. Patients with Burkitt types of lymphoma should have a bone marrow aspiration and biopsy and a diagnostic lumbar puncture. All patients should be screened for hepatitis B, because the exacerbation of this virus by the use of rituximab or chemotherapy can be prevented by screening patients for hepatitis B surface antigen and hepatitis B core antibody and treating those found to have positive results. Hepatitis B surface antigen–positive patients or patients who have a history of hepatitis B with

Table 44-3 Ann Arbor Staging Classification for Hodgkin Lymphoma

Stage	Characteristics
I	Involvement of a single lymph node region (I) or a single extralymphatic organ or site (IE).
II	Involvement of two or more lymph node regions on the same side of the diaphragm (II) or localized involvement of an extralymphatic organ or site (IIE).
III	Involvement of lymph node regions on both sides of diaphragm (III) or localized involvement of an extralymphatic organ or site (IIIE) or spleen (IIIS) or both (IIISE).
IV	Diffuse or disseminated involvement of one or more extralymphatic organs with or without associated lymph node involvement. The organ(s) involved should be identified by a symbol: A, asymptomatic; B, fever, sweats, weight loss >10% of body weight.

Data from Carbone PP, Kaplan HS, Mushoff K, et al. Report of the Committee on Hodgkin's Disease Staging. *Cancer Res.* 1971;31:1860-1861.

a positive e antigen should be treated for hepatitis B prior to the administration of rituximab. For those with only positive core antibodies, measurements of HBV DNA and of the presence or absence of anti–hepatitis B surface antibodies are important in guiding the decision to intervene ([42]).

Before HAART, the presence of an opportunistic infection, less than 100 CD4+ cells/μL of blood, bone marrow involvement, and increased age predicted for a poor survival, with patients often suboptimally treated due to poor tolerance to standard doses of chemotherapy. After HAART, two factors have become predictors of poor survival: a CD4+ cell count of less than 100 cells/μL and high-intermediate International Prognostic Index scores ([43]).

Therapy for Acquired Immunodeficiency Syndrome–Related Systemic Non-Hodgkin Lymphoma

Prior to HAART, all regimens had in common reduced doses of chemotherapy. After 1996, it became clear that patients on HAART can receive standard doses of chemotherapy. The outcomes of treatment in the presence of HAART are related to the subtype of lymphoma and the specific treatment rather than the immunodeficiency status of the patient (Table 44-4). Vigorous prevention of infections with prophylactic antibiotics, aggressive use of growth factors (G-CSF and pegylated G-CSF), and rituximab where indicated have improved the outcomes for these patients (Table 44-5). Although investigators were originally concerned that rituximab

Table 44-4 Summary of Selected HIV-Related Lymphoma Trials

Chemotherapy Regimen	No. of Patients	Median CD4 Cell Count at Enrollment (/μL)	CR (%)	ORR (%)	HAART	OI (%)	OS	Year (ref.)
Modified m-BACOD	98	100	41	69	NR	22	35 weeks	1997 ([81])
vs								
m-BACOD+GM-CSF	94	107	52	78	NR	23		
MTX/LV	29	132	46	77	AZT	NR	12 months	1997 ([82])
CHOP-HAART	24	190	50	NR	Yes	18	62% at 8.5 months	2001 ([44])
vs								
CHOP	80	146	36					
G-CSF+CHOP-R	95	133 total	58	NR	NR	NR	Median follow-up	2003 ([45])
vs								
G-CSF+CHOP	47		50				26 weeks	
Infusional CDE	62	NR	48	74	NR	NR	2.7 years	2002 ([46])
G-CSF+CDE-R	30	132	86	90	Yes	7	80% at 2 years	2002 ([47])
EPOCH	39	198	74	87	Held during chemotherapy	[a]	60% at 53 months	2003 ([48])

AZT, azidothymidine; CDE, cyclophosphamide, doxorubicin, and etoposide; CHOP, cyclophosphamide, doxorubicin, vincristine, and prednisone; CR, complete response; EPOCH, etoposide, prednisone, vincristine, cyclophosphamide, and doxorubicin hydrochloride; G-CSF, granulocyte colony-stimulating factor; GM-CSF, granulocyte-macrophage colony-stimulating hormone; HAART, highly active antiretroviral therapy; m-BACOD, methotrexate with leucovorin, bleomycin, doxorubicin, cyclophosphamide, vincristine, and dexamethasone; MTX/LV, methotrexate and leucovorin; NR, not reported; OI, opportunistic infection; ORR, overall response rate; OS, overall survival; R, rituximab.

[a]0% during chemotherapy, 9% after.

Table 44-5 Suggested Supportive Care for the Patient With HIV Infection and Lymphoma or Other Malignancies

Indication	Drug(s)
Primary infection prophylaxis	
Pneumocystis carinii, Toxoplasma	Trimethoprim-sulfamethoxazole 1 DS daily. Alternatives for patients with allergy to Bactrim-DS are dapsone 100mg PO once a day or atovaquone 1500mg once a day with food.
Oral and/or esophageal candidiasis	Fluconazole 100 mg daily
MAI complex (CD4 <50 cells/μL)	Azithromycin 1,200 mg weekly
Secondary infection prophylaxis	
Herpes simplex infections	Acyclovir 400 mg bid or 200 mg tid
Cytomegalovirus infection	Ganciclovir 1 g tid
Mycobacterium avium complex	Clarithromycin 500 mg bid plus ethambutol
	15 mg/kg daily, with or without rifabutin 300 mg daily
Toxoplasma gondii	Sulfadiazine 1-1.5 g q6h, pyrimethamine 25-75 mg daily
	Leucovorin 10-25 mg daily-qid
Cryptococcus neoformans	Fluconazole 200 mg daily
Salmonella bacteremia	Ciprofloxacin 500 mg bid
Hematopoietic growth factors	
For selected patients in whom the risk of febrile neutropenia ≥40%	G-CSF 5 μg/kg or GM-CSF 250 μg/m² SC daily beginning after completion of chemotherapy and continuing until neutrophil recovery
Antiretroviral agents	
Selecting patients for therapy	[a]Follow NIH guidelines
Role of therapy in controlling malignancy	
Kaposi sarcoma	Essential
Lymphoma	Unknown
Other tumors	Unknown
May be used with myelosuppressive drugs	General principles of HIV treatment: An INSTI, NNRTI, or PI combined with 2 NRTIs. First Choice: NRTIs: emtricitabine/tenofovir (Truvada) or abacavir/lamivudine (Epzicom); with an INSTIs: dolutegravir or raltegravir. Second choice: NNRTIs: rilpivirine (weak CYP3A4 inducer); efavirenz. Efavirenz can be combined with emtricitabine/tenofovir in a single capsule (Atripla). Strong inducer of CYP34A.
Avoid with myelosuppressive drugs/regimens	Zidovudine
Avoid with neurotoxic drugs/regimens	Didanosine, zalcitabine, stavudine
May alter the metabolism of cytotoxic drugs metabolized by cytochrome P-450 enzymes	All PIs and NNRTIs

bid, two times daily; DS, double strength; G-CSF, granulocyte colony-stimulating factor; GM-CSF, granulocyte-macrophage colony-stimulating factor; INSTI, integrase strand transfer inhibitor; MAI, *Mycobacterium avium-intracellulare*; NIH, National Institutes of Health; NNRTI, nonnucleoside reverse transcriptase inhibitor; NRTIs, nucleoside reverse transcriptase inhibitors; PI, protease inhibitor; tid, three times daily; qid, four times daily; SC, subcutaneous.
Reproduced with permission from Sparano JA. Clinical aspects and management of AIDS-related lymphoma, *Eur J Cancer* 2001 Jul;37(10):1296-1305.

might compromise the immune status of patients with CD20⁺ B-cell lymphomas, studies have demonstrated that rituximab can safely be used for patients with ≥50 CD4⁺ cells/μL of blood.

Regimens commonly used to treat patients with AIDS-related DLBCL include CHOP (cyclophosphamide, doxorubicin, vincristine, and prednisone) or rituximab plus CHOP (R-CHOP), R-CDE (rituximab, cyclophosphamide, doxorubicin, and etoposide), and dose-adjusted EPOCH (etoposide, prednisone, vincristine, cyclophosphamide, and doxorubicin hydrochloride) or dose-adjusted EPOCH plus rituximab (EPOCH-R).

Progression-free survival rates at 2 years for these different treatment regimens are 70% for R-CHOP and R-CDE and approximately 90% for dose-adjusted EPOCH-R ([44-50]). In the case of Burkitt lymphoma, CHOP and similar regimens are not recommended because the response is poor. Burkitt lymphoma should be treated with R-HyperCVAD (rituximab plus cyclophosphamide, vincristine, doxorubicin, and dexamethasone) ([51, 52]) or R-CODOX-M/IVAC (rituximab plus cyclophosphamide, doxorubicin, vincristine, methotrexate/ifosfamide, etoposide, high-dose cytarabine) ([53]). Either protocol can achieve remissions of more than 92% and a 2-year overall survival rate of 49% (Figs. 44-3 and 44-4). Recent data suggest that dose-adjusted EPOCH-R also has excellent activity against Burkitt lymphoma, establishing this regimen as a potential new standard of care. This regimen known as SC(for short)-RR (Rituximab days 1 and 5)-DA-EPOCH for HIV-related Burkitt lymphoma consists of a 4-day infusion of etoposide (50 mg/m²/d), vincristine (0.4 mg/d), and doxorubicin (10 mg/m²/d) admixed in the same solution, along with prednisone, at a dose of 60 mg/m²/d orally on days 1 to 5. Cyclophosphamide is given at a dose of 750mg/m² as 2-hour infusion on day 5. Rituximab is given at a standard dose of 375 mg/m² on days 1 and 5. Filgrastim is given subcutaneously starting on day 6 until the absolute neutrophil count is 5,000/μL (post nadir). Cyclophosphamide is increased or decreased from the previous course dose if the absolute neutrophil count nadir is over 500/μL or less than 500/μL ANC, respectively. Importantly, only cyclophosphamide is dose-adjusted for hematologic toxicity. Patients receive one cycle after complete remission is established for a minimum of three cycles and a maximum of six cycles (Table 44-6). All patients receive intrathecal chemotherapy ([54]). For patients with relapsed or refractory lymphoma, R-ICE (rituximab, ifosfamide, carboplatin, and etoposide) or R-ESHAP (rituximab, etoposide, methylprednisolone, cytarabine, and cisplatin) can be of value. Patients with disease responsive to salvage therapy can be considered for high-dose chemotherapy and autologous stem-cell transplantation or experimental therapies ([55]).

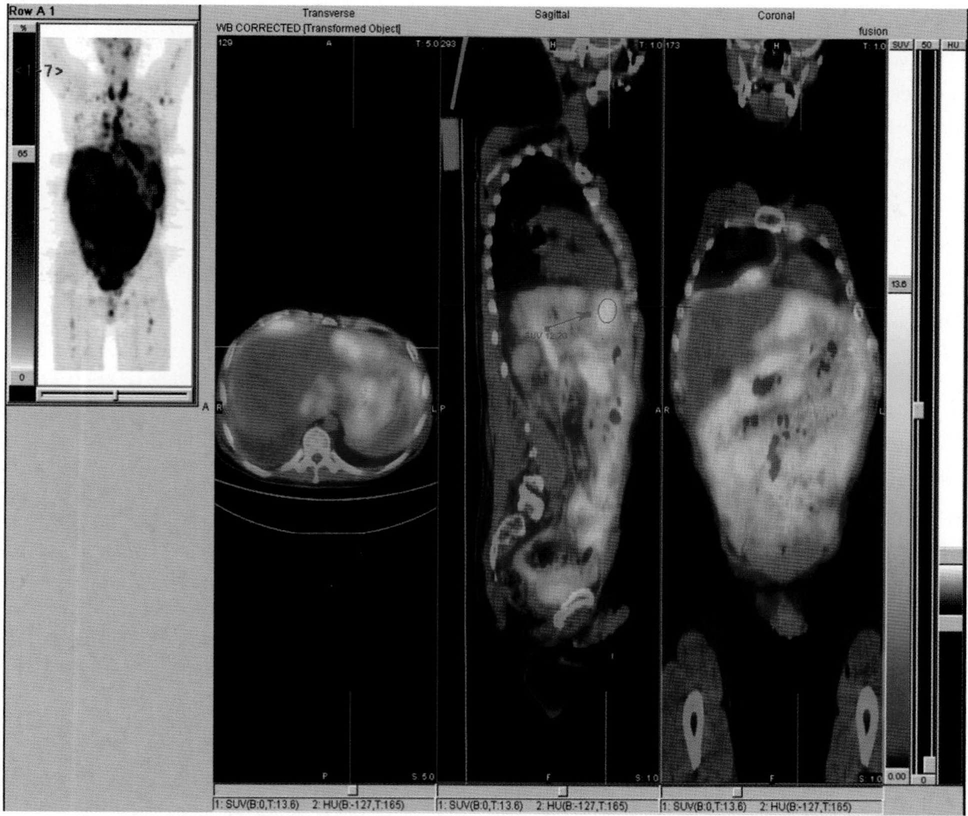

FIGURE 44-3 Computed tomography positron emission tomography scan in a 51-year-old HIV-positive patient demonstrating extensive involvement by Burkitt lymphoma of the chest, abdomen, and pelvis.

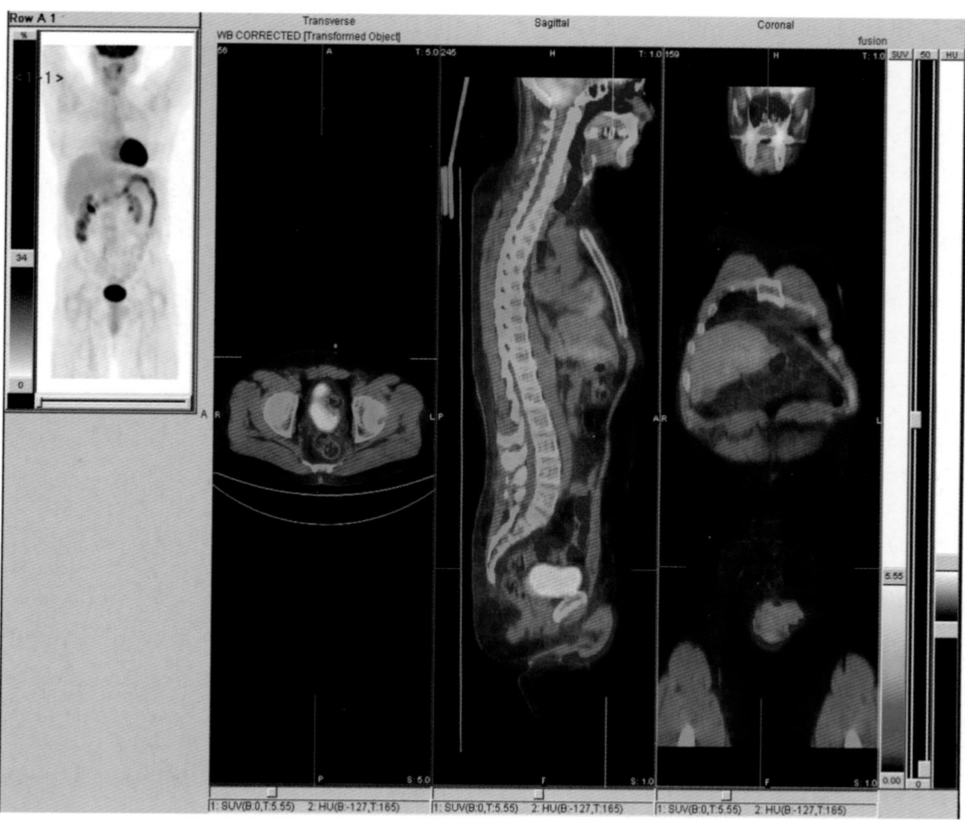

FIGURE 44-4 Same patient as in Fig. 44-3. The computed tomography positron emission tomography scan after four courses of hyperfractionated cyclophosphamide, vincristine, doxorubicin, and dexamethasone (hyperCVAD) alternated with high-dose methotrexate-ara-C an leucovorin rescue, reveals a dramatic improvement with no residual hypermetabolic activity. The patient went on to complete eight courses of treatment with hyperCVAD-HD methotrexate-Ara-C-leucovorin rescue. He remains in complete remission of the Burkitt lymphoma 4 years after treatment and on highly active antiretroviral therapy.

Acquired Immunodeficiency Syndrome–Related Non-Hodgkin Lymphoma: Primary Central Nervous System Lymphoma

Epidemiology and Pathogenesis

Primary CNS lymphoma became an AIDS-defining malignancy in 1983. Primary CNS lymphoma accounted for up to 15% of NHLs in HIV-infected patients compared to only 1% of NHLs in the general population. In the pre-HAART era, typical patients were men who were younger (median age, 40 years) than their immunocompetent counterparts, with $CD4^+$ cell counts of less than 50 cells/μL of blood. The impact of HAART was evidenced by a significant decrease in the disease incidence after 1996 (from 313.2 per 100,000 person-years to 77.4 per 100,000 person-years) ([3]). The development of PCNSL is related to the effect of HIV immunodeficiency on the activity of EBV. The virus does not replicate in CNS tissue. Thus, infected B cells most likely reach the CNS in increased numbers as a result of the progression of the HIV infection. There is loss of capacity by specific T cells for the production of IFN-γ in response to EBV peptides with increased expression of EBNA-2, LMPs, and EBERs (EBV latency type III). This pattern is seen when EBV transforms primary B cells in vitro. The expression of type III latency upregulates genes involved in transformation, including *Bcl-2* and *IRF-7*, and inactivation of *p53* and *Rb* tumor suppressor gene products ([56]).

Clinical Presentation and Diagnosis

Patients with AIDS and PCNSL present with acute organic brain syndrome, in contrast to immunocompetent patients, in whom neurologic deterioration can be slow and progressive. Headaches, seizures, and focal neurologic signs and symptoms are common. Personality changes are frequent, and nausea and vomiting indicate an increased intracranial pressure. When the rare comatose state occurs, it indicates

Table 44-6 Short-Course Dose-Adjusted EPOCH[a]

Drug	Dose	Route	Treatment Days
Infused agents[b]			
Etoposide	50 mg/m^2/d	CIV	1, 2, 3, 4 (96 h)
Doxorubicin	10 mg/m^2/d	CIV	1, 2, 3, 4 (96 h)
Vincristine[c]	0.4 mg/m^2/d	CIV	1, 2, 3, 4 (96 h)
Bolus agents			
Cyclophosphamide (cycle 1)	750 mg/m^2/d	IV	5
Cyclophosphamide dose adjustment (after cycle 1)[d] nadir ANC <500/μL or platelets <25,000/μL for 2 to 4 days.	↓ 187 mg/m^2. Route and treatment days remains unchanged. below previous cycle	NA	NA
If the nadir ANC <500/μL or platelets <25,000/μL for more than 5 days, reduce cyclophosphamide by 50% of the initial full dose.	375 mg/m^2 below previous cycle. Under route and Treatment Days put NA.		
Prednisone	60mg/m^2/d	PO	1,2,3,4,5.
Rituximab	375 mg/m^2	IVPB	1 and 5.
Filgrastim	5 μg/kg/d	SC	6→ANC >5000/μL past nadir)
Next cycle[e]			Day 21

Intrathecal therapy: Intrathecal therapy with 12 mg of methotrexate or 100 mg of cytarabine is administered intrathecally on days 1 and 5 every 3 weeks beginning in cycle 3 for eight doses for patients without central nervous system involvement. For patients with central nervous involvement please refer to original reference.
ANC, absolute neutrophil count; BSA, body surface area; CIV, continuous intravenous infusion; EPOCH, etoposide, prednisone, vincristine, cyclophosphamide, and doxorubicin hydrochloride; IV, intravenous; IVPB, intravenous piggyback; NA, not applicable; PO, oral; SC, subcutaneous.
[a]Data are for cycle 1 except where noted in "cyclophosphamide dose adjustment."
[b]Etoposide, doxorubicin, and vincristine can be admixed in the same solution. Etoposide, doxorubicin, and vincristine are never dose-adjusted for hematologic toxicity.
[c]Vincristine dose should never be routinely capped.
[d]Dose based on previous cycle ANC nadir (complete blood count) twice-weekly) maximum cyclophosphamide dose, 750 mg/m^2.
[e]Begin day 21 if ANC ≥1,000/μL and platelets ≥75,000/μL.
Data from Dunleavy K, Pittaluga S, Shovlin M. et al. Low-intensity therapy in adults with Burkitt's lymphoma. *N Engl J Med*. 2013;369:1915-1925.

an acute intracranial catastrophe, such as intratumoral hemorrhage.

Patients with a primary lesion in the brain and no history of systemic lymphoma usually have a brain lesion as the sole manifestation of the disease (Fig. 44-5). Radiologic diagnostic methods paired with analysis of the cerebrospinal fluid are the cornerstones of the diagnosis of PCNSL. Diagnostic MRI of the brain is preferred to CT scan because of the capacity of the former to detect small lesions. Whenever MRI is not available, CT scan is acceptable because it allows detection of larger lesions (≥1 cm) and provides information about safety of performing a lumbar puncture. Prior to and after HAART, the most important differential diagnosis of PCNSL has been cerebral toxoplasmosis, the most frequent cause of cerebral infection and masses in severely HIV-immunosuppressed patients ([57]). In both PCNSL and cerebral toxoplasmosis, multiple lesions can occur, and both can also have enhancing ring lesions, so distinction between the two can be difficult. A positive serology for toxoplasmosis can be helpful if titers are >1:256. If the toxoplasmosis serology is negative, the presence of EBV DNA by PCR in the cerebral spinal fluid and a positive single-photon emission CT–thallium scan of the brain have high specificity for diagnosis of the PCNSL ([58, 59]). More recently, flow cytometry examination of the cerebrospinal fluid has been used to detect occult disease ([60]).

During the early years of the AIDS pandemic, it was difficult to perform invasive procedures in patients afflicted by an infectious process of which little was known and much was feared. These difficulties resulted in a series of practices borne out of necessity rather than rational approaches to the management and treatment of these patients such as the routine empirical treatment of brain lesions with anti-toxoplasmosis therapy and gauging the diagnosis of the patient based on the clinical response to the anti-toxoplasmosis treatment. Today, there is little room for continuation of such practices, and they should be avoided. They cause unnecessary delays in diagnosis and complicate the patient's management because there are potential side effects associated with treatment for an illness the patient may not have. Therefore, unless there is an absolute contraindication, the standard of care for a patient with a brain lesion and AIDS is the performance of a stereotactic biopsy of the brain, particularly in patients with a negative serology for toxoplasmosis.

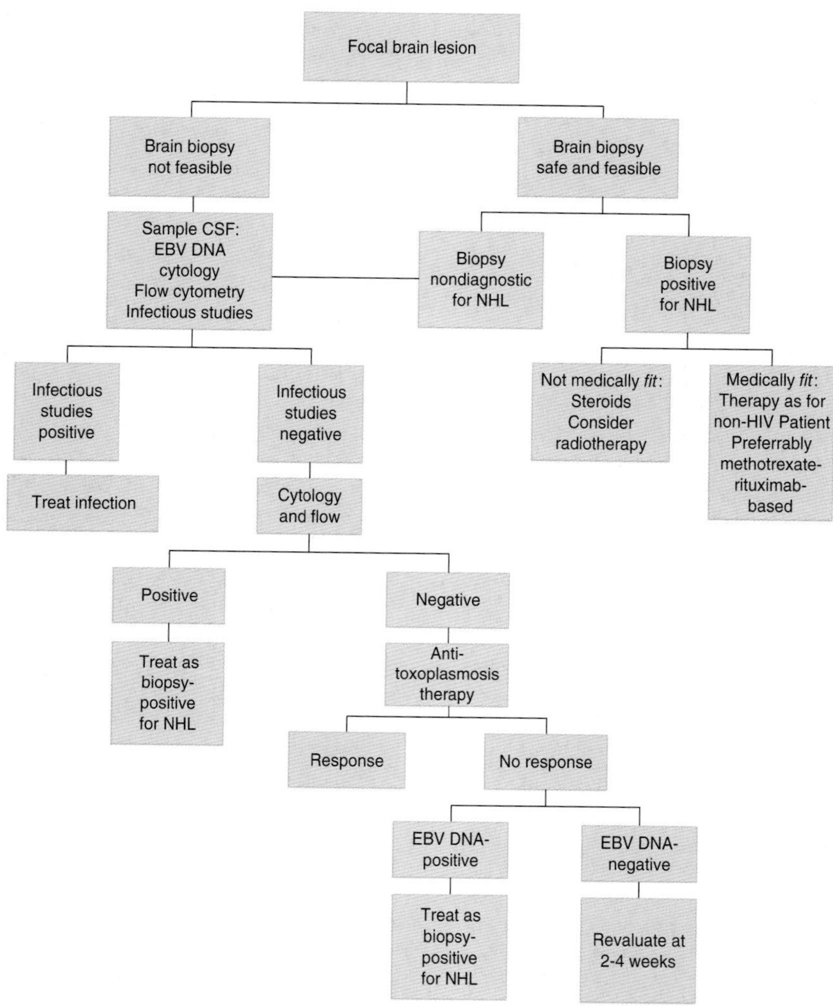

FIGURE 44-5 Evaluation of brain lesions in patients with human immunodeficiency virus (HIV) disease. CSF, cerebrospinal fluid; EBV, Epstein-Barr virus; NHL, non-Hodgkin lymphoma. (Adapted with permission, from Sparano JA. Clinical aspects and management of AIDS-related lymphoma. *Eur J Cancer.* 2001;37:1296-1305.)

Treatment of Primary Central Nervous System Lymphoma

Highly active antiretroviral therapy is the first step in the treatment of these patients. There is a clear correlation between the immune status of the patient and prognosis. The use of steroids and anticonvulsants is debated among some investigators concerned with the potential of steroids to confound the histologic diagnosis. However, a few days of steroids (4-5 days) can be of clinical benefit, particularly when there is an obvious mass effect. Anticonvulsive therapy administered for a few days can allow the stabilization of the neurologic condition of the patient controlling the risk of focal or grand mal seizures. Even solitary lesions of PCNSL tend to infiltrate surrounding tissues. Thus, there is no role for surgical resection in the treatment of this disease.

Before HAART, whole-brain radiotherapy was standard of care for PCNSL, until replaced by best comfort measures, as the brains of severely immunocompromised patients tolerated poorly the administration of radiotherapy. Similarly to immunocompetent patients with PCNSL, high-dose methotrexate and rituximab have replaced the administration of radiotherapy in patients with HIV and PCNSL. Investigators have suggested a modification of a standard regimen used for the treatment of patients without HIV, which includes rituximab 500 mg/m^2 on day 1 and methotrexate 3.5 g/m^2 and vincristine 1.4 mg/m^2 given only on day 2. Leucovorin rescue is given in standard fashion, and HAART treatment is initiated or continued. This modified regimen is administered for five to six cycles depending on the tolerance of the patient followed by four courses of monthly maintenance with radiotherapy administered in a stereotactic manner at the discretion of the treating physician ([61]).

Hodgkin Lymphoma: An Aids-Defining Illness?

Epidemiology, Clinical Features, and Therapy

People infected with HIV have a 10-fold higher risk of developing HL than do HIV-seronegative persons. However, in contrast to KS and NHL, the risk is more pronounced in patients with HIV who only have moderate immunosuppression. In general, patients with HIV have a higher incidence of an unfavorable histology, including mixed cellularity and lymphocyte depletion subtypes of HL, when compared with that seen in patients without HIV infection. Instead of observing a decrease in HL in patients in the post-HAART era, as with certain NHL subtypes, investigators have noted an increase in the incidence of HL in HIV patients ([62]). This observation has made the relationship between immunodeficiency and HL uncertain. Despite the WHO inclusion as an AIDS-defining malignancy, HL is not considered by most experts as a true AIDS-associated disease. From the pathogenesis point of view, EBV is often associated with HIV-related HL, in the range of 80% to 100%. The Reed-Sternberg cells of HIV-related HL express the EBV-encoded LMP-1, known to have oncogenic properties ([63]). In the post-HAART era, it has been postulated that an increase in $CD4^+$ cells as a result of antiretroviral therapy fosters the development of the appropriate cellular milieu seen in HL in patients without HIV infection. These $CD4^+$ cells, generated as a result of immune reconstitution by HAART, produce ligands for membrane receptors in the Reed-Sternberg cells that activate the classical NF-κB pathway ([63]).

Clinically, patients with HIV and HL are young and have stage III or IV disease with B symptoms (fever, night sweats, and loss of >10% of body weight). Bone marrow involvement is frequent at the time of diagnosis ([64]). In the pre-HAART era, the immunodeficiency of the patients limited the use of standard chemotherapeutic regimens in patients with HL. In the post-HAART era, the standards of care applicable to patients without HIV disease and HL have been applied successfully to patients with AIDS and HL once the HIV disease is controlled. Prior to HAART, Levine and colleagues in the ACTG evaluated the efficacy of ABVD (doxorubicin, bleomycin, vinblastine, and dacarbazine) with G-CSF in 21 HIV-seropositive patients. There was an overall response rate of 62%, with 43% complete response and 19% partial response. The median survival in this cohort was 1.5 years. Almost half the patients experienced grade 4 neutropenia, and 29% of patients developed opportunistic infections ([65]). In this study, patients did not receive antiretroviral therapy while on treatment. Following the introduction of HAART during treatment, investigators reported that ABVD induced a 91% complete remission rate and a median time to relapse of over 36 months ([66]). Other investigators used the Stanford V regimen, administering only short-term chemotherapy (12 weeks) with adjuvant radiotherapy. Of 59 patients who received this therapy, 69% completed the treatment without dose reduction or delays in the administration of the chemotherapy. Eighty-one percent of the patients achieved a complete remission, and with a median follow-up of 17 months, 33 (56%) of 59 patients were alive and free of disease ([67]). After the introduction of HAART, the response rates for patients treated with ABVD or BEACOPP (bleomycin, etoposide, doxorubicin, cyclophosphamide, vincristine, procarbazine, prednisone) became essentially similar, irrespective of the patient's stage of the disease. However, more treatment-related mortality occurred in patients who received BEACOPP ([68]). The available data suggest that ABVD with HAART should be the initial treatment of choice for HIV-related HL. High-dose chemotherapy and autologous stem cell transplantation are being explored for patients who have disease progression while on treatment or relapse after remission induction. Thus, because of HAART, patients with HL and HIV disease can be treated with standard-of-care options that are similar to those used for HL patients who do not have HIV.

OTHER MALIGNANCIES AFFECTING HUMAN IMMUNODEFICIENCY VIRUS–INFECTED PATIENTS

Cervical Neoplasms

Epidemiology

In the early 1980s, reports appeared signaling an increased association between HIV infection and cervical intraepithelial neoplasia in HIV-infected women. It was not until 1993 that cervical cancer was officially added to WHO recommendations as an AIDS-related malignancy ([69]). Women with HIV disease have a higher incidence of infection with multiple types of oncogenic HPV and higher incidence of dysplastic changes of the cervix than women without HIV disease, events that can culminate in the development of cervical cancer (Table 44-7). There is no obvious association between the level of $CD4^+$ cell count and cervical cancer, and the statistical correlations between the association of HIV and HPV-induced cervical cancer remains moderately

Table 44-7 Traditional Factors for Cervical Cancer Risk

History of more than six sexual partners
Cigarette smoking
Early age of first intercourse
History of sexually transmitted disease
Immunosuppression
Human papillomavirus

Data from Stier E. Cervical neoplasia and the HIV-infected patient. *Hematol Oncol Clin North Am.* 2003;17:873-887.

strong at best. The decline observed for KS and PCNSL after HAART has not been seen in the incidence of HPV-related malignancies.

There are reasons why HPV, the etiologic agent of cervical cancer, causes this disease regardless of the immune status of the infected host. Human papillomavirus infects the basal keratinocytes of the stratified epithelium, and its replication is coupled to the process of keratinocyte differentiation in the infected squamous epithelium. From an initial low-copy number episome in basal keratinocytes, there is a dramatic increase in the concentrations of proteins E1 and E2 by the time the keratinocytes differentiate and enter the stratum spinosum layer of the epithelium. In addition, for oncogenic strains of HPV such as 16, 18, and 31, there is also an increase in the expression of E6 and E7, which have a high oncogenic capacity manifested by the functional inactivation of p53 and Rb ([70,71]). Regardless, this is a slow process, and it takes several years for an HPV-induced cervical lesion to transform into cancer. For these reasons, there is uncertainty regarding the relationship between HIV and cervical cancer as an AIDS-related malignancy.

Despite controversies regarding the relationship between HIV, HPV, and cervical cancer, the increased incidence of infections by oncogenic HPV types in patients with HIV in contrast to non–HIV-infected women highlights the importance of mandatory cervical screening of HIV-infected women. However, recent studies have suggested that HIV-infected women are not being offered cervical screening, even though older women without HIV for whom the relevance of the screening may not be considered as important are routinely screened. Clearly, educational efforts are necessary as the number of HIV-infected woman increases in the United States and elsewhere.

Cervical Cytology and Screening

Papanicolaou tests in HIV-infected women have a high prevalence of cytologic abnormalities, ranging from 20% to 40%. Women with negative Pap smears will, over the course of 3 to 5 years, develop cytologic abnormalities at a higher rate than will HIV-negative women, and there is evidence of a higher rate of progression to cervical cancer following the longevity induced by HAART ([72]). Therefore, it is imperative that patients with HIV infection be screened appropriately with Pap smears, colposcopy, and biopsy when needed for the early detection of cervical cancer. Pap smears interpreted as demonstrating "atypical squamous cells" cannot exclude a high-grade squamous intraepithelial lesion (HGSIL) and must be evaluated with colposcopic examination (see Fig. 44-4). Current US Public Health Service (USPHS) and Infectious Diseases Society of America (IDSA) guidelines recommend Pap smears every 6 months during the first year after HIV diagnosis; if both tests are normal, annual screening is suggested ([73]) (Fig. 44-6).

Treatment for Cervical Cancer

Because they rarely progress and often go away on their own, the American Society for Colposcopy and Cervical Cytopathology recommends close observation for cervical intraepithelial neoplasia (CIN) grade 1 lesions. However, treatment of invasive cervical cancer is the same as for HIV-seronegative women: surgery in early stages and a combination of surgery and chemoradiotherapy in intermediate stages. For CIN grade 2, the preferred mode of treatment is the loop electrosurgical excision procedure. Cryotherapy and laser surgery can also be used, although these methods are usually reserved for larger lesions. Chemotherapy alone is used for more advanced cases, although the immune status of the patient can influence the response to treatment ([74]).

One of the most important advances against HPV-induced cervical cancer has been the development of preventive HPV vaccines. The HPV vaccines made of viral-like particles display a remarkable structural and antigenic similitude to HPV virions and can induce the production of high titers of neutralizing antibodies. Two versions of HPV viral-like particle vaccines are available for immunization of humans against HPV. Gardasil (Merck, Sharp, and Dohme) has viral-like particles of HPV subtypes 16 and 18 (oncogenic subtypes) and 6 and 11 (the causes of genital warts). Cervarix (GlaxoSmithKline) contains viral-like particles of HPV subtypes 16 and 18. They are both administered intramuscularly and have demonstrated almost 100% protection in clinical trials prior to their approval by the FDA. They should be used prior to the initiation of sexual activity, and neither have demonstrated therapeutic efficacy in the treatment of preexisting infections. Future work is aimed at increasing the immunogenicity of the viral-like particles and expanding the number of HPV oncogenic subtypes available for vaccination ([75]).

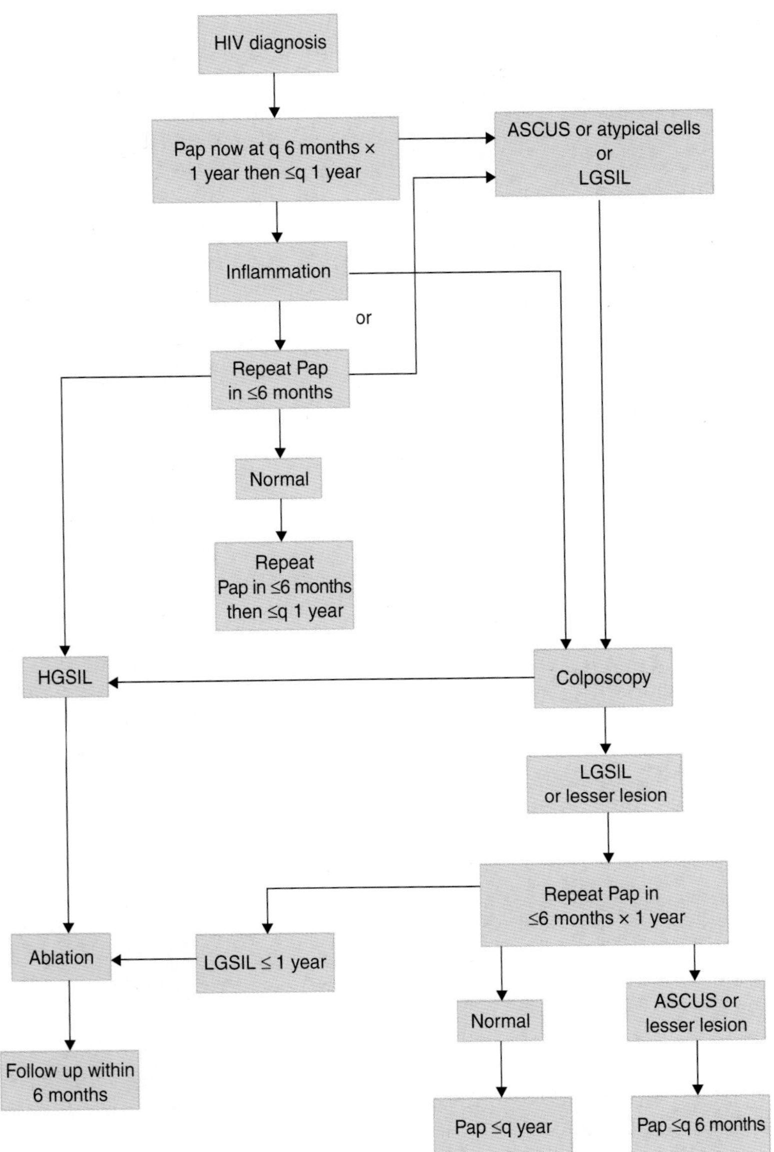

FIGURE 44-6 Screening/treatment algorithm for cervical cancer. ASCUS, atypical squamous cells of undetermined significance; HGSIL, high-grade squamous intraepithelial lesion; LGSIL, low-grade squamous intraepithelial lesion; q, every.

Anorectal Carcinoma

Infection of the anogenital tract in men with oncogenic strains of HPV has the same consequence as it does in women. After HAART, the incidence of this disease has increased as patients live longer and the biological characteristics unique to the HPV oncogenic transformation are expressed over time (Table 44-8). The incidence of anal cancer has increased from 19.0 per 100,000 person-years in the pre-HAART era (1992-1995) to 48.3 persons per 100,000 person-years in the immediate post-HAART period (1996-1999) to 78.2 per 100,000 person-years more recently (2000-2003, $P < .001$) ([76]).

The same subtypes of HPV and pathogenic mechanisms involved in the oncogenic activity of HPV in women apply to men. The screening and treatment of CIN 2 and 3 is of relevance in these patient populations. There has been a greater understanding of the need for anal screening of both men and women with HIV disease ([77]) (Fig. 44-7). The treatment of HGSILs includes the use of local therapies such as podophyllotoxin, liquid nitrogen, and laser surgery (Fig. 44-8). Investigators have recommended that men with HIV infection and

Table 44-8 Risk Factors for AIDS-Associated Anal Carcinoma

HIV seropositivity
Low CD4 cell count
Persistent HPV infection
High-risk HPV genotypes
Multiple HPV genotypes
History of anal intercourse
Cigarette smoking
Immunosuppression

AIDS, acquired immunodeficiency syndrome; HIV, human immunodeficiency virus; HPV, human papillomavirus.
Data from Martin F, Bowers M. Anal intraepithelial neoplasia in HIV-positive people. *Sex Transm Inf.* 2001;77:327-331.

anal HPV-related lesions undergo screening with Pap smears every 6 months the first year following diagnosis and yearly thereafter. Invasive lesions are treated as in the general population with the use of chemoradiotherapy followed by salvage surgery when there is no response or relapse after initial treatment ([78]).

Other Malignancies

Patients with HIV can develop other malignancies not necessarily associated with HIV. For example, lung cancer continues to increase in its incidence in this population. In general, smoking is one of the most important negative factors predicting for poor survival in HIV patients even in the presence of HAART. Patients with HIV who develop malignant tumors often do so at an earlier age and tend to have atypical presentations, and frequently their tumors follow a very aggressive course.

IMMUNE RECONSTITUTION INFLAMMATORY SYNDROME

In patients with advanced HIV disease (<100 CD4$^+$ cells/μL of blood), the initiation of HAART can be accompanied by a paradoxical worsening of established infections or appearance of new ones. This phenomenon is most frequent in patients who have tuberculosis or cryptococcal disease as their opportunistic infection but can happen with any other type of infection. This syndrome is known as immune reconstitution inflammatory syndrome (IRIS). The management of IRIS consists of the administration of specifically indicated therapies and a short course of steroids for 1 to 2 weeks with a rapid taper. The recommended dose of prednisone is 1 to 2 mg/kg/d. Antiretroviral therapy should only be interrupted in severe cases as most patients respond to the use of steroid or anti-inflammatory agents depending on the severity of the IRIS. Because the management of patients with AIDS-related malignancies involves a multidisciplinary team and given the importance of the use of HAART in the management of patients with AIDS and malignancies, treating oncologists must be familiar with this condition to avoid unnecessary delays or interruptions in the HAART of their patients ([79]).

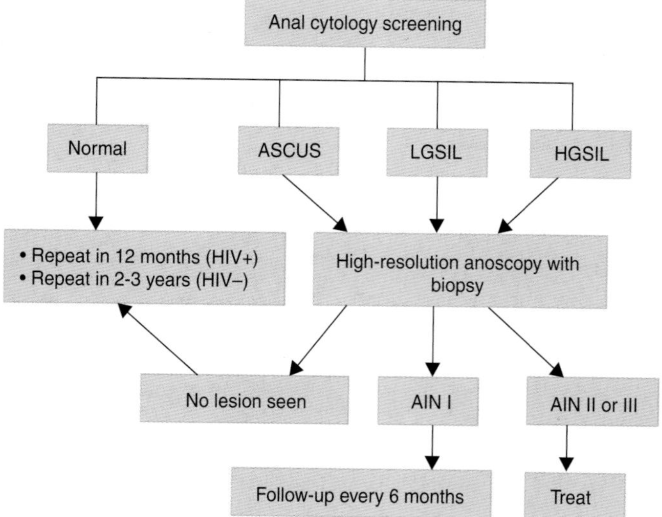

FIGURE 44-7 Protocol for screening anal intraepithelial neoplasia (AIN). ASCUS, atypical squamous cells of indeterminate significance; HGSIL, high-grade squamous intraepithelial lesion; HIV, human immunodeficiency virus; LGSIL, low-grade squamous intraepithelial lesion. (Reproduced, with permission, from Chin-Hong PV, Palefsky JM. Natural history and clinical management of anal human papillomavirus disease in men and women infected with human immunodeficiency virus. *Clin Infect Dis.* 2002;35(9):1127-1134.)

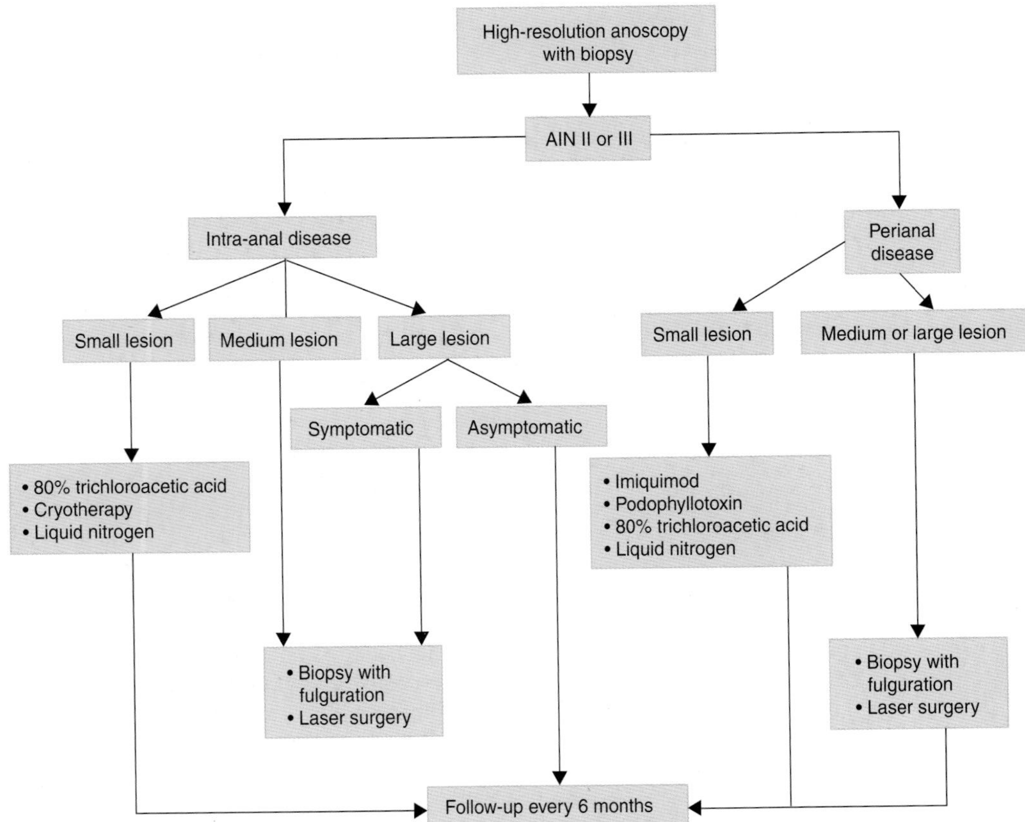

FIGURE 44-8 Treatment of anal intraepithelial neoplasia (AIN) II and III. Imiquimod and podophyllotoxin have not been approved by the US Food and Drug Administration for this indication. (Reproduced, with permission, from Chin-Hong PV, Palefsky JM. Natural history and clinical management of anal human papillomavirus disease in men and women infected with human immunodeficiency virus. *Clin Infect Dis.* 2002;35:1127-1134.)

MD ANDERSON CANCER CENTER AND THE ACQUIRED IMMUNODEFICIENCY SYNDROME PANDEMIC

When the AIDS pandemic began, Houston quickly became an AIDS epicenter, occupying the fourth place among cities with the highest number of AIDS cases in the United States for several years. The Department of Epidemiology, under the leadership of Peter W. Mansell and its Director, Guy Newell, took a leading role in studying methods for prevention of AIDS and public education efforts. Their work, together with the collaboration of R. Palmer Beasley, Dean of the University of Texas Health Science Center School of Public Health, the Department of Immunology and Biological Therapy, under the direction of Evan Hersh, and the collaboration of immunologists and virologists including James M. Reuben and Blaine F. Hollinger, was recognized with one of the first AIDS Treatment Evaluation Units Grants awarded for basic science and clinical research in AIDS. This work led to the creation of the Institute for Immunological Disorders under the direction of Peter W. Mansell and Adan Rios. Although the institute was ahead of its time, it opened doors for a humane treatment of AIDS patients and the development of new therapies and strategies for research of the disease. This base of knowledge was instrumental in development of community strategies subsequently applied in management and treatment of AIDS in the state of Texas. This effort extends to current times with the pioneering work done at the institution in the treatment of Burkitt lymphoma in HIV patients by Drs. Jorge Cortes, Debbie Thomas and Houston AIDS community physicians using what is considered today a standard strategy for treatment of AIDS-related malignancies: the use of HAART in combination with the best known strategy for the treatment of the malignancy.

CONCLUSIONS

The complexities of the AIDS pandemic are captured in the history of the AIDS-related malignancies (Table 44-9). The introduction of effective anti-HIV therapy or HAART in 1996 brought a profound change in the overall management of cancer in HIV patients. One important predictor of good outcomes in the therapy of cancer and HIV is the administration of HAART ([80]). The common goals for treatment of patients with AIDS and cancer are to treat HIV with HAART and the cancer with the same standards of care that exists for patients without HIV

Table 44-9 AIDS-Associated Cancers[a]

Cancer Type	Observed Cases	Expected Cases	Relative Risk	Etiologic or Contributing Factors
Kaposi sarcoma				KSHV
Men	5,583	57.3	97.5[b]	
Women	200	1.0	202.7[b]	
Non-Hodgkin lymphoma				EBV and KSHV
Men	2,434	65	37.4	
Women	342	6.3	54.6	
Cervical, invasive				HPV
Women	133	14.7	9.1	
Hodgkin lymphoma				EBV
Men	160	20	8	
Women	20	3.1	6.4	
Tongue				HPV and EBV
Men	17	9.3	1.8	
Women	5	0.7	7.1	
Rectal, rectosigmoidal, and anal				HPV (anal carcinoma)
Men	75	22.7	3.3	
Women	9	3.0	3.0	
Liver (primary only)				HCV,[c] HBV, alcohol
Men	36	7.1	5.1	
Tracheal, bronchial, and lung				Smoking[d]
Men	217	66.1	3.3	
Women	50	6.7	7.5	
Brain and CNS				EBV for CNS lymphoma
Men	42	13.4	3.1	
Women	7	2.0	3.4	
Skin, excluding Kaposi saroma				HPV[e] and ultraviolet light exposure
Men	133	6.4	20.8	
Women	8	1.1	7.5	
Melanoma, skin				
Men	24	17.3	1.4	
Testicular				
Men	38	25.6	1.5	
Colon				
Men	32	38.2	0.8	
Women	5	6.3	0.8	
Prostate				

(Continued)

Table 44-9 AIDS-Associated Cancers[a] (*Continued*)

Cancer Type	Observed Cases	Expected Cases	Relative Risk	Etiologic or Contributing Factors
Men	37	53.7	0.7	
Breast				
Women	47	59.9	0.8	
Ovarian				
Women	6	7.8	0.8	

AIDS, acquired immunodeficiency syndrome; CNS, central nervous system; EBV, Epstein-Barr virus; HBV, hepatitis B virus; HCV, hepatitis C virus; HPV, human papillomavirus; KSHV, Kaposi sarcoma-associated herpesvirus.

[a]Data are based on the observed number of cases in HIV-positive individuals (men and women age 15-69 years), expected cases based on the incidence in a nonimmunocompromised population in New York State (NYS), relative risk, and etiologic factors. Data from the AIDS/Cancer Matched Cohort NYS, 1981-1991.

[b]Relative risk for Kaposi sarcoma (KS) is lower than in other studies, probably because the background population in NYS is enriched with population groups (eg, Italians, Greeks, and Jews) that have an increased risk for classic KS.

[c]HCV contributes to increased incidence of liver cancer, particularly in HIV-infected men with hemophilia, and in intravenous drug users.

[d]The increase in lung cancer might be confounded by the fact that HIV-infected individuals have been reported to smoke more cigarettes per day than HIV-negative individuals.

[e]In Africa, HPV and ultraviolet light exposure have been implicated in the high incidence of conjunctival squamous carcinoma, and HPV is also implicated as the cause of skin cancers seen after an organ transplant. Misdiagnosis of KS might also contribute to increased risk of skin cancer.

Reproduced with permission from Boshoff C, Weiss R: AIDS-related malignancies, *Nat Rev Cancer*. 2002 May;2(5):373-382.

disease, along with vigorous prophylaxis of opportunistic infections, supportive therapy including growth factors, and appropriate nutritional and emotional support.

REFERENCES

1. Hogg RS, Heath KV, Yip B, et al. Improved survival among HIV-infected individuals following initiation of anti-retroviral therapy. *JAMA*. 1998;279:450-454.
2. Sepkowitz KA. AIDS—the first 20 years. *N Engl J Med*. 2001;344:1764-1772.
3. Biggar RJ, Anil K, Chaturvedi AK, et al. AIDS-related cancer and severity of immunosuppression in persons with AIDS. *J Natl Cancer Inst*. 2007;99:962-972.
4. Stebbing J, Duru O, Bower M. Non-AIDS-defining cancers. *Curr Opin Infect Dis*. 2009;22:7-10.
5. Centers for Disease Control and Prevention. Pneumocystis pneumonia—Los Angeles. *MMWR Morb Mortal Wkly Rep*. 1981;30:250-252.
6. Gottlieb MS. AIDS—past and future. *N Engl J Med*. 2001;344:1788-1791.
7. Farge D, Lebbé C, Marjanovic Z, et al. Human herpes virus-8 and other risk factors for Kaposi's sarcoma in kidney transplant recipients. Groupe Cooperatif de Transplantation d'Ile de France (GCIF). *Transplantation*. 1999;67:1236-1242.
8. Barré-Sinoussi F, Chermann JC, Rey F, et al. Isolation of a T-lymphotropic retrovirus from a patient at risk for acquired immune deficiency syndrome (AIDS). *Science*. 1983;220:868-871.
9. Hahn BH, Shaw GM, De Cock KM, et al. AIDS as a zoonosis: scientific and public health implications. *Science*. 2000;287:607-614.
10. WHO/UNAIDS. The importance of simple/rapid assays in HIV testing. *Wkly Epidemiol Rec*. 1998;73:321-328.
11. WHO/UNAIDS. AIDS epidemic update. Available at: http://data.unaids.org/pub/Report/2014/JC1700_ Epi_Update_2014_en.pdf. Accessed May 6, 2015
12. Parrish NF, Gao F, Li H, et al. Phenotypic properties of transmitted founder HIV-1. *Proc Natl Acad Sci USA*. 2013;110:6626-6633.
13. Santiago ML, Montano M., Benitez R, et al. Apobec3 encodes Rfv3, a gene influencing neutralizing antibody control of retrovirus infection. *Science*. 2008;321:1343-1346.
14. Centers for Disease Control and Prevention. Kaposi's sarcoma and pneumocystis pneumonia among homosexual men—New York City and California. *MMWR Morb Mortal Wkly Rep*. 1981;30:305.
15. Chang Y, Cesarman E, Pessin MS, et al. Identification of herpesvirus-like DNA sequences in AIDS-associated Kaposi's sarcoma. *Science*. 1994;266:1865-1869.
16. Moore PS, Boshoff C, Weiss RA, et al. Molecular mimicry of human cytokine and cytokine response pathways genes by KSHV. *Science*. 1996;274:1739-1744.
17. Nicholas J. Human herpesvirus 8-encoded proteins with potential roles in virus-associated neoplasia. *Front Biosci*. 2007;12:265-281.
18. Dezube BJ. Clinical presentation and natural history of AIDS-related Kaposi's sarcoma. *Hematol Oncol Clin North Am*. 1996;5:1023-1029.
19. Cattelan AM, Calabró ML, Gasperini P, et al. Acquired immunodeficiency syndrome-related Kaposi's sarcoma regression after highly active antiretroviral therapy: biologic correlates of clinical outcome. *J Natl Cancer Inst Monogr*. 2001;28:44-49.
20. Cattelan AM, Calabró ML, De Rossia A, et al. Long-term clinical outcome of AIDS-related Kaposi's sarcoma during highly active antiretroviral therapy. *Int J Oncol*. 2005;3:779-785.
21. Quesada JR, Reuben J, Manning JT, et al. Alpha interferon for induction of remission in hairy-cell leukemia. *N Engl J Med*. 1984;310:15-18.
22. Krown SE. The role of interferon in the therapy of epidemic Kaposi's sarcoma. *Semin Oncol*. 1987;14(2 Suppl 3):27-33.
23. Rios A, Mansell PW, Newell GR, et al. Treatment of acquired immunodeficiency syndrome-related Kaposi's sarcoma with lymphoblastoid interferon. *J Clin Oncol*. 1985;4:506-512.
24. Carbone A, Cesarman E, Spina M, et al. HIV-associated lymphomas and gamma-herpesviruses. *Blood*. 2009;113:1213-1224.
25. National Cancer Institute sponsored study of classifications of non-Hodgkin's lymphomas: summary and description of a working formulation for clinical usage. The Non-Hodgkin's Lymphoma Pathologic Classification Project. *Cancer*. 1982;49:2112-2135.
26. Barclay LR, Buskin SE, Kahle EM, et al. Clinical and immunologic profile of AIDS-related lymphoma in the era of highly active antiretroviral therapy. *Clin Lymphoma Myeloma*. 2007;4:272-279.
27. Jaffe ES, Harris NL, Stein H, et al. *World Health Organization*

Classification of Tumors: Pathology & Genetics: Tumors of Haematopoietic and Lymphoid Tissues. Lyon, France: IARC Press; 2001.
28. Levine AM. Acquired immunodeficiency-syndrome related lymphoma. *Blood*. 1992;80:8-20.
29. Vajdic CM, van Leeuwen MT. What types of cancers are associated with immune suppression in HIV? Lessons from solid organ transplant recipients. *Curr Opin HIV/AIDS*. 2009;1:35-41.
30. Pelicci P, Knowles DM, Arlin ZA, et al. Multiple monoclonal B cell expansions and c-myc oncogene rearrangements in acquired immune deficiency syndrome-related lymphoproliferative disorders. *J Exp Med*. 1986;164:2049-2076.
31. Carbone A, Gloghini A. AIDS-related lymphomas: from pathogenesis to pathology. *Br J Haematol*. 2005;130:662-670.
32. Angeletti PC, Luwen Z, Wood C. The viral etiology of AIDS-associated malignancies. *Adv Pharmacol*. 2008;56:509-557.
33. Vaghefi P, Martin A, Prévot S, et al. Genomic imbalances in AIDS-related lymphomas: relation with tumoral Epstein-Barr virus status. *AIDS*. 2006;20:2285-2291.
34. Gaidano G, Pastore C, Lanza C, et al. Molecular pathology of AIDS-related lymphomas. Biologic aspects and clinicopathologic heterogeneity. *Ann Hematol*. 1994;69:281-290.
35. Knowles DM. Molecular pathology of acquired immunodeficiency syndrome-related non-Hodgkin's lymphoma. *Semin Diagn Pathol*. 1997;1:67-82.
36. Voelkerding KV, Sandhaus LM, Kim HC, et al. Plasma cell malignancy in the acquired immune deficiency syndrome. *Am J Clin Pathol*. 1989;92:222-228.
37. Levine AM, Sadeghi S, Espina B, et al. Characteristics of indolent non-Hodgkin lymphoma in patients with type 1 human immunodeficiency virus infection. *Cancer*. 2002;94:1500-1506.
38. Goldstein J, Becker N, Delrowe J, et al. Cutaneous T-cell lymphoma in a patient infected with human immunodeficiency virus type 1. Use of radiation therapy. *Cancer*. 1990;66:1130-1132.
39. Tsimberidou AM, Medina J, Cortes J, et al. Chronic myeloid leukemia in a patient with acquired immune deficiency syndrome: complete cytogenetic response with imatinib mesylate: report of a case and review of the literature. *Leuk Res*. 2004;6:657-660.
40. Ziegler JL, Beckstead JA, Volberding PA, et al. Non-Hodgkin's lymphoma in 90 homosexual men. Relation to generalized lymphadenopathy and the acquired immunodeficiency syndrome. *N Engl J Med*. 1984;311:565-570.
41. Rossi G, Donisi A, Casari S, et al. The International Prognostic Index can be used as a guide to treatment decisions regarding patients with human immunodeficiency virus-related systemic non-Hodgkin lymphoma. *Cancer*. 1999;86:2391-2397.
42. Francisci D, Falcinelli F, Schiaroli E, et al. Management of hepatitis B virus reactivation in patients with hematological malignancies treated with chemotherapy. *Infection*. 2010;38:58-61.
43. Bower M, Gazzard B, Mandallia S, et al. A prognostic index for systemic AIDS-related non-Hodgkin lymphoma treated in the era of highly active antiretroviral therapy. *Ann Intern Med*. 2005;143(4):265-273.
44. Vaccher E, Spina M, di Gennaro G, et al. Concomitant cyclophosphamide, doxorubicin, vincristine, and prednisone chemotherapy plus highly active antiretroviral therapy in patients with human immunodeficiency virus-related, non-Hodgkin lymphoma. *Cancer*. 2001;91(1):155-163.
45. Kaplan LD, Scadden DT. No benefit from rituximab in a randomized phase III trial of CHOP with or without rituximab for patients with HIV-associated non-Hodgkin's lymphoma: AIDS malignancies consortium study 010 [abstract]. *Proc Am Soc Clin Oncol*. 2003;2268.
46. Sparano JA, Weller E, Nazeer T, et al. Phase II trial of infusional cyclophosphamide, doxorubicin, and etoposide in patients with poor-prognosis, intermediate-grade non-Hodgkin lymphoma: an Eastern Cooperative Oncology Group trial (E3493). *Blood*. 2002;100(5):1634-1640.
47. Tirelli U, Spina M, Jaeger U, et al. Infusional CDE with rituximab for the treatment of human immunodeficiency virus-associated non-Hodgkin's lymphoma: preliminary results of a phase 1/II study. *Recent Results Cancer Res*. 2002;159:149-153.
48. Little RF, Pittaluga S, Grant N, et al. Highly effective treatment of acquired immunodeficiency syndrome-related lymphoma with dose-adjusted EPOCH: impact of antiretroviral therapy suspension and tumor biology. *Blood*. 2003;101(12):4653-4659.
49. Sparano JA. Clinical aspects and management of AIDS-related lymphoma. *Eur J Cancer*. 2001;37(10):1296-1305.
50. Antinori A, Cingolani A, Alba L, et al. Better response to chemotherapy and prolonged survival in AIDS-related lymphomas responding to highly active antiretroviral therapy. *AIDS*. 2001;15:1483-1491.
51. Levine AM. Management of AIDS-related lymphoma. *Curr Opin Oncol*. 2008;20:522-528.
52. Cortes J, Thomas D, Rios A, et al. Hyperfractionated cyclophosphamide, vincristine, doxorubicin, and dexamethasone and highly active antiretroviral therapy for patients with acquired immunodeficiency syndrome-related Burkitt lymphoma/leukemia. *Cancer*. 2002;94:1492-1499.
53. Wang ES, Straus DJ, Teruya-Feldstein J, et al. Intensive chemotherapy with cyclophosphamide, doxorubicin, high dose methotrexate/ifosfamide, etoposide, and high-dose cytarabine (CODOX-M/IVAC) for human immunodeficiency virus associated Burkitt lymphoma. *Cancer*. 2003;98:1196-1205.
54. Dunleavy K, Pittaluga S, Shovlin M, et al. Low-intensity therapy in adults with Burkitt lymphoma. *N Engl J Med*. 2013;369:1915-1925.
55. Krishnan A, Molina A, Zaia J, et al. Durable remissions with autologous stem cell transplantation for high risk HIV associated lymphomas. *Blood*. 2004;105:874-878.
56. Pagano JS. Epstein-Barr virus: the first human tumor virus and its role in cancer. *Proc Assoc Am Phys*. 1999;111:573-580.
57. Wong SY, Israeliski DM, Remington JS. AIDS-associated toxoplasmosis, in Sande MA, Volberding PA, (eds): *The Medical Management of AIDS*, 4th ed. Philadelphia: WB Saunders; 1995:460.
58. Lorberboym M, Wallach F, Estok L, et al. Thallium-201 retention in focal intracranial lesions for differential diagnosis of primary lymphoma and nonmalignant lesions in AIDS patients. *J Nucl Med*. 1998;39:1366-1369.
59. Corcoran C, Rebe K, van de Plas H, Myer L, Hardie DR. The predictive value of cerebrospinal fluid Epstein-Barr viral load as a marker of primary central nervous system lymphoma in HIV-infected persons. *J Clin Virol*. 2008;42:433-436.
60. Broomberg JEC, Breems DA, Kran J, et al. CSF flow cytometry greatly improves diagnostic accuracy in CNS hematologic malignancies. *Neurology*. 2007;68:1674-1679.
61. Shah GD, Yahalom J, Correa DD, et al. Combined immunochemotherapy with reduced whole-brain radiotherapy for newly diagnosed primary CNS lymphoma. *J Clin Oncol*. 2007;25:4730-4735.
62. Carbone A, Gloghini A, Serraino D, et al. HIV-associated Hodgkin lymphoma. *Curr Opin HIV/AIDS*. 2009;4:3-10.
63. Carbone A, Gloghini A, Dotti G: EBV-associated lymphoproliferative disorders: classification and treatment. *Oncologist*. 2008;13:577-585.
64. Vaccher E, Spina M, Tirelli U. Clinical aspects and management of Hodgkin's disease and other tumours in HIV-infected individuals. *Eur J Cancer*. 2001;37:1306-1315.
65. Hessol NA, Katz MH, Liu JU, et al. Increased incidence of Hodgkin's disease in homosexual men with HIV infection. *Ann Intern Med*. 1992;117:309-311.
66. Levine AM, Li P, Cheung T, et al. Chemotherapy consisting of doxorubicin, bleomycin, vinblastine, and dacarbazine with granulocyte-colony-stimulating factor in HIV-infected patients

with newly diagnosed Hodgkin's disease: a prospective, multi-institutional AIDS clinical trials group study (ACTG 149). *J AIDS*. 2000;15:444-450.

67. Berenguer J, Miralles P, Ribera JM, et al. Characteristics and outcome of AIDS-related Hodgkin's lymphoma before and after the introduction of highly active antiretroviral therapy. *J Acquire Immune Defic Syndr*. 2008;47:422-428.
68. Spina M, Gabarre J, Rossi G, et al. Stanford V regimen and concomitant HAART in 59 patients with Hodgkin's disease and HIV infection. *Blood*. 2002;100:1984-1991.
69. Stier E. Cervical neoplasia and the HIV-infected patient. *Hematol Oncol Clin North Am*. 2003;17:873-887.
70. Chow LT, Brooker TR. Papillomavirus DNA replication. *Intervirology*. 1994;37:150-158.
71. Munger K, Phelps WC, Bubb V, et al. The E6 and E7 genes of the human papillomavirus type 16 together are necessary and sufficient for transformation of primary human keratinocytes. *J Virol*. 1989;63:4417-4421.
72. Ellerbrock TV, Chiasson MA, Bush TJ, et al. Incidence of cervical squamous intraepithelial lesions in HIV-infected women. *JAMA*. 2000;282:1031-1037.
73. US Preventive Services Task Force. Screening for cervical cancer. In: AHRQ Publication No. 03–515A, January 2003. Rockville, MD: Agency for Healthcare Research and Quality; 2003.
74. NCCN Clinical Practice Guidelines in Oncology: Cervical cancer version 1.2010. National Comprehensive Cancer Network, 2010. Available at: http://www.nccn.org/professionals/physician_gls/ PDF/cervical.pdf. Accessed January 15, 2015.
75. zur Hausen H. Papillomaviruses and cancer: from basic studies to clinical application. *Nat Rev Cancer*. 2002;2:342-350.
76. Martin F, Bowers M. Anal intraepithelial neoplasia in HIV-positive people. *Sex Transm Inf*. 2001;77:327-331.
77. Chin-Hong PV, Palefsky JM. Natural history and clinical management of anal human papillomavirus disease in men and women infected with human immunodeficiency virus. *HIV/AIDS*. 2002;35:1127-1134.
78. NCCN Clinical Practice Guidelines in Oncology: Anal cancer version 1.2011. National Comprehensive Cancer Network, 2010. Available at: http://www.nccn.org/professionals/physician_ gls/PDF/anal.pdf. Accessed January 15, 2011.
79. French MA. Immune reconstitution syndrome: A reappraisal. *Clin Infect Dis*. 2009;48:101-107.
80. Valencia Ortega ME. AIDS-related malignancies: a new approach. *AIDS Rev*. 2008;10:125-127.
81. Kaplan LD, Straus DJ, Testa MA, et al. Low-dose compared with standard-dose m-BACOD chemotherapy for non-Hodgkin's lymphoma associated with human immunodeficiency virus infection. National Institute of Allergy and Infectious Diseases AIDS Clinical Trials Group. *N Engl J Med*. 1997;336:1641-1648.
82. Tosi P, Gherlinzoni F, Mazza P, et al. 3′-Azido-3′-deoxythymidine plus methotrexate as a novel antineoplastic combination in the treatment of human immunodeficiency virus-related non-Hodgkin's lymphomas. *Blood*. 1997;89:419-425.

Section XIII

Novel and Other Cancer Topics of Interest

Section Editors: Apostolia-Maria Tsimberidou and Nizar M. Tannir

第十三篇 前沿和其他有趣的肿瘤话题

45

Carcinoma of Unknown Primary

第四十五章　原发灶不明的转移癌

Gauri R. Varadhachary

中文导读

原发灶不明的转移癌临床表现形式多种多样，在诊断评估和治疗方面均提出了挑战。在过去的40年里，人们对于原发灶不明的转移癌的认识有了重大转变。本章阐述了原发灶不明的转移癌的诊断评估和治疗策略，根据表现部位和组织病理学的不同，还讨论了不同的病史特点。本章首先概述了流行病学的现况，影像学技术的进步使原发灶不明的转移癌发病率有所下降。在生物学、染色体异常及基因组学部分介绍了原发灶不明癌在以上层面的表现特性。该病临床表现形式多种多样，一些症状和体征与已知来源的晚期肿瘤患者相似。在诊断评估部分包括了体检与实验室检查、诊断影像与内镜检查、组织病理特征评估和分子生物学研究等内容。在特殊临床病理亚型部分，着重介绍了以孤立性脑转移为首发表现的原发灶不明癌，原发灶不明的转移性子宫颈腺癌、原发灶不明的女性孤立腋窝淋巴结转移癌、以孤立性胸腔积液/恶性腹水为首发的原发灶不明癌、原发灶不明的孤立骨转移癌、原发灶未明的肝转移癌、原发灶不明的神经内分泌肿瘤等特点及处理原则。在化疗策略部分，介绍了一些临床试验的研究结果，以及目前的治疗推荐。最后在未来趋势方面做了简明指引，通过运用基因组工具来识别单个肿瘤的驱动基因，在肿瘤个体化治疗方面将产生广泛的推动作用。

OVERVIEW

Carcinomas of unknown primary (CUPs), with their heterogeneous presentations, pose a challenge on the diagnostic and therapeutic fronts. Depending on the extent of evaluation, CUP comprises 3% to 5% of all tumors diagnosed ([1-3]). A working definition for CUP is biopsy-proven metastatic cancer with no identifiable primary source by history; physical examination; chest radiography; complete blood cell count; chemistry; computed tomography (CT) of the chest, abdomen and pelvis; prostate-specific antigen (PSA) in men; and mammography in women ([2]). The natural history of disease for CUP is diverse and is dependent on multiple variables, such as, age, number of metastatic sites, dominant area of disease, and histology. This considerable heterogeneity presents a challenge to the systematic study of CUPs. In addition, the emergence of sophisticated imaging, robust immunohistochemistry (IHC), and genomic and proteomic tools have challenged the "unknown" designation. Depending on histologic features, sites of disease, and performance status, a small but significant minority of patients will be long-term survivors, and it is important to identify these groups of patients ([4, 5]).

This chapter discusses the evaluation of patients with CUP and optimal therapeutic strategies in the era of sophisticated diagnostics. The differing natural histories in CUP, depending on both the sites of disease and histology, are also discussed. Studies showed that, in this population, a search for the primary tumor beyond "routine" evaluation is unrewarding in the majority of patients ([5]). This fact has caused much consternation for both patients and physicians. The foundation for cancer treatment traditionally relies on identification of the tumor origin, thereby allowing treatment to be chosen based on the known natural history as well as specific therapies that have been proven effective for the cancer; this is becoming even more important with the rapid emergence of targeted therapies. Without knowledge of the primary site, the oncologist is often hesitant to recommend therapy, especially given the disease heterogeneity. Although most patients with metastatic CUP have tumors that respond poorly to current treatments and will consequently have a poor prognosis, it has become evident over the last two decades that subsets of patients with CUP have a favorable prognosis and respond to chemotherapy or can be successfully treated with regional therapy alone. The current era of sophisticated diagnostics and introduction of targeted therapies has been particularly important in the CUP setting; this cancer entity is the epitome of personalized therapy.

EPIDEMIOLOGY

The incidence of CUP cancers as estimated from the cancer registries and databases of "unknown and unspecified cancers" is reported to be approximately 3%-4% of all cancers ([6]). This is probably an overestimation because this group includes a mix of patients: those with true CUP, those with primaries not yet diagnosed at the time of death, and those with difficult-to-diagnose tumors. Further, improved imaging allowing identification of small primary tumors suggests that the incidence of true CUP is decreasing.

A minority of patients (10%) with CUP have a history of an antecedent cancer. In autopsies performed before the advent of CT, the occult primary tumor was identified in 60% to 80% of cases. In one autopsy series, the two most commonly identified primary sites were the pancreas (20%) and lungs (18%) ([7, 8]). Given the current high-quality CT imaging and positron emission tomographic (PET) scans, it is unclear whether these cancer profiles are still the majority.

The classification of CUP continues to evolve. The last four decades have seen a shift in our understanding of CUP. First, improved imaging increased our confidence for the entity termed *occult primary*. Later, "favorable" CUP subsets were determined, based primarily on histopathology, the pattern of spread of select CUP cancers, and serum markers. Subsequently, with the advent of novel IHC markers and advances in diagnostic pathology, tissue of origin (ToO) profiles were described that assigned additional putative primary sites to CUP cancers based on IHC patterns. Current research involves the application of proteomic and genomic tools to CUP cancers.

BIOLOGY, CHROMOSOMAL ABERRATIONS, AND MUTATIONAL PROFILING

Carcinomas of unknown primary, despite their heterogeneity, are a clinically unique oncologic entity; as such, they share many common features that set them apart from other malignancies. The central unifying clinical feature of CUP is the absence of a detectable primary tumor. Previous studies have shown that, even after an autopsy, the primary site will not be identified in 20% to 40% of cases; that number is likely much lower with significant improvements in imaging. At present, it is not known why primary carcinomas exhibit this unique biological behavior. One current hypothesis is that the acquisition of a "metastatic phenotype" is an early event in CUPs, soon after oncogenesis, thus enabling cells to metastasize early, before the development of a clinically detectable tumor ([9]). It has also been hypothesized that the primary tumors may regress or involute before the metastases become clinically evident, attributed to a host immunologic response. A third hypothesis is that the primary tumor is exposed to antiangiogenic factors locally, whereas the metastases acquire the angiogenic phenotype after a period of dormancy ([10]).

Several studies have demonstrated a specific nonrandom pattern of chromosomal aberrations that seems to be unique to CUPs. These data suggest that some of these genetic changes may be the underlying cause of the metastatic phenotype. Carcinoma of unknown primary is characterized by greater genetic instability, with massive GAs, when compared with other distant metastases. In a study by Pantou and colleagues ([11]), cytogenetic profiling of tumors from 20 patients with CUP was performed, revealing an average of 11 chromosomal changes per case. Of the three histologic subtypes in this study, adenocarcinomas had not only the highest number of cytogenetic changes (16 vs 3) but also involvement of distinct sites (4q31, 6q15, 10q25, and 13q22) when compared with carcinomas or undifferentiated malignancies. The latter group was distinguished by the involvement of changes at 11q22. Overall, the most commonly rearranged chromosomal regions were 1q21, 3p13, 6q21-23, 7q22, 11p15-12, and 11q14-24. The number of cytogenetic alterations was found to be prognostically relevant. Median survival was significantly greater for patients with five or fewer cytogenetic changes compared with those with more than five changes (3 vs 18 months, $P = .003$). An older study of 12 CUP cell lines also demonstrated a preponderance of chromosome 1 abnormalities. These changes were observed on both the long arm (eg, 1p deletion, isochromosome 1p, and translocations with a 1p breakpoint) and on the short arm (1q21), suggesting the importance of chromosome 1 in the biology of CUPs ([12]). Chromosome 1p aberrations are also commonly associated with advanced malignancies.

Chromosome 12 abnormalities have also been shown in CUP. This is of particular interest because one of the observed alterations, isochromosome 12p (i12p), is present in as many as 80% of germ cell tumors. Motzer and colleagues reported that 30% of patient tumors in their series had either i12p or 12q deletions. The presence of either of these two cytogenetic abnormalities was found to be predictive of a complete response to cisplatin-based chemotherapy (75% vs 17%, $P = .002$) ([13, 14]). In the current era of sophisticated IHC, we rarely miss a patient with an extragonadal presentation and seldom order cytogenetics to inform therapeutic plans.

The tumor suppressor gene *p53* is commonly mutated in human cancers, especially in advanced malignancies. Paradoxically, this does not seem to be true in CUP. Bar-Eli and colleagues found *p53* mutations to be less frequent than expected (26%) in CUP after evaluating 15 biopsy specimens and 8 cell lines ([15]). However, work by other researchers evaluating IHC studies of *p53* in CUP has found this protein to be highly expressed in 70% of the tumors examined ([16, 17]). Nevertheless, *p53* expression has not been found to have prognostic relevance. Molecular studies have also demonstrated the overexpression of other oncogenes, such as c-*myc*, *ras*, *bcl-2*, and *Her2/neu*, in CUPs, but none have been found to have any correlation with either survival or response to chemotherapy ([18]).

More recent data with next-generation sequencing likely has therapeutic implications for patients with CUP, and it is exciting times for CUP researchers to extend the therapeutic envelope. In a recent study, Ross and colleagues presented results from a retrospective study of 200 consecutive CUP tumor specimens that that underwent comprehensive genomic profiling (CGP) using the hybrid-capture–based Foundation-One 10 assay ([19]). The DNA extracted from these CUP tumor specimens was analyzed after hybridization capture of 3,769 exons from 236 cancer-related genes and 47 introns of 19 genes commonly rearranged in cancer. There were 125 adenocarcinomas of unknown primary site (ACUPs) and 75 nonadenocarcinomas (non-ACUPs). The authors reported that a large number of CUP samples (85%) harbored at least one clinically relevant genomic alteration (GA) with the potential to influence and personalize therapy. The mean number of GAs was 4.2 GAs per tumor. The ACUP tumors were more frequently driven by GAs in the receptor tyrosine kinase (RTK)/Ras/mitogen-activated protein kinase (MAPK) signaling pathway than non-ACUP tumors. The authors concluded that CGP can identify novel treatment paradigms and suggested that early testing may have utility in CUP management. These data do illustrate some important considerations in the management of CUP cancers, as discussed in this chapter.

NATURAL HISTORY AND CLINICAL PRESENTATION

The clinical course of patients with CUP varies widely. Median survival in large retrospective studies has ranged from 11 weeks to 11 months. In the University of Texas MD Anderson Cancer Center study, the 5-year overall survival (OS) rate was only 11%. Although survival is poor as a whole, there are certain prognostic variables that correlate with longer survival, including disease limited to one organ site, involvement of lymph nodes only, and histologic diagnoses of squamous or neuroendocrine carcinoma. Variables suggestive of a poor prognosis include male sex, histologic diagnosis of adenocarcinoma, and metastatic involvement of the liver, lungs, bone, pleura, or brain (Table 45-1) ([4]).

CHAPTER 45

Table 45-1 Favorable- Versus Poor-Prognosis Carcinoma of Unknown Primary

Favorable Prognosis	Poor Prognosis
Extragonadal germ cell syndrome	Liver metastases (nonneuroendocrine)
Isolated single small metastasis	Pleural or lung metastases
Papillary peritoneal adenocarcinoma (women)	Adrenal metastases
Isolated axillary adenocarcinoma (women)	Multiple brain metastases
Cervical adenopathy (squamous cell)	
Isolated inguinal adenopathy	
Neuroendocrine histology	

By performing multivariate analyses on a consecutive series of 1,000 patients with CUP with classification and regression tree (CART) analysis, Hess and colleagues ([4]) were able to more closely study the interactions between different clinical variables and how this influenced survival.

Patients with CUP present with symptoms and signs similar to those of patients with advanced malignancies of known origin. In one review, the most common symptoms at presentation of CUP were general deterioration (73%), digestive symptoms (58%), liver enlargement (58%), abdominal pain (56%), respiratory symptoms (45%), ascites (26%), and node enlargement (16%) ([20]). Most patients with CUP present with multiple metastases, with three or more organs involved. In patients with a dominant (or single) site of metastasis, the most common reported sites were liver (25%), bone (22%), lungs (20%), lymph nodes (15%), pleural space (10%), and brain (5%).

DIAGNOSTIC EVALUATION

In the past, minimalist diagnostic strategies had been advocated, limiting the scope of initial evaluations to differentiate only between treatable and untreatable disease. Others have supported a more aggressive approach, wherein a complete assessment of the extent of the disease and detection of the primary tumor site are attempted. In our experience, a more pragmatic approach is better. Extensive evaluation of all patients presenting with metastases is an expensive and wasteful extreme that does not benefit patients. In one study, the average cost of evaluating a patient with CUP was $17,973 and much higher with recent testing ([21, 22]). In that study, mean survival was 8.1 months, representative of the natural history of CUP, with only 18% of patients surviving 1 year. However, a strictly minimalist approach may result in the oversight of treatable and potentially curable neoplasms.

An important determinant of the appropriate extent of evaluation for any patient with CUP is whether the data obtained by a diagnostic test will influence treatment decisions. If a treatable or potentially curable cancer is strongly suspected (eg, a germ cell tumor or lymphoma or oligometastatic disease treated with surgery or multimodality therapy), further investigation should proceed until a precise clinical diagnosis can be made, provided that therapy is not unreasonably delayed. The recommended general approach at the present time is thus one of a directed evaluation based on clinical presentation and pathologic findings; predictions of tumor origin or mutations from molecular profiling techniques may also play a role in streamlining the scope of evaluation.

Physical Examination and Laboratory Tests

A thorough medical history should be obtained, and a physical examination, including a digital prostate examination in men and a breast and pelvic examination in women, should be performed. Determination of the patient's performance status, nutrition, and the presence or absence of concomitant medical illnesses and malignancy-related complications (eg, paraneoplastic syndromes or painful metastases) that may affect patient care is required.

Laboratory tests should include routine biochemical and hematologic surveys. The role of tumor markers in the evaluation of patients with CUP is often not diagnostic. Most tumor markers are nonspecific and are not useful for identifying a primary site or for prognostic purposes. Adenocarcinoma markers (eg, carcinoembryonic antigen [CEA], cancer antigen 125 [CA 125], CA 15-3, and CA 19-9) are often elevated in patients with CUP and cannot be reliably used to identify a specific primary site or to predict either OS or the exact burden of metastatic disease ([23-25]). Serum tumor markers may play a role in helping to evaluate patients for responses to therapy, although levels are not always predictive of response to chemotherapy.

Their selective use in a directed approach is more helpful than ordering a large battery of tumor markers on all patients who present with CUP. Men who present with metastatic adenocarcinoma and osteoblastic bone metastases CUP should have PSA and prostatic acid phosphatase levels measured. In all men with undifferentiated (or poorly differentiated) midline carcinomas, beta-human chorionic gonadotropin and alpha-fetoprotein levels should be measured, especially if the clinical presentation suggests an extragonadal germ cell tumor. In patients with hepatic tumors, alpha-fetoprotein levels should also be measured if there are risk factors or pathologic characteristics that suggest a possibility of primary hepatocellular carcinoma.

Diagnostic Imaging and Invasive Studies

In the absence of contraindications, a baseline intravenous contrast CT scan of the chest, abdomen, and pelvis is the standard of care, as supported by the National Comprehensive Cancer Network and National Institute for Health and Clinical Excellence CUP radiology guidelines [26, 27]. Patients with CUP should then be approached in a "directed" fashion. Endoscopy of the upper and lower gastrointestinal (GI) tract is indicated for patients with abdominal complaints, ascites, liver metastases, or other findings in the initial workup and pathology that are indicative of a possible GI primary tumor.

All women with CUP and adenocarcinoma should undergo mammography. In cases of suspicious findings on a breast examination and negative mammography findings, patients should have breast sonography and a biopsy as indicated. Because both the sensitivity (23%-29%) and specificity (71%-73%) of mammography in detecting an occult carcinoma are low, breast magnetic resonance imaging (MRI) has been evaluated as an alternative in patients with a high suspicion for breast primary cancer. In the setting of isolated axillary adenopathy, MRI is sensitive in detecting occult primary breast cancers (>75%) and should be performed in women with isolated axillary adenopathy and negative mammography findings [28-33]. Women with adenocarcinoma presenting with metastatic sites other than cervical or axillary adenopathy that are compatible with breast cancer (ie, bone, liver, or lungs) may also undergo breast MRI if the mammography findings are negative [32, 33].

Patients with upper or midcervical adenopathy with a squamous cell carcinoma on pathology should undergo a thorough head and neck evaluation, including panendoscopy (ie, laryngoscopy, bronchoscopy, and esophagoscopy) with random biopsies. Ipsilateral or (more often) bilateral tonsillectomy has also been recommended as part of the staging process because this has been shown to identify an occult primary lesion deep in the tonsillar crypts in up to 30% of patients with this presentation of CUP [34-36]. Computed tomography of the head and neck region is routinely done as part of the initial workup. In addition, the utility of 18-fluorodeoxyglucose positron emission tomography (FDG-PET) has been well documented in patients with squamous carcinoma and cervical adenopathy; small prospective and retrospective studies suggest that a primary head and neck tumor is identified in 25% to 30% of these patients [36-42]. A recent retrospective review found that the primary tumor site was identified in 44% of these patients undergoing PET-CT fusion scans, and this modality appears to be emerging as a superior alternative to either PET or CT alone [38, 39].

Outside the indication given previously, the role of PET-CT is unclear. Several small studies have evaluated the utility of PET in CUP patients [43, 44]. Moller et al reviewed [18] FDG-PET as a diagnostic tool for patients with extracervical CUP [44]. They identified four publications (152 patients); these studies were retrospective and heterogeneous in their inclusion criteria, study design, and diagnostic workup prior to FDG PET-CT. The primary tumor was detected by FDG PET-CT in 39% of patients with extracervical CUP. Lung was the most commonly detected primary tumor site (≈50%). Pooled estimates of sensitivity, specificity, and accuracy of FDG PET-CT in the detection of the primary tumor site were 87%, 88%, and 87.5%, respectively. They concluded that FDG PET-CT may have a role in identification of the primary tumor in extracervical CUP; however, prospective studies with more uniform inclusion criteria are warranted. Although not studied prospectively, PET-CT scans may be useful in selected patients with solitary metastases prior to definitive locoregional therapies and in follow-up of patients with predominant bone disease [2].

Histopathologic Evaluation

All pathologic material obtained at biopsy from a patient with CUP should be evaluated by an experienced pathologist who is familiar with CUP workup. The pathologist should also be informed of the patient's pertinent history and clinical findings so that he or she can recommend further analysis on the basis of this information. In the CUP world, pathology trumps radiology. Collaboration between the pathologist and treating oncologist is critical. Adequate tissue sampling is essential.

The CUP cancers include adenocarcinoma, poorly differentiated adenocarcinoma (60%); poorly differentiated carcinoma (PDC), undifferentiated carcinoma, or undifferentiated neoplasm (30%); squamous cell carcinoma (5%); and neuroendocrine cancer (2%). Rarely (2%), CUP can present as mixed tumors, including sarcomatoid, basaloid, and adenosquamous carcinomas (Table 45-2).

Adequacy of tissue is essential, especially when the pathologist has to make a diagnosis on deep fine-needle aspirations and there is insufficient tissue for IHC staining. The diagnosis of a poorly differentiated neoplasm implies that the pathologist is unable to classify it into any of the general neoplastic categories (carcinoma, lymphoma, melanoma, or sarcoma). Subsequent evaluation of this group of poorly

Table 45-2 Major Histologies in Carcinoma of Unknown Primary

Histology	Proportion (%)
Well to moderately differentiated adenocarcinoma	55
Poorly differentiated adenocarcinoma	30
Squamous	6
Neuroendocrine	4
Undifferentiated malignancy	5

differentiated lesions by means of special IHC techniques is warranted because some of these patients will have tumors that are potentially curable and very responsive to treatment. Many IHC reagents are at the disposal of the pathologist, making the histologic classification of the tumor easier (Table 45-3).

Especially useful are the antibodies to common leukocyte antigens present in lymphoma and the antibodies to PSA present in most prostate cancers. Other useful IHC markers include cytokeratin CK7, CK20, and thyroid transcription factor (TTF-1). Thyroid transcription factor is a nuclear transcription factor that is normally expressed in lung and thyroid tissues and in their neoplasms. Staining for TTF-1 is frequently positive in lung cancer, especially in adenocarcinomas (60%-75%) and small cell lung cancers (66%-87%); however, it is inconsistently expressed in squamous cell carcinoma. Among the various monoclonal antibodies against various cytokeratins, CK7 and CK20 can help differentiate between different solid tumors. (For instance, CK7 is more commonly associated with pulmonary or gynecologic malignancies, whereas CK20 is frequently seen in GI adenocarcinomas.) The CK7+/CK20- immunophenotype, in conjunction with TTF-1 staining, is suggestive of a lung primary and is a highly sensitive and specific method for differentiating primary pulmonary adenocarcinomas from metastatic extrapulmonary adenocarcinomas (Fig. 45-1) ([45-49]). In contrast, the CK7-/CK20+ immunophenotype is suggestive of a colorectal primary site. CK7+ and CK20+ dual staining suggest a malignancy of urothelial origin. Using light microscopy and IHC, a putative primary tumor may be assigned in up to a third of CUP cases. Immunohistochemistry can also suggest biomarker studies with potential therapeutic impact (eg, Kras, epidermal growth factor receptor [EGFR], Her2, and ALK mutations).

Hep par 1 is an antigen whose expression is confined to benign and malignant hepatocytes and aids in the diagnosis of hepatocellular carcinoma in patients with CUP presenting with liver lesions. In women, depending on the pathology and pattern of metastasis,

Table 45-3 Commonly Utilized Immunoperoxidase Stains to Assist in the Differential Diagnosis of Poorly Differentiated Neoplasms

Stain	Likely Primary Site
Estrogen/progesterone receptor, gross cystic disease fluid protein-15 (GCDFP-15), low molecular weight cytokeratin (CK)	Breast cancer
Thyroid transcription factor (TTF-1), CK7, CK20, surfactant protein A precursor (SP-A1)	Lung cancer
Prostate-specific antigen (PSA), epithelial membrane antigen (EMA), alpha-methylacyl coenzyme A racemase/P504S (AMACR/P504S)	Prostate cancer
Leukocyte common antigen (LCA), CD3, CD4, CD5, CD20, CD45	Lymphoma
Vimentin, desmin,[a] factor VIII[b]	Sarcoma
Chromogranin/synaptophysin, neuron-specific enolase, cytokeratin	Neuroendocrine tumor
EMA, β-hCG, AFP, placental alkaline phosphatase (PLAP)	Germ cell tumor
CK7, CK20,[c] uroplakin III	Urothelial malignancies
S100, vimentin, HMB-45, neuron-specific enolase	Melanoma
CK7, CK20,[c] CDX-2, carcinoembryonic antigen (CEA)	Colorectal cancer

Abbreviations: AFP, alpha-fetoprotein; β-hCG, beta-human chorionic gonadotrophin; CDX-2, Caudal type homeobox-2; HMB-45, Human melanomablack-45.
[a]Positive in desmoid tumors, rhabdomyosarcomas, and leiomyosarcomas.
[b]Positive in angiosarcomas.
[c]Whereas a CK7+/CK20- staining pattern is typical of lung neoplasms, CK7-/CK20+ is suggestive of a colorectal primary. Dual CK7+/CK20+, however, is suggestive of urothelial primary.

estrogen receptor and progesterone receptor staining is done to look for a breast primary. Another marker for a breast primary is gross cystic disease fluid protein 15 (GCDFP-15), which is present in 62% to 72% of breast cancers.

Dennis and colleagues ([50]) have identified other novel molecular markers using a bioinformatics approach. All publicly available gene expression data from various adenocarcinomas were pooled together, and four novel proteins not previously recognized as tumor markers were found to be significantly upregulated. This was confirmed by reverse transcription–polymerase chain reaction. One example was lipophilin B, which was found to be restricted to breast, ovarian, and prostate cancers.

The use of cytogenetic analysis in the diagnosis of CUPs is limited. Specific chromosomal abnormalities

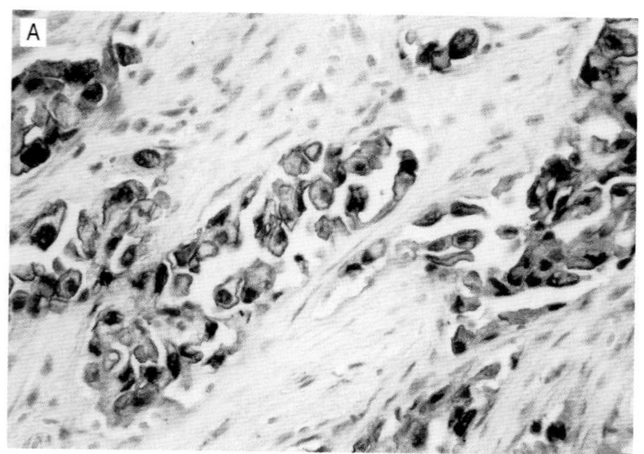

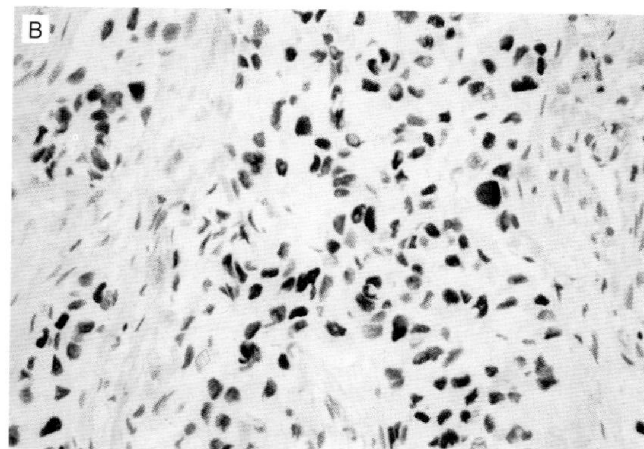

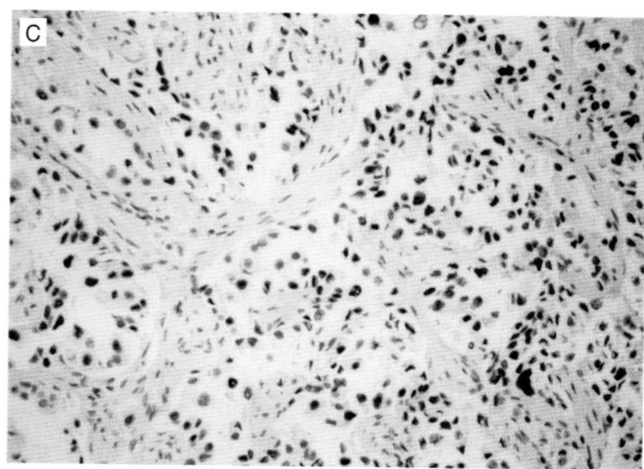

FIGURE 45-1 Immunohistochemical stains performed on the biopsy specimen from a patient with primary metastatic adenocarcinoma to a supraclavicular lymph node. Immunoperoxidase stains were positive for CK-7 (A) and TTF-1 (B) but negative for CK-20, (C), thus suggestive of metastatic non–small cell lung cancer. (Used with permission from Dr. Nelson Ordoñez, Department of Pathology, MDACC.)

have been identified in several types of lymphoma (8; 14 translocation in small non–cleaved-cell non-Hodgkin lymphoma), germ cell tumors (i12p), and Ewing sarcoma (t11; 22 or t21; 22). In the cytogenetic study by Pantou et al ([11]), lymphoma was diagnosed in four patients with CUP on the basis of the presence of immunoglobulin (Ig) H/Alk-1 rearrangement, which was identified by fluorescence in situ hybridization. In addition, one patient was diagnosed with Ewing sarcoma due to detection of characteristic rearrangement of chromosomes 11 and 22. In the era of novel and sophisticated IHC, cytogenetics is rarely ordered to help with therapy decisions. Most useful are patterns and groups of IHC used in an effective algorithm that can prove to be clinically appropriate and cost effective, although the approach to this is not uniform in the community ([51, 52]).

Molecular Profiling of Carcinomas of Unknown Primary

Tissue of origin molecular profiling using DNA microarray and reverse transcription–polymerase chain reaction (RT-PCR) is a promising technique to establish the putative primary diagnosis in patients with CUP ([53, 54]) The performance of these assays in known cancers has been validated using independent blinded sets of tumor samples, with an accuracy of approximately 90% ([55-57]). The feasibility of using formalin-fixed small biopsy or fine-needle aspiration samples makes this practical for use in the clinic setting.

Messenger RNA– or microRNA-based ToO assays have been studied in prospective and retrospective CUP trials. In CUP, these assays suggest a specific primary tumor in about 70% of patients studied ([58-64]). Because, by definition, the primary tumor site is not known in CUP, validation of site prediction in CUP remains a challenge. Results from multiple small studies suggest that ToO predictions are likely accurate. Indicators include (1) concordant results of ToO testing and the appearance of a latent primary during the course of the patient's illness (or many years later); (2) strong correlation between ToO assay results and diagnostic IHC (both suggesting a single putative primary); (3) a prospective study demonstrating that patients treated with ToO-based site-directed therapy had survival similar to those with the corresponding known primary ([65]).

In the United States, there are currently three commercially available Medicare-approved tests. They differ in the platform used, number of potential cancers identified, the size and histologic samples of the training set, and the reporting format. All three assays report on identifying a putative primary in about 75%-85% of patients with CUP. No comparative studies have been conducted, although in our personal experience when IHC is diagnostic, all three tests usually give similar results.

At present, the only *outcomes*-based study is a prospective single-arm study evaluating the role of the 92-gene assay to predict the ToO and assay-directed site-specific therapy in patients with CUP ([65]). The authors concluded that the median OS of 12.5 months (95% CI, 9.1 to 15.4 months) for patients who received assay-directed site-specific therapy compares favorably with previous studies using empiric therapy. Biliary and urothelial profiles were 33% of the predictions. Unfortunately, firm conclusions of therapeutic impact cannot be drawn from this study given the nonrandomized design; statistical biases; confounding variables, including use of subsequent lines of (empiric) therapy; and the heterogeneity of the CUP cancers.

At this time, we lack randomized controlled trials to gauge the therapeutic impact of ToO molecular profiling assays. Creative trial designs are urgently needed to study CUP subsets and impact of these assays on survival and quality of life of patients with CUP.

Two prospectively defined blinded studies of difficult-to-diagnose primary cancers (several poorly differentiated) have reported on the cost effectiveness of ToO molecular profiling over IHC. Samples were evaluated by IHC/morphology analysis or the ToO molecular profiling test ([66]). Accuracy was defined based on comparison with pathology of known primary. In one, the assay demonstrated overall accuracy of 79% for tumor classification versus 69% for IHC/morphology analysis (P = .019). Mean IHC use was 7.9 stains per case (range 2 to 15). The other study also confirmed similar findings ([67]); the assay accurately identified 89% of specimens, compared with 83% accuracy using IHC (P = .013). In the subset of poorly differentiated and undifferentiated carcinomas, assay accuracy exceeded that of IHC (91% to 71%, P = .023). These results have important implications for management of CUP cancers and warrant a study of an integrated algorithm evaluating ToO molecular profiling complementing IHC in select patients. At this time, we lack randomized controlled trials to gauge the therapeutic impact of ToO molecular profiling assays. Creative trial designs are urgently needed to study CUP subsets and impact of these assays on survival and quality of life of patients with CUP.

MANAGEMENT OF SPECIFIC CLINICOPATHOLOGIC SUBGROUPS

Carcinomas of Unknown Primary Presenting as Isolated Brain Metastases

In up to 15% of patients presenting with brain metastases, the primary site remains unknown ([68, 69]). The important factor in treating patients with brain lesions is to distinguish patients with metastatic disease from those with primary brain tumors. Once this distinction has been made, patients with single metastatic lesions should be considered for surgery, and those with multiple lesions should receive radiotherapy. In a recent small prospective study, patients with CUP who had single brain metastases treated with gross total resection and subsequent whole-brain radiotherapy (WBRT) had a median survival of 13 months. Patients with CUP who had multiple brain metastases and who underwent either WBRT alone or gross resection of symptomatic lesions followed by adjuvant WBRT had a median survival of only 6 to 8 months ([69]). Stereotactic brain radiation is often used in the CUP setting using the same principles as for brain metastases from known primary cancers.

Carcinomas of Unknown Primary Presenting as Metastatic Cervical Adenopathy

In this subgroup, patients present with high-to-midcervical or -supraclavicular adenopathy; on histopathology, these tumors are squamous cell or PDCs. For squamous cell carcinoma, the primary site is eventually identified during follow-up in approximately 20% of patients, with the tonsil being the most common site, followed by the pyriform sinus and base of the tongue.

Adenocarcinoma is much less common and is generally from either metastatic nonpapillary thyroid carcinoma or advanced malignant disease from a distant site (GI, lung, or breast carcinoma presenting as a metastatic supraclavicular node). Of all malignancies of the head and neck, only 5% to 10% are classified as unknown primary after imaging and panendoscopy. The prognosis for patients with cervical CUP overall is better than that for other CUP clinical subgroups, but even within this group, significant heterogeneity exists. Yalin et al ([70]), in a retrospective study of 107 patients with cervical CUP (62% PDC, 24% squamous carcinoma, and 14% adenocarcinoma), reported a 5-year OS rate of 35.5%. In another retrospective study by Issing et al ([71]), 5- and 10-year OS rates were 42.7% and 30.6%, respectively. The prognosis is significantly worse in the presence of any of the following: adenocarcinoma, level III/IV lymphadenopathy, multiple lymph nodes, and bulky disease.

Patients with supraclavicular adenopathy have a far worse prognosis than those with adenopathy in other lymph node–bearing areas. Carcinoma affecting supraclavicular lymph nodes on the right most commonly arises from occult primary tumors of the lungs and breast. When disease affects the lymph nodes on the left side, spread from intra-abdominal malignancies by way of the thoracic duct (Virchow node) is an additional possibility.

The management of patients with cervical CUP has become increasingly controversial, primarily because of the question of postoperative radiation therapy. The notion of adjuvant irradiation of all potential mucosal sites has been questioned because of the absence of any demonstrated survival benefit in randomized studies. To date, postoperative radiation therapy in cervical CUP significantly improves locoregional control, but this does not translate into improved OS. This being said, combined-modality therapy (surgery and radiation therapy) is better than either modality alone ([72]). Most patients with only cervical or supraclavicular involvement should have regional therapy consisting of surgery, postoperative radiation therapy, and close follow-up. Patients who undergo an excisional biopsy for diagnosis usually do not need additional surgery if no gross disease is left behind, only a single lymph node measuring less than 6 cm is involved, and no extracapsular extension is noted on pathologic review. If any of these features is present, a neck dissection is indicated. In addition, for patients with squamous cell carcinoma, unilateral tonsillectomy ipsilateral to the presenting neck mass is commonly advocated as part of the surgical treatment because occult tonsillar carcinomas are usually found in 18% to 39% of patients who undergo tonsillectomy ([71, 72]). Identification of the primary site would thereby reduce morbidity by limiting the field of radiation and would improve surveillance.

In patients with N1 or N2a disease (squamous cell), it is unclear whether postoperative radiation improves local control because studies have been contradictory. In this case, close surveillance would also be an acceptable option after surgery. All other patients should receive postoperative radiation to the bilateral neck covering all potential occult primary sites (ie, nasopharynx, oropharynx, and hypopharynx). The 3-year survival rate after radical neck dissection or radical neck irradiation ranges from 35% to 60%. Within this group, patients with N1 disease have a better prognosis; patients with N3 disease, regardless of the local treatment modality used (surgery, radiotherapy, or both), fail to achieve complete remission in 65% of cases.

Although the role of chemotherapy in patients with cervical CUP remains poorly defined, extrapolation of phase II/III data in head and neck cancer indicates a role in patients with advanced nodal disease (N3). A recent large meta-analysis of more than 10,000 patients in 63 trials with head and neck squamous cell carcinoma demonstrated a small but significant absolute survival benefit of 4% at 5 years for chemotherapy ([73]). Intensive concurrent chemoradiotherapy in unresectable squamous cell head and neck cancers with cisplatin/5-fluorouracil–based and cetuximab-based regimens has resulted in improved complete response rates, locoregional control, and preservation of organ function, albeit at the cost of significant toxicities.

Women With Carcinomas of Unknown Primary and Isolated Axillary Adenopathy

Women who present with adenocarcinoma in the axillary lymph nodes compose another subset with a more favorable prognosis. These patients are often managed as women with stage II breast cancer. Isolated axillary adenopathy is an uncommon presentation of breast cancer, accounting for only 1 to 3 of every 1,000 diagnosed breast cancers. Mammography and ultrasound should be performed, and biopsies should be performed on any identified lesions. If mammography findings are normal, additional imaging of the breast with MRI is indicated because of its greater ability to detect small primary breast tumors (70%-95% sensitivity). Magnetic resonance imaging has a very low false-negative rate. Of approximately 40 women reported in the literature with isolated axillary adenocarcinoma and negative breast MRI findings, only 4 were found to have breast cancer at surgery or during follow-up ([74]).

The present recommended management of women with CUP of the axilla includes axillary dissection, axillary radiotherapy for those at high risk of local recurrence (eg, extracapsular invasion or more than four positive lymph nodes), and appropriate systemic therapy for breast cancer, depending on age and menopausal status. If breast MRI findings are negative, neither mastectomy nor breast irradiation is recommended ([75-77]). If the breast MRI is positive or suspicious, radiation to the breast is usually recommended. The prognosis is not as favorable in men who present with axillary adenopathy only ([75]).

This management paradigm is changing as molecular profiling complements pathology as a diagnostic tool in this subset of patients. All women with axillary adenopathy do not have occult breast cancer. Profiling for ToO can help with treatment decisions especially if the IHC does not correlate with breast cancer and ER, PR, and Her-2 status is negative.

Carcinomas of Unknown Primary Presenting as Isolated Inguinal Adenopathy

A few patients with CUP present with inguinal adenopathy. Undifferentiated (anaplastic) carcinoma is identified in at least half of these cases. Some of these anaplastic "carcinomas" appear to be melanomas with no obvious primary skin lesion. The remaining patients have squamous cell carcinomas arising from the skin, genitourinary tract, anus, or pelvis. A detailed investigation for primary lesions in these areas is important because curative therapy is available for carcinomas of the anus, vulva, vagina, and cervix even with spread to regional lymph nodes. In patients with carcinomas and PDCs confined to the groin nodes, where no primary site was identified, a superficial groin dissection should be performed with or without radiation therapy. Bimodality therapy with surgery and radiation may increase the risk of significant lymph edema and requires careful planning. Chemotherapy, before definitive therapy and in the context of a clinical trial, may be offered to patients with bulky locoregional adenopathy and is not an uncommon practice in the clinic.

Carcinomas of Unknown Primary and Isolated Pleural Effusions

Most patients with isolated pleural effusions have adenocarcinomas, which may sometimes be difficult to differentiate from mesotheliomas. Newer IHC markers (eg, calretinin, CK 5/6, and WT1 [Wilms Tumor-1]) that are more sensitive in differentiating epithelioid malignant mesothelioma from pulmonary adenocarcinoma can assist in the diagnosis ([78]). Additional IHC markers, including TTF-1, CK 7/20, and breast markers, should routinely be done as first- and second-tier diagnostics to aid in treatment. If the effusion reaccumulates quickly, pleurodesis may be attempted to slow the rate of fluid reaccumulation, or as done more often currently, a pleural catheter with daily aspirations is preferred (this can be removed after chemotherapy response is noted and the flow decreases). Chemotherapy is initiated in most patients based on their IHC profile and taxane plus carboplatin versus gemcitabine plus cisplatin are commonly used doublets.

Carcinomas of Unknown Primary Presenting as Malignant Ascites

Patients with malignant ascites usually belong to one of two subsets, each with a very different natural history of disease. The first group consists of patients with mucin-producing adenocarcinoma, who may present with ascitic fluid that contains signet-ring cells. These patients often have multiple peritoneal implants, with the primary site most likely being the GI tract (ie, stomach, small bowel, appendix, colon, or pancreaticobiliary). Given the current armamentarium of drugs available for treatment of metastatic colon cancer and the improved survival, it is important to consider those combinations for patients with IHC suggestive of colon profile (CK20$^+$, CK 7$^-$, and CDX-2$^+$). The second subset is composed of women patients with primary serous papillary peritoneal carcinomatosis. This disease is often also associated with pelvic adenopathy or masses. These patients may have elevated CA 125 levels but do not have detectable ovarian cancer. Some investigators consider these patients to have true unknown primary ovarian tumors or primary serous carcinomas of the peritoneum ([79, 80]). Disease management should be the same as for women with ovarian carcinoma. A prolonged median survival of 13 months, with 25% of patients having a progression-free survival lasting more than 2 years, was reported for paclitaxel/carboplatin-based chemotherapy in patients with peritoneal carcinomatosis. In this study, a high overall response rate (ORR) and number of complete responses were reported for this subgroup of patients with CUP (68.4% and 20%, respectively).

Carcinomas of Unknown Primary Presenting as Isolated Bony Metastases

When bone metastases are detected, men should be evaluated for prostate cancer and women for breast cancer given that they may be candidates for hormonal therapy, which is relatively easier compared to cytotoxic therapies. Other cancer profiles include lung, cholangiocarcinoma, renal, and rarely melanoma. Patients with a single bony metastasis may be candidates for surgery or radiation and then monitored. Patients with disease at multiple sites and good performance status and whose tumors progress after radiation therapy should be offered a trial of chemotherapy. Many experimental agents are currently available in ongoing clinical trials. Therapy with bone-seeking radioisotopes (eg, strontium 89) may be useful in the treatment of disseminated painful bone metastases in a few patients. Bisphosphonates are routinely used as in other malignancies, such as multiple myeloma, breast cancer, and prostate cancer. Often, PET-CT is the imaging modality of choice to follow response to therapy for disseminated osseous metastatic disease.

Carcinomas of Unknown Primary Presenting as Hepatic Metastases

Patients with hepatic metastases constitute 30% to 40% of people with CUPs; they compose a clinical subgroup with a relatively poor prognosis, with reported median OS between 49 days and 7 months. The most important diagnostic considerations in this class are to distinguish primary liver and biliary tumors (hepatocellular carcinoma and cholangiocarcinoma) from cancers that have metastasized to the liver and to identify patients with neoplasms of a more indolent nature (eg, neuroendocrine tumors). A careful pathologic review with IHC of liver biopsy specimens is therefore essential. The two most common histologies in primary CUP of the liver are adenocarcinoma (55%) and poorly differentiated/undifferentiated carcinoma (30%). The recommended initial therapy for unresectable disease is systemic chemotherapy, and surgery may be considered an option for those with resectable disease.

Neuroendocrine Tumors of Unknown Primary Site

Neuroendocrine tumors compose about 4% of all CUPs and commonly present with diffuse liver or bone metastases. Histologically, neuroendocrine tumors can be well differentiated or low grade, with features that are typical of carcinoid or islet cell tumors exhibiting a more indolent behavior. Management of these tumors should be similar to established guidelines for metastatic low-grade neuroendocrine tumors from a known primary site. In patients with limited disease, surgical resection or chemoembolization may be appropriate. If not amenable to local therapy, then targeted therapy is considered with (anti–vascular endothelial growth factor [anti-VEGF] agents, including sunitinib, or mammalian target of rapamycin [mTOR] inhibitors, including everolimus.

A second group involves high-grade neuroendocrine tumors that may present as PDC by light microscopy but have strong neuroendocrine features revealed by IHC (ie, neuron-specific enolase, chromogranin A, and synaptophysin positive). These high-grade neuroendocrine tumors are treated like small cell lung carcinoma with etoposide plus platinum or irinotecan plus platinum combinations, with high reported response rates.

Carcinomas of Unknown Primary and Extragonadal Germ Cell Syndrome

As a group, patients who have undifferentiated carcinoma or PDC are younger than 50 years and present with rapidly growing midline tumors involving the lymph nodes, mediastinum, or retroperitoneum; their tumors have been found to be very responsive to chemotherapy, particularly to platinum-containing regimens. It is believed that these patients have poorly differentiated extragonadal germ cell tumors. They have response rates to chemotherapy of 35% to 50%, and those who achieve a complete response often enjoy a durable remission. In a prospective study by Hainsworth and colleagues of 220 patients with PDC or poorly differentiated adenocarcinoma (PDAC) treated between 1978 and 1989 with cisplatin-based chemotherapy regimens, approximately half of the patients had a predominant tumor location in the mediastinum, retroperitoneum, or peripheral lymph nodes. The ORR was 63%, with 26% complete responses and an actuarial 10-year disease-free survival rate of 16%.

However, this was not found to be true by Lenzi and colleagues ([4]), who retrospectively reviewed the clinical outcomes of 337 patients with PDC/PDAC. No prolonged survival was observed in this cohort of patients, and no significant survival advantage resulted from cisplatin-based chemotherapy. Moreover, elevated serum levels of alpha-fetoprotein or beta-human chorionic gonadotropin, contrary to other reports in the literature, were not found to be predictive of an improved median OS. This discrepancy may have resulted from several confounding factors.

First, older studies of extragonadal germ cell syndrome included patients with PDCs who in actuality did not have CUP but had other highly treatable malignancies ([4]). In a study by Hainsworth et al ([81]), of the 36 long-term survivors, 20% were subsequently found to have either lymphoma ([5]), testicular cancer ([1]), or leiomyosarcoma ([1]). Conversely, in the study by Lenzi, patients in whom the primary site was identified were excluded from the analysis. Most of these patients were found to have highly treatable malignancies, such as lymphoma (6%), breast cancer (8%), ovarian cancer (3%), germ cell tumors (2%), and prostate cancer (1%). Exclusion of these patients would significantly reduce response and median survival rates.

Second, even among patients with PDC/PDAC of unknown primary, significant heterogeneity exists. In the study by Lenzi, CART analysis of 337 patients revealed different groups with widely discrepant survival times. The group with the longest median OS (40 months) included patients with PDC, lymph node involvement, and only one or two metastatic sites. By contrast, patients with non–lymph node metastases had a very poor prognosis, with a median OS of only 7 months ([4]).

Carcinomas of Unknown Primary and Single Sites Discovered Incidentally on Resection

Carcinomas of unknown primary are notorious for unusual, isolated presentations. Such lesions may appear on the skin, in single isolated lymph nodes removed during surgery for benign unrelated conditions, and at other, even more unusual sites. Patients should be examined for primary tumors and other sites of metastasis, as described previously. If no primary tumor and no additional sites of metastasis are found, complete removal of the lesion must be ensured; this often requires additional excision with wider margins (if skin or subcutaneous). The patient may then be monitored without therapy and in selected cases are candidates for radiation. Many such patients may enjoy prolonged survival. Patients with isolated skin lesions may have an undifferentiated primary integumentary tumor with a potential for cure after adequate local surgical treatment.

CHEMOTHERAPEUTIC STRATEGIES FOR CARCINOMAS OF UNKNOWN PRIMARY

Combination regimens using newer chemotherapeutic agents have demonstrated greater benefit than did older single-agent therapies for CUP cancers. Several difficulties arise when survival and response rates reported in different chemotherapy trials are compared. For example, histologic criteria for patient selection often varied from study to study. Moreover, in older studies, IHC methods were not used to evaluate pathologic specimens. Despite these difficulties, no study has firmly established any chemotherapy regimen as the "gold standard" in CUP. The median survival in most studies, regardless of regimen, has ranged between 5 and 13 months, with response rates of less than 30% and without a significant improvement in survival (Table 45-4).

Nevertheless, patients with certain clinical subtypes (eg, peritoneal carcinomatosis and lymph node–predominant disease) do benefit from chemotherapy. Historically, cisplatin-based combination chemotherapy regimens were frequently used to treat patients with CUP. Response rates in the literature range from 12% to 26% and median survival from 5 to 7 months. Combining paclitaxel with carboplatin has modestly improved both survival and response rates. In patients with widespread metastases and poor performance status, however, systemic chemotherapy is unlikely to be beneficial, and only supportive therapy is usually indicated.

In a phase II study by Hainsworth and colleagues, patients with CUP (n = 55) received paclitaxel (200 mg/m^2 day 1), carboplatin (AUC = 6 day 1), and oral etoposide (50 mg alternating with 100 mg days 1-10) every 21 days ([82]). Most were previously untreated, with only four having received prior chemotherapy. Most patients had moderately to well-differentiated adenocarcinoma (55%) or PDC/PDAC (38%), with squamous (2%) and neuroendocrine (5%) histologies less prevalent. The dominant sites of disease were lymph nodes (25%), liver (16%), and lungs (16%). Approximately 24% of patients in the study had multiple sites of disease, with 42% of patients having more than two metastatic sites. Response rates were equivalent in all histologic subgroups, with a reported ORR of 47% and a median OS of 13.4 months. This regimen was well tolerated, with myelosuppression the most common grade 3/4 toxicity. No treatment-related deaths were reported.

Briasoulis and colleagues ([83]) found equivalent response rates and median OS in CUP with carboplatin (AUC = 6) and paclitaxel (200 mg/m^2) without oral etoposide. In this phase II trial, patients (n = 77) were given a maximum of eight cycles of chemotherapy. In addition, granulocyte colony-stimulating factor was administered on days 5 to 12. The proportions of differing histologic subtypes were comparable to those in the Hainsworth study: adenocarcinoma (61%), undifferentiated (35%), and squamous (4%). Three distinct clinical subsets were present in this study: peritoneal carcinomatosis (25%, mostly women); visceral or bony metastases (43%); and predominant nodal or pleural disease (30%). The reported ORR, median response duration, and median OS were 38.7%, 6 months, and 13 months, respectively. Although response rates were equivalent for adenocarcinoma and undifferentiated carcinoma, significant differences were seen among the three clinical subsets: liver/bone or disseminated metastases (ORR, 15.1%; median OS, 10 months); nodal/pleural disease (ORR, 47.8%; median OS, 13 months); and peritoneal (ORR, 68.4% [75% for women]; median OS, 15 months), $P = .01$. Three patients with nodal-predominant disease had durable responses lasting longer than 2 years. Grade 3/4 neutropenia was only 4%, with two reported septic deaths.

The results of docetaxel in combination with carboplatin in one small phase II study appear to be inferior to those of paclitaxel/carboplatin in the trials mentioned. The ORR was 22%, the median OS was 8 months, and the 1-year OS rate was 29%. Differences in sites of disease and histology among these three studies may account for the discrepancy. Severe grade 3/4 myelosuppression was more frequent with docetaxel (50%) than with paclitaxel, with two reported septic deaths ([84]).

Patients with undifferentiated or PDCs not fitting into the extragonadal germ cell or neuroendocrine clinical subgroups have traditionally been given a trial of a cisplatin-based regimen. Patients with squamous cell carcinomas who require chemotherapy are also often treated effectively using a cisplatin-based regimen.

The role of salvage chemotherapy in CUP is poorly defined. Gemcitabine has been published as second-line therapy in patients with previously treated CUP. In a phase II study by Hainsworth and colleagues ([85]), gemcitabine was administered weekly at 1,000 mg/m^2 (on days 1, 8, and 15 of a 28-day cycle). All patients (n = 39) received two cycles and were then evaluated for response. Chemotherapy was continued for a maximum of six cycles for either an objective response or stable disease. Approximately 90% of patients had failed a prior regimen containing platinum and a taxane. Most patients had either adenocarcinoma (59%) or PDC/PDAC (31%). Median time to progression was 5 months. Gemcitabine was well tolerated, with 92% of patients receiving two or more cycles. The most common grades 3 to 4 toxicities were fatigue/weakness and mucositis/esophagitis.

Hainsworth et al ([86]) reported on a combination-targeted therapy trial of bevacizumab and erlotinib in 51 patients; 25% were chemotherapy naïve with advanced bone or liver metastases, and 75% had been

Table 45-4 Selected Phase II Studies in Carcinoma of Unknown Primary

Overall Survival									
Author	n	Chemotherapy Regimen	Two or More Metastatic Sites (%)	ORR (%)	Median TTP (Months)	Median (Months)	1 Year (%)	2 Years (%)
Assersohn et al.	45	5-FU versus	44	11.6	4.1	6.6	28	NR
	43	5-FU+ Mi		20	3.6	4.7	21	NR
Culine et al.	82	AC →EP, alt q14d + GCSF	68	39	NR	10		
McDonald et al.	31	Mi/P/CI 5-FU	52	27	3.4	7.7	28	
Greco et al.	120	Gem/Cb/Pac	65	25	NR	9	42	23
Saghatchian et al.	33	PDC/PDAC: EP × 2 → BI	57	40	8.1	9.4	NR	28
	18	Adeno: P/ CI-5-FU/IFNα	44	44	8.6	16.1	NR	39
Hainsworth et al.	39	Gem	NR	33	5	NR		
Dowell et al.	17	Pac + 5-FU/ leucovorin versus	59	19	NR	8.4		
	17	CbE	65	19		6.5		
Briasoulis et al.	77	Cb + Pac	22% with 3 or more	38.7	6	13		
Greco et al.	23	DP versus	73	29	NR	8	42	
	40	DCb	68	22		8	29	
Culine et al.	20	HDCT + AutoSCT versus	80	42	NR	11		
	40	AC alt with EP	75	39		8		
Falkson et al.	43	Mi/Epi/P versus	53	50	4.5[a]	9.4[a]		
	41	Mi	44	17	2.0	5.4		
Warner et al.	33	Cb + E (PO)		91	23	NR	5.6	NR
Hainsworth et al.	55	Pac/Cb/E (PO)	67	47	NR	13.4	58	NR
Hainsworth et al.	220	BEvP +/− Doxo; after 1985: BEP	74	63	NR			10-year survival: 16%
Van der Gaast et al.	34	BEP × 4 → EP × 2	53	53	NR	NR		
Eagen et al.	28	MiA → CAM versus	NR	14	NR	5.5	19	8
	27	MiAP → CAM		26		4.6	12	0

A, doxorubicin; Adeno, adenocarcinoma; alt, alternating; AutoSCT, autologous stem cell transplant; B, bleomycin; C, cyclophosphamide; Cb, carboplatin; CI, continuous infusion; D, docetaxel; Doxo, doxorubicin; E, etoposide; Epi, epirubicin; 5-FU, 5-flurouracil; Gem, gemcitabine; GCSF, granulocyte colony-stimulating factor; HDCT, high-dose chemotherapy; I, ifosfamide; IFN, interferon; M, methotrexate; Mi, mitomycin; Neuro, neuroendocrine; NR, not reported; ORR, overall response rate; P, cisplatin; Pac, paclitaxel; PDC/PDAC, poorly differentiated carcinoma/adenocarcinoma; TTP, time to progression; Undif, undifferentiated malignancy; v, vinblastine.
[a]Statistically significant difference $P = .05$.

treated with one or two chemotherapy regimens. Responses were noted in 4 patients (8%), and 30 patients (59%) experienced stable disease or a minor response. The median OS duration was 8.9 months, with 42% of patients alive at 1 year.

These combination therapy trials have been a significant contribution in the post 5-flurouracil and cisplatin era of second-generation chemotherapeutic agents. They have certainly served their function in allowing the access to several broad-spectrum chemotherapies in patients with CUP and helped us understand the responses to these therapies. Although evaluation of empiric regimens was the preferred approach in the past, with the emergence of modern molecular diagnostic trials that help define CUP subtypes, our focus has shifted from empiric combinations to more tailored regimens, especially as directed by IHC and where helpful ToO or mutational profiles. Further, as therapies for known cancers improve and become more selective based on evolving predictive markers, the newer therapeutic approaches should be evaluated in the appropriate CUP subtypes as well.

SUMMARY AND FUTURE TRENDS

All patients with CUP should undergo a directed diagnostic evaluation for the primary tumor and a detailed pathologic evaluation of the metastatic specimen. A subset of patients defined by clinicopathologic criteria and considered to have favorable prognosis benefit significantly from selective or aggressive treatments. For most patients who present with advanced disseminated CUP, the prognosis remains poor, and no unique empiric combination therapy of established efficacy is available. We have moved away from the paradigm of one treatment fits all to a more focused approach that integrates clinical presentation, pathologic evaluation, and the evolving diagnostic tools. Our current focus is to study the impact of molecular profiling and next-generation sequencing-based studies that help individualize CUP treatments. More broadly, there is an extensive push toward personalizing cancer care through the use of genomic tools to identify driver mutations in an individual tumor. For this approach to be successful, it will require both additional molecular insights and novel drugs that are effective against specific mutations.

REFERENCES

1. van de Wouw AJ, Janssen-Heijnen ML, Coebergh JW, et al. Epidemiology of unknown primary tumours; incidence and population-based survival of 1,285 patients in Southeast Netherlands, 1984-1992. *Eur J Cancer*. 2002;38(3):409-413.
2. Varadhachary GR, Raber MN. Cancer of unknown primary site. *N Engl J Med*. 2014;371:757-765.
3. Greco FA, Burris HA III, Erland JB, et al. Carcinoma of unknown primary site. *Cancer*. 2000;89(12):2655-2660.
4. Hess KR, Abbruzzese MC, Lenzi R, et al. Classification and regression tree analysis of 1000 consecutive patients with unknown primary carcinoma. *Clin Cancer Res*. 1999;5(11):3403-3410.
5. Briasoulis E, Tolis C, Bergh J, Pavlidis N. ESMO minimum clinical recommendations for diagnosis, treatment and follow-up of cancers of unknown primary site (CUP). *Ann Oncol*. 2005;16(Suppl 1):i75-i76.
6. Siegel R, Naishadham D, Jemal A. Cancer statistics, 2013. CA Cancer J Clin. 2013;63;1:11-30.
7. Le Chevalier T, Cvitkovic E, Caille P, et al. Early metastatic cancer of unknown primary origin at presentation. A clinical study of 302 consecutive autopsied patients. *Arch Intern Med*. 1988;148(9):2035-2039.
8. Abbruzzese JL, Abbruzzese MC, Lenzi R, et al. Analysis of a diagnostic strategy for patients with suspected tumors of unknown origin. *J Clin Oncol*. 1995;13(8):2094-2103.
9. van de Wouw AJ, Jansen RL, Speel EJ, et al. The unknown biology of the unknown primary tumour: a literature review. *Ann Oncol*. 2003;14(2):191-196.
10. Naresh KN. Do metastatic tumours from an unknown primary reflect angiogenic incompetence of the tumour at the primary site? A hypothesis. *Med Hypoth*. 2002;59(3):357-360.
11. Pantou D, Tsarouha H, Papadopoulou A, et al. Cytogenetic profile of unknown primary tumors: Clues for their pathogenesis and clinical management. *Neoplasia*. 2003;5(1):23-31.
12. Atkin NB. Chromosome 1 aberrations in cancer. *Cancer Genet Cytogenet*. 1986;21(4):279-285.
13. Motzer RJ, Rodriguez E, Reuter VE, et al. Molecular and cytogenetic studies in the diagnosis of patients with poorly differentiated carcinomas of unknown primary site. *J Clin Oncol*. 1995;13(1):274-282.
14. Motzer RJ, Rodriguez E, Reuter VE, et al. Genetic analysis as an aid in diagnosis for patients with midline carcinomas of uncertain histologies. *J Natl Cancer Inst*. 1991;83(5):341-346.
15. Bar-Eli M, Abbruzzese JL, Lee-Jackson D, et al. *p53* gene mutation spectrum in human unknown primary tumors. *Anti-cancer Res*. 1993;13(5A):1619-1623.
16. Pavlidis N, Briassoulis E, Bai M, et al. The expression of *cmyc, ras,* and c-erbB-2 in patients with carcinoma of unknown primary [Abstr 1374]. *Proc Am Soc Clin Oncol*. 1994;13.
17. Soong R, Robbins PD, Dix BR, et al. Concordance between p53 protein overexpression and gene mutation in a large series of common human carcinomas. *Hum Pathol*. 1996;27(10):1050-1055.
18. Hainsworth JD, Lennington WJ, Greco FA. Overexpression of Her-2 in patients with poorly differentiated carcinoma or poorly differentiated adenocarcinoma of unknown primary site. *J Clin Oncol*. 2000;18(3):632-635.
19. Ross JS, Wang K, Gay L, et al. Comprehensive genomic 8 profiling of carcinoma of unknown primary site reveals 9 new routes to targeted therapies. *JAMA Oncol*. Epub February 12, 2015;1(1):40-49.
20. Mayordomo JI, Guerra JM, Guijarro C, et al. Neoplasms of unknown primary site: A clinicopathological study of autopsied patients. *Tumori*. 1993;79(5):321-324.
21. Schapira DV, Jaret AR. Cost of diagnosis and survival of patients with unknown primary cancer [Abstr 481]. *Proc Am Soc Clin Oncol*. 1994;13.
22. Nystrom SJ, Hornberger JC, Varadhachary GR, et al. Clinical utility of gene-expression profiling for tumor-site origin in patients with metastatic or poorly differentiated cancer: impact on diagnosis, treatment, and survival. 2012. *Oncotarget*. 3(6):620-628.
23. Milovic M, Popov I, Jelic S. Tumor markers in metastatic disease from cancer of unknown primary origin. *Med Sci Monit*. 2002;8(2):MT25-MT30.
24. Bates SE. Clinical applications of serum tumor markers. *Ann Intern Med*. 1991;115(8):623-638.
25. Abbruzzese JL, Raber MN, Frost P. The role of CA-125 in

patients with unknown primary tumors [Abstr 39]. *Proc Am Soc Clin Oncol.* 1991;10.

26. Varadhachary GR. Carcinoma of unknown primary: focused evaluation. *J Natl Compr Canc Netw.* 2011;9:1406-1412.
27. National Comprehensive Cancer Network. *Occult Primary (Cancer of Unknown Primary) 2013*, version 1. http://www.nccn.org/professionals/physician_g/s/f_guidelines.asp#occult; December 2015.
28. Bedrosian I, Mick R, Orel SG, et al. Changes in the surgical management of patients with breast carcinoma based on pre-operative magnetic resonance imaging. *Cancer.* 2003;98(3):468-473.
29. Schelfout K, Kersschot E, Van Goethem M, et al. Breast MR imaging in a patient with unilateral axillary lymphadenopathy and unknown primary malignancy. *Eur Radiol.* 2003;13(9):2128-2132.
30. Henry-Tillman RS, Harms SE, Westbrook KC, et al. Role of breast magnetic resonance imaging in determining breast as a source of unknown metastatic lymphadenopathy. *Am J Surg.* 1999;178(6):496-500.
31. Schorn C, Fischer U, Luftner-Nagel S, et al. MRI of the breast in patients with metastatic disease of unknown primary. *Eur Radiol.* 1999;9(3):470-473.
32. Olson JA Jr, Morris EA, Van Zee KJ, Linehan DC, Borgen PI. Magnetic resonance imaging facilitates breast conservation for occult breast cancer. *Ann Surg Oncol.* 2000;7:411–415.
33. Lu H, Xu YL, Zhang SP, et al. Breast magnetic resonance imaging in patients with occult breast carcinoma: evaluation on feasibility and correlation with histopathological findings. *Chin Med J (Engl).* 2011;124;12:1790-1795.
34. Koch WM, Bhatti N, Williams MF, et al. Oncologic rationale for bilateral tonsillectomy in head and neck squamous cell carcinoma of unknown primary source. *Otolaryngol Head Neck Surg.* 2001;124:331-333.
35. Lassen U, Daugaard G, Eigtved A, et al. 18F-FDG whole body positron emission tomography (PET) in patients with unknown primary tumours (UPT). *Eur J Cancer.* 1999;35(7):1076-1082.
36. Regelink G, Brouwer J, de Bree R, et al. Detection of unknown primary tumours and distant metastases in patients with cervical metastases: value of FDG-PET versus conventional modalities. *Eur J Nucl Med Mol Imaging.* 2002;29:1024-1030.
37. Rusthoven KE, Koshy M, Paulino AC. The role of fluorodeoxyglucose positron emission tomography in cervical lymph node metastases from an unknown primary tumor. *Cancer.* 2004;101:2641-2649.
38. Waltonen JD, Ozer E, Hall NC, et al. Metastatic carcinoma of the neck of unknown primary origin. *Arch Otolaryngol Head Neck Surg.* 2009;135:1024-1029.
39. Rudmik L, Lau HY, Matthews TW, et al. Clinical utility of PET/CT in the evaluation of head and neck squamous cell carcinoma with an unknown primary: a prospective clinical trial. *Head Neck.* 2011;33;7:935-940.
40. Johansen J, Eigtved A, Buchwald C, et al. Implication of 18F-fluoro-2-deoxy-D-glucose positron emission tomography on management of carcinoma of unknown primary in the head and neck: a Danish cohort study. *Laryngoscope.* 2002;112(11):2009-2014.
41. Delgado-Bolton RC, Fernandez-Perez C, Gonzalez-Mate A, et al. Meta-analysis of the performance of 18F-FDG PET in primary tumor detection in unknown primary tumors. *J Nucl Med.* 2003;44(8):1301-1314.
42. Alberini JL, Belhocine T, Hustinx R, et al. Whole-body positron emission tomography using fluorodeoxyglucose in patients with metastases of unknown primary tumours (CUP syndrome). *Nucl Med Commun.* 2003;24(10):1081-1086.
43. Joshi U, van der Hoeven JJ, Comans EF, Herder GJ, Teule GJ, Hoekstra OS. In search of an unknown primary tumour presenting with extracervical metastases: the diagnostic performance of FDG-PET. *Br J Radiol.* 2004;77:1000-1006.
44. Moller AK, Loft A, Berthelsen AK, et al. 18F-FDG PET/CT as a diagnostic tool in patients with extracervical carcinoma of unknown primary site: a literature review. *Oncologist.* 2011;16;4:445-451.
45. Wu M, Wang B, Gil J, et al. p63 and TTF-1 immunostaining. A useful marker panel for distinguishing small cell carcinoma of lung from poorly differentiated squamous cell carcinoma of lung. *Am J Clin Pathol.* 2003;119(5):696-702.
46. Ng WK, Chow JC, Ng PK. Thyroid transcription factor-1 is highly sensitive and specific in differentiating metastatic pulmonary from extrapulmonary adenocarcinoma in effusion fluid cytology specimens. *Cancer.* 2002;96(1):43-48.
47. Chhieng DC, Cangiarella JF, Zakowski MF, et al. Use of thyroid transcription factor 1, PE-10, and cytokeratins 7 and 20 in discriminating between primary lung carcinomas and metastatic lesions in fine-needle aspiration biopsy specimens. *Cancer.* 2001;93(5):330-336.
48. Reis-Filho JS, Carrilho C, Valenti C, et al. Is TTF1 a good immunohistochemical marker to distinguish primary from metastatic lung adenocarcinomas? *Pathol Res Pract.* 2000;196(12):835-840.
49. DeYoung BR, Wick MR, Immunohistologic evaluation of metastatic carcinomas of unknown origin: an algorithmic approach. *Semin Diagn Pathol.* 2000;17:184-193.
50. Dennis JL, Vass JK, Wit EC, et al. Identification from public data of molecular markers of adenocarcinoma characteristic of the site of origin. *Cancer Res.* 2002;62(21):5999-6005.
51. Dennis JL, Hvidsten TR, Wit EC, et al. Markers of adenocarcinoma characteristic of the site of origin: development of a diagnostic algorithm. *Clin Cancer Res.* 2005;11:3766-3772.
52. Ramaswamy S, Tamayo P, Rifkin R, et al. Multiclass cancer diagnosis using tumor gene expression signatures. *Proc Natl Acad Sci U S A.* 2001;98:15149-15154.
53. Su AI, Welsh JB, Sapinoso LM, et al. Molecular classification of human carcinomas by use of gene expression signatures. *Cancer Res.* 2001;61:7388-7393.
54. Tothill RW, Kowalczyk A, Rischin D, et al. An expression-based site of origin diagnostic method designed for clinical application to cancer of unknown origin. *Cancer Res.* 2005;65:4031-4040.
55. Kerr SE, Schnabel CA, Sullivan PS, et al. Multisite validation study to determine performance characteristics of a 92-gene molecular cancer classifier. *Clin Cancer Res.* 2012;18:3952-3960.
56. Pillai R, Deeter R, Rigl CT, et al. Validation and reproducibility of a microarray-based gene expression test for tumor identification in formalin-fixed, paraffin-embedded specimens. *J Mol Diagn.* 2011;13:48-56.
57. Meiri E, Mueller WC, Rosenwald S, et al. A second-generation microRNA-based assay for diagnosing tumor tissue origin. *Oncologist.* 2012;17:801-812.
58. Varadhachary GR, Spector Y, Abbruzzese JL, et al. Prospective gene signature study using microRNA to identify the tissue of origin in patients with carcinoma of unknown primary. *Clin Cancer Res.* 2011;17:4063-4070.
59. Oien KA, Dennis JL. Diagnostic work-up of carcinoma of unknown primary: from immunohistochemistry to molecular profiling. *Ann Oncol.* 2012;23:271-277.
60. Pentheroudakis G, Golfinopoulos V, Pavlidis N. Switching benchmarks in cancer of unknown primary: from autopsy to microarray. *Eur J Cancer.* 2007;43:2026-2036.
61. Bloom G, Yang IV, Boulware D, Kwong KY, et al. Multi-platform, multi-site, microarray-based human tumor classification. *Am J Pathol.* 2004;164:9-16.
62. Ferracin M, Pedriali M, Veronese A, et al. MicroRNA profiling for the identification of cancers with unknown primary tissue-of-origin. *J Pathol.* 2011;225:43-53.
63. Horlings HM, van Laar RK, Kerst JM, et al. Gene expression profiling to identify the histogenetic origin of metastatic adenocarcinomas of unknown primary. *J Clin Oncol.* 2008;26:4435-4441.

64. Greco FA, Spigel DR, Yardley DA, Erlander MG, Ma XJ, Hainsworth JD. Molecular profiling in unknown primary cancer: accuracy of tissue of origin prediction. *Oncologist.* 2010;15:500-506.
65. Hainsworth JD, Rubin MS, Spigel DR, et al. Molecular gene expression profiling to predict the tissue of origin and direct site-specific therapy in patients with carcinoma of unknown primary site: a prospective trial of the Sarah Cannon Research Institute. *J Clin Oncol.* 2013;31:217-223.
66. Handorf CR, Kulkarni A, Grenert JP, et al. A multicenter study directly comparing the diagnostic accuracy of gene expression profiling and immunohistochemistry for primary site identification in metastatic tumors. *Am J Surg Pathol.* 2013;37(7):1067-1075.
67. Weiss L, Chu P, Schroeder BE, et al. Immunohistochemistry (IHC) vs a 92-gene cancer classifier in the diagnosis of primary site in metastatic tumors: a blinded comparator study. *J Mol Diagn.* 2013;15(2):263-269.
68. Soffietti R, Ruda R, Mutani R. Management of brain metastases. *J Neurol.* 2002;249(10):1357-1369.
69. Ruda R, Borgognone M, Benech F, et al. Brain metastases from unknown primary tumour: a prospective study. *J Neurol.* 2001;248(5):394-398.
70. Yalin Y, Pingzhang T, Smith GI, et al. Management and outcome of cervical lymph node metastases of unknown primary sites: a retrospective study. *Br J Oral Maxillofac Surg.* 2002;40(6):484-487.
71. Issing WJ, Taleban B, Tauber S. Diagnosis and management of carcinoma of unknown primary in the head and neck. *Eur Arch Otorhinolaryngol.* 2003;260:436-443.
72. Zuur CL, van Velthuysen ML, Schornagel JH, et al. Diagnosis and treatment of isolated neck metastases of adenocarcinomas. *Eur J Surg Oncol.* 2002;28(2):147-152.
73. Pignon JP, Bourhis J, Domenge C, et al. Chemotherapy added to locoregional treatment for head and neck squamous-cell carcinoma: three meta-analyses of updated individual data. MACH-NC Collaborative Group. Meta-analysis of chemotherapy on head and neck cancer. *Lancet.* 2000;355(9208):949-955.
74. Olson JA Jr., Morris EA, Van Zee KJ, et al. Magnetic resonance imaging facilitates breast conservation for occult breast cancer. *Ann Surg Oncol.* 2000;7(6):411-415.
75. Foroudi F, Tiver KW. Occult breast carcinoma presenting as axillary metastases. *Int J Radiat Oncol Biol Phys.* 2000;47(1):143-147.
76. Bugat R, Bataillard A, Lesimple T, et al. Standards, options and recommendations for the management of patient with carcinoma of unknown primary site. *Bull Cancer.* 2002;89(10):869-875.
77. Jackson B, Scott-Conner C, Moulder J. Axillary metastasis from occult breast carcinoma: diagnosis and management. *Am Surg.* 1995;61(5):431-434.
78. Ordonez NG. The immunohistochemical diagnosis of mesothelioma: a comparative study of epithelioid mesothelioma and lung adenocarcinoma. *Am J Surg Pathol.* 2003;27(8):1031-1051.
79. Gershenson DM, Silva EG. Serous ovarian tumors of low malignant potential with peritoneal implants. *Cancer.* 1990;65(3):578-585.
80. Strnad CM, Grosh WW, Baxter J, et al. Peritoneal carcinomatosis of unknown primary site in women. A distinctive subset of adenocarcinoma. *Ann Intern Med.* 1989;111(3):213-217.
81. Hainsworth JD, Johnson DH, Greco FA. Cisplatin-based combination chemotherapy in the treatment of poorly differentiated carcinoma and poorly differentiated adenocarcinoma of unknown primary site: results of a 12-year experience. *J Clin Oncol.* 1992;10(6):912-922.
82. Hainsworth JD, Erland JB, Kalman LA, et al. Carcinoma of unknown primary site: treatment with 1-hour paclitaxel, carboplatin, and extended-schedule etoposide. *J Clin Oncol.* 1997;15(6):2385-2393.
83. Briasoulis E, Kalofonos H, Bafaloukos D, et al. Carboplatin plus paclitaxel in unknown primary carcinoma: a phase II Hellenic Cooperative Oncology Group Study. *J Clin Oncol.* 2000;18(17):3101-3107.
84. Greco FA, Erland JB, Morrissey LH, et al. Carcinoma of unknown primary site: phase II trials with docetaxel plus cisplatin or carboplatin. *Ann Oncol.* 2000;11(2):211-215.
85. Hainsworth JD, Burris HA III, Calvert SW, et al. Gemcitabine in the second-line therapy of patients with carcinoma of unknown primary site: a phase II trial of the Minnie Pearl Cancer Research Network. *Cancer Invest.* 2001;19(4):335-339.
86. Hainsworth JD, Spigel DR, Farleg C et al. Phase II trial of bevacizumab and erlotimis in Carcinomas of unknown primary site: The Minnie Pearl Cancer Research Network. *J Clin Oncol.* 2007; 25(13):1747-1752.

46 Pediatric Cancers

第四十六章　儿童肿瘤

Ryuma Tanaka
Patrick A. Zweidler-McKay

中文导读

本章首先指出了儿童肿瘤的治疗挑战。接下来本章列举了一些儿童中常见的肿瘤类型，包括急性淋巴细胞白血病、霍奇金淋巴瘤、骨肉瘤、增生性小圆细胞肿瘤、髓母细胞瘤、低级别胶质瘤、扩散型内因性脑桥神经胶质瘤、高级别胶质瘤，并分别阐述了相应的治疗策略和进展。在急性淋巴细胞白血病部分，介绍了MRC R3为复发后标准治疗方案，靶向治疗也是一种有效的治疗手段，CD19 CAR-T在复发的B细胞急性淋巴细胞白血病也表现出巨大潜力。在霍奇金淋巴瘤部分，介绍了复发性/难治性霍奇金淋巴瘤患者的标准治疗是挽救性化疗后序贯自体干细胞移植，CD30单抗本妥昔单抗具备巨大前景。在骨肉瘤部分描述了放射性核素及免疫调节治疗等新型治疗手段。在增生性小圆细胞肿瘤部分，简述了ganitumab、帕唑帕尼等可能有效的药物，以及广泛外科切除序贯腹腔内热化疗对腹腔播散的控制作用。在髓母细胞瘤部分，介绍了基因层面的4种分型，并讲述了标危、高危、复发肿瘤的治疗方式，以及MD安德森癌症中心正在探索的一系列新的治疗手段。在低级别胶质瘤部分，介绍了化疗方案，并重点讲解了靶向BRAF突变的治疗方式。在扩散型内因性脑桥神经胶质瘤部分，介绍了目前的标准治疗依然是放疗，靶向治疗也有相关临床研究。在高级别胶质瘤部分，手术切除及术后放疗并辅以同步口服替莫唑胺是目前标准治疗方式，对于复发肿瘤，替莫唑胺、贝伐单抗、伊立替康都是可选药物，靶向治疗也在研究中。

INTRODUCTION

Fortunately, pediatric cancers are rare, with only 1 in 300 children being diagnosed before 18 years of age. And, with overall survival (OS) approaching 80%, there is hope for most of these children and for their families. However, just as in adults, if their cancer is metastatic at diagnosis, if the cancer does not respond to standard therapies, or if they suffer a relapse, the prognosis is universally grim. Despite intensified therapies, the survival for most children with relapsed cancer has not improved in decades. In large part, this is due to the toxicities of such regimens as we have likely reached the tolerable limit with most chemotherapeutic agents. Thus, as is the case for adults with cancer, there has been a focus on understanding the underlying biology of the disease to find targetable lesions and to develop novel agents and treatment regimens to improve survival in children with relapse. However, there are multiple challenges we face. First, the spectrum of pediatric cancers is distinctly different from adults (Fig. 46-1), with acute lymphoblastic leukemia (ALL), medulloblastoma and gliomas, neuroblastoma, Hodgkin and non-Hodgkin lymphomas, and sarcomas the most common cancers in children as opposed to the most common carcinomas of the prostate, breast, lung, colon, and so on in adults. Second, the relative rarity of these cancers results in less preclinical research to find and develop potential therapeutic targets and limited patient numbers to enroll and test novel therapeutic strategies.

One of our approaches has been to study the pediatric cancers in parallel with similar adult tumors and to enroll patients on early adult trials to give children access to promising agents and to provide some data on safety and efficacy to support the development of pediatric-specific trials. In this chapter, we present a few examples of tumor types seen commonly in children and describe some of the therapeutic advances and promising strategies for treating children with relapsed cancers.

SALVAGE STRATEGIES

Acute Lymphoblastic Leukemia

Acute lymphoblastic leukemia is the most common cancer diagnosis in children, accounting for 25% of cancer diagnoses in children 15 years old or less. An estimated 3,000 new cases of childhood ALL are diagnosed yearly in the United States. After a peak incidence of 90 cases per million per year at age 2 to

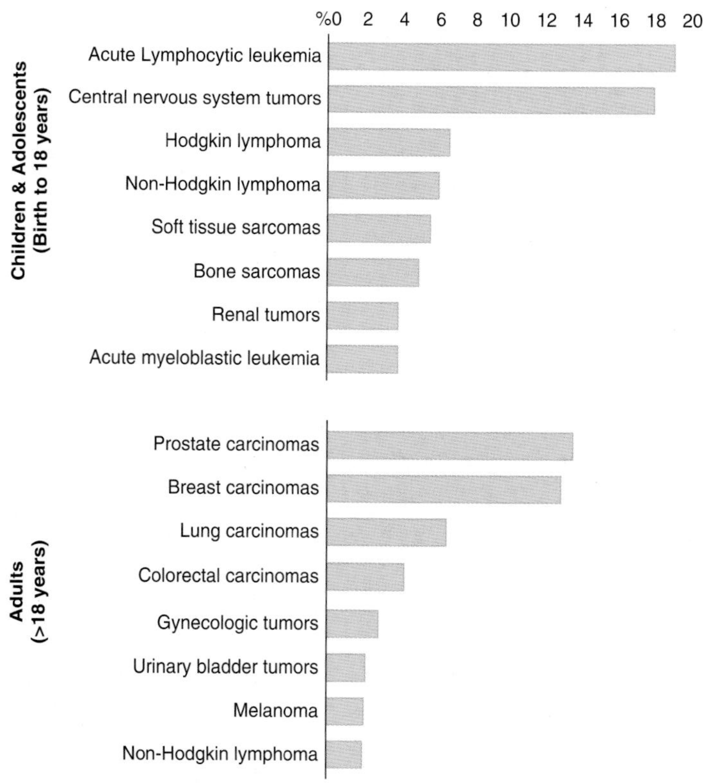

FIGURE 46-1 Spectrum of Pediatric and Adult Cancers.

3 years, ALL incidence rates decrease steadily into adolescence. Initial complete remission (CR) rates are 95%, and survival in childhood ALL is approaching 90% through the application of reliable prognostic factors that permit use of risk-oriented treatment protocols. However, relapse occurs in approximately 20%, with higher rates of relapse in adolescents and young adults as well as children less than 1 year of age (ie, "infants"). Despite excellent outcomes overall, relapsed patients with ALL outnumber nearly all other childhood malignancies. With traditional intensive combination chemotherapy and allogeneic hematopoietic stem cell transplantation, 30% to 40% of all children with relapsed ALL can be cured. The factors that effect salvage rate are timing of relapse (18-36 months from diagnosis), site of relapse (bone marrow, central nervous system [CNS]/testicular, combined), and immunophenotype (T cell vs B cell). Unfortunately, most children still die from relapsed ALL despite aggressive chemoradiotherapy approaches, including transplantation, and novel salvage regimens are needed ([1]).

For children with first relapse of childhood ALL, the mitoxantrone-based Medical Research Council (MRC) ALL R3 relapsed protocol has relatively better outcomes than other common regimens and is currently our standard reinduction regimen ([2]). Promising CR2 rates have also been seen with the addition of the proteasome inhibitor bortezomib to the MRC ALL R3 backbone, with 80% (16/20) CR/CRi in B-ALL patients ([3]), as well as the addition of bortezomib to the more traditional four-drug reinduction regimen in COG AALL07P1, with 64% (63/99) of B-ALL patients achieving CR2. Surprisingly, AALL07P1 showed similar CR2 rates of 68% (15/22) in T-ALL patients ([4]). The current first relapse regimen under study in the COG is testing the substitution of the CD19-targeting bispecific engaging antibody blinatumomab to the MRC ALL R3 relapsed protocol.

With attainment of CR2 in 70% to 85% (<1% minimal residual disease by flow cytometry), we offer transplant to most children with relapsed ALL, with very late relapses and isolated CNS relapses as typical exceptions. We offer a variety of transplant trials, including cord blood and haploidentical, as well as addition of anti-CD19 chimeric antigen receptor (CAR) T cells, natural killer (NK) cells, and so on. Failure to respond adequately to first-relapse regimens leads to a variety of second-line regimens. We commonly offer clofarabine/cyclophosphamide/etoposide (CR2 rates of 44% [[5]]), mitoxantrone/cytarabine (CR2 rate of 57% [[6]]) or one of several targeted agents with the institutional adult ALL regimen hyper-CVAD ([7]), or promising single agents when available. With recently published complete responses in children ([8]), we are testing the combination of anti-CD22 immunotoxin inotuzumab with hyper-CVAD (without anthracycline), with some dramatic responses in children. In addition, the combination of the mTOR inhibitor everolimus and Hyper-CVAD is being tested. For T-cell ALL specifically, we have used nelarabine in combination with hyper-CVAD ([9]), a trial testing a 5-day continuous infusion of nelarabine (NCT01094860), and a single agent Notch-inhibiting gamma secretase inhibitor BMS-906024 phase I trial (NCT01363817), based on multiple responses in adults ([10]).

Targeting ALL blasts with antibodies, both unconjugated and conjugated to toxins, has been shown to be an effective therapeutic strategy. Monoclonal antibodies to surface antigens such as CD19, CD20, CD22, and CD52 have been used in unconjugated form (eg, rituximab and epratuzumab), conjugated to immunotoxins or chemotherapeutic drugs (eg, moxetumomab, inotuzumab ozogamicin), or in the form of bispecific antibodies (eg, blinatumomab). The incorporation of rituximab (CD20) into the hyper-CVAD regimen showed improved outcome in adults younger than 60 years with more than 5% CD20-positive, *BCR-ABL1*–negative B lymphoblastic leukemia ([11]). Recent significant success with the anti-CD19–anti-CD3 bispecific T-cell engaging (BiTE) antibody blinatumomab has led to responses in about 50% of patients with relapsed pediatric B-ALL.

Recent therapeutic advances in ALL have also included the use of adoptive immunotherapies. Anti-CD19 CAR-expressing T cells have shown dramatic success in patients with relapsed B-ALL, with up to 90% remission rates reported ([12]). We have developed a unique nonretroviral approach utilizing the Sleeping Beauty transposon system to transfect T cells with CAR constructs, opening this technology to rapid translation of targetable tumor markers ([13]).

Patients with *BCR-ABL1*–positive ALL had poor prognoses. When tyrosine kinase inhibitors targeting *ABL1* are added to multidrug chemotherapy, CR rates are more than 90%, and event-free survival (EFS) is superior to that in historical controls. Recent work has discovered that a subset (~10%) of children with *BCR-ABL1*–negative ALL have gene expression patterns similar to those with *BCR-ABL1*–positive ALL. Most children and adults with this "Ph-like" ALL harbor a range of novel kinase translocations (including *ABL1, ABL2, PDGFRB, EPOR, JAK2, JAK1*, etc.), some of which are targetable clinically. Thus, we and others have begun to screen for these lesions and to target these cases with appropriate kinase inhibitors (dasatinib, ruxolitinib) and chemotherapy in the clinical trial setting ([14, 15]).

Hodgkin Lymphoma

Hodgkin lymphoma (HL) is one of the first malignancies cured by a combination of chemotherapy and radiation therapy (RT). With appropriate staging and evaluation of treatment response using positron emission tomographic (PET) scanning, current treatment for HL achieves a 5-year EFS of 80% and 5-year OS of more than 90% ([16]). The standard of care for patients with relapsed or refractory HL is salvage chemotherapy followed by autologous stem cell transplantation (SCT), which can induce long-term remissions in approximately 50% of patients. The malignant Hodgkin's Reed-Sternberg cells of classical HL are characterized by the expression of CD30, a member of the tumor necrosis factor T cells, and eosinophils; it represents an ideal target for monoclonal antibody therapy. Brentuximab vedotin (SGN-35) is an antibody-drug conjugate (ADC) comprising an anti-CD30 antibody conjugated by a protease-cleavable linker to the potent antimicrotubule agent monomethyl auristatin E (MMAE). Binding of the ADC to CD30 on the cell surface initiates internalization of the ADC-CD30 complex, which then disrupts the microtubule network, induces cell cycle arrest, and results in apoptotic death of the CD30-expressing tumor cell. Brentuximab vedotin is currently approved by the Food and Drug Administration (FDA) for HL after failure of autologous SCT or failure of two chemotherapy regimens with patients who are not candidates for autologous SCT ([17]). Use of brentuximab vedotin at an earlier treatment time is under investigation with multiple clinical trials. Phase I study of brentuximab vedotin with standard chemotherapy of doxorubicin, bleomycin, vincristine, and decarbazine (ABVD) and modified standard chemotherapy with doxorubicin, vincrisitine, and decarbazine (AVD) as first-line treatment for advanced-stage HL showed significantly increased pulmonary toxicity associated with the combination of brentuximab vedotin and bleomycin. This study confirmed the dose of brentuximab vedotin was safely escalated to 1.2 mg/kg and showed a remarkable response rate of 95% to 96% to the therapy ([18]).

Osteosarcoma

Osteosarcoma is the most common malignant bone tumor of childhood. Osteosarcoma typically affects pubertal adolescents, with a peak incidence in childhood of 12 years. Risk stratification can be made using tumor stage, location, and response to therapy. Survival of patients with nonmetastatic disease at the time of diagnosis has improved dramatically over the past 30 years due to advances in chemotherapy and surgery, with 60% to 65% of patients surviving more than 10 years. However, patients who present with metastatic disease at the diagnosis or those who have recurrent disease have a poor prognosis, with OS rates of less than 20% ([19]).

Treatment of metastatic or relapsed osteosarcoma is challenging, although multiple novel approaches are being tested. One approach under investigation is targeting the bone-forming behavior of this tumor through treatment with radioactive samarium 153–EDTMP or more recently radium 223 dichloride, which concentrated in bone-producing osteosarcoma ([20]). As another approach, we have introduced immunemodulators into osteosarcoma therapy. Based on its potent immunestimulatory properties, liposomal muramyl tripeptide phosphatidylethanolamine (L-MTP-PE) was added to standard osteosarcoma chemotherapy. Although the statistical benefit to survival was not clear in the largest US trial, the European Medicines Evaluation Agency approved this therapy for patients with pulmonary metastases of osteosarcoma; however, it is not currently available in the United States. More recently, we have used aerosolized interleukin (IL) 2 to enhance local immune responses against pulmonary metastases. Preclinical evidence demonstrates that aerosolized gemcitabine upregulates *Fas* expression in pulmonary metastases, leading to immune sensitivity ([21]).

Desmoplastic Small Round Cell Tumor

Desmoplastic small round cell tumor (DSRCT) is an extremely rare undifferentiated mesechymal tumor that affects about 100 children, adolescents, and young adults annually in the United States. It is an aggressive tumor that may show a response to multimodal frontline therapy, although OS rates remain below 30%. The t(11;22) *EWS-WT1* translocation is seen in the majority of cases, confirming the unique pathobiology of this disease.

For patients with relapsed DSRCT, few chemotherapeutics have shown activity, and targeted agents have had limited success as well. However, the insulin-like growth factor (IGF) 1R–inhibiting antibody ganitumab showed one partial response, and there were 3 patients with prolonged stable disease (>24 weeks) of 16 patients with DSRCT. Individual partial responses have been seen with other agents (eg, the multikinase inhibitor pazopanib, the novel agent tasisulam, etc.). Unfortunately, DSRCT frequently disseminates throughout the peritoneal cavity. For these cases, we have used the approach of combining extensive surgical resection followed by hyperthermic intraperitoneal chemotherapy (HIPEC), which has shown promise ([22]).

Medulloblastoma

Medulloblastoma is the most common pediatric malignant CNS tumor, with a peak age of incidence at 5 years and with 80% of medulloblastomas occurring before the age of 15 years. Medulloblastoma is known to be associated with familial cancer syndrome in less than 1% of patients; Gorlin (*PTCH* mutation, SHH receptor) and Turcot (mismatch repair genes) syndromes are the most common. Age less than 3 years at diagnosis, residual tumor after resection, anaplastic histology, *MYC* amplification, 17p loss, and metastatic disease may predict poor outcome. Children with localized disease have a greater than 80% 5-year EFS comparing to those with disseminated disease, who have less than 40% EFS. Treatment typically is multidisciplinary, including surgery, chemotherapy, and RT in newly diagnosed children more than 3 years old.

Recent genomic studies have identified four subtypes of medulloblastoma with distinct cellular origins, namely, WNT, SHH, group 3, and group 4, with the WNT and group 3 subtypes having the best and worst prognosis, respectively. Recurrent mutations in *CTNNB1, PTCH1, MLL2, SMARCA4, DDX3X, CTDNEP1, KDM6A, and TBR1* have been identified ([23]). The pathways of current clinical interest for medulloblastoma include *VEGF, SHH, WNT, Notch, and ERBB* with therapeutic implications ([24]).

For standard-risk medulloblastoma, Packer et al reported that 421 patients between 3 and 21 years of age with nondisseminated medulloblastoma were prospectively randomly assigned to treatment with 23.4 Gy of craniospinal RT, 55.8 Gy of posterior fossa RT, plus one of two adjuvant chemotherapy regimens: lomustine (CCNU), cisplatin, and vincristine or cyclophosphamide, cisplatin, and vincristine. The results of this study disclosed an 81% 5-year EFS rate for children older than 3 years of age with nondisseminated disease ([25]). Proton beam–based radiation is currently being investigated as an alternative to conventional irradiation (NCT01063114).

For high-risk medulloblastoma in children under the age of 3, a German group conducted a study for new diagnoses of medulloblastoma treated with postoperative chemotherapy alone, consisting of cyclophosphamide, methotrexate, vincristine, carboplatin, and etoposide. Forty-three children were treated according to the protocol. In children who had complete resection (17 patients), residual tumor (14), and macroscopic metastases (12), the 5-year progression-free survival (PFS) and OS rates (+/– SE) were 82% +/– 9% and 93% +/– 6%, 50% +/– 13% and 56 +/– 14 %, and 33% +/– 14% and 38% +/– 15%, respectively ([26]).

An alternate treatment approach for patients less than 3 years old is to avoid radiation and use high-dose chemotherapy and autologous stem cell rescue. Dhall et al reported the result for 21 patients with nonmetastatic disease. The 5-year EFS and OS rates (+/– SE) for all patients, patients with gross total resection, and patients with residual tumor were 52% +/– 11% and 70% +/– 10%, 64% +/– 13% and 79% +/– 11%, and 29% +/– 17% and 57% +/– 19%, respectively. The 5-year EFS and OS (+/–SE) for patients with desmoplastic and classical medulloblastoma were 67% +/– 16% and 78% +/– 14%, and 42% +/– 14% and 67% +/– 14%, respectively ([27]). There were four treatment-related deaths. The majority of survivors (71%) avoided irradiation completely. Mean intellectual functioning and quality of life for children surviving without irradiation was within average range for a majority of survivors tested.

For relapsed medulloblastoma, the combination of irinotecan and temozolomide showed some efficacy, with an objective response rate 33.3%; 68.3% experienced clinical benefit, and median survival was 16.7 months ([28]).

In MD Anderson, our focus is to profile novel therapy for relapsed brain tumors. Focusing on locoregional and immunotherapy, we have begun to infuse methotrexate into a catheter placed in the fourth ventricle to target posterior fossa tumors (medulloblastoma, ependymoma, and ATRT; NCT02458339) ([29]). Extending this approach of targeting the posterior fossa tumors, we now infuse autologous ex vivo expanded NK cells (NCT02271711). Another area of interest is target therapy; we are testing an SHH inhibitor for relapsed medulloblastoma.

Low-Grade Gliomas

Approximately half of pediatric CNS tumors are gliomas and are associated with two cancer predisposition syndromes: neurofibromatosis 1 (*NF1* mutations) and tuberous sclerosis syndrome (*TSC* mutations). Gliomas occur in both children and adults; however, the majority of pediatric gliomas are low-grade gliomas (LGGs), with indolent pilocytic astrocytomas the most common subtype. Surgical resection, if feasible, is the most effective therapeutic option, with complete resection of an LGG leading to greater than 90% survival, while less than total resection leads to an about 60% survival. The management of pediatric LGGs that cannot be completely resected has evolved considerably during the last two decades. Although radiation used to be the standard treatment for incompletely resected or unresectable LGGs, chemotherapy and observation have now progressively become the most commonly used options after initial diagnosis, depending on several factors, including tumor location, amount of residual tumor, age, or association with NF1.

The most widely used first-line chemotherapy is a combination of vincristine and carboplatin. In a study of children with newly diagnosed LGGs with evidence of progression, 56% had an objective response to vincristine/carboplatin, and PFS was 68% +/– 7% at 3 years ([30]). Multiple chemotherapies are proven to be effective as treatment of LGGs, including vinblastine, temozolomide, irinotecan, and bevacizumab ([31]). However, some of the short-term and long-term adverse effects are not negligible: severe myelosuppression that requires transfusion and growth factors, hearing loss, or infertility. The COG study showed that a procarbazine, thioguanine, lomustine, and vincristine combination had similar EFS as a combination of vincristine and carboplatin ([32]). Any of the chemotherapies mentioned can be used as relapse treatment if not used as frontline treatment. Although there is no single standard of care, tolerability and long-term adverse effects are considered to be major factors to determine the treatment plan.

Importantly, translocations of *BRAF* occur in 70% of pilocytic astrocytomas ([33]), and the *BRAF* V600E-activating mutation occurs in 5% to 10% of pediatric pilocytic astrocytomas. Although the *BRAF* V600E mutation is not frequently seen with pediatric gliomas, there are case reports that gliomas with *BRAF* V600E mutation showed a dramatic response to vemurafenib ([34]). We offer screening of the mutation and have been experiencing cases with great responses. Because adult melanoma studies showed that most of the patients develop resistance to vemurabenib after a certain period, development of resistance to vemurafenib is also concerning with pediatric gliomas. To overcome this resistance, mTOR inhibitor (everolimus) has been combined with vemurafinib in a phase I trial at MD Anderson (NCT01596140). Alternatively, MEK1 inhibitor, when combined with BRAF inhibitor in melanoma patients, showed improvement of EFS and overcame single-drug resistance ([35]).

Diffuse Intrinsic Pontine Glioma

Diffuse intrinsic pontine glioma (DIPG) comprises 70% to 80% of brainstem tumors in children, with an annual incidence of nearly 300 in the United States. Despite the collaborative efforts and advancement in the multimodality management of brain tumors, the prognosis of these tumors has remained dismal over the last two decades and poses therapeutic challenges. The median OS has remained 9 to 12 months. These tumors occur commonly between the ages of 5 and 10 years, arising from the pons and causing its diffuse enlargement. Stereotactic biopsy of these tumors was first reported in 1978. There have been arguments against biopsy as this is thought to have poor yield and biology of the limited sample would not be truly representative of the entire tumor. Treatment strategies based on clinical trials in adults with high-grade gliomas (HGGs) did not translate into increased OS of DIPG. Today, focal RT given over 6 weeks remains the standard of care for newly diagnosed DIPG ([36]).

Recently, whole-genome, whole-exome, or transcriptome sequencing identified recurrent somatic mutations in *ACVR1* exclusively in DIPGs (32%), in addition to previously reported frequent somatic mutations in histone H3 genes *TP53* and *ATRX* ([37]). Structural variants generating fusion genes were found in 47% of DIPGs, with recurrent fusions involving the neurotrophin receptor genes *NTRK1* and *NTRK2*. Mutations targeting receptor tyrosine kinase–RAS-PI3K signaling, histone modification or chromatin remodeling, and cell cycle regulation were found in 68%, 73%, and 59% of pediatric HGGs, respectively, including in DIPGs. There have been multiple trials with target therapies, imatinib, sunitinib; however, none of them showed increased OS. There is also always concern of drug penetration to the tumor in the pons area. Currently, a COG phase I/II study is investigating use of suberoylanilide hydroxamic acid (SAHA) along with RT and maintenance therapy with SAHA for newly diagnosed DIPG. For relapsed DIPG, the tumors that respond to radiation once and show progression after a certain period, multiple target therapies such as SAHA and everolimus are under consideration for clinical trials. Re-irradiation is also an option for patients who maintain stable disease for a certain period.

High-Grade Gliomas

The outcome for children with HGGs remains poor despite the use of multimodal therapy with surgery, RT, and chemotherapy. Although RT does prolong time to progression slightly, adjuvant chemotherapy has had little impact on survival in children with HGGs. In the first study by the Children's Cancer Group (CCG 943), RT with chemotherapy consisting of chloroethyl-cyclohexyl nitrosourea (CCNU), vincristine, and prednisone following surgical therapy showed a 5-year EFS of 46%, compared to 18% in patients with RT only. Then, the CCG 945 study showed no improvement in survival for patients treated with the 8-in-1drug regimen compared to the CCNU/vincristine/prednisone regimen. Five-year PFS was 19% +/– 3%, while those who did not have a GTR had a 5-year PFS of 11% +/– 4% ([38]). The COG ACNS0126 study used temozolomide as a radiosensitizer followed by 10 cycles of temozolomide at 200 mg/m^2/d for 5 days of every 28-day cycle. The 3-year EFS and OS were 11% +/– 3% and 22% +/– 5%, respectively ([39]). The results with temozolomide given during RT and as an adjuvant therapy were similar to CCG 945 ($P = .98$). ACNS0126 demonstrated comparable survival with less toxicity than in studies utilizing prior nitrosourea-based regimens, which made temozolomide a de facto standard treatment.

Recently, the COG study conducted a randomized "pick-the-winner" approach to determine if either of the two experimental treatment arms (bevacizumab or vorinostat during chemoradiotherapy) had a higher nominal 1-year EFS than the standard treatment arm (temozolomide during chemoradiotherapy). A preliminary report showed that there was no significant benefit from choosing bevacizumab or vorinostat over temozolomide ([40]). From adult studies and small pediatric studies, using bevacizumab along with temozolomide as adjuvant therapy is tolerable therapy, and this was used as a backbone neoadjuvant therapy in this study ([41]).

For relapse HGGs, adult studies for glioblastoma multiforme (GBM) suggest bevacizumab and protracted temozolomide for recurrent/progressive disease even after prior temozolomide exposure ([42]). Multiple adult studies with recurrent HGGs showed activity of bevacizumab with or without irinotecan ([43]). Bevacizumab in patients with recurrent GBM is approved by the FDA. To date, robust identification and correlation of dysfunctional genes with the tumorigenesis have not been performed—a likely reason for continuing therapeutic failure. There is a dire need to treat these patients as they come for therapy after having exhausted treatment options. To understand the genetic landscape of relapsed brain tumors, we enroll our patients in the CM50 study, which is a sequencing study of 50 genes commonly altered in cancers, with at least 50% of those genes pertinent to pediatric brain cancers. We are currently opening a phase I targeted therapy trial for pediatric HGG. The trial is using a combination of dasatinib (PDGFR and SRC inhibitor) and temsirolimus (mTOR inhibitor) and metronomic cyclophosphamide (antiangiogenesis) for targeting the most common driving pathways in pediatric HGG: AKT and angiogenesis (NCT02389309) ([61]).

Table 46-1 Current Successful Treatments

Cancer Type	Salvage Therapy	Targeted Therapy
Acute lymphoblastic leukemia	MRC R3 protocol	Blinatumomab, CAR19 T cell
Hodgkin lymphoma	High-dose chemo with autologous SCT	Brentuximab
Osteosarcoma	Ifosfamide, etoposide	Radium 223, aerosolized IL-2
Desmoplastic small round cell tumor	HIPEC	Ganitumab, pazopanib
Medulloblastoma	Irinotecan + temozolomide, fourth-ventricle methotrexate, IT: intrathecal lipo-AraC	Fourth ventricle NK cell
Low-grade glioma	Vinblastine, irinotecan, temozolomide	Vemurafenib
Diffuse intrinsic pontine glioma	Reradiation	Vorinostat, everolimus
High-grade glioma	Temzolomide, bevacizumab, Irinotecan	Vemurafenib

FINAL WORD

Although OS for children with cancer is excellent, children with relapsed disease still face dismal outcomes. Several recent successes (Table 46-1) have allowed us to make significant progress for specific subsets of patients, although much more work must be done. We still face the challenges of increasing knowledge of the biology of these tumors, and through increasing access to novel therapeutic agents, we are hopeful that we will be able to make a brighter future for our young patients.

REFERENCES

1. Locatelli F, Schrappe M, Bernardo ME, et al., How I treat relapsed childhood acute lyphoblastic leukemia. *Blood.* 2012;120(14):2807-2816.
2. Parker C, Waters R, Leighton C, et al., Effect of mitoxantrone on outcome of children with first relapse of acute lymphoblastic leukaemia (ALL R3): an open-label randomised trial. *Lancet.* 2010;376:2009-2017.
3. Messinger YH, Gaynon PS, Sposto R, et al., Bortezomib with chemotherapy is highly active in advanced B-precursor acute lymphoblastic leukemia: Therapeutic Advances in Childhood Leukemia & Lymphoma (TACL) study. *Blood.* 2012;120(2):285-290.
4. Horton T, Lu X, O'Brien M, et al., Bortezomib with reinduction chemotherapy for first relapse pediatric ALL. A Children's Oncology Group study. Paper presented at: SIOP2014, 46th Congress of the International Society of Pediatric Oncology; October 25, 2014; Toronto, Canada.
5. Hijiya N, Thomson B, Isakoff MS, et al., Phase 2 trial of clofarabine in combination with etoposide and cyclophosphamide in pediatric patients with refractory or relapsed acute lymphoblastic leukemia. *Blood.* 2011;118(23):6043-6049.
6. Wells RJ, Odom LF, Gold SH, et al., Cytosine arabinoside and mitoxantrone treatment of relapsed or refractory childhood leukemia: initial response and relationship to multidrug resistance gene 1. *Med Pediatr Oncol.* 1994;22(4):244-249.
7. Rytting ME, Thomas DA, O'Brien SM, et al., Augmented Berlin-Frankfurt-M€unster therapy in adolescents and young adults (AYAs) with acute lymphoblastic leukemia (ALL). *Cancer.* 2014;120:3660-3668.
8. Rytting M, Triche L, Thomas D, et al., Initial experience with CMC-544 (inotuzumab ozogamicin) in pediatric patients with relapsed B-cell acute lymphoblastic leukemia. *Pediatr Blood Cancer.* 2014;61:369-372.
9. Jain P, Kantarjian H, Ravandi F, et al., The combination of hyper-CVAD plus nelarabine as frontline therapy in adult T-cell acute lymphoblastic leukemia and T-lymphoblastic lymphoma: MD Anderson Cancer Center experience. *Leukemia.* 2014;28(4):973-975.
10. Hernandez Tejada FN, Galvez Silva JR, Zweidler-McKay PA., The challenge of targeting Notch in hematologic malignancies.

Front Pediatr. 2014;10(2):54.

11. Thomas DA, O'Brien S, Faderl S, et al., Chemoimmunotherapy with a modified hyper-CVAD and rituximab regimen improves outcome in de novo Philadelphia chromosome-negative precursor B-lineage acute lymphoblastic leukemia. *J Clin Oncol*. 2010;28(24):3880-3889.
12. Maude SL, Frey N, Shaw PA, et al., Chimeric antigen receptor T cells for sustained remissions in leukemia. *N Engl J Med*. 2014;371:1507-1517.
13. Singh H, Moyes JS, Huls MH, et al., Manufacture of T cells using the Sleeping Beauty system to enforce expression of a CD19-specific chimeric antigen receptor. *Cancer Gene Ther*. 2015;22:95-100.
14. Den Boer ML, van Slegtenhorst M, De Menezes RX, et al., A subtype of childhood acute lymphoblastic leukaemia with poor treatment outcome: a genome-wide classification study. *Lancet Oncol*. 2009;10:125-134.
15. Roberts KG, Li Y, Payne-Turner D, et al., Targetable kinase-activating lesions in Ph-like acute lymphoblastic leukemia. *N Engl J Med*. 2014;371:1005-1015.
16. Schwartz CL, Constine LS, Villaluna D, et al., Arisk-adapted, response-based approach usingABVE-PC for children and adolescents with intermediate- and high-risk Hodgkin lymphoma: the results of P9425. *Blood*. 2009;114:2051-2059.
17. Moskowitz CH, Nademanee A, Masszi T, et al., Brentuximab vedotin as consolidation therapy after autologous stem-cell transplantation in patients with Hodgkin's lymphoma at risk of relapse or progression (AETHERA): a randomised, double-blind, placebo-controlled phase 3 trial. *Lancet*. 2015;385:1853-1862.
18. Younes A, Gopal AK, Smith SE, et al., Results of a pivotal phase II study of brentuximab vedotin for patients with relapsed or refractory Hodgkin's lymphoma. *J Clin Oncol*. 2012;30:2183-2189.
19. Janeway KA, Grier HE, Sequelae of osteosarcoma medical therapy: a review of rare acute toxicities and late effects. *Lancet Oncol*. 2010;11:670-678.
20. Anderson PM, Subbiah V, Rohren E., Bone-seeking radiopharmaceuticals as targeted agents of osteosarcoma: samarium-153-EDTMP and radium-223. *Adv Exp Med Biol*. 2014;804:291-304.
21. Gordon N, Kleinerman ES., Aerosol therapy for the treatment of osteosarcoma lung metastases: targeting the Fas=FasL pathway and rationale for the use of gemcitabine. *J Aerosol Med Pulm Drug Deliv*. 2010;23(4):189-196.
22. Hayes-Jordan A, Green HL, Lin H, et al., Complete cytoreduction and HIPEC improves survival in desmoplastic small round cell tumor. *Ann Surg Oncol*. 2014;21(1):220-224.
23. Jones DT, Jager N, Kool M, et al., Dissecting the genomic complexity underlying medulloblastoma. *Nature*. 2012;488(7409):100-105.
24. Gopalakrishnan V, Tao RH, Dobson T, et al., Medulloblastoma development: tumor biology informs treatment decisions. *CNS Oncol*. 2015;4(2):79-89.
25. Packer RJ, Gajjar A, Vezina G, et al., Phase III study of craniospinal radiation therapy followed by adjuvant chemotherapy for newly diagnosed average-risk medulloblastoma. *J Clin Oncol*. 2008;24:4202-4208.
26. Rutkowski S, Bode U, Deinlein F, et al., Treatment of early childhood medulloblastoma by postoperative chemotherapy alone. *N Engl J Med*. 2005;352:978-986.
27. Dhall G, Grodman H, Ji L, et al., Outcome of children less than three years old at diagnosis with non-metastatic medulloblastoma treated with chemotherapy on the "Head Start" I and II protocols. *Pediatr Blood Cancer*. 2008;50(6):1169-1175.
28. Grill J, Geoerger B, Gesner L, et al., Phase II study of irinotecan in combination with temozolomide (TEMIRI) in children with recurrent or refractory medulloblastoma: a joint ITCC and SIOPE brain tumor study. *Neuro-Oncology*. 2013;15(9):1236–1243.
29. Sandberg DI, Peet MM, Johnson MD, et al., Chemotherapy administration directly into the fourth ventricle in a nonhuman primate model. *J Neurosurg Pediatr*. 2012. 9(5):530-41.
30. Packer RJ, Ater J, Allen J, et al., Carboplatin and vincristine chemotherapy for children with newly diagnosed progressive low-grade gliomas. *J Neurosurg*. 1997;86:747-754.
31. Packer RJ, Jakacki R, Horn M, et al., Objective response of multiply recurrent low-grade gliomas to bevacizumab and irinotecan. *Pediatr Blood Cancer*. 2009;52(7):791-795.
32. Ater JL, Zhou T, Holmes E, et al., Randomized study of two chemotherapy regimens for treatment of low-grade glioma in young children: a report from the Children's Oncology Group. *J Clin Oncol*. 2012;30:2641-2647.
33. Korshunov A, Meyer J, Capper D, et al., Combined molecular analysis of BRAF and IDH1 distinguishes pilocytic astrocytoma from diffuse astrocytoma. *Acta Neuropathol*. 2009;118(3):401-405.
34. Rush S, Foreman N, Liu A., Brainstem ganglioglioma successfully treated with vemurafenib. *J Clin Oncol*. 2013;10(31):159-160.
35. Long GV, Stroyakovskiy D, Gogas H, et al., Combined BRAF and MEK inhibition versus BRAF inhibition alone in melanoma. *N Engl J Med*. 2014;371:1877-1888.
36. Khatua S, Zaky W., Diffuse intrinsic pontine glioma: time for therapeutic optimism. *CNS Oncol*. 2014;3(5):337-348.
37. Wu G, Diaz AK, Paugh BS, et al., The genomic landscape of diffuse intrinsic pontine glioma and pediatric non-brainstem high-grade glioma. *Nat Genet*. 2014;46(5):444-450.
38. Sands SA, Zhou T, O'Neil SH, et al., Long-term follow up of children treated for high-grade gliomas: Children's Oncology Group L991 final study report. *J Clin Oncol*. 2012;30(9):943-949.
39. Cohen KJ, Pollack IF, Zhou T, et al., Temozolomide in the treatment of high-grade gliomas in children: a report from the Children's Oncology Group. *Neuro Oncol*. 2011;13(3):317-323.
40. Hoffman LM, Geller J, Leach J, et al., A feasibility and randomized phase II study of vorinostat, bevacizumab, or temozolomide during radiation followed by maintenance chemotherapy in newly-diagnosed pediatric high-grade glioma: Children's Oncology Group Study ACNS0822. Paper presented at: 2015 Pediatric Neuro-Oncology: Basic and Translational Rsearch Conference of Society of Neuro-Oncology; May 7-8, 2015; San Diego, CA.
41. Friedman GK, Spiller SE, Harrison DK, et al., Treatment of children with glioblastoma with conformal radiation, temozolomide, and bevacizumab as adjuncts to surgical resection. *J Pediatr Hematol Oncol*. 2013;35:123-126.
42. Kamiya-Matsuoka C, Gilbert MR., Treating recurrent glioblastoma: an update. *CNS Oncol*. 2015;4(2):91-104.
43. Vredenburgh JJ, Desjardins A, Reardon DA, et al., The addition of bevacizumab to standard radiation therapy and temozolomide followed by bevacizumab, temozolomide, and irinotecan for newly diagnosed glioblastoma. *Clin Cancer Res*. 2011;17(12):4119-4124.

47

Cancer Genomics

第四十七章　肿瘤基因组学

Jennifer B. Goldstein
Zhijing Zhang
Andy Futreal

中文导读

过去的50年，有关肿瘤基因组测序的大量研究已经帮助人们逐渐了解到癌症发生发展过程的基因改变。本章首先以基因发现过程中具有里程碑意义的病毒癌基因SRC基因、原癌基因HRAS基因和肿瘤抑制基因RB基因为例，回顾了人类对肿瘤基因的认识过程。本章后续着重阐述了肿瘤基因组学方面的一些重要突破及认识。其中包括二代测序等测序技术的发展、肿瘤突变负荷的概述、染色体异常（获得、丢失和易位）与癌症发生的关系、肿瘤异质性的发展理论、多阶段肿瘤进展模型、ctDNA这一新型生物标志物等。随后本章指出肿瘤基因组学的发展帮助开发出许多突破性的靶向药物，并详细列举了当前美国食品和药物管理局（FDA）批准的主要靶向治疗药物。而基因检测技术的普及也使主要基于分子特征的一系列靶向治疗篮子临床试验应运而生。本章最后也对未来肿瘤基因组学的研究方向和发展前景进行了展望。

CANCER GENES

Over the past 50 years, multiple discoveries have had an impact on our understanding of key genomic events that influence the development of malignant growth. After many large-scale sequencing projects of cancer genomes, we now understand that many genetic alterations in specific cancer genes are responsible for the development and progression of the disease. These alterations may occur at the level of the patient's germline, predisposing to inherited forms of cancer that may develop in many tissues throughout the body. Genetic alterations may also be somatic, or newly acquired changes within the genes of an individual cell or group of cells over time and due to environmental stresses. Somatic alterations may come in many forms, including single-base substitutions; insertions or deletions of DNA fragments; rearrangements and rejoining of DNA from alternative locations in the genome; and copy number increases and reductions. Should these alterations effect key cancer genes, malignancy may develop.

In the early 1970s, when studying retroviruses that reverse transcribe RNA into DNA, it was found that ([1]) certain retroviruses, when incorporated into host cells, have the ability to transform normal cells into rapidly dividing tumors. Rous sarcoma virus (RSV), isolated by Peyton Rous, was the first retrovirus found to cause sarcoma in chickens ([2]). Later, hybridization studies proved that the RSV gene, termed *v-src*, was homologous to a highly conserved eukaryotic gene, *c-src*. *Src* became the first known viral oncogene ([3]). In contrast to highly transforming retroviruses, weakly transforming viruses can insert into the genome near proto-oncogenes, normal genes that when mutated give rise to an oncogene, and induce cancer. Activation of proto-oncogenes to oncogenes, through activating point mutations, gene amplification, or chromosomal translocation events, can occur independent of retroviral transformation and cause cancer.

In 1981, Shih and colleagues showed that normal NIH3T3 mouse fibroblast cells could be made cancerous by introduction of total genomic DNA from human cancers ([4]). Isolation of the specific DNA segment responsible for this transforming activity led to the identification of the first naturally occurring, human cancer-causing sequence change—the single-base G > T substitution that causes a glycine-to-valine substitution in codon 12 of the *HRAS* gene ([5]). These experiments demonstrated the causal relationship between oncogenic mutations and cancer. The discovery of *HRAS* and many other oncogenes altered our understanding of cancer and expanded our knowledge of driver mutations that can be targeted to treat disease.

Another commonly referred to class of cancer genes is tumor suppressor genes. These genes are frequently involved in cell cycle regulation, inhibition of cellular proliferation, and DNA repair. When functioning normally, they act as barriers to unregulated tumor growth. However, dysfunction of both copies of the gene are usually required to initiate tumor development as only one functioning copy is needed to regulate the cell. Alfred Knudson, in 1971, was the first to theorize about the role of tumor suppressor genes in cancer development ([6]). He described the two-hit hypothesis: The development of cancer was due to the loss of inherited regulatory genes that functioned to suppress tumor formation, subsequently followed by the somatic loss of the normal homologous allele. In non-hereditary forms, both alleles would be somatically affected ([6,7]).

The first tumor suppressor gene to be identified was the retinoblastoma (*RB*) gene, found to cause childhood cancers of the retina. In the hereditary form, one copy of the *RB* gene is usually defective, with a second mutation or deletion of the normal gene leading to early cancer development. Hereditary forms frequently affect the bilateral eyes. Sporadic retinoblastoma is much rarer and occurs when there is homozygous deletion or somatic mutation of both normal copies of the gene. Sporadic retinoblastoma usually presents later in life than the hereditary form and usually effects only one eye.

In the mid-1980s, Webster Cavanee localized the retinoblastoma gene to a small region on chromosome 13 and found that both the inherited and sporadic varieties had the same secondary abnormalities leading to homozygosity of mutations in the *RB* region ([8]). In 1986, Stephen Friend isolated human complementary DNA mapping to the *RB* gene ([9]). The following year, Wen-Hwa Lee and Yuen-Kai Fung both cloned *RB* using chromosome walking ([10, 11]). Huei-Jen Su Huang and colleagues later proved a causative relationship between the defective *RB* gene and cancer by performing rescue experiments of the neoplastic phenotype in *RB*-mutated retinoblastoma cells with wild-type *RB* ([12]). Aside from retinoblastoma, many tumors have subsequently been found to have defects in the *RB* gene, which may play a role in the establishment of these cancers.

NEXT-GENERATION SEQUENCING

Completion of the Human Genome Project in April 2003 and subsequent publication of a human reference genome provided new opportunities for analyzing cancer. Early on, many groups conducted these studies by sequencing large segments of polymerase chain reaction (PCR) products to detect substitutions and small insertions and deletions. More recently, second-generation sequencing, or next-generation sequencing, has revolutionized the field of oncology by allowing for the entire sequencing of whole genomes in a relatively timely and economic manner ([13]). Commonly used next-generation platforms include the Illumina and Ion Torrent systems. In just over a week, a solitary run on an Illumina HiSeq 2000 sequencer can generate 200 gigabases of data. Over the past decade, there has been a dramatic decrease in sequencing cost with an increase in sequencing capacity that has outpaced Moore's law of technology ([14]). Deep sequencing and single-cell sequencing has allowed us to identify mutations in highly admixed samples. In addition, next-generation sequencing has allowed us to query multiple genomic alterations at a time, such as somatic mutations, copy number variations, as well as some structural information common to cancer ([15]).

MUTATIONAL BURDEN OF CANCER

Some cancers may be driven by a single mutation alone; however, other tumors may contain alterations in multiple driver genes, leading to overproliferation. On the low end of the range, leukemias and liquid malignancies harbor far fewer coding single mutations, about 9.6 per tumor that would alter protein-coding sequence, on average ([16, 17]). Some more common solid tumors, such as colon, breast, brain, or pancreas, contain 33 to 66 genes, on average, with coding somatic mutations ([16]). The large majority, about 95% of mutations, are single-base substitutions (90.7% missense, 7.6% nonsense, and 1.7% alterations of splice sites or untranslated regions), the minority being insertions or deletions of one or more bases ([16]).

Toxic environmental factors may cause some tumors to have markedly more mutations than others with distinct mutational signatures. In addition, defects in DNA repair proteins such as dysfunction in the Fanconi pathway, the DNA mismatch repair pathway (Lynch syndrome), or the proofreading domains of DNA polymerases *POLE* or *POLD1* may increase mutational burden ([18, 19]). Recently, it was also found that the median frequency of mutations varies within cancer types as well. In 2013, Lawrence et al published a study examining 27 different cancer types. This study showed a wide variance in the frequency of nonsynonymous mutations that ranged more than 1,000-fold across cancers within a given subtype (Fig. 47-1) ([20]). As previously described, this study showed a high frequency of mutations in melanoma and lung cancer, thought to be caused by UV radiation and tobacco carcinogen exposure, respectively, with over 100 mutations/Mb. The frequency of mutations in melanoma and lung cancers

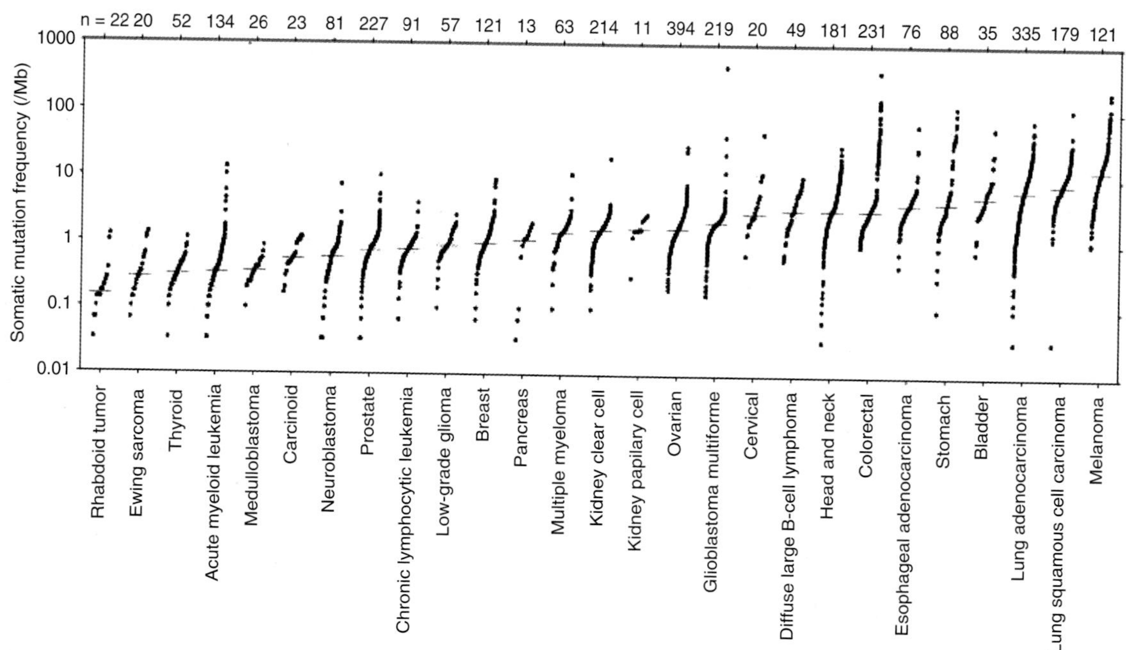

FIGURE 47-1 Whole-exome somatic mutation frequencies in 3,083 tumor-normal pairs. Each dot represents a tumor-normal pair. The *y* axis is the total somatic mutation frequency. Tumor types are ordered on the *x* axis (lowest to highest) by their median somatic mutation frequency. (Reproduced with permission from Lawrence MS, Stojanov P, Polak P, et al: Mutational heterogeneity in cancer and the search for new cancer-associated genes, *Nature*. 2013 Jul 11;499(7457):214-218.)

was also quite variable, however, ranging from 0.1 to 100 mutations/Mb. Although less extreme than the latter cancers, acute myelogenous leukemia's (AML's) frequency of mutations also ranged widely from 0.01 to 10 mutations/Mb. This was despite the overall low number of mutations (0.37/Mb) ([20]). Alexandrov and colleagues analyzed the sequencing data from 7,042 cancers and demonstrated that these tumors exhibited greater than 20 discrete mutational signatures. Some signatures could be found across cancer types (ie, APOBEC cytidine deaminase signature), and other signatures were found in a single cancer class. Kataegis, or regional hypermutation, was also found in many cancers ([21]).

Despite the number of mutations present, not all mutations contribute to the production and growth of tumor cells. Identifying the background mutation rates for tumors as described previously was integral to our understanding of those genes that play a key role in the development of the tumor and confer a selective growth advantage. These alterations in genes are termed *driver* mutations. Those genes that are present within the tumor but do not contribute to tumor formation are deemed *passenger* mutations ([22]). Driver mutations may not all contribute to tumor growth in the same manner, and some driver mutations may be integral to certain steps of tumor development (proliferation vs invasion). Common driver mutations that occur in cancer genes include *PTEN*, *EGFR*, *TP53*, *IDH1*, *RB1*, *KRAS*, and *BRAF* ([23]). In addition, some mutations originally deemed passenger mutations may become drivers once treatment leads to eradication of sensitive clones and provides a niche for already present, resistant, clones to develop ([24]). Work is currently under way to target these genes for treatment options.

CHROMOSOMAL GAINS, LOSSES, AND TRANSLOCATIONS

Chromosomal gains, losses, and translocations are some commonly observed hallmarks of cancer alterations. Somatic copy number alterations may span the entire chromosome or one arm of a chromosome, although they may be limited to particular regions of the genome ([25]). It has been reported that an average cancer cell may have gains or losses involving a quarter of its chromosomes, with smaller, local events affecting about 10% of the genome ([26]). Many of these focal events occur in "peak" regions, affecting a median of 6 to 7 genes (although up to 150-200 genes in some cases). Due to the broader effect of amplification and deletion events, it is difficult to interpret which genetic alterations contribute to carcinogenesis ([15, 27]).

Chromosomal translocations are associated with both liquid and solid malignancies, particularly leukemias, lymphomas, and sarcomas. In some tumors, translocations can result in the fusion of genes normally found at a distance from each other or bring genes closer to enhancer or promoter elements, resulting in alteration in their normal expression patterns. The number of translocations may differ between cancers depending on their degree of genomic instability ([28]). As discussed further in the chapter, translocations can become targets for cancer treatment.

TUMOR HETEROGENEITY

Not only have tumors been found to have a varied number of mutations, but also tumors display intertumoral heterogeneity, with diverse mutations within a given tumor type. In melanoma, for example, *BRAF* mutations are present in about 50% to 60% of patients, allowing for the majority, but not all, patients to benefit from *BRAF* inhibitors ([29, 30]). Intertumoral heterogeneity therefore may have an impact on treatment of patients as each individual patient's tumor may respond to a drug differently. Currently, sequencing is used to correlate mutation status with disease response in individual patients and may be used as a biomarker to stratify patients in a clinical trial. Large-scale sequencing projects by groups such as The Cancer Genome Atlas and the International Cancer Genome Consortium have set out to characterize the mutational landscape of various tumors to obtain a better understanding for the degree of tumor diversity ([31, 32]).

As mutations may vary among individuals with the same type of cancer, individual tumors or their metastatic lesions may also have cells with distinct mutations and, by extension, phenotypes. This is termed *intratumoral heterogeneity* ([33]). This added complexity may account for partial responses to treatment and therapeutic resistance within an individual when treated with chemotherapy or targeted agents. Two classically described theories regarding the development of intratumoral heterogeneity include the cancer stem cell hypothesis and the clonal evolution model. In the cancer stem cell hypothesis, it is suggested that a small, distinct population of cells retain the ability to grow and divide. These cells are responsible for the maintenance of the tumor. As is seen with noncancerous stem cells throughout the body, epigenetic modifications can cause these cells to differentiate into their biologically diverse nonrenewable constituents. These diverse, differentiated cancer cells compose the bulk of tumor, yet do not necessarily contribute to its expansion and tumorigenic potential ([34]). In the clonal evolution model, with time, genetic and epigenetic events accumulate in cells; if these changes confer a competitive advantage, they will allow selective growth of distinct clones that survive over others ([34]). It is possible that both phenomena can occur in the same tumor. Figure 47-2 depicts the two models ([35]).

The expansion of subclones may occur in a linear or branched fashion ([36]). In 2012, Gerlinger and colleagues published a paper in the *New England Journal of Medicine* using multiregional whole-exome sequencing of four renal cell carcinoma samples to elucidate the subclonal architecture and branched evolution of the disease. They found that the majority of driver alterations were subclonal, which acted as a confounder when identifying pertinent driver mutations. This study also demonstrated the unconventional pattern of mutations with regional patterns of heterogeneity. Mutational convergence was also seen with multiple subclonal mutations found in the same driver genes, however at different loci ([33]).

In stark contrast to the former study, in 2015, Zhang and colleagues and Bruin and colleagues published two studies concurrently in *Science* examining multiregional samples from lung cancer specimens ([37, 38]). Unlike renal cell carcinoma, mutational architecture showed more limited branching of subclones with the majority of driver mutations being truncal. Patients who relapsed also had a higher degree of subclonal mutations than those who did not. Smoking-related mutations decreased over time, despite an increase in APOBEC-associated mutations. This may speak to an etiology of treatment resistance due to increased diversity of alterations ([38]). These studies show the vast differences between the patterns of intratumoral heterogeneity between cancer subtypes and the need for greater understanding of heterogeneity to personalize cancer therapy.

MULTISTEP CANCER PROGRESSION

There are multiple theories on how the development and progression of cancer occurs. Some have explained this process with the use of a multistep cancer progression model. Cancer growth occurs due the acquisition and subsequent selection of mutations that give a selective advantage to the cells in which they occur. In Fig. 47-3, we show how this model has been used to describe the acquisition of mutations during progression of myeloproliferative neoplasia and how this has an impact on clinical outcomes ([39]). Here, for example, myeloproliferative neoplasms have been classified as *JAK2* or *TET2* mutation positive or negative. Those positive for both mutations can then be further examined to assess whether the order of mutation acquisition has an impact on phenotype, clinical presentation, and outcomes. The *TET2*-first tumors gain a self-renewal advantage but do not overdivide. Secondary *JAK2* mutants then compete with the *TET2*-alone clones, leading to overpopulation of terminal cells. When *JAK2* homozygosity occurs as a last event, this clone has limited space to expand. This may account for the slower clinical presentation of *TET2*-first mutants. The *JAK2*-first mutants produce excess

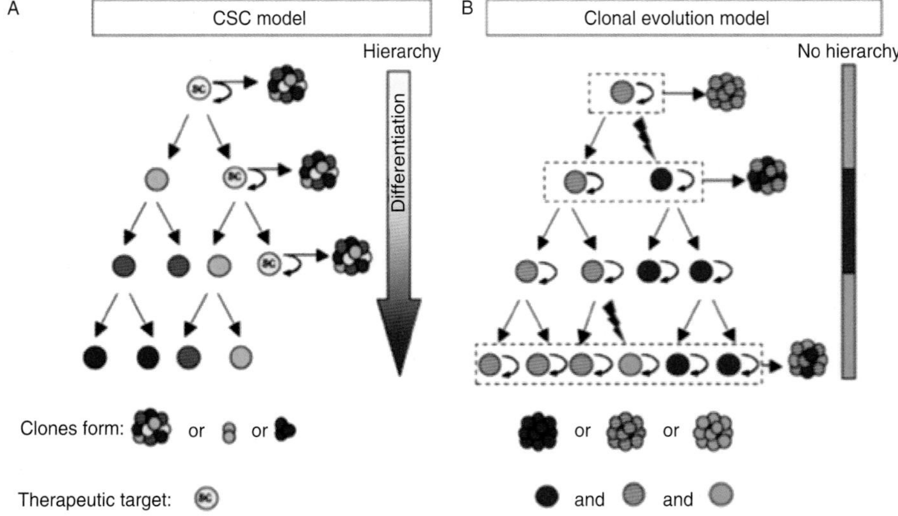

FIGURE 47-2 Models of intratumoral heterogeneity: A. The cancer stem cell model: a specialized subpopulation of cancer cells possesses the capacity of self-renewal and differentiation. This leads to formation of a hierarchical lineage system of subclones (B). The clonal evolution model: genetic mutations lead to multiple cell populations without distinct cellular hierarchy. Most cells are assumed to retain self-renewing capacity. CSC: Cancer Stem Cell. (Adapted with permission from Laks DR, Visnyei K, Kornblum HI: Brain tumor stem cells as therapeutic targets in models of glioma, Yonsei Med J. 2010 Sep;51(5):633-640.)

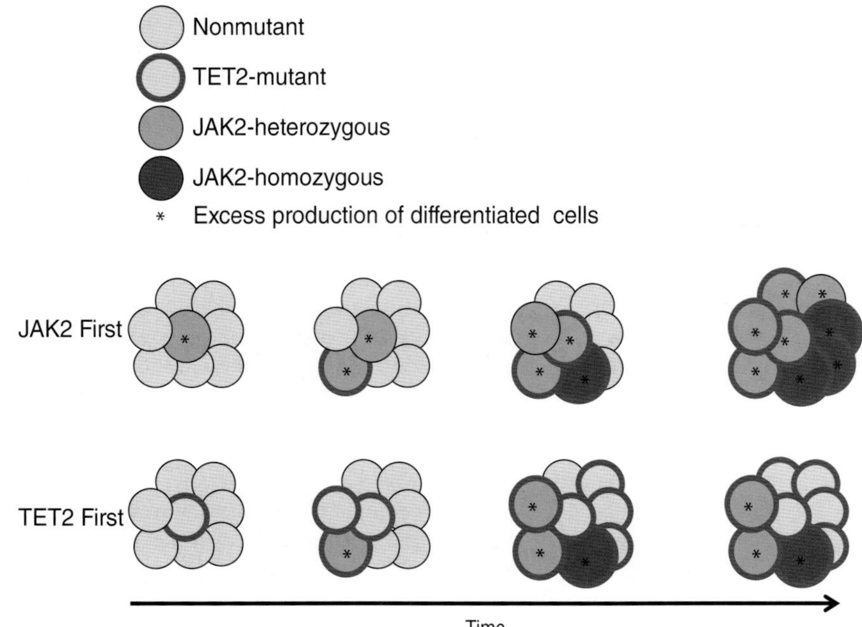

FIGURE 47-3 Multistep cancer progression of myeloproliferative neoplasia: order of mutation acquisition influences the evolution of disease. This model depicts single hematopoietic units acquiring mutations over time.

differentiated cells. After secondary *TET2* mutation acquisition, stem cells obtain a self-renewal advantage, and *JAK2–TET2*–mutant cells expand.

Loss of heterozygosity of *JAK2* V617F (either before or after *TET2* mutation) leads to expansion and resultant excess of differentiated cells. Subsequently, *JAK2*-first patients present more frequently as having polycythemia vera and have an elevated risk of thrombotic events. The understanding of the sequence of mutational events has allowed us to build more reliable tumor models that recapitulate the evolution of the disease from benign to malignant. Also, knowing what are the initial mutational events dictating a cancer's history will help with development of screening efforts against early disease. Further studies of disease biology have shown that this model may be too simplified, and that tumor progression and acquisition of mutations may be happening concomitantly.

CIRCULATING DNA

Although serum-based biomarkers are commonly used to diagnose and track cancer progression, these indicators are often not elevated or are nonspecific. In addition, they are often prognostic rather than predictive of response to therapy. DNA sequencing has allowed for the discovery of multiple cancer-associated genes that may be correlated to cancer development and metastasis. Depending on tumor location and the patient's clinical status, however, it is often difficult to serially biopsy or surgically remove tumor specimens for sequencing. This is particularly a problem with solid tumors. Circulating tumor cells or cell-free DNA have been found in blood specimens as a noninvasive source for sequencing ([40]). This information can then be used as a surrogate for analysis of the tumor itself ([41]). In 2008, Maheswaran et al demonstrated the ability to detect epidermal growth factor receptor (EGFR) mutations in circulating lung cancer cells ([42]). They showed that deleterious EGFR activating mutations could be detected in circulating tumor cells from 92% of patients and in 33% of matched free-plasma DNA. In more recent years, circulating tumor cells and cell-free DNA have become surrogate markers in clinical trials ([43]).

CURRENT TARGETED THERAPIES

With the advent of second-generation sequencing, as well as improvements in molecular biology (immunohistochemistry, fluorescent in situ hybridization, PCR), our ability to characterize tumors has improved. This expansion in our knowledge base has led to many breakthroughs in drug development of targeted agents. One of the first breakthroughs for targeted therapy was the discovery of the BCR-ABL translocation as the main driver for a majority of chronic myelogenous leukemia (CML) cases and a smaller subset of acute lymphoblastic leukemia ([44, 45]). In the 1990s, while performing a high-throughput screen for tyrosine kinase inhibitors, Novartis developed the compound STI-571 (imatinib). In collaboration with Moshe Talpaz and Charles Sawyers, Brian Druker conducted the first clinical trial of STI-571, demonstrating its ability to inhibit proliferation of BCR-ABL–positive CML ([46]). This trial paved the way for imatinib's approval by the Food and Drug Administration (FDA) in 2001 for CML.

After the success of imatinib, many more targeted therapies were presented to the FDA for approval. In 1998, the targeted monoclonal antibody trastuzumab was approved to treat metastatic breast cancer ([47]). In 2011, the small molecule inhibitor vemurafenib was approved by the FDA to treat metastatic melanoma ([48]). These agents, and many more, are discussed in detail throughout the manual; they are highlighted here in Table 47-1, which includes a list of the current FDA-approved targeted cancer therapies. Note that this table does not include targeted immunotherapies, hormonal agents, or cell cycle inhibitors discussed in other chapters.

BASKET CLINICAL TRIALS

At MD Anderson, we routinely send gene panels to assess the mutational profile of individual patients. These panels include commonly mutated, validated cancer driver genes. A patient's tumor samples are sequenced using next-generation sequencing technology, and then results undergo an analytic process to determine which of these mutations are deemed actionable. The results of these studies can then be used to direct physicians on treatment decision making or for referral to clinical trial based on the aberrations. Recently, the FDA required biomarker testing in conjunction with efficacy results for targeted therapy approval. One way to develop trials in line with new FDA standards is the creation of basket clinical trials.

Basket trials are a relatively new clinical trial design theory; recruitment is based on the molecular aberration rather than the underlying tumor histology. In these trials, patients with multiple different tumor types may be receiving the same treatment. The MD Anderson Battle Umbrella trials have been conducted with a similar principle; patients with late-stage lung

CHAPTER 47

Table 47-1 Current FDA-Approved Targeted Therapies

Agent	Target(s)	FDA-Approved Indication(s)
Ado-trastuzumab emtansine (Kadcyla)	HER2 (ERBB2/neu)	Breast cancer (HER2+)
Afatinib (Gilotrif)	EGFR (HER1/ERBB1), HER2 (ERBB2/neu)	Non–small cell lung cancer (EGFR exon 19 deletions or exon 21 substitution [L858R] mutations)
Axitinib (Inlyta)	KIT, PDGFRβ, VEGFR1/2/3	Renal cell carcinoma
Bevacizumab (Avastin)	VEGF ligand	Cervical cancer Colorectal cancer Ovarian and fallopian cancer Glioblastoma Non–small cell lung cancer Peritoneal cancer Renal cell carcinoma
Bosutinib (Bosulif)	ABL	Chronic myelogenous leukemia (Philadelphia chromosome positive)
Cabozantinib (Cometriq)	FLT3, KIT, MET, RET, VEGFR2	Medullary thyroid cancer
Ceritinib (Zykadia)	ALK	Non–small cell lung cancer (ALK fusion)
Cetuximab (Erbitux)	EGFR (HER1/ERBB1)	Colorectal cancer (KRAS wild type) Squamous cell cancer of the head and neck
Crizotinib (Xalkori)	ALK, MET	Non–small cell lung cancer (ALK fusion)
Dabrafenib (Tafinlar)	BRAF	Melanoma (*BRAF* V600 mutation)
Dasatinib (Sprycel)	ABL	Chronic myelogenous leukemia (Philadelphia chromosome positive) Acute lymphoblastic leukemia (Philadelphia chromosome positive)

(Continued)

Table 47-1 Current FDA-Approved Targeted Therapies (*Continued*)

Agent	Target(s)	FDA-Approved Indication(s)
Erlotinib (Tarceva)	EGFR (HER1/ERBB1)	Non–small cell lung cancer Pancreatic cancer
Everolimus (Afinitor)	mTOR	Pancreatic neuroendocrine tumor Renal cell carcinoma Nonresectable subependymal giant cell astrocytoma associated with tuberous sclerosis Breast cancer (HR^+, $HER2^-$)
Gefitinib (Iressa)	EGFR (HER1/ERBB1)	Non–small cell lung cancer with known prior benefit from gefitinib (limited approval)
Ibrutinib (Imbruvica)	BTK	Mantle cell lymphoma Chronic lymphocytic leukemia Waldenstrom's macroglobulinemia
Idelalisib (Zydelig)	PI3Kδ	Chronic lymphocytic leukemia Follicular B-cell non–Hodgkin lymphoma Small lymphocytic lymphoma
Imatinib (Gleevec)	KIT, PDGFR, ABL	Gastrointestinal stromal tumor (KIT^+) Dermatofibrosarcoma protuberans Multiple hematologic malignancies, including Philadelphia chromosome-positive ALL and CML
Lapatinib (Tykerb)	HER2 (ERBB2/neu), EGFR (HER1/ERBB1)	Breast cancer ($HER2^+$)
Lenvatinib (Lenvima)	VEGFR2	Thyroid cancer
Nilotinib (Tasigna)	ABL	Chronic myelogenous leukemia (Philadelphia chromosome positive)
Olaparib (Lynparza)	PARP	Ovarian cancer (BRCA mutation)
Panitumumab (Vectibix)	EGFR (HER1/ERBB1)	Colorectal cancer (KRAS wild type)
Pazopanib (Votrient)	VEGFR, PDGFR, KIT	Renal cell carcinoma
Pertuzumab (Perjeta)	HER2 (ERBB2/neu)	Breast cancer ($HER2^+$)
Ponatinib (Iclusig)	ABL, FGFR1-3, FLT3, VEGFR2	Chronic myelogenous leukemia Acute lymphoblastic leukemia (Philadelphia chromosome positive)
Ramucirumab (Cyramza)	VEGFR2	Gastric cancer or gastroesophageal junction (GEJ) adenocarcinoma Non–small cell lung cancer
Regorafenib (Stivarga)	KIT, PDGFRβ, RAF, RET, VEGFR1/2/3	Colorectal cancer Gastrointestinal stromal tumors
Ruxolitinib (Jakafi)	JAK1/2	Myelofibrosis
Sorafenib (Nexavar)	VEGFR, PDGFR, KIT, RAF	Hepatocellular carcinoma Renal cell carcinoma Thyroid carcinoma
Temsirolimus (Torisel)	mTOR	Renal cell carcinoma
Trametinib (Mekinist)	MEK	Melanoma (BRAF V600 mutation)
Trastuzumab (Herceptin)	HER2 (ERBB2/neu)	Breast cancer ($HER2^+$) Gastric cancer ($HER2^+$)
Vandetanib (Caprelsa)	EGFR (HER1/ERBB1), RET, VEGFR2	Medullary thyroid cancer
Vemurafenib (Zelboraf)	BRAF	Melanoma (*BRAF* V600 mutation)
Vismodegib (Erivedge)	PTCH, Smoothened	Basal cell carcinoma
Ziv-aflibercept (Zaltrap)	PIGF, VEGFA/B	Colorectal cancer
Axitinib (Inlyta)	KIT, PDGFRβ, VEGFR1/2/3	Renal cell carcinoma

cancer are assigned to an arm of therapy based on their biomarker profile. This has allowed for testing of multiple targeted therapies in a more timely fashion. In the phase I department of MD Anderson, there are basket trials under way currently that are sponsored by a pharmaceutical company.

In 2015, the National Cancer Institute (NCI) launched the NCI-MATCH (Molecular Analysis for Therapy Choice) trial, with plans to enroll 1,000 patients on targeted drug combination therapies, based on molecular alterations by pathway rather than on tumor histology. Patients will be randomly assigned to receive a drug specific for that genetic alteration or a treatment unknown to be particularly effective on that pathway ([49]).

FUTURE DIRECTIONS

In the future, we hope to use our knowledge of mutational alterations to find novel therapeutic targets. Through our understanding of altered driver pathways and their inherent sensitivities, we may be able to build on rational combination therapies already in existence. With the decreasing cost of sequencing, there will be an expansion in genetic testing of tumors to characterize their mutational profiles and to better understand their underlying biology. Deep sequencing as well as single-cell sequencing has enabled us to understand the evolution of cancer and the complexity of intratumoral heterogeneity and mechanisms of tumor resistance. Currently, the majority of targeted therapies are being developed and tested in the metastatic setting. Understanding the developmental process may allow us to screen for cancers earlier in the disease process. In addition, better understanding of the interplay between genomics and the immune system will allow us to design trials that are synergistic with our body's own defenses. In conclusion, our expanded understanding of the mutational landscape of cancer has greatly affected our ability to treat and even cure malignancy. It is important to continue to develop this knowledge and translate genomics research to improve patient care.

REFERENCES

1. Varmus HE. Form and function of retroviral proviruses. *Science*. 1982;216:812-820.
2. Rous P. A transmissible avian neoplasm. (Sarcoma of the common fowl) by Peyton Rous, M.D., *Experimental Medicine* for Sept. 1, 1910, vol. 12, pp. 696-705. *J Exp Med*. 1979;150:738-753.
3. Frame MC. Src in cancer: deregulation and consequences for cell behaviour. *Biochim Biophys Acta*. 2002;1602:114-130.
4. Shih C, Padhy LC, Murray M, Weinberg RA. Transforming genes of carcinomas and neuroblastomas introduced into mouse fibroblasts. *Nature*. 1981;290:261-264.
5. Reddy EP, Reynolds RK, Santos E, Barbacid M. A point mutation is responsible for the acquisition of transforming properties by the T24 human bladder carcinoma oncogene. *Nature*. 1982;300:149-152.
6. Knudson AG Jr. Mutation and cancer: statistical study of retinoblastoma. *Proc Natl Acad Sci U S A*. 1971;68:820-823.
7. Knudson AG Jr, Strong LC. Mutation and cancer: a model for Wilms' tumor of the kidney. *J Natl Cancer Inst*. 1972;48:313-324.
8. Cavenee WK, Dryja TP, Phillips RA, et al. Expression of recessive alleles by chromosomal mechanisms in retinoblastoma. *Nature*. 1983;305:779-784.
9. Friend SH, Bernards R, Rogelj S, et al. A human DNA segment with properties of the gene that predisposes to retinoblastoma and osteosarcoma. *Nature*. 1986;323:643-646.
10. Lee WH, Bookstein R, Hong F, et al. Human retinoblastoma susceptibility gene: cloning, identification, and sequence. *Science*. 1987;235:1394-1399.
11. Fung YK, Murphree AL, T'Ang A, et al. Structural evidence for the authenticity of the human retinoblastoma gene. *Science*. 1987;236:1657-1661.
12. Huang HJ, Yee JK, Shew JY, et al. Suppression of the neoplastic phenotype by replacement of the *RB* gene in human cancer cells. *Science*. 1988;242:1563-1566.
13. Campbell PJ, Stephens PJ, Pleasance ED, et al. Identification of somatically acquired rearrangements in cancer using genome-wide massively parallel paired-end sequencing. *Nat Genet*. 2008;40:722-729.
14. Pettersson E, Lundeberg J, Ahmadian A. Generations of sequencing technologies. *Genomics*. 2009;93:105-111.
15. Chin L, Hahn WC, Getz G, Meyerson M. Making sense of cancer genomic data. *Genes Dev*. 2011;25:534-555.
16. Vogelstein B, Papadopoulos N, Velculescu VE, et al. Cancer genome landscapes. *Science*. 2013;339:1546-1558.
17. Miller DG. On the nature of susceptibility to cancer. The presidential address. *Cancer*. 1980;46:1307-1318.
18. Cancer Genome Atlas N. Comprehensive molecular characterization of human colon and rectal cancer. *Nature*. 2012;487:330-337.
19. Palles C, Cazier JB, Howarth KM, et al. Germline mutations affecting the proofreading domains of POLE and POLD1 predispose to colorectal adenomas and carcinomas. *Nat Genet*. 2013;45:136-144.
20. Lawrence MS, Stojanov P, Polak P, et al. Mutational heterogeneity in cancer and the search for new cancer-associated genes. *Nature*. 2013;499:214-218.
21. Alexandrov LB, Nik-Zainal S, Wedge DC, et al. Signatures of mutational processes in human cancer. *Nature*. 2013;500:415-421.
22. Greenman C, Stephens P, Smith R, et al. Patterns of somatic mutation in human cancer genomes. *Nature*. 2007;446:153-158.
23. Tamborero D, Gonzalez-Perez A, Perez-Llamas C, et al. Comprehensive identification of mutational cancer driver genes across 12 tumor types. *Sci Rep*. 2013;3:2650.
24. Roche-Lestienne C, Soenen-Cornu V, Grardel-Duflos N, et al. Several types of mutations of the Abl gene can be found in chronic myeloid leukemia patients resistant to STI571, and they can preexist to the onset of treatment. *Blood*. 2002;100:1014-1018.
25. Sebat J, Lakshmi B, Troge J, et al. Large-scale copy number polymorphism in the human genome. *Science*. 2004;305:525-528.
26. Beroukhim R, Mermel CH, Porter D, et al. The landscape of somatic copy-number alteration across human cancers. *Nature*. 2010;463:899-905.
27. Garraway LA, Lander ES. Lessons from the cancer genome. *Cell*. 2013;153:17-37.
28. Bunting SF, Nussenzweig A. End-joining, translocations and cancer. *Nat Rev Cancer*. 2013;13:443-454.
29. Davies H, Bignell GR, Cox C, et al. Mutations of the BRAF gene in human cancer. *Nature*. 2002;417:949-954.

30. Curtin JA, Fridlyand J, Kageshita T, et al. Distinct sets of genetic alterations in melanoma. *N Engl J Med*. 2005;353:2135-2147.
31. Cancer Genome Atlas Research N. Comprehensive genomic characterization defines human glioblastoma genes and core pathways. *Nature*. 2008;455:1061-1068.
32. Wood LD, Parsons DW, Jones S, et al. The genomic landscapes of human breast and colorectal cancers. *Science*. 2007;318:1108-1113.
33. Gerlinger M, Rowan AJ, Horswell S, et al. Intratumor heterogeneity and branched evolution revealed by multiregion sequencing. *N Engl J Med*. 2012;366:883-892.
34. Shackleton M, Quintana E, Fearon ER, Morrison SJ. Heterogeneity in cancer: cancer stem cells versus clonal evolution. *Cell*. 2009;138:822-829.
35. Laks DR, Visnyei K, Kornblum HI. Brain tumor stem cells as therapeutic targets in models of glioma. *Yonsei Med J*. 2010;51:633-640.
36. Swanton C. Intratumor heterogeneity: evolution through space and time. *Cancer Res*. 2012;72:4875-4882.
37. Zhang J, Fujimoto J, Zhang J, et al. Intratumor heterogeneity in localized lung adenocarcinomas delineated by multiregion sequencing. *Science*. 2014;346:256-259.
38. de Bruin EC, McGranahan N, Mitter R, et al. Spatial and temporal diversity in genomic instability processes defines lung cancer evolution. *Science*. 2014;346:251-256.
39. Ortmann CA, Kent DG, Nangalia J, et al. Effect of mutation order on myeloproliferative neoplasms. *N Engl J Med*. 2015;372:601-612.
40. Nagrath S, Sequist LV, Maheswaran S, et al. Isolation of rare circulating tumour cells in cancer patients by microchip technology. *Nature*. 2007;450:1235-1239.
41. Cristofanilli M, Budd GT, Ellis MJ, et al. Circulating tumor cells, disease progression, and survival in metastatic breast cancer. *N Engl J Med*. 2004;351:781-791.
42. Maheswaran S, Sequist LV, Nagrath S, et al. Detection of mutations in EGFR in circulating lung-cancer cells. *N Engl J Med*. 2008;359:366-377.
43. Janku F, Angenendt P, Tsimberidou AM, et al. Actionable mutations in plasma cell-free DNA in patients with advanced cancers referred for experimental targeted therapies. *Oncotarget*. 2015;6:12809-12821.
44. Nowell PC, Hungerford DA. A minute chromosome in human chronic granulocytic leukemia. *Science*. 1960;132:1488-1501.
45. Kurzrock R, Gutterman JU, Talpaz M. The molecular genetics of Philadelphia chromosome-positive leukemias. *N Engl J Med*. 1988;319:990-998.
46. Druker BJ, Talpaz M, Resta DJ, et al. Efficacy and safety of a specific inhibitor of the BCR-ABL tyrosine kinase in chronic myeloid leukemia. *N Engl J Med*. 2001;344:1031-1037.
47. Slamon DJ, Leyland-Jones B, Shak S, et al. Use of chemotherapy plus a monoclonal antibody against HER2 for metastatic breast cancer that overexpresses HER2. *N Engl J Med*. 2001;344:783-792.
48. Chapman PB, Hauschild A, Robert C, et al. Improved survival with vemurafenib in melanoma with BRAF V600E mutation. *N Engl J Med*. 2011;364:2507-2516.
49. Redig AJ, Janne PA. Basket trials and the evolution of clinical trial design in an era of genomic medicine. *J Clin Oncol*. 2015;33:975-977.

48 Immuno-Oncology

第四十八章　肿瘤免疫治疗

Sangeeta Goswami
James P. Allison
Padmanee Sharma

中文导读

本章首先回顾了肿瘤免疫治疗的探索历程。肿瘤免疫学的基本理论包括免疫监视、免疫编辑和免疫耐受，人体免疫系统也包括抗肿瘤与促肿瘤两种不同功能的免疫细胞及细胞因子。本章主要从细胞免疫治疗、肿瘤疫苗及抗体/受体免疫治疗3个方面阐述肿瘤的免疫治疗。细胞免疫治疗包含在体外大量扩增肿瘤浸润淋巴细胞并回输的过继性T细胞治疗，另一种为嵌合抗原受体T细胞（CART）治疗。针对肿瘤细胞表面特异性表达的抗原制备肿瘤疫苗是一种免疫刺激性治疗，主要针对抗原包括前列腺特异性抗原（PSA）、人类表皮生长因子受体2（HER2）及个体化抗原等。针对抗体/受体的免疫治疗可能通过刺激免疫实现T细胞活化，或者解除T细胞功能“关闭”而实现。前者包括树突状细胞免疫刺激治疗和T细胞免疫刺激治疗，如TLR激动药等。而后者以抗CTLA4、抗PD1或抗PDL1为代表的免疫检查点抑制剂已在多种实体瘤中显示了卓越的疗效。本章最后指出肿瘤免疫治疗未来将从转移性疾病向围手术期推进，并鼓励合理的联合治疗，针对特殊不良反应进行管理减少毒性，制定合理的免疫治疗策略。

PROMISE OF IMMUNOTHERAPY

The ability of the immune system to recognize and eradicate cancer was first postulated in the 19th century; however, proof of principle remained elusive until the 20th century. The effect of infection on tumor regression was observed as early as 1884 by Anton Chekov ([1]); following this, William Coley developed a mixture of killed bacteria that were used to treat various types of cancer between the 1890s and 1960s with mixed clinical benefit. In addition, the concept of using bacterial elements was validated with Food and Drug Administration (FDA) approval of intravesical administration of BCG, which is an FDA-approved therapy that leads to nonspecific inflammatory immune responses and clinical benefit for patients with superficial bladder cancer ([2]). The discovery of the major histocompatibility complex (MHC) and T-cell receptor (TCR) in the 1980s provided insight into T-cell function that led to a number of clinical trials ([3, 4]). Unfortunately, many of the early clinical trials failed due to incomplete understanding of T-cell function. Further research led to understanding of costimulatory and coinhibitory molecules, which led to improved strategies in the field of cancer immunotherapy, including chimeric antigen receptor (CAR) T cells and immune checkpoint therapies, resulting in clinical success that turned the tide in favor of immunotherapy.

The basic principles that guide cancer immunology are (a) immune surveillance, (b) immune editing, and (c) immune tolerance ([5]). Immune surveillance involves scanning and eliminating the transformed nascent cells by the immune system. This theory was bolstered by the finding of tumor-specific antigen that could be identified by cytotoxic T cells ([6]). Immune editing is a process that involves elimination in which the immune system acts as an extrinsic tumor suppressor (similar to the original concept of immunosurveillance); second, *equilibrium* occurs, in which tumor cells survive but are held in check by the immune system; and third, in *escape*, tumor cell variants with either reduced immunogenicity or the capacity to attenuate or subvert immune responses grow into clinically apparent cancers. Escape theory also gave credence to the concept of immune tolerance by which cancer cells exploit the body's immune system and use it for their continuous immune evasion and subsequent growth and proliferation.

The immune compartments that aid in tumor elimination and promote tumor evasion are listed in Table 48-1. The guiding theory for development of immunotherapy is to promote antitumor immune factors and attenuate protumor factors.

CELL-BASED THERAPY

Immune cells, such as cytotoxic T cells, are one of the main effector mechanisms of tumor killing and elimination. Cell-based therapy involves increasing the number and efficiency of immune cells that are capable of recognizing and killing the tumor cells

Adoptive T-Cell Therapy

Adoptive T-cell therapy (ACT) involves adoptive transfer of autologous tumor-infiltrating lymphocytes (TILs) to the tumor-bearing host ([7, 8]). It involves isolation and ex vivo rapid expansion of TILs from tumor, followed by infusion of large numbers of expanded autologous TILs as depicted in Fig. 48-1. Therapy with TILs has been especially promising for patients with stage III and IV unresectable melanoma, and its efficacy has been further increased with combined interleukin (IL) 2 therapy and preconditioning of the host with chemotherapy agents such as Cytoxan and fludaribine. Objective response has been reported in more than 50% of patients ([8, 9]). The transition of ACT into the clinical setting, however, has not been without difficulties. These can be considered in two groups: factors relating to difficulties in generating appropriate

Table 48-1 Anti and Protumor Arms of the Immune System

	Antitumor	Protumor
	Innate: Mature dendritic cell Tumor-associated macrophage (M1 phenotype) Tumor-associated neutrophil (N1)	Innate: Immature dendritic cell Tumor-associated macrophage (M2 phenotype) Tumor-associated neutrophil (N2)
Cellular compartment	NK cells Adaptive: CD8+ T cells CD4+ T cells: Th-1, Th-9, Th-17	Adaptive: CD4+ T cells: Th-9, Th-17 T-regulatory cells
Soluble factors (cytokines)	Granzyme B, IL-1 a,b, IL-2, IL-6, IFN-g, IL-12, IL-17	TGF-b, IL-2, IL-4, IL-6, IL-10, IL-17, IL-23

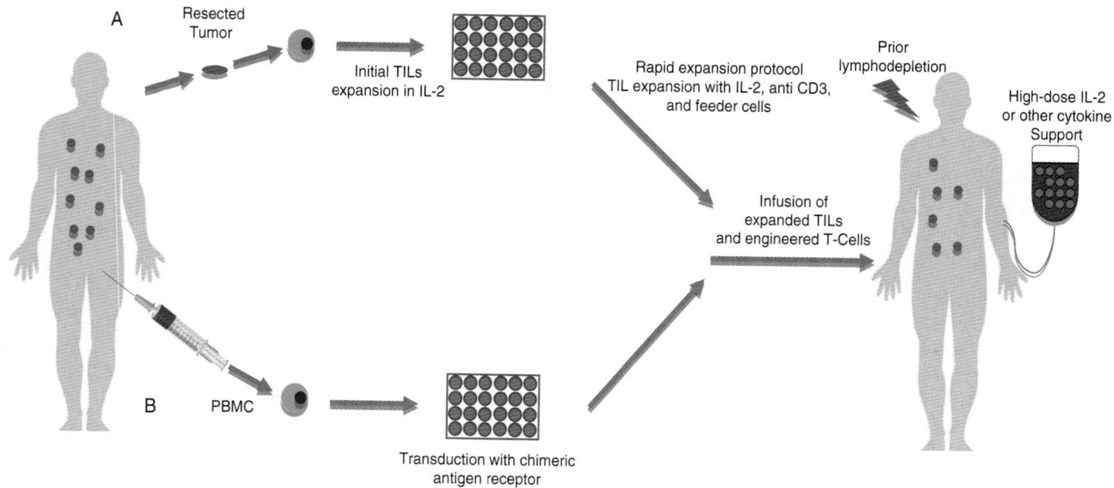

FIGURE 48-1 Adoptive T-cell therapy. There are currently two major sources of T cells used in adoptive cell therapy for melanoma and other cancers. A. The first form of therapy uses tumor-infiltrating lymphocytes (TILs) expanded ex vivo from surgically resected metastatic tumors. The TILs are initially expanded ex vivo using anti-CD3 activation in the presence of irradiated PBMC feeder cells and IL-2. The final product is infused into the patient. B. The second major approach for adoptive T-cell therapy uses T cells expanded from autologous PBMCs that undergo one of three possible manipulations to enrich the cells for tumor antigen-specific T cells.

products for adoptive transfer and factors relating to host or tumor resistance to transferred populations. Recent advances in development of artificial antigen-presenting cells (aAPCs) have helped to overcome many technical issues with rapid TIL expansion ([10]). Further, TIL therapy has been shown to be particularly beneficial in patients pretreated with other immunotherapy agents such as IL-2 or checkpoint blockade like anti-CTLA4 (anti–cytotoxic T lymphocyte-associated antigen 4) ([8]).

Chimeric Antigen Receptor T Cell

In an effort to increase the affinity of T cells to tumor antigen, CAR T cells are engineered that contain a synthetic antigen receptor with specificity to a tumor cell marker coupled with T-cell signaling domain, resulting in high-affinity recognition of the tumor antigen ([11]). The CAR T cells are particularly effective against cancer with known tumor antigen. The CAR T cells with specificity for CD19 have shown activity in chronic lymphocytic lymphoma ([12]). Recently, a phase III study demonstrated the CD19-coupled CAR T cells were particularly effective against relapsed refractory acute lymphoblastic leukemia (ALL) ([13, 14]). Autologous T cells transduced with lentiviral vector expressing a chimeric antigen receptor with specificity for the B-cell antigen CD19, coupled with CD137/4-1 BB (a costimulatory receptor in T cells) and CD3-zeta (a signal transduction component of the T-cell antigen receptor) signaling domains were infused in patients with relapsed or refractory ALL and resulted in complete remission in 90% of cases. A potential drawback of CAR T-cell therapy is exaggerated immune response against normal tissue expressing the antigen; therefore, careful dose escalation studies are necessary to predict the therapeutic window. Further, in many cancers the tumor antigen is not known, making CAR T-cell therapy ineffective against undefined tumor antigens.

CANCER VACCINE

Tumors express a vast array of antigens. Cancer vaccines typically consist of a known tumor antigen with an immunostimulatory formulation that could activate the tumor antigen-specific lymphocyte population, leading to eradication of cells expressing this antigen.

Although therapeutic cancer vaccines have impressive antitumor activity in various animal models, their clinical benefit in cancer patients has to date been minimal ([15]). However, optimization of a cancer vaccine with a combinatorial strategy resulted in significant success of the cancer vaccine, most notably two prostate cancer vaccines: Provenge and Prostvac ([16, 17]). Provenge (sipuleucel-T) is a cancer vaccine based on dendritic cells (DCs) that was approved in 2010. Provenge is prepared from patient's peripheral blood mononuclear cells (PBMCs) pulsed with a fusion protein of granulocyte-macrophage colony-stimulating factor (GM-CSF) and the prostate cancer antigen prostatic acid phosphatase (PAP), with the rationale that on injection GM-CSF–

activated DCs will present the antigen (PAP) to T cells in a more efficient manner. Provenge increased the median survival by 4.1 months compared to placebo in metastatic prostate cancer. Prostvac is another prostate cancer vaccine that is composed of vaccinia and fowlpox vector that contain the transgenes for prostate-specific antigen (PSA) and multiple T-cell costimulatory molecules (TRICOM) ([18]). The TRICOM consists of costimulatory molecules B7.1, leukocyte function-associated antigen 3 (LFA-3), and intercellular adhesion molecule 1 (ICAM-1). The PSA-TRICOM vaccines infect antigen-presenting cells (APCs) and generate proteins that are expressed on the surface of APCs that present antigen to T cells, resulting in antigen-specific tumor killing. E75 (nelipepimut-S) is a human leukocyte antigen (HLA) A2/A3–restricted immunogenic peptide derived from the HER2 protein, which was used in a phase I/II trial involving patients with node-positive or high-risk node-negative breast cancer expressing any level of Her-2 to prevent recurrence ([19]).

Although there remains significant room for improvement in the design and delivery of cancer vaccines, these clinical successes have led to the proof of principle that cancer vaccines are effective. Few of the cancer vaccines that are approved or are currently in clinical trials are listed in Table 48-2.

ANTIBODY-/RECEPTOR-BASED THERAPY

Immunostimulatory Agents

Dendritic cells are professional APCs that are critical for effective T-cell stimulation. Both DCs and T cells possess an array of stimulatory molecules that are necessary for sustained and durable immune response, making them potential therapeutic targets.

Dendritic Cell–Based Immunostimulatory Agents

Toll-like receptors (TLRs) are a group of 13 receptors present in DCs that have distinct ligands, and the receptor-ligand interaction leads to the activation of DCs, inducing the expression of type I interferons, cytokines (eg, IL-12), and costimulatory molecules (eg, CD80, CD86, and CD40) that are critical for T-cell activation ([20, 21]). Clinical trials with TLR agonists have shown promise, particularly in combination with other therapeutic modalities. The imidazoquinolone Imiquimod ligates TLR7; in several clinical trials, topical application resulted in an 80% to 90% clearance rate for superficial basal cell carcinoma ([22, 23]). Systemic administration of TLR7 and TLR9 agonist as monotherapy in melanoma and renal cell carcinoma had a strong immune response but failed to demonstrate objective clinical response ([24, 25]). Although they failed as monotherapy, their capacity to boost the immune system makes them a suitable adjuvant therapy. Both CpG and imiquimod induced increased levels of tumor antigen-specific T cells in patients with melanoma and prostate cancer vaccinated with recombinant protein tumor antigen NY-ESO1 showing promise in combination therapy ([26, 27]).

Another attractive target for enhancing DC function is CD40, which is present on APCs, including DCs, and ligation of CD40 with its ligand CD40L present on T cells is critical for T-cell priming ([28]). CD40 targeting agents as monotherapy showed modest clinical benefit in non-Hodgkins lymphoma and melanoma ([29]). To increase its efficacy, a novel approach utilized electroporation to introduce messenger RNA encoding CD40

Table 48-2 List of Cancer Vaccines

Types of Cancer	Target Antigen	Formulation
Breast	Her-2/Neu	E75, a human leukocyte antigen (HLA) A2/A3-restricted HER-2/neu (HER2) peptide and granulocyte-macrophage colony-stimulating factor.
Breast	Mammoglobin-A	A plasmid encoding the mammaglobin-A gene with potential immunostimulating and antineoplastic activities
Prostate	PAP	Autologous PBMC loaded with GM-CSF+PAP fusion protein
Prostate	PSA	Vaccinia and fowlpox virus encoding PSA and CD86, ICAM-1, and LFA3
Follicular B cell Lymphoma	Idiotype	Autologous tumor Ig Idiotype conjugated to KLH, given with GM-CSF
Vulvar neoplasia: HPV16 E6/E7 Melanoma	gp100	Overlapping long peptides of HPV E6/E7 proteins emulsified in IFA gpl00.209-217(210M) peptide emulsified in IFA

ligand, constitutively active TLR4, CD70, and multiple melanoma tumor antigens into autologous DCs (TriMix-DC). Tumor regressions were observed in 6 of 17 patients who had received interferon-α-2b in combination with TriMix-DC ([30]). Further, combination of anti-CD40 antibody and the chemotherapy agent gemcitabine showed tumor regression in both humans and mice ([31]).

T-Cell Based Immunostimulatory Agents

Engagement of the TCR on T cells with MHC serves as a first signal for T-cell activation; the second signal is mediated by the binding of costimulatory molecules on the T-cell surface to B7 proteins (such as CD80 or CD86) on APCs. Both signals are critical for effective T-cell activation, proliferation, and migration, making costimulatory molecules an interesting therapeutic target for sustained immune response ([32, 33]).

Greater attention has been focused on 41BB (CD137) and OX40 (CD134). Preclinical studies with antimouse anti-CD137 have shown promising activity in combination with antitumor antibody. Most recently, it was shown that targeting anti-CD137 increases the efficacy of cetuximab (anti–epidermal growth factor receptor monoclonal antibody [mAb]) in murine xenograft models, making it another suitable target for combination therapy ([34]). Clinical studies with PF-05082566 (Pfizer, anti-CD-137) in combination with rituximab in B-cell Lymphoma and MK-3475 (anti–programmed cell death 1 [PD-1]) in solid tumor are ongoing. Further, a phase I clinical trial using a mouse mAb that agonizes human OX40 signaling in patients with advanced cancer showed that patients treated with one course of the anti-OX40 mAb (9B12) had an acceptable toxicity profile and regression of at least one metastatic lesion in 12 of 30 patients ([35]).

Immune Checkpoint Blockade

T-cell activation is tightly controlled by immune-suppressive cells and cytokines as well as by the coinhibitory molecules present in T cells, such as CTLA-4 or PD-1 (see Fig. 48-2) ([36]). The CTLA-4 is expressed by activated CD4 and CD8 T cells, and it competes with costimulator CD28 for binding to its ligands (B7 proteins). Binding of CTLA-4 to B7 proteins interrupts CD28 costimulatory signals and serves as a negative regulator of T-cell responses.

For many years, it was widely accepted that T-cell responses can be turned "on" via T-cell receptor and CD28

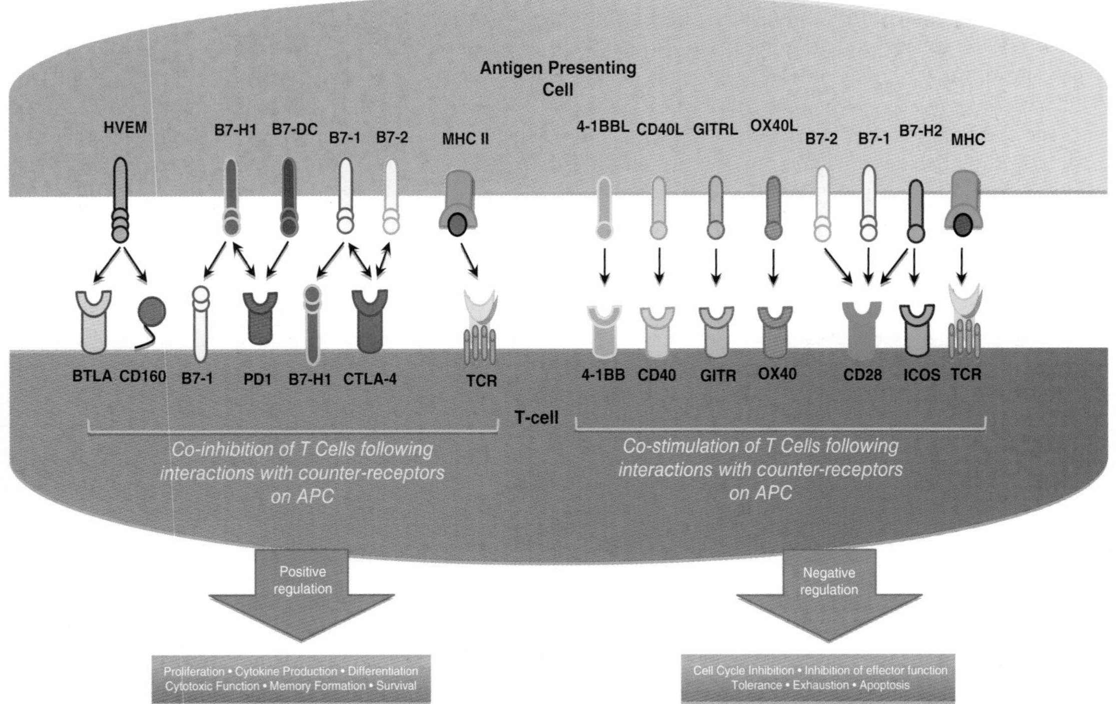

FIGURE 48-2 T-cell activation begins with interaction of the T-cell receptor (TCR) on a T cell with major histocompatibility complex (MHC) bound to antigen on an antigen-presenting cell (APC) (signal 1); activation of the T cell requires additional signals that are provided by the interaction between CD28 and other costimulatory molecules (signal 2). T-cell activation is inhibited by coinhibitory molecules such as CTLA4, PD-1.

costimulation, but the concept of turning "off" T-cell responses did not exist until the discovery of CTLA-4. It was a paradigm shift in cancer immunotherapy to move away from vaccine strategies aimed at turning on T-cell responses to immunotherapy strategies aimed at turning off T-cell inhibitory pathways [37]. Preclinical studies with anti-CTLA-4 antibodies demonstrated rejection of syngeneic transplanted tumors in mice.

These preclinical studies led to the eventual development of an antibody to block human CTLA-4 (ipilimumab), which was subsequently shown in a phase III randomized, controlled trial in patients with metastatic melanoma to improve the median overall survival [38]. Importantly, additional studies have shown that a subset of patients treated with anti-CTLA-4 had durable clinical responses lasting 10 or more years [39]. This trial led to the approval of ipilimumab by the FDA in March 2011 for the treatment of patients with metastatic melanoma. A number of factors have been proposed to potentially serve as biomarkers for response to ipilimumab therapy. Recent studies suggest that an increase in TILs correlates with clinical response of anti-CTLA-4 therapy [40]. In addition, sustained Inducible T-cell COStimulator (ICOS) expression on CD4 T cells has also been observed to correlate with survival of patients with melanoma treated with anti-CTLA-4 therapy [41].

Consistent with this observation, increased frequency of ICOS$^+$ CD4 T cells can also serve as a pharmacodynamic biomarker for anti-CTLA-4 therapy [42]. ICOS is one of the costimulatory receptors of T cells. A preclincial study showed that engagement of the ICOS pathway markedly enhanced efficacy of CTLA-4 blockade in cancer immunotherapy [43]. This finding provides a potential mechanism for future clinical studies with agonistic signaling through ICOS in combination with blockade of CTLA-4.

Programmed cell death 1 is another negative regulator of T-cell response that is mainly expressed by activated CD4 and CD8 T cells as well as APCs [44]. In preclinical studies, blocking antibodies against PD-1 resulted in reduction of tumor metastasis and growth in a number of experimental tumor models [45,46]. These preclinical results led to many clinical trials. In a phase I clinical trial, a fully human immunoglobulin (Ig) G4 anti-PD-1 mAb (nivolumab) was evaluated in patients with relapsed or refractory Hodgkin's lymphoma and demonstrated objective responses in 20 patients (87%), including 17% with a complete response [47].

A randomized, controlled, phase III clinical study compared nivolumab versus dacarbazine (chemotherapy) in patients with previously untreated melanoma (without the *BRAF* mutation), and the overall response rate favored nivolumab (40% vs 14%) [48]. Another phase III clinical trial compared nivolumab versus chemotherapy (dacarbazine or carboplatin plus paclitaxel) in patients with ipilimumab-refractory advanced melanoma induced an overall response rate of 32% versus 11%, respectively, leading to the accelerated FDA approval of nivolumab for patients with unresectable or metastatic melanoma no longer responding to other drugs [49].

Pembrolizumab is another humanized IgG4 mAb targeting PD-1 that demonstrated an overall response rate of 26% in patients with ipilimumab-refractory advanced melanoma in a phase I clinical trial, which prompted its accelerated FDA approval [50]. Nivolumab also had an overall response rate of 87% in patients with Hodgkin's lymphoma who had failed brentuximab vedotin [47]. These studies show that nivolumab and pembrolizumab have significant clinical activity in a variety of heavily pretreated patients with solid tumor malignancies as well as patients with hematological malignancies.

Programmed cell death 1 has two ligands, PD-L1 and PD-L2, with distinct expression profiles. The PD-L1 ligand is expressed not only on APCs but also on T cells, B cells, and nonhematopoietic cells, including tumor cells. Expression of PD-L2 is largely restricted to APCs, including macrophages and myeloid DCs, as well as mast cells. Promising clinical results were observed with drugs targeting PD-L1. A phase I trial with anti-PD-L1 (human IgG4 mAb; BMS-936559) demonstrated an objective response rate of 6% to 17% in patients with advanced non–small cell lung cancer (NSCLC), melanoma, and Renal Cell Carcinoma (RCC) [51]. Another agent targeting PD-L1, MPDL3280A (human IgG1), was engineered with a modification in the Fc domain that eradicates antibody-dependent cellular cytotoxicity. MPDL3280A showed objective response rates of 13% to 26% in multiple solid tumor malignancies, including NSCLC, melanoma, RCC, colorectal cancer, gastric cancer, and head and neck squamous cell carcinoma [52]. Remarkably, MPDL3280A also had a 26% objective response rate in bladder cancer [53].

Because anti-CTLA-4 and anti-PD-1 target distinct inhibitory pathways in T cells, preclinical studies have shown that concurrent targeting of CTLA-4 and PD-1 significantly improves therapeutic efficacy when compared to the monotherapies [54]. A phase I clinical trial evaluated the concurrent treatment of advanced melanoma with ipilimumab plus nivolumab using various doses of both drugs (four cohorts). The objective response rate was 40% when all four cohorts were included and 53% in the cohort representing the maximum dose that was associated with an acceptable level of toxicities. This latter cohort was also associated with unprecedented 1- and 2-year overall survival rates of 94% and 88%, respectively [55]. These results show that drugs targeting the immune checkpoints, CTLA-4, PD-1, and PD-L1 as monotherapy or in combinations, are likely to become the standard of care in various solid as well as hematologic malignancies.

FUTURE DIRECTION

Recent success with immunotherapy in the management of cancer has given credence to the long-held belief that the immune system can be used to treat cancer. Most immunotherapies currently approved or in clinical trials are being used in the metastatic setting. More clinical trials are warranted to test the efficacy of immunotherapy in the presurgical or neoadjuvant setting. The potential for immunotherapies augmenting the effects of conventional chemotherapy or radiotherapy also requires further exploration. Combinational immunotherapy and the combination of immunotherapy with conventional therapy will be the theme of future cancer treatment. The identification of multiple other immune pathways that can be targeted has led to the development of numerous immunotherapy agents that will require testing as monotherapy and combination therapy in the clinic. Furthermore, this new class of cancer treatment also brings a unique set of side effects, which will require close monitoring of patients and additional work to understand predictive biomarkers of toxicities, as well as studies to guide rational development of combination strategies for optimal patient benefit.

REFERENCES

1. Gresser I. A. Chekhov, M.D., and Coley's toxins. *N Engl J Med.* 1987;317(7):457.
2. Lamm DL, et al. A randomized trial of intravesical doxorubicin and immunotherapy with bacille Calmette-Guerin for transitional-cell carcinoma of the bladder. *N Engl J Med.* 1991;325(17):1205-1209.
3. Bjorkman PJ, et al. Structure of the human class I histocompatibility antigen, HLA-A2. *Nature.* 1987;329(6139):506-512.
4. Allison JP, McIntyre BW, Bloch D. Tumor-specific antigen of murine T-lymphoma defined with monoclonal antibody. *J Immunol.* 1982;129(5):2293-2300.
5. Mittal D, et al. New insights into cancer immunoediting and its three component phases—elimination, equilibrium and escape. *Curr Opin Immunol.* 2014;27:16-25.
6. van der Bruggen, P, et al. A gene encoding an antigen recognized by cytolytic T lymphocytes on a human melanoma. *Science.* 1991;254(5038):1643-1647.
7. Dudley ME, et al. Cancer regression and autoimmunity in patients after clonal repopulation with antitumor lymphocytes. *Science.* 2002;298(5594):850-854.
8. Rosenberg SA, et al. Durable complete responses in heavily pretreated patients with metastatic melanoma using T-cell transfer immunotherapy. *Clin Cancer Res.* 2011;17(13):4550-4557.
9. Dudley ME, et al. Adoptive cell transfer therapy following non-myeloablative but lymphodepleting chemotherapy for the treatment of patients with refractory metastatic melanoma. *J Clin Oncol.* 2005;23(10):2346-2357.
10. Ye Q, et al. Engineered artificial antigen presenting cells facilitate direct and efficient expansion of tumor infiltrating lymphocytes. *J Transl Med.* 2011;9:131.
11. Yun C.O, et al. Targeting of T lymphocytes to melanoma cells through chimeric anti-GD3 immunoglobulin T-cell receptors. *Neoplasia.* 2000;2(5):449-459.
12. Porter DL, et al. Chimeric antigen receptor-modified T cells in chronic lymphoid leukemia. *N Engl J Med.* 2011;365(8):725-733.
13. Grupp SA, et al. Chimeric antigen receptor-modified T cells for acute lymphoid leukemia. *N Engl J Med.* 2013;368(16):1509-1518.
14. Maude, S.L, et al. Chimeric antigen receptor T cells for sustained remissions in leukemia. *N Engl J Med.* 2014. 371(16):1507-17.
15. Rosenberg SA, Yang JC, Restifo NP. Cancer immunotherapy: moving beyond current vaccines. *Nat Med.* 2004;10(9):909-915.
16. Kantoff PW, et al. Sipuleucel-T immunotherapy for castration-resistant prostate cancer. *N Engl J Med.* 2010;363(5):411-422.
17. Kantoff PW, et al. Overall survival analysis of a phase II randomized controlled trial of a Poxviral-based PSA-targeted immunotherapy in metastatic castration-resistant prostate cancer. *J Clin Oncol.* 2010;28(7):1099-1105.
18. Madan RA, et al. Prostvac-VF: a vector-based vaccine targeting PSA in prostate cancer. *Expert Opin Investig Drugs.* 2009;18(7):1001-1011.
19. Mittendorf EA, et al. Final report of the phase I/II clinical trial of the E75 (nelipepimut-S) vaccine with booster inoculations to prevent disease recurrence in high-risk breast cancer patients. *Ann Oncol.* 2014;25(9):1735-1742.
20. Iwasaki A, Medzhitov R. Regulation of adaptive immunity by the innate immune system. *Science.* 2010;327(5963):291-295.
21. Banchereau J, Steinman RM. Dendritic cells and the control of immunity. *Nature.* 1998;392(6673):245-252.
22. Geisse J, et al. Imiquimod 5% cream for the treatment of superficial basal cell carcinoma: results from two phase III, randomized, vehicle-controlled studies. *J Am Acad Dermatol.* 2004;50(5):722-733.
23. Schulze HJ, et al. Imiquimod 5% cream for the treatment of superficial basal cell carcinoma: results from a randomized vehicle-controlled phase III study in Europe. *Br J Dermatol.* 2005;152(5):939-947.
24. Pashenkov M, et al. Phase II trial of a toll-like receptor 9-activating oligonucleotide in patients with metastatic melanoma. *J Clin Oncol.* 2006;24(36):5716-5724.
25. Thompson JA, et al. Safety and efficacy of PF-3512676 for the treatment of stage IV renal cell carcinoma: an open-label, multicenter phase I/II study. *Clin Genitourin Cancer.* 2009;7(3):E58-E65.
26. Karbach J, et al. Efficient in vivo priming by vaccination with recombinant NY-ESO-1 protein and CpG in antigen naive prostate cancer patients. *Clin Cancer Res.* 2011;17(4):861-870.
27. Adams, S, et al. Immunization of malignant melanoma patients with full-length NY-ESO-1 protein using TLR7 agonist imiquimod as vaccine adjuvant. *J Immunol.* 2008;181(1):776-784.
28. Vonderheide RH. Prospect of targeting the CD40 pathway for cancer therapy. *Clin Cancer Res.* 2007;13(4):1083-1088.
29. Advani R, et al. Phase I study of the humanized anti-CD40 monoclonal antibody dacetuzumab in refractory or recurrent non-Hodgkin's lymphoma. *J Clin Oncol.* 2009;27(26):4371-4377.
30. Wilgenhof S, et al. Therapeutic vaccination with an autologous mRNA electroporated dendritic cell vaccine in patients with advanced melanoma. *J Immunother.* 2011;34(5):448-456.
31. Beatty GL, et al. CD40 agonists alter tumor stroma and show efficacy against pancreatic carcinoma in mice and humans. *Science.* 2011;331(6024):1612-1616.
32. Watts TH. TNF/TNFR family members in costimulation of T cell responses. *Annu Rev Immunol.* 2005;23:23-68.
33. Melero I, et al. Immunostimulatory monoclonal antibodies for cancer therapy. *Nat Rev Cancer.* 2007;7(2):95-106.
34. Kohrt HE, et al. Targeting CD137 enhances the efficacy of cetuximab. *J Clin Invest.* 2014;124(6):2668-2682.
35. Curti BD, et al. OX40 is a potent immune-stimulating target in late-stage cancer patients. *Cancer Res.* 2013;73(24):7189-7198.
36. Peggs KS, Quezada SA, Allison JP. Cancer immunotherapy: co-stimulatory agonists and co-inhibitory antagonists. *Clin Exp Immunol.* 2009;157(1):9-19.
37. Leach DR, Krummel MF, Allison JP. Enhancement of antitumor

immunity by CTLA-4 blockade. *Science*. 1996;271(5256):1734-1736.

38. Hodi FS, et al. Improved survival with ipilimumab in patients with metastatic melanoma. *N Engl J Med*. 2010;363(8):711-723.
39. Robert C, et al. Efficacy and safety of retreatment with ipilimumab in patients with pretreated advanced melanoma who progressed after initially achieving disease control. *Clin Cancer Res*. 2013;19(8):2232-2239.
40. Hamid O, et al. A prospective phase II trial exploring the association between tumor microenvironment biomarkers and clinical activity of ipilimumab in advanced melanoma. *J Transl Med*. 2011;9:204.
41. Liakou CI, et al. CTLA-4 blockade increases IFNgamma-producing CD4+ICOShi cells to shift the ratio of effector to regulatory T cells in cancer patients. *Proc Natl Acad Sci U S A*. 2008;105(39):14987-14992.
42. Ng Tang D, et al. Increased frequency of ICOS+ CD4 T cells as a pharmacodynamic biomarker for anti-CTLA-4 therapy. *Cancer Immunol Res*. 2013;1(4):229-234.
43. Fan X, et al. Engagement of the ICOS pathway markedly enhances efficacy of CTLA-4 blockade in cancer immunotherapy. *J Exp Med*. 2014;211(4):715-725.
44. Keir ME, et al. PD-1 and its ligands in tolerance and immunity. *Annu Rev Immunol*. 2008;26:677-704.
45. Iwai Y, Terawaki S, Honjo T. PD-1 blockade inhibits hematogenous spread of poorly immunogenic tumor cells by enhanced recruitment of effector T cells. *Int Immunol*. 2005;17(2):133-144.
46. Nomi T, et al. Clinical significance and therapeutic potential of the programmed death-1 ligand/programmed death-1 pathway in human pancreatic cancer. *Clin Cancer Res*. 2007;13(7):2151-2157.
47. Ansell SM, et al. PD-1 blockade with nivolumab in relapsed or refractory Hodgkin's lymphoma. *N Engl J Med*. 2015;372(4):311-319.
48. Robert C, et al. Nivolumab in previously untreated melanoma without BRAF mutation. *N Engl J Med*. 2015;372(4):320-330.
49. Weber JS, et al. Safety, efficacy, and biomarkers of nivolumab with vaccine in ipilimumab-refractory or -naive melanoma. *J Clin Oncol*. 2013;31(34):4311-4318.
50. Robert C, et al. Anti-programmed-death-receptor-1 treatment with pembrolizumab in ipilimumab-refractory advanced melanoma: a randomised dose-comparison cohort of a phase 1 trial. *Lancet*. 2014;384(9948):1109-1117.
51. Brahmer JR, et al. Safety and activity of anti-PD-L1 antibody in patients with advanced cancer. *N Engl J Med*. 2012;366(26):2455-2465.
52. Herbst RS, et al. Predictive correlates of response to the anti-PD-L1 antibody MPDL3280A in cancer patients. *Nature*. 2014;515(7528):563-567.
53. Powles T, et al. MPDL3280A (anti-PD-L1) treatment leads to clinical activity in metastatic bladder cancer. *Nature*. 2014;515(7528):558-562.
54. Curran MA, et al. PD-1 and CTLA-4 combination blockade expands infiltrating T cells and reduces regulatory T and myeloid cells within B16 melanoma tumors. *Proc Natl Acad Sci U S A*. 2010;107(9):4275-4280.
55. Wolchok JD, et al. Nivolumab plus ipilimumab in advanced melanoma. *N Engl J Med*. 2013;369(2):122-133.

49 Targeted Therapy in Cancer

第四十九章　肿瘤靶向治疗

Apostolia-Maria Tsimberidou

中文导读

随着新药研发手段的进步，精准医疗的治疗理念正加速推广。针对特异性的分子靶点如生长因子受体、肿瘤细胞特异性代谢酶等是抗肿瘤治疗的重要发展方向。本章着重阐述了多个参与肿瘤发生与发展的重要信号通路、致癌基因与分子，包括：RAS-RAF-MEK通路，PI3K-AKT-mTOR通路，上皮生长因子受体（EGFR）家族、KIT基因、CDK4/6、BRCA基因等。在每一小节中，首先对不同的通路及分子的定义及功能进行了总结，之后总结了已经在临床上使用的靶向药物的作用机制以及在不同瘤种中的临床研究数据，另外也对目前肿瘤靶向治疗的临床研究现状和方向进行了详细的综述。本章的最后也提出抗肿瘤靶向治疗未来的研发方向，需要根据肿瘤的基因组学、表观遗传学以及肿瘤微环境的特征，借助计算机学、生物信息学以及合理的临床研究设计恶性肿瘤的治疗带来更多希望。

INTRODUCTION

The Human Genome Project has enabled sequencing of human DNA and led to advancements in technologies that detect genomic, transcriptional, proteomic, and epigenetic changes. These technologies, combined with novel drug development, have accelerated the implementation of personalized medicine. Personalized medicine uses concepts of the genetic and environmental bases of disease to individualize prevention, diagnosis, and treatment ([1, 2]). Optimization of treatment using targeted therapy—molecules targeting specific enzymes, growth factor receptors, and signal transducers, thereby interfering with a variety of oncogenic cellular processes—and other strategies made possible by advances in translational medicine holds the promise of improving patient care ([3]).

This chapter focuses on targeted therapy in cancer therapeutics. The material is organized according to the key drivers of carcinogenesis in humans and summarizes the current state-of-the-art applications of personalized medicine.

RAS-RAF-MEK PATHWAY

Upregulation of the mitogen-activated protein kinase (MAPK) cascades RAF (rapidly accelerated fibrosarcoma) and MEK (MAPK/extracellular signal-regulated kinase [ERK]) contributes to carcinogenesis. Several cell surface molecules activate RAS (KRAS, NRAS, and HRAS), a family of guanine triphosphatases (GTPases) that activate downstream RAF protein kinases (BRAF, CRAF, and ARAF). The most important substrates of RAF kinases are MEK1 and MEK2 (MAPK/ERK kinases). The MEK kinases have one main substrate, ERK ([4]). Activation of ERK leads to modifications in gene expression mediated by transcription factors that control cell cycle progression, differentiation, metabolism, survival, migration, and invasion. This pathway regulates apoptosis by the posttranslational phosphorylation of apoptotic regulatory molecules (Bad, Bim, Mcl-1, and caspase 9). RAS is a downstream effector of the epidermal growth factor receptor (EGFR). Activation of ERK promotes upregulated expression of EGFR ligands and an autocrine loop critical for tumor growth ([5]). The frequency of molecular alterations in major pathway components is shown in the COSMIC (Catalogue of Somatic Mutations in Cancer) database (http://www.sanger.ac.uk/genetics/CGP/cosmic/).

Melanoma

Mutations in *BRAF* are found in 62% to 72% of patients with metastatic melanoma ([6]) and are less frequent in the radial growth phase (10%) and in situ (5.6%) melanomas ([7]). Mutations of *NRAS* occur in 5.2% of melanomas ([7]). In conjunctival melanoma, *BRAF* and *NRAS* mutations were identified in 29% and 18% of patients, respectively ([8]). Alterations of KIT were found in 36% and 39% of patients with acral and mucosal melanoma, respectively ([9]). Alterations of GNAQ and GNA11 were found in 45% and 32% of patients with uveal melanoma, respectively ([10]).

Inhibitors of BRAF and MEK have been approved by the US Food and Drug Administration (FDA) based on their significant antitumor activity and tolerability in patients with melanoma. The FDA-approved drugs and selected investigational agents by molecular target/pathway are listed in Table 49-1.

Vemurafenib and Dabrafenib

Vemurafenib was the first BRAF FDA-approved inhibitor for metastatic melanoma with a *BRAF* V600E mutation. A phase III trial demonstrated a 3.7-month improvement in progression-free survival (PFS) in the vemurafenib arm compared to the dacarbazine arm (median PFS 5.3 months and 1.6 months, respectively). The median overall survival (OS) was not reached in the vemurafenib arm and was 7.9 months in the control arm ([11]). Dabrafenib is also FDA approved for patients with unresectable or metastatic melanoma with a *BRAF* V600E mutation, based on the results of a phase III study that compared dabrafenib with dacarbazine. The median PFS was 5.1 months and 2.7 months in the dabrafenib and the dacarbazine arms, respectively ([12]). Vemurafenib ([13]) and dabrafenib ([14]) have antitumor activity in patients with melanoma and brain metastases.

Trametinib

Trametinib is a MEK1/MEK2 kinase inhibitor that was approved by the FDA as a single agent or combined with dabrafenib for unresectable or metastatic melanoma with a *BRAF* V600E or V600K mutation. Approval was based on the results of a randomized trial, which demonstrated longer PFS with trametinib than with chemotherapy consisting of either dacarbazine or paclitaxel in patients with stage IIIc or IV melanoma and a BRAF V600E or V600K mutation ([15]). The median PFS durations were 4.8 and 1.5 months in the trametinib and chemotherapy arms, respectively (hazard ratio [HR], 0.47; $P < .0001$). The 6-month OS rates were 81% and 67%, respectively ([15]).

In a phase I and II study of dabrafenib plus trametinib or dabrafenib monotherapy in patients with melanoma and a *BRAF* V600E or V600K mutation, the objective response (complete response [CR] and partial response [PR]) rates were 76% and 54%, respectively ($P = .03$) ([16]). Cutaneous squamous cell

Table 49-1 FDA-Approved and Selected Investigational Targeted Agents by Molecular Target/Pathway

Pathway/Target	FDA-Approved Drugs	Investigational Agents
RAS-RAF-MEK pathway		
BRAF	Dabrafenib (Tafinlar)	Encorafenib (LGX818)
	Vemurafenib (Zelboraf)	GDC-0879
		PLX-4720
MEK	Trametinib (Mekinist)	Cobimetinib (GDC-0973)
		Selumetinib (AZD6244)
RAS		Tipifarnib
		Lonafarnib
PI3K/AKT/mTOR pathway		
mTOR	Everolimus (Afinitor)	MLN0128
	Temsirolimus (Torisel)	JNK128
		AZD8055
		Ridaforolimus
PI3K		BKM120
		Copanlisib (BAY 80-6946)
		XL-147
		GDC-0032 (Taselisib)
		INK1117
		BYL719
		GDC-0941
PI3K and mTOR		BEZ235
		XL-765
		BGT-226
		GDC-0980
		PF4691502
AKT		MK2206
		GSK2141795
		BAY1125976
		GDC-0068
p70S6K/AKT		MSC2363318A
BRCA		
PARP	Olaparib (Lynparza)	ABT-888 (Veliparib)
		PF-01367338 (Rucaparib)
		BMN 673 (Talazoparib)
EGFR	Cetuximab (Erbitux)	CO-1686 (Rociletinib)
	Erlotinib (Tarceva)	
	Afatinib (Gilotrif)	
	Panitumumab (Vectibix)	
EGFR, RET, VEGFR2	Vandetanib (Caprelsa)	
HER2	Pertuzumab (Perjeta)	
	Trastuzumab (Herceptin)	
HER2 and EGFR	Lapatinib (Tykerb)	

(*Continued*)

Table 49-1 FDA-Approved and Selected Investigational Targeted Agents by Molecular Target/Pathway (*Continued*)

Pathway/Target	FDA-Approved Drugs	Investigational Agents
ALK	Ceritinib (Zykadia)	Alectinib
	Crizotinib (Xalkori)	AP26113 (Brigatinib)
		ASP3026
		PF-06463922
		X-396
NOTCH		Tarextumab (OMP-59R5)
		OMP-21M18 (Demcizumab)
		MK-0752
		RO4929097
		PF-03084014
KIT, PDGFR, ABL	Imatinib (Gleevec)	Bosutinib (Bosulif)
	Dasatinib (Sprycel)	
	Ponatinib (Iclusig)	
KIT, PDGFRβ, RAF, RET, VEGFR1/2/3	Regorafenib (Stivarga)	Dovitinib
	Sorafenib (Nexavar)	
VEGF ligand	Bevacizumab (Avastin)	
Receptor tyrosine kinase (RTK) inhibitor	Sunitinib (Sutent)	
VEGF	Nintedanib (Ofev)	Brivanib (BMS-540215)
MET		AMG102 (Rilotumumab)
		AV-299 (Ficlatuzumab)
		MetMab (Onartuzumab)
		LY-2875358
		h224G11A
		DN30
		MGCD-265
		Tivantinib (ARQ197)
		JNJ-38877605
		AMG 337
		AMG 208
		PF-04217903
		EMD-1214063
		LY-2801653
		INC-280
		Foretinib (GSK1363089)
		Cabozantinib (Cometriq)
FGF		Brivanib
		Dovitinib (TKI258)
		AZD4547
		BAY1187982
		Lucitanib
		Ponatinib (Iclusig)
		TAS-120
		Debio 1347 (CH5183284)

(*Continued*)

Table 49-1 FDA-Approved and Selected Investigational Targeted Agents by Molecular Target/Pathway (*Continued*)

Pathway/Target	FDA-Approved Drugs	Investigational Agents
		BAY1163877
		FGF401
		BGJ398
		Nintedanib (BIBF1120)
		JNJ-42756493
		GSK3052230
		ARQ 087
		BAY1179470
		FPA144
P53 MDM2		DS-3032b
		RO6839921
		RO5045337
		RO5503781
		HDM201

carcinoma (SCC), an adverse event associated with BRAF inhibitors, was less common in the dabrafenib plus trametinib group than in the dabrafenib group (7% vs 19%, respectively) ([16]).

Other MEK inhibitors are in clinical trials. In a randomized phase II study in patients with BRAF-mutated advanced melanoma, selumetinib (MAP2K1/MAP2K2 inhibitor) plus dacarbazine was associated with longer PFS compared to dacarbazine (5.6 vs 3 months), but no improvement in OS was noted ([17]).

Lung Cancer

Mutations in *BRAF* occur in 1% to 4% of patients with non–small cell lung cancer (NSCLC). Molecular alterations in *EGFR, ALK, ROS1, NRAS,* and *KRAS* are also involved in the pathogenesis of lung cancer. We have noted responses in patients with NSCLC and *BRAF* V600E mutation treated with vemurafenib. A study of dabrafenib with or without trametinib in *BRAF* V600E–mutant NSCLC is ongoing.

Mutations of *KRAS* are more common in smokers. In metastatic NSCLC, mutated *KRAS* is associated with a worse prognosis than mutated *EGFR*. Mutation of *KRAS* was associated with shorter PFS in patients receiving maintenance erlotinib. No difference was noted in OS between mutated and wild-type *KRAS* ([18]). In colorectal cancer (CRC), *KRAS* mutations are associated with resistance to cetuximab. In a phase II study, selumetinib combined with docetaxel was associated with a higher response rate (37%, all PRs) in patients with *KRAS*-mutant NSCLC compared to docetaxel plus placebo (0%) ([19]). Other clinical trials evaluating MEK inhibitors combined with chemotherapy in *KRAS*-mutant NSCLC have been completed (NCT01192165, NCT01362296). In a phase II randomized study of trametinib compared to docetaxel in patients with *KRAS*-mutant NSCLC ([20]), the rates of response and PFS were similar in the two arms (response, 12% [all PR]; median PFS, trametinib: 12 weeks; docetaxel: 11 weeks). Other studies of RAS-RAF-MEK inhibitors are ongoing.

PI3K-AKT-mTOR PATHWAY

The phosphatidylinositol 3-kinase (PI3K) signaling pathway is involved in the survival, growth, metabolism, motility, and progression of cancer and is a critical pathway in cancer ([21]). The PI3K family of proteins catalyzes the phosphorylation of phosphatidylinositols (PtdIns) at their 3′ position and consists of classes I, II, and III. Only class IA signaling aberrations are involved in human cancers ([22]). The class IA PI3Ks are composed of heterodimers of regulatory subunits (p85α, p85β, p50α, p55α, and p55γ) and catalytic subunits (p110α, p110β, p110δ). Three genes encode the regulatory subunits: PIK3R1 encodes p85α ([22]), and PIK3R2 and PIK3R3 encode the p85β and p55γ isoforms of the p85 regulatory subunit, respectively. Three genes, PIK3CA, PIK3CB, and PIK3CD, encode the highly homologous p110 catalytic subunit isoforms p110α, p110β, and p110δ and share a similar five-domain structure. At the amino terminus, there is an adapter-binding domain that interacts with the p85 regulatory subunit, followed by a RAS-binding domain that mediates interaction with RAS.

The class I PI3Ks can phosphorylate the 3′ position of PtdIns, PI-4-P, and PI-4,5-P_2 though PI-4,5-P_2. This phosphorylation generates the second-messenger phosphatidylinositol (3,4,5) triphosphate (PIP_3). Cytosolic proteins, such as the AKT family of protein-serine/threonine kinases, bind to PIP_3 and localize to the plasma membrane in response to PI3K activation [23]. In the absence of stimulated growth conditions, baseline levels of PIP_3 are undetectable in mammals. The PIP_3 levels at the plasma membrane are regulated by the tumor suppressor phosphatase and tensin (PTEN) homolog, whose lipid phosphatase activity converts PIP_3 to PI-4,5-P_2. Loss of PTEN function through inactivating mutations, deletion, chromosomal translocation, or epigenetic silencing is the second most common initiating event in cancer after p53 mutations.

Mutations or amplifications of the PI3K catalytic subunits p110α (*PIK3CA*) and p110β (*PIK3CB*), the PI3K regulatory subunits p85α (*PIK3R1*) and p85β (*PIK3R2*), and AKT (*AKT1*) can activate the PI3K pathway. Mutations, deletions, or epigenetic changes in negative regulators of the PI3K axis (PTEN and inositol polyphosphate-4-phosphatase, type II) may modify tumor cell sensitivity to chemotherapy or targeted therapies [24]. AKT is the main effector of PI3K activation and has three isoforms: AKT1, AKT2, and AKT3. AKT signaling plays a significant role in cell hypertrophy, survival, hyperplasia, and metabolism. Mammalian target of rapamycin (mTOR) is the catalytic subunit of mTOR complex 1 (mTORC1) and mTOR complex 2 (mTORC2), which are distinguished by their accessory proteins, regulatory-associated protein of mTOR (RAPTOR) and rapamycin-insensitive companion of mTOR (RICTOR) [25].

Several studies focused on targeting the PI3K-AKT-mTOR pathway. Rapamycin analogues (rapalogs) have antitumor activity in various tumors and are frequently combined with other anticancer agents [26]. Everolimus is approved for the treatment of subependymal giant cell astrocytoma; hormone receptor (HR)-positive, HER2 (human epidermal growth factor receptor 2)-negative breast cancer (in combination with exemestane); neuroendocrine pancreatic tumors; tuberous sclerosis–associated subependymal giant cell astrocytoma; and renal cell carcinoma (sunitinib or sorafenib refractory). Temsirolimus is approved for renal cell carcinoma. The efficacy of rapalogs combined with endocrine therapy for advanced breast cancer was evident in the BOLERO-2 trial, which showed a median PFS of 6.9 months for everolimus and exemestane versus 2.8 months for exemestane alone [27].

PI3K Inhibitors

The first generation of class I pan-PI3K inhibitors targeted PI3Kα, PI3Kβ, PI3Kγ, and PI3Kδ. Wortmannin and LY294002 had limited activity. Ongoing studies are evaluating new pan-PI3K inhibitors with improved pharmacokinetic profiles and target specificity. Their antitumor activity is primarily cytostatic. Novel agents that inhibit both PI3K and mTOR may improve the antitumor activity of either agent.

GDC-0941

GDC-0941 is a selective oral class I PI3K inhibitor and at high concentrations also an mTOR inhibitor. It is being investigated in clinical trials in patients with metastatic breast cancer (NCT00960960, NCT01437566) and advanced NSCLC. Initial studies of GDC-0941 demonstrated PRs in patients with melanoma and ovarian, cervical, and estrogen receptor (ER)–positive/HER-negative breast cancer [28-30]. At the maximum tolerated dose (MTD), dose-limiting toxicities (DLTs) included grade 3 macular rash and asymptomatic T-wave inversion on electrocardiograms, grade 3 thrombocytopenia, and grade 4 hyperglycemia [29, 30]. Ongoing studies evaluating GDC-0941 include a phase II study in patients with untreated advanced or recurrent NSCLC treated with carboplatin/paclitaxel or carboplatin/paclitaxel/bevacizumab with or without GDC-0941 (NCT01493843). In a phase I/II study, GDC-0941 and cisplatin are being studied in patients with androgen receptor (AR)–negative, triple-negative, metastatic breast cancer, and in a phase II study, patients with advanced/metastatic breast cancer resistant to aromatase inhibitor therapy are being treated with GDC-0941 or GDC-0980 with fulvestrant versus fulvestrant alone (NCT01437566). Clinical trials are also investigating combinations of PI3K inhibitors taselisib (GDC-0032) or pictilisib (GDC-0941) with other targeted agents (eg, palbociclib, a cyclin-dependent kinase 4 and 6 [CDK4/6] inhibitor) in advanced solid tumors or breast cancer (NCT02389842).

BKM120

BKM120 is an oral pyrimidine-derived pan-PI3K inhibitor with activity against all class I PI3K isoforms. A phase I study demonstrated that BKM120 was well tolerated, with a dose-dependent safety profile [31]. Adverse events included hyperglycemia, rash, nausea, fatigue, and mood alterations. Hyperglycemia is a typical adverse event associated with the use of PI3K/AKT/mTOR pathway inhibitors. Another study demonstrated that in colorectal, breast, lung, and endometrial cancers treated with BKM120, two of 77 patients had a PR (triple-negative breast cancer with

KRAS and *p53* mutations, n = 1; and ER-positive/HER-negative metastatic breast cancer, n = 1; both had tumor *PIK3CA* mutations), and 58% of patients had stable disease (SD).

BAY 80-6946

BAY 80-6946 is a pan–class I PI3K inhibitor with activity against PI3Kα, PI3Kβ, PI3Kδ, and PI3Kγ. A phase I study demonstrated that the MTD of BAY 80-6946 was 0.8 mg/kg intravenously weekly (3 weeks on, 1 week off). Adverse events included hyperglycemia, fatigue, nausea, diarrhea, and mucositis. Clinical benefit was reported in patients with advanced breast, endometrial, and gastric cancers.

BEZ235

BEZ235 is an oral, reversible, and selective inhibitor of PI3K and TORC1/2. Preclinical data demonstrated antitumor activity in melanoma, breast, CRC and sarcoma. BEZ235 suppresses cell proliferation, induces G1 cell cycle arrest, and promotes autophagy by inhibiting the activity of AKT, S6K, S6, and 4EBP1 target proteins. BEZ235 has been investigated in phase I/II clinical trials in patients with advanced cancer alone ([32]) or in combination with paclitaxel, trastuzumab, everolimus, or MEK162. In a phase IB study, BEZ235 combined with trastuzumab in 15 patients with HER2-positive metastatic breast cancer with altered PI3K/PTEN status was tolerable. Stable disease and PR were reported in four and one patients, respectively ([33]). An improved formulation of BEZ235 was used as a monotherapy or combined with trastuzumab, and SD was noted in 40% of patients with advanced cancer. The most common adverse events were nausea, diarrhea, elevated transaminases, and headache. The DLTs were fatigue, asthenia, grade 3 thrombocytopenia, and grade 3 mucositis ([32]). A clinical trial of BEZ235 and everolimus in advanced cancer is ongoing (NCT01628913).

In prostate cancer, PTEN loss may be associated with resistance to castration ([34, 35]). BEZ235 causes growth arrest in PTEN-negative prostate cancers, but inhibition of the PI3K pathway leads to activation of AR signaling (inhibition of AR appears to result in promotion of PI3K activity) ([35]).

Other p110α Isoform-Specific Inhibitors

Other p110α isoform-specific inhibitors, such as BYL719, GDC-0032, and INK1117, are being investigated in various solid tumors. BYL719 was associated with less hyperglycemia than the pan-PI3K inhibitor BKM120 ([36]). In a phase I study, BYL719 induced tumor reduction in 33% of patients with ER-positive, metastatic breast cancer and a PIK3CA mutation ([37]). Multiple studies are investigating the role of BYL719 in solid tumors as a single agent or in combination with targeted agents and cytotoxics. Although preclinical data demonstrated that PIK3CA alterations are the best biomarkers for predicting sensitivity to BYL719, p110α inhibitors are not effective in PIK3CA-mutated cells that also have a PTEN deletion ([37]).

AKT Inhibitors

The AKT inhibitors may induce the PI3K-stimulating receptor tyrosine kinase HER3 in breast cancer cell lines and may increase IGF-1R and the insulin receptor, thereby leading to the development of escape pathways and resistance mechanisms. Combination therapies that block the feedback response may overcome resistance to AKT inhibitors. Several studies have investigated or are investigating AKT inhibitors (such as MK2206, GSK2141795, and BAY1125976) as single agents or in combination with targeted therapies or chemotherapy in specific tumor types (examples are NCT01333475, NCT01902173, NCT01979523, and NCT01915576). Other drugs, such as MSC2363318A, a dual p70S6K/AKT inhibitor, are in clinical trials (NCT01971515).

Based on the increase in tumor inhibition with combined MEK/PI3K targeting and the tolerability of drugs targeting each pathway individually, early-phase trials combining GDC-0941 (PI3K inhibitor) with GDC-0973 (MEK inhibitor) and combining BKM120 (PI3K inhibitor) with GSK1120212 (MEK inhibitor) have been completed ([38, 39]). The latter study demonstrated promising antitumor activity in patients with *KRAS*-mutant ovarian cancer.

Conclusions

In summary, molecular alterations in the PI3K/AKT/mTOR pathway have been identified in multiple tumor types, emphasizing the critical role of this pathway in tumorigenesis and disease progression. The PI3K inhibitors, as single agents, have mostly cytostatic activity. Several escape mechanisms are involved in resistance to PI3K/AKT/mTOR inhibitors. Clinical trials are exploring the role of PI3K, AKT, or mTOR inhibitors in combination with other targeted or cytotoxic agents. In our experience, patients with molecular alterations in the PI3K/AKT/mTOR pathway treated with targeted therapies have shorter survival compared to patients with alterations in the RAS/RAF/MEK or EGFR/HER/other pathways treated with the matched targeted agents, perhaps due to less-effective therapies than those for other pathways or intrinsic resistance (unpublished data). Carefully designed clinical trials, patient selection, and the elucidation of mechanisms of response and resistance to PI3K/AKT/mTOR pathway inhibitors, including protein and phosphoprotein expression with signatures of sensitivity/resistance, may improve clinical outcomes.

EPIDERMAL GROWTH FACTOR RECEPTOR

Epidermal growth factor receptor (ErbB1, HER1) is a cell surface transmembrane receptor that belongs to the EGF family of extracellular protein ligands. It is a member of the ErbB receptor family, which consists of four receptor tyrosine kinases: EGFR, HER2 (ErbB2), HER3 (ErbB3), and HER4 (ErbB4). The EGF binds to EGFR, stimulating ligand-induced dimerization, receptor dimerization, and signaling through tyrosine kinase activity, leading to activation of multiple pathways involved in cell proliferation, survival, metastases, and neoangiogenesis ([40]).

Epidermal Growth Factor Receptor–Targeted Therapies

Therapies that target EGFR include tyrosine kinase inhibitors (TKIs) and monoclonal antibodies. Gefitinib was the first selective EGFR inhibitor and was approved by the FDA in 2003 for NSCLC, but in 2005 the FDA withdrew this approval for use in new patients because gefitinib did not improve survival compared to placebo in previously treated patients ([41]).

Erlotinib

Erlotinib targets the EGFR tyrosine kinase and is approved by the FDA for first-line treatment of patients with metastatic NSCLC with tumor *EGFR* exon 19 deletions or exon 21 (L858R) substitution mutations; maintenance therapy of patients with NSCLC and no evidence of disease progression after four cycles of platinum-based first-line chemotherapy; and treatment of NSCLC after failure of one or more prior chemotherapy regimens. It is approved as first-line treatment, in combination with gemcitabine, of patients with locally advanced/metastatic pancreatic cancer. In NSCLC, erlotinib demonstrated a significant improvement in median PFS and OS compared to placebo ([42]). Mutations in the *EGFR* kinase domain predicted response to EGFR TKIs ([43, 44]). In patients with *EFGR* alterations, the response rate to EGFR TKIs ranged from 48% to 90% ([45, 46]). Randomized trials demonstrated that the use of gefitinib or erlotinib is associated with longer PFS compared to platinum doublets in patients with lung adenocarcinoma and activating EGFR mutations. However, no OS benefit was noted ([47-51]), perhaps partially due to crossover after disease progression.

In a randomized study of erlotinib versus placebo as maintenance therapy in patients with advanced NSCLC who had an objective response or SD after four cycles of a platinum-based doublet, erlotinib was associated with superior PFS in patients with adenocarcinoma or SCC. Survival benefit was noted only in patients with SCC ([52]). The role of EGFR TKIs in patients with wild-type EGFR is unclear ([53]).

The role of adjuvant erlotinib in patients with resected NSCLC and EGFR molecular alterations was investigated in a phase III trial (comparing placebo vs erlotinib) (NCT00373425) ([54]). In 973 randomized patients, there was no difference in disease-free survival between the two arms (HR, 0.90; P = .32). In a subset analysis of 161 patients with deletion 19 or L858R EGFR mutations, the median disease-free survival was 46.4 months in the erlotinib arm versus 28.5 months in the placebo arm (HR, 0.61; P = .04) ([55, 56]). In a phase II study (RTOG 1306, NCT01822496), patients with stage III EGFR-mutant lung cancer or ALK-positive NSCLC were randomized to erlotinib followed by concurrent chemoradiation, crizotinib followed by concurrent chemoradiation, or chemoradiation alone.

Afatinib

Newer agents irreversibly inhibit EGFR and target additional EGFR members, such as HER2 and HER4. Afatinib is a selective, oral inhibitor of EGFR/ErbB1, HER2, and HER4. In a phase III study of afatinib or cisplatin plus pemetrexed in patients with metastatic lung adenocarcinoma with EGFR mutations, afatinib was associated with longer PFS compared to standard doublet chemotherapy (11.1 months vs 6.9 months, respectively; P = .001) ([57]). In patients with exon 19 deletions or L858R mutations, the median PFS was 13.6 months. Development of resistance is attributed to additional *EGFR* mutations (T790M on exon 20, 50% of patients) ([58]) or *PIK3CA* mutations; *MET* or *HER2* amplification; epithelial-to-mesenchymal transformation; or transformation to small cell lung cancer. Novel third-generation EGFR TKIs that target T790M mutations such as CO-1686 (rociletinib) are being investigated.

Cetuximab

Cetuximab is a chimeric mouse-human immunoglobulin 1 monoclonal antibody against EGFR. It is indicated for the treatment of advanced SCC of the head and neck (combined with radiation therapy); recurrent or metastatic SCC of the head and neck (combined with platinum-based therapy with 5-fluorouracil); and recurrent or metastatic SCC of the head and neck that progresses after platinum-based therapy. Cetuximab with FOLFIRI (irinotecan, fluorouracil, and leucovorin) is indicated for the first-line treatment of K-RAS wild-type, EGFR-positive metastatic CRC and cetuximab with irinotecan for irinotecan-refractory patients; cetuximab monotherapy is indicated for patients with oxaliplatin- and irinotecan-refractory CRC or patients with irinotecan intolerance.

The role of cetuximab in lung cancer has not been determined. In a phase III study, the addition of cetuximab to taxane/carboplatin did not significantly improve PFS or OS ([59]). In another phase III study in patients with advanced EGFR-expressing NSCLC, the addition of cetuximab to cisplatin and vinorelbine was associated with improved OS compared to the cisplatin and vinorelbine arm (median OS, 11.3 months vs 10.1 months, respectively; *P* = .04) ([60]). The SWOG 0819 trial comparing carboplatin/paclitaxel with and without bevacizumab (in eligible patients) and/or cetuximab in stage IV or recurrent NSCLC has been suspended (NCT00946712).

Mutations and overexpression of EGFR are frequent in patients with CRC ([61]). In patients with irinotecan-refractory CRC, cetuximab demonstrated significant antitumor activity as monotherapy (overall response rate [ORR], 10.8%; median time to progression, 1.5 months; median OS, 6.9 months) or combined with irinotecan (22.9%; 4.1 months and 8.6 months, respectively) ([61]). In a phase III study, cetuximab was associated with improved survival compared to best supportive care in patients with refractory metastatic CRC (6.1 months vs 4.6 months) ([62]). In another phase III study, first-line treatment with cetuximab plus FOLFIRI reduced the risk of progression compared to FOLFIRI alone in patients with metastatic CRC, but the benefit of cetuximab was limited to patients with KRAS wild-type tumors ([63]).

In patients with previously untreated metastatic CRC, cetuximab plus FOLFOX-4 (oxaliplatin, leucovorin, and fluorouracil) was associated with a higher ORR (43% vs 36%) compared to FOLFOX-4 alone ([64]). In patients with KRAS wild-type CRC, cetuximab plus FOLFOX-4 compared to FOLFOX-4 alone was associated with a higher ORR (61% vs 37%; *P* = .01) and a lower risk of disease progression (HR, 0.57; *P* = .02). This study demonstrated that KRAS mutational status is a highly predictive selection criterion for the addition of cetuximab to FOLFOX-4 in this setting ([64]).

Panitumumab

Panitumumab is a fully humanized IgG2 anti-hEGFR antibody indicated for the treatment of patients with wild-type *KRAS* (exon 2 in codons 12 or 13) metastatic CRC as first-line therapy in combination with FOLFOX and monotherapy in fluoropyrimidine-, oxaliplatin-, and irinotecan-refractory patients. In a phase III study of panitumumab with FOLFOX4 versus FOLFOX4 alone as first-line therapy in patients with wild-type *KRAS* metastatic CRC, the addition of panitumumab to FOLFOX4 resulted in higher rates of overall response (57% vs 48%; *P* = .02), PFS (10 vs 8.6 months; *P* = .01), and OS (HR, 0.83; *P* = .03) ([65]). In a randomized study of panitumumab versus cetuximab in patients with chemotherapy-refractory wild-type *KRAS* exon 2 metastatic CRC, panitumumab was not inferior to cetuximab, and the OS benefit was similar (median OS, 10.4 vs 10 months, respectively; HR, 0.97) ([66]).

KIT

The tyrosine-protein kinase KIT (c-Kit or CD117) is a receptor tyrosine kinase protein that is encoded by the *KIT* gene. KIT regulates cell differentiation and proliferation, resists cell apoptosis, and plays an important role in tumorigenesis and migration by activating downstream signaling molecules following interaction with stem cell factor (SCF). Complete loss of KIT activity results in in utero or perinatal death; "loss of function" leads to failure of particular stem cell populations to migrate and survive. Activating mutations of *KIT* occur in almost all patients with systemic mastocytosis. In gastrointestinal stromal tumors (GISTs), activating mutations of KIT occur in more than 80% of patients; two-thirds of *KIT* mutations occur in exon 11, resulting in dysfunction of the intracellular autoinhibitory juxtamembrane domain. The majority of these mutations are indels. Deletion of exon 11 is associated with shorter PFS and OS in patients with GIST ([67]). Approximately 10% to 15% of *KIT* mutations in GIST occur in the extracellular region encoded by exon 9 (primarily in intestinal GIST). Mutations in *KIT* occur in core binding factor leukemias (17% of acute myeloid leukemia [AML]), in up to 26% of patients with testicular seminomas, and in 30% of patients with unilateral ovarian dysgerminomas ([68]). Activating *KIT* mutations and amplifications have been reported in 5% of patients with melanoma. In melanoma, *KIT* mutations occur as follows: exon 9 (5%), exon 11 (45%), exon 13 (25%), exon 17 (10%), and exon 18 (15%); more than 90% of these mutations are missense mutations. Therefore, KIT inhibition is an attractive therapeutic strategy in patients with tumor aberrations of the SCF/c-KIT signaling pathway.

Gastrointestinal Stromal Tumor

Imatinib binds directly to the ATP-binding site within KIT, competitively inhibiting ATP binding and stabilizing the kinase in the inactive conformation. In the preimatinib era, the median survival of patients with advanced GIST was less than 1.5 years. The use of imatinib in advanced GIST is associated with a median survival of approximately 5 years ([69]). In the adjuvant setting, imatinib was associated with decreased risk of relapse after surgery with curative intent. The reintroduction of imatinib after disease relapse is associated with results inferior to those for continued imatinib therapy, suggesting that imatinib should not be interrupted ([69]). Primary resistance to imatinib is noted in 10% of patients with GIST and is attributed to the type of *KIT* mutation (exon 9 mutations have a threefold higher risk of resistance than exon 11 mutations) or to suboptimal dose in patients with *KIT* exon 9 mutations ([70]). Secondary resistance is attributed to acquired mutations in the ATP-binding site (exons 13/14) that interfere with imatinib binding or in the activation loop (exons 17/18) that stabilize the active conformation of KIT ([71]). In patients with imatinib-resistant GIST tumors, sunitinib (TKI/anti-VEGF agent) demonstrated significant improvement in the median time to progression compared to placebo, leading to FDA approval for this indication ([72]). The efficacy of sunitinib in imatinib-secondary resistance is attributed to structural and enzymatic characteristics of sunitinib. Other tyrosine kinases targeted by sunitinib may play a role in its efficacy.

Regorafenib is FDA approved for TKI-resistant GIST. In a phase III study, regorafenib was associated with longer PFS than placebo (median PFS, 4.8 months vs 0.9 months, respectively; $P < .0001$) ([73]). Although antitumor activity was noted with dasatinib and sorafenib, the use of nilotinib has not shown significant antitumor activity in the third-line setting ([74]).

Inhibitors of *KIT* combined with other targeted agents may improve the outcomes of patients with *KIT* alterations and overcome resistance. A phase I study of dasatinib and ipilimumab for unresectable or metastatic GIST or other sarcomas is ongoing (NCT01643278).

Melanoma

In patients with melanoma and a *KIT* alteration, the use of imatinib was associated with an ORR of 23.3% ([75]). Patients whose disease responds to imatinib typically have activating mutations in exons 11 (L576p; response, 64%) and 13 (K462E; response, 43%). Other mutations in exon 11 (eg, V559X, V560D) are also sensitive to imatinib. Wild-type KIT amplification is not sensitive to imatinib. In smaller studies, sunitinib or nilotinib also had antitumor activity ([76, 77]).

Mastocytosis

One of the indications of imatinib is the treatment of adults with systemic mastocytosis and a non-*KIT* D816V mutation (or unknown *KIT* mutation status). A *KIT* D816V mutation, which occurs in most patients with mastocytosis, is resistant to imatinib. In a phase II clinical trial, dasatinib was associated with symptomatic benefit in patients with mastocytosis harboring a *KIT* D816V mutation ([78]). In this setting, responses have been reported with midostaurin (NCT00782067).

HUMAN EPIDERMAL GROWTH FACTOR RECEPTOR 2

As previously discussed, the HER family includes four receptors: HER1, HER2, HER3, and HER4. HER2 is involved in the regulation of proliferation and survival of epithelial cells and is considered an orphan receptor because it has no known ligand. HER1, HER3, and HER4 receptors have ligands and form homodimers or heterodimers on ligand binding. HER2 can heterodimerize with any of the other receptors and is the preferred dimerization partner, leading to autophosphorylation of tyrosine residues within the cytoplasmic domain of the receptors and initiating signal transduction via the PI3K/AKT and RAS/MAPK pathways ([79]). In breast cancer, amplification and overexpression of the *HER2* oncogene is a poor prognostic factor ([80]). Overexpression of HER2 occurs in approximately 15% to 20% of early-stage breast cancer and was historically associated with poor clinical outcomes.

Studies combining HER2-targeted therapies with other agents (PI3K, mTOR inhibitors) or immunotherapy and combinations of two or more HER2-targeted therapies (trastuzumab and TDM1; trastuzumab and pertuzumab followed by TDM1) have been completed or are ongoing (examples are NCT02073487, NCT02073916, NCT01835236, and NCT02252887).

Trastuzumab

Trastuzumab is a recombinant DNA-derived humanized monoclonal antibody that selectively binds with high affinity to the extracellular domain of HER2 protein. The antibody is an IgG1 kappa that contains human framework regions with the complementarity-determining regions of a murine antibody that binds to HER2. Trastuzumab is indicated as monotherapy for patients with metastatic breast cancer whose tumors overexpress HER2 protein and had one or more chemotherapy regimen(s) and combined with paclitaxel for patients with metastatic breast cancer whose tumors overexpress HER2 protein and who have not received chemotherapy for their metastatic disease. Approximately 15% of patients develop disease recurrence after trastuzumab therapy. Resistance to trastuzumab has been attributed to altered receptor-antibody interaction, activation of the downstream pathways by increased signaling from other members of the HER family or other receptors, or constitutive activation of downstream elements. Prospective studies are assessing the role of trastuzumab in patients whose breast cancers do not overexpress HER2.

Lapatinib

Lapatinib, a dual TKI of EGFR and HER2, has antitumor activity in trastuzumab-refractory breast cancer. Lapitinib is FDA approved in combination with capecitabine for patients with advanced or metastatic breast cancer whose tumors overexpress HER2 and who have received prior therapy, including anthracycline, taxane, and trastuzumab therapy, and letrozole for postmenopausal women with hormone receptor-positive metastatic breast cancer that overexpresses the HER2 receptor and for whom hormonal therapy is indicated.

Trastuzumab Emtansine

Trastuzumab emtansine (ado-trastuzumab emtansine, T-DM1) is an antibody-drug conjugate consisting of trastuzumab linked to the cytotoxic agent mertansine (DM1). Trastuzumab inhibits the growth of cancer cells by binding to HER2, and mertansine enters and destroys cells by binding to tubulin. T-DM1 is specifically toxic to tumor cells because it targets HER2, which is overexpressed in cancer cells. In patients with HER2-positive, trastuzumab-resistant breast cancer, T-DM1 improved survival by 5.8 months compared to lapatinib and capecitabine combination therapy ([81]). This study led to the FDA approval of T-DM1, which is indicated as monotherapy for patients with HER2-positive, metastatic breast cancer previously treated with trastuzumab with or without a taxane. Patients receiving T-DM1 should have received prior therapy for metastatic disease or developed disease recurrence during or within 6 months of completing adjuvant therapy.

Pertuzumab

Pertuzumab is a humanized monoclonal antibody that binds to the HER2 receptor and inhibits the interaction between HER2 and other HER family members (HER1, HER3, and HER4) on the surface of cancer cells. Pertuzumab is FDA approved in combination with trastuzumab and docetaxel as a neoadjuvant treatment for patients with HER2-positive breast cancer and as a treatment for patients with HER2-positive metastatic breast cancer. Clinical trials are evaluating the role of pertuzumab or T-DM1, combined with standard chemotherapy and trastuzumab, for early-stage breast cancer in the adjuvant setting.

CDK4/6 INHIBITORS

In many cancer cells, CDK4 and CDK6 mediate cell cycle control. Randomized phase II trials in patients with ER-positive metastatic breast cancer demonstrated that CDK4/6 inhibition combined with first-line endocrine treatment can improve PFS. Clinical trials with CDK4/6 inhibitors as single agents or combined with other drugs are ongoing.

ANDROGEN RECEPTOR INHIBITION

The AR is expressed in the vast majority of ER-positive breast cancers. Interestingly, a subset of ER-negative tumors also expresses AR. Ongoing clinical trials will define the role of androgen deprivation and AR blockade in ER-positive and ER-negative tumors.

BRCA1 AND *BRCA2*

Hereditary *BRCA1* and *BRCA2* mutations are associated with an increased risk of developing breast and ovarian cancer. *BRCA1/2* mutations lead to impaired double-strand DNA repair. PARP1 plays an important role in repairing single-strand breaks, and PARP1 inhibitors result in the formation of multiple double-strand breaks. Thus, the use of PARP inhibitors in tumors with *BRCA1*, *BRCA2*, or *PALB2* mutations renders the cells unable to efficiently repair DNA and makes them vulnerable to apoptosis. In phase II studies in *BRCA*-associated breast cancer, the use of PARP inhibitors was associated with clinical responses ([82]). Ongoing studies are comparing PARP inhibitors with standard chemotherapy in women with *BRCA1/2*-mutated advanced breast cancer. Clinical trials of PARP inhibitors in patients with deleterious *BRCA1/2* mutations have been completed or are ongoing in breast and ovarian cancer and in other tumor types (examples are NCT01989546, NCT02326844). The PARP inhibitors in clinical testing include olaparib (as a single agent or in combination with the PI3K inhibitors BKM120 or BYL713), veliparib, rucaparib, and talazoparib as single agents or in combination with cytotoxics.

C-MET

c-MET (or MET) is a receptor tyrosine kinase with specificity for a single ligand, the hepatocyte growth factor (HGF). Binding of HGF to MET leads to receptor dimerization and autophosphorylation of MET on its intracellular kinase domain and subsequent phosphorylation of its C-terminal docking site and juxtamembrane domain. These phosphorylation events enable activation of multiple downstream effector proteins, such as the adaptor proteins Grb2 and Gab1, leading to activation of the PI3K, Ras/RAF/MEK/ERK, PLC-γ, STATs, and FAK signaling pathways. c-MET plays a role in promoting the proliferation, survival, motility, and invasion of normal and tumor cells. It is thought c-MET promotes metastasis through increased production of HGF by hepatocytes, leading to enhanced paracrine signaling and clonal selection of metastatic cells with high MET expression ([83, 84]). c-MET promotes angiogenesis, and it is involved in the development of resistance to cytotoxic chemotherapy and VEGF or EGF receptor inhibitors. c-MET and phospho-c-MET have been associated with poor clinical outcomes in patients with CRC and lung cancer and with disease progression in patients with breast cancer and melanoma. The intracellular pathways activated by c-MET interact with receptors such as EGFR, HER2, WNT, and the insulinlike growth factor receptor 1 (IGFR1). Activation of EGFR leads to c-MET phosphorylation and activation. Activation of the WNT-β-catenin pathway results in *MET* transcription ([85]). c-MET activation can promote other growth receptor pathways, including the HER3-PI3K-AKT signaling pathway ([86]). The c-MET mutations are usually a result of sporadic somatic alterations acquired during cancer development ([83, 84, 86, 87]). Germline *MET* mutations are found in papillary renal cell carcinoma, familial gastric cancer, and CRC. Development of resistance to sunitinib ([88]), gefitinib ([86]), and erlotinib ([87]) has been in part attributed to c-MET activation. Paired analysis of tumors from patients with lung cancer whose disease stopped responding to gefitinib or erlotinib identified MET amplification as an acquired resistance mechanism in selected patients ([86]).

Targeted therapy against the HGF/MET pathway includes small-molecule inhibitors and antibodies against either HGF or MET. Cabozantinib is a small-molecule inhibitor that inhibits c-Met and VEGFR2 and is FDA approved for medullary thyroid cancer. Monoclonal antibodies include rilotumumab and ficlatuzumab. Rilotumumab was in development, but all clinical trials in advanced gastric cancer (including two phase III studies) were closed after a randomized trial demonstrated an increased death rate in the rilotumumab and chemotherapy combination arm compared to the chemotherapy arm. A phase II randomized, double-blind study is comparing ficlatuzumab plus erlotinib with placebo plus erlotinib in patients with previously untreated, metastatic, EGFR-mutated NSCLC and "BDX004-positive label" (NCT02318368). Onartuzumab is a monovalent humanized monoclonal antibody produced in *Escherichia coli* that binds to the Sema domain on the extracellular part of MET to block HGF binding. A phase III study that compared onartuzumab plus erlotinib versus erlotinib plus placebo in patients with MET-positive advanced NSCLC was discontinued owing to the lack of clinically meaningful efficacy in an interim analysis.

Clinical trials have been completed or are in development for the monoclonal antibodies against c-MET, such as LY-2875358, h224G11A, and DN30. Synthetic small-molecule unselective (crizotinib, foretinib, cabozatinib, MGCD-265) and selective (tivantinib, JNJ-38877605, AMG337, AMG208, PF-04217903, EMD-1214063, LY-2801653, and INC-280) c-MET TKIs are being investigated. A phase III trial of tivantinib plus erlotinib for the treatment of patients with locally advanced or metastatic, nonsquamous NSCLC was discontinued because it did not meet its primary end point of prolonging OS.

ANAPLASTIC LYMPHOMA KINASE

Gene rearrangements of ALK occur in 2% to 7% of patients with NSCLC. In these patients, the use of the ALK inhibitor crizotinib as first-line therapy was associated with longer PFS and less toxicity compared to chemotherapy ([89, 90]). Crizotinib is a small-molecule inhibitor initially developed to target c-MET (and is highly specific in this targeting) that is FDA approved for the treatment of ALK-positive NSCLC. A phase II trial is evaluating the role of crizotinib in predefined tumor types in patients whose tumors are harboring specific alterations in ALK or MET (NCT01524926). The next-generation ALK inhibitors were developed to overcome resistance to crizotinib, which is attributed to secondary mutations within the ALK-TK domain; EML4-ALK amplification; bypass activation of alternative signaling pathways (EGFR, c-KIT, KRAS, IGF1 receptor); and progression/occurrence of central nervous system (CNS) metastases.

Ceritinib

Ceritinib is an ATP-competitive ALK inhibitor that showed greater antitumor potency than crizotinib in preclinical studies. Ceritinib is FDA approved (accelerated process) for patients with ALK-positive NSCLC previously treated with crizotinib. In a phase I study in patients with ALK-rearranged NSCLC (n = 114) who had received 400 mg or more of ceritinib, the response rate was 58%, and the median PFS was 7 months. The response rate for crizotinib-pretreated patients was 56%. The median PFS was longer in crizotinib-naïve (10.4 months) than in crizotinib-pretreated (6.9 months) patients ([91]). In an expansion cohort of 246 patients with ALK-rearranged metastatic NSCLC treated with the MTD of 750 mg orally daily, the response rate was 58.5% (ALK inhibitor pretreated, 54.6%; ALK inhibitor naïve, 66.3%), and the median PFS was 8.2 months (6.9 months and not reached, respectively). Central nervous system responses were noted in some patients with untreated lesions.

A randomized trial for patients with ALK-rearranged metastatic NSCLC previously untreated or treated with chemotherapy and crizotinib is comparing ceritinib with pemetrexed/cisplatin or pemetrexed/carboplatin (NCT01828099). A phase III trial is comparing ceritinib with standard chemotherapy in patients with ALK-rearranged NSCLC. Other studies are investigating ceritinib as monotherapy in cholangiocarcinoma with ROS1 or ALK overexpression or in anaplastic/undifferentiated thyroid cancer with ALK alterations or in combination with targeted therapies or chemotherapy, such as with everolimus, in solid tumors and ALK-rearranged NSCLC, with chemotherapy in pancreatic cancer, with LEE011 in ALK-positive NSCLC, and with nivolumab in NSCLC.

Alectinib

Alectinib is another second-generation ALK inhibitor. In a phase I/II study of alectinib in ALK inhibitor-naïve patients with metastatic ALK-rearranged NSCLC, no DLTs were noted up to doses of 300 mg twice daily, and the response rate was 93.5%. In another phase I/II study in patients with ALK-rearranged tumors who had progressed on crizotinib treatment, the MTD of alectinib was 600 mg twice daily. The response rate during the dose escalation part of the study was 55%. In patients with known CNS metastases treated with alectinib, the response rate was 52% within the CNS. No patient initially free of CNS metastases developed new CNS lesions during treatment. A phase III trial is comparing alectinib to crizotinib in treatment-naïve patients with advanced ALK-rearranged NSCLC.

Other ALK Inhibitors

Another ALK inhibitor with antitumor activity in NSCLC is AP26113, which has activity against ALK and mutant isoforms of EGFR without activity against wild-type EGFR. Preliminary data from a phase I/II trial in crizotinib-pretreated patients demonstrated a response rate of 63%. ASP3026 is a selective, ATP-competitive ALK inhibitor with activity against wild-type ALK and against the most frequent crizotinib resistance-mediating gatekeeper mutation, L1196 M. In a phase I trial, the MTD was 125 mg, and 44% of patients with crizotinib-resistant ALK-rearranged NSCLC had a PR. TSR-011 is an inhibitor with antitumor activity against ALK and tropomyosin-related kinase. PD-06463922 is a TKI with activity against ALK and ROS1, which appears to retain its signal-blocking effects even when several ALK mutations, leading to crizotinib resistance, are present. X-396 is a small-molecule TKI blocking ALK signaling in the wild-type conformation and with considerable activity against at least two of the crizotinib resistance-mediating ALK point mutations (L1196 M and C1156Y). An ongoing phase I study demonstrated promising activity (NCT01625234). The heat shock protein 90 (HSP90) inhibitors have also demonstrated activity against ALK-rearranged NSCLC in early clinical trials. In a phase II trial of the HSP90 inhibitor ganetespib, PRs were noted in 4 of 98 patients ([92]). The HSP90-inhibiting compound AUY922 has shown promising activity.

NOTCH

Notch was identified as an oncogene in T-cell acute lymphoblastic leukemia (T-ALL) in which the (7;9) chromosomal translocation fuses the N-terminal region of the T-cell receptor beta (TCRβ) to the C-terminus of Notch1. This leads to expression of a truncated Notch1 protein that lacks the extracellular subunit and is thus constitutively active ([93]). The intracellular forms of all four Notch proteins are potentially oncogenic and capable of transforming normal cells. Deregulated expression of Notch proteins, ligands, and targets has been described in various solid tumors, including cervical, head and neck, endometrial, renal, lung, pancreatic, breast, ovarian, prostate, esophageal, hepatocellular, and gastric carcinomas; osteosarcoma; mesothelioma; melanoma; glioma; medulloblastoma; and rhabdomyosarcoma. They have also been found in T-ALL, Hodgkin lymphoma, anaplastic large-cell non–Hodgkin lymphoma (NHL), AML, B-cell chronic lymphocytic leukemia (CLL), and multiple myeloma. Notch may contribute to carcinogenesis by inhibiting differentiation, inhibiting apoptosis, or promoting proliferation. The intracellular forms of Notch induce transformation when it is expressed with oncoproteins that disable the G1-S checkpoint, such as adenovirus E1A, human papillomavirus E6 and E7, Ras, Myc, or SV40 large T antigen. Notch can activate the expression of several oncogenic pathways via direct or indirect induction of cyclins D1, D3, and A; SKP2; and c-Myc or via activation of PI3K-AKT-mTOR, nuclear factor (NF) κB and NF-κB2, β-catenin, or signal transducer and activator of transcription 3. Notch can also cooperate with oncogenic pathways such as WNT or HER2/Neu.

In addition to its cell-autonomous effects on oncogenic pathways, Notch is involved in tumor-stroma interactions and has a tumor suppressor effect in the epidermis. Notch activity has been reported in cancer stemlike cells (CSCs), which constitute a small subset of cancer cells with a stemlike phenotype that are a reservoir of self-sustaining cells with the ability to self-renew, presumably leading to recurrence. The stemlike phenotype is characterized by enhanced resistance to chemotherapy and radiotherapy, supporting the role of Notch signaling in the maintenance of breast CSCs. Neutralizing monoclonal antibodies directed against Notch 1, 2, and 3 have been used in the clinic. A phase I study of OMP-59R5, a humanized monoclonal antibody that blocks Notch 2 and Notch 3 signaling, was followed by two phase Ib/II trials: the ALPINE trial (Antibody Therapy in First-Line Pancreatic Cancer Investigating Anti-Notch Efficacy and Safety), which is testing OMP-59R5 with gemcitabine and abraxane as first-line therapy in patients with advanced pancreatic cancer, and the PINNACLE trial (Phase Ib/II Investigation of Anti-Notch Antibody Therapy With Cisplatin and Etoposide in Small Cell Lung Carcinoma Efficacy and Safety), which is testing OMP-59R5 combined with cisplatin and etoposide as first-line therapy in patients with extensive-stage small cell lung cancer.

Soluble Dll4-Fc fusion proteins, which bind Notch receptors and prevent their activation by endogenous Dll4, inhibit Notch signaling in endothelial cells, causing disorganized angiogenesis and inhibiting tumor growth. Clinical trials using the OMP-21M18 antibody are ongoing for patients with pancreatic cancer (as first-line therapy with or without abraxane), small cell lung cancer (with carboplatin and pemetrexed), and platinum-resistant ovarian cancer (with paclitaxel).

Nonselective γ-secretase inhibitors (GSIs) are also known as "Notch inhibitors." The GSI MK-0752 is being investigated in clinical trials in solid tumors and T-ALL. In a phase I trial, MK-0752 was combined with gemcitabine in patients with pancreatic ductal adenocarcinoma.

In a phase Ib trial of the GSI RO4929097 combined with exemestane in metastatic, ER-positive breast cancer, treatment was tolerable, and responses were noted (NCT01149356). The development of RO4929097 has been hampered by its pharmacokinetic liability due to the autoinduction of hepatic metabolism. GSI PF-03084014 is currently in phase I clinical trials for T-ALL and various solid tumors (NCT01981551).

In summary, deregulation of Notch proteins has been associated with cancer development and progression and with the self-propagation of CSCs. Notch-targeted therapies include nonselective GSIs, but various other agents are in development. In HER2-positive breast cancer, the effect of Notch inhibition was recurrence prevention rather than tumor volume decrease.

FIBROBLAST GROWTH FACTOR RECEPTOR

The fibroblast growth factor receptor (FGFR) family comprises four main members (*FGFR1-FGFR4*) and encodes membrane tyrosine kinase receptors involved in signaling by interacting with fibroblast growth factors. Activating mutations *FGFR3* and *FGFR4* exist ([94, 95]), but amplification of *FGFR3* and *FGFR4* has been described rarely in cancer. According to the public Cancer Genome Atlas (http://cancergenome.nih.gov), *FGFR1* amplification occurred in 3.4% of 10,648 patients and *FGFR2* amplification occurred in 0.9% of 8,352 patients. The amplifications were found in lung (16.9%), breast (13.4%), and gastric (5.1%) cancer. Amplification of *FGFR1* has been found in lung cancer, SCC of the head and neck, esophageal SCC, and breast and pancreatic cancer. Amplification of *FGFR2* has been found in gastric and breast cancer and NSCLC. In a meta-analysis, it was shown that amplification of *FGFR1* or *FGFR2* may be associated with poor OS in various cancers ([95e]). Amplification of *FGFR1* was also associated with shorter disease-free survival.

In a phase II study of brivanib (an oral, multitargeted TKI with activity against VEGF and FGFR) in recurrent or persistent endometrial cancer, the ORR was 18.6% (8 of 43 patients; CR, n = 1; PR, n = 7), and 13 patients were progression free at 6 months ([96]). Dovitinib (TKI258) is a TKI that inhibits FGFR, VEGFR, and platelet-derived growth factor receptor ([97]). In a phase II study of dovitinib in metastatic renal cell carcinoma, of 67 patients enrolled, 82.1% were previously treated with one or more VEGFR TKI and one or more mTOR inhibitor. The rates of 8-week overall response and disease control were 1.8% and 52.7%, respectively. The median PFS and the median OS were 3.7 and 11.8 months, respectively ([97]). In a phase II trial of dovitinib in 81 patients with metastatic breast cancer, unconfirmed response or SD for more than 6 months was observed in five (25%) and one (3%) patient(s), respectively, with FGFR1-amplified/HR-positive or FGFR1-nonamplified/HR-positive breast cancer. Other FGFR inhibitors that are being investigated in clinical trials include AZD4547, BAY1187982, BIBF1120, lucitanib (VEGFR-FGFR inhibitor), ponatinib, TAS-120, Debio 1347 (CH5183284), BAY1163877 (pan-FGFR inhibitor), FGF401, BGJ398 (as monotherapy or combined with BYL719), nintedanib, JNJ-42756493, GSK3052230 (combined with paclitaxel and carboplatin or docetaxel or as monotherapy), ARQ 087, BAY1179470, and FPA144. Clinical trials that set FGFR copy number as an inclusion criterion and standardization of FGFR amplification testing may improve these trials ([95]).

INSULIN-LIKE GROWTH FACTOR RECEPTOR

Insulin like growth factor (IGF) signaling plays a critical role in the growth and survival of many types of human cancer cells. Although preclinical data of several inhibitors of GF1R were promising in early-phase clinical trials, serious toxicities were observed. Larger randomized phase III trials targeting this pathway failed and led to termination of the anti-IGF1R programs ([98]).

P53 MDM2 INHIBITORS

Clinical trials with other inhibitors, such as the murine double minute 2 (MDM2) inhibitor DS-3032b; RO6839921; RO5045337 in combination with doxorubicin in soft tissue sarcoma; RO5503781; HDM201 in combination with LEE011 in liposarcoma; and HDM201 in TP53 wild-type advanced tumors, are ongoing or have been completed. To date, they have demonstrated limited, if any, antitumor activity.

FUTURE PERSPECTIVES

Breakthroughs in technology and the discovery of effective drugs have led to epic advances in the war against cancer. We first demonstrated that, in early-phase clinical trials across tumor types, targeted therapy is associated with high rates of response, PFS, and survival in patients with one targetable molecular alteration ([1, 99, 100]). Next-generation sequencing, circulating DNA and tumor cells, and other profiling will improve our understanding of tumor biology in individual patients. Currently, there is a gap between the plethora of preclinical data and the lack of effective therapies, which is at least partially due to suboptimal drug development for "driver" alterations of human cancer, the high cost of clinical trials and available drugs, and limited access of patients to clinical trials. The complexity of the development of anticancer drugs is evidenced by the high rate of failure of phase III clinical trials of various agents that showed promising results in early-phase studies. Ongoing clinical trials with innovative adaptive study design hold the promise of expediting effective drug development (NCT02152254, NCT01827384, NCT01771458, NCT01248247, NCT01042379, NCT02117167).

Further advances in cancer therapy will be associated with improved technology and bioinformatic analyses to understand dynamic changes in biology and tumor plasticity. Vertical access (changes in time) of cancer biological components to address molecular evolution and horizontal access (changes by site of disease involvement) to address tumor heterogeneity, the interaction between the cancer genome and the epigenome, and the surrounding microenvironment need to be considered. The computational sciences are expected to accelerate drug development by establishing methods to characterize the molecular interactions and analyze a large amount of data about activated pathways, cross talk, and interactions between various components of the cancer intracellular machinery. The power of computational medicine and data sharing is stimulating investigators to develop promising projects that involve the implementation of both bioinformatics and big data analyses. Finally, the development of effective therapeutic strategies, carefully designed clinical trials, and collaborative efforts among key stakeholders in cancer therapy ultimately hold the promise of curing cancer.

REFERENCES

1. Tsimberidou AM, Iskander NG, Hong DS, et al. Personalized medicine in a phase I clinical trials program: the MD Anderson Cancer Center initiative. *Clin Cancer Res*. 2012;18(22):6373-6383.
2. Von Hoff DD, Stephenson JJ Jr, Rosen P, et al. Pilot study using molecular profiling of patients' tumors to find potential targets and select treatments for their refractory cancers. *J Clin Oncol*. 2010;28(33):4877-4883.
3. Tsimberidou AM, Eggermont AM, Schilsky RL. Precision cancer medicine: the future is now, only better. *Am Soc Clin Oncol Educ Book*. 2014;34:61-69.
4. Tidyman WE, Rauen KA. The RASopathies: developmental syndromes of Ras/MAPK pathway dysregulation. *Curr Opin Genet Dev*. 2009;19(3):230-236.
5. Roberts PJ, Der CJ. Targeting the Raf-MEK-ERK mitogen-activated protein kinase cascade for the treatment of cancer. *Oncogene*. 2007;26(22):3291-3310.
6. Dong J, Phelps RG, Qiao R, et al. BRAF oncogenic mutations correlate with progression rather than initiation of human melanoma. *Cancer Res*. 2003;63(14):3883-3885.
7. Poynter JN, Elder JT, Fullen DR, et al. BRAF and NRAS mutations in melanoma and melanocytic nevi. *Melanoma Res*. 2006;16(4):267-273.
8. Griewank KG, Westekemper H, Murali R, et al. Conjunctival melanomas harbor BRAF and NRAS mutations and copy number changes similar to cutaneous and mucosal melanomas. *Clin Cancer Res*. 2013;19(12):3143-3152.
9. Curtin JA, Busam K, Pinkel D, Bastian BC. Somatic activation of KIT in distinct subtypes of melanoma. *J Clin Oncol*. 2006;24(26):4340-4346.
10. Van Raamsdonk CD, Griewank KG, Crosby MB, et al. Mutations in GNA11 in uveal melanoma. *N Engl J Med*. 2010;363(23):2191-2199.
11. Chapman PB, Hauschild A, Robert C, et al. Improved survival with vemurafenib in melanoma with BRAF V600E mutation. *N Engl J Med*. 2011;364(26):2507-2516.
12. Hauschild A, Grob JJ, Demidov LV, et al. Dabrafenib in BRAF-mutated metastatic melanoma: a multicentre, open-label, phase 3 randomised controlled trial. *Lancet*. 2012;380(9839):358-365.

13. Rochet NM, Kottschade LA, Markovic SN. Vemurafenib for melanoma metastases to the brain. *N Engl J Med.* 2011;365(25):2439-2441.
14. Long GV, Trefzer U, Davies MA, et al. Dabrafenib in patients with Val600Glu or Val600Lys BRAF-mutant melanoma metastatic to the brain (BREAK-MB): a multicentre, open-label, phase 2 trial. *Lancet Oncol.* 2012;13(11):1087-1095.
15. Flaherty KT, Robert C, Hersey P, et al. Improved survival with MEK inhibition in BRAF-mutated melanoma. *N Engl J Med.* 2012;367(2):107-114.
16. Flaherty KT, Infante JR, Daud A, et al. Combined BRAF and MEK inhibition in melanoma with BRAF V600 mutations. *N Engl J Med.* 2012;367(18):1694-1703.
17. Robert C, Dummer R, Gutzmer R, et al. Selumetinib plus dacarbazine versus placebo plus dacarbazine as first-line treatment for BRAF-mutant metastatic melanoma: a phase 2 double-blind randomised study. *Lancet Oncol.* 2013;14(8):733-740.
18. Brugger W, Triller N, Blasinska-Morawiec M, et al. Prospective molecular marker analyses of EGFR and KRAS from a randomized, placebo-controlled study of erlotinib maintenance therapy in advanced non-small-cell lung cancer. *J Clin Oncol.* 2011;29(31):4113-4120.
19. Janne PA, Shaw AT, Pereira JR, et al. Selumetinib plus docetaxel for KRAS-mutant advanced non-small-cell lung cancer: a randomised, multicentre, placebo-controlled, phase 2 study. *Lancet Oncol.* 2013;14(1):38-47.
20. Blumenschein G Jr, Smit EF, Planchard D, et al. A randomized phase 2 study of the MEK1/MEK2 inhibitor trametinib (GSK1120212) compared with docetaxel in KRAS-mutant advanced non-small cell lung cancer (NSCLC). *Ann Oncol.* 2015;26(5):894-901.
21. Cantley LC. The phosphoinositide 3-kinase pathway. *Science.* 2002;296(5573):1655-1657.
22. Zhao L, Vogt PK. Helical domain and kinase domain mutations in p110alpha of phosphatidylinositol 3-kinase induce gain of function by different mechanisms. *Proc Natl Acad Sci U S A.* 2008;105(7):2652-2657.
23. Stephens L, Anderson K, Stokoe D, et al. Protein kinase B kinases that mediate phosphatidylinositol 3,4,5-trisphosphate-dependent activation of protein kinase B. *Science.* 1998;279(5351):710-714.
24. Kim JS, Yun HS, Um HD, et al. Identification of inositol polyphosphate 4-phosphatase type II as a novel tumor resistance biomarker in human laryngeal cancer HEp-2 cells. *Cancer Biol Ther.* 2012;13(13):1307-1318.
25. Hara K, Maruki Y, Long X, et al. Raptor, a binding partner of target of rapamycin (TOR), mediates TOR action. *Cell.* 2002;110(2):177-189.
26. Hanahan D, Weinberg RA. The hallmarks of cancer. *Cell.* 2000;100(1):57-70.
27. Baselga J, Campone M, Piccart M, et al. Everolimus in postmenopausal hormone-receptor-positive advanced breast cancer. *N Engl J Med.* 2012;366(6):520-529.
28. Wagner AJ, Von Hoff DH, Lorusso PM, et al. A first-in-human phase I study to evaluate the pan-PI3K inhibitor GDC-0941 administered QD or BID in patients with advanced solid tumors. Paper presented at: ASCO Annual Meeting Proceedings. doi:10.1200/JCO.2008.18.5918 2009, Orlando Florida.
29. Moreno Garcia V, Baird RD, Shah KJ, et al. A phase I study evaluating GDC-0941, an oral phosphoinositide-3 kinase inhibitor, in patients with advanced solid tumors or multiple myeloma. *J Clin Oncol.* [ASCO Annual Meeting Proceedings] 2011;29: 3021.
30. Von Hoff DD, LoRusso P, Demetri GD, et al. A phase I dose-escalation study to evaluate GDC-0941, a pan-PI3K inhibitor, administered QD or BID in patients with advanced or metastatic solid tumors. *J Clin Oncol.* [ASCO Annual Meeting Proceedings] 2011;29:3052. doi:10.1200/JCO.2011. 36. 57422011
31. Bendell JC, Rodon J, Burris HA, et al. Phase I, dose-escalation study of BKM120, an oral pan-Class I PI3K inhibitor, in patients with advanced solid tumors. *J Clin Oncol.* 2012;30(3):282-290.
32. Arkenau H-T, Jones SF, Kurkjian C, et al. The PI3K/mTOR inhibitor BEZ235 given twice daily for the treatment of patients (pts) with advanced solid tumors. *J Clin Oncol.* [ASCO Annual Meeting Proceedings] 2012;30:abstr. 3097.
33. Krop IE, Saura C, Ahnert JR, et al. A phase I/IB dose-escalation study of BEZ235 in combination with trastuzumab in patients with PI3-kinase or PTEN altered HER2+ metastatic breast cancer. *J Clin Oncol.* [ASCO Annual Meeting Proceedings] 2012;30:abstr. 508. doi:10.1200/JCO.2011.40.5902 2012
34. Carver BS, Chapinski C, Wongvipat J, et al. Reciprocal feedback regulation of PI3K and androgen receptor signaling in PTEN-deficient prostate cancer. *Cancer Cell.* 2011;19(5):575-586.
35. Reid AH, Attard G, Ambroisine L, et al. Molecular characterisation of ERG, ETV1 and PTEN gene loci identifies patients at low and high risk of death from prostate cancer. *Br J Cancer.* 2010;102(4):678-684.
36. Fritsch C, Huang A, Chatenay-Rivauday C, et al. Characterization of the novel and specific PI3Kalpha inhibitor NVP-BYL719 and development of the patient stratification strategy for clinical trials. *Mol Cancer Ther.* 2014;13(5):1117-1129.
37. Juric D, Argiles G, Burris HA, et al. Phase I study of BYL719, an alpa-specific PI3K inhibitor, in patients with PIK3CA mutant advanced solid tumors: preliminary efficacy and safety in patients with PIK3CA mutant ER-positive metastatic breast cancer. *Cancer Res.* 2012;72(24 Suppl): Abstr. nr P6-10-07.
38. Hoeflich KP, Merchant M, Orr C, et al. Intermittent administration of MEK inhibitor GDC-0973 plus PI3K inhibitor GDC-0941 triggers robust apoptosis and tumor growth inhibition. *Cancer Res.* 2012;72(1):210-219.
39. Bedard PL, Tabernero J, Janku F, et al. A phase Ib dose-escalation study of the oral pan-PI3K inhibitor buparlisib (BKM120) in combination with the oral MEK1/2 inhibitor trametinib (GSK1120212) in patients with selected advanced solid tumors. *Clin Cancer Res.* 2015;21(4):730-738.
40. Ciardiello F, Tortora G. EGFR antagonists in cancer treatment. *N Engl J Med.* 2008;358(11):1160-1174.
41. Thatcher N, Chang A, Parikh P, et al. Gefitinib plus best supportive care in previously treated patients with refractory advanced non-small-cell lung cancer: results from a randomised, placebo-controlled, multicentre study (Iressa Survival Evaluation in Lung Cancer). *Lancet.* 2005;366(9496):1527-1537.
42. Shepherd FA, Rodrigues Pereira J, Ciuleanu T, et al. Erlotinib in previously treated non-small-cell lung cancer. *N Engl J Med.* 2005;353(2):123-132.
43. Lynch TJ, Bell DW, Sordella R, et al. Activating mutations in the epidermal growth factor receptor underlying responsiveness of non-small-cell lung cancer to gefitinib. *N Engl J Med.* 2004;350(21):2129-2139.
44. Paez JG, Janne PA, Lee JC, et al. EGFR mutations in lung cancer: correlation with clinical response to gefitinib therapy. *Science.* 2004;304(5676):1497-1500.
45. Sequist LV, Martins RG, Spigel D, et al. First-line gefitinib in patients with advanced non-small-cell lung cancer harboring somatic EGFR mutations. *J Clin Oncol.* 2008;26(15):2442-2449.
46. Cappuzzo F, Ligorio C, Janne PA, et al. Prospective study of gefitinib in epidermal growth factor receptor fluorescence in situ hybridization-positive/phospho-Akt-positive or never smoker patients with advanced non-small-cell lung cancer: the ONCOBELL trial. *J Clin Oncol.* 2007;25(16):2248-2255.
47. Mok TS, Wu YL, Thongprasert S, et al. Gefitinib or carboplatin-paclitaxel in pulmonary adenocarcinoma. *N Engl J Med.* 2009;361(10):947-957.
48. Mitsudomi T, Morita S, Yatabe Y, et al. Gefitinib versus cisplatin plus docetaxel in patients with non-small-cell lung cancer harbouring mutations of the epidermal growth factor receptor

(WJTOG3405): an open label, randomised phase 3 trial. *Lancet Oncol*. 2010;11(2):121-128.

49. Maemondo M, Inoue A, Kobayashi K, et al. Gefitinib or chemotherapy for non-small-cell lung cancer with mutated EGFR. *N Engl J Med*. 2010;362(25):2380-2388.
50. Zhou C, Wu YL, Chen G, et al. Erlotinib versus chemotherapy as first-line treatment for patients with advanced EGFR mutation-positive non-small-cell lung cancer (OPTIMAL, CTONG-0802): a multicentre, open-label, randomised, phase 3 study. *Lancet Oncol*. 2011;12(8):735-742.
51. Rosell R, Carcereny E, Gervais R, et al. Erlotinib versus standard chemotherapy as first-line treatment for European patients with advanced EGFR mutation-positive non-small-cell lung cancer (EURTAC): a multicentre, open-label, randomised phase 3 trial. *Lancet Oncol*. 2012;13(3):239-246.
52. Cappuzzo F, Ciuleanu T, Stelmakh L, et al. Erlotinib as maintenance treatment in advanced non-small-cell lung cancer: a multicentre, randomised, placebo-controlled phase 3 study. *Lancet Oncol*. 2010;11(6):521-529.
53. Garassino MC, Martelli O, Broggini M, et al. Erlotinib versus docetaxel as second-line treatment of patients with advanced non-small-cell lung cancer and wild-type EGFR tumours (TAILOR): a randomised controlled trial. *Lancet Oncol*. 2013;14(10):981-988.
54. Altorki NK, O'brien MER, Eberhardt WEE, et al. Adjuvant erlotinib versus placebo for completely resected stage IB-IIIA EGFR-positive non-small cell lung cancer: RADIANT results. *Int J Radiat Oncol*. 2014;90:S2-S3.
55. Richardson F, Richardson K, Sennello G, et al. Biomarker analysis from completely resected NSCLC patients enrolled in an adjuvant erlotinib clinical trial (RADIANT). *ASCO Meeting Abstracts*. 2009;27(15S):7520.
56. Neal JW, Pennell NA, Govindan R, et al. The SELECT study: a multicenter phase II trial of adjuvant erlotinib in resected epidermal growth factor receptor (EGFR) mutation-positive non-small cell lung cancer (NSCLC). *ASCO Meeting Abstracts*. 2012;30(15 Suppl):7010.
57. Sequist LV, Yang JC, Yamamoto N, et al. Phase III study of afatinib or cisplatin plus pemetrexed in patients with metastatic lung adenocarcinoma with EGFR mutations. *J Clin Oncol*. 2013;31(27):3327-3334.
58. Sequist LV, Waltman BA, Dias-Santagata D, et al. Genotypic and histological evolution of lung cancers acquiring resistance to EGFR inhibitors. *Sci Transl Med*. 2011;3(75):75ra26.
59. Lynch TJ, Patel T, Dreisbach L, et al. Cetuximab and first-line taxane/carboplatin chemotherapy in advanced non-small-cell lung cancer: results of the randomized multicenter phase III trial BMS099. *J Clin Oncol*. 2010;28(6):911-917.
60. Pirker R, Pereira JR, Szczesna A, et al. Cetuximab plus chemotherapy in patients with advanced non-small-cell lung cancer (FLEX): an open-label randomised phase III trial. *Lancet*. 2009;373(9674):1525-1531.
61. Cunningham D, Humblet Y, Siena S, et al. Cetuximab monotherapy and cetuximab plus irinotecan in irinotecan-refractory metastatic colorectal cancer. *N Engl J Med*. 2004;351(4):337-345.
62. Jonker DJ, O'Callaghan CJ, Karapetis CS, et al. Cetuximab for the treatment of colorectal cancer. *N Engl J Med*. 2007;357(20):2040-2048.
63. Licitra L, Storkel S, Kerr KM, et al. Predictive value of epidermal growth factor receptor expression for first-line chemotherapy plus cetuximab in patients with head and neck and colorectal cancer: analysis of data from the EXTREME and CRYSTAL studies. *Eur J Cancer*. 2013;49(6):1161-1168.
64. Bokemeyer C, Bondarenko I, Makhson A, et al. Fluorouracil, leucovorin, and oxaliplatin with and without cetuximab in the first-line treatment of metastatic colorectal cancer. *J Clin Oncol*. 2009;27(5):663-671.
65. Douillard JY, Siena S, Cassidy J, et al. Final results from PRIME: randomized phase III study of panitumumab with FOLFOX4 for first-line treatment of metastatic colorectal cancer. *Ann Oncol*. 2014;25(7):1346-1355.
66. Price TJ, Peeters M, Kim TW, et al. Panitumumab versus cetuximab in patients with chemotherapy-refractory wild-type KRAS exon 2 metastatic colorectal cancer (ASPECCT): a randomised, multicentre, open-label, non-inferiority phase 3 study. *Lancet Oncol*. 2014;15(6):569-579.
67. Andersson J, Bumming P, Meis-Kindblom JM, et al. Gastrointestinal stromal tumors with KIT edeletions are associated with poor prognosis. *Gastroenterology*. 2006;130(6):1573-1581.
68. Corless CL, Heinrich MC. Molecular pathobiology of gastrointestinal stromal sarcomas. *Annu Rev Pathol*. 2008;3:557-586.
69. Patel S. Long-term efficacy of imatinib for treatment of metastatic GIST. *Cancer Chemother Pharmacol*. 2013;72(2):277-286.
70. Heinrich MC, Corless CL, Demetri GD, et al. Kinase mutations and imatinib response in patients with metastatic gastrointestinal stromal tumor. *J Clin Oncol*. 2003;21(23):4342-4349.
71. Corless CL, Barnett CM, Heinrich MC. Gastrointestinal stromal tumours: origin and molecular oncology. *Nat Rev Cancer*. 2011;11(12):865-878.
72. Demetri GD, van Oosterom AT, Garrett CR, et al. Efficacy and safety of sunitinib in patients with advanced gastrointestinal stromal tumour after failure of imatinib: a randomised controlled trial. *Lancet*. 2006;368(9544):1329-1338.
73. Demetri GD, Reichardt P, Kang YK, et al. Efficacy and safety of regorafenib for advanced gastrointestinal stromal tumours after failure of imatinib and sunitinib (GRID): an international, multicentre, randomised, placebo-controlled, phase 3 trial. *Lancet*. 2013;381(9863):295-302.
74. Reichardt P, Blay JY, Gelderblom H, et al. Phase III study of nilotinib versus best supportive care with or without a TKI in patients with gastrointestinal stromal tumors resistant to or intolerant of imatinib and sunitinib. *Ann Oncol*. 2012;23(7):1680-1687.
75. Guo J, Si L, Kong Y, et al. Phase II, open-label, single-arm trial of imatinib mesylate in patients with metastatic melanoma harboring c-Kit mutation or amplification. *J Clin Oncol*. 2011;29(21):2904-2909.
76. Minor DR, Kashani-Sabet M, Garrido M, O'Day SJ, Hamid O, Bastian BC. Sunitinib therapy for melanoma patients with KIT mutations. *Clin Cancer Res*. 2012;18(5):1457-1463.
77. Cho JH, Kim KM, Kwon M, Kim JH, Lee J. Nilotinib in patients with metastatic melanoma harboring KIT gene aberration. *Invest New Drugs*. 2012;30(5):2008-2014.
78. Verstovsek S, Tefferi A, Cortes J, et al. Phase II study of dasatinib in Philadelphia chromosome-negative acute and chronic myeloid diseases, including systemic mastocytosis. *Clin Cancer Res*. 2008;14(12):3906-3915.
79. Jeselsohn R, Yelensky R, Buchwalter G, et al. Emergence of constitutively active estrogen receptor-alpha mutations in pretreated advanced estrogen receptor-positive breast cancer. *Clin Cancer Res*. 2014;20(7):1757-1767.
80. Slamon DJ, Clark GM, Wong SG, Levin WJ, Ullrich A, McGuire WL. Human breast cancer: correlation of relapse and survival with amplification of the HER-2/neu oncogene. *Science*. 1987;235(4785):177-182.
81. Mustacchi G, Biganzoli L, Pronzato P, et al. HER2-positive metastatic breast cancer: A changing scenario. *Crit Rev Oncol Hematol*. 2015;95(1):78-87.
82. Tutt A, Robson M, Garber JE, et al. Oral poly(ADP-ribose) polymerase inhibitor olaparib in patients with BRCA1 or BRCA2 mutations and advanced breast cancer: a proof-of-concept trial. *Lancet*. 2010;376(9737):235-244.
83. Di Renzo MF, Olivero M, Giacomini A, et al. Overexpression and amplification of the met/HGF receptor gene

during the progression of colorectal cancer. *Clin Cancer Res.* 1995;1(2):147-154.

84. Di Renzo MF, Olivero M, Martone T, et al. Somatic mutations of the MET oncogene are selected during metastatic spread of human HNSC carcinomas. *Oncogene.* 2000;19(12):1547-1555.
85. Boon EM, van der Neut R, van de Wetering M, Clevers H, Pals ST. Wnt signaling regulates expression of the receptor tyrosine kinase met in colorectal cancer. *Cancer Res.* 2002;62(18):5126-5128.
86. Engelman JA, Zejnullahu K, Mitsudomi T, et al. MET amplification leads to gefitinib resistance in lung cancer by activating ERBB3 signaling. *Science.* 2007;316(5827):1039-1043.
87. Bean J, Brennan C, Shih JY, et al. MET amplification occurs with or without T790M mutations in EGFR mutant lung tumors with acquired resistance to gefitinib or erlotinib. *Proc Natl Acad Sci U S A.* 2007;104(52):20932-20937.
88. Shojaei F, Lee JH, Simmons BH, et al. HGF/c-Met acts as an alternative angiogenic pathway in sunitinib-resistant tumors. *Cancer Res.* 2010;70(24):10090-10100.
89. Shaw AT, Kim DW, Nakagawa K, et al. Crizotinib versus chemotherapy in advanced ALK-positive lung cancer. *N Engl J Med.* 2013;368(25):2385-2394.
90. Shaw AT, Yeap BY, Solomon BJ, et al. Effect of crizotinib on overall survival in patients with advanced non-small-cell lung cancer harbouring ALK gene rearrangement: a retrospective analysis. *Lancet Oncol.* 2011;12(11):1004-1012.
91. Shaw AT, Mehra R, Kim D-W, et al. Clinical activity of the ALK inhibitor LDK378 in advanced, ALK-positive NSCLC. *J Clin Oncol.* 2013;31(Suppl): Abstr 8010.
92. Socinski MA, Goldman J, El-Hariry I, et al. A multicenter phase II study of ganetespib monotherapy in patients with genotypically defined advanced non-small cell lung cancer. *Clin Cancer Res.* 2013;19(11):3068-3077.
93. Greenwald I. Structure/function studies of lin-12/Notch proteins. *Curr Opin Genet Dev.* 1994;4(4):556-562.
94. Rugo HS, Olopade O, DeMichele A, et al. Veliparib/carboplatin plus standard neoadjuvant therapy for high-risk breast cancer: first efficacy results from the I-SPY 2 TRIAL. Paper presented at the 36th Annual San Antonio Breast Cancer Symposium; December 13, 2013; Abstract S5-02.
95. Chang J, Liu X, Wang S, et al. Prognostic value of FGFR gene amplification in patients with different types of cancer: a systematic review and meta-analysis. *PloS One.* 2014;9(8):e105524.
96. Powell MA, Sill MW, Goodfellow PJ, et al. A phase II trial of brivanib in recurrent or persistent endometrial cancer: an NRG Oncology/Gynecologic Oncology Group Study. *Gynecol Oncol.* 2014;135(1):38-43.
97. Escudier B, Grunwald V, Ravaud A, et al. Phase II results of Dovitinib (TKI258) in patients with metastatic renal cell cancer. *Clin Cancer Res.* 2014;20(11):3012-3022.
98. Yee D. Insulin-like growth factor receptor inhibitors: baby or the bathwater? *J Natl Cancer Inst.* 2012;104(13):975-981.
99. Tsimberidou AM, Ringborg U, Schilsky RL. Strategies to overcome clinical, regulatory, and financial challenges in the implementation of personalized medicine. *Am Soc Clin Oncol Educ Book.* 2013:118-125.
100. Tsimberidou AM, Wen S, Hong DS, et al. Personalized medicine for patients with advanced cancer in the phase I program at MD Anderson: validation and landmark analyses. *Clin Cancer Res.* 2014;20(18):4827-4836.

50 Applied Biostatistics

第五十章　应用生物统计学

Xuelin Huang

中文导读

本章首先从MD安德森癌症中心临床研究概况、肿瘤相关临床研究的特点以及对生物统计日益增加的需求等方面强调了生物统计中心在临床研究中扮演的重要角色。然后从临床研究设计、数据分析以及统计学预测模型建立3个方面介绍了生物统计学的进展。在临床研究设计部分，本章主要讲述了一种自适应性Ⅱ/Ⅲ期临床研究设计方法的研发背景、理论基础及应用，介绍了一种根据疗效动态调整随机方式及样本量的方法及其应用价值，这为早期药物临床研究设计尤其是样本量计算提供了新的思路；在数据分析部分，主要讲述了生物统计学在肿瘤复发、肿瘤监测以及生物标志物研究中的应用及其进展；预测模型部分主要阐述了MD安德森癌症中心的两部分工作，一是通过该中心建立TKI治疗下慢性髓系白血病患病率预测模型的过程讲述了在特定治疗模式下预测肿瘤患病率的方法，二是介绍该中心通过受试者生物标志物的变化以预测肿瘤复发及生存，并不断调整预测模型增加准确率的过程，同时讲述了生物统计学在预测模型建立中的应用价值。

INTRODUCTION

The Department of Biostatistics at the University of Texas MD Anderson Cancer Center works on developing innovative designs for clinical trials and biological experiments, analysis of complex data, and consulting and collaborating with clinical and biological investigators. Thousands of clinical trials are conducted at MD Anderson Cancer Center each year. Most of them are phase I/II trials, and a small number are phase III trials organized by biopharmaceutical companies. A large fraction of these phase I/II trials are initiated by MD Anderson investigators. Faculty members in the Department of Biostatistics are responsible for the statistical designs of these trials.

Although many statistical designs have been developed for phase I/II trials, most were not developed specifically for oncology clinical trials. Oncology trials usually have a small sample size due to the heterogeneity of patients, the large number of competing trials, and the fact that each particular subtype of cancer is a rare disease. Oncology trials need to consider multiple end points, such as tumor response, patient survival, and toxicity. To accommodate the special needs of oncology trials, the biostatisticians develop innovative adaptive designs to maximize the benefits of both patients participating in the trial and future patients, to make the most efficient use of patients as a valuable resource for competing trials, and to accelerate the drug development, discovery, and testing processes.

STATISTICAL RESEARCH ON CLINICAL TRIAL DESIGN

Faculty in the Department of Biostatistics advocate adaptive clinical trial designs ([1-7]) and other innovative early-phase designs ([8-15]). Some examples of adaptive designs are discussed next. We developed a statistical design for phase II clinical trials that better selects drug candidates for phase III trials ([11]). Currently, most phase II oncology trials use complete remission (CR) of the cancer as the primary end point. Drugs associated with higher CR rates are evaluated in subsequent phase III trials, which are usually required to demonstrate that the drug increases the patient's survival time. Although achieving CR is necessary to prolong survival, it is not a sufficient measurement because patients may experience cancer relapse shortly after achieving CR. This discrepancy is one of the major reasons for the high failure rates (60%) of phase III trials ([15]). Thus, it is desirable to evaluate survival outcomes in phase II trials. Based on these considerations, our phase II design uses information on both CR and survival. There are several innovative features of this design. It makes full use of the information that accumulates in all stages of the trial and thus saves valuable patient resources. Interim stopping rules for toxicity, futility, and efficacy are defined. To evaluate the efficacy of treatments, patients are assigned to therapy in a randomized adaptive fashion. This means that patients in the trial tend to receive the more effective treatment, and the important aspects of the dose-response relationship are determined in an efficient manner. In particular, simulation studies show that the design has better operating characteristics than traditional trial designs.

The statistical aspects of this innovative design were published in *Statistics in Medicine* ([11]), and results of the actual trial were published in *Leukemia & Lymphoma* ([16]). Free computer software to implement this design is available on the website of the Department of Biostatistics for public use. Since the software was posted in 2009, it has been downloaded hundreds of times by people around the world, and the authors have replied to numerous e-mail inquiries. The URL for the software website is https://biostatistics.mdanderson.org/SoftwareDownload/.

We developed another statistical design to make the results of phase II or III clinical trials more reliable ([6]). In clinical trials with a relatively small sample size, patient characteristics among different treatment arms may not be well balanced. This may lead to an invalid inference. For trials that utilize response-adaptive randomization, this problem may be even more severe than for trials that use equal randomization. We developed a patient allocation scheme to adjust this imbalance during response-adaptive randomization. This design ensures that the observed differences between different treatments are real, rather than being due to an imbalance of patient characteristics between the different treatment groups. Because individuals with cancer are highly heterogeneous and oncology trials usually have relatively small sample sizes (compared with trials for some other diseases), clinical investigators have always had the concerns described. This design solves this important problem. The related research has been published in *Statistics in Medicine* ([6]).

Innovative statistical designs can help conduct clinical trials more ethically and more efficiently. For example, the Department of Leukemia at MD Anderson conducted a randomized phase II study of clofarabine alone versus clofarabine in combination with low-dose cytarabine (ara-c) in previously untreated patients who were 60 years of age or older and who had acute myeloid leukemia (AML) or high-risk myelodysplastic syndrome (MDS). The maximum sample size was set to be 108. The first 20 patients were equally randomized to the two treatment arms. After that, we designed an algorithm to assign more patients to the better-performing treatment arm. The trial would be stopped early if at any time the probability that one arm was superior was greater than or equal to 95%. Using this early stopping rule, the trial was stopped after 70 patients became evaluable for response. At that time, the treatment arm of clofarabine alone had 16 patients, 5 of whom (31%) had CR. The combination arm had 54 patients, 34 of whom (63%) had CR. By using this innovative statistical design, we not only reduced the sample size (from 108 to 70), but also assigned more patients (54 vs 16) to the treatment that showed better performance. These results were published in *Blood* ([17]). Many such efficient and ethical clinical trials have been conducted ([18-30]).

DATA ANALYSIS

Faculty in the Department of Biostatistics devote great effort into genomic research ([31-48]), imaging data analysis ([49-53]), survival analysis ([54-61]), biomarker data analysis ([62, 63]), drug interactions ([64]), causal inference ([65-67]), epidemiology studies ([68-72]), and many other diverse topics. Next is a discussion of some issues in the analyses of disease recurrence, cancer screening, and biomarker studies.

Although curing cancer remains a challenge, medical advancements have successfully transitioned many types of cancer from a rapidly fatal disease to a chronic disease. After their initial treatments, patients may experience a few disease recurrences and receive different salvage treatments after each such recurrence. That is, cancer patients usually experience the following process:

> Initial treatment ➔ Disease recurrence ➔ Salvage treatment ➔ Another disease recurrence ➔ Another salvage treatment …

This is a long and complicated process. For many forms of cancer, a number of therapeutic options are available at the initial and at subsequent salvage treatment stages. In these circumstances, instead of considering only the effect of a treatment on the time to the next disease recurrence, it is important to understand the long-term effects of each treatment on the overall survival time. Optimizing treatment decisions during this process can minimize treatment toxicity, reduce drug resistance, prolong the survival time, and enhance the patient's quality of life.

The duration of disease-free survival is commonly used in medical research to compare different treatments. This method considers the time to disease recurrence or death, whichever happens first. Equating death with disease recurrence in this manner does not give sufficient penalty to treatments associated with high death rates. This is a serious problem when the lifetime after disease recurrence can be substantial. Consequently, disease-free survival is not the best basis for making treatment decisions.

A number of statistical methods have been developed to address the shortcomings of methods based on the end point of disease-free survival ([73-78]). We have been using frailty models to analyze recurrent events and a terminal event, such as death ([73-75]). We provide estimation of the effects on survival by treatment sequence ([76]). We provide new and easily implemented statistical approaches to optimize treatment sequences for recurrent diseases ([77, 78]). The optimized treatment sequences are personalized; that is, treatment decisions depend on a patient's previous response, current disease status, characteristics, and genetic biomarkers. These methods can be applied to data from randomized or nonrandomized studies.

The importance of dealing with the problem of informative censoring is well known in statistics, but it remains a challenge. We have developed a frailty model for informative censoring ([79]) and a test for informative censoring in clustered survival data ([80]). They can be used to test the presence of informative censoring, to estimate the degree of association between censoring and the risks affecting survival, and to estimate treatment effects while accounting for the informative censoring. This model can also be used to assess the correlation between different competing risks. We have developed a method for conducting sensitivity tests for survival analysis ([81]).

Screening for risk factors or early evidence of disease is important for cancer prevention. The distribution of the preclinical duration of cancer is unobservable, but knowledge of this distribution would be of great help in many situations. For example, such knowledge can help in making recommendations about optimal cancer-screening frequencies. We have developed a nonparametric method to estimate the preclinical duration distribution using data from a randomized early cancer detection trial ([82]). This estimation method is expected to have good practical use.

An important aspect of modern cancer research is the identification of molecular and genetic markers that predict an individual's cancer risk and future response to a treatment and the validation of these identified markers. We have provided a method to use in building and validating a prognostic index for biomarker studies ([83]). This method is especially useful when there are many markers under consideration, which is currently true of typical biomarker trials because of the use of high-throughput arrays and other modern biomedical technologies.

The statistical analyses we have conducted for numerous biomarker studies are crucial for the translation of laboratory research results into clinical innovations, with a frequent goal of replacing toxic chemotherapies with safe and effective targeted therapies. A good example of targeted therapy is the use of tyrosine kinase inhibitors (TKIs, such as imatinib) to successfully control chronic myeloid leukemia (CML). Working with the Department of Leukemia, we found that CCL3 (MIP-1a) plasma levels were associated with the risk of disease progression in chronic lymphocytic leukemia (CLL) ([84]). Then, we helped design a phase I/II study to determine the effects of an Syk-JAK inhibitor on this biomarker. We also found that DNA methylation predicted survival and response to therapy in patients with MDS ([28]). Another finding was that the gene that produces the protein survivin was highly expressed in leukemic stem cells and predicted poor clinical outcomes in AML ([85]). These are examples of the biomarker discoveries to which we have contributed ([86-94]).

STATISTICAL PREDICTION

Another important branch of statistics is prediction. We developed a new method for estimating the future prevalence of a particular type of cancer when it is brought under therapeutic control ([95]). This was motivated by the success of TKIs therapy, introduced around the year 2001. Since then, the all-cause annual mortality rate for CML has been reduced to 2%. More people are surviving with CML; therefore, the prevalence of CML is increasing over time.

Estimating CML prevalence in the coming years and its plateau prevalence is important for the implementation of health-care strategies and future therapeutic trials. The Department of Leukemia at MD Anderson raised this question and provided a data set of all patients with CML who have been treated at MD Anderson since 2001. With about 10 years of data, we needed to estimate the prevalence in the next 20 to 40 years. Considering the short time span covered by the data and the long time span of the prediction, this was a difficult task. Different projection methods will yield dramatically different results. To solve this problem, we first realized that using only the CML data set was not sufficient. We needed other data sources, such as the life tables of the general US population provided by the census. Our analysis integrated many factors and indicated that the prevalence of CML will continue to increase for about 40 years before reaching a near-plateau prevalence of 35 times the current annual incidence. The report of this study was published in *Cancer* ([95]). Details of this prediction are given next.

We made various attempts to conduct sensible predictions. Our first idea was to use parametric models to extrapolate to a future time. That is, we fit the 10 years (from 2001 to 2010) of survival data of patients with CML who received imatinib by using a Weibull model and then extended the model beyond 10 years. Unfortunately, this approach did not give sensible prediction results. One indication of a nonsensible prediction was that although the model fit the 10-year data well, its prediction result showed that patients with CML will have better life expectancies than the normal population of the same age mixture. We then recognized that this unrealistic outcome was not surprising because, no matter how well a parametric model fits the first 10 years of data, there is no rationale for how it would extend beyond 10 years.

Although our attempts to use parametric models failed, they provided us with important information. That is, we needed to use the life tables of the normal population to set a boundary for the survival of patients with CML. The annual all-cause mortality rate of patients with CML treated with imatinib is about 1% to 2% in the first 8 to 10 years of follow-up ([95]). This estimate is based on a patient population that has a median age of 40 to 50 years. However, as patients age, the all-cause mortality rate is anticipated to increase. Because the follow-up time for patients with CML who were treated with imatinib is only 10 years, an extrapolation is necessary for the prediction of survival beyond 10 years. We therefore compared the mortality rates of 415 patients with newly diagnosed CML who were referred to MD Anderson from 2001 to 2010 with that of the general population with the same age distribution. We used a Cox proportional hazards model to estimate the hazard ratio between these two populations. Our calculation of the hazard ratio of patients with CML (in their first 10 years since the diagnosis of CML) versus the general population with the same age distribution was 1.53. We then assumed that this trend will remain the same for the rest of the lifetimes of these two populations. Based on the hazard rates of a general population by age group, we extrapolated the mortality rates for patients with CML for all the years after their diagnosis. This approach allowed us to obtain predictions that are in a reasonable range, in contrast to our previous attempts with parametric models that yielded predictions that were totally out of range. Exploring prediction methods and comparing them to determine the best approaches for different scenarios is an interesting topic of research.

Another important prediction task is to use a patient's biomarker history to predict future disease relapse and survival time. After a cancer patient receives treatment, during each follow-up visit, new measurements are taken for many disease-related biomarkers. It would be appealing to update the patient's prognosis in a real-time fashion based on both the historical and current biomarker measurements for that individual. This task is called dynamic prediction. Landmark analysis is a tool commonly used for such a task. However, it requires a data set with a large of number of patients who have biomarker measurements taken at the same time (measured from the beginning of each patient's treatment). That is, for example, it requires patients in the data set to have follow-up visits and the appropriate measurements made on a precise posttreatment schedule, such as at exactly 3-month intervals. However, this level of follow-up precision is rarely possible. All types of conflicts and constraints commonly result in patient follow-up times that are scattered throughout the time between 3 and 6 months, 6 and 9 months, and so on. Another popular statistical tool, the Cox proportional hazard model, can be applied with biomarker measurements taken during follow-up visits as time-dependent covariates. However, this model also needs to impute biomarker values during its parameter estimation, so we face the same difficulty in its application.

To make better use of such biomarker data collected from somewhat irregular follow-up visits, we designed a new method for dynamic prediction. The idea is to start the model on the basis of a simple case and then allow it to evolve to handle complex situations. First, if we ignore all the patient characteristics and biomarker data, we may simply use the Kaplan-Meier estimator $S(t)$ to perform predictions. At any follow-up visit time u, the chance a patient will survive an additional v years is $S(u + v)/S(u)$. Then, if we would like to conduct this prediction for different subgroups of patients, such as groups defined by gender, race, disease subtypes, or other information that is available at the time of diagnosis, we may use a Cox proportional hazards model with these factors as (time-independent) covariates. This will give each patient number k an individual survival function of $S_k(t)$. Similarly, at any follow-up visit time u, the chance this patient will survive an additional v years is $S_k(u + v)/S_k(u)$. This should yield a more accurate prediction than the first method given by $S(u + v)/S(u)$.

Next, we consider using each patient's historical and current biomarkers to make the prediction even more accurate. To do this, we first need to find out what kind of summary statistics have good predictive power, such as current biomarker values or changing slopes of biomarkers. We denote these summary statistics at time t for patient number k by $Z_k(t)$. Then, we postulate a model on the patient's future survival, conditional on the patient being alive at time u, which assumes that the patient's probability of surviving at least v additional years is $\{S_k(u + v)/S_k(u)\}$ being raised to the power of $\exp\{\beta(u)' Z_k(u)\}$. We use time-varying effects $\beta(u)$, which may be specified as a fractional polynomial or cubic spline function. The only parameters we need to estimate here are those in $\beta(u)$ since $S_k(u + v)/S_k(u)$ has already been estimated from the model. This eliminates the requirement to obtain biomarker measurements from all the patients at the same time and makes the computation easy to implement.

REFERENCES

1. Berry DA. Bayesian approaches for comparative effectiveness research. *Clin Trials*. 2012;9(1):37-47. e-Pub 8/30/2011. PMID: 21878446.
2. Berry DA. Adaptive clinical trials in oncology. *Nat Rev Clin Oncol*. 2012;9(4):199-207. e-Pub 11/8/2011. PMID: 22064459.
3. Berry DA. Commentary on Hey and Kimmelman. *Clin Trials*. 1740774515569011, first published February 3, 2015, as doi:10.1177/1740774515569011
4. Lee JJ. Commentary on Hey and Kimmelman. *Clin Trials*. 1740774514568875, first published February 3, 2015, as doi:10.1177/1740774514568875
5. Thall PF, Nguyen HQ, Braun TM, Qazilbash MH. Using joint utilities of the times to response and toxicity to adaptively optimize schedule-dose regimes. *Biometrics*. 2013;69(3):673-682. e-Pub 8/19/2013. PMCID: PMC3963428.
6. Ning J, Huang X. Response-adaptive randomization for clinical trials with adjustment for covariate imbalance. *Stat Med*. 2010;29(17):1761-178. PMCID: PMC2911996.
7. Yuan Y, Huang X, Liu S. A Bayesian response-adaptive covariate-balanced randomization design with application to a leukemia clinical trial. *Stat Med*. 2011;30(11):1218-1229. e-Pub 3/2011. PMCID: PMC3086983.
8. Hobbs BP, Carlin BP, Mandrekar SJ, Sargent DJ. Hierarchical commensurate and power prior models for adaptive incorporation of historical information in clinical trials. *Biometrics*. 2011;67(3):1047-1056. e-Pub 3/2011. PMCID: PMC3134568.
9. Hobbs BP, Carlin BP, Sargent DJ. Adaptive adjustment of the randomization ratio using historical control data. *Clin Trials*. 2013;10(3):430-440. PMCID: PMC3856641.
10. Huang X, Biswas S, Oki Y, Issa JP, Berry DA. A parallel phase I/II clinical trial design for combination therapies. *Biometrics*. 2007;63(2):429-436.
11. Huang X, Ning J, Li Y, Estey E, Issa JP, Berry DA. Using short-term response information to facilitate adaptive randomization for survival clinical trials. *Stat Med*. 2009;28(12):1680-1689. PMCID: PMC2883264.
12. Thall PF, Szabo A, Nguyen HQ, Amlie-Lefond CM, Zaidat OO. Optimizing the concentration and bolus of a drug delivered by continuous infusion. *Biometrics*. 2011;67(4):1638-1646. e-Pub 3/14/2011. PMCID: PMC3137757.
13. Braun TM, Thall PF, Nguyen H, de Lima M. Simultaneously optimizing dose and schedule of a new cytotoxic agent. *Clin Trials*. 2007;4(2):113-124. PMID: 17456511.
14. Liu S, Pan H, Xia J, Huang Q, Yuan Y. Bridging continual reassessment method for phase I clinical trials in different ethnic populations. *Stat Med*. 2015 Jan 28. doi:10.1002/sim.6442
15. Ji Y, Liu P, Li Y, Bekele BN. A modified toxicity probability interval method for dose-finding trials. *Clin Trials*. 2010;7(6):653-663. PMID: 20935021.
16. Borthakur G, Huang X, Kantarjian H, et al. Report of a phase 1/2 study of a combination of azacitidine and cytarabine in acute myelogenous leukemia and high-risk myelodysplastic syndromes. *Leuk Lymphoma*. 2010;51(1):73-78. PMCID: PMC2876330.
17. Faderl S, Ravandi F, Huang X, et al. A randomized study of clofarabine versus clofarabine plus low-dose cytarabine as front-line therapy for patients aged 60 years and older with acute myeloid leukemia and high-risk myelodysplastic syndrome. *Blood*. 2008;112(5):1638-1645. e-Pub 6/2008.

18. Kantarjian H, Oki Y, Garcia-Manero G, et al. Results of a randomized study of 3 schedules of low-dose decitabine in higher-risk myelodysplastic syndrome and chronic myelomonocytic leukemia. *Blood*. 2007;109(1):52-57. e-Pub 8/2006.
19. Kantarjian HM, O'Brien S, Huang X, et al. Survival advantage with decitabine versus intensive chemotherapy in patients with higher risk myelodysplastic syndrome: comparison with historical experience. *Cancer*. 2007;109(6):1133-1137. PMCID: PMC2952542.
20. O'Brien S, Ravandi F, Riehl T, et al. Valganciclovir prevents cytomegalovirus reactivation in patients receiving alemtuzumab-based therapy. *Blood*. 2008;111(4):1816-1819. e-Pub 11/2007.
21. Faderl S, Ferrajoli A, Wierda W, et al. Clofarabine combinations as acute myeloid leukemia salvage therapy. *Cancer*. 2008;113(8):2090-2096.
22. Garg R, Faderl S, Garcia-Manero G, et al. Phase II study of rabbit anti-thymocyte globulin, cyclosporine and granulocyte colony-stimulating factor in patients with aplastic anemia and myelodysplastic syndrome. *Leukemia*. 2009;23(7):1297-1302. e-Pub 2/2009.
23. Ravandi F, Aribi A, O'Brien S, et al. Phase II study of alemtuzumab in combination with pentostatin in patients with T-cell neoplasms. *J Clin Oncol*. 2009;27(32):5425-5430. e-Pub 10/2009.
24. Kadia TM, Borthakur G, Garcia-Manero G, et al. Final results of the phase II study of rabbit anti-thymocyte globulin, ciclosporin, methylprednisone, and granulocyte colony-stimulating factor in patients with aplastic anaemia and myelodysplastic syndrome. *Br J Haematol*. 2012;157(3):312-320. e-Pub 2/2012. PMCID: PMC3924750.
25. Jabbour E, Garcia-Manero G, Cortes J, et al. Twice-daily fludarabine and cytarabine combination with or without gentuzumab ozogamicin is effective in patients with relapsed/refractory acute myeloid leukemia, high-risk myelodysplastic syndrome, and blast- phase chronic myeloid leukemia. *Clin Lymphoma Myeloma Leuk*. 2012;12(4):244-251. e-Pub 4/2012. PMCID: PMC3859239.
26. Faderl S, Ravandi F, Huang X, et al. Clofarabine plus low-dose cytarabine followed by clofarabine plus low-dose cytarabine alternating with decitabine in acute myeloid leukemia frontline therapy for older patients. *Cancer*. 2012;118(18):4471-4477. e-Pub 1/2012. PMCID: PMC3907176.
27. Nazha A, Kantarjian H, Ravandi F, et al. Clofarabine, idarubicin, and cytarabine (CIA) as frontline therapy for patients ≤; 60 years with newly diagnosed acute myeloid leukemia (AML). *Am J Hematol*. 2013;88(11):961-966. e-Pub 9/2013. PMCID: PMC4110914.
28. Issa JP, Garcia-Manero G, Huang X, et al. Results of phase II randomized study of low-dose decitabine with or without valproic acid in patients with myelodysplastic syndrome and acute myelogenous leukemia. *Cancer*. 2015;121(4):445-561.
29. Burger JA, Keating MJ, Wierda WG, et al. Safety and activity of ibrutinib plus rituximab for patients with high-risk chronic lymphocytic leukaemia: a single-arm, phase 2 study. *Lancet Oncol*. 2014;15(10):1090-1099. e-Pub 8/2014. PMCID: PMC4174348.
30. Doecke JD, Chekouo T, Stingo FC, Do K-A. miRNA target gene identification: sourcing miRNA-target gene relationships for the analyses of TCGA Illumina miSeq and RNA-Seq Hiseq platform data. *Int J Hum Gen*. 2014;14(1):17-22.
31. Chavez-Macgregor M, Liu S, De Melo-Gagliato D, et al. Differences in gene and protein expression and the effects of race/ethnicity on breast cancer subtypes. *Cancer Epidemiol Biomarkers Prev*. 2014;23(2):316-323. e-Pub 12/2/2013. PMCID: PMC3946290.
32. Liu Y, Zhou R, Baumbusch LO, et al. Genomic copy number imbalances associated with bone and non-bone metastasis of early-stage breast cancer. *Breast Cancer Res Treat*. 2014;143(1):189-201. e-Pub 12/2013. PMID: 24305980.
33. Gorlov IP, Yang JY, Byun J, et al. How to get the most from microarray data: advice from reverse genomics. *BMC Genomics*. 2014;15:223. e-Pub 3/21/2014. PMCID: PMC3997969.
34. Leon-Novelo LG, Mueller P, Arap W, Sun J, Pasqualini R, Do KA. Bayesian decision theoretic multiple comparison procedures: an application to phage display data. *Biomed J*. 2013;55(3):478-489. e-Pub 12/2012. PMCID: PMC3840910.
35. Leon-Novelo LG, Mueller P, Arap W, et al. Semiparametric Bayesian Inference for Phage Display Data. *Biometrics*. 2013;69(1):174-183. e-Pub 1/2013. PMCID: PMC3622196.
36. Wang W, Baladandayuthapani V, Morris JS, Broom BM, Manyam G, Do KA. iBAG: integrative Bayesian analysis of high-dimensional multi-platform genomics data. *Bioinformatics*. 2013;29(2):149-159. e-Pub 11/9/2012. PMCID: PMC3546799.
37. Wang W, Baladandayuthapani V, Holmes CC, Do KA. Integrative network-based Bayesian analysis of diverse genomics data. *BMC Bioinformatics*. 2013;14(Suppl 13):S8. e-Pub 10/2013. PMCID: PMC3849715.
38. Bonato V, Baladandayuthapani V, Broom BM, Sulman EP, Aldape KD, Do KA. Bayesian ensemble methods for survival prediction in gene expression data. *Bioinformatics*. 2011;27(3):359-367. e-Pub 12/2010. PMCID: PMC3031034.
39. Hess KR, Wei C, Qi Y, Iwamoto T, Symmans WF, Pusztai L. Lack of sufficiently strong informative features limits the potential of gene expression analysis as predictive tool for many clinical classification problems. *BMC Bioinformatics*. 2011;12(463). PMCID: PMC3245512.
40. Hu J, He X. Searching for alternative splicing with a joint model on probe measurability and expression intensities. *J Am Stat Assoc*. 2012;107(499):935-945.
41. Maadooliat M, Huang JZ, Hu J. Analyzing multiple-probe microarray: estimation and application of gene expression indexes. *Biometrics*. 2012;68(3):784-792. e-Pub 7/2012. PMCID: PMC3989902.
42. Guindani M, Sepúlveda N, Paulino CD, Müller P. A Bayesian semi-parametric approach for the differential analysis of sequence counts data. *J R Stat Soc Ser C Appl Stat*. 2014;63(3):385-404. PMCID: PMC4017673.
43. Ni Y, Stingo FC, Baladandayuthapani V. Integrative Bayesian network analysis of genomic data. *Cancer Inform*. 2014;2:39-48. PMCID: PMCPMC4179606.
44. Stingo FC, Guindani M, Vannucci M, Calhoun VD. An integrative Bayesian modeling approach to imaging genetics. *J Am Stat Assoc*. 2013;108(105):876-891. PMCID: PMC3843531.
45. Stingo FC, Chen YA, Tadesse MG, Vannucci M. Incorporating biological information into linear models: a Bayesian approach to the selection of pathways and genes. *Ann Appl Stat*. 2011;5(3):1978-2002. PMCID: PMC3650864.
46. Stingo FC, Vannucci M. Variable selection for discriminant analysis with Markov random field priors for the analysis of microarray data. *Bioinformatics*. 2011;27(4):495-501. e-Pub 12/14/2010. PMCID: PMC3105481.
47. Stingo FC, Chen YA, Vannucci M, Barrier M, Mirkes PE. A Bayesian graphical modeling approach to microRNA regulatory network inference. *Ann Appl Stat*. 2010;4(4):2024-2048. PMCID: PMC3740979.
48. Baladandayuthapani V, Ji Y, Talluri R, Nieto-Barajas LE, Morris JS. Bayesian random segmentation models to identify shared copy number aberrations for array CGH data. *J Am Stat Assoc*. 2010;105(492):1358-1375. PMCID: PMC3079218.
49. Zhu H, Brown PJ, Morris JS. Robust classification of functional and quantitative image data using functional mixed models. *Biometrics*. 2012;68(4):1260-1268. e-Pub 6/6/2012. PMCID: PMC3443537.

50. Zhu H, Brown PJ, Morris JS. Robust, adaptive functional regression in functional mixed model framework. *J Am Stat Assoc.* 2011;106(495):1167-1179. PMCID: PMC3270884.
51. Morris JS, Baladandayuthapani V, Herrick RC, Sanna P, Gutstein H. Automated analysis of quantitative image data using isomorphic functional mixed models, with application to proteomics data. *Ann Appl Stat.* 2011;5(2A):894-923. PMCID: PMC3298181.
52. Morris JS, Clark BN, Wei W, Gutstein HB. Evaluating the performance of new approaches to spot quantification and differential expression in 2-dimensional gel electrophoresis studies. *J Proteome Res.* 2010;9(1):595-604. e-Pub 12/2009. PMCID: PMC2802214.
53. Zhang L, Guindani M, Vannucci M. Bayesian models for fMRI data analysis. *WIREs Comput Stat.* 2015;7:21-41. NIHMSID: NIHMS657892.
54. Hess KR. Comparing survival curves using an easy to interpret statistic. *Clin Cancer Res.* 2010;16(20):4912-4913. e-Pub 8/2010. PMID: 20732962.
55. Qin J, Ning J, Liu H, Shen Y. Maximum likelihood estimations and EM algorithms with length-biased data. *J Am Stat Assoc.* 2011;106(496):1434-1449. PMCID: PMC3273908.
56. Ning J, Qin J, Shen Y. Score estimating equations from embedded likelihood functions under accelerated failure time model. *J Am Stat Assoc.* 2014;109(508):1625-1635. PMID: 25663727
57. Shen Y, Qin J, Costantino JP. Inference of tamoxifen's effects on prevention of breast cancer from a randomized controlled trial. *J Am Stat Assoc.* 2007;102(480):1235-1244. PMCID: PMC2721282.
58. Qin J, Shen Y. Statistical methods for analyzing right-censored length-biased data under Cox model. *Biometrics.* 2010;66(2): 382-392. e-Pub 6/2009. PMCID: PMC3035941.
59. Liu H, Shen Y. A semiparametric regression cure model for interval-censored data. *J Am Stat Assoc.* 2009;104(487):1168-1178. PMCID: PMC2846840.
60. Choi S, Huang X. A semiparametric inverse-Gaussian model and inference for survival data with a cured proportion. *Can J Stat.* 2014;42(4):635-649. doi:10.1002/cjs.11226
61. Choi S, Huang X. Maximum likelihood estimation of semiparametric mixture component models for competing risks data. *Biometrics.* e-Pub 4/2014. doi:10.1111/biom.12167. PMID: 24734912.
62. Zheng Y, Cai T, Jin Y, Feng Z. Evaluating prognostic accuracy of biomarkers under competing risk. *Biometrics.* 2012;68(2):388-396. e-Pub 12/7/2011. PMCID: PMC3694786.
63. Huang Y, Fong Y, Wei J, Feng Z. Borrowing information across populations in estimating positive and negative predictive values. *J R Stat Soc Ser C Appl Stat.* 2011;60(5):633-653. PMCID: PMC3196635.
64. Kong M, Lee JJ. A semiparametric response surface model for assessing drug interaction. *Biometrics.* 2008;64(2):396-405. e-Pub 9/26/2007. PMID: 17900314.
65. Li Y, Mueller P, Lin X. Center-adjusted inference for a nonparametric Bayesian random effect distribution. *Stat Sin.* 2011;21(3):1201-1223.
66. Li L, Hu B, Kattan MW. Modeling potential time to event data with competing risks. *Lifetime Data Anal.* 2014;20(2):316-334. e-Pub 9/24/2013. PMID: 24061908.
67. Li L, Greene T. A weighting analogue to pair matching in propensity score analysis. *Int J Biostat.* 2013;9(2):215-234. e-Pub 7/2013. PMID: 23902694.
68. Wang J, Yu, R, Shete S. Comparison of multilevel modeling and the family-based association test (FBAT) for identifying genetic variants associated with systolic and diastolic blood pressure using GAW18 simulated data. *BMC Proc.* 2014;8(Suppl 1):S30.
69. Wang J, Yu R, Shete S. X-chromosome genetic association test accounting for X-inactivation, skewed X-inactivation, and escaping of X-inactivation. *Genet Epidemiol.* 2014;38(6):483-493. PMCID: PMC4127090.
70. Talluri R, Shete S. Gaussian graphical models for phenotypes using pedigree data and exploratory analysis using networks with genetic and non-genetic factors in GAW18 data. *BMC Proc.* 2014;8(Suppl 1):S99.
71. Talluri R, Wang J, Shete S. Calculation of exact p-values when SNPs are tested using multiple genetic models. *BMC Genet.* 2014;15(1):10.1186/1471-2156-15-75. PMCID: PMC4076502.
72. Talluri R, Wilkinson A, Spitz M, Shete S. A risk prediction model for smoking experimentation in Mexican American youth. *Cancer Epidemiol Biomarkers Prev.* 2014;23(10):2165-2174. PMCID: PMC4184980.
73. Liu L, Wolfe RA, Huang X. Shared frailty model for recurrent events and a terminal event. *Biometrics.* 2004;60(3):747-656.
74. Liu L, Huang X, O'Quigley J. Analysis of longitudinal data in the presence of informative observational times and a dependent terminal event, with application to medical cost data. *Biometrics.* 2008;64(3):950-958. e-Pub 12/2007.
75. Liu L, Huang X. Joint analysis of correlated repeated measures and recurrent events processes in the presence of death, with application to an AIDS study. *J R Stat Soc Ser C Appl Stat.* 2009;58(1):65-81.
76. Huang X, Cormier JN, Pisters PW. Estimation of the causal effects on survival of two-stage nonrandomized treatment sequences for recurrent diseases. *Biometrics.* 2006;62(3): 901-909.
77. Huang X, Ning J. Analysis of multi-stage treatments for recurrent diseases. *Stat Med.* 2012;31(24):2805-2821. e-Pub 7/2012. PMCID: PMC3500149.
78. Huang X, Ning J, Wahed AS. Optimization of individualized dynamic treatment regimes for recurrent diseases. *Stat Med.* 2014;33(14):2363-2378. e-Pub 2/2014. PMCID: PMC4043865.
79. Huang X, Wolfe RA. A frailty model for informative censoring. *Biometrics.* 2002;58(3):510-520.
80. Huang X, Wolfe RA, Hu C. A test for informative censoring in clustered survival data. *Stat Med.* 2004;23(13):2089-2107.
81. Huang X, Zhang N. Regression survival analysis with an assumed copula for dependent censoring: a sensitivity analysis approach. *Biometrics.* 2008;64(4):1090-1099. e-Pub 2/2008.
82. Shen Y, Huang X. Nonparametric estimation of asymptomatic duration from a randomized prospective cancer screening trial. *Biometrics.* 2005;61(4):992-999.
83. Huang X, Biswas S, Estey EH, Berry DA. Building and validating a prognostic index for biomarker studies. *Cancer Biomark.* 2006;2(3-4):97-101.
84. Sivina M, Hartmann E, Kipps TJ, et al. CCL3 (MIP-1a) plasma levels and the risk for disease progression in chronic lymphocytic leukemia. *Blood.* 2011;117(5):1662-1669. e-Pub 11/2010. PMCID: PMC3318778.
85. Carter BZ, Qiu Y, Huang X, et al. Survivin is highly expressed in CD34(+)38(-) leukemic stem/progenitor cells and predicts poor clinical outcomes in AML. *Blood.* 2012;120(1):173-180. e-Pub 5/2012. PMCID: PMC3390955.
86. Konoplev S, Rassidakis GZ, Estey E, et al. Overexpression of CXCR4 predicts adverse overall and event-free survival in patients with unmutated FLT3 acute myeloid leukemia with normal karyotype. *Cancer.* 2007;109(6):1152-1156.
87. Anaya DA, Xing Y, Feng L, et al. Adjuvant high-dose interferon for cutaneous melanoma is most beneficial for patients with early stage III disease. *Cancer.* 2008;112(9):2030-2037.
88. Konoplev S, Huang X, Drabkin HA, et al. Cytoplasmic localization of nucleophosmin in bone marrow blasts of acute myeloid leukemia patients is not completely concordant with NPM1 mutation and is not predictive of prognosis. *Cancer.* 2009;115(20):4737-4744.
89. Walter RB, Kantarjian HM, Huang X, et al. Effect of complete remission and responses less than complete remission on survival in acute myeloid leukemia: a combined Eastern Cooperative

Oncology Group, Southwest Oncology Group, and M.D. Anderson Cancer Center study. *J Clin Oncol.* 2010;28(10):1766-1771. e-Pub 2/2010. PMCID: PMC2849766.

90. Chen Y, Cortes J, Estrov Z, et al. Persistence of cytogenetic abnormalities at complete remission after induction in patients with acute myeloid leukemia: prognostic significance and the potential role of allogeneic stem-cell transplantation. *J Clin Oncol.* 2011;29(18):2507-2513. e-Pub 5/2011.
91. Kojima K, McQueen T, Chen Y, et al. p53 activation of mesenchymal stromal cells partially abrogates microenvironment-mediated resistance to FLT3 inhibition in AML through HIF-1α-mediated down-regulation of CXCL12. *Blood.* 2011;118(16):4431-4439. e-Pub 8/2011. PMCID: PMC3204912.
92. Ravandi F, Jorgensen JL, Thomas DA, et al. Detection of MRD may predict the outcome of patients with Philadelphia chromosome-positive ALL treated with tyrosine kinase inhibitors plus chemotherapy. *Blood.* 2013;122(7):1214-1221. e-Pub 7/2013. PMCID: PMC3976223.
93. Pierceall WE, Kornblau SM, Carlson NE, et al. BH3 profiling discriminates response to cytarabine-based treatment of acute myeloid leukemia. *Mol Cancer Ther.* 2013;12(12):2940-2949. e-Pub 10/2013. PMCID: PMC3881173.
94. Mak PY, Mak DH, Mu H, et al. Apoptosis repressor with caspase recruitment domain is regulated by MAPK/PI3K and confers drug resistance and survival advantage to AML. *Apoptosis.* 2014;19(4):698-707. PMCID: PMC3943601.
95. Huang X, Cortes J, Kantarjian H. Estimations of the increasing prevalence and plateau prevalence of chronic myeloid leukemia in the era of tyrosine kinase inhibitor therapy. *Cancer.* 2012;118(12):3123-3217. e-Pub 1/2012. PMCID: PMC3342429.

Section XIV

Supportive Care

Section Editor: Karen H. Lu

第十四篇　支持治疗

51

Fungal and Viral Infections in Cancer Patients

第五十一章　肿瘤患者的真菌和病毒感染

Bruno P. Granwehr
Roy F. Chemaly
Dimitrios P. Kontoyiannis

中文导读

真菌和病毒感染是癌症患者发病率和死亡率的重要原因，因此，癌症感染的现代管理需要了解真菌和病毒感染方面的具体知识。本章分别介绍了真菌感染和病毒感染两个方面的内容。真菌感染部分，首先概括介绍了肿瘤患者接触真菌感染的自体因素及环境因素，活检、影像等诊断手段，以及癌症患者发生真菌感染的高危因素。接着分别详细阐述了假丝酵母菌、曲霉、隐球菌、镰刀菌、毛霉以及一些罕见特有真菌（如组织胞浆菌病、球孢子菌病）等不同真菌感染的流行病学、发病机制、临床表现以及治疗方面的内容，最后针对真菌感染的辅助治疗手段如白细胞输注、细胞因子治疗、手术切除等方面进行了简要的推荐。病毒感染部分，本章分别对人类疱疹病毒、单纯疱疹病毒、带状疱疹病毒、巨细胞病毒、人类疱疹病毒6、EB病毒、社区呼吸道病毒、肝炎病毒、腺病毒、细小病毒B19及多瘤病毒感染的流行病学、发病机制、高危因素、临床表现及治疗手段以及预后方面进行了解析。

INTRODUCTION

Fungal and viral infections remain a significant cause of morbidity and mortality in patients with cancer. Modern management of infections in cancer requires knowledge of the epidemiology, pathogenesis, treatment, and prevention of such infections. Fungal infections range from nosocomial infections with *Candida* spp to endemic fungi acquired outside the hospital, such as *Histoplasma capsulatum*. Opportunistic fungi, especially molds, have emerged as a leading cause of death in patients with leukemia or hematopoietic stem cell transplant (HSCT) ([1]). Viral infections such as varicella zoster virus (VZV), herpes simplex virus (HSV), or cytomegalovirus (CMV), have been associated with increased morbidity and mortality in patients with cancer, including patients with multiple myeloma or chronic lymphocytic leukemia (CLL), and in HSCT recipients ([2-5]). Respiratory viruses, such as respiratory syncytial (RSV), adenovirus, and influenza, are increasingly recognized as significant pathogens in patients with cancer, particularly as molecular diagnostic methods improve. In addition, viruses such as novel influenza H1N1, West Nile virus, bocaviruses, and noroviruses have emerged as newly recognized pathogens in patients with cancer.

FUNGAL INFECTIONS

Fungal infections pose a continuing challenge for oncology patients. Exposure to fungi is common, with exposure typically occurring in the environment. Patients with cancer are susceptible not only to new infection with endemic fungi (such as *Histoplasma capsulatum*), but also to reactivation of latent infections. Opportunistic molds, such as *Fusarium* spp, *Scedosprorium* spp, and Zygomycetes cause devastating disease in hematologic patients. Cases of nosocomial infection due to molds are reported in the setting of hospital construction, leading to routine air sampling and filtration. In contrast, *Candida* spp are a common component of the patient's or health-care workers' endogenous microbial flora. Manifestations of infection may not present until the patient receives chemotherapy or undergoes HSCT.

Diagnosis of invasive fungal infections is problematic as well, despite increased use of fungal biomarkers ([6]). The skin and lungs are accessible areas for examination and biopsy as they are commonly affected by fungal pathogens. In our institution, a retrospective study of skin biopsies in patients with leukemia suggested that ulcerated or necrotic skin lesions in the context of bacteremia or fungemia were predictive of infection ([7]). Of note, skin biopsy revealed infection in 39% of all patients undergoing biopsy and 55% of those with severe neutropenia ([7]). Of patients with biopsy-proven skin infection, 39% of those infections were fungal, led by *Candida* species (25%), *Fusarium* (19%), Mucorales (13%), *Aspergillus* species (9%), *Alternaria* (6%), and *Curvularia* (3%) ([7]).

In the setting of pulmonary nodules, lung biopsy, utilizing open biopsy or computed tomographic (CT)–guided percutaneous biopsy, has also proven useful in diagnosis. Studies of CT-guided biopsy show a yield of approximately 60% for a specific diagnosis ([8]). In a study at our center of patients with hematologic malignancy, 34% of the specific diagnoses with CT-guided biopsy were previously unidentified infection, predominantly fungal ([9]). A recent retrospective study of open lung biopsy revealed 19% previously undiagnosed infectious etiologies ([8]). Identified organisms included 58% endemic molds (*Histoplasma*, *Coccidioides*), 14% *Aspergillus* species, and 7% *Cryptococcus* species ([9]).

Despite these efforts, diagnosis is often a challenge if infection is more diffuse or thrombocytopenia is too severe to safely permit biopsy. Autopsy, unfortunately after all diagnostic and treatment efforts failed, has historically been an approach to ultimate diagnosis of etiology, but autopsy rates have fallen almost 90% from 0.63/100 deaths in 1989 to 1993 to 0.06/100 deaths in 2004 to 2008 at our institution ([10]). Diagnosis of fungal infections, often manifesting as pulmonary nodules or skin lesions, is challenging, but important, given the modification of therapy that may occur based on identification of a particular species of fungus or discovery of coinfection, malignancy, or other alternative diagnosis. Figure 51-1 suggests an approach to identification of fungal (and other) pulmonary pathogens at our institution.

Risk Factors

Severe neutropenia, particularly prolonged, has long been associated with invasive fungal infections. Chemotherapy resulting in prolonged and severe CD4 lymphocytopenia can also result in infections similar to those seen in patients with untreated human immunodeficiency virus (HIV) or AIDS, such as cryptococcosis and reactivation of endemic fungi, including histoplasmosis and coccidiomycosis. In addition, conditioning regimens for stem cell transplant and immunosuppressives to treat or prevent graft-versus-host disease (GVHD) result in deficient cell-mediated immunity, increasing risk for invasive fungal infection ([4, 10]). Disruption of mucocutaneous barriers predisposes to invasive candidal infection, exemplified by catheter-related bloodstream infections caused by *Candida* spp ([11]).

A recent study from Italy utilized a retrospective cohort of patients with hematologic malignancy to develop a risk prediction score for invasive fungal infections ([4]). The score emphasizes the central roles played by lymphopenia, relapsed or refractory malignancy, prolonged neutropenia (>10 days), and prior history of invasive fungal infection in identifying patients at highest risk of invasive fungal infection. Of interest, the authors found that posaconazole prophylaxis was exclusively beneficial to the group with highest risk of invasive fungal infection ([4]).

Finally, another aspect of importance is the change in flora that takes place with broad-spectrum antibacterial and antifungal therapy. The latter may result in suppression of normal bacterial flora and candidal overgrowth in the oropharynx and gastrointestinal (GI) tract. Antifungal therapy or prophylaxis may result in breakthrough infection with non–*Candida albicans* species, such as *Candida krusei* (resistant to fluconazole) ([11]). Aside from non–*Candida albicans* species, prophylaxis with non–mold active antifungals (eg, fluconazole) may predispose to infection with molds, such as aspergillosis.

CANDIDIASIS

Candidiasis remains the most common invasive fungal infection in patients with cancer. Modern medical care is increasingly complex, involving frequent antimicrobial use and device utilization that alter patient flora and disrupt the mucocutaneous barrier. *Candida* spp commonly arise from the patient's endogenous flora, but rare hospital-acquired cases have been reported due to contaminated equipment, solutions, and hospital personnel. Manifestations of candidiasis range from local infection of the skin or oral mucosa to candidemia and widely disseminated infection.

Superficial Candidiasis

Oral Infection

Thrush is the most common superficial candidal infection among patients with cancer, typically those with cancers involving the head and neck undergoing chemoradiation ([12]). Oropharyngeal candidiasis is characterized by whitish plaques on the buccal mucosa, palate, or tongue (Fig. 51-2) that may be painful if removed, exposing the erythematous base. Oral thrush may also be a manifestation of esophagitis ([12]). The diagnosis is commonly made clinically but is confirmed by finding yeast and pseudohyphae on scraping or culture.

Esophagitis

Esophageal candidiasis may cause dysphagia, retrosternal pain, and odynophagia in patients with cancer ([13]). Serious complications of this infection can occur, including chronic esophageal strictures, broncho-esophageal fistulas, and mediastinitis. Esophagoscopy with biopsy and culture are necessary to confirm the diagnosis of candidal esophagitis ([11]). Unfortunately, thrombocytopenia often makes esophagoscopy challenging, so empiric therapy is often used. Esophageal

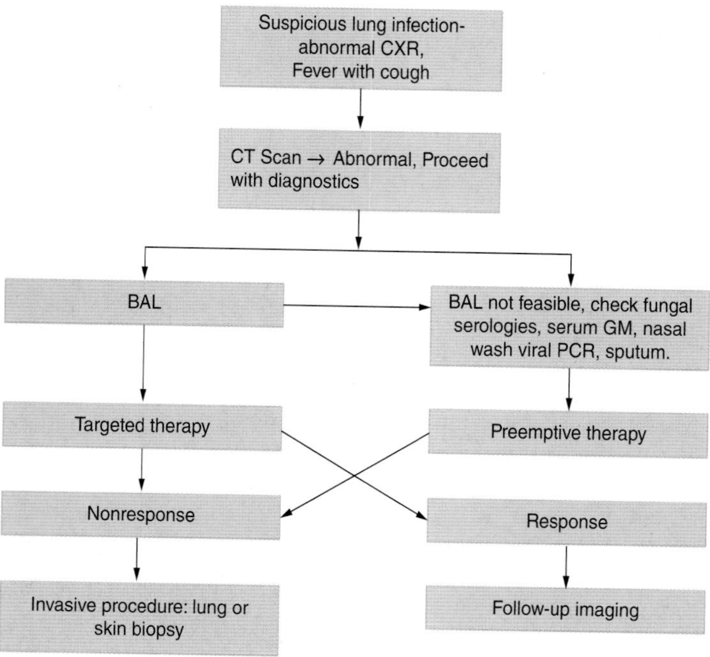

FIGURE 51-1 Evaluation of suspicion of lung infection. CXR, chest x-ray; PCR, polymerase chain reaction. ; BAL, bronchoalveolar lavage; GM, galactomannan.

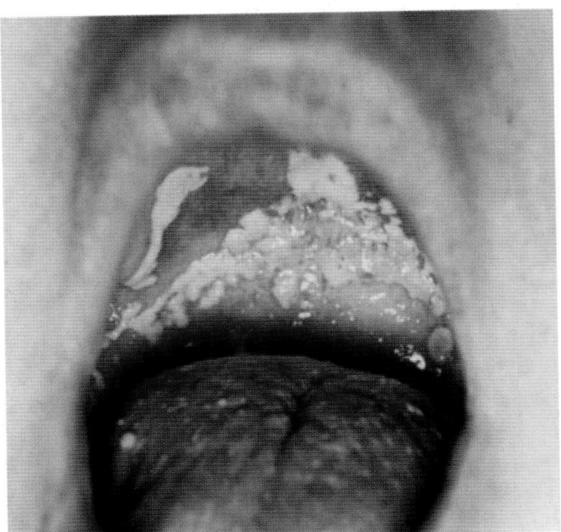

FIGURE 51-2 Typical appearance of oropharyngeal candidiasis on palatal and buccal mucosa.

candidiasis requires systemic therapy, typically utilizing fluconazole as initial therapy ([11]). Caspofungin or other echinocandins may be used if fluconazole fails or is not well tolerated, but it is available only as an intravenous preparation ([11]). Itraconazole, voriconazole, posaconazole, or amphotericin B formulations are rarely indicated for these infections ([11]).

Urinary Tract Infection

Patients with cancer, as with many other hospitalized patients, may develop primary infections of the urinary tract in the settings of urinary obstruction and particularly urinary catheters. Differentiating between colonization and infection is challenging in the presence of urinary catheters. Urinalysis may be normal, and high organism counts are not sufficient to confirm infection. In febrile neutropenic patients, candiduria should be considered as a harbinger of disseminated candidiasis. Recent guidelines recommend treatment with fluconazole, with amphotericin B formulations used for resistant *Candida* spp ([11]). Of note, echinocandins fail to penetrate the urinary tract, so they should not be used in this setting. Relapse of infection, however, will be likely unless the urinary catheter is removed.

Candidemia

Neutropenia, presence of colonization of oropharynx and other sites, steroid use, presence of central venous catheters, and persistent fever in the setting of broad-spectrum antibacterial therapy suggest the diagnosis of candidemia ([14]). A study from a multicenter database demonstrated that *C. albicans* now represents a minority of candidemia infections (45.6%) ([15]). In that study, candidemia resulted in an overall 12-week crude mortality of 35.2%, with highest mortality rate associated with *C. krusei* (52.9%) and lowest with *Candida parapsilosis* (23.7%) ([15]). *Candida parapsilosis* candidemia has been associated with central venous catheters ([15]). Patients with *C. parapsilosis*, including nononcology patients from a multicenter database, were less likely to be neutropenic and immunosuppressed, perhaps explaining the lower mortality rate ([15]). *Candida krusei* has been associated with prior antifungal use, hematologic malignancy (including stem cell transplant), neutropenia, and steroid use. These host factors associated with infection suggest why *C. krusei* exhibits the highest mortality rate of species causing candidemia (52.9%) ([15]).

Disseminated Candidiasis

Disseminated candidiasis is difficult to differentiate from other disseminated fungal and bacterial infections. Persistent fever in the setting of antibacterial therapy and liver dysfunction may suggest consideration of disseminated candidiasis ([15]). In patients with cancer, disseminated candidiasis typically originates from the GI tract or central venous catheters. Dissemination affects multiple organs, such as the kidneys, heart, GI tract, lung, liver, spleen, and skin ([16]). *Candida tropicalis* is more likely to cause the characteristic skin lesions associated with disseminated candidiasis and occasionally causes a syndrome of skin lesions and painful myositis ([17]). Lesions may appear as clusters of pustules or larger nodules and may even develop necrotic centers similar to ecthyma gangrenosum ([18]). Common presentation is nontender, firm, nonblanching, raised nodules that are pink to red in color (Fig. 51-3).

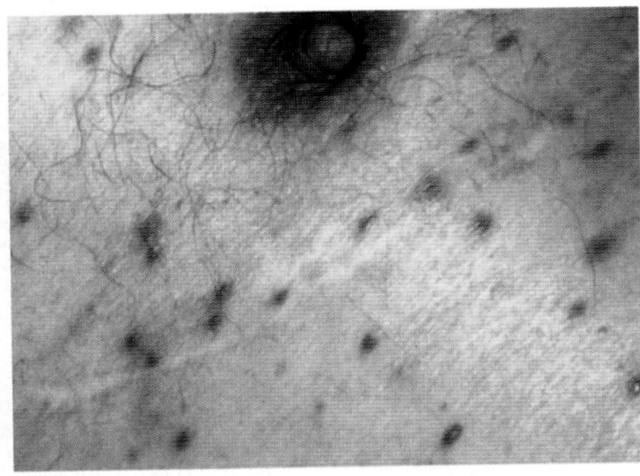

FIGURE 51-3 Widespread nodular skin lesions in a patient with disseminated candidiasis.

Diagnosis

The diagnosis of disseminated candidiasis may be difficult to establish because culture of the organism from sputum, urine, and feces may be positive in patients without infection. On the other hand, 40% of patients with widespread infection demonstrated at autopsy examination had multiple negative blood cultures ([16]). Given the challenge of appropriate diagnosis and morbidity associated with failure to treat the severely immunocompromised, empiric therapy is commonly given for those who continue to be ill in the setting of broad-spectrum antibacterial therapy.

Therapy

Therapy for candidiasis includes three classes of medications: azoles (eg, voriconazole), echinocandins (eg, caspofungin), and the polyenes (eg, amphotericin B). Dosing regimens, major toxicities, and general considerations for antifungal agents are shown in Tables 51-1 through 51-3, respectively. Timely appropriate therapy is necessary because the mortality rate for candidemia ranges from 24% for candidemia caused by *C. parapsilosis* to as high as 53% for *C. krusei* ([15]). *Candida glabrata* exhibits decreased susceptibility to fluconazole ([14]). Mortality, however, is not significantly different from *C. albicans* candidemia ([14]). *Candida krusei*, inherently resistant to fluconazole, is increasingly isolated in institutions where fluconazole is commonly used for prophylaxis ([19]). *Candida lusitaniae*, more commonly seen in patients with stem cell transplant or neutropenia, is of concern due to amphotericin B resistance ([20]).

Recently published guidelines suggest that echinocandins be utilized as first-line therapy in neutropenic patients with candidemia, with lipid formulations of amphotericin B as second-line therapy ([11]). Species-specific recommendations, however, are provided, given inherent differences in resistance. The guidelines emphasize that if a therapeutic approach is resulting in clinical improvement, then current therapy can be continued. For *C. glabrata*, an echinocandin or lipid formulation of amphotericin B is recommended ([11]). For infection with *C. parapsilosis*, an azole or lipid formulation of amphotericin B is recommended. For *C. krusei*, fluconazole is contraindicated due to innate resistance ([11]). For neutropenic patients with invasive candidiasis (but not candidemia), lipid formulations of amphotericin B, echinocandins, or voriconazole are recommended ([11]). In candidemia and invasive candidiasis, fluconazole may be used in patients who have no prior exposure to azoles and are not critically ill ([11]). If fluconazole is used, the initial recommended dose is 12 mg/kg/d. The guidelines recommend the use of lipid formulations of amphotericin B, rather than amphotericin B deoxycholate (D-AMB), to avoid nephrotoxicity ([11]).

Caspofungin was the first echinocandin approved by the Food and Drug Administration (FDA), showing broad-spectrum activity against *Candida* spp. In comparison to D-AMB in a study of invasive candidiasis (80% of which was candidemia), caspofungin showed similar outcomes with fewer adverse events ([11]). Of note, however, few patients were neutropenic in this study. The three currently available echinocandins (caspofungin, micafungin, and anidulafungin) are comparable in their efficacies, although only one study in patients

Table 51-1 Dosage Regimens for Serious Fungal Infections

Drug	Loading Dose	Daily Dose	Route
D-AMB	—	1-1.5 mg/kg	IV only
Lipid AMB	—	3-5 mg/kg	IV only
Fluconazole	800 mg	400-800 mg	IV, Oral
Itraconazole IV	200 mg bid × 2 days	200 mg	IV
Itraconazole solution	200 mg bid × 2 days	200 mg	Oral
Posaconazole tabs	300 mg bid × 2 doses	300 mg	Oral
Posaconazole IV	300 mg bid × 2 doses	300 mg	IV
Posaconazole (susp)	—	200 mg every 6h	Oral
Voriconazole IV	6 mg/kg every 12 h × 2 doses	4 mg/kg every 12 h	IV
Voriconazole tabs	—	200 mg every 12 h (>40 kg)	Oral
		100 mg every 12 h (<40 kg)	
Caspofungin	70 mg × 1 dose	50 mg	IV
Micafungin	—	150 mg	IV
Anidulafungin	200 mg × 1 dose	100 mg	IV

D-AMB, amphotericin B deoxycholate; IV, intravenous; susp, suspension; tabs, tablets.

CHAPTER 51

Table 51-2 Major Toxicities of Antifungal Agents

Amphotericin B	Infusion related (headache, chills, hypotension, etc); nephrotoxicity; hypokalemia, hypomagnesemia; anemia
Fluconazole	Nausea, vomiting; headache; hepatotoxicity (rare); drug interactions
Itraconazole	Nausea, vomiting; headache; hepatotoxicity (rare); pulmonary edema; drug interactions
Posaconazole	Hepatotoxicity (rarely requires discontinuation)
Voriconazole	Visual disturbances; rash; nausea, vomiting; headache; hepatotoxicity; drug interactions
Echinocandins (eg, caspofungin)	Fever; nausea; flushing; rash; some drug interactions; phlebitis

with nononcologic candidemia directly compared micafungin and caspofungin and showed equivalent outcomes ([21]).

The management of catheter-related bloodstream infections is controversial. Debate exists with respect to need for catheter removal. Patients with indwelling intravascular catheters typically require them for chemotherapy or supportive care. The removal of surgically implanted catheters is particularly difficult, given thrombocytopenia is often present in this patient population and also the high costs of placement. Studies suggest a role for catheter removal, particularly if it is clear that the catheter is the source or in the setting of persistent candidemia without another source. Removal of the catheter may improve response rates and reduce duration of candidemia ([11]). Infection with *C. parapsilosis*, in particular, is associated with persistent candidemia without catheter removal ([11]).

In brief, *Candida* causes a wide spectrum of syndromes, from superficial oral candidiasis to candidemia, in patients with cancer. The therapeutic approach should take into consideration host risk factors, medication interactions, antifungal toxicities, and comorbidities when selecting a particular agent.

ASPERGILLOSIS

One of the most common and important invasive fungal infections is aspergillosis. *Aspergillus* spp are the most common invasive mold infections in patients with hematologic cancer ([22]). *Aspergillus fumigatus* is the species most commonly associated with infection, although *Aspergillus terreus* and *Aspergillus flavus,* more

Table 51-3 Therapeutic Options for Disseminated and Major Organ Candidiasis

Regimen	Advantages	Disadvantages
Amphotericin B deoxycholate (D-AMB)	Broad-spectrum activity.	Acute chronic toxicities; minimally effective in patients with neutropenia and with chronic disseminated candidiasis; Intravenous preparations only.
Lipid formulations of AMB	Broad-spectrum activity, reduced nephrotoxicity. Higher doses can be administered.	Only prospective randomized trial showed no advantage in efficacy over D-AMB despite higher doses. More expensive. Intravenous preparations only.
Fluconazole	Oral and intravenous preparation. As effective as AMB in randomized trials of nonneutropenic individuals. Minimal toxicity. More effective for chronic disseminated candidiasis. Little experience in neutropenic patients but appears to be as effective as AMB.	Variable activity against *C. glabrata* and *C. dubliniensis*; inactive against *C. krusei*. Some drug-drug interactions.
Echinocandins (eg, caspofungin)	Broad-spectrum activity. Minimal toxicity. In randomized trials, as active as amphotericin B and fluconazole. Limited experience in neutropenic patients.	No oral preparation.
Flucytosine	Synergistic with AMB and fluconazole. Combination of flucytosine and AMB may be superior to AMB alone for chronic disseminated candidiasis and *C. tropicalis* infection.	No intravenous preparation. Causes myelosuppression. Often need monitoring of serum concentrations. Emergence of resistance if used alone.

resistant *Aspergillus* spp, are becoming increasingly common ([22]). Infections are typically acquired by spore inhalation, but construction in hospitals and surrounding areas have been associated with infection ([23]). The most important risk factor is prolonged neutropenia ([22]). In patients with stem cell transplants, reported risk factors for increased mortality include poor baseline pulmonary status, high doses of steroids (≥2 mg/kg/d), disseminated aspergillosis, proved invasive aspergillosis, increased bilirubin, increased creatinine, HLA-mismatched stem cells, and invasive aspergillosis occurring 40 or more days after transplant ([24]). A recent retrospective study suggested that elevated serum galactomannan index (GMI), but not bronchoalveolar lavage GMI, is associated with increased mortality ([25]).

Pulmonary Infection

The most common syndrome associated with aspergillosis is pneumonia. Due to the angioinvasive nature of the infection, symptoms suggesting pulmonary involvement (eg, pulmonary embolism, pleuritic chest pain, fever, hemoptysis, and friction rub) are occasionally encountered ([26]). Initial chest x-ray may be unremarkable, with fever proceeding in the setting of broad-spectrum antibacterials ([26]).

Radiologic findings are variable, with wedge-shaped infarcts, necrotizing bronchopneumonia, lobar consolidation, or diffuse infiltrates noted ([26]). If suspicion is high for infection, early CT scan of the thorax is essential, potentially demonstrating a halo sign (area of low attenuation surrounding a nodular infiltrate), an important early sign that disappears in 75% of cases within the first week ([26]) (Fig. 51-4). Analysis of radiologic studies from a clinical trial suggested that patients with the halo sign had an improved response to treatment and also improved mortality compared to those who did not exhibit the halo sign ([27]). Cavitation occurs as the infection progresses, with lesions often increasing in size until neutrophil recovery occurs. Differentiation from infection with other molds (ie, mucormycosis) can be difficult. A study suggested that CT of the thorax with greater than 10 nodules and pleural effusion are more often seen in pulmonary mucormycosis rather than invasive pulmonary aspergillosis ([27]).

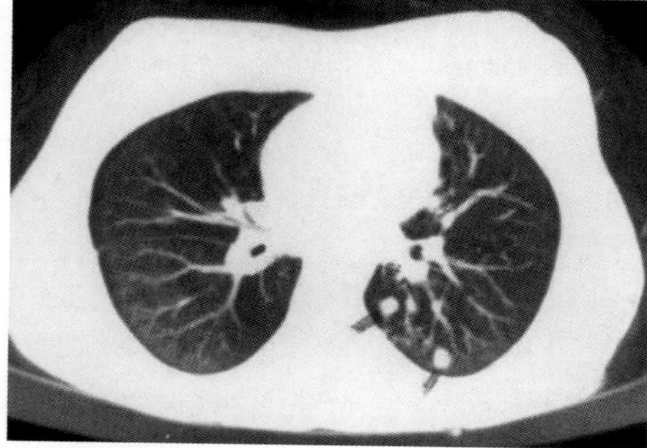

FIGURE 51-4 Computed tomographic scan showing nodular lesions in lung of patient on high-dose adrenal corticosteroid therapy who developed sudden onset of pleuritic chest pain and a pleural friction rub due to pulmonary aspergillosis. The chest roentgenogram was normal.

Sinusitis

Immunocompromised patients may exhibit acute sinusitis as a component of invasive diseases, occurring in 15% to 20% of neutropenic patients ([28]). Fever, headache, cough, epistaxis, and sinus discharge are signs and nonspecific symptoms suggestive of fungal sinusitis ([28]). On exam, necrotic lesions may be seen in the nose or palate (Fig. 51-5), with accurate diagnosis improved by examination and confirmed by biopsy by experienced otolaryngologists ([29]). Imaging of the sinuses by CT or magnetic resonance imaging scan may show opacification of the sinuses or bony destruction. Mortality may be as high as 20% in patients with leukemia in remission to 100% for those with invasive sinusitis who have refractory leukemia or are undergoing HSCT ([28]).

Skin Infection

Aspergillosis as part of dissemination is discussed in the next section, although primary cutaneous infection occurs with direct inoculation. These infections are rarely associated with a central venous access device ([30]). The mechanism of spread is presumed to be via inoculation during catheter insertion or possibly dressing changes or application. Initially, lesions may appear as erythematous plaques, progressing to necrotic ulcers with black eschars ([30]). *Aspergillus flavus* is the most common cause of cutaneous invasive aspergillosis.

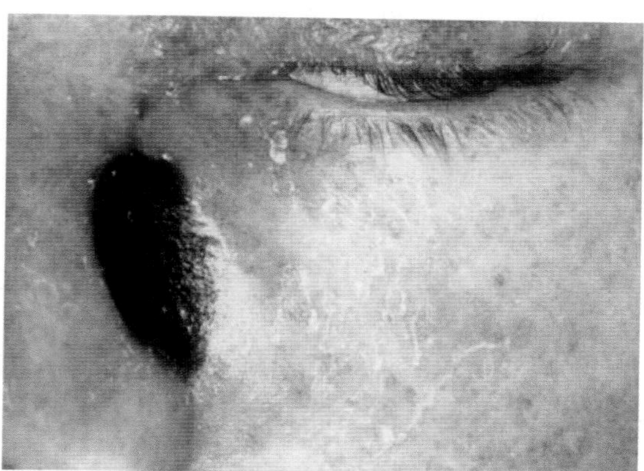

FIGURE 51-5 Black eschar on bridge of the nose in a patient with *Aspergillus* sinusitis.

Disseminated Infection

Given the angioinvasive nature of aspergillosis, hematogenous dissemination occurs in approximately 20% of patients with active hematologic malignancy or HSCT [31]. Common sites of dissemination include the central nervous system (CNS), GI tract, and skin. Gastrointestinal involvement is apparent in 40% to 50% of cases, affecting the esophagus and large bowel [32]. Perforation or massive hemorrhage may occur in this setting. Skin infection may also occur, evolving from erythematous plaques to ulcers that ultimately may be covered by black eschar [33]. Given the broad differential diagnosis of skin lesions in this patient population, skin biopsy is critical.

Diagnosis

A continuing challenge in management of aspergillosis is early and reliable diagnosis [26]. Tissue biopsies from infected tissue may reveal invading hyphae. Paradoxically, cultures of the biopsy specimens fail to grow the fungus in over 50% of cases, although histology and pathology correlate with culture in 78% of those cases [34]. Similarly, blood cultures will rarely (except in the case of *A. terreus*) demonstrate the organism, in contrast to fusariosis [35]. Unfortunately, *Aspergillus* spp fail to grow well from sputum or bronchoscopy, with only 30% of biopsy-proven aspergillosis cases growing mold in sputum cultures [36]. Due to these challenges of diagnosis, patients commonly receive empiric antifungal therapy while undergoing workup.

To increase the likelihood of detection of aspergillosis, various non–culture-based tests have been developed. Available tests detect circulating antigens or immune complexes. Galactomannan and 1,3-β-D-glucan are the most commonly used tests. Via a sandwich enzyme-linked immunosorbent assay used to detect the polysaccharide cell wall component of *Aspergillus* spp, galactomannan can be detected in the serum, and more recently bronchoalveolar lavage fluid, of infected patients [26]. Sensitivity ranges from 67% to 100% and specificity from 86% to 99%, but the test has been studied primarily in patients with hematologic malignancy with profound neutropenia. The positive predictive value of this test is poor in patients with solid tumor and other cancer [26]. An additional challenge occurs in interpreting a galactomannan in the context of prophylaxis with antimold activity. A recent study suggested up to 86% false-positive results for those on active antimold therapy [37].

1,3-β-D-Glucan is an integral component of the cell wall of several yeasts and fungi [26]. Sensitivity ranges from 67% to 100% and specificity 84% to 100%, but false positives are noted due to cirrhosis, hemodialysis, and some chemotherapeutic agents [26].

Therapy

Early diagnosis of aspergillosis utilizing the various available tools has allowed for earlier treatment, but challenges continue in assessing the impact of various treatments, given categorization of infection as proven, probable, or possible [29]. Table 51-4 describes various principles for management of aspergillosis. Persistence of neutropenia is a host factor that is critical in determining the outcome of infection, regardless of therapy. In fact, in a study of patients with acute myeloid leukemia (AML), mortality was 90% in those patients who failed to recover from neutropenia [38].

Voriconazole is currently recommended as first-line therapy of invasive pulmonary aspergillosis [28]. A randomized trial comparing voriconazole to D-AMB for patients with definite or probable aspergillosis showed decreased mortality in the voriconazole group (71% vs 58%). Both oral and intravenous formulations are available, with decreased nephrotoxicity compared to amphotericin B. Voriconazole does, however, cause visual disturbances, hallucinations, and liver dysfunction in a subset of patients.

Posaconazole, the newest FDA-approved azole, was previously only available as an oral solution. Posaconazole tablets are now available, with considerably improved absorption, with minimal impact from food, mucositis, or elevated gastric pH [39]. Despite resultant elevated liver function tests due to dramatically increased posaconazole levels in tablet form, no clinically significant hepatotoxicity occurred [39]. Posaconazole was associated with increased response to therapy and decreased mortality compared to Liposomal Amphotericin B (L-AMB) with or without caspofungin [40]. In addition, nephrotoxicity and change in liver function tests were more likely in the L-AMB–containing regimens.

Lipid formulations of amphotericin B are now recommended in lieu of D-AMB, given the decreased risk of nephrotoxicity. In a randomized study of early treatment of aspergillosis in neutropenic patients, doses of 10 mg/kg/d were compared with 3 mg/kg/d with

Table 51-4 Principles of Therapy for Aspergillosis

Early, aggressive treatment with high doses of voriconazole or a lipid formulation of amphotericin B deoxycholate (D-AMB)
Rapid tapering of dose of adrenal corticosteroids if possible
Consideration for G-CSF-primed granulocyte transfusions in select cases
Long-term antifungal therapy, which should be individualized based on response
Debridement of necrotic tissue of localized disease (onychomycosis, sinusitis, abscess)

comparable outcomes (46% high dose vs 50% low dose), but the higher dose resulted in greater nephrotoxicity (32% vs 20%) ([28]).

Echinocandins inhibit the synthesis of β-(1,3)-D-glucan, an essential component of the fungal cell wall. A disadvantage of echinocandins is that they are available only as an intravenous preparation ([28]). In a noncomparative trial of 90 patients with definite or probable aspergillosis who had failed other therapy, a complete or partial response occurred in 45% ([41]). Responses were observed in 50% of patients with pulmonary infection but in only 26% of those with neutropenia ([41]).

Treatment of Invasive Aspergillosis (IA) is challenging, particularly in the setting of prolonged neutropenia. This has led to the use of combination therapy. In a recent randomized, placebo-controlled trial of HSCT and patients with hematologic malignancy, voriconazole combined with placebo or anidulafungin failed to demonstrate a difference in overall or 6-week mortality ([42]). In a subgroup with radiographic findings consistent with IA and elevated serum galactomannan, the mortality was significantly higher in the monotherapy group (15.7% vs 27.3%, $P = .037$) ([42]).

Antifungal agents utilized for prophylaxis against aspergillosis in high-risk patients have included posaconazole, itraconazole, voriconazole, aerosolized or nebulized formulations of amphotericin B, and micafungin ([22, 28]). Posaconazole is the only agent currently FDA approved for the indication of prevention of invasive aspergillosis in patients with acute leukemia and high-risk stem cell transplant recipients, but significant expense continues to limit the utility of this agent ([41]).

CRYPTOCOCCOSIS

Cryptococci are encapsulated yeasts that have a worldwide distribution, with a dramatic increase in incidence corresponding with the advent of HIV/AIDS ([43]). *Cryptococcus neoformans* is the most common pathogen, found in pigeon excretions, with infection acquired by inhalation into the lungs. Patients with HIV/AIDS had the highest incidence of infection prior to the initiation of highly active antiretroviral therapy ([43]). Factors associated with cryptococcosis in patients with cancer include lymphopenia, chemotherapy, and steroid use less than 1 month prior to diagnosis ([44]). Those at particular risk include those with lymphoma or CLL. Risk in patients with hematologic malignancy is low because of widespread use of fluconazole and other agents for antifungal prophylaxis.

Pneumonia

Given inhalation as the mechanism of entry, the lung typically serves as the primary site of infection. Despite this fact, less than 40% of patients present with symptoms suggestive of pneumonia ([43]). Symptoms may, however, include chest pain, fever, or dyspnea. Chest radiographic findings may include single or multiple nodules, airspace consolidation, reticular patterns, ground-glass opacities, cavitary lesions, and occasionally pleural effusions, with all findings unilateral or bilateral ([43]). Cryptococcal pneumonia can rapidly progress, resulting in higher mortality in patients with cancer. For susceptible patients, finding of this organism in a patient with chest radiography and symptoms consistent with infection is sufficient indication for therapy. In a series from a cancer center, fine-needle aspiration, bronchoalveolar lavage, and open lung biopsy had a yield of over 90% on culture ([44]).

Central Nervous System Infection

Many series showed a predominance of CNS infection in patients with cancer, primarily with meningoencephalitis, but rarely with meningitis alone or with cryptococcoma. Depending on degree of immunosuppression, patients may exhibit an indolent course, with initial symptoms of fever and headache ([43]). As the disease progresses, symptoms may include nausea, vomiting, dizziness, somnolence, irritability, confusion, photophobia, or obtundation. Absence of nuchal rigidity (a finding exhibited in only 15% of patients) does not rule out infection ([43]). Patients infected with *Cryptococcus gatti* can include those with no apparent immunosuppression but with high predeliction for CNS involvement ([43]). In patients with CNS disease, findings include elevated opening pressure, decreased glucose, and high protein concentration. Leukocyte count may also be elevated, with lymphocyte predominance ([44]). Available diagnostic tests include India ink, serum cryptococcal antigen, and fungal culture. India ink detects 50% of infections, whereas serum cryptococcal antigen is positive in 90% of cerebrospinal fluid (CSF) and 70% of blood in patients with CNS infection.

Disseminated Infection

Multiple organs, including the liver, prostate, eyes, skin, and bone, may serve as sites of dissemination. Serum cryptococcal antigen has greater than 90% sensitivity and specificity for invasive cryptococcal disease ([43]). Skin lesions, present in only approximately 10% of patients, tend to be painless and located on the face, neck, and scalp ([43]). The lesions may appear as papules, plaques, ulcerations, acneiform eruptions, lesions, or even draining sinuses. With wide use of antifungal prophylaxis, skin, soft tissue, and osteoarticular lesions appear to be less common ([43]).

Therapy

Treatment of cryptococcal disease depends largely on site of infection. Combination of D-AMB with flucytosine is the traditional approach of choice for severe pulmonary cryptococcosis and CNS disease in non–HIV-infected immunocompromised patients as induction therapy ([43]). Flucytosine is available only as an oral preparation with myelosuppressive toxicity (see Tables 51-1 and 51-2). The recommended dose is D-AMB 0.7 to 1.0 mg/kg/d plus flucytosine 100 mg/kg/d for 2 weeks, as induction therapy, consolidation with fluconazole 400 to 800 mg daily for 8 weeks, and then 200 mg daily maintenance therapy for 6 to 12 months ([43]). In mild-to-moderate cases of pulmonary disease, fluconazole 400 mg daily alone may be given for 6 to 12 months ([43]). Of note, synergy has been noted between some antifungal agents and calcineurin inhibitors, associated with improved outcomes for solid-organ transplant patients ([45]), potentially of relevance in patients with HSCT although not established.

Management of cryptococcal meningitis requires monitoring of CSF pressure and appropriate measures if elevated pressures are noted to prevent complications and reduce mortality ([43]). Complications of elevated intracranial pressures (>200 mm H_2O) include papilledema, hearing loss, vision loss, severe headache, and cognitive impairment. Therefore, management is aggressive, including daily lumbar puncture or, if necessary, ventricular shunt placement ([43]). Timely intervention is necessary to prevent irreversibile neurologic complications or death.

FUSARIOSIS

Humans are exposed to various *Fusarium* spp found in the air and soil. Superficial (cutaneous, keratitis, onychomycosis), locally invasive, and disseminated infection syndromes are included. The most common species that causes human disease is *Fusarium solani* (approximately 50% of cases), but others include *F. moniliforme, F. oxysporum,* and *F. dimerum* ([46]). Entry points for infection by *Fusarium* spores are typically skin, onychomycosis, and respiratory tract. Risk factors for invasive fusariosis among patients with hematologic malignancy include uncontrolled cancer (71%), stem cell transplant (47%), and neutropenia (82%) ([46]). Mortality was highest in one retrospective study in patients with fungemia, with an abysmal 6% survival at 12 weeks ([46]). All-cause mortality was 66%, but 50% was attributable to fusariosis.

Sinus infection and pneumonia occur in 80% of patients, and blood cultures are positive in 50% to 70% of cases ([47]). In neutropenic patients, dissemination occurs 75% of the time and is characterized by multiple skin lesions ([48]). Skin lesions may appear as red or gray macules, pustules, or classically papules with central necrosis or eschar (Fig. 51-6). Lesions may also appear to be different types of lesions at different stages of evolution ([48]). Myalgias or subcutaneous lesions are also noted in disseminated fusariosis. In nonneutropenic patients with less-severe immunocompromise, infection may be relatively localized, with paronychia, erythematous nodules, hemorrhagic bullae, or trauma-associated tender, necrotic lesions ([47]).

Therapy

The significance of in vitro susceptibility results is unclear, with conflicting reports of species-specific susceptibility to amphotericin B in some series, whereas others do not demonstrate such an association. Azoles, particularly voriconazole and posaconazole, exhibit variable in vitro activity against different *Fusarium* species ([47]). Posaconazole and voriconazole have both been used as salvage therapy after initial monotherapy with high-dose lipid formulations of amphotericin B failed ([47]). Combination therapy has been used with anecdotal success, but definitive evidence of effectiveness is lacking. In neutropenic patients, however, neutrophil recovery is the critical component improving outcomes ([46]).

MUCORMYCOSIS

Mucormycosis is an infection caused by molds of the order Mucorales present in the environment, acquired by inhalation of spores ([41]). These molds, similar to *Aspergillus* spp, are angioinvasive, causing thrombosis and infarction. Macrophages and neutrophils are key components of the immune response to mucormycosis. Patients with acute leukemia, diabetic ketoacidosis, or iron overload; HSCT recipients; and those treated

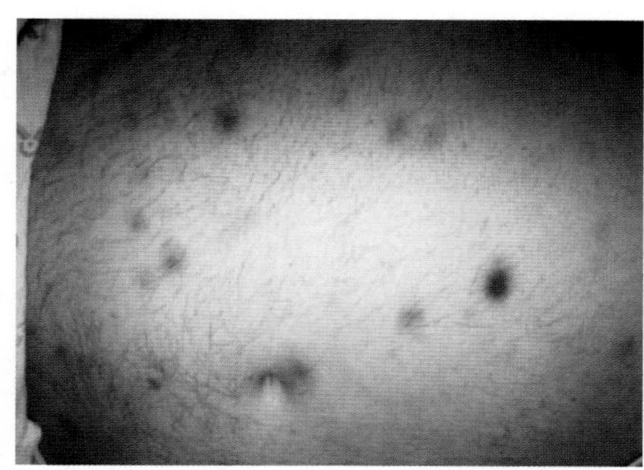

FIGURE 51-6 Skin lesions in a patient with disseminated fusariosis.

CHAPTER 51

with adrenal corticosteroids ([41]) may be affected by mucormycosis. Syndromes include rhinocerebral, pulmonary, GI, and cutaneous involvement ([49]). Patients with hematologic malignancy tend to have pulmonary or disseminated disease, whereas those with diabetes have predominantly sinus involvement ([50]).

Overall mortality is 44%, but patients with cancer with definite or probably mucormycosis have a mortality rate of 71% ([41]). Patients with neutropenia are more likely to have disseminated disease, which has a mortality over 90%.

Therapy

Amphotericin B, more recently in lipid formulations, has been the most commonly used approach to treatment of mucormycosis ([49, 50]). High doses of amphotericin B (5-10 mg/kg/d) can be provided with lipid formulations ([50]). Other modalities that have been used include hyperbaric oxygen, iron-chelating agents (deferasirox), surgical intervention, immunomodulatory therapy with granulocyte-macrophage colony-stimulating factor (GM-CSF) or interferon gamma and granulocyte transfusions ([50]). The addition of posaconazole typically occurs in transition to oral therapy, but rarely may be used as a frontline agent if there is a contraindication to amphotericin B formulations or relatively mild, localized disease that has been surgically resected ([50]). In addition to monotherapy with amphotericin B formulations, various combinations of antifungals, including echinocandins, are given with any or all of the modalities mentioned ([50]). A review of the common nonendemic fungi and associated syndromes is provided in Table 51-5.

ENDEMIC FUNGI

The list of common endemic fungi that may infect patients with cancer in North America includes *Coccidioides immitis* and *Histoplasma capsulatum* ([51]). The distribution of these organisms is determined by climate and geography. These may infect patients without severe immunosuppression and may manifest as lung lesions that may even be confused with malignancy, such as lung cancer, or as disseminated disease ([51]). In patients with hematologic malignancies with cellular immunity impaired by the disease process or by treatments, including steroids (eg, CLL), these infections may represent reactivation of latent infection ([51]).

Histoplasmosis

Presentation of histoplasmosis is with pulmonary lesions in patients with solid tumor, but predominantly is disseminated disease in patients with hematologic malignancy ([51]). In the United States, histoplasmosis is most common in the Ohio and Mississippi River valleys. Hepatosplenomegaly and mucocutaneous ulcerations, particularly in the oral cavity, may be present ([51]). Histoplasmosis is identified by culture from infected tissues, including respiratory samples

Table 51-5 Major Fungal Infections and Syndromes

Organism	Infections/Syndromes	Comments
Candida	Thrush Esophageal candidiasis Urinary tract infection Candidemia Disseminated candidiasis	*C. parapsilosis* resistant to echinocandins *C. krusei* fluconazole resistant *C. glabrata* fluconazole resistant
Aspergillus	Pulmonary Sinusitis Skin infection Disseminated	Bronchoscopy or biopsy of nodules Head and neck surgery evaluation, debridement Biopsy skin; rare blood culture positive
Cryptococcus	Pneumonia CNS Disseminated	Check serum *Cryptococcus* Low threshold for lumbar puncture in immunocompromised
Fusarium	Sinus infection Pneumonia Skin infection Dissemination	Bronchoscopy or biopsy of nodules Head and neck surgery evaluation, debridement Biopsy skin; blood culture positive
Mucormycosis	Rhinocerebral Pulmonary Gastrointestinal Cutaneous	Urgent debridement of rhinocerebral disease Bronchoscopy or biopsy of nodules Hyperbaric oxygen

and rarely the bloodstream on culture. Histoplasmosis antigen testing can be used to detect evidence of histoplasmosis in urine ([52]). Recent guidelines suggest utilizing liposomal amphotericin B (3-5 mg/kg/d) for severe pulmonary or disseminated disease, followed by itraconazole (200 mg twice daily for 2 days, then 200 mg daily) ([52]). For most infections requiring treatment, therapy is provided for 6 to 9 months ([52]). Severely immunocompromised patients may require even more prolonged therapy. Successful therapy with voriconazole has been used for histoplasmosis ([53]).

Coccidioidomycosis

Coccidioides immitis is reported to cause fever, hypoxemia, and diffuse pulmonary infiltrates in immunocompromised patients ([51]). In the United States, coccidioidomycosis is endemic to western Texas, central California, southern New Mexico, and southern Arizona. Disseminated infection may involve the skin and bone. In patients with hematologic malignancy, serologic tests may be negative. In most cases, specimens from the lung, CSF, or other tissue provide the best approach for diagnosis ([54]). Current guidelines recommend therapy for severe pulmonary or severe disseminated infection should begin with an amphotericin B formulation, D-AMB (0.7-1.0 mg/kg/d) or liposomal amphotericin B (3-5 mg/kg/d). For meningitis, guidelines recommend fluconazole (400 to 800 mg/d), possibly combined with intrathecal amphotericin B ([54]). After completing initial aggressive therapy according to syndrome on presentation, fluconazole (400 mg/d) or itraconazole (400 mg/d) is continued for at least a year for most cases and indefinitely for immunocompromised patients ([54]). Lifelong therapy with fluconazole or voriconazole, which penetrate the CNS, are recommended for those with meningitis ([54]).

ADJUVANT THERAPY FOR FUNGAL INFECTIONS

White Blood Cell Transfusions

Recovery of neutropenia is essential for recovery from invasive fungal infection. Almost five decades ago, transfusions of leukocytes were first utilized to assist neutropenic patients in recovery. Some studies have suggested that this approach could be effective in management of invasive fungal infection, but doubts remain. Issues include the challenge of the dose of cells and the length of time during which they remain active ([55]). Administration of granulocyte colony-stimulating factor (G-CSF) has allowed healthy volunteers to provide adequate numbers of cells ([55]). The effectiveness of this approach may be as a bridge to recovery of bone marrow. Finally, clinical issues with granulocyte transfusions include an initial worsening of respiratory symptoms, although skin and soft tissue infections appear to improve.

Cytokines

Proinflammatory cytokines, exemplified by interferon gamma (IFN-γ), tumor necrosis factor alpha (TNF-α), and interleukin (IL) 2, are produced by Th1 lymphocytes, activating effector immune cells ([56]). Treatment with IFN-γ, sometimes in combination with GM-CSF, has been used to stimulate the immune response to fungal infections ([56]). The IFN-γ enhances hyphal damage to fungal pathogens by neutrophils and monocytes ([56]).

The duration and depth of neutropenia can be decreased using colony-stimulating factors, including G-CSF (filgrastim) and GM-CSF (sargramostim, molgramostim) ([41]). Here, GM-CSF may be of particular use because it not only increases the number of granulocytes but also improves the function of macrophages and granulocytes ([56]). Case reports and case series have suggested the potential benefit of several of these adjunct therapies, although data are not adequate to make firm recommendations for use of these immunomodulators.

Surgical Resection

The role of surgical resection is characterized for fungal infection by organism, but a recent study described patients undergoing resection as a component of therapy for a broad array of fungal infections from 1984 through 2009; the study provided insight into use of this approach ([57]). Patients with hematologic malignancy and suspected pulmonary invasive fungal infection on appropriate systemic antifungal therapy underwent resection in select circumstances. These included progression of fungal infection despite therapy, with neutropenia not considered a contraindication. Platelets were transfused over 50 times 10^9/L. After surgery, nearly 90% of patients underwent further chemotherapy or stem cell transplant, with mortality of 7% and 48% at 30 days and 1 year, respectively ([57]). Fungal organisms isolated were predominantly *Aspergillus* species (88%) and Mucorales (8%). Bacterial infection was noted in 8% of patients, with lung infarction in another 3%, with no evidence of fungal infection, obviating the need for active antimold therapy. Over the time of the retrospective study, the surgical procedures became less invasive, shifting from lobectomy and open limited resections to video-assisted thoracoscopic procedures ([57]). Surgical resection, via open or video-assisted thoracoscopy, presents a viable option for management of focal fungal infection that fails to respond to antifungal therapy alone, even with patients with hematologic malignancies. In fact, these procedures have successfully been followed by subsequent chemotherapy and stem cell transplant.

VIRAL INFECTIONS

Viral infections are an important cause of morbidity and mortality in patients with cancer. Although morbidity and mortality are greater for patients with hematologic malignancies or after HSCT, viral infections, such as norovirus or influenza virus, can increase length of hospital stay and delay chemotherapy, radiation, or surgery in a broad patient population. The most common viral infections are respiratory viral infections, including adenovirus, influenza, parainfluenza, RSV, rhinovirus, and human metapneumovirus ([5]). DNA viruses, such as herpes simplex, varicella, and CMV, are well known to cause serious infections in patients with hematologic malignancies or after HSCT, resulting in intense monitoring and prophylaxis directed against such viruses ([58]). Patients with hematopoeitic stem cell transplant are at particular risk for severe viral infections. Modern tools of diagnosis can quickly identify infection, but treatment options are limited for many viral infections. The following sections provide an overview of viral infections in patients with cancer. Special focus is placed on those with hematologic malignancies and patients after HSCT because this population is uniquely susceptible to viral infections.

Human Herpesviruses

Human herpesviruses are among the most common causes of viral infections in immunocompetent as well as in immunocompromised patients. Morbidity and mortality from these viruses are high among immunosuppressed patients. Herpesviruses are double-stranded DNA viruses. The herpesvirus group has eight members, six of which are important pathogens in immunosuppressed patients (ie, patients with hematologic malignancies and solid-organ or stem cell transplant recipients) ([58, 59]). This group of pathogens includes HSV 1 and 2, VZV, CMV, Epstein-Barr virus (EBV), and human herpesvirus 6 (HHV-6).

Herpesviruses establish a latent phase after primary infection. The reactivation of these DNA viruses can be triggered by several stimuli; this is perhaps best recognized in the recurrent blisters and ulcers associated with HSV. The likelihood of reactivation of these viruses is increased during profound T-cell immunosuppression, as host defenses against these viruses are dependent on virus-specific helper and cytotoxic T lymphocytes. Over the past decade, substantial improvements have been made in the techniques used to detect these infections, such as real-time polymerase chain reaction (PCR), as well as the development of effective antiviral agents and the use of different strategies for prophylaxis and treatment.

Herpes Simplex Viruses

Among the most common causes of mucocutaneous lesions in immunocompromised patients are HSV types 1 and 2 ([59]). Approximately 40% to 60% of seropositive patients undergoing induction chemotherapy for leukemia or conditioning for HSCT will experience HSV reactivation, usually in early stages, when immunosuppression is most intense ([59]). Reactivation of HSV may cause severe disease during neutropenia. Patients with a CD4 count less than 50 who received purine analogs or alemtuzumab are at highest risk of reactivation ([59]). Oropharyngeal and esophageal disease is usually but not exclusively caused by HSV-1. The clinical manifestations of oropharyngeal HSV disease can range from gingivitis to stomatitis and cheilitis. Esophagitis from HSV may occur from local spread. Clinical presentation ranges from fever, malaise, myalgia, dysphagia, and bleeding to severe oral pain and odynophagia. Disease caused by HSV-2 is more likely to cause genital and anal disease.

CHAPTER 51

Diagnosis

The diagnosis of HSV infection can be made by isolating the virus in culture or by performing a biopsy showing the characteristic inclusions by immunohistochemistry. Direct detection methods of the virus in clinical specimens are generally not as sensitive as culture methods but offer the advantage of a rapid diagnosis. Direct or indirect immunofluorescence can be used to detect HSV-1, HSV-2, and VZV from specimens of cutaneous lesions.

Prophylaxis

Antiviral prophylaxis should be strongly considered in HSV-seropositive patients at risk for reactivation during intensive chemotherapy for acute leukemia and during early stages of HSCT ([58, 59]). Oral acyclovir and valacyclovir are the agents of choice for prophylaxis. If patients are receiving intravenous foscarnet or ganciclovir for treatment of another viral infection, then they do not need to continue acyclovir prophylaxis ([60]). Guidelines suggest that continuing prophylaxis for over a year post-HSCT significantly reduces reactivation, with a finding that this may even decrease the risk of acyclovir-resistant HSV ([59-61]).

Therapy

The available antiviral agents for the treatment of HSV disease include acyclovir, valacyclovir, famciclovir, foscarnet, and cidofovir (Tables 51-6 and 51-7) ([58, 60]). The bioavailability of oral valacyclovir and famciclovir is three to five times superior to that of oral acyclovir. All of these drugs are dependent on the virus-encoded thymidine kinase for their intracellular phosphorylation for activity.

Established HSV disease can be treated either orally or intravenously. The most commonly used drug is acyclovir. Immunosuppressed patients with disseminated or severe HSV disease should be treated with intravenous acyclovir (5-10 mg/kg every 8 h). Otherwise, an oral regimen can be used for milder HSV disease (famciclovir, 500 mg three times a day, or valacyclovir, 1 g three times a day) ([58, 59]). Foscarnet and cidofovir can be used for resistant disease but are only available in intravenous formulations ([60]).

Varicella Zoster Virus

Reactivation of VSV occurs primarily in elderly individuals, seropositive organ transplant and HSCT recipients, patients with cancer, and those with AIDS. Disseminated VZV infection can be life threatening in HSCT recipients and patients receiving intensive corticosteroid therapy ([59]).

The clinical manifestations of VZV infection are primary varicella infection (chickenpox) and herpes zoster. The clinical presentation includes low-grade fever, malaise, and a vesicular rash that evolves to scabs. Constitutional symptoms usually develop after the onset of rash and include pruritus, anorexia, and listlessness. Primary VZV infection (chickenpox) occurs mainly in children under 10 years of age.

Reactivation of latent VZV or herpes zoster is frequently observed among patients with cancer, mainly patients with leukemia or lymphoma, as well as in HSCT recipients ([58, 59]). Visceral herpes zoster may follow cutaneous dissemination in immunocompromised patients and can result in pneumonia, encephalitis, retinal necrosis, hepatitis, and small bowel disease. Cutaneous VZV eruption can be complicated by secondary bacterial infections, thrombocytopenia, and vasculitis (Fig. 51-7).

Diagnosis

Immunocompromised patients may exhibit single dermatomal disease, but more commonly develop multidermatomal or disseminated cutaneous disease, which can make the clinical diagnosis less certain on visual inspection alone. The diagnosis can be established within hours by the direct method of immunofluorescent staining on material collected from a skin lesion or from a skin biopsy. Viral culture should also be performed. In some cases, a biopsy is required to establish the diagnosis because other diseases can mimic VZV, such as streptococcal impetigo, GVHD, and various noninfectious bullous diseases.

Therapy

The treatment of choice for chickenpox or VZV in immunocompromised patients is high-dose intravenous acyclovir (10 mg/kg every 8 h) (see Tables 51-6 and 51-7). Early initiation of acyclovir is paramount because it may reduce progression to end-organ disease

Table 51-6 Antiviral Compounds

Antiviral	Dosage	Mechanism of Action	Active Against
Acyclovir	5-10 mg/kg IV every 8 h	Inhibits DNA polymerase	HSV, VZV
Famciclovir	500 mg by mouth every 8 h	Inhibits DNA polymerase	HSV, VZV
Valacyclovir	0.5-1 g every 8-12 h	Inhibits DNA polymerase	HSV, VZV
Ganciclovir	5 mg/kg every 12 h	Inhibits DNA polymerase	CMV
Foscarnet	60 mg/kg IV every 8 h	Inhibits DNA polymerase	CMV, HSV, VZV, HHV-6
Cidofovir[a]	5 mg/kg IV once a week	Inhibits DNA polymerase	CMV, ADV, HSV, VZV, BK
Ribavirin	Oral or aerosolized	Inhibits viral replication	HCV, RSV
Amantadine	100 mg by mouth every 12 h or 200 mg by mouth daily	Inhibits M2 protein	Influenza A only
Ramantadine	100 mg by mouth every 12 h	Inhibits M2 protein	Influenza A only
Oseltamivir	75 mg by mouth every 12 h	Neuraminidase inhibitor	Influenza A and B
Peramavir	600 mg IV daily	Neuraminidase inhibitor	Influenza A and B
Zanamivir	2 inhalations every 12 h (IV formulation available, clinical trial)	Neuraminidase inhibitor	Influenza A and B

ADV, adenovirus; CMV, cytomegalovirus; HCV, hepatitis C virus; HSV, herpes simplex viruses; IV, intravenous; RSV, respiratory syncytial virus; VZV, varicella zoster virus.
[a] Licensed for CMV retinitis.

Table 51-7 Common and Serious Toxicities of Antivirals

Acyclovir	Transient renal insufficiency (IV), nausea, vomiting, agitation, confusion, TTP (rare)
Famciclovir	Headache, somnolence, nausea, diarrhea
Valacyclovir	Headache, nausea, vomiting, TTP (rare)
Ganciclovir	Anemia, neutropenia (more common), thrombocytopenia, fever, phlebitis, anorexia
Foscarnet	Nephrotoxicity (major toxicity), electrolyte disturbances (hypocalcemia, hypophosphatemia, hyperphosphatemia, hypomagnesemia, hypokalemia), diarrhea, nausea, vomiting
Cidofovir	Headache, rash, severe nephrotoxicity, metabolic acidosis, decreased intraocular pressure, neutropenia
Ribavirin	Fatigue, headache, nausea, rash, pruritus, conjunctivitis (risk of toxicity to healthcare workers during administration), hemolytic anemia (cardiac and pulmonary events have occurred), worsening respiratory status, including death (inhalation)
Oseltamivir	Insomnia, vertigo, nausea, vomiting (most common), bronchitis
Zanamivir	Headache, nausea, diarrhea, cough, bronchospasm, decline in lung function (some fatal outcomes)

IV, intravenous; TTP, thrombotic thrombocytopenia purpura

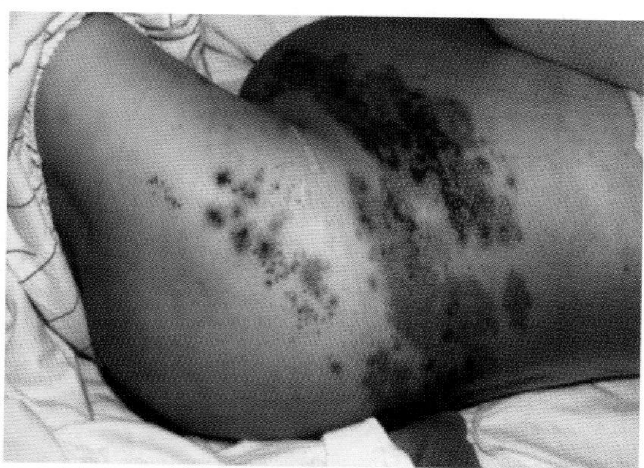

FIGURE 51-7 Hemorrhagic vesicular lesions of herpes zoster.

and usually prevents death in patients with reactivated disease. Therapy can be changed to an oral agent once clinical improvement has occurred, including resolution of fever or healing/crusting of lesions. The options for an oral regimen for treatment of localized herpes zoster among patients with mild immunosuppression include acyclovir (rarely used because of bioavailability and pill burden), valacyclovir, and famciclovir ([62]).

Prevention of Infection

Varicella zoster virus can be transmitted from person to person, and this can become problematic in a hospital or clinic setting. To prevent nosocomial transmission, immunocompromised patients with cutaneous lesions suspicious of VZV eruption and those with disseminated zoster should be placed under contact and respiratory isolation. In addition, it is recommended that the family members, caregivers, and visitors of patients scheduled to undergo transplant be vaccinated against VZV, preferably at least 4 weeks prior to conditioning regimen ([59, 60]).

Immunosuppressed patients with negative VZV titers and no history of chickenpox should be offered VZV immune globulin after being in close contact with individuals with either chickenpox or herpes zoster. Close contact includes prolonged face-to-face contact, a household or playmate contact, or exposure to a roommate in a shared hospital room. Varicella zoster immune globulin, if available, should be administered within 96 h of exposure to be most effective in preventing infection ([59]).

Immunocompromised persons should avoid contact with individuals who developed a rash after receiving zoster vaccine. No additional precautions are required if a rash has not developed ([59, 60]). A study of an inactivated varicella vaccine in HSCT patients resulted in decreased incidence and severity of zoster but is not commercially available ([59]).

Cytomegalovirus

Evidence of prior CMV infection is present in approximately 85% of the US population ([59]). Therefore, reactivation of latent CMV infection is the primary concern in the hematologic malignancy and HSCT patient populations ([59, 60]). Reactivation can manifest as viremia alone, a mononucleosis-like syndrome with lymphadenopathy, or more severe disease with end-organ damage. Other symptoms of CMV reactivation include fever, lymphadenopathy, splenomegaly, lymphocytosis, and polyradiculopathy. Manifestations of end-organ disease include retinitis, encephalitis, and hepatitis, but pneumonitis and GI disease are the most common and can be life threatening ([59]).

The most common sites of CMV infection in the GI tract are the esophagus and colon. The hallmarks of CMV colitis are abdominal pain and diarrhea. Esophagitis caused by CMV is associated with pain and dysphagia. On upper GI endoscopy, ulcerations can be seen in the esophagus, and a biopsy must be obtained to rule out other infectious etiologies, such as HSV or candida esophagitis. As with esophagitis, the diagnosis of colitis requires biopsy. In a retrospective study at our institution, 72% of patients diagnosed with GI CMV disease had hematologic malignancies, 25% had AIDS, and overall CMV-attributable mortality rate was 42% ([63]). Independent predictors of mortality were disseminated CMV and diagnosis of AIDS ([63]).

Cytomegalovirus pneumonitis is associated with a mortality rate of 80% to 100% in patients with high-risk leukemia and HSCT ([59]). Pneumonitis typically presents with severe dyspnea, hypoxia, and interstitial disease on chest radiograph. Similar to GI disease, finding of CMV from bronchoscopy specimens without accompanying pathology is of unclear significance. The thrombocytopenia present in most patients with leukemia and HSCT often prevents acquisition of a biopsy specimen that can accurately confirm diagnosis of CMV pneumonitis. A study of autopsy-proven CMV pneumonia in patients with HSCT and hematologic malignancy showed that incidence decreased over the time of the study (from 1990 to 2004) ([64]).

Risk Factors

Patients with HSCT and hematologic malignancies are at highest risk for CMV infection and reactivation. In patients with leukemia, those at highest risk include patients who have received purine analogues (eg, fludarabine) and T-cell–depleting monoclonal antibodies (eg, alemtuzumab) ([59]). Reactivation can occur in almost 5% of those receiving purine analogues and in 15% to 66% of those receiving alemtuzumab, with the highest risk period for the latter group being in the first 1 to 3 months after therapy ([59]). Reactivation in the setting of alemtuzumab therapy, however, was significantly reduced (0% vs 35% in the control arm) with prophylaxis utilizing valganciclovir 450 mg orally twice per day when compared to 500 mg daily valacyclovir ([65]).

In patients with HSCT, the highest-risk group is the CMV-seropositive recipient, regardless of donor serostatus, followed by the CMV-seronegative recipient with seropositive donor ([59]). Nonmyeloablative regimens for HSCT patients have resulted in decreased risk of CMV reactivation, although cases have occurred later after transplant ([66]). The period of highest risk is in the first 100 days after transplant, although prophylaxis and preemptive strategies have resulted in CMV infections after day 100 from transplantation ([67]). Risk factors for late disease in HSCT patients include GVHD, CMV reactivation before day 100 posttransplant, steroid use, low CD4 count (<50), use of unmatched stem cells, cord blood, T-cell–depleted stem cells, and receipt of allograft-negative donors in CMV-positive recipients ([60, 68]). Also, CMV can be transmitted to HSCT recipients from seropositive donors and from blood products ([59]). The utilization of CMV-seronegative blood for transfusions and leukoreduction of blood products has resulted in significantly reduced CMV infection ([59]).

Diagnosis

Diagnosis of CMV depends on the site of infection. For detection of disseminated infection or reactivation, two types of tests are available and recommended for diagnosis of CMV: pp65 testing and detection of DNA ([60]). Serologic testing is not useful, except for donor selection for transplant, because CMV antibodies demonstrate evidence of prior exposure, rather than active infection. For detection of end-organ disease such as in the liver and lungs, the recommended approach is biopsy with detection of viral inclusions on histopathology or by immunohistochemistry (Fig. 51-8), which has greater sensitivity. If available, in situ PCR and nucleic acid hybridization are also useful diagnostic tools for biopsy samples. Detection of CMV DNA is a widely available test in transplant centers, utilizing quantitative real-time polymerase chain reaction (RT-PCR) for CMV DNA detection ([59, 60, 69]).

Therapy

Antiviral agents are used for prevention and treatment of CMV infection. Available agents are described in Tables 51-6 and 51-7. Strategies for utilization of these agents include treatment of established disease, preemptive therapy, or prophylaxis ([59]). The last two strategies focus on disease prevention in high-risk HSCT patients. At MD Anderson Cancer Center, prophylaxis with ganciclovir or foscarnet used to be the strategy in high-risk HSCT patients; now, preemptive therapy is used in all HSCT patients at risk for reactivation.

A recent study compared daily oral 900 mg valganciclovir to placebo (paired with preemptive therapy)

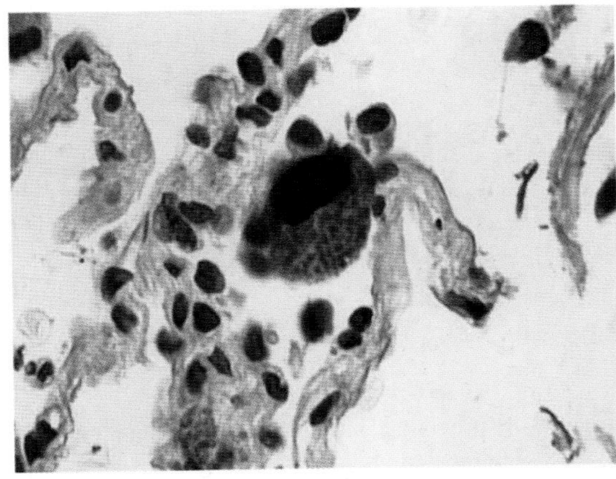

FIGURE 51-8 Typical cytomegalovirus inclusions in the lung parenchyma of a patient with lymphoma with pneumonia.

for prophylaxis against late CMV infection after allo-BMT. The study failed to show the impact of valganciclovir on reduction in mortality, CMV disease, or other invasive infections, although less CMV infection was detected ([67]). Another multicenter study compared a novel anti-CMV agent, letermovir, targeted against the viral terminase complex, to placebo for prophylaxis for allo-BMT patients. In the modified intention-to-treat analysis, a dose-dependent reduction of 30% in CMV reactivation was noted in the letermovir group, without any noted adverse hematologic events ([70]). A similar study in allo-BMT patients showed a 27% reduction in CMV events with CMX001, a lipid acyclic nucleoside phosphatase. Diarrhea was the most common adverse effect of the study medication ([71]).

Ganciclovir functions as a competitive inhibitor of viral DNA polymerase. Its major side effect is myelosuppression, limiting its use as a prophylactic agent and requiring frequent blood count monitoring ([59]). Dosing for treatment is 5 mg/kg intravenously every 12 hours ([59]). Valganciclovir, a prodrug of ganciclovir available in capsule form, is significantly better absorbed than its prodrug ganciclovir in oral form ([59]). A common induction dose is 900 mg twice daily by mouth.

An alternative agent, foscarnet, functions as a noncompetitive inhibitor of the pyrophosphate-binding site of CMV DNA polymerase, which does not require phosphorylation to become active ([59]). Foscarnet is typically used when resistance to ganciclovir is suspected or bone marrow suppression is excessive with ganciclovir. It is also useful in patients with delayed engraftment ([69]). Side effects of foscarnet include nephrotoxicity, azotemia, and electrolyte abnormalities.

Cidofovir, a nucleotide analogue, has been approved for treatment of CMV retinitis in patients with HIV. It works as a competitive inhibitor of the CMV DNA polymerase. Its role in treatment or prophylaxis of CMV in immunocompromised patients, however, is limited due to nephrotoxicity. The long half-life not only makes once-weekly administration possible, but also results in a lasting impact of adverse effects ([69]). Modalities used to reduce risk of nephrotoxicity include hydration and probenicid.

Human Herpesvirus 6

Human herpesvirus 6 is a beta-herpesvirus with two subtypes (A and B). Primary infection with HHV-6 is common in children. Exanthem subitum, the most common cause of fever and hospitalization of infants less than 1 year of age, is caused by HHV-6 subtype B ([58, 59]). In addition to fever, children present with mild upper respiratory symptoms and a classic diffuse maculopapular exanthem. It is unclear whether HHV-6 subtype A causes any primary infection. In immunosuppressed individuals, typically patients with AIDS and transplant recipients, HHV-6 may cause opportunistic viral infections. As this infection is common early in life, positive titers are found in more than 95% of adults. In immunosuppressed individuals, especially HSCT recipients, this virus occasionally may cause interstitial pneumonia, fever, encephalitis, hepatitis, and delayed engraftment ([60]). Up to 40% to 60% of HSCT patients may demonstrate viremia by PCR, but the significance of this finding is unclear, so routine surveillance is not currently recommended ([58-60]).

Therapy

Both ganciclovir and foscarnet are used to treat HHV-6 infections, but this is based on in vitro studies only because clinical experience is minimal. Both ganciclovir and foscarnet have been reported to be effective against HHV-6 meningoencephalitis after HSCT in a small number of patients ([58]).

CHAPTER 51

Epstein-Barr Virus

Epstein-Barr virus infection is common in the adult population. It is the cause of infectious mononucleosis and has also been linked to several geographically defined cancers. Posttransplant lymphoproliferative disorder (PTLD) associated with EBV is an important cause of morbidity and mortality in HSCT and solid-organ transplant recipients. Posttransplant lymphoproliferative disorder is reported in 0.45% to 29% of HSCT patients, depending on the source of hematopoietic cells (cord blood with the higher risk), manipulation of those cells, and immunosuppressive regimen ([72]). Although variable in incidence, PTLD can be fulminant and lethal. The disease results from suppression of cytotoxic T-cell function.

The first step in the management of PTLD is to reduce the dose of any immunosuppressive therapy if possible. Another therapeutic approach using the anti-CD20 monoclonal antibody (rituximab) has been tested for therapy for EBV-induced PTLD. It has been successful for the treatment or prevention of PTLD in solid-organ transplant and HSCT recipients as well as those with proven EBV lymphomas ([58, 59]). Another approach is utilization of EBV-cytotoxic T lymphocytes (CTL), typically derived from EBV-positive stem cell donors or from third-party donors ([72]). There is no apparent role for antivirals in treatment of EBV-associated PTLD. Treatment with rituximab and EBV-targeted CTLs has resulted in over 85% survival, compared with less than 20% before these modalities were available ([72]).

Community Respiratory Viral Infections

Infections caused by community respiratory viruses (CRVs) were not considered to be a significant problem for patients with cancer until the early 1990s. Since then, it has been recognized that they represent a threat to patients undergoing chemotherapy for acute leukemia and to HSCT recipients, especially recipients of allogeneic transplants ([73]). Early surveys indicated that about 30% of respiratory illnesses occurring during the winter and spring among these patient populations were due to CRVs. Recent studies have reported CRVs as the cause of as few as 5% to as many as 48% of respiratory infections ([73]). Although many patients acquire only upper respiratory infections (URIs), some develop pneumonias, which may be fatal. In a retrospective study conducted at our institution, progression from URI to pneumonia was noted in 35% of patients with HSCT and hematologic malignancy ([73]). Many of these pneumonias may be due to bacterial or fungal pathogens and not attributed to the virus. For example, it has been recognized for many years that influenza can predispose to bacterial pneumonia.

Epidemics of CRV have occurred on leukemia and transplant units, where the virus may be transmitted by patients, visitors, and hospital personnel. Clinics may serve as an important starting point for epidemics. Also, epidemics may occur among these susceptible patients in the absence of a recognized epidemic in the community. An additional problem is that these immunocompromised patients may have prolonged viral shedding (in some cases >100 days) after resolution of symptoms ([59, 74]). Shedding of influenza virus continued despite antiviral therapy, halting only when lymphopenia resolved ([59, 74]).

The most commonly reported viruses causing infection are influenza A and B (predominantly influenza A), RSV, and parainfluenza virus (almost entirely type 3) ([5]). Rhinoviruses are the most common cause of community respiratory illnesses but are identified infrequently in most surveys of patients with cancer, suggesting that they are underdiagnosed. Rhinoviruses have been associated with pneumonia in HSCT patients, but commonly are accompanied by bacterial coinfection ([75]). Influenza, RSV, and parainfluenza types 1 and 2 occur during the winter and spring, whereas parainfluenza 3 infection occurs throughout the year. Some patients may be infected by multiple viruses simultaneously or have multiple episodes of the same viral infection separated by only a few weeks. There is considerable variability in the relative frequency of the three major viruses in different geographical areas and in different years, most likely reflecting the relative prevalence of the infections within the community.

A study of parainfluenza virus pneumonia in HSCT patients pointed to high oxygen requirement, low monocyte counts, and high-dose steroids as predisposing to mortality, ranging from 13% to 55% ([76]). A retrospective study conducted at our center emphasized relapsed or refractory malignancy, high APACHE (Acute Physiology and Chronic Health Evaluation) II score, and high-dose steroids as predictors of mortality in a mixed population of patients with leukemia and HSCT ([77]). Human metapneumovirus is a paramyxovirus similar to RSV that was first described in children but has now been described in immunocompetent and immunocompromised adults ([78, 79]). Fatal cases in HSCT patients were reported from Seattle, Washington, with mortality rates as high as 43% ([80]), but HSCT patients from France demonstrated a low mortality rate, even with lower respiratory tract infection ([81]). One of the continuing challenges in comparison of mortality between studies is the degree to which individual investigators consider viral infection the cause or major contributor to death, particularly when considering the significant underlying disease in the oncology populations studied to date ([81]).

Finally, influenza virus infection is associated with different presentation and natural course of disease in severely immunocompromised hosts. In a recent study at the US National Institutes of Health, immunocompromised hosts exhibited less prominent symptoms, such as cough, chills, myalgias, or dyspnea than hosts who were not immunocompromised ([74]). Physical exam findings demonstrating pulmonary compromise were also more common in nonimmunocompromised hosts, but radiographic abnormalities on chest imaging were more common in immunocompromised hosts ([74]). Finally, immunocompromised patients exhibited more severe disease, despite similar cytokine profiles, with prolonged viral shedding and higher risk of developing drug-resistant influenza virus ([74]).

Predisposing Factors

Several important predisposing factors for these infections have been identified in HSCT recipients and patients with hematologic malignancies. These include age more than 65 years, severe neutropenia, severe lymphopenia, allogeneic transplantation, transplant conditioning regimen, GVHD, and adrenal corticosteroid therapy (over 1 mg/kg body weight) ([58, 73, 79, 82]). Recipients of HSCT are at greatest risk within the first 100 days posttransplant, although nonmyeloablative transplant has resulted in an increase in disease occurring after this initial period ([58, 82]). Neutropenia, lymphopenia, marrow or cord blood as source of transplant, age over 65 years, GVHD, smoking history, and allogeneic HSCT were risk factors for progression from RSV URI to pneumonia ([5, 73]).

An immunodeficiency scoring system developed at MD Anderson has been useful in estimating outcomes and appropriate focus of expensive therapy for RSV infection ([83]). Factors given the most weight are neutropenia, lymphopenia, and age 40 years or older, followed by other factors such as GVHD, corticosteroid use, myeloablative conditioning regimen, and preengraftment or within 30 days of engraftment ([83]). Without therapy, those patients in the highest-risk category all progressed to pneumonia, compared to 15% of those who received antiviral therapy. The subsequent mortality in untreated high-risk patients who progressed to pneumonia was 100%, compared to 50% for those who received antiviral therapy ([83]).

Pneumonia

There is great variability in the frequency of viral pneumonia in different studies, ranging from 15% to over 70%, but most surveys have reported only small patient populations. Fatality rates from viral pneumonia vary widely in different reports, but most include only small numbers of cases. In our institution, mortality in patients with hematologic malignancies was 15%, although reports in HSCT patients range as high as 50% to 70% ([73]). The same factors that predispose for pneumonia may predispose to fatal outcome.

Diagnosis

The diagnosis of CRV infection is established from nasopharyngeal wash, sputum, swab, or bronchoalveolar lavage specimens ([73]). Rapid antigen detection tests are available for influenza and RSV, whereas tissue cell cultures are used for detecting parainfluenza and rhinoviruses. Modern tools for diagnosis include available multiplex PCR platforms that are capable of detecting multiple respiratory viruses simultaneously with improved sensitivity compared to cell culture or direct fluorescent antibody ([84]).

Therapy

Therapy for these infections has been limited (see Tables 51-6 and 51-7). At present, there is no demonstrably effective therapy for parainfluenza infection, with DAS-181, a fusion protein inhibitor, under evaluation ([5]). Neuraminidase inhibitors, inhaled zanamavir, oral oseltamavir, and intravenous peramavir are currently approved antivirals against influenza ([85, 86]). In the pandemic 2009 H1N1 influenza A outbreak, early therapy was shown to be critical in improving mortality in patients with cancer ([5]). Viral resistance to these agents developed in some patients during therapy, particularly among those with lymphopenia, who may shed the viruses for weeks to months ([74]). Given the predisposition to prolonged shedding in immunocompromised hosts, innovative approaches to treatment are required to prevent poor outcomes and antiviral resistance ([74, 86]). Considerations have included immunomodulatory medications from statins to naproxen to mTOR inhibitors ([86]). Steroids should be used with caution because they may prolong the duration of shedding, leading to emerging resistance. Steroids are also associated with increased risk of secondary fungal and bacterial infections ([86]).

Ribavirin is available for therapy for RSV infection (Fig. 51-9). Ribavirin is administered by aerosolization 2 to 3 hours every 8 hours or continuously over 18 hours, requiring the patient to be confined in a tent ([87]). In patients with leukemia, lack of aerosolized ribavirin and high APACHE II scores were independent predictors of developing pneumonia in this population ([83]). Use of aerosolized ribavirin was suggested to be the key predictor of progression to pneumonia and mortality in allo-HSCT recipients in a study conducted at our center ([88]). Ribavirin may also be combined with immunoglobulin (Ig) therapy when the infection progresses to the lower tract ([5]). Palivizumab, a humanized monoclonal antibody directed against the F glycoprotein of RSV, is currently available and approved for prophylaxis of RSV infection in high-risk pediatric patients ([5]). Most patients with RSV pneumonia are being treated with combination therapy, but the limited numbers of patients and lack of clinical trial data reported make interpretation of results difficult.

Hepatitis Viruses

Hepatitis B

Hepatitis B virus (HBV) and hepatitis C virus (HCV) infections are common in many countries. There is a global epidemic of HBV infections, affecting more than 350 million people worldwide. Chronic HBV or HCV infections lead to progressive liver disease, cirrhosis, and hepatocellular cancer. Hepatitis can be a serious problem in patients with cancer for various reasons. Chemotherapy-induced immunosuppression may lead to reactivation and fulminant infection in patients with chronic HBV infection. Furthermore, the presence of hepatitis may require substantial delays in the administration of antineoplastic therapy. In HSCT patients, reactivation is more likely in those who have received high-dose steroids, fludarabine, rituximab, or alemtuzumab ([60]).

Hepatitis C

Hepatitis C is the most common chronic blood-borne infection. In the United States, 4 million individuals (1.6% of the population) have been infected ([89]). It is the leading indication for liver transplantation. Transmission of HCV occurs primarily through exposure to infected blood. It can be acquired from intravenous drug

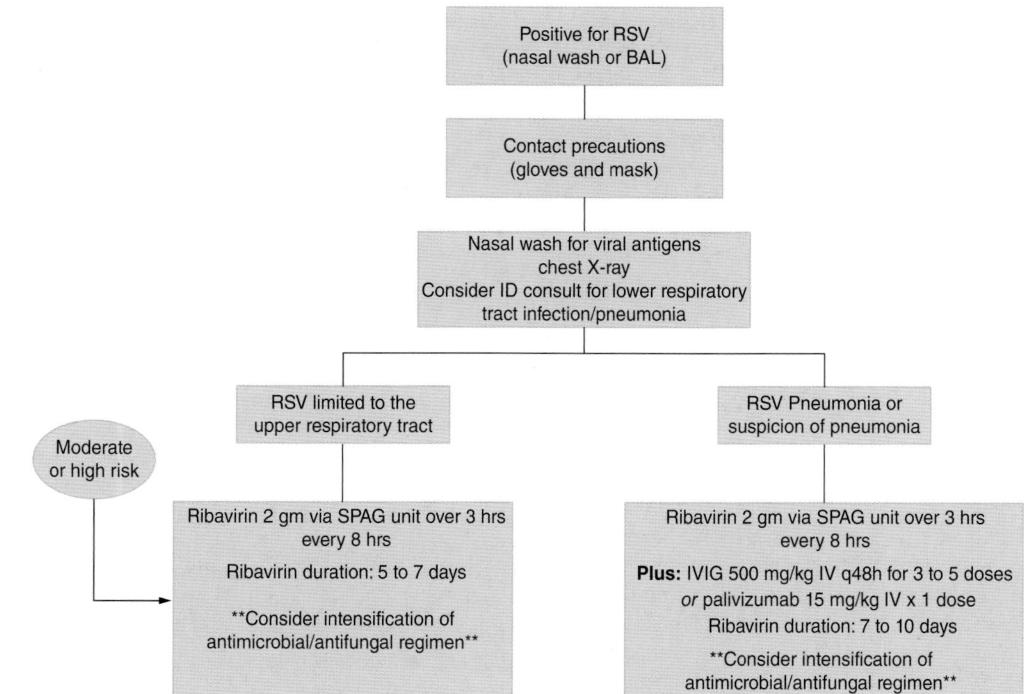

FIGURE 51-9 Management of RSV infection after hematopoietic stem cell transplantation. ID, infectious disease; IVIG, intravenous immunoglobulin; RSV, respiratory syncytial virus SPAG, small particle aerosol generator; BAL, bronchoalveolar lavage.

abuse, blood transfusion before 1992, solid-organ transplantation from infected donors, unsafe medical practices, occupational exposure to infected blood, birth to an infected mother, sexual contact with an infected person, and possibly via intranasal cocaine use ([58]).

Antibody testing should be used first to assess exposure to HCV, but in cases of persistent liver disease with immunocompromised status that may prevent adequate response, HCV RNA testing should be undertaken ([89]). Patients who are seropositive for HCV should be tested for HCV RNA to determine if virus is circulating ([89]). If virus is circulating, then the MD Anderson algorithm (Fig. 51-10), can be used for further management ([89]). The combination of pegylated INF-α plus ribavirin produced sustained virologic responses (SVRs) in only 4% of genotype 1 infections ([89]). Notably, even treated patients without SVR exhibited slower progression to cirrhosis and portal hypertension ([89]). The authors also cited an important link between HCV infection and various cancers, including hepatocellular carcinoma, lymphomas, and esophageal, prostate, and thyroid cancers ([89]).

This intriguing suggestion points to an expanded role for testing and treatment of HCV infection in prevention or treatment of malignancy. The treatment of HCV is also being revolutionized by new directly acting antivirals (DAAs) that are being rapidly introduced and promise to reduce the complications associated with HCV infection as well as improve outcomes. Treatment is uniformly recommended for HCV-infected HSCT recipients, although timing should be at least 2 years after transplant with no evidence of GVHD and off immunosuppression ([60]). At present, no active or passive immunizations are available for HCV.

Adenovirus

Adenoviruses are a common cause of self-limited respiratory and GI infections in normal individuals. Transmission occurs by aerosolized droplets or the oral-fecal route. Adenovirus infections have been recognized in patients undergoing intensive chemotherapy for hematologic and occasionally other malignancies, but they are especially prevalent among HSCT recipients ([58]). The frequency of infection among HSCT recipients has varied from 3% to 21%, and it is more prevalent among children than adults. There is no seasonal variation, and the onset of infection from time of transplantation can be variable, although the median interval is about 50 days ([58]).

Important risk factors have been identified for adenovirus infection, including childhood, allogeneic transplantation (particularly umbilical cord blood),

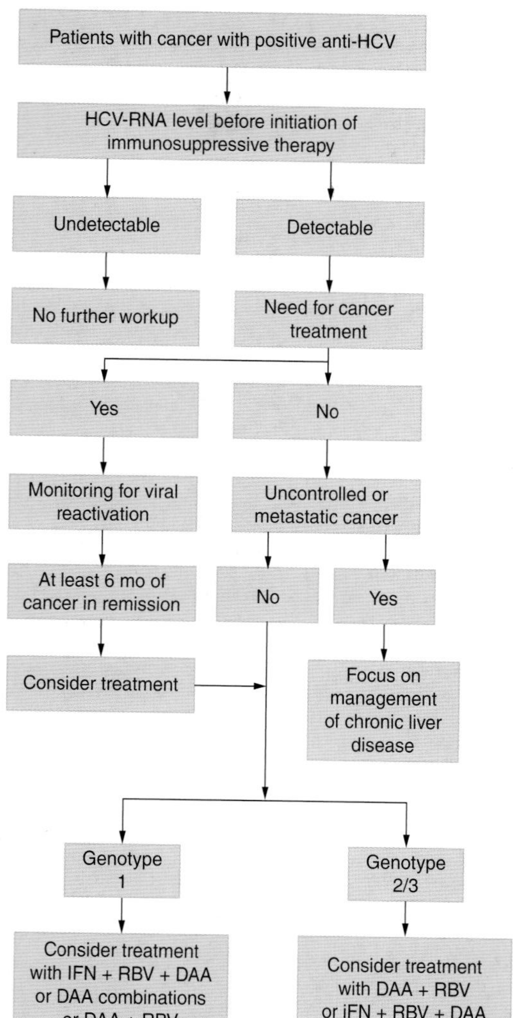

FIGURE 51-10 Management of hepatitis C viral infection. IFN, pegylated IFN; RBV, ribavirin; DAA, direct-acting antivirals.

GVHD, total-body irradiation (in children), T-cell–depleting conditioning regimens, alemtuzumab, corticosteroid therapy, and lymphopenia ([58]).

Immunocompromised patients may have asymptomatic infection, single-organ disease, or disseminated disease ([58]). The most common disease is gastroenteritis, presenting as fever and diarrhea, which may become bloody. Infections of the respiratory tract may vary from mild URI to severe pneumonitis with respiratory failure. Adenovirus may cause nephritis, and as many as 50% of patients with positive urine cultures develop hemorrhagic cystitis. Hepatitis may lead to liver failure and death. Other types of infection include encephalitis, pancreatitis, and disseminated infection with multiple- organ failure.

Diagnosis

The virus may be identified from nasopharyngeal washings, throat swabs, lower respiratory specimens, urine, stool, blood, and infected tissues. The diagnosis can be established by culture or more rapidly by the use of commercially available tests for antigen detection. Positive cultures are most often obtained from stool or urine specimens. Polymerase chain reaction is a useful diagnostic tool, particularly in screening those HSCT recipients at highest risk ([58]). Unfortunately, however, there is no threshold for viral load that definitively correlate with clinically relevant infection.

Outcome

The mortality rate from symptomatic infection is about 25%, but it is 60% to 75% in patients with disseminated disease ([90]). Death is mainly due to pneumonitis, hepatitis, or multiorgan failure. Many patients who die have other concomitant infections. There is no established therapy for these infections. In one series of 45 patients, intravenous cidofovir produced successful results in 69% and was as effective in asymptomatic patients as in those with definite disease ([91]). Lipid esters of cidofovir have been developed to improve bioavailability and reduce toxicity associated with this compound ([92]) and are currently under evaluation in immunocompromised patients with either localized or disseminated infection. Immunotherapy with adenovirus-specific cytotoxic T-lymphocyte infusions is a promising future approach ([58]).

Parvovirus B19 Infection

Parvovirus B19 causes erythema infectiosum in children. It has been associated with aplastic crises in diseases in which the life span or production of red blood cells is reduced ([93]). Anti-B19 IgG has been found to be more prevalent among patients with cancer undergoing chemotherapy than among the general population. In this study, 63% of the seropositive patients with cancer had unexplained anemia ([94]). Prolonged erythroid aplasia in childhood acute lymphocytic leukemia was associated with detection of B19 DNA in the bone marrow. Several patients with CLL have developed severe parvovirus B19 infection, manifested by a flulike illness followed by anemia owing to pure red cell aplasia in the bone marrow. The infection may be followed by an incapacitating polyarthritis. Intravenous Ig is a treatment available for this infection, but with significant risk of relapse ([95]). A concern is the potential risk posed for infection or reactivation with parvovirus B19 for patients on dasatinib (a tyrosine kinase inhibitor) ([96]).

CHAPTER 51

Polyoma Viruses Infection

BK Virus

Polyoma hominis, or BK virus, infects 80% of the general population without causing clinical manifestations ([58]). It persists in the genitourinary tract and is a major cause of hemorrhagic cystitis among HSCT recipients. About 60% to 80% of these patients have persistent viruria, and 5% to 15% develop hemorrhagic cystitis ([58]). Risk is higher in allo-HSCT recipients ([58]). Patients with hemorrhagic cystitis have higher viral loads in the urine, as detected by PCR ([60]). The disease may vary from asymptomatic microscopic hematuria to severe dysuria, frequency, and passage of clots, which may cause outflow obstruction and renal failure. Symptomatic therapy includes red blood cell and platelet transfusions, saline bladder irrigations, and cauterization. The use of quinolones is of unclear benefit. Intravenous cidofovir has been utilized, and successful treatment of refractory cystitis with hyperbaric oxygen therapy was reported ([97]), but no specific therapy is currently recommended ([58]).

JC Virus

Progressive multifocal leukoencephalopathy (PML) is a demyelinating disease of the brain caused by the JC virus, a polyomavirus that is related to BK virus ([98]). The disease results from reactivation of latent infection. About 80% of normal adults demonstrate JC virus antibodies by middle age. Progressive multifocal leukoencephalopathy was first described in patients with CLL and Hodgkin's disease. Subsequent reports centered on patients with HIV, who currently account for 80% of new PML cases ([98]). Symptoms include visual disturbances, speech defects, and mental deterioration leading to dementia and coma. The mortality rate is 80% at 1 year, and the mean time from diagnosis to death is 4 months. An association has been reported with steroid use, fludarabine, cyclophosphamide, methotrexate, mycophenolate, and, more recently, monoclonal antibodies, including rituximab ([98, 99]). Therapeutic choices are limited, with individual and combination therapy attempted with cytarabine, cidofovir, IL-2, IFN-α, Ig, zidovudine, ganciclovir, donor lymphocyte infusion, and if possible, discontinuation of GVHD prophylaxis ([100]). No consistently effective therapy is available.

REFERENCES

1. Bodey GP. Fungal infections complicating acute leukemia. *J Infect Dis*. 1966;19:667-687.
2. Egerer G, Hensel M, Ho AD. Infectious complications in chronic lymphoid malignancy. *Curr Treat Options Oncol*. 2001;2:237-244.
3. Dearden C. Disease-specific complications of chronic lymphocytic leukemia. *Hematology Am Soc Hematol Educ Program*. 2008:450-456.
4. Stanzani M, Lewis RE, Fiacchini M, et al. A risk prediction score for invasive mold disease in patients with hematological malignancies. *PloS One*. 2013;8:e75531.
5. Chemaly RF, Shah DP, Boeckh MJ. Management of respiratory viral infections in hematopoietic cell transplant recipients and patients with hematologic malignancies. *Clin Infect Dis*. 2014;59(Suppl 5):S344-S351.
6. Marchetti O, Lamoth F, Mikulska M, Viscoli C, Verweij P, Bretagne S. ECIL recommendations for the use of biological markers for the diagnosis of invasive fungal diseases in leukemic patients and hematopoietic SCT recipients. *Bone Marrow Transplant*. 2012;47:846-854.
7. Farmakiotis D, Ciurea AM, Cahuayme-Zuniga L, Kontoyiannis DP. The diagnostic yield of skin biopsy in patients with leukemia and suspected infection. *J Infect*. 2013;67:265-272.
8. Lewis RE, Albert NP, Liao G, Wang W, Prince RA, Kontoyiannis DP. High-dose induction liposomal amphotericin B followed by de-escalation is effective in experimental *Aspergillus terreus* pneumonia. *J Antimicrob Chemother*. 2013;68:1148-1151.
9. Gupta S, Sultenfuss M, Romaguera JE, et al. CT-guided percutaneous lung biopsies in patients with haematologic malignancies and undiagnosed pulmonary lesions. *Hematol Oncol*. 2010;28:75-81.
10. Lewis RE, Cahyame-Zuniga L, Leventakos K, et al. Epidemiology and sites of involvement of invasive fungal infections in patients with haematological malignancies: a 20-year autopsy study. *Mycoses*. 2013;56:638-645.
11. Pappas PG, Kauffman CA, Andes D, et al. Clinical practice guidelines for the management of candidiasis: 2009 update by the Infectious Diseases Society of America. *Clin Infect Dis*. 2009;48:503-535.
12. Samonis G, Skordilis P, Maraki S, et al. Oropharyngeal candidiasis as a marker for esophageal candidiasis in patients with cancer. *Clin Infect Dis*. 1998;27:283-286.
13. Roseff SA. Oral and esophageal candidiasis. In: Bodey GP, ed. *Candidiasis: Pathogenesis, Diagnosis, and Treatment*. 2nd ed. New York, NY: Raven Press; 1993:185-203.
14. Klevay MJ, Horn DL, Neofytos D, Pfaller MA, Diekema DJ, Alliance P. Initial treatment and outcome of *Candida glabrata* versus *Candida albicans* bloodstream infection. *Diagn Microbiol Infect Dis*. 2009;64:152-157.
15. Horn DL, Neofytos D, Anaissie EJ, et al. Epidemiology and outcomes of candidemia in 2019 patients: data from the prospective antifungal therapy alliance registry. *Clin Infect Dis*. 2009;48:1695-1703.
16. Maksymiuk AW, Thongprasert S, Hopfer R, Luna M, Fainstein V, Bodey GP. Systemic candidiasis in cancer patients. *Am J Med*. 1984;77:20-27.
17. Kontoyiannis DP, Vaziri I, Hanna HA, et al. Risk factors for *Candida tropicalis* fungemia in patients with cancer. *Clin Infect Dis*. 2001;33:1676-1681.
18. Bae GY, Lee HW, Chang SE, et al. Clinicopathologic review of 19 patients with systemic candidiasis with skin lesions. *Int J Dermatol*. 2005;44:550-555.
19. Hachem R, Hanna H, Kontoyiannis D, Jiang Y, Raad I. The changing epidemiology of invasive candidiasis: *Candida glabrata* and *Candida krusei* as the leading causes of candidemia in hematologic malignancy. *Cancer*. 2008;112:2493-2499.
20. Atkinson BJ, Lewis RE, Kontoyiannis DP. *Candida lusitaniae* fungemia in cancer patients: risk factors for amphotericin B failure and outcome. *Med Mycol*. 2008;46:541-546.
21. Pappas PG, Rotstein CM, Betts RF, et al. Micafungin versus caspofungin for treatment of candidemia and other forms of invasive candidiasis. *Clin Infect Dis*. 2007;45:883-893.
22. Leventakos K, Lewis RE, Kontoyiannis DP. Fungal infections

in leukemia patients: how do we prevent and treat them? *Clin Infect Dis*. 2010;50:405-415.
23. Vonberg RP, Gastmeier P. Nosocomial aspergillosis in outbreak settings. *J Hosp Infect*. 2006;63:246-254.
24. Upton A, Kirby KA, Carpenter P, Boeckh M, Marr KA. Invasive aspergillosis following hematopoietic cell transplantation: outcomes and prognostic factors associated with mortality. *Clin Infect Dis*. 2007;44:531-540.
25. Fisher CE, Stevens AM, Leisenring W, Pergam SA, Boeckh M, Hohl TM. The serum galactomannan index predicts mortality in hematopoietic stem cell transplant recipients with invasive aspergillosis. *Clin Infect Dis*. 2013;57:1001-1004.
26. Kontoyiannis DP, Bodey GP. Invasive aspergillosis in 2002: an update. *Eur J Clin Microbiol Infect Dis*. 2002;21:161-172.
27. Georgiadou SP, Sipsas NV, Marom EM, Kontoyiannis DP. The diagnostic value of halo and reversed halo signs for invasive mold infections in compromised hosts. *Clin Infect Dis*. 2011;52:1144-1155.
28. Walsh TJ, Anaissie EJ, Denning DW, et al. Treatment of aspergillosis: clinical practice guidelines of the Infectious Diseases Society of America. *Clin Infect Dis*. 2008;46:327-360.
29. De Pauw B, Walsh TJ, Donnelly JP, et al. Revised definitions of invasive fungal disease from the European Organization for Research and Treatment of Cancer/Invasive Fungal Infections Cooperative Group and the National Institute of Allergy and Infectious Diseases Mycoses Study Group (EORTC/MSG) Consensus Group. *Clin Infect Dis*. 2008;46:1813-1821.
30. Allo MD, Miller J, Townsend T, Tan C. Primary cutaneous aspergillosis associated with Hickman intravenous catheters. *N Engl J Med*. 1987;317:1105-1108.
31. Patterson TF, Kirkpatrick WR, White M, et al. Invasive aspergillosis. Disease spectrum, treatment practices, and outcomes. I3 Aspergillus Study Group. *Medicine (Baltimore)*. 2000;79:250-260.
32. Young RC, Bennett JE, Vogel CL, Carbone PP, DeVita VT. Aspergillosis. The spectrum of the disease in 98 patients. *Medicine (Baltimore)*. 1970;49:147-173.
33. Mays SR, Bogle MA, Bodey GP. Cutaneous fungal infections in the oncology patient: recognition and management. *Am J Clin Dermatol*. 2006;7:31-43.
34. Shah AA, Hazen KC. Diagnostic accuracy of histopathologic and cytopathologic examination of *Aspergillus* species. *Am J Clin Pathol*. 2013;139:55-61.
35. Kontoyiannis DP, Sumoza D, Tarrand J, Bodey GP, Storey R, Raad II. Significance of aspergillemia in patients with cancer: a 10-year study. *Clin Infect Dis*. 2000;31:188-189.
36. Tarrand JJ, Lichterfeld M, Warraich I, et al. Diagnosis of invasive septate mold infections. A correlation of microbiological culture and histologic or cytologic examination. *Am J Clin Pathol*. 2003;119:854-858.
37. Duarte RF, Sanchez-Ortega I, Cuesta I, et al. Serum galactomannan-based early detection of invasive aspergillosis in hematology patients receiving effective antimold prophylaxis. *Clin Infect Dis*. 2014;59:1696-1702.
38. Pagano L, Caira M, Candoni A, et al. Invasive aspergillosis in patients with acute myeloid leukemia: SEIFEM-2008 registry study. *Haematologica*. 2010;95(4):644-650.
39. Jung DS, Tverdek FP, Kontoyiannis DP. Switching from posaconazole suspension to tablets increases serum drug levels in leukemia patients without clinically relevant hepatotoxicity. *Antimicrob Agents Chemother*. 2014;58:6993-6995.
40. Raad II, Hanna HA, Boktour M, et al. Novel antifungal agents as salvage therapy for invasive aspergillosis in patients with hematologic malignancies: posaconazole compared with high-dose lipid formulations of amphotericin B alone or in combination with caspofungin. *Leukemia*. 2008;22:496-503.
41. Kontoyiannis DP, Lewis RE. Treatment Principles for the Management of Mold Infections. *Cold Spring Harbor Perspect Med*. 2014;5(4). pii. a019737.
42. Marr KA, Schlamm HT, Herbrecht R, et al. Combination antifungal therapy for invasive aspergillosis: a randomized trial. *Ann Intern Med*. 2015;162:81-89.
43. Perfect JR, Dismukes WE, Dromer F, et al. Clinical practice guidelines for the management of cryptococcal disease: 2010 update by the Infectious Diseases Society of America. *Clin Infect Dis*. 2010;50:291-322.
44. Kontoyiannis DP, Peitsch WK, Reddy BT, et al. Cryptococcosis in patients with cancer. *Clin Infect Dis*. 2001;32:E145-E150.
45. Kontoyiannis DP, Lewis RE, Alexander BD, et al. Calcineurin inhibitor agents interact synergistically with antifungal agents in vitro against *Cryptococcus neoformans* isolates: correlation with outcome in solid organ transplant recipients with cryptococcosis. *Antimicrob Agents Chemother*. 2008;52:735-738.
46. Campo M, Lewis RE, Kontoyiannis DP. Invasive fusariosis in patients with hematologic malignancies at a cancer center: 1998-2009. *J Infect*. 2010;60:331-337.
47. Lionakis MS, Kontoyiannis DP. Fusarium infections in critically ill patients. *Semin Respir Crit Care Med*. 2004;25:159-169.
48. Bodey GP, Boktour M, Mays S, et al. Skin lesions associated with *Fusarium* infection. *J Am Acad Dermatol*. 2002;47:659-666.
49. Roden MM, Zaoutis TE, Buchanan WL, et al. Epidemiology and outcome of zygomycosis: a review of 929 reported cases. *Clin Infect Dis*. 2005;41:634-653.
50. Spellberg B, Walsh TJ, Kontoyiannis DP, Edwards J Jr, Ibrahim AS. Recent advances in the management of mucormycosis: from bench to bedside. *Clin Infect Dis*. 2009;48:1743-1751.
51. Torres HA, Rivero GA, Kontoyiannis DP. Endemic mycoses in a cancer hospital. *Medicine*. 2002;81:201-212.
52. Wheat LJ, Freifeld AG, Kleiman MB, et al. Clinical practice guidelines for the management of patients with histoplasmosis: 2007 update by the Infectious Diseases Society of America. *Clin Infect Dis*. 2007;45:807-825.
53. Freifeld A, Proia L, Andes D, et al. Voriconazole use for endemic fungal infections. *Antimicrob Agents Chemother*. 2009;53:1648-1651.
54. Galgiani JN, Ampel NM, Blair JE, et al. Coccidioidomycosis. *Clin Infect Dis*. 2005;41:1217-1223.
55. Drewniak A, Kuijpers TW. Granulocyte transfusion therapy: randomization after all? *Haematologica*. 2009;94:1644-1648.
56. Safdar A. Strategies to enhance immune function in hematopoietic transplantation recipients who have fungal infections. *Bone Marrow Transplant*. 2006;38:327-337.
57. Nebiker CA, Lardinois D, Junker L, et al. Lung resection in hematologic patients with pulmonary invasive fungal disease. *Chest*. 2012;142:988-995.
58. Tomblyn M, Chiller T, Einsele H, et al. Guidelines for preventing infectious complications among hematopoietic cell transplantation recipients: a global perspective. *Biol Blood Marrow Transplant*. 2009;15:1143-1238.
59. Angarone M, Ison MG. Prevention and early treatment of opportunistic viral infections in patients with leukemia and allogeneic stem cell transplantation recipients. *J Natl Compr Canc Netw*. 2008;6:191-201.
60. Zaia J, Baden L, Boeckh MJ, et al. Viral disease prevention after hematopoietic cell transplantation. *Bone Marrow Transplant*. 2009;44:471-482.
61. Erard V, Wald A, Corey L, Leisenring WM, Boeckh M. Use of long-term suppressive acyclovir after hematopoietic stem-cell transplantation: impact on herpes simplex virus (HSV) disease and drug-resistant HSV disease. *J Infect Dis*. 2007;196:266-270.
62. Tyring S, Barbarash RA, Nahlik JE, et al. Famciclovir for the treatment of acute herpes zoster: effects on acute disease and postherpetic neuralgia. A randomized, double-blind, placebo-controlled trial. Collaborative Famciclovir Herpes Zoster Study Group. *Ann Intern Med*. 1995;123:89-96.
63. Torres HA, Kontoyiannis DP, Bodey GP, et al. Gastrointestinal

cytomegalovirus disease in patients with cancer: a two decade experience in a tertiary care cancer center. *Eur J Cancer*. 2005;41:2268-79.
64. Torres HA, Aguilera E, Safdar A, et al. Fatal cytomegalovirus pneumonia in patients with haematological malignancies: an autopsy-based case-control study. *Clin Microbiol Infect*. 2008;14:1160-1166.
65. O'Brien S, Ravandi F, Riehl T, et al. Valganciclovir prevents cytomegalovirus reactivation in patients receiving alemtuzumab-based therapy. *Blood*. 2008;111:1816-1819.
66. Boeckh M, Murphy WJ, Peggs KS. Recent advances in cytomegalovirus: an update on pharmacologic and cellular therapies. *Biol Blood Marrow Transplant*. 2015;21:24-29.
67. Boeckh M, Nichols WG, Chemaly RF, et al. Valganciclovir for the prevention of complications of late cytomegalovirus infection after allogeneic hematopoietic cell transplantation: a randomized trial. *Ann Intern Med*. 2015;162:1-10.
68. Fries BC, Riddell SR, Kim HW, et al. Cytomegalovirus disease before hematopoietic cell transplantation as a risk for complications after transplantation. *Biol Blood Marrow Transplant*. 2005;11:136-148.
69. Boeckh M, Ljungman P. How we treat cytomegalovirus in hematopoietic cell transplant recipients. *Blood*. 2009;113:5711-5719.
70. Chemaly RF, Ullmann AJ, Stoelben S, et al. Letermovir for cytomegalovirus prophylaxis in hematopoietic-cell transplantation. *New Engl J Med*. 2014;370:1781-1789.
71. Marty FM, Winston DJ, Rowley SD, et al. CMX001 to prevent cytomegalovirus disease in hematopoietic-cell transplantation. *N Engl J Med*. 2013;369:1227-1236.
72. Styczynski J, Einsele H, Gil L, Ljungman P. Outcome of treatment of Epstein-Barr virus-related post-transplant lymphoproliferative disorder in hematopoietic stem cell recipients: a comprehensive review of reported cases. *Transpl Infect Dis*. 2009;11:383-392.
73. Chemaly RF, Ghosh S, Bodey GP, et al. Respiratory viral infections in adults with hematologic malignancies and human stem cell transplantation recipients: a retrospective study at a major cancer center. *Medicine*. 2006;85:278-287.
74. Memoli MJ, Athota R, Reed S, et al. The natural history of influenza infection in the severely immunocompromised vs nonimmunocompromised hosts. *Clin Infect Dis*. 2014;58:214-24.
75. Jacobs SE, Soave R, Shore TB, et al. Human rhinovirus infections of the lower respiratory tract in hematopoietic stem cell transplant recipients. *Transpl Infect Dis*. 2013;15:474-486.
76. Seo S, Xie H, Campbell AP, et al. Parainfluenza virus lower respiratory tract disease after hematopoietic cell transplant: viral detection in the lung predicts outcome. *Clin Infect Dis*. 2014;58:1357-1368.
77. Chemaly RF, Hanmod SS, Rathod DB, et al. The characteristics and outcomes of parainfluenza virus infections in 200 patients with leukemia or recipients of hematopoietic stem cell transplantation. *Blood*. 2012;119:2738-2745; quiz 969.
78. Walsh EE, Peterson DR, Falsey AR. Human metapneumovirus infections in adults: another piece of the puzzle. *Arch Intern Med*. 2008;168:2489-2496.
79. Boeckh M. The challenge of respiratory virus infections in hematopoietic cell transplant recipients. *Br J Haematol*. 2008;143:455-467.
80. Renaud C, Xie H, Seo S, et al. Mortality rates of human metapneumovirus and respiratory syncytial virus lower respiratory tract infections in hematopoietic cell transplantation recipients. *Biol Blood Marrow Transplant*. 2013;19:1220-1226.
81. Godet C, Le Goff J, Beby-Defaux A, et al. Human metapneumovirus pneumonia in patients with hematological malignancies. *J Clin Virol*. 2014;61:593-596.
82. Schiffer JT, Kirby K, Sandmaier B, Storb R, Corey L, Boeckh M. Timing and severity of community acquired respiratory virus infections after myeloablative versus non-myeloablative hematopoietic stem cell transplantation. *Haematologica*. 2009;94:1101-1108.
83. Shah DP, Ghantoji SS, Ariza-Heredia EJ, et al. Immunodeficiency scoring index to predict poor outcomes in hematopoietic cell transplant recipients with RSV infections. *Blood*. 2014;123:3263-3268.
84. Wolfromm A, Porcher R, Legoff J, et al. Viral respiratory infections diagnosed by multiplex PCR after allogeneic hematopoietic stem cell transplantation: long-term incidence and outcome. *Biol Blood Marrow Transplant*. 2014;20:1238-1241.
85. Chemaly RF, Torres HA, Aguilera EA, et al. Neuraminidase inhibitors improve outcome of patients with leukemia and influenza: an observational study. *Clin Infect Dis*. 2007;44:964-967.
86. Dunning J, Baillie JK, Cao B, Hayden FG, International Severe Acute Respiratory and Emerging Infection Consortium (ISARIC). Antiviral combinations for severe influenza. *Lancet Infect Dis*. 2014;14:1259-1270.
87. Torres HA, Aguilera EA, Mattiuzzi GN, et al. Characteristics and outcome of respiratory syncytial virus infection in patients with leukemia. *Haematologica*. 2007;92:1216-1223.
88. Shah JN, Chemaly RF. Management of RSV infections in adult recipients of hematopoietic stem cell transplantation. *Blood*. 2011;117:2755-2763.
89. Torres HA, Mahale P, Blechacz B, et al. Effect of hepatitis C virus infection in patients with cancer: addressing a neglected population. *J Natl Compr Canc Netw*. 2015;13:41-50.
90. La Rosa AM, Champlin RE, Mirza N, et al. Adenovirus infections in adult recipients of blood and marrow transplants. *Clin Infect Dis*. 2001;32:871-876.
91. Ljungman P, Ribaud P, Eyrich M, et al. Cidofovir for adenovirus infections after allogeneic hematopoietic stem cell transplantation: a survey by the Infectious Diseases Working Party of the European Group for Blood and Marrow Transplantation. *Bone Marrow Transplant*. 2003;31:481-486.
92. Ison MG. Adenovirus infections in transplant recipients. *Clin Infect Dis*. 2006;43:331-339.
93. Chisaka H, Morita E, Yaegashi N, Sugamura K. Parvovirus B19 and the pathogenesis of anaemia. *Rev Med Virol*. 2003;13:347-359.
94. Kuo SH, Lin LI, Chang CJ, Liu YR, Lin KS, Cheng AL. Increased risk of parvovirus B19 infection in young adult cancer patients receiving multiple courses of chemotherapy. *J Clin Microbiol*. 2002;40:3909-3912.
95. Eid AJ, Brown RA, Patel R, Razonable RR. Parvovirus B19 infection after transplantation: a review of 98 cases. *Clin Infect Dis*. 2006;43:40-48.
96. Torres HA, Chemaly RF. Viral infection or reactivation in patients during treatment with dasatinib: a call for screening? *Leuk Lymphoma*. 2007;48:2308-2309.
97. Hosokawa K, Yamazaki H, Nakamura T, et al. Successful hyperbaric oxygen therapy for refractory BK virus-associated hemorrhagic cystitis after cord blood transplantation. *Transpl Infect Dis*. 2014;16:843-846.
98. Carson KR, Focosi D, Major EO, et al. Monoclonal antibody-associated progressive multifocal leucoencephalopathy in patients treated with rituximab, natalizumab, and efalizumab: a review from the Research on Adverse Drug Events and Reports (RADAR) Project. *Lancet Oncol*. 2009;10: 816-824.
99. Garcia-Suarez J, de Miguel D, Krsnik I, Banas H, Arribas I, Burgaleta C. Changes in the natural history of progressive multifocal leukoencephalopathy in HIV-negative lymphoproliferative disorders: impact of novel therapies. *Am J Hematol*. 2005;80:271-281.
100. Pelosini M, Focosi D, Rita F, et al. Progressive multifocal leukoencephalopathy: report of three cases in HIV-negative hematological patients and review of literature. *Ann Hematol*. 2008;87:405-412.

52

Endocrine and Metabolic Complications of Cancer Therapy

第五十二章　肿瘤治疗的内分泌和代谢并发症

Levent Ozsari
Naifa L. Busaidy
Mouhammed A. Habra

中文导读

随着抗肿瘤新药的不断问世及肿瘤患者生存时间延长，内分泌和代谢并发症逐渐被发现并得以重视，同时为医生的临床诊治带来了挑战。本章从肿瘤治疗的代谢并发症和内分泌并发症两大方面进行介绍。首先着重阐述了几种肿瘤治疗中常见的代谢并发症，其中包括：糖代谢异常并发症、脂代谢异常并发症、水和电解质代谢异常并发症、骨和骨矿物质代谢异常并发症。这部分简述了产生以上并发症的药物种类及产生机制等内容。随后详细阐述了肿瘤治疗常见内分泌器官受损导致的并发症，主要包括：垂体和下丘脑功能异常并发症、甲状腺功能异常并发症、肾上腺功能异常并发症、性腺功能异常并发症，这部分主要介绍了产生以上器官损伤相关内分泌并发症的药物类型、机制、临床表现和治疗。本章最后着重探讨了在肿瘤幸存者中进行肿瘤治疗所致内分泌和代谢并发症的监测，强调需要关注肿瘤治疗所产生并发症的长期影响，提出早发现和及时处理极为重要。本章对采用不同治疗手段、不同人群（成年或儿童）、不同治疗药物、不同内分泌和代谢并发症监测的内容、时间间隔等给予了相应的推荐。

In the past two decades, cancer research has rapidly advanced, spurred by the development of high-throughput technology and the maturation of genomic and proteomic research methods. These advances have resulted in treatments that have substantial effects on the outcomes of certain cancers. The continuous development of new antineoplastic agents adds increasing challenges for practicing physicians.

Current cancer treatments include surgery, radiation, cytotoxic chemotherapy, hormonal therapy, bio-immunotherapy, and targeted therapy. Adverse effects of antineoplastic agents on the endocrine system are caused by several different mechanisms and can range from a subtle laboratory abnormality with limited clinical significance to potentially lethal clinical syndromes. Antineoplastic agents in general can be cytotoxic to endocrine cells and result in glandular dysfunction. Antineoplastic agents can also interfere with the synthesis or postsynthesis processing of hormones at different levels (ie, transcription, translation, or posttranslation). An agent may inhibit or induce secretion of a hormone by interacting with receptors, perturbing intracellular second messenger metabolism, or may affect hormone delivery by changing carrier protein levels in serum or by competing for binding on the carrier protein. Finally, antineoplastic agents can interact with signal transduction pathways to inhibit or enhance hormonal action in the end organs.

In this chapter, we summarize the major and common endocrine complications of cancer therapy and discuss screening and surveillance of these complications in cancer patients and survivors.

METABOLIC DISORDERS

Glucose Metabolism Disorders

Diabetes Mellitus

Serum glucose is under continuous complex regulation. Many processes can affect glucose levels, including gut absorption, cellular uptake, gluconeogenesis, and glycogenolysis. Multiple hormones also play important roles in overall glucose homeostasis, including insulin, glucagon, growth hormone (GH), cortisol, somatostatin, and incretins.

Glucocorticoids are frequently used with many chemotherapy protocols and can have profound effects on glucose levels by increasing insulin resistance. Glucocorticoids can unmask preexisting prediabetic states by precipitating overt diabetes or make diabetes more difficult to control. The severity may range from asymptomatic hyperglycemia to nonketotic hyperosmolar coma. Most patients taking glucocorticoids with elevated glucose require insulin therapy to achieve blood glucose control, especially when given high-dose steroids. Long-acting and intermediate-acting insulin formulations are often combined with mealtime rapid-acting or short-acting insulins. Currently, there emerging studies about the management of steroid-induced diabetes mellitus in cancer patients by using multiple daily injections including mealtime short-acting insulin to counteract postprandial glucose excursions. Recent concerns about the promotion of malignancy by the mitogenic effect of insulin ([1]) and especially insulin analogs ([2]) that cross-activate insulin-like growth factor 1 (IGF-1) receptors ([3]), in combination with conflicting clinical study results on insulin glargine and cancer, have brought attention to the gap in knowledge about proper diabetes management for maximization of survival in cancer patients and survivors. A large cohort study showed that insulin analogs including insulin glargine are associated with a lower risk of cancer in general than human insulin ([4]).

Mammalian target of rapamycin (mTOR) inhibitors, L-asparaginase, streptozocin, and interferon-α (IFN-α) have also been associated with impaired glucose homeostasis and frank diabetes mellitus ([5]).

Phosphoinositide-3 (PI3) kinase/Akt/mTOR pathway–targeted therapy can cause hyperglycemia. Inhibition of this pathway results in peripheral insulin resistance, increased gluconeogenesis, and hepatic glycogenolysis ([5]). Everolimus, a tyrosine kinase inhibitor, is used in patients with advanced breast cancer, progressive neuroendocrine tumors of pancreatic origin, and advanced renal cell carcinoma. Fifty percent of patients taking everolimus have hyperglycemia (Table 52-1) ([6]). Temsirolimus is another kinase inhibitor used in patients with advanced renal cell carcinoma. The incidence of hyperglycemia in patients using this drug is 26% ([7]). The mechanism by which temsirolimus leads to diabetes may be similar to that of tacrolimus, which decreases glucose-stimulated insulin release in the pancreatic islets by reducing adenosine triphosphate (ATP) production and glycolysis ([8]).

Idelalisib, a PI3 kinase inhibitor, is indicated in patients with chronic lymphocytic leukemia. One of the idelalisib's emergent laboratory abnormalities is hyperglycemia, which occurred in 54% of patients taking both idelalisib and rituximab in a phase III study ([9, 10]). Another study showed that idelalisib alone in different dose regimens increased serum glucose in 40% of patients ([11]).

L-Asparaginase is used mainly to treat hematologic malignancies. The risk of hyperglycemia associated with pegylated *Escherichia coli* asparaginase has been reported to be similar to the risk associated with native asparaginase; in one study, the risk was about 20% in children with acute lymphoblastic leukemia treated with either agent. The exact mechanism of L-asparaginase–associated hyperglycemia is not known, although it has been postulated that inhibition of insulin, insulin receptor synthesis, or both may be the cause, leading to a combined insulin deficiency–insulin resistance syndrome ([12]). Pancreatitis, which can occur with L-asparaginase therapy, is another possible mechanism for hyperglycemia. Pancreatitis can cause islet cell destruction, and some patients might require insulin therapy ([13]). One potential complication is hypoglycemia after cessation of L-asparaginase; thus, close monitoring of blood glucose is recommended. Diabetic ketoacidosis has been reported during L-asparaginase therapy. Long-term insulin therapy may not be needed in some cases of L-asparaginase–induced diabetes mellitus ([12]).

Streptozocin, used primarily to treat malignant islet cell tumors and other neuroendocrine tumors, is an *N*-nitrosourea derivative of glucosamide. Streptozocin's effect on islet cells is species specific and dose related; rat islet cells appear to be more susceptible to the cytotoxic effects of streptozocin than human islet cells. Most of streptozocin's effects are reversible upon discontinuation of the drug. Although the reported incidence of glucose intolerance varies from 6% to 60%, most cases are mild to moderate in severity ([14]).

Interferon therapy activates immune system cells to fight some cancers and certain infections. According to a survey on IFN therapy in Japan, some patients may experience earlier development of type 1 diabetes, resulting in initiation of insulin therapy ([15]). These patients were positive for islet cell antibody and anti-glutamic acid decarboxylase antibodies ([16]).

We recommend monitoring of fasting serum glucose levels prior to the start of and during these therapies and possibly determining the levels of anti-islet autoantibodies before IFN therapy in patients with family history of type 1 diabetes mellitus ([15]).

Glucosuria

Some antineoplastic drugs (eg, ifosfamide and mercaptopurine) cause a proximal tubular defect and lower the renal threshold for glucosuria without affecting glucose metabolism. Glucosuria has been detected with an increased incidence in 67% of adult and 75% of pediatric patients treated with high-dose ifosfamide, cisplatin, and high-dose methotrexate, compared to the early postchemotherapy assessment (13% adults and 29% children) ([17]).

Lipid Disorders

Lipid disorders are seldom evaluated in the process of active anticancer therapy, because patients are often encouraged to maintain a positive metabolic balance via liberal oral intake. Investigation or treatment of mild lipid abnormalities is often overlooked because the focus is on maintaining a positive caloric balance during cancer treatment. Some lipid disorders may be short-lived without clear clinical consequences, but some may be of clinical importance and need to be detected and treated. In general, triglyceride levels higher than 1,000 mg/dL increase the rate of complications, including pancreatitis.

Lipid disorders are among the main side effects of vitamin A derivatives, which are commonly used in dermatologic disorders. One vitamin A derivative, bexarotene, has been used against malignancies like cutaneous T-cell lymphoma, acute promyelocytic leukemia, and head and neck cancer. Bexarotene is an agonist of retinoid X receptors, a family of peroxisome proliferator-activated receptors that are upregulated by the binding of bexarotene to a receptor on the nucleus.

Table 52-1 Select Small-Molecule Kinase Inhibitors With Metabolic Adverse Effects

Drug	Type	Mechanism	Main Indications	Endocrine Adverse Effect(s) (rate)
Everolimus	Rapamycin analog	Inhibits mTOR	Advanced hormone receptor–positive, HER2-negative breast cancer; progressive neuroendocrine tumors of pancreatic origin; and advanced renal cell carcinoma	Hyperglycemia (50%) Hypercholesterolemia (76%) Hypertriglyceridemia (71%)
Temsirolimus	Rapamycin analog	Inhibits mTOR	Advanced renal cell carcinoma	Hyperglycemia (26%) Hypercholesterolemia (24%)
Idelalisib	Small-molecule inhibitor	Inhibits PI3 kinase selectively	Chronic lymphocytic leukemia	Hyperglycemia (54%)

HER2, human epidermal growth factor receptor; mTOR, mammalian target of rapamycin.

This upregulation not only regulates lipid metabolism but also affects thyroid hormone synthesis ([18]). Hypothyroidism contributes to lipid disorders in patients receiving bexarotene. Because bexarotene causes hypertriglyceridemia in approximately 40% of patients, lipid levels and thyroid functions should be checked before bexarotene therapy. If triglyceride levels are 200 to 400 mg/dL, dietary modifications are recommended. If triglyceride levels are 400 to 1,000 mg/dL, omega-3 fatty acids with fibrates or nicotinic acid should be started. Lipid levels should be checked after initiation of therapy, because triglyceride levels over 1,000 mg/dL increase the risk of acute pancreatitis ([19]).

Hypercholesterolemia is the second most common side effect of bexarotene, having been reported in 48% of treated patients ([20]). The long-term significance of drug-induced hypercholesterolemia is unclear; however, atorvastatin has been successfully used to treat bexarotene-associated hypercholesterolemia in patients at the University of Texas MD Anderson Cancer Center (MDACC).

Mitotane, an analog of the insecticide dichlorodiphenyltrichloroethane, is used in patients with adrenocortical carcinoma as adjuvant therapy. The potential side effects of this therapy include hypercholesterolemia. Although the exact mechanisms of hypercholesterolemia remain unclear, mitotane stimulates hydroxymethylglutarate–coenzyme A reductase. A study from MDACC showed that mitotane increases high-density lipoprotein cholesterol, low-density lipoprotein (LDL) cholesterol, and triglyceride levels ([21]). Patients with adrenocortical carcinoma usually have a poor prognosis, making the clinical significance of mild to moderate elevation of cholesterol uncertain. However, in long-term survivors on adjuvant mitotane therapy, hyperlipidemia can lead to early development of atherosclerotic disease. The benefits of treating mitotane-induced lipid abnormalities in long-term survivors have not been established.

Mammalian target of rapamycin inhibitors have metabolic side effects that include hypercholesterolemia and hypertriglyceridemia (see Table 52-1). Although the mechanisms of these side effects are unclear, hypercholesterolemia can be caused by dysregulation of sterol regulatory element binding proteins in the mTOR pathway ([22]). Another possible mechanism is reduction in lipid clearance from the bloodstream ([23]).

Before starting mTOR inhibitor therapy, baseline fasting glucose, LDL cholesterol, and triglyceride levels should be checked. The lipid profile should be monitored for every cycle. The goals of lipid-reducing therapy are to keep fasting LDL cholesterol at or below 190 mg/dL and triglycerides at or below 300 mg/dL, if life expectancy is >1 year. Therapeutic lifestyle changes are the first appropriate approach for patients with hyperlipidemia. If such lifestyle changes fail to reduce LDL cholesterol to ≤190 mg/dL, statin therapy should be started. The goals of LDL cholesterol reduction vary with patients' cardiovascular risk factors. Patients with triglyceride levels above 1,000 mg/dL have an increased risk for acute pancreatitis. Fibrate, omega-3 acid esters, niacin, and combination therapy are the treatment options for hypertriglyceridemia ([5]).

Water and Electrolyte Disorders

Serum osmolality is tightly regulated, primarily by interaction between the hypothalamic osmoreceptors that regulate secretion of antidiuretic hormone from cells in the paraventricular and supraoptic nuclei, the hypothalamic thirst center, and the kidneys. Disruption of any of these regulators may lead to a disturbance in free water clearance and subsequent abnormalities in serum sodium levels.

Syndrome of Inappropriate Antidiuretic Hormone Secretion and Hyponatremia

Hyponatremia is a relatively common electrolyte abnormality in patients with cancer. The syndrome of inappropriate antidiuretic hormone secretion (SIADH) is one of the most common underlying causes for hyponatremia in this patient population. In addition to its association with hyponatremia, SIADH is characterized by low serum osmolality and an inappropriately high urine osmolality with elevated urine sodium. SIADH is a diagnosis of exclusion after ruling out hypovolemia, heart failure, renal insufficiency, cirrhosis, adrenal insufficiency, hypothyroidism, salt-wasting syndrome, and the use of diuretics. In patients with cancer, SIADH may be caused by ectopic antidiuretic hormone production by a variety of tumors. Syndrome of inappropriate antidiuretic hormone secretion is most commonly seen in patients with small cell lung cancer. Other tumors described (less commonly) in association with SIADH include malignant thymoma, oral squamous cell carcinoma, prostate carcinoma, and pancreatic carcinoma. Chemotherapy-induced lysis of antidiuretic hormone–containing cancer cells may lead to severe hyponatremia at the time of chemotherapy induction.

Other factors that may increase antidiuretic hormone secretion include nausea, pain, narcotics, and nicotine. Antineoplastic agents such as high-dose intravenous cyclophosphamide, vincristine, vinblastine, and cisplatin can also increase antidiuretic hormone secretion.

In cases of hyponatremia secondary to SIADH, urine osmolality is higher than plasma osmolality, and urine sodium is determined by sodium intake. In patients with SIADH, urine sodium is usually higher than 40 mEq/L. Fluid restriction (usually 500-1,500 mL of free water a day), an increase in salt intake, and occasionally, loop diuretics are attempted first in most cases of SIADH when the patient is asymptomatic or has mild symptoms. In the presence of severe symptoms (seizures or obtundation), hypertonic saline infusions might be needed with close and frequent monitoring of sodium levels to avoid rapid correction and possible osmotic demyelination syndrome (previously called central pontine myelinolysis). Demeclocycline (600-1,200 mg/d) can be used in cases in which hyponatremia does not respond to more fluid restriction. Vasopressin receptor (V2) antagonists (tolvaptan and conivaptan) have been approved by the US Food and Drug Administration for treatment of clinically significant hypervolemic or euvolemic hyponatremia associated with heart failure or SIADH ([24]).

Diabetes Insipidus and Hypernatremia

Central diabetes insipidus can occur after surgery for brain tumors and occasionally in cases of tumors near the sella or the hypothalamus that invade the neurohypophysis or disrupt the pituitary stalk. These cases are often recognized by a clinical presentation of polyuria or polydipsia and are usually treated with 1-deamino-8-D-arginine vasopressin (subcutaneously, intranasally, or orally) to control the symptoms and correct the associated hypernatremia.

Nephrogenic diabetes insipidus can also occur in patients with cancer, and multiple antineoplastic agents have been described in association with this syndrome. Ifosfamide is well known to induce damage to the proximal renal tubule and, to a lesser extent, the distal renal tubule, and thereby induce nephrogenic diabetes insipidus. Streptozocin has also been reported to cause nephrogenic diabetes insipidus.

In addition to being associated with diabetes insipidus, hypernatremia in patients with cancer is commonly caused by insufficiency of free water, especially when patients are on parenteral or tube feeding regimens or are too debilitated to obtain water for themselves.

DISORDERS OF BONE AND BONE MINERAL METABOLISM

Osteoporosis

Normal bone remodeling requires a delicate balance between bone formation by osteoblasts and bone resorption by osteoclasts. Antineoplastic therapy may affect this balance by increasing the activity of osteoclasts (eg, interleukin-2) and sometimes by having direct toxic effects on osteoblast function. Hormones and cytokines (ie, parathyroid hormone [PTH], PTH-related peptide, and interleukin-1) can also affect the overall bone turnover rate.

Bone mineral loss is one of the side effects of cancer treatment. Hormone-suppressive therapies, chemotherapeutics, and corticosteroids can cause osteoporosis in cancer patients ([25]). Improved oncologic treatments and patient longevity have increased the importance of skeletal health in cancer patients.

Breast cancer patients are at high risk for osteoporosis after hormone-suppressive therapy ([26]). Aromatase inhibitors, including anastrozole and letrozole, have been shown to decrease bone density and increase the rate of fractures in postmenopausal women. This is in sharp contrast to the positive effect on bone (both bone mineral density and fracture rates) seen with tamoxifen, a selective estrogen receptor modulator (Fig. 52-1). In the ATAC (Arimidex [anastrozole], Tamoxifen, Alone or in Combination) trial, 9,366 postmenopausal women with invasive operable breast cancer who had completed primary therapy were randomly assigned to receive anastrozole, tamoxifen, or both. More fractures were seen in patients receiving anastrozole compared with patients on tamoxifen ([27]). According to these findings, patients should undergo bone mineral density testing prior to treatment with aromatase inhibitors, and annual follow-up should be conducted thereafter. Antiresorptive therapy is usually

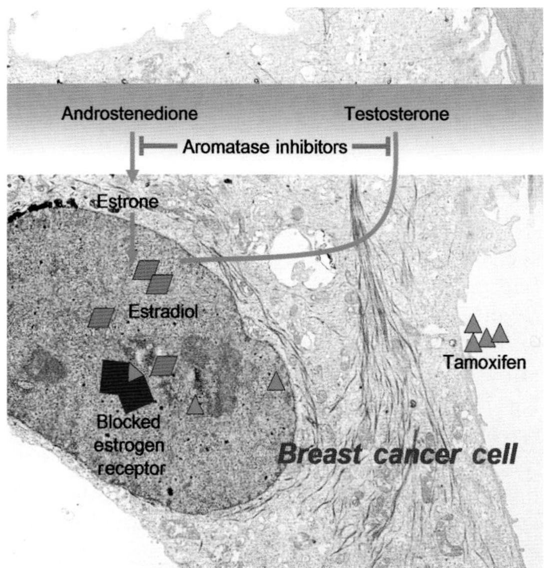

FIGURE 52-1 Mechanism of action of selective estrogen receptor modulators and aromatase inhibitors. Aromatase inhibitors, including anastrozole and letrozole, inhibit conversion of androstenedion or testosterone to estrone, which causes a decrease in bone mineral density. Tamoxifene, a selective estrogen receptor modulator, has a positive effect on bone.

added if a patient's bone density is within the osteoporotic range (T score ≤ −2.5) before treatment or if a significant decline in bone mineral density was seen during follow-up.

Osteoporosis can also occur in prostate cancer patients treated with androgen deprivation therapy (ADT), which can consist of gonadotropin-releasing hormone (GnRH) agonists, nonsteroidal antiandrogens, bilateral orchiectomy, and/or androgen blockers. These therapies can result in bone mineral loss and fractures ([28]) due to hypogonadism that increases bone resorption. The risk of fractures is higher in prostate cancer patients undergoing ADT than in those not undergoing ADT ([29]).

Patients with prostate cancer should be evaluated with dual-energy x-ray absorptiometry before starting ADT. Patients with fragility fractures or osteoporosis should be offered antiosteoporosis treatment. Before such treatment, nonpharmacologic approaches such as lifestyle modifications and calcium and vitamin D supplementation can be helpful ([30]).

Antineoplastic agents have also been implicated in chemotherapy-associated osteoporosis. Prolonged therapy with oral methotrexate for acute lymphoblastic leukemia has led to distal extremity pain, severe osteoporosis, and associated fractures, with significant improvement after cessation of methotrexate therapy ([31]). Other agents reported to reduce bone density include cisplatin and carboplatin. In addition, many chemotherapy protocols include corticosteroids, which are known to decrease bone density and increase the risk of fractures.

Patients who have undergone bone marrow transplantation have been reported to have low bone mass. The reduced bone density is likely to be secondary to the long-term side effects of bone marrow radiation, chemotherapy, corticosteroids, and hypogonadism.

Osteoblasts and osteoclasts are under the influence of many hormonal and signaling pathways, including tyrosine kinase receptors for platelet-derived growth factor (PDGF receptors α and β) and c-Abl. Activation of the PDGF pathway improves bone mineral density in ovariectomized rats and accelerates fracture healing. The absence of c-Abl is associated with impaired osteoblast maturation, leading to an osteoporosis phenotype ([32]).

Multikinase inhibitors such as sorafenib, sunitinib, and imatinib, among others, can inhibit pathways that affect bone remodeling. Not much is known about the clinical effects of tyrosine kinase inhibitors, small molecules with variable receptor affinity and an intracellular signal blocking effect, on bone. Imatinib has been the best studied and will be discussed here.

After 2 to 4 years of treatment with imatinib in patients with chronic myelogenous leukemia, a significant increase in the volume of the trabecular bone in the iliac crest has been observed ([33]). Pre-osteoblast cells exposed to imatinib undergo suppression of PDGF-induced PI3 kinase/Akt activation with upregulation of genes associated with osteoblast differentiation and bone formation.

More studies are needed to determine the effects of imatinib and other tyrosine kinase inhibitors on bone and bone mineral metabolism.

Osteomalacia and Rickets

Osteomalacia occurs when normal mineralization of the organic bone matrix fails. In children, abnormal mineralization and maturation of the growth plate at the epiphysis is called rickets. Nutritional deficiency (especially vitamin D deficiency) and renal wasting of phosphorus leading to hypocalcemia or hypophosphatemia are among the common causes of osteomalacia. Other contributing factors include drugs such as anticonvulsants or aluminum and systemic acidosis. Antineoplastic agents can also cause or worsen osteomalacia.

Ifosfamide-induced tubular damage leads to renal phosphate wasting, hypophosphatemia, and rickets. Although renal and skeletal consequences of ifosfamide therapy have been well described in children, only four adult patients with osteomalacia have been reported ([34]). Another antineoplastic agent, the estrogen derivative estramustine, used in prostate cancer metastatic to bone, can cause hypocalcemia, hypophosphatemia, secondary hyperparathyroidism, and osteomalacia with normal vitamin D levels ([35]).

Hypercalcemia

Calcium homeostasis is normally maintained by the interplay of PTH, calcitonin, phosphorus, and vitamin D metabolites in several target organs, including bones, parathyroid glands, intestines, and kidneys. In patients with cancer, multiple factors can affect this delicate balance, including nutritional status, medications, and tumor secretion of cytokines, hormones, or other humoral factors.

Hypercalcemia occurs in 5% to 10% of all patients with advanced cancer, and severe hypercalcemia (calcium level >12 mg/dL) is seen in about 0.5% of all patients with cancer ([36]). Squamous carcinoma, renal cell carcinoma, non–small cell lung carcinoma, breast carcinoma, leukemia, non-Hodgkin lymphoma, and multiple myeloma are among the most common malignancies associated with hypercalcemia. Retinoic acid derivatives have been reported to induce hypercalcemia in treatment of acute promyelocytic leukemia ([37]).

Hyperparathyroidism occurs 2.5 to 3 times more often in patients treated with low-dose (2-7.5 Gy) external radiation to the head and neck area than in the age-matched control population. Hyperparathyroidism after high-dose irradiation is uncommon. Radiation exposure from radioactive iodine treatment has also been reported in association with hyperparathyroidism ([38]).

Hypocalcemia

Many factors can increase a cancer patient's risk of hypocalcemia. These factors include the patient's nutritional status, the antineoplastic agents used, and the type of surgical procedures performed (eg, neck dissection). Cytotoxic chemotherapy can result in tumor lysis syndrome and its resultant hypocalcemia, as commonly seen in treatment of hematologic malignancies. Hyperphosphatemia, hyperkalemia, hypocalcemia, and hyperuricemia can occur after induction chemotherapy; it is of vital importance to prevent the complications of tumor lysis by hydration, alkaline diuresis, inhibition of uric acid synthesis, and administration of oral calcium or aluminum-based compounds to bind intestinal phosphate and enhance calcium absorption. Intravenous calcium administration can potentially cause calcium phosphate precipitation in the presence of severe hyperphosphatemia and should be used with extreme caution. Dialysis may be needed in cases of symptomatic hypocalcemia and serum phosphorus levels higher than 10 mg/dL.

Cisplatin has been associated with hypocalcemia. One proposed mechanism of cisplatin's ability to induce hypocalcemia is through hypomagnesemia resulting in decreased PTH secretion ([39]). Other theories include inhibition of 1,25-dihydroxy-vitamin D formation by hypomagnesemia or cisplatin inhibition of mitochondrial function in the proximal renal tubule. Other agents reported to induce hypocalcemia include dactinomycin, carboplatin, doxorubicin, and cytarabine. Hypocalcemia has been seen following administration of bisphosphonates (zoledronic acid and pamidronate) or denosumab (a monoclonal antibody that inhibits receptor activator of nuclear factor-κB ligand [RANKL]), both used to reduce skeletal complications in treatment and prevention of advanced malignancies involving the bone ([40]). Serum calcium levels and 25-hydroxyvitamin D levels should be checked prior to and during therapy with bisphosphonates or denosumab.

Hypomagnesemia

Hypomagnesemia is a well-known side effect in patients receiving platinum-based chemotherapy. Cisplatin has toxic effects on the kidneys, causing morphologic changes and necrosis in the proximal tubule, a major site of magnesium reabsorption. Hypomagnesemia is a frequent complication of cisplatin chemotherapy, affecting up to 90% of patients; 10% of these patients have symptoms of muscle weakness, tremulousness, and dizziness. A recent study showed that premedication with magnesium reduced cisplatin-induced nephrotoxicity in patients with thoracic cancers ([41]).

Carboplatin, a second-generation platinum compound, was developed to reduce the side effects of cisplatin. However, hypomagnesemia has been seen with increasing frequency and severity at higher doses of carboplatin.

Oxaliplatin, a third-generation platinum derivative that has become an integral part of various chemotherapy protocols, particularly in advanced colorectal cancer, has dose-limiting cumulative sensory neurotoxicity similar to that of cisplatin. Oxaliplatin chelates to calcium and decreases magnesium levels. Hypomagnesemia was seen in 11% of patients with advanced epithelial ovarian cancer treated with oxaliplatin in a phase II trial ([42]). Oxaliplatin is considered to carry a lower risk for hypomagnesemia compared with cisplatin and carboplatin.

Cetuximab, a monoclonal antibody against the epithelial growth factor receptor (EGFR), is used to treat metastatic colon cancer. Because EGFR is common in the loop of Henle, cetuximab blocks reabsorption of magnesium in the kidneys. Increased renal wasting of magnesium can cause supplement-resistant hypomagnesemia. Magnesium levels should be checked before and during cetuximab therapy. Cetuximab-induced hypomagnesemia is also used as a marker of worse overall survival ([43]).

PITUITARY AND HYPOTHALAMIC DISORDERS

Hypothalamic-pituitary damage leading to single or multiple hormonal deficiencies can occur in patients treated with cranial or craniospinal irradiation or intracranial surgery. Cranial radiation therapy is often used to treat leukemia and lymphoma, nonpituitary brain tumors, pituitary tumors, nasopharyngeal carcinoma, and skull base tumors ([44]). The hypothalamus appears to be more radiosensitive than the pituitary gland and may be damaged by low radiation doses (<40 Gy), but high radiation doses are likely to damage both hypothalamic and pituitary functions. Deficiency in one or more pituitary hormones occurs following irradiation (>40 Gy) of the hypothalamic-pituitary area in about 90% of patients 5 years after radiation treatment (Fig. 52-2) ([45]).

Ipilimumab, an immunoglobulin G1 antibody that blocks cytotoxic T lymphocyte-associated antigen 4

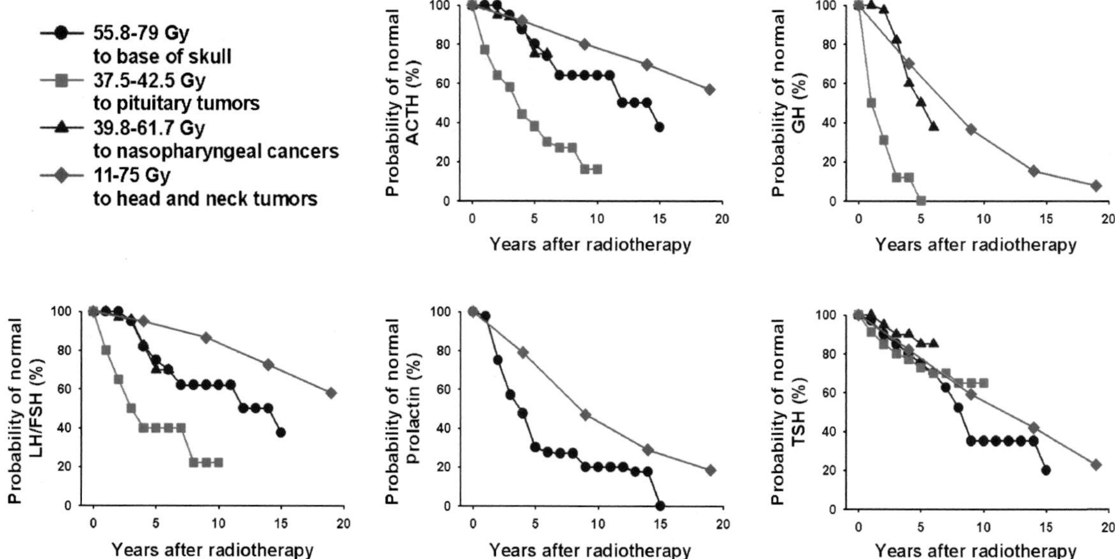

FIGURE 52-2 Probability of normal pituitary hormone secretion over time after irradiation of the hypothalamic-pituitary area. The data are from four studies: Pai et al ([55]), in which 55.8 to 79 Gy was administered to the base of the skull; Shalet et al ([45]), in which pituitary tumors were treated with 37.5 to 42.5 Gy; Appelman-Dijkstra et al ([54]), in which nasopharyngeal carcinoma was treated with 39.8 to 61.7 Gy; and Samaan et al ([56]), in which 11 to 75 Gy was administered to treat head and neck tumors. ACTH, adrenocorticotropic hormone; FSH, follicle-stimulating hormone; GH, growth hormone; LH, luteinizing hormone; TSH, thyroid-stimulating hormone.

(CTLA4), is used to treat melanoma and renal cell carcinoma. Ipilimumab-induced autoimmune hypophysitis was reported in 11% of patients in a retrospective study (Table 52-2) ([46]). The risk factors for ipilimumab-induced hypophysitis are male gender and old age ([47]). The typical clinical presentation includes headache, fatigue, and nausea. Magnetic resonance imaging (MRI) may reveal pituitary gland and stalk enlargement. After cessation of the drug, pituitary morphology returns to normal (Fig. 52-3) ([48]). The earliest and most frequently affected hormone is adrenocorticotropic hormone (ACTH), but other hormones can also be affected; the effects often disappear after drug cessation. Physicians should be aware of hypopituitarism symptoms and test for adrenal insufficiency, hypogonadism, and hypothyroidism.

Growth Hormone Deficiency

Growth hormone deficiency is frequently noted after cranial irradiation. In children, isolated GH deficiency can occur after low radiation doses, but high doses may produce panhypopituitarism. Hypopituitarism appears to be dose dependent. At low doses (20-24 Gy), the only effect may be an altered pulsatile secretory pattern. At doses higher than 30 Gy, deficient GH secretion and growth retardation are observed in more than a third of patients (Fig. 52-4). Children who receive cranial irradiation require long-term follow-up ([49]).

Growth hormone deficiency is also common in adults who have undergone cranial radiation

Table 52-2 Novel Immunotherapeutic Agents With Endocrine Adverse Effects

Drug	Type	Mechanism	Endocrine Adverse Effects
Ipilimumab	IgG1 monoclonal antibody	Blocks CTLA4 receptor	Hypophysitis Thyroiditis Graves disease
Pembrolizumab	IgG4 monoclonal antibody	Blocks PD-1 receptor	Hypothyroidism Transient thyrotoxicosis

CTLA4, cytotoxic T lymphocyte-associated antigen 4; Ig, immunoglobulin; PD, programmed death.

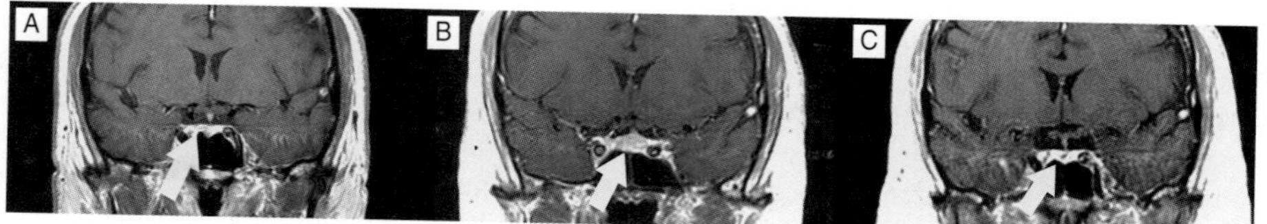

FIGURE 52-3 Magnetic resonance images of a patient before (A), during (B), and 8 weeks after (C) ipilimumab therapy.

therapy. In those patients, GH deficiency is thought to cause decreased bone and muscle mass, fatigue, impaired sense of well-being, lowered exercise capacity, increased volume of adipose tissue, and altered myocardial function. In addition, patients with GH deficiency may have a higher occurrence of atherosclerotic plaques and an increased risk for cardiovascular diseases. GH replacement in these patients can restore normal adipose tissue composition, bone metabolism, quality of life, sense of well-being, lipid profile, and cardiac function. Despite the apparent benefits, data on the effect of GH replacement in long-term cancer survivors are still lacking. Growth hormone replacement is contraindicated in any patient with an active malignant condition, but it can be initiated in an adult in whom malignant disease has been absent for at least 5 years. Another treatment reported to result in GH deficiency is long-term intrathecal opioids. Patients receiving this treatment have about a 15% elevation in the risk of developing GH deficiency ([50]).

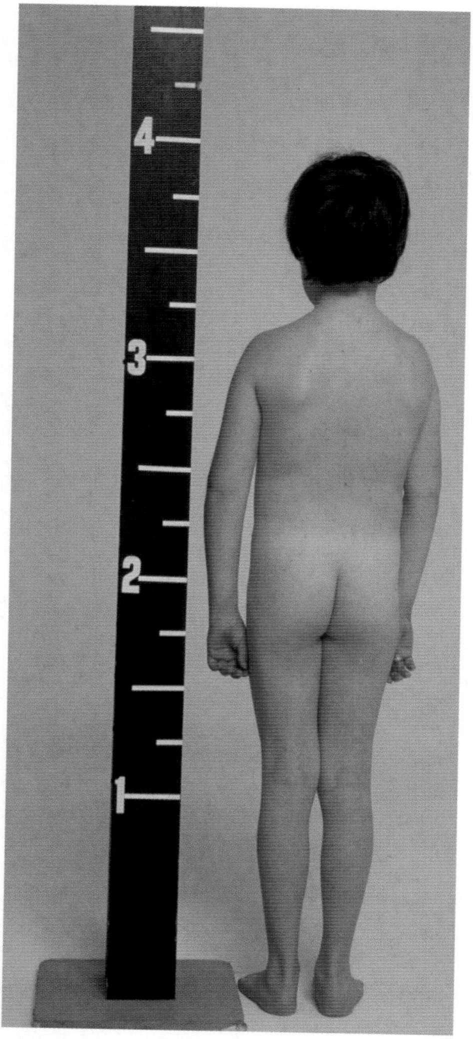

FIGURE 52-4 A patient with short stature due to growth hormone deficiency resulting from radiation treatment of a brain tumor.

Central Hypothyroidism

Radiation therapy can cause immediate and long-term effects. One such effect, central hypothyroidism, may be a result of the possible effects of brain or head and neck irradiation on hypothalamic and pituitary regulation of thyroid-stimulating hormone (TSH) secretion. Not only cranial irradiation but also craniospinal irradiation can cause central hypothyroidism. In one study, central hypothyroidism was detected a year after the end of radiation treatment in 6% of patients ([51]). In that study, 15% to 20% of patients who had undergone cranial irradiation had diminished TSH secretion 5 years after the end of treatment, and approximately 35% of those patients had it after 10 years. Because of the combined effect of irradiation on the thyroid gland and the hypothalamic-pituitary axis, we suggest measuring patients' levels of both serum free thyroxine and TSH concentrations yearly or if the patients is having symptoms suggestive of hypothyroidism to replace thyroid hormones when necessary.

Chemotherapy may enhance the deleterious effect of radiation. Children with brain tumors (not involving the hypothalamic-pituitary axis) who receive vincristine, carmustine, lomustine, or procarbazine in combination with brain irradiation have a 35% incidence of hypothyroidism, compared with a 10% incidence in children who undergo brain irradiation alone ([52]).

Bexarotene was found to cause central hypothyroidism in 40% of patients with cutaneous T-cell lymphoma ([20]). Reversible, retinoid X receptor–mediated suppression of TSH secretion is one explanation for this side effect. Bexarotene patients often require higher levothyroxine dose compared with patients with other causes of hypothyroidism. This observation is related to bexarotene-related increase in thyroid hormone metabolic clearance ([53]).

Hypogonadotropic Hypogonadism

Brain surgery and irradiation of the skull carry the potential for hypothalamic-pituitary damage, including hypogonadotropic hypogonadism. Hypogonadism occurs within 7 years after cranial irradiation for non-pituitary neoplasia in 25% of patients. Hypogonadism is transient in the presence of hyperprolactinemia and is treated with antidopaminergic therapy ([54]). Hyperprolactinemia is the most commonly reported hormonal abnormality in patients who have undergone head and neck irradiation, occurring in more than 66% of patients ([55, 56]). Hyperprolactinemia inhibits gonadotropin secretion from the pituitary gland and decreases the responsiveness of the pituitary gland to GnRH, causing secondary hypogonadism. In children, inadequate sexual development, delayed puberty, and absent menarche are significant problems, whereas in adults, gonadotropin deficiency may cause sex steroid hormone deficiency, infertility, and loss of axillary and pubic hair (Fig. 52-5). Sex steroid hormone deficiency lowers libido and may have deleterious effects on bone and lipid metabolism.

Early or even precocious puberty has also been reported in patients with acute lymphoblastic leukemia treated with combined chemotherapy and cranial irradiation and in patients with brain tumors treated with cranial irradiation. This phenomenon is more common in girls. Coexisting GH deficiency is frequently noted. In a recent study of male cancer survivors (excluding those who had undergone treatment that may have otherwise affected gonadal function), chronic opioid therapy, given in morphine-equivalent daily doses of at least 200 mg daily, was associated with secondary hypogonadism ([57]).

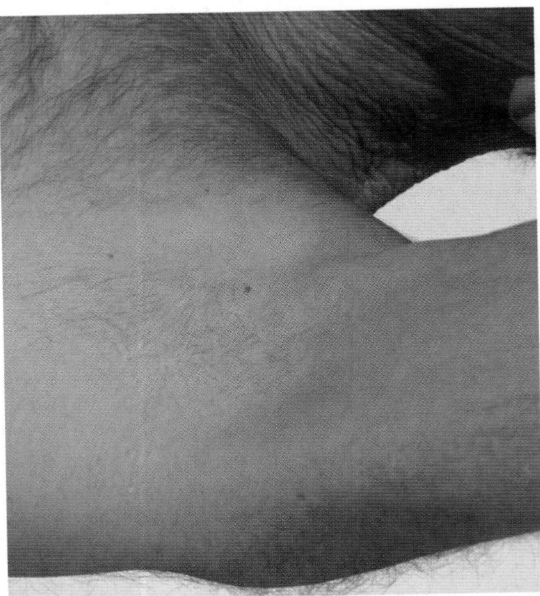

FIGURE 52-5 Loss of axillary hair in a patient who developed secondary hypogonadism after cranial irradiation.

THYROID DISORDERS

Thyroid Neoplasms

Ionizing radiation is implicated in the etiology of thyroid cancer. Irradiation of the thyroid, especially in children and young adults (such as young patients with Hodgkin disease), increases the risk of papillary thyroid carcinoma ([58]).

Hyperthyroidism

Radiation-induced hyperthyroidism has been described but is far less common than radiation-induced hypothyroidism.

Radiation-induced silent thyroiditis with transient thyrotoxicosis has been reported in patients treated with radiation. Thyroiditis-induced thyrotoxicosis occurs within a few months of radiation therapy in most cases; hypothyroidism occurs several months later. The risk of Graves disease increases following radiation therapy. Patients with lymphoma treated with radiation constitute the largest number of patients who have developed Graves disease after radiation therapy; this finding raises the possibility of a relationship between the two clinical entities. Patients treated with radiation for nasopharyngeal, breast, and/or laryngeal carcinomas may also develop Graves disease. Cytokines have also been reported to lead to Graves disease. Interferon is known to induce the production of autoantibodies and can lead to autoimmune thyroid disease, such as autoimmune primary hypothyroidism, transient thyrotoxicosis, or more rarely, Graves disease. Women have a higher risk than men of developing autoimmune thyroid disease upon starting IFN treatment ([59]). It is important to distinguish the cases in which IFN induces transient thyrotoxicosis followed by hypothyroidism from the cases in which IFN induces Graves disease. Thyroid scans showing increased homogeneous uptake in the presence of hyperthyroidism are highly suggestive of Graves disease and warrant treatment with antithyroid medications (eg, methimazole).

Systemic therapies can also be linked to hyperthyroidism. Monoclonal antibodies directed against CTLA4 (ipilimumab and tremelimumab) and anti-CD52 antibody (alemtuzumab) are associated with painful thyroiditis and Graves disease ([60]). Interleukin-2 (denileukin diftitox) treatment alone causes transient hyperthyroidism followed by hypothyroidism in about 50% of patients ([61]). The mechanism of interleukin-2–induced autoimmune thyroid dysfunction is unclear, although interleukin-2–induced disruption of self-tolerance has been suggested as a mechanism. Tyrosine kinase inhibitors can cause transient thyrotoxicosis via destructive thyroiditis ([60]). Pembrolizumab treatment caused hyperthyroidism in 1 of 135 patients in a safety study ([62]).

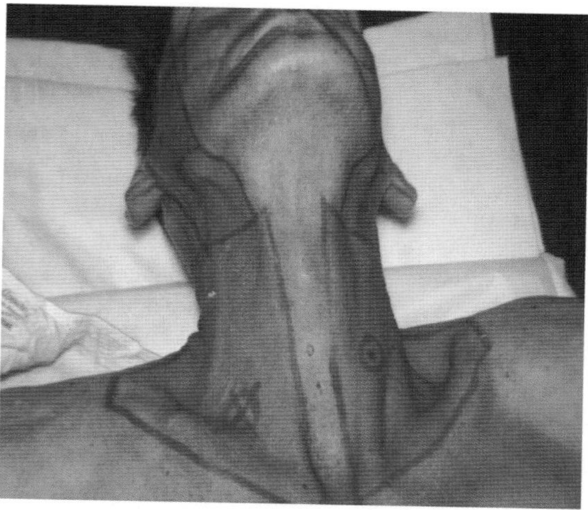

FIGURE 52-6 Mapping of radiation ports on a patient with squamous cell cancer of the head and neck. The patient developed primary hypothyroidism 2 years after radiation therapy.

Hypothyroidism

Head and neck irradiation frequently causes dysfunction of the thyroid gland. Radiation can induce primary hypothyroidism when given in doses higher than 25 Gy to the region near the thyroid gland (Fig. 52-6). Secondary and tertiary hypothyroidism can be seen with doses of 40 Gy or higher to the hypothalamic-pituitary area. Most cases of primary hypothyroidism occur about 5 years after radiation therapy. The probability of hypothyroidism is dose related and increases with duration of follow-up after radiation treatment. In a study of 1,677 patients with Hodgkin disease whose thyroid had been irradiated, the risk of thyroid disease was 52% and 67% after 20 and 26 years, respectively ([63]). Four hundred eighty-six patients (29%) received thyroxine therapy because of elevated serum TSH concentrations, and 27 (2%) had transient elevations in serum thyrotropin level that were not treated. A recent review estimated the rate of hypothyroidism after thyroid irradiation to be 20% to 30%, with half of the cases occurring within the first 5 years ([63]).

A significant number of patients develop subclinical hypothyroidism (elevated TSH with normal thyroxine levels), not overt hypothyroidism, when less than 40 Gy of radiation is administered. Subclinical hypothyroidism (20%) is more frequent than overt hypothyroidism (5%) 5 years after chemotherapy and radiation therapy ([64]). Multiple factors increase the risk for hypothyroidism, including high doses of radiation to the head and neck, combined radiation and surgical treatments, time interval since therapy, and failure to shield midline structures. Other risk factors include thyroid resection during a laryngectomy or disruption of the vascular supply of the thyroid gland during surgery.

The use of iodine-131 (^{131}I) may result in thyroid dysfunction. The use of ^{131}I-metaiodobenzylguanidine in treatment of metastatic pheochromocytoma carries the possibility of inducing primary hypothyroidism and requires routine use of potassium perchlorate to block the thyroid ^{131}I uptake.

Interferon therapy is associated with primary hypothyroidism in about 10% of treated patients and was not related to IFN dosage ([65]). The presence of pretreatment serum antithyroid antibodies in patients treated with IFN therapy increases the risk for development of IFN-induced thyroid disease. During 6 years of observation after IFN therapy, the absence of thyroid autoantibodies at the end of IFN treatment was found to be a protective factor against development of thyroiditis, whereas positivity for thyroid antibodies at high titers at the end of IFN treatment was significantly related to chronic subclinical hypothyroidism. Interferon-related thyroid autoimmunity is not a completely reversible phenomenon, because some patients develop chronic thyroiditis, especially in the presence of high autoantibody titers.

Interleukin-2 causes painless thyroiditis with acute onset, with initial hyperthyroxinemia followed by primary hypothyroidism. The hypothyroidism may last months but is occasionally permanent; 9% of patients require replacement thyroid hormone therapy ([66]).

Patients treated with multiple antineoplastic agents (with or without radiation) also have a higher than normal incidence of primary hypothyroidism. Fifteen percent of patients who received a combination of cisplatin, bleomycin, dactinomycin, vinblastine, and etoposide developed elevated TSH levels with normal free triiodothyronine (T_3) and free thyroxine (T_4), compatible with subclinical primary hypothyroidism, in contrast to the control group ([67]).

The targeted therapy has also been linked to development of a variety of thyroid abnormalities. For example, autoimmune thyroid disease has been seen in 23% of patients receiving alemtuzumab [68].

Imatinib use was reported to increase levothyroxine requirements in thyroidectomized patients, whereas nonthyroidectomized patients had no significant alterations of their thyroid functions. These data suggest that imatinib and maybe tyrosine kinase inhibitors in general may accelerate the clearance of levothyroxine, leading to clinical hypothyroidism in patients who are dependent on exogenous levothyroxine [69].

Thyroid dysfunction was reported in 21% of renal cell carcinoma patients receiving sorafenib [70]. Prospective studies estimated the risk of thyroid dysfunction to reach 68%; however, only 6% of patients had clinical symptoms requiring thyroid hormone replacement [71]. Sorafenib-related thyroiditis has been suggested as a mechanism of thyroid dysfunction in some of the patients, but it is unclear if thyroid dysfunction represents an autoimmune process or a manifestation of vascular endothelial growth factor blockade affecting the thyroid blood supply.

Sorafenib also affects the thyroid hormone replacement dose requirement in thyroidectomized patients with differentiated or medullary thyroid cancer. In one study, the dose of L-thyroxin had to be changed in 42% of the patients using sorafenib [72]. Another study showed that the daily dose of L-thyroxin was increased in 19% of patients and decreased in 16% of patients with anorexia and weight loss [73].

Similarly, thyroid dysfunction was reported in 62% of patients receiving sunitinib, including 36% of patients who had persistent elevation of TSH, which was suggestive of primary hypothyroidism, especially in patients with longer sunitinib use. Destructive thyroiditis has been suggested as an explanation, although some patients became athyrotic on sunitinib after having normal thyroid function at baseline [74]. Another study showed that thyroid size was reduced to 59% after 12 months of sunitinib use in patients with renal cell carcinoma [75]. Other prospective studies found that 27% of patients receiving sunitinib had elevated TSH requiring hormone replacement [76]. Some patients were reported to present with thyrotoxic phase preceding hypothyroidism, which further supports the theory of sunitinib-related destructive thyroiditis leading to hypothyroidism in these patients [77]. Impaired iodine uptake and inhibition of peroxidase activity were also suggested as potential mechanisms to explain hypothyroidism [78,79].

Ipilimumab-induced activation of T cells results in not only antitumor activity but also immune infiltration of endocrine glands. The major endocrine glands affected by ipilimumab are the pituitary and thyroid glands. Although hypophysitis causes central hypothyroidism, thyroiditis causes primary hypothyroidism [80].

Pembrolizumab is an anti-programmed cell death (PD)-1 antibody that blocks interaction of PD-1 with the PD-L1 or PD-L2 ligand (see Table 52-2). Although PD-1 is expressed by T lymphocytes, PD-L1 or PD-L2 on tumor cells inhibits T-lymphocyte action. Anti-PD-1 antibody reverses this inhibition. The US Food and Drug Administration granted the approval to use pembrolizumab in patients with unresectable or metastatic melanoma. Primary hypothyroidism has been reported to occur in 8.3% of patients receiving pembrolizumab, with median time to onset being 3.5 months (range, 0.7 weeks to 19 months). Because the timing of the onset of thyroid dysfunction varies widely, patients who have received pembrolizumab should be monitored closely for changes in thyroid function [62].

Abnormalities in Thyroid Hormone-Binding Proteins

Thyroid hormones are preferentially bound to thyroid hormone–binding globulin (TBG) (65%-70%), transthyretin (15%-20%), and albumin (10%-15%). Multiple factors can affect the levels of these binding proteins and the subsequent levels of bound thyroid hormones. In patients with malignancies, changes in sex hormone levels, glucocorticoids, narcotics, nutritional status, and some antineoplastic agents are the major factors affecting the protein-binding properties. Overall, the level of total T_3 and T_4 may be affected, but in general, the levels of free (biologically active) hormones are normal. The effect on TBG synthesis or clearance is usually reversible. Not only are estrogens known to increase TBG and total thyroid hormone levels, but tamoxifen also causes elevated plasma concentrations of TBG in postmenopausal women with breast cancer after 6 months of therapy. Nonsteroidal aromatase inhibitors (anastrozole and letrozole) are known to lower estrogen levels, but the effect on TBG has still not been fully documented in the literature; when letrozole was given at 2.5 mg/d, however, there was a statistically significant decrease in total T_4 but not total T_3 levels [81].

Glucocorticoids are frequently used in combination with chemotherapy and are known to suppress TSH secretion and inhibit TBG synthesis. L-Asparaginase can inhibit the synthesis of albumin and TBG, which affects serum thyroid hormone levels. 5-Fluorouracil increases total T_3 and T_4 levels and maintains a normal free thyroxine index, suggesting that this agent increases serum thyroid hormone–binding proteins, resulting in normal thyroid function [82].

Mitotane increases the levels of hormone-binding globulins, but the increase in TBG is less remarkable than mitotane's effect on corticosteroid-binding globulin.

ADRENAL DISORDERS

Primary Adrenal Insufficiency

Mitotane is an orphan drug mostly used to treat adrenocortical carcinoma. Mitotane has selective toxicity to both normal and malignant adrenocortical cells. It also causes an increase in serum levels of cortisol-binding globulin [83]. Glucocorticoid replacement therapy is needed when mitotane is used; high doses are required because of the increased levels of binding globulin and enhanced metabolic clearance of corticosteroids by mitotane.

Animal studies found cases of adrenal necrosis associated with sunitinib use, leading the Food and Drug Administration to recommend monitoring adrenal functions in patients receiving sunitinib. However, there was no evidence of adrenal hemorrhage or clinical evidence of adrenal insufficiency in subsequent clinical safety data [84].

Secondary Adrenal Insufficiency

Prolonged glucocorticoid treatment is the most common cause of adrenal dysfunction in patients with cancer. Secondary (central) adrenal insufficiency may develop up to 2 years after discontinuation of glucocorticoids and can persist for months. Irradiation of the hypothalamic-pituitary region causes ACTH deficiency with resultant secondary adrenal insufficiency in 19% to 42% of patients. The median time to development of adrenal insufficiency after radiation therapy is 5 years, but onset can occur in as little as 2 years. The 1-μg cosyntropin stimulation test has been proposed to screen central adrenal insufficiency in cancer survivors who received >30 Gy of radiation to hypothalamic and pituitary areas [85].

Prolonged therapy with busulfan was initially reported to cause a reversible clinical syndrome resembling central adrenal insufficiency as evidenced by metyrapone testing. No recent reports have corroborated this finding. Long-term intrathecal opioid therapy for intractable nonmalignant pain resulted in central adrenal insufficiency in 15% of patients tested for insulin-induced hypoglycemia [50].

Megestrol acetate is used to stimulate appetite in patients with cancer, but its prolonged use can lead to a Cushing-like syndrome, and sudden withdrawal after prolonged treatment may result in adrenal insufficiency. Megestrol shows glucocorticoid-like effects with an acute suppressive effect on the hypothalamic-pituitary axis and ACTH secretion, leading to central adrenal insufficiency as determined with the 1-μg cosyntropin stimulation test [86, 87]. Secondary adrenal insufficiency can be diagnosed by a variety of tests with varying sensitivity and specificity, but in our practice, we frequently use a combination of basal (8:00 AM) serum cortisol and ACTH measurement as well as1-μg cosyntropin stimulation testing. Rarely, insulin-induced hypoglycemia is used to assess the overall cortisol and GH response to hypoglycemia when evaluating patients for panhypopituitarism.

GONADAL DISORDERS

Direct radiation exposure and cytotoxic chemotherapeutic agents are common causes of hypogonadism and infertility in cancer survivors. Because of the considerable differences between female and male gametogeneses, cancer therapy can have a variety of effects on fertility and gonadal functions in the two sexes.

Female Gonadal Disorders

Oogenesis occurs during embryonic life, and oocytes remain quiescent most of their lifespan; it is this property that makes oocytes resistant to the adverse effects of cytotoxic chemotherapy. However, because the number of oocytes is limited, damage to oocytes may in effect shorten a woman's reproductive period. Granulosa cells are also susceptible to cytotoxic drugs, as evidenced by the results of ovarian biopsies performed after chemotherapy (Fig. 52-7). Infertility may occur as a result of impairment of either granulosa cells or oocytes.

With advances in cancer treatment, an increasing number of women survive malignancies to face reproductive disorders. It is of vital importance to discuss fertility issues before radiation or systemic chemotherapy, because these modalities carry significant risks for ovarian dysfunction and infertility. The effects of radiation treatment on the ovaries differ with patient age, radiation dose, and field of treatment. Radiation treatment that includes the pelvis increases the risk of infertility more than radiation treatment that includes only the abdomen [88]. Pregnancy rates decrease at doses between 5 and 10 Gy [89]. Fractionated radiation

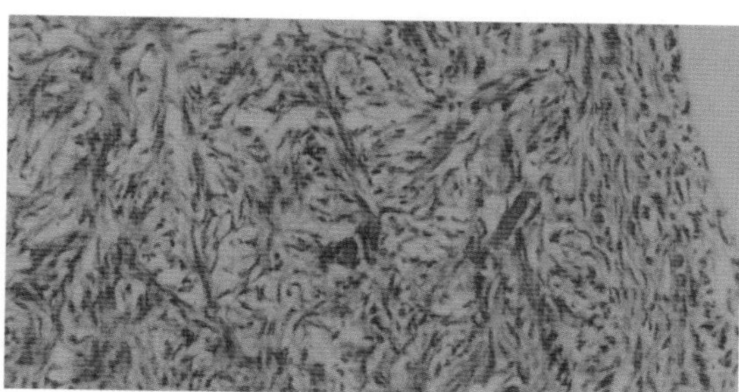

FIGURE 52-7 Hematoxylin and eosin staining of a biopsy sample showing atrophy of ovarian tissue after cytotoxic chemotherapy.

seems to carry less risk for permanent sterility. When possible, fractionated radiation should be used with shielding of the gonads, and restriction of radiation fields reduces the risk of ovarian failure. Ovarian transposition (oophoropexy) to the paracolic gutters before pelvic irradiation has been suggested to preserve ovarian function in women less than 40 years of age with cervical carcinoma less than 3 cm in diameter ([90]). Ovarian transposition can also be used prior to pelvic irradiation in other diseases, including lymphoma. This procedure can be done by either a laparotomy or a laparoscopy with the intent of preventing radiation-induced (but not chemotherapy-induced) ovarian failure. Assisted fertilization is often needed after this procedure.

Oocyte cryopreservation has been proposed as a means of preserving fertility in women treated for cancer, but it has been less successful in humans than in animal models. Ovarian tissue cryopreservation and transplantation have also been proposed for patients before cancer treatment.

The ethical issues behind these techniques are still being disputed, and there is still the concern of potential disease recurrence from residual disease in autografted ovarian tissues. Obtaining unilaminar follicles from cryopreserved, thawed tissue and growing them in vitro has been proposed to reduce the risk of recurrence. The cytotoxic effects of chemotherapeutic agents are seen more in rapidly dividing cells than in cells at rest, which led to the hypothesis ([91]) that GnRH agonists would suppress the hypothalamic-pituitary-ovary axis and make the ovaries less susceptible to the cytotoxic effects of chemotherapy. In animal models, GnRH agonist therapy lowered cyclophosphamide-induced but not radiation-induced ovarian toxicity. Some studies have reported encouraging results of the use of this approach in women with breast cancer, leukemia, and lymphoma ([91]). Another study showed that GnRH agonist therapy may protect ovarian reserve but does not decrease the risk of premature ovarian failure in patients treated for lymphoma ([92]).

In premenopausal women with breast cancer treated with regimens based on anthracyclines (5-fluorouracil, epirubicin, and cyclophosphamide), the rate of chemotherapy-related amenorrhea is 93%. At the end of therapy, menstrual periods resumed in 24% of the patients ([93]).

Alkylating agents, which are non–cell-cycle specific, are generally highly gonadotoxic. Mechlorethamine is usually used in combination with vincristine, procarbazine, and prednisone. This combination is highly gonadotoxic, but the exact contribution of mechlorethamine to the gonadotoxicity is difficult to evaluate. Chlorambucil, melphalan, busulfan, and cyclophosphamide also carry a high risk of ovarian damage. Ovarian failure with alkylating agents was found to impose the highest risk with an estimated odds ratio (relative to no treatment) of 3.98 ([94]). The extent of cisplatin toxicity in women is less well defined, with an odds ratio (relative to no treatment) of 1.77. Temporary amenorrhea developed in 2 of 12 female patients in whom cisplatin (0.4-0.6 g/m^2) was used in combination with bleomycin and vinblastine to treat ovarian germ cell tumors; the amenorrhea lasted from 12 to 15 months after the cessation of chemotherapy ([94]).

Transient and permanent ovarian failure has been reported with etoposide use ([95]).

Antimetabolites, which are cell-cycle specific, may exert few toxic effects on the ovaries. As a single agent, doxorubicin has few, if any, adverse effects on ovarian function, although a synergistic effect of the combination of doxorubicin and cyclophosphamide is a concern.

Vinblastine has been known to cause reversible and dose-related amenorrhea when combined with alkylating agents ([96]).

Male Gonadal Disorders

Spermatogenesis occurs in a continuous cycle of meiosis, mitosis, differentiation, and maturation. Germ cells and spermatogonia, in contrast to Leydig or Sertoli cells, are sensitive to cytotoxic agents. If sufficient germ cells remain after cytotoxic chemotherapy, resumption of spermatogenesis usually occurs; the longer the duration of azoospermia, the lower is the likelihood of spermatogenesis recovery ([97]).

Radiation damage to the gonads is dose dependent. Low-dose testicular irradiation leads to a transient suppression of sperm counts with a recovery time proportional to the radiation dose ([98]). However, permanent infertility was reported in patients who received fractionated radiation doses of more than 2 Gy (Fig. 52-8), whereas clinically significant Leydig cell impairment occurs rarely with doses of less than 20 Gy ([99]).

Therapy with alkylating agents such as cyclophosphamide or chlorambucil administered alone may result in reversible but prolonged azoospermia. Chlorambucil causes azoospermia at cumulative doses of 400 to 800 mg; recovery may take 3 to 4 years after a mean total dose of about 750 mg/m^2 ([100]). Cyclophosphamide affects spermatogenesis more than Leydig cell function, causing reduced sperm count with normal testosterone levels.

Antineoplastic agents causing azoospermia in humans can be classified in four groups. The first group consists of chemotherapeutics that cause prolonged azoospermia: chlorambucil, cyclophosphamide, procarbazine, melphalan, and cisplatin. The chemotherapeutics in the second group, carmustine and lomustine, cause azoospermia in adults who had chemotherapy treatment prior to puberty. The agents in the third group cause prolonged azoospermia when given with other sterilizing agents; this group consists of busulfan, ifosfamide, nitrogen mustard, and dactinomycin. The agents in the fourth group have additive and temporary effects on azoospermia when combined with agents from the other three groups; this group consists of doxorubicin, thiotepa, cytosine arabinoside, and vinblastine ([101]).

Multiple methods of preventing or reversing infertility in men treated for cancer have been suggested. In rats, fertility can be restored by suppressing testosterone with GnRH agonists or antagonists, either before or after cytotoxic therapy. This approach does not protect survival of stem cells in the testes but enhances the ability of the testes to maintain differentiation of type A spermatogonia ([102]). It would be premature to apply this method to everyday clinical practice, as the limited data from human trials did not show this benefit. Semen cryopreservation before starting gonadotoxic therapy followed by assisted fertilization is another strategy to preserve fertility in men with cancer.

SURVEILLANCE FOR COMPLICATIONS IN CANCER SURVIVORS

Primary care physicians and oncologists should be aware of the major long-term consequences of cancer therapy for early detection and management of treatment-related side effects. Long-term follow-up is frequently needed because many of the complications occur years after treatment and can have subtle clinical presentations.

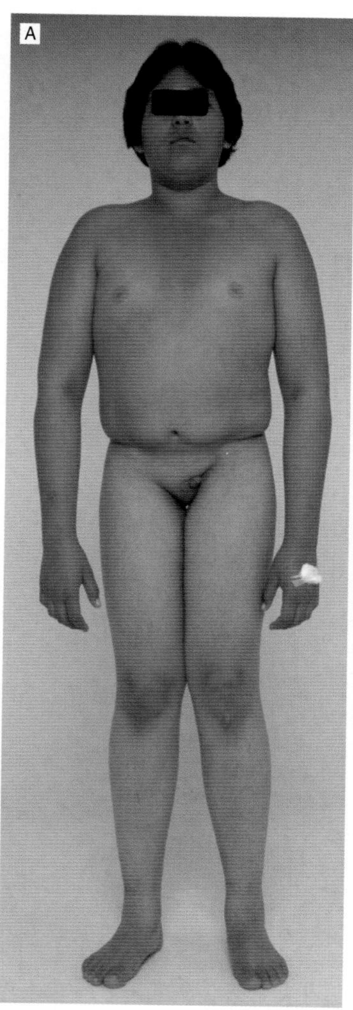

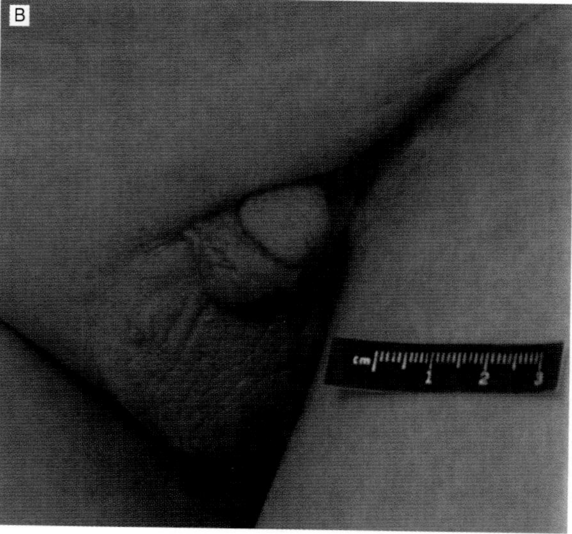

FIGURE 52-8 A young male patient after therapeutic irradiation of the left testicle for a testicular tumor. Note the loss of body hair, hypogonadal facial puffiness, decreased muscle mass, and increased body fat (A). The left testicle was small and firm (B). The patient was infertile.

For long-term cancer survivors who were treated with streptozocin, L-asparaginase, or partial pancreatectomy, screening for delayed development of diabetes mellitus is recommended.

In children with a history of cranial irradiation or craniospinal irradiation, the growth rate should be assessed at 6-month intervals. A more detailed evaluation, including measurement of the levels of GH and IGF-1, thyroid function tests, and bone age assessments, should be performed when there is evidence of an abnormal growth pattern. The T_4 and TSH measurements should be performed annually for the first 5 years and less frequently thereafter. Careful physical examination should be performed annually to detect thyroid nodules, and if any are detected, a more detailed examination should be performed using ultrasound and, if necessary, fine-needle aspiration biopsy.

In adults who have undergone cranial irradiation with >20 Gy, clinical monitoring with measurement of serum cortisol, ACTH, free T_4, IGF-1 (if the patient is a candidate for GH replacement), prolactin, luteinizing hormone, follicle-stimulating hormone, and serum testosterone and documentation of menstrual history should be undertaken annually for 15 years and then every 2 years for another 15 years ([54]).

In survivors of childhood malignancies, bone mass may be assessed in the early 30s, an age at which peak bone mass has been attained in most people. It is also important to consider the possibility of bone loss in androgen- or estrogen-deficient adults. If bone mass is normal, no further evaluation is needed beyond the usual recommendations for prevention of osteoporosis. In those with low bone mass, an active program of calcium and vitamin D supplementation, exercise, and occasionally, medical therapy (bisphosphonates or recombinant parathyroid hormone) should be combined with assessment of bone mass every 12 to 18 months.

Patients who have been treated with chemotherapeutic agents that cause hypophosphatemia, hypomagnesemia, or hypocalcemia, such as ifosfamide, platinum compounds, fludarabine, or estramustine, are particularly at risk for osteomalacia and should undergo an evaluation of serum calcium, phosphorus, magnesium, alkaline phosphatase, and vitamin D metabolite levels.

Patients who have been treated with aromatase inhibitors should have bone mineral density measurements before and during treatment and should be given calcium and vitamin D. Patients can be given bisphosphonates if deemed necessary. Because multitarget tyrosine kinase inhibitors can cause thyroid dysfunction, thyroid hormone levels should be checked before treatment begins. During treatment, thyroid hormone levels should be checked periodically to adjust thyroxine replacement. Multitarget tyrosine kinase inhibitors can cause new-onset hypothyroidism or increase the levothyroxine requirements in patients on chronic thyroid hormone replacement.

REFERENCES

1. Kim EH, Kim HK, Bae SJ, et al. Fasting serum insulin levels and insulin resistance are associated with colorectal adenoma in Koreans. *J Diabetes Investig.* 2014;5:297-304.
2. Weinstein D, Simon M, Yehezkel E, Laron Z, Werner H. Insulin analogues display IGF-I-like mitogenic and anti-apoptotic activities in cultured cancer cells. *Diabetes Metab Res Rev.* 2009;25:41-49.
3. Pierre-Eugene C, Pagesy P, Nguyen TT, et al. Effect of insulin analogues on insulin/IGF1 hybrid receptors: increased activation by glargine but not by its metabolites M1 and M2. *PloS One.* 2012;7:e41992.
4. Ruiter R, Visser LE, van Herk-Sukel MPP, et al. Risk of cancer in patients on insulin glargine and other insulin analogues in comparison with those on human insulin: results from a large population-based follow-up study. *Diabetologia.* 2012;55:51-62.
5. Busaidy NL, Farooki A, Dowlati A, et al. Management of metabolic effects associated with anticancer agents targeting the PI3K-Akt-mTOR pathway. *J Clin Oncol.* 2012;30:2919-2928.
6. Motzer RJ, Escudier B, Oudard S, et al. Efficacy of everolimus in advanced renal cell carcinoma: a double-blind, randomised, placebo-controlled phase III trial. *Lancet.* 2008;372:449-456.
7. Hudes G, Carducci M, Tomczak P, et al. Temsirolimus, interferon alfa, or both for advanced renal-cell carcinoma. *N Engl J Med.* 2007;356:2271-2281.
8. Radu RG, Fujimoto S, Mukai E, et al. Tacrolimus suppresses glucose-induced insulin release from pancreatic islets by reducing glucokinase activity. *Am J Physiol Endocrinol Metab.* 2005;288:E365-E371.
9. Furman RR, Sharman JP, Coutre SE, et al. Idelalisib and rituximab in relapsed chronic lymphocytic leukemia. *N Engl J Med.* 2014;370:997-1007.
10. Furman RR, Sharman JP, Coutre SE, et al. Idelalisib and rituximab in relapsed chronic lymphocytic leukemia. *N Engl J Med.* 2014;370:997-1007.
11. Flinn IW, Kahl BS, Leonard JP, et al. Idelalisib, a selective inhibitor of phosphatidylinositol 3-kinase-delta, as therapy for previously treated indolent non-Hodgkin lymphoma. *Blood.* 2014;123:3406-3413.
12. Lowas SR, Marks D, Malempati S. Prevalence of transient hyperglycemia during induction chemotherapy for pediatric acute lymphoblastic leukemia. *Pediatr Blood Cancer.* 2009;52:814-818.
13. Raja RA, Schmiegelow K, Albertsen BK, et al. Asparaginase-associated pancreatitis in children with acute lymphoblastic leukaemia in the NOPHO ALL2008 protocol. *Br J Haematol.* 2014;165:126-133.
14. Schein PS, Oconnell MJ, Blom J, et al. Clinical antitumor activity and toxicity of streptozotocin (Nsc-85998). *Cancer.* 1974;34:993-1000.
15. Nakamura K, Kawasaki E, Imagawa A, et al. Type 1 diabetes and interferon therapy: a nationwide survey in Japan. *Diabetes Care.* 2011;34:2084-2089.
16. Yamazaki M, Sato A, Takeda T, Komatsu M. Distinct clinical courses in type 1 diabetes mellitus induced by peg-interferon-alpha treatment for chronic hepatitis C. *Intern Med.* 2010;49:403-407.
17. Ferrari S, Pieretti F, Verri E, et al. Prospective evaluation of renal function in pediatric and adult patients treated with high-dose ifosfamide, cisplatin and high-dose methotrexate. *Anticancer*

Drugs. 2005;16:733-738.
18. Lilley JS, Linton MF, Fazio S. Oral retinoids and plasma lipids. *Dermatol Ther*. 2013;26:404-410.
19. Klor HU, Weizel A, Augustin M, et al. The impact of oral vitamin A derivatives on lipid metabolism: what recommendations can be derived for dealing with this issue in the daily dermatological practice? *J Dtsch Dermatol Ges*. 2011;9:600-606.
20. Duvic M, Martin AG, Kim Y, et al. Phase 2 and 3 clinical trial of oral bexarotene (Targretin capsules) for the treatment of refractory or persistent early-stage cutaneous T-cell lymphoma. *Arch Dermatol*. 2001;137:581-593.
21. Shawa H, Deniz F, Bazerbashi H, et al. Mitotane-induced hyperlipidemia: a retrospective cohort study. *Int J Endocrinol*. 2013;2013:624962.
22. Cho DC, Atkins MB. Serum cholesterol and mTOR inhibitors: surrogate biomarker or epiphenomenon? *Clin Cancer Res*. 2012;18:2999-3001.
23. Morrisett JD, Abdel-Fattah G, Hoogeveen R, et al. Effects of sirolimus on plasma lipids, lipoprotein levels, and fatty acid metabolism in renal transplant patients. *J Lipid Res*. 2002;43:1170-1180.
24. Elhassan EA, Schrier RW. Hyponatremia: diagnosis, complications, and management including V2 receptor antagonists. *Curr Opin Nephrol Hypertens*. 2011;20:161-168.
25. Drake MT. Osteoporosis and cancer. *Curr Osteoporos Rep*. 2013;11:163-170.
26. Spangler L, Yu O, Loggers E, Boudreau DM. Bone mineral density screening among women with a history of breast cancer treated with aromatase inhibitors. *J Womens Health*. 2013;22:132-140.
27. Baum M, Budzar AU, Cuzick J, et al. Anastrozole alone or in combination with tamoxifen versus tamoxifen alone for adjuvant treatment of postmenopausal women with early breast cancer: first results of the ATAC randomised trial. *Lancet*. 2002;359:2131-2139.
28. Smith MR. Androgen deprivation therapy for prostate cancer: new concepts and concerns. *Curr Opin Endocrinol Diabetes Obes*. 2007;14:247-254
29. Smith MR, Boyce SP, Moyneur E, Duh MS, Raut MK, Brandman J. Risk of clinical fractures after gonadotropin-releasing hormone agonist therapy for prostate cancer. *J Urol*. 2006;175:136-139; discussion 139.
30. Gralow JR, Biermann JS, Farooki A, et al. NCCN Task Force Report: bone health in cancer care. *J Natl Compr Cancer Netw*. 2013;11(Suppl 3):S1-50; quiz S51.
31. D'Angelo P, Conter V, Di Chiara G, Rizzari C, Memeo A, Barigozzi P. Severe osteoporosis and multiple vertebral collapses in a child during treatment for B-ALL. *Acta Haematol*. 1993;89:38-42.
32. Li BJ, Boast S, de los Santos K, et al. Mice deficient in Abl are osteoporotic and have defects in osteoblast maturation. *Nat Genet*. 2000;24:304-308.
33. Fitter S, Dewar AL, Kostakis P, et al. Long-term imatinib therapy promotes bone formation in CML patients. *Blood*. 2008;111:2538-2547.
34. Church DN, Hassan AB, Harper SJ, Wakeley CJ, Price CG. Osteomalacia as a late metabolic complication of ifosfamide chemotherapy in young adults: illustrative cases and review of the literature. *Sarcoma*. 2007;2007:91586.
35. Stava CJ, Jimenez C, Hu MI, Vassilopoulou-Sellin R. Skeletal sequelae of cancer and cancer treatment. *J Cancer Surviv*. 2009;3:75-88.
36. Vassilopoulou-Sellin R, Newman BM, Taylor SH, Guinee VF. Incidence of hypercalcemia in patients with malignancy referred to a comprehensive cancer center. *Cancer*. 1993;71:1309-1312.
37. Yamamoto T, Tashiro H, Sugao T, et al. [Hypercalcemia due to the administration of all-trans retinoic acid for acute promyelocytic leukemia: report of two cases]. *Nihon Naika Gakkai Zasshi*. 2010;99:828-830.
38. Tsuchiya T, Ito K, Murata M. [An evaluation of the incidence of hyperparathyroidism after 131I treatment for Basedow disease (Part I)]. *Kaku Igaku*. 1996;33:729-735.
39. Liamis G, Milionis HJ, Elisaf M. A review of drug-induced hypocalcemia. *J Bone Miner Metab*. 2009;27:635-642.
40. Jones SG, Dolan G, Lengyel K, Myers B. Severe increase in creatinine with hypocalcaemia in thalidomide-treated myeloma patients receiving zoledronic acid infusions. *Br J Haematol*. 2002;119:576-577.
41. Yoshida T, Niho S, Toda M, et al. Protective effect of magnesium preloading on cisplatin-induced nephrotoxicity: a retrospective study. *Jpn J Clin Oncol*. 2014;44:346-354.
42. Sundar S, Symonds RP, Decatris MP, et al. Phase II trial of oxaliplatin and 5-fluorouracil/leucovorin combination in epithelial ovarian carcinoma relapsing within 2 years of platinum-based therapy. *Gynecol Oncol*. 2004;94:502-508.
43. Vickers MM, Karapetis CS, Tu D, et al. Association of hypomagnesemia with inferior survival in a phase III, randomized study of cetuximab plus best supportive care versus best supportive care alone: NCIC CTG/AGITG CO.17. *Ann Oncol*. 2013;24:953-960.
44. Darzy KH. Radiation-induced hypopituitarism after cancer therapy: who, how and when to test. *Nat Clin Pract Endocrinol Metab*. 2009;5:88-99.
45. Shalet SM, Clayton PE, Price DA. Growth and pituitary function in children treated for brain tumours or acute lymphoblastic leukaemia. *Horm Res*. 1988;30:53-61.
46. Iwama S, De Remigis A, Callahan MK, Slovin SF, Wolchok JD, Caturegli P. Pituitary expression of CTLA-4 mediates hypophysitis secondary to administration of CTLA-4 blocking antibody. *Sci Transl Med*. 2014;6:230ra245.
47. Faje AT, Sullivan R, Lawrence D, et al. Ipilimumab-induced hypophysitis: a detailed longitudinal analysis in a large cohort of patients with metastatic melanoma. *J Clin Endocrinol Metab*. 2014;99:4078-4085.
48. Chodakiewitz Y, Brown S, Boxerman JL, Brody JM, Rogg JM. Ipilimumab treatment associated pituitary hypophysitis: clinical presentation and imaging diagnosis. *Clin Neurol Neurosurg*. 2014;125:125-130.
49. Toogood AA. Endocrine consequences of brain irradiation. *Growth Horm IGF Res*. 2004;14(Suppl A):S118-S124.
50. Abs R, Verhelst J, Maeyaert J, et al. Endocrine consequences of long-term intrathecal administration of opioids. *J Clin Endocrinol Metab*. 2000;85:2215-2222.
51. Schmiegelow M, Feldt-Rasmussen U, Rasmussen AK, Poulsen HS, Muller J. A population-based study of thyroid function after radiotherapy and chemotherapy for a childhood brain tumor. *J Clin Endocrinol Metab*. 2003;88:136-140.
52. Ogilvy-Stuart AL, Shalet SM, Gattamaneni HR. Thyroid function after treatment of brain tumors in children. *J Pediatr*. 1991;119:733-737.
53. Sherman SI. Etiology, diagnosis, and treatment recommendations for central hypothyroidism associated with bexarotene therapy for cutaneous T-cell lymphoma. *Clin Lymph*. 2003;3:249-252.
54. Appelman-Dijkstra NM, Malgo F, Neelis KJ, Coremans I, Biermasz NR, Pereira AM. Pituitary dysfunction in adult patients after cranial irradiation for head and nasopharyngeal tumours. *Radiother Oncol*. 2014;113:102-107.
55. Pai HH, Thornton A, Katznelson L, et al. Hypothalamic/pituitary function following high-dose conformal radiotherapy to the base of skull: demonstration of a dose-effect relationship using dose-volume histogram analysis. *Int J Radiat Oncol*. 2001;49:1079-1092.
56. Samaan NA, Schultz PN, Yang KP, et al. Endocrine complications after radiotherapy for tumors of the head and neck. *J Lab Clin Med*. 1987;109:364-372.

57. Rajagopal A, Vassilopoulou-Sellin R, Palmer JL, Kaur G, Bruera E. Hypogonadism and sexual dysfunction in male cancer survivors receiving chronic opioid therapy. *J Pain Symptom Manag.* 2003;26:1055-1061.
58. Nikiforov YE. RET/PTC rearrangement in thyroid tumors. *Endocr Pathol.* 2002;13:3-16.
59. Prummel MF, Laurberg P. Interferon-alpha and autoimmune thyroid disease. *Thyroid.* 2003;13:547-551.
60. Hamnvik OP, Larsen PR, Marqusee E. Thyroid dysfunction from antineoplastic agents. *J Natl Cancer Inst.* 2011;103:1572-1587.
61. Ho VT, Zahrieh D, Hochberg E, et al. Safety and efficacy of denileukin diftitox in patients with steroid-refractory acute graft-versus-host disease after allogeneic hematopoietic stem cell transplantation. *Blood.* 2004;104:1224-1226.
62. Hamid O, Robert C, Daud A, et al. Safety and tumor responses with lambrolizumab (anti-PD-1) in melanoma. *N Engl J Med.* 2013;369:134-144.
63. Jereczek-Fossa BA, Alterio D, Jassem J, Gibelli B, Tradati N, Orecchia R. Radiotherapy-induced thyroid disorders. *Cancer Treat Rev.* 2004;30:369-384.
64. Demirkaya M, Sevinir B, Saglam H, Ozkan L, Akaci O. Thyroid functions in long-term survivors of pediatric Hodgkin's lymphoma treated with chemotherapy and radiotherapy. *J Clin Res Pediatr Endocrinol.* 2011;3:89-94.
65. Dalgard O, Bjoro K, Hellum K, et al. Thyroid dysfunction during treatment of chronic hepatitis C with interferon alpha: no association with either interferon dosage or efficacy of therapy. *J Intern Med.* 2002;251:400-406.
66. Krouse RS, Royal RE, Heywood G, et al. Thyroid dysfunction in 281 patients with metastatic melanoma or renal carcinoma treated with interleukin-2 alone. *J Immunother Emphasis Tumor Immunol.* 1995;18:272-278.
67. Stuart NS, Woodroffe CM, Grundy R, Cullen MH. Long-term toxicity of chemotherapy for testicular cancer--the cost of cure. *Br J Cancer.* 1990;61:479-484.
68. Investigators CT, Coles AJ, Compston DAS, et al. Alemtuzumab vs. interferon beta-1a in early multiple sclerosis. *N Engl J Med.* 2008;359:1786-1801.
69. Dora JM, Leie MA, Netto B, et al. Lack of imatinib-induced thyroid dysfunction in a cohort of non-thyroidectomized patients. *Eur J Endocrinol.* 2008;158:771-772.
70. Tamaskar I, Bukowski R, Elson P, et al. Thyroid function test abnormalities in patients with metastatic renal cell carcinoma treated with sorafenib. *Ann Oncol.* 2008;19:265-268.
71. Miyake H, Kurahashi T, Yamanaka K, et al. Abnormalities of thyroid function in Japanese patients with metastatic renal cell carcinoma treated with sorafenib: a prospective evaluation. *Urol Oncol.* 2010;28:515-519.
72. Schneider TC, Abdulrahman RM, Corssmit EP, Morreau H, Smit JW, Kapiteijn E. Long-term analysis of the efficacy and tolerability of sorafenib in advanced radio-iodine refractory differentiated thyroid carcinoma: final results of a phase II trial. *Eur J Endocrinol.* 2012;167:643-650.
73. Hoftijzer H, Heemstra KA, Morreau H, et al. Beneficial effects of sorafenib on tumor progression, but not on radioiodine uptake, in patients with differentiated thyroid carcinoma. *Eur J Endocrinol.* 2009;161:923-931.
74. Desai J, Yassa L, Marqusee E, et al. Hypothyroidism after sunitinib treatment for patients with gastrointestinal stromal tumors. *Ann Intern Med.* 2006;145:660-664.
75. Kitajima K, Takahashi S, Maeda T, et al. Thyroid size change by CT monitoring after sorafenib or sunitinib treatment in patients with renal cell carcinoma: comparison with thyroid function. *Eur J Radiol.* 2012;81:2060-2065.
76. Wolter P, Stefan C, Decallonne B, et al. The clinical implications of sunitinib-induced hypothyroidism: a prospective evaluation. *Br J Cancer.* 2008;99:448-454.
77. Grossmann M, Premaratne E, Desai J, Davis ID. Thyrotoxicosis during sunitinib treatment for renal cell carcinoma. *Clin Endocrinol (Oxf).* 2008;69:669-672.
78. Mannavola D, Coco P, Vannucchi G, et al. A novel tyrosine-kinase selective inhibitor, sunitinib, induces transient hypothyroidism by blocking iodine uptake. *J Clin Endocrinol Metab.* 2007;92:3531-3534.
79. Wong E, Rosen LS, Mulay M, et al. Sunitinib induces hypothyroidism in advanced cancer patients and may inhibit thyroid peroxidase activity. *Thyroid.* 2007;17:351-355.
80. Hodi FS, O'Day SJ, McDermott DF, et al. Improved survival with ipilimumab in patients with metastatic melanoma. *N Engl J Med.* 2010;363:711-723.
81. Bajetta E, Zilembo N, Dowsett M, et al. Double-blind, randomised, multicentre endocrine trial comparing two letrozole doses, in postmenopausal breast cancer patients. *Eur J Cancer.* 1999;35:208-213.
82. Ferster A, Glinoer D, Vanvliet G, Otten J. Thyroid function during l-asparaginase therapy in children with acute lymphoblastic leukemia: difference between induction and late intensification. *Am J Pediat Hematol.* 1992;14:192-196.
83. Vanseters AP, Moolenaar AJ. Mitotane increases the blood-levels of hormone binding proteins. *Acta Endocrinol.* 1991;124:526-533.
84. Goodman VL, Rock EP, Dagher R, et al. Approval summary: sunitinib for the treatment of imatinib refractory or intolerant gastrointestinal stromal tumors and advanced renal cell carcinoma. *Clin Cancer Res.* 2007;13:1367-1373.
85. Patterson BC, Truxillo L, Wasilewski-Masker K, Mertens AC, Meacham LR. Adrenal function testing in pediatric cancer survivors. *Pediatr Blood Cancer.* 2009;53:1302-1307.
86. Meacham LR, Mazewski C, Krawiecki N. Mechanism of transient adrenal insufficiency with megestrol acetate treatment of cachexia in children with cancer. *J Pediatr Hematol Oncol.* 2003;25:414-417.
87. Raedler TJ, Jahn H, Goedeken B, Gescher DM, Kellner M, Wiedemann K. Acute effects of megestrol on the hypothalamic-pituitary-adrenal axis. *Cancer Chemother Pharmacol.* 2003;52:482-486.
88. Sudour H, Chastagner P, Claude L, et al. Fertility and pregnancy outcome after abdominal irradiation that included or excluded the pelvis in childhood tumor survivors. *Int J Radiat Oncol.* 2010;76:867-873.
89. Green DM, Kawashima T, Stovall M, et al. Fertility of female survivors of childhood cancer: a report from the Childhood Cancer Survivor Study. *J Clin Oncol.* 2009;27:2677-2685.
90. Le Bouedec G, Rabishong B, Canis M, Achard JL, Pomel C, Dauplat J. [Ovarian transposition by laparoscopy in young women before curietherapy for cervical cancer]. *J Gynecol Obstet Biol Reprod (Paris).* 2000;29:564-570.
91. Recchia F, Saggio G, Amiconi G, et al. Gonadotropin-releasing hormone analogues added to adjuvant chemotherapy protect ovarian function and improve clinical outcomes in young women with early breast carcinoma. *Cancer.* 2006;106:514-523.
92. Demeestere I, Brice P, Peccatori FA, et al. Gonadotropin-releasing hormone agonist for the prevention of chemotherapy-induced ovarian failure in patients with lymphoma: 1-year follow-up of a prospective randomized trial. *J Clin Oncol.* 2013;31:903-909.
93. Berliere M, Dalenc F, Malingret N, et al. Incidence of reversible amenorrhea in women with breast cancer undergoing adjuvant anthracycline-based chemotherapy with or without docetaxel. *BMC Cancer.* 2008;8:56.
94. Meirow D, Nugent D. The effects of radiotherapy and chemotherapy on female reproduction. *Hum Reprod Update.* 2001;7:535-543.
95. Choo YC, Chan SY, Wong LC, Ma HK. Ovarian dysfunction in patients with gestational trophoblastic neoplasia treated

with short intensive courses of etoposide (VP-16-213). *Cancer.* 1985;55:2348-2352.

96. van Beek RD, van den Heuvel-Eibrink MM, Laven JS, et al. Anti-Mullerian hormone is a sensitive serum marker for gonadal function in women treated for Hodgkin's lymphoma during childhood. *J Clin Endocrinol Metab.* 2007;92:3869-3874.
97. Sieniawski M, Reineke T, Nogova L, et al. Fertility in male patients with advanced Hodgkin lymphoma treated with BEACOPP: a report of the German Hodgkin Study Group (GHSG). *Blood.* 2008;111:71-76.
98. Shanei A, Baradaran-Ghahfarokhi M. Evaluation of testicular dose and associated risk from common pelvis radiation therapy in Iran. *Phys Med.* 2014;30:867-870.
99. Howell SJ, Shalet SM. Effect of cancer therapy on pituitary-testicular axis. *Int J Androl.* 2002;25:269-276.
100. Cheviakoff S, Calamera JC, Morgenfeld M, Mancini RE. Recovery of spermatogenesis in patients with lymphoma after treatment with chlorambucil. *J Reprod Fertil.* 1973;33:155-157.
101. Meistrich ML. Effects of chemotherapy and radiotherapy on spermatogenesis in humans. *Fertil Steril.* 2013;100:1180-1186.
102. Meistrich ML, Shetty G. Suppression of testosterone stimulates recovery of spermatogenesis after cancer treatment. *Int J Androl.* 2003;26:141-146.

53 Oncologic Emergencies

第五十三章　肿瘤急症

Sai-Ching Jim Yeung
Ellen F. Manzullo

中文导读

本章按照人体不同系统，从症状、体征、病因、治疗等方面对肿瘤急症进行讨论。在神经系统急症中对脊髓压迫、颅内压升高、软脑膜疾病、癫痫发作与精神状态改变进行了系统讲解，描述了脊髓压迫、颅内占位的影像学表现，介绍了癫痫发作和精神状态改变的诊疗方法。在心血管系统急症中讲解了心脏压塞、上腔静脉综合征与心肌缺血的病因和处理方法。在血液系统急症中介绍了高黏滞综合征、高白细胞血症、静脉血栓形成以及出血，其中重点介绍了静脉血栓形成的临床表现和诊疗路径，以及引起出血的病因和弥散性血管内凝血的治疗原则。在泌尿生殖系统、呼吸系统、代谢与消化系统急症中分别简述了出血性膀胱炎和尿路梗阻、气道梗阻和咯血、肿瘤溶解综合征和高钙血症、消化道出血和盲肠炎等急症的病因及治疗要点。同时本章也简要介绍了化疗药物外渗的处理方法。肿瘤急症可以因肿瘤本身或抗肿瘤治疗引起。本章指出，由于肿瘤患者常合并免疫、代谢及血液学方面的缺陷，且其他共存疾病也可以引起急症，要对肿瘤急症有全面的了解才能迅速识别病情并及时给予治疗。

Oncologic emergencies can result from either the cancer or its treatment. Cancer patients often have immunologic, metabolic, and hematologic defects, which can lead to complex emergency conditions when they present to an emergency center. In addition, emergencies resulting from comorbid conditions also occur in cancer patients. It is important for practitioners who treat patients with cancer to be aware of the various oncologic emergencies so that they can be recognized and treated promptly. This chapter discusses many of these emergencies, including their signs and symptoms, causes, and management.

NEUROLOGIC EMERGENCIES

Spinal Cord Compression

Spinal cord compression is a serious complication of cancer progression, affecting about 2.5% of cancer patients overall ([1]). It is not immediately life-threatening unless it involves the first three cervical vertebrae, but involvement in the rest of the spine leads to significant morbidity ([2]). The spinal cord is compressed at the thoracic vertebrae in 70% of patients, cervical vertebrae in 10% of patients, and lumbar vertebrae in 20% of patients. In 10% to 38% of cases, spinal cord compression occurs at multiple levels ([3]). Such compression is predominantly due to metastatic tumors, with lung, breast, and prostate cancer comprising 50% of these. Other tumors that commonly metastasize to the spine are multiple myeloma, renal cell carcinoma, melanoma, lymphoma, sarcoma, and gastrointestinal (GI) cancers. The mechanisms by which tumors can appear in the spine are hematogenous spread of tumor cells to the vertebral bodies, metastasis of primary lesions to the posterior spinal elements, and direct extension of paraspinal tumors. Spinal cord compression is caused by epidural metastases in 75% of cases and bony collapse in 25% of cases ([4]).

The most common presentation of spinal cord compression is back pain, occurring in over 90% of patients. Depending on the location of the tumor in the spinal canal, the pain can be unilateral or bilateral following dermatomal patterns. Patients typically report that their pain is worse when they are supine and better when they are upright. Ataxia due to compression of the spinocerebellar tracts can be confused with cerebellar metastasis, overmedication with analgesics, or other disorders. Metastasis to the spinal cord can precede spinal cord compression by weeks or months. The patient may also note sensory symptoms, including numbness or tingling in the toes, which can progress proximally. Preexisting peripheral neuropathy must be differentiated from spinal cord compression and acute worsening of existing symptoms or experienced new numbness or tingling. Motor symptoms are the second most common complaint after pain; difficulty walking, buckling under of the legs, and a feeling of heaviness in the legs are all frequent symptoms. The last symptoms to appear are autonomic symptoms, such as urinary retention and constipation. Autonomic symptoms are late findings in spinal cord compression and must be distinguished from the effects of chemotherapy, pain medicines, and antihistamines. It is important to remember that the patient may present with intractable pain only, so a high level of suspicion for spinal cord compression is important in treating cancer patients.

The physical examination usually reveals tenderness to percussion over the affected level of the spine, but the spine might not be tender if there is no bone involvement. Other possible findings are urinary retention, decreased rectal sphincter tone, and muscle weakness. The patient might have pain at a referred site; for instance, patients with L1 compression might have pain in the sacroiliac area. Sensory changes are more difficult to diagnose than motor deficits and can either precede or accompany motor effects. The patient might have decreased sensation in the lower extremities, which may ascend to the level of spinal cord involvement with dorsal column deficits, including loss of light touch sensation, proprioception, and position sense. When the cauda equina is compressed, the sensory changes are dermatomal, with loss of sensation in the perineal area, the posterior thigh, or lateral leg.

The differential diagnosis of spinal cord compression includes osteoarthritis, degenerative disk disease, spinal abscess, hematoma/bleeding, hemangioma, chordoma, meningioma, and neurofibroma. A standard x-ray is generally ordered first to analyze the area of the spine within which compression is suspected. However, simple roentgenography yields false-negative results in 10% to 17% of cases, in part because approximately 30% to 50% of the bone must be destroyed before bony lesions can be seen on x-ray films ([5]). Magnetic resonance imaging (MRI) is the imaging technique of choice today for suspected spinal cord compression (Fig. 53-1).

For patients with suspected spinal cord compression, physicians should consider imaging the entire spine because spinal epidural disease is often multifocal. Findings for the whole spine can help the physician optimize the type and extent of therapy needed. For any patient with rapidly progressive neurologic symptoms, diagnostic imaging should be performed on an emergency basis. Magnetic resonance imaging of the spine is the diagnostic study of choice. Gadolinium enhancement will be helpful in detecting other causes of neurologic symptoms such as epidural abscess or leptomeningeal metastasis. Patients who are not able to undergo MRI (eg, the presence of paramagnetic cerebral aneurysm clips, or cardiac pacemakers) can undergo computed tomography (CT) myelogram.

Clinical guidelines for diagnosis and management of spinal cord compression are available ([6, 7]). Corticosteroid is a temporizing measure to stabilize or even improve neurologic function until definitive treatment. Conventionally, dexamethasone is initially given at 10 to 100 mg intravenously and then 4 to 24 mg every 4 to 6 hours ([8]). The duration of therapy with high-dose glucocorticoids should be minimized to prevent complications of steroid use.

Surgery is indicated for recurrent or progressive disease at an area with previous maximal radiotherapy, spinal mechanical instability, an unknown tissue diagnosis of malignancy, or for compression of the spinal cord by bony structure/fragment ([6, 7]). Currently, anterior decompression with spinal stabilization is the surgery of choice, allowing removal of the affected vertebral body and stabilization above and below the vertebrae by metal hardware. Surgical resection followed by radiotherapy may improve ambulation ability and survival better than radiotherapy alone ([9]). Benefit from decompressive surgery is evident in ambulatory patients with poor prognostic factors for radiotherapy and in paralyzed patients with a single spinal area of compression, paraplegia less than 48 hours, non-radiosensitive tumors, and an expected survival of more than 3 months ([10]). If surgery is not indicated, radiation therapy can be used for radiosensitive tumors; the most common dosage is 3,000 cGy delivered in 10 fractions ([3]). The incidence of myelopathy, which can occur as a complication of radiation therapy, increases with increasing total dosage of therapy and can appear from months to several years after such therapy is given. Palliative radiotherapy is recommended for those with paraplegia longer than 48 hours, expected to live for fewer than 3 months, unable to tolerate surgery, and with multiple areas of compression. An ambulatory patient with a stable spine may be considered for radiation

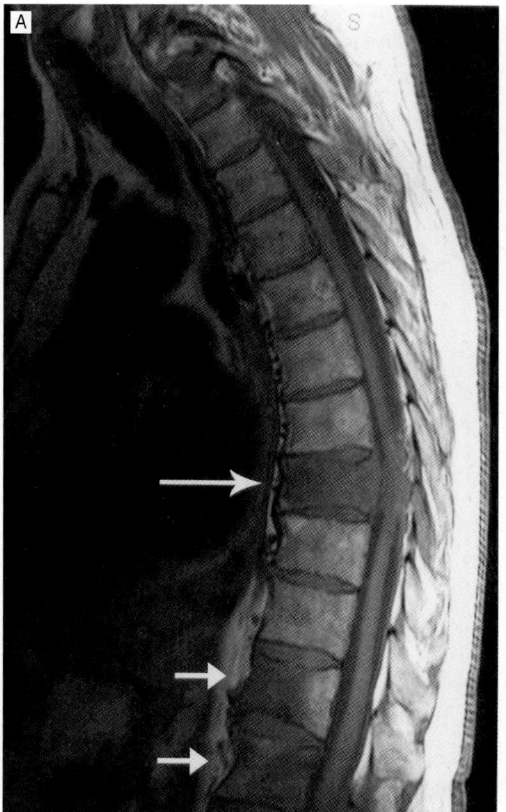

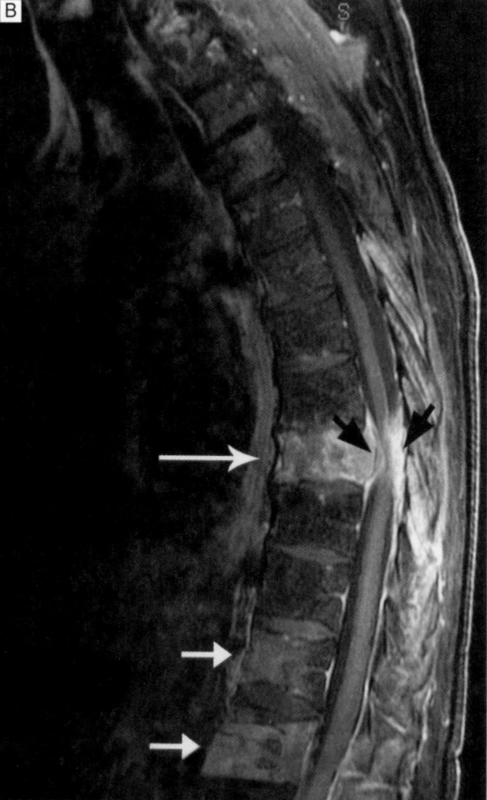

FIGURE 53-1 A. Precontrast T1-weighted magnetic resonance image (MRI) of thoracic cord compression at the T8 level produced by an epidural tumor from vertebral body metastasis (*large arrow*). Smaller *arrows* point to other sites of bony metastasis. The patient is a 67-year-old man with melanoma and back pain. B. Postcontrast T1-weighted MRI of the same patient. The epidural tumor is visualized better with contrast (*black arrows*). (Used with permission from Dr. Ashok Kumar, MD Anderson Cancer Center.)

treatment ([8]). Chemotherapy is occasionally used for chemotherapy-sensitive tumors, such as Hodgkin disease, neuroblastoma, non-Hodgkin lymphoma, germ cell tumors, and breast cancer.

One of the most important prognostic factors at diagnosis is the patient's neurologic function. Of patients who are ambulatory at the time of presentation, approximately three-fourths will be able to regain their strength with treatment. By contrast, only a small percentage of patients who are paralyzed at the time of presentation are likely to walk again. This difference illustrates why it is imperative to diagnose spinal cord compression at an early stage. A scoring system based on tumor type, interval between tumor diagnosis and spinal cord compression, other bone or visceral metastases, ambulatory status, and duration of paralysis can estimate survival ([11]). The median overall survival following the first episode of spinal cord compression is about 3 months ([1]).

Increased Intracranial Pressure

Increased intracranial pressure in cancer patients is commonly due to hemorrhage (from thrombocytopenia or tumor bleeding), brain metastasis with vasogenic edema and mass effect, or hydrocephalus due to obstruction of the flow of cerebrospinal fluid (CSF). Increased intracranial pressure can also be caused by tumor treatments, such as radiation therapy and surgery. The normal CSF pressure is less than 10 mm Hg. As intracranial pressure increases, herniation syndromes may develop, including uncal, central, and tonsillar herniation. Uncal herniation is caused by unilateral supratentorial lesions that push brain tissue through the tentorial notch. Signs and symptoms include ipsilateral pupil dilation, decreased consciousness, and hemiparesis, first contralateral and then ipsilateral to the mass. Central herniation involves bilateral supratentorial lesions that displace tissue symmetrically and bilaterally. Signs and symptoms of central herniation include decreased consciousness leading to coma and Cheyne-Stokes respiration, followed by central hyperventilation, midposition unreactive pupils, and posturing. Tonsillar herniation involves increased pressure in the posterior fossa, which forces the cerebellar tonsil through the foramen magnum, thereby compressing the medulla. Signs and symptoms of tonsillar herniation include decreased consciousness and respiratory abnormalities leading to apnea. Headache is the most frequent symptom reported in increased intracranial pressure. Headache is a common symptom in any patient population, but in cancer patients, the clinician must always maintain a high index of suspicion for increased intracranial pressure. Headaches due to increased intracranial pressure are typically present on waking in the morning, recur throughout the day, and are increased with Valsalva maneuver; they can be associated with nausea and vomiting, altered mental status, vision changes, seizures, or focal neurologic deficits. On physical examination, the patient might have papilledema, focal neurologic deficits, or a decreased level of consciousness.

The diagnosis of increased intracranial pressure can be ascertained from CT scans of the brain. Noncontrast CT imaging of the brain is superior to MRI in detecting acute hemorrhage (Fig. 53-2).

Computed tomography scans with contrast will usually reveal cerebral metastasis and occasionally leptomeningeal disease (LMD). Contrast-enhanced MRI is more sensitive than CT in revealing cerebral neoplasms and metastases as small as 3 mm (Fig. 53-3), LMD (Fig. 53-4), and early strokes (Fig. 53-5). Lumbar puncture should not be used to diagnose increased intracranial pressure, because this can lead to brain herniation.

The differential diagnosis of increased intracranial pressure includes bleeding, tumor edema, hydrocephalus, postradiation effects, postradiosurgery effects, brachytherapy-induced changes, benign tumor effects, subdural hematomas, meningitis, encephalitis, and abscess formation.

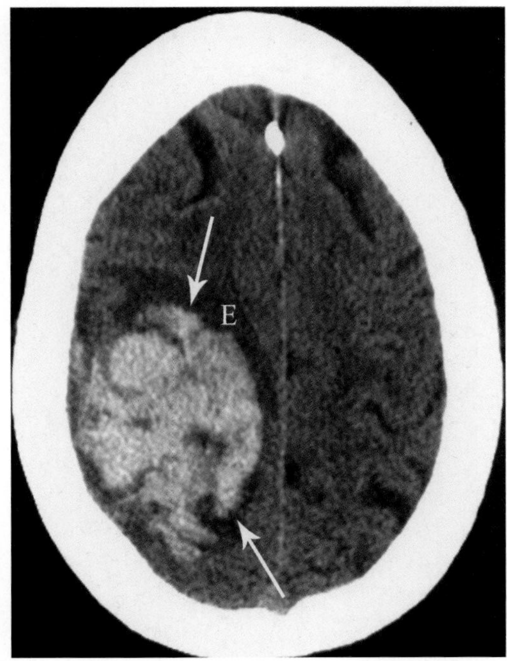

FIGURE 53-2 Acute intracranial hemorrhage within the right frontoparietal lobe (*arrows*) with edema (E) in a 79-year-old woman with ovarian cancer. The hemorrhage was revealed by noncontrast computed tomography imaging. This modality is superior to magnetic resonance imaging in detecting acute hemorrhage. (Used with permission from Dr. Ashok Kumar, MD Anderson Cancer Center.)

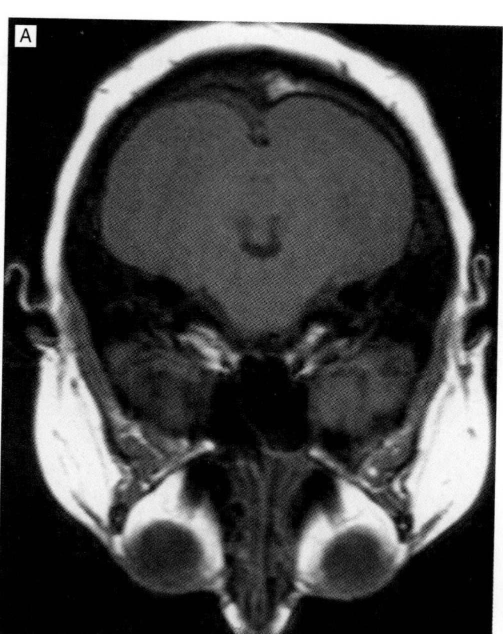

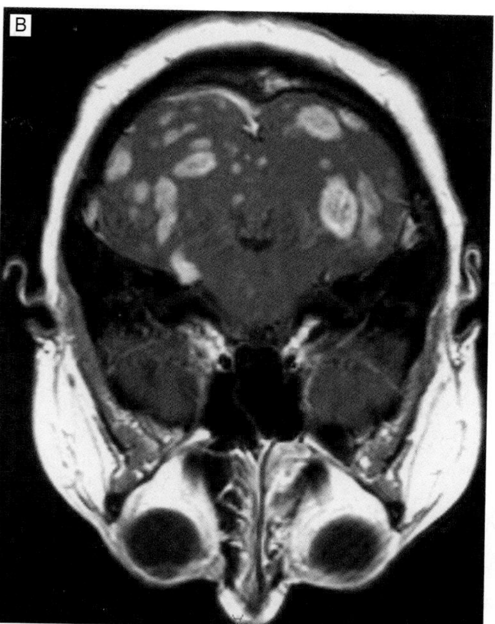

FIGURE 53-3 A. Precontrast T1-weighted magnetic resonance images in a 40-year-old woman with breast cancer and multiple cerebellar metastases. B. Postcontrast images of the same patient reveal dramatic enhancement of the cerebellar metastases.

Brain metastases may develop in 10% to 40% of cancer patients ([12]). Leptomeningeal disease occurs in 5% of all patients with cancer ([13]). Two-thirds to three-quarters of brain metastases are recognized as multiple lesions on MRI. Lung cancer is the neoplasm that most frequently metastasizes to the brain, followed by breast cancer and melanoma. Other cancers that commonly metastasize to the brain are colorectal, kidney, prostate, testicular, and ovarian cancers and sarcomas, although any systemic cancer can metastasize

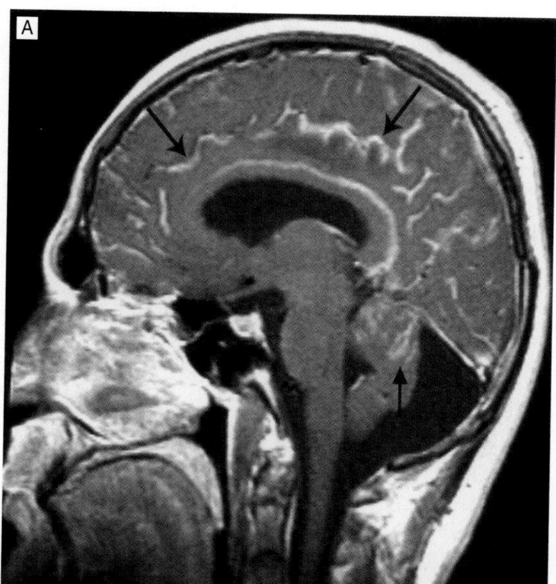

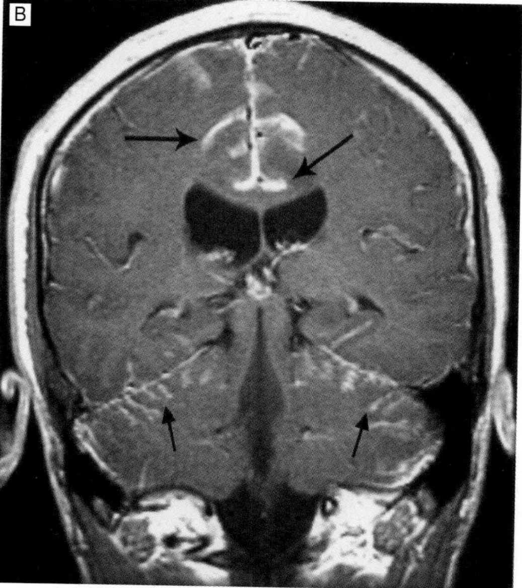

FIGURE 53-4 A. Sagittal postcontrast T1-weighted magnetic resonance imaging (MRI) showing subarachnoid spread of melanoma metastasis to the brain in a 29-year-old man. Abnormal enhancement of the cortical sulci (*large arrows*) and cerebellar sulci (*small arrows*) is noted. B. Coronal postcontrast T1-weighted MRI in the same patient. (Used with permission from Dr. Ashok Kumar, MD Anderson Cancer Center.)

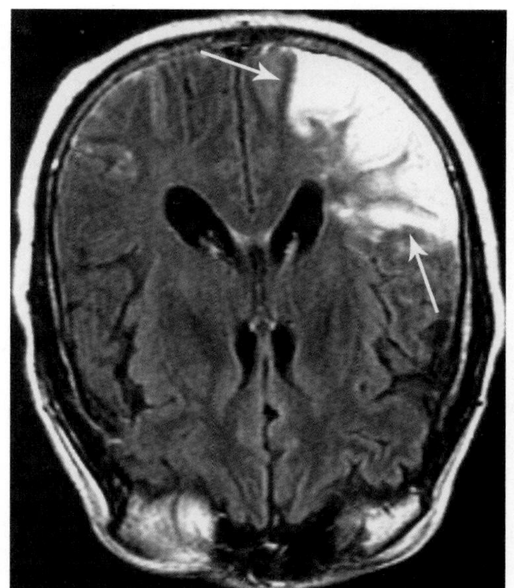

FIGURE 53-5 Acute infarction involving the territory of the right middle cerebral artery in a 58-year-old patient with renal cell carcinoma. Magnetic resonance imaging (MRI; fluid-attenuated inversion recovery [FLAIR] image) demonstrates abnormal thickening, with a T2-weighted increase in signal intensity (*arrows*) involving the right temporo-occipital lobe cortex and subcortical white matter. MRI is more sensitive than computed tomography in detecting early stroke. (Used with permission from Dr. Ashok Kumar, MD Anderson Cancer Center.)

to the brain. Melanomas have the highest propensity to metastasize to the brain, with up to 40% of cases behaving in this manner at some point. Tumors most commonly metastasize to the gray-white junction where the vessels are small and narrow and tumor emboli can be trapped. Eighty percent of tumors metastasize to the cerebral hemispheres, 15% to the cerebellum, and 5% to the brainstem. Pelvic tumors have an increased propensity to metastasize to the posterior fossa, possibly by means of venous drainage of these tumors through Batson plexus ([14]). The tumors that are most often hemorrhagic include melanoma, renal cell carcinoma, and choriocarcinoma.

The treatment for increased intracranial pressure depends on the underlying etiology ([15]). Infectious sources, such as meningitis, should be treated with antibiotics, and brain abscesses should be drained. Hydrocephalus should be treated with surgical shunting or ventriculostomy, and subdural hematomas should be either drained or, if small, monitored under the guidance of a neurosurgeon. Edema associated with brain tumors is initially treated with oral dexamethasone at a dosage of 16 mg/d or 4 mg every 6 hours ([16]). For patients with impending herniation, very large doses of intravenous (IV) dexamethasone can be used, initially 40 to 100 mg intravenously and subsequently 40 to 100 mg/d ([3]). Dexamethasone is the steroid of choice because of its lack of mineralocorticoid effect. Steroids may not be needed in asymptomatic brain lesions ([17]).

For life-threatening edema or brain herniation, emergency treatments include hyperventilation and administration of mannitol in addition to steroids ([15]). Hyperventilation after intubation to achieve a partial pressure of carbon dioxide of 25 to 30 mm Hg is the most rapid way to decrease intracranial pressure, but the benefit is generally short lived, and equilibration may occur within a few hours. Mannitol is a hyperosmotic agent that can shift water out of brain cells and into the vessels. The recommended dose of mannitol is a 20% to 25% solution at 0.5 to 2.0 g/kg administered intravenously over 10 to 30 minutes. Mannitol has a rapid onset of action and lasts for hours, but prolonged use can lead to hyperosmolarity and an inadvertent increase in intracranial pressure ([3]). Further treatment in intensive care may include IV infusion of hypertonic saline, propofol, and hypothermia ([4]). Neurosurgical intervention such as placement of a ventricular drain or decompressive craniectomy may be necessary if the patient has neurologic deterioration despite appropriate medical management.

Radiation therapy can be used to treat brain metastasis. The dosage for whole-brain radiation therapy (WBRT) typically ranges between 20 Gy over 1 week and 50 Gy over 4 weeks. Treatment with WBRT can increase survival in patients by 3 to 6 months relative to no treatment ([16]). Increased intracranial pressure should be treated before WBRT is instituted because radiotherapy can further increase pressure. Common side effects of WBRT are nausea and vomiting, alopecia, headache, hearing loss, loss of taste, and fever. Possible delayed complications of WBRT are progressive leukoencephalopathy with dementia, ataxia, apraxia, and incontinence syndrome, which can mimic normal-pressure hydrocephalus. This dreaded side effect can occur as long as 1 year after therapy, and elderly patients are more susceptible.

Surgery can be used to treat accessible brain metastases. A stereotactic biopsy can be performed for the patient with multiple brain metastases, which are then generally treated with radiation ([18]). Surgery is generally not indicated for patients with widespread systemic disease, poor functional status, or tumors in critical or hard-to-access locations ([16]). In selected patients with good functional status, even when multiple brain metastases are present, survival time is longer for patients who have all tumors removed than for those who do not. Consequently, it is common for the neurosurgeons at our institution to remove up to four metastatic lesions at a time ([17]). Patients with single brain metastases who underwent WBRT after surgery had longer survival than those who had surgery alone ([19]).

For patients with brain lesions that are not amenable to surgery, stereotactic radiosurgery can be used in single doses as high as 1,400 cGy. This approach is typically used for brain tumors less than 4 cm in diameter and has the benefit of being noninvasive and relatively fast acting ([5]). Brachytherapy can be used on larger tumors, but this approach requires that radioactive seeds be invasively implanted in the designated area and left for 5 or 6 days, delivering approximately 6,000 cGy to the area. Brachytherapy may cause radiation necrosis in up to 50% of patients 6 months after treatment. No treatment exists for radiation necrosis, although the symptoms may respond to corticosteroids.

Chemotherapy can be used in some patients with brain metastasis. Dexamethasone, which is thought to aid in reestablishing the blood-brain barrier, should not be used if possible, so that the selected chemotherapeutic agent(s) can reach the tumor cells. Cancers for which chemotherapy has been used include choriocarcinoma, small cell cancer of the lungs, and breast cancer ([16, 20, 21]).

Leptomeningeal Disease

Leptomeningeal disease can involve invasion of the brain, the spinal parenchyma, the nerve roots, and blood vessels of the nervous system. The cancers that most commonly result in LMD are breast and lung cancer, melanoma, non-Hodgkin lymphoma, and leukemia. Patients present with a variety of symptoms depending on the location of the leptomeninges affected, but they can include headache, altered mental status, cranial nerve palsies (in about 50% of patients), incontinence, back pain, sensory changes, seizures, isolated neurologic findings, and even a stroke-like presentation ([5, 21]). Leptomeningeal metastases occur in 0.8% to 8% of all cases of cancer ([5]).

The diagnosis of LMD can be difficult. Computed tomography scans will occasionally be suggestive of LMD. Magnetic resonance imaging scanning has better sensitivity than CT for detecting LMD, including leptomeningeal enhancement, hydrocephalus, and cortical nodules. However, MRI results are not diagnostic. Inflammation of the meninges can also be found in cases of meningitis, trauma, infection, and hematoma formation. Lumbar puncture and evaluation of the CSF is the gold standard for diagnosing LMD, although multiple lumbar taps may be required to make the diagnosis because only 50% of patients will have positive cytologic evidence of LMD on the first CSF evaluation ([5, 22]). Cerebrospinal fluid findings consistent with LMD include a high opening pressure, low glucose and high protein levels, and a mononuclear pleocytosis ([5]). Among patients with normal values for CSF protein, glucose, and opening pressure and cytology negative for LMD, fewer than 5% will have LMD ([22]).

The treatment of LMD can include chemotherapy through an implanted subcutaneous reservoir and ventricular catheter (SRVC) or through lumbar puncture instillation. Lumbar tap administration does not require placement of a catheter, but 10% to 15% of the subarachnoid space might be missed using this technique. Chemotherapeutic agents frequently used are methotrexate and thiotepa. Cytarabine can also be used in patients with leukemias and lymphomas, but it is generally not effective against solid tumors. Radiation therapy is commonly used for localized LMD or in areas of nerve root involvement where intrathecal chemotherapy is not likely to reach adequate concentrations. Fixed neurologic deficits caused by LMD are not likely to improve with therapy, but encephalopathy may ([22]). The prognosis of patients with LMD is poor, with a median survival of 3 to 6 months and only a 15% to 25% chance of surviving longer than 1 year ([5]).

Seizures

Seizures are the presenting symptom in 15% to 20% of patients with brain metastases ([21]). In cancer patients presenting with seizures, metabolic, infectious, and coagulopathic causes should also be considered. The initial laboratory work should include analysis of glucose level, electrolytes, blood urea nitrogen (BUN), creatinine, liver enzymes, calcium, urine analysis, prothrombin time (PT), activated partial thromboplastin time (PTT), and toxicology screening if indicated (Fig. 53-6).

Patients can have seizures during withdrawal from high-dose, short-acting benzodiazepines (such as alprazolam), alcohol, antibiotics (such as the carbapenems), pain medicines (such as meperidine), and many other medicines. The patient's family can be helpful in sorting out the etiology of seizures by providing information about the patient's medications, social history, and preceding symptoms, such as fever or headache. Computed tomography without and with contrast is also helpful and can identify increased intracranial pressure, bleeding, or brain metastasis. Electroencephalography (EEG) is also helpful in the evaluation of seizures and can determine whether an epileptic focus is present. Lumbar tap for CSF analysis can be helpful if the seizures are suspected to be secondary to infection or LMD, provided that there are no contraindications on brain imaging (signs of increased intracranial pressure or impending herniation) and that the convulsions have stopped.

Status epilepticus occurs when a patient has prolonged seizures with continuous seizure activity lasting >5 minutes or two or more sequential seizures

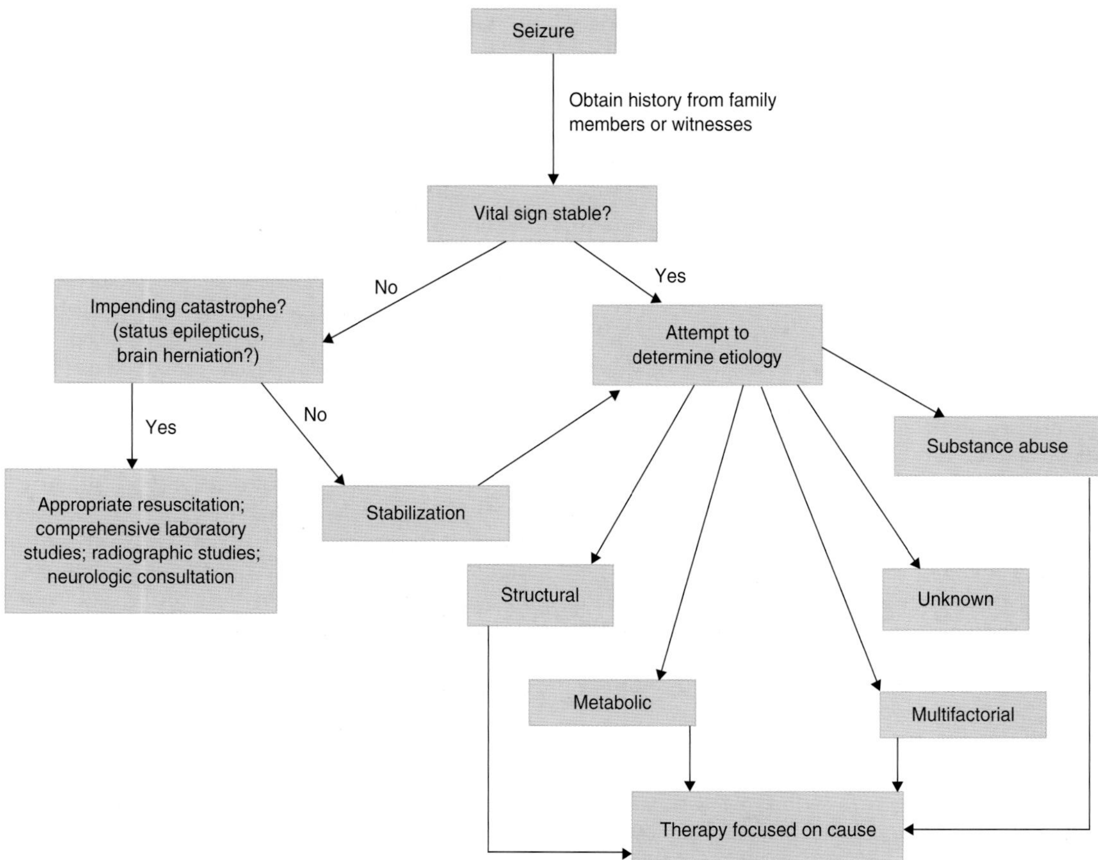

FIGURE 53-6 Algorithm for the evaluation of seizure. (Adapted with permission from Yeung SJ, Escalante CP [eds]: *Oncologic Emergencies*. Hamilton, Ontario, Canada: BC Decker; 2002.)

without full recovery of consciousness between seizures. When patients present with status epilepticus, airway, breathing, and circulation should be assessed immediately ([23, 24]). Initial care for patients with status epilepticus includes placing the patient in a safe environment, administering 100% oxygen by nonrebreather mask, monitoring with a continuous pulse oximeter providing suction, and administering IV fluids (normal saline). Priority should be placed on exclusion of hypoglycemia, protecting the airway, and terminating the convulsions. Anticonvulsant therapy with IV benzodiazepines (eg, diazepam, 0.2 mg/kg at 5 mg/min, up to 10 mg, or lorazepam, 0.1 mg/kg at 2 mg/min, up to 4 mg) should be administered to halt seizure activity. For patients with continuing seizures, therapy can be escalated in steps; second-line therapy includes fosphenytoin IV at15 to 20 mg of phenytoin equivalents (PE) per kilogram. Patients with refractory seizures might require high-dose anticonvulsant therapy (eg, pentobarbital, thiopental, propofol, midazolam) with complete sedation, intubation/ventilator support, EEG, and careful monitoring in the intensive care unit.

It is the general consensus of the American Academy of Neurology that routine use of prophylactic antiepileptic drugs (AEDs) for patients with brain metastases who have not experienced a seizure is not indicated ([16]). Once new-onset seizure in a cancer patient has been controlled, the patient should be placed on an AED. Several drugs can be used, including phenytoin, carbamazepine, clonazepam, gabapentin, lamotrigine, phenobarbital, primidone, topiramate, and valproate. Because of no significant interaction with antineoplastic drugs, some clinicians prefer levetiracetam in cancer patients.

Altered Mental Status

Altered mental status is a common neurologic complaint in cancer patients, with metabolic encephalopathy being the most common cause. Altered mental status can range from a slight decrease in normal intellectual functioning to coma. A cancer patient's mental status may change in response to several factors, such as infections/sepsis, metabolic derangements, bleeding, medications, hypoxemia, cancer therapies, paraneoplastic neurologic syndromes, and intracranial events, such as brain metastases. Organ failure, whether hepatic, renal, adrenal, thyroid, or pulmonary, can also produce fluctuations in mental status. The most common metabolic deficiencies causing such alterations are hyponatremia, hypercalcemia, hypoglycemia, and vitamin B_1 deficiency. The causes of altered mental status are numerous; an extensive history and physical examination can help to identify the underlying cause and determine appropriate therapy (Fig. 53-7). The differential diagnosis and diagnostic evaluation are beyond the scope of this chapter, but a few entities are unique to cancer patients.

For instance, cancer therapy is a common cause of altered mental status. Many neurologic manifestations, such as dementia, cognitive decline, and encephalopathy, can result from chemotherapy. Table 53-1 highlights some of the common neurologic complications of chemotherapy ([5, 17, 25]).

Radiation therapy can also cause complications, among them leukoencephalopathy, radiation necrosis, and decreased memory and mental functioning. (The preceding section on increased intracranial pressure provides a fuller discussion of the cognitive side effects of radiation therapy.) Other possible causes of cognitive decline are narcotics (commonly prescribed for pain), infections (pneumonia, sepsis, urinary tract infection), and cerebral infarction.

Paraneoplastic syndromes are unique to cancer patients and should be considered in cases of altered mental status. In many instances, the paraneoplastic syndrome will precede the cancer diagnosis. Paraneoplastic syndromes must be differentiated from symptoms caused by progression of cancer or the side effects of cancer therapy. The two common paraneoplastic syndromes that cause mental status change through electrolyte abnormalities are hypercalcemia of malignancy and hyponatremia due to syndrome of inappropriate antidiuretic hormone (SIADH). Paraneoplastic neurologic syndromes associated with mental status changes and neurophysiologic abnormalities are paraneoplastic cerebellar degeneration and Lambert-Eaton myasthenic syndrome ([5]).

CARDIAC EMERGENCIES

Cardiac Tamponade

Tumors involving the heart are much more frequently metastatic than primary. The tumors that most often metastasize to the heart are lung, breast, and GI tract cancers; leukemia; lymphoma; melanoma; and sarcoma. Metastatic involvement of the heart has also been noted in leukemia and lymphoma patients. Certain therapies can also affect the myocardium and cause pericardial disease, especially cyclophosphamide and ifosfamide at high doses, all-*trans*-retinoic acid (ATRA), doxorubicin, and radiation therapy ([26]). Cardiac tamponade occurs when pericardial fluid accumulates and presses on the heart, increasing diastolic pressure in the ventricles and thereby decreasing stroke volume. The patient develops decreased cardiac output and systemic arterial pressure and can present with a shock-like syndrome. Most patients with pericardial effusions report no symptoms, but patients with cardiac tamponade present with shortness of breath, cough, hoarseness, epigastric pain, or chest pain that is made worse by lying down or leaning forward. On examination, the patient typically has distended neck veins, low systemic blood pressure, and low pulse pressure, and can have a pericardial rub or decreased heart sounds. The presence of pulsus paradoxus, which is an inspiratory decline in systolic blood pressure of >10 mm Hg, should be ruled out. Pulsus paradoxus can also occur in chronic obstructive pulmonary disease (COPD), pulmonary embolism, right ventricular infarction, and shock. Chest x-ray often reveals a "water bottle" configuration if the effusion has accumulated slowly, but the cardiac silhouette can appear normal if the effusion accumulates rapidly. Prior chest x-ray images can be useful in determining changes in the size of the cardiac silhouette. The electrocardiogram (ECG) might reveal electrical alternans (a variation of voltage in individual QRS complexes) and low-voltage or ST-segment and T-wave changes. Transthoracic echocardiography is the best test to determine whether tamponade exists. If cardiac tamponade is present, echocardiography can help determine whether the effusion is localized or loculated, and it can also aid in planning pericardiocentesis. On echocardiograms, tamponade can be evidenced by collapse of the right ventricle and atria in diastole (Fig. 53-8).

Treatment of tamponade includes the administration of oxygen, IV fluids, and vasopressors if necessary. Pericardiocentesis can be performed under ultrasound guidance and is relatively safe. A scoring system may help to decide whether pericardiocentesis needs to be performed emergently ([27]). At the University of Texas MD Anderson Cancer Center (MDACC), a drainage catheter is commonly placed in patients with tamponade, with drainage performed daily. When the total volume of fluid drained is less than 50 mL/d, the catheter can be removed. Fibrinolytic agents may be used to unclog the catheter to avoid repeat pericardiocentesis or replacement of the catheter ([28]). Long-term management focuses on preventing reaccumulation of fluid. Creation of a pleuropericardial window can prevent

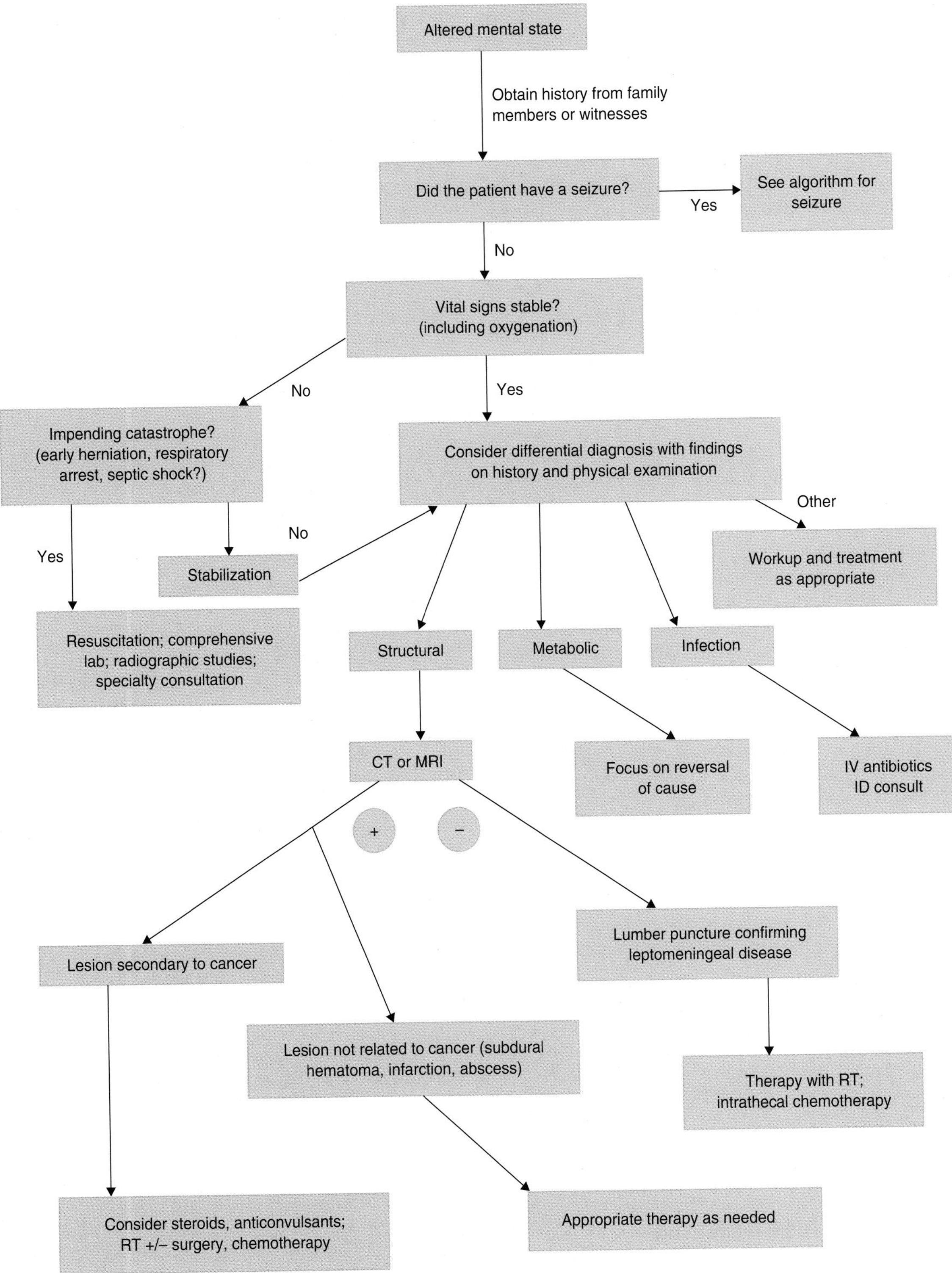

FIGURE 53-7 Algorithm for the evaluation and treatment of altered mental status. CT, computed tomography; ID, infectious disease; IV, intravenous; MRI, magnetic resonance imaging; RT, radiation therapy. (Adapted with permission from Yeung SJ, Escalante CP [eds]: *Oncologic Emergencies*. Hamilton, Ontario, Canada: BC Decker; 2002.)

Table 53-1 Neurologic Complications of Chemotherapy

Chemotherapy	Seizure	Neuropathy or Sensory Changes	Encephalopathy	Cerebellar Symptoms	Vascular Events/ Stroke	Cognitive/ Dementia Nerve Palsy	Cranial	Visual Changes/ Loss	Myelopathy	Other
BCNU (carmustine)	+		+		+	+	+	+		
Busulfan	+									
Cisplatin	+	+	+		+					Ototoxicity
Cytarabine		+	+	+		+			+	
Dacarbazine	+									
Docetaxel		+								
Doxorubicin								+		
Etoposide	+									
Fludarabine			+							
5-Fluorouracil			+	+						
Gemcitabine		+								
Ifosfamide	+	+	+	+						
Interferon	+		+			+				
Interleukin-2			+							
L-Asparaginase	+		+		+					
Methotrexate	+		+	+	+	+	+		+	
Paclitaxel	+									Gait abnormality
Procarbazine		+	+	+						
Tamoxifen			+					+		
Taxol		+								
Teniposide		+								
Thalidomide		+								
Thiotepa									+	
Vincristine	+	+		+		+	+	+		Vertigo, autonomic neuropathy
Vinorelbine		+								

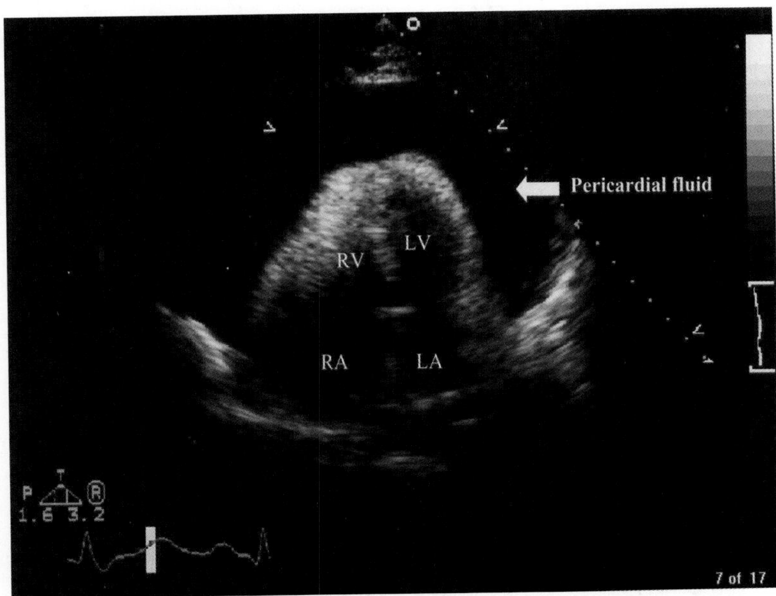

FIGURE 53-8 Two-dimensional echocardiogram in the apical four-chamber view demonstrating a large pericardial effusion. The right ventricle is not well visualized because of acoustic shadowing, which commonly occurs with large effusions. (Used with permission from Dr. Joseph Swafford, MD Anderson Cancer Center.)

reaccumulation of fluid and avoid repeated pericardiocentesis. Radiation therapy and chemotherapy can also be used to prevent reaccumulation of fluid, as can sclerosis of the pericardial sac.

Superior Vena Cava Syndrome

Superior vena cava (SVC) syndrome is characterized by low blood flow from the SVC to the right atrium. Malignancy is by far the most common cause of SVC syndrome, although nonmalignant causes, such as indwelling central venous catheters, aneurysms, and goiters, can also cause this syndrome ([2]). Lung cancer is the most common malignant neoplasm causing SVC syndrome, but lymphoma, breast and GI cancers, sarcomas, melanomas, prostate cancer, and any mediastinal tumor can also cause this disorder. Among mechanisms that can lead to this syndrome are extrinsic compression by tumor, intrinsic compression by tumor or clot, or fibrosis. Patients may present with headache; dizziness; confusion; swelling of the upper extremities, face, and neck; shortness of breath; and dysphagia. Physical examination often reveals engorgement of veins and collaterals in the upper extremities due to elevated pressure in the venous system.

Diagnosis of SVC syndrome requires imaging ([28a]). Routine chest x-rays will often reveal mediastinal widening, a right-side chest mass, or a mediastinal mass. Computed tomography scanning of the chest using IV contrast is an excellent means of delineating the cause of the obstruction and any associated finding (Fig. 53-9). If IV iodine contrast is contraindicated, radionuclide venography and MRI are alternatives. Doppler ultrasound may be helpful to evaluate for the presence of a clot.

The treatment of SVC syndrome depends on the nature of the obstruction. Patients might respond to elevation of the head, corticosteroids if the intracranial pressure is increased, and occasionally diuretics. If thrombosis is present, local lytic therapy or anticoagulation can be used. Intravascular stenting with metallic stents can be used, as can angioplasty. Stent placement has been associated with a faster resolution of symptoms relative to radiation therapy ([29]) (Fig. 53-10).

Stenting may be first-line treatment of SVC syndrome ([29, 30]), especially in emergent situations of impending airway obstruction or increased intracranial pressure ([31]).

It is important to obtain a tissue specimen of the tumor if its type is not known, so that it can be treated adequately. For patients with tumors that are chemotherapy sensitive, such as small cell lung cancer, chemotherapy can be instituted. Patients with non–small cell lung cancer will often respond to radiation therapy, and SVC syndrome symptoms begin to improve in about 1 week. Radiotherapy is also justified if a histologic diagnosis cannot be established in a timely manner. Surgical treatment with

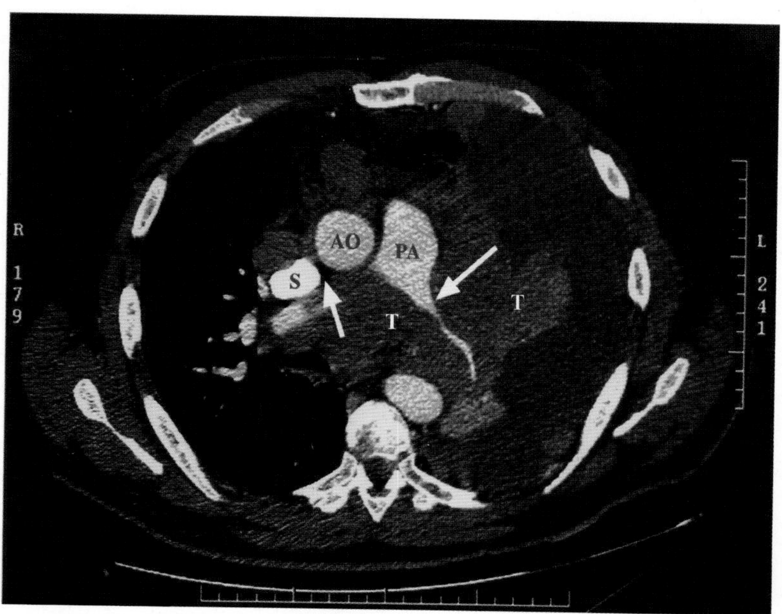

FIGURE 53-9 Computed tomography scan revealing superior vena cava (SVC) syndrome from extrinsic compression of the SVC in a patient with non–small cell lung cancer. ***Large arrow*** **indicates compression of the left pulmonary artery;** ***small arrow*** **indicates obliteration of the right pulmonary artery. AO, aorta; PA, main pulmonary artery; S, superior vena cava; T, tumor.** (Used with permission from Dr. Joel Dunnington, MD Anderson Cancer Center.)

reconstruction is also possible for certain tumor types or selected patients ([32]).

Myocardial Ischemia

Patients with cancer can present to the emergency center with myocardial ischemia. A full discussion of ischemic heart disease is beyond the scope of this chapter, but there are special considerations in cancer patients that should be mentioned.

Many cancer patients have thrombocytopenia due to chemotherapy, radiation therapy, or bone marrow infiltration with tumor. Despite platelet counts in the single or double digits, these patients can still present with acute cardiac syndrome. Although the practitioner might feel uncomfortable giving aspirin to these patients, cardiologists at MDACC have found that patients with platelet counts less than 50,000/μL who have cardiac ischemia and are treated with aspirin have a better 24-hour survival rate than those who are not given aspirin.

Certain chemotherapeutic agents can predispose patients to myocardial ischemia, including 5-fluorouracil (5-FU), interferons, and presumably capecitabine, which is a metabolite of 5-FU. Radiation therapy can also be a predisposing factor ([26]). It is important to consider myocardial ischemia in patients who have undergone any of these therapies, especially those who otherwise have no risk factors for ischemic heart disease.

The cardiac markers troponin, creatine phosphokinase (CPK), and CPK-MB are useful in diagnosing myocardial infarction. Cardiac troponins are more sensitive and specific markers for ischemic heart disease than CPK-MB, which can be influenced by skeletal muscle injury; however, cardiac troponin levels can also be raised by chronic renal insufficiency (CRI), cardiomyopathy with severe congestive heart failure, myocarditis, and massive pulmonary embolism. In one small study evaluating 24 patients with submassive pulmonary embolism, troponin levels were higher than normal in 5 patients ([33]). In this study, patients who presented with chest pain and for whom a ventilation/perfusion (V/Q) scan revealed a high probability of submassive pulmonary embolism were analyzed. High troponin was defined as a level >0.4 μg/L, and myocardial infarction was evidenced by a level >2.3 μg/L. It was found that four of the five patients with submassive pulmonary embolism had slightly elevated troponin levels and the fifth patient had a troponin level of 11.1 μg/L. The study was limited in that it did not investigate the possibility of underlying ischemia in patients with documented pulmonary embolism. Such patients commonly present with chest pain, and pulmonary embolism and ischemic heart disease are both in the differential diagnosis of myocardial infarction. In patients with small increases of troponin, pulmonary embolism (even submassive)

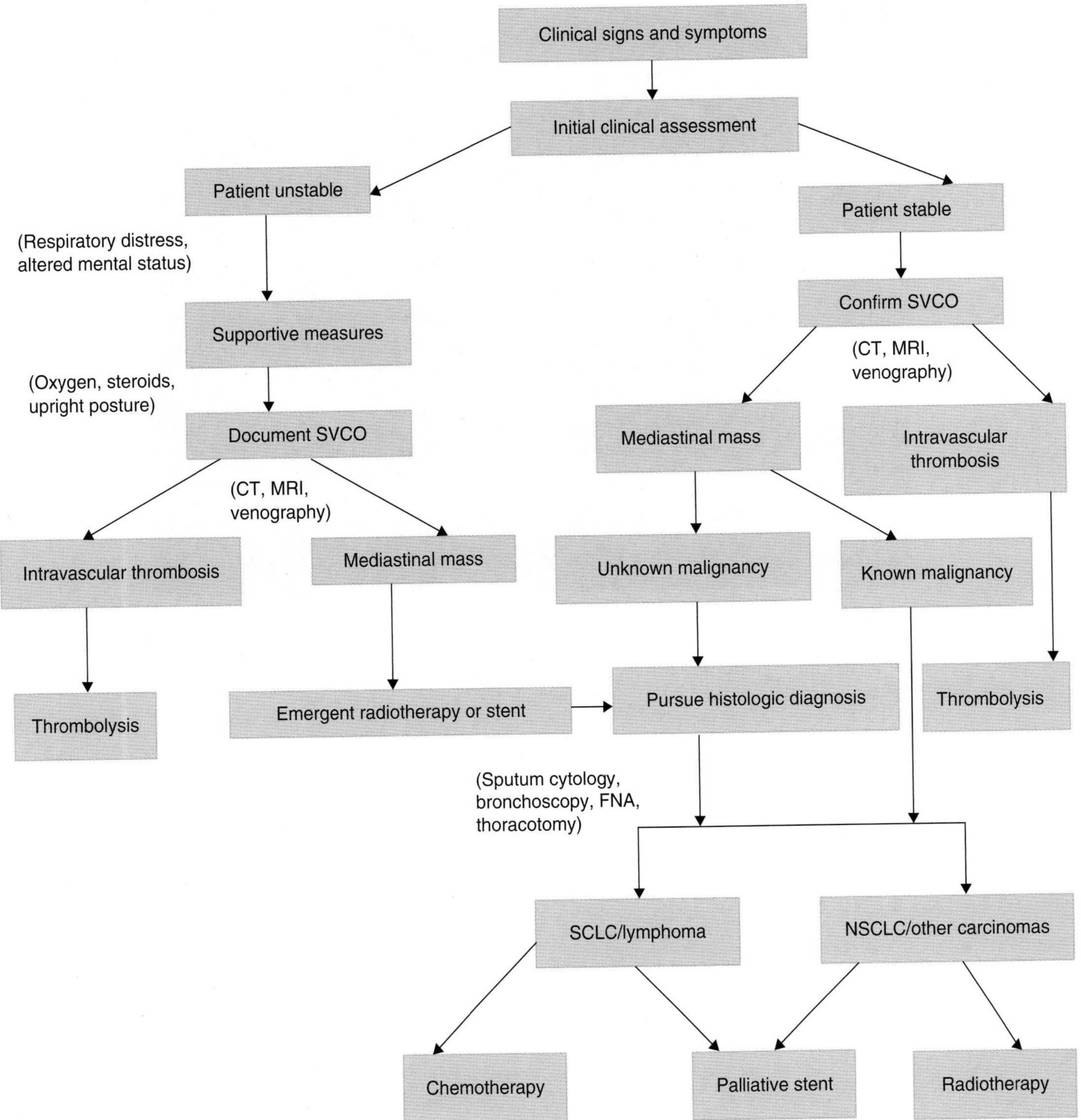

FIGURE 53-10 Algorithms for the diagnosis and management of superior vena cava syndrome. CT, computed tomography; FNA, fine-needle aspiration; MRI, magnetic resonance imaging; NSCLC, non–small cell lung cancer; SCLC, small cell lung cancer; SVCO, superior vena cava obstruction. (Adapted with permission from Yeung SJ, Escalante CP [eds]: *Oncologic Emergencies*. Hamilton, Ontario, Canada: BC Decker; 2002.)

can be the cause, rather than ischemic heart disease; this possibility should be considered in patients presenting with chest pain.

HEMATOLOGIC EMERGENCIES

Hyperviscosity Syndrome

Hyperviscosity syndrome is due to abnormally high concentrations of paraproteins in the serum, which increase viscosity and cause red blood cell (RBC) sludging and low oxygen delivery to the tissues. This disorder occurs in 15% of patients with Waldenström macroglobulinemia, which is characterized by the presence of high-molecular-weight (IgM) macromolecules and thus predisposes patients to this syndrome. Aggregation of IgG macromolecules and polymerization of IgA macromolecules, as well as purely light-chain myeloma, are also capable of causing this syndrome ([34]). Other conditions that can cause hyperviscosity syndrome are polycythemia vera, dysproteinemias, and occasionally leukemias.

Hyperviscosity syndrome can present with either bleeding due to abnormal platelet functioning or thrombosis due to hyperviscosity. Visual complaints, headache, dizziness, alterations in mental status, and mucosal bleeding are all symptoms of hyperviscosity syndrome. Patients can also develop retinal hemorrhages, congestive heart failure due to increased plasma volume, peripheral neuropathy, weakness, and fatigue ([34]). Funduscopic examination can reveal venous dilatation, retinal vein occlusion, or papilledema (Fig. 53-11).

The diagnosis is made on the basis of a high serum viscosity. Normal serum viscosity ranges between 1.4 and 1.8 Ostwald units (relative to water, at 1). Patients start to develop symptoms when serum viscosity exceeds 4.0 Ostwald units ([34-36]).

The treatment for hyperviscosity syndrome includes the administration of IV fluids followed by diuresis. Plasma exchange can decrease symptoms quickly and can be followed by chemotherapy.

Hyperleukocytosis

Hyperleukocytosis is typically defined as a white blood cell (WBC) count in the peripheral blood higher than 100,000/μL. Acute myelogenous leukemia (AML), chronic myelogenous leukemia (CML), and less frequently (because of the smaller size of the lymphocytes) acute and chronic lymphocytic leukemia (CLL) are associated with leukostasis. From 5% to 30% of adult patients with acute leukemias present with leukostasis that requires prompt recognition and initiation of therapy to prevent respiratory failure or intracranial hemorrhage ([35]). The WBC count in acute lymphocytic leukemia (ALL) typically must be greater than 400,000/μL before leukostasis will develop. The highest rate of mortality is in patients with AML who have high blast counts.

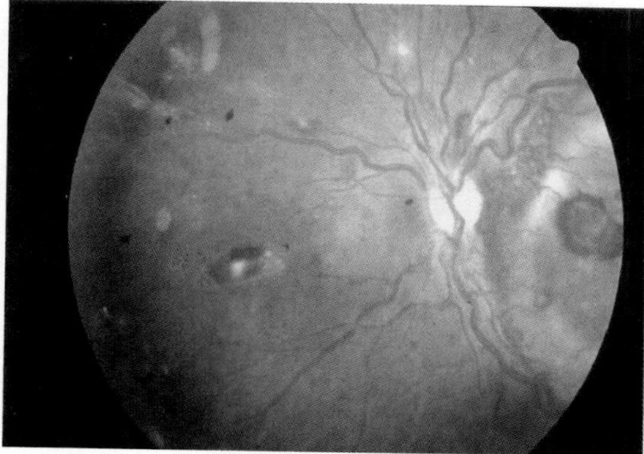

FIGURE 53-11 Funduscopic examination revealing a Roth spot (the white-centered retinal hemorrhage). The Roth spot is the hallmark of leukemic retinopathy. (Used with permission from Dr. Bita Esmaeli, MD Anderson Cancer Center.)

Symptoms of hyperleukocytosis are headache, dizziness, vertigo, shortness of breath, altered mental status, and hemoptysis. WBCs are poorly deformable and can become lodged in the microvasculature of the kidneys, lungs, brain, and other organs. The pulmonary and neurologic systems are most critically affected in hyperleukocytosis syndrome. In the lungs, WBCs can get caught in the pulmonary circulation, causing adult respiratory distress syndrome (ARDS), or can mimic pulmonary embolism because of WBC stasis in the pulmonary vasculature, thereby causing a V/Q mismatch ([36]). Patients with the latter condition should not be given diuretics, because this will further increase stasis. Most patients with leukemia are anemic; this condition can offset the WBC elevation, so hyperviscosity is not as common in these patients. It is important not to give these patients blood transfusions unless absolutely necessary, because this treatment can exacerbate hyperleukocytosis and increase the RBC mass without changing the total blood volume. Patients can present with decreased mental status, which can be caused by endothelial leakage from the small vessels of the brain or hemorrhage, but other causes of altered mental status should also be considered, including infection, LMD from leukemia, and metabolic sources. Imaging studies, such as CT scan and MRI, as well as lumbar tap should be performed when indicated ([3]).

The treatment of hyperleukocytosis involves lowering the WBC count, which can be accomplished with leukapheresis or chemotherapy. Leukapheresis can lower the WBC count by 30% to 60% from pretreatment levels. These effects can be transient; therefore, repeat leukapheresis might be necessary. Patients undergoing leukapheresis should also be monitored closely to prevent tumor lysis syndrome.

Thrombosis

Venous thromboembolism (VTE) is influenced by Virchow triad: venous stasis, higher than normal coagulability, and intimal injury. Patients with cancer have a high risk of VTE, and up to 15% of patients will develop VTE because of hypercoagulability, the use of central venous catheters, and high stasis ([37]). Cancer patients can have increased serum viscosity due to dehydration or, less frequently, hyperviscosity syndrome (described previously). Stasis and intimal injury can be caused by numerous events—for example, tumor encroachment on blood vessels or indirect effects of cancer, such as spinal cord compression, brain metastasis, dehydration, or impaired ambulation. Some chemotherapeutic cancer agents can also induce VTE, among them tamoxifen, cisplatin, cyclophosphamide, methotrexate, and 5-FU ([37]).

Symptoms of pulmonary embolism (PE) include chest pain, shortness of breath, palpitations, fever up to 102°F, and syncope in the case of massive PE. Electrocardiogram findings can include T-wave inversion in the precordial leads, sinus tachycardia, right bundle branch block, or rightward movement of the QRS axis. Chest roentgenograms can be normal or might reveal a pleural effusion or elevation of the diaphragm on the involved side. Physical examination can reveal tachypnea, tachycardia, and leg edema or erythema in the case of associated deep vein thrombosis.

Diagnosis of PE can be made by V/Q scanning, spiral CT angiography, pulmonary angiography, or MRI (Fig. 53-12).

Ventilation/perfusion scans are noninvasive, and the results are useful in patients with a high probability of PE, which can be treated as VTE; normal results on V/Q scans can rule out PE. Clinical suspicion based on the patient's risk factors and results of other tests can guide the clinician regarding the patient's pretest probability of PE. Patients with indeterminate result from V/Q scans who are strongly suspected of having a PE can undergo further testing, such as spiral CT angiography, pulmonary angiography, or MRI. Spiral CT scanning and MRI can detect segmental PE but not necessarily subsegmental PE. Both of these tests are useful in that they give further information about the condition of the lung, such as whether pneumonia is present, tumor size, and impingement on the bronchial airways; this additional information is helpful in determining the cause of the patient's symptoms. Pulmonary angiography remains the gold standard in detecting PE, although it requires more dye than other contrast methods and has a greater risk of renal complications. The alveolar-arterial gradient (A-a gradient) from an arterial blood gas (ABG) can serve to corroborate the diagnosis of PE, but a normal A-a gradient does not rule out a PE. The upper limit of normal of an A-a gradient is equal to patient age/4 + 4, but this value can also increase when the patient is supine. In the PIOPED (Prospective Investigation of Pulmonary Embolism Diagnosis) study, ABGs were normal in 14% of patients with preexisting cardiopulmonary disease and in 38% of patients with no underlying cardiopulmonary disease despite the presence of pulmonary emboli [38] (Fig. 53-13).

The diagnosis of peripheral VTE can be made by Doppler ultrasound, impedance plethysmography, venography, nuclear venogram, or magnetic resonance (MR) venography (Fig. 53-14).

The D-dimer test can also be used in the evaluation of VTE; normal results are associated with a significantly lower likelihood of VTE than high values [37]. D-Dimer has a high negative predictive value for pulmonary embolism in cancer patients, and a normal D-dimer can be used to exclude pulmonary embolism in cancer patients. Combining D-dimer with clinical symptoms and signs did not substantially change negative predictive value, positive predictive value, sensitivity, or specificity [39]. Because D-dimer is commonly high in patients with cancer, an elevated D-dimer is not useful in diagnosing VTE.

First-line treatment for VTE consists of either unfractionated heparin (UFH) or low-molecular-weight

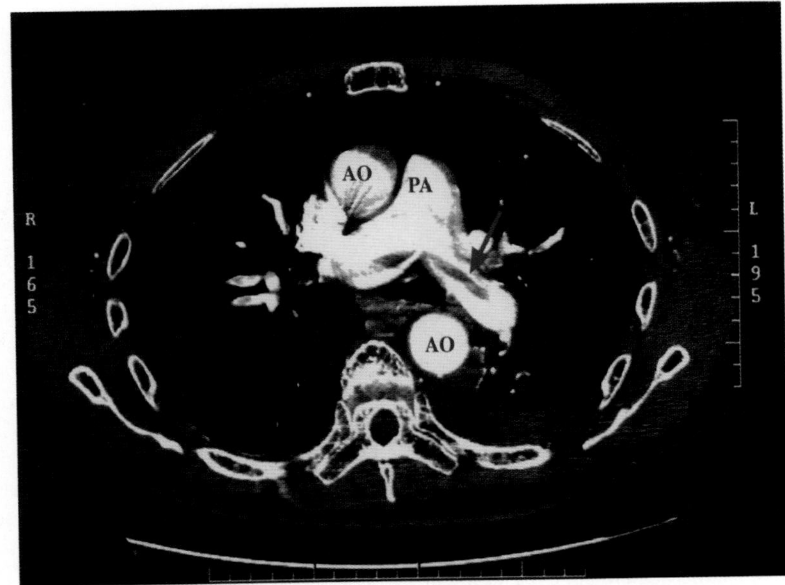

FIGURE 53-12 Spiral computed tomography angiogram in a patient with a saddle pulmonary embolism (*arrow*). AO, aorta; PA, main pulmonary artery. (Used with permission from Dr. Joel Dunnington, MD Anderson Cancer Center.)

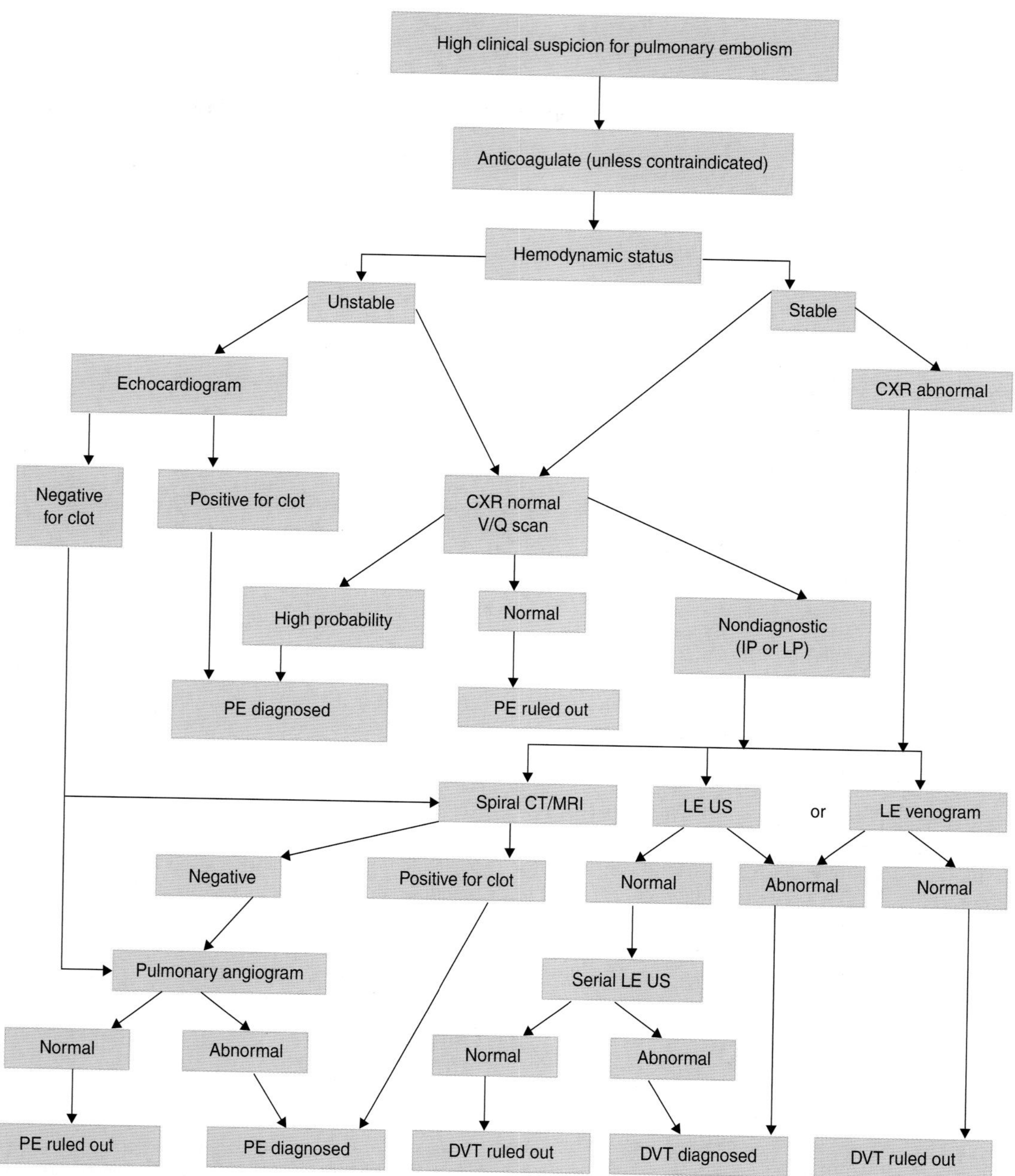

FIGURE 53-13 Suggested algorithm for the evaluation of pulmonary embolism. CXR, chest x-ray; DVT, deep venous thrombosis; IP, intermediate probability; LE US, lower extremity ultrasound; LE venogram, lower extremity venogram; LP, low probability; PE, pulmonary embolism; V/Q scan, ventilation/perfusion scan. (Adapted with permission from Yeung SJ, Escalante CP [eds]: *Oncologic Emergencies*. Hamilton, Ontario, Canada: BC Decker; 2002.)

heparin (LMWH). Low-molecular-weight heparin has the advantage that factor Xa levels usually do not have to be monitored because protein binding is low. It also has a longer half-life than UFH and thus can be given less frequently (once or twice per day). The LMWHs enoxaparin, tinzaparin, and dalteparin are all different and cannot be used interchangeably. Monitoring may be required for patients with obesity and renal insufficiency, because LMWH is cleared by the kidneys. When monitoring is necessary, the Xa level should be measured 4 hours after the injection, with a target level ranging from 0.6 to 1.0 IU/mL for twice-daily dosing. For daily dosing, the Xa level should range between 1.9 and 2.0 IU/mL ([40]). For patients who will

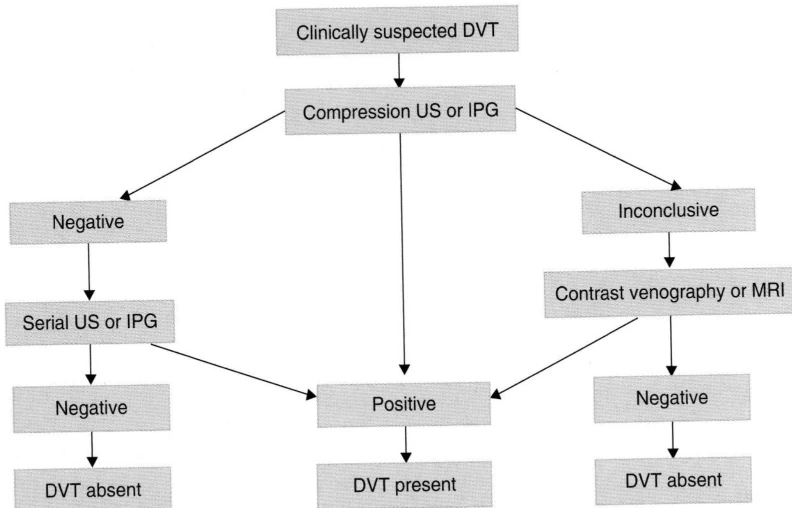

FIGURE 53-14 Diagnostic approach to patients with suspected acute deep venous thrombosis (DVT). IPG, impedance plethysmography; MRI, magnetic resonance imaging; US, ultrasound. (Adapted with permission from Yeung SJ, Escalante CP [eds]: *Oncologic Emergencies*. Hamilton, Ontario, Canada: BC Decker; 2002.)

be transitioned to warfarin treatment, there should be an overlap of at least 5 days with LMWH.

In a study, 672 cancer patients with VTE were randomized to dalteparin with oral anticoagulation (OA) versus dalteparin alone ([41]). The OA group was given warfarin and dalteparin 200 IU/kg subcutaneously every day for 5 to 7 days until the international normalized ratio (INR) reached 2 to 3. At that point, dalteparin was discontinued and the warfarin continued for 6 months. In the OA group, the goal INR was 2.5. The dalteparin group was given dalteparin 200 IU/kg subcutaneously every day for 1 month and then 150 IU/kg subcutaneously every day for the remaining 5 months. The patients in the dalteparin group had a lower rate of recurrent VTE at 6 months (8.8%) than those in the OA group (17.4%). There were no significant differences in major or minor bleeding between the two groups. The study investigators concluded that the occurrence of recurrent VTE can be decreased by the use of dalteparin rather than warfarin ([41]).

Although VTE can often be treated on an outpatient basis, patients not eligible for outpatient treatment are those with active bleeding, major comorbid illnesses, a history of heparin-induced thrombocytopenia, hypertensive emergencies, major surgery or trauma within the previous 2 weeks, recent GI bleeding, stroke or transient ischemic attack, severe renal dysfunction, or a platelet count below 100,000/μL ([42]). Table 53-2 shows the dosing schedule.

Most patients are treated for at least 3 to 6 months. Patients from whom the central venous catheter has been removed can undergo repeat testing using such techniques as Doppler ultrasound or nuclear venous flow study to determine whether the clot has resolved, so that cessation of anticoagulation therapy may be considered. For patients with small clots at the distal tip, manifested by the inability of the central line to work, tissue plasminogen activator (t-PA) can be given carefully provided that there are no contraindications.

Inferior vena cava filters can be used for patients who cannot tolerate anticoagulation therapy. Inferior vena cava filters do not decrease peripheral edema from deep venous thrombosis (DVT) and, in fact, can serve as a nidus for further clot formation. Inferior vena cava filters can prevent life-threatening pulmonary emboli. Patients

Table 53-2 Heparin Dosage Schedule for Venous Thromboembolism

Low-molecular-weight heparin	
Enoxaparin	1 mg/kg subcutaneously every 2 h or 1.5 mg/kg subcutaneously every 24 h
Dalteparin	200 IU/kg subcutaneously every 24 h or in a divided dose every 12 h; maximum dosage = 18,000 IU
Tinzaparin	175 anti-Xa antibody IU/kg subcutaneously every 24 h
Unfractionated heparin	
IV unfractionated heparin	80 IU/kg bolus, with a maintenance dose of 18 IU/kg/d; this should be adjusted to keep PTT at 1.5-2.5× the normal range

PTT, partial thromboplastin time.

with massive pulmonary emboli may require thrombolysis or embolectomy. See Table 53-3 for a synopsis of the relative and absolute contraindications for thrombolytic therapy and Table 53-4 for thrombolytic doses.

Patients with cancer and VTE should be treated indefinitely if the cancer remains active or for at least 3 to 6 months after resolution of the VTE if the cancer is no longer active ([43, 44]). For patients who are treated with warfarin but who experience warfarin failure as evidenced by the recurrence or progression of clot formation, the INR range can be increased from 2 to 3, to 3 to 3.5, the patient can be switched to twice-daily UFH, or the patient can be switched to LMWH ([45]). Thrombectomy should be used only for patients with massive PE who are hemodynamically unstable and who either have contraindications for thrombolytic therapy or have previously failed thrombolytic therapy ([37]).

Bleeding

Bleeding in cancer patients is most commonly due to thrombocytopenia induced by chemotherapy, marrow infiltration, disseminated intravascular coagulopathy (DIC), extensive radiation therapy, splenic sequestration, peripheral destruction, or infection. Thrombocytopenia usually manifests as mucocutaneous bleeding, such as gum oozing, epistaxis, and gynecologic or GI bleeding ([37]). At MDACC, all patients generally receive platelet transfusions if their platelet count falls to ≤10,000/μL. If the patient has active bleeding and the platelet count is between 20,000/μL and 50,000/μL, a platelet transfusion will also be given. A patient will also receive a platelet transfusion if an invasive procedure is planned and his or her platelet count is below 50,000/μL. The American Society of Clinical Oncology (ASCO) recommends prophylactic platelet transfusions for patients being treated for leukemia and those receiving bone marrow transplants if their platelet counts are below 10,000/μL. Transfusion thresholds may be higher for patients with fever, hyperleukocytosis, a rapid fall in platelet count, coagulation abnormalities, or active bleeding. In addition, ASCO recommends that patients with chronic stable thrombocytopenia who are not undergoing active treatment, such as those with aplastic anemia and patients with myelodysplastic syndrome (MDS), be monitored and given platelets only for active bleeding, even if their platelet count is below 10,000/μL. For patients with solid tumors, prophylactic platelet transfusions should be given if the platelet counts are below 10,000/μL unless the tumor is necrotic or is located in the bladder and undergoing treatment; in those cases, the threshold for transfusion should be 20,000/μL. According to ASCO's guidelines, platelet counts of 50,000/μL should be sufficient for invasive procedures, such as surgery. For lumbar puncture, the platelet count should be above 20,000/μL. Patients with AML commonly receive multiple transfusions and can develop alloimmunization against human leukocyte antigens (HLAs). Approximately 25% to 35% of patients with AML will become alloimmunized and refractory to nonhistocompatible platelet transfusions, predominantly through their exposure to leukocytes. Random-donor platelets are derived from pooled platelet concentrates from whole-blood donations, whereas single-donor

Table 53-3 Absolute and Relative Contraindications to Thrombolysis

Absolute Contraindications to Thrombolysis
Major intracranial surgery or trauma within prior 2 months
Cerebrovascular hemorrhage within prior 3-6 months
Active intracranial neoplasm
Major internal hemorrhage within prior 6 months
Severe bleeding diatheses, including those associated with severe liver or renal disease
Relative Contraindications to Thrombolysis
Prolonged cardiopulmonary resuscitation
Pregnancy or postpartum period within prior 10 days
Nonhemorrhagic stroke within prior 2 months
Major trauma or surgery (excluding that of the central nervous system) within prior 10 days
Thrombocytopenia (platelet count <100,000/μL)
Hemorrhagic retinopathy
Allergies to thrombolytic agents
Minor surgery to noncompressible vessels within prior 10 days
Tissue biopsy within prior 10 days
Peptic ulceration within prior 3 months
Infective endocarditis/pericarditis
Uncontrolled hypertension (systolic BP ≥200 mm Hg or diastolic BP ≥110 mm Hg)
Aortic aneurysm

BP, blood pressure.
Adapted with permission from Yeung SJ, Escalante CP [eds]: *Oncologic Emergencies*. Hamilton, Ontario, Canada: BC Decker; 2002.

Table 53-4 Dosages of Thrombolytics

Streptokinase	250,000 IU intravenous load over 30 min, then 100,000 IU/h for 24 h for pulmonary embolism or 72 h for deep vein thrombosis
Urokinase	4,400 IU/kg intravenous load over 10 min, then 4,400 IU/kg/h for 12 h
Alteplase	100 mg intravenous infusion over 2 h; initiate heparin at the end of alteplase infusion

platelets are obtained from one donor by platelet pheresis. The likelihood of alloimmunization can be decreased by using single-donor platelets, leukocyte-depleted platelets, leukocyte filters, and ultraviolet-irradiated platelets. The ASCO guidelines recommend that patients who are platelet refractory not receive platelet transfusions unless they are hemorrhaging or HLA-compatible platelets are available [45].

Disseminated intravascular coagulopathy can cause bleeding and thrombosis. Disseminated intravascular coagulopathy should be suspected in a patient who has an unexplained elevation in PT, PTT, or thrombocytopenia with associated bleeding or thrombosis. Although bleeding is most often noted in patients with DIC, it is the thrombosis of small (and occasionally large) blood vessels that leads to the most serious complications [46]. Collaborative laboratory findings are high D-dimer and fibrin split product levels, low levels of fibrinogen and thrombin-antithrombin III (TAT), or the presence of schistocytes [46]. It is important to remember that DIC is a clinical diagnosis based on the entire clinical scenario, and results for these laboratory tests might not be abnormal. Patients can also have mildly abnormal test results in cases of subclinical DIC, and these patients should be monitored closely for conversion to overt DIC.

Tumors can cause DIC, especially adenocarcinomas of the breast, prostate, stomach, lungs, and colon. In this instance, the disorder is believed to be stimulated by mucin produced from these cancers. Leukemia, especially acute promyelocytic leukemia (APL), is associated with DIC in up to 85% of patients because of a tissue factor in APL that has procoagulant activity. Other tumors associated with DIC are melanoma, lymphoma, and ovarian and pancreatic cancers. Other causes of DIC are sepsis, acidosis, extensive burns, the use of Denver catheters or LeVeen shunts in patients with malignant ascites, hemolytic blood transfusion reactions, polycythemia rubra vera, and amniotic fluid embolism [37, 46].

Patients who have both DIC and bleeding can present with oozing from multiple sites, such as arterial or venous punctures or the mucous membranes, or with epistaxis. Thrombotic complications can be visible on the skin in the form of hemorrhagic bullae, acral cyanosis, or even gangrene [46]. Microvascular thrombosis most commonly affects the lungs, brain, and kidneys. The patient may develop shortness of breath, pleuritic chest pain, and ARDS. The kidneys can become clogged with microemboli, in which case patients often present with oliguria, anuria, hematuria, or proteinuria. The small vessels of the brain also can receive microemboli, causing strokes, seizures, altered mental status, or coma. As the patient deteriorates, hypotension, acidosis, and hypoxia can develop [46].

The treatment of DIC should focus on reversing the underlying cause or trigger, such as treating an underlying infection. Acidosis, high catecholamine release, vasoconstriction, and corticosteroid use can exacerbate thrombosis associated with DIC [46]. Additional therapeutic measures for thrombosis can include heparin administration at 15 U/kg/h by continuous infusion. When the patient is bleeding, blood components (including platelets) can be transfused to correct coagulation abnormalities. Platelet transfusions are indicated to maintain platelet counts of at least 50,000/μL. Cryoprecipitate should only be used for severe hypofibrinogenemia <50 mg/dL, or <100 mg/dL if the patient is actively bleeding. Cryoprecipitate can be given at 0.2 bags per kilogram of body weight, and the fibrinogen level should be tested 20 to 60 minutes after the infusion and every 6 hours thereafter until the bleeding has stopped. Fresh frozen plasma (FFP) can be transfused at 10 to 15 mg/kg to correct abnormalities in PT. Other products that might be needed are prothrombin complex, antithrombin concentrates, or washed RBCs. For patients with persistent bleeding, fibrinolytic inhibitors such as ε-aminocaproic acid (EACA) can be given. ε-Aminocaproic acid should always be given with heparin to prevent thrombosis; because EACA can cause hypotension, ventricular arrhythmias, and hypokalemia, it should be used with caution. Tranexamic acid is a newer fibrinolytic inhibitor that has fewer side effects and has been used successfully in DIC associated with APL.

GENITOURINARY EMERGENCIES

Hemorrhagic Cystitis

Hemorrhagic cystitis is inflammation or bleeding of the bladder; it can be due to radiation therapy, viral infection, or chemotherapy. Radiation-induced bladder bleeding can present as early as 3 months or as late as 5 years after the termination of radiation therapy. Chemotherapeutic agents associated with hemorrhagic cystitis are cyclophosphamide and ifosfamide (because of the liver metabolites secreted during use of these compounds, namely acrolein and chloroacetaldehyde). The mechanism by which cyclophosphamide and ifosfamide metabolites are toxic to the urinary bladder is not known, but they have been implicated as the cause of hematuria in some patients [47]. Mesna is a thiol compound that binds acrolein, chloroacetaldehyde, and other metabolites of cyclophosphamide and ifosfamide; when it is administered before the patient receives the chemotherapeutic agents, the incidence of bladder toxicity can be decreased [47]. Forced diuresis and adequate hydration complement mesna administration [47].

In addition to radiation therapy and chemotherapy-inducing hemorrhagic cystitis, the BK virus (a polyomavirus) can become activated in immunocompromised patients undergoing bone marrow transplantation and cause hematuria ([47]).

Treatment of hemorrhagic cystitis involves gentle bladder irrigation to remove any clots and decompress the bladder. Any coagulopathy, such as thrombocytopenia, should be corrected, as should manifestations of DIC, such as low fibrinogen levels or an elevated PT or PTT. For patients with persistent bleeding, prostaglandins E_2 or F_2, 1% alum, or formalin can be instilled. Formalin instillation is painful and requires general or spinal anesthesia. To correct continued bleeding, some patients require surgery, hypogastric artery embolization, or open surgical intervention.

Urinary Tract Obstruction

Obstructive uropathy can be secondary to outflow obstruction or impingement on the ureters or kidneys; it can also be due to tumor invasion, radiotherapy-induced changes, or indirect effects of the tumor, such as ascites, lymphadenopathy, or fibrosis. A patient who is unable to urinate should have a small Foley catheter, such as a 14-F, placed. In patients with benign prostatic hypertrophy (BPH), a coudé catheter can often be inserted more easily ([47]). The catheter should not be forced, and if the bladder cannot be accessed, a suprapubic catheter can be used. A lack of residual urine in the absence of severe dehydration usually indicates either obstruction at a more proximal level in the urinary system or acute anuric renal failure. Patients who have residual urine may be unable to urinate because of a mechanical cause, such as BPH, urethral stricture, tumor impingement, or stone obstruction. Other possible causes of acute urinary retention are infection, spinal cord compression, viral radiculomyelitis, postsurgical effects interrupting bladder innervation, or medicines such as pain medications and antihistamines ([47]). In each case, the underlying disorder should be treated. Patients with BPH can undergo a trial of α-blockers, such as terazosin, prazosin, doxazosin, or finasteride, a type II 5-α-reductase inhibitor. Transurethral resection of the prostate can be considered for patients who do not respond to medical treatments.

Laboratory values are also useful in differentiating prerenal, postrenal, and renal failure. Patients with prerenal failure typically have a high ratio of BUN to creatinine of more than 20:1, although upper tract GI bleeding, corticosteroid use, and high protein intake can also increase the BUN-to-creatinine ratio. Acute urinary obstruction can present as flank pain, whereas chronic obstruction is often painless, with patients presenting with anuria or decreased urine output. The tumors most likely to cause ureteral obstruction are cervical, prostate, bladder, ovarian, breast, and GI cancers as well as lymphoma ([47]). Patients with infected urine and obstruction may also present with symptoms of urosepsis, including fever, confusion, and a high WBC count.

Computed tomography scanning of the abdomen is good for evaluating the cause of ureteral obstruction in that it can elucidate the nature of the obstruction. Other tests that can be used are MRI, renal ultrasound, IV urography, retrograde pyelography, and radionuclide renography ([47]). Helical CT scanning of the abdomen has the added benefit of avoiding the use of IV contrast. Urinary obstruction can be managed with ureteral stents or percutaneous nephrostomy tubes with or without internal stents; the stents or tubes are typically placed under guidance by interventional radiology. Many patients with stents develop infection, which often requires hospitalization, IV antibiotics, and stent replacement. Other possible complications are stent clogging and stent migration. The "double J" stent, which is now most frequently used, is anchored in the bladder and the renal pelvis, so that stent migration is less common than it once was. Open surgical procedures are much less frequently performed now than in the past and are generally reserved for patients in whom endourologic procedures have failed ([47]).

RESPIRATORY EMERGENCIES

Airway Obstruction

Airway obstruction can be caused by intraluminal tumor growth or compression of the airway by an extraluminal tumor. The oral cavity should be quickly visualized to exclude foreign body aspiration. In most cases of upper airway obstruction, the clinical examination provides the diagnosis. Computed tomography of the neck and/or chest is helpful in diagnosing obstruction by tumors. For lower airway obstruction, chest radiographs identify the obstruction in 75% of cases. Rigid or flexible bronchoscopy can be used to both diagnose and treat airway obstruction.

Patients with severe respiratory distress and airway obstruction should undergo endotracheal intubation distal to the obstruction before the obstruction is treated. Laryngoscope or bronchoscope may be used to guide intubation ([48]). Once the airway has been stabilized, the obstruction can be treated. Patients with obstructions in the upper third of the trachea may need a low tracheotomy.

The methods that can be used to provide expedient relief of central airway obstruction include laser treatment, argon plasma coagulation (APC), electrocautery, endobronchial balloon dilation, and stent placement. Argon plasma coagulation can be achieved through flexible or rigid bronchoscopy at a relatively low cost and degrades the obstructive tissue by increasing its temperature. Electrocautery is also relatively inexpensive and can provide immediate relief of the obstruction, but side effects can include fire, hemorrhage, and electric shock. Rigid bronchoscopy can be used to treat extraluminal tumors by metal or silicone stent placement; this technique is most useful for tracheal or main bronchial disease. Metal stents can promote the growth of granulomatous tissue, whereas silicone stents are more likely to develop mucous plugging and to migrate. Laser therapy can also be used for endobronchial lesions, with the possible side effects of hemorrhage, pneumothorax, and pneumomediastinum. Laser therapy is more expensive than the other techniques and requires a skilled technician. Other methods that can be used for airway obstruction are cryotherapy, external beam radiotherapy, brachytherapy, and photodynamic therapy, CT-guided radiofrequency ablation, and surgical debulking or resection.

Hemoptysis

Massive hemoptysis (about 5% of hemoptysis episodes) ([49]) is defined as the expectoration of >100 mL of blood in a single episode or bleeding into the airway at a rate of >600 mL/d. Some 7% to 10% of patients with lung cancer will develop massive hemoptysis, which carries a poorer prognosis than massive hemoptysis associated with other cancers. In addition to structural abnormalities in the lungs, bleeding can be due to chemotherapy or other medications, sepsis, fungal infections, and thrombocytopenia. Death from this type of hemorrhage usually results from asphyxiation rather than anemia or blood loss.

The cardiopulmonary status should be initially supported by IV fluid and supplemental oxygen. The most important aspect of managing massive hemoptysis is protecting the airway. The American College of Chest Physicians guidelines recommend endotracheal intubation with a single-lumen tube and emergent bronchoscopy ([50]). If the right lung is affected, the left lung can be selectively intubated through bronchoscopy. Use of a rigid bronchoscope allows removal of the tumor or clots, whereas flexible bronchoscopy allows access to the more distal airways. If the left lung is affected, the right lung should not be selectively intubated because inadvertent collapse of the right upper lobe can ensue. A single-lumen endotracheal tube is easier to place than a double-lumen tube and allows a larger area for evacuation of blood and clots. The patient should lie on the side of the bleeding lung to promote aeration of the unaffected lung. Any coagulopathy should be corrected, and cough suppressed with codeine or other agents. If a tumor is causing the bleeding and it can be localized, the patient can undergo bronchial artery embolization or tumor resection. If the tumor is unresectable, external beam radiation therapy can be used. If only the location of the bleeding can be determined, endobronchial interventions may also include administration of topical agents (thrombin), iced saline lavage, injection of epinephrine 1:20,000, laser treatment, electrocautery, APC, photocoagulation, or balloon tamponade.

Bronchial artery embolization is becoming increasingly important for massive or recurrent hemoptysis. An algorithm for management of massive hemoptysis has been proposed ([51]), in which CT angiography provides information about the tumor, bleeding site, and vascular anatomy for planning the embolization. The bleeding vessel may be embolized with Gianturco steel coils, isobutyl-2-cyanoacrylate, polyvinyl alcohol foam, or absorbable gelatin pledgets. Failure of embolization to stop bleeding may require emergency radiotherapy or lung resection ([52]).

CHEMOTHERAPY-INDUCED EXTRAVASATIONS

Extravasation injuries due to chemotherapy can produce a variety of symptoms ranging from skin irritation to skin ulceration, tissue necrosis, nerve damage, and (rarely) loss of limbs. Vesicant chemotherapy agents, including the alkylating agents (mechlorethamine, cisplatin, mitomycin C), DNA intercalating agents (doxorubicin, daunorubicin), and plant alkaloids (vinblastine, vincristine, vinorelbine), can cause the most severe reactions. Irritant chemotherapy extravasations are generally not severe, causing only pain, erythema, and inflammation at the extravasated site ([53]).

The goal is to prevent chemotherapy extravasations. The patient should be told to inform the staff of any discomfort, swelling, or erythema over the infusion site. Nursing staff should evaluate the IV infusion site carefully by administering IV fluids before chemotherapy agents are infused, and they should monitor the patient frequently for any evidence of extravasation. Intravenous lines should be placed carefully; areas that have a poor blood supply or overlie a joint should be avoided. If an extravasation does occur, the infusion should be stopped immediately with the catheter left in place, and the staff should attempt to withdraw any remaining chemotherapy agents. Cold compresses should then be placed on the involved site except when the agents are plant alkaloids, in which case warm compresses should be applied ([54, 55]).

Topical dimethylsulfoxide in a 50% solution can relieve extravasations when applied at a volume of 1.5 mL to the site every 6 hours for 7 to 14 days. Dimethylsulfoxide is commonly used to treat extravasations caused by mitomycin C and the anthracyclines ([53-57]).

For extravasations caused by plant alkaloids (vinblastine, vincristine, vinorelbine) and epidophyllotoxins (etoposide, teniposide), a solution of 150 units of hyaluronidase in 1 to 3 mL of saline can be injected into the needle and subcutaneously around the extravasated site [54, 55].

A 0.17-mol/L solution of sodium thiosulfate can be injected into mechlorethamine-induced extravasation sites. Sodium thiosulfate is thought to work by creating an alkaline-rich site to which the vesicant binds instead of the skin. The by-product is then excreted in the urine [55]. There is some evidence that sodium thiosulfate can also be used for extravasations caused by carmustine, cisplatin, carboplatin, cyclophosphamide, dacarbazine, and oxaliplatin [53]. Table 53-5 lists selected chemotherapeutic agents and their antidotes.

If local measures fail to contain symptoms in all patients with anthracycline-induced extravasations, a plastic surgeon should be consulted. Surgery can consist of debridement, excision of dead tissues, and, in severe cases, skin graft placement. In patients with doxorubicin-induced extravasation, the drug remains in the tissue for a long period, perhaps being released by dying or dead cells and spreading over time.

Patients who have had previous extravasation reactions can also experience a "recall reaction" when the same chemotherapy is received later, causing ulcerations or burns to reappear at the previously affected area.

METABOLIC EMERGENCIES

Tumor Lysis Syndrome

Tumor lysis syndrome (TLS) is a result of excessive tumor breakdown, causing hypocalcemia, hyperphosphatemia, hyperkalemia, elevated uric acid, and

Table 53-5 Chemotherapeutic Extravasations and Their Antidotes

Chemotherapy Agent	Irritant/ Vesicant	Sodium Thiosulfate	DMSO	Hyaluronidase	Cool	Warm
Carboplatin	I	+			+	
Carmustine	I/V	+		+		Dry warm
Cisplatin	I/V	+			+	
Cyclophosphamide	I	+			+	
Dacarbazine	I/V	+				
Dactinomycin	I/V				+	
Daunorubicin	I/V		+		+	
Docetaxel	I				+	Warm soaks
Doxorubicin	I/V		+		+	
Epirubicin	I/V		+		+	
Etoposide	I/V			+		+
Idarubicin	I/V		+		+	
Ifosfamide	I				+	
Mechlorethamine	I/V	+				
Mitomycin C	V		+		+	
Oxaliplatin	I/V	+				
Paclitaxel	I/V			+		
Plicamycin	I/V					
Streptozocin	I/V					
Teniposide	I/V			+		+
Topotecan					+	
Vinblastine	I/V			+		+
Vincristine	I/V			+		+
Vindesine	I/V			+		+
Vinorelbine	I/V			+		+

DMSO, dimethylsulfoxide.

occasionally acute renal failure. Risk factors for TLS include high tumor burden, chronic renal insufficiency, and certain tumor types (Burkitt lymphoma, lymphoblastic lymphoma, diffuse large cell lymphoma, undifferentiated lymphoma, and leukemia) ([2]). Tumor lysis syndrome usually presents during chemotherapy, but it can also occur after radiation therapy, corticosteroid treatment for sensitive tumors, or administration of hormonal agents.

Patients with TLS can present with nausea and vomiting, diarrhea, constipation, low urine output, weight gain, acute renal failure, weakness, cramps, seizures, tetany, or arrhythmias.

A scoring system for predicting TLS has been derived from acute myelocytic leukemia patients ([58, 59]). The score may guide prophylaxis for TLS. Preventive measures for patients at risk are hydration with IV crystalloid fluid up to 3 L/m^2/d to maintain a urine output >100 mL/h and allopurinol (100-300 mg/d orally).

Alkalinizing the urine to increase uric acid solubility in the urine is no longer recommended for prophylaxis. To prevent TLS, patients with leukemia and high WBC counts may be treated with leukapheresis or hydroxyurea before chemotherapeutic agents are administered.

Once TLS is diagnosed based on the Cairo-Bishop definition ([60, 61]) patients with severe TLS should be monitored in intensive care. Rasburicase is a highly soluble IV recombinant form of urate oxidase that converts uric acid to allantoin and is highly efficacious in prevention or treatment of hyperuricemia. Rasburicase (150-200 μg/kg IV daily or one-time dosing with a rescue dose as needed) may be used to prevent or treat urate nephropathy ([62]). Increased IV fluid hydration may be coupled with diuretics. Urinary alkalinization by IV infusion of sodium bicarbonate or acetate should only be considered in cases of severe hyperuricemia when rasburicase cannot be obtained.

Hyperkalemia should be monitored closely and treated with insulin plus dextrose, calcium, and bicarbonate intravenously along with oral potassium ion exchange resins (sodium polystyrene sulfonate). In hyperphosphatemic patients with hypocalcemia, oral calcium compounds will reduce phosphate absorption and enhance calcium absorption. Some patients with refractory electrolyte abnormalities might require dialysis if conservative measures fail. An indication for dialysis is symptomatic hypocalcemia in the presence of hyperphosphatemia (serum phosphorus >3.3 mmol/L [>10.2 mg/dL]). Other indications for dialysis include persistent or refractory azotemia, volume overload, hyperuricemia, acidemia, and refractory hyperkalemia. Dialysis should be continued until biochemical abnormalities resolve.

Hypercalcemia

Hypercalcemia is present in 10% to 20% of patients with advanced cancer ([2]). The most common cancers include squamous cell cancer of the lungs, breast cancer, multiple myeloma, and lymphoma ([2]). The two major mechanisms of hypercalcemia include the secretion of a parathyroid-related peptide (PTHrP) and abnormal 1,25-vitamin D production (which occurs in Hodgkin disease and non-Hodgkin lymphoma).

Symptoms of hypercalcemia are altered mental status, polyuria, polydipsia, nausea, vomiting, anorexia, constipation, and seizures ([2]). Measured serum calcium levels should be adjusted according to the albumin level for accurate estimation. A low albumin level should be subtracted from 4, and the difference should be multiplied by 0.8. This product should be added to the serum calcium level to arrive at the estimated calcium. Alternatively, ionized calcium can be measured, which assesses the active calcium in the serum and is more accurate.

The choice of treatment for hypercalcemia depends on the patient's calcium level and symptoms. Calcium is a potent diuretic, and patients with mild hypercalcemia can be treated by IV fluids. Patients with a calcium level greater than 14 mg/dL should be treated with additional measures. Patients who have symptoms of hypercalcemia and a calcium level between 12 and 14 mg/dL should also receive additional treatment to lower the calcium level.

Bisphosphonates are the drugs of choice in treating hypercalcemia. Pamidronate can be given intravenously over 2 to 24 hours. A 60-mg dose corrects hypercalcemia 60% of the time, and a 90-mg dose does so 100% of the time ([2]). Bisphosphonates do not work immediately but have an onset of action after 12 to 48 hours ([2]). Zoledronic acid, a relatively new agent, can be infused more rapidly than pamidronate; the recommended dose is 4 mg intravenously over 15 minutes. Bisphosphonates are useful in not only reducing serum calcium levels but also helping to decrease bone pain and treat skeletal complications in cancer patients with bone metastases ([63]).

Calcitonin can also be used to treat hypercalcemia; it has an onset of action of 2 to 4 hours, but its effects are transient because tachyphylaxis develops after 3 days. Patients may develop nausea, abdominal cramps, or hypersensitivity reactions to calcitonin ([2]).

Corticosteroids can be helpful in some patients with hypercalcemia—for instance, those with lymphoma and myeloma. Dialysis is reserved for patients who are unable to tolerate hydration. Furosemide can be used, but only after the patient has been hydrated adequately. Gallium nitrate and plicamycin are rarely used because of the high risk of toxic effects.

GASTROINTESTINAL EMERGENCIES

Gastrointestinal Bleeding

Patients with cancer can present with GI bleeding due to direct tumor invasion, effects of chemotherapy agents or corticosteroids, thrombocytopenia, coagulopathy, side effects of radiation therapy, or Mallory-Weiss tears from intractable nausea and vomiting. Other possible causes of GI bleeding are gastritis, peptic ulcer disease, duodenal ulcers, arteriovenous malformations, and diverticulosis. Patients who have undergone bone marrow transplantation can present with GI bleeding as a manifestation of graft-versus-host disease, which typically presents as ulcerations in the small intestine. For patients bleeding from the upper GI tract, a nasogastric tube should be inserted and the tract lavaged with normal saline until the bleeding clears. If the bleeding does not clear, emergent upper GI endoscopy may be considered. Patients with small tumors rarely have significant bleeding, and patients with large tumors tend to ooze and bleed. However, relief of bleeding by endoscopic measures is usually temporary, and these tumors tend to bleed repeatedly. Endoscopic interventions can include electrocoagulation, epinephrine injections, and argon plasma laser treatment. For patients with persistent bleeding, arteriography and embolization are occasionally successful. If all other interventions have failed, surgery can be considered. Patients with bleeding should have any coagulopathy corrected, including deficits in the platelet count, which should be greater than 60,000/μL. Somatostatin or vasopressin can be used to control bleeding of esophageal varices. The patient should receive either an H_2 blocker or a proton pump inhibitor intravenously. Nausea should be controlled using IV antiemetics, and the patient should receive nothing by mouth. The patient should also receive maintenance IV fluid. If hypotensive, the patient should be volume resuscitated with IV crystalloid fluid and/or transfusion.

Typhlitis

Typhlitis is a syndrome of bowel inflammation, edema, and wall thickening involving the proximal large bowel in patients with neutropenic fever. It commonly affects the cecum but can also affect the ascending colon and occasionally the transverse colon. Typhlitis can occur in conjunction with any cancer but is most common in patients with leukemia ([26]). The organisms most often isolated in cases of typhlitis are *Clostridium* and gram-negative bacilli ([64]).

Patients with typhlitis present with fever, pain in the right lower quadrant of the abdomen, and sometimes diarrhea, which may be bloody. The patient with typhlitis is neutropenic, and plain abdominal x-ray films are often inconclusive. The diagnosis of typhlitis is made based on clinical suspicion and CT or MRI findings that reveal bowel inflammation, edema, wall thickening, and possibly air formation or, in severe cases, free air (Fig. 53-15).

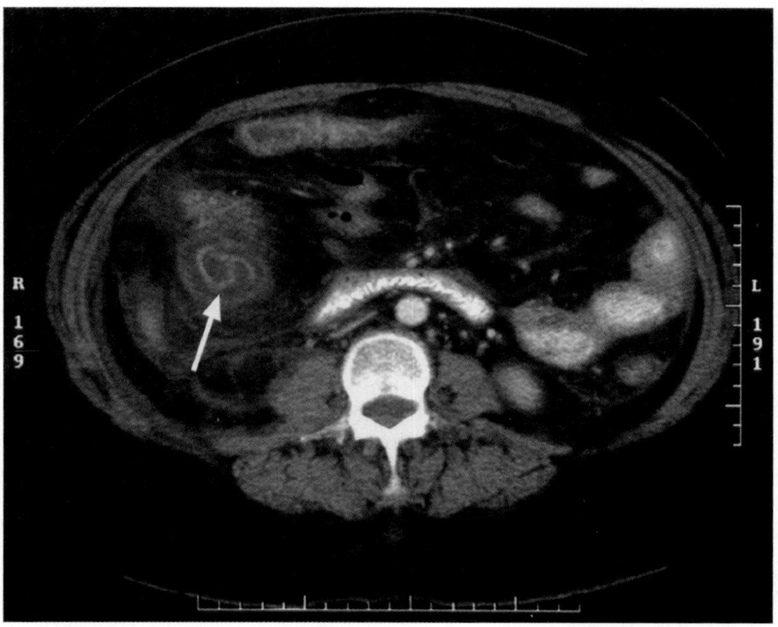

FIGURE 53-15 Inflammation of the cecum and ascending colon in a 45-year-old patient with typhlitis. The *arrow* points to inflammation and edema of the cecum. (Used with permission from Dr. Stephanie Mundy, MD Anderson Cancer Center.)

CHAPTER 53

Typhlitis is managed by bowel rest and IV administration of broad-spectrum antibiotics, including anaerobic coverage. Patients rarely require surgery unless they develop intractable bleeding or bowel perforation or do not respond to conservative measures.

REFERENCES

1. Loblaw DA, Laperriere NJ, Mackillop WJ. A population-based study of malignant spinal cord compression in Ontario. *Clin Oncol (R Coll Radiol)* 2003;15(4):211-217.
2. Krimsky WS, Behrens RJ, Kerkvliet GJ. Oncologic emergencies for the internist. *Cleve Clin J Med*. 2002;69(3):209-210, 213-214, 216-217.
3. Quinn JA, DeAngelis LM. Neurologic emergencies in the cancer patient. *Semin Oncol*. 2000;27(3):311-321.
4. Saarto T, Janes R, Tenhunen M, et al. Palliative radiotherapy in the treatment of skeletal metastases. *Eur J Pain*. 2002;6(5):323-330.
5. Schiff D, Batchelor T, Wen PY. Neurologic emergencies in cancer patients. *Neurol Clin*. 1998;16(2):449-483.
6. National Institute for Health and Care Excellence. Metastatic spinal cord compression: diagnosis and management of patients at risk of or with metastatic spinal cord compression. www.nice.org.uk/guidance/CG75/. Accessed November 2, 2015.
7. O'Phelan KH, Bunney EB, Weingart SD, Smith WS. Emergency neurological life support: spinal cord compression (SCC). *Neurocrit Care*. 2012;17(Suppl 1):S96-S101.
8. Vaillant B, Loghin M. Treatment of spinal cord tumors. *Curr Treat Options Neurol*. 2009;11(4):315-324
9. Lee CH, Kwon JW, Lee J, et al. Direct decompressive surgery followed by radiotherapy versus radiotherapy alone for metastatic epidural spinal cord compression: a meta-analysis. *Spine*. 2014;39:E587-E592.
10. George R, Jeba J, Ramkumar G, et al. Interventions for the treatment of metastatic extradural spinal cord compression in adults. *Cochrane Database Syst Rev*. 2008;(4):CD006716.
11. Rades D, Dunst J, Schild SE. The first score predicting overall survival in patients with metastatic spinal cord compression. *Cancer*. 2008;112(1):157-161.
12. Kaal EC, Taphoorn MJ, Vecht CJ. Symptomatic management and imaging of brain metastases. *J Neurooncol*. 2005;75(1):15-20.
13. Chamberlain MC. Leptomeningeal metastasis. *Curr Opin Neurol*. 2009;22(6):665-674.
14. Soffietti R, Ruda R, Mutani R. Management of brain metastases. *J Neurol*. 2002;249(10):1357-1369.
15. Stevens RD, Huff JS, Duckworth J, Papangelou A, Weingart SD, Smith WS. Emergency neurological life support: intracranial hypertension and herniation. *Neurocrit Care*. 2012;17(Suppl 1): S60-S65.
16. Arnold SM, Patchell RA. Diagnosis and management of brain metastases. *Hematol Oncol Clin North Am*. 2001;15(6):1085-1107.
17. Sawaya R. Considerations in the diagnosis and management of brain metastases. *Oncology (Williston Park)*. 2001;15(9):1144-1154, 1157-1158; discussion 1158, 1163-1165.
18. Wen PY, Loeffler JS. Brain metastases. *Curr Treat Options Oncol*. 2000;1(5):447-458.
19. Patchell RA, Tibbs PA, Regine WF, et al. Postoperative radiotherapy in the treatment of single metastases to the brain: a randomized trial. *JAMA*. 1998;280(17):1485-1489.
20. Ewend MG, Carey LA, Morris DE, et al. Brain metastases. *Curr Treat Options Oncol*. 2001;2(6):537-547.
21. Davey P. Brain metastases: treatment options to improve outcomes. *CNS Drugs*. 2002;16(5):325-338.
22. Grossman SA, Krabak MJ. Leptomeningeal carcinomatosis. *Cancer Treat Rev*. 1999;25(2):103-119.
23. Brophy GM, Bell R, Claassen J, et al. Guidelines for the evaluation and management of status epilepticus. *Neurocrit Care*. 2012;17:3-23.
24. Claassen J, Silbergleit R, Weingart SD, Smith WS. Emergency neurological life support: status epilepticus. *Neurocrit Care*. 2012;17(Suppl 1):S73-S78.
25. Demopoulos A, DeAngelis LM. Neurologic complications of leukemia. *Curr Opin Neurol*. 2002;15(6):691-699.
26. Shanholtz C. Acute life-threatening toxicity of cancer treatment. *Crit Care Clin*. 2001;17(3):483-502.
27. Ristic AD, Imazio M, Adler Y, et al. Triage strategy for urgent management of cardiac tamponade: a position statement of the European Society of Cardiology Working Group on Myocardial and Pericardial Diseases. *Eur Heart J*. 2014;35:2279-2284.
28. Johnson KK, Soundarraj D, Patel P. Tenecteplase for malignant pericardial effusion. *Pharmacotherapy*. 2007;27:303-305.
28a. Yu JB, Wilson LD, Detterbeck FC. Superior vena cava syndrome–a proposed classification sytem and algorithm for management. J Thoracic Oncol. 3:811-814. 2008.
29. Smayra T, Otal P, Chabbert V, et al. Long-term results of endovascular stent placement in the superior caval venous system. *Cardiovasc Intervent Radiol*. 2001;24:388-394.
30. Fagedet D, Thony F, Timsit JF, et al. Endovascular treatment of malignant superior vena cava syndrome: results and predictive factors of clinical efficacy. *Cardiovasc Intervent Radiol*. 2013;36:140-149.
31. Rachapalli V, Boucher LM. Superior vena cava syndrome: role of the interventionalist. *Can Assoc Radiol J*. 2014;65:168-176.
32. Lanuti M, De Delva PE, Gaissert HA, et al. Review of superior vena cava resection in the management of benign disease and pulmonary or mediastinal malignancies. *Ann Thorac Surg*. 2009;88:392-397.
33. Douketis JD, Crowther MA, Stanton EB, et al. Elevated cardiac troponin levels in patients with submassive pulmonary embolism. *Arch Intern Med*. 2002;162(1):79-81.
34. Blumenthal DT, Glenn MJ. Neurologic manifestations of hematologic disorders. *Neurol Clin*. 2002;20(1):265-281, viii.
35. Majhail NS, Lichtin AE. Acute leukemia with a very high leukocyte count: confronting a medical emergency. *Cleve Clin J Med*. 2004;71(8):633-637.
36. Kaminsky DA, Hurwitz CG, Olmstead JI. Pulmonary leukostasis mimicking pulmonary embolism. *Leuk Res*. 2000;24(2):175-178.
37. DeSancho MT, Rand JH. Bleeding and thrombotic complications in critically ill patients with cancer. *Crit Care Clin*. 2001;17(3):599-622.
38. Tissue plasminogen activator for the treatment of acute pulmonary embolism. A collaborative study by the PIOPED Investigators. *Chest*. 1990;97(3):528-533.
39. King V, Vaze AA, Moskowitz CS, et al. D-dimer assay to exclude pulmonary embolism in high-risk oncologic population: correlation with CT pulmonary angiography in an urgent care setting. *Radiology*. 2008;247(3):854-861.
40. Nazario R, Delorenzo LJ, Maguire AG. Treatment of venous thromboembolism. *Cardiol Rev*. 2002;10(4):249-259.
41. Levine MN. Can we optimise treatment of thrombosis? *Cancer Treat Rev*. 2003;29(Suppl 2):19-22.
42. Garcia DA, Spyropoulos AC. Update in the treatment of venous thromboembolism. *Semin Respir Crit Care Med*. 2008;29(1):40-46.
43. Levine MN. Managing thromboembolic disease in the cancer patient: efficacy and safety of antithrombotic treatment options in patients with cancer. *Cancer Treat Rev*. 2002;28(3):145-149.
44. Lee AY. Treatment of venous thromboembolism in cancer patients. *Thromb Res*. 2001;102(6):V195-V208.
45. Schiffer CA, Anderson KC, Bennett CL, et al. Platelet transfusion for patients with cancer: clinical practice guidelines

of the American Society of Clinical Oncology. *J Clin Oncol.* 2001;19(5):1519-1538.
46. Bick RL. Disseminated intravascular coagulation: a review of etiology, pathophysiology, diagnosis, and management: Guidelines for care. *Clin Appl Thromb Hemost.* 2002;8(1):1-31.
47. Russo P. Urologic emergencies in the cancer patient. *Semin Oncol.* 2000;27(3):284-298.
48. Patel A, Pearce A. Progress in management of the obstructed airway. *Anaesthesia.* 2011;66(Suppl 2):93-100.
49. Ibrahim WH. Massive haemoptysis: the definition should be revised. *Eur Respir J.* 2008;32:1131-1132.
50. Simoff MJ, Lally B, Slade MG, et al. Symptom management in patients with lung cancer: Diagnosis and management of lung cancer, 3rd ed: American College of Chest Physicians evidence-based clinical practice guidelines. *Chest.* 2013;143:e455S-497S.
51. Noe GD, Jaffe SM, Molan MP. CT and CT angiography in massive haemoptysis with emphasis on pre-embolization assessment. *Clin Radiol.* 2011;66:869-875.
52. Jougon J, Ballester M, Delcambre F, et al. Massive hemoptysis: what place for medical and surgical treatment. *Eur J Cardiothorac Surg.* 2002;22:345.
53. Alley E, Green R, Schuchter L. Cutaneous toxicities of cancer therapy. *Curr Opin Oncol.* 2002;14(2):212-216.
54. Dorr RT. Antidotes to vesicant chemotherapy extravasations. *Blood Rev.* 1990;4(1):41-60.
55. Kassner E. Evaluation and treatment of chemotherapy extravasation injuries. *J Pediatr Oncol Nurs.* 2000;17(3):135-148.
56. Fenchel K, Karthaus M. Cytotoxic drug extravasation. *Antibiot Chemother.* 2000;50:144-148.
57. Valks R, Garcia-Diez A, Fernandez-Herrera J. Mucocutaneous reactions to chemotherapy. *J Am Acad Dermatol.* 2000;42(4):699.
58. Montesinos P, Lorenzo I, Martin G, et al. Tumor lysis syndrome in patients with acute myeloid leukemia: identification of risk factors and development of a predictive model. *Haematologica.* 2008;93:67-74.
59. Mato AR, Riccio BE, Qin L, et al. A predictive model for the detection of tumor lysis syndrome during AML induction therapy. *Leuk Lymphoma.* 2006;47:877-883.
60. Cairo MS, Bishop M. Tumour lysis syndrome: new therapeutic strategies and classification. *Br J Haematol.* 2004;127:3-11.
61. Wilson FP, Berns JS. Tumor lysis syndrome: new challenges and recent advances. *Adv Chronic Kidney Dis.* 2014;21:18-26.
62. Mahmoud HH, Leverger G, Patte C, Harvey E, Lascombes F. Advances in the management of malignancy-associated hyperuricaemia. *Br J Cancer.* 1998;77:18-20.
63. Janjan N. Bone metastases: approaches to management. *Semin Oncol.* 2001;28(4 Suppl 11):28-34.
64. Davila ML. Neutropenic enterocolitis. *Curr Treat Options Gastroenterol.* 2006;9(3):249-255.

Onco-Cardiology

第五十四章　肿瘤心脏学

Elie Mouhayar
Danielle El-Haddad
Peter Kim
Kara Thompson

中文导读

本章首先回顾了肿瘤心脏学的发展史，由于肿瘤发病率的升高及肿瘤患者的生存期不断延长，这个交叉学科也日益受到重视。在介绍肿瘤心脏学的病理生理机制以后，着重阐述了几个在肿瘤患者中观察到的心血管综合征，其中包括：心肌功能失常、肿瘤相关缺血性动脉疾病、心率失常、心包疾病、高血压和肿瘤管理以及放疗相关的心血管毒性。在心肌功能失常部分，包括了急性心肌病、化疗相关心肌病和基础心脏病的定义、发病机制和诊疗内容。在肿瘤相关缺血性动脉疾病部分，描述了病因和机制以及治疗推荐。在心率失常部分，根据缓慢心律失常和快速心律失常的不同，讲述了不同的处理原则。在心包疾病部分，按照进行心包炎和心包积液两个话题分别进行病因、诊断和治疗的解析。在高血压和肿瘤管理部分，简述了抗肿瘤药导致高血压的原因以及如何选择不同类型的降血压药治疗。最后在放疗相关的心血管毒性部分，对有纵隔放疗史的患者如何进行长期随访也做了简明的指引。

INTRODUCTION

Onco-cardiology is a fast-growing medical subspecialty focused on the management of heart diseases in patients with cancer. Although cancer remains a leading cause of morbidity and mortality worldwide, the survival rate of patients with cancer has increased in the last 25 years. In the United States, the 5-year relative survival rate of patients diagnosed with cancer between 1975 and 1977 was 50%; it increased to 68% between 1999 and 2005. The US National Cancer Institute estimates that at least 13.7 million cancer survivors were alive in the United States in 2012 ([1]). With the survival improvement, the long-term adverse treatment effects have also become more apparent. A survey of 1,807 cancer survivors with a 7-year follow-up found that 33% died of heart diseases and 51% died of cancer ([2]). Historically, since the late 1970s, the interest in chemotherapy-induced cardiotoxicity was focused on cardiomyopathy related to few chemotherapeutic agents. As the field of cancer therapies has expanded, so has the finding of other cardiovascular side effects such as transient left ventricular dysfunction, hypertension (HTN), cardiac arrhythmias, pericardial effusions, and arterial ischemia. Patients with known or subclinical cardiac disease are more susceptible to the cardiotoxic side effects of cancer therapy, and those with known cardiac disease often need to alter their cardiac management to allow for the treatment of cancer. This can be associated with significant cardiovascular risks. Onco-cardiology has evolved to address the cardiovascular needs of patients whose optimal outcome mandates close and collaborative efforts between cardiologists and oncologists in a multidisciplinary approach. Involvement of cardiologists in cancer patients' care has changed from focusing on management of the cardiovascular complications of therapy to an overall assistance in the care of these patients from the initial cancer diagnosis to survivorship as outlined in Fig. 54-1.

PATHOPHYSIOLOGY

Clinical knowledge and basic science discoveries in onco-cardiology have grown over the last decade. There is better understanding of molecular mechanisms of cardiac toxicity of several cancer drugs. An example is the observation that the Bruton tyrosine kinase receptor is expressed in the atria of human heart tissue ([3]). This tyrosine kinase receptor is the target of a novel drug, ibrutinib, used in certain hematologic malignancies including chronic lymphocytic leukemia. Ibrutinib has been associated with a significant incidence of atrial arrhythmias, potentially mediated by its on-target effect and more specifically by inhibiting the PI3K-Akt signaling pathway ([3]). Similarly, trastuzumab targets ErbB2 in breast cancer cells and has been shown to improve outcome and prolong survival in HER2+/ErbB2 breast cancer. The same receptors within the cardiac myocyte are responsible for normal

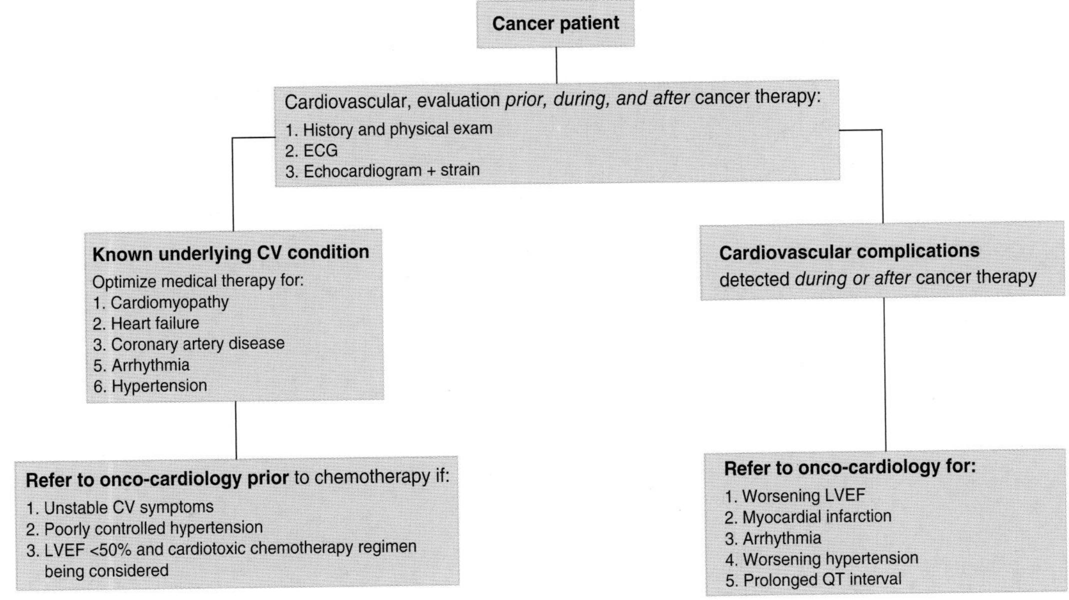

FIGURE 54-1 Algorithm for the general role of onco-cardiology. CV, cardiovascular; ECG, electrocardiogram; LVEF, left ventricular ejection fraction.

cell function and myocyte repair. When affected by ErbB2 inhibitors like trastuzumab, secondary mitochondrial dysfunction can be observed ([4]). Other mechanisms of toxicities have recently been reported with older conventional chemotherapeutic drugs like the anthracyclines; cardiovascular toxicity of this drug has been recently linked to inhibition of topoisomerase IIβ ([5]). This enzyme is responsible for normal myocyte function, and its inhibition partially explains the cardiovascular toxicity of doxorubicin. In addition to the benefit of improving strategies to prevent drug toxicities, a better understanding of these biologic pathways may also provide better understanding of certain heart diseases and their management. For example, the discovery of the key role of ErbB2 in normal cardiac function and its relation to trastuzumab toxicity was followed by the discovery of the benefit of an ErbB2 agonist called neuregulin-1 in the animal models of heart failure ([6]). Neuregulin-1 is currently being studied for the treatment of heart failure in humans.

CARDIOVASCULAR SYNDROMES OBSERVED IN CANCER PATIENTS

Aside from the direct cardiac toxic effect of certain cancer drugs (Fig. 54-2), many aspects of the cardiovascular system can be affected by cancer or cancer therapy (Fig. 54-3), resulting in a variety of cardiovascular syndromes.

Myocardial Dysfunction

Onco-cardiologists are often asked to assess patients with cancer and clinical heart failure (HF) symptoms. Although the most feared etiology is the progressive, permanent, and irreversible myocardial damage related to anthracycline toxicity, this in fact constitutes only a small percentage of patients with clinical HF. The majority of patients with new-onset HF in the setting of cancer and cancer therapy have their symptoms triggered by mechanisms other than anthracycline toxicity. Despite some overlap, a clinically useful approach is to divide patients into two groups based on the initial clinical presentation (Table 54-1). The first group includes patients presenting with sudden and new-onset acute HF with associated systolic dysfunction. These patients include those with cardiomyopathy related to sepsis, stress cardiomyopathy, and myocarditis (toxic or infectious). The second group includes patients presenting with subacute or chronic HF symptoms and includes those with underlying structural heart disease, those with chemotherapy-induced cardiomyopathy, and those with infiltrative myocardial conditions related to their underlying malignancies or to cancer therapy (amyloidosis, iron overload).

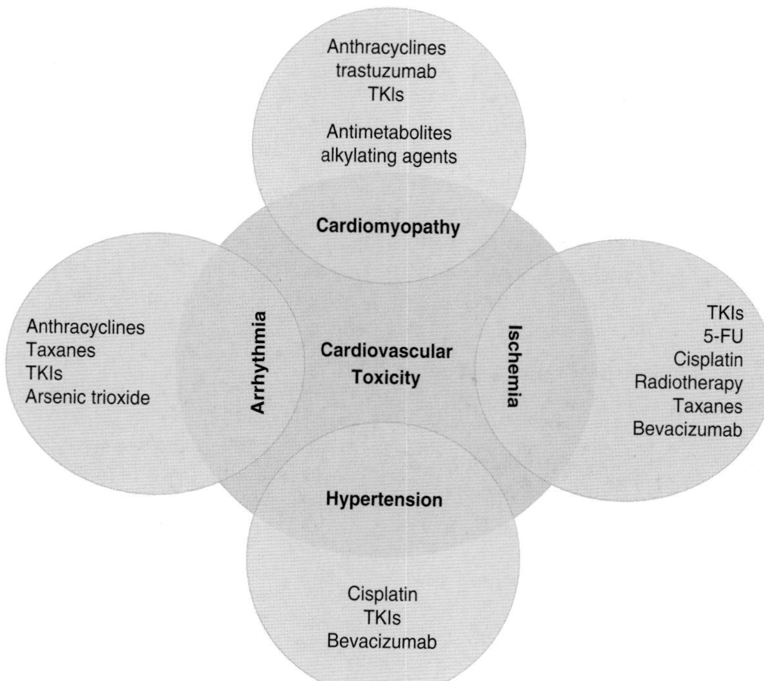

FIGURE 54-2 Cardiovascular syndromes associated with certain chemotherapy agents. 5-FU, 5-fluorouracil; TKI, tyrosine kinase inhibitor.

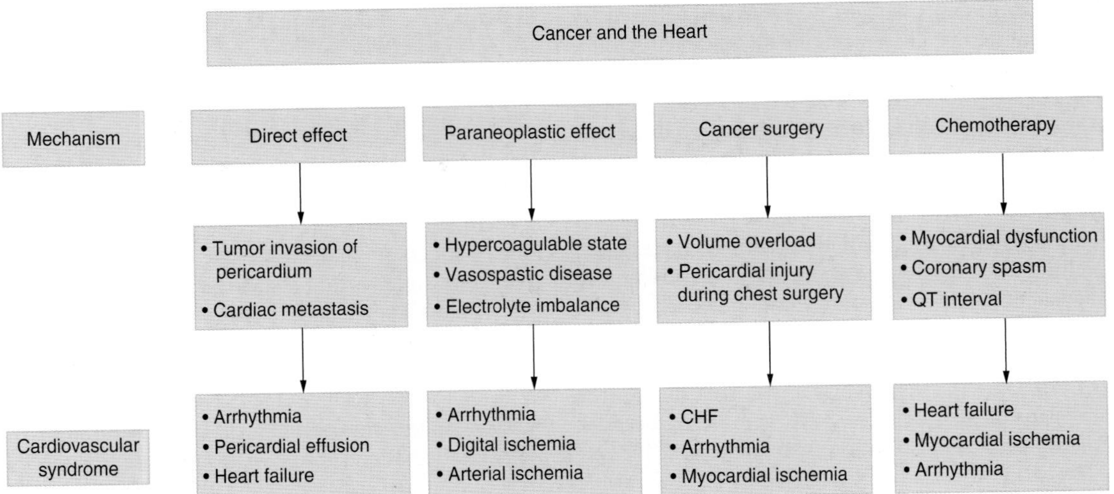

FIGURE 54-3 Mechanisms and etiology of some cardiovascular syndromes observed in cancer patients. CHF, congestive heart failure.

Evaluation of these patients typically includes obtaining a two-dimensional echocardiogram, brain natriuretic peptide, troponin, thyroid function tests, iron/ferritin level, ischemia assessment, and occasionally endomyocardial biopsy.

Acute Cardiomyopathy

Most of these cases are related to conditions referred to as reversible myocardial dysfunction or stress cardiomyopathy. This is a phenomenon typically triggered by sepsis, but also occurs in a wide range of acute illnesses (see Table 54-1). Myocardial dysfunction has been documented in up to 40% of patients with sepsis and is a major predictor of mortality in this population [7, 8]. During the course of the malignancy management, patients are at risk of these acute illnesses, especially during chemotherapy with secondary neutropenic sepsis. Physiologically, both left and right ventricular systolic functions are diminished with variable degrees of myocardial depression. This is typically reversed within 7 to 10 days. The exact mechanism for myocardial dysfunction is not well defined, and multiple theories have been suggested including the possibility of altered microcirculatory flow, mitochondrial dysfunction, myofibrillary dysfunction, autonomic dysregulation, altered calcium cellular transportation, and others [7, 9] (Fig. 54-4). Clinically, patients with reversible myocardial dysfunction/stress cardiomyopathy are recognized when evidence of new-onset left ventricular (LV) dysfunction is documented in the appropriate clinical setting (see Table 54-1). It is frequently associated with repolarization abnormalities on electrocardiogram (ECG) and minimal rise in cardiac troponins. Echocardiographic findings of severe LV dysfunction are typically out of proportion to the ECG changes and the cardiac biomarkers rise. The severity of LV dysfunction, however, correlates well with the brain natriuretic peptide (BNP) and N-terminal proBNP (NT-proBNP) levels [7, 9]. The management is focused on stabilizing the patient's blood pressure using vasopressors if shock is present and transitioning to cardioprotective drugs like angiotensin-converting enzyme (ACE) inhibitors and β-blockers after the patient is weaned off of pressure support and when blood pressure is stable for 24 to 48 hours. Improvement and recovery of myocardial dysfunction are typically observed within 7 to 10 days [7]. Persistent LV dysfunction beyond 2 weeks should raise suspicion of possible underlying ischemic heart disease or viral myocarditis in these typically immunocompromised

Table 54-1 Etiologies of Left Ventricular Systolic and Diastolic Heart Failure in Cancer Patients

Acute Left Ventricular Systolic Dysfunction	Subacute/Chronic Left Ventricular Dysfunction

Stress cardiomyopathy
Sepsis
Myocarditis
  Viral
  Chemotherapy
Myocardial infarction
Metabolic derangement
  Hypocalcemia
	Preexistent cardiomyopathy
	  Ischemic heart disease
	  Nonischemic cardiomyopathy
	Hypertensive heart disease
	Chemotherapy
	Infiltrative cardiomyopathy
	  Amyloid heart disease
	  Iron overload

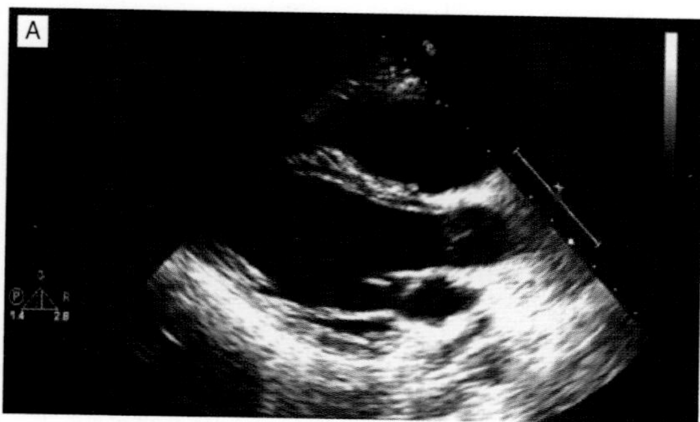

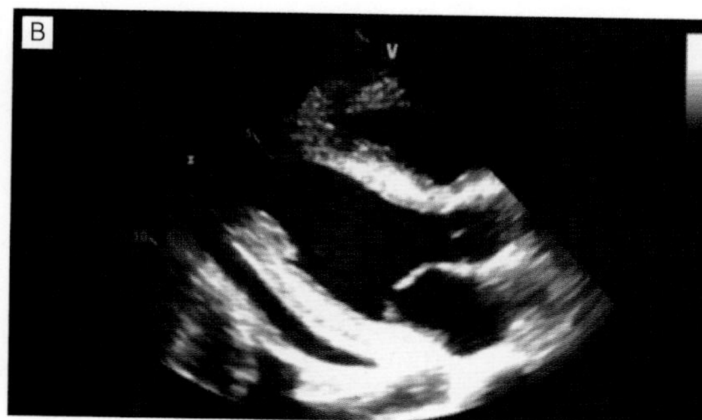

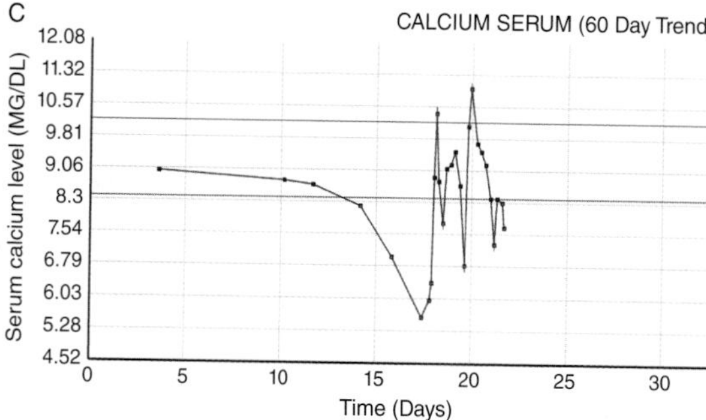

FIGURE 54-4 Acute severe cardiomyopathy with shock following chemotherapy for ovarian cancer complicated by severe hypocalcemia. Echocardiographic studies showing (A) baseline normal left ventricular systolic function and (B) severely depressed systolic function with small pericardial effusion 48 hours after developing severe hypocalcemia. (C) Severe hypocalcemia following chemotherapy.

patients. These two conditions are associated with significant rise in cardiac biomarkers like troponin and creatine kinase (CK)-MB. Patients with suspected ischemic heart disease should undergo evaluation and management of coronary artery disease. The diagnosis of viral myocarditis is more challenging because viral cultures and antibody titers have limited diagnostic accuracy. Myocardial biopsy is the gold standard in the general population for diagnosis of viral myocarditis despite its limited diagnostic yield (60% and 80% sensitivity and specificity, respectively) ([10]). This can be more challenging and risky in patients with cancer because they often have coagulopathy with risk of procedure-related complications (bleeding, myocardial perforation). The use of empiric therapy with intravenous immunoglobulin for its antiviral and immunomodulatory effect in this setting is controversial, especially with the limited data to support the benefit of such intervention in the adult population ([11]). It is also typically associated with high-volume fluid shift, which can exacerbate HF. Figure 54-5 summarizes a suggested algorithm for evaluation of new-onset cardiomyopathy and HF in patients with cancer.

Chemotherapy-Induced Cardiomyopathy

Definition

A large number of chemotherapeutic agents have been linked to cytotoxic myocardial injury. Table 54-2 lists several groups of chemotherapeutic agents known to be associated with LV systolic dysfunction or HF. The ones most commonly associated with cardiomyopathy include anthracyclines, alkylating agents, and tyrosine kinase inhibitors (TKIs). Cardiotoxicity in general is defined as a drop in LV ejection fraction (LVEF) by 5% or more, to less than 55% in the presence of HF symptoms, or an asymptomatic drop in LVEF by 10% or more to less than 55% ([12]). Myocardial toxicity is also classified into type I and type II based on the nature of myocyte injury.

CHAPTER 54

Type I Myocardial Toxicity

Anthracyclines are the prototype of drugs causing type I, irreversible myocyte damage. Histologic findings include myofibrillar disarray, disruption of cellular organelles, myofibrillar loss, and myocyte death ([13]). Myocardial toxicity is dose dependent, with <5% chance of cardiomyopathy observed at a cumulative dose of <400 mg/m^2 in the case of doxorubicin (150 mg/m^2 for idarubicin and 900 mg/m^2 for epirubicin). This risk increases to 26% at a cumulative dose of 550 mg/m^2 ([14]). Anthracycline-related cardiotoxicity has also been classified as acute or chronic. The acute form manifests as nonspecific ECG changes, arrhythmia, myopericarditis, and transient LV dysfunction. The more feared chronic form is marked by LV systolic dysfunction occurring many months to years following exposure and manifests as progressive HF. It is not clear whether the acute form of anthracycline cardiotoxicity is the prodrome of the more delayed cardiomyopathy form, because it has been shown that myocyte dysfunction can be observed even after the first dose of the drug. It is plausible that myocardial reserve allows normal cardiac function despite initial injury and until a second insult leads to further myocardial cell loss and subsequent systolic dysfunction.

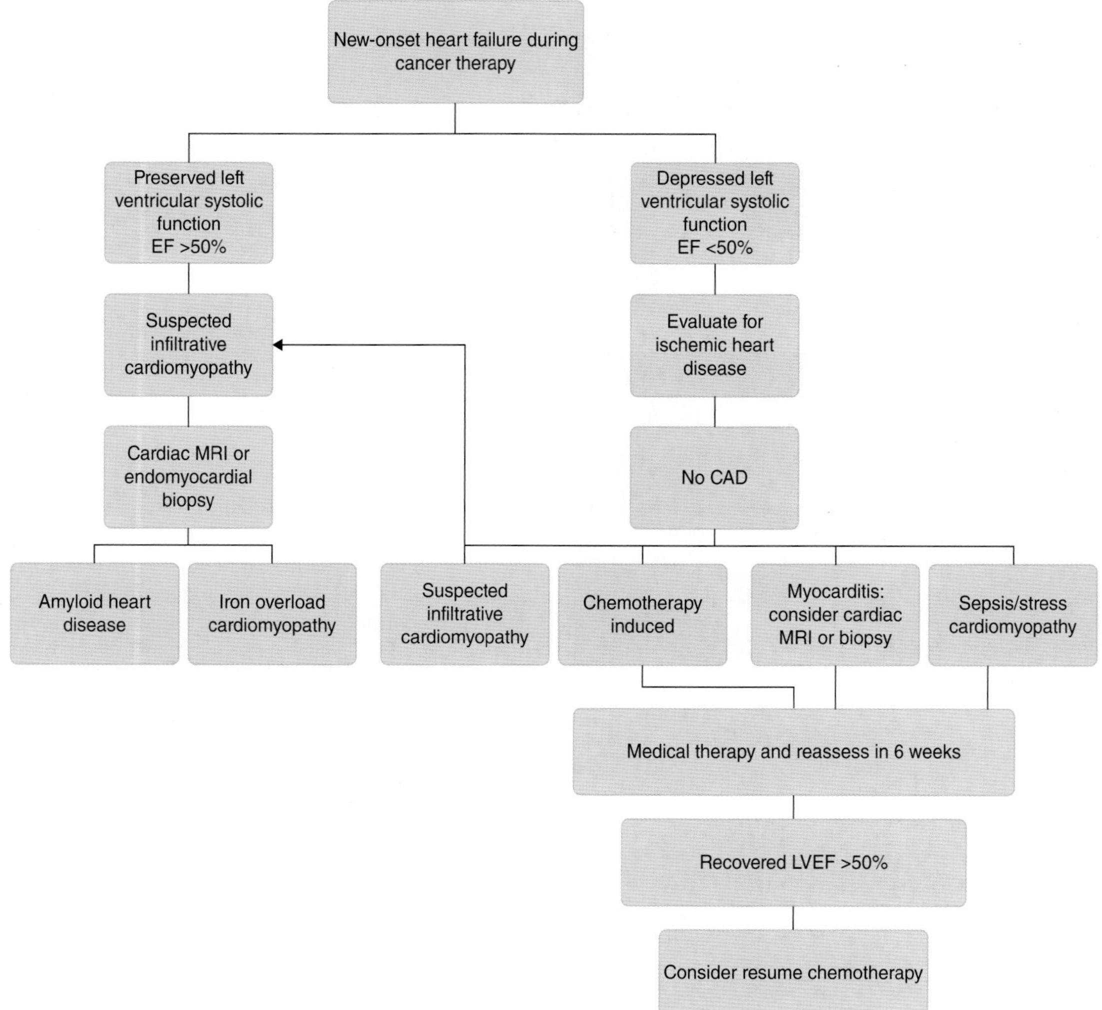

FIGURE 54-5 Algorithm for evaluation of patients with acute cardiomyopathy during cancer therapy. CAD, coronary artery disease; EF, ejection fraction; LVEF, left ventricular ejection fraction; MRI, magnetic resonance imaging.

The long-term prognosis of chemotherapy-induced cardiomyopathy is much worse compared to other etiologies ([15]). For years, the understood mechanism has been based on the free radical and iron hypothesis. The addition of an electron to the quinone moiety of anthracyclines within the cardiomyocytes leads to the generation of excess reactive oxygen species (ROS) and subsequent mitochondrial and intracellular protein damage. This toxicity is further increased when ROS interact with iron, generating a surge of oxidative stress ([16]). More recently, topoisomerase IIβ was found to be a key mediator of anthracycline-induced cardiomyocyte toxicity. Anthracycline-mediated inhibition of topoisomerase IIβ causes double-stranded DNA breaks, which can lead to cardiomyocyte death ([5]). The use of topoisomerase IIβ level in peripheral blood leukocytes has recently been reported to be of potential benefit for risk stratification and as a surrogate biomarker for individual susceptibility for anthracycline-induced cardiotoxicity ([17]). In a small study, the level of topoisomerase IIβ was significantly higher in the anthracycline-sensitive group. Close cardiac monitoring with early recognition and treatment of LV dysfunction using β-blockers and ACE inhibitors within the first 6 months of onset has been shown to be associated with stabilization and even recovery of cardiac function ([18]). These observations are the basis for the current recommendations of routine cardiac monitoring during anthracycline therapy. Different diagnostic tools have been useful in monitoring these patients including the use of cardiac biomarkers and/or cardiac imaging studies ([19]). There is no consensus regarding

Table 54-2 Most Commonly Used Chemotherapeutic Agents Known to Be Associated With Left Ventricular Systolic Dysfunction or Heart Failure

Chemotherapeutic Agent	Mechanism of Toxicity	Cardiomyopathy Incidence	Other Cardiovascular Toxicity
Anthracyclines • Doxorubicin • Epirubicin • Idarubicin	Oxidative stress Inhibition of topoisomerase IIβ	5% at 400 mg/m² 18% at 700 mg/m² 4% at 900 mg/m² 15% at 1 g/m² 5%	Arrhythmia Pericarditis Arrhythmia
Anthracyclines analogues • Mitoxantrone		2.6%	Arrhythmia Hypertension
Monoclonal antibodies • Rituximab • Cetuximab • Alemtuzumab • Trastuzumab • Bevacizumab	No direct toxicity Hypomagnesemia-related arrhythmia Infusion-related hemodynamic effect ErbB2 receptor–mediated myocyte dysfunction VEGF inhibition Hypertension-mediated cardiomyopathy	<0.5% 2%-28% 1.7%-3%	Arrhythmia Hypotension Arterial thrombosis Hypertension
Alkylating agents (at high dose) • Cyclophosphamide (>1.5 mg/m²) • Busulfan • Ifosfamide (>1 g/m²)	Myocarditis Myocardial fibrosis Myocarditis	3%-25% Rare 17%	Tamponade Pericardial effusion Myocardial infarction, arrhythmia
Antimetabolites • Gemcitabine • 5-Fluorouracil	Noncardiogenic pulmonary edema	7.1% 2%	Ischemia
Antimicrotubule agents • Vinca alkaloids (vincristine, vinblastine)	Impairment of myocardial metabolism	3%	Coronary spasm Hypertension
Oral tyrosine kinase inhibitors • Dasatinib • Lapatinib • Pazopanib • Sorafenib • Sunitinib • Vandetanib	Mitochondrial toxicity Dysregulation of cellular energy Mitochondrial toxicity	1%-4% heart failure Up to 10%-28% left ventricular systolic dysfunction	Hypertension QT prolongation Arterial thrombosis Arrhythmia Fluid retention

VEGF, vascular endothelial growth factor.

the best approach and optimal timing for testing. At the University of Texas MD Anderson Cancer Center (MDACC), we rely on serial imaging with two-/three-dimensional echocardiograms with myocardial strain to monitor these patients (Figs. 54-1 and 54-6).

Multiple primary preventive measures may be needed to lower the risks of anthracycline-induced cardiomyopathy. Continuous infusions instead of repetitive boluses are associated with a lower incidence of myocyte damage ([20]). Drug peak plasma level correlates with the degree of myocyte toxicity, whereas the area under the curve determines antitumor efficacy. Modified preparations of anthracyclines such as liposomal doxorubicin are associated with lower risk. Dexrazoxane is thought to lower risk through iron chelation and interference with the topoisomerase IIβ complex by preventing it from binding to anthracyclines. Finally, the use of β-blockers and ACE inhibitors or angiotensin receptor blockers has been associated with mixed results in small prospective studies ([21, 22]). It is not clear if they exert a potential cell protection effect or if they only have a beneficial hemodynamic effect. Their role in primary prevention of chemotherapy-induced cardiotoxicity is uncertain.

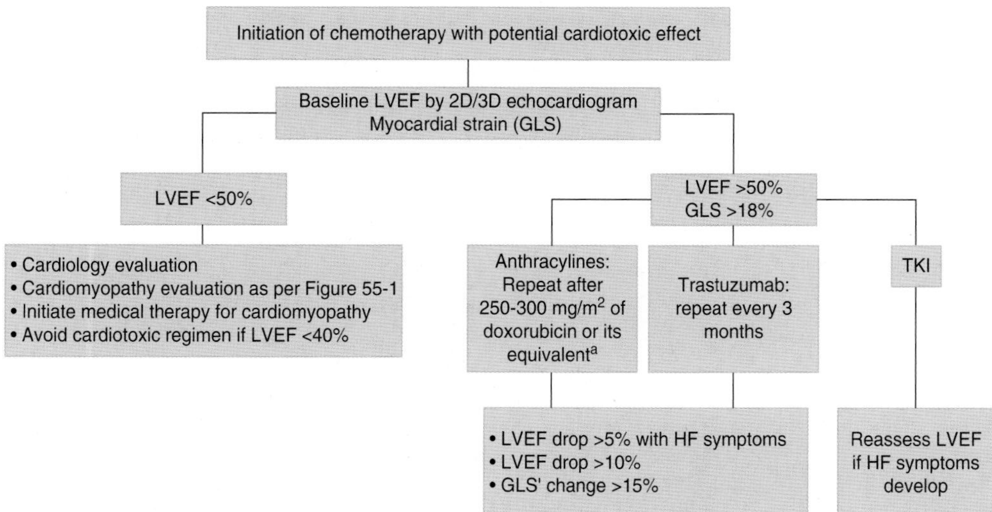

FIGURE 54-6 Algorithm for cardiac monitoring and management of patients receiving potentially cardiotoxic chemotherapy. 2D/3D, two-dimensional/three-dimensional; GLS, global longitudinal strain; HF, heart failure; LVEF, left ventricular ejection fraction; TKI, tyrosine kinase inhibitor. [a]Equivalent cardiotoxicity dose to 300 mg/m^2 of doxorubicin = 150 mg/m^2 of idarubicin = 900 mg/m^2 of epirubicin.

CHAPTER 54

Type II Myocardial Toxicity

This toxicity is associated with reversible disruption of myocyte contractile function. Trastuzumab is the prototype drug. Other targeted chemotherapy agents, including several small-molecule oral TKIs, are also suspected to exert type II cardiotoxicity. The mechanism involves disruption of signaling pathways responsible for tumor growth and also for cardiac cell repair (ErbB2 in the case of trastuzumab), resulting in myocyte dysfunction but not cell death ([23]). Up to a third of patients treated with trastuzumab develop evidence of LV systolic dysfunction or HF symptoms that are often reversible upon discontinuation of this agent ([24]). Re-initiation or continuation of trastuzumab after LV systolic function recovery is usually well tolerated. The US Food and Drug Administration (FDA) recommends monitoring LV function with imaging every 3 months during therapy. Not all patients are at the same risk, and several predisposing factors increase susceptibility for trastuzumab cardiotoxicity. These include concomitant use of anthracyclines, advanced age, and HTN or other underlying structural heart disease. There is an incremental increase in the incidence of LV systolic dysfunction or HF as the number of risk factors increases. For example, the risk of myocardial dysfunction increases from <1% in young women with no risk factors to 27% in elderly patients receiving concomitant anthracyclines ([12]). A clinical risk stratification model (National Surgical Adjuvant Breast and Bowel Project cardiac risk score) has been proposed to help risk stratify patients, but it needs to be validated ([25]).

Tyrosine kinase inhibitor–related LV dysfunction has been reported since early phase I and II studies. The mechanisms of toxicity are not fully understood, and several theories have been proposed, including apoptotic versus nonapoptotic cell death, dysregulation of cellular energy hemostasis through inhibition of 5-AMPK ([26]), mitochondrial toxicity, and HTN-mediated LV dysfunction ([27]). The incidence of TKI-related cardiomyopathy and HF varies widely with different drugs (mostly reported with sunitinib, sorafenib, imatinib, nilotinib, and ponatinib) and differs between studies by almost 10-fold. This is partially related to the fact that cancer trials typically do not have cardiovascular events as outcomes, and this likely leads to an underestimation of the incidence of such events. Also, the usual clinical HF symptoms of fatigue, dyspnea, and leg edema are nonspecific in patients with cancer, leading to limitations in clinical diagnostic accuracy. The incidence of symptomatic HF necessitating medical therapy varies between 1.5% and 15%, and the rate of reported drop in LVEF is between 7% and 28% ([27-31]). Time to onset of cardiomyopathy varies from a few weeks to several months after initiation of TKIs. Evidence of reversibility of significant LV dysfunction was seen in half of the patients after TKIs were discontinued.

Management

When clinical HF or LV systolic dysfunction is confirmed, patients typically are taken off of the TKI, and HF drugs are initiated (ACE inhibitors, β-blockers, and diuretics). Depending on the patient risk factors and clinical presentation, workup for other possible etiologies of cardiomyopathy should be performed when appropriate (ie, ischemic heart disease, HTN). In the absence of strong prospective data, there is not enough information to support the routine use of cardiac imaging to monitor asymptomatic patients. It is common practice to obtain a baseline two-dimensional echocardiogram study before initiating these drugs, with a low clinical threshold to obtain repeated echocardiographic studies if dyspnea or fluid retention symptoms develop on TKIs.

Preexisting Cardiac Dysfunction

This is usually observed in patients with underlying diastolic or systolic LV dysfunction including hypertensive heart disease, ischemic heart disease, or nonischemic cardiomyopathy. Decompensated HF symptoms are often triggered by large amounts of intravenous fluids given during certain chemotherapy infusions (eg, cisplatin). Patients typically respond well to withholding fluids and using diuretics. Standard HF therapy, including β-blockers and ACE inhibitors, is indicated if LV systolic dysfunction is present [32].

Other Forms of Cardiomyopathies Observed in Cancer Patients

Infiltrative processes are another cause of cardiomyopathies commonly encountered. Examples include amyloidosis and secondary hemochromatosis. In patients with myelodysplastic syndrome, myocardial iron overload develops from frequent blood transfusions (ie, >100 units).

Ischemic Arterial Disease in Cancer

The association between malignancy and ischemic arterial diseases is well established. The clinical presentation and management of arterial ischemic events vary based on the arterial bed and the organ involved. The clinical spectrum includes stroke, myocardial infarction, and visceral and limb ischemia. In two large separate cohorts of patients with cancer, Khorana et al reported a 1.5% to 3.1% incidence of arterial ischemic events [33, 34]. The most common events were cardiac, and less than 0.5% of events involved limb ischemia. The rate of arterial ischemic events is higher in specific cancer populations such as those with myeloproliferative disorders or hematologic malignancies with secondary amyloidosis. To assess the significance and outcome of these arterial events, Khorana et al prospectively followed 4,466 patients receiving active chemotherapy. Thromboembolism was a leading cause of death (9.2%) [35], with a higher rate of death from arterial events compared to venous events.

Etiology and Mechanisms

In addition to the usual causes and the traditional risk factors typically associated with arterial ischemia in the general population, patients with underlying malignancy have added increased risks for arterial ischemic events related to the inherent thrombophilia associated with the cancer and its therapy (Table 54-3). From the clinical perspective, it is useful to divide these cancer-related etiologies into two broad categories; the first category includes mechanisms, and the second group includes cancer etiologies.

Specific Mechanisms of Arterial Ischemia

Hypercoagulability

Multifactorial mechanisms have been implicated in the pathogenesis of hypercoagulability and thrombosis. As shown in Fig. 54-7, circulating and in situ cancer cells can enhance activity of tissue factor and other cancer procoagulant factors and can activate platelets. These mediators can then trigger coagulation in previously damaged vessels like the coronary arteries or peripheral arteries or even in previously healthy vessels [36]. The end result is cancer-enhanced thrombosis, which manifests as (1) low-grade disseminated intravascular coagulation, (2) venous thrombophlebitis, (3) arterial thrombosis, (4) accelerated ischemic cardiac and peripheral vascular disease, and (5) nonbacterial thrombotic endocarditis. Another subgroup of patients with a hypercoagulable condition present with digital ischemia with no evidence of large-vessel involvement (Fig. 54-8). The mechanism is thought to be due to capillary deposition of antigen-mediated antibody complexes from tumor cells. This paraneoplastic syndrome is usually very difficult to treat; symptoms do not respond to usual vascular therapy until the cancer is fully controlled [37].

Table 54-3 List of Potential Causes of Arterial Ischemic Events in Patients With and Without Malignancy

Noncancer Patients	Cancer Patients	
Atherosclerosis Atrial fibrillation Aortic arch plaques Mitral stenosis Valvular prosthesis Infective endocarditis Thrombophilia Antiphospholipid syndrome Antithrombin deficiency Protein C and S deficiency	Paraneoplastic syndrome Tumor invasion Tumor embolization Paradoxical embolization	Leukemia Amyloidosis Myeloproliferative disorders Chemotherapy Radiation therapy

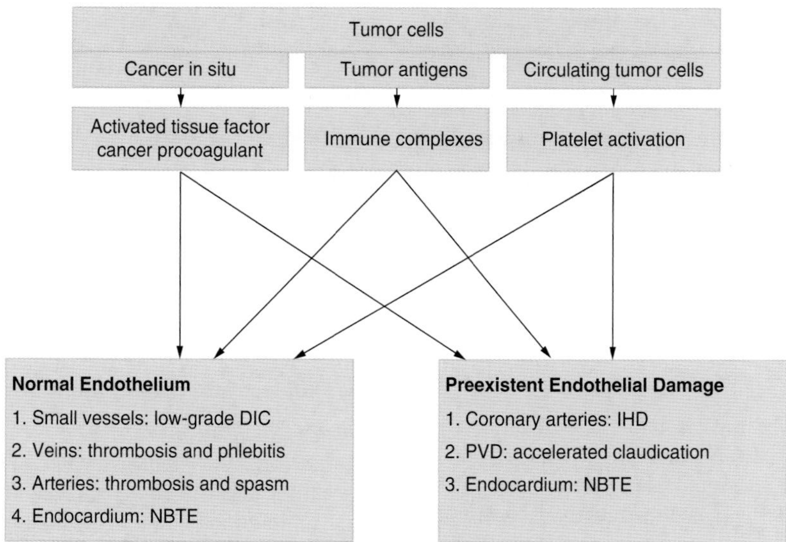

FIGURE 54-7 Suggested mechanism for the enhanced thrombosis observed in cancer patients. DIC, disseminated intravascular coagulation; IHD, ischemic heart disease; NBTE, nonbacterial thrombotic endocarditis; PVD, peripheral vascular disease.

Other Mechanisms

Other reported etiologies include radiation therapy, tumor embolization, arterial wall invasion by tumor, and paradoxical embolization. Often, a specific cause is never identified. In our cohort of 74 patients ([38]) with acute arterial limb ischemia, 24 confirmed pathology samples were available. The majority of patients (67%) had thrombus, and 21% had associated underlying significant atherosclerotic disease. Tumor invasion of the artery was observed in two cases, and only one patient with leukemia had leukemic cell aggregates (Fig. 54-9).

Thrombotic Events Associated With Specific Malignancies and Cancer Therapy

Myeloproliferative Disorders

Myeloproliferative disorders, such as polycythemia vera and essential thrombocythemia, are associated with vascular events characterized by microcirculatory dysregulation and thrombosis in various central and peripheral terminal arterial beds leading to ischemic strokes and acute coronary syndrome ([39, 40]). The incidence of thrombosis at diagnosis of polycythemia vera and essential thrombocythemia is 9.7% and 38.6%, respectively, in various studies, with 64% to 96.7% of these being arterial events ([41]). Primary prevention of thrombosis in myeloproliferative disorder involves the use of aspirin ([42]).

Acute Leukemia

Although hemorrhage is the typical complication in acute leukemia, arterial ischemic events due to thrombosis can occur. De Stefano et al reported a 1.4% incidence of thrombosis at presentation in acute lymphoblastic leukemia and a 9.6% incidence in acute promyelocytic

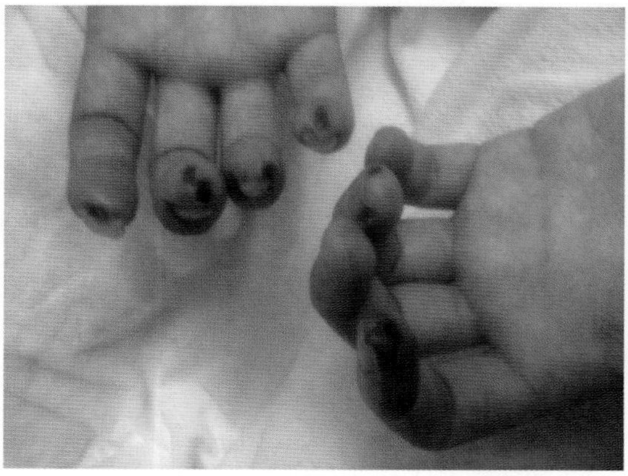

FIGURE 54-8 Digital ischemia in a 54-year-old male with small cell lung cancer.

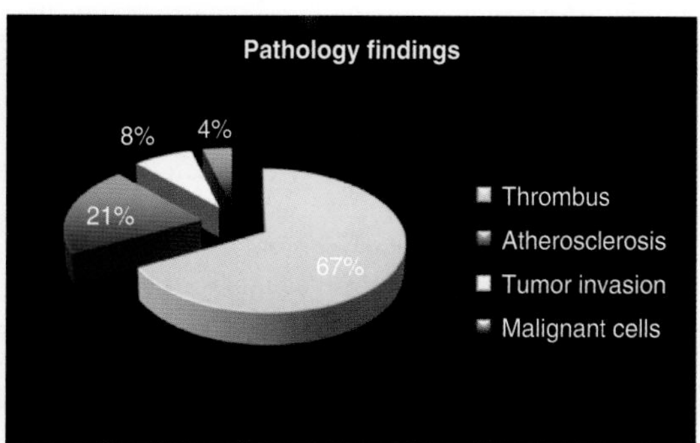

FIGURE 54-9 Etiology of acute arterial ischemia at the University of Texas MD Anderson Cancer Center. (Data from Chow SF, McKenna CH. Ovarian cancer and gangrene of the digits: case report and review of the literature, Mayo Clinic Proc 1996 Mar;71(3):253-258).

leukemia ([43]). Thromboembolism was reported as the presenting manifestation in more than half of the patients in this study, with 80% venous thromboembolisms and 20% arterial ischemic events. Options for management include leukapheresis, immediate chemotherapy, and sometimes revascularization of large-vessel occlusion.

Cardiac Amyloidosis

Primary amyloidosis, particularly AL type, has been associated with intracardiac thrombosis and thromboembolic events despite preserved LVEF and absence of cardiac arrhythmias, with an incidence ranging from 26% to 33% ([44, 45]) and arterial thromboembolism–related mortality of 26% in one study ([45]). A variety of mechanisms have been proposed for this phenomenon including endothelial dysfunction, endomyocardial damage ([46]), direct myocardial toxic effect ([47]), and hypercoagulability ([48]). In managing these patients, the benefit of prophylactic anticoagulation needs to be balanced against the risk of hemorrhage from fragile blood vessels with amyloid deposition ([49]).

Arterial Ischemic Events Related to Cancer Management and Therapy

Certain chemotherapeutic agents are known to have a stronger association with arterial ischemic events due to specific pathophysiological mechanisms. These drugs can be divided into two categories (Table 54-4). The first category includes several standard chemotherapeutic agents like L-asparaginase, cisplatin, 5-fluorouracil, capecitabine, and gemcitabine. In a study by De Stefano et al, the incidence of thrombosis in a population with acute lymphoblastic leukemia was shown to increase from 1.4% to 10.6% with L-asparaginase treatment ([43]). Cisplatin is known to induce thrombosis by causing endothelial damage ([50]) and increasing monocyte tissue factor activity and platelet activation with a reported 12% to 17.6% ([51]) incidence of thrombosis, including strokes, recurrent peripheral arterial events, and aortic thrombosis ([52]). 5-Fluorouracil leads to a decrease in protein C and endothelial independent vasoconstriction via protein kinase C ([53]). Gemcitabine has been associated with vascular events including systemic capillary leaks, thrombotic microangiopathy with digital ischemia, and venous thromboembolism ([54]).

The second category of cancer drugs associated with arterial ischemia includes the group of angiogenesis inhibitors like thalidomide and several targeted therapy drugs also known as the vascular signaling pathway inhibitors. These include bevacizumab and several TKIs like sunitinib, sorafenib, axitinib, pazopanib, and ponatinib. Thalidomide is associated with a risk of vascular thrombosis due to its anti-angiogenic effects and modulation of adhesion molecules ([55, 56]). In a prospective cohort of 195 patients with multiple myeloma, 11 patients developed an arterial ischemic event over a period of 522 patient-years (5.6%) ([57]). Several of these patients developed arterial thrombosis while receiving anticoagulation therapy. Bevacizumab has been linked to serious arterial ischemic events ([58, 59]) through mechanisms such as endothelial damage and overexpression of proinflammatory genes ([60-62]). In patients receiving concurrent bevacizumab and chemotherapy, Scappaticci et al reported the absolute rate of arterial events as 5.5 events per 100 person-years ([63]). Pereg and Lishner reported the efficacy of low-dose aspirin in preventing cardiovascular complications in patients 65 years of age or older who had a prior history of thromboembolic events and were receiving bevacizumab ([58]). The mechanism of vascular toxicities associated with TKIs is not well understood and is thought to be partially mediated by nitric oxide inhibition versus accelerated atherosclerosis and possible interference with platelet function. In a meta-analysis by Choueiri et al, the incidence of arterial ischemia was 4% with a three-fold increase in risk in patients treated with sunitinib or sorafenib ([64]). Arterial ischemia with ponatinib has been reported to be greater than 20%, leading to the implementation of major restrictions on indications and monitoring by the FDA ([65]).

Table 54-4 Chemotherapeutic Agents Associated With Arterial Ischemic Events

Cisplatin
L-Asparaginase
Fluorouracil
Gemcitabine
Capecitabine
Angiogenesis inhibitors: Thalidomide Bevacizumab Sunitinib Sorafenib Ponatinib

Management

The management strategy should be tailored to the patient's clinical condition and the cancer type. Primary preventive strategies include life-long antiplatelet therapy and statins for radiation-induced and known underlying atherosclerotic disease, aspirin and/or hydroxyurea for myeloproliferative disorders ([66]), and aspirin for patients with a history of prior cardiovascular events or who are over age 65 and receiving bevacizumab ([58]). Treatment of the acute event varies by type of organ involved (cardiac, central nervous system, limb, or bowel ischemia) and is aimed at reversing ischemia and minimizing organ damage, followed by long-term therapy and secondary prevention. The decision to use medical therapy versus a surgical or percutaneous approach for revascularization is determined by the general condition of the patient and availability of local expertise. Management of these patients is often a challenge because of the bleeding risks, especially in the setting of associated thrombocytopenia. Although acute coronary intervention has been shown to be reasonably safe in these patients ([67]), there is a significant concern regarding the need for dual antiplatelet therapy for an extended period of time. Drug-eluting coronary stents pose a special problem in this setting and should be avoided. We typically recommend using bare metal stents because many patients end up receiving more chemotherapy and/or surgery for the management of cancer. The type of long-term anticoagulation recommended for secondary prevention depends on the underlying mechanism and etiology. Table 54-5 summarizes some of the therapeutic interventions for arterial ischemic events observed in the setting of malignancy or hematologic disorders.

Table 54-5 Therapeutic Interventions of Potential Benefit for Arterial Ischemic Events Observed in the Setting of Malignancy or Hematologic Disorders

Arterial Ischemic Events Associated With:	Treatment Options
Acute leukemia	Chemotherapy and leukapheresis Surgical thromboembolectomy
Radiation therapy	Antiplatelet therapy Statin therapy Percutaneous angioplasty with or without stenting Surgery
Paradoxical embolization	Systemic anticoagulation PFO closure for recurrent events
Myeloproliferative disorders	Aspirin (for primary and secondary prevention) Cell reduction therapy (ie, phlebotomy, hydroxyurea, anagrelide, interferon-α)
Cardiac amyloidosis	Systemic anticoagulation
Bevacizumab	Aspirin (for primary prevention in patients over 65 years of age or with a history of cardiovascular events)
NBTE	Systemic anticoagulation

NBTE, nonbacterial thrombotic endocarditis; PFO, patent foramen ovale.

Cardiac Arrhythmia

Introduction

Patients with cancer have complex comorbidities that predispose to certain arrhythmias and limit the therapeutic options when using antiarrhythmic drugs. Patients with underlying malignancy can develop cardiac arrhythmia as a consequence of the malignancy itself or its therapy (Fig. 54-10). When patients present with cardiac rhythm disturbances, they typically have associated complex comorbidities. The presence of a rapid heart rate or rhythm irregularity can be simply a sign of a more complicated and severe acute illness (eg, atrial tachycardia or fibrillation in the setting of acute pulmonary embolism, polymorphic ventricular tachycardia triggered by severe metabolic derangements and electrolyte imbalance while on a QT-prolonging agent). Adequate patient management necessitates accurate diagnosis and identification of the potential etiologies and mechanisms that triggered the arrhythmias.

Diagnosis and Management

The management of cardiac arrhythmia should follow the well-established standard-of-care guidelines ([68, 69]). Treatment can sometimes differ slightly from those without malignancy. The difference is mainly related to the choice of antiarrhythmic drugs and atrioventricular-blocking agents and the timing and safety of anticoagulation. The choice of these drugs should take into consideration the possibility of drug-drug interactions. Cardizem and verapamil are potent cytochrome P inhibitors that can alter the pharmacokinetics of many chemotherapeutic agents. Several classes of antiarrhythmic drugs can potentiate QT prolongation observed with many cancer-targeted therapies. The decision for short- and long-term anticoagulation for atrial fibrillation or flutter should be tailored carefully in each case, because many patients face higher risks of bleeding in the setting of thrombocytopenia secondary to the malignancy or its therapy.

Bradyarrhythmias

Bradyarrhythmias can generally be categorized as sick sinus syndrome or heart block. The most common presenting symptoms of bradyarrhythmias include fatigue, lightheadedness, dizziness, or syncope. Many different causes have been linked to bradyarrhythmias. These include myocardial infiltration, atrioventricular nodal blocking drugs such as antiemetics, and certain chemotherapies. like paclitaxel and thalidomide.

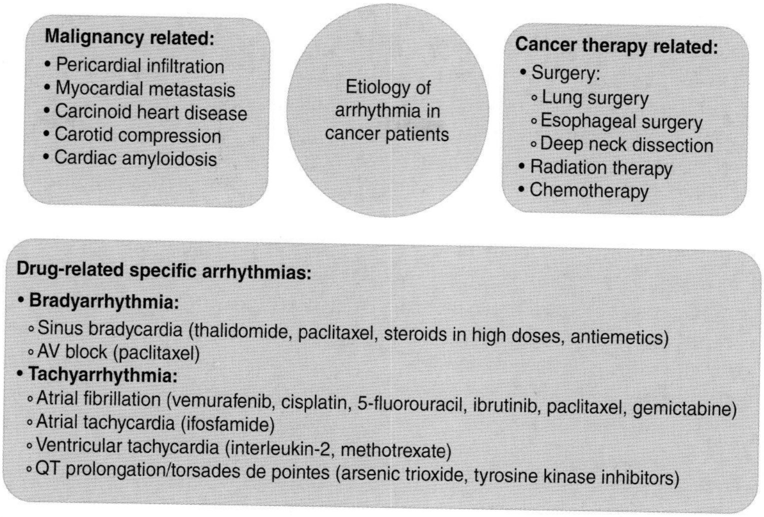

FIGURE 54-10 Etiology and mechanism of cardiac arrhythmia related to cancer and its management. AV, atrioventricular.

Possible suggested mechanisms include direct effect on the Purkinje system and extracardiac autonomic controls. The incidence of bradycardia with paclitaxel is as high as 30%. A less common but equally important cause of bradycardia is baroreflex failure. This is typically characterized by volatility of heart rate and blood pressure, including profound and severe bradycardia necessitating the use of a permanent pacemaker. This is most often seen in patients who undergo extensive head and neck surgery or receive neck radiation therapy causing dysregulation of the autonomic system at the level of the vascular baroreceptors, the glossopharyngeal or vagal nerves, or the brainstem ([70]).

Treatment

Treatment of bradyarrhythmias begins with identifying and removing any potentially offending agents that can exacerbate bradycardia. For severely symptomatic patients, urgent medical therapy with atropine or an intravenous inotrope, such as dopamine or epinephrine, may be used. In emergency situations, transcutaneous or transvenous pacemaker therapy may be required to maintain hemodynamic support. Long-term support with permanent pacing will depend on the severity of the symptoms related to the bradyarrhythmia and whether it is reversible.

Tachyarrhythmias

These are typically classified into four different categories:

1. Irregular tachycardia: atrial fibrillation, atrial flutter, multifocal atrial tachycardia
2. Regular narrow QRS complex tachycardia: sinus tachycardia, atrial tachycardia, supraventricular tachycardia
3. Wide QRS complex tachycardia: ventricular tachycardia, supraventricular tachycardia with aberrancy, preexcited tachycardia
4. Polymorphic ventricular tachycardia

Sinus tachycardia is by far the most common cause of rapid heart rate. It is usually secondary to other concomitant acute illnesses (eg, infection, pneumonia, pulmonary embolism, surgery). Evaluation and treatment of the primary etiology and the precipitating causes are effective.

Atrial fibrillation has been shown in several epidemiologic studies to be more prevalent in patients with cancer compared to the general population ([71]). Guzzetti et al reported a three-fold increase in the prevalence of atrial fibrillation in patients hospitalized with colon cancer compared to those admitted for nonneoplastic diseases ([72]). The highest incidence of malignancy-related atrial fibrillation has been reported in patients undergoing thoracic (6%-32%) ([73]) and esophageal (9.2%) ([74]) cancer surgery. Postoperative atrial fibrillation appears to be associated with higher in-hospital length of stay, intensive care unit admissions, and more importantly, higher short- and long-term mortality ([72]).

Acute management of atrial fibrillation follows the general recommendations of urgent cardioversion for the hemodynamically unstable patient and initial rate control for stable patients. Ventricular rate control can be achieved using atrioventricular-blocking agents like digoxin, β-blockers, or the nondihydropyridine calcium channel antagonists (diltiazem hydrochloride

[Cardizem] or verapamil). Amiodarone can also be considered for rate control in patients with marginal blood pressure or LV dysfunction. For the subgroup of patients with previously known and documented permanent atrial fibrillation, controlling the heart rate and reversing the cause of acute decompensation should suffice.

The clinical decision for short- and long-term anticoagulation for atrial fibrillation is challenging and should be tailored individually because patients can be at high thromboembolic risk based on the standard risk scores used in cardiology and concomitantly at high risks of bleeding in the setting of thrombocytopenia secondary to the malignancy or its therapy. On the other hand, a patient with low thromboembolic risks based on these same scores can still be at high risk secondary to an acquired hypercoagulable state related to cancer or its therapy. Figure 54-11 shows a suggested algorithm to help risk stratify patients for anticoagulation in the setting of atrial fibrillation, based on their thromboembolic and bleeding risk scores. (This algorithm has not been validated.)

Patients with cancer require special consideration due to the risk of QT prolongation and torsades de pointes from both chemotherapeutic agents and adjunctive medications. QT intervals as measured by ECG reflect the total duration of the action potential at the cellular level. QT prolongation is associated with increased risk for polymorphic ventricular tachycardia, also known as torsades de pointes, and subsequent sudden cardiac death. The corrected QT interval is considered prolonged when it is greater than 480 milliseconds in women and 470 milliseconds in men. The QT interval varies with the cardiac rate and is typically reported as corrected QT interval (QTc) after correction for the patient heart rate. Current ECG technology and digital diagnostic algorithms can generate immediate measurement of the QTc interval. It is important to recognize that an accurate measurement and interpretation of QTc is essential to minimize the chances of inappropriate drug discontinuation or overestimation of the true incidence of QT prolongation with these drugs.

In the cancer population, there are several risk factors predisposing to QT prolongation and subsequent torsades de pointes. These include electrolyte imbalance (hypomagnesemia, hypokalemia, hypocalcemia), metabolic derangements (hypothyroidism), and certain cancer therapies including chemotherapeutic agents (Table 54-6). It is of clinical importance to correct any concomitant contributing factors that may predispose to or worsen QT interval prolongation. Cancer treatment interruption is typically advised

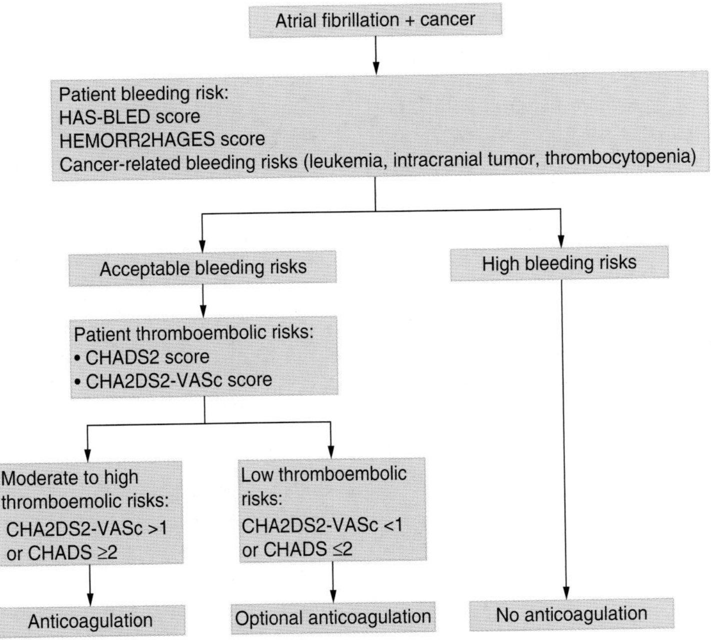

FIGURE 54-11 Algorithm for decision making regarding antithrombotic therapy in cancer patient with atrial fibrillation. Thromboembolic risk scores: CHA2DS2VASc is the acronym for congestive heart failure, age 2 (if >75 years), diabetes, stroke, vascular disease, age (65-74 years), sex category; CHADS2 is the acronym for congestive heart failure, age (if >75 years), diabetes, stroke. Bleeding risk scores: HAS-BLED is the acronym for hypertension, abnormal renal/liver function, previous stroke, prior major bleeding, labile international normalized ratio, elderly (age >65 years), drugs/alcohol use; HEMORR2HAGES is the acronym for hepatic or renal disease, ethanol use, malignancy, older age (>75 years), reduced platelets, rebleeding, hypertension (uncontrolled), anemia, genetic factor, elevated risk of fall, stroke.

Table 54-6 Drugs Associated With QT Prolongation

Chemotherapy Agents	Nonchemotherapy Agents
BRAF inhibitors	Antiemetics
Vemurafenib	Ondansetron
HDAC inhibitors	Promethazine
Depsipeptide	Antimicrobials
Vorinostat	Voriconazole
Tyrosine kinase inhibitors	Ciprofloxacin
Dasatinib	Moxifloxacin
Lapatinib	Erythromycin
Nilotinib	Clarithromycin
Pazopanib	Analgesics
Sunitinib	Methadone
Vandetanib	
Others	
Arsenic trioxide	

HDAC, histone deacetylase.

when a QT interval is above 500 milliseconds, and permanent treatment discontinuation is recommended if QT prolongation recurs or is associated with ventricular tachycardia or syncope. Figure 54-12 shows a useful algorithm to screen and monitor patients being considered for therapy with agents associated with potential QT prolongation or torsades de pointes.

Among TKIs, a high incidence of QT prolongation has been reported with several of these drugs, leading to an FDA black box warning mandating close ECG monitoring and management recommendations (Table 54-7).

Pericardial Diseases

Pericardial diseases are common in patients with cancer and can manifest as acute pericarditis, pericardial effusion, cardiac tamponade, or constrictive pericarditis. Triggers of pericardial diseases include infections, tumor invasion of the pericardium, and cancer therapy, specifically chest radiation or chemotherapy (Table 54-8). The lack of randomized clinical trials makes the management of these syndromes mainly empirical, based on expert opinion and limited data extrapolated from the few trials in noncancer populations ([75,76]).

Acute Pericarditis

The diagnosis of pericarditis is based on the findings of pleuritic chest pain, fever, and ST elevation detected by ECG. Patients are typically hospitalized after they present with acute pericarditis if they show evidence of high fever, suspected myopericarditis, and/or the presence of a large (>20 mm in diameter) pericardial effusion or have tamponade physiology detected by echocardiography. Nonsteroidal anti-inflammatory drugs (NSAIDs) and aspirin are the mainstay of therapy for acute pericarditis. Intermediate to high doses of NSAIDs are typically used for 10 to 15 days followed by a slow taper over an additional 1 to 2 weeks. Colchicine is often added to the regimen at a dose of 0.6 mg daily for 3 months to help minimize recurrence ([77,78]). It is a well-tolerated drug with few side effects. However, the few contraindications to the use of colchicine are common in patients with cancer, particularly in recent stem cell transplant recipients. Contraindications include significant interactions with several drugs, including antifungal agents, antibiotics, and immunosuppressants such

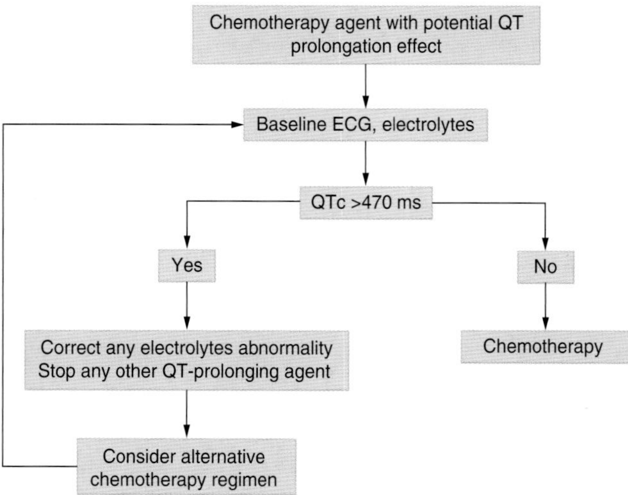

FIGURE 54-12 Suggested algorithm for the initial assessment and management of patients being considered for potential QT-prolonging chemotherapeutic agents. ECG, electrocardiogram.

Table 54-7 Monitoring Recommendations for Small-Molecule TKIs Associated With Prolonged QT Interval

Drug	Monitoring
Pazopanib (Votrient) Bosutinib (Bosulif) Crizotinib (Xalkori) Dasatinib (Sprycel) Lapatinib (Tykerb)	Use caution in patients at risk for QT prolongation, including patients with long QT syndrome; patients taking antiarrhythmic medications or other medications that lead to QT prolongation or potassium-wasting diuretics; and patients taking cumulative high-dose anthracycline therapy and with conditions that cause hypokalemia or hypomagnesemia. Correct hypokalemia and hypomagnesemia before initiation of therapy.
In addition to the general recommendations listed above, the ECG monitoring guidelines listed below must be followed when patients take certain TKI agents.	
Vandetanib (Caprelsa)	1. Do not initiate treatment unless the Fridericia-corrected QT interval (QTcF) is <450 ms. 2. Order an ECG at baseline, at 2-4 weeks, at 8-12 weeks, and every 3 months thereafter. 3. During treatment, if QTcF >500 ms, withhold vandetanib and resume at a reduced dose when QTcF is <450 ms.
Nilotinib (Tasigna)	Monitor ECG and QT_c at baseline, at 7 days, with dose change, and periodically. 1. QTc >480 ms: Withhold treatment, monitor and correct potassium and magnesium levels; review concurrent medications. 2. If QTcF returns to <450 ms and to within 20 ms of baseline within 2 weeks, resume at prior dose. 3. If QTcF returns to 450-480 ms after 2 weeks, reduce dose to 400 mg once daily. 4. If QTcF >480 ms after dosage reduction to 400 mg once daily, discontinue treatment.
Vemurafenib (Zelboraf)	1. Do not initiate treatment if baseline QTc >500 ms. 2. Monitor ECG at baseline, at 15 days, then monthly for 3 months, and then every 3 months and with dosage adjustments. 3. During treatment, if QTc >500 ms, temporarily interrupt treatment; may reinitiate with a dose reduction once QTc falls to <500 ms. 4. Discontinue (permanently) if, after correction of risk factors, the QTc continues to increase >500 ms.

ECG, electrocardiogram; TKI, tyrosine kinase inhibitor.

as tacrolimus. These drugs can alter colchicine metabolism such that the level is significantly increased.

The use of corticosteroids is typically discouraged in noncancer patients because of significant side effects and the association with an increased incidence of recurrent pericarditis. The situation is reversed in patients with cancer due to the numerous contraindications to the use of aspirin and NSAIDs. Steroids are typically used in patients with low platelet counts or patients with blood dyscrasias when NSAIDs cannot be used. The evidence comparing the effectiveness of low-dose versus high-dose steroids is weak. High-dose prednisone of 1.0 to 1.5 mg/kg (or its equivalent) over many weeks with a slow taper is associated with the lowest rate of recurrence but with a high rate of steroid-related side effects. A lower dose of prednisone of 0.2 to 0.5 mg/kg is associated with fewer side effects but a higher relapse rate. Because there are no strong data to support one option over the other, we typically use the protocol summarized in Fig. 54-13.

Table 54-8 Etiologies of Pericardial Diseases in Cancer Patients

Etiology
Infection
Tumor invasion
Radiation
Chemotherapy Purine analogues (ie, fludarabine) Antimetabolites (ie, capecitabine) Anthracyclines (ie, doxorubicin) Alkylating agents (ie, cyclophosphamide) Histone deacetylase (HDAC) inhibitors (ie, mocetinostat)

Pericardial Effusion

Pericardial effusion is a common finding and has been reported in up to 34% of autopsies performed on patients with cancer. Its management is guided by three main factors: (1) clinical significance of the effusion (presence or absence of associated symptoms), (2) effusion size, and (3) etiology of the effusion

Etiology

Up to two-thirds of pericardial effusions are nonmalignant. The mechanism of effusion in this setting is likely related to loss of adequate lymphatic drainage of the pericardial sac secondary to lymphangitic spread of the malignancy or mediastinal irradiation. Other etiologies include infection, radiation, and certain drugs

Medical (Therapy)

NSAIDs:

- Ibuprofen: 400-800 mg TID 1-2 weeks, taper to off over 1-2 weeks
- Indomethacin: 50 mg TID 1-2 weeks, taper to off over 1-2 weeks
- Aspirin: 600-800 TID 1-2 weeks if known CAD

Colchicine:

- 0.6 mg BID day 1 then QD × 3-6 months

Prednisone:

- ***Avoid***: Use only if NSAIDs contraindicated
- High dose: 1 mg/kg for 2 days then taper over 1 week
- Low dose: 0.5 mg/kg for 2 weeks then taper to off over 2 weeks
- Add NSAIDs or colchicine when tapering off, if possible

A) Recurrent pericarditis

- Resume same drug at the lowest effective dose that suppressed symptoms.
- Add colchicine for 3-6 months.
- If steroids used, *slow* taper over 3 months.

B) Steroids *Slow* taper

- >50 mg: 10 mg/d every 1-2 weeks
- 50-25 mg: 5 mg/d every 1-2 weeks
- 25-15 mg: 2.5 mg/d every 2-4 weeks
- <15 mg: 1-2.5 mg/d every 2-6 weeks

FIGURE 54-13 Medical management of acute pericarditis. BID, twice a day; CAD, coronary artery disease; NSAIDs, nonsteroidal anti-inflammatory drugs; QD, every day; TID, three times a day.

(see Table 54-8). Clarifying the specific etiology of an effusion not only helps to define the treatment modality, but also helps to determine prognosis because malignant effusions are associated with a dismal prognosis (1-year survival rate of 16% compared with 55% with nonmalignant effusions) ([79]).

Diagnosis

Patients with a pericardial effusion may be asymptomatic but may also present with mild symptoms of chest pain, cough, and/or dyspnea. Extreme cases can present with frank tamponade and shock. Clinicians should be very careful when relying on vital signs to guide the management in patients with a pericardial effusion. Stroke volume and cardiac output drop at an early stage (as the effusion builds up). Blood pressure (BP), however, is maintained by a progressive increase in heart rate until it reaches a plateau, after which a threshold is reached and a severe drop in BP follows. Waiting for these clinical findings to manifest (ie, rapid heart rate and drop in BP) may cause treatment to occur too late, and the patient can rapidly progress to shock. Echocardiography is the main diagnostic tool to confirm the diagnosis of a pericardial effusion and detect tamponade physiology. Pericardial effusion size is classified as small, moderate, or large (large effusions are >2 cm in diameter). Helpful echocardiographic findings to detect early tamponade physiology include the presence of chamber collapse and/or of significant respiratory variation in the mitral or tricuspid valve inflow; these features manifest much earlier than BP drop and heart rate increase.

Management

There is no evidence that medical therapy plays any role in the management of an effusion, except in the case of concomitant inflammation (ie, pericarditis). At MDACC, the three main indications for pericardial fluid drainage are large effusion (>2 cm in diameter), diagnostic purposes, and the presence of clinical or echocardiographic evidence of tamponade physiology. As shown in Fig. 54-14, the first step following the detection of a moderate to large pericardial effusion is to assess for clinical or echocardiographic evidence of tamponade. If there is no sign of tamponade, the effusion size dictates the next step in management. Small to moderate effusions (<2 cm in diameter) are monitored clinically and with serial echocardiograms; larger effusions (>2 cm in diameter) require drainage because about one-third of patients progress to tamponade ([80]).

Draining a pericardial effusion can be achieved percutaneously or surgically by creating a pericardial window and, in some centers, by thoracoscopy. Surgery is preferred in the setting of recurrent effusions, purulent effusions, or high-output drainage (>100 mL/d for 5-7 days following percutaneous pericardiocentesis). The percutaneous approach is preferred in the majority of cases at MDACC, especially if the patient has hypotension or a coagulopathy. Following pericardiocentesis, pericardial fluid is sent for analysis (chemistry,

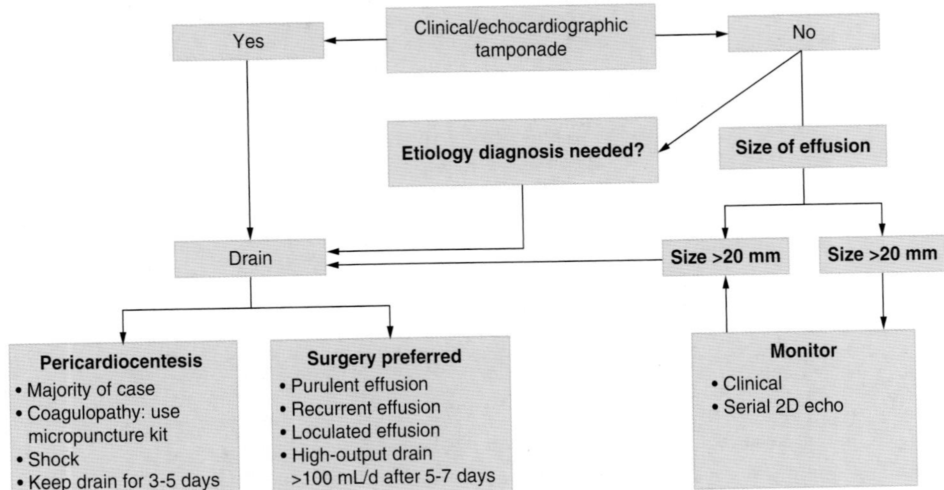

FIGURE 54-14 Management algorithm for pericardial effusion. 2D echo, two-dimensional echocardiography.

microbiology, cytology, flow cytometry, and sometimes to check for tumor markers) ([81]). A pericardial draining catheter is typically left in place for 5 days because this approach has shown to lower the effusion recurrence rate by two-thirds. Sometimes the catheter is removed early if drainage output is less than 25 mL over 24 hours and if there is no significant residual effusion on an echocardiogram. When performed by experienced teams, pericardiocentesis is safe with a low complication rate (<5%) and a high success rate (98%) ([82]). Recently, we demonstrated the feasibility and safety of this approach in a cohort of patients with severe thrombocytopenia related to leukemia or chemotherapy ([83]). Following initial pericardiocentesis, 25% of patients will develop recurrent effusions. Chemical pericardiodesis can be considered, but this approach can be complicated by severe pain, risk of infection, and long-term constrictive physiology, in addition to a 10% recurrence rate despite chemical pericardiodesis ([79]).

Hypertension and Cancer Management

Hypertension is known to be the most commonly diagnosed comorbidity in patients with cancer (37%). Its prevalence prior to chemotherapy exposure is similar to that reported in the general population (29%). A higher rate has been reported in association with certain cancer therapies including alkylating agents, angiogenesis inhibitors, immunosuppressants, and hormones like steroids, erythropoietin, and some TKIs (eg, ponatinib) (Table 54-9) ([84-86]).

Etiology and Pathophysiology

The most common chemotherapeutic agents known to cause HTN include several of the angiogenesis inhibitors, also referred to as vascular signaling pathway (VSP) inhibitors. These drugs include anti–vascular endothelial growth factor (VEGF) antibody (bevacizumab) and several TKIs (sunitinib, sorafenib,

Table 54-9 Cancer Therapies Associated With New-Onset or Worsening Hypertension

Medications	Overall Incidence of HTN (%)
Anti-VEGF antibody	
Bevacizumab	4-35
Tyrosine kinase inhibitors	
Pazopanib	40-47
Sorafenib	17-43
Sunitinib	15-34
Vandetanib	33
Alkylating agents	
Busulfan	36
Cisplatin	39
Calcineurin inhibitors	
Cyclosporine	60-80
Tacrolimus	30
Immunosuppressants	
Mycophenolate mofetil	28-78
mTOR inhibitors	
Sirolimus	45-49
Others	
Steroids	20
Erythropoietin	13.7-27.7

HTN, hypertension; mTOR, mammalian target of rapamycin; VEGF, vascular endothelial growth factor.

pazopanib, vandetanib, and ponatinib). Hypertension is one of the most common side effects of these drugs. Vascular endothelial growth factor normally plays an important role in maintaining a balanced vascular tone by regulating nitric oxide (NO) production in endothelial cells. Hypertension develops when NO bioavailability is reduced, leading to vasoconstriction, increased endothelin production, capillary rarefaction, and increased peripheral resistance ([86, 87]). New-onset or worsening HTN with these agents can develop very early (within 24 hours) after initiation but is typically observed within the first few weeks. Blood pressure usually returns to baseline shortly after therapy has been discontinued. Several previous limited observations raised the interesting concept of using HTN as a biomarker of cancer response to VSP inhibitors ([88]). More data are needed to further clarify the clinical significance of such observation.

Other classes of chemotherapeutic agents are known to cause HTN. The incidence and time to hypertensive effect for the VSP inhibitors and other agents used in cancer therapy are provided in Table 54-9. Alkylating agents are commonly used in a large number of oncology protocols to treat various solid tumors and blood cancers. Hypertension is frequent with these agents and is commonly seen with cisplatin and busulfan and much less often with cyclophosphamide. Their effect has been observed both acutely as well as years after therapy has been discontinued. The mechanism is thought to be the result of endothelial dysfunction and arterial vasoconstriction ([84]). Calcineurin inhibitors, used for the treatment of graft-versus-host disease, are also associated with a high incidence of HTN. Cyclosporine and tacrolimus are the major drugs in this class. Their effects are generally seen within the first 6 weeks of therapy and are thought to be the result of sympathetic system activation and an increase in endothelin-1 synthesis leading to vasoconstriction ([86]). Following transplant, many patients receive immunosuppression with mycophenolate mofetil and the mammalian target of rapamycin inhibitor sirolimus. The mechanism by which these agents cause HTN is not well understood. Corticosteroids are frequently used and have been associated with variable rates of dose-dependent HTN. The mechanism by which they cause HTN is complex but likely involves increased production of angiotensinogen that induces salt and fluid retention, activation of the sympathetic nervous system, and an increase in patient sensitivity to vasoactive substances. Patients receiving erythropoietin for anemia are also at risk for experiencing severe HTN. The driving mechanism behind the HTN is complex and goes beyond just volume expansion. It is also the result of an activation of the renin-angiotensin system and an increase in endothelin-1 with a decrease in NO production due to changes in the erythropoietin receptor ([86]).

Diagnosis and Management

Because HTN is a risk factor for chemotherapy-induced cardiotoxicity and poorly controlled HTN can lead to discontinuation of certain cancer therapies, a prompt and adequate intervention is essential to prevent potential irreversible damage. The Investigational Drug Steering Committee of the National Cancer Institute established a panel of experts to address the concern regarding VSP inhibitor–induced HTN. The recommendations published in 2010 focused on the evaluation, surveillance, and management of BP problems in patients receiving VSP inhibitors ([89]). Treatment of HTN should begin at the time of diagnosis, without a concern of negatively impacting cancer treatment outcomes.

The choice of a pharmacologic regimen to manage HTN should take into consideration several factors. For example, the underlying pathophysiology leading to BP elevation in calcineurin-induced HTN is caused by excessive vasoconstriction that responds well to dihydropyridine calcium channel blockers. Diuretic agents can help relieve fluid retention associated with steroid-related HTN. Clonidine has been recommended for the management of severe BP swings in patients with baroreflex failure. Other important factors that need to be considered include the risk of drug-drug interactions. It is also important to consider agents that may have compelling indications in specific types of cancer. Several recent epidemiologic studies reported potential oncologic benefit of β-blockers in melanoma, breast, lung, and colon cancers with the mechanism suspected to be mediated by altering β-adrenergic signaling in cancer ([90]). It is also important to consider the risks and benefits of medications that target NO or angiotensin II production when determining management strategies for patients on specific agents like the VSP inhibitors. Because these anticancer agents cause vasoconstriction in part through a decrease in NO production, medications such as nitrates, phosphodiesterase-5 inhibitors, and nebivolol, an NO-producing β-blocker, would in theory seem beneficial. However, there is a theoretical concern that by targeting this pathway these anti-HTN medications might compromise the efficacy of the antitumor therapy.

Radiation Therapy–Related Cardiovascular Toxicity

Radiation therapy to the mediastinum, left breast area, and neck region is a risk factor for premature coronary and carotid atherosclerotic disease (Fig. 54-15). The risk of arterial ischemic events depends on the radiation dose, technique, extent of vasculature exposed, and type of cancer ([91]). Radiation therapy can accelerate atherosclerosis by triggering oxidative stress leading to

CHAPTER 54

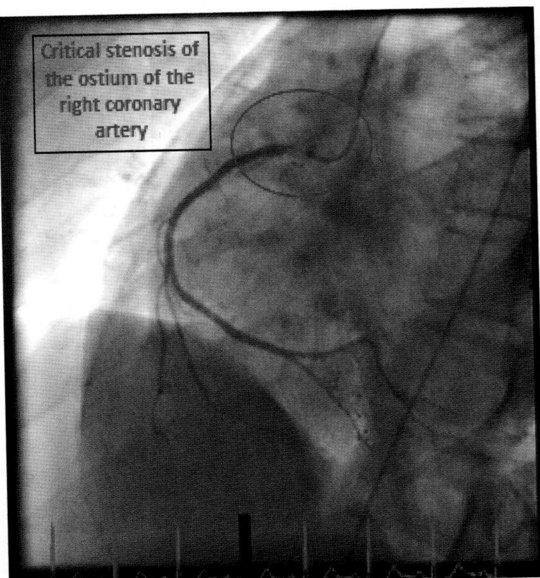

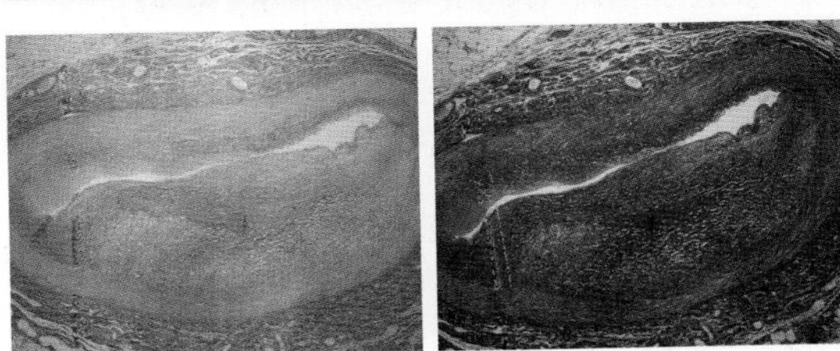

FIGURE 54-15 Coronary angiogram showing critical near occlusion of the ostium of the right coronary artery in a 36-year-old patient with prior chest radiation for lymphoma at the age of 5. Pathology findings shown below are consistent with radiation arteritis.

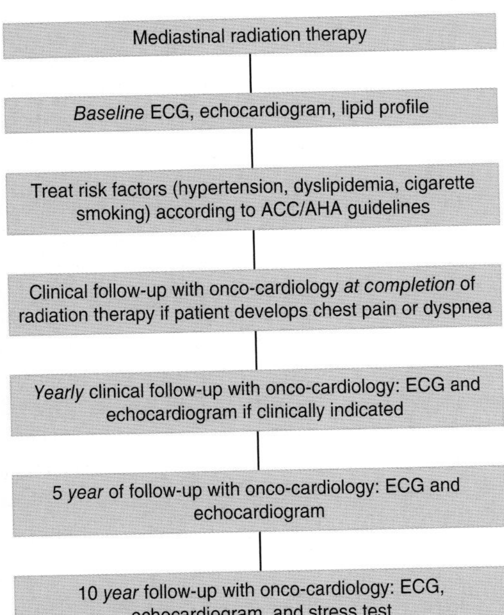

FIGURE 54-16 The University of Texas MD Anderson Cancer Center Department of Cardiology recommended algorithm for cardiac monitoring of patients following radiation therapy to the mediastinal area. ACC/AHA, American College of Cardiology/American Heart Association; ECG, electrocardiogram.

endothelial damage (92). The acute injury during therapy is sustained for a long period of time via activation of nuclear factor-κB (93). Symptoms typically manifest after a long latent period of 5 to 10 years following exposure. Mediastinal exposure is also responsible for a spectrum of cardiovascular syndromes including acute pericarditis, chronic constrictive pericardial disease, valvular heart disease, and myocardial dysfunction with restrictive cardiomyopathy. There is no defined threshold level below which radiation therapy is safe to the cardiovascular system. Modification of radiation protocols (including field planning and breath-holding techniques) is currently being done to reduce radiation dose to the cardiovascular system. The challenge in managing these patients is the long latency period between exposure and clinical manifestation, with many affected patients being no longer under the care of a treating oncologist. The 2013 expert consensus by the American Society of Echocardiography and the European Association of Cardiovascular Imaging recommends yearly clinical evaluation, with a history and physical exam, and echocardiogram studies in symptomatic patients. They also recommend a screening echocardiogram at 10 years after chest radiation and every 5 years thereafter. Primary prevention in patients with documented atherosclerosis following radiation therapy includes management of traditional atherosclerotic risk factors (49). Lifelong antiplatelet therapy and statin therapy are recommended for their anti-inflammatory and antithrombotic effects on the irradiated endothelium (94). Radiation-induced scarring makes surgical intervention difficult; hence percutaneous angioplasty with or without stenting is becoming the preferred revascularization method with encouraging results for radiation-induced renal, iliac, and femoral arterial disease (95). Figure 54-16 shows our recommended algorithm for management and monitoring of these patients.

REFERENCES

1. Siegel R, DeSantis C, Virgo K, et al. Cancer treatment and survivorship statistics, 2012. *CA Cancer J Clin*. 2012;62(4):220-241.
2. Ning Y, Shen Q, Herrick K, et al. Cause of death in cancer survivors [abstract]. *Cancer Res*. 2012;72:LB–339.
3. McMullen JR, Boey EJ, Ooi JY, Seymour JF, Keating MJ, Tam CS. Ibrutinib increases the risk of atrial fibrillation, potentially through inhibition of cardiac PI3K-Akt signaling. *Blood*. 2014;124(25):3829-3830.

4. Sawyer DB, Zuppinger C, Miller TA, Eppenberger HM, Suter TM. Modulation of anthracycline-induced myofibrillar disarray in rat ventricular myocytes by neuregulin-1beta and anti-erbB2: potential mechanism for trastuzumab-induced cardiotoxicity. *Circulation*. 2002;105(13):1551-1554.
5. Zhang S, Liu X, Bawa-Khalfe T, et al. Identification of the molecular basis of doxorubicin-induced cardiotoxicity. *Nat Med*. 2012;18(11):1639-1642.
6. Gao R, Zhang J, Cheng L, et al. A phase II, randomized, double-blind, multicenter, based on standard therapy, placebo-controlled study of the efficacy and safety of recombinant human neuregulin-1 in patients with chronic heart failure. *J Am Coll Cardiol*. 2010;55(18):1907-1914.
7. Blanco J, Muriel-Bombin A, Sagredo V, et al. Incidence, organ dysfunction and mortality in severe sepsis: a Spanish multicentre study. *Crit Care*. 2008;12(6):R158.
8. Romero-Bermejo FJ, Ruiz-Bailen M, Gil-Cebrian J, Huertos-Ranchal MJ. Sepsis-induced cardiomyopathy. *Curr Cardiol Rev*. 2011;7(3):163-183.
9. Merx MW, Weber C. Sepsis and the heart. *Circulation*. 2007;116(7):793-802.
10. Hauck AJ, Kearney DL, Edwards WD. Evaluation of postmortem endomyocardial biopsy specimens from 38 patients with lymphocytic myocarditis: implications for role of sampling error. *Mayo Clin Proc*. 1989;64(10):1235-1245.
11. Robinson JL, Hartling L, Crumley E, Vandermeer B, Klassen TP. A systematic review of intravenous gamma globulin for therapy of acute myocarditis. *BMC Cardiovasc Disord*. 2005;5(1):12.
12. Seidman A, Hudis C, Pierri MK, et al. Cardiac dysfunction in the trastuzumab clinical trials experience. *J Clin Oncol*. 2002;20(5):1215-1221.
13. Friedman MA, Bozdech MJ, Billingham ME, Rider AK. Doxorubicin cardiotoxicity. Serial endomyocardial biopsies and systolic time intervals. *JAMA*. 1978;240(15):1603-1606.
14. Swain SM, Whaley FS, Ewer MS. Congestive heart failure in patients treated with doxorubicin: a retrospective analysis of three trials. *Cancer*. 2003;97(11):2869-2879.
15. Felker GM, Thompson RE, Hare JM, et al. Underlying causes and long-term survival in patients with initially unexplained cardiomyopathy. *N Engl J Med*. 2000;342(15):1077-1084.
16. Link G, Tirosh R, Pinson A, Hershko C. Role of iron in the potentiation of anthracycline cardiotoxicity: identification of heart cell mitochondria as a major site of iron-anthracycline interaction. *J Lab Clin Med*. 1996;127(3):272-278.
17. Vejpongsa P, Yeh ETH. Topoisomerase 2[beta]: a promising molecular target for primary prevention of anthracycline-induced cardiotoxicity. *Clin Pharmacol Ther*. 2014;95(1):45-52.
18. Cardinale D, Colombo A, Lamantia G, et al. Anthracycline-induced cardiomyopathy: clinical relevance and response to pharmacologic therapy. *J Am Coll Cardiol*. 2010;55(3):213-220.
19. Plana JC, Galderisi M, Barac A, et al. Expert consensus for multimodality imaging evaluation of adult patients during and after cancer therapy: a report from the American Society of Echocardiography and the European Association of Cardiovascular Imaging. *J Am Soc Echocardiogr*. 2014;27(9):911-939.
20. Valdivieso M, Burgess MA, Ewer MS, et al. Increased therapeutic index of weekly doxorubicin in the therapy of non-small cell lung cancer: a prospective, randomized study. *J Clin Oncol*. 1984;2(3):207-214.
21. Bosch X, Rovira M, Sitges M, et al. Enalapril and carvedilol for preventing chemotherapy-induced left ventricular systolic dysfunction in patients with malignant hemopathies: the OVERCOME trial (preventiOn of left Ventricular dysfunction with Enalapril and caRvedilol in patients submitted to intensive ChemOtherapy for the treatment of Malignant hEmopathies). *J Am Coll Cardiol*. 2013;61(23):2355-2362.
22. Kalay N, Basar E, Ozdogru I, et al. Protective effects of carvedilol against anthracycline-induced cardiomyopathy. *J Am Coll Cardiol*. 2006;48(11):2258-2262.
23. Ewer MS, Lippman SM. Type II chemotherapy-related cardiac dysfunction: time to recognize a new entity. *J Clin Oncol*. 2005;23(13):2900-2902.
24. Ewer MS, Vooletich MT, Durand JB, et al. Reversibility of trastuzumab-related cardiotoxicity: new insights based on clinical course and response to medical treatment. *J Clin Oncol*. 2005;23(31):7820-7826.
25. Romond EH, Jeong JH, Rastogi P, et al. Seven-year follow-up assessment of cardiac function in NSABP B-31, a randomized trial comparing doxorubicin and cyclophosphamide followed by paclitaxel (ACP) with ACP plus trastuzumab as adjuvant therapy for patients with node-positive, human epidermal growth factor receptor 2-positive breast cancer. *J Clin Oncol*. 2012;30(31):3792-3799.
26. Kerkela R, Woulfe KC, Durand JB, et al. Sunitinib-induced cardiotoxicity is mediated by off-target inhibition of AMP-activated protein kinase. *Clin Transl Sci*. 2009;2(1):15-25.
27. Chu TF, Rupnick MA, Kerkela R, et al. Cardiotoxicity associated with tyrosine kinase inhibitor sunitinib. *Lancet*. 2007;370(9604):2011-2019.
28. Khakoo AY, Kassiotis CM, Tannir N, et al. Heart failure associated with sunitinib malate: a multitargeted receptor tyrosine kinase inhibitor. *Cancer*. 2008;112(11):2500-2508.
29. Di Lorenzo G, Autorino R, Bruni G, et al. Cardiovascular toxicity following sunitinib therapy in metastatic renal cell carcinoma: a multicenter analysis. *Ann Oncol*. 2009;20(9):1535-1542.
30. Schmidinger M, Zielinski CC, Vogl UM, et al. Cardiac toxicity of sunitinib and sorafenib in patients with metastatic renal cell carcinoma. *J Clin Oncol*. 2008;26(32):5204-5212.
31. Telli ML, Witteles RM, Fisher GA, Srinivas S. Cardiotoxicity associated with the cancer therapeutic agent sunitinib malate. *Ann Oncol*. 2008;19(9):1613-1618.
32. Yancy CW, Jessup M, Bozkurt B, et al. 2013 ACCF/AHA guideline for the management of heart failure: a report of the American College of Cardiology Foundation/American Heart Association Task Force on Practice Guidelines. *J Am Coll Cardiol*. 2013;62(16):e147-e239.
33. Khorana AA, Francis CW, Culakova E, Fisher RI, Kuderer NM, Lyman GH. Thromboembolism in hospitalized neutropenic cancer patients. *J Clin Oncol*. 2006;24(3):484-490.
34. Khorana AA, Francis CW, Blumberg N, Culakova E, Refaai MA, Lyman GH. Blood transfusions, thrombosis, and mortality in hospitalized patients with cancer. *Arch Intern Med*. 2008;168(21):2377-2381.
35. Khorana AA, Francis CW, Culakova E, Kuderer NM, Lyman GH. Thromboembolism is a leading cause of death in cancer patients receiving outpatient chemotherapy. *J Thromb Haemost*. 2007;5(3):632-634.
36. Naschitz JE, Yeshurun D, Abrahamson J. Arterial occlusive disease in occult cancer. *Am Heart J*. 1992;124(3):738-745.
37. Chow SF, McKenna CH. Ovarian cancer and gangrene of the digits: case report and review of the literature. *Mayo Clinic Proc*. 1996;71(3):253-258.
38. Mouhayar E, Tayar J, Fasulo M, et al. Outcome of acute limb ischemia in cancer patients. *Vasc Med*. 2014;19(2):112-117.
39. Rossi C, Randi ML, Zerbinati P, Rinaldi V, Girolami A. Acute coronary disease in essential thrombocythemia and polycythemia vera. *J Intern Med*. 1998;244(1):49-53.
40. Marchioli R, Finazzi G, Landolfi R, et al. Vascular and neoplastic risk in a large cohort of patients with polycythemia vera. *J Clin Oncol*. 2005;23(10):2224-2232.
41. Landolfi R, Di Gennaro L, Falanga A. Thrombosis in myeloproliferative disorders: pathogenetic facts and speculation. *Leukemia*. 2008;22(11):2020-2028.

42. Harrison CN, Campbell PJ, Buck G, et al. Hydroxyurea compared with anagrelide in high-risk essential thrombocythemia. *N Engl J Med*. 2005;353(1):33-45.
43. De Stefano V, Sora F, Rossi E, et al. The risk of thrombosis in patients with acute leukemia: occurrence of thrombosis at diagnosis and during treatment. *J Thromb Haemost*. 2005;3(9):1985-1992.
44. Roberts WC, Waller BF. Cardiac amyloidosis causing cardiac dysfunction: analysis of 54 necropsy patients. *Am J Cardiol*. 1983;52(1):137-146.
45. Feng D, Edwards WD, Oh JK, et al. Intracardiac thrombosis and embolism in patients with cardiac amyloidosis. *Circulation*. 2007;116(21):2420-2426.
46. Berghoff M, Kathpal M, Khan F, Skinner M, Falk R, Freeman R. Endothelial dysfunction precedes C-fiber abnormalities in primary (AL) amyloidosis. *Ann Neurol*. 2003;53(6):725-730.
47. Liao R, Jain M, Teller P, et al. Infusion of light chains from patients with cardiac amyloidosis causes diastolic dysfunction in isolated mouse hearts. *Circulation*. 2001;104(14):1594-1597.
48. Browne RS, Schneiderman H, Kayani N, Radford MJ, Hager WD. Amyloid heart disease manifested by systemic arterial thromboemboli. *Chest*. 1992;102(1):304-307.
49. Yood RA, Skinner M, Rubinow A, Talarico L, Cohen AS. Bleeding manifestations in 100 patients with amyloidosis. *JAMA*. 1983;249(10):1322-1324.
50. Walsh J, Wheeler HR, Geczy CL. Modulation of tissue factor on human monocytes by cisplatin and adriamycin. *Br J Haematol*. 1992;81(4):480-488.
51. Numico G, Garrone O, Dongiovanni V, et al. Prospective evaluation of major vascular events in patients with nonsmall cell lung carcinoma treated with cisplatin and gemcitabine. *Cancer*. 2005;103(5):994-999.
52. Grenader T, Shavit L, Ospovat I, Gutfeld O, Peretz T. Aortic occlusion in patients treated with cisplatin-based chemotherapy. *Mt Sinai J Med*. 2006;73(5):810-812.
53. Alter P, Herzum M, Soufi M, Schaefer JR, Maisch B. Cardiotoxicity of 5-fluorouracil. *Cardiovasc Hematol Agents Med Chem*. 2006;4(1):1-5.
54. Dasanu CA. Gemcitabine: vascular toxicity and prothrombotic potential. *Expert Opin Drug Saf*. 2008;7(6):703-716.
55. Fanelli M, Sarmiento R, Gattuso D, et al. Thalidomide: a new anticancer drug? *Expert Opin Investig Drugs*. 2003;12(7):1211-1225.
56. Baz R, Li L, Kottke-Marchant K, et al. The role of aspirin in the prevention of thrombotic complications of thalidomide and anthracycline-based chemotherapy for multiple myeloma. *Mayo Clin Proc*. 2005;80(12):1568-1574.
57. Libourel EJ, Sonneveld P, van der Holt B, de Maat MP, Leebeek FW. High incidence of arterial thrombosis in young patients treated for multiple myeloma: results of a prospective cohort study. *Blood*. 2010;116(1):22-26.
58. Pereg D, Lishner M. Bevacizumab treatment for cancer patients with cardiovascular disease: a double edged sword? *Eur Heart J*. 2008;29(19):2325-2326.
59. Grivas AA, Trafalis DT, Athanassiou AE. Implication of bevacizumab in fatal arterial thromboembolic incidents. *J BUON*. 2009;14(1):115-117.
60. Yoon S, Schmassmann-Suhijar D, Zuber M, Konietzny P, Schmassmann A. Chemotherapy with bevacizumab, irinotecan, 5-fluorouracil and leucovorin (IFL) associated with a large, embolizing thrombus in the thoracic aorta. *Ann Oncol*. 2006;17(12):1851-1852.
61. Ferrara N. Vascular endothelial growth factor: basic science and clinical progress. *Endocr Rev*. 2004;25(4):581-611.
62. Kilickap S, Abali H, Celik I. Bevacizumab, bleeding, thrombosis, and warfarin. *J Clin Oncol*. 2003;21(18):3542; author reply 3543.
63. Scappaticci FA, Skillings JR, Holden SN, et al. Arterial thromboembolic events in patients with metastatic carcinoma treated with chemotherapy and bevacizumab. *J Natl Cancer Inst*. 2007;99(16):1232-1239.
64. Choueiri TK, Schutz FA, Je Y, Rosenberg JE, Bellmunt J. Risk of arterial thromboembolic events with sunitinib and sorafenib: a systematic review and meta-analysis of clinical trials. *J Clin Oncol*. 2010;28(13):2280-2285.
65. Bair SM, Choueiri TK, Moslehi J. Cardiovascular complications associated with novel angiogenesis inhibitors: emerging evidence and evolving perspectives. *Trends Cardiovasc Med*. 2013;23(4):104-113.
66. Landolfi R, Marchioli R, Kutti J, et al. Efficacy and safety of low-dose aspirin in polycythemia vera. *N Engl J Med*. 2004;350(2):114-124.
67. Iliescu C, Durand JB, Kroll M. Cardiovascular interventions in thrombocytopenic cancer patients. *Tex Heart Inst J*. 2011;38(3):259-260.
68. Shen H, Guo JH. [ACC/AHA/ESC treatment guideline for supraventricular arrhythmia]. *Zhongguo Wei Zhong Bing Ji Jiu Yi Xue*. 2004;16(9):513-514.
69. Hirsch AT, Haskal ZJ, Hertzer NR, et al. ACC/AHA 2005 practice guidelines for the management of patients with peripheral arterial disease (lower extremity, renal, mesenteric, and abdominal aortic): a collaborative report from the American Association for Vascular Surgery/Society for Vascular Surgery, Society for Cardiovascular Angiography and Interventions, Society for Vascular Medicine and Biology, Society of Interventional Radiology, and the ACC/AHA Task Force on Practice Guidelines (Writing Committee to Develop Guidelines for the Management of Patients With Peripheral Arterial Disease): endorsed by the American Association of Cardiovascular and Pulmonary Rehabilitation; National Heart, Lung, and Blood Institute; Society for Vascular Nursing; TransAtlantic Inter-Society Consensus; and Vascular Disease Foundation. *Circulation*. 2006;113(11):e463-e654.
70. Robertson D, Hollister AS, Biaggioni I, Netterville JL, Mosqueda-Garcia R, Robertson RM. The diagnosis and treatment of baroreflex failure. *N Engl J Med*. 1993;329(20):1449-1455.
71. Farmakis D, Parissis J, Filippatos G. Insights into onco-cardiology: atrial fibrillation in cancer. *J Am Coll Cardiol*. 2014;63(10):945-953.
72. Guzzetti S, Costantino G, Sada S, Fundaro C. Colorectal cancer and atrial fibrillation: a case-control study. *Am J Med*. 2002;112(7):587-588.
73. Imperatori A, Mariscalco G, Riganti G, Rotolo N, Conti V, Dominioni L. Atrial fibrillation after pulmonary lobectomy for lung cancer affects long-term survival in a prospective single-center study. *J Cardiothorac Surg*. 2012;7:4.
74. Bhave PD, Goldman LE, Vittinghoff E, Maselli J, Auerbach A. Incidence, predictors, and outcomes associated with postoperative atrial fibrillation after major noncardiac surgery. *Am Heart J*. 2012;164(6):918-924.
75. Imazio M, Brucato A, Cemin R, et al. A randomized trial of colchicine for acute pericarditis. *N Engl J Med*. 2013;369(16):1522-1528.
76. Maisch B, Seferovic PM, Ristic AD, et al. Guidelines on the diagnosis and management of pericardial diseases executive summary; the task force on the diagnosis and management of pericardial diseases of the European Society of Cardiology. *Eur Heart J*. 2004;25(7):587-610.
77. Imazio M, Brucato A, Cemin R, et al. Colchicine for recurrent pericarditis (CORP): a randomized trial. *Ann Intern Med*. 2011;155(7):409-414.
78. Imazio M, Bobbio M, Cecchi E, et al. Colchicine in addition to conventional therapy for acute pericarditis: results of the COlchicine for acute PEricarditis (COPE) trial. *Circulation*. 2005;112(13):2012-2016.
79. McDonald JM, Meyers BF, Guthrie TJ, Battafarano RJ, Cooper JD, Patterson GA. Comparison of open subxiphoid pericardial drainage with percutaneous catheter drainage for symptomatic pericardial effusion. *Ann Thorac Surg*. 2003;76(3):811-815;

discussion 816.

80. Sagrista-Sauleda J, Angel J, Permanyer-Miralda G, Soler-Soler J. Long-term follow-up of idiopathic chronic pericardial effusion. *N Engl J Med.* 1999;341(27):2054-2059.
81. Karatolios K, Maisch B, Pankuweit S. [Tumor markers in the assessment of malignant and benign pericardial effusion]. *Herz.* 2011;36(4):290-295.
82. Tsang TS, Seward JB, Barnes ME, et al. Outcomes of primary and secondary treatment of pericardial effusion in patients with malignancy. *Mayo Clin Proc.* 2000;75(3):248-253.
83. Manoukian G, Mouhayar E, LeBeau J, et al. Cardiac tamponade in cancer patients with severe thrombocytopenia-management and outcomes. In: *Society for Cardiovascular Angiography and Interventions Scientific Sessions.* Washington, DC: Society for Cardiovascular Angiography and Interventions; 2013.
84. Meinardi MT, Gietema JA, van der Graaf WT, et al. Cardiovascular morbidity in long-term survivors of metastatic testicular cancer. *J Clin Oncol.* 2000;18(8):1725-1732.
85. Escudier B, Eisen T, Stadler WM, et al. Sorafenib in advanced clear-cell renal-cell carcinoma. *N Engl J Med.* 2007; 356(2):125-134.
86. Rossi GP, Seccia TM, Maniero C, Pessina AC. Drug-related hypertension and resistance to antihypertensive treatment: a call for action. *J Hypertens.* 2011;29(12):2295-2309.
87. Aparicio-Gallego G, Afonso-Afonso FJ, Leon-Mateos L, et al. Molecular basis of hypertension side effects induced by sunitinib. *Anticancer Drugs.* 2011;22(1):1-8.
88. Rini BI, Cohen DP, Lu DR, et al. Hypertension as a biomarker of efficacy in patients with metastatic renal cell carcinoma treated with sunitinib. *J Natl Cancer Inst.* 2011;103(9):763-773.
89. Maitland ML, Bakris GL, Black HR, et al. Initial assessment, surveillance, and management of blood pressure in patients receiving vascular endothelial growth factor signaling pathway inhibitors. *J Natl Cancer Inst.* 2010;102(9):596-604.
90. Cole SW, Sood AK. Molecular pathways: beta-adrenergic signaling in cancer. *Clin Cancer Res.* 2012;18(5):1201-1206.
91. Jurado JA, Bashir R, Burket MW. Radiation-induced peripheral artery disease. *Catheter Cardiovasc Interv.* 2008;72(4):563-568.
92. Riley PA. Free radicals in biology: oxidative stress and the effects of ionizing radiation. *Int J Radiat Biol.* 1994;65(1):27-33.
93. Weintraub NL, Jones WK, Manka D. Understanding radiation-induced vascular disease. *J Am Coll Cardiol.* 2010;55(12):1237-1239.
94. Gaugler MH, Vereycken-Holler V, Squiban C, Vandamme M, Vozenin-Brotons MC, Benderitter M. Pravastatin limits endothelial activation after irradiation and decreases the resulting inflammatory and thrombotic responses. *Radiat Res.* 2005;163(5):479-487.
95. Jurado J, Thompson PD. Prevention of coronary artery disease in cancer patients. *Pediatr Blood Cancer.* 2005;44(7):620-624.

55 Pulmonary Complications of Cancer Therapy

第五十五章　癌症治疗的肺部并发症

Saadia A. Faiz
Horiana B. Grosu
Vickie R. Shannon

中文导读

本章主要回顾了与癌症及其治疗相关的肺部并发症。首先概述了其常见的疾病模式、易感因素和有效的治疗模式。本章分别介绍了化疗所致肺损伤、放疗引起的肺损伤、干细胞移植导致的非感染性肺部并发症、血管疾病、恶性中央气道阻塞以及癌症本身相关的胸膜疾病及癌症治疗引起的睡眠障碍。化疗所致肺损伤部分包括：间质性肺炎、过敏性肺炎、非心源性肺水肿和弥漫性肺泡损害/急性呼吸窘迫综合征、胸腔积液、肺血管疾病、呼吸道疾病和药物所致呼吸道疾病。在间质性肺炎部分，简述了病因、后期发展的不良结果，重点分析了博来霉素引起间质性肺炎的机制及治疗。在过敏性肺炎部分，阐述了病因、易发时间及治疗方法。在非心源性肺水肿和弥漫性肺泡损害/急性呼吸窘迫综合征部分，描述了两者的关系、背景、病因及其治疗建议。在肺血管疾病部分，描述了静脉血栓栓塞和肺动脉高压的风险因素及治疗推荐。在呼吸道疾病部分，描述了药物可能引起的输液反应，并介绍其诱发因素和预防措施。在放疗所致肺损伤部分，介绍了病因、疾病特征和治疗。在造血干细胞移植引起的非感染性肺并发症部分，分别描述了早期和晚期的风险因素、临床症状及治疗。在血管疾病部分，介绍了静脉血栓栓塞症病因、诊断、预防和治疗。在恶性中央气道阻塞部分，简介了常见症状，病因及治疗。在胸膜疾病部分，对复发性恶性胸腔积液的检查诊断及其治疗处理提供了可选方式。本章最后对癌症引起的睡眠障碍进行分析，介绍了病因和治疗思路。

Chest medicine is inextricably intertwined with cancer medicine as a result of the propensity for cancer therapy or the disease itself to affect the lungs. Pulmonary complications in the cancer patient may manifest as injury to the pulmonary interstitium, alveolar-capillary membrane, pleura, pulmonary circulation, or airways, or, alternatively, may involve multiple intrathoracic structures. This chapter will review cancer-related pulmonary complications, including lung toxicities associated with aggressive chemotherapy and radiotherapy regimens, noninfectious lung disorders arising in the post–stem cell transplant setting, and cancer-related pleural disease, pulmonary vascular disease, and sleep disorders. The focus of this review is to identify, discuss, and provide practical algorithms for the diagnosis and treatment of these complications with emphasis on those issues in which early diagnosis may have a significant impact on patient management and outcome.

CHEMOTHERAPY-INDUCED LUNG INJURY

Injury to the lung due to cancer therapy results in stereotyped histopathologic disease patterns and syndromes (Tables 55-1 and 55-2). Lung toxicity has been described following exposure to conventional chemotherapy as well as molecularly targeted agents and immune modulators. Interstitial and alveolar lung injury patterns are the most frequent. Pleural effusions, pulmonary vascular disease, and, less frequently, drug-induced granulomatous disease and lymphadenopathy have also been described. In addition to direct lung injury, chemotherapy-induced immune suppression may predispose patients to life-threatening pneumonias.

The diagnosis of drug-induced lung injury is hampered by the frequent use of multiagent and multimodality therapies. In addition, overlapping clinical, radiographic, and pathologic manifestations of lung injury caused by infections, aspiration, cancer relapse, radiation, and cancer-induced cardiac disease confound clinical distinctions between these entities and render precise estimates of drug-induced lung injury (DILI) difficult. Other conditions that may mimic DILI include pneumonia, aspiration pneumonitis, diffuse alveolar hemorrhage, and cardiogenic pulmonary edema [1, 2]. Predisposing factors, such as older age, cumulative dose, concomitant or sequential radiotherapy, oxygen administration, prior lung injury, and the use of multidrug regimens, not only increase the risk of DILI, but also may shorten the latency period between drug exposure and the development of clinical symptoms.

The diagnosis of DILI is suggested by a temporal association between drug exposure and the development of compatible clinical, radiographic, and laboratory evidence of lung injury, coupled with the exclusion of competing diagnoses. Interstitial and mixed alveolar-interstitial opacities, manifested as ground-glass opacities, reticular lines, septal thickening, and mosaic attenuation, typically localize to the peripheral and lower lung zones on chest imaging studies. Upper lobe predominant disease may be seen with hypersensitivity reactions and be accompanied by skin rash and wheezing. Bronchoscopy with performance of bronchoalveolar lavage (BAL) and/or transbronchial biopsies may be helpful in excluding infection or background disease. For example, findings of BAL eosinophilia of greater than 25% are supportive of drug-induced eosinophilic pneumonia. Increased numbers of hemosiderin-laden macrophages on BAL fluid and/or progressively bloody saline aliquots on sequential BAL samples is supportive of diffuse alveolar hemorrhage. A BAL lymphocytosis of greater than 50% with decreased CD4/CD8 ratios on BAL fluid is suggestive of interstitial lung disease; however, these findings are not sufficient to distinguish interstitial lung disease caused by drug toxicity from other causes. Although none of these histopathologic findings are pathognomonic of DILI, a few drugs produce characteristic patterns of involvement. For example, methotrexate, ipilimumab, everolimus, and interferon-γ may cause an acute granulomatous inflammation that mimics opportunistic infection. Histopathologic changes consistent with bronchiolitis obliterans with organizing pneumonia may be seen after exposure to several drugs, including bleomycin, cyclophosphamide, cetuximab, panitumumab, thalidomide, bortezomib, interferon-γ, and methotrexate (Table 55-3).

Clinical manifestations drug-induced interstitial lung disease include low-grade fever, dry cough, and dyspnea, which typically develop insidiously, usually within weeks to a few months after initiation of the first or subsequent cycles of therapy [3, 4]. Pulmonary fibrosis may immediately ensue or occur as a late manifestation of DILI months to years after exposure to some agents, such as bleomycin, busulfan, cyclophosphamide, gemcitabine, and carmustine (BCNU). Bronchospasm and allergic reactions are common manifestations of infusion reactions, which typically occur within minutes to hours of therapy.

Evidence-based guidelines in the management of DILI are limited. In most cases, drug withdrawal is recommended once sufficient evidence to implicate the culprit agent with pneumotoxicity is established. Systemic corticosteroids have proven efficacy in the treatment of DILI patterns such as hypersensitivity pneumonitis, eosinophilic pneumonia, and bronchiolitis obliterans organizing pneumonia. In other

Table 55-1 Histopathologic Patterns of Lung Injury Following Conventional Chemotherapy

	Agent Class						
Pulmonary Syndrome	**Alkylating Agents**	**Antimetabolites**	**Cytotoxic Antibiotics**	**Topoisomerase Inhibitors**	**Podophyllotoxins**	**Taxanes Microtubule Inhibitors**	**Other**
Parenchymal Disease							
Interstitial pneumonitis/ pulmonary fibrosis	Busulfan BCNU CCNU Cyclophosphamide Ifosphamide Temazolamide Oxaliplatin Melphalan	Methotrexate Azathioprine Cytarabine Fludarabine Azacitabine Gemcitabine	Bleomycin Mitomycin C	Topotecan Irinotecan Amrubicin Daunorubicin Liposomal Doxorubicin		Paclitaxel Docetaxel	ATRA Arsenic trioxide Procarbazine
Eosinophilic pneumonia	Busulfan, Cyclophosphamide, oxaliplatin,	Methotrexate Cytarabine Fludarabine Gemcitabine Pentostatin	Bleomycin		Etoposide	Paclitaxel Docetaxel	
DAD/ARDS/NCPE/ DAH	Busulfan, Cyclophosphamide, Ifosphamide, Temazolamide, Oxaliplatin Melphalan	Methotrexate Azathioprine Cytarabine Fludarabine Azacitabine Gemcitabine Pentostatin Pemetrexed Zinostatin	Bleomycin Mitomycin C	Topotecan	Etoposide	Paclitaxel Docetaxel Vincristine Vinblastine Vindesine Vinorelbine Ixabepilone	ATRA Arsenic trioxide
Radiation recall pneumonitis		Gemcitabine	Bleomycin	Amrubicin Daunorubicin Liposomal Doxorubicin		Paclitaxel Docetaxel	
Granuloma formation	Oxaliplatin	Methotrexate					

(*Continued*)

Table 55-1 Histopathologic Patterns of Lung Injury Following Conventional Chemotherapy (Continued)

	Agent Class						
Pulmonary Syndrome	**Alkylating Agents**	**Antimetabolites**	**Cytotoxic Antibiotics**	**Topoisomerase Inhibitors**	**Podophyllotoxins**	**Taxanes Microtubule Inhibitors**	**Other**
Airway Disease							
Infusion reaction/ bronchospasm	Cyclophosphamide Ifosphamide Carboplatin Cisplatin Oxaliplatin	Methotrexate Gemcitabine Pemetrexed	Bleomycin Mitomycin C	Amrubicin Daunorubicin Liposomal Doxorubicin	Etoposide Teniposide	Paclitaxel Docetaxel Vincristine Vinblastine Vindesine Vinorelbine	L-asparaginase
BOOP	Busulfan, Cyclophosphamide Ifosphamide Oxaliplatin	Methotrexate	Bleomycin	Topotecan			L-asparaginase
Vascular Disease							
Pulmonary hypertension		Zinostatin	Bleomycin Mitomycin C				
VTE/DVT							ATRA
Pleural Disease							
Pleural effusion	Cyclophosphamide	Methotrexate Gemcitabine				Docetaxel Paclitaxel	ATRA Arsenic trioxide Procarbazine
Pleural thickening							
Other							
Opportunistic infections	Temozolamide	Methotrexate Fludarabine					
MetHemoglobinemia	Cyclophosphamide Ifosphamide						

ARDS, acute respiratory distress syndrome; ATRA, all-*trans*-retinoic acid; BCNU, carmustine; BOOP, bronchiolitis obliterans organizing pneumonia; CCNU, lomustine; DAD, diffuse alveolar damage; DAH, diffuse alveolar hemorrhage; DVT, deep venous thrombosis; NCPE, noncardiogenic pulmonary edema; VTE, venous thromboembolism.

Table 55-2 Histopathologic Patterns of Lung Injury Following Targeted Therapies

	Agent Class				
Pulmonary Syndrome	**Monoclonal Antibodies**	**Tyrosine Kinase Inhibitors**	**Rapamycin Inhibitors**	**Proteosome Inhibitors**	**Immunomodulators**
Parenchymal Disease					
Interstitial pneumonitis/ pulmonary fibrosis	Cetuximab Panitumumab Alemtuzumab Rituximab	Gefitinib Erlotinib Imatinib Dasatinib Sorafenib Sunitunib Vandetanib Idelalisib Trametinib Crizotinib	Everolimus Temsirolimus	Bortezomib Carlfizomib	Thalidomide IL-2
Eosinophilic Pneumonia					
DAD/ARDS/NCPE/DAH	Cetuximab Panitumumab Alemtuzumab Rituximab Ofatumumab Ibritumomab Trastuzumab Pertuzumab Gemtuzumab	Gefitinib Erlotinib Imatinib Sorafenib Vandetanib Crizotinib Ruxolitinib	Everolimus Temsirolimus	Bortezomib	Thalidomide Lenolidomide
Radiation recall pneumonitis	Panitumumab	Erlotinib Vemurafenib		Bortezomib	
Granuloma formation	Ipilumumab		Everolimus		IFN-γ
Hemoptysis	Bevacizumab Alemtuzumab Rituximab	Sorafenib Sunitunib Pazopanib			IL-2 TNF IFN-γ
Airway Disease					
Infusion reaction/ bronchospasm	Cetuximab Panitumumab Bevacizumab Alemtuzumab Rituximab Obinutuzumab Ofatumumab Ibritumomab Trastuzumab Pertuzumab Gemtuzumab Ipilumumab				
BOOP	Cetuximab Panitumumab			Bortezomib	Thalidomide IFN-γ
Vascular Disease					
Pulmonary hypertension				Bortezomib Carlfizomib	IL-2 IFN-γ
VTE/DVT	Bevacizumab	Dasatinib Ponatinib Pazopanib Crizotinib			Thalidomide Lenolidomide

(Continued)

CHAPTER 55

Table 55-2 Histopathologic Patterns of Lung Injury Following Targeted Therapies (Continued)

	Agent Class				
Pulmonary Syndrome	**Monoclonal Antibodies**	**Tyrosine Kinase Inhibitors**	**Rapamycin Inhibitors**	**Proteosome Inhibitors**	**Immunomodulators**
Pleural Disease					
Pleural effusion	Panitumumab	Imatinib Dasatinib Bosutinib			IL-2 IFN-γ
Pleural Thickening					
Other					
Opportunistic infections	Ofatumumab Ibritumomab	Idelalisib Trametinib Crizotinib Vemurafenib Ruxolitinib	Everolimus		
MetHemoglobinemia					

ARDS, acute respiratory distress syndrome; BOOP, bronchiolitis obliterans organizing pneumonia; DAD, diffuse alveolar damage; DAH, diffuse alveolar hemorrhage; DVT, deep venous thrombosis; IFN, interferon; IL-2, interleukin-2; NCPE, noncardiogenic pulmonary edema; TNF, tumor necrosis factor; VTE, venous thromboembolism.

Table 55-3 Cytologic and Histopathologic Changes on BAL or Lung Tissue Biopsies and Suggested Diagnosis

Suggested Diagnosis	Histopathologic Findings
Eosinophilic pneumonia	BAL eosinophilia (>25%)
Diffuse alveolar hemorrhage	Increased hemosiderin-laden macrophages (>20%)
Diffuse alveolar hemorrhage	Progressively bloody saline aliquots on sequential BAL samples
Hypersensitivity pneumonitis	Increased lymphocytes and plasma cell on BAL fluid; variable numbers of giant cells; small, noncaseating granulomas on biopsy specimens
Interstitial lung disease	BAL lymphocytosis (>50%) with decreased CD4/CD8 ratio; interstitial fibrosis, destruction of type I pneumocytes with proliferation of type II pneumocytes following some drug exposures
Bronchiolitis obliterans with organized pneumonia	Organized polypoid inflammatory granulation tissue in the small airways
Sarcoid-like reactions/ Granulomatous pneumonitis	Granulomatous inflammation without necrosis

BAL, bronchoalveolar lavage.

entities (pulmonary fibrosis, bronchiolitis obliterans), no beneficial role has been established. Steroid therapy should be considered in patients with progressive, steroid-responsive, and/or advanced-stage lung injury patterns. No guidelines for corticosteroid management in DILI are currently available. General recommendations include starting doses of prednisone at 40 to 60 mg or weight-based dosing at 0.75 to 1 mg/kg daily with tapers over a 1- to 3-month time period, pending response to therapy. With few exceptions (see below), drug rechallenge is not recommended. Several of the specific drugs causing DILI deserve separate mention and are discussed below.

Interstitial Lung Disease

Nonspecific interstitial pneumonitis (NSIP) is the most common morphologic pattern of interstitial lung disease. Dry cough and progressive dyspnea develop insidiously, over weeks to months following drug exposure. Radiographic findings may include pleural-based, lower lobe ground-glass attenuations, reticular lines, mosaic patterns, and nodules. Injury to epithelial and endothelial cells leads to alveolar edema and diffuse alveolar damage early on, which may progress to end-stage fibrotic lung disease, despite drug withdrawal and corticosteroid therapy.

Bleomycin-induced interstitial pneumonitis (BIP) has been well studied. This cytotoxic antibiotic is widely used in the treatment of germ cell tumors, lymphomas, and a variety of squamous cell carcinomas, particularly those of head and neck and esophageal origin. The lungs and skin are targets of bleomycin-induced lung injury due to the lack of the inactivating enzyme, bleomycin hydrolase, in these two organ systems. Bleomycin-induced interstitial pneumonitis is the most common pattern of bleomycin lung injury, occurring in up to 20% of treated patients, typically 4 to 10 weeks after bleomycin administration (Fig. 55-1) ([5]). Risk factors for BIP include age greater than 70 years, cumulative dose greater than 400 U, concomitant or sequential radiation therapy, uremia, multiagent therapy, and high inspired oxygen administration ([6, 7]). Evidence suggesting an association between hyperoxia and increased BIP risk and/or severity is largely anecdotal. Questions regarding the threshold dose of oxygen and duration of oxygen therapy that confer an increased risk of bleomycin lung toxicity are unknown. In addition, the latency period between bleomycin and high oxygen exposure that mitigates the risk of increased toxicity has not been established. Nonetheless, general recommendations regarding supplemental oxygen therapy in bleomycin-exposed patients includes titration to achieve oxygen saturations at or above 89% to 92%. Declining values of diffusing capacity of the lung for carbon monoxide (DL_{CO}) are thought to be early markers of bleomycin lung injury, although threshold cut-offs for drug withdrawal based on declining DL_{CO} have not been established. Pulmonary function tests (PFTs) with DLCO should be considered in patients with known lung disease and/or abnormal lung function at baseline. Serial monitoring of DL_{CO} is recommended as cumulative doses of bleomycin approach 400 U. Drug withdrawal is the mainstay of therapy with or without the institution of corticosteroids. The grade of pneumotoxicity should be used to guide the need for corticosteroid therapy. In patients with moderate (grade 2 or greater) interstitial pneumonitis, prednisone dosed at 0.75 to 1 mg/kg/d or its equivalent is recommended.

Rates of DILI following BCNU approach 50% among patients receiving cumulative doses of this drug in excess of 1,500 mg/m^2. Carmustine toxicity is unique in its predilection for middle and upper lobe disease, which may occur years after BCNU exposure. Late-onset pneumonitis and fibrosis have also been described following cyclophosphamide and busulfan administration. Gemcitabine and paclitaxel are also known causes of interstitial pneumonitis, which may be fatal in some cases. Among the molecular targeted therapies, the mammalian target of rapamycin (mTOR) inhibitors (everolimus, temsirolimus) and epidermal growth factor receptor (EGFR) inhibitors (gefitinib, erlotinib, cetuximab, panitumumab) are most frequently implicated in the development of interstitial pneumonitis ([8-11]).

Hypersensitivity Pneumonitis

Hypersensitivity pneumonitis (HP)-like reactions typically occur after repeated drug exposure to an offending agent Associated symptoms of fever dyspnea, dry cough, and rash typically occur over the first 3 to 4 weeks following drug exposure and may wax and wane without adjustments in therapy. Poorly formed granulomas and BAL lymphocytosis are common histopathologic findings. Upper lobe predominant disease is characteristic, particularly in chronic forms of the disease. Methotrexate is the prototype agent associated with HP, which may develop following oral, intravenous, intrathecal, and intramuscular routes of methotrexate administration. Drug withdrawal and steroid therapy typically produce favorable outcomes, with complete resolution of clinical signs and symptoms in most cases.

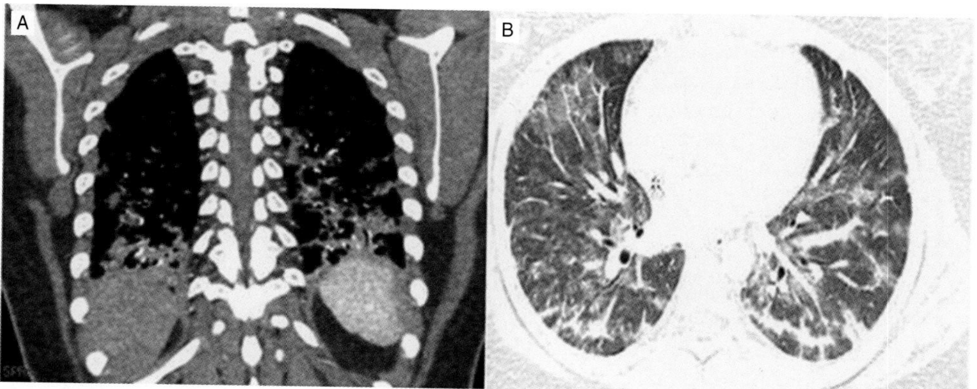

FIGURE 55-1 Bleomycin lung injury. A 26-year-old woman with progressive shortness of breath, hypoxia, and decline in diffusing capacity of the lung for carbon monoxide on lung function testing following the fifth cycle of bleomycin-based chemotherapy for Hodgkin lymphoma. Sagittal (A) and standard (B) views on chest computed tomography imaging showed bilateral, lower lobe predominant ground-glass opacities and parenchymal consolidation. Bronchoalveolar lavage cultures showed no growth. The patient was treated with high-dose steroids for presumed bleomycin-induced lung injury but succumbed to respiratory failure.

Noncardiogenic Pulmonary Edema and Diffuse Alveolar Damage/Acute Respiratory Distress Syndrome

Drug-induced injury to the alveolar-capillary membranes may result in capillary leak and a permeability (noncardiogenic) pulmonary edema. Acute respiratory distress syndrome (ARDS) and its histologic hallmark, diffuse alveolar damage (DAD), may ensue as the disease progresses. These reactions may be unrelated to drug dosage or duration of therapy. Busulfan, bleomycin, cyclophosphamide, molecularly targeted agents (gefitinib, erlotinib, cetuximab), antilymphocyte monoclonal antibodies (rituximab, alemtuzumab, ofatumumab), and rapamycin inhibitors (everolimus, temsirolimus) are most often implicated in the development of drug-induced noncardiogenic pulmonary edema (NCPE). Noncardiogenic pulmonary edema leading to ARDS has been described following ruxolitinib, a novel JAC1/2 inhibitor, as a result of a cytokine rebound reaction. This reaction is mitigated with the preemptive use of corticosteroids and supportive therapy ([12, 13]). Cytokine storm has also been described following all-*trans*-retinoic acid (ATRA) and arsenic trioxide therapies in the treatment of acute promyelocytic leukemia (APL). The so-called differentiation syndrome occurs in up to 25% of APL patients undergoing induction therapy, which is characterized by potentially fatal NCPE and ARDS. Unlike many of the lung injury processes, in patients with ATRA- and arsenic-related differentiation syndrome, de-escalation of drug dose, rather than drug withdrawal, along with systemic steroid therapy has been associated with successful resolution of toxicity in patients with mild to moderate forms of this syndrome ([14, 15]). Diffuse alveolar hemorrhage (DAH) is typically seen as sequela of alveolar-capillary membrane injury and, thus, in the setting of ARDS/DAD. Occasionally, bland alveolar hemorrhage has been described in the absence of DAD following rituximab and alemtuzumab therapy ([12, 16]). Massive, and sometimes fatal, bleeding has been reported during bevacizumab therapy for treatment of central airway tumors ([17]).

Pleural Effusions

Drug-induced pleural effusions may occur as an isolated toxicity to the pleura (following methotrexate, dasatinib, bosutinib, docetaxel, ATRA, or granulocyte colony-stimulating factor [GCSF] administration) or as a manifestation of a generalized pleuroparenchymal abnormality ([18, 19]). These small to moderate-sized effusions are typically exudative and lymphocyte predominant and may be unilateral or bilateral. Withdrawal of the offending agent may result in spontaneous resolution in some cases.

Pulmonary Vascular Disorders

The development of thromboembolic disease, pulmonary hypertension, and pulmonary veno-occlusive disease (PVOD) has been described following conventional chemotherapeutic, molecularly targeted, and immune-modulating agents. Increased rates of venous thromboembolism (pulmonary embolism and deep venous thrombosis) have been reported with the ALK inhibitor crizotinib, the Bcr-Abl inhibitor ponatinib, and the vascular endothelial growth factor (VEGF) inhibitors bevacizumab, sunitinib, sorafenib, and pazopanib ([17, 20-23]). In addition, the angiogenesis inhibitors (thalidomide, lenalidomide, pomalidomide) in combination with steroids, doxorubicin, or BCNU are associated with a 14% to 43% increased risk of thromboembolic events. Other agents, including hormonal therapies, growth factors, and erythropoietic agents, contribute to cancer-associated venous thromboembolism. The development of pulmonary arterial hypertension (PAH) has been associated with several drugs, including bleomycin, busulfan, BCNU, interferon, and dasatinib. Severe PAH following dasatinib, a multikinase Bcr-Abl tyrosine kinase inhibitor (TKI) is well described. Once dasatinib-associated PAH develops, drug withdrawal without rechallenge is recommended. There have been no reports of PAH following exposure to the more selective Bcr-Abl–targeted TKIs (imatinib and nilotinib), which may be safely used in dasatinib-induced PAH ([24-27]). Bleomycin and BCNU have also been implicated in the development of PVOD, an irreversible and often fatal form of pulmonary hypertension that is characterized by fibrous obliteration of pulmonary venules.

Drug-Induced Airway Disease

Virtually all chemotherapeutic and targeted agents may trigger an infusion reaction (IR), a sometimes life-threatening acute reaction that may be associated with dry cough, dyspnea, wheezing, chest pain, and hypoxia. Infusion reactions may manifest as IgE-mediated, type 1 hypersensitivity reactions (carboplatin, oxaliplatin, and L-asparaginase) or as anaphylactoid reactions, mediated by cytokine release. The latter reaction is often seen following the administration of many of the monoclonal antibodies (mAbs). Infusion reactions may be triggered by the drug itself or in response to the vehicle in which the drug is formulated. This is particularly true of the taxane class of drugs. For example, paclitaxel is formulated in Cremophor EL, a highly allergenic polyoxyethylated castor oil solvent. Docetaxel is formulated in polysorbate 80. Both vehicles may induce mast cell/basophil activation and subsequent hypersensitivity reaction. Other drugs that are formulated in Cremophor EL (cyclosporine, teniposide, ixabepilone) or polysorbate 80 (etoposide) may trigger similar reactions and should be avoided in patients with a history of IRs following taxane administration ([28, 29]). Histamine receptor antagonists and steroids are recommended as standard prophylaxis prior to taxane administration, which has reduced the incidence of taxane-induced bronchospasm from 30% to 2% ([30, 31]). Infusion reactions may occur within minutes to several hours following drug exposure. Close monitoring during and immediately following drug infusion is critical, as breakthrough IRs may occur despite prophylaxis. Although vinca alkaloids are rarely associated with lung toxicity, severe bronchospasm has been described when these agents are given with concurrent or sequential administration of mitomycin therapy.

RADIATION-INDUCED LUNG INJURY

Clinically significant radiation-induced lung injury (RILI) is the most common dose-limiting complication of thoracic radiation therapy (RT), occurring in 5% to 20% of patients. Recent advances in radiation techniques and delivery systems, such as proton therapy, three-dimensional conformal RT (CRT), intensity-modulated RT (IMRT), and stereotactic body RT (SBRT), purport lower lung injury rates while delivering higher target doses of radiation to the lung. Factors associated with radiation delivery (total radiation dose, dose per fraction, volume of irradiated lung, and beam characteristics and arrangements) as well as clinical factors (preexisting lung disease, underlying poor pulmonary reserve, prior radiotherapy, multimodality regiments, rapid steroid withdrawal) all potentiate the appearance and severity of radiation pneumotoxicity. Radiographically apparent lung injury is common with total doses of radiation that exceed 40 Gy and is rare at doses below 20 Gy ([32, 33]). Hyperfractionated radiation doses delivered to the smallest lung volume is recommended.

Acute clinical radiation pneumonitis, heralded by dyspnea, low-grade fever, and dry cough, develops insidiously over 1 to 3 months after completion of radiation. Radiographic changes typically precede clinical symptoms, appearing 3 to 4 weeks following RT. Discrete ground-glass opacities, ill-defined patchy nodules, or consolidation with air bronchograms and volume loss within the irradiated field are common early findings that evolve over the ensuing 6 to 23 months, leaving a linear scar. Regional fibrosis is seen in nearly all patients, including those without clinical symptoms, and is characterized by the appearance of a well-demarcated area of volume loss, linear densities, bronchiectasis, retraction of the lung parenchyma, tenting and elevation of the hemidiaphragm, and ipsilateral pleural thickening within the irradiated field (Fig. 55-2). Postradiation volume loss, bronchiectasis,

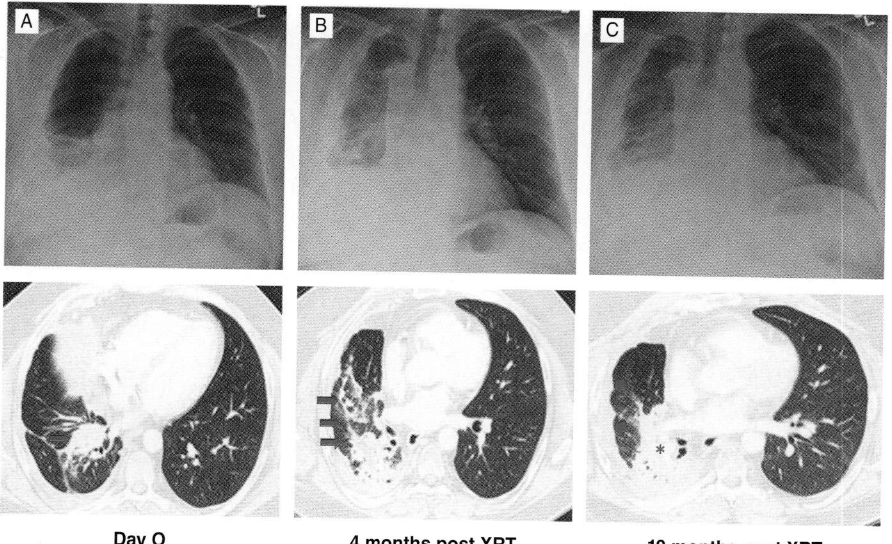

FIGURE 55-2 Radiation-induced lung injury. Chest radiographs (*top row*) and computed tomography (CT) images (*bottom row*) of evolving radiation injury to the lung in a 44-year-old man with primary lung adenocarcinoma. Baseline images **(A)** showed a large right-sided pleural effusion. The right lower lobe mass seen on CT (*arrows*) is obscured by the right-sided pleural effusion and pleural thickening. Ground-glass opacities and dense consolidations within the treatment field are noted 4 months after completing radiation therapy. The pleura appears thickened. Well-demarcated linear areas of consolidation and volume loss are seen and continue to evolve over time (*arrows*) **(B)**. By 10 months after radiotherapy (XRT), further consolidation* and pleural thickening, *volume loss, and radiation fibrosis within the treatment field are seen **(C)**.

and consolidation may occur following the newer modes of RT delivery, but typically are less extensive than injury patterns following conventional radiation.

Radiation recall pneumonitis (RRP) is a rare inflammatory reaction that develops within a previously irradiated field following certain chemotherapy and molecularly targeted therapies. This reaction has been most often observed following taxane- and anthracycline-based therapies. Gemcitabine, etoposide, vinorelbine, trastuzumab, and erlotinib may also trigger this disease [34, 35]. Clinically, RRP is signaled by dry cough, fever, and dyspnea, and accompanied by ground-glass opacities and areas of consolidation that conform to the prior radiation treatment portal. Radiation recall pneumonitis may develop during the first or subsequent course of therapy with the inciting agent, which may be weeks to years following completion of RT. Drug withdrawal and corticosteroid therapy may mitigate symptoms of radiation pneumonitis but have not been shown to be of benefit in the treatment of radiation fibrosis. Drug reintroduction has been successful in some cases [35, 36].

Pleural effusions may develop as early (within 6 months) and late (1–5 years) sequelae of RT. Effusions are typically small and ipsilateral or bilateral. Reactive mesothelial cells with negative pleural fluid cytology are common. Most radiation-induced pleural effusions are asymptomatic, although pleuritic chest pain and dyspnea are occasionally presenting symptoms. Radiation-related organizing pneumonia and eosinophilic pneumonia have been described in patients with breast cancer and may involve nonirradiated areas of the lung [37, 38]. These lung injury patterns are characterized by migratory pulmonary opacities that develop 1 to 3 months after completing RT. A prior history of asthma or atopy, coupled with blood or tissue eosinophilia, supports the diagnosis of radiation-induced eosinophilic pneumonia. Both lung injury patterns are typically steroid responsive.

NONINFECTIOUS PULMONARY COMPLICATIONS OF HEMATOPOIETIC STEM CELL TRANSPLANTATION

Pulmonary complications remain a formidable threat to the success of hematopoietic stem cell transplantation (HSCT). Posttransplant lung injury occurs in up to 60% of patients as a consequence of direct toxicities from conditioning regimens, delayed bone marrow recovery, prolonged immunosuppressive therapy, and graft-versus-host disease (GVHD). Recipients of allogeneic HSCT are at increased risk of infectious complications, due to the increased rates of GVHD and the protracted need for immunosuppressive therapy in this group of patients. Antimicrobial prophylaxis has emerged as a standard protocol following HSCT, effectively reducing the rates of transplant-related infections. Noninfectious pulmonary complications, however, remain a major cause of post-HSCT morbidity and mortality [39, 40]. Infectious and noninfectious pulmonary complications following HSCT are temporally related to immune recovery and the development of GVHD (Fig. 55-3).

Early-onset pulmonary complications occur within the first 100 days after transplant and include diffuse pulmonary edema, DAH, periengraftment respiratory distress syndrome (PERDS), idiopathic pneumonia syndrome (IPS), delayed pulmonary toxicity syndrome, and PVOD. Bronchiolitis obliterans syndrome (BOS), cryptogenic organizing pneumonitis, and posttransplant lymphoproliferative disorder (PTLD) compose the late-onset pulmonary complications, which typically occur more than 100 days after HSCT (Table 55-4). Each of these entities is briefly discussed below.

Early-Onset Noninfectious Pulmonary Complications

Early-onset pulmonary complications are characterized by nonspecific symptoms of acute dyspnea, cough, and fever with associated diffuse pulmonary infiltrates. The exclusion of a competing diagnosis such as infection, cardiac disease, and renal failure along with documentation of diffuse infiltrates are supportive findings. Diffuse pulmonary edema may develop as a result of increased hydrostatic capillary pressure or permeability pulmonary edema and is one of the most common early complications of HSCT. Hydrostatic and permeability etiologies of HSCT may coexist and overlap with other early-onset pulmonary complications, which confounds diagnosis. The diagnosis is supported by diffuse bilateral pulmonary infiltrates with or without bilateral pleural effusions and coupled with the absence of competing diagnoses, such as infection on diagnostic evaluation. Diffuse alveolar hemorrhage may occur as a result of widespread alveolar injury in association with PERDS, DAD, or IPS, or as a separate syndrome. Bronchoscopic findings of DAH include sequential aliquots of progressively bloody BAL fluid. Cytologic evidence of >20% hemosiderin-laden macrophages on BAL fluid is also supportive. Hemoptysis only occurs in approximately 20% to 25% of patients with DAH. Diffuse alveolar hemorrhage may develop independent of thrombocytopenia or coagulopathy. Supportive therapy is standard. The benefits of steroid therapy have not been definitely proven. Periengraftment respiratory distress syndrome may develop following both allogeneic and autologous transplants and is characterized by fever, hypoxemia, noncardiogenic pulmonary edema, erythematous skin rash, and weight gain arising during the periengraftment period. Diffuse alveolar hemorrhage complicates PERDS in approximately one-third of patients ([41-43]). Growth factor administration, infusion of increased numbers of CD34$^+$ cells, prolonged neutropenia, and peripheral blood source of stem cells all confer an increased risk of PERDS. Reductions in morbidity and mortality have been noted following steroid therapy in several small studies ([44, 45]). Another early-onset diffuse lung disease,

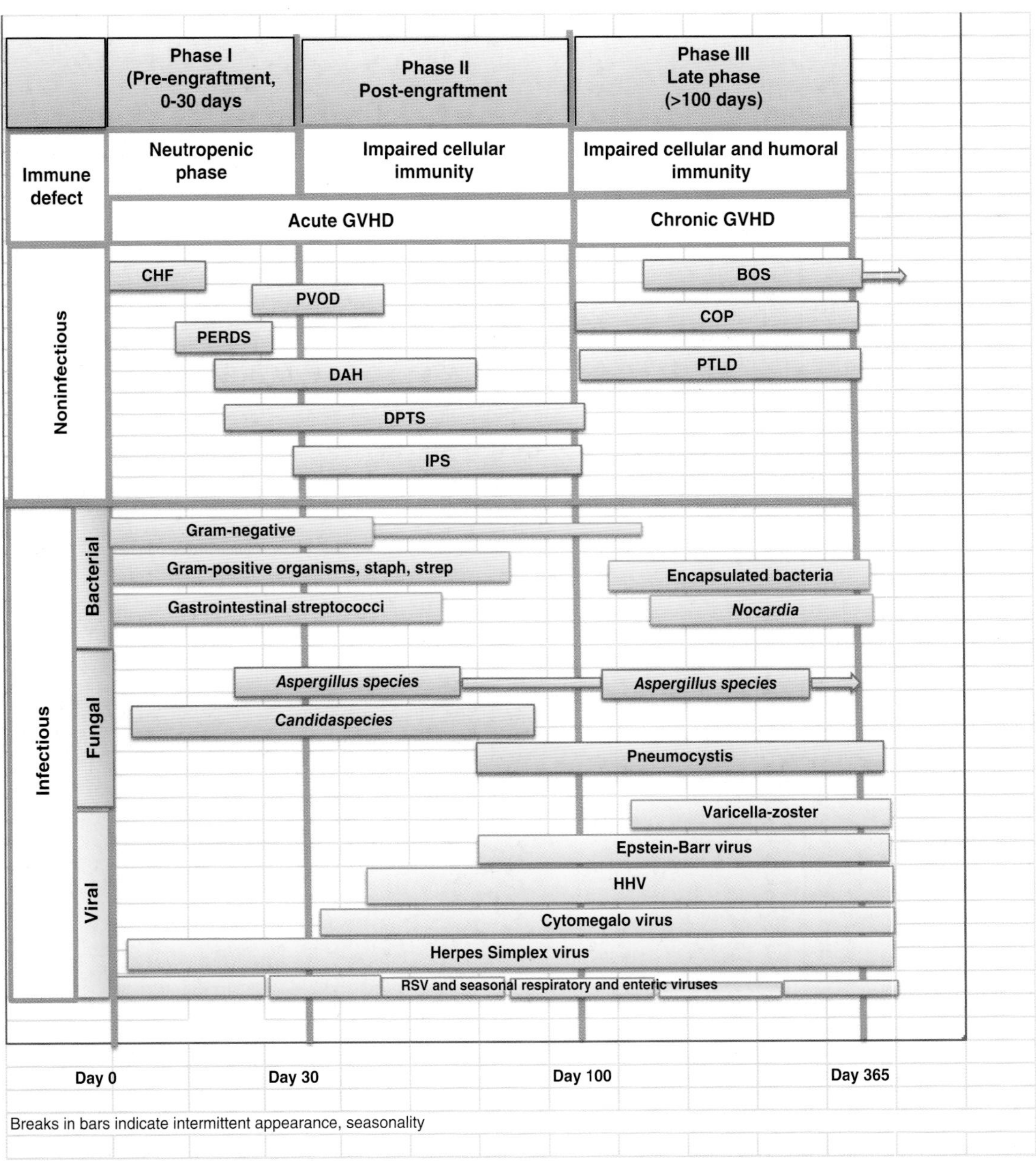

FIGURE 55-3 Temporal relationship of infectious and noninfectious complications following hematopoietic stem cell transplantation. BOS, bronchiolitis obliterans syndrome; CHF, congestive heart failure; COP, cryptogenic organizing pneumonia; DAH, diffuse alveolar hemorrhage; DPTS, delayed pulmonary toxicity syndrome; GVHD, graft-versus-host disease; HHV, human herpesvirus; IPS, idiopathic pneumonia syndrome; PERDS, periengraftment respiratory distress syndrome; PTLD, posttransplant lymphoproliferative disorder; PVOD, pulmonary veno-occlusive disease; RSV, respiratory syncytial virus. Breaks in bars indicate intermittent appearance or seasonality.

Table 55-4 Comparison of Early and Late Pulmonary Complications Following HSCT

	Early Complications (<100 days)					Late Complications (>100 days)	
	DAH	PERDS	DPTS	IPS	PVOD	BOS	COP
Incidence	5%-12%	33%	29%-64%	3%-15%	1%	2%-30%	2%
Transplant type	Autologous = allogeneic	Autologous	Autologous	Allogeneic	Allogeneic > autologous	Allogeneic	Allogeneic
Onset post HSCT	1-3 months	Within 5-7 days of neutrophil engraftment	5 weeks-3 months	1-3 months	3 weeks-3 months	4-24 months	3-12 months
Risk factors	Prolonged neutropenia	Growth factor use Infusion of CD34+ cel1s; Prolonged neutropenia; Peripheral blood HSCT source	Preconditioning regimens containing BCNU, cyclophosphamide and cisplatin radiotherapy?	GVHD, HLA disparity, CMV seropositivity; Increased age, TBI HSCT for cancer other than leukemia	Conditioning regimens containing cyclophosphamide?	GVHD	GVHD
Clinical symptoms/ signs	Cough, progressive dyspnea, hemoptysis rare (<25%) Progressively bloody lavage fluid on BAL	Fever, dyspnea, dry cough, skin rash, weight gain, edema	Fever, dyspnea, dry cough,	Fever, cough dyspnea, hypoxemia	Progressive dyspnea	Cough, dyspnea Progressive dyspnea, wheezing, obstructive findings on PFTs; DL_{CO} may be normal; Usually clinical diagnosis	Fever, dyspnea, dry cough, skin rash, weight gain, edema; Restrictive findings on PFTs; DL_{CO} reduced; Usually requires surgical lung biopsy for diagnosis
Histopathologic pattern	20% hemosiderin-laden macrophages in BAL fluid	BAL neutrophilia; Diffuse alveolar damage	Type II pneumocyte dysplasia, intra-alveolar edema, increased alveolar macrophages	Diffuse alveolar damage	Fibrous intimal proliferation of pulmonary venules and occasionally arterioles	Bronchiolitis obliterans (BO); cellular and constrictive bronchiolitis; Neutrophil-predaninant BAL fluid	Organizing pneumonia intraluminal organizing fibrosis in distal airspares; mild interstitial inflammation; BAL lymphocytosis

Radiographic findings	Diffuse infiltrates; may be central early on; ground-glass, linear, and nodular opacities may be seen	Bilateral infiltrates; pleural effusions; findings range from mild NCPE to ARDS	Ground-glass, linear, and nodular opacities may be seen	Bilateral interstitial infiltrates; ground-glass, opacities most common	Cardiomegaly, enlarged pulmonary arteries on CXR or CT	Hyperinflation on CXR; otherwise routinely normal; CT findings include mosaic attenuation (early) and air trapping, bronchiectasis (late)	Bilateral, patchy airspace disease with ground-glass appearance; may be nodular
Treatment	Supportive; response to steroids variable	Excellent; steroid responsive	Excellent; steroid responsive	Supportive; poor response to steroids	Supportive; no benefit from steroids	Supportive; immunosuppressive therapy; Variable response to steroids;	Steroid responsive disease
Prognosis	Less favorable prognosis when advanced; may progress to multi-organ system failure, sepsis and death	Favorable	Favorable	Poor	Poor	Poor; progressive disease with respiratory failure may occur	Favorable; potentially reversible disease

ARDS, acute respiratory distress syndrome; BAL, bronchoalveolar lavage; BCNU, carmustine; BOS, bronchiolitis obliterans syndrome; CMV, cytomegalovirus; COP, cryptogenic organizing pneumonitis; CT, computed tomography; CXR, chest x-ray; DAH, diffuse alveolar hemorrhage; DLCO, diffusing capacity of the lung for carbon monoxide; DPTS, delayed pulmonary toxicity syndrome; GVHD, graft-versus-host disease; HLA, human leukocyte antigen; HSCT, hematopoietic stem cell transplantation; IPS, idiopathic pneumonia syndrome; NCPE, noncardiogenic pulmonary edema; PERDS, periengraftment respiratory distress syndrome; PFT, pulmonary function test; PVOD, pulmonary veno-occlusive disease; TBI, total-body irradiation.

IPS, typically develops 14 to 90 days after transplant. The presence of GVHD, cytomegalovirus seropositivity, older age, total-body radiation, transplant type, human leukocyte antigen (HLA) disparity, and transplantation for malignancy other than leukemia are possible risk factors ([46, 47]). High-dose steroids, broad-spectrum antibiotics, and supportive care are the mainstays of treatment. Mortality rates may exceed 50% at 5 years, despite aggressive therapy. Pulmonary veno-occlusive disease (PVOD) is a rare complication of HSCT, which results in intractable dyspnea associated with severe pulmonary hypertension. Symptoms of dyspnea and fatigue develop insidiously, several weeks to month following HSCT. Treatment options are limited, with 2-year mortality approaching 100%. Delayed pulmonary toxicity syndrome occurs in 29% to 64% of autologous transplant recipients who received BCNU-, cyclophosphamide-, or cisplatin-based pretransplant conditioning regimens. This syndrome is heralded by dry cough, dyspnea, and bilateral pulmonary infiltrates, which typically occur 45 days after HSCT. Corticosteroid therapy leads to complete resolution of symptoms in 92% of patients ([48]).

Late-Onset Noninfectious Complications

Chronic GVHD, an immunologic posttransplant disorder in which donor cells attack healthy host tissue, is the most common late complication of allogeneic HSCT ([49, 50]). Involvement of GVHD in the lung results in BOS, a nonspecific lung injury causing inflammation, smooth muscle hypertrophy, and concentric intraluminal fibrosis of the small airways. The clinical hallmark of BOS is airflow limitation ([49, 50]). Patients are often asymptomatic during the early stages of BOS, leading to delays in diagnosis. At presentation during late stages of the disease, wheezing, dry cough, and dyspnea on exertion predominate as airflow obstruction progresses. Recurrent sinusitis and antecedent "cold" symptoms are common prior to diagnosis. Hyperinflation may be seen on plain chest radiographs, which are otherwise normal ([51, 52]). The lack of precise definition and uniform diagnostic criteria, along with a paucity of knowledge regarding the pathogenesis of BOS and delays in diagnosis, represent distinct challenges in management. The National Institutes of Health recently provided consensus guidelines in the diagnosis of BOS that require: (1) evidence of airflow obstruction (forced expiratory volume in 1 second [FEV_1]/forced vital capacity [FVC] <0.7 and FEV_1 <75% of predicted), with evidence of air trapping on PFT; (2) increased residual volume (>120% predicted); (3) air trapping, small airway thickening, or bronchiectasis on expiratory computed tomography (CT) or lung biopsy or pathologic confirmation of constrictive bronchiolitis; and (4) absence of any infectious process on radiographic, laboratory, or clinical testing ([53]). The prognosis of BOS is poor, with 5-year survival estimates of only 13%. Immunosuppressive therapy with corticosteroids and calcineurin inhibitors composes the mainstay of treatment. Recent studies have demonstrated stabilization of FEV_1 with high-dose inhaled corticosteroids. Other agents, including azithromycin, montelukast, azathioprine, sirolimus, and antithymocyte globulin, have been shown to have some benefit by PFT in small clinical trials and observational studies ([54-56]). Early disease recognition is crucial to improvements in therapy and survival.

Cryptogenic organizing pneumonia, previously known as idiopathic bronchiolitis obliterans organizing pneumonia, is seen almost exclusively among allogeneic HSCT recipients with GVHD. Presenting symptoms of dry cough, dyspnea, and fever may be accompanied by a restrictive defect on PFTs and bilateral patchy infiltrates on chest imaging studies. Cryptogenic organizing pneumonia is typically steroid responsive, although no evidence-based guidelines regarding dosage and duration of corticosteroid therapy are currently available. Normalization of chest radiographs and PFTs may be seen within 1 to 3 months of therapy ([57-60]).

Posttransplant lymphoproliferative disorder is a well-recognized complication of both solid organ transplantation and allogeneic HSCT. The disease is characterized by uncontrolled B-cell proliferation of donor-derived, Epstein-Barr virus–infected lymphocytes. Major risk factors include the use of T-cell–depleted donor stem cells, unrelated or HLA-mismatched related donor cells, and antithymocyte globulin. Posttransplant lymphoproliferative disorder complicates approximately 1% of allogeneic HSCTs, but may increase to 22% in patients with two or more risk factors. The lymph nodes, liver, spleen, and lungs are primary targets of PTLD. Dyspnea and fever typically develop 4 to 12 months following transplant, accompanied by interstitial and intra-alveolar infiltrates and ill-defined nodules. Reduction of immunosuppressive agents and administration of anti-CD20 (rituximab) therapy represent primary therapy ([50, 61]). The prognosis is generally poor.

VASCULAR DISEASE

Venous thromboembolism (VTE) is a well-recognized complication of cancer and its therapy. The manifestations of VTE, pulmonary embolism (PE), and deep venous thrombosis (DVT) are seen in 20% of cancer patients. Cancer is associated with a four- to seven-fold increased risk of VTE. Evidence suggests that tumor type and stage as well as specific cancer therapies influence the absolute risk of thromboembolism. Furthermore, surgery, immobility, hormonal therapy, growth factors, angiogenesis inhibitors, erythropoietic agents, and central venous catheters all impact the overall likelihood of thrombotic complications ([62, 63]). Rates of VTE as high as 28% to 43% have been reported in patients treated with combination antiangiogenic therapies, such as thalidomide and steroids or certain cancer chemotherapies (doxorubicin or BCNU). Unprovoked VTE may herald an impending diagnosis of cancer in patients without known malignancy. D-Dimer assays and scoring systems developed to estimate the pretest probability of VTE are neither sufficiently specific nor sensitive enough to rule out VTE ([64]). Computed tomographic pulmonary angiography (CTA) is the standard imaging technique for diagnosing PE and permits evaluation of competing diagnoses (Fig. 55-4). In unstable patients, echocardiography may provide rapid bedside assessment. Findings of right ventricle dilatation, right ventricle hypokinesis, tricuspid regurgitation, septal flattening, paradoxical septal wall motion, pulmonary artery hypertension, and lack of inspiratory collapse of the inferior vena cava are suggestive findings in the diagnosis of hemodynamically significant PE. Incidental PE is occasionally identified on CTAs performed for other reasons. Limited data support treatment of these asymptomatic PEs with full-dose anticoagulant therapy ([65]). Guidelines for VTE prophylaxis and treatment in the cancer setting have been established (Fig. 55-5). Low-molecular-weight heparin (LMWH) is the preferred agent, based on superior efficacy and safety data. In patients with impaired renal function, unfractionated heparin, or alternatively, fondaparinux should be considered. Recommendations include a 7- to 10-day course of LMWH for cancer patients undergoing surgery, which should be started preoperatively. Among patients at high risk for VTE, 4 weeks of LMWH are recommended. Thromboprophylaxis is not warranted in the routine management of the ambulatory cancer patient. This recommendation is based on analysis of the known risk of bleeding among patients with cancer and potential benefits of anticoagulant therapy in this setting. However, once hospitalized, VTE prophylaxis should be considered. Conversely, prophylactic LMWH is recommended for the ambulatory patient with multiple myeloma who is receiving thalidomide- or lenalidomide-based combination therapy. Prophylactic anticoagulation to prevent catheter-associated thrombosis is not recommended. Once established, full anticoagulant therapy should be initiated ([66-70]). Thrombolytic therapy for management of massive PE should be considered, although its efficacy and safety in the cancer setting have not been systematically studied. In all cases, contraindications to anticoagulant therapy should be weighed against the potential benefits of therapy ([71]).

A variety of conditions in the cancer setting may be associated with pulmonary hypertension (PH), defined as an elevated mean pulmonary artery pressure (mPAP) ≥25 mm Hg at rest. These conditions are represented in all five categories of the revised 2013 World Health Organization classification scheme for PH (Table 55-5). For example, chemotherapeutic agents, such as dasatinib, and PVOD caused by chemotoxins, thoracic radiation, and stem cell transplantation are known causes of PAH (group 1). Cancer treatment–related left heart disease is a common cause of PH (group 2). Hypoxemic pleuroparenchymal disease due to tumor infiltration, infection, and chemotoxicity are well known sources of group 3 PH. Increased rates of acute and chronic PE as well as splenectomy in the cancer setting are associated with chronic thromboembolic PH (group 4). Finally, myeloproliferative disorders and entrapment/compression of large pulmonary vessels by infection and treatment-related mediastinal fibrosis, adenopathy, or neoplasms are recognized risk factors of group 5 PH ([72-76]). The development of significant PH in cancer portends a worse prognosis. Dyspnea, nonproductive cough, and hypoxemia develop insidiously in cancer-related PH and may progress to respiratory

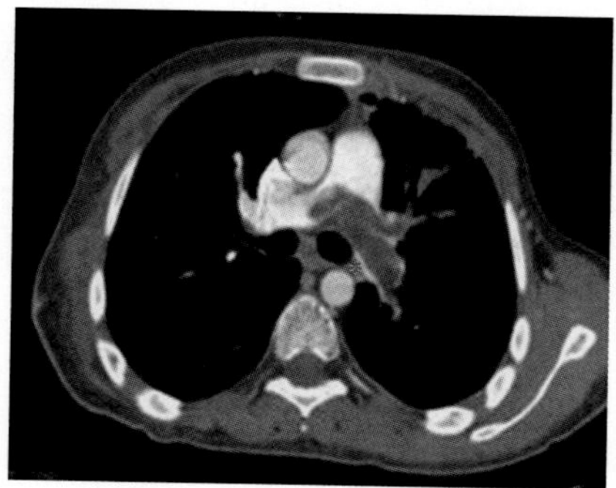
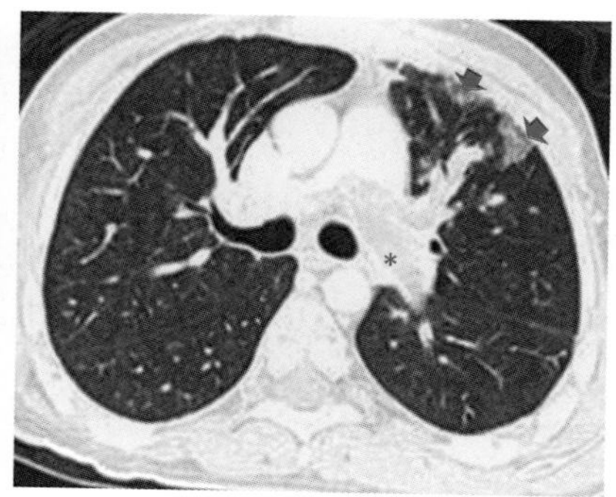

FIGURE 55-4 Pulmonary embolism. A 25-year-old man presented to the emergency room with acute pleuritic chest pain and shortness of breath. Computed tomography angiogram confirmed a large saddle embolus with extension of clot into the left interlobar and lingular arteries (*). Subpleural ground-glass opacities (*arrows*) likely represent pulmonary infarction or hemorrhage.

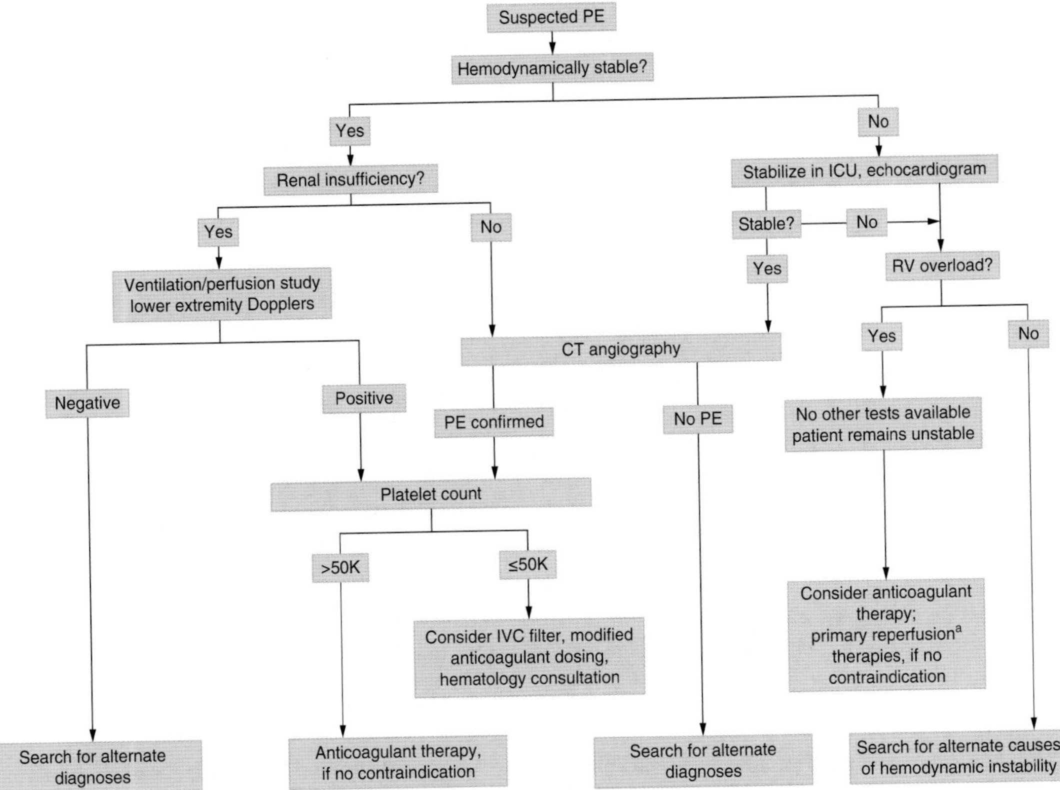

FIGURE 55-5 Algorithm for approach to assessment and management of pulmonary embolism (PE) in the cancer setting. CT, computed tomography; ICU, intensive care unit; IVC, inferior vena cava; RV, right ventricle. [a]Systemic thrombolytic therapy, surgical pulmonary embolectomy, percutaneous catheter-directed thrombolysis.

failure and death. Supportive care and treatment of the underlying disease are the mainstays of therapy. The utility of pulmonary vasodilator agents, including treatment strategies that target nitric oxide, endothelin, and prostaglandin pathways in the management of cancer-related PH has not been definitively studied. Vasodilator therapy in the setting of cancer-related PVOD should be used with extreme caution, because fatal pulmonary edema precipitated by vasodilator therapy in this setting has been reported (73, 74, 77).

MALIGNANT CENTRAL AIRFLOW OBSTRUCTION

Malignant central airway obstruction refers to obstruction at the level of the trachea, mainstem bronchi, and/or bronchus intermedius. Cough, stridor, wheezing, dyspnea, atelectasis, and recurrent or persistent postobstructive pneumonia are common presenting symptoms. Hemoptysis, which can be massive and life threatening, may also occur. Stridor signals a more proximal level of obstruction at the level of the trachea or larynx, whereas focal wheezing is typically due to obstruction distal to the main carina. Tracheal stenosis resulting in airway narrowing of 50% or greater is associated with a 16-fold increase in flow resistance. Thus, obstructive symptoms typically develop with airway occlusions of 50% or more (78). Tracheal diameters of 8 mm are associated with dyspnea on exertion. Resting dyspnea occurs with tracheal diameters of 5 mm or less. Confounding factors, such as chronic obstructive pulmonary disease, mucosal edema, and increased airway secretions may precipitate inexorable dyspnea even in patients with only moderate tumor-related airflow limitation. Compromised airway caliber by tumor may be due to endoluminal tumor, extrinsic compression, or direct extension through the airway wall. Optimization of therapy is predicated on the location and extent of airway disease and quantification of airflow limitation. With the exception of rare findings of tracheal deviation on plain films, chest radiographs are of limited value in defining the anatomic extent of airway tumor. Blunting of the flow-volume loop on PFT is an insensitive signal of upper airway obstruction, which typically only occurs once tracheal caliber is

Table 55-5 Revised Classification of Pulmonary Hypertension

Class	Subclass
1. Pulmonary arterial hypertension (PAH)	1.1. Idiopathic PAH 1.2. Heritable PAH 1.3. Drug- and toxin-induced 1.4. Associated with 1.4.1. Connective tissue disease 1.4.2. HIV infection 1.4.3. Portal hypertension 1.4.4. Congenital heart diseases 1.4.5. Schistosomiasis 1.5. Pulmonary veno-occlusive disease and/or pulmonary capillary hemangiomatosis 1.6. Persistent pulmonary hypertension of the newborn
2. Pulmonary hypertension due to left heart disease	2.1. Left ventricular systolic dysfunction 2.2. Left ventricular diastolic dysfunction 2.3. Valvular heart disease 2.4. Congenital/acquired left heart inflow/outflow tract obstruction and congenital cardiomyopathies
3. Pulmonary hypertension due to lung disease or hypoxia	3.1. COPD 3.2. Interstitial lung disease 3.3. Other pulmonary disease with mixed restrictive and obstructive pattern 3.4. Sleep-disordered breathing 3.5. Alveolar hypoventilation disorders 3.6. Chronic exposure to high altitude 3.7. Developmental lung diseases
4. Chronic thromboembolic pulmonary hypertension (CTEPH)	
5. Pulmonary hypertension with unclear or multifactorial etiologies	5.1. Hematologic disorders: chronic hemolytic anemia, myeloproliferative disorders, splenectomy 5.2. Systemic disorders: sarcoidosis, pulmonary histiocytosis, lymphangiomyomatosis 5.3. Metabolic disorders: glycogen storage disease, Gaucher disease, thyroid disorders 5.4. Others: tumoral obstruction, fibrosing mediastinitis, chronic renal failure

COPD, chronic obstructive pulmonary disease; HIV, human immunodeficiency virus.

reduced to less than 10 mm (Fig. 55-6) ([79]). The use of spirometry in patients with severe airway obstruction is not recommended because it may precipitate frank respiratory failure.

Bronchoscopic examination is central to diagnosis and treatment of malignant central airflow obstruction. Characterization and histologic confirmation of the tumor as well as the extent of obstruction attributable to endoluminal and/or extraluminal disease at bronchoscopy are important findings that help to guide treatment decisions (Fig. 55-7). Therapeutic strategies for predominant endoluminal disease include surgical resection and mechanical debulking using the rigid bronchoscope. Balloon bronchoplasty and endobronchial argon plasma coagulation (APC) and/or laser therapy, electrocautery, cryotherapy, brachytherapy, and photodynamic therapy are additional therapeutic options for predominant endobronchial disease and may be performed during rigid bronchoscopy. Stent placement and RT are reasonable treatment options for patients with predominant extraluminal disease. A multimodality approach that includes endobronchial debulking and stent placement is common, as many patients present with mixed endo- and extraluminal disease (Fig. 56-8). Treatment options are based on the type of obstruction.

PLEURAL DISEASES IN THE CANCER SETTING

Nearly 50% of all cancer patients develop pleural effusions. These may be malignant pleural effusions (MPEs) or paramalignant pleural effusions. The latter result from direct or indirect effects of tumor on the pleural space and include bronchial obstruction, infiltration of mediastinal lymph nodes, superior vena cava syndrome, trapped lung PE, and atelectasis. Paramalignant

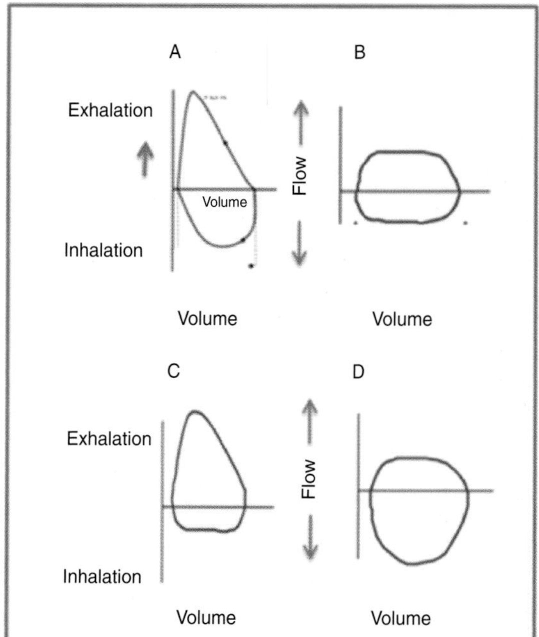

FIGURE 55-6 Flow-volume loops in upper airway obstruction. A. Normal. B. Flattening of both the inspiratory and expiratory limbs of the flow-volume loop, consistent with fixed upper airway obstruction with flow limitation. C. Flattening of the inspiratory limb consistent with dynamic (variable, nonfixed) extrathoracic obstruction with flow limitation. D. Flattening of the expiratory limb consistent with dynamic (variable, nonfixed) intrathoracic obstruction.

effusions occur on the involved side and are typically small to moderate in size, with negative pleural fluid cytology. Malignant pleural effusions rank second as the leading cause of exudative effusions, after parapneumonic effusions. Malignant pleural effusions may be quite large. In contrast to parapneumonic effusions, pleural fluid cytology is positive in more than 60% of patients with MPE ([80]). Malignant pleural involvement may also occur in the absence of pleural fluid in patients with primary pleural tumors or metastatic disease to the pleura ([81]).

Fifty percent of all cancer-related pleural effusions are due to lung cancer. Breast carcinoma and effusions due to hematologic malignancies, including lymphoma and leukemias, are also common causes. Progressive dyspnea and dry cough are presenting symptoms in most patients, which may be accompanied by constitutional symptoms of malaise, anorexia, and weight loss with advanced disease. Preprocedure imaging is an important component in the diagnostic workup and treatment planning. Standard chest radiographs and bilateral decubitus films provide critical information regarding effusion size, position of the mediastinum and diaphragms, presence of fluid loculations, and characteristics of the underlying lung parenchyma. Patients with large pleural effusions and associated contralateral shift of the mediastinum should undergo prompt therapeutic thoracentesis. A centered or ipsilateral shift of the mediastinum with associated pleural effusion may signify frozen mediastinum, tumor encasement of the ipsilateral mainstem bronchus, or extensive parenchymal involvement due to lymphangitic spread of tumor, infection, or other infiltrative lung diseases. Any of these diagnoses may cause ipsilateral opacification of the lung and simulate a large pleural effusion (Fig. 55-9). Pleural effusions in this setting should therefore be approached with caution ([82]).

Transthoracic ultrasonography is a well-established and validated imaging tool that has gained an increasing role in diagnostic and therapeutic pleural interventions. Pleural ultrasonography is easy to learn and interpret and provides valuable information regarding optimal site localization for thoracentesis and other invasive pleural procedures, as well as information

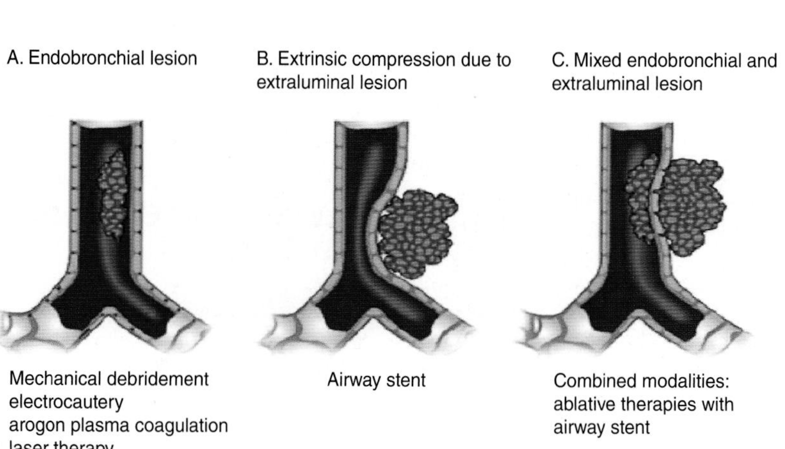

FIGURE 55-7 Approach to malignant central airway obstruction using interventional bronchoscopic therapies.

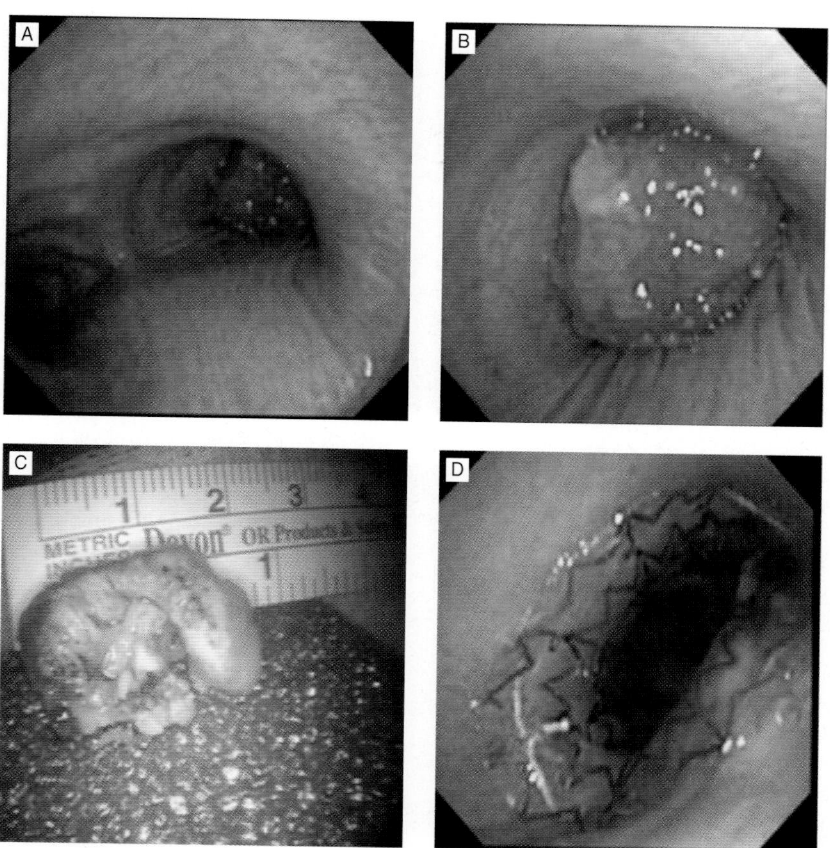

FIGURE 55-8 Complete occlusion of the right mainstem bronchus due to a large endobronchial bronchogenic carcinoma (**A**, **B**). The 2-cm tumor was removed using an electrocautery snare (**C**) followed by airway stent placement (**D**).

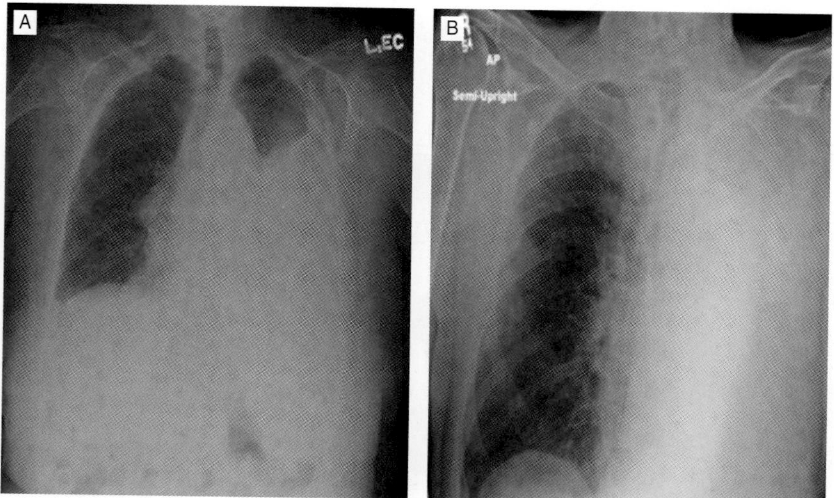

FIGURE 55-9 Large pleural effusion causing shift of the mediastinum to the contralateral side (**A**). Patient **B** also has a large effusion; however, the mediastinum is shifted ipsilaterally due to central airway obstruction caused by tumor, resulting in non-expandable lung.

regarding pleural fluid characteristics such as the presence of loculations, fibrin strands, and pleural metastases (Fig. 55-10). Computed tomography provides valuable anatomic information of the visceral and parietal pleura, chest wall, lung parenchyma, and mediastinal structures and is particularly useful in characterizing the pleural fluid and identifying competing diagnoses [83]. Findings on positron emission tomography (PET)-CT and conventional CT imaging, such as irregular, thickened, or nodular pleural surface, suggest malignancy. Pleural enhancement with intravenous contrast material is also suggestive of malignancy, although pleural inflammation may be associated with similar findings. Recent studies have shown that PET imaging with 18-fluorodeoxyglucose is useful in delineating pleural tumors and extrapleural extension of disease in patients with malignant pleural mesothelioma (MPM). Magnetic resonance imaging (MRI) of the pleural space is also valuable in displaying pleural tumors. This imaging strategy provides excellent soft tissue contrast and delineation of extrapleural invasion of the chest wall, spine, nerves, and mediastinal vascular structures [83]. This information is complementary to chest CT imaging and markedly enhances surgical planning for patients with MPM.

Nearly all MPEs are categorized as exudates using Light's criteria [84]. The cytologic or histologic confirmation of malignant cells on pleural fluid or biopsy is key to diagnosis, although pleural cytology is only positive in 62% of patients [80]. Flow cytometry with identification of tumor markers may improve the diagnostic yield of cytologically negative effusions by 33%. This diagnostic strategy has proved particularly useful when pleural effusions associated with lymphoma, leukemia, or multiple myeloma are suspected [85, 86]. A definitive diagnosis is yielded after closed pleural biopsy in only 44% of patients, but increases to 77% [80] with the addition of pleural fluid cytology. More recent advances in pleuroscopic and image-guide biopsy techniques have improved the diagnostic yield as compared to traditional closed-needle biopsy in the diagnosis of pleural malignancy (Fig. 55-11). For example, pleuroscopy and CT-guided pleural biopsies exhibit 95% and 87% sensitivity in the diagnosis of pleural malignancies, respectively. The addition of pleural fluid cytology to pleuroscopy offers only a marginal increase in the diagnostic yield [85].

With few exceptions, the presence of MPE portends a poor prognosis, with mean survival measured in months. Therefore, treatment is focused on palliation. Our approach to the management of MPEs is outlined in Fig. 55-12. Factors such as associated symptoms, performance status, volume of fluid evacuated, whether symptom palliation and lung reexpansion were achieved with prior thoracenteses, time course for recurrence, and tumor response to systemic therapy should be considered in management options. Among patients with newly diagnosed chemo- or radiosensitive tumors (lymphoma, breast, small-cell lung cancer, prostate, thyroid, germ cell), simple thoracentesis while awaiting response to definitive therapy is reasonable. Most MPEs will recur with 30 days of the prior thoracentesis. Repeated thoracentesis is also recommended in patients with slowly reaccumulating pleural effusions and short life expectancy (1-3 months). Poor performance status is predictive of limited survival among patients with recurrent malignant pleural effusions [87]. Evacuation of pleural fluid is ideally ultrasound guided, which is associated with lower rates of pneumothorax. In a recent consensus statement, the American Thoracic Society and the European Respiratory Society endorsed symptom-limited pleural fluid evacuation, not to exceed 1.0 to 1.5 L of fluid in one sitting [81]. In our experience, symptom-limited evacuation of up to 2.0 to 2.5 L of pleural fluid in one sitting is safe among patients with contralateral mediastinal shift associated

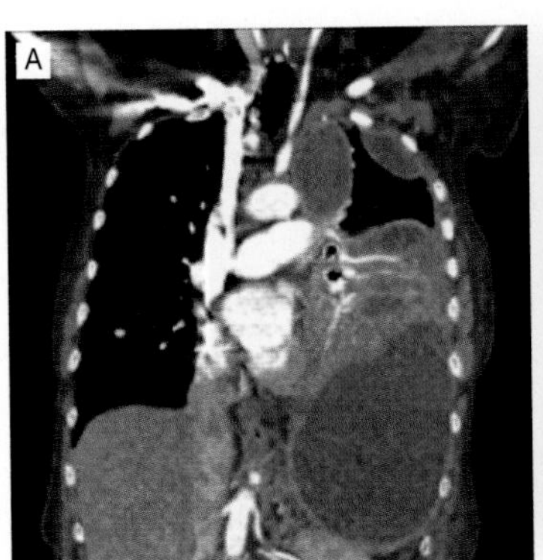

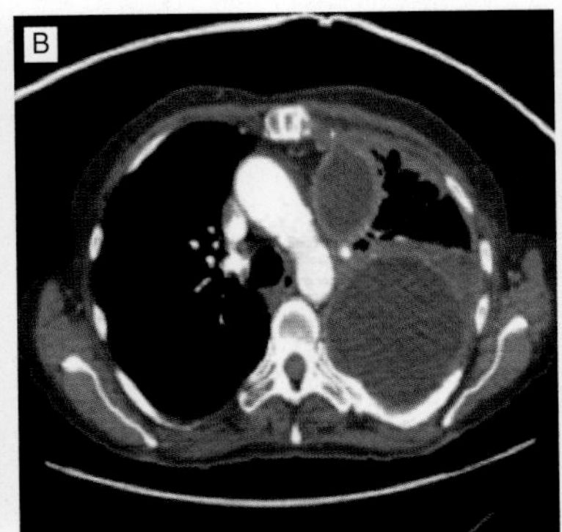

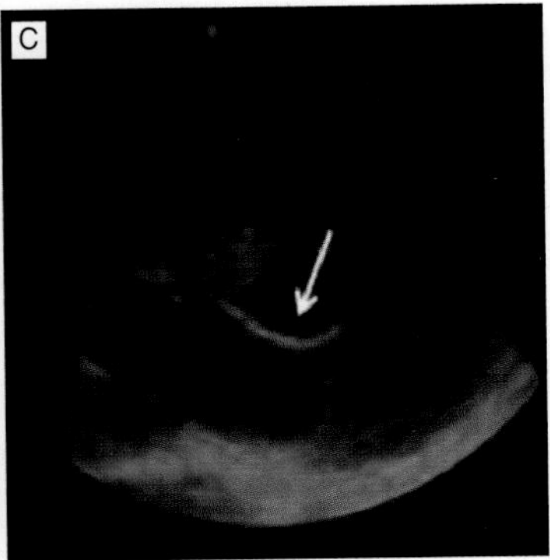

FIGURE 55-10 Coronal (A) and axial (B) views on computed tomography evaluation of a large multiloculated, left-sided pleural effusion in a patient with malignant mesothelioma. The loculations are caused by thick-walled adhesions (*arrow*), seen on ultrasound evaluation (C).

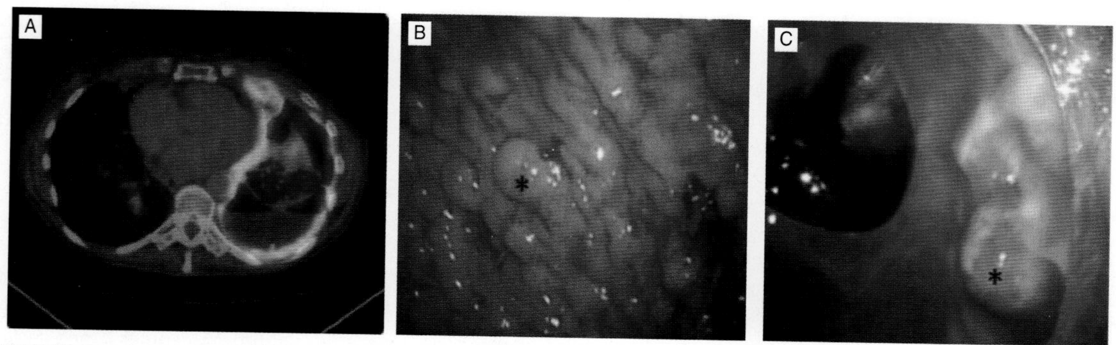

FIGURE 55-11 Positron emission tomography/computed tomography imaging (A) showing a fluorodeoxyglucose (FDG)-avid rind of thickened, nodular pleural deposits encasing the left lung. Extensive nodularity along the visceral pleural surface (*) was seen at pleuroscopy (B, C). Pathologic analysis of the biopsied nodules was consistent with malignant mesothelioma.

with a large pleural effusion. Chest pain, cough, and dyspnea are limiting symptoms that should prompt discontinuation of the procedure. Cautious evacuation of large volumes of pleural fluid is recommended in patients with centered or ipsilateral shift of the mediastinum. Pleural pressure measurements during thoracentesis have not been shown to be superior to symptom-limited pleural drainage in reducing the risk of procedure-related complications [88].

Indwelling pleural catheter (IPC) placement is an increasingly viable palliative option for patients with recurrent MPEs. Patients whose life expectancy exceeds 30 days and those in whom symptomatic improvement was achieved on prior thoracenteses are ideal candidates for IPC placement. Symptom improvement may occur without imaging evidence of lung reexpansion following thoracentesis due to other physiologic and mechanical changes that occur in the chest post large volume thoracentesis. Most catheters are placed in the outpatient setting. Designated family members and/or caretakers are then trained on the proper use of the catheter. Daily home drainage is recommended initially, followed by every other day drainage as pleural fluid volume decreases. In our experience, 94% of patients reported symptom relief, and in 52%, effective pleurodesis with subsequent removal

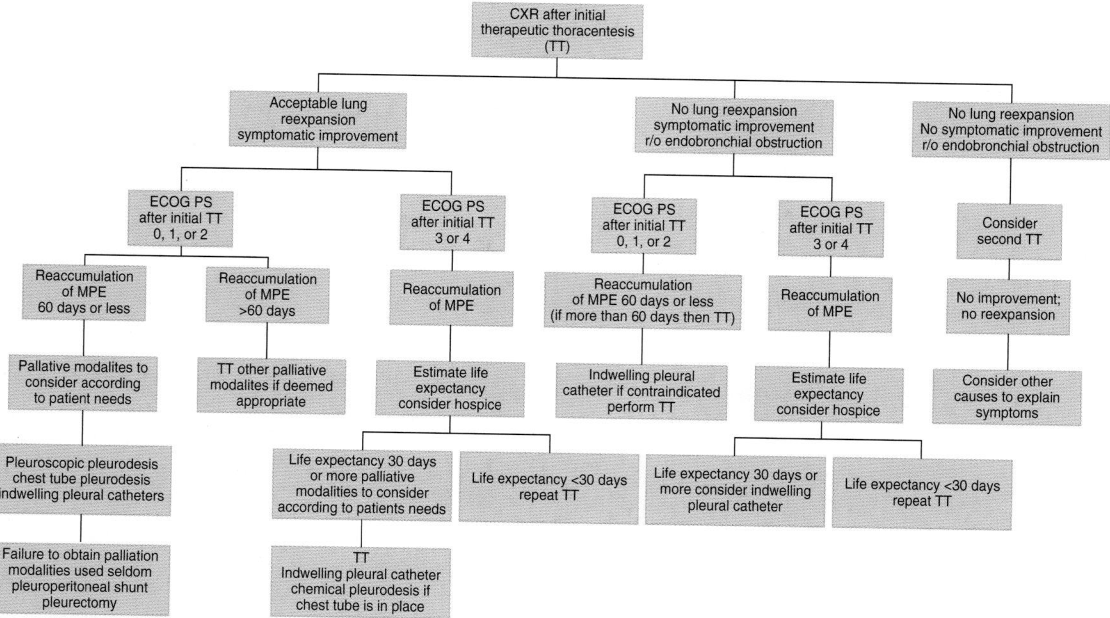

FIGURE 55-12 Management of malignant pleural effusions (MPEs). CXR, chest x-ray; ECOG PS, Eastern Cooperative Oncology Group performance status.

of the catheter was achieved. The average time from catheter insertion to removal was 32 days. Empyema and persistent pain at the insertion site were rare complications of IPC placement in our review. Recurrent effusion has also been rarely described in a small group of patients following catheter removal ([89]).

Chemical pleurodesis using asbestos-free talc is a widely used strategy in the management of MPE. Several studies suggest that talc is superior to other sclerosants (bleomycin, tetracycline) in achieving pleurodesis. Eligible patients for this procedure should have a good performance status (Eastern Cooperative Oncology Group performance status of 0 to 2) and report symptomatic relief and lung reexpansion following prior thoracentesis. Pleuroscopic talc poudrage and talc slurry instillation via small-bore chest tube are both viable methods of chemical pleurodesis.

The management of recurrent chylous effusions is a particular challenge because of the potential for severe lymphopenia, nutritional depletion, and water and electrolyte loss from prolonged loss of chyle. These effusions, when cancer-related, require treatment of the underlying malignancy. Parenteral alimentation, talc pleurodesis, and indwelling pleural catheter placement represent reasonable alternatives in the management of recalcitrant effusions ([90]). Pleuroperitoneal shunt placement is an attractive treatment option that permits reabsorption of chyle in the peritoneum, which mitigates the risk of malnourishment and immune suppression. However, small-volume shunt removal and increased potential for pump obstruction limit the utility of this treatment modality. Embolization of the thoracic duct has not been definitively studied but appears well tolerated.

SLEEP DISTURBANCES IN CANCER THERAPY

Nearly half of all patients with cancer develop sleep disturbances. Insomnia, poor sleep efficiency, early awakening, excessive daytime sleepiness, and restless legs may occur during all phases of cancer care and persist for many months to years after completion of cancer therapy. The biochemical changes inherent to cancer growth, anticancer therapies, and cancer-related symptoms of fatigue, pain, and depression may all adversely impact sleep quality.

Sleep disturbance may occur due to a myriad of causes and may have important implications in cancer treatment, prevention, and survivorship (Fig. 55-13). For example, sleep duration appears to influence cancer risk. Excess cancer prevalence has been demonstrated among insomniacs with sleep times of less than 5 hours per night and patients undergoing 9 or more hours of sleep nightly ([91]). In the American Nurse Health Study, a relative increased risk of breast cancer was demonstrated among nurses working rotating shifts for many years ([92, 93]). In another study, cancer mortality increased by five-fold among patients with a protracted history of severe sleep apnea ([94]).

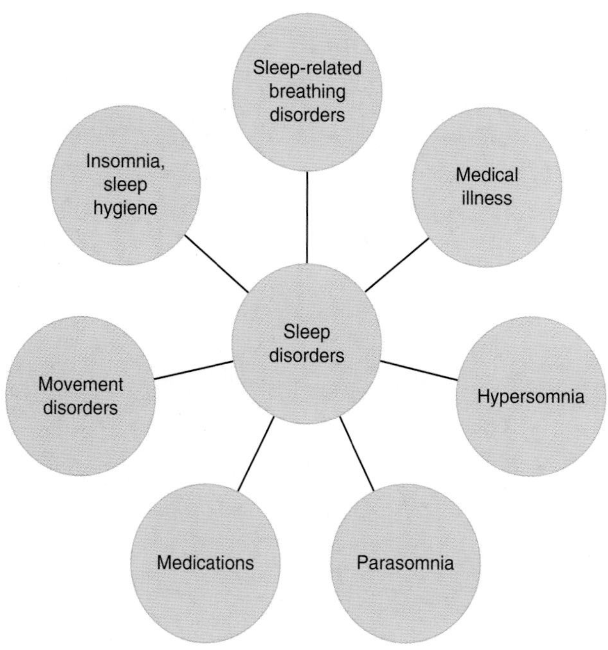

FIGURE 55-13 Causes of sleep disorders.

A detailed history and physical examination may elucidate a single etiology or multiple etiologies for sleep disturbance. Two frequent causes of sleep disturbance in the cancer setting include sleep-related breathing disorders and insomnia. The incidence of sleep-related breathing disorders may be increased in the cancer setting due to the cancer itself or as a sequela of cancer therapy. For example, higher rates of obstructive sleep apnea have been reported among patients with head and neck cancers ([95]). Increased rates of central sleep apnea in the cancer setting have been attributed to the frequent use of opioid medications ([96]). In addition, RT, pain medications, and chest wall deformities caused by cancer or its treatment may exacerbate sleep-related hypoventilation. Supplemental oxygen and positive airway pressure therapy are the mainstays of therapy for sleep-related breathing disorders. Cessation of sedating medications should be considered along with optimization of underlying pulmonary and cardiac disease.

Insomnia is a common problem in the cancer setting that impacts cancer treatment as well as survival. In one study, reported rates of insomnia among cancer patients completing their first cycle of chemotherapy were three-fold higher than the general population ([97]). Sleep loss, and in particular rapid eye movement (REM) sleep deprivation, is hyperanalgesic. Thus, insomnia, which is common in the cancer setting, may confer an increased sensitivity to pain ([98]). Insomnia is a major contributing factor to cancer-related fatigue, and the prevalence and association of these two disorders may vary greatly during the course of cancer care ([99-101]). Cognitive behavioral therapy is the mainstay of therapy, which may improve insomnia, optimize sleep hygiene, decrease sedative-hypnotic medication use, and improve quality of life among these patients. Treatment of other potential etiologies for cancer-related fatigue, including pain, anemia, and thyroid disorders, may also help to improve symptoms of insomnia.

REFERENCES

1. Camus P, Fanton A, Bonniaud P, Camus C, Foucher P. Interstitial lung disease induced by drugs and radiation. *Respiration.* 2004;71(4):301-326.
2. Camus P, Kudoh S, Ebina M. Interstitial lung disease associated with drug therapy. *Br J Cancer.* 2004;91(Suppl 2):S18-S23.
3. Vahid B, Marik P. Pulmonary complications of novel antineoplastic agents for solid tumors. *Chest.* 2008;133(2):528-538.
4. Vahid B, Marik P. Infiltrative lung diseases: complications of novel antineoplastic agents in patients with hematological malignancies. *Can Respir J.* 2008;15(4):211-216.
5. Yousem SA. The histological spectrum of pulmonary graft-versus-host disease in bone marrow transplant recipients. *Hum Pathol.* 1995;26:668-675.
6. Sleijfer S. Bleomycin-induced pneumonitis. *Chest.* 2001;120(2): 617-624.
7. Donat SM, Levy DA. Bleomycin associated pulmonary toxicity: is perioperative oxygen restriction necessary? *J Urol.* 1998;160(4):1347-1352.
8. Duran I, Goebell PJ, Papazisis K, et al. Drug-induced pneumonitis in cancer patients treated with mTOR inhibitors: management and insights into possible mechanisms. *Expert Opin Drug Saf.* 2014;13(3):361-372.
9. Gartrell BA, Ying J, Sivendran S, et al. Pulmonary complications with the use of mTOR inhibitors in targeted cancer therapy: a systematic review and meta-analysis. *Target Oncol.* 2014;9(3):195-204.
10. Dabydeen DA, Jagannathan JP, Ramaiya N, et al. Pneumonitis associated with mTOR inhibitors therapy in patients with metastatic renal cell carcinoma: incidence, radiographic findings and correlation with clinical outcome. *Eur J Cancer.* 2012;48:1569-1524.
11. Maroto J, Hudes G, Dutcher JP, et al. Drug-related pneumonitis in patients with advanced renal cell carcinoma treated with temsirolimus. *J Clin Oncol.* 2011;29(13):1750-1756.
12. Tefferi A, Pardanani A. Serious adverse events during ruxolitinib treatment discontinuation in patients with myelofibrosis. *Mayo Clin Proc.* 2011;86(12):1188-1191.
13. Beauverd Y, Samii K. Acute respiratory distress syndrome in a patient with primary myelofibrosis after ruxolitinib treatment discontinuation. *Int J Hematol.* 2014;100(5):498-501.
14. Rogers J, Yang D. Differentiation syndrome in patients with acute promyelocytic leukemia. *J Oncol Pharm Pract.* 2012;18(1):109-114.
15. Luesink M, Jansen JH. Advances in understanding the pulmonary infiltration in acute promyelocytic leukaemia. *Br J Haematol.* 2010;151(3):209-220.
16. Sachdeva A, Matuschak G. Diffuse alveolar hemorrhage following alemtuzumab. *Chest.* 2008;33(6):1476-1478.
17. Sandler A. Bevacizumab in non-small cell lung cancer. *Clin Cancer Res.* 2007;45:2321-2335.
18. Huggins JT, Sahn SA. Drug-induced pleural disease. *Clin Chest Med.* 2004;25(1):141-153.
19. Wohlrab J, Liu M, Anderson E, Kia Noury D. Docetaxel induced pleural effusions [abstract]. *Chest.* 2002;122:94S-95S.
20. Socinski MA, Novello S, Sanchez JM, et al. Efficacy and safety of sunitinib in previously treated, advanced non-small cell lung cancer (NSCLC): preliminary results of a multicenter phase II trial [abstract]. *J Clin Oncol.* 2006;24:7001.
21. Procopio G, Verzoni E, Gevorgyan A, et al. Safety and activity of sorafenib in different histotypes of advanced renal cell carcinoma. *Oncology.* 2007;73(3-4):204-209.
22. Keefea D, Bowena J, Gibson R, et al. Noncardiac vascular toxicities of vascular endothelial growth factor inhibitors in advanced cancer: a review. *Oncologist.* 2011;16:432-444.
23. Nalluri S, Chu D, Keresztes R, Zhu X, Wu S. Risk of venous thromboembolism with the angiogenesis inhibitor bevacizumab in cancer patients: a meta-analysis. *JAMA.* 2008;300(19): 2277-2285.
24. Godinas L, Guignabert C, Seferian A, et al. Tyrosine kinase inhibitors in pulmonary arterial hypertension: a double-edge sword? *Semin Respir Crit Care Med.* 2013;34(5):714-724.
25. Montani D, Bergot E, Gunther S, et al. Pulmonary arterial hypertension in patients treated by dasatinib. *Circulation.* 2012;125:2128-2137.
26. Abratt RP, Morgan GW. Lung toxicity following chest irradiation in patients with lung cancer. *Lung Cancer.* 2002;35(2):103-109.
27. Force T. Double-edged sword of the new cancer therapeutics. *Circulation.* 2012;125:2057-2058.
28. Szebeni J, Alving CR, Savay S, et al. Complement activation-related pseudoallergy caused by liposomes, micellar carriers of intravenous drugs, and radiocontrast agents. Formation of

complement-activating particles in aqueous solutions of Taxol: possible role in hypersensitivity reactions. *Crit Rev Ther Drug Carrier Syst*. 2001;18(6):567-606.
29. Kang S, Saif M. Infusion-related and hypersensitivity reactions of monoclonal antibodies used to treat colorectal cancer: identification, prevention, and management. *J Support Oncol*. 2007;5:451-457.
30. Markman M. Management of toxicities associated with the administration of taxanes. *Expert Opin Drug Saf*. 2003; 2(2):141-146.
31. Engels FK, Mathot RA, Verweij J. Alternative drug formulations of docetaxel: a review. *Anticancer Drugs*. 2007;18(2):95-103.
32. Marks LB, Yu X, Vujaskovic Z, Small W Jr, Folz R, Anscher MS. Radiation-induced lung injury. *Semin Radiat Oncol*. 2003;13(3):333-345.
33. Movsas B, Raffin TA, Epstein AH, Link CJ Jr. Pulmonary radiation injury. *Chest*. 1997;111(4):1061-1076.
34. Schweitzer VG, Juillard GJ, Bajada CL, RG. P. Radiation recall dermatitis and pneumonitis in a patient treated with paclitaxel. *Cancer*. 1995;76(6):1069-1072.
35. Schwarte S, Wagner K, Karstens JH, Bremer M. Radiation recall pneumonitis induced by gemcitabine. *Strahlenther Onkol*. 2007;183:215-217.
36. Ding K, Ji W, Li J, et al. Radiation recall pneumonitis induced by chemotherapy after thoracic radiotherapy for lung cancer. *Radiat Oncol*. 2011;6(24):1-6.
37. Cottin V, Frognier R, Monnot H, et al. Chronic eosinophilic pneumonia after radiation therapy for breast cancer. *Eur Respir J*. 2004;23(1):9-13.
38. Cornelissen R, Senan S, Antonisse IE, et al. Bronchiolitis obliterans organizing pneumonia (BOOP) after thoracic radiotherapy for breast carcinoma. *Radiat Oncol*. 2007;2:2.
39. Diab KJ, Yu Z, Wood KL, et al. Comparison of pulmonary complications after nonmyeloablative and conventional allogeneic hematopoietic cell transplant. *Biol Blood Marrow Transplant*. 2012;18(12):1827-1834.
40. Shioyama Y, Tokuuye K, Okumura T, et al. Clinical evaluation of proton radiotherapy for non-small-cell lung cancer. *Int J Radiat Oncol Biol Phys*. 2003;56(1):7-13.
41. Capizzi SA, Kumar S, Huneke NE, et al. Peri-engraftment respiratory distress syndrome during autologous hematopoietic stem cell transplantation. *Bone Marrow Transplant*. 2001;27(12):1299-1303.
42. Afessa B, Tefferi A, Litzow MR, Krowka MJ, Wylam ME, Peters SG. Diffuse alveolar hemorrhage in hematopoietic stem cell transplant recipients. *Am J Respir Crit Care Med*. 2002;166(5):641-645.
43. Soubani A, Miller K, Hassoun P. Pulmonary complications of bone marrow transplantation. *Chest*. 1996;109(4):1066-1077.
44. Spitzer TR. Engraftment syndrome following hematopoietic stem cell transplantation. *Bone Marrow Transplant*. 2001;27(9): 893-898.
45. Afessa B, Peters S. Major complications following hematopoietic stem cell transplantation. *Semin Respir Crit Care Med*. 2006;27(3):297-309.
46. Yanik G, Hellerstedt B, Custer J, et al. Etanercept (Enbrel) administration for idiopathic pneumonia syndrome after allogeneic hematopoietic stem cell transplantation. *Biol Blood Marrow Transplant*. 2002;8(7):395-400.
47. Panoskaltsis-Mortari A, Griese M, Madtes DK, et al. An official American Thoracic Society research statement: noninfectious lung injury after hematopoietic stem cell transplantation: idiopathic pneumonia syndrome. *Am J Respir Crit Care Med*. 2011;183(9):1262-1279.
48. Cao TM, Negrin RS, Stockerl-Goldstein KE, et al. Pulmonary toxicity syndrome in breast cancer patients undergoing BCNU-containing high-dose chemotherapy and autologous hematopoietic cell transplantation. *Biol Blood Marrow Transplant*. 2000;6(4):387-394.
49. Chien JW, Martin PJ, Gooley TA, et al. Airflow obstruction after myeloablative allogeneic hematopoietic stem cell transplantation. *Am J Respir Crit Care Med*. 2003;168(2):208-214.
50. Kotloff RM, Ahya VN, Crawford SW. Pulmonary complications of solid organ and hematopoietic stem cell transplantation. *Am J Respir Crit Care Med*. 2004;170(1):22-48.
51. Panoskaltsis-Mortari A, Tram KV, Price AP, Wendt CH, Blazar BR. A new murine model for bronchiolitis obliterans post-bone marrow transplant. *Am J Respir Crit Care Med*. 2007;176(7):713-723.
52. Soubani AO, Uberti JP. Bronchiolitis obliterans following haematopoietic stem cell transplantation. *Eur Respir J*. 2007;29(5):1007-1019.
53. Filipovich AH, Weisdorf D, Pavletic S, et al. National Institutes of Health consensus development project on criteria for clinical trials in chronic graft-versus-host disease: I. Diagnosis and staging working group report. *Biol Blood Marrow Transplant*. 2005;11(12):945-956.
54. Bashoura L, Gupta S, Jain A, et al. Inhaled corticosteroids stabilize constrictive bronchiolitis after hematopoietic stem cell transplantation. *Bone Marrow Transplant*. 2008;41(1):63-67.
55. Bergeron A, Belle A, Chevret S, et al. Combined inhaled steroids and bronchodilators in obstructive airway disease after allogeneic stem cell transplantation. *Bone Marrow Transplant*. 2007;39(9):547-553.
56. Khalid M, Al Saghir A, Saleemi S, et al. Azithromycin in bronchiolitis obliterans complicating bone marrow transplantation: a preliminary study. *Eur Respir J*. 2005;25(3):490-493.
57. Afessa B, Litzow MR, Tefferi A. Bronchiolitis obliterans and other late onset non-infectious pulmonary complications in hematopoietic stem cell transplantation. *Bone Marrow Transplant*. 2001;28(5):425-434.
58. Yoshihara S, Yanik G, Cooke KR, et al. Bronchiolitis obliterans syndrome (BOS), bronchiolitis obliterans organizing pneumonia (BOOP), and other late-onset noninfectious pulmonary complications following allogeneic hematopoietic stem cell transplantation. *Biol Blood Marrow Transplant*. 2007;13(7):749-759.
59. Nakasone H, Onizuka M, Suzuki N, et al. Pre-transplant risk factors for cryptogenic organizing pneumonia/bronchiolitis obliterans organizing pneumonia after hematopoietic cell transplantation. *Bone Marrow Transplant*. 2013;48(10):1317-1323.
60. Freudenberger TD, Madtes DK, Curtis JR, et al. Association between acute and chronic graft-versus-host disease and bronchiolitis obliterans organizing pneumonia in recipients of hematopoietic stem cell transplants. *Blood*. 2003;102(10):3822-3828.
61. Rasche L, Kapp M, Einsele H, et al. EBV-induced post transplant lymphoproliferative disorders: a persisting challenge in allogeneic hematopoietic SCT. *Bone Marrow Transplant*. 2014;49(2):163-167.
62. Timp JF, Braekkan SK, Versteeg HH, et al. Epidemiology of cancer-associated venous thrombosis. *Blood*. 2013;122: 1712-1723.
63. Prandoni P, Lensing AW, Piccioli A, et al. Recurrent venous thromboembolism and bleeding complications during anticoagulant treatment in patients with cancer and venous thrombosis. *Blood*. 2002;100(10):3484-3488.
64. ten Wolde M, Kraaijenhagen RA, Prins MH, et al. The clinical usefulness of D-dimer testing in cancer patients with suspected deep venous thrombosis. *Arch Intern Med*. 2002;162(16):1880-1884.
65. Moores LK, Jackson WL Jr, Shorr AF, Jackson JL. Meta-analysis: outcomes in patients with suspected pulmonary embolism managed with computed tomographic pulmonary angiography. *Ann Intern Med*. 2004;141(11):866-874.

66. Connors J. Prophylaxis against venous thromboembolism in ambulatory patients with cancer. *N Engl J Med*. 2014;370(26):2515-2519.
67. Lyman GH, Khorana AA, Kuderer NM, et al. Venous thromboembolism prophylaxis and treatment in patients with cancer: American Society of Clinical Oncology clinical practice guideline update. *J Clin Oncol*. 2013;31(17):2189-2204.
68. Kahn SR, Lim W, Dunn AS, et al. Prevention of VTE in nonsurgical patients: Antithrombotic Therapy and Prevention of Thrombosis, 9th ed: American College of Chest Physicians Evidence-Based Clinical Practice Guidelines. *Chest*. 2012;141 (2 Suppl):195S-226S.
69. Kearon C, Akl EA, Comerota AJ, et al. Antithrombotic therapy for VTE disease: Antithrombotic Therapy and Prevention of Thrombosis, 9th ed: American College of Chest Physicians Evidence-Based Clinical Practice Guidelines. *Chest*. 2012;141 (2 Suppl):419S-494S.
70. Jasti N, Streiff MB. Prevention and treatment of thrombosis associated with central venous catheters in cancer patients. *Expert Rev Hematol*. 2014;7(5):599-616.
71. Konstantinides S, Torbicki A, Agnelli G, et al. 2014 ESC guidelines on the diagnosis and management of acute pulmonary embolism (Engl Ed). *Rev Esp Cardiol* . 2015; 68(1):10-16.
72. Trobaugh-Lotrario AD, Greffe B, Deterding R, Deutsch G, Quinones R. Pulmonary veno-occlusive disease after autologous bone marrow transplant in a child with stage IV neuroblastoma: case report and literature review. *J Pediatr Hematol Oncol*. 2003;25(5):405-409.
73. Swift G, Gibbs A, Campbell I. Pulmonary veno-occlusive disease and Hodgkin's lymphoma. *Eur Respir J*. 1993;6: 596-598.
74. Gagnadoux F, Capron F, Lebeau B. Pulmonary veno-occlusive disease after neoadjuvant mitomycin chemotherapy and surgery for lung carcinoma. *Lung Cancer*. 2002;36:213-215.
75. Simonneau G, Gatzoulis MA, Adatia I, et al. Updated clinical classification of pulmonary hypertension. *J Am Coll Cardiol*. 2013;62:D34-41.
76. Dingli D, Utz JP, Krowka MJ, Oberg AL, Tefferi A. Unexplained pulmonary hypertension in chronic myeloproliferative disorders. *Chest*. 2001;120(3):801-808.
77. Trobaugh-Lotrario AD, Greffe B, Deterding R, et al. Pulmonary veno-occlusive disease after autologous bone marrow transplant in a child with stage IV neuroblastoma: case report and literature review. *J Pediatr Hematol Oncol*. 2003;25:405-409.
78. Brouns M, Jayaraju ST, Lacor C, et al. Tracheal stenosis: a flow dynamics study. *J Appl Physiol (1985)*. 2007;102(3):1178-1184.
79. Miller RD, Hyatt RE. Evaluation of obstructing lesions of the trachea and larynx by flow-volume loops. *Am Rev Respir Dis*. 1973;108(3):475-481.
80. Loddenkemper R. Thoracoscopy—state of the art. *Eur Respir J*. 1998;11(1):213-221.
81. Antony VB, Loddenkemper R, Astoul P, et al. Management of malignant pleural effusions. *Eur Respir J*. 2001;18(2):402-419.
82. Sahn S. Pleural diseases related to metastatic malignancies. *Eur Respir J*. 1997;10:1907-1913.
83. Evans AL, Gleeson FV. Radiology in pleural disease: state of the art. *Respirology*. 2004;9(3):300-312.
84. Bellingan GJ. The pulmonary physician in critical care * 6: the pathogenesis of ALI/ARDS. *Thorax*. 2002;57(6):540-546.
85. Porcel JM, Vives M, Esquerda A, Salud A, Perez B, Rodriguez-Panadero F. Use of a panel of tumor markers (carcinoembryonic antigen, cancer antigen 125, carbohydrate antigen 15-3, and cytokeratin 19 fragments) in pleural fluid for the differential diagnosis of benign and malignant effusions. *Chest*. 2004;126(6):1757-1763.
86. O'Hara MF, Cousar JB, Glick AD, Collins RD. Multiparameter approach to the diagnosis of hematopoietic-lymphoid neoplasms in body fluids. *Diagn Cytopathol*. 1985;1(1):33-38.
87. Burrows CM, Mathews WC, Colt HG. Predicting survival in patients with recurrent symptomatic malignant pleural effusions: an assessment of the prognostic values of physiologic, morphologic, and quality of life measures of extent of disease. *Chest*. 2000;117(1):73-78.
88. Villena V, Lopez-Encuentra A, Pozo F, De-Pablo A, Martin-Escribano P. Measurement of pleural pressure during therapeutic thoracentesis. *Am J Respir Crit Care Med*. 2000;162(4 Pt 1): 1534-1538.
89. Alinsonorin CY, Jimenez CA, Ersoy YM, Haque SA, Keus L, Morice RC. Indwelling pleural catheters for management of recurrent malignant pleural effusions. *Am J Respir Crit Care Med*. 2003;167(7 Suppl):A901.
90. Mares DC, Mathur PN. Medical thoracoscopic talc pleurodesis for chylothorax due to lymphoma: a case series. *Chest*. 1998;114(3):731-735.
91. Tamakoshi A, Ohno Y, JACC Study Group. Self-reported sleep duration as a predictor of all-cause mortality: results from the JACC study, Japan. *Sleep*. 2004;27:51-54.
92. Schernhammer ES, Laden F, Speizer FE, et al. Rotating night shifts and risk of breast cancer in women participating in the nurses' health study. *J Natl Cancer Inst*. 2001;93:1563-1568.
93. Schernhammer ES, Schulmeister K. Melatonin and cancer risk: does light at night compromise physiologic cancer protection by lowering serum melatonin levels? *Br J Cancer*. 2004;90:941-943.
94. Nieto FJ, Peppard PE, Young T, et al. Sleep-disordered breathing and cancer mortality: results from the Wisconsin Sleep Cohort study. *Am J Respir Crit Care Med*. 2012;186:190-194.
95. Faiz SA, Balachandran D, Hessel AC, et al. Sleep-related breathing disorders in patients with tumors in the head and neck region. *Oncologist*. 2014;19:1200-1206.
96. Farney RJ, Walker JM, Cloward TV, et al. Sleep-disordered breathing associated with long-term opioid therapy. *Chest*. 2003;123:632-639.
97. Palesh O. Prevalence, demographics and psychological associations of sleep disruption in patients with cancer. *J Clin Oncol*. 2010;28:292-298.
98. Roehrs T, Hyde M, Blaisdell B, et al. Sleep loss and REM sleep loss are hyperalgesic. *Sleep*. 2006;29:145-151.
99. Bower JE, Ganz PA, Aziz N, Fahey JL. Fatigue and proinflammatory cytokine activity in breast cancer survivors. *Psychosom Med*. 2002;64:604-611.
100. Savard J, Simard S, Blanchet J, Ivers H, Morin CM. Prevalence, clinical characteristics, and risk factors for insomnia in the context of breast cancer. *Sleep*. 2001;24:583-590.
101. Ancoli-Israel S, Moore PJ, Jones V. The relationship between fatigue and sleep in cancer patients: a review. *Eur J Cancer Care*. 2001;10:245-255.

56 Cancer-Associated Thrombosis

第五十六章　癌症相关性血栓形成

Rachel A. Sanford
Michael H. Kroll

中文导读

癌症相关性血栓形成是一种备受关注的重要并发症，与疾病本身及抗肿瘤治疗措施都可能相关。本章主要分4部分阐述。第一部分为静脉栓塞，对其临床表现（肺栓塞及深静脉血栓）、流行病学、诊断方法、预防措施、治疗措施、如何预防血栓复发等进行了细致阐述，此外，还特别对合并有血小板减少症的癌症患者的抗凝治疗给出指导，同时，对发生率高达50%的置管相关血栓形成处理进行了阐述，而关于抗凝治疗的出血也给出了处理建议，最后简介了口服抗凝血药治疗。第二部分内容为癌症相关性血栓微血管病，阐述了其发病机制，如新生血栓性血小板减少性紫癜、补体介导血栓形成微血管病、血管性血友病因子ADAMTS-13及补体交互作用微血管病；癌症相关性血栓微血管病综合征与多种因素相关，如药物、造血干细胞移植、副肿瘤血栓性微血管病等，本章指出由于癌症相关性血栓微血管病诊断的异质性，需要努力辨明发病机制，建立诊断标准，开展个体化治疗。第三部分对血管综合征进行了描述，包括可能导致静脉血栓栓塞症的抗肿瘤药类型、骨髓增生性肿瘤相关血栓形成时应注意门静脉血栓和布加综合征、特劳梭综合征等内容。第四部分指导了动脉血栓形成的处理。

VENOUS THROMBOEMBOLISM

Scope of the Problem

Pulmonary embolism (PE) and deep venous thrombosis (DVT) are manifestations of venous thromboembolism (VTE). Approximately 20% of all VTEs are associated with cancer, and cancer increases the risk for VTE four- to sixfold. Surgery, chemotherapy, hormonal therapy, growth factors, angiogenesis inhibitors, immunomodulators, erythropoietic agents, and central venous catheters (CVCs) contribute to cancer-associated VTE ([1]). Risk of VTE is associated with the type of cancer and its clinical stage, with glioblastoma, stomach cancer, pancreatic cancer, lung cancer, gynecologic cancer, and leukemia frequently associated with VTE, and early-stage breast cancer, prostate cancer, and melanoma least commonly associated with VTE ([1]). Cancer-associated VTE is rarely lethal within 6 months of diagnosis and treatment ([2]), but it is often undiagnosed, and its onset can be associated with considerable mortality. Venous thromboembolism was the death certificate–attributed cause of death for 0.21% of patients with cancer in a large population-based death certificate review ([3]), the cause of 3.5% of 141 deaths recorded among 4,466 community hospital–treated ambulatory patients with cancer ([4]), and the objectively documented cause of death among 1.5% of all patients with cancer managed by a single cancer center ([5]).

Diagnosis

Clinical presentations of VTE are not specific. Most patients with DVT have unilateral leg swelling and tenderness, and most patients with PE have abrupt-onset dyspnea and pleuritic chest pain. These symptoms are nonspecific, especially in patients who have cancer. Scoring systems developed to estimate pretest probability of DVT and PE (like the Well's scores) can be used to rule out VTE in patients with cancer, but the likelihood of finding a normal D-dimer level among patients with cancer is less than 30%, and elevated D-dimers are of no positive predictive value ([6]). Doppler/compression ultrasound is the preferred method to diagnose DVT, although magnetic resonance imaging (MRI) and computed tomography (CT) may be required in special circumstances, such as internal iliac vein or vena cava thrombosis. High-resolution CT or CT angiography is the best method for diagnosing PE ([7]), and it offers the advantage of providing additional information regarding synchronous thoracic pathology that may confound the diagnosis of PE. Conversely, up to 5% of all chest CTs done for cancer staging, monitoring, and surveillance show asymptomatic incidental PEs ([8]).

Prevention

Pharmacological VTE prophylaxis should be considered in every hospitalized patient with cancer for whom there is no contraindication ([8]). Contraindications to pharmacological anticoagulation are absolute (recent central nervous system bleed, intracranial or spinal lesion at high risk for bleeding, or major active bleeding: more than 2 units transfused in 24 hours) or relative (chronic, clinically significant measurable bleeding >48 hours; platelets <50,000/μL; platelet dysfunction [uremia, medications, dysplastic hematopoiesis]; recent major operation at high risk for bleeding; underlying hemorrhagic coagulopathy; high risk for falls; neuraxial anesthesia/lumbar puncture). Enoxaparin 40 mg, dalteparin 5,000 IU, or fondaparinux 2.5 mg subcutaneously once per day can be used for VTE prevention in patients with cancer.

Patients with cancer undergoing abdominal or pelvic surgery should receive low molecular weight heparin (LMWH) prophylaxis extended for 4 weeks ([9]). Routine pharmacological prophylaxis in ambulatory patients with cancer receiving chemotherapy is recommended only for patients with myeloma receiving thalidomide or lenalidomide as part of combination chemotherapy, although outpatient pharmacological prophylaxis can be considered in high-risk patients receiving systemic chemotherapy, such as those with pancreatic or gastric cancers ([10]).

Treatment

Routine VTE induction therapy is used to treat symptomatic VTE or incidental PE. Incidental PEs, including those found in the subsegmental branches of the pulmonary artery, appear to have a recurrence risk similar to symptomatic PE and should be managed similarly. Preference is for LMWH—for example, enoxaparin 1 mg/kg/12 hours or dalteparin 200 IU/kg/24 hours—but infused unfractionated heparin should be used for patients with renal failure or nonsevere hemorrhage. Thrombolysis can be considered in cases of massive PE (defined as associated with systolic blood pressure <90 mm Hg lasting for more than 15 minutes), and an inferior vena cava (IVC) filter should be placed when anticoagulation is contraindicated. If the contraindication is temporary, a retrievable IVC filter is preferred.

Maintenance therapy is different from that for patients without cancer, however, as it is with LMWH because LMWH is better than warfarin at preventing recurrences ([2]). When tolerated, maintenance therapy should be continued indefinitely for most patients with active cancer ([8, 11]). The risk of recurrent cancer-associated DVT after stopping anticoagulation can be stratified by examining residual venous thrombosis 6 months into treatment: Only 3/105 patients without residual venous thrombosis had recurrent DVT after stopping LMWH anticoagulation. The recurrence rate among those with residual venous thrombosis was high (49/242), and continuing anticoagulation for 6 months did not significantly affect the risk of recurrence ([12]).

The reason why LMWH is better than warfarin for maintaining anticoagulation (and may be better than the new oral anticoagulants [NOACs]) in patients with cancer is not clear. Preclinical data indicate that LMWH, but not warfarin or fondaparinux, inhibits tumor procoagulant activity by blocking mucin binding to endothelial, leukocyte, and platelet selectins. The LMWH also stimulates endothelial cell release of the potent natural anticoagulant protein *tissue factor pathway inhibitor* and binds to soluble inflammatory cytokines, thereby preventing their effect of shifting the endothelium toward an inflamed prothrombotic phenotype ([13]).

Recurrence

Recurrence of VTE on anticoagulation therapy is common in patients with cancer. The Comparison of Low-Molecular-Weight Heparin versus Oral Anticoagulant Therapy for the Prevention of Recurrent Venous Thromboembolism in Patients with Cancer (CLOT) trial from 2003 showed a best-case scenario of 9% recurrence at 6 months among those treated with LMWH maintenance ([2]). The more recent CATCH trial showed that we have not made great progress in the intervening decade: The recurrence rate was 6.9% at 6 months among patients receiving LMWH maintenance ([14]).

Optimal management of VTE recurrence remains uncertain. If the anti-FXa level drawn 4 hours after injection is not in the therapeutic range, the dose of LMWH should be adjusted, aiming toward the therapeutic peak anti-FXa level. If the anti-FXa level is therapeutic, one can increase the dose of LMWH by 20%, change to another anticoagulant, or place an IVC filter ([11]).

Anticoagulation in Patient With Thrombocytopenia

Mild thrombocytopenia (platelets <50,000/μL) is presented as a relative contraindication for anticoagulation by the American Society of Clinical Oncology and the National Comprehensive Cancer Network despite the lack of data about the risk of anticoagulation in patients with thrombocytopenia. There are, however, fairly consistent data that thrombocytopenia preventing pharmacological prophylaxis is a critical factor in the large risk of VTE and its recurrence among patients with acute leukemia ([15]) and following stem cell transplant (SCT) ([16]).

To address this conundrum, the Subcommittee on Haemostasis and Malignancy for the Scientific and Standardization Committee of the International Society of Thrombosis and Haemostasis has developed consensus guidelines ([11]). One recommendation is that patients with chronic thrombocytopenia be given dose-adjusted LMWH, with full-dose LMWH when the platelet count is greater than 50,000/μL; half-dose LMWH when the platelet count is between 25,000 and 50,000/μL; and no anticoagulation when the platelet count is less than 25,000/μL. Such an approach can also be considered for patients with cyclical thrombocytopenia from chemotherapy.

Catheter Thrombosis

Catheter thrombosis may affect almost 50% of patients who have CVCs, although fewer than 5% of catheters are associated with symptomatic occlusive DVTs ([17]). In addition to all the other risk factors for DVT development in patients with cancer, the catheter type (peripherally inserted central catheter > centrally inserted catheters > implanted ports) and location (femoral > jugular > subclavian) affect the risk of developing a catheter-related DVT.

There is no evidence that anticoagulation prevents catheter-associated thrombosis, and all guidelines currently recommend against it. The diagnosis and treatment of catheter-associated DVT are, however, similar to the diagnosis and treatment of lower-extremity DVTs, with two special considerations. The first is that the catheter can be maintained in place during anticoagulation if it is functional and useful. In this case, therapeutic anticoagulation should be maintained for as long as the catheter is in place. The second is how to manage anticoagulation when a catheter has been removed because it is infected or no longer needed. Clinical guidelines recommend 3 months of anticoagulation after catheter removal.

Bleeding Complications

Bleeding while on anticoagulation is common. During the first 6 months of treatment, about 3% of all patients with cancer will have major bleeding (generally defined as a fall in hemoglobin of 2 g over 24 hours, the need for 2 units of packed red blood cell transfusion over 24 hours, or bleeding into a vital organ or eye), and another 10% will have nonmajor bleeding ([14]). These rates may double during the next 6 months of anticoagulation. After the first year, they appear to stabilize ([18]).

Bleeding often develops unexpectedly at the beginning of treatment when LMWH unmasks a previously unrecognized bleeding threat ([8]). When major bleeding occurs, it is essential to stop anticoagulation, reverse it when appropriate (Table 56-1), and place an IVC filter.

Direct Oral Anticoagulants

The use of the DOACs—rivaroxaban, apixaban, and dabigatran—for cancer-associated VTE is generally

CHAPTER 56

Table 56-1 Rapid Reversal of the Effects of Low Molecular Weight Heparins (LMWHs)

LMWH	Reversal Agent	Dosage	Comments
Enoxaparin (Lovenox[a]) ½ life: 4.5-7 h	Protamine % Xa activity neutralized: Enoxaparin 54.2% Dalteparin 74%	Administer 1 mg of protamine for each 1 mg of enoxaparin or 100 IU of dalteparin IV slowly over 10 min or as a continuous infusion over 30 min. Rate should not exceed 5 mg/min. If enoxaparin/dalteparin was used greater than 8 h ago, then reduce dose by half (0.5 mg/1 mg enoxaparin)(0.5 mg/100 units of dalteparin). A second dose (0.5 mg/1 mg enoxaparin)(0.5 mg/100 IU dalteparin) of protamine may be given 2-4 h after the completion of the first dose. Single dose of protamine should not exceed 50 mg. Half-life is 10 min so repeat dosing may be needed.	Hypersensitivity reactions may occur in patients with known hypersensitivity to fish Monitoring: aPTT and anti-Xa Possible side effects of protamine: severe hypotension, anaphylaxis, dyspnea, bradycardia, flushing, a feeling of warmth especially when given too rapidly
Dalteparin (Fragmin®) ½ life: 4-8 h	Recombinant factor VIIa (Novo-Seven®): ½ life: 2.6-3.1 h	For life-threatening bleed that persists despite protamine administration: 20-30 µg/kg IV times 1 dose Repeat in 2 hours if needed Round to the nearest 1 mg	Monitoring: monitor for evidence of hemostasis A "normal" INR may not mean successful reversal Accepted by most Jehovah's Witness patients

Rapid reversal of the effects of low molecular weight heparins can be accomplished in bleeding patients using protamine and, if necessary, recombinant activated factor VII.
[a]PTT, activated partial thromboplastin time; INR, international normalized ratio.

discouraged, as few patients with cancer were included in the major trials of these agents, and there are no established procedures for monitoring or reversing their effects ([19]). Clinical trials are ongoing to determine the therapeutic index of these agents when they are used to prevent or treat cancer-associated VTE.

THROMBOTIC MICROANGIOPATHIES

Cancer-associated thrombotic microangiopathies (TMAs) are a group of disorders identified mainly by descriptive clinical characteristics, always involving the presence of circulating schistocytes associated with intravascular hemolysis (elevated lactate dehydrogenase LDH and indirect bilirubin), anemia, and when the bone marrow is healthy, elevated reticulocytes. Anemia and thrombocytopenia are the principle clinical manifestations, but there may also be end-organ dysfunction from microvascular thrombosis, particularly in the kidneys. Cancer-associated TMAs are distinguished from disseminated intravascular coagulation (DIC) by normal coagulation studies and D-dimer levels.

Pathogenesis of Cancer-Associated Thrombotic Microangiopathy

The molecular pathogenesis of cancer-associated TMAs is barely understood, and ignorance about pathophysiological mechanisms is coupled to inadequate diagnostic measures and a paucity of effective evidence-based clinical therapeutics. Most of the approaches utilized derive from those used to manage patients with two of the well-characterized TMAs: de novo thrombotic thrombocytopenic purpura (TTP) and hereditary complement-mediated TMA (also referred to as familial atypical hemolytic uremic syndrome [aHUS]) ([20]). Because some forms of cancer-associated TMA almost certainly result from an overlap of pathophysiological elements present in TTP and complement-mediated TMA (Fig. 56-1), a brief overview of each is presented.

De Novo Thrombotic Thrombocytopenic Purpura

Thrombotic thrombocytopenic purpura is an autoimmune disorder leading to severely deficient (<5%) activity of the primary von Willebrand factor (VWF) cleaving protease ADAMTS-13 (the thirteenth member of the protein family designated "a disintegrin

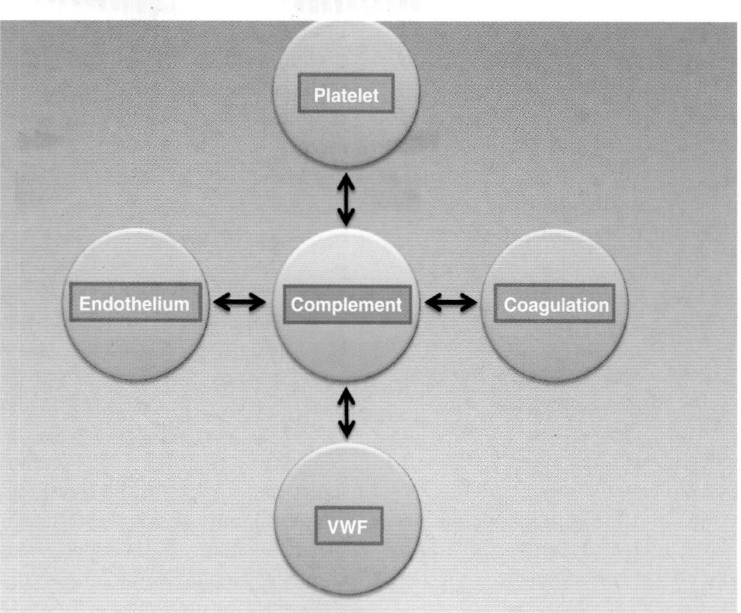

FIGURE 56-1 Cancer-associated thrombotic microangiopathies represent a pathophysiological nexus involving von Willebrand factor (VWF), platelets, the soluble coagulation system, perturbed vascular endothelium, and the complement system. Identifying and ranking the major predisposing and triggering elements is the clinical challenge that one must confront with each individual case.

and metalloproteinase with thrombospondin-type 1 motif"). Anti-ADAMTS-13 antibodies cause its dysfunction or rapid clearance, and this results in absent cleavage of ultralarge VWF multimers that are synthesized and secreted by vascular endothelium. The ultralarge VWF multimers are adhesive, and when they circulate systemically, they attach to platelet glycoprotein Ib in the microcirculation, leading to in vivo platelet activation and aggregation, microvascular thrombosis, and end-organ ischemia accompanied by microangiopathic hemolytic anemia. This is a hematological emergency with considerable mortality when it is unrecognized and untreated. Treatment targets the antibody (immune suppression with corticosteroids and urgent plasmapheresis) and restoring normal ADAMTS-13 activity (immediate plasma infusion). Factors separate from ADAMTS-13 deficiency (eg, numerous infections) are involved in triggering the onset and relapse of TTP, suggesting that there is more than a single pathophysiological element driving the development of this TMA ([21]).

Complement-Mediated Thrombotic Microangiopathy

The aHUS is characterized by microangiopathic hemolytic anemia, thrombocytopenia, and renal impairment. It is distinguished from typical hemolytic uremic syndrome by the absence of infection with Shiga-like toxin-producing bacteria ([22]). The most common etiological element in both inherited and sporadic aHUS is a deficiency of the alternative complement pathway regulatory protein factor H. Factor H binds indirectly to endothelial surfaces and engages C3b, serving as an essential allosteric cofactor for C3b cleavage by factor I. Factor I cleavage of C3b shuts down the proteolytic cascade of complement activation, thereby preventing the formation of the membrane attack complex on intact vascular endothelium. In the absence of factor H, there is unregulated complement activation and deposition of the membrane attack complex on the vascular endothelium, leading to endothelial injury and its shift from an antithrombotic to a prothrombotic surface. The reason why the renal compartment is the primary target for thrombosis in aHUS is poorly understood, although one hypothesis is that the fenestrated endothelium of the glomerulus makes the kidney particularly vulnerable to complement attack ([22]). The aHUS is treated with the anti-C5 antibody eculizumab.

Cross Talk Between von Willebrand factor, ADAMTS-13, and Complement

A story relevant to the pathogenesis of cancer-associated TMAs is rapidly developing: Recent data indicate that de novo TTP involves complement activation, and that aHUS involves abnormalities in the VWF/ADAMTS-13 axis ([23, 24]). Furthermore, mechanisms of cross talk between these two prototypical pathogenic elements have been identified and include direct interactions between factor H, VWF, and ADAMTS-13 [25, 26]. These molecular interactions provide a conceptual framework from which to explore mechanisms of cancer-associated TMAs. Innovations in diagnosis and treatment will only become possible when pathogenic elements can be identified and their clinical significance elucidated and ranked.

Syndromes of Cancer-Associated Thrombotic Microangiopathy

There are rare but predictable clinical associations between TMA and some malignancies and their treatments. These may provide general clarity about pathogenesis, and their recognition often provides a useful management strategy for patients with microangiopathic hemolytic anemia and thrombocytopenia, particularly when the TMA is due to a drug that can be replaced with an effective alternative agent.

Drugs

Several antineoplastic drugs have been repeatedly associated with TMA [27]. These include mitomycin C, gemcitabine, interferons, pentostatin, sunitinib, bevacizumab, oxaliplatin, and docetaxol. Also, TMA is predictably associated with drugs used routinely in the management of SCT: the calcineurin inhibitors cyclosporine and tacrolimus and the m-TOR inhibitors sirolimus and evirolimus. End-organ injury, should it occur, mainly involves the kidneys and is reversible after stopping the drug [28].

Hematopoietic Stem Cell Transplantation

Perhaps 25% of all recipients of SCT develop TMA [29]. Risk factors include conditioning programs (total body irradiation, busulfan, fludarabine, and platinum compounds); graft-versus-host disease; infections (especially *Aspergillus*, cytomegalovirus, and adenovirus); and medications (especially calcineurin inhibitors). The pathogenesis of post-SCT TMA focuses primarily on vascular endothelial injury (directly from drugs or irradiation or indirectly by inflammatory cytokines) as the trigger (see Fig. 56-1). Genetic or acquired abnormalities of the VWF/ADAMTS-13 axis or complement are theorized as predisposing factors that drive the development of overt TMA in susceptible individuals suffering a triggering event.

Diagnosis is based on scoring systems that have been weakly validated, only one of which includes acute renal failure, which is the primary and most threatening clinical consequence of post-SCT TMA [29]. Renal biopsy, while diagnostic, is rarely employed because comorbidities increase risks—especially bleeding—associated with it. Treatment with plasma exchange or any other active intervention is rarely effective, but discontinuing a calcineurin inhibitor can often arrest (and sometimes reverse) kidney injury. The long-term prognosis of post-SCT TMA is unfavorable; there is an increased risk of hypertension, chronic kidney disease, end-stage kidney disease, cardiac disease, and death.

Paraneoplastic Thrombotic Microangiopathy

Thrombotic microangiopathy may develop in patients with solid tumors. The most likely development pattern for patients is gastric > breast > prostate > lung > lymphoma > unknown primary cancer. Paraneoplastic TMA almost always develops in patients with bone marrow metastases and can involve a DIC-like coagulation picture. It rarely involves any end-organ injury and appears to be treatable only with effective chemotherapy, although plasma infusion followed by plasma exchange (if needed because of TMA progression despite plasma infusion) is often employed along with anticancer therapy [30].

Summary

In patients with cancer, TMAs are a heterogeneous group of diagnoses, almost all of which have common clinical correlates and a final common pathway of microvascular thromboses that threaten or injure the kidneys. Dissecting established pathophysiological elements of de novo TTP (VWF and ADAMTS-13) and aHUS (complement over activity); putative pathophysiological elements of chemotherapy and post-SCT TMA (direct endothelial toxicity and cytokine "storms"); and vague pathophysiological elements of paraneoplastic TMA (myelophthisis and coagulation system activation) may someday allow clinicians to establish diagnostic criteria and treatments that are based on a hierarchy of pathophysiological factors driving each individual case.

VASCULAR SYNDROMES

Chemotherapy-Induced Thrombosis

A number of medications used to treat cancer have been documented to increase the risk of venous thromboembolic events. These are reviewed individually. It is worth noting, however, that the use of any chemotherapeutic agent has consistently been demonstrated to increase thrombotic risk. In 2008, Khorana et al developed a predictive model for chemotherapy-associated thrombosis. In their derivation cohort of 2,701 patients, 60 patients (2.2%) developed VTE; of these events, 75% of the VTEs occurred within the first two cycles of chemotherapy [31]. A 2009 review identified systemic chemotherapy as carrying a two- to sixfold increased risk of VTE ([32-34]).

The most common oncologic medications that carry an increased risk of thrombosis include thalidomide and its derivatives when combined with steroids or chemotherapy; bevacizumab and other angiogenesis-inhibiting tyrosine kinase inhibitors (TKIs); L-asparginase; and tamoxifen. Tamoxifen raises the risk of thromboembolic events particularly in the first 2 years of use; its procoagulant effect is amplified by coadministration with chemotherapy ([35, 36]). The 2011 meta-analysis of the Early Breast Cancer Trialists' Collaborative Group found a small but real increase in VTE, including fatal PE, in patients with estrogen receptor–positive breast cancer treated with tamoxifen who were followed for 10 years. This risk was higher in patients over 55 years of age (14 fatal VTEs in 2,386 woman >55 years treated with 5 years of tamoxifen and followed for 10 years versus 1 fatal VTE in 2,289 women >55 years who did not receive tamoxifen) ([37]). In a premenopausal patient with breast cancer, a history of VTE may be an indication to consider alternative antiestrogen therapy with ovarian suppression and an aromatase inhibitor.

Bevacizumab and other angiogenesis-inhibiting TKIs have been associated with an increase in arterial thrombotic events; there are mixed data on whether the risk of venous thrombotic events is also increased ([38]). Mechanistically, it is thought that these drugs disturb the endothelial lining of the vasculature, providing a nidus for thrombus formation. Given the risk for both thrombotic and hemorrhagic complications with these medications, prophylactic anticoagulation is not recommended.

Thalidomide and its derivatives (lenalidomide, pomalidomide) increase the risk of VTE when administered in combination with steroids or chemotherapy; the highest risk is when thalidomide is combined with doxorubicin. This is thought to be due to direct endothelial damage caused by both thalidomide and doxorubicin, in addition to alterations in the coagulation cascade ([8]). Thalidomide alone does not raise the risk of VTE. Patients with multiple myeloma treated with combination therapy containing thalidomide have a risk of VTE approaching 20%. Therefore, pharmacologic VTE prophylaxis is indicated with aspirin, LMWH, or warfarin. The Myeloma Working Group has proposed a risk stratification model including factors such as obesity, recent surgery, history of VTE, and type of therapy to help determine which agent to use for VTE prophylaxis. Patients with no or one risk factor should receive aspirin (81 mg or 325 mg), and patients with two or more risk factors should receive LMWH (enoxaparin 40 mg subcutaneous daily) ([39]).

Myeloproliferative Neoplasm–Associated Thrombosis With Attention to Portal Vein Thrombosis and Budd-Chiari Syndrome

The Philadelphia chromosome–negative myeloproliferative neoplasms (Ph^- MPN), including polycythemia vera (PV), essential thrombocytosis (ET), and primary myelofibrosis (PMF), are clonal disorders of myeloid lineage stem cells associated with *JAK2*, *MPL*, or *CALR* mutations. These disorders carry an increased risk of both arterial and venous thrombotic events, as well as increased risk of hemorrhagic events. The mechanism of thrombophilia in Ph^- MPN is complex. Proposed factors include increased total volume of erythrocytes, activated/adhesive platelets and erythrocytes, inflammation leading to endothelial damage, inhibition of anticoagulant pathways, and secretion of procoagulant factors ([40]). Thrombotic events contribute significantly to disease-specific morbidity and mortality, causing 45% of all disease-specific fatal events ([41]). Venous thrombosis in an unusual location (ie, portal vein thrombosis [PVT]) may be the presenting symptoms of Ph^- MPN, and *JAK2* mutation testing should be strongly considered in a patient presenting with a first thrombosis in an unusual location.

A number of studies have sought to stratify patients with PV and ET into those with high- versus low-risk of thrombotic events, with conflicting results. Patients over age 60 or with a history of thrombosis are considered high risk. High-risk patients should be managed with low-dose aspirin, phlebotomy to a goal hematocrit of less than 45%, and cytoreduction with hydroxyurea or interferon alpha to normalize platelet count (for ET) or if phlebotomy alone is unable to produce the target hematocrit level (for PV) ([42]). Additional factors to be considered in evaluating the individual patient include *JAK2* mutation status and allele burden, leukocytosis, inflammatory markers, and any history of bleeding, particularly the presence of an acquired von Willebrand syndrome. Traditional risk factors for arterial and venous thrombotic events (smoking, hyperlipidemia, and diabetes and immobility, respectively) should be managed aggressively ([43]). The role of ruxolitinib and other *JAK* inhibitors in the prevention of thrombotic events is uncertain at this time.

Management of the acute VTE in a patient with Ph^- MPN includes anticoagulation with LMWH, heparin, fondaparinux, warfarin, or a new oral anticoagulant (NOAC); LMWH is the preferred agent. The duration of anticoagulation remains controversial; a minimum of 3 to 6 months is required, with longer duration to be guided by the clinician's estimate of risk of recurrence. Risk of recurrence is influenced by MPN disease burden, advanced age, and prior history of VTE. Bleeding complications must also be considered. If the decision is made to continue anticoagulation beyond

3 to 6 months, the risk and benefit of anticoagulation should be reassessed frequently. Aggressive management of the MPN, with attention to achieving goal complete blood cell count values, is an integral component of the management of VTE in the patient with MPN. Concurrent use of anticoagulation and antiplatelet therapy increases the risk of bleeding events ([44]). After VTE, monotherapy with an antiplatelet agent reduces the risk of both recurrent venous and arterial events; therefore, a reasonable course of action for the patient with MPN and a new VTE is 3 to 6 months of LMWH followed by long-term low-dose aspirin with optimal cytoreduction. Patient-specific factors (a life-threatening VTE or life-threatening bleeding) must always be considered.

As noted, the diagnosis of MPN may be heralded by development of a VTE in an unusual location, including the portal vein or the hepatic vein; the latter may result in venous congestion and hepatocyte damage (Budd-Chiari syndrome). The management of portal vein thrombosis (PVT) is dictated by the acuity of the thrombus. Acute PVT, in which symptoms precede the diagnosis of PVT by less than 60 days and there is no evidence of cirrhosis, is managed with therapeutic anticoagulation. The diagnosis is made with abdominal ultrasound, which has a 98% negative predictive value ([45]). Chronic PVT, and patients with PVT and cirrhosis, should not be anticoagulated as the likelihood of recanalization of the blood vessel in this setting is low, and the sequelae of PVT-related portal hypertension (gastric and esophageal varices) increase the risk of life-threatening bleeding with anticoagulation. Making the diagnosis of MPN at the time of chronic PVT diagnosis may be hindered by portal hypertension causing gastrointestinal blood loss or hypersplenism resulting in platelet sequestration, falsely suppressing hematocrit and platelet levels; a high index of suspicion is required.

Budd-Chiari syndrome can be classified as fulminant, acute, sub-acute or chronic. Unless there are clear contraindications, anticoagulation should be started promptly upon diagnosis and continued indefinitely. Although a stepwise approach is warranted with medical management alone first, a number of interventions for patients with MPN-associated Budd-Chiari syndrome are available including endovascular stenting, transjugular intrahepatic portosystemic shunt (TIPS procedure), and even orthotopic liver transplant for patients with good-prognosis ET and PV ([46]).

Trousseau's Syndrome

Trousseau's sign is the appearance of superficial thrombophlebitis heralding the diagnosis of malignancy, named after the French physician Armand Trousseau, who noted the phenomenon in 1865. Trousseau's syndrome is used more broadly to describe the hypercoagulable state associated with malignancy. The pathogenesis of Trousseau's syndrome is multifactorial and likely to involve all three components of Virchow's triad (stasis of blood flow, activation of the coagulation cascade, and damage to endothelial cells of the blood vessel) ([47, 48]). Mouse models of MET oncogene-driven hepatocellular carcinoma have demonstrated a relationship between MET-driven malignancies and the development of a thrombohemorrhagic phenotype similar to Trousseau's syndrome, mediated by cyclooxygenase-2 (COX-2) and plasminogen activator type 1 (PAI-1) genes ([49]).

ARTERIAL THROMBOSIS

The management of patients with malignancy-associated thrombocytopenia and acute coronary syndrome (ACS) poses a unique challenge; the cardioprotective effect of antiplatelet agents must be balanced with the increased risk of bleeding. A retrospective analysis of 70 patients demonstrated marked improvement in seven-day survival in patients with ACS and thrombocytopenia who received aspirin. Patients with ACS and thrombocytopenia who received aspirin had a 90% survival rate at seven-days, compared with only 6% for those with ACS and thrombocytopenia who did not receive aspirin (P <0.0001). Platelet counts in the thrombocytopenic group ranged from 4,000 to 100,000, and no major bleeding events (defined as major gastrointestinal bleeding, intracranial bleeding, or fatal bleeding) were reported ([50]). In an appropriately monitored setting and in the absence of clear contraindications, aspirin should not be withheld from the patient with malignancy-associated thrombocytopenia and acute coronary syndrome.

REFERENCES

1. Timp JF, Braekkan SK, Versteeg HH, Cannegieter SC. Epidemiology of cancer-associated venous thrombosis. *Blood.* 2013;122:1712-1723.
2. Lee AY, Levine MN, Baker RI, et al. Low-molecular-weight heparin versus a coumarin for the prevention of recurrent venous thromboembolism in patients with cancer. *N Engl J Med.* 2003;349:146-153.
3. Stein PD, Beemath A, Meyers FA, et al. Pulmonary embolism as a cause of death in patients who died of cancer. *Am J Med.* 2006;119:163-165
4. Khorana AA, Francis CW, Culakova E, Kuderer NM, Lyman GH. Thromboembolism is a leading cause of death in cancer patients receiving outpatient chemotherapy. *J Thromb Haemost.* 2007;5:632-634.
5. Pemmaraju N, Kroll SJ, Oo T, Afshar-Kharghan V, Kroll MH. Mortality from cancer-associated venous thromboembolism. *Blood.* 2014;124(Suppl 1):A4829.
6. ten Wolde M, Kraaijenhagen RA, Prins MH, et al. The clinical usefulness of D-dimer testing in cancer patients with suspected

deep venous thrombosis. *Arch Intern Med*. 2002;162:1880-1884.

7. Agnelli G, Becattini C. Acute pulmonary embolism. *N Engl J Med*. 2010;363:266-274
8. Lyman GH, Khorana AA, Falanga A, et al. American Society of Clinical Oncology guideline: recommendations for venous thromboembolism prophylaxis and treatment in patients with cancer. *J Clin Oncol*. 2007;25:5490-505.
9. Bergqvist D, Agnelli G, Cohen AT, et al. Duration of prophylaxis against venous thromboembolism with enoxaparin after surgery for cancer. *N Engl J Med*. 2002;346:975-980.
10. Connor JM. Prophylaxis against venous thromboembolism in ambulatory patients with cancer. *N Engl J Med*. 2014;370:2515-2519.
11. Carrier M, Khorana AA, Zwicker J, Noble S, Lee AY; Subcommittee on Haemostasis and Malignancy for the SSC of the ISTH. Management of challenging cases of patients with cancer-associated thrombosis including recurrent thrombosis and bleeding: guidance from the SSC of the ISTH. *J Thromb Haemost*. 2013;11:1760-1765.
12. Napolitano M, Saccullo G, Malato A, et al. Optimal duration of low molecular weight heparin for the treatment of cancer-related deep vein thrombosis: the Cancer-DACUS Study. *J Clin Oncol*. 2014;32:3607-3612.
13. Varki A. Trousseau's syndrome: multiple definitions and multiple mechanisms. *Blood*. 2007;110:1723-1729.
14. Lee AYY, Kamphuisen PW, Meyer G, et al. A randomized trial of long-term tinzaparin, a low molecular weight heparin, versus warfarin for treatment of acute venous thromboembolism (VTE) in cancer patients—the CATCH study. *Blood*. 2014;124 (Suppl 1):LBA-2.
15. Vu K, Luong NV, Hubbard J, et al. A retrospective study of venous thromboembolism in acute leukemia patients treated at the University of Texas MD Anderson Cancer Center. *Cancer Medicine* 2015;4(1):27-35. doi:10.1002/cam4.332
16. Gerber DA, Segal JB, Levy MY, Kane J, Jones RJ, Streiff MB. The incidence of and risk factors for venous thromboembolism (VTE) transplantation: implications for VTE prevention and bleeding among 1514 patients undergoing hematopoietic stem cell transplantation. *Blood*. 2008;112:504-510.
17. Geerts W. Central venous catheter-related thrombosis. Hematology Am Soc Hematol Educ Program. 2014;2014(1):306-311.
18. Chee CE, Ashrani AA, Marks RS, Petterson TM, et al. Predictors of venous thromboembolism recurrence and bleeding among active cancer patients: a population-based cohort study. *Blood*. 2014;123:3972-3978.
19. Yeh CH, Gross PL, Weitz JI. Evolving use of new oral anticoagulants for treatment of venous thromboembolism. *Blood*. 2014;124:1020-1028.
20. George JN, Nester CM. Syndromes of thrombotic microangiopathy. *N Engl J Med*. 2014;371:654-666.
21. Verbij FC, Fijnheer R, Voorberg J, Sorvillo N. Acquired TTP: ADAMTS13 meets the immune system. *Blood Rev*. 2014;28:227-234.
22. Noris M, Remuzzi G. Atypical hemolytic–uremic syndrome. *N Engl J Med*. 2009;361:1676-1687.
23. Feng S, Kroll MH, Nolasco L, Moake J, Afshar-Kharghan V. Complement activation in thrombotic microangiopathies. *Br J Haematol*. 2013;160:404-406.
24. Feng S, Eyler SJ, Zhang Y, et al. Partial ADAMTS13 deficiency in atypical hemolytic uremic syndrome. *Blood*. 2013;122:1487-1493.
25. Feng S, Liang X, Cruz MA, et al. The interaction between factor H and Von Willebrand factor. *PLoS One*. 2013;8(8):e73715. doi:10.1371
26. Feng S, Liang X, Kroll MH, Chung DW, Afshar-Kharghan V. Von Willebrand factor is a cofactor in complement regulation. *Blood*. 2015;125(6):1034-1037.
27. Al-Nouri ZL, Reese JA, Terrell DR, Vesely SK, George JN. Drug-induced thrombotic microangiopathy: a systematic review of published reports. *Blood*. 2015;125(4):616-618.
28. Jhaveri KD, Shah HH, Calderon K, Campenot ES, Radhakrishnan J. Glomerular diseases seen with cancer and chemotherapy: a narrative review. *Kidney Int*. 2013;84:34-44.
29. Laskin BL, Goebel J, Davies SM, Jodele S. Small vessels, big trouble in the kidneys and beyond: hematopoietic stem cell transplantation-associated thrombotic microangiopathy. *Blood*. 2011;118:1452-1462.
30. Lechner K, Obermeier HL. Cancer-related microangiopathic hemolytic anemia: clinical and laboratory features in 168 reported cases. *Medicine (Baltimore)*. 2012;91:195-205.
31. Khorana AA, Kuderer NM, Culakova E, et al. Development and validation of a predictive model for chemotherapy-associated thrombosis. *Blood*. 2008;111(10):4902-4907.
32. Khorana AA, Connolly GC. Assessing risk of venous thromboembolism in the patient with cancer. *J Clin Oncol*. 2009;27(29):4839-4847.
33. Blom JW, Vanderschoot JP, Oostindiër MJ, et al. Incidence of venous thrombosis in a large cohort of 66,329 cancer patients: results of a record linkage study. *J Thromb Haemost*. 2006;4(3):529-535
34. Heit JA, Silverstein MD, Mohr DN, et al. Risk factors for deep vein thrombosis and pulmonary embolism: a population-based case-control study. *Arch Intern Med*. 2000;160(6):809-815.
35. Fisher B, Costantino JP, Wickerham DL, et al. Tamoxifen for prevention of breast cancer: report of the National Surgical Adjuvant Breast and Bowel Project P-1 Study. *J Natl Cancer Inst*. 1998;90(18):1371-1388.
36. Cuzick J, Forbes J, Edwards R, et al. First results from the International Breast Cancer Intervention Study (IBIS-I): a randomised prevention trial. *Lancet*. 2002;360(9336):817-824.
37. Early Breast Cancer Trialists' Collaborative. Relevance of breast cancer hormone receptors and other factors to the efficacy of adjuvant tamoxifen: patient-level meta-analysis of randomised trials. *Lancet*. 2011;378(9793):771-784.
38. Zangari M, Fink LM, Elice F, et al. Thrombotic events in patients with cancer receiving antiangiogenesis agents. *J Clin Oncol*. 2009;27(29):4865-4873.
39. Palumbo A, Rajkumar SV, Dimopoulos MA, et al. Prevention of thalidomide- and lenalidomide-associated thrombosis in myeloma. *Leukemia*. 2008;22(2):414-423.
40. Kroll MH, Michaelis LC, Verstovsek S. Mechanisms of thrombogenesis in polycythemia vera. *Blood Rev*. 2015;29(4):215-221. doi:http://dx.doi.org/10.1016/j.blre.2014.12.002
41. Marchioli R, Finazzi G, Landolfi R, et al. Vascular and neoplastic risk in a large cohort of patients with polycythemia vera. *J Clin Oncol*. 2005;23(10):2224-2232.
42. Barbui T, Barosi G, Birgegard G, et al. Philadelphia-negative classical myeloproliferative neoplasms: critical concepts and management recommendations from European LeukemiaNet. *J Clin Oncol*. 2011;29(6):761-770.
43. Kreher S, Ochsenreither S, Trappe RU, et al. Prophylaxis and management of venous thromboembolism in patients with myeloproliferative neoplasms: consensus statement of the Haemostasis Working Party of the German Society of Hematology and Oncology (DGHO), the Austrian Society of Hematology and Oncology (OGHO) and Society of Thrombosis and Haemostasis Research (GTH e.V.). *Ann Hematol*. 2014;93(12):1953-1963.
44. De Stefano V, Za T, Rossi E, et al. Recurrent thrombosis in patients with polycythemia vera and essential thrombocythemia: incidence, risk factors, and effect of treatments. *Haematologica*. 2008;93(3):372-380.
45. Parikh S, Shah R, Kapoor P. Portal vein thrombosis. *Am J Med*. 2010;123(2):111-119.
46. Menon KV, Shah V, Kamath PS. The Budd-Chiari syndrome. *N Engl J Med*. 2004;350(6):578-585.

47. Dammacco F, Vacca A, Procaccio P, et al. Cancer-related coagulopathy (Trousseau's syndrome): review of the literature and experience of a single center of internal medicine. *Clin Exp Med*. 2013;13(2):85-97.
48. Varki A. Trousseau's syndrome: multiple definitions and multiple mechanisms. *Blood*. 2007;110(6):1723-1729.
49. Boccaccio C, Sabatino G, Medico E, et al. The MET oncogene drives a genetic programme linking cancer to haemostasis. *Nature*. 2005;434(7031):396-400.
50. Sarkiss MG, Yusuf SW, Warneke CL, et al. Impact of aspirin therapy in cancer patients with thrombocytopenia and acute coronary syndromes. *Cancer*. 2007;109(3):621-627.

Section XV

Palliative Care and Symptom Management

Section Editors: Eduardo Bruera and Michael Fisch

第十五篇 姑息治疗和症状管理

57

Palliative and Supportive Care

第五十七章　姑息和支持治疗

David Hui
Eduardo Bruera

中文导读

本章首先阐述了姑息和支持治疗的重要性。由于肿瘤本身和抗肿瘤治疗可导致一系列的症状和不良反应以及社会心理层面的需求，姑息和支持治疗对于肿瘤患者很有必要。在简单介绍了医院内咨询团队、急性姑息治疗团队、门诊和社区姑息治疗团队的分工和作用后，本章列举了支持早期进行姑息治疗的证据。在如何获得姑息治疗这部分内容中，本章提到了初级、二级和三级姑息治疗团队所发挥的不同作用和获得不同级别姑息治疗的途径，并指出初级姑息治疗团队接受进一步培训的必要性。在谈到如何解决姑息治疗推行困难的部分，本章列举了来自肿瘤学团队、患者和健康护理团队的障碍，并提出可通过常规的症状监测、使用类似“怎样开车才能更顺利到达目的地”的比喻来宣教患者、将姑息治疗更名为支持治疗来克服医患的误解、提高肿瘤学医生对于支持治疗的意识等方法来解决。

THE NEED FOR PALLIATIVE CARE

Despite significant progress in our understanding of cancer biology and the development of novel therapeutics, most patients with advanced cancer still die of their disease ([1]). In addition to the significant mortality, cancer contributes to significant morbidity for cancer patients and their families.

The growth of cancer can result in multiple symptoms by direct invasion, obstruction, compression, inflammation, effusions, and paraneoplastic syndromes. Moreover, cancer predisposes patients to various complications, such as infections, bleeding, thrombosis, and fractures. Cancer treatments such as surgery, radiation, chemotherapy-targeted agents, and immunotherapy can also cause multiple adverse effects involving the cardiac, pulmonary, gastrointestinal, hematologic, musculoskeletal, neurological, endocrine, and dermatologic systems. Living with cancer also means that patients not only have to face their own mortality but also have to deal with many psychosocial stresses related to the uncertainties along the disease trajectory. They have to cope with changes in their bodily function, body image, ability to engage in daily activities, and family dynamics. Finally, many patients and families express significant existential issues and financial concerns. Taken together, the direct cancer effects, cancer treatments, and psychosocial issues all contribute to a large number of physical and psychological symptoms, resulting in a decrease in quality of life and increase in caregiver burden ([2]).

The literature has consistently demonstrated that cancer patients, particularly those with advanced disease, experience an average of 8 to 12 symptoms ([3, 4]), suggesting that many symptoms are underrecognized, underdiagnosed, and undertreated. In addition to physical, psychological, and existential concerns, patients and families often have informational and decision-making needs ([4]).

Over the past few decades, palliative care has matured as a discipline that specializes in addressing the multidimensional care needs of patients and their families. Palliative care

> *is an approach that improves the quality of life of patients and their families facing the problem associated with life-threatening illness, through the prevention and relief of suffering by means of early identification and impeccable assessment and treatment of pain and other problems, physical, psychosocial and spiritual. … Palliative care is applicable early in the course of illness, in conjunction with other therapies that are intended to prolong life, such as chemotherapy or radiation therapy, and includes those investigations needed to better understand and manage distressing clinical complications.* ([5])

The key domains of palliative care include the following: building relationships and rapport, assessing and managing symptoms, addressing coping, establishing illness understanding, discussing cancer treatments, discussing end-of-life planning, and engaging family members ([6]).

Multiple studies have demonstrated improved patient outcomes associated with palliative care. In a meta-analysis, Higginson et al found that palliative care was associated with a significant improvement in pain (odds ratio [OR], 0.38; 95% CI, 0.23-0.64) and other symptoms (OR, 0.51; CI, 0.30-0.88) ([7]). Recent randomized controlled trials also demonstrated that palliative care involvement was associated with improvement in health-related quality of life compared to routine oncologic care ([8, 9]). Evidence also supports the role of palliative care in enhancing patient satisfaction ([10]) and caregiver satisfaction ([11]). Through facilitating end-of-life discussions, providing spiritual care, and offering an alternative to aggressive care, palliative care also contributes to improved quality of end-of-life care ([12-14]). This in turn leads to a reduction in the cost of care in the last days of life ([15]).

Setting of Palliative Care

Specialist palliative care is provided in four care settings: inpatient consultation teams, acute palliative care units, outpatient clinics, and community-based palliative care. Inpatient consultation teams represent the backbone of palliative care in the United States, with 92% of cancer centers designated by the National Cancer Institute (NCI) and 74% of non–NCI-designated cancer centers reporting their presence ([16]). Acute palliative care units provide intensive symptom control for patients and families in severe distress and facilitate transition of care ([17-19]). The mortality rate varies widely, but the average is approximately 30% ([20]). Outpatient clinics are present in 59% of NCI-designated cancer centers and in 22% of non–NCI-designated cancer centers ([16]). They are key to early palliative care access and provide longitudinal supportive care concurrent with active cancer treatments ([21]). There is growing emphasis to increase the availability of these programs. Finally, the community branch of palliative care is tailored for patients as they approach the end of life (ie, 6 months or less) ([22]), when they often have decreased ability to travel back and forth to the hospital. These individuals may benefit from outreach by the palliative care team in the form of home palliative care or a transition to home-based or inpatient hospice programs.

Evidence to Support Early Palliative Care

In the 1990s, several first-generation randomized controlled trials compared palliative care interventions to usual care; however, they did not consistently demonstrate improved outcomes ([23-25]). A systematic review revealed significant methodological limitations among these studies, such as contamination, underpowered sample size, attrition, and poor adherence ([11]). The variable timing of introduction of palliative care, the lack of standardization of palliative care programs, the heterogeneous study duration, and the inconsistent outcome measures all made it difficult to clearly identify the intervention effect associated with palliative care.

Over the past decade, second-generation studies with improved designs have provided more evidence to support not only the need for specialist palliative care but also the early involvement for patients with advanced cancer. We review the key studies supporting involvement of palliative care early in the disease trajectory.

Temel et al conducted a landmark randomized controlled trial involving 151 patients with stage IV non–small cell lung cancer comparing routine oncology care with or without early palliative care referral ([8]). Patients were eligible if they were within 8 weeks of diagnosis of metastatic cancer and had an Eastern Cooperative Oncology Group (ECOG) performance status of 0 to 2. Early palliative care involvement was associated with significant improvement in the primary outcome Trial Outcome Index in the Functional Assessment of Cancer Therapy–Lung (FACT-L) scale at 12 weeks (59 vs 53, $P = .009$). The secondary outcomes, including the Lung Cancer Subscale (21 vs 19, $P = .04$); FACT-L total score (98 vs 92, $P = .03$); Hospital Anxiety and Depression Scale (HADS) depression (16% vs 39%, $P = .01$); Patient Health Questionnaire 9 (PHQ-9) (4% vs 17%, $P = .04$); aggressive end-of-life care (33% vs 54%, $P = .05$); documentation of resuscitation preferences (53% vs 28%, $P = .05$); and overall survival (11.6 months vs 9.8 months; hazard ratio 0.59, $P = .01$) also improved significantly. Largely based on this study, the American Society of Clinical Oncology published a provisional clinical opinion in 2012 supporting the integration of palliative care into standard oncologic care ([26]).

Bakitas et al examined the effect of a nurse-led palliative care intervention in a randomized controlled trial ([9]). A total of 322 patients within 8 to 12 weeks of their diagnosis of advanced lung, gastrointestinal, genitourinary, or breast cancer were randomized to the intervention arm or usual care arm. Specifically, the study intervention was led by advanced practice nurses and consisted of four structured educational and problem-solving sessions followed by monthly telephone follow-up sessions addressing various aspects of care, such as symptom management, crisis prevention, communication strategies, advance care planning, and timely referral to palliative care and hospice teams. Over time, palliative care was associated with a significant improvement in health-related quality of life (Functional Assessment of Chronic Illness Therapy for Palliative Care [FACIT-PC], $P = .02$), depression (Center for Epidemiological Studies Depression Scale [CES-D], $P = .03$). However, symptom burden (Edmonton Symptom Assessment Scale [ESAS], $P = .06$), resource use at the end of life (intensive care unit admission, $P > .99$; emergency room visits, $P = .53$), and palliative care team referral ($P = .32$) were not significant different between the intervention and control groups. Because the study intervention was primarily nursing based, the lack of involvement of other disciplines, such as medicine, may have contributed to the lack of a significant difference in some observed outcomes.

Zimmermann et al randomized, using a cluster randomized design, 461 patients in 24 medical oncology clinics to either early involvement of palliative care or routine oncology care ([10]). Unlike the two previous clinical trials that enrolled patients from time of diagnosis, patients in this study had stage III/IV lung, gastrointestinal, genitourinary, breast, or gynecological cancer with an estimated survival of 6-24 months. The primary outcome, Functional Assessment of Chronic Illness Therapy–Spiritual Well-Being (FACIT-Sp) at 3 months, improved in the early palliative care arm (1.6) and decreased in the control arm (−2.0), although the difference was not statistically significant (3.6, $P = .07$). At 4 months, a significant improvement was observed (2.5 vs −4.0, difference = 6.4, $P = .006$). Secondary outcomes also favored early palliative care by 4 months, including Quality of Life at the End of Life (QUAL-E) scale (3.0 vs −0.5, difference = 3.5, $P = .003$), symptom burden measured by the ESAS (−1.3 vs 3.2, difference = −4.4, $P = .05$), and patient satisfaction with care assessed by FAMCARE-P16 (3.7 vs −2.4, difference = 6.0, $P < .0001$). The median survival in the early palliative care arm was 340 days, suggesting that these patients accessed palliative care relatively early in the disease trajectory.

Because the studies mentioned compared early palliative care to routine oncologic care, it was unclear if late palliative care was as effective as early palliative care. This question was partly addressed in a recent retrospective cohort study examining the quality of end-of-life care indicators in the last 30 days of life among patients who died of advanced cancer at MD Anderson Cancer Center ([14]). Patients referred to palliative care 3 months or more before death had significantly lower rates of emergency room visits (39% vs 68%, $P < .001$), hospital admission (48% vs 81%, $P < .001$), and hospital death (17% vs 31%, $P = .004$) compared with a patient seen by the same palliative care team less than 3 months before death. Similar differences were also reported using 6 months as the cutoff. Moreover, outpatient palliative care consultation was associated with significantly improved outcomes compared with inpatient palliative care consultation

(Table 57-1). In multivariate analysis, improved quality of end-of-life care was associated with female gender (OR, 1.63; $P = .027$), palliative care outpatient referral (OR, 2.4; $P < .001$), and nonhematologic malignancies (OR, 2.6; $P = .02$).

Taken together, these studies suggest that early outpatient palliative care is associated with improved health-care outcomes. Table 57-2 summarizes some key questions related to palliative care delivery.

Access to Palliative Care

The delivery of palliative care can be categorized as primary, secondary, and tertiary ([27, 28]). Primary palliative care is the provision of basic symptom management and psychosocial care by oncology teams and primary care clinicians. Because these clinicians see patients in the frontline setting, it is crucial that they are all equipped with core palliative care competencies. Secondary palliative care refers to consultation services provided by interdisciplinary specialist palliative care teams. Often, patients have more complex supportive care needs, such as severe pain not relieved by first-line strong opioids. A growing number of countries, such as the United Kingdom, the United States, and Canada, have formal board accreditation for palliative medicine ([29]). Tertiary palliative care denotes the situation when palliative care becomes the primary coordinating team. For example, patients admitted to acute palliative care units are followed by tertiary palliative

Table 57-1 Outpatient Palliative Care Consultation Is Associated With Improved Quality of End-of-Life Care[a]

Within the Last 30 Days of Life	Outpatient Referral, n = 169 (%)	Inpatient Referral, n = 199 (%)	*P* Value
Any emergency room visit	80 (48)	135 (68)	<.001
2 or more emergency room visits	18 (11)	51 (26)	<.001
Any hospital admission	87 (52)	171 (86)	<.001
2 or more hospital admissions	17 (10)	47 (24)	.001
More than 14 days of hospitalization	14 (8)	40 (20)	.002
Hospital death	30 (18)	67 (34)	.001
Any ICU admission	7 (4)	28 (14)	.001
ICU death	3 (2)	10 (5)	.15
Chemotherapy and targeted agent use	41 (25)	55 (28)	.55

ICU, intensive care unit.
[a]Modified with permission from Hui D, Kim SH, Roquemore J, et al. Impact of timing and setting of palliative care referral on quality of end-of-life care in cancer patients, *Cancer* 2014 Jun 1;120(11):1743-1749.

Table 57-2 The Delivery of Palliative Care

Question	Answer
Who should receive palliative care?	According to the National Comprehensive Cancer Network guideline, all patients with significant physical, psychological, social, or spiritual concerns should be considered for referral to a palliative care team. Additional triggers include comorbidities, caregiver distress, and professional distress ([49]).
When should palliative care be provided?	The literature supports early introduction of palliative care from the time of diagnosis of advanced cancer.
Who should deliver palliative care?	All oncologists and primary care teams should be prepared to provide core palliative care skills. At the same time, specialized interdisciplinary palliative care teams should be available to provide further support and guidance, particularly for patients with significant distress.
How should palliative care be delivered?	Comprehensive palliative care interventions, including outpatient and inpatient components, should be used.
Where should patients receive palliative care?	Outpatient palliative care facilitates early involvement and is ideal for initial consultation and longitudinal follow-up. Inpatient palliative care is appropriate for hospitalized patients who are acutely ill. Community-based palliative care is particularly helpful for patients who are too frail to make repeated visits to the hospital.

care teams. Tertiary palliative care teams are often actively involved in education and research.

In delivering primary palliative care, oncologists generally feel the need for their active involvement in the provision of symptom management and supportive care ([30]). A 1998 survey of 3,227 medical, radiation, surgical, and pediatric oncologists revealed that 90% learned palliative care by trial and error. A majority also reported that they had inadequate coaching in discussing prognosis and symptom control ([31]). In another survey of 895 medical oncologists in Europe, only 36% agreed that a palliative care specialist is the best person to coordinate palliative care of patients with advanced cancer; however, only 37% reported that most medical oncologists they know are expert in symptom management ([30]). A more recent survey of US oncology trainees showed they still received limited core palliative care training, with less than half reporting having explicit training in the management of depression at the end of life and opioid rotation ([32]). To date, only approximately 25% of oncology fellows have routine palliative care rotations ([16, 32]). To enhance the level of primary palliative care delivery, oncology fellowships should incorporate a greater degree of didactic and clinical training related to palliative care, ideally with role modeling and clinical rotations. Recognizing this important gap in knowledge, multiple organizations, such as the American Society of Clinical Oncology (ASCO) and the European Society of Medical Oncology (ESMO), are taking active measures to increase the level of core palliative care skills among oncology professionals through conferences, continuing medication education, and web-based learning ([33]).

For secondary and tertiary palliative care, access to specialized teams can be measured in several ways: (1) What is the level of availability of palliative care in cancer centers? (2) Among cancer centers that offer palliative care programs, how many patients with advanced cancer see palliative care before they die? (3) Among patients who have had a palliative care consultation, when was the time of referral?

Although most US cancer centers reported having a palliative care service, the infrastructure of these programs varied widely, ranging from a single nurse practitioner to a comprehensive interdisciplinary team ([34]). Cancer center executives, particularly in NCI-designated cancer centers, generally supported the expansion of palliative care in their centers. On a global scale, the development of palliative care has recently been outlined in the Worldwide Hospice Palliative Care Alliance (WPCA) Global Atlas of Palliative Care, demonstrating higher level of development in developed nations and areas for improvement in developing nations ([35]).

The proportion of cancer patients who had palliative care consultations is another measure of access, although the denominator is not easily defined because not all patients may benefit from palliative care. We examined the timing of referral for patients who died of advanced cancer at MD Anderson Cancer Center during a 6-month period and found that only 366 of 816 (45%) had a palliative care consultation ([36]). The percentage of referral varied significantly among tumor types. Over 60% of patients with gynecology malignancies had a palliative care consultation before death compared to only slightly over 30% in patients with hematologic malignancies. Older patients and those who were married were more likely to have a referral ([36]). The timing of palliative care referral was also examined in this study. A majority of patients were referred to palliative care late in the disease trajectory, ranging from 1 to 2 months before death for patients with solid tumors to 0.4 months before death for hematologic malignancies ([36]). In a US national survey, the median time from referral to death was 90 days for outpatient palliative care clinics and 7 days for inpatient palliative care programs ([16]).

Overcoming Barriers to Palliative Care Access

Despite the evidence to support early palliative care, there remain significant barriers to accessing specialist palliative care. These barriers can be categorized as oncology team–related barriers, patient-related barriers, and health-care system–related barriers (Table 57-3) ([36-39]). In particular, the lack of emphasis of supportive care needs and the stigma associated with palliative care represent barriers common to both patients and oncology teams. A number of interventions, such as routine symptom screening, use of the goals of car analogy (discussed further in the chapter), and name change to supportive care may facilitate early palliative care access early in the disease trajectory.

To increase the awareness of supportive care needs, routine symptom screening using validated questionnaires in the oncology setting is essential. The ESAS examines 10 symptoms (pain, fatigue, nausea, depression, anxiety, drowsiness, appetite, well-being, dyspnea, and sleep). The intensity of each symptom is documented using a one-item numeric rating scale that ranges from 0 to 10 (0 is no symptom, 10 is worst possible intensity) ([40, 41]). Other symptom batteries include the Memorial Symptom Assessment Scale and Palliative Care Outcome Scale ([42, 43]). Routine symptom screening allows the oncology team to obtain patient-reported outcomes, which would help bring significant symptoms to their attention that would otherwise be missed. Once symptoms are identified, the oncology team may initiate treatments or make a referral to specialist palliative care. Repeat screening in future visits

Table 57-3 Barriers to Palliative Care Referral

Types of Barriers	Examples
Oncology team related	• Oncology professionals' perception that they should be the team providing most of the supportive care to their patients • Oncology professionals' misconception that palliative care should only be delivered late in the disease trajectory • Stigma associated with palliative care (a referral denotes hopelessness) • Lack of routine symptom screening leads to lack of recognition of supportive care needs • Lack of time to discuss palliative care referral
Patient related	• Unaware that palliative care is available as a service • Misconception that palliative care should only be received late in the disease trajectory • Stigma associated with palliative care (a referral denotes hopelessness) • Unwillingness to discuss symptom burden to maximize chances to receive cancer treatments • Lack of time to discuss symptom concerns • Financial constraints (eg, insurance copay, transportation, parking)
Health-care system related	• Lack of resources to support palliative care teams • Fragmentation of health-care system means patients with supportive care needs receive heterogeneous referral • Financial barriers for patients (eg, parking, transportation)

allows symptoms to be monitored longitudinally and symptom response to be assessed [44].

Another approach to increase the awareness of supportive care needs is to educate patients using the analogy of the goals of the use of a car (Fig. 57-1) [45]. Some patients focus on seeking cancer treatments and do not want to worry about addressing their supportive care issues, such as symptom management, psychological distress, and advance care planning. This is similar to a hopeful and unrealistic driver who only wants to get to the destination without worrying about the potential hazards on the road and the possibility of accidents. In contrast, a hopeful and realistic driver knows the need to prepare for the road trip ahead—seat belts, insurance policies, suspensions, and cushions are essential to help arrive at the destination comfortably and safely. Because patients with advanced cancer inevitably develop symptom burden along the disease trajectory, it is important for the hopeful and realistic patient to maximize supportive care while receiving cancer treatments. Optimal supportive care would help to maximize symptom control and function, which may help in tolerating cancer treatments and deriving a treatment response.

Because palliative care is often felt to be synonymous with hospice care and end-of-life care, many clinicians and patients may have the impression that palliative care is not compatible with early referrals. To overcome this misconception, the term *supportive care* has been proposed to facilitate early palliative care referral. Supportive care is defined as "the provision of the necessary services for those living with or affected by cancer to meet their informational, emotional, spiritual, social or physical needs during their diagnostic, treatment, or follow-up phases encompassing issues of health promotion and prevention, survivorship, palliation and bereavement" [28]. Thus, palliative care is, by definition, supportive care for patients with advanced diseases. We previously conducted a survey of oncology specialists at our cancer center to examine clinicians' beliefs toward the palliative care and supportive care. Compared to supportive care, oncology specialists were significantly more likely to feel that the service name palliative care decreases hope in patients and families, is synonymous with hospice and end of life, and is a barrier for referral (Table 57-4) [46]. This led our program to change its name from Palliative Care to Supportive Care in 2007. We found an increased number of referrals and earlier referral among outpatients after the name change, supporting the hypothesis that supportive care facilitates palliative care access (Table 57-5) [47].

Finally, it is important to help oncologists understand how integration of palliative care with oncology can help them care for their patients. The everyday oncology practice consists of management of cancer, such as diagnosis, staging, and treatment decisions, as well as management of supportive care issues such as pain, fatigue, anxiety, and care planning. There are three approaches to address these increasingly complex issues (Fig. 57-2). In the solo practice model, the oncologist manages all the issues. Because of lack of time to conduct routine symptom screening, inability to keep up with the growing literature on supportive care, and absence of an interdisciplinary team, those in solo practice may not provide the optimal level of supportive care. In the congress model, the oncologist focuses on cancer-related issues and involves many different services, each focusing on one particular aspect

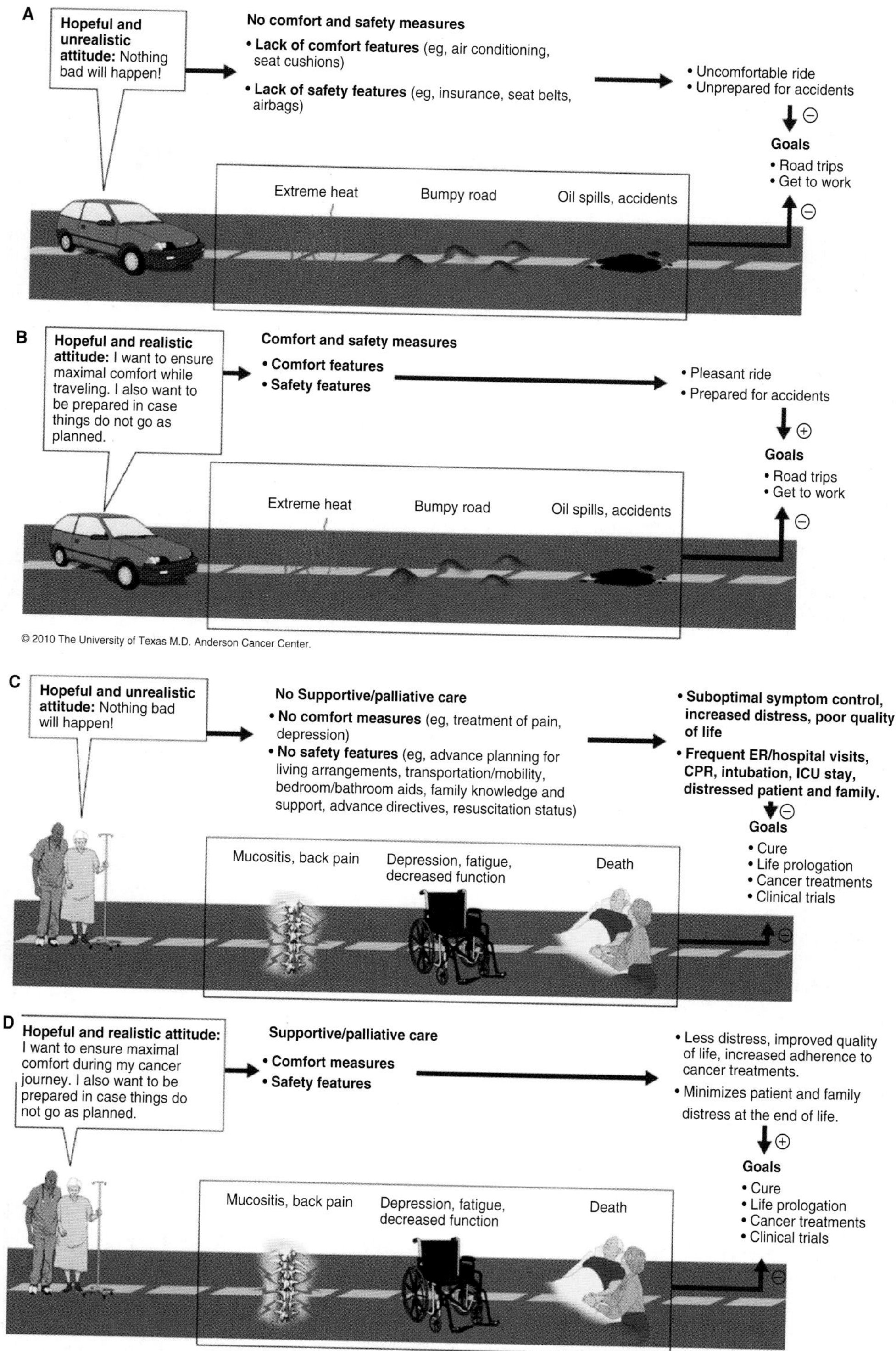

FIGURE 57-1 **Goals of care. The use of a car is an analogy for setting goals of care. (A). A hopeful and unrealistic driver wishes that nothing bad will happen on the road. This is in contrast to (B), the hopeful and realistic driver who knows the importance of comfort measures and of being prepared for the trip ahead. (C). A hopeful and unrealistic patient focuses on cancer cure and life-prolongation measures without paying attention to her symptoms and advance care needs. This results in unnecessary distress for patients and families. This is in contrast to (D), a hopeful and realistic patient, who has the same goals for cancer control but is better equipped to manage symptoms and prepared for crisis because of the concurrent use of supportive/palliative care. ER, emergency room; CPR, cardiopulmonary resuscitation; ICU, intensive care unit.** (Reproduced with permission from The University of Texas MD Anderson Cancer Center.)

Table 57-4 Perception of the Names *Palliative Care* and *Supportive Care*[a]

Perception	Supportive Care, n (%)	Palliative Care, n (%)	*P* value
Service name is a barrier for me to refer patients	9 (7)	32 (23)	<.0001
Service name is synonymous with hospice and end of life	21 (15)	78 (57)	<.0001
Service name can decrease hope in patient and families	15 (11)	61 (44)	<.0001
Service name is associated with treatment of chemotherapy side effects	85 (61)	20 (15)	<.0001

[a]Adapted with permission from Fadul N, Elsayem A, Palmer JL, et al. Supportive versus palliative care: what's in a name?: a survey of medical oncologists and midlevel providers at a comprehensive cancer center, *Cancer* 2009 May 1;115(9):2013-2021.

Table 57-5 Growth in New Patient Activity Before and After Name Change[a]

Program	Before Name Change (January 1, 2006, to August 31, 2007), n	After Name Change (January 1, 2008, to August 31, 2009), n	% Change
Supportive care program	1,950	2,751	41%
Division of Cancer Medicine	17,009	21,325	25%
Hospital overall	58,540	66,608	14%

[a]Data from Dalal S, Palla S, Hui D, et al. Association between a name change from palliative to supportive care and the timing of patient referrals at a comprehensive cancer center, *Oncologist* 2011;16(1):105-111.

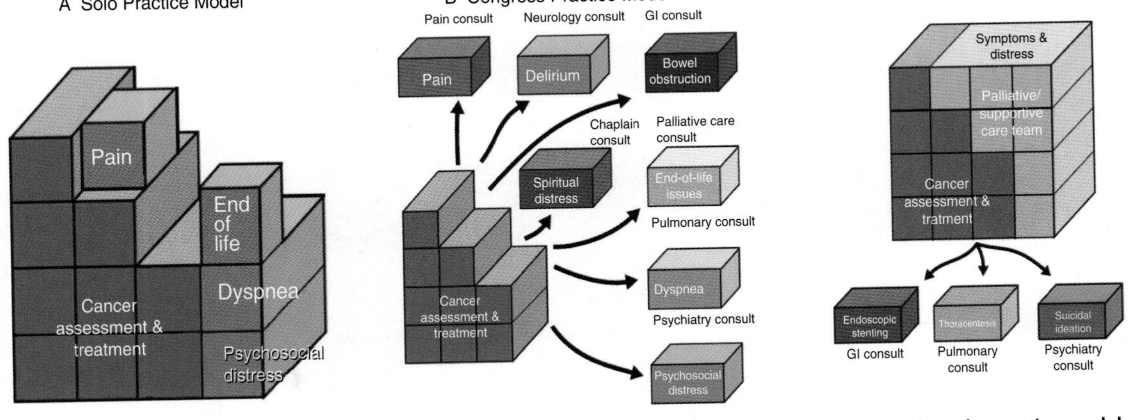

FIGURE 57-2 Conceptual model for integration of palliative and supportive care in oncology. A. In the solo practice model, the oncologist attempts to take care of all patient-related issues. B. In the congress practice model, the oncologist focuses on cancer assessment and treatment and refers the patient to various subspecialties for other concerns. C. In the integrated-care model, the oncologist collaborates closely with the interdisciplinary supportive/palliative care team to provide comprehensive cancer care. GI, gastrointestinal. (Reproduced with permission from The University of Texas MD Anderson Cancer Center.)

of supportive care. This could potentially result in fragmentation of care, sometimes-conflicting recommendations, and added care costs. In the integrated care model, the oncologist addresses cancer management and involves the supportive/palliative team early in the disease trajectory. Patients thus would receive timely and comprehensive supportive care. A study showed that consultation to palliative care saves the oncologist on average 170 minutes of patient encounter ([48]).

In summary, cancer patients experience significant symptom burden and have information and decision-making needs. Palliative care is now an accredited discipline that addresses these issues to improve patients' quality of life. There is a growing body of evidence to support that early referral to palliative care improves patient outcomes, including symptom control, quality of life, quality of end-of-life care, patient and caregiver satisfaction, and possibly survival. However, there remain many barriers to palliative care access. Innovative models and approaches are needed to overcome these barriers and to maximize patient outcomes.

REFERENCES

1. Siegel R, Ma J, Zou Z, et al. Cancer statistics, 2014. *CA Cancer J Clin*. 2014;64:9-29.
2. Hui D, Bruera E. Supportive and palliative oncology: a new paradigm for comprehensive cancer care. *Hematol Oncol Rev*. 2013;9:68-74.
3. Portenoy RK, Thaler HT, Kornblith AB, et al. Symptom prevalence, characteristics and distress in a cancer population. *Qual Life Res*. 1994;3:183-189.
4. Whelan TJ, Mohide EA, Willan AR, et al. The supportive care needs of newly diagnosed cancer patients attending a regional cancer center. *Cancer*. 1997;80:1518-1524.
5. World Health Organization. *WHO Definition of Palliative Care*. Geneva, Switzerland: World Health Organization. http://www.who.int/cancer/palliative/definition/en/. Last accessed 12/3/2015.
6. Yoong J, Park ER, Greer JA, et al. Early palliative care in advanced lung cancer: a qualitative study. *JAMA Intern Med*. 2013;173:283-290.
7. Higginson IJ, Finlay IG, Goodwin DM, et al. Is there evidence that palliative care teams alter end-of-life experiences of patients and their caregivers? *J Pain Symptom Manage*. 2003;25:150-168.
8. Temel JS, Greer JA, Muzikansky A, et al. Early palliative care for patients with metastatic non-small-cell lung cancer. *N Engl J Med*. 2010;363:733-742.
9. Bakitas M, Lyons KD, Hegel MT, et al. Effects of a palliative care intervention on clinical outcomes in patients with advanced cancer: the Project ENABLE II randomized controlled trial. *JAMA*. 2009;302:741-749.
10. Zimmermann C, Swami N, Krzyzanowska M, et al. Early palliative care for patients with advanced cancer: a cluster-randomised controlled trial. *Lancet*. 2014;383:1721-1730.
11. Zimmermann C, Riechelmann R, Krzyzanowska M, et al. Effectiveness of specialized palliative care: a systematic review. *JAMA*. 2008;299:1698-1709.
12. Wright AA, Zhang B, Ray A, et al. Associations between end-of-life discussions, patient mental health, medical care near death, and caregiver bereavement adjustment. *JAMA*. 2008;300:1665-1673.
13. Balboni TA, Paulk ME, Balboni MJ, et al. Provision of spiritual care to patients with advanced cancer: associations with medical care and quality of life near death. *J Clin Oncol*. 2010;28:445-452.
14. Hui D, Kim SH, Roquemore J, et al. Impact of timing and setting of palliative care referral on quality of end-of-life care in cancer patients. *Cancer*. 2014;120:1743-9.
15. Morrison RS, Penrod JD, Cassel JB, et al. Cost savings associated with US hospital palliative care consultation programs. *Arch Intern Med*. 2008;168:1783-1790.
16. Hui D, Elsayem A, De la Cruz M, et al. Availability and integration of palliative care at US cancer centers. *JAMA*. 2010;303:1054-1061.
17. Hui D, Dos Santos R, Chisholm G, et al. Symptom expression in the last 7 days of life among cancer patients admitted to acute palliative care units. *J Pain Symptom Manage*. 2015;50(4):488-494.
18. Hui D, Elsayem A, Li Z, et al. Antineoplastic therapy use in patients with advanced cancer admitted to an acute palliative care unit at a comprehensive cancer center: a simultaneous care model. *Cancer*. 2010;116:2036-2043.
19. Lagman R, Rivera N, Walsh D, et al. Acute inpatient palliative medicine in a cancer center: clinical problems and medical interventions—a prospective study. *Am J Hosp Palliat Care*. 2007;24:20-28.
20. Hui D, Elsayem A, Palla S, et al. Discharge outcomes and survival of patients with advanced cancer admitted to an acute palliative care unit at a comprehensive cancer center. *J Palliat Med*. 2010;13:49-57.
21. Yennurajalingam S, Kang JH, Hui D, et al. Clinical response to an outpatient palliative care consultation in patients with advanced cancer and cancer pain. *J Pain Symptom Manage*. 2012;44:340-350.
22. Hui D, Nooruddin Z, Didwaniya N, et al. Concepts and definitions for "actively dying," "end of life," "terminally ill," "terminal care," and "transition of care": a systematic review. *J Pain Symptom Manage*. 2014;47:77-89.
23. McWhinney IR, Bass MJ, Donner A. Evaluation of a palliative care service: problems and pitfalls. *BMJ*. 1994;309:1340-1342.
24. Grande GE, Todd CJ, Barclay SI, et al. Does hospital at home for palliative care facilitate death at home? Randomised controlled trial. *BMJ*. 1999;319:1472-1475.
25. Hughes SL, Cummings J, Weaver F, et al. A randomized trial of the cost effectiveness of VA hospital-based home care for the terminally ill. *Health Serv Res*. 1992;26:801-817.
26. Smith TJ, Temin S, Alesi ER, et al. American Society of Clinical Oncology provisional clinical opinion: the integration of palliative care into standard oncology care. *J Clin Oncol*. 2012;30:880-887.
27. von Gunten CF. Secondary and tertiary palliative care in US hospitals. *JAMA*. 2002;287:875-881.
28. Hui D. Definition of supportive care: does the semantic matter? *Curr Opin Oncol*. 2014;26:372-379.
29. von Gunten CF, Lupu D. Development of a medical subspecialty in palliative medicine: progress report. *J Palliat Med*. 2004;7:209-219.
30. Cherny NI, Catane R; European Society of Medical Oncology Taskforce on Palliative and Supportive Care. Attitudes of medical oncologists toward palliative care for patients with advanced and incurable cancer: report on a survery by the European Society of Medical Oncology Taskforce on Palliative and Supportive Care. *Cancer*. 2003;98:2502-2510.
31. Ferris FD, Bruera E, Cherny N, et al. Palliative cancer care a decade later: accomplishments, the need, next steps. *J Clin Oncol*. 2009;27:3052-3058.
32. Buss MK, Lessen DS, Sullivan AM, et al. Hematology/oncology fellows' training in palliative care: results of a national survey. *Cancer*. 2011;117:4304-4311.
33. Von Roenn JH, Voltz R, Serrie A. Barriers and approaches to the successful integration of palliative care and oncology practice. *J Natl Compr Canc Netw*. 2013;11(Suppl 1):S11-S16.
34. Bruera E, Hui D. Conceptual models for integrating palliative care at cancer centers. *J Palliat Med*. 2012;15:1261-1269.
35. Alliance WHPC. *WHO Global Atlas on Palliative Care at the End of Life*. WHPCA; 2014.
36. Hui D, Kim SH, Kwon JH, et al. Access to palliative care among patients treated at a comprehensive cancer center. *Oncologist*. 2012;17:1574-1580.
37. Alesi ER, Fletcher DS. Integrating palliative care into oncology care: confronting the barriers. *Oncology*. 2013;27(1). pii: 168739.
38. Miyashita M, Hirai K, Morita T, et al. Barriers to referral to inpatient palliative care units in Japan: a qualitative survey with content analysis. *Support Care Cancer*. 2006;16:217-222.
39. Schenker Y, Crowley-Matoka M, Dohan D, et al. Oncologist factors that influence referrals to subspecialty palliative care clinics. *J Oncol Pract*. 2014;10(2):e37-e44.
40. Bruera E, Kuehn N, Miller MJ, et al. The Edmonton Symptom Assessment System (ESAS): a simple method for the assessment of palliative care patients. *J Palliat Care*. 1991;7:6-9.
41. Chang VT, Hwang SS, Feuerman M: Validation of the Edmonton Symptom Assessment Scale. *Cancer*. 2000;88:2164-2171.
42. Portenoy RK, Thaler HT, Kornblith AB, et al. The Memorial Symptom Assessment Scale: an instrument for the evaluation of

symptom prevalence, characteristics and distress. *Eur J Cancer.* 1994;30A:1326-1336.

43. Hearn J, Higginson IJ. Development and validation of a core outcome measure for palliative care: the palliative care outcome scale. Palliative Care Core Audit Project Advisory Group. *Qual Health Care.* 1999;8:219-227.
44. Kang JH, Kwon JH, Hui D, et al. Changes in symptom intensity among cancer patients receiving outpatient palliative care. *J Pain Symptom Manage.* 2013;46(5):652-660.
45. Bruera E, Hui D. Integrating supportive and palliative care in the trajectory of cancer: establishing goals and models of care. *J Clin Oncol.* 2010;28:4013-4017.
46. Fadul N, Elsayem A, Palmer JL, et al. Supportive versus palliative care: what's in a name? A survey of medical oncologists and midlevel providers at a comprehensive cancer center. *Cancer.* 2009;115:2013-2021.
47. Dalal S, Palla S, Hui D, et al. Association between a name change from palliative to supportive care and the timing of patient referrals at a comprehensive cancer center. *Oncologist.* 2011;16:105-111.
48. Muir JC, Daly F, Davis MS, et al. Integrating palliative care into the outpatient, private practice oncology setting. *J Pain Symptom Manage.* 2010;40:126-135.
49. Levy MH, Adolph MD, Back A, et al. *NCCN Clinical Practice Guidelines in Oncology. Palliative Care.* National Comprehensive Cancer Network; 2014.

58 Pain Management and Symptom Control

第五十八章　疼痛管理和症状控制

Kaoswi Shih
Rony Dev
Suresh K. Reddy

中文导读

本章集中讲述多种肿瘤相关症状的评估与控制策略。首先重点介绍了肿瘤疼痛的病理生理过程、评估和管理原则，并详细阐明了药物治疗的原则、便秘的预防和治疗、阿片类药物的剂量转换、疼痛辅助用药以及非药物治疗方法。随后本章介绍了肿瘤相关疲乏的评估和管理、恶心/厌食/恶液质的病因管理与营养咨询，以及呼吸困难的处理原则。本章接着介绍了临床常见的精神和神经系统异常，不仅强调了谵妄的临床表现、评估、处理原则和姑息镇静，还简要介绍了抑郁、沟通（传递坏消息等）、精神困扰等诸多方面内容。本章最后强调，上述肿瘤相关症状的管理应当尽早进行，并应贯穿于肿瘤患者的治疗全程。

INTRODUCTION

Cancer is frequently associated with a host of distressing physical and psychosocial symptoms that can occur throughout the disease trajectory ([1]). Access to a multidisciplinary supportive care service is imperative for patients with cancer experiencing distressing symptoms, including fatigue, pain, anorexia, nausea, dyspnea, anxiety, depression, and weight loss, to improve the quality of life of patients. Without optimal symptom control, administration of anticancer therapies may be delayed or discontinued (Table 58-1).

CANCER PAIN

Uncontrolled pain has been reported by 42% of patients seen in the outpatient cancer center ([1]) and 50% of hospitalized patients with cancer ([2]). Pain was the most common symptom (82%) among patients with cancer referred to a palliative care service ([3]). In patients with cancer, pain may be the only symptom present prior to diagnosis and can indicate the recurrence or spread of the disease.

As many as 30% to 50% of patients receiving active anticancer therapy experience pain ([1]). Pain resulting from the tumor burden occurs in approximately 65% to 85% of patients with advanced cancer ([4]). In addition, treatment-related pain is reported by approximately 15% to 25% of patients, and 3%-10% of patients with cancer develop chronic nonmalignant pain syndromes similar to the general population (eg, low back pain associated with degenerative disk disease).

Pathophysiology

The pathophysiologic classification of pain forms the basis for therapeutic choices. Pain may be broadly divided into those associated with ongoing tissue damage (nociceptive) and those resulting from nervous system dysfunction (neuropathic). Nociceptive pain can be classified as either somatic or visceral and results from the activation of nociceptors in cutaneous or deep tissues. Nociceptive pain is described by patients as localized aching, throbbing, and gnawing discomfort. Visceral pain is the result of activation of nociceptors resulting from distention, stretching, and inflammation of internal organs. It is often poorly localized discomfort, described as a deep aching or cramping or a pressure-like sensation. An example of visceral pain is abdominal pain due to pancreatic cancer. Breakthrough pain is defined as a transitory exacerbation of discomfort that occurs on a background of stable persistent chronic pain. Causes of breakthrough pain include end-of-dose failure of opioids and pain exacerbation by activity or spontaneous occurrence. Breakthrough pain is also characterized by a short duration, often less than 3 minutes in 43% of cases according to previous prospective surveys ([5]).

Classification of pain can help guide selection of appropriate interventions to improve pain control; however, they have not been universally accepted. Pain mechanism, incidental occurrences, psychological distress, addictive behavior, and cognitive dysfunction have been indicated as factors associated with higher ratings of pain intensity ([6]). The revised Edmonton Classification System for Cancer Pain (Fig. 58-1) characterizing these factors has been used at our institution to guide pain management.

Table 58-1 Symptoms in Advanced Cancer[a]

• Pain (80%-85%)
• Fatigue (90%)
• Weight loss (80%)
• Lack of appetite (80%)
• Nausea, vomiting (80%-90%)
• Anxiety (25%)
• Shortness of breath (50%)
• Confusion/agitation (80%)

[a]Reproduced with permission from Elsayem A, Driver LC, Bruera E. *The MD Anderson Palliative Care Handbook*. Houston, TX: MD Anderson Cancer Center; 2002.

Pain Assessment

Pain can be measured by using visual, analogue, verbal, or numerical scales and, in the research setting, complex pain questionnaires ([7]). The Edmonton Symptom Assessment Scale is a useful assessment tool that allows patients to rate pain between 0 and 10 over the past 24 hours, where 0 signifies no pain and 10 is the worst pain imaginable. Effective pain assessments can be converted into graphic displays of pain and incorporated with other symptoms, allowing quick dissemination of information regarding a patient's symptom burden to all health-care providers (Fig. 58-2). Pain assessment needs to take into account other symptoms experienced by patients with cancer because they are often are interconnected.

In 1984, the World Health Organization (WHO) proposed an analgesic ladder for the pharmacologic management of cancer pain ([8]) and has shown that the simple principle of escalating from nonopioid to strong opioid analgesics is safe and effective (Fig. 58-3). Other guidelines have been published, such as the Analgesic Quantification Algorithm and National Comprehensive Cancer Network guidelines for treating cancer pain ([9]).

Principles of Management

- Assess pain syndromes and other symptoms accurately.
- Respect and accept the complaint of pain as real.
- Treat pain appropriately.
- Treat underlying disorders.
- Address psychosocial concerns.
- Multidisciplinary approach is essential.

PHARMACOTHERAPY

Principles of Pharmacotherapy

- Match the drug to the pain syndrome.
- Low threshold to prescribe opioids for cancer pain.
- Use sustained-release formulations for constant, chronic pain and short acting for breakthrough discomfort.
- Use adjunct medications for certain pain syndromes.
- Use an oral route for analgesics if possible.
- Use an intravenous route for acute titration.
- Sequential opioid trials are often beneficial.
- Become familiarized with equianalgesic dosing.
- Become familiarized with the pharmacokinetics of opioids.
- Differentiate between tolerance, physical dependence, and addiction.
- Use caution with opioid and adjuvant drug titration in the setting of renal impairment.

Constipation Prevention and Treatment

A bowel regimen should always be prescribed with an opioid prescription because of the constipation opioids induce.

- Always include stimulant laxatives to prevent opioid-induced constipation.
- Preferred choices include sennosides and polyethylene glycol.
- Decreased motility, gastroparesis, is a common side effect of opioids and can be treated with metoclopramide.
- Activity and adequate hydration are important.
- Bulking agents without a prokinetic may worsen constipation.
- Refractory constipation may be managed with lactulose 30 mL by mouth every 6 h until a large bowel movement occurs.
- Intractable cases may require a suppository or enema.
- Proximal impaction may require oral laxatives.
- In rare cases of hard stools present in the vault, manual disimpaction may be necessary.
- Constipation may be evaluated with imaging to assess the degree of severity of constipation (Fig. 58-4).

Opioid Rotation

Opioid rotation is the switching from one type of opioid to another in the setting of opioid neurotoxicity. The following are reasons to rotate opioids:

- Uncontrolled pain despite escalating opioid doses

1. Mechanism of pain	
No	No pain syndrome
Nc	Nociceptive pain
Ne	Neuropathic pain with or without nociceptive pain
Nx	Insufficient information to classify
2. Incident pain	
Io	No incident pain
Ii	Incident pain Present
Ix	Insufficient information to classify
3. Psychological distress	
Po	No psychological distress
Pp	Psychological distress present
Px	Insufficient information to classify
4. Addictive behavior	
Ao	No addictive behavior
Aa	Addictive behavior present
Ax	Insufficient information to classify
5. Cognitive function	
Co	No cognitive impairment
Ci	Partial cognitive impairment[1]
Cu	Total cognitive impairment[2]
Cx	Insufficient information to classify

[1] Sufficient impairment to affect patients ability to provide accurate present and/or past pain history.
[2] Patient unresponsive, delirious, or demented to the stage of being unable to provide and present and past pain history.

FIGURE 58-1 Edmonton System of Classification for Cancer Pain.

No Pain	0	1	2	3	4	5	6	7	8	9	10	Worst Possible Pain
No Fatigue	0	1	2	3	4	5	6	7	8	9	10	Worst Possible Fatigue
No Nausea	0	1	2	3	4	5	6	7	8	9	10	Worst Possible Nausea
No Depression	0	1	2	3	4	5	6	7	8	9	10	Worst Possible Depression
No Anxiety	0	1	2	3	4	5	6	7	8	9	10	Worst Possible Anxiety
No Drowsiness	0	1	2	3	4	5	6	7	8	9	10	Worst Possible Drowsiness
No Shortness of Breath	0	1	2	3	4	5	6	7	8	9	10	Worst Possible Shortness of Breath
Best Appetite	0	1	2	3	4	5	6	7	8	9	10	Worst Possible Appetite
Best Sleep	0	1	2	3	4	5	6	7	8	9	10	Worst Possible Sleep
Best Feeling of Well-Being	0	1	2	3	4	5	6	7	8	9	10	Worst Possible Feeling or Well-being
No Financial Distress	0	1	2	3	4	5	6	7	8	9	10	Worst Financial Distress
No Spiritual Pain	0	1	2	3	4	5	6	7	8	9	10	Worst Spiritual Pain

Completed By: Patient Family

0 = No Symptom; Best 10 = Worst Imaginable on average in the past 24 hours

FIGURE 58-2 Edmonton Symptom Assessment Scale.

- Development of tolerance or dose-limiting side effects of opioid neurotoxicity (hallucinations, confusion, myoclonus)
- Hyperalgesia as a result of the production of excitatory amino acids from the opioid itself
- Cost necessitating switching of opioid

Opioid rotation has been shown to not only improve pain control, resolve delirium, and alleviate myoclonus, but also may improve other symptoms, including depression and insomnia ([10]).

In a recent study of an outpatient population of 114 patients with cancer at MD Anderson Cancer Center with mean Eastern Cooperative Oncology Group (ECOG) performance status of 1, opioid rotation for side effects or uncontrolled pain achieved improved symptom control successfully in 65% of the patient population ([10]).

Individual variability of opioid activation of multiple subtypes of opioid receptors accounts for the benefits of opioid rotation that should be considered when managing uncontrolled pain ([11, 12]). In difficult cases, this may include rotation on two or three occasions to reduce opioid neurotoxicity and improve pain control.

The following are general guidelines for opioid rotation:

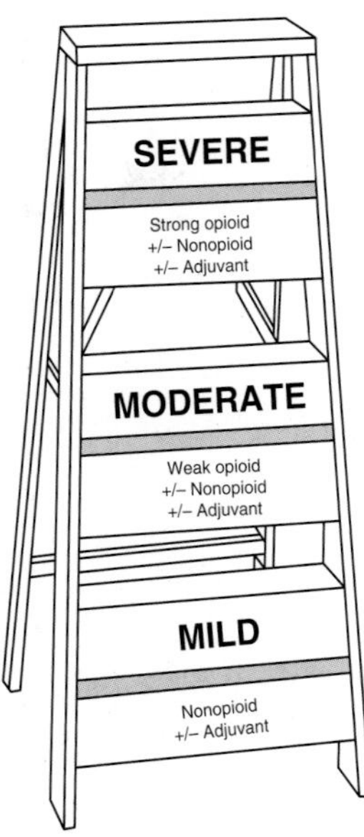

FIGURE 58-3 World Health Organization three-step ladder for oral analgesic management of pain. Adapted with permission from the World Health Organization.

1. Calculate total daily dose.
2. Calculate dose of new opioid using opioid conversion table (Tables 58-2 and 58-3).
3. Reduce dose of new opioid by 30% to 50% to account for incomplete cross tolerance.

Codeine

Codeine is a prodrug used to treat mild-to-moderate pain, diarrhea, and intractable coughing spells. It is the second most common alkaloid in opium and is hypothesized to be 200 times less potent than morphine. Metabolism by the liver converts 90% of the drug to inactive metabolites and 10% as morphine. The cytochrome oxidase 2D6 (CYP2D6) gene is responsible for the conversion to morphine and, in some groups, may not be fully active, while others may express multiple copies of the gene and be considered ultrarapid metabolizers ([13]). These ultrarapid metabolizers have greater risk of opioid neurotoxicity due to codeine rapidly metabolizing into morphine, especially in the pediatric population. On the other hand,

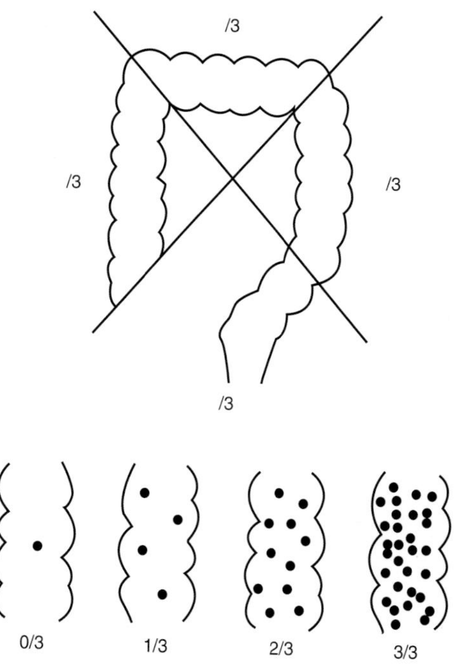

On a flat abdominal x-ray, draw two diagonal lines intersecting at the umbilicus as shown here. This transects the abdomen into four quadrants corresponding to the ascending, transverse, descending, and rectosigmoid colons. Then, assess the amount of stool in each of the four quadrants using the following scoring system: 0 = no stool; 1 = stool occupying <50% of the lumen of colon; 2 = stool occupying >50% of the lumen; 3 = stool completely occupying the lumen. The total score will therefore range from 0 to 12. A score of 7 indicates severe constipation and requires immediate intervention.

FIGURE 58-4 How to calculate a "constipation score" using a flat abdominal x-ray. (Reproduced with permission from Elsayem A, Driver LC, Bruera E. *The MD Anderson Palliative Care Handbook*. Houston, TX: MD Anderson Cancer Center; 2002.)

CHAPTER 58

Table 58-2 Opioid Analgesics

Drug	Usual Starting Dosages
Full opioid agonists	
Morphine[a]	15-30 mg by mouth every 3-4 h
Morphine extended release (MScontin)	30-60 mg by mouth every 8-12 h
Hydromorphone (Dilaudid)	2-4 mg by mouth every 4-6 h
Hydromorphone ER (Exalgo)	8-16 mg by mouth every 12-24 h
Fentanyl (Duragesic)	25-50 μg/h transdermally every 3 days
Codeine	15-30 mg by mouth every 3-4 h
Oxycodone (Percodan and others)	5-10 mg by mouth every 3-4 h
Methadone hydrochloride (Dolophine)[b]	5-10 mg by mouth every 3-4 h
Partial agonists and mixed agonists/antagonists[c]	
Nalbuphine (Nubain)	10 mg IV every 3-4 h
Butorphanol (Stadol)	0.5-2 mg IV every 3-4 h 1-2 mg SL three times a day
Dezoncine (Dalgan)	10 mg IV every 3-4 h
Pentazocine (Talwin)	50 mg by mouth every 4-6 h

[a]Morphine can be given as an immediate-release or sustained-release preparation. It is recommended that a relatively rapid onset, short-acting opioid preparation (such as immediate-release morphine) be given to patients who take sustained-release morphine to provide rescue medication for breakthrough pain.
[b]Methadone is 10 to 15 times more potent than morphine. Expertise is needed to use it.
[c]This class of drugs is *not* recommended for the management of chronic cancer pain because these drugs will reverse analgesia when coadministered with full opioid agonists and precipitate withdrawal in physically dependent individuals.

Table 58-3 Opioid Conversion Table[a,b]

Intravenous MO	Oral MO	1:2.5
Intravenous HM	Oral HM	1:2
Oral HM	Oral MO	1:5
Intravenous HM	Intravenous MO	1:5
Oral oxymorphone	Oral MO	1:3
Oral oxycodone	Oral MO	1:1.5
Oral HCD	Oral MO	1:1 at ≥40 mg HCD/d
Oral HCD	Oral MO	1:1.5 at <40 mg HCD/d
Fentanyl patch	Oral MO	Fentanyl patch × 2 = Oral MO
Intravenous fentanyl	Intravenous MO	1:100

HCD, hydrocodone; HM, hydromorphone; MO, morphine.
[a]Reproduced with permission from Elsayem A, Driver LC, Bruera E. *The MD Anderson Palliative Care Handbook*. Houston, TX: MD Anderson Cancer Center; 2002.
[b](1) Take the total amount of opioid that effectively controls pain in 24 h.
(2) Multiply by conversion factor in table; give 30% less of the new opioid to avoid partial cross tolerance.
(3) Divide by the number of doses per day.

patients who have decreased metabolization may experience ineffective analgesia with the drug.

In addition, some medications are CYP2D6 inhibitors and block conversion of codeine to morphine when coadministered. These include the antidepressants paroxetine, fluoxetine, buproprion, and diphenhydramine. Medications known to increase CYP2D6, such as dexamethasone, should also be used with caution with codeine (Fig. 58-5).

Hydrocodone

Hydrocodone has historically been considered a weak opioid on the WHO ladder. It is manufactured commonly in combination with acetaminophen or ibuprofen. It is a semisynthetic opioid derived from codeine and is metabolized by the liver and excreted in the urine. Hydrocodone is metabolized by cytochrome P450 2D6 to hydromorphone. Recent studies have shown that hydrocodone, when taken at doses of less than 40 mg per day, is equivalent to one and half the strength of morphine; however, the ratio of morphine to hydrocodone at doses greater than or equal to 40 mg per day have been shown to be closer to 1:1 ([14]) (Fig. 58-6).

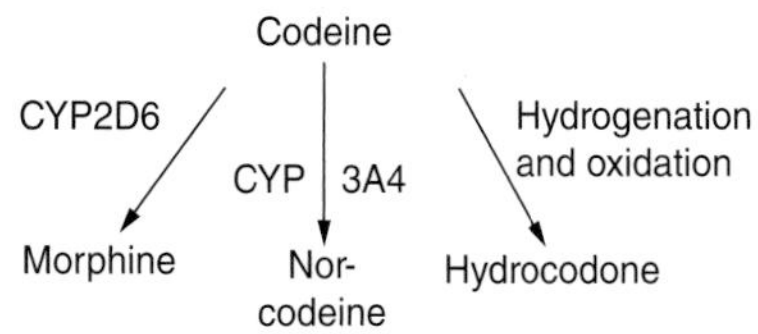

FIGURE 58-5 Codeine metabolism.

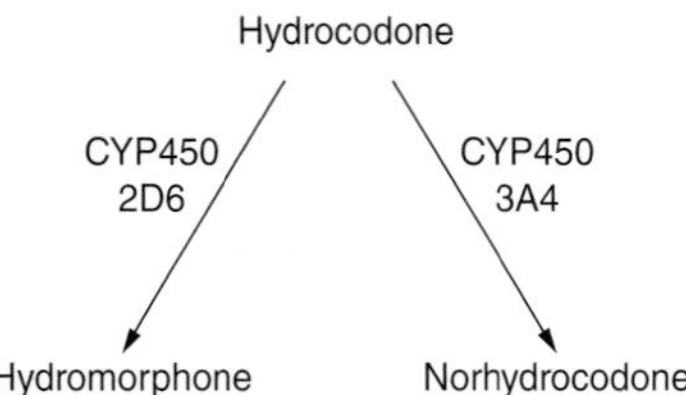

FIGURE 58-6 Hydrocodone metabolization.

Morphine

Morphine is commonly used as a standard prototype drug for opioid pain management. It is a naturally occurring opioid purified from opium poppy seeds and is available in short- and long-acting preparations. In the liver, it is converted to morphine-3-glucoronide and morphine-6-glucoronide (M3G and M6G, respectively) by glucuronyl transferase. Morphine-3-glucoronide is responsible for excitatory neurotoxic side effects, including myoclonus, hallucinations, seizures, and confusion and accumulates with renal insufficiency. Morphine is available as oral, rectal, intramuscular, intravenous, and sublingual preparations (Fig. 58-7).

Hydromorphone

Hydromorphone is a semisynthetic opioid derived from morphine and is five to seven times more potent. It is available for administration via all routes, including neuroaxial. It may be an alternative to morphine when dose-limiting side effects require rotation to a more potent opioid. Long-acting formulations are available, known by the trade name Exalgo, but are expensive.

Oxycodone

Oxycodone is another semisynthetic opioid derived from thebaine, a minor natural component of opium similar to morphine and codeine. Oxycodone has been known to be 1.5 times more potent than morphine. Previously, its dosage was limited by its combination with acetaminophen or aspirin, but now it is commonly available as oxycodone by itself as a pill in the United States. It has a higher bioavailability than morphine and exists both as extended-release and short-acting formulations.

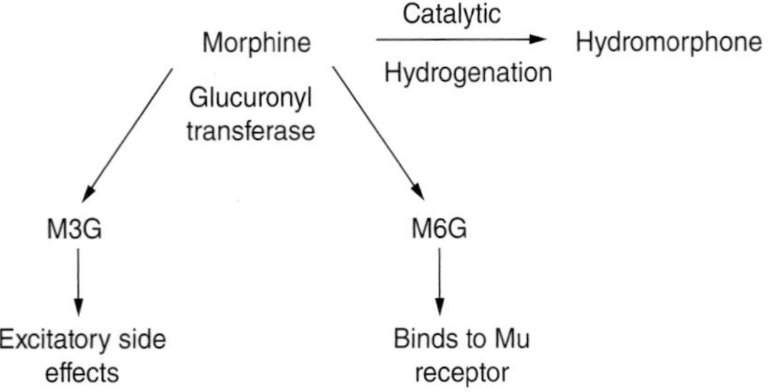

FIGURE 58-7 Metabolism of morphine in the liver.

Oxymorphone

Oxymorphone is produced after the CYP2D6 metabolism of oxycodone. It is a semisynthetic opioid and, like oxycodone, is also derived from thebaine. It has a low bioavailability orally and is three times more potent than morphine. Its maximum serum concentration is reached in 30 minutes, and the effects of immediate-release tablets may last up to 6 to 8 hours. Extended-release oxymorphone effects last 12 hours, and it should be dosed as such due to its long half-life of 14 hours. Oxymorphone should be given on an empty stomach because coadministration with food can result in increased absorption and result in opioid toxicities.

Meperidine

Meperidine (Demerol) is a weaker opioid with a potency 1/10 that of morphine. Dose escalation is limited by the risk of accumulation of the metabolite normeperidine, metabolized by the liver. Both meperidine and nor-meperidine cause central nervous system toxicity, including convulsions, especially in renal impairment and in the geriatric population. Due these risks, it is becoming less commonly used.

Fentanyl

Fentanyl is a synthetic opioid that is 80 to 100 times more potent than morphine and has a rapid onset and short duration of analgesia. It is used often in the setting of acute or incidental breakthrough pain. Transdermal sustained-release formulations, fentanyl patches, are a good choice for stable pain and are changed every 72 hours. Fentanyl patches are convenient in patients with oral routes that are limited or unavailable. Oral transmucosal fentanyl has been used for breakthrough pain; however, fentanyl has a very rapid onset of action, which makes it difficult to calculate total dose delivered, and erratic equianalgesic dosing often raises safety concerns.

Methadone

Methadone is a synthetic opioid. Recent research ([15]) has characterized appropriate equianalgesic dosing ([16, 17]), and advantages include low cost, less-active metabolites, good bioavailability, and *N*-methyl-D-aspartate antagonism, which may account for the absence of the development of tolerance associated with chronic use. Methadone potency can be 10 to 15 times that of morphine; thus, caution should be exercised when rotating to methadone. Close monitoring when initiated is necessary due to its tendency to accumulate as time advances before reaching a steady state. The half-life varies with the individuals; it can be between 15 and 190 hours. Clinicians prescribing methadone should be aware of potential drug interactions due to metabolism via the cytochrome P450 system, with these drugs including antifungals, antiretrovirals, and selective serotonin inhibitors ([18]). Methadone also has been associated with QTc interval prolongation ([19, 20]), so proper cardiac monitoring is indicated. Prospective studies at MD Anderson Cancer Center found it to be safe in advanced cancer ([21]). It is being researched as a viable first-line treatment option for pain management ([22]) and is especially useful in refractory cancer pain ([23]).

Adjuvant Medications

Although opioids are often first-line analgesics, adjuvant medications are useful for pain control in some settings, such as neuropathic pain. Due to the delay in onset as well as side effects with some drug groups, adjuvant drugs may be best reserved after optimal trials of opioids. Of the tricyclic antidepressants drug class, nortriptyline is felt to be the most efficacious and has less cardiovascular side effects. Tricyclic antidepressants are limited by anticholinergic and sedative side effects. Anticonvulsants are helpful in treating brachial and lumbosacral plexopathies. Side effects and safety limit their wide use. For the adjuvant treatment of neuropathic pain, gabapentin has been shown to be effective but does require dose adjustment in renal failure. Pregabalin has been used as an alternative to gabapentin but is costly and has not shown greater efficacy (Table 58-4).

Table 58-4 Adjuvant Analgesics

Nonsteroidal anti-inflammatory drugs
Acetaminophen Aspirin Ibuprofen Naproxen Celecoxib Ketorolac Diclofenac
Tricyclic antidepressants
Amitriptyline Nortriptyline Doxepin
Antiepileptic drugs
Gabapentin Topiramate Levetiracetam Tiagabine Oxcarbazepine Lamotrigine Felbamate
Local anesthetics
Lidocaine
***N*-Methyl-D-aspartate receptor antagonists**
Ketamine Methadone Dextromethorphan Haldol
Topical analgesics
Capsaicin Lidocaine patches

Nonpharmacologic Treatment

Adjuvant nonpharmacological treatments include nerve blocks, neurosurgical procedures, and radiation therapy. Physical and psychological interventions to treat pain include counseling, psychotherapy, relaxation techniques, massage therapy, music therapy, and acupuncture. Addressing psychosocial and spiritual distress for both patients and family may be needed for patients with cancer experiencing complex, total pain at the end of life (Table 58-5).

CANCER-RELATED FATIGUE

Fatigue is among the most common and distressing symptoms encountered in approximately 60% to 90% of patients with cancer ([24]). The National Comprehensive Cancer Network defines cancer-related fatigue as a persistent subjective sense of physical, emotional, as well as cognitive tiredness or exhaustion related to cancer or cancer treatment that is not proportional to recent activity and is both distressing and interferes with usual function ([25]). Fatigue may include a lack of interest and difficulty maintaining attention, concentration, or motivation in objects or activities (Table 58-6). Patients may present with depressed mood, have a flat affect,

Table 58-5 Anesthetic Procedures[a]

• Celiac plexus/splanchnic block for abdominal visceral pain (eg, pancreatic cancer pain)
• Subarachnoid neurolytic block for extremity and thoracic wall pain in terminally ill patients
• Epidural/intrathecal opioids +/– local anesthetic (eg, for neuropathic or plexopathy pain)
• Cordotomy for intractable lower-extremity pain
• Vertebroplasty (injection of cement into a vertebral body) for metastatic spinal pain involving one or two vertebrae

[a]Reproduced with permission from Elsayem A, Driver LC, Bruera E. *The MD Anderson Palliative Care Handbook*. Houston, TX: MD Anderson Cancer Center; 2002.

CHAPTER 58

Table 58-6 *International Classification of Diseases, Tenth Revision*, Criteria for Cancer-Related Fatigue

Criteria	Yes	No
Fatigue, decreased energy, increased need to rest[a]		
Generalized weakness/limb heaviness		
Diminished concentration or attention		
Decreased motivation/interest to engage in usual activities		
Insomnia/hypersomnia		
Sleep unrefreshing or nonrestorative		
Struggle to overcome inactivity		
Emotional reactivity to feeling fatigue: sadness/frustration/irritability		
Difficulty completing daily tasks		
Problems with short-term memory		
Postexertional fatigue lasting several hours		

[a]Reproduced with permission from Elsayem A, Driver LC, Bruera E. *The MD Anderson Palliative Care Handbook*. Houston, TX: MD Anderson Cancer Center; 2002.

and appear lethargic or somnolent. Rest or sleep does not eliminate or alleviate symptoms of cancer-related fatigue.

Fatigue may be experienced at any point in the cancer trajectory and often worsens at the end of life. Cancer-related fatigue may render patients unable to tolerate physical or mental activity, resulting in an inability to complete activities of daily living, impairment in social and occupational function, and diminished overall quality of life. Fatigue may also heighten other symptoms associated with cancer.

The etiology of cancer-related fatigue is often multifactorial (Fig. 58-8), including not only the underlying cancer itself but also treatments such as chemotherapy or radiation therapy. Fatigue may be exacerbated by other underlying metabolic abnormalities, such as hypothyroidism or hypogonadism, and can be amplified by psychosocial distress (see Fig. 58-8).

Fatigue Assessment

Assessment of fatigue requires a multidimensional approach. Fatigue severity is included on the Edmonton Symptom Assessment Scale, where 0 equals no fatigue and 10 equals the worst fatigue imaginable (see Fig. 58-2). Other numeric and verbal rating scales have been validated for fatigue, including the Functional Assessment of Cancer Therapy–Fatigue, Piper Fatigue Scale, Schwartz Cancer Fatigue Scale, Fatigue Symptom Inventory, and Functional Assessment of Chronic Illness Therapy–Fatigue (FACIT-F).

Significant fatigue, diminished energy, or increased need to rest disproportionate to any recent change in activity level must be present in addition to five or more of the other symptoms present daily or nearly every day during the same 2-week period in the past month ([26]).

Cancer-related fatigue should not primarily be a consequence of comorbid psychiatric disorders, which must be excluded, including major depression, somatization disorder, somatoform disorder, or delirium.

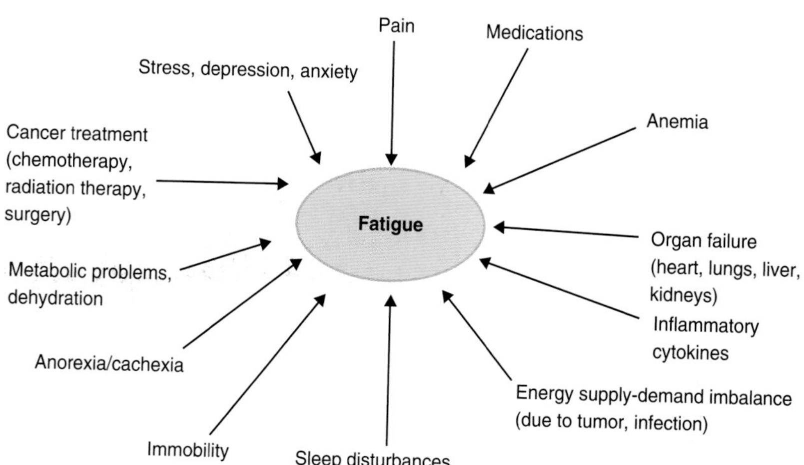

FIGURE 58-8 Multifactorial etiologies of fatigue. (Reproduced with permission from Elsayem A, Driver LC, Bruera E. *The MD Anderson Palliative Care Handbook*. Houston, TX: MD Anderson Cancer Center; 2002.)

Fatigue Management

The initial assessment of fatigue should focus on contributing factors that can be corrected, such as hypothyroidism, anemia, B_{12} deficiency, and renal insufficiency. Treatment of cancer-related fatigue should be considered only after correction of underlying etiologies ([27, 28]). Treatment of pain, depression, anxiety, sleep disturbances, dehydration, and cancer anorexia-cachexia syndrome are critical to improve symptoms of fatigue. Medications that exacerbate fatigue should be reviewed and, if indicated, discontinued; underlying infections should be aggressively treated; and patients with symptomatic anemia should receive blood transfusions when appropriate ([28]).

Corticosteroids

Low-dose steroids may alleviate some symptoms of fatigue. Recent studies have confirmed their short-term benefit; however, more studies are required to determine the optimal dose ([29]).

Methylphendiate

Psychostimulants such as methylphenidate may be useful if the patient is experiencing concomitant problems, such as depression or drowsiness related to opioids ([30-32]). However, a recent randomized trial examining methylphenidate reported no significant difference in median FACIT-F scores in regard to cancer-related fatigue when compared with a placebo ([33]).

Antidepressants

Selective serotonin reuptake inhibitors (SSRIs) may improve fatigue; however, their benefit has not been proven and may be indirectly related to the treatment of underlying mood disorder. A Cochrane review that included two double-blind, placebo-controlled studies (n = 645) using paroxetine in a meta-analysis did not show any significant improvement in fatigue in patients with cancer ([34]).

Testosterone Replacement

Recently, there has been evidence that patients with cancer with hypogonadism on chronic opioid therapy may benefit from testosterone replacement ([35]). A pilot study of testosterone replacement at 4 weeks in hypogonadal males with advanced cancer did not have significant improvement of fatigue as measured with FACIT-F, although there was a trend for improvement with longer duration of treatment ([36]).

Homeopathic Dietary Supplements

Studies have evaluated dietary supplements for treatment of fatigue. Ginseng has been used medicinally in the Far East for several millennia and is a widely used supplement to treat fatigue in the United States. The composition of the active ingredients of ginseng root (ginsenosides and saponins) varies, and standardization can be problematic. A recent double-blind, randomized controlled trial of 132 patients with either a mixed solid tumor or cancer survivors has shown significant improvement in fatigue scores when patients were prescribed American ginseng, 2,000 mg daily, for at least 4 weeks ([37]). Other potentially promising homeopathic supplements include guarana extract and L-carnitine.

Integrative Nonpharmacological Interventions

Exercise therapy, such as brisk walking, may help with fatigue. In a recent meta-analysis of randomized trials examining supervised exercise therapy supported exercise improving cancer-related fatigue. These findings suggest that combined aerobic and resistance exercise regimens, with or without stretching, should be included as part of rehabilitation programs for patients with cancer ([38]). Yoga has also been studied for the treatment of cancer-related fatigue with some positive results, although level of bias and inconsistent methods in previous randomized studies may have influenced results ([39]). Indirect natural light ([40]) and massage therapy may also help to reduce fatigue.

In addition, treatment of fatigue should address underlying psychosocial factors such as depression, anxiety, as well as other symptoms, including pain, cachexia, or dyspnea, to be effective. Cognitive-behavioral therapy, in treating psychosocial distress or insomnia, may indirectly improve symptoms of fatigue. In the future, multimodality treatment of cancer-related fatigue should be personalized for each individual cancer patient, and more research is needed to develop successful interventions.

NAUSEA, ANOREXIA, AND CACHEXIA

The anorexia-cachexia syndrome (Figs. 58-9 and 58-10) is characterized by a loss of appetite coinciding with significant weight loss; loss in lean body mass, including muscle wasting; loss of fat; fatigue; immune dysfunction; and metabolic derangements. Cancer cachexia has been defined as a multifactorial syndrome of ongoing skeletal muscle mass atrophy with or without the loss of fat mass that cannot be fully reversed by conventional nutritional support and leads to progressive functional impairment. Diagnosis of cachexia has been agreed on by a panel of experts as a weight loss greater than 5% or weight loss greater than 2% in individuals already with a body mass index (BMI) less than 20 ([41]). Studies have shown that even a loss of 5% or more of premorbid weight prior to chemotherapy is associated with shorter survival ([42]).

Cachexia is found in the majority of patients with advanced cancer and is a major contributing factor to death in about 50% of these patients ([42]). Complex interactions between tumor and host lead to an aberrant immune response, neurohormonal dysfunction, and endocrine dysregulation. Both cachexia and fatigue are associated with increased proinflammatory cytokines (interleukin [IL] 1, IL-6, tumor necrosis factor alpha), low testosterone levels, abnormal cortisol secretion, and resistance to insulin and ghrelin ([43]). These cellular derangements are associated with increased production of acute-phase proteins in the liver and loss of muscle protein due to proteolysis and lipolysis and results in elevated triglycerides and decreased high-density lipoproteins.

Unfortunately, neither nutritional supplementation nor artificial feeding reverses the cancer anorexia-cachexia syndrome ([43]). Multiple studies have examined the role of total parenteral and enteral nutrition in patients with cancer and have reported limited benefits. Artificial feeding of patients with cancer with cachexia was found to increase acute-phase protein production without influencing the rate of albumin synthesis ([44]). Other contributory factors resulting in weight loss (ie, depression, nausea, dysphagia, bowel obstruction, or constipation) should be treated aggressively.

Treating patients in the early stages of weight loss may be important to maintain or increase lean body mass because it is difficult to reverse cachexia in late stages ([43]). A comprehensive history, including recent changes in weight and diet patterns, is important. Simple and inexpensive tests are available to assess body composition, such as anthropometric measurements, skinfold thickness, arm muscle circumference and area, and weight and BMI. Laboratory markers such as

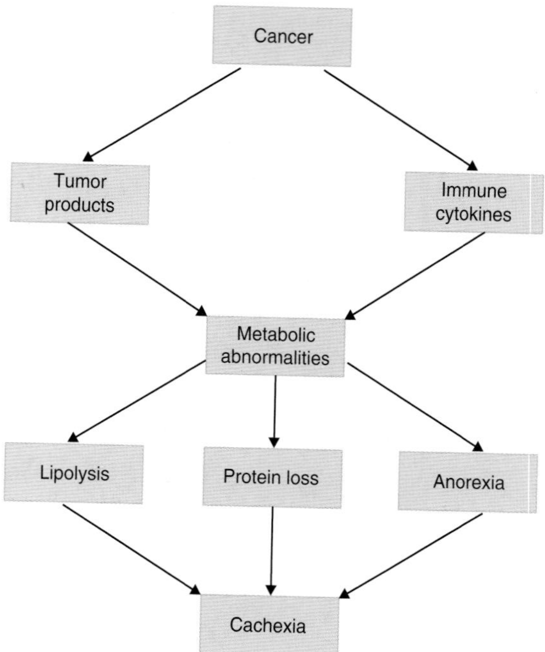

FIGURE 58-10 Mechanism of cachexia. (Reproduced with permission from Elsayem A, Driver LC, Bruera E. *The MD Anderson Palliative Care Handbook*. Houston, TX: MD Anderson Cancer Center; 2002.)

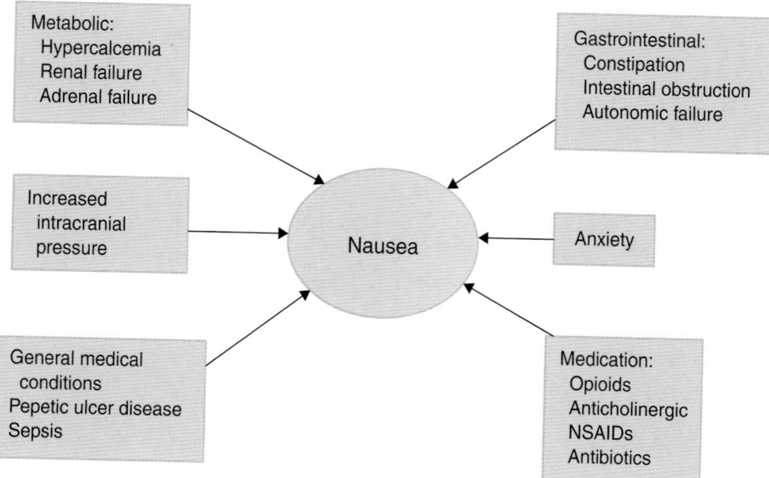

FIGURE 58-9 Causes of nausea. (Reproduced with permission from Elsayem A, Driver LC, Bruera E. *The MD Anderson Palliative Care Handbook*. Houston, TX: MD Anderson Cancer Center; 2002.)

electrolytes, serum albumin, transferrin, and prealbumin may also be useful.

Management

For management, identify etiology and treat the underlying cause:

- Treat nausea/early satiety: metoclopramide 5 to 10 mg every 4 to 6 hours (renal adjustment required) (see Table 58-7 for nausea agents)
- Progestational agents
  - Megestrol acetate: 40 to 120 mg by mouth four times a day (risk of thromboembolism, hypogonadism, and adrenal suppression)
- Corticosteroids
  - Dexamethasone: 4 mg by mouth twice a day (lower mineralocorticoid effect than other steroids ([43])
- For patients with cancer with depression: use antidepressants such as tricyclic antidepressants and SSRIs (ie, mirtazapine 15 mg by mouth at bedtime)

Nutritionist Consultation

Counseling and psychosocial support for cachectic patients and their family caregivers are critical at the end of life and will decrease patient-family conflict. Counseling should emphasize the pleasure of eating as well as promote the social participation of patients in family meals as opposed to increasing caloric intake. Counseling should highlight the normal loss of appetite as patients, who are often not hungry, approach the end of life, and family caregivers should not pressure patients to eat, which can result in nausea and psychological distress.

DYSPNEA

Dyspnea is a subjective symptom defined as an "uncomfortable awareness of breathing" ([45]). It is often described as a sensation of air hunger, suffocation, choking, or heavy breathing. Dyspnea may be related to underlying tumor progression, altered by psychosocial factors, including anxiety, and exacerbated by preexisting pulmonary comorbidities. Shortness of breath can develop in response to pain or a mismatch between perceived ventilation rate and respiratory drive. Dyspnea is considered refractory when it persists at rest or with minimal activity and is distressful despite optimal medical therapy ([46]).

Dyspnea in patients with advanced cancer is an indicator of poor prognosis ([47, 48]). The etiology of dyspnea is often multifactorial. It is postulated that in the brain, the cortical-limbic network is responsible for dyspnea

Table 58-7 Nausea Treatments[a]

Drug[b]	Main Receptor	Main Indication	Starting PO Dose/Route	Equivalent Price[c]	Side Effects
Metoclopramide	D2	Opioid induced, gastric stasis	10 mg q4h PO, SC, IV	1	EPS (akathisia, dystonia, dyskinesia)
Prochlorperazine	D2	Opioid induced	10 mg q6h PO, IV	3	Sedation, hypotension
Cyclizine	H1	Vestibular causes, intestinal obstruction	25-50 mg q8h PO, SC, PR		Sedation, dry mouth, blurred vision
Promethazine	H1	Vestibular, motion sickness, obstruction	12.5 mg q4h PO, PR, IV	2	Sedation
Haloperidol	D2	Opioid, chemical, metabolic	1-2 mg bid PO, IV, SC	1	Rarely EPS
Ondansetron	5 HT_3	Chemotherapy	4-8 mg q8h PO, IV	84	Headache, constipation
Diphenhydramine	H1, Ach	Intestinal obstruction, vestibular, ICP	25 mg q6h PO, IV, SC	0.2	Sedation, dry mouth, blurred vision
Hyoscine	Ach	Intestinal obstruction, colic, secretions	0.2-0.4 mg q4h SL, SC, TD	0.4	Dry mouth, blurred vision, urine retention, agitation

Ach, acetylcholine; D2, dopamine; EPS, extrapyramidal symptoms; H1, histamine; ICP, intracranial pressure; PR, per rectum; SL, sublingual; TD, transdermal.
[a] From chapter 58 file
[b] Corticosteroids are not included because they vary in dosage and have limited indications (see text).
[c] Prices are compared to metoclopramide 10-mg tablets orally for 10 days based on the formulary prices at MD Anderson Cancer Center, November 2001.

perception. Recent research reported that the anterior cingulate cortex and the dorsolateral prefrontal cortex are involved in sensing dyspnea ([49]). In addition, the insular cortex is modulated by sensations of dyspnea, and studies of patients with asthma have shown that it is downregulated in patients experiencing dyspnea as well as pain ([50]).

Treatment of Dyspnea

The aim of treatment of dyspnea is to improve the patient's perception of shortness of breath and involves not only treating the underlying cause but also palliating symptoms of air hunger. Treating the underlying etiologies can vary from thoracentesis for a pleural effusion, blood transfusions for anemic patients, corticosteroids for systemic inflammation or lymphangitic carcinomatosis, or antibiotics for pneumonia.

Symptomatic relief may include oxygen therapy, bilevel positive airway pressure, or high-flow oxygen therapy ([51]). In patients with chronic obstructive pulmonary disease (COPD), long-term oxygen therapy has shown mortality reduction but does not necessarily improve dyspnea. Palliative oxygenation is often prescribed irrespective of oxygen saturations. Oxygen delivery by nasal cannula does not always equate to relief of dyspnea in nonhypoxemic patients with advanced illness when compared with room air.

Pharmacological interventions for dyspnea include opioids, benzodiazepines, and corticosteroids and are often utilized when medical therapy fails to improve the perception of dyspnea. Opioids, when titrated carefully, will often improve dyspnea without reducing oxygenation or causing respiratory depression ([49]). Immediate-release, short-acting, and sustained-release morphine have been used in clinical trials of dyspnea management. The American Thoracic Society and the Canadian Thoracic Society advocate opioid dose titration to achieve the lowest effective dose based on patient ratings of shortness of breath ([49]).

Corticosteroids are most useful in situations of lymphangitic spread or inflammation causing obstruction of airways ([52]). Bronchodilators may also play a role when dyspnea is related to bronchospasm and reduce airway smooth muscle tone, thereby improving airflow and deflating an overinflated lung ([49]). Tachycardia is a common side effect of bronchodilators.

Integrative approaches may also be effective, such as relaxation techniques or guided imagery, for patients with anticipatory or anxiety-driven dyspnea. Low-dose benzodiazepines in conjunction with opioids may have a role in the treatment of dyspnea complicated by severe anxiety, but they have the potential to cause delirium and decrease respiratory drive ([53]). Acupuncture has also been researched for the treatment of dyspnea. In a study by Jones and colleagues ([54]), one 45-minute session of transcutaneous electrical nerve stimulation at acupuncture sites resulted in improvement of dyspnea, increased FEV_1 (forced expiratory volume in first second of expiration) and blood levels of β-endorphin compared with placebo. Suzuki and colleagues reported exertional dyspnea was reduced in patients with COPD after receiving acupuncture once a week for 12 weeks compared to placebo ([55]). Assist devices can be used to minimize muscular effort: postural drainage, a fan with airflow directed to the face ([56]). Incentive spirometry can also help in certain settings.

DELIRIUM

Delirium, an acute state of encephalopathy, results from diffuse organic brain dysfunction. The prevalence of delirium is approximately 10% in hospitalized medical and surgical patients and is noted in 26% to 44% of patients with advanced cancer at the time of hospital admission. Roughly half of these cases may be reversible. In patients with advanced cancer, over 80% of patients will develop delirium at the end of life ([57]). Delirium is often misdiagnosed and associated with increased morbidity and mortality ([58]). It complicates assessment of pain and other symptoms and results in distress for patients, family caregivers, and health-care providers.

Clinical Presentation of Delirium

Delirium is characterized by waxing-and-waning mentation. The main diagnostic criteria, according to the *Diagnostic and Statistical Manual of Mental Disorders* (Fourth Edition, Text Revision) (*DSM-IV-TR*), include a disturbance of consciousness with reduced ability to focus, sustain, or shift attention; a change in cognition (disorientation/language disturbance) or the development of a perceptual disturbance that is not better accounted for by a preexisting dementia; and a disturbance that develops over a short period of time (hours to days) and fluctuates during the course of the day. Three clinical variants of delirium have been designated based on type of arousal disorder: hypoactive, hyperactive, and mixed.

Delirium Assessment

Delirium is often misdiagnosed as anxiety, insomnia, worsening pain, or mood disturbance, resulting in inappropriate treatment with anxiolytics or hypnotics, inappropriate increase in opioids, or use of antidepressants, which can worsen symptoms. Maintaining a high index of suspicion can help to avoid misdiagnosis of delirium, and routine use of screening tools such as the Memorial Delirium Assessment Scale or Mini-Mental State Examination is recommended. Clinicians should pay attention to metabolic derangements that may precipitate delirium, such as liver or renal failure. Medications may be the cause as well and include opioids (responsible for almost 60% of cases in patients with cancer [59]), benzodiazepines, some antiemetics, and corticosteroids (Fig. 58-11).

Delirium Management

1. Provide patients a safe environment, including fall precautions; minimize noise and excessive light; place patients in a familiar setting with visible clock and calendar; and have family at bedside to help reorient patients.
2. Treat underlying causes, such as hypercalcemia or pneumonia.
3. Treat agitation (Table 58-8).
4. To treat severe agitation secondary to delirium, it may be necessary to give haloperidol more frequently initially. In patients refractory to haloperidol, a combination of haloperidol and a benzodiazepine may be necessary. However, in a study by Brietbart ([60]), lorazepam alone was ineffective in the treatment of delirium and actually contributed to its worsening and increased cognitive impairment in terminal patients with HIV. Newer atypical antipsychotics may be just as effective as typical antipsychotics but are more expensive. Olanzapine may be more sedating. Sometimes, acute dystonia and extrapyramidal side effects are seen with haloperidol, in which case benztropine

Table 58-8 Treatment of Agitation

Haloperidol[a]	IV/Oral/IM	Start 1-2 mg every 6 h and 1-2 mg every 2 h prn
Olanzapine	Oral/ODT/IM	2.5-5 mg daily, titrated to 5–10 mg daily
Risperidone	Oral/ODT/IM	0.25-0.5 mg every 12 h titrated to 1.5 mg every 12 h
Quetiapine	Oral/IM	12.5-25 mg by mouth every 12 h titrated to 100 mg every 12 h
Chlorpromazine	IV/Oral/IM	Start 10-25mg daily and 10-25 mg every 2 h prn
Ativan	IV/Oral/IM	0.5-1 mg every hour until calm; recommend against use as single agent

[a] The oral bioavailability is approximately 60%-70% when converting from oral to parenteral.

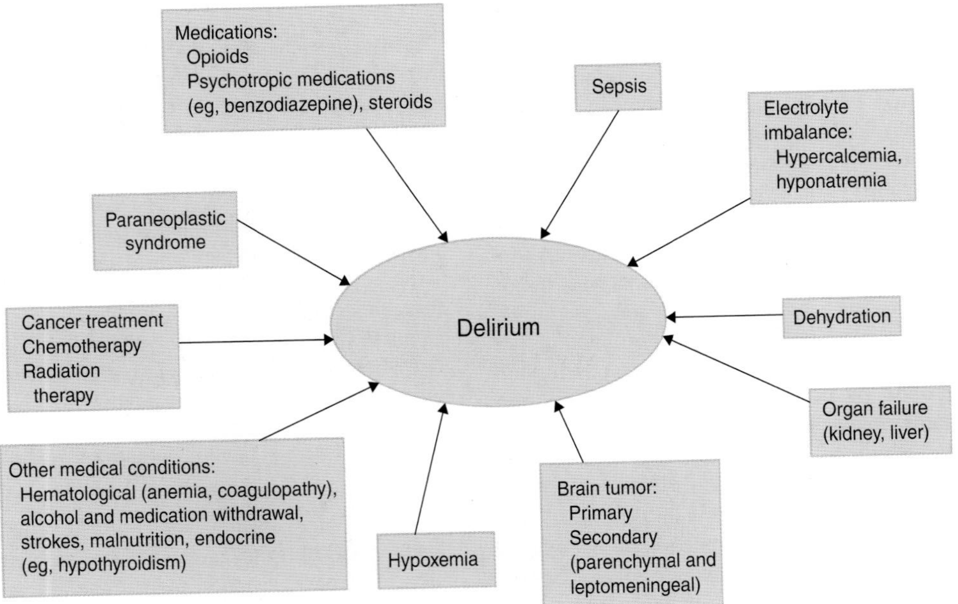

FIGURE 58-11 Delirium management. (Reproduced with permission from Elsayem A, Driver LC, Bruera E. *The MD Anderson Palliative Care Handbook*. Houston, TX: MD Anderson Cancer Center; 2002.)

can be administered. Once symptoms are under control, reducing haloperidol to the minimal effective dose is recommended ([61, 62]).

5. Counseling a patient's family caregivers and healthcare providers regarding the patient's expression of previously well-controlled physical symptoms by grimacing or moaning may be inhibition of emotions due to delirium. In such cases, treatment should be directed at controlling delirium and not inappropriately increasing opioids (Fig. 58-12).

Palliative Sedation

Instances of refractory delirium, as well as other uncontrolled symptoms at the end of life, may require palliative sedation. Palliative sedation is defined as the monitored use of sedative medication to reduce patients' awareness of intractable and refractory symptoms near the end of life when other interventions have failed to control them ([63]). It is important to ensure all available symptomatic measures, including consulting palliative medicine specialists, have been tried before deeming symptoms refractory. The goal of palliative sedation is to control symptoms, not hasten death, which is differentiated from physician-assisted euthanasia. Therefore, it is imperative to discuss this with the patient and family caregivers to avoid misunderstanding. Midazolam, titrated to control symptoms, is often used for palliative sedation. Patients need regular assessments, including use of the Richmond Agitation Sedation Scale, to monitor for excessive sedation. If underlying symptoms have improved or been controlled, sedatives may be decreased and even discontinued.

DEPRESSION

Clinical depression is a common mood disorder encountered in patients with cancer and can affect from 25% to 35% of the patient population ([64]). Clinical depression increases in frequency in advanced disease ([65]), and diagnosis can be challenging in these patients. For instance, symptoms often strongly associated with clinical depression in healthy individuals

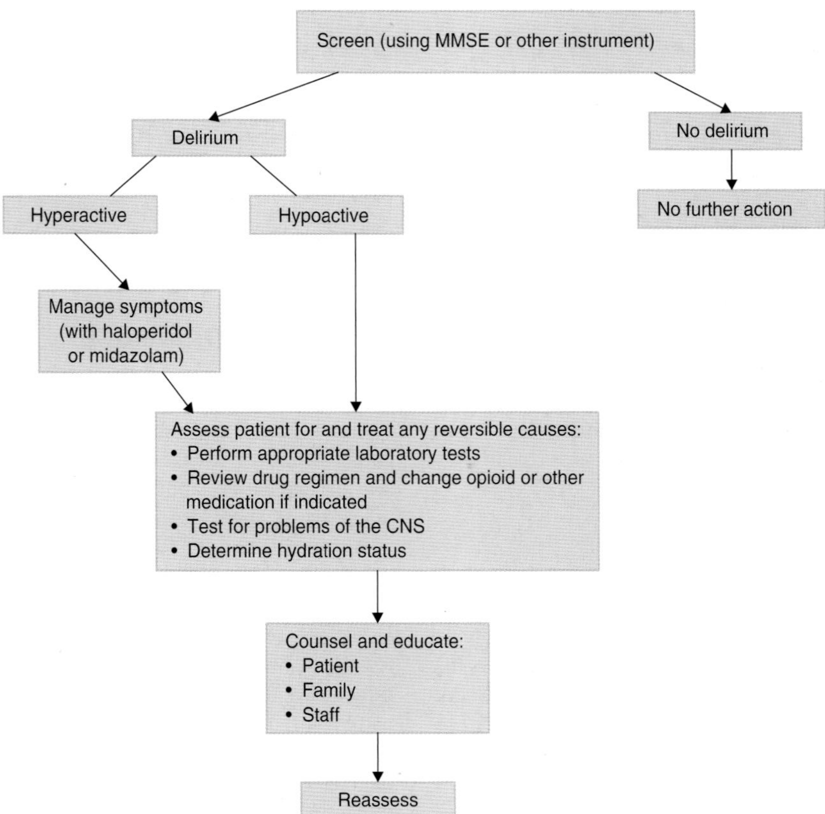

FIGURE 58-12 Algorithm for treating delirium. (Reproduced with permission from Elsayem A, Driver LC, Bruera E. *The MD Anderson Palliative Care Handbook*. Houston, TX: MD Anderson Cancer Center; 2002.)

CHAPTER 58

(including fatigue, impaired decision-making ability, insomnia, and poor appetite) are frequently commonly encountered in patients with advanced disease. Per *DSM-IV* criteria ([66]), the cardinal features of clinical depression include anhedonia; feelings of guilt, hopelessness, or worthlessness; and suicidal ideation, and a thorough patient history directed at assessment for these symptoms is needed.

In addition, the diagnosis of clinical depression can be difficult to differentiate from adjustment disorder, anticipatory grief, or delirium. Validated measures of assessing depression in the primary care setting include the WHO-5 well-being index ([67]), PHQ-9 screening test ([68]), Hamilton Rating Scale for Depression (HAM-D) ([69]), and Montgomery-Asberg Depression Rating Scale ([70]) (MADRS). Other factors that increase the risk of depression include a history of substance abuse, family history of depression and suicide, concurrent life stressors, and poor social support.

Common antidepressants and their common initial doses are as follows ([78]):

- Nortriptyline 25 mg/d (at bedtime)
- Amitriptyline 25 mg/d (at bedtime)
- Fluoxetine 10 to 20 mg/d
- Paroxetine 10 mg/d
- Sertraline 20 mg/d
- Citalopram 20 mg/d
- Venlafaxine 37.5 mg/d
- Mirtazapine 15 mg/d (at bedtime)
- Methylphenidate 5 to 10 mg in the morning and 5 mg at noon

Escitalopram has a lower side-effects profile and works slightly faster than other first-generation SSRIs. Side effects include reduced appetite, nausea, and anxiety. Antidepressants should be given for a trial of 6 weeks for beneficial effects, and if there is no significant improvement, they may need adjustment of dose or a change to an alternate medication. In patients with cancer with unclear criteria for clinical depression or suicidal ideation, consultation with a psychiatrist is indicated.

COMMUNICATION

The majority of chronically ill patients in the United States want to be informed about their prognosis ([74]) and appreciate being told the truth ([72]). Health-care providers' ability to accurately prognosticate life expectancy of patients with cancer is still limited. In addition, a patient's acceptance of information regarding prognosis and end-of-life issues is heavily influenced by the manner in which this information is conveyed. It is common that health-care professionals feel uncomfortable with discussing prognosis and other end-of-life issues. Reasons include lack of training, stress, feeling rushed and not having enough time to address emotional needs of patients, fear of upsetting the patient or family, or reluctance to diminish hope with regard to the unavailability of further curative treatment. Avoidance of end-of-life discussions can lead to patient dissatisfaction and further psychological distress.

There are few trials testing the effectiveness of different strategies in delivering bad news ([74]). Most recommendations on discussing bad news agree on the following key features: preparing for the discussion, addressing the message content, dealing with the patient's responses, and ending the encounter ([74]) (Table 58-9).

Important guidelines regarding end-of-life discussions have emphasized the following: identify the reason for discussion and patients' expectations, elicit their knowledge of the situation, consider cultural awareness and preferences in regard to information, validate feelings and take an empathetic approach, explain information using language without medical jargon, use easy-to-understand terms, explain the limitations of prognostication and end-of-life information, and avoid exact timelines ([75]).

Family meetings are championed by health-care professionals as a tool to improve communication and can be helpful to inform, deliberate, clarify goals, and mediate difficult end-of-life discussions that family members might have in regard to the care of the patient. They can help to formulate acceptable care plans between patient, family caregivers, and health-care providers ([75]) and clarify goals of care so everyone is on the "same page" ([76]) (see Table 58-9).

SPIRITUAL DISTRESS

Spirituality has generally been defined as a way an individual seeks and expresses meaning and purpose in life and how one experiences connectedness to the moment, self, others, nature, and the significant or sacred. While religiosity has been defined as the active participation in an organized religion ([77]), recent studies conducted at MD Anderson have indicated that a majority of our patients identify themselves as being spiritual or religious. Almost all patients report that their spirituality or religious faith is a source of strength and assists with coping with a life-threatening illness. Caregivers have also shown similar patterns of identification with spirituality and religiosity. Caregivers expressed that their spirituality had helped them cope with their loved one's illness and had a positive impact on their loved one's physical and emotional well-being ([77]). Patients with increased spiritual distress tend to have an association with a higher physical

Table 58-9 SPIKES Protocol (Setup/Patient's Perception/Invitation/Knowledge/Emotions/Support)[a]

Step 1: Setting Up the Interview	
Goals	*Purpose*
To prepare yourself for the interview To establish rapport with the patient and put the patient at ease To facilitate information exchange	Reflect on the task at hand. Arrange for uninterrupted time. Decide who should be present. Determine whether the patient is ready. Sit down when you speak to the patient. Have facial tissues handy. Maintain eye contact.
Step 2: Find Out the Patient's Perception of the Illness	
Goals	*Purpose*
To determine what the patient understands To assess denial in the patient/family To promote rapport through listening To understand the patient's expectations and concerns	Ask open-ended questions; ie, "Tell me what you've been told," or "I'd like to make sure you understand the reason for the tests." Correct misinformation and misunderstanding. Address denial. Address unrealistic expectation. Define your role.
Step 3: Get an Invitation to Give Information	
Goals	*Purpose*
To determine how much information the patient wants and when he or she is ready to hear it To acknowledge that patient information needs may change over time To resolve conflicts with families regarding information disclosure	Ask "Are you the type of person who wants information in detail?" Explore sources of family concern.
Step 4: Giving the Patient Knowledge and Information	
Goals	*Purpose*
To prepare the patient for the bad news To ensure patient understanding	"Forecast" the arrival of bad news; ie, "I'm afraid I have some bad news..." Give the information in small parcels. Check periodically for understanding. Avoid using medical jargon. Address all questions.
Step 5: Responding to Patient Emotions	
Goals	*Purpose*
To address emotional responses To facilitate emotional recovery To acknowledge our own emotions	Anticipate emotional reactions. Resist the temptation to try and make the bad news better than it really is. Support the patient by using emphatic response to expressions of emotion such as crying. Clarify emotions about which you are not sure. Validate the patient's feelings.
Supporting the Patient	
Be prepared, and have a strategy (escape is not a strategy). Have someone with you if it will be difficult. Shift to a supportive role. Give the patient time to emote. Have facial tissue ready.	Sit down and get close if you can. Respond to any emotions with one of the following: Empathic statements Validating statements Exploratory questions

[a]Reproduced with permission from Elsayem A, Driver LC, Bruera E. *The MD Anderson Palliative Care Handbook*. Houston, TX: MD Anderson Cancer Center; 2002.

symptom burden. Acknowledging and addressing spiritual needs can be of value for improved quality of life in patients with advanced cancer.

MODELS OF PALLIATIVE CARE

Health care has traditionally been delivered in a dichotomous model with a focus on curative or life-prolonging treatment followed by an abrupt transition to palliative or hospice care in anticipation of death. In recent years, there has been a renewed emphasis on improving quality of life and integration of supportive care and palliative medicine earlier in the disease trajectory and concurrent with life-prolonging treatments. Integrating palliative care into the current best practice of cancer treatment allows for the prevention and relief of suffering while ensuring dignity during significant illness for both cancer survivors and patients at the end of life.

CONCLUSION

Patients with cancer will encounter distressing symptoms that can diminish a their quality of life and interfere with the ability to receive cancer therapy. Physical and emotional symptoms are encountered at any point during the illness trajectory from diagnosis, treatment, survivorship, or end of life. An oncologist may be overwhelmed with the challenges of cancer treatment when patients have uncontrolled symptoms. In collaboration with an interdisciplinary palliative care team, health-care providers may simultaneously treat cancer aggressively while maintaining the integrity of human life and diminishing unnecessary suffering.

There is an urgent need to incorporate assessment and treatment of physical and emotional symptoms facing patients with cancer and integrating a palliative medicine team into the delivery of cancer care. For patients with complex symptoms, early adoption of interdisciplinary palliative care can aggressively treat symptoms to prevent the sequelae of physical and emotional pain. In addition, an open dialogue with patients and family caregivers regarding issues of treatment options, prognosis, and end-of-life care, including a transition from focus on curing cancer to care directed at controlling symptoms, is needed along the continuum of cancer treatment.

REFERENCES

1. Portenoy RK, Lesage P. Management of cancer pain. *Lancet.* 1999;353(9165):1695-1700.
2. Holtan A, Aass N, Nordoy T, et al. Prevalence of pain in hospitalized cancer patients in Norway: a national survey. *Palliat Med.* 2007;21(1):7-13.
3. Krech RL, Walsh D. Symptoms of pancreatic cancer. *J Pain Symptom Manage.* 1991;6:360-367.
4. Foley KM. The treatment of cancer pain. *N Engl J Med.* 1984;313:84-95.
5. Portenoy RK, Hagen NA. Breakthrough pain: definition, prevalence, and characteristics. *Pain.* 1990;41:273-281.
6. Arthur J, Yennurajalingam S, Nguyen L, et al. The routine use of the Edmonton Classification System for Cancer Pain in an outpatient supportive care center. *Palliat Support Care.* 2014 Oct 14:1-8.
7. Bruera E, Kuehn N, Miller MJ, et al. The Edmonton Symptom Assessment System: a simple method for the assessment of palliative care patients. *J Palliat Care.* 1991;7:6-9.
8. World Health Organization. *Cancer Pain Relief.* Geneva, Switzerland: World Health Organization; 1986.
9. Patrick DL, Cleeland CS, von Moos R, et al. Pain outcomes in patients with bone metastases from advanced cancer: assessment and management with bone-targeting agents. *Support Care Cancer.* 2015;23(4):1157-1168.
10. Reddy A, Yennurajalingam S, Pulivarthi K, et al. Frequency, outcome, and predictors of success within 6 weeks of an opioid rotation among outpatients with cancer receiving strong opioids. *Oncologist.* 2013;18(2):212-220.
11. Galer BS, Coyle N, Pasternak GW, et al. Individual variation in the response to different opiods—report of five cases. *Pain.* 1992;49:87-91.
12. Hanks G, Forbes K. Opioid responsiveness. *Acta Anesthesiol Scand.* 1997;41:154-158.
13. Prommer E. Role of codeine in palliative care. *J Opioid Manage.* 2011;7(5):401-406.
14. Reddy A, Yennurajalingam S, Desai H, et al. The opioid rotation ratio of hydrocodone to strong opioids in cancer patients. *Oncologist.* 2014;19(11):1186-1193.
15. Davis MP, Walsh D. Methadone for relief of cancer pain: a review of pharmakokinetics, pharmacodynamics, drug interactions and protocols of administration. *Support Care Cancer.* 2001;9:63-83.
16. Ripamonti C, Groff L, Brunelli C, et al. Switching from morphine to oral methadone in treating cancer pain: what is the equianalgesic dose ratio? *J Clin Oncol.* 1998;16(10):3216-3221.
17. Ripamonti C, de Conno F, Groff L, et al. Equianalgesic dose/ratio between methadone and other opioid agonists in cancer pain: comparison of two clinical experiences. *Ann Oncol.* 1998;9:79-83.
18. Tarumi Y, Pereira J, Watanabe S. Methadone and fluconazole: respiratory depression by drug interaction. *J Pain Symptom Manage.* 2002;23(2):148-153.
19. Andersen G, Christrup L, Sjogren P. Relationships among morphine metabolism, pain and side effects during long-term treatment: an update. *J Pain Symptom Manage.* 2003;25(1):74-91.
20. Cruciani RA, Sekine R, Homel P, et al. Measurement of QTc in patients receiving chronic methadone therapy. *J Pain Symptom Manage.* 2005;29(4):385-391.
21. Reddy S, Hui D, El Osta B, et al. The effect of oral methadone on the QTc interval in advanced cancer patients: a prospective pilot study. *J Palliat Med.* 2010;13(1):33-38.
22. Rhondali W, Tremellat F, Ledoux M, et al. Methadone rotation for cancer patients with refractory pain in a palliative care unit: an observational study. *J Palliat Med.* 2013;16(11):1382-1387.
23. Salpeter RS, Buckley JS, Bruera E. The use of very-low-dose methadone for palliative pain control and the prevention of opioid hyperalgesia. *J Palliat Med.* 2013;616(6):616-622.
24. Yennu S, Urbauer D, Bruera E. Factors associated with the severity and improvement of fatigue in patients with advanced cancer presenting to an outpatient palliative care clinic. *BMC Palliat Care.* 2012;11:16.
25. Piper BF, Cella D. Cancer-related fatigue: definitions and clinical subtypes. *J Natl Compr Cancer Netw.* 2010;8(8):958-966.

26. Cella D, Peterman A, Passik S, et al. Progress toward guidelines for the management of fatigue. *Oncology*. 1998;12:369-377.
27. Portenoy RK, Itri LM. Cancer-related fatigue: guidelines for evaluation and management. *Oncologist*. 1999;4:1-10.
28. Demetri GD, Kris M, Wade J, et al. Quality of life benefit in chemotherapy patients treated with epoetin alfa is independent of disease response or tumor type: results from a prospective community oncology study. *Oncology*. 1998;16:3412-3425.
29. Yennurajalingam S, Bruera E. Role of corticosteroids for fatigue in advanced incurable cancer: is it a "wonder drug" or "deal with the devil." *Curr Opin Support Palliat Care*. 2014;8(4):346-351.
30. Bruera E, Yennurajalingam S, Palmer J, et al. Methylphenidate and/or a nursing telephone intervention for fatigue in patients with advanced cancer: a randomized, placebo-controlled, phase II trial. *J Clin Oncol*. 2013;31(19):2421-2427.
31. Bruera E, Brenneis C, Paterson AH, et al. Use of methylphenidate as an adjuvant to narcotic analgesics in patients with advanced cancer. *J Pain Symptom Manage*. 1989;4:3-6.
32. Breitbart W, Mermelstein H. An alternative psychostimulant for the management of depressive disorders in cancer patients. *Psychosomatics*. 1992;33:352-356.
33. Katon W, Raskind M. Treatment of depression in the medically ill elderly with methylphenidate. *Am J Psychiatry*. 1980;137:963-965.
34. Minton O, Richardson A, Sharpe M, Hotopf M, Stone P. Drug therapy for the management of cancer related fatigue. *Cochrane Database Syst Rev*. 2010;(7):CD006704.
35. Rajagopal A, Vassilopoulou-Sellin R, Palmer JL, et al. Symptomatic hypogonadism in male survivors of cancer with chronic exposure to opioids. *Cancer*. 2004;100(4):851-858.
36. Del Fabbro E, Garcia JM, Dev R, et al. Testosterone replacement for fatigue in hypogonadal ambulatory males with advanced cancer: a preliminary double-blind placebo-controlled trial. *Support Care Center*. 2013;21(9):2599-2607.
37. Yennurajalingam S, Bruera E. Review of clinical trials of pharmacologic interventions for cancer-related fatigue focus on psychostimulants and steroids. *Cancer J*. 2014;20:319-324.
38. Meneses-Echávez J, Gonza lez-Jimenez E, Ramirez-Velez R. Supervised exercise reduces cancer-related fatigue: a systematic review. *J Physiother*. 2015;61(1):3-9.
39. Sadja J, Mills PJ. Effects of yoga interventions on fatigue in cancer patients and survivors: a systematic review of randomized controlled trials. *Explore (NY)*. 2013;9(4):232–243.
40. Liu L, Da M, Rissling M, et al. Fatigue and circadian activity rhythms in breast cancer patients before and after chemotherapy: a controlled study. *Fatigue*. 2013;1(1-2): 12–26.
41. Fearon K, Strasser F, Anker S, et al. Definition and classification of cancer cachexia: an international consensus. *Lancet Oncol*. 2011;12:489–495.
42. Dewys WD, Begg C, Lavin PT, et al. Prognostic effect of weight loss prior to chemotherapy in cancer patients. Eastern Cooperative Oncology Group. *Am J Med*. 1980;69:491-497.
43. Egidio Del Fabbro, Shalini Dalal, Eduardo Bruera. Symptom control in palliative care—part II: cachexia/anorexia and fatigue. *J Palliat Med*. 2006;9(2):409-421.
44. Barber MD, Fearon KC, McMillan DC, et al. Liver export protein synthetic rates are increased by oral meal feeding in weight losing cancer patients. *Am J Physiol Endocrinol Metab*. 2000;279:707E-E714E.
45. Wasserman K, Casaburi R. Dyspnea and physiological and athophysiological mechanisms. *Annu Rev Med*. 1988;39:503-515.
46. Mahler DA, Selecky PA, Harrod CG. Management of dyspnea in patients with advanced lung or heart disease: practical guidance from the American College of Chest Physicians consensus statement. *Polish Arch Intern Med*. 2010;120(5):160-166.
47. Hardy JR, Turner R, Saunders M, et al. Prediction of survival in a hospital-based continuing care unit. *Eur J Cancer*. 1994;30:284-288.
48. Escalante CP, Martin CG, Elting LS, et al. Dyspnea in cancer patients: etiology, resource utilization, and survival. *Cancer*. 1996;78:1314-1319.
49. Mahler DA, O'Donnell DE. Recent advances in dyspnea. *Chest*. 2015;147(1):232-241.
50. von Leupoldt A, Sommer T, Kegat S, et al. Down-regulation of insular cortex responses to dyspnea and pain in asthma. *Am J Respir Crit Care Med*. 2009;180(3):232-238.
51. Hui D, Morgado M, Chisholm G, et al. High-flow oxygen and bi-level positive airway pressure for persistent dyspnea in patients with advanced cancer: a phase II randomized trial. *J Pain Symptom Manage*. 2013;46(4):463-473.
52. Weir DC, Gove RI, Robertson AS, et al. Corticosteroids trials in nonasthmatic chronic airflow obstruction: A comparison of oral prednisolone and inhaled bechomethasone diproprionate. *Thorax*. 1991;45:112-117.
53. Allcroft P, Margitanovic V, Greene A, et al. The role of benzodiazepines in breathlessness: a single site, open label pilot of sustained release morphine together with clonazepam. *J Palliat Med*. 2013;16(7):741-744.
54. Jones AY, Ngai SP, Hui-Chan CW, Yu HP. Acute effects of Acu-TENS on FEV1 and blood b–endorphin level in chronic obstructive pulmonary disease. *Altern Ther Health Med*. 2011;17(5):8-13.
55. Suzuki M, Muro S, Ando Y, et al. A randomized, placebo-controlled trial of acupuncture in patients with chronic obstructive pulmonary disease (COPD): the COPD-acupuncture trial (CAT). *Arch Intern Med*. 2012;172(11):878-886.
56. Galbraith S, Fagan P, Perkins P, Lynch A, Booth S. Does the use of a handheld fan improve chronic dyspnea? A randomized controlled, crossover trial. *J Pain Symptom Manage*. 2010;39(5):831-838.
57. Bruera E, Bush SH, Willey J, et al. Impact of delirium and recall on the level of distress in patients with advanced cancer and their family caregivers. *Cancer*. 2009;115(9):2004-2012.
58. de la Cruz M, Fan J, Yennu S, et al. The frequency of missed delirium in patients referred to palliative care in a comprehensive cancer center. *Support Care Cancer*. 2015;23(8):2427-2433.
59. Centeno C, Sanz A, Bruera E. Delirum in advanced cancer patients. *Palliat Med*. 2004;18(3):184-194.
60. Briebart W, Marotta R, Platt MM, et al. A double-blinded trial of haloperidol, chlorazepam, and lorazepam in the treatment of delirium in the hospitalized AIDS patients. *Am J Psychiatry*. 1996;153:231-237.
61. Hui D, Bush SH, Gallo LE, et al. Neuroleptic dose in the management of delirium in patients with advanced cancer. *J Pain Symptom Manage*. 2010;39(2):186-196.
62. Elsayem A, Bush SH, Munsell MF, et al. Subcutaneous olanzapine for hyperactive or mixed delirium in patients with advanced cancer: a preliminary study. *J Pain Symptom Manage*. 2010;40(5):774-782.
63. Sanft T, Hauser J, Rosielle D, et al. Coyle N. Physical pain and emotional suffering: the case for palliative sedation. *J Pain*. 2009;10(3):238-242.
64. Derogatis LR, Marrow GR, Fettig J, et al. The prevalence of psychiatric disorders among cancer patients. *JAMA*. 1983;249:751-757.
65. Wilson KG, Chochinov HM, de Faye B, et al. Diagnosis and management of depression in palliative care. In: Chochinov HM, Breitbart W, eds. *Handbook of Psychiatry in Palliative Care*. Oxford, UK: Oxford University Press; 2000:25-49, 106.
66. American Psychiatric Association. *Diagnostic and Statistical Manual of Mental Disorders*, 4th ed. Washington, DC: American Psychiatric Association; 1994.
67. Bonsignore M, Barkow K, Jessen F, et al. Validity of the five item WHO Well Being Index (WHO-5) in an elderly population. *Eur Arch Psychiatry Clin Neurosci*. 2001;251(suppl 2):II27-II31.

68. Kroenke K, Spitzer RL, Williams JB. The PHQ-9: validity of a brief depression severity measure. *J Gen Intern Med*. 2001;16:606-613.
69. Hamilton M. A rating scale for depression. *J Neurol Neurosurg Psychiatry*. 1960;23:56-62.
70. Montgomery S, Asberg MA. A new depression scale designed to be sensitive to change. *Br J Psychiatry*. 1979;134:382-389.
71. Christakis NA. Predicting patient survival before and after hospice enrollment. *Hosp J*. 1998;13:71-87.
72. Parkes CM. Accuracy of predictions of survival in later stages of cancer. *Br Med J*. 1972;2:29-3.
73. Girgis A, Sanson-Fisher RW. Breaking bad news: consensus guidelines for medical practitioners. *J Clin Oncol*. 1995;13:2449-2456.
74. Ptacek JT, Eberhardt TL. Breaking bad news: a review of the literature. *JAMA*. 1996;276:496-502.
75. Clayton JM, Hancock KM, Butow PN, et al. Clinical practice guidelines for communicating prognosis and end-of-life issues with adults in the advanced stages of a life-limiting illness, and their caregivers. *Med J Aust*. 2007;186(12 Suppl):S77, S79, S83-S108.
76. Hudson P, Quinn K, O'Hanlon B, Aranda S. Family meetings in palliative care: multidisciplinary clinical practice guidelines. *BMC Palliative Care*. 2008;7:12.
77. Delgado-Guay M, Parsons H, Hui D, et al. Spirituality, religiosity, and spiritual pain among caregivers of patients with advanced cancer. *Am J Hospice Palliat Med*. 2012;30(5):455-461.
78. Elsayem A, Driver LC, Bruera E. *The MD Anderson Palliative Care Handbook*. Houston, TX: MD Anderson Cancer Center; 2002.

59 Rehabilitation

第五十九章　康复

Sunny S. Dhah
Jack B. Fu
Ki Y. Shin

中文导读

癌症本身及其相关治疗是导致身体损伤甚至残疾的主要原因。近年来，随着癌症治疗中取得的成功，人们越来越关注癌症患者的生活质量，特别是康复方面。本章首先梳理了癌症康复学的基本概念，包括癌症康复的不同阶段、在MD安德森癌症中心康复治疗的情况以及康复相关的功能指标。随后本章分别从癌症康复的实际操作、紧急的癌症康复治疗、脑转移患者的康复、淋巴水肿患者的康复、癌症相关脊髓损伤患者的康复、患者整体的体能失调和虚弱情况的康复、耐用医疗设备、压疮、血小板减少症、癌症患者的运动、障碍消除、终末期的康复以及癌症康复学的未来发展进行了详细阐述。在脑转移患者康复的部分，分别介绍了在神经运动损害、共济失调、失语症、认知缺陷、吞咽困难、强直、膀胱功能障碍等方面的康复治疗。在脊髓损害部分，则分别从膀胱功能处理、肠道功能处理及强直状态等方面进行讲解。在癌症患者运动的部分，详细介绍了如何保证癌症患者运动时的安全以及对于癌症患者如何给予运动相关的处方。在障碍消除中，则详细阐述了该如何处理影响重返职场的癌症相关的残疾。对于癌症康复未来的发展方向，癌症幸存者的康复、对于癌症康复概念认知度的增加、运动及癌症生存、运动的抗炎作用以及癌症患者由于急症再次回到初级急症护理服务等在未来可能会得到更多的关注。

GENERAL PRINCIPLES

Cancer and its treatments are a major cause for impairments and disability. Because cancer treatments have become increasingly successful and have improved survival, there has been an increasing focus on quality of life and, in particular, rehabilitation. Cancer rehabilitation is practiced in outpatient clinics, oncology wards, inpatient rehabilitation units, skilled nursing facilities, nursing homes, long-term acute care centers, palliative care units, and hospices. Common diagnoses addressed include asthenia, deconditioning, hemiplegia, spinal cord injury, peripheral neuropathy, somatic and neuropathic pain, steroid myopathy, lymphedema, bowel/bladder management, limb amputation, and limb dysfunction.

The major goal of cancer rehabilitation is to improve quality of life by minimizing the disability caused by cancer and its treatments and decreasing the "burden of care" needed by patients with cancer and their caregivers. The more patients can do for themselves, the more personal dignity they are able to maintain and the less help they require from those around them.

In 1978, Justus Lehmann, supported by the National Cancer Institute (NCI), screened 805 randomly selected patients with cancer, identifying multiple problems in the population of patients with cancer who are amenable to rehabilitation interventions along with barriers limiting the delivery of rehabilitation care. More than 30 years later, many of Lehmann's remediable cancer rehabilitation problems and barriers to rehabilitation care remain the same (Table 59-1).

These problems are familiar to rehabilitation professionals because many are also found in traditional noncancer rehabilitation patients. Lehman also described major barriers to the delivery of cancer rehabilitation care, including the lack of identification of these problems by oncologists and the lack of referral to rehab professionals for a rehabilitation intervention. In addition, there are multiple patient-related factors that can affect the successful rehabilitation of the patient with cancer. Several reported by DeLisa include reduced life expectancy, extensive comorbidities, degree of pain, the dynamic nature of cancer lesions, the demands of anticancer therapies, and the desire to spend remaining time with loved ones ([1]).

Phases of Cancer Rehabilitation

In 1980, Dietz categorized cancer rehabilitation into four stages: preventive, restorative, supportive, and palliative ([2]). Preventive rehabilitation occurs before or immediately after a treatment to prevent loss of function or disability. An example would include preamputation stump care teaching and ambulation with a walker in a patient with a lower extremity sarcoma. In 2001, Courneya described a concept called "buffering" whereby a patient with cancer undergoes exercises and therapies to increase the patient's physical and functional reserves before cancer treatment ([3]).

Restorative rehabilitation occurs in patients who are believed to be disease free or will have an anticipated relatively stable disease course. Taking our previous example, a patient with lower extremity sarcoma with no known metastatic disease following amputation undergoes prosthetic rehabilitation. These first two stages are not significantly different from conventional nononcologic rehabilitation. Fortunately, as survivorship has increased, restorative rehabilitation has become more prominent in addressing issues in this population, including disability, return to work, and lymphedema management.

If patients are unable to achieve or maintain a state of remission, supportive rehabilitation is performed to sustain function and provide symptom management.

Table 59-1 Remediable Rehabilitation Problems and Barriers to Delivery of Rehabilitation Care

Remediable Rehabilitation Problems		Barriers to Delivery of Rehabilitation Care
Psychological/psychiatric impairments	Lymphedema management	Lack of identification of patient problems
Generalized weakness	Musculoskeletal difficulties	Lack of appropriate referral by physicians unfamiliar with the concept of rehabilitation
Impairments in activities of daily living	Swallowing dysfunction	Patient too ill to participate
Pain	Impaired communication	Patient denies need
Impaired gait/ambulation	Skin management	Cancer prognosis too limited
Disposition/housing issues	Vocational assessments	Rehabilitation unavailable
Neurologic impairments	Impaired nutrition	No financial resources
Vocational assessments	Lymphedema management	
Impaired nutrition		

Data from Lehmann JF, DeLisa JA, Warren CG, et al. Cancer rehabilitation: assessment of need, development, and evaluation of a model of care. *Arch Phys Med Rehabil.* 1978;59:410-419.

CHAPTER 59

Expanding on our example, a patient with metastatic sarcoma may be provided therapies and durable medical equipment (DME) to promote functional independence while receiving chemoradiation.

Unfortunately, patients may succumb to their malignancy, or its accompanying morbidities, and efforts to maximize function may require a transition to focusing on quality of life. Palliative rehabilitation is provided to reduce discomfort and improve independence in patients with advanced disease. Our example patient with sarcoma and advancing metastatic disease may have failed multiple treatment regimens and now requires rehabilitation to return home with some degree of assistance. The emphasis of palliative rehabilitation is typically to get the patient home safely as soon as possible. The patient likely has limited time to live and the costs of a lengthy inpatient rehabilitation stay must be taken into consideration. Goals once the the patient is home in a safe environment focus on family and transfer training. Higher-level goals should be addressed as an outpatient or through home health therapy.

The last two stages described by Dietz ([1]) are relatively unique to cancer rehabilitation. The typical course for a patient in conventional rehabilitation (eg, after a stroke) is continued improvement after the inciting event. In the patient with cancer with persistent disease, however, the war continues with brief victories followed by declines as the disease progresses ([3]) (Fig. 59-1).

Multiple studies have established a need for rehabilitation in the population of patients with cancer ([4, 5]). Functional improvements of patients in cancer rehabilitation have been demonstrated in a number of settings, including inpatient ([6-9]) and palliative care ([10, 11]), on a consultation basis ([12]), in a hospice setting ([13, 14]), and for outpatient settings ([15]). The maintenance of physical activity and exercise has been implicated in increasing survival, with the greatest quantity of evidence in patients with breast and colon cancer. Multiple mechanisms may exist, and some have proposed these findings to be related to levels of insulin/c-peptide, along with the positive effects of buffering on physiological reserves, potentially allowing for more treatment ([16, 17]). Cancer physiatrists must also address medical sequelae and complications that are unique to this patient population. With limited training in general medical and surgical fields, these comorbidities may serve as a significant challenge and require frequent communication between the primary oncology and rehabilitation teams. The transfer rate from inpatient rehabilitation to acute care teams is high compared to other rehabilitation diagnoses ([18]).

Rehabilitation goals are accomplished by the efforts of a comprehensive interdisciplinary team of health-care professionals, including the rehabilitation physician, rehabilitation nurse, physical therapist, occupational therapist, speech therapist, dietitian, pharmacist, chaplain, social worker, and case manager. Each member of the team has specific expertise in assisting the patient with a care plan of maximizing medical stability, function, financial resources, and caregiver involvement for a discharge that is as safe and meaningful as possible (Fig. 59-2).

Rehabilitation at MD Anderson

At the University of Texas MD Anderson Cancer Center (MDACC), our cancer rehabilitation practice includes seven physical medicine and rehabilitation physicians and a rehabilitation therapy staff of over 100 physical therapy and occupational therapy clinicians. Rehabilitation therapists see over 300 inpatients and 100 outpatients per day. Patients include those with most of the different tumor types seen in the institution, the most common being brain, spine, lung, breast, hematologic, genitourinary, gastrointestinal, and head and neck tumors. The most common inpatient rehabilitation diagnoses included asthenia, gait abnormality, dyspnea, hemiparesis, spinal cord injury, and neurogenic bowel and bladder. Common outpatient rehabilitation diagnoses include lymphedema, myofascial pain, rotator cuff dysfunction, peripheral neuropathy, and low back pain. Inpatient and outpatient electromyograms are performed for neuropathic and myopathic diagnoses and spasticity management.

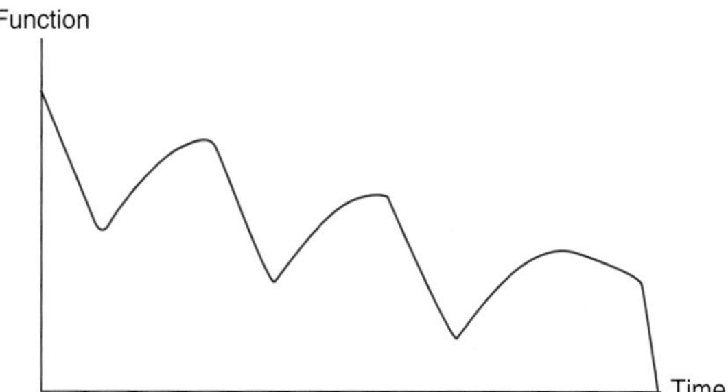

FIGURE 59-1 Function/time graph of cancer patient.

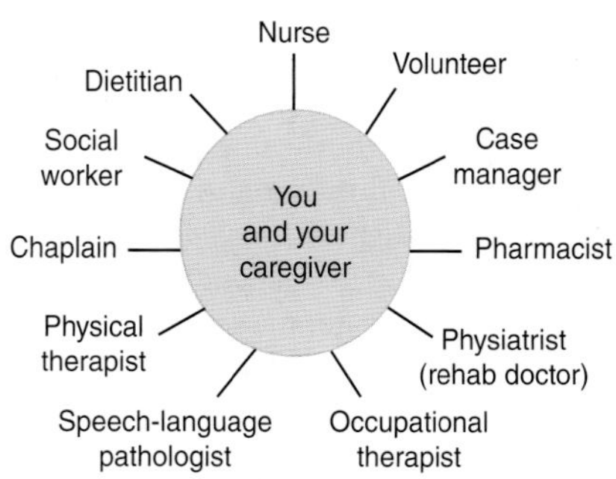

FIGURE 59-2 Rehabilitation team.

Functional Metrics

When describing the functional status of a patient with cancer, the Karnofsky Performance Scale is often used. It is the most widely used scale both clinically and in research in oncology patients ([19]). It is an easy and quick generalized measurement of a patient's function. Weaknesses of the scale include overgeneralization (unable to measure specific tasks) and poor correlation with cognition ([20]).

In rehabilitation, the outcome scale most often used is the Functional Independence Measure (Fig. 59-3). This multidimensional scale addresses 18 items from a scale of 1 (total assistance) to 7 (complete independence). Items are subdivided into self-care, sphincter control, transfers, locomotion, communication, and social cognition. An aggregate score is also often useful out of a total of 126. Criticisms of the scale include that it is too general and omits items that are important for specific populations, such as those with spinal cord injuries ([21]).

PRACTICAL ASPECTS OF CANCER REHABILITATION

Physiatry is a holistic specialty that accounts for medical needs while focusing on a patient's functional issues. Safety is a primary concern of rehabilitation health-care professionals. The first question a physiatrist often asks is, What is the minimum level of safe function for this patient to be discharged? That "safe" functional level goal depends on the patient's current functional level, strength, cognition, amount of supervision or assistance available on discharge, accessibility of home conditions, and financial resources. Physiatrists must ask patients and their caregivers detailed social questions.

Common obstacles confronted are a lack of assistance or supervision at home. This often is due to the patient's significant other being required to work during the day, the significant other's inability either physically or mentally (eg, dementia) to care for the patient, or having no one available to care for them.

One of the most practical and simple rehabilitation techniques that an inpatient must learn is to transfer. A transfer is a change in station or position from sitting in bed to standing or from sitting in bed to sitting in a chair. A person must transfer to get into a wheelchair or into a car seat. Patients cannot effectively mobilize until this is accomplished. Depending on the patient's level of disability, a transfer may be performed to sit to stand, to stand and pivot, with a sliding board, or with a lift requiring total assistance. After basic transfers are mastered, ambulation may be the next goal to increase mobility. Weakness from paresis, deconditioning, neuropathy, or brain injury can also make self-care difficult. Practical skills such as feeding, grooming, bathing, and dressing are taught or relearned to improve independence.

ACUTE CANCER REHABILITATION

Rehabilitation begins when a patient is admitted into the hospital. Impairments are identified, and based on the practical considerations mentioned previously, realistic and suitable rehabilitation goals are set. If a patient is medically stable with unmet functional and safety goals, the patient's activity tolerance and performance trajectory are used to guide determination of the appropriate intensity and location for additional rehabilitation.

REHABILITATION OF INDIVIDUALS WITH BRAIN TUMORS

Primary brain tumors are less than 2% of all malignancies but are the second leading cause of death from neurologic disorders after stroke ([22]). One-half to two-thirds of intracranial tumors have been reported to be primary tumors ([23]). Primary brain tumors are classified by cell of origin; the primary system of classification is that of the World Health Organization (WHO), which divides tumors into nine categories. The most common categories include tumors that displace brain parenchyma of the intracranial supratentorial compartment. Of these tumors, the most common in adults are the astrocytomas, in particular grade IV astrocytoma, otherwise known as glioblastoma multiforme (GBM) ([24]). The median survival for a patient with GBM has been reported between 7 and 17 months ([25]).

In addition to primary brain tumors, brain metastases are estimated to occur in 20% to 40% of patients with cancer. The most common mechanism of metastasis to the brain is through hematogenous spread. Most of the metastases are located in the cerebral hemispheres, followed by the cerebellum and then the brainstem. The incidence of brain tumor metastases is rising, possibly due to the increasing length of survival of a patient with cancer ([26]), increasing ability to diagnose a tumor with improved radiographic imaging ([27]), and possibly recent chemotherapy agents, which may weaken the blood-brain barrier ([28]).

Normal brain parenchyma can be destroyed or compressed by the tumor, and the location of the tumor determines the resultant neurologic deficit. Surgical resection may exacerbate these deficits by creating inflammation or peritumoral infarct ([29]). Radiation

FIM™ Instrument

Levels		
	7 Complete Independence (timely, safely) 6 Modified Independence (device)	No helper
	Modified Dependence 5 Supervision (subject = 100%) 4 Minimal Assistance (subject = 75%+) 3 Moderate Assistance (subject = 50%+) **Complete Dependence** 2 Maximal Assistance (subject = 25%+) 1 Total Assistance (subject = less than 25%+)	Helper

	Admission	Discharge	Follow-up
Self-Care			
A. Eating			
B. Grooming			
C. Bathing			
D. Dressing - Upper Body			
E. Dressing - Lower Body			
F. Toileting			
Sphincter Control			
G. Bladder Management			
H. Bowel Management			
Transfers			
I. Bed, Chair, Wheelchair			
J. Toilet			
K. Tub, Shower			
Locomotion			
L. Walk/Wheelchair	W Walk C Wheelchair B Both	W Walk C Wheelchair B Both	W Walk C Wheelchair B Both
M. Stairs			
Motor Subtotal Score			
Communication			
N. Comprehension	A Auditory V Visual B Both	A Auditory V Visual B Both	A Auditory V Visual B Both
O. Expression	A Auditory V Visual B Both	A Auditory V Visual B Both	A Auditory V Visual B Both
Social Cognition			
P. Social Interaction			
Q. Problem Solving			
R. Memory			
Cognitive Subtotal Score			
Total FIM™ Score			

Note: Leave no blanks. Enter 1 if patient is not testable due to risk.

FIGURE 59-3 Functional Independence Measure (FIM) instrument.

treatment has long been an integral part of brain tumor treatments and often results in collateral damage. Early acute radiation leukoencephalopathy is likely due to increased cerebral edema. Late delayed radiation reactions include focal cerebral radiation necrosis, diffuse cerebral radiation injury (DCRI), and combined-therapy diffuse white matter injury/leukoencephalopathy. Clinical DCRI has been reported in 2% to 5% of patients with metastases and 19% of 1-year survivors after whole-brain radiation ([30, 31]).

The most common neurologic deficits include impaired cognition (80%), weakness (78%), visual-perceptual deficits (53%), sensory loss (38%), and bowel/bladder dysfunction (37%). Other deficits include cranial nerve palsy, dysarthria, dysphagia, aphasia, ataxia, and diplopia, which are less common. Approximately 75% of patients with a brain tumor have three or more neurologic deficits concurrently, and 39% have five or more deficits ([32]). Because of the diverse nature of these neurologic deficits, comprehensive multidisciplinary inpatient rehabilitation is often necessary for these patients. In rehabilitation medicine, the physical impairments that could result in functional deficits are primarily addressed.

Patients who have impairments resulting in functional decline that could affect bed mobility, ambulation, transferring from sitting or lying to a standing position, or activities of daily living (ADLs) (eg, eating, grooming, dressing, bathing, and toileting) can benefit from comprehensive inpatient rehabilitation. Comprehensive cancer rehabilitation services are not widely available for these patients ([33]). Because of this, many patients with a brain tumor receive their rehabilitation at general rehabilitation facilities alongside patients with stroke and traumatic brain injury. Patients with a brain tumor have similar efficiencies of improvement when compared to traumatic brain injury, stroke, and between brain tumor types. Lengths of stay tend to be shorter among patients with a brain tumor, possibly secondary to a need to return the patients home sooner given their shorter life expectancies ([34-38]). However, some notable differences between these populations should be noted (eg, physiatrists may need to be cognizant of the continued decline of patients with progressive tumors).

Neurologic Motor Impairment

Motor impairment can be due to hemiparesis, ataxia, and apraxia. Motor impairment may lead to an unsafe gait pattern creating a higher risk for falls and a need for inpatient rehabilitation transfer. In inpatient rehabilitation, the patient will be seen by physical and occupational therapists. Physical therapy would focus on gait and transfers. To address transfers, efforts could be focused on sliding board transfer or stand pivot transfers. With respect to mobility, physical therapists focus on wheelchair mobility and gait with or without an assistive device (eg, a single-point cane, quad cane, rolling walker, hemiwalker). Occupational therapy would focus on problems with ADLs. Commonly addressed basic ADLs include dressing, bathing, toileting, grooming, eating, and the like. The occupational therapist and physical therapist are also aware of the cognitive component necessary for mobility and ADLs. Once a patient is functionally safe using an assistive device such as a rolling walker, he or she can be discharged home. Then, the patient can continue with outpatient rehabilitation, gradually improving his or her ambulation with an assistive device and further strengthening weakened muscles by way of a progressive resistance exercise program.

The pattern of recovery of muscle strength and function does not always follow the pattern of recovery observed in patients with stroke. However, the stroke recovery pattern is often used as a guideline for patients with brain tumors. The recovery of strength occurs in a proximal-to-distal direction, with flaccidity and decreased muscle tone progressing to spasticity and increased muscle tone. The spasticity in the affected limbs can evolve into flexor or extensor synergy patterns. Recovery of muscle movement may plateau at any stage or may progress to isolated coordinated volitional motor movement ([39, 40]).

Several techniques and exercises are used for neuromuscular facilitation in patients with stroke. Often, a combination of procedures and techniques from the various programs are used in patients with cancer with neuromuscular weakness. Proprioceptive neuromuscular facilitation developed by Kabat, Knott, and Voss relies on several mechanisms, such as spiral diagonal movement patterns of the extremities and quick stretch. Brunnstrom movement therapy facilitates the use of the synergy patterns mentioned as a means of developing voluntary control. Rood proposed that cutaneous sensory stimulation in the form of superficial stroking, tapping, brushing, vibrating, or icing provides facilitatory or inhibitory inputs ([41]).

In addition to the traditional range-of-motion and strengthening exercises as well as neuromuscular facilitation techniques, functional electrical stimulation can also be incorporated into the rehabilitation program for neuromuscular weakness. It uses a low-level electrical current that stimulates motor nerves or reflex sensory nerves to produce muscle contraction. The goal of functional electric stimulation is to produce purposeful, functional movements in paretic or paralytic muscles ([42]).

Sometimes, owing to weakness of the ankle dorsiflexors, it is necessary to use an ankle-foot orthosis (AFO) to improve hemiparetic gait. There are two major types of AFOs: the double metal upright AFO attached to an orthopedic shoe and the molded plastic AFO, which is more commonly used. With the plastic AFO, the footplate sits within the shoe and extends upward behind the calf. The advantages of a plastic AFO over a double metal upright AFO include better cosmesis, lighter weight, and the freedom to wear different shoes.

Shoulder subluxation, predominantly inferior, which is caused by the loss of normal motor control of the shoulder stabilizers, including the deltoid and supraspinatus muscle, is often seen in the hemiparetic patient [43]. It can often be the cause of shoulder pain in hemiplegic patients [44, 45]. Other possible causes of shoulder pain in this patient population include complex regional pain syndrome, traction injury of the brachial plexus, rotator cuff tendinitis or tear, subacromial or subdeltoid bursitis, adhesive capsulitis, or heterotopic ossification. Diagnosis of glenohumeral subluxation is made through physical examination and radiographic evaluation. The acromiohumeral interval is compared on each side with the arms in an unsupported position during physical examination, and radiographic evaluation is used to quantify the amount of subluxation. Radiographic studies can provide an early evaluation for subluxation with slight gapping of the superior aspect of the glenohumeral joint [46].

Treatment of hemiparetic shoulder subluxation involves proper positioning of the arm, physical modalities, and exercise. The use of an arm sling can help maintain proper positioning and posture during ambulation. However, this is discouraged when the patient is seated, and its overuse may contribute to compromise of superficial blood flow as well as to joint contracture. Arm troughs and lapboards are used while patients are seated [47]. Other interventions include biofeedback and functional electrical stimulation.

Hemisensory deficit and homonymous hemianopsia may be seen with hemiparesis. Visual or somatic hemineglect is more frequently seen when the nondominant cerebral hemisphere is affected. Hemispatial neglect has a negative effect on sitting balance, visual perception, wheelchair mobility safety awareness, and risk of falling [42]. Patients with neglect have difficulty with hygiene and self-care activities on the affected side. Rehabilitation programs must address the issue of hemispatial neglect through focused measures led by speech therapists, occupational therapists, and physical therapists. Family training and education are important in this setting as well.

Ataxia

Cerebellar ataxia may be seen with mass effect within the posterior fossa. Of note, cerebellar ataxia can also be seen in paraneoplastic cerebellar degeneration and with high-dose administration of cytarabine (ara-C) or 5-fluorouracil (5-FU) [48, 49]. Involvement of the cerebellum can produce intention tremors, dysmetria, and dysdiadochokinesis as patients lose the ability to coordinate the agonist and antagonist muscle groups [50]. The response to pharmaceutical management has been poor; consequently, physical and occupational therapy has been the mainstay of treatment for ataxia. This includes the teaching of compensatory techniques for performing basic self-care and occupational activities and the possible use of weighted bracelets or similar devices to help decrease the oscillations. Physical therapy directed at gait training with the use of assistive devices can help improve mobility in ataxic individuals [51].

Aphasia

Depending on its location, a tumor may be associated with deficits in speech, which can vary in severity and type. Often, one can diagnose the type of aphasia from a comprehensive neurologic examination, including speech comprehension, fluency, and repetition. These include Broca's aphasia, Wernicke's aphasia, anomic aphasia, global aphasia, conduction aphasia, and the transcortical motor and sensory aphasias.

A speech pathologist will implement treatment approaches, including melodic intonation therapy, Amer-Ind Code treatment, functional communication treatment, stimulation approach, and Promoting Aphasics' Communication Effectiveness (PACE) therapy [52].

Cognitive Deficits

Cognitive deficits often are more problematic than motor deficits. They can arise from direct injury to the brain tissue due to the tumor itself, from surgical resection, radiation, chemotherapy, depression/anxiety, as well as medications, particularly steroids and anticonvulsants [28]. Impairments most commonly seen involve limited memory and attention, decreased initiation, and psychomotor retardation [53].

The rehabilitation physician will assess the patient's cognitive status as part of the physical examination. This assessment is needed to formulate a rehabilitation program involving speech pathologists. Specific deficits in language and cognition can further be delineated through specific testing performed by a speech pathologist. However, it is sometimes necessary to have formal neuropsychological testing done, especially if the patient wishes to return to work.

Dysphagia

A disruption in the swallowing process can also occur in patients with brain tumors or following craniotomies. It is important to determine, through clinical assessment, whether dysphagia is present because there is the potential for serious complications, such as malnutrition and aspiration pneumonia, if dysphagia remains undetected. Often, its presence can be established from a history and neurologic examination. If dysphagia is suspected, a speech pathologist is consulted; then, daily swallowing therapy and exercises are incorporated into the therapeutic milieu.

Treatments include dietary modifications and dysphagia exercise and facilitation techniques (54). Depending on the results from a clinical swallowing evaluation or videofluoroscopic evaluation, food can be modified to different consistencies, including puree, semisolid, or solid. Liquids may also have to be thickened using various thickening (55).

Exercises and facilitation techniques are employed to aid and strengthen various components of the swallowing process. These include exercises employed for treatment for the lips to facilitate the ability to prevent food or liquid from leaking out of the oral cavity. There are exercises to assist the pharyngeal swallow by improving tongue base retraction. Vocal cord adduction exercises are instituted to strengthen weak cords to prevent aspiration.

Compensatory strategies include proper head and trunk positioning, which for most patients is to be seated upright with head midline, trunk erect, and the neck slightly flexed forward. Other techniques include the chin-tuck method and head turning and tilting during swallowing.

After dysphagia has been identified and measures are implemented for its treatment, regular follow-up to assess for improvement is required. This again can be done through clinical examination or radiographically. If improvement is noted, the diet may be advanced appropriately.

Spasticity

Spasticity is defined as velocity-dependent resistance to passive movement across a joint. It is an abnormality involving increased muscle tone and is one of the positive findings of the upper motor neuron syndrome. Spasticity must be distinguished from soft tissue contractures. Soft tissue contractures result from scar tissue formation and may be the result of a number of causes, including uncontrolled spasticity.

Often, brain tumors can cause muscle spasticity. This can affect the gait pattern or ADLs and, in severe cases, can cause pain and joint contractures as well as being a detriment to hygiene of the involved areas. Sometimes, spasticity may be beneficial, as when a patient may use knee extensor spasticity to assist in transferring from a sitting to a standing position. Indications for the treatment of spasticity include the need to decrease pain, improve hygiene, improve gait and transfers, minimize contractures, and improve self-care.

Treatment measures for spasticity include physical and medical interventions. Proper positioning, passive range-of-motion exercises, serial casting, splints, and braces are some of the physical interventions used in treating spasticity. Oral medications may also be used, including tizanidine, dantrolene sodium, and baclofen. Because these medications work systemically, the most common limiting side effects are excessive drowsiness and cognitive changes. Tizanidine or dantrolene is recommended by most clinicians for treating spasticity stemming from primary brain pathology (55). Often, because of the cognitive side effects of these oral medications, botulinum toxin injections, phenol injections, or intrathecal baclofen pumps may be useful. These medications act locally but are harder to administer and more invasive.

Bladder Dysfunction

As in patients with stroke, bladder incontinence may be present in patients with brain tumors. The causes of bladder incontinence can be multifactorial and include an untreated urinary tract infection, inability to ambulate to the bathroom, and altered cognitive status. If the pontine micturition center is preserved, patients with brain tumors can have upper motor neuron bladder dysfunction, which is characterized by bladder hyperreflexia with reflex or urge incontinence and complete emptying (56). Postvoid residual volumes are generally low in the absence of bladder outlet obstruction. Persistent areflexia and retention may occur with bilateral lesions (57).

Treatment first involves identifying the cause of the bladder dysfunction. Obtaining a urinalysis with cultures and sensitivities and then starting appropriate antibiotics is the treatment for urinary tract infections. Using a bedside commode or a urinal is of benefit for patients who have weakness or inability to safely ambulate to the bathroom. A timed voiding program that has the patient urinate at set times throughout the day, before the bladder can contract, can be of help for patients with hyperreflexic urgency. Anticholinergic medications such as oxybutynin (Ditropan) or tolterodine tartrate (Detrol) can be used for persistent incontinence in this setting of a hyperreflexic detrusor (57). If the patient's blood pressure can tolerate it, a trial of an alpha-adrenergic agent (eg, tamsulosin, terazosin) may be useful in reducing urinary resistance in older male patients who are experiencing symptoms of urinary retention.

LYMPHEDEMA

Physiatrists are often asked to assist with the care of patients with lymphedema. Malignancy (including breast, melanoma, gynecologic, lymphoma, and urologic cancers) is the number one cause of secondary lymphedema in the United States. The lymphedema can be caused by a combination of the cancer, surgical treatments, and radiation treatments. Breast cancer is the leading cause of upper extremity lymphedema in the United States and develops in 2% to 40% of patients after surgery, radiation, or both [58, 59].

The majority of lymphedema cases are diagnosed clinically. The differential diagnosis would include deep venous thrombosis (DVT), venous insufficiency, myxedema, lipedema, heart failure, kidney failure, and hypoproteinemia. In difficult-to-diagnose cases, lymphoscintigraphy is the gold standard.

The treatment of lymphedema typically starts with conservative treatments consisting of manual lymph drainage, compression sleeves, and sometimes pneumatic compression sleeves. Over one or two sessions by lymphedema-trained physical therapists, patients are taught a lymphedema regimen to do at home. Measurements are often taken, and the patients are followed up periodically to ensure that they are completing the regimen as prescribed and to measure changes in their lymphedema. Progression of lymphedema can be measured using a number of techniques, including volumetric/circumferential measurements, bioelectric impedance, tonometry, and perometry. In patients with severe or difficult-to-treat lymphedema, a number of surgical options are available, including microsurgery, liposuction, and debulking procedures.

REHABILITATION OF CANCER-RELATED SPINAL CORD INJURY

Spinal cord injury in the patient with cancer has several etiologies. These involve primary spinal cord tumor or metastatic lesions. Primary tumors such as meningiomas, neurofibromas, and gliomas are relatively rare, and the majority of tumors involving the spinal cord are metastatic. The metastatic lesions that cause nerve root or spinal cord compression can be paravertebral, extradural, intradural, or intramedullary; however, 95% of metastatic lesions are extradural. These lesions most often originate from primary tumors of the breast, lung, and prostate. Other tumors that metastasize to the spine include renal, melanoma, myeloma, and thyroid. Most extradural metastases arise from the vertebral body and result in compression of the anterior spinal cord. Approximately 70% of spinal metastases occur in the thoracic spine, which has a smaller ratio of canal-to-cord diameter than the other two spinal segments [60].

Pain worse at night and in the supine position is a common clinical presentation. Weakness and sensory loss, along with the development of bowel or bladder incontinence, may indicate spinal cord compromise. Rapid progression of paraparesis over only a few hours indicates arterial compromise by tumor invasion or pressure; slowly evolving symptoms suggest gradual cord impingement and may respond to steroids and radiotherapy [61].

Corticosteroids can alleviate pain and improve neurologic function, and radiation therapy is the treatment of choice with most cases of cord compression. If the tumor involves two or three columns of the spine, spinal stability is of concern; consequently, treatment is aimed toward stabilization of the spinal column. This can be done with cervical orthoses. Sternal occipital mandibular immobilization is well tolerated and provides adequate flexion and extension as well as stability to the lower cervical segments. Philadelphia collars provide stability in flexion and extension for higher levels but do not restrict rotation and lateral bending in the lower cervical segments. The "clamshell" thoracic lumbar-spinal orthosis is used to provide thoracic and lumbar support but may not be an option in patients with friable or intolerant skin following chemotherapy or steroid use. Therefore, the Taylor-Knight brace, which limits spinal extension, and the Jewitt brace, which limits spinal flexion, can be used to provide thoracic and lumbar support [62].

Surgery is also indicated sometimes with instability and neurologic compromise; indications include pathologic fracture and dislocation, failure of radiation therapy, and rapidly progressing myelopathic signs and symptoms. Surgical stabilization can frequently alleviate the need for external bracing, which is an added benefit.

Once spinal stabilization is achieved, comprehensive inpatient rehabilitation can address the impairments, functional limitations, and disabilities associated with spinal cord compression and injury due to cancer. Individuals with nontraumatic spinal cord injuries can achieve significant gains in functional independence measurements during inpatient rehabilitation [10]. It has also been suggested that due to the limited prognosis of patients with cancer with spinal cord compression, an expedited inpatient rehabilitation stay with the focus on family training and home safety should be emphasized.

Bladder Management

For all patients with cancer with neurologic involvement and those with profound deconditioning, it is prudent to check postvoid residuals for signs of bladder dysfunction. This can be performed noninvasively by an ultrasound-mediated bladder scanner or, more accurately, by straight catheterization and measurement postvoid. If the postvoid volumes are 100 to

150 mL or greater, an intermittent catheterization program is initiated.

Tumors involving the spinal cord cause suprasacral neurogenic bladder problems, which typically result in a hyperreflexic detrusor; this is characterized by low urinary volumes, high bladder pressures, and diminished bladder compliance. Incomplete lesions may produce the supraspinal pattern, with urgency and adequate emptying, while patients with complete lesions have reflex incontinence and incomplete voiding due to detrusor-sphincter dyssynergia ([57]). Some patients have hypocontractile or areflexic bladders, with urinary retention and associated overflow incontinence if the lesion involves the sacral micturition center. Sometimes, there is a mixed picture of upper motor neuron dysfunction, hyperreflexic bladder and lower motor neuron dysfunction, and areflexic bladder.

Management of lower motor neuron bladder dysfunction involves the use of a condom catheter for men or an indwelling catheter for women if sphincter tone is diminished with normal or compromised detrusor tone. When the sphincter tone is competent but the bladder tone diminished, an intermittent catheterization program is instituted. This can frequently be seen in patients with sacral tumors such as chordomas and chondromas. The management of upper motor neuron bladder dysfunction involves the use of an anticholinergic medication such as oxybutynin to decrease detrusor tone and allow for greater capacity; then, an intermittent catheterization program can be instituted.

An intermittent catheterization program first involves daily measurements of postvoid residuals or the volume of urine left in the bladder after a void. If the postvoid volumes are 100 to 150 mL or greater, the patient is catheterized initially every 4 hours. The goal is to have the catheterized volumes not exceed 400 to 500 mL. If the volumes remain consistently below those numbers, the frequency of catheterization can be decreased to every 6 hours.

In addition, management of bladder dysfunction in this population involves assessing for urinary tract infections, which can be common. Appropriate antibiotics should be started based on urinalysis, cultures, and sensitivities.

It is important to note that, in the cancer population, life expectancy often plays a part in rehabilitation management. Intermittent catheterization is the preferred method of management for the scenarios mentioned; however, a Foley catheter is sometimes used instead for ease and comfort in those patients with limited prognosis.

Bowel Management

Typically, with lesions above the conus medullaris, an upper motor neuron bowel dysfunction is present, with the muscles of the external anal sphincter and pelvic floor becoming spastic. The connection between the spinal cord and the colon remain intact and bowel and stool can be propelled by reflex activity. With lesions below the conus medullaris, an areflexic lower motor neuron bowel dysfunction is present, with the myenteric plexus intrinsically moving stool slowly ([62]).

A complicating matter with patients with cancer is opioid-induced constipation. This and other premorbid factors and current bowel function must be ascertained before instituting a bowel program. Often, a plain x-ray of the abdomen is obtained to assess for obstipation before beginning a bowel program. If obstipation is present, suppositories or enemas can be given to clean out the bowels and especially to evacuate the rectal vault.

The goals of a bowel management program are to prevent fecal impaction and to facilitate bowel evacuation on a routine schedule compatible with one's daily activities. This is a logical, structured program based initially on evaluation of the current bowel pattern. A bowel management program begins with a proper diet, which should contain adequate amounts of fluid and fiber to create soft bulky stools, which can decrease bowel transit time. Fatty foods can increase transit time. Medication management involves the introduction of a stimulant such as senna. A bisacodyl suppository can be used as an adjunct.

In stepwise fashion, a bowel program begins with an x-ray to determine whether evacuation by enemas is necessary; then, an appropriate diet is begun, along with stool softeners or stimulants. To take advantage of the gastrocolic reflex, the patient is placed on the commode approximately 30 minutes after a meal, preceded by a bisacodyl suppository 10 minutes before the patient is placed on the commode. In addition, manual digital stimulation 20 minutes after suppository insertion can induce the rectocolic reflex ([57]).

Spasticity

Similar to brain injury, many patients with spinal cord injury suffer from spasticity, which is an abnormality of muscle tone and is velocity-dependent resistance to passive movement across a joint. In addition, they experience muscle flexor spasms, which also respond to the same treatment strategies as those used for spasticity.

Treatment begins with proper positioning and can also involve splinting, casting, stretching, range-of-motion exercises, and the use of medications. In contrast to spasticity originating from brain pathology, spasticity associated with spinal cord injury is treated medically, primarily with baclofen. Tizanidine is also an appropriate choice. In addition, chemical neurolysis, botulinum toxin, and—for severe cases—an intrathecal baclofen pump may be used.

REHABILITATION OF GENERALIZED DECONDITIONING AND ASTHENIA

Generalized weakness and deconditioning are common problems in patients with cancer, and they simply imply a loss of their prior state of conditioning. Asthenia is also a common diagnosis in patients engaging in inpatient cancer rehabilitation. It implies a combination of weakness and decreased exercise tolerance arising from a number of factors, including muscle wasting, disuse atrophy, malnutrition, anemia, and cardiac or pulmonary comorbidities. Functional impact from asthenia can include difficulty with transfers and ambulation, difficulty with ADLs, and decreased balance with risk for falls.

Rehabilitation treatment can begin with increased sitting time and gentle range-of-motion exercises. This is followed by a progressive increase in exercise dose, duration, and intensity, along with instruction in fatigue management and balance training. It is also important to address other medical conditions, such as anemia, malnutrition, sleep, pain, and mood disorders. Short-term inpatient rehabilitation can be effective in improving functional status after an acute decline, and outpatient therapy can help in maintaining or more slowly improving functional performance. However, if the primary malignancy progresses, functional performance will likely deteriorate.

To better grasp these concepts, an understanding of basic muscle physiology is important. There are three types of muscle fibers. Type I muscle fibers are the slow-twitch oxidative metabolism fibers, which have slow fatigability and are used for prolonged activity. Type IIB fibers are the fast-twitch fibers, which use glycolytic anaerobic metabolism and have rapid fatigability. Type IIA is an intermediate fiber.

Prolonged bed rest can result in muscle weakness. In a classic study by Mueller, the muscles of a person on strict bed rest can decrease approximately 1.0% to 1.5% of their initial strength per day, corresponding to approximately a 10% to 20% loss of strength per week ([63]). Antigravity muscles like the gastrocnemius and back extensor muscles tend to lose strength disproportionately, with larger muscles losing strength more quickly than smaller muscles; handgrip strength is unaffected ([64, 65]). Type I fibers are more affected than type II fibers ([66]).

These effects on muscles can be counteracted by a daily stretching program, which delays muscle atrophy ([67]). In addition, daily isometric muscle contractions of 10% to 20% of maximal tension for 10 seconds can help maintain muscle strength ([64]). Electrical stimulation of muscles can also be used. In general, it may take two or more times as long as the period of immobilization to recover muscle strength ([68]).

Joint contracture is an abnormal limitation of passive joint range of motion and can be caused by prolonged immobilization. Typical contractures from immobilization include hip flexion, knee flexion, elbow flexion, and internally rotated shoulder contractures as well as ankle plantar flexion contractures. Once they have developed, contractures are treated with range-of-motion exercises. For more severe cases, deep heating followed by range-of-motion exercises and serial casting may be necessary. One goal of nursing and inpatient therapy should be to prevent joint contractures before they occur. Hip flexion contractures can be prevented with the avoidance of an overly soft mattress and lying occasionally in a prone position. Dorsiflexion exercises and footboards can help prevent ankle plantar flexion contractures.

Immobilization can also affect the bones. Wolff's law states that the ratio of formation to resorption is influenced by the stresses to which bones are subjected. The primary stress on most bones is weight bearing, which causes a buildup of bone; a lack of stress on bones leads to a predominance of bone resorption. Weight bearing is eliminated when lying in bed in a supine position and can lead to disuse osteoporosis. This is best treated with preventive measures such as active muscle contraction and active weight-bearing exercises. Exercises conducted in bed are not particularly effective ([69]). Activities involving getting out of bed to a chair are encouraged as soon as possible.

There are cardiovascular effects from prolonged bed rest. The first such form of cardiac deconditioning is resting tachycardia. After a period of bed rest, the heart rate can increase by about one-half beat per minute each day for the first 3 to 4 weeks of immobilization ([70]). In addition, there are decreased diastolic filling times, with resultant decreased myocardial perfusion, decreased stroke volume with submaximal and maximal exercises, decline in cardiac output at submaximal exercise, and deleterious hemodynamic and orthostatic changes.

The treatment of the cardiovascular effects is mainly aimed at prevention. Sitting in a chair prevents deterioration of $\dot{V}_{O_2max}$ (maximum oxygen consumption) and orthostatic intolerance. Isometric exercise minimizes decreases in $\dot{V}_{O_2max}$ ([71]). Cardiovascular deconditioning can be reversed by a progressive increase in activity and regaining an upright posture. Orthostatic intolerance can be helped by range-of-motion exercises, progressive ambulation, abdominal strengthening, and leg exercises to reverse venous stasis. In addition, supportive treatments for orthostatic intolerance include the use of a tilt table, supportive garments, leg stockings, abdominal binders, and medications such as ephedrine, midodrine, and fludrocortisone acetate (Florinef Acetate).

Thrombotic complications, such as the development of a DVT or a pulmonary embolism (PE), are a risk of immobility. Virchow's triad states that hypercoagulability, endothelial injury, and stasis of blood flow are factors that can contribute to clot formation. Rehabilitation often begins after a prolonged state of immobility, and it is imperative we take measures to prevent DVT or PE development. Patients should be mobilized, encouraged to ambulate, provided with external intermittent leg compression devices, and administered low-dose anticoagulation when contraindications are not present ([70]).

DURABLE MEDICAL EQUIPMENT

Patients with cancer may have a number of rehabilitation-related DME needs, both as inpatients and outpatients. Many are covered by Medicare and third-party payers when patients demonstrate appropriate need. These can include, but are not limited to, artificial limbs; braces (arm, leg, back, and neck); canes; commode chairs; continuous passive motion machines; crutches; orthotics; patient lifts; prosthetic devices; reachers; tub benches; walkers; wheelchairs; and other power mobility devices. Table 59-2 lists several commonly prescribed pieces of equipment with a few of their most common indications. Many variations exist within the categories of orthotics and DME mentioned. Thus, consultation between a trained a physiatrist, therapist, and orthotist may be required to ensure adequate performance, safe mobility, and optimization of self-care.

Table 59-2 Commonly Prescribed Orthotics and DME

Prescribed Equipment	Common Indications
• Ankle-foot orthosis	• Ankle dorsiflexion weakness or "foot drop"
• Neutral wrist-hand orthosis	• Median neuropathy at the wrist or "carpal tunnel syndrome"
• Shoulder sling	• Hemiparesis with shoulder pain due to glenohumeral subluxation
• Thoracic-lumbar-sacral orthosis	• Mild spinal instability or vertebral compression fractures
• Rolling walker	• Impaired mobility, balance, or proprioception
• Hemiwalker	• Hemiparesis with impaired mobility or balance
• Manual wheelchair	• Unsafe gait, poor endurance
• Bedside commode	• Impaired transfers to/from toilet
• Sliding board	• Impaired transfers in/out of bed or chair
• Tub transfer chair	• Impaired transfers in/out of shower
• Shower chair	• Poor endurance, impaired ADLs
• Reacher	• Impaired mobility or ADLs

PRESSURE ULCERS

According to the National Pressure Ulcer Advisory Panel (NPUAP), a pressure ulcer is an area of unrelieved pressure over a defined area, usually over a bony prominence, resulting in ischemia, cell death, and tissue necrosis. Incidence of pressure ulcers in the acute care setting is 7% to 9%; long-term care incidence is estimated to be between 3% and 31%; estimates for home care incidence are 0% to 17%. Patients with cancer have a number of risk factors that can place them at risk of developing pressure ulcers (Table 59-3).

The NPUAP staging system for pressure ulcers includes the following:

- Stage I: intact skin with nonblanchable redness of a localized area, usually over a bony prominence.
- Stage II: partial-thickness loss of dermis presenting as a shallow open ulcer with a red-pink wound bed, without slough.
- Stage III: full-thickness tissue loss; subcutaneous fat may be visible but bone, tendon, or muscle is not exposed.
- Stage IV: full-thickness tissue loss with exposed bone, tendon, or muscle.

In suspected deep-tissue injury, there is localized discolored intact skin or a blood-filled blister due to damage of underlying soft tissue from pressure or shear. An ulcer that cannot be staged is described as full-thickness tissue loss with slough or eschar covering the wound bed. The mainstay of pressure ulcer treatment is the off-loading of pressure. This is frequently accomplished

Table 59-3 Risk Factors for Pressure Ulcer Development

• Impaired proprioception	• Decreased activity	• Impaired mobility
• Decreased nutrition	• Friction/shear forces	• Advanced age
• Male gender	• Low body mass index	• Urinary or fecal incontinence
• Fever/sepsis	• Hypotension	• Dehydration
• Anemia	• Immunosuppression	• Renal failure

by a turning schedule if the patient cannot get out of bed. If the patient is a wheelchair user, frequent position changes (up to every 20 minutes) are recommended.

Other interventions include the use of appropriate support surfaces for the bed and wheelchair, nutritional consultation, physical and occupational therapy consultation for mobility issues, and addressing incontinence. Topical dressings may be used based on wound characteristics (Table 59-4). Surgical treatment can include sharp debridement of devitalized tissue if the patient's immune status allows, and plastic surgery may be able to assist with flap coverage. If available, wound care nursing specialists can also assess the wound and help guide treatment recommendations.

Pressure ulcer healing will also depend on improvement in the patient's overall health and medical condition. Healed ulcers can have decreased tissue tolerance and are at risk for reinjury without ongoing prevention measures. Patients should be monitored throughout cancer treatment for signs of skin compromise or wound degradation.

THROMBOCYTOPENIA

Thrombocytopenia, along with the suppression of other cell lines, is commonly seen in patients with cancer. These findings are especially frequent in patients receiving chemotherapy or extensive irradiation, with resulting myelosuppression, bone marrow infiltration, and splenomegaly. Hematologic malignancies introduce a variety of associated complications, which previously limited implementation of intensive rehabilitation programs with patients at greatest risk. A rehabilitation program or exercise in a severely thrombocytopenic patient remains somewhat controversial. The major concern in this situation is the development of a spontaneous intracranial hemorrhage.

Table 59-4 Wound Characteristics and Topical Dressings

Wound Characteristic	Type of Topical Dressing
• Scant or small amounts of drainage	• Foam dressing, hydrocolloid, gel/gauze dressing, composite dressing, transparent film
• Moderate drainage	• Foam dressing, calcium alginate, hydrofiber
• Deep wounds	• "Filler" dressing followed by a cover dressing
• High drainage	• Negative-pressure drainage management system, calcium alginate/foam dressing combination; increase the frequency of dressing changes

Dimeo et al monitored patients during a 6-week intensive aerobic exercise program after high-dose chemotherapy and autologous stem cell transplantation. The investigators did not exclude for neutropenia, anemia, or thrombocytopenia, but in the end, they observed no adverse effects. Based on this initial study, the authors proposed utilizing lower-limit thresholds of 20,000/μL for platelet counts and 1,500/μL for leukocyte counts prior to safely engaging in a rehabilitation program ([72]). With platelet counts over 5,000/mm^3, another study found fatal intracranial hemorrhage in only 1 of 92 patients receiving chemotherapy ([73]).

No clear guidelines exist, but one recommendation is to allow nonresistive activities at platelet counts between 5,000 and 10,000/mm^3 and light resistive exercises with counts above 10,000/mm^3, with ambulation allowed with counts above 5,000/mm^3 ([74]). Clinicians must use their own judgment with individual patients. In addition, platelet transfusions with counts below 10,000 should be performed in patients undergoing comprehensive rehabilitation.

EXERCISE IN CANCER

Long considered a time to decrease physiologic burden, treatment algorithms for many patients with cancer often neglected to incorporate physical exercise as a primary component of care. More recently, however, many studies have emerged not only quelling the idea of exercise causing significant undue harm but also substantiating the short- and long-term benefits of a well-constructed exercise program. Along the time spectrum of cancer prevention, treatment, and survivorship, patients may benefit from an individualized exercise regimen at each stage.

As the prevalence of cancer continues to climb, researchers have developed an increased interest in prevention strategies. According to the International Agency for Research on Cancer, obesity and a sedentary lifestyle may contribute to a quarter of new cancer cases. Women are at greatest risk, with nearly three times the rate of overweight- and obesity-related cancer ([75]).

In addition to reducing the burden of primary risk factors, physical activity may serve as a cancer prevention strategy by directly improving musculoskeletal strength, endurance, balance, and flexibility, while indirectly enhancing the performance of the body's cardiovascular, pulmonary, neurologic, and immune systems. A systematic review performed by Rajarajeswaran ([76]) found convincing evidence for average risk reduction in colon (40%-50%) and breast (30%-40%) cancers. Additional evidence suggesting reduced risk for the development of prostate, endometrial, lung, and many other cancers has also been identified, but the relatively sparse quantity of evidence available for review continues to limit the strength of our recommendations.

In addition to the more obvious direct effects, there is an increasing body of research demonstrating improved cancer- and treatment-related symptoms with moderate increases in activity ([77]). Rehabilitation regimens including a combination of aerobic and resistance training have demonstrated improvements in body weight, body composition, flexibility, strength, fatigue, depression, anxiety, rigor, anger, mood, self-esteem, perception of well-being, pain, nausea, diarrhea, functional capacity, and life satisfaction ([78]). Many patients with cancer experience significant amounts of weight loss, particularly involving lean tissues. This problem may be exacerbated by hormone or chemotherapy treatments used to combat their primary malignancy and may contribute to generalized weakness and fatigue. Cornie et al ([79]) evaluated the potential to reduce factors leading to treatment-related deconditioning while promoting those that would maintain or improve fitness. In a randomized controlled trial among 63 men with prostate cancer receiving androgen-deprivation therapy, participants performed at least weekly 150 minutes of moderate-intensity training during a 3-month period. Compared to the control group, the exercise group demonstrated preserved appendicular lean mass and prevented gains in whole-body fat and trunk fat mass. Between-group analyses also demonstrated significant improvements in peak oxygen consumption, muscle strength, cholesterol levels, sexual function, and fatigue.

Speck et al ([80]) performed a comprehensive meta-analysis of 82 studies involving 6,838 cancer survivors and assessing 60 different outcome measures. Of the studies reviewed with high internal validity, nearly all demonstrated positive effects of exercise on their respective primary outcome measures (Table 59-5). Additional studies also demonstrated positive effects on lean body mass, lower body flexibility, vigor/vitality, IFG-BP-III levels, pain, breast cancer subscale, and immune parameters such as neutrophil count, natural killer cell activity, C-reactive protein, and cytokines.

Significantly improved weighted mean effect sizes of outcomes were stratified by timing of rehabilitation administration ([79]).

CHAPTER 59

Table 59-5 Outcome Measures Improved With Exercise

Outcome Improvements *During* Treatment	Outcome Improvements *Post* treatment
• Physical activity	• Physical activity
• Aerobic fitness	• Aerobic fitness
• Upper body strength	• Upper body strength
• Lower body strength	• Lower body strength
• Body weight	• Body weight
• Body fat percentage	• Body fat percentage
• Functional quality of life	• BMI
• Mood	• Overall quality of life
• Anxiety	• Breast cancer–specific concerns
• Self-esteem	• Perception of physical condition
	• Mood disturbance
	• Confusion
	• Body image
	• Fatigue
	• General symptoms and side effects
	• Insulinlike growth factor 1 levels

Safety of Exercise in Cancer

The reason for the limited numbers of intensive exercise regimens for patients with cancer is likely multifactorial but may often emanate from patient and provider fears. Cheville ([81]) interviewed a group of patients with late-stage non–small cell lung cancer and identified potential exercise barriers that included fear of harm and a lack of direction from their physician. Patients were found to be less receptive to guidance from ancillary health professionals, but early expert consultation with a physiatrist may prove helpful in formulating an individualized rehabilitation program with medical monitoring as it may alleviate some potential barriers.

Reported adverse events following a structured rehabilitation program are primarily limited to musculoskeletal injuries. Patients with breast cancer and survivors are among the most commonly studied, and population-specific concern exists for exacerbation of lymphedema ([82]). However, evidence suggests breast cancer survivors undergoing a strength training protocol demonstrate a reduced risk of lymphedema exacerbations, while improving strength and bone mineral density ([83, 84]).

Hayes et al ([85]) allocated patients following stem cell transplantation to a control group receiving a stretching program and an intervention group receiving an aerobic and resistance program performed three times a week over 3 months. Similar to findings of studies in solid tumor populations, results demonstrated increased recovery of fat-free mass and no significant body weight differences at the conclusion of the intervention period.

Prescribing Exercise in Cancer

With growing amounts of data supporting the benefits of exercise along the cancer diagnosis and treatment continuum, there has grown an emerging need for expert clinical exercise guidelines. The 2008 US Department of Health and Human Services

(US DHHS) report of physical activity guidelines for Americans provides a generic foundation for patients with cancer to follow. The report recommends patient participation in physical activities as their abilities and conditions permit, with a goal weekly duration of 150 minutes of moderate intensity or 75 minutes of vigorous intensity (Fig. 59-4) ([86]).

In 2009, the American College of Sports Medicine (ACSM) assembled an expert panel of 13 researchers and clinicians to evaluate the available evidence of safety and benefits of exercise in cancer. In the ACSM report, studies were stratified by cancer type, and the strength of evidence was assessed on the basis of several outcome measures. Many risks specific to particular cancer types have been outlined, but the experts concluded that exercise testing and prescriptions are safe and efficacious for patients with cancer. The authors recommended utilization of 2008 US DHHS guidelines for aerobic training and supported the addition of resistance training exercises for a comprehensive rehabilitation program ([88]).

Current research is demonstrating improved mortality in patients with cancer participating in an exercise program. However, due to the observational nature of many of these studies, significant variability exists in the prescribed intensity, frequency, duration, and combination of exercises. A clear dose response has yet to be established, and future research may require a more detailed evaluation of tumor marker expression and a patient's immunologic, hormonal, and metabolic factors, much in the same way targeted medical therapies are based on host factors ([89, 90]).

ELIMINATING BARRIERS

In the face of chronic disease or acute illness, the goal of rehabilitation is to restore a meaningful transition back to one's previous state of health and level of functional performance. The absence of function invokes the term *disability*. The WHO defines disability as "a complex phenomenon, reflecting the interaction between features of a person's body and features of the society in which he or she lives." To better elucidate such problems, health-care providers must first seek to identify a problem within a particular body structure or system, defined as the "impairment." Some impairments may directly or indirectly result in difficulty performing a specific task or action, coined an "activity limitation" or alternatively, a "disability." If an individual is unable to perform a specific activity in his or her normal environment or community, the individual is described as having a "participation restriction" ([91]).

Identifying each patient's unique set of impairments, activity limitations, and participation restrictions is an initial step in defining functional concerns. Unfortunately, such concerns are often missed by many primary and consulting providers. On reviewing 6 months of previous electronic medical record notes, Cheville et al found oncology patient-reported symptoms to be fairly well documented in the medical record, while activity limitations were very unlikely to be noted. Referrals for such problems were yet rarer, leaving a significant gap in functional problems requiring further assessment and those that were addressed ([92]).

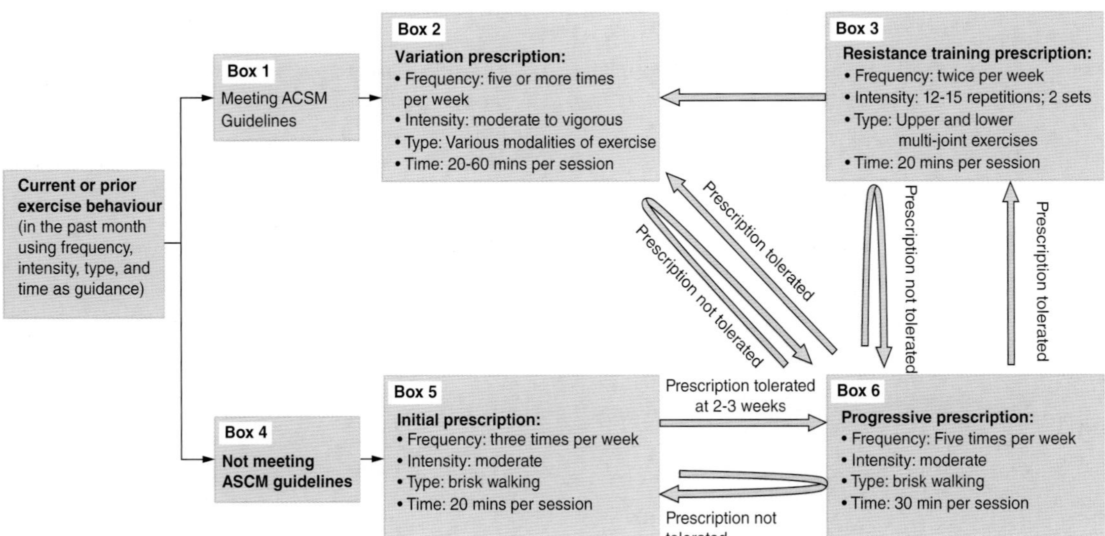

FIGURE 59-4 A model for prescribing an appropriate exercise regimen for a cancer patient. Reproduced with permission from Jones LW, Eves ND, Peppercorn J: Pre-exercise screening and prescription guidelines for cancer patients, *Lancet Oncol* 2010 Oct;11(10):914-916.

Physiatrists are optimally trained to help facilitate a patient's transition from illness, and its associated medical care, to home with functional restoration. With the appropriate tools and resources, we can modify, support, or remove impairments to focus on strengths and abilities. In general, musculoskeletal injuries are among the most common causes of debility and contribute to a great deal of functional impairment. In a population of patients with cancer, these injuries may be overlooked due to more serious illnesses, but a well-trained physiatrist is well equipped to detect, diagnose, and treat them. If resolution of an impairment is feasible and presents relatively low risk, treatment should be pursued to alleviate activity limitations (Table 59-6). If treatment is inappropriate or not feasible, a physiatrist may employ alternative strategies, such as orthotics or

Table 59-6 Adjunctive Diagnostic and Treatment Interventions Which May Be Employed by a Trained Physiatrist[a]

Procedure	Indication	Common Sites
• Botulinum toxin injection for chemodenervation	• Upper motor neuron or mixed motor neuron injury leading to spasticity or dystonia • Migraine headache • Spasmodic torticollis • Trismus • Postmastectomy syndrome • Postradiation muscle spasms	• Shoulder internal rotators • Upper and lower extremity flexors • Lower extremity adductors • Facial and suboccipital musculature • Sternocleidomastoid, scalene, trapezius, levator scapularis musculature • Muscles of mastication • Shoulder adductors and internal rotators • Location dependent
• Phenol injection for chemical neurolysis	• Upper motor neuron or mixed motor neuron injury leading to spasticity or dystonia • Painful neuroma • Trigeminal neuralgia • Spasmodic torticollis	• Terminal motor branch of femoral, obturator, tibial nerves • Morton's (intermetatarsal) neuroma • Postamputation neuroma • Terminal branch of trigeminal nerve • Sternocleidomastoid, scalene, trapezius, levator scapularis musculature
• Corticosteroid injection	• Arthritis • Rotator cuff tendinopathy • Bursitis • Adhesive capsulitis • Carpal tunnel syndrome	• Shoulder and knee joints • Subacromial or glenohumeral space • Subacromial and trochanteric bursae • Shoulder • Wrist
• Hyaluronic acid injection	• Degenerative arthritis	• Knee joint
• Trigger point injection	• Muscle spasm with painful trigger points	• Trapezius, levator scapularis, rhomboid musculature
• Prolotherapy	• Tendinopathy • Fasciitis • Enthesopathy	• Achilles or patellar tendons • Plantar fascia • Origin of extensor carpi radialis brevis (ECRB) musculature for "tennis elbow"
• Electrodiagnostic study	• Foot drop • Carpal tunnel syndrome • Ulnar neuropathy • Radiculopathy • Brachial plexopathy • Guillain-Barre syndrome • Peripheral mono- or polyneuropathy of unknown origin	• Nerve conductions and needle electromyography of upper and/or lower extremities +/− Paraspinal musculature
• Diagnostic dynamic ultrasound	• Tendinopathy • Enthesopathy • Bursitis • Baker's cyst • Carpal tunnel syndrome	• Rotator cuff, Achilles, gluteus medius, patellar tendons • ECRB • Subacromial, greater trochanteric, pes anserine bursae • Popliteal fossa • Median nerve proximal to and within carpal tunnel

[a]Not intended to serve as an exhaustive list.

DME, to reduce the burden of activity limitations and participation restrictions.

Employment-Related Disability Management

Impairment and disability evaluations are complicated by the fact that there are considerable variations between objectively measured impairments and subjectively reported disability. Psychological, social, and behavioral factors must be recognized as significant contributors to the relationship between impairment and disability.

Increasing survivorship among patients with cancer has led to an increased focus on disability. Many cancer survivors are unable to work secondary to the effects of chemotherapy, operations, the tumor itself, and symptoms associated with the tumor, including chronic pain and fatigue. The patient may have been cured of the cancer, but the patient must live with the sequelae of those treatments. It has been reported that 38% of cancer survivors are working age ([93]). Survivors frequently wish to return to work for continued insurance benefits, income, and self-esteem. Quality-of-life assessments show that employed cancer survivors have a higher quality of life. It provides a sense of normalcy and control when cancer takes control away from other aspects of their lives ([94]). Survivors may report an inability to work for a variety of reasons, including fatigue, physical limitations, emotional problems, changing personal priorities, cognitive deficits, awkward interaction with coworkers, and unsympathetic employers ([95]).

Yankelovich surveyed 200 supervisors of cancer survivors in two studies. Of the supervisors, 66% were concerned about the cancer survivor's ability to work. Prior to the survivor returning to work after cancer treatment, 33% believed the survivor would not be able to handle the job, and 31% believed the survivor needed to be replaced. After the survivor returned to work, 34% of supervisors and 43% of coworkers were less concerned regarding the survivor's ability to work. About 50% of supervisors admitted that a cancer diagnosis would affect their decision to hire ([96]). Ferrell surveyed 662 fellow employees of cancer survivors. Of these fellow employees, 14% felt that cancer survivors probably would not be able to do their job, and 27% of workers felt that they would have to pick up the slack of their cancer survivor colleague ([97]).

Of patients with cancer, 20% report some cancer-related disability. However, most working patients with cancer do return to work after treatment. At 1 year, 73% are employed, and 84% are at 4 years. Patients with central nervous system, head and neck, and stage IV hematologic cancer had the highest risk of disability. Also, patients who were involved in more physically demanding work, were less educated, were women, and were of older age were less likely to return to work after treatment. Also, 87% reported that their employer was accommodating ([98]). Of employed cancer survivors, 54% reported having to adjust their work schedule during their cancer treatment ([99]). The Americans With Disabilities Act of 1990 brought legislative protection to cancer survivors with disabilities. It requires employers to make "reasonable accommodation" for employees with disabilities and prevents discrimination in pay, hiring, firing, fringe benefits, and working conditions. It also requires employers to make accommodations for family members that are not an "undue hardship." Accommodations can include extended leave, flexible work schedules, permitting working from home, changing work environment, and allowing rest periods.

If there is uncertainty regarding whether a cancer survivor can return to work, several options are available. If the primary concern is energy and endurance, the cancer survivor's hours are gradually increased each week, with the patient reporting any difficulties to the physician. When issues of coordination, strength, or endurance are uncertain, a functional capacity evaluation can be performed by a physical or occupational therapist. The evaluation can be useful for determining tolerance for lifting, bending, squatting, and the like. Often, the therapist is able to replicate the duties of the patient and recommend ergonomic or environmental modifications if necessary.

Without proper physiatric training and experience, a variety of impairments may serve as barriers to initiating or maintaining exercise programs for patients with cancer. There is no doubt that social, economic, and psychological factors often also present significant problems for the successful implementation of a rehabilitation program. The involvement of a multidisciplinary team is essential to adequately address such problems. The assistance of a social worker, case manager, chaplain, registered dietician, registered nurse, and the appropriate therapists working with a physiatrist as an experienced team can be a great asset for a patient or family with multidisciplinary needs.

REHABILITATION AT THE END OF LIFE

Mackey described caregiver concerns, which can include fear of hurting the patient physically by moving the patient, fear of hurting themselves when moving or transferring the patient, and a lack of clarity regarding how hard to push the patient. Family education in transfer training and positioning can decrease caregiver stress of providing care and also the patient's concern about being a burden.

The practices of cancer rehabilitation and palliative care share several similarities. Both support qualify of life and relieving discomfort. The framework for intervention can be similar with a multidisciplinary team to adequately assess and treat the patient. Both have an emphasis not only on the disease process but also on physical symptoms, limitations of the patient, and how to improve or relieve them. Both emphasize the family in patient care and education. Rehabilitation interventions at the end of life can include mobility and ADL training, positioning and pressure relief techniques, chest physiotherapy, swallow therapy, edema management, and physical modalities to treat pain and bracing and splinting to relieve pain and assist with mobility.

FUTURE OF CANCER REHABILITATION

Survivorship

There are 13.7 million Americans who are cancer survivors. That number is expected to increase to 18 million by 2022 ([100]). According to the National Coalition for Cancer Survivorship, a cancer survivor is any person diagnosed with cancer from the time of initial diagnosis until his or her death ([101]). This definition includes patients receiving active treatment for malignant disease. The numbers of long-term cancer survivors without evidence of disease is also growing. These growing numbers of long-term cancer survivors suffer from a multitude of disabilities that were acquired during cancer treatment. Rehabilitation can help patients with hemiparesis ([102]), neuropathy/plexopathy ([103]), myopathy ([104]), chronic fatigue ([105]), radiation fibrosis syndrome ([106]), postmastectomy pain syndrome, cognitive deficits ([107]), lymphedema ([108]), spasticity ([109]), cervical dystonia ([110]), trismus ([111]), and chronic musculoskeletal pain ([112]). Once the focus has been changed from surviving the cancer to quality of life, rehabilitation often plays an integral role. The bulk of the growth in the field of cancer rehabilitation over the past two decades has been surrounding the growth in the numbers of long-term cancer survivors. This rehabilitation is predominantly provided in outpatient clinics.

Increasing Recognition

Cancer rehabilitation has suffered from underreferrals by oncologists and lack of availability at many cancer centers ([113]). Cancer rehabilitation education is still lacking in PM&R departments ([114]). However, the field has experienced tremendous growth and increasing acceptance over the past 5 to 10 years. Cancer rehabilitation has become increasingly viewed as important by physiatry academic departments across the United States ([114]). Furthermore, cancer rehabilitation research publications have grown at a significantly faster rate than the whole field of rehabilitation ([115]).

Exercise and Cancer Survival

Most of the prior research in the field of cancer rehabilitation has shown improvements in quality of life, function, symptoms, and cardiopulmonary and muscular strength benefits. It has been noted that patients with a lower functional status have a higher risk of graft-versus-host disease and reduced survival ([116-120]). Some studies have shown possible beneficial effects of exercise programs on medical outcomes of patients with cancer, including survival ([121]). The mechanisms for improved survival could be because performance status does have an impact on treatment decisions, treatment completion rates, treatment response, disease progression, and death from other causes ([122]). This has led some to call exercise a cancer "medicine" that should be discussed with all oncology patients.

In 1980, Dietz described four types of cancer rehabilitation. The first was called preventive rehabilitation ([123]). This concept has been more recently coined as "prehabilitation." While the concept of prehabilitation is not unique to cancer, it has become of great interest to cancer researchers. Several studies have been published in the recent past, mostly regarding patients receiving oncologic surgery. The results suggest better medical and surgical outcomes with prehabilitation programs ([124-128]). However, further study is needed.

The Anti-Inflammatory Effects of Exercise

The anti-inflammatory effects of physical activity may also contribute to improved survival. The role of inflammation in cancer symptoms has been well established in multiple studies. Exercise has been shown to reduce cancer symptoms, including fatigue, appetite, and cognitive dysfunction, presumably through an anti-inflammatory mechanism. A hyperinflammatory state has been shown to be involved in the development of several maladies, including cardiovascular disease, Alzheimer's dementia, and cancer. Inflammation also plays a role in tumor progression and proliferation ([129, 130]). This has resulted in an increased interest in anti-inflammatory treatments. Research has identified the anti-inflammatory effects of exercise in different patient populations, including those with cancer ([131, 132]).

Return to the Primary Acute Care Service

It has been shown that cancer rehabilitation inpatients are transferred back to the primary acute care service more frequently than patients without cancer ([133]). The medical fragility of these patients has led to interest in identifying predictors of medical complications while on inpatient rehabilitation. Published research has identified a number of factors in general oncology patients ([134,135]) and more specific groups, including those with lymphoma ([136]), leukemia ([137]), or hematopoietic stem cell transplantation ([138]). The presence of antimicrobial agents, elevated creatinine, and thrombocytopenia at the time of inpatient rehabilitation transfer have been identified as possible predictors of transfer back to the primary acute care service.

REFERENCES

1. DeLisa JA, ed. *Rehabilitation Medicine, Principles and Practice*. 6th ed. Philadelphia, PA: Lippincott; 1993.
2. Dietz JH Jr. Adaptive rehabilitation of the cancer patient. *Curr Probl Cancer*. 1980;5:1-56.
3. Courneya KS, Friedenreich CM. Framework PEACE: an organizational model for examining physical exercise across the cancer experience. *Ann Behav Med*. 2001;23:263-272.
4. Fu J. Palliative Rehabilitation: Optimizing Function at End of Life. Paper presented at: American Academy of Physical Medicine & Rehabilitation Medicine Annual Assembly; 2009; Austin, TX; F415.
5. Houts PS, Yasko JM, Harvey HA, et al. Unmet needs of persons with cancer in Pennsylvania during the period of terminal care. *Cancer*. 1988;62:627-634.
6. Morasso G, Capelli M, Viterbori P, et al. Psychological and symptom distress in terminal cancer patients with met and unmet needs. *J Pain Symptom Manage*. 1999;17:402-409.
7. Marciniak CM, Sliwa JA, Spill G, et al. Functional outcome following rehabilitation of the cancer patient. *Arch Phys Med Rehabil*. 1996;77:54-57.
8. Sliwa JA, Marciniak C. Physical rehabilitation of the cancer patient. *Cancer Treat Res*. 1999;100:75-89.
9. Cole RP, Scialla SJ, Bednarz L. Functional recovery in cancer rehabilitation. *Arch Phys Med Rehabil*. 2000 October;81:623-627.
10. McKinley WO, Conti-Wyneken AR, Vokac CW, et al. Rehabilitative functional outcome of patients with neoplastic spinal cord compressions. *Arch Phys Med Rehabil*. 1996;77:892-895.
11. Scialla S, Cole R, Scialla T, et al. Rehabilitation for elderly patients with cancer asthenia: making a transition to palliative care. *Palliat Med*. 2000;14:121-127.
12. Oldervoll LM, Loge JH, Paltiel H, et al. The effect of a physical exercise program in palliative care: a phase II study. *J Pain Symptom Manage*. 2006;31:421-430.
13. Sabers SR, Kokal JE, Girardi JC, et al. Evaluation of consultation-based rehabilitation for hospitalized cancer patients with functional impairment. *Mayo Clin Proc*. 1999;74:855-861.
14. Yoshioka H. Rehabilitation for the terminal cancer patient. *Am J Phys Med Rehabil*. 1994;73:199-206.
15. Cheville A. Rehabilitation of patients with advanced cancer. *Cancer*. 2001;92:1039-1048.
16. Porock D, Kristjanson LJ, Tinnelly K, et al. An exercise intervention for advanced cancer patients experiencing fatigue: a pilot study. *J Palliat Care*. 2000;16:30-36.
17. Newton RU, Galvao DA. Exercise in prevention and management of cancer. *Curr Treat Options Oncol*. 2008;9:135-146.
18. Friedenreich CM, Gregory J, Kopciuk KA, et al. Prospective cohort study of lifetime physical activity and breast cancer survival. *Int J Cancer*. 2009;124:1954-1962.
19. Guo Y, Persyn L, Palmer JL, et al. Incidence of and risk factors for transferring cancer patients from rehabilitation to acute care units. *Am J Phys Med Rehabil*. 2008;87:647-653.
20. Karnofsky D, Burchenal JH. Clinical evaluation of chemotherapeutic agents in cancer. In: Macleod CM, ed. *Evaluation of Chemotherapy Agents*. New York, NY: Columbia University Press, 1949:191-205.
21. Meyers CA, Weitzner MA. Neurobehavioral functioning and quality of life in patients treated for cancer of the central nervous system. *Curr Opin Oncol*. 1995;7:197-200.
22. Meyers CA. Neuropsychological aspects of cancer and cancer treatment. In: Garden FH, Grabois M, eds. *Physical Medicine and Rehabilitation: State of the Art Reviews*. Philadelphia, PA: Hanley & Belfus; 1994:229-241.
23. Radhakrishnan K, Bohnen NI, Kurland L. Epidemiology of brain tumors. In: Morantz RA, Walsh JW, eds. *Brain Tumors: A Comprehensive Text*. New York, NY: Dekker; 1994:1-18.
24. Osborn A. *Diagnostic Neuroradiology*. St. Louis, MO: Mosby; 1994.
25. Berger MS, Leibel SA, Bruner JM, et al. Primary cerebral tumors. In: Levin VA, ed. *Cancer in the Nervous System*. 2nd ed. New York, NY: Oxford University Press; 2002:75–134.
26. Shawl EG, Seiferheld W, Scott C, et al. Re-examining the radiation therapy oncology group (RTOG) recursive partitioning analysis (RPA) for glioblastoma multiforme (GBM) patients. *Int J Radiat Oncol Biol Phys*. 2003;57:S135-S136.
27. Nugent JL, Bunn PA Jr, Matthews MJ, et al. CNS metastases in small cell bronchogenic carcinoma: increasing frequency and changing pattern with lengthening survival. *Cancer*. 1979;44:1885-1893.
28. Bell KR, O'Dell MW, Barr K, et al. Rehabilitation of the patient with brain tumor. *Arch Phys Med Rehabil*. 1998;79:S-37-S-47.
29. Greenberg MS. *Handbook of Neurosurgery*. Vol 1. Lakeland, FL: Greenberg Graphics; 1997:240-322.
30. Ulmer S, Braga TA, Barker FG 2nd, et al. Clinical and radiographic features of peritumoral infarction following resection of glioblastoma. *Neurology*. 2006;67:1668-1670.
31. Dropcho EJ. Central nervous system injury by therapeutic irradiation. *Neurol Clin*. 1991;9:969-988.
32. DeAngelis LM, Delattre JY, Posner JB. Radiation-induced dementia in patients cured of brain metastases. *Neurology*. 1989;39:789-796.
33. Mukand JA, Blackinton DD, Crincoli MG, et al. Incidence of neurologic deficits and rehabilitation of patients with brain tumors. *Am J Phys Med Rehabil*. 2001;80:346-350.
34. Meyers CA, Boake C, Levin VA, et al. Symptom management, rehabilitation strategies, and improved quality of life for patients with brain tumors. In Levin VA, ed. *Cancer in the Nervous System*. New York, NY: Churchill Livingstone; 1996:449-459.
35. Marciniak CM, Sliwa JA, Heinemann AW, et al. Functional outcomes of persons with brain tumors after inpatient rehabilitation. *Arch Phys Med Rehabil*. 2001;82:457-463.
36. Huang ME, Cifu DX, Keyser-Marcus L. Functional outcome after brain tumor and acute stroke: a comparative analysis. *Arch Phys Med Rehabil*. 1998;79:1386-1390.
37. Huang ME, Cifu DX, Keyser-Marcus L. Functional outcomes in patients with brain tumor after inpatient rehabilitation: comparison with traumatic brain injury. *Am J Phys Med Rehabil*. 2000;79:327-335.
38. Huang ME, Wartella J, Kreutzer J, et al. Functional outcomes and quality of life in patients with brain tumours: a review of the literature. *Brain Inj*. 2001;15:843-856.
39. O'Dell MW, Barr K, Spanier D, et al. Functional outcome of inpatient rehabilitation in persons with brain tumors. *Arch Phys Med Rehabil*. 1998;79:1530-1534.
40. Twitchell TE. The restoration of motor function following hemiplegia in man. *Brain*. 1951;74:443-480.
41. Sawner K, LaVigne J. *Brunstromm's Movement Therapy in*

Hemiplegia: A Neurophysiological Approach. 2nd ed. Philadelphia, PA: Lippincott; 1992.

42. Roth EJ, Harvey RL. Rehabilitation of stroke syndromes. In: Braddom RL, ed. *Physical Medicine and Rehabilitation*. Philadelphia, PA: Saunders; 1996:1053–1099.
43. Kraft GH. New methods for the assessment and treatment of the hemiplegic arm and hand. *Phys Med Rehabil Clin North Am*. 1991;2:579.
44. Chaco J, Wolf E. Subluxation of the glenohumeral joint in hemiplegia. *Am J Phys Med*. 1971;50:139-143.
45. Calliet R. *The Shoulder in Hemiplegia*. Philadelphia, PA: Davis; 1980.
46. Van Ouwenaller C, Laplace PM, Chantraine A. Painful shoulder in hemiplegia. *Arch Phys Med Rehabil*. 1986;67:23-26.
47. Shai G, Ring H, Costeff H, et al. Glenohumeral malalignment in the hemiplegic shoulder. An early radiologic sign. *Scand J Rehabil Med*. 1984;16:133-136.
48. Garrison SJ, Rolak LA. Rehabilitation of patients with completed stroke. In: DeLisa JA, ed. *Rehabilitation Medicine, Principles and Practice*. 2nd ed. Philadelphia, PA: Lippincott; 1993:801.
49. Macdonald DR. Neurologic complications of chemotherapy. *Neurol Clin*. 1991;9:955-967.
50. Posner JB. Paraneoplastic syndromes. *Neurol Clin*. 1991;9:919-936.
51. Diener HC, Dichgans J. Pathophysiology of cerebellar ataxia. *Mov Disord*. 1992;7:95-109.
52. Silver KH, Fishman P, Speed J. Movement disorders. In: O'Young BJ, Young MA, Steins SA, eds. *Physical Medicine and Rehabilitation Secrets*. 2nd ed. Philadelphia, PA: Hanley & Belfus; 2002:182–193.
53. Rao PR. Adult communication disorders. In: Braddom RL, ed. *Physical Medicine and Rehabilitation*. Philadelphia, PA: Saunders; 1996:43–65.
54. Gillis TA, Yadav R, Guo Y. Rehabilitation of patients with neurologic tumors and cancer-related central nervous system disabilities. In: Levin VA, ed. *Cancer in the Nervous System*. 2nd ed. New York, NY: Oxford University Press; 2002:470–492.
55. Noll S, et al. Rehabilitation of patients with swallowing disorders. In: Braddom RL, ed. *Physical Medicine and Rehabilitation*. 2nd ed. Philadelphia, PA: Saunders; 2000:535–557.
56. Kaplan M. Upper motor neuron syndrome and spasticity. In: Woo BH, Nesathurai S, eds. *The Rehabilitation of People With Traumatic Brain Injury*. Malden, MA: Blackwell Science; 2000:85–99.
57. Cardenas DD, Mayo ME, King JC. Urinary tract and bowel management in the rehabilitation setting. In: Braddom RL, ed. *Physical Medicine and Rehabilitation*. Philadelphia, PA: Saunders; 1996:555–579.
58. Noll SF, Bender CE, Nelson MC, Stroke rehabilitation. In: Nesathurai S, Blaustein D, eds. *Essentials of Inpatient Rehabilitation*. Malden, MA: Blackwell Science; 2000:117–126.
59. Logan V. Incidence and prevalence of lymphedema: a literature review. *J Clin Nurs*. 1995;4:213-219.
60. Ozalslan C, Kuru B. Lymphedema after treatment of breast cancer. *Am J Surg*. 2004;187:69-72.
61. Gilbert RW, Kim JH, Posner JB. Epidural spinal cord compression from metastatic tumor: diagnosis and treatment. *Ann Neurol*, 1978;3:40-51.
62. Garden FH, Gillis TA. Principles of cancer rehabilitation. In: Braddom RL, ed. *Physical Medicine and Rehabilitation*. Philadelphia, PA: Saunders; 1996:1199–1214.
63. Bergman SB. Bowel management. In: Nesathurai S, ed. *The Rehabilitation of People With Spinal Cord Injury*. 2nd ed. Malden, MA: Blackwell Science; 2000:53–58.
64. Muller EA. Influence of training and of inactivity on muscle strength. *Arch Phys Med Rehabil*. 1970;51:449-462.
65. Deitrick JE, Whedon GD, Shorr E. Effects of immobilization upon various metabolic and physiologic functions of normal men. *Am J Med*. 1948;4:3-36.
66. Greenleaf JE, Van Beaumont W, Convertino VA, et al. Handgrip and general muscular strength and endurance during prolonged bedrest with isometric and isotonic leg exercise training. *Aviat Space Environ Med*. 1983;54:696-700.
67. Appell HJ. Muscular atrophy following immobilisation. A review. *Sports Med*. 1990;10:42-58.
68. Baker JH, Matsumoto DE. Adaptation of skeletal muscle to immobilization in a shortened position. *Muscle Nerve*. 1988;11:231-244.
69. Houston ME, Bentzen H, Larsen H. Interrelationships between skeletal muscle adaptations and performance as studied by detraining and retraining. *Acta Physiol Scand*. 1979;105:163-170.
70. Buschbacher RM. Deconditioning, conditioning, and the benefits of exercise. In: Braddom RL, ed. *Physical Medicine and Rehabilitation*. Philadelphia, PA: Saunders; 1996:687–707.
71. Taylor HL, Henschel A, et al. Effects of bed rest on cardiovascular function and work performance. *J Appl Physiol*. 1949;2:223-239.
72. Stremel RW, Convertino VA, Bernauer EM, et al. Cardiorespiratory deconditioning with static and dynamic leg exercise during bed rest. *J Appl Physiol*. 1976;41:905-909.
73. Dimeo FC, Tilmann MH, Bertz H, Kanz L, Mertelsmann R, Keul J. Aerobic exercise in the rehabilitation of cancer patients after high dose chemotherapy and autologous peripheral stem cell transplantation. *Cancer*. 1997;79(9):1717-1722.
74. Gaydos LA, Freireich EJ, Mantel N. The quantitative relation between platelet count and hemorrhage in patients with acute leukemia. *N Engl J Med*. 1962;266:905-909.
75. Sayre R, Marcoux B. Exercise and autologous bone marrow transplants. *Clin Manage Phys Ther*. 1992;12:78-82.
76. Arnold M, Pandeya N, Byrnes G, et al. Global burden of cancer attributable to high body-mass index in 2012: a population-based study. *Lancet Oncol*. 2015;16(1):36-46.
77. Rajarajeswaran P, Vishnupriya R. Exercise in cancer. *Indian J Med Paediatr Oncol*. 2009;30(2):61-70.
78. Cheville A. Rehabilitation of patients with advanced cancer. *Cancer*. 2001;92(4 Suppl):1039-1048.
79. Rajarajeswaran P, Vishnupriya R. Exercise in cancer. *Indian J Med Paediatr Oncol*. 2009;30(2):61-70.
80. Cormie P, Galvao DA, Spry N, et al. Can supervised exercise prevent treatment toxicity in patients with prostate cancer initiating androgen-deprivation therapy: a randomised controlled trial. *BJU Int*. 2015;115(2):256-266.
81. Speck RM, Courneya KS, Masse LC, Duval S, Schmitz KH. An update of controlled physical activity trials in cancer survivors: a systematic review and meta-analysis. *J Cancer Surviv*. 2010;4(2):87-100.
82. Cheville AL, Dose AM, Basford JR, Rhudy LM. Insights into the reluctance of patients with late-stage cancer to adopt exercise as a means to reduce their symptoms and improve their function. *J Pain Symptom Manage*. 2012;44(1):84-94.
83. Schmitz KH, Ahmed RL, Troxel A, et al. Weight lifting in women with breast-cancer-related lymphedema. *N Engl J Med*. 2009;361(7):664-673.
84. Winters-Stone KM, Dobek J, Nail L, et al. Strength training stops bone loss and builds muscle in postmenopausal breast cancer survivors:a randomized, controlled trial. *Breast Cancer Res Treat*. 2011;127(2):447-456.
85. Winters-Stone KM, Dobek J, Nail LM, et al. Impact + resistance training improves bone health and body composition in prematurely menopausal breast cancer survivors: a randomized controlled trial. *Osteoporos Int*. 2013;24(5):1637-1646.
86. Hayes S, Davies PS, Parker T, Bashford J. Total energy expenditure and body composition changes following peripheral blood stem cell transplantation and participation in an exercise programme. *Bone Marrow Transplant*. 2003;31(5):331-338.
87. Physical Activity Guidelines Advisory Committee report,

2008. To the Secretary of Health and Human Services. Part A:executive summary. *Nutr Rev*. 2009;67(2):114-120.

88. Jones LW, Eves ND, Peppercorn J. Pre-exercise screening and prescription guidelines for cancer patients. *Lancet Oncol*. 2010;11(10):914-916.
89. Schmitz KH, Courneya KS, Matthews C, et al. American College of Sports Medicine Roundtable on Exercise Guidelines for Cancer Survivors. *MedSci Sports Exerc*. 2010;42(7):1409-1426..
90. Jones LW, Eves ND, Haykowsky M, Freedland SJ, Mackey JR. Exercise intolerance in cancer and the role of exercise therapy to reverse dysfunction. *Lancet Oncol*. 2009;10(6):598-605.
91. Meyerhardt JA, Ogino S, Kirkner GJ, et al. Interaction of molecular markers and physical activity on mortality in patients with colon cancer. *Clin Cancer Res*. 2009;15(18):5931-5936.
92. World Health Organization. Disabilities. 2015. http://www.who.int/topics/disabilities/en/. Accessed on 12/5/2014.
93. Cheville AL, Beck LA, Petersen TL, Marks RS, Gamble GL. The detection and treatment of cancer-related functional problems in an outpatient setting. *Support Care Cancer*. 2009;17(1):61-67.
94. Hoffmann B. The Employment and Insurance Concerns of Cancer Survivors. In: Ganz PA, *Cancer Survivorship: Today and Tomorrow*. New York: Springer; 2007:273.
95. Frazier LM, Miller VA, Horbelt DV, et al. Employment and quality of survivorship among women with cancer:domains not captured by quality of life instruments. *Cancer Control*. 2009;16:57-65.
96. Chapman SA. The experience of returning to work for employed women with breast cancer. Paper presented at: Academy for Health Services Research and Health Policy meeting. June 25-27, 2000; Los Angeles, CA. 17.
97. Yankelovich CS. Cerenex survey on cancer patients in the workplace: breaking down discrimination barriers. Unpublished. 1992.
98. Ferrell BR, Grant MM, Funk B, et al. Quality of life in breast cancer survivors as identified by focus groups. *Psychooncology*. 1997;6:13-23.
99. Short PF, Vasey JJ, Tunceli K. Employment pathways in a large cohort of adult cancer survivors. *Cancer*. 2005;103:1292-1301.
100. Bradley CJ, Bednarek HL. Employment patterns of long-term cancer survivors. *Psychooncology*. 2002;11:188-198.
101. DeSantis CE, Lin CC, Mariotto AB, Siegel RL, Stein KD, Kramer JL, Alteri R, Robbins AS, Jemal A. Cancer treatment and survivorship statistics, 2014. *CA Cancer J Clin*. 2014 Jul-Aug;64(4):252-71.
102. Centers for Disease Control. 2015. *http://www.cdc.gov/cancer/survivorship/what_cdc_is_doing/research/survivors_article.htm*. Accessed on 12/16/2015.
103. Fu JB, Parsons HA, Shin KY, et al. Comparison of functional outcomes in low- and high-grade astrocytoma rehabilitation inpatients. *Am J Phys Med Rehabil*. 2010;89(3):205-212.
104. Stubblefield MD, McNeely ML, Alfano CM, Mayer DK. A prospective surveillance model for physical rehabilitation of women with breast cancer: chemotherapy-induced peripheral neuropathy. *Cancer*. 2012;118(8 Suppl):2250-2260.
105. Morishita S, Kaida K, Yamauchi S, et al. Relationship between corticosteroid dose and declines in physical function among allogeneic hematopoietic stem cell transplantation patients. *Support Care Cancer*. 2013;21(8):2161-2169.
106. Meneses-Echavez JF, Gonzalez-Jimenez E, Ramirez-Velez R. Supervised exercise reduces cancer-related fatigue: a systematic review. *J Physiother*. 2015;61(1):3-9.
107. Stubblefield MD, Levine A, Custodio CM, Fitzpatrick T. The role of botulinum toxin type A in the radiation fibrosis syndrome: a preliminary report. *Arch Phys Med Rehabil*. 2008;89(3):417-421.
108. Gehring K, Roukema JA, Sitskoorn MM. Review of recent studies on interventions for cognitive deficits in patients with cancer. *Expert Rev Anticancer Ther*. 2012;12(2):255-269.
109. Ochalek K, Gradalski T, Szygula A. Five-year assessment of maintenance combined physical therapy in postmastectomy lymphedema. *Lymphat Res Biol*. 2015;13(1):54-58.
110. Fu J, Gutierrez C, Bruera E, Guo Y, Palla S. Use of injectable spasticity management agents in a cancer center. *Support Care Cancer*. 2013;21(5):1227-1232.
111. Jinnah HA, Factor SA. Diagnosis and treatment of dystonia. *Neurol Clin*. 2015;33(1):77-100.
112. Hartl DM, Cohen M, Julieron M, Marandas P, Janot F, Bourhis J. Botulinum toxin for radiation-induced facial pain and trismus. *Otolaryngol Head Neck Surg*. 2008;138(4):459-463.
113. Stubblefield MD. Radiation fibrosis syndrome: neuromuscular and musculoskeletal complications in cancer survivors. *PM R*. 2011;3(11):1041-1054.
114. Cheville AL. Cancer rehabilitation. *Semin Oncol*. 2005;32(2):219-224.
115. Raj VS, Balouch J, Norton JH. Cancer rehabilitation education during physical medicine and rehabilitation residency: preliminary data regarding the quality and quantity of experiences. *Am J Phys Med. Rehabil*. 2014;93(5):445-452.
116. Ugolini D, Neri M, Cesario A, et al. Scientific production in cancer rehabilitation grows higher: a bibliometric analysis. *Support Care Cancer*, 2012;20(8):1629-1638.
117. Terwey TH, Hemmati PG, Martus P, Dietz E, et al. A modified EBMT risk score and the hematopoietic cell transplantation-specific comorbidity index for pre-transplant risk assessment in adult acute lymphoblastic leukemia. *Haematologica*. 2010;95(5):810-818.
118. Rotta M, Storer BE, Sahebi F, et al. Long-term outcome of patients with multiple myeloma after autologous hematopoietic cell transplantation and nonmyeloablative allografting. *Blood*. 2009;113(14):3383-3391.
119. Guilfoyle R, Demers A, Bredeson C, et al. Performance status, but not the hematopoietic cell transplantation comorbidity index (HCT-CI), predicts mortality at a Canadian transplant center. *Bone Marrow Transplant*. 2009;43(2):133-139.
120. Sorror M, Storer B, Sandmaier M, et al. Hematopoietic cell transplantation-comorbidity index and Karnofsky performance status are independent predictors of morbidity and mortality after allogeneic nonmyeloablative hematopoietic cell transplantation. *Cancer*. 2008;112(9):1992-2001.
121. Artz AS, Pollyea DA, Kocherginsky M, et al. Performance status and comorbidity predict transplant-related mortality after allogeneic hematopoietic cell transplantation. *Biol Blood Marrow Transplant*. 2006;12(9):954-964.
122. Courneya KS, Friedenreich CM, Franco-Villalobos C, et al. Effects of supervised exercise on progression-free survival in lymphoma patients: an exploratory follow-up of the HELP Trial. *Cancer Causes Control*. 2015;26(2):269-276.
123. Courneya KS, Jones LW, Fairey AS, et al. Physical activity in cancer survivors: Implications for recurrence and mortality. *Cancer Ther*. 2004;(2):1-12.
124. Dietz JH Jr. Adaptive rehabilitation of the cancer patient. *Curr Probl Cancer*. 1980;5(5):1-56.
125. Santa Mina D, Clarke H, Ritvo P, et al. Effect of total-body prehabilitation on postoperative outcomes: a systematic review and meta-analysis. *Physiotherapy*. 2014;100(3):196-207.
126. Gillis C, Li C, Lee L, et al. Prehabilitation versus rehabilitation: a randomized control trial in patients undergoing colorectal resection for cancer. *Anesthesiology*. 2014;121(5):937-947.
127. West MA, Loughney L, Lythgoe D, et al. Effect of prehabilitation on objectively measured physical fitness after neoadjuvant treatment in preoperative rectal cancer patients: a blinded interventional pilot study. *Br J Anaesth*. 2015;114(2):244-251.
128. Jensen BT, Petersen AK, Jensen JB, Laustsen S, Borre M. Efficacy

of a multiprofessional rehabilitation programme in radical cystectomy pathways: a prospective randomized controlled trial. *Scand J Urol.* 2015;49(2):133-141.
129. Santa Mina D, Matthew AG, Hilton WJ, et al. Prehabilitation for men undergoing radical prostatectomy: a multi-centre, pilot randomized controlled trial. *BMC Surg.* 2015;14:89.
130. Coussens LM, Werb Z. Inflammation and cancer. *Nature.* 2002;420(6917):860-867.
131. Grivennikov SI, Greten FR, Karin M. Immunity, inflammation, and cancer. *Cell.* 2010;140(6):883-899.
132. Jones SB, Thomas GA, Hesselsweet SD, Alvarez-Reeves M, Yu H, a Irwin ML. Effect of exercise on markers of inflammation in breast cancer survivors: the Yale exercise and survivorship study. *Cancer Prev Res (Phila).* 2013;6(2):109-118.
133. Lof M, Bergstrom K, a Weiderpass E. Physical activity and biomarkers in breast cancer survivors: a systematic review. *Maturitas.* 2012;73(2):134-142.
134. Alam E, Wilson RD, Vargo MM. Inpatient cancer rehabilitation: a retrospective comparison of transfer back to acute care between patients with neoplasm and other rehabilitation patients. *Arch Phys Med Rehabil.* 2008;89(7):1284-1289.
135. Asher A, Roberts PS, Bresee C, Zabel G, Riggs RV, Rogatko A. Transferring inpatient rehabilitation facility cancer patients back to acute care (TRIPBAC). *PM R.* 2014;6(9):808-813.
136. Guo Y, Persyn L, Palmer JL, Bruera E. Incidence of and risk factors for transferring cancer patients from rehabilitation to acute care units. *Am J Phys Med Rehabil.* 2008;87(8):647-653.
137. Fu JB, Lee J, Smith DW, Shin K, Guo Y, Bruera E. Frequency and reasons for return to the primary acute care service among patients with lymphoma undergoing inpatient rehabilitation. *PM R.* 2014;6(7):629-634.
138. Fu JB, Lee J, Smith DW, Bruera E. Frequency and reasons for return to acute care in patients with leukemia undergoing inpatient rehabilitation: a preliminary report. *Am J Phys Med Rehabil.* 2013;92(3):215-222.
139. Fu JB, Lee J, Smith DW, Guo Y, Bruera E. Return to primary service among bone marrow transplant rehabilitation inpatients: an index for predicting outcomes. *Arch Phys Med Rehabil.* 2013;94(2):356-361.

60 Long-Term Survivorship in Adult and Pediatric Cancer

第六十章　儿童和成人肿瘤长期生存者的随访

Ravin Ratan
Joann Ater
Alyssa G. Rieber
Maria A. Rodriguez

中文导读

随着肿瘤治疗手段的进步、疗效的提高和患者生存期的延长，长期生存者数量不断增加。一些儿童时期罹患肿瘤的患者在治疗后可取得超过数十年的生存。因此，对于这些患者的随访十分重要，将有利于评估肿瘤本身以及抗肿瘤治疗带来的持续终身的影响。本章介绍了对长期生存者随访研究的结果，并着重阐述了3个方面的关键内容：一是在这些人群中积极筛查第二原发性或继发性肿瘤，并就危险度分层、检查方法和检查频率进行了介绍；二是监控肿瘤治疗带来的长期副反应，包括疼痛等躯体症状以及对心血管系统、呼吸系统、内分泌系统、认识功能和生殖功能的影响，并简述了目前在该领域的研究现状；三是阐述了疾病和治疗对患者心理状态和生活方式的影响，并强调了良好心理状态和生活方式对于整体预后和生存质量的积极意义。

INTRODUCTION

Over the last four decades, substantial improvements in treatment effectiveness for childhood and adult cancers have resulted in cure or increased survival for these populations. Over 80% of all patients diagnosed with cancer before the age of 20 years will be surviving at 5 years. As a consequence of both improved survival rates and increasing incidence of childhood cancer, the number of long-term survivors of childhood cancer in the United States is rapidly increasing. An estimated 320,000 or more childhood cancer survivors are living in the United States, and at least 75% of these survivors are now adults. Of these, 24% have survived more than 30 years ([1, 2]). These individuals are living long enough to demonstrate the lifelong consequences of the cancer and treatments ([3, 4]). The numbers of adult cancer survivors are growing as well, with an estimated 18 million adult survivors in the United States by 2022 (Fig. 60-1).

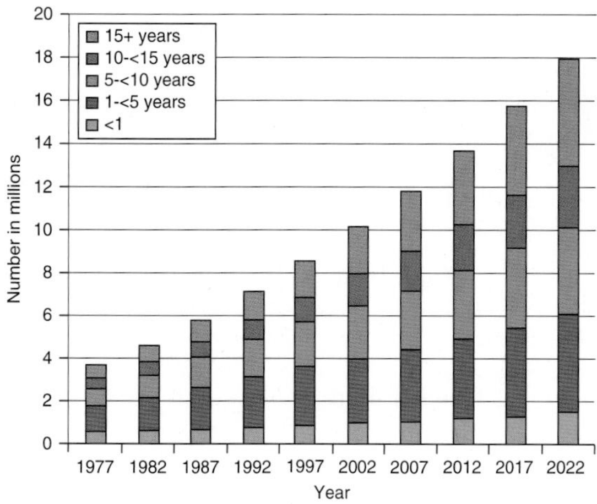

FIGURE 60-1 Estimated and projected number of cancer survivors in the United States. Reproduced with permission from de Moor JS, Mariotto AB, Parry C, et al: Cancer survivors in the United States: prevalence across the survivorship trajectory and implications for care, *Cancer Epidemiol Biomarkers Prev* 2013 Apr;22(4):561-570.

In 2006, the Institute of Medicine published *From Cancer Patient to Cancer Survivor: Lost in Transition* (Hewitt M, Greenfield S, Stovall E. *From Cancer Patient to Cancer Survivor: Lost in Transition*. Washington, DC: National Academies; 2006). This seminal report defined the "essential" components of survivorship care as (1) prevention of recurrent and new cancers; (2) surveillance for recurrence, secondary cancers, and medical effects of treatment; (3) intervention for the sequelae of cancer and its treatment; and (4) coordination of care between specialists and primary care providers. Other chapters address disease-specific surveillance; this chapter expands on the first three components of the report.

SCREENING FOR SECONDARY MALIGNANCIES

Patients who have been treated for a cancer are at higher risk for a second primary cancer or recurrence of their primary tumor, most particularly at the time of their transition from active cancer treatment to survivorship. In fact, second- and higher-order cancers accounted for as many as 16% of incident cancers in the SEER (Surveillance, Epidemiology, and End Results Program) database as of 2003 ([5]). The reasons for this are varied based on malignancy and include factors related to previous therapy (radiation, chemotherapy, hormonal therapies); previous or ongoing exposure to carcinogens; predisposing conditions (tobacco, alcohol, sun exposure, dietary influences, immunologic dysfunction); and familial genetic syndromes, including the *BRCA1* and *BRCA2* breast cancer syndromes, Bloom's syndrome, Cowden's syndrome, Li-Fraumeni, Lynch syndrome, and others ([6]). The confluence of these factors, which are increased in their incidence in the population of cancer survivors, necessitates a careful approach to screening for second malignancies. In some cases, this entails increased surveillance for patients who have known risk factors related to their previous cancer or its treatment. For others, the cancer survivorship care provider must pay close attention to the best-practice screening guidelines that already exist for the greater population at large.

In survivors of childhood cancer, these issues are magnified. As childhood cancer survivors progress through adulthood, the risk of subsequent malignant neoplasms (SMNs) increases. Among 14,359 individuals who were 5-year survivors of childhood cancer at median of 30 years (range 5-56 years) the cumulative incidence was 20.5% at 30 years for subsequent neoplasm, representing a sixfold increased incidence compared to the age-adjusted general population (standardized incidence ratio, SIR) ([7]). The most frequent subsequent malignancies were nonmelanoma skin cancer and breast cancer. Patients treated in childhood for Hodgkin's lymphoma and Ewing sarcoma had the highest risk (SIR 8.7 and 8.5, respectively). While the majority of SMNs are diagnosed within the first 10 years, they can occur up to 30 years after the original cancer diagnosis, with secondary leukemia having shorter latency than solid tumors (Table 60-1). Of solid tumors, the highest risks were observed for bone cancer (SIR 19), thyroid cancer (SIR 10.9), breast cancer (SIR 9.8), central nervous system (CNS) malignancies (SIR 10.4), and soft tissue sarcoma (SIR 8.1). In addition, survivors are at increased risk for other cancers, such as head and neck, kidney, bladder, lung, gastrointestinal and colon, and genitourinary cancers.

The increased risk of second malignancies is particularly well described in survivors of Hodgkin's lymphoma ([8-11]). Radiation therapy, particularly when delivered in adolescence, is known to be a predisposing factor for a host of second cancers in the radiation field, including cancers of the skin, breast, lung, and connective tissue ([8]). Moreover, there is evidence to suggest that receiving chemotherapy in addition to radiation may increase the risk of subsequent development of solid tumors. Thus, it is not surprising that the risk of acute myeloid leukemia is also increased, likely due to both radiation exposure and the use of alkylating agents during treatment ([11]).

The recognition that patients who have received mantle radiation have a higher risk of malignancy has led to the tailoring of screening recommendations, particularly those regarding breast cancer, to address this increased susceptibility ([12]). While formal guidelines for screening for cancer at sites other than the breasts in the involved fields do not exist, a key function of interval updates to history and physical exam during survivorship care is to focus on these important possible late complications of cancer treatment.

Like survivors of Hodgkin's lymphomas, there is significant literature regarding the importance of second cancers in patients with primary head and neck neoplasms ([13, 14]). The human papilloma virus (HPV) is an important causative agent of oral and oropharyngeal cancers and also anal, vaginal, and cervical cancers. That said, there is little literature regarding synchronous or metachronous primary tumors of the anus or uterine cervix in patients with oral index tumors. Perhaps more important, tobacco use is a major risk factor for this category of cancers, as well as for cancers of the lung, bladder, and other sites. Consequently, as many as a third of deaths in patients with head and neck cancers are attributable to second primary cancers, a larger number than those that die from distant metastases from the first tumor. In a recent analysis based on SEER data, the incidence and type of second cancers varied based on the site of primary tumor. Patients with index oral and oropharyngeal cancers had more second head and neck tumors, while patients with hypopharyngeal and laryngeal cancers had more lung cancers as their second primary, likely reflecting the diminished importance of HPV infection and increased contribution of tobacco exposure as a cause of cancer at these sites.

Table 60-1 Screening for Subsequent Malignant Neoplasms in Childhood Cancer Survivors

Second Malignant Neoplasm	Risk Factors	Screening Recommendations
Skin cancer	10%-20% of patients; increased risk in irradiated skin	Annual skin exams by dermatologist; close monitoring of irradiated skin and palms and soles
Breast cancer	Risk in women younger than 30 years is elevated 5 to 54 times depending on radiation dose to thorax	Yearly mammograms or magnetic resonance imaging of breasts beginning 8 years after radiation or age 25 years, whichever occurs later, for women who had chest radiation
Thyroid cancer	Increased risk with radiation to head, neck, or chest	Annual history and physical examination; free thyroxine, thyroid-stimulating hormone tested yearly; thyroid ultrasound every 3-4 years after treatment completion or sooner if nodule is found
Leukemia (acute myeloid leukemia/ myelodysplastic syndrome)	Increased risk with exposure to alkylating agents, topoisomerase inhibitors	Annual history and physical examination, including complete blood cell count with differential and platelet count (highest risk first 5 years after exposure)
Brain tumors	Increased risk with cranial radiation; the younger the age at primary diagnosis, the greater the risk; received cranial radiation for brain tumor, acute lymphoblastic leukemia, some head and neck sarcomas	Latency period 9 to 10 years after radiation; monitor with annual history and physical examination, including yearly neurological exam (more often if indicated by examination or symptoms)
Other carcinomas	Can occur in patients who have or have not undergone radiation therapy	Latency period 5 to 30 years, median 15 years; yearly history and physical examination; if abdominal radiation: colon cancer screening with colonoscopy every 10 years beginning 15 years after completion of treatment or at age 35 years, whichever is later

While the volume of literature regarding second tumors in survivors of other cancers varies, the survivorship care provider must understand that any survivor of cancer or cancer treatment may be at risk. Like primary tumors, occurrence of second cancers is due to a confluence of environmental exposures, behavioral influences, and genetic milieu.

Site-Specific Screening for Second Tumors

Breast Cancer Screening

The most important factor modifying breast cancer screening (Fig. 60-2) in cancer survivors is a history of radiation exposure to the chest. Of women who received radiation therapy involving the breast during childhood and adolescence, 13% to 20% will go on to develop a breast malignancy by the age of 40 to 45 years. This risk is most pronounced for women who received 20 Gy or more of radiation to breast tissue, but the increased risk is measurable even among women who received 1 to 9 Gy. International consensus guidelines recommend starting screening at age 25 or 8 years after treatment, whichever comes last, for women who received 20 Gy or more of radiation, with individualization of the screening approach for women who received lower doses of radiation. Our approach at MD Anderson involves starting at age 25 or 8 to 10 years after exposure to radiation, whichever comes first, and we alternate annual mammograms and annual magnetic resonance imaging (MRI) every 6 months, with clinical breast exam done annually. While we acknowledge that data to support the use of MRI as the optimal approach in these patients is still in evolution, this modality has the added benefit of sparing additional radiation exposure while providing excellent imaging detail. Thus, the use of MRI in breast cancer screening has greatly increased over the last decade, particularly in the pool of high-risk women ([15]).

Similarly, for those patients who are diagnosed with predisposing familial syndromes during the workup for their breast cancers, we recommend annual MRI and mammograms, alternating every 6 months, with clinical breast exams every 6 to 12 months. The recommendations are similar for women with a lifetime breast cancer risk of 20% or more based on models that take into account family history. While screening recommendations for other survivors of breast cancer without identified predispositions do not materially differ from those for the general population, it is acknowledged that these women represent a higher-risk pool, and as such, adherence to screening regimens is of increased importance.

Colon Cancer

Colon cancer screening is also of increased importance among cancer survivors. There are several familial

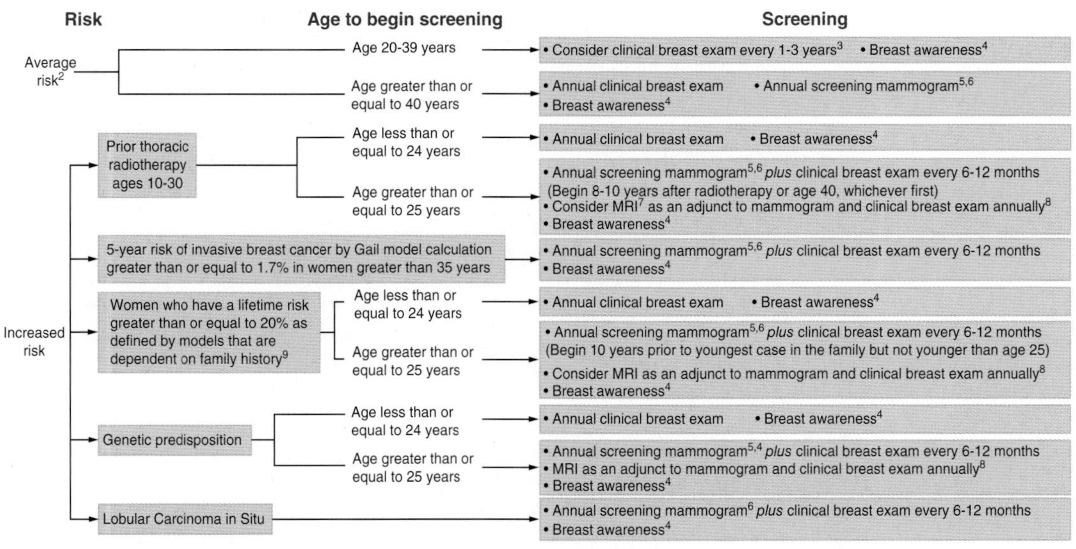

[1]Please see the Breast Cancer Treatment or Survivorship algorithms for the management of women with a personal history of breast cancer.

[2]Women who do not meet one of the increased risk categories.

[3]Effectiveness of clinical breast exams has not been assessed in women 20-39 years of age.

[4]Women should be familiar with their breasts and promptly report changes to their healthcare provider.

[5]Augmented breasts need additional views for complete assessment.

[6]3D screening mammography is not yet standard of care but may be considered as a supplement to 2D mammography.

[7]Risk of breast cancer begins to increase 8-10 years after thoracic exposure. The optimal age to begin MRI screening in this high risk population is not currently known.

[8]Current practice at M.D. Anderson is to alternate the mammogram and breast MRI every 6 months. While there are no data to suggest that this is the optimal approach, it is done with the expectation that interval cancers may be identified earlier. Other screening regimens, such as breast MRI done at the time of the annual mammogram, are also acceptable.

[9]Risk models that are largely dependent on family history include Tyrer-Cuzick and Claus.

Department of Clinical Effectiveness V5
Approved by the Executive Committee of Medical Staff 09/30/2014

FIGURE 60-2 MD Anderson breast cancer screening algorithm.

syndromes that predispose to both primary and second colon cancers, including the Lynch syndrome and familial adenomatous polyposis (FAP). In addition, environmental, dietary, and immunologic factors may contribute to an increased risk of second colonic primary in patients with a previous history of colorectal cancer or polyps. Thus, patients with a history of colon cancer require increased frequency of screening for second colorectal primary tumors indefinitely. In the MD Anderson colorectal screening guidelines, we suggest screening colonoscopy every 5 years in long-term survivors. For patients with adenomas at the time of colonoscopy, more frequent screening is recommended (Fig. 60-3).

Colonoscopy

For patients with a diagnosis of Lynch syndrome, some of whom may have a history of gynecologic or other solid tumors, colorectal cancer screening is recommended starting at age 25 or 10 years prior to the earliest colorectal cancer in the immediate family, with colonoscopies every 1 to 2 years thereafter.

Cervical Cancer

The decreased incidence of cervical cancer–related mortality in the United States is related primarily due to widespread screening for premalignant lesions by Papanicolaou testing. Screening for cervical cancer is logically important in survivors of HPV-associated malignancies, including cervical, anal, and oral cancers as these patients likely have a history of high-risk HPV exposures, in addition to possible immunocompromised or other risk factors. In addition, tobacco exposure is an important risk factor that may predispose survivors of other tobacco-related tumors to cervical cancer. Screening for this disease may be particularly important in survivors of adolescent and young adult cancers. In a recent study based on SEER data, it was noted that survivors of pediatric and young adult cancers seem to have a younger age of onset for cervical cancer than the overall population (33 vs 40 years). It is possible that this effect is explained by a surveillance bias. Survivors of pediatric cancer are likely to receive more frequent screening examinations, but this effect deserves further study ([16]).

The cervical cancer screening guidelines of MD Anderson do not change for patients with a history of previous cancer. We recommend a liquid-based Papanicolaou test every 3 years for women from ages 21 to 29. Starting at age 30 until age 65, we recommend a liquid-based Papanicolaou test with high-risk HPV testing. If high-risk HPV testing is done and negative, repeat tests should be done every 5 years. If high-risk HPV testing is not done, the screening interval is every 3 years. For patients with abnormal Papanicolaou tests or positive high-risk HPV, appropriate workup according to diagnostic algorithms is recommended.

Ultimately, screening procedures for these and other malignancies will continue to evolve as additional information becomes available. The key point for the provider caring for the cancer survivor is that having a previous malignancy may predispose to additional cancers in the future and certainly is not protective against subsequent primaries. Therefore, attention to cancer screening is of critical importance in preventing or mitigating morbidity and mortality in survivors of a first cancer.

Screening in Survivors of Childhood Cancers

As in adults, the reasons for increased incidence are related to the survivors' exposure to radiation, chemotherapy, and possible increased genetic predisposition ([17]). Therefore, screening for certain types of cancers is recommended to begin earlier in survivors of childhood cancer than in the general population, as shown in Table 60-1. As discussed previously in this chapter, screening for breast cancer in women who had chest radiation is especially important because magnitude of risk by age 50 is comparable to carriers of *BRCA* mutations ([18]). In addition, children treated with abdominal radiation had increased risk of gastrointestinal cancers (SIR 11.2), warranting earlier screening colonoscopies ([19]).

Screening in Patients With Genetic Predisposition to Cancer

Children and adults with a genetic predisposition to a second malignancy, such as those with neurofibromatosis, Li-Fraumeni syndrome, von Hippel–Lindau syndrome, Beckwith-Wiedemann syndrome, FAP, retinoblastoma germline mutations, or multiple endocrine neoplasia syndromes, should be followed in specialty clinics for these disorders or in a childhood cancer survivor clinic. At the MD Anderson Cancer Center (MDACC), a new program led by the Genetics Department is the LEAD (Li-Fraumeni Syndrome Education and Early Detection) program for patients and family members who have germline *p53* mutations. Individuals in the program undergo periodic biochemical and imaging surveillance, modeled after the published program that showed significantly improved survival of patient with Li-Fraumeni syndrome who had screening ([20]).

LATE EFFECTS OF TREATMENT

Cancer and its treatment can have myriad effects on the overall well-being of cancer survivors. Not surprisingly, patients with cancer rate themselves as having

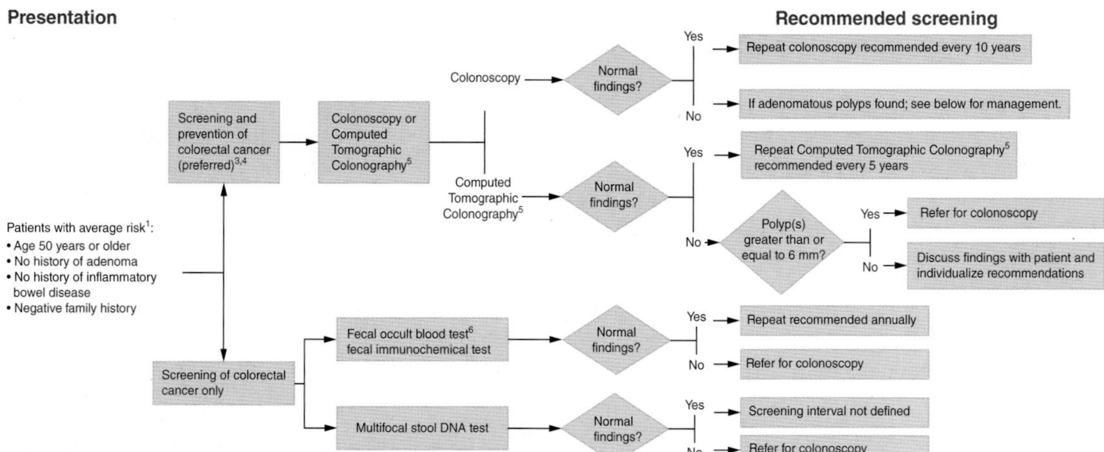

[1]African Americans have had a higher risk of large polyps and tumors from ages 50-56 years, thus it is important to start screening this population at age 50. Follow-up frequency would be based on colonoscopy findings
[2]See the Colorectal Cancer Treatment or Survivorship algorithms for the management of individuals with a personal history of colorectal cancer.
[3]While there is good evidence to support Fecal Occult Blood Test, tests that both screen for and prevent colon cancer are the preferred screening modality. Annual Fecal Occult Blood Tests should not be performed if colonoscopy or CT colonography isused as the screening measure in an average-risk patient.
[4]Flexible sigmoidoscopy is an alternate option, but is not the preferred endoscopic modality as the entire colon is not visualized.
[5]Preauthorization with one's insurance carrier is always advised.
[6]High sensitivity Fecal Occult Blood Test (guaic-based or immunochemical).

Department of Clinical Effectiveness V4
Approved by the Executive Committee of Medical Staff 09/31/2014

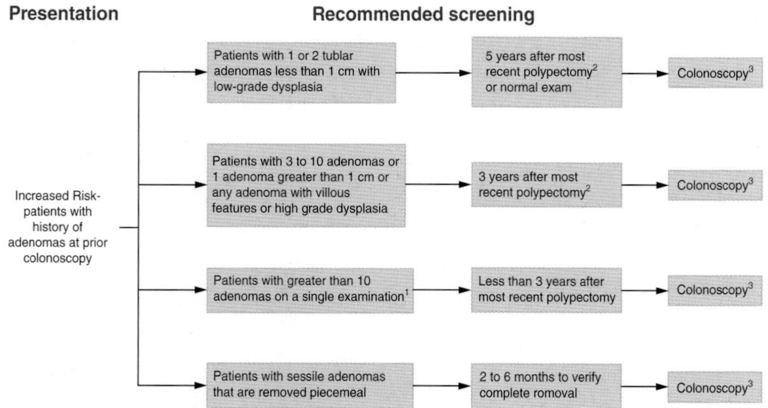

[1]Consider familial syndrome
[2]Precise timing based on clinical factors, patient and physician preference.
[3]Subsequent follow-up is based on the number and size of polyps at the time of colonoscopy as well as the degree of dysplasia. If the follow-up colonoscopy is negative for adenomatous polyps, follow-up in 5 years is recommended.
[4]Surveillance individualized based on endoscopist's judgment

Department of Clinical Effectiveness V4
Approved by the executive committee of medical staff 03/31/2015

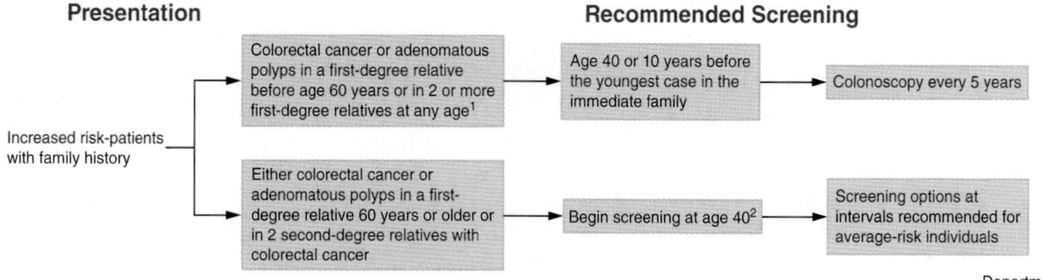

Department of Clinical Effectiveness V4
Approved by the executive committee of medical staff 03/31/2015

[1]Consider familial syndrome
[2]Screening should begin at an earlier age, but individuals may be screened with any recommended from of testing.

FIGURE 60-3 MD Anderson algorithm for colorectal screening for patients with adenomas on prior colonoscopy.

CHAPTER 60

poorer health-related quality of life than noncancer survivors, with a significant component of this being physical impairment ([21]). Broadly, a history of cancer and cancer treatment can have an impact on every system in the body, with common long-term issues that include painful or nonpainful neuropathy, sexual dysfunction, persistent fatigue, lymphedema, surgical disfigurement, and bowel and bladder dysfunction, among other symptoms.

As with the risk of second primaries, the risk of late effects of treatment is particularly important to the survivor of childhood cancers. Over the last 40 years, considerable literature has documented the late effects of cancer treatments in this group. In a report from the Childhood Cancer Survivor Study (CCSS) of 14,359 survivors of childhood cancer with a median follow-up of 24.5 years after diagnosis (range 5 to 39.3 years), cumulative incidence of a severe, disabling, life-threatening, or fatal condition was 53.6% for survivors compared to 19.8% in siblings by age 50 ([22]). The most common severe chronic conditions were congestive heart failure, second malignant neoplasm, cognitive dysfunction, coronary artery disease, cerebrovascular accident, renal failure, major joint replacement, hearing loss, legal blindness, and ovarian failure ([3, 23]). New onset of these conditions continued to occur at higher incidence than for siblings in every decade for over 35 years from diagnosis. Among survivors who reached age 35 years without a previous grade 3 or 4 condition, 25.9% experienced a subsequent grade 3 to 5 condition (renal failure, stroke, heart attack, congestive heart failure, and pulmonary fibrosis) within 10 years compared with 6.0% of siblings ($P < .001$) ([4]). The overall cumulative mortality rate of 20,483 survivors (over 5 years from diagnosis at enrollment) in the CCSS study was 18.1% at 30 years from diagnosis, with the most frequent causes of mortality second malignant neoplasm, cardiac death, and pulmonary death—largely due to treatment-related causes ([24]).

These late effects threaten both quality and length of life. With over 80% of children with cancer surviving more than 5 years, there is a need to screen for, and if possible prevent, late-occurring problems. With this in mind, the Children's Oncology Group in 2003 developed evidence-based guidelines that recommend follow-up screening and care of survivors of childhood cancer who are at risk for late effects. These guidelines are risk based depending on the specific exposures to surgery, radiation, and chemotherapy and are designed to begin when a child enters a survivorship clinic at either 5 years from diagnosis or 2 years off therapy when the child is cancer free and without recurrence. They are based on treatment rather than diagnosis and are available to the public (http://www.survivorshipguidelines.org). In our Childhood Cancer Survivor Clinic at MDACC, we follow these guidelines and use them to recommend the standard of care for follow-up in an individualized "Passport for Care."

CARDIOVASCULAR LATE EFFECTS

Cardiotoxicity is one of the most serious chronic complications of treatment of cancer for both adults and children, but children are particularly vulnerable. Thirty-year survivors of childhood cancer have been shown to have a 15 times higher rate of heart failure, a 10 times higher rate of other cardiovascular diseases, and a 9 times higher risk of stroke than age-matched sibling controls. This risk can persist for 30 or more years after completion of treatment and represents an important source of excess morbidity in patients with cancer ([25]). The most common causes of cardiotoxicity are anthracycline-based chemotherapy or radiation therapy to the neck and mediastinum.

Anthracyclines are a class of antineoplastic agents that are highly efficacious in the treatment of pediatric and adult hematologic cancers, including acute myeloid leukemia, acute lymphoblastic leukemia (ALL), Hodgkin's disease, and non-Hodgkin lymphoma, as well as solid tumors, sarcomas, and ovarian cancer. Among children in the United States who are survivors of childhood cancer, approximately 50% have received anthracyclines. Cumulative dose-related cardiac adverse effects may become apparent at the time that the first dose is administered, and clinical data suggest that deterioration of cardiac function is sustained throughout treatment and may become apparent many years after treatment is completed ([26]).

Known risk factors for anthracycline-induced cardiac adverse effects include high cumulative doses of anthracycline, high anthracycline dose intensity, female sex, age younger than 5 years at diagnosis, radiation therapy, and combining anthracyclines with other cardiotoxic chemotherapy. Patients who were treated for lymphoma, Hodgkin's lymphoma, sarcomas, or myeloid leukemia generally have the highest risk of cardiotoxicity because of the high doses of anthracyclines they usually receive, often accompanied by radiation. Higher-than-expected occurrences of cardiac adverse effects are observed in patients who receive anthracyclines in combination with new targeted drugs, such as the human epidermal growth factor receptor 2 antibody trastuzumab. These risk factors are helpful in establishing monitoring guidelines, as has been done for children, although they do not predict the risk of cardiac adverse effects for all patients. A new scoring system based on CCSS data provides a score of individual risk for the survivors ([27]).

Medications such as enalopril and carvedilol can support cardiac function when signs of deterioration in left ventricular function are noted on echocardiograms. While MD Anderson cardiologists prescribe these medications for survivors with decreased ejection fraction and have seen benefit for individuals, the long-term benefit in survivors of childhood cancer has not yet been proven and needs further investigation ([28]). In adults, these medications have been shown to be effective in preventing chemotherapy-induced left ventricular systolic dysfunction in a randomized trial of adults undergoing aggressive chemotherapy and stem cell transplantation (SCT) ([29]).

In 2003, the Children's Oncology Group released risk-based, exposure-related guidelines for children treated with anthracyclines. These guidelines include recommendations for echocardiograms every 1 to 5 years depending on exposure (http://survivorshipguidelines.org). These recommendations differ substantially from those given for patients treated for cancer during adulthood and should be followed. They have been found to be cost effective ([30]).

Stroke is another late vascular effect of radiation to the head and neck. Survivors of brain tumor and leukemia who received cranial radiation as well as survivors of Hodgkin's disease who had radiation to the neck have increased risk of cerebral vascular accident when compared to siblings ([31]). In addition, once a survivor has had a stroke, the risk of having another is significant; therefore, aggressive preventive treatment is recommended ([32]).

PULMONARY LATE EFFECTS

Bleomycin or pulmonary radiation is associated with abnormal pulmonary function in 44% of survivors of childhood cancer referred for pulmonary function tests. They were found to have restrictive pulmonary function impairments and decreased diffusion capacity ([33]). Pulmonary fibrosis may also occur after treatment with high doses of cyclophosphamide, busulfan, or nitrosourea-based drugs. Pulmonary function studies will reveal a diffuse interstitial fibrosis, restrictive pulmonary disease, and arterial hypoxemia. A chest x-ray will show a pattern of diffuse interstitial fibrosis with patchy basilar infiltrates. In the chronic stage, pulmonary fibrosis associated with treatment with cyclophosphamide or nitrosourea-based drugs also manifests as diffuse interstitial and intra-alveolar fibrosis. Whole-lung radiation even at low doses is associated with pulmonary fibrosis and increased risk of spontaneous pneumothorax many years later ([33, 34]). Patients who receive cranial-spinal radiation for CNS are also at risk for late pulmonary complications. Rates of emphysema, asthma, chronic cough, and need for oxygen were significantly higher for long-term CNS survivors than for their siblings ([35]).

Our pediatric survivorship guidelines (those developed by the Children's Oncology Group in 2013) recommend a chest x-ray and pulmonary function tests at entry to the survivorship clinic in patients treated with bleomycin, busulfan, nitrosoureas, chest radiation, and allogenic bone marrow transplantation/SCT with chronic graft-versus-host disease (cGVHD). Following these guidelines strictly, one clinic found that the screening yielded 84% with abnormal findings in survivors followed an average of 10 years from diagnosis ([36]). Such guidelines are not available for adults entering survivorship, but awareness of the possible late pulmonary effects of chemotherapy, radiation, and surgery is important for the survivorship care provider.

ENDOCRINE LATE EFFECTS

Because growth and development to become a normal adult is one of our important goals of survivors of childhood cancer, hormonal screening and treatment are essential. Pediatric/adult endocrinologists often comanage patients in the Childhood Cancer Survivor Clinic. Pituitary hormone insufficiency can occur within months to many years from surgery involving the pituitary or radiation to the brain. Hormonal insufficiency can develop for survivors of brain tumor, even in tumors outside the pituitary/hypothalamic axis ([37]). Thyroid hormone deficiency is common after radiation either directly or indirectly to the thyroid. Because this problem is readily treated with oral replacement, thyroid screening in at-risk patients is an essential part of survivorship care. Thyroid cancer is also one of the most common second malignant neoplasms due to either radiation to the neck or chemotherapy.

Hormonal deficiencies, if untreated, can lead to short stature, early or delayed puberty, cortisol insufficiency with insufficient stress response, or thyroid deficiency. Patients with growth hormone deficiency require treatment with the hormone for adequate growth before they pass through puberty and the growth plates have fused. Some have also advocated for adult hormone replacement in patients with metabolic syndrome uncontrolled by other medications. Although there has been concern, growth hormone treatment has not been associated with increased risk of recurrence or of second neoplasms ([38]). Patients with brain tumors that involved the pituitary/hypothalamic axis are also at risk for diabetes insipidis. The most common diagnoses associated with this problem are hypothalamic astrocytoma, CNS germ cell tumors, and craniopharyngioma. In this setting, panhypopituitarism and the associated risks are lifelong and can lead to early death if not managed appropriately. Unfortunately, endocrine deficits and cognitive impairment can occur in the same patient, making these patients a challenge to manage if they do not have the support of a parent or caretaker.

COGNITIVE DEFICITS

The younger the patient when the radiation is administered, the greater the damage that can occur. This is especially important when the CNS or head are radiated ([34]). Children, especially those who receive radiation at age under 7 years, are at risk for cognitive deficits that include decrease in IQ, poor attention, poor memory, and deficits in executive functioning and mental speed. The degree of the deficit varies with individuals and the dose of radiation, size of the field, and critical structures within the radiation field. Young children treated with Total Body Irradiation (TBI) also have risk of decreased cognitive function ([39]). Very young children who receive whole-brain radiation are less likely to achieve independence in adulthood. In addition, older children treated with lower doses of radiation, such as CNS prophylaxis for childhood ALL, still have risk of intellectual decline in later life ([40]). Cognitive impairment after whole-brain radiation in adults for metastatic disease or prophylaxis is also well known to have myriad long-term side effects, ranging from mild decline in memory, mood, or concentration all the way to dementia.

The patients at the highest risk are those who live for longer than a year, those who had concurrent chemotherapy, or those who received high fractional doses ([41]). Many protocols for treatment of brain tumors such as both medulloblastoma and leukemia have attempted to decrease or eliminate radiation doses, with some success, without sacrificing decrease in cure rate. Now, methods such as proton radiation help decrease the radiation to normal tissues. It is yet to be proven that proton radiation will improve cognitive outcomes, although short-term results show some promise, but with radiation to left temporal lobe/hippocampus still leading to significant cognitive declines in young children ([42]). Developing interventions for cancer-related cognitive dysfunction in childhood cancer survivors is a priority ([40]).

PAIN

Approximately 33% of cancer survivors report some element of chronic pain after the completion of treatment ([43]). Chronic postoperative pain is an often-encountered sequela of lumpectomy or mastectomy for breast cancer treatment, with 50% to 60% of patients reporting some element of pain after surgery ([44, 45]). The causes for this are complex and include nerve damage, phantom pains, intercostobrachial neuralgia, lymphedema, and psychological contributions. Predictors for postoperative pain in one large survey study of patients with breast cancer included young age, axillary lymph node dissection (ALND), adjuvant radiotherapy, and pain complaints at other sites in the body ([44]). Postthoracotomy pain relating to damage to intercostal nerves can complicate the course of up to 50% of patients. Other postoperative pain syndromes can include phantom limb pain and post–neck dissection pain for head and neck tumors ([43]).

Radiation can also predispose to a host of pain syndromes, including plexopathies, osteonecrosis, nerve entrapment, and chronic colitis and cystitis ([43, 46]). Brachial plexopathies are most common in women who have received radiation for breast cancer and also occur in patients treated for lymphoma and lung cancer. Symptoms can start anywhere from 6 months to 20 years after radiation therapy and manifest as paras-thesias, weakness, and pain. Lumbar plexopathies are less common but can be seen with treatment of gynecologic and colorectal tumors ([46]).

Hormonal therapies are an underconsidered cause of pain. As we transition to a period during which prolonged hormonal blockade is a favored therapy for patients with hormone receptor–positive breast cancer, these symptoms are more likely to be managed in the setting of cancer survivorship. Of women taking aromatase inhibitors, 47% and 44% report joint pain and stiffness, respectively. This typically manifests as symmetric small-joint arthralgia involving the hands and feet ([47]). Interestingly, there is also an increased incidence of carpal tunnel syndrome in patients on aromatase inhibitors ([48, 49]). Most often, these symptoms are attributed to the acute decrease in estrogen levels, as perimenopausal women can report similar symptoms, although interestingly, the incidence of arthralgias is more common in patients who have received taxanes ([47, 50]). It is important to address these symptoms as the occurrence of arthralgia leads to discontinuation of the aromatase inhibitor in up to 20% of cases ([51]), despite the fact that these symptoms may be predictive of better efficacy ([52]).

Chemotherapy-induced peripheral neuropathy (CIPN) is perhaps the most characteristic cancer pain syndrome, due to both its high prevalence and the difficulty that can be experienced in successfully treating it. This most often presents as a burning or pins-and-needles sensation that occurs in a stocking-and-glove distribution. The most common implicated agents include platinum-containing agents, taxanes, vinka alkaloids, bortezomib, thalidomide and its derivatives, and ixabepilone. The duration of persistence of neuropathy after discontinuation of the drug varies by agent but can be indefinite ([46]). Unfortunately, effective treatment of CIPN has been elusive, although there are several recent promising preliminary studies. Randomized trials have been conducted for gabapentin, amitriptyline, nortriptyline, and lamotrigine, all of which are used to varying degrees for non–chemotherapy-related peripheral neuropathy. Unfortunately, these have not been definitively shown to be effective for CIPN ([46]).

That said, there are several agents currently under investigation that have shown some activity in early trials. In a phase II single-arm study of pregabalin in 23 patients with oxaliplatin-induced peripheral neuropathy, 48% of patients described some improvement in their neurologic symptoms ([53]). A multicenter randomized phase III trial of duloxetine versus placebo in patients with at least grade 2 CIPN showed a statistically significant reduction in pain and improvement in function ([54]). Similarly, venlafaxine has been shown to be of interest in treating oxaliplatin-induced peripheral neuropathy in the acute setting, although its role in treating chronic CIPN is less clear ([55]). Another recently reported study suggested that a topical combination of ketamine, amitriptyline, and baclofen may also be of some utility in treating painful sensory as well as motor neuropathy ([56]).

Ultimately, pain in survivors of cancer is often a complex problem, with nociceptive, neuropathic, and inflammatory components. As such, its treatment often requires a multimodality approach, including μ-agonists, nonsteroidal anti-inflammatory agents, neuropathy-directed therapy, procedures, and physical rehabilitation to help with pain and maximize function and quality of life.

FATIGUE

Fatigue is a nearly universal issue in patients undergoing active treatment of cancer. Even after treatment ends, persistent fatigue can remain a disabling problem for survivors of cancer, with up to 29% of patients reporting some degree of fatigue ([57]). A variety of contributing factors may exist, including deconditioning and psychological issues. Immune dysregulation and evidence of persistent inflammation have also been implicated as contributing to persistent cancer-related fatigue ([58, 59]). Our own survivorship algorithms as well as those of the National Comprehensive Cancer Network emphasize screening for fatigue, as this can be an underdiagnosed and undermanaged issue that remains distressing for patients.

Several interventions have been examined as options for the treatment of cancer-related fatigue. Behavioral counseling to promote energy conservation can be of utility in the immediate posttreatment period ([60]) but is of questionable utility in long-term survivors. In these patients, more evidence supports the use of increased physical activity as a way to improve endurance, emotional well-being, and health-related quality of life ([61, 62]). Cognitive-behavioral therapy (CBT), on the other hand, is a validated approach to improving cancer-related fatigue, with evidence to suggest that positive effects on level of fatigue can be observed up to 2 years after completion of therapy.

Studies of pharmacologic treatment of cancer-related fatigue must be interpreted carefully, as more than half of patients may experience improvement in their symptoms with placebo ([63]). Several stimulants have been examined as possible treatments of cancer-related fatigue in survivors. A recent meta-analysis of five randomized trials of methylphenidate for cancer-related fatigue found limited evidence to support its use ([64]). Modafinil has also been of interest, with several small, uncontrolled trials supporting its use. Unfortunately, two randomized controlled trials have now failed to show any benefit over placebo for this agent in patients with cancer-related fatigue ([65, 66]). However, psychostimulants may still have a role in treating contributing conditions such as narcotic-related fatigue and depression ([67]).

SEXUAL DYSFUNCTION

Infertility is a non–life-threatening late effect of treatment that for young adult survivors, and in their 20s and early 30s is one of their greatest concerns. Fortunately, most survivors have normal sexual function, but exposures to alkylating chemotherapy or brain or gonadal radiation can lead to sterility. In a CCSS study of female survivors of childhood cancer who were currently 18 to 39 years old and who had been sexually active, 16% had total infertility. Increasing doses of uterine radiation and alkylating chemotherapy were strongly associated with female infertility ([68]). In a similar study of men, 46% reported infertility, but of these, 37% reported at least one pregnancy with a female partner that resulted in a live birth. The best way to preserve fertility is to bank sperm or ovum/embryos before chemotherapy. Unfortunately, this is not generally available to children and is difficult in adolescent females.

Many chemotherapeutic drugs have the potential to cause gonadal failure or impairment. Alkylating agents, particularly cyclophosphamide and ifosfamide, can damage the testes, resulting in sterility or lack of testosterone production. The risk is greater in pubescent boys than in younger boys. The ovaries can also be damaged in pubescent girls. This may result in infertility, lack of estrogen production, or premature menopause. Damage to the gonads may manifest as delayed puberty, amenorrhea (in girls), and absence of secondary sexual characteristics, growth retardation, or infertility. Levels of follicle-stimulating hormone, luteinizing hormone, and insulin-like growth factor should be determined, semen analysis performed (in boys and girls), and testosterone or estrogen levels checked. A referral to a fertility expert is always indicated if pregnancy is desired. Conceptions achieved by "infertile" long-term survivors, both male and female, have been reported in survivors of cancer. If these survivors have children, an increased risk of birth defects has not been found.

Other forms of sexual dysfunction can vary based on the patient's tumor type and the therapies use to treat it. Among the increasing numbers of women on selective estrogen receptor modulators or aromatase inhibitors, loss of libido, vaginal atrophy, and dyspareunia are common complaints ([69]). Women who have undergone pelvic surgery may suffer from painful intercourse due to vaginal shortening; nerve damage from pelvic surgery, resulting in anorgasmia; or the psychological consequences of disfigurement ([70,71]).

Similarly, treatment of prostate cancer can result in sexual dysfunction among men. The majority of patients receiving surgery or radiotherapy report some degree of erectile dysfunction 2 years after completing treatment, and this increases with time, likely due to increasing age and possible additional cancer-directed therapy ([72]). In one study, men younger than 50 at the time of radical prostatectomy were more than twice as likely as men older than 70 to recover sexual function ([73]).

Survivors of breast, genitourinary, and gynecologic cancer are prone to sexual dysfunction, but this an issue common to almost all cancers. Nerve damage due to pelvic surgery for colon cancer can cause erectile dysfunction and anorgasmia, and body image issues related to ileostomy or colostomies can also be distressing ([69]). Even for patients undergoing SCT, where the anatomical issues are less obvious, survivors report lower sexual satisfaction than patients without cancer histories. Perhaps not surprisingly, this finding was associated with the presence of cGVHD.

Treatments of sexual dysfunction also vary based on the etiology. For men with erectile dysfunction, the most commonly used treatments are the PDE5 inhibitors. Other treatments, such as vacuum pumps and penile implants, are also available and effective, although less commonly used ([74]).

Pharmacologic therapies for female sexual dysfunction have been less successful. Studies examining the use of testosterone supplementation and PDE5 inhibitors have been disappointing ([75,76]). One recent development is the availability of a Selective Estrogen Receptor Modulation (SERM), ospemifene, which has been shown in a phase III randomized controlled trial to be effective in the treatment of vaginal dryness. There is little evidence regarding the safety of this intervention in cancers that are breast and other hormone receptor positive, but this may be a useful therapy for women with a history of other malignancies. Another important approach is counseling regarding vaginal care, including the use of lubricants and dilators to increase blood flow and treat or prevent atrophy ([77]). Psychoeducational training, including elements of CBT, may also be of utility in treating female sexual arousal disorder in survivors of cancer ([78]).

LYMPHEDEMA

Lymphedema is generally a postsurgical complication that can take place at any site where a downstream lymphadenectomy is performed. Survivors of breast cancer are likely the most visible group of patients with lymphedema, with up to 49% of women who undergo ALND reporting some element of lymphedema at 20 years after treatment ([79]). The practice of doing a sentinel lymph node biopsy prior to proceeding to ALND if necessary can decrease the incidence and severity of this complication, but a significant fraction of women still require ALND for locally advanced disease and are at risk for this long-term complication. Moreover, while patients with breast cancer may represent the most visible group of patients with lymphedema, this complication is also seen in patients who have undergone lymph node dissection for head and neck cancers, melanoma, gynecological malignancies, and others.

Treatment of most afflicted patients is conservative, including modalities like elevation of affected extremity, compressive therapy, or lymphedema-specific manual lymphatic drainage massage. These are effective in patients with mild-to-moderate lymphedema, but are also highly dependent on patient compliance. Benzopyrones, drugs that are believed to decrease vascular permeability, have little convincing evidence for their use ([80]). Surgical techniques are also available for patients who have failed less-invasive interventions. Microsurgical lymphovenous bypass is the most commonly reported procedure, with one large study demonstrating subjective symptom improvement in 87% of patients and 83% of patients demonstrating improvement in volume measurements ([81]).

At MD Anderson, we more commonly use a subtype of this procedure, lymphaticovenular bypass. In this procedure, distal lymphatics, which are typically less affected by lymphedema changes and consequently more available for bypass, are anastomosed to subdermal venules, which are under lower pressure and thus may result in less backflow into the lymphatic system and better long-term effect. A small prospective study at our institution demonstrated subjective benefit in 95% of patients undergoing the procedure, although long-term follow-up is needed to illustrate the durability of these results over time ([82]).

PSYCHOSOCIAL CONSEQUENCES OF CANCER TREATMENT

Financial difficulty can contribute considerably to the well-being of cancer survivors and is an important source of distress. Adult patients with cancer are more likely to be retired or unemployed than their siblings without cancer, although the likelihood increases as patients get further away from their diagnosis ([83, 84]). Patients with breast cancer, male genital cancers, and skin cancers more likely to return to work than patients with lung or gastrointestinal cancers ([83]). Not surprisingly, the risk of not returning to work is higher for patients with higher-stage tumors and patients who required extensive surgery ([85]). Even among those who do return to work, productivity can suffer due to physical and cognitive limitations. While it is important for the survivorship care provider to be aware of these issues, there is little guidance regarding effective interventions. Even though employer education and policy initiatives are likely to be of utility, most evidence to date focuses on intensive multidisciplinary evaluation and guidance for patients. A recent Cochrane review found moderate evidence to support interventions with physical, psychological, and vocational components ([83]).

Another cause of psychological concern among patients with cancer is altered body image related to surgery, weight changes, or other sequelae of treatment. This in turn is a predictor for depression in survivors ([86]). Patients with male genitourinary cancers have variable outcomes. One study found that orchiectomy in older survivors of testicular cancer was not associated with worsened body image regardless of whether a prosthesis was placed, as long as sexual function was preserved. Among younger patients, however, concern over scars made many patients report feeling less attractive. Encouragingly, 88.2% of spouses in the same study did not report any decrease in attraction to their partners. For patients with prostate cancer, hormonal therapy is associated with worsening body image, and over 50% of patients report a decrease in perception of body image over 2 years. Moreover, the decrease seems to be associated in a decrease in quality-of-life metrics ([87]).

The financial and physical concerns relating to cancer survivorship can lead to distress, defined as depression and anxiety that may lead to somatic symptoms. Interestingly, while older cancer patients seem to be at higher risk for suicide, there is a suggestion that adolescent and young adult patients are at higher risk for long-term distress ([88, 89]). At particular risk seems to be patients that are younger at diagnosis, female, those with late effects, those with lower education, and those with less perceived parental support ([89]).

Childhood survivors of cancer represent an important subgroup within survivors of cancer in general. Although many survivors of childhood cancer show tremendous resilience and strength in overcoming the trauma of cancer at a young age, a significant proportion report more symptoms of global distress and poorer physical function than controls. Other reported late effects include anxiety, depression, and posttraumatic stress. These factors can significantly hinder attainment of lifetime educational, social, and vocational goals. As a result, survivors are less likely to be married, have a higher risk of experiencing unemployment and legal difficulties, and are likely to attain lower educational achievements than other adults. Survivors who have had cranial radiation or surgery are at the highest risk of experiencing psychosocial problems and are likely to face problems related to motor, sensory, and behavioral disturbances, often culminating in social isolation and failure to attain independence ([40, 90]). In addition, survivors who experienced psychological problems as adolescents have an increased risk of developing poor health behaviors in adulthood. In our clinic, we frequently refer patients to our vocational counselors, psychologists, and psychiatrists for psychosocial support and advice about school and careers ([91, 92]).

The most feared complication of distress in patients with cancer is suicide. The risk of suicide is highest in patients recently diagnosed and is more common among patients with poor prognoses. Completed suicide is more common within 3 to 6 months of diagnosis; however, excess risk seems to persist past 5 years. In a Finnish study of 60 patients with cancer who committed suicide, 25 were patients who were in a remission. Most of these suicides were of patients with mental illness or other comorbidities. Other risk factors for suicide that have been identified include male sex and a history of previous suicide attempts. A study of adult survivors of childhood cancer found suicidal ideation among survivors of childhood cancer was reported in 12.6% of respondents, with occurrence in the general population estimated at 2.65% to 3.3%. Interestingly, in addition to depression, a history of cranial radiation was described as a risk factor in this study, possibly due to cognitive or cosmetic sequelae ([93]).

HEALTHY LIFESTYLES IN CANCER PATIENTS

Management of risk factors for heart disease takes on special important in survivors of cancer. Survivors should be encouraged to have a healthy lifestyle with exercise and a healthy diet to prevent other known risk factors for cardiovascular disease, such as obesity and hyperlipidemia. The combination of elements of metabolic syndrome and exposure to anthracyclines or chest radiation increase the risk of a serious cardiac event ([94]). Therefore, control of weight, hypertension, cholesterol, and diabetes is especially important in all survivors of cancer, particularly those treated as children or adolescents. In one study, among survivors of childhood cancer, adherence to a heart-healthy lifestyle was associated with lower risk of metabolic syndrome. Even after adjusting for known treatment and demographic risk factors, failure to follow a heart-healthy lifestyle was associated with a more than two-fold increased risk of developing metabolic syndrome. Additional work is needed to evaluate the impact of lifestyle interventions on risk for metabolic syndrome among survivors of childhood cancer, especially in individuals predisposed to adverse cardiovascular outcomes because of their treatment of childhood cancer ([95]). Female survivors, adolescents and young adults, and survivors of cancers of the CNS and lymphoma are the highest-risk populations for poor dietary behaviors, sedentary behaviors, and poor health-related quality of life ([96]).

Physical activity has been linked to improved all-cause mortality in survivors of cancer with a variety of tumor types ([97, 98]). While a decreased cardiovascular risk profile is likely the explanation for much of this effect, there is also noted to be a decrease in the risk of cancer recurrence and disease-specific mortality in patients with many tumor types, including breast and prostate cancers ([99]). Exercise also leads to improvements in overall quality of life, including decreased anxiety, depression, and fatigue and improved body image ([99]).

Diet is another component of a healthy lifestyle that has been examined in patients with cancer. The largest studies to date are the Women's Interventional Nutrition Study (WINS) and the Women's Healthy Eating and Living (WHEL) Study, both of which were done in women with early breast cancer ([99]). The WINS study compared women placed on a low-fat diet with a control group of women. The dietary intervention group experienced weight loss and an increased disease-free survival, with a median survival of 5.6 years ([100]). The WHEL study similarly prescribed a low-fat diet that increased fruit and vegetable intake and dietary fiber. At 7.3 years, there was no difference in recurrence rates between the dietary intervention and control groups. Consequently, the intervention in the WINS trial has been attributed to the observed weight loss rather than the lower fat content of the diet in the experimental group ([99]).

A continued emphasis on smoking cessation, which should begin prior to a cancer diagnosis, remains important in the survivorship setting. Patients who continue to smoke after being diagnosed with early-stage lung cancer have increased all-cause mortality as well as increased recurrence rates compared to patients who do not smoke after being diagnosed. This has also been demonstrated in patients with esophageal cancer. Smoking while drinking moderate amounts of alcohol (at least 7 alcoholic beverages a week) seemed to amplify the increased risk of cancer recurrence.

REFERENCES

1. Mariotto AB, Rowland JH, Yabroff KR, et al. Long-term survivors of childhood cancers in the United States. *Cancer Epidemiol Biomarkers Prev*. 2009;18:1033-1040.
2. Ward E, DeSantis C, Robbins A, Kohler B, Jemal A. Childhood and adolescent cancer statistics. *Cancer*. 2014;64:83-103.
3. Hudson MM, Ness KK, Gurney JG, et al. Clinical ascertainment of health outcomes among adults treated for childhood cancer. *JAMA*. 2013;309:2371-81.
4. Armstrong GT, Kawashima T, Leisenring W, et al. Aging and risk of severe, disabling, life-threatening, and fatal events in the Childhood Cancer Survivor Study. *J Clin Oncol*. 2014;32:1218-1227.
5. Travis LB, Rabkin CS, Brown LM, et al. Cancer survivorship—genetic susceptibility and second primary cancers: research strategies and recommendations. *J Natl Cancer Inst*. 2006;98:15-25.
6. Ng AK, Travis LB. The epidemiology of second primary cancers. In: Miller KD, ed. *Medical and Psychosocial Care of the Cancer Survivor*. Sudbury, MA: Jones and Bartlett; 2010:211-231.
7. Friedman DL, Whitton J, Leisenring W, et al. Subsequent neoplasms in 5-year survivors of childhood cancer: the Childhood Cancer Survivor Study. *J Natl Cancer Inst*. 2010;102:1083-1095.
8. Daniels LA, Krol AD, Schaapveld M, et al. Long-term risk of secondary skin cancers after radiation therapy for Hodgkin's lymphoma. *Radiother Oncol*. 2013;109:140-145.
9. Foss Abrahamsen A, Andersen A, Nome O, et al. Long-term risk of second malignancy after treatment of Hodgkin's disease: the influence of treatment, age and follow-up time. *Ann Oncol*. 2002;13:1786-1791.
10. Ng AK, Bernardo MV, Weller E, et al. Second malignancy after Hodgkin disease treated with radiation therapy with or without chemotherapy: long-term risks and risk factors. *Blood*. 2002;100:1989-1996.
11. van Leeuwen FE, Klokman WJ, Veer MB, et al. Long-term risk of second malignancy in survivors of Hodgkin's disease treated during adolescence or young adulthood. *J Clin Oncol*. 2000;18:487-497.
12. Mulder RL, Kremer LC, Hudson MM, et al. Recommendations for breast cancer surveillance for female survivors of childhood, adolescent, and young adult cancer given chest radiation: a report from the International Late Effects of Childhood Cancer Guideline Harmonization Group. *Lancet Oncol*. 2013;14:e621-e629.
13. Jin L, Sturgis EM, Zhang Y, et al. Genetic variants in p53-related genes confer susceptibility to second primary malignancy in patients with index squamous cell carcinoma of head and neck. *Carcinogenesis*. 2013;34:1551-1557.
14. Morris LG, Sikora AG, Patel SG, Hayes RB, Ganly I. Second primary cancers after an index head and neck cancer: subsite-specific trends in the era of human papillomavirus-associated oropharyngeal cancer. *J Clin Oncol*. 2011;29:739-746.
15. Stout NK, Nekhlyudov L, Li L, et al. Rapid increase in breast magnetic resonance imaging use: trends from 2000 to 2011. *JAMA*. 2014;174:114-121.

16. Ojha RP, Jackson BE, Tota JE, Offutt-Powell TN, Hudson MM, Gurney JG. Younger age distribution of cervical cancer incidence among survivors of pediatric and young adult cancers. *Gynecol Oncol*. 2014;134:309-313.
17. Choi DK, Helenowski I, Hijiya N. Secondary malignancies in pediatric cancer survivors: perspectives and review of the literature. *Int J Cancer*. 2014;135:1764-1773.
18. Moskowitz CS, Chou JF, Wolden SL, et al. Breast cancer after chest radiation therapy for childhood cancer. *J Clin Oncol*. 2014;32:2217-2223.
19. Henderson TO, Oeffinger KC, Whitton J, et al. Secondary gastrointestinal cancer in childhood cancer survivors: a cohort study. *Ann Intern Med*. 2012;156:757-766, W-260.
20. Villani A, Tabori U, Schiffman J, et al. Biochemical and imaging surveillance in germline TP53 mutation carriers with Li-Fraumeni syndrome: a prospective observational study. *Lancet Oncol*. 2011;12:559-567.
21. Weaver KE, Forsythe LP, Reeve BB, et al. Mental and physical health-related quality of life among US cancer survivors: population estimates from the 2010 National Health Interview Survey. *Cancer Epidemiol Biomarkers Prev*. 2012;21:2108-2117.
22. Robison LL, Armstrong GT, Boice JD, et al. The Childhood Cancer Survivor Study: a National Cancer Institute-supported resource for outcome and intervention research. *J Clin Oncol*. 2009;27:2308-2318.
23. Oeffinger KC, Mertens AC, Sklar CA, et al. Chronic health conditions in adult survivors of childhood cancer. *N Engl J Med*. 2006;355:1572-1582.
24. Armstrong GT, Liu Q, Yasui Y, et al. Long-term outcomes among adult survivors of childhood central nervous system malignancies in the Childhood Cancer Survivor Study. *J Natl Cancer Inst*. 2009;101:946-958.
25. Mulrooney DA, Yeazel MW, Kawashima T, et al. Cardiac outcomes in a cohort of adult survivors of childhood and adolescent cancer: retrospective analysis of the Childhood Cancer Survivor Study cohort. *BMJ*. 2009;339:b4606.
26. Lipshultz SE, Cochran TR, Franco VI, Miller TL. Treatment-related cardiotoxicity in survivors of childhood cancer. *Nat Rev Clin Oncol*. 2013;10:697-710.
27. Chow EJ, Chen Y, Kremer LC, et al. Individual prediction of heart failure among childhood cancer survivors. *J Clin Oncol*. 2015;33(5):394-402.
28. Sieswerda E, van Dalen EC, Postma A, Cheuk DK, Caron HN, Kremer LC. Medical interventions for treating anthracycline-induced symptomatic and asymptomatic cardiotoxicity during and after treatment for childhood cancer. *Cochrane Database Syst Rev*. 2011:CD008011.
29. Bosch X, Rovira M, Sitges M, et al. Enalapril and carvedilol for preventing chemotherapy-induced left ventricular systolic dysfunction in patients with malignant hemopathies: the OVERCOME trial (preventiOn of left Ventricular dysfunction with Enalapril and caRvedilol in patients submitted to intensive ChemOtherapy for the treatment of Malignant hEmopathies). *J Am Coll Cardiol*. 2013;61:2355-2362.
30. Wong FL, Bhatia S, Landier W, et al. Cost-effectiveness of the Children's Oncology Group long-term follow-up screening guidelines for childhood cancer survivors at risk for treatment-related heart failure. *Ann Intern Med*. 2014;160:672-683.
31. Mueller S, Fullerton HJ, Stratton K, et al. Radiation, atherosclerotic risk factors, and stroke risk in survivors of pediatric cancer: a report from the Childhood Cancer Survivor Study. *Int J Radiat Oncol Biol Phys*. 2013;86:649-655.
32. Mueller S, Sear K, Hills NK, et al. Risk of first and recurrent stroke in childhood cancer survivors treated with cranial and cervical radiation therapy. *Int J Radiat Oncol Biol Phys*. 2013;86:643-648.
33. Mulder RL, Thonissen NM, van der Pal HJ, et al. Pulmonary function impairment measured by pulmonary function tests in long-term survivors of childhood cancer. *Thorax*. 2011;66:1065-1071.
34. Armstrong GT, Stovall M, Robison LL. Long-term effects of radiation exposure among adult survivors of childhood cancer: results from the Childhood Cancer Survivor Study. *Radiat Res*. 2010;174:840-850.
35. Huang TT, Chen Y, Dietz AC, et al. Pulmonary outcomes in survivors of childhood central nervous system malignancies: a report from the Childhood Cancer Survivor Study. *Pediatr Blood Cancer*. 2014;61:319-325.
36. Landier W, Armenian SH, Lee J, et al. Yield of screening for long-term complications using the children's Oncology Group long-term follow-up guidelines. *J Clin Oncol*. 2012;30:4401-4408.
37. Clement SC, Meeteren AY, Kremer LC, van Trotsenburg AS, Caron HN, van Santen HM. High prevalence of early hypothalamic-pituitary damage in childhood brain tumor survivors: need for standardized follow-up programs. *Pediatr Blood Cancer*. 2014;61:2285-2289.
38. Patterson BC, Chen Y, Sklar CA, et al. Growth hormone exposure as a risk factor for the development of subsequent neoplasms of the central nervous system: a report from the Childhood Cancer Survivor Study. *J Clin Endocrinol Metab*. 2014;99:2030-2037.
39. Willard VW, Leung W, Huang Q, Zhang H, Phipps S. Cognitive outcome after pediatric stem-cell transplantation: impact of age and total-body irradiation. *J Clin Oncol*. 2014;32:3982-3988.
40. Castellino SM, Ullrich NJ, Whelen MJ, Lange BJ. Developing interventions for cancer-related cognitive dysfunction in childhood cancer survivors. *J Natl Cancer Inst*. 2014;106(8). pii: dju186.
41. Shaw MG, Ball DL. Treatment of brain metastases in lung cancer: strategies to avoid/reduce late complications of whole brain radiation therapy. *Curr Treat Options Oncol*. 2013;14:553-567.
42. Greenberger BA, Pulsifer MB, Ebb DH, et al. Clinical outcomes and late endocrine, neurocognitive, and visual profiles of proton radiation for pediatric low-grade gliomas. *Int J Radiat Oncol Biol Phys*. 2014;89:1060-1068.
43. Pachman DR, Barton DL, Swetz KM, Loprinzi CL. Troublesome symptoms in cancer survivors: fatigue, insomnia, neuropathy, and pain. *J Clin Oncol*. 2012;30:3687-3696.
44. Gartner R, Jensen MB, Nielsen J, Ewertz M, Kroman N, Kehlet H. Prevalence of and factors associated with persistent pain following breast cancer surgery. *JAMA*. 2009;302:1985-1992.
45. Meretoja TJ, Leidenius MH, Tasmuth T, Sipila R, Kalso E. Pain at 12 months after surgery for breast cancer. *JAMA*. 2014;311:90-92.
46. Paice JA. Chronic treatment-related pain in cancer survivors. *Pain*. 2011;152:S84-S89.
47. Crew KD, Greenlee H, Capodice J, et al. Prevalence of joint symptoms in postmenopausal women taking aromatase inhibitors for early-stage breast cancer. *J Clin Oncol*. 2007;25:3877-3883.
48. Mieog JS, Morden JP, Bliss JM, Coombes RC, van de Velde CJ. Carpal tunnel syndrome and musculoskeletal symptoms in postmenopausal women with early breast cancer treated with exemestane or tamoxifen after 2-3 years of tamoxifen: a retrospective analysis of the Intergroup Exemestane Study. *Lancet Oncol*. 2012;13:420-432.
49. Sestak I, Sapunar F, Cuzick J. Aromatase inhibitor-induced carpal tunnel syndrome: results from the ATAC trial. *J Clin Oncol*. 2009;27:4961-4965.
50. Crew KD, Capodice JL, Greenlee H, et al. Randomized, blinded, sham-controlled trial of acupuncture for the management of aromatase inhibitor-associated joint symptoms in women with early-stage breast cancer. *J Clin Oncol*. 2010;28:1154-1160.
51. Niravath P. Aromatase inhibitor-induced arthralgia: a review.

Ann Oncol. 2013;24:1443-1449.
52. Cuzick J, Sestak I, Cella D, Fallowfield L. Treatment-emergent endocrine symptoms and the risk of breast cancer recurrence: a retrospective analysis of the ATAC trial. *Lancet Oncol*. 2008;9:1143-1148.
53. Saif MW, Syrigos K, Kaley K, Isufi I. Role of pregabalin in treatment of oxaliplatin-induced sensory neuropathy. *Anticancer Res*. 2010;30:2927-2933.
54. Smith EM, Pang H, Cirrincione C, et al. Effect of duloxetine on pain, function, and quality of life among patients with chemotherapy-induced painful peripheral neuropathy: a randomized clinical trial. *JAMA*. 2013;309:1359-1367.
55. Durand JP, Deplanque G, Montheil V, et al. Efficacy of venlafaxine for the prevention and relief of oxaliplatin-induced acute neurotoxicity: results of EFFOX, a randomized, double-blind, placebo-controlled phase III trial. *Ann Oncol*. 2012;23:200-205.
56. Barton DL, Wos EJ, Qin R, et al. A double-blind, placebo-controlled trial of a topical treatment for chemotherapy-induced peripheral neuropathy: NCCTG trial N06CA. *Support Care Cancer*. 2011;19:833-941.
57. Wang XS, Zhao F, Fisch MJ, et al. Prevalence and characteristics of moderate to severe fatigue: a multicenter study in cancer patients and survivors. *Cancer*. 2014;120:425-432.
58. Alfano CM, Imayama I, Neuhouser ML, et al. Fatigue, inflammation, and omega-3 and omega-6 fatty acid intake among breast cancer survivors. *J Clin Oncol*. 2012;30:1280-1287.
59. Bower JE, Ganz PA, Aziz N, Fahey JL, Cole SW. T-cell homeostasis in breast cancer survivors with persistent fatigue. *J Natl Cancer Inst*. 2003;95:1165-1168.
60. Barsevick AM, Dudley W, Beck S, Sweeney C, Whitmer K, Nail L. A randomized clinical trial of energy conservation for patients with cancer-related fatigue. *Cancer*. 2004;100:1302-1310.
61. Mishra SI, Scherer RW, Geigle PM, et al. Exercise interventions on health-related quality of life for cancer survivors. *Cochrane Database Syst Rev*. 2012;8:CD007566.
62. McMillan EM, Newhouse IJ. Exercise is an effective treatment modality for reducing cancer-related fatigue and improving physical capacity in cancer patients and survivors: a meta-analysis. *Appl Physiol Nutr Metab*. 2011;36:892-903.
63. de la Cruz M, Hui D, Parsons HA, Bruera E. Placebo and nocebo effects in randomized double-blind clinical trials of agents for the therapy for fatigue in patients with advanced cancer. *Cancer*. 2010;116:766-774.
64. Gong S, Sheng P, Jin H, et al. Effect of methylphenidate in patients with cancer-related fatigue: a systematic review and meta-analysis. *PloS One*. 2014;9:e84391.
65. Spathis A, Fife K, Blackhall F, et al. Modafinil for the treatment of fatigue in lung cancer: Results of a placebo-controlled, double-blind, randomized trial. *J Clin Oncol*. 2014;32:1882-1888.
66. Jean-Pierre P, Morrow GR, Roscoe JA, et al. A phase 3 randomized, placebo-controlled, double-blind, clinical trial of the effect of modafinil on cancer-related fatigue among 631 patients receiving chemotherapy: a University of Rochester Cancer Center Community Clinical Oncology Program Research base study. *Cancer*. 2010;116:3513-3520.
67. Ruddy KJ, Barton D, Loprinzi CL. Laying to rest psychostimulants for cancer-related fatigue? *J Clin Oncol*. 2014;32:1865-1867.
68. Barton SE, Najita JS, Ginsburg ES, et al. Infertility, infertility treatment, and achievement of pregnancy in female survivors of childhood cancer: a report from the Childhood Cancer Survivor Study cohort. *Lancet Oncol*. 2013;14:873-881.
69. Bober SL, Varela VS. Sexuality in adult cancer survivors: challenges and intervention. *J Clin Oncol*. 2012;30:3712-3719.
70. Aerts L, Enzlin P, Vergote I, Verhaeghe J, Poppe W, Amant F. Sexual, psychological, and relational functioning in women after surgical treatment for vulvar malignancy: a literature review. *J Sex Med*. 2012;9:361-371.
71. Aerts L, Enzlin P, Verhaeghe J, Vergote I, Amant F. Sexual and psychological functioning in women after pelvic surgery for gynaecological cancer. *Eur J Gynaecol Oncol*. 2009;30:652-656.
72. Resnick MJ, Koyama T, Fan KH, et al. Long-term functional outcomes after treatment for localized prostate cancer. *N Engl J Med*. 2013;368:436-445.
73. Kundu SD, Roehl KA, Eggener SE, Antenor JA, Han M, Catalona WJ. Potency, continence and complications in 3,477 consecutive radical retropubic prostatectomies. *J Urol*. 2004;172:2227-2231.
74. Tal R, Jacks LM, Elkin E, Mulhall JP. Penile implant utilization following treatment for prostate cancer: analysis of the SEER-Medicare database. *J Sex Med*. 2011;8:1797-1804.
75. Barton DL, Wender DB, Sloan JA, et al. Randomized controlled trial to evaluate transdermal testosterone in female cancer survivors with decreased libido; North Central Cancer Treatment Group protocol N02C3. *J Natl Cancer Inst*. 2007;99:672-679.
76. Caruso S, Intelisano G, Lupo L, Agnello C. Premenopausal women affected by sexual arousal disorder treated with sildenafil: a double-blind, cross-over, placebo-controlled study. *BJOG*. 2001;108:623-628.
77. Carter J, Goldfrank D, Schover LR. Simple strategies for vaginal health promotion in cancer survivors. *J Sex Med*. 2011;8:549-559.
78. Brotto LA, Heiman JR, Goff B, et al. A psychoeducational intervention for sexual dysfunction in women with gynecologic cancer. *Arch Sex Behav*. 2008;37:317-329.
79. Sackey H, Magnuson A, Sandelin K, et al. Arm lymphoedema after axillary surgery in women with invasive breast cancer. *Br J Surg*. 2014;101:390-397.
80. Doscher ME, Herman S, Garfein ES. Surgical management of inoperable lymphedema: the re-emergence of abandoned techniques. *J Am Coll Surg*. 2012;215:278-283.
81. Campisi C, Bellini C, Accogli S, Bonioli E, Boccardo F. Microsurgery for lymphedema: clinical research and long-term results. *Microsurgery*. 2010;30:256-260.
82. Chang DW. Lymphaticovenular bypass for lymphedema management in breast cancer patients: A prospective study. *Plast Reconstr Surg*. 2010;126:752-758.
83. Mehnert A, de Boer A, Feuerstein M. Employment challenges for cancer survivors. *Cancer*. 2013;119(Suppl 11):2151-2159.
84. Sesto ME, Faatin M, Wang S, Tevaarwerk AJ, Wiegmann DA. Employment and retirement status of older cancer survivors compared to non-cancer siblings. *Work*. 2013;46:445-453.
85. Roelen CA, Koopmans PC, Groothoff JW, van der Klink JJ, Bultmann U. Sickness absence and full return to work after cancer: 2-year follow-up of register data for different cancer sites. *Psychooncology*. 2011;20:1001-1006.
86. Aguado Loi CX, Baldwin JA, McDermott RJ, et al. Risk factors associated with increased depressive symptoms among Latinas diagnosed with breast cancer within 5 years of survivorship. *Psychooncology*. 2013;22:2779-2788.
87. Taylor-Ford M, Meyerowitz BE, D'Orazio LM, Christie KM, Gross ME, Agus DB. Body image predicts quality of life in men with prostate cancer. *Psychooncology*. 2013;22:756-761.
88. Misono S, Weiss NS, Fann JR, Redman M, Yueh B. Incidence of suicide in persons with cancer. *J Clin Oncol*. 2008;26:4731-4738.
89. Gianinazzi ME, Rueegg CS, Wengenroth L, et al. Adolescent survivors of childhood cancer: are they vulnerable for psychological distress? *Psychooncology*. 2013;22:2051-2058.
90. Armstrong GT. Long-term survivors of childhood central nervous system malignancies: the experience of the Childhood Cancer Survivor Study. *Eur J Paediatr Neurol*. 2010;14:298-303.
91. Zeltzer LK, Recklitis C, Buchbinder D, et al. Psychological status in childhood cancer survivors: a report from the Childhood Cancer Survivor Study. *J Clin Oncol*. 2009;27:2396-2404.
92. Krull KR, Huang S, Gurney JG, et al. Adolescent behavior and

adult health status in childhood cancer survivors. *J Cancer Surviv*. 2010;4:210-217.

93. Recklitis CJ, Lockwood RA, Rothwell MA, Diller LR. Suicidal ideation and attempts in adult survivors of childhood cancer. *J Clin Oncol*. 2006;24:3852-3857.
94. Armstrong GT, Oeffinger KC, Chen Y, et al. Modifiable risk factors and major cardiac events among adult survivors of childhood cancer. *J Clin Oncol*. 2013;31:3673-3680.
95. Smith WA, Li C, Nottage KA, et al. Lifestyle and metabolic syndrome in adult survivors of childhood cancer: A report from the St. Jude Lifetime Cohort Study. *Cancer*. 2014;120:2742-2750.
96. Badr H, Chandra J, Paxton RJ, Ater JL, Urbauer D, et al. Health-related quality of life, lifestyle behaviors, and intervention preferences of survivors of childhood cancer. *J Cancer Surviv*. 2013;7:523-534.
97. Campbell PT, Patel AV, Newton CC, Jacobs EJ, Gapstur SM. Associations of recreational physical activity and leisure time spent sitting with colorectal cancer survival. *J Clin Oncol*. 2013;31:876-885.
98. Lee IM, Wolin KY, Freeman SE, Sattlemair J, Sesso HD. Physical activity and survival after cancer diagnosis in men. *J Phys ActHealth*. 2014;11:85-90.
99. Ligibel J. Lifestyle factors in cancer survivorship. *J Clin Oncol*. 2012;30:3697-3704.
100. Pfeiler G, Konigsberg R, Fesl C, et al. Impact of body mass index on the efficacy of endocrine therapy in premenopausal patients with breast cancer: an analysis of the prospective ABCSG-12 trial. *J Clin Oncol*. 2011;29:2653-2659.

图书在版编目（C I P）数据

MD 安德森肿瘤学：第 3 版：双语版：汉、英文 / [美] 海格 M.坎塔尔简（Hagop M. Kantarjian），[美] 罗伯特 A.沃尔夫（Robert A. Wolff）主编；詹启敏等编译. —长沙：湖南科学技术出版社，2020.10
（西医经典名著集成）
ISBN 978-7-5710-0724-9

Ⅰ. ①M… Ⅱ. ①海… ②罗… ③詹… Ⅲ. ①肿瘤学—汉、英文 Ⅳ. ①R73

中国版本图书馆 CIP 数据核字（2020）第 155681 号

Hagop M. Kantarjian, Robert A. Wolff
The MD Anderson Manual of Medical Oncology, Third Edition
ISBN9780071847944

著作权合同登记号 18-2020-193

西医经典名著集成
MD ANDESEN ZHONGLIUXUE
MD 安德森肿瘤学 第 3 版 （双语版）
主　　编：[美]海格 M. 坎塔尔简（Hagop M. Kantarjian），[美]罗伯特 A. 沃尔夫（Robert A. Wolff）
编 译 者：詹启敏等
责任编辑：李　忠
出版发行：湖南科学技术出版社
社　　址：长沙市湘雅路 276 号
　　　　　http://www.hnstp.com
印　　刷：湖南天闻新华印务有限公司
　　　　　（印装质量问题请直接与本厂联系）
厂　　址：湖南望城·湖南出版科技园
邮　　编：410219
版　　次：2020 年 10 月第 1 版
印　　次：2020 年 10 月第 1 次印刷
开　　本：787mm×1092mm　1/16
印　　张：80.5
字　　数：3310 千字
书　　号：ISBN 978-7-5710-0724-9
定　　价：590.00 元